INTRODUCING

Classroom Preparation Resources (Learning Object Gallery)

- **New and Unique!**
  Correlation to Today's Nursing Standards!
  - Correlation guides link book and supplement content to nursing standards such as the *2010 ANA Scope and Standards of Practice, QSEN, National Patient Safety Goals, AACN Essentials of Baccalaureate Education* and more!

- **New and Unique!**
  Pearson Nursing Lecture Series
  - Highly visual, fully narrated and animated, these short lectures focus on topics that are traditionally difficult to teach and difficult for students to grasp
  - All lectures accompanied by case studies and classroom response questions for greater interactivity within even the largest classroom
  - Useful as lecture tools, remediation material, homework assignments and more!

- **Textbook Resources for Educators**
  - Find assets such as **videos, animations, lecture starters, classroom and clinical activities** and more!
  - **Add selected resources** to presentations that can be shown online or exported to PowerPoint™ or HTML pages
  - Organized by topic and **fully searchable** by type and keyword
  - **Upload your own resources** to keep everything in one place
  - **Rate resources** and view other instructor ratings!

- **Pearson Nursing Question Bank**
- Even **more** accessible with both pencil and paper and online delivery options
  - **All NCLEX®-style** questions
  - **Complete rationales** for both correct and incorrect answers mapped to learning outcomes

Book-specific resources also available to instructors including:

- Instructor's Manual and Resource Guide
- Image library

REAL NURSING SIMULATIONS

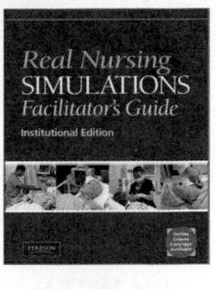

- 25 simulation scenarios that span the nursing curriculum
- Consistent format includes learning objectives, case flow, set-up instructions,
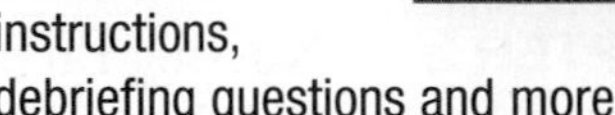
debriefing questions and more!
- Companion online course cartridge with student pre- and post-simulation activities, videos, skill checklists and reflective discussion questions

Brief Contents

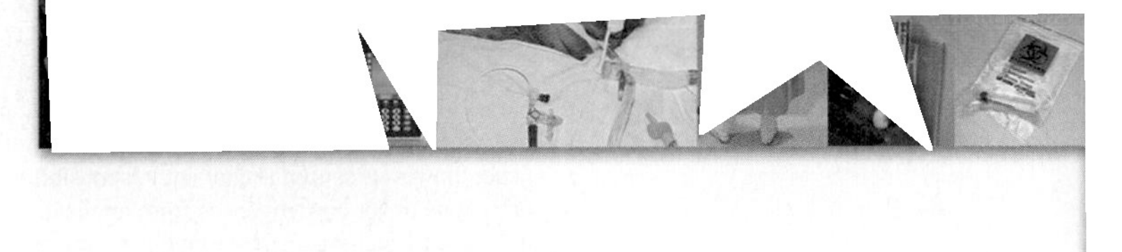

Eighth Edition

Clinical Nursing Skills

Basic to Advanced Skills

Sandra F. SMITH

President, National Nursing Review; Los Altos, California

Donna J. DUELL

Consultant to Deans and Directors of Nursing; California

Barbara C. MARTIN

Professor of Nursing, The University of Tulsa; Tulsa, Oklahoma

Pearson

Boston Columbus Indianapolis New York San Francisco Upper Saddle River
Amsterdam Cape Town Dubai London Madrid Milan Munich Paris Montreal Toronto
Delhi Mexico City Sao Paulo Sydney Hong Kong Seoul Singapore Taipei Tokyo

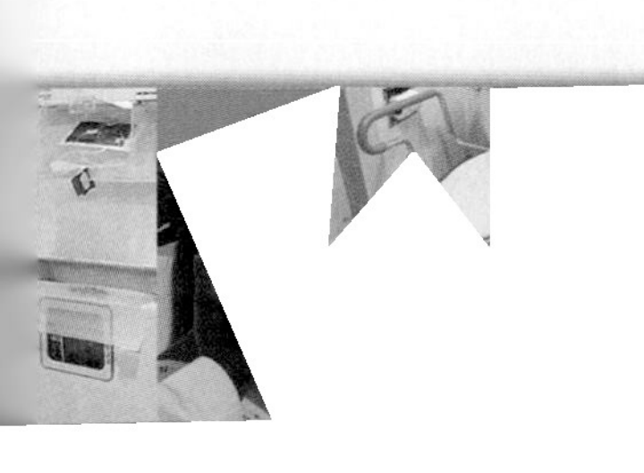

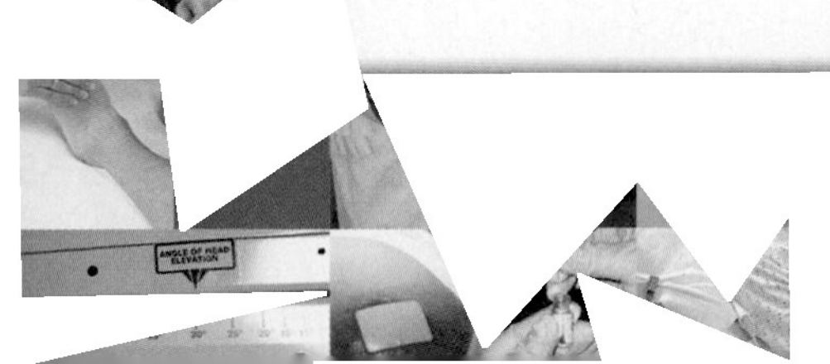

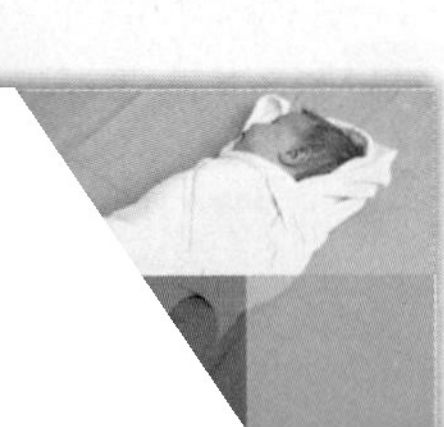

Cataloging-in-Publication data on file with the Library of Congress.

Notice: Care has been taken to confirm the accuracy of the information presented in this book. The authors, editors, and the publisher, however, cannot accept any responsibility for errors or omissions or for consequences from application of the information in this book and make no warranty, express or implied, with respect to its contents.

The authors and the publisher have exerted every effort to ensure that drug selections and dosages set forth in this text are in accord with current recommendations and practice at time of publication. However, in view of ongoing research, changes in government regulations, and the constant flow of information relating to drug therapy and drug reactions, the reader is urged to check the package inserts of all drugs for any change in indications of dosage and for added warnings and precautions. This is particularly important when the recommended agent is a new and/or infrequently employed drug.

The authors and publisher disclaim all responsibility for any liability, loss, injury, or damage incurred as a consequence, directly or indirectly, of the use and application of any of the contents of this volume.

Publisher: Julie Levin Alexander
Publisher's Assistant: Regina Bruno
Senior Acquisitions Editor: Kelly Trakalo
Assistant Editor: Lauren Sweeney
Development Editor: Karen Hoxeng
Managing Production Editor: Patrick Walsh
Production Liaison: Yagnesh Jani
Production Editor: Tracy Duff, PreMedia Global
Manufacturing Manager: Ilene Sanford
Manager, Design Development: John Christiana
Interior and Cover Design: Laura Gardner
Director of Marketing: David Gesell
Marketing Manager: Phoenix Harvey
Marketing Specialist: Michael Sirinides
Media Product Manager: Travis Moses—Westphal
Media Project Managers: Rachel Collett / Leslie Brado
Composition: PreMediaGlobal
Printer/Binder: RR Donnelley/Von Hoffman
Cover Printer: Lehigh-Phoenix Color
Cover photos: Ronald May, Celina Burkhart, Rick Brady

Credits and acknowledgments borrowed from other sources and reproduced, with permission, in this textbook appear on appropriate page within text.

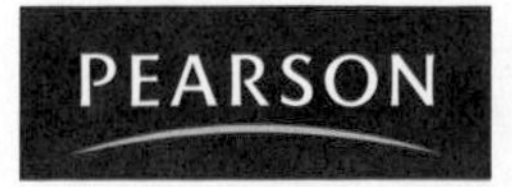

www.pearsonhighered.com

10 9 8 7 6 5 4 3 2 1
ISBN 13: 978-0-13-511473-5
ISBN 10: 0-13-511473-X

Acknowledgments

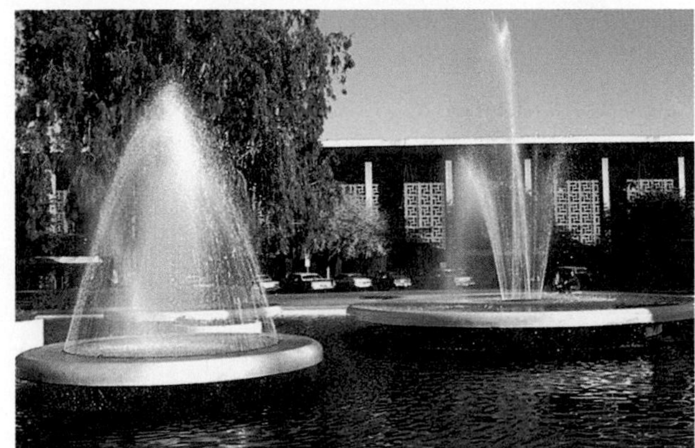

Stanford University Hospital

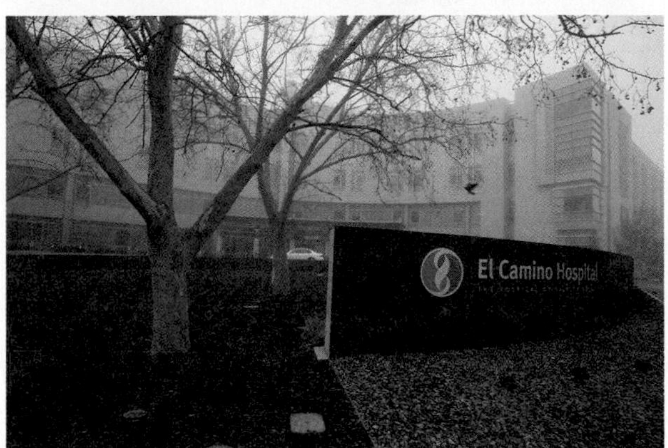

El Camino Hospital

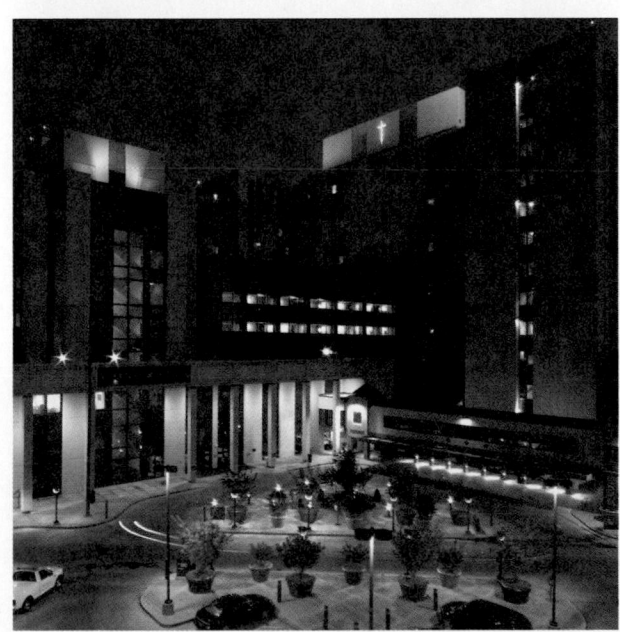

St. John Medical Center, Tulsa, OK

The authors express their thanks to the many people who assisted with the editorial and production phases of this edition of *Clinical Nursing Skills*, with special thanks to Kelly Trakalo, Nursing Editor, and the Team at PreMedia Inc. We especially wish to thank our Developmental Editor, Karen Hoxeng, for support, guidance, and editorial advice. We also thank our photographers, Rick Brady and Celina Burkhart, and models Heather Wright, Wendy Ogden, Virginia Williams, Christine Lieso, Jeff Sevey. In addition, we thank Cathy Patton and June Brown and the Nursing Education Department at El Camino for their consulting expertise, time and support.

The authors also express their sincere appreciation to the hospitals and staff who have so generously offered their assistance and support for our extensive photography in the appropriate clinical environment. We especially thank Stanford University Medical Center, Stanford, CA; El Camino Hospital, Mountain View, CA; Regional Medical Center, San Jose, CA; St. John Health System, Tulsa, OK; Sutter Hospital, Santa Cruz, CA; and Salinas Valley Medical Center, Salinas, CA.

Once again, we thank our families and friends for their encouragement and support while we were preparing this new edition.

Thank You

A special thank you to all of the nurse educators and practicing nurses who have spent their time reviewing and contributing to this new edition.

CONTRIBUTORS TO CURRENT AND PREVIOUS EDITIONS

Theresa Britt, RN, MSN
Director of Nursing, Lab and Clinical Assessment
University of Tennessee Health Science Center, Memphis, TN

Shirley S. Chang, RN, MS, PhD
Professor, Evergreen Valley College
San Jose, CA

Janet W. Cook, RN, MS
formerly Assistant Professor,
University of North Carolina
Greensboro, NC

Deborah Denham, RN, MS, PhD
Research Project Coordinator,
Good Samaritan Medical Center
San Jose, CA

Jacqueline Dowling, RN, MS
Professor, University of Massachusetts
Lowell, MA

Lou Ann Emerson, RN, MSN
Assistant Professor, University of Cincinnati
Cincinnati, OH

Rachel Faiano, RN, MS
Clinical Simulation Coordinator,
Salinas Valley Memorial Healthcare System
Salinas, CA

Patricia J. Rahnema, RN, MSN, FNP
Nurse Practitioner Southwest Cardiovascular Associates
Bullhead City, AZ

Sally Talley, RN
ET Specialist in Enterostomal Therapy
San Jose, CA

Jean O. Trotter, RN, C, MS
Assistant Professor, University of Maryland
Baltimore, MD

REVIEWERS

Traci Ashcraft, BSN, RN, BC
Ruby Memorial Hospital
Morgantown, WV

Lawrette Axley, PhD, RN, CNE
University of Memphis
Memphis, TN

Katherine Balkema MM, BSN, BA, RRT, RN, CMSRN
Holland Hospital
Holland, MI

Billie E Blake, EdD, MSN, BSN, RN
St. John's River CC
Orange Park, FL

Staci M. Boruff, PhD (C), MSN, RN
Walters State CC
Morristown, TN

Michelle Bussard, MSN, RN, ANCS-BC, CNE
Firelands Regional Medical Center
Sandusky, OH

Dr. Victor Ching, M.D. MD, MBA, FACS
Loma Linda School of Medicine
Loma Linda, CA

Mary Davis, RN, MSN, MPA, CRNI
Hartnell College
Salinas, CA

Cindy Fong, RN, MSN
Loma Linda Hospital
Loma Linda, CA

Erin Heleen Discenza, MSN, RN
Cuyahoga CC—Metropolitan
Cleveland, OH

Denise R. Doliveira, RN, MSN
CCAC Boyce
Monroeville, PA

Mary Farrell MSN/Ed, RN
Huron School of Nursing
East Cleveland, OH

Mary A. Gers, MSN, CNS, RNC
Northern Kentucky University
Highland Heights, KY

Theresa A. Glanville, RN, MS, CNE
Springfield Technical CC
Springfield, MA

Denise Isibel, RN, MSN
Old Dominion University
Norfolk, VA

Kathleen C. Jones, MSN, RN, CNS
Walters State CC
Morristown, TN

Fran Kamp, RN, MSN
Mercer University
Atlanta, GA

Susan M. Koos, MS, RN, CNE
Heartland CC
Normal, IL

Cheryl M. Lantz, PhD, RN
Dickinson State University
Dickinson, ND

Kathleen McManus, RN, MSN, CNE
Central Maine CC
Auburn, ME

Joshua Meringa, MPA, MHA, BSN, RN, ONC
Spectrum Health Hospitals
Grand Rapids, MI

Nancy Renzoni, RN, MS
Trocaire College
Buffalo, NY

Vicki Simpson RN, MSN, CHES, PhD
Purdue University
West Lafayette, IN

Charlotte Stephenson, RN, DSN, CLNC
Texas Woman's University
Houston, TX

Patricia Taylor, RN, MSN, Ed
Kapiolani CC
Honolulu, HI

Donna Woshinsky, RN, MSN, CNE
Springfield Technical CC
Springfield, MA

PHOTO CONSULTANTS

June Brown, RN, BSN

Arnold Failano, RN, BSN

Wendy Ogden, RN, MS

Ann O'Neill, RN, MS

Cathy Patton, RN, BSN, MA

Debbie Salerno, RN, MS

Diana Soria, RN, BSN

Constance Troolines, RN, BSN

Virginia Williams, RN, MS

Preface

A highly acclaimed skills book since its first edition in 1982, *Clinical Nursing Skills* applies to all levels of nursing education. It is also used as a procedure manual by many hospitals systems. Current with both the National Council Test Plan for RN and the NCLEX®, this textbook offers faculty a format for teaching nursing skill content that is both progressive and innovative. Content flows from the most basic to the more complex skills, and teaches the student how to assess the client, formulate nursing diagnoses, perform the procedure according to accepted and safe protocols, evaluate the outcomes and document the pertinent data.

The content continues to be organized around the nursing process and is both theoretical, as an introduction to the skills, and practical. Within each of the 34 chapters, skills are grouped together into units. Nursing process data is then provided for each unit. Unlike other skill textbooks, *Clinical Nursing Skills* conceptualizes the nursing process data for each unit (including Assessment, Planning, Implementation, and Evaluation) so that it does not have to be repeated with every skill. This avoidance of repetition allows us to offer more than 800 complete nursing skills, significantly more than other skills textbooks. Each skill includes a list of equipment necessary to perform the skill, preparation, and step-by-step nursing interventions. Critical steps include relevant rationale for the nursing action.

The clear and concise format of the eighth edition enables the student to easily access key material for immediate reference in the clinical area. Extensive color photographs and drawings within each unit illustrate the concepts presented and enable students to visualize each step that must be performed.

NEW TO THIS EDITION

- **More than 800 new and updated skills** provide the most up-to-date nursing techniques recommended by current standards of practice.
- **New! Chapter on Neurological Management.** As head trauma and neurological conditions require a high level of nursing competence, this chapter provides the skills to achieve this objective.
- **Expanded! Evidence-Based Nursing Practice** boxes that present specific scientific studies that validate the skills protocols. Research studies are included to emphasize new information related to improving client care.
- **Expanded! Legal Alerts,** which assist nurses in recognizing legal pitfalls so that when performing nursing actions they are aware of the actions that constitute legal malpractice.
- **New! New Trends** feature presents new equipment and systems that are being incorporated in 21st century nursing care.
- **Expanded! Critical Thinking Strategies** in the form of case studies have been expanded at the end of each chapter to assist students to apply critical thinking principles to clinical situations. The **Critical Thinking Application section** includes Expected Outcomes, Unexpected Outcomes, and Alternative Actions.

HALLMARK FEATURES

Clinical Nursing Skills' all-inclusive, clear, and concise format teaches the student to:

- Learn each skill from basic to advanced in a contextual framework.
- Understand the theoretical concepts that serve as a foundation for skills.
- Apply this knowledge to a clinical situation with a "client need" focus.
- Use critical thinking to assess and evaluate the outcome of the skill and consider unexpected outcomes.
- Appreciate cultural diversity principles as they apply to client situations.
- Validate clinical skills by applying evidence-based nursing practice data and studies.
- Function in, and adapt to, the professional role by understanding management responsibilities.

Our primary goal in writing *Clinical Nursing Skills* is to produce a relevant, useful, and comprehensive text that is flexible for various education programs and learning needs of students. Further, we hope that faculty will find this textbook a valuable teaching tool and reference for clinical practice.

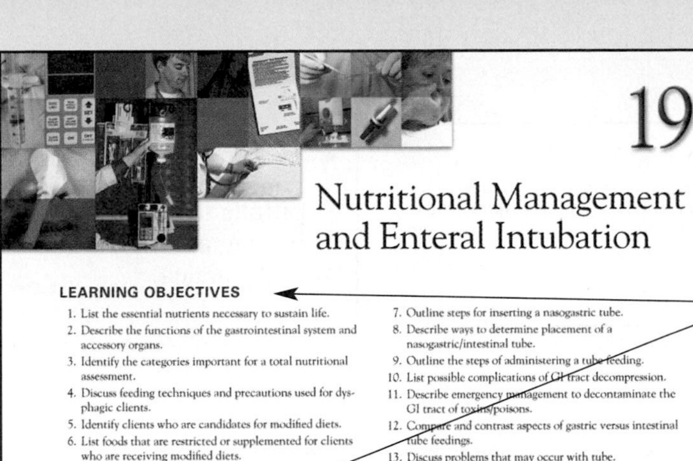

19

Nutritional Management and Enteral Intubation

LEARNING OBJECTIVES

1. List the essential nutrients necessary to sustain life.
2. Describe the functions of the gastrointestinal system and accessory organs.
3. Identify the categories important for a total nutritional assessment.
4. Discuss feeding techniques and precautions used for dysphagic clients.
5. Identify clients who are candidates for modified diets.
6. List foods that are restricted or supplemented for clients who are receiving modified diets.
7. Outline steps for inserting a nasogastric tube.
8. Describe ways to determine placement of a nasogastric/intestinal tube.
9. Outline the steps of administering a tube feeding.
10. List possible complications of GI tract decompression.
11. Describe emergency management to decontaminate the GI tract of toxins/poisons.
12. Compare and contrast aspects of gastric versus intestinal tube feedings.
13. Discuss problems that may occur with tube.

Each chapter opens with **Learning Objectives** and a **Chapter Outline** for easy reference and review of chapter contents.

CHAPTER OUTLINE

Skill procedures within each chapter are grouped together in **Units** and organized around a Nursing Process Framework.

TERMINOLOGY

Alimentary of or pertaining to nutrition.
Anabolism reaction in which small molecules are put together to form larger ones—repairing or building up cells.
Anorexia loss of appetite for food.
Aspirate to remove fluids or gases by suction.
Aspiration accidental inspiration of fluid or a foreign body into the airway.
Calorie the amount of heat necessary to raise the temperature of 1 kilogram of water 1°C. This is the "small" calorie. The dietary, or large, Calorie represents 1,000 of these calories, or 1 kilocalorie.
Carbohydrates a group of chemical substances, including sugars, glycogen, starches, dextrins, and celluloses, that contain only carbon, oxygen, and hydrogen.
Cardio prefix pertaining to the heart.
Carina point at which the trachea divides into the right and left bronchi.
Cardiovascular term that pertains to the heart and blood vessels as cardiovascular system.
Gavage introduction of nourishment into the GI tract by mechanical means.
Gastrointestinal term that pertains to the stomach and intestines.
Hematemesis vomitus containing blood.
Hydrogenation a chemical process by which hydrogens are added to monounsaturated or polyunsaturated fats, making the fats more saturated, termed *trans fats*.
Hyperalimentation the process of nourishing the body through parenteral means.
Hyperglycemia condition characterized by an increase in blood sugar.
Hypertonic solution having a higher osmotic pressure or tonicity than a solution to which it is compared.
Hypoglycemia condition characterized by a deficiency of sugar or glucose in the blood.
Ileus obstruction of the intestine caused by paralysis of the intestinal muscles.
Ingest the process of taking material into the gastrointestinal tract.

Key **Terminology** is included at the beginning of the chapter for easy review. ▶

Cultural Awareness

Cultural Accommodations for Special Diets

When a special diet is prescribed, it should be consistent with the client's cultural preferences and religious practices. For example, Jewish people do not combine certain foods. So, to comply with kosher laws, do not combine meat and dairy products at the same meal.

Food Is One of the Most Interesting Aspects About Any Culture

- American acculturation tends to *replace* traditional habits, tastes, and preferences with a detrimental *switch* to highly processed foods.
- This may account for increased rates of illness and death from heart disease and cancer in some populations.
- While not all cultural food habits are healthy, they are *usually* higher in fiber and vitamins than the typical American diet and should be encouraged.

General Recommendations

- Food preferences should be maintained.
- Focus education on food practices and preparation, possible health hazards, and importance of role modeling for children.

◀ Expanded! **Cultural Awareness** sections remind nurses of issues surrounding diversity and providing culturally responsive client care.

Legal Considerations

Nimodipine capsules were dispensed to clinical area where they were used for patients who could not swallow. In one case, a nurse softened the gelatin capsule in hot water, withdrew the medication into a parenteral syringe, and the dose was inadvertently administered as IV instead of via a feeding tube. Subsequently, the patient died. A boxed warning has now been added to the nimodipine labeling to caution about this type of administration error.

Source: ISMP Medication Safety Alert, *Nurse Adviser*, April 2010.

◄ **Legal Considerations** boxes highlight legal pitfalls and make nurses aware of legal malpractice.

New! **New Trends** feature presents new equipment and systems that are being incorporated in 21st century nursing care. ►

New Trends—Electronic Stethoscope

A new electronic stethoscope is now available. It measures a client's blood pressure via Bluetooth-Enabled Cardioscan and sends the results directly into the client's computer record for immediate evaluation.

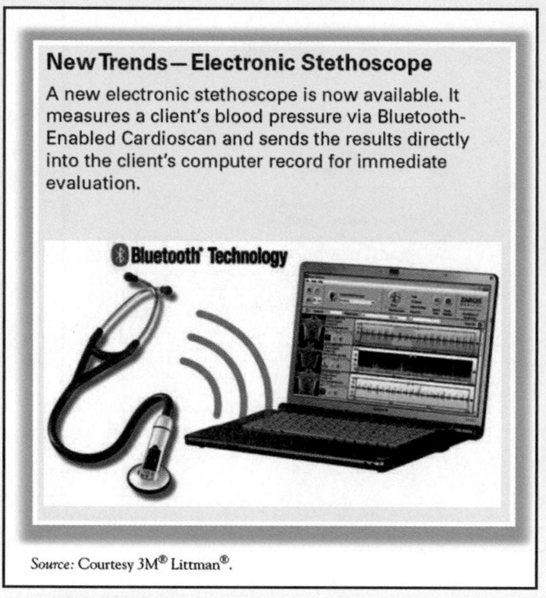

Source: Courtesy 3M® Littman®.

NURSING DIAGNOSES

The following nursing diagnoses are appropriate to use on client care plans when the components are related to nutritional problems or nutritional health maintenance.

NURSING DIAGNOSIS	RELATED FACTORS
Aspiration, Risk for	CVA, neuromuscular disease, NG intubation, artificial airway, decreased level of consciousness, oral/cervical surgery
Dentition, Impaired	Poor oral hygiene, oral surgery, injury, ill-fitting dentures
Knowledge, Deficient	Lack of appropriate dietary information, misinterpretation of information, cognitive limitation, inadequate motivation
Noncompliance	Chronic illness, disease-related symptoms, side effects of therapy, financial status, cultural practices
Imbalanced Nutrition: Less than Body Requirements	Impaired swallowing, faulty metabolism, altered level of consciousness, inadequate absorption, eating disorders
Imbalanced Nutrition: More than Body Requirements	Lack of basic nutritional knowledge, excessive intake in relation to metabolic requirements, decreased activity patterns, decreased metabolic needs, eating disorders
Impaired swallowing	Esophageal obstructive disorder, chronic neurologic disorder (multiple sclerosis, ALS, myasthenia gravis), muscle disfunction (stroke, dementia, Parkinson's dsisease)

CLEANSE HANDS The single most important nursing action to decrease the incidence of hospital-based infections is hand hygiene. *Remember to wash your hands or use antibacterial gel before and after each and every client contact.*

IDENTIFY CLIENT Before every procedure, check two forms of client identification, not including room number. These actions prevent errors and conform to the Joint Commission standards.

◄ **Nursing Diagnoses** for each chapter give quick and clear guidelines for appropriate use of nursing diagnoses in client care plans.

Chapter 19

UNIT ❸

Nasogastric Tube Therapies

Nursing Process Data

ASSESSMENT Data Base

- Validate order for NG tube type and purpose.
- Assess overall status necessitating NG decompression (gastric surgery, intestinal obstruction).
- Assess status of GI function (presence of nausea, vomiting, abdominal distention, presence/absence of passage of flatus or bowel movement).
- Assess patency of nares.
- Assess risk for aspiration.
- Assess client's I&O balance and relevant lab data (electrolytes, hemoglobin and hematocrit, coagulation studies).
- Assess type of IV fluid replacement therapy client is receiving.

PLANNING Objectives

- To remove fluid and gas from the gastrointestinal tract
- To maintain decompression tube patency
- To perform gastric lavage to remove blood, fluid, or particles, or to prevent digestion and absorption of poison

IMPLEMENTATION Procedures

EVALUATION Expected Outcomes

- NG tube is placed without complication.
- NG tube functions effectively (gastric contents are decompressed).
- Toxic substances are removed by lavage/not absorbed.

Pearson Nursing Student Resources

Find additional review materials at **nursing.pearsonhighered.com**

Prepare for success with NCLEX®-style practice questions and Skill Checklists

◄ Within each chapter, **Units** open with a complete overview of the Nursing Process Data that applies to the Procedures.

New! The **Online Student Resources** for each unit contains competency checklists for each procedure and NCLEX® review questions. (Visit nursing.pearsonhighered.com)

…sogastric (NG) Tube

…single-lumen tube)
…men Salem sump
…n.)

Water-soluble lubricant
Tape (2.5 cm or 1 in.) or commercial tube holder
pH chemstrip or Gastroccult test card and developer
Towel
Emesis basin
Tissues
Safety pin and rubber band
Tongue blade
Glass of water with straw
50-mL catheter-tip syringe
Clean gloves
Indelible pen or piece of tape for marking tube
Spindle adapter
Suction tubing and suction source

Preparation

1. Check physician's order and client care plan for inserting an NG tube.
2. Check client's Ident-A-Band and have client state name and birth date.
3. Discuss procedure with client. ▸ *Rationale:* Demonstration and display of items to be used helps to allay client's fear and to gain cooperation.
4. Provide privacy.
5. Gather equipment.

Procedure

1. Perform hand hygiene. Don clean gloves.
2. Position client at 45° angle or higher with head of bed elevated.
3. Examine nostrils, and select the most patent nostril by having client breathe through each one. ▸ *Rationale:* The nostril with greater airflow should be chosen for insertion.
4. Place a towel over client's chest, an emesis basin and tissues within reach; establish a cueing signal for client to use to stop you momentarily. ▸ *Rationale:* Client may experience discomfort or gag during tube insertion.

Clinical Alert

Nurses never insert or withdraw an NG tube for clients recovering from gastric surgery. The suture line could be interrupted, and hemorrhage could occur. The physician should be notified of dislodgement.

Never insert an NG tube in a client after nasal, craniofacial, or hypophysectomy surgery.

Gastric (Salem) Sump Tube

This gastric tube is a double-lumen radiopaque plastic tube. One lumen is used for decompression. The blue lumen with a blue pigtail provides an air vent to allow atmospheric pressure to enter the stomach to prevent tube adherence to gastric mucosa when the tube is attached to suction. It is NOT used for irrigation, obtaining a specimen, etc. However, if the vent lumen is blocked and requires flushing, after the flush, the pigtail should be cleared with an injection of 20 mL air. The pigtail should be kept above the level of the client's stomach to prevent stomach contents from siphoning into the air vent lumen, making it dysfunctional.

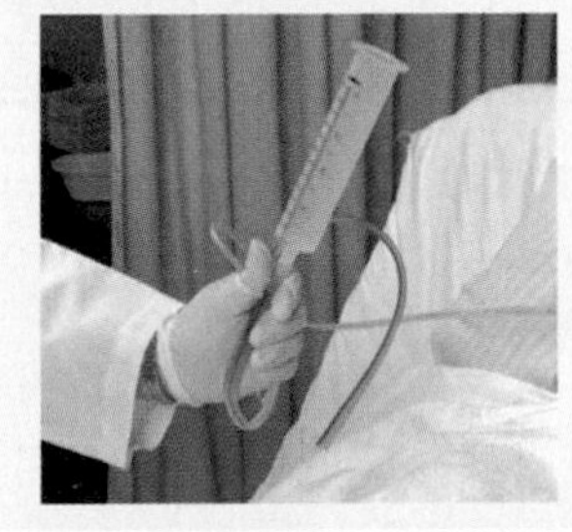

Salem Sump Tube With Gientri Port

This nasogastric system has selector knobs to allow a change in modes for suctioning (decompression), feeding, irrigating, and medication administration all through one closed port. The anti-reflux valve/air vent lumen allows atmospheric air to enter the stomach similar to the way the double lumen tube with blue pigtail functions.

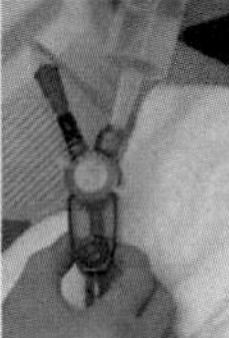

▲ Salem Sump w/Gentri port.

Step-by-Step Skills. More than 250 full-color photographs, line drawings, charts, and tables depict step-by-step nursing procedures. Clear, concise skills complete with rationales provide nurses of all levels the ability to visualize, perform, and evaluate skills in any clinical setting. ►

Clinical Alerts throughout the skills call attention to safety issues, essential information, nursing judgment and actions that require critical decision making. ►

EVIDENCE-BASED PRACTICE

Determining Proper NG Tube Placement

A number of methods have been proposed to determine whether a tube has been inadvertently placed into the pulmonary tree, including air insufflation, observation of respiratory symptoms, pH testing of aspirated fluid, visual inspection of aspirated fluid, detection of carbon dioxide in the tube, and x-ray tube location verification. The best method of confirming the location of a blindly inserted gastrointestinal tube is by chest/abdominal x-ray.

Rauen, C. A., Chulay, M., Bridges, E., Vollman, K. M., & Arbour, R. (2008). Seven evidence-based practice habits: putting some sacred cows out to pasture. *Critical Care Nurse*, *28*(2), 98–123.

◄ Expanded! **Evidence-Based Practice** boxes present specific scientific studies that validate skill protocols.

Each unit ends with **Documentation** to remind nurses to document important data regarding the skill, the outcome, and the client response. ►

DOCUMENTATION for Nasogastric Tube Therapies

- Type of tube inserted
- Technique used to assess NG tube placement
- Character and amount of drainage
- Type of suction and pressure setting used
- Frequency and solution used for flush or irrigation
- Gastrointestinal assessment findings (e.g., passage of flatus, bowel movement)
- Net return for lavaged client (amount of irrigant instilled subtracted from amount of aspirated return).
- Frequent vital signs (if indicated)
- Nasal and oral hygiene measures
- Client's tolerance of decompression
- Results of gastric specimen testing (blood, pH)
- Decontaminating agents instilled

CRITICAL THINKING Application

Expected Outcomes

- NG tube is placed without complication.
- NG tube functions effectively (gastric contents are decompressed).
- Toxic substances are removed by lavage/not absorbed.

Unexpected Outcomes	Alternative Actions
NG tube is difficult to advance.	• Select more patent nostril: Have client compress each nostril and breathe in to determine which is more patent. • Rotate tube or withdraw slightly, then try to advance, but do not force. • Relubricate tube and try again. • Curl tube around fist and hold under warm running water to soften for easier insertion. • Have client hold ice chips in mouth for a few minutes to numb nasal passage and suppress gag reflex.
Client coughs, is unable to speak and becomes cyanotic during tube insertion.	• Remove tube immediately as these indicate that tube is being advanced into client's airway.
Salem sump pigtail leaks gastric contents.	• Flush pigtail with normal saline, then with air to clear. • Keep blue pigtail at level above client's stomach. • Maintain antireflux valve plug insertion (blue side into blue pigtail lumen).
Client has ingested a large number of tablets which cannot be removed by lavage.	• Whole bowel irrigation is more effective for ingestion of enteric coated or sustained-release tablets. • Repeated dose of activated charcoal may be indicated to speed drug elimination. • Prepare for possible arrangement for hemodialysis.

◄ **Critical Thinking Applications** review Expected Outcomes, and provide Alternative Actions to take with Unexpected Outcomes.

GERONTOLOGIC Considerations

Dietary Needs of the Elderly

Energy (caloric) requirement: 2,000–2,400 kcal/day (may adjust to energy expenditure and physical activity).

Protein: 10% of energy requirement, increases to 20% of energy requirement during periods of stress (surgery, infection, burn).

Fiber: 20–35 g/day of fiber (five servings of fruit per day).

Fluids: 1,500–2,000 mL of water/day or 30 mL/kg body weight.

Vitamins: same as for younger adult except for vitamins D, B_6, and B_{12}. *Significant deficiencies in serum levels of vitamins and minerals are rare in healthy older adults.*

Vitamin D requirement is 10 mg/day for adults 51–70 and 15 mg/day for those over age 70.

Vitamin B_6 intake should be 1.7 mg/day for men and 1.5 mg/day for women over age 51 (25% of elderly are deficient in vitamin B_6).

Vitamin B_{12} intake should be 2.4 mg for all adults over age 51 (about 15% of elderly are deficient in vitamin B_{12}).

Minerals: increased need—10 mg/day of iron.

The elderly are at high risk for malnutrition due to age-related physiologic changes, healthcare status, and lifestyle factors.

Physiologic Changes Associated with Aging

- Between ages 25 and 70, percentage of body fat doubles and lean body mass decreases by about one third.
- Metabolic rate decreases 20% in men and 13% in elderly

Health Status Factors

- Poor dentition (up to 37% of elderly are edentulous). Loss of dentition is not due to the normal aging process but to improper oral hygiene and or inadequate nutrition beginning at an earlier age.
- Ill-fitting dentures causing pain limiting variety and quantity of intake.
- Swallowing or self-care deficit disorders (e.g., neuromuscular disorders, Parkinson's, Alzheimer's).
- Psychological changes (depression, cognitive impairment).
- Effect of medications (altered metabolism, anorexia, nausea, diarrhea, cognitive disturbance).
- Inappropriate diet prescription (low-salt, low-cholesterol, or low-calorie diet).
- Medical conditions (e.g., COPD, heart failure, cancer resulting).

Lifestyle Factors

- Alcoholism
- Inadequate income
- Decreased physical activity, lack of transport, isolation
- Cultural values
- Lack of monitoring/caregiving

  Assessment parameters for nutritional status of the elderly client in addition to the above risk factors include:
- Anthropometric values:

  Ideal body weight = men should weigh 106 lb for 5 feet

◄ **Gerontologic Considerations** help nurses consider special adaptations for care of the older adult.

MANAGEMENT Guidelines

Each state legislates a Nurse Practice Act for RNs and LVN/LPNs. Healthcare facilities are responsible for establishing and implementing policies and procedures that conform to their state's regulations. Verify the regulations and role parameters for each healthcare worker in your facility.

Delegation

- Each state identifies the scope of practice for RNs and LVN/LPNs. Several states have identified that the LVN/LPN has a specific role in IV therapy, but the scope of practice is always dictated by each agency (e.g., initiating, regulating, discontinuing IVs). The LPN/LVN educated in IV therapy is the minimum level practitioner to assist in tasks delegated by the RN for the delivery of IV therapy. The RN may be assisted by an LVN/LPN educated in IV therapy, but the RN remains responsible for the care given.
- Policies outlining the responsibility of the IV nurse vary significantly among agencies. A written policy should clearly outline all aspects of this role, and all staff should be familiar with its scope. Policies and procedures should follow national guidelines and standards of practice established by the Centers for Disease Control and Prevention, the American Association of Blood Banks, and the IV Nurses Society. All nurses must be aware of the many physical hazards associated with IV therapy and related OSHA rules to be observed.
- Central line catheter management must be done by an RN.
- The nurse who delivers IV therapy must be qualified by specific knowledge and experience to perform such highly specialized skills. Many agencies utilize a team of specialty educated and experienced certified IV nurses who focus their attention solely on aspects of IV therapy (initiation, drug preparation, fluid/blood/drug administration, regular client assessment and site care, as well as monitoring product integrity). While these nurses are freed from other care responsibilities, the professional nurse must provide for ongoing client care and ensure client safety.
- TPN and lipids may be administered only by an RN according to specific physician orders.
- The CNA/UAP providing personal hygiene must understand that the IV system is a closed one and must be able to give care without disrupting the system. The components of the CVAD system must never be disconnected. Doing so places the client at risk for infection and air embolism. The CNA/UAP should receive training in changing the client's gown without disrupting the CVAD system.
- For the client with a CVAD allowed to shower, the RN should disconnect infusion lines, place a dry sterile gauze (4 × 4) over the dressed site and exposed tubing(s), then cover all with a large transparent dressing for waterproofing. Post-shower removal of the covering and inspection of the dressing should also be performed by the RN.

Communication Matrix

While the professional monitors the IV infusion site regularly, the CNA/UAP provides vital data to the professional nurse by immediately reporting:

- Observations of redness or swelling around the CVAD insertion site (signs of possible infiltration, hematoma, sepsis).
- Presence of crepitus (bubble-wrap feeling) on the client's chest (sign of possible subcutaneous emphysema that can lead to respiratory distress).
- Observations of respiratory distress in any client with recent (24 hr) placement of a central line (symptoms of possible pneumothorax).
- Any client complaint of arm, shoulder, or neck pain (symptom of possible thrombosis or infiltration).
- Temperature elevation (fever—sign of possible catheter-related infection if otherwise unexplainable).
- Infusion device alarms to prompt the professional to further assess the client.
- Presence of blood backup in the catheter.
- A loose or soiled/wet dressing.

Management Guidelines include a **Delegation** section which teaches nurses to delegate tasks within safe, legal, and appropriate parameters. A **Communication Matrix** section helps nurses learn to prioritize and communicate relevant client information to members of the healthcare team. ◄

CRITICAL THINKING Strategies

Scenario 1

Mr. John Baker is a 68-year-old retired pharmacist who has just returned from surgery after placement of a tunneled CVAD with a Groshong valve. He will be started on a long-term intermittent chemotherapy regimen for acute lymphocytic leukemia. His wife is a retired RN who worked in the operating room for many years.

1. Identify at least three advantages for inserting the tunneled catheter for his treatment.
2. His wife is very concerned about the initial care of the catheter. What explanation will you give her?
3. After the explanation regarding the care of the catheter, Mrs. Baker asks you how they can prevent an infection of the catheter.
4. The client needs to be instructed on how to flush the catheter. What are the most important directions you should provide to him?
5. Mrs. Baker asks you to describe what symptoms require reporting to the physician. What is your best response to this question?

Scenario 2

Seth Eley, age 24, has been admitted to your unit with the diagnosis of inflammatory bowel disease (Crohn's disease) with exacerbation of fever, severe diarrhea, right lower quadrant pain, weight loss, and anemia. Short-term total parenteral nutrition and bowel rest are planned. A triple-lumen central venous catheter has been placed for these purposes.

1. Based on these data, what generalizations can you make about the purpose of hyperalimentation for this client?
2. Why is central venous access necessary?
3. Develop several scenarios about the most common complications of central catheter placement.
4. How does TPN affect fluid and electrolyte balance?

Critical Thinking Strategies provide case scenarios that help nurses develop clinical reasoning skills.

NCLEX® Review Questions. NCLEX®-style questions have been included at the end of each chapter and reflect the Practice Analysis of newly Licensed Registered Nurses upon which the NCLEX® is based. Answers with complete rationales are in the Answers Appendix.

NCLEX® Review Questions

Unless otherwise specified, choose only one (1) answer.

1. Trans fats are polyunsaturates and monounsaturates that:
   1. Have been hydrogenated.
   2. Are unsaturated.
   3. Primarily come from vegetables, nuts, and seeds.
   4. Come from animal sources.
2. Which of the following clients would mostly likely be placed on a potassium restricted diet?
   1. Heart failure client
   2. Renal failure client
   3. COPD client
   4. Burn client
3. Which of the following are helpful for the dysphagic client?
   Select all that apply.
   1. Swallowing liquid foods.
   2. Eating food accompanied by liquids.
   3. Swallowing thickened liquids.
   4. Eating food without accompanying liquid.
   5. Using a straw for liquids.
   6. Being fed with a syringe.
4. The purpose of the Salem NG decompression tube's blue lumen is to:
   1. Prevent esophageal reflux of gastric contents.
   2. Allow siphoning of gastric contents if they stagnate.
   3. Provide a port for continuous feeding.
   4. Prevent tube adherence to the gastric mucosa.
5. Which of the following is the least reliable indicator of the return of bowel function?
   1. Appetite
   2. Bowel sounds
   3. Presence of flatus
   4. Bowel movement
6. The best way to determine NG tube placement with continuous feeding is to:
   1. Auscultate for injected air sound over the epigastrium.
   2. Aspirate secretions and check for an acid pH.
   3. Note the character of aspirated secretions.
   4. Use capnography to detect presence of carbon dioxide.
7. An intermittent NG tube feeding should be withheld if the residual volume is:
   1. 50 mL.
   2. 100 mL.
   3. 150 mL.
   4. >200 mL.
8. The best way to prevent clogging of a small bore feeding tube is to:
   1. Flush frequently with cola.
   2. Flush frequently with cranberry juice.
   3. Flush frequently with warm water.
   4. Replace the tube weekly.
9. The most effective way to promote small bore feeding tube advancement into the small intestine is to:
   1. Place the client right side-lying.
   2. Place the client left side-lying.
   3. Administer prokinetic medication before tube insertion.
   4. Reinsert guidewire to advance the tube.
10. The most appropriate method for extended nutritional support is:
    1. Nasogastric tube feeding.
    2. Nasointestinal tube feeding.
    3. Gastrostomy tube feeding.
    4. Parenteral nutrition.

Contents

1

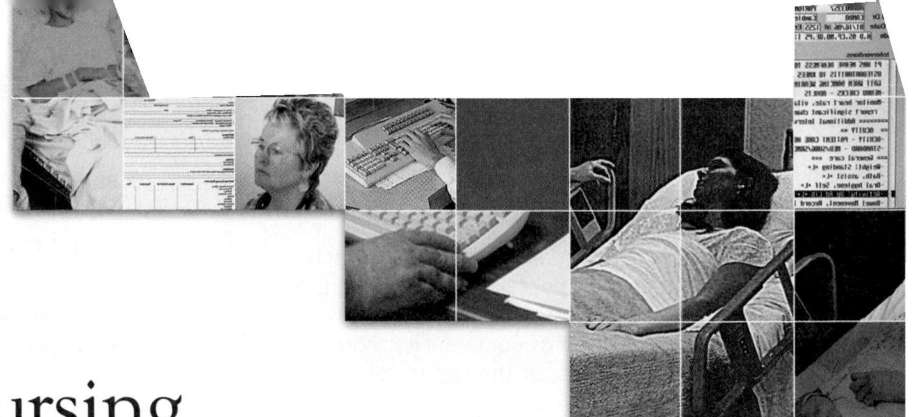

Professional Nursing

LEARNING OBJECTIVES

1. Discuss what is meant by the concept "professional role of the nurse."
2. Discuss the ANA Code of Ethics.
3. Define the purpose of "A Code of Academic and Clinical Conduct."
4. Define professional nursing.
5. Define the term *accountable*.
6. List three ways you can assist the client to assume and adapt to the client role.
7. Identify the guidelines that will assist the nurse to convey nursing competence to the clients.
8. Describe the purpose of the Nurse Practice Act.
9. Discuss major sections of the Nurse Practice Act.
10. Define the term *nurse licensure*.
11. State four functions of the Board of Registered Nursing.
12. Discuss four grounds for licensure revocation for professional misconduct.
13. Explain the legal issues of drug administration.
14. Describe what is meant by "clients' rights."
15. Explain what is meant by "Advance Directives."
16. List four actions or guidelines that you need to complete to prepare for daily client care.
17. Describe the steps of planning for client care.

CHAPTER OUTLINE

PROFESSIONAL ROLE

As you enter the profession of nursing, you will experience some of the most frustrating and some of the most rewarding situations of your life. To decrease the frustrations and increase the positive experiences, this chapter introduces you to the role of the nurse. Emphasis is placed on those procedures that will assist you to become a functioning member of the health team, even with limited experience.

The information in this chapter will help you through the first few critical days of your clinical experience. In addition, legal aspects of the nursing profession are discussed to help you become aware of the far-reaching consequences of nursing actions. Clients' rights and the Nurse Practice Act (also called the Nursing Practice Act in some states) are also presented for your information.

Nurses must function within the Nurses' Code of Ethics. The Code of Ethics is a set of formal guidelines for governing professional action. It assists the nurse in problem solving where judgment is required. More emphasis is now being placed on the professional organizations to uphold the Code of Ethics and to admonish those nurses who violate the code. The Code of Ethics was revised in June 2001 by the American Nurses Association (ANA). The Code should be reviewed as you progress in the program. The National Student Nurses Association, Inc., also developed a Code of Academic and Clinical Conduct in April 2001. The Code provides guidance for nursing students in the personal development of an ethical foundation as both a nurse and human being.

American Nurses Association: Code of Ethics for Nurses

1. The nurse in all professional relationships practices with compassion and respect for the inherent dignity, work, and uniqueness of every individual, unrestricted by considerations of social or economic status, personal attributes, or the nature of health problems.
2. The nurse's primary commitment is to the patient, whether an individual, family, group or community.
3. The nurse promotes, advocates for, and strives to protect the health, safety, and rights of the patient.
4. The nurse is responsible and accountable for individual nursing practice and determines the appropriate delegations of tasks consistent with the nurse's obligation to provide optimum patient care.
5. The nurse owes the same duties to self as to others, including the responsibility to preserve integrity and safety, to maintain competence, and to continue personal and professional growth.
6. The nurse participates in establishing, maintaining, and improving healthcare environments and conditions of employment conducive to the provision of quality health care and consistent with the values of the profession through individual and collective action.
7. The nurse participates in the advancement of the profession through contributions to practice, education, administration, and knowledge development.
8. The nurse collaborates with other health professionals and the public in promoting community, national, and international efforts to meet health needs.
9. The profession of nursing, as represented by associations and their members, is responsible for articulating nursing values, for maintaining the integrity of the profession and its practice, and for shaping social policy.

Source: Fowler, M. (Ed.) (2008). *American Nurses Association, Guide to the Code of Ethics for Nurses: Interpretation and Application.* Silver Spring, MD: American Nurses Association.

Definition of Professional Nursing

The American Nurses Association in 2003 defined professional nursing as the protection, promotion, and optimization of health and abilities, prevention of illness and injury, alleviation of suffering through the diagnosis and treatment of human responses, and advocacy in the care of individuals, families, communities, and populations.

ANA's Nursing's Social Policy Statement, second edition in 2003, identifies six essential features of professional nursing. These features include:

- Provision of a caring relationship that facilitates health and healing.
- Attention to the range of human experiences and responses to health and illness within the physical and social environments.
- Integration of objective data with knowledge gained from an appreciation of the patient's or group's subjective experience.
- Application of scientific knowledge to the processes of diagnosis and treatment through the use of judgment and critical thinking.
- Advancement of professional nursing knowledge through scholarly inquiry.
- Influence on social and public policy to promote social justice.

American Nursing Association. (2010). *Scope and Standards of Practice* (2nd ed.). Silver Spring, MD.

Assuming the Nursing Role

Your actions, both verbal and nonverbal, influence the client's feelings and ideas regarding your level of competence, the role of nursing in administering care, and the client's overall adaptation to healthcare facilities. Assuming a professional role means that you behave as a professional person. Following the guidelines below will assist you to convey nursing competence, not only to clients, but also to your peers and other nursing staff.

- Always dress neatly in appropriate, clean attire, and follow the dress code of your school or facility.
- Cover visible tattoos and body piercing with clothing or band-aid/dressing according to nursing program policies and procedures.
- Keep hair off collar and fingernails cut short. Wear clear nail polish, not colored polish. Synthetic nails are not allowed as they harbor bacteria and fungus.
- Speak in correct English without slang or inappropriate language, using medical terminology appropriate to the situation.
- Relate to the clients as worthwhile individuals who deserve respect and consideration. Call the client by his or her surname, and use the appropriate honorific (Mr., Ms., Miss, Mrs.). Do not use nicknames (such as "grannie" or "sweetie") or first names.
- Do not "talk down" to or patronize the client. Remember that the client knows more about his or her own body, symptoms, feelings, and responses than anyone else. Listen and pay attention to what the client says about himself or herself or the underlying feelings that are not expressed.
- Remain in a professional role at all times. Do not socialize with the clients. Clients should view you as a knowledgeable professional who brings healing, caring, and teaching roles to the relationship.
- Use yourself as a therapeutic tool to convey caring and healing. Use body language to reinforce honest and direct verbalization, not to contradict it.
- Be accountable and answerable for your behavior and nursing actions and the nursing care you are expected to provide. If you do not understand what is expected, seek assistance from a staff member or your instructor. Your responsibility is to remain reliable, honest, and trustworthy in administering nursing care.
- Maintain client confidentiality. Do not talk about clients in public areas. Follow HIPAA standards (see "HIPAA" section later in this chapter).

A Code of Academic and Clinical Conduct

As students are involved in the clinical and academic environments, we believe that ethical principles are a necessary guide to professional development. Therefore, within these environments, we:

1. Advocate for the rights of all clients.
2. Maintain client confidentiality.
3. Take appropriate action to ensure the safety of clients, self, and others.
4. Provide care for the client in a timely, compassionate, and professional manner.
5. Communicate client care in a truthful, timely, and accurate manner.
6. Actively promote the highest level of moral and ethical principles and accept responsibility for our actions.
7. Promote excellence in nursing by encouraging lifelong learning and professional development.
8. Treat others with respect and promote an environment that respects human rights, values, and choice of cultural and spiritual beliefs.
9. Collaborate in every reasonable manner with the academic faculty and clinical staff to ensure the highest quality of client care.
10. Use every opportunity to improve faculty and clinical staff understanding of the learning needs of nursing students.
11. Encourage faculty, clinical staff, and peers to mentor nursing students.
12. Refrain from performing any technique or procedure for which the student has not been adequately trained.
13. Refrain from any deliberate action or omission of care in the academic or clinical setting that creates unnecessary risk of injury to the client, self, or others.
14. Assist the staff nurse or preceptor in ensuring that there is full disclosure and that proper authorizations are obtained from clients regarding any form of treatment or research.
15. Abstain from the use of alcoholic beverages or any substances that impair judgment in the academic and clinical setting.
16. Strive to achieve and maintain an optimal level of personal health.
17. Support access to treatment and rehabilitation for students who are experiencing impairments related to substance abuse and mental or physical health issues.
18. Uphold school policies and regulations related to academic and clinical performance, reserving the right to challenge and critique rules and regulations as per school grievance policy.

Source: National Student Nurses' Association, Inc. April 6, 2001.

The Client Role

Assisting the client to adapt to hospitalization and ensuring that the client is as comfortable as possible will assist him or her to be less anxious and more open to receiving treatment during hospitalization. The nurse can assist in adaptation by understanding that all clients have individual needs, concerns, and perceptions that require discussion and planning as they take on the role of client in the healthcare setting. You must accept the client's perceptions of his or her new surroundings. If possible, try to accommodate client's wishes, assess previous concepts of illness and hospitalization, and discuss previous experiences. Be aware that anxiety is a natural reaction to an unfamiliar setting, to new procedures, and to new people. If, for example, a client is extremely fatigued or overwhelmed by traveling to the hospital and the admission procedure, you can help him or her adapt to the surroundings, regain a sense of control and identity, and accept the changed circumstances.

Another way to assist the client to retain his or her identity and uniqueness is to communicate with the client as an individual. Ask questions and observe verbal responses as well as nonverbal cues. Provide ways to care for a client's personal possessions, clothing, and physical comfort so that the client adapts more easily to the change in environment and feels more secure and in control.

Be aware that the medical condition is only one part of the client's life and that the changes that have led up to admission affect other areas of his or her well-being. Clients may have concerns about new routines, financial matters, their families, or their future. By responding to clients' total needs at the time of admission, you can help them establish a positive attitude toward their total care.

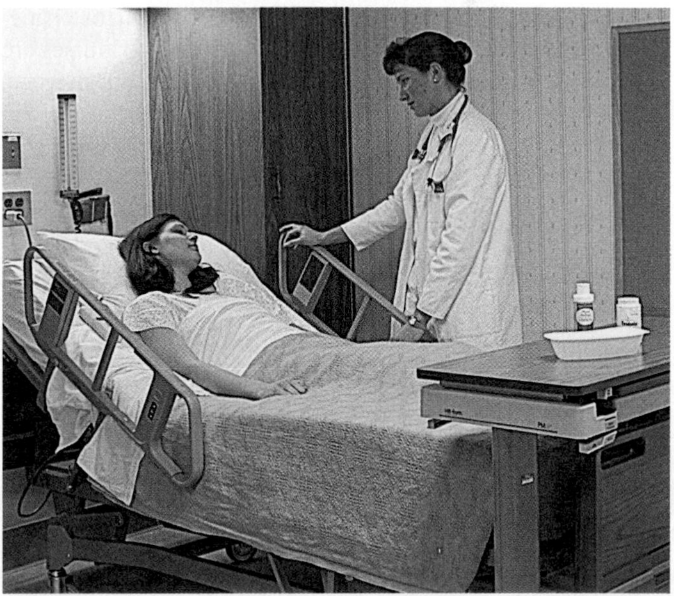

▲ Relate to clients as worthwhile individuals who deserve respect and consideration.

Acknowledge and accept any statements or behavior the client uses to adapt to his or her new surroundings. Even though various cultures and groups differ in their response to illness and some responses may differ from your personal beliefs, acknowledge the client's individuality. These specific groups often utilize their own identified and respected traditional healthcare providers. Concepts of illness, wellness, and health are part of the client's total belief system and must be recognized by the nurse as part of what makes the client an individual. Support the client's beliefs and behavior as long as they do not increase the risk of injury or illness. Be sensitive to any past healthcare experiences that may influence the client's feelings at the time of admission. A prior experience in the hospital may determine how a client responds to the current environment and how he or she accepts treatment. If they are present and the client is negative or fearful, allow time for the client to discuss these feelings. Try to answer questions they may have about this hospitalization in light of earlier adminssions.

STANDARDS AND STATUTES

Legal issues and regulations play a dominant role in nursing practice today. The law provides a framework for establishing nursing actions in the care of clients. Laws determine and set boundaries and maintain a standard of nursing practice.

The Nurse Practice Act defines professional nursing practice and recommends those actions that the nurse can practice independently and those actions that require a physician's order before completion. Individual states allow other healthcare providers who have prescriptive rights—such as nurse practitioners, physician assistants, dentists, and so on—to write orders.

Each state has the authority to regulate and administrate healthcare professionals. Although the provisions of Nurse Practice Acts are quite similar from state to state, it is imperative that the nurse know the licensing requirements and the grounds for license revocation defined by the state in which he or she works.

Legal and ethical standards for nurses are complicated by a myriad of federal and state statutes and the continually changing interpretation of them by the courts of law. Nurses are faced today with the threat of legal action based on negligence, malpractice, invasion of privacy, and other grounds. This chapter covers the basic legal issues and topics, from clients' rights and nurses' liability in the administration of drugs to grounds for proceedings to address professional misconduct.

The Nurse Practice Act

The Nurse Practice Act is a series of statutes enacted by a state to regulate the practice of nursing in that state. Subjects covered by Nurse Practice Acts include definition of the scope of practice, education, licensure, and grounds for disciplinary actions. Nurse Practice Acts are quite similar throughout the United States, but the professional nurse is held legally responsible for the specific requirements for licensure and regulations of practice as defined by the state in which she or he works.

The responsibilities of the professional nurse involve a level of performance for a defined range of healthcare services. These services include assessment, planning, implementation, and evaluation of nursing action, as well as teaching and related services, such as counseling. Skills and functions that professional nurses perform in daily practice include:

- Providing direct and indirect client care services.
- Performing and delivering basic healthcare services.
- Implementing testing and prevention procedures.
- Observing signs and symptoms of illness.
- Administering treatments per physician's order.
- Monitoring treatment reactions and responses.
- Administering medications per physician's order.
- Monitoring medication responses and any side effects.
- Observing general physical and mental conditions of individual clients.
- Providing client and family teaching.
- Acting as a client advocate when needed.
- Documenting nursing care.
- Supervising allied nursing personnel.
- Coordinating members of the healthcare team.

Nurse Licensure

The authorization to practice nursing is defined legally as the right to practice nursing by an individual who holds an active license issued by the state in which she or he intends to work. The licensing process is administered by the Board of Registered Nursing, frequently called the BRN (or BON). This board may also grant endorsement or reciprocity to an applicant who holds a current license in another state. The applicant for RN licensure must have attended an accredited school of nursing, be a qualified nursing professional or paraprofessional, or have met specific prerequisites if licensed in a foreign country. Paraprofessionals can sit for the NCLEX if they meet all of the requirement (one example is a medic, in some states).

Board of Registered Nursing Functions

- Establishes and oversees educational standards
- Establishes professional standards
- Determines the candidates' qualifications and checks the candidates paperwork/applications
- Registers and renews nurses' licenses
- Conducts investigations into violations of the statutes and regulations
- Issues citations
- Holds disciplinary hearings for possible suspension or revocation of the license
- Imposes penalties following disciplinary hearings
- Establishes and oversees diversion programs in some states

Standards of Clinical Nursing Practice

The American Nurses Association first published these standards in 1973. The standards were revised in 1991 and updated in 2010. The standards apply to all registered nurses working in

Standards of Clinical Nursing Practice

Standards of Care

- Assessment
- Diagnosis
- Outcome Identification
- Planning
- Implementation
- Coordination of Care
- Health Teaching and Health Promotion
- Consultation
- Prescriptive Authority and Treatments
- Evaluation

Standards of Professional Performance

- Quality of Practice
- Education
- Professional Practice Evaluation
- Collegiality
- Collaboration
- Ethics
- Research
- Resource Utilization

clinical practice regardless of clinical specialty, practice setting, or educational preparation. These standards have shaped nursing practice and have helped both nurses and others understand what nursing is and does.

The standards describe a competent level of professional nursing care and professional performance common to all nurses engaged in clinical practice. This includes descriptions of the responsibility and accountability of the professional.

The standards of practice consist of two segments: Standards of Care, which describe the six standards of Clinical Nursing Practice using the nursing process; and the eight Standards of Professional Performance. These eight standards describe a competent level of behavior in the professional role.

Nurses in specialty nursing practice, such as critical care nursing or neonatal nursing, practice under standards that further define the responsibilities in these settings. The nursing specialties and appropriate groups, with the American Nurses Association, determine these standards.

Nurses practicing at an advanced level are accountable for meeting and maintaining the basic standards of clinical nursing practice in addition to the Scope and Standards of Advanced Practice Registered Nursing.

Standards of Care (Example)

Standard II. Diagnosis

The nurse analyzes the assessment data in determining diagnoses.

Measurement Criteria

1. Diagnoses are derived from the assessment data.
2. Diagnoses are validated with the patient, family, and other healthcare providers, when possible and appropriate.
3. Diagnoses are documented in a manner that facilitates the determination of expected outcomes and plan of care.

American Nurses Association Standards of Professional Performance

I. Quality of Practice: The nurse systematically enhances the quality and effectiveness of nursing practice.

II. Education: The nurse attains knowledge and competency that reflects current nursing practice.

III. Professional Practice Evaluation: The nurse evaluates one's own nursing practice in relation to professional practice standards and guidelines, relevant statutes, rules, and regulations.

IV. Collegiality: The nurse interacts with, and contributes to, the professional development of peers and colleagues.

V. Collaboration: The nurse collaborates with the patient, family, and others in the conduct of nursing practice.

VI. Ethics: The nurse integrates ethical provisions in all areas of practice.

VII. Research: The nurse integrates research findings into practice.

VIII. Resource Utilization: The nurse considers factors related to safety, effectiveness, cost, and impact on practice in planning and delivery of nursing services.

Source: American Nurses Association. (2010). *Nursing Scope and Standards of Practice*. Washington, DC.

Liability and Legal Issues

Each state defines and regulates the grounds for professional misconduct. Even though many states have similar standards, the practicing nurse must know how his or her state defines professional misconduct. The penalties for professional misconduct include probation, censure and reprimand, suspension of license, or revocation of license. The state's Board of Registered Nursing (BRN/BON) has the authority to impose any of these penalties for professional misconduct. Any one of the following actions would be considered professional misconduct:

- Obtaining an RN license through misrepresentation or fraudulent methods.
- Giving false information on application for license.
- Practicing in an incompetent or gross negligent manner.
- Practicing when ability to practice is severely impaired.
- Being habitually under the influence of drugs and/or alcohol.
- Furnishing controlled substances to himself or herself or to another person.
- Impersonating another certified or licensed practitioner or allowing another person to use his or her license for the purpose of nursing.
- Being convicted of or committing an act constituting a crime under federal or state law.
- Refusing to provide healthcare services on the grounds of race, color, creed, national origin, religion, or beliefs different from your own.

- Permitting or aiding an unlicensed person to perform activities requiring a license.
- Practicing nursing while license is suspended.
- Practicing medicine without a license.
- Procuring, aiding, or offering to assist at a criminal abortion.
- Holding oneself out to the public as a "nurse practitioner" without being certified by the BRN/BON as a nurse practitioner.

Drugs and the Nurse

In their daily work, most nurses handle a wide variety of drugs. Failure to give the correct medication or improper handling of drugs may result in serious problems for the nurse due to strict federal and state statutes relating to drugs. The Comprehensive Drug Abuse Prevention Act of 1970 provides the fundamental federal regulations for compounding, selling, and dispensing narcotics, stimulants, depressants, and other controlled items. Each state has a similar set of regulations for the same purpose.

Noncompliance with federal or state drug regulations can result in liability. Violation of the state drug regulations or licensing laws are grounds for the Board of Registered Nursing to initiate disciplinary action.

Negligence/Malpractice

The doctrine of negligence rests on the duty of every person to exercise due care in his or her conduct toward others from which injury may result. Negligence includes doing something that the reasonable and prudent person would not do. Anyone, including nonmedical persons, can be liable for negligence. Professionals (nurses) are held to a higher standard of care than nonprofessionals. The doctrine of negligence consists of the following elements: a duty owed to the client, a breach of that duty, damages to the client, and a causal relationship between the damages and the breach of duty. To find liability, it is necessary to identify a breach of duty to act with care, or a failure to act as a reasonable and prudent person (or nurse) would act under similar circumstances.

The standards referenced above form the basis for negligence or malpractice. Malpractice addresses a professional standard of care as well as the professional status of the caregiver. To be liable for malpractice, the person committing the civil wrong must be a professional. Courts define malpractice as any professional misconduct, unreasonable lack of skill, or fidelity in professional or judiciary duties that results in unnecessary suffering, injury, or death to the person.

Gross negligence is the intentional failure to perform a duty in reckless disregard of the consequences affecting the client. It is viewed as a gross lack of care to such a level as to be considered willful and wanton. Gross negligence can be due to improper use of restraints, client falls, or medication errors that lead to a client injury.

Criminal negligence also consists of a duty on the part of the nurse and an act that is the proximate cause of the injury or death of a client. This type of negligence is usually defined by statute and as such is punishable as a crime. The punishable act represents a flagrant and reckless disregard to the safety of others and/or a willful disregard to the injury liable to follow so as to convert the act into a crime when it results in personal injury or death. One is not "negligent" unless he or she fails to exercise the degree of reasonable care that would be exercised by a person of ordinary prudence under all the existing circumstances in view of probable danger of injury. The death or serious injury of a client after a medication or IV error can result in criminal negligence.

Malpractice is any professional misconduct that is an unreasonable lack of skill or fidelity in professional duties. In a more specific sense it means bad, wrong, or injurious treatment of a client resulting in injury, unnecessary suffering, or death to a client, proceeding from ignorance; carelessness; lack of professional skill; disregard of established rules, protocols, principles, or procedures; neglect; or a malicious or criminal intent.

Civil Law	Criminal Law
Contract	Assault
Unintentional tort	Battery
Intentional tort	Murder
Negligence	Manslaughter

The Joint Commission states "Malpractice is a cause of action for which damages are allowed."

Source: The Joint Commission's Sentinel Event Glossary of Terms, n.d. http://www.jointcommission.org/SentinelEvents/se_glossary.htm

It is the nurse's legal duty to provide competent, reasonable care to clients. To ensure that this occurs, the nurse must know the standards of care, develop consistent patterns of practice that meet the standards, and reflect his or her action in accurate

Guidelines for Drug Administration

- Nurses must not administer a specific drug unless allowed to do so by the particular state's Nurse Practice Act.
- Nurses must not administer any drug without a specific physician order.
- Nurses are to take every safety precaution in whatever they are doing.
- Nurses are to be certain that employer's policy allows them to administer a specific drug.
- Nurses must not administer a controlled substance if the physician's order is outdated.
- A drug may not lawfully be administered unless all the above items are in effect.
- Nurses are not permitted to fill prescriptions and in most states cannot write prescriptions, except in the case of nurse practitioners in some states.
- General rules for drug dispensing:
  - Check two forms of client identification before administering medications.
  - Never leave prepared medicines unattended.
  - Always report errors immediately.
  - Send labeled bottles or packages that are unintelligible back to the pharmacist for relabeling.
  - Store internal and external medicines separately if possible.

and complete documentation. Legal action against nurses has been increasing over the last decade. Nursing actions that constitute a breach of a standard of care that can lead to injury of a client include such actions as not inserting a Foley catheter correctly, not taking appropriate steps to decrease a client's temperature, not reporting unusual or worsening condition of the client to his or her physician, and not preventing falls. All of these situations can lead to malpractice suits.

Most lawsuits against nurses are for alleged violations of tort law. A tort is defined as an action or omission that harms someone. Malpractice refers to a tort committed by a professional acting in his/her professional capacity.

Legal doctrine holds that an employer may also be liable for negligent acts of employees in the course and scope of employment. Physicians, hospitals, clinics, and other employers may be held liable for negligent acts of their employees. This doctrine does not support acts of gross negligence or acts that are outside the scope of employment.

HIPAA

The Health Insurance Portability and Accountability Act (HIPAA), enacted into law in 1996 and phased in gradually, requires the Secretary of Health and Human Services (HHS) to devise standards to improve Medicare and Medicaid programs and the efficiency and effectiveness of the healthcare system. It ensures continuing healthcare insurance if the client has had existing group insurance and the client either changes or loses his/her job, proposes standards for electronic transactions and security signatures, and ensures privacy of individual health information.

The privacy rule component went into effect on April 14, 2003. The Privacy Rule applies to health plans, to healthcare clearinghouses, and to any healthcare provider who transmits health insurance information in electronic form. This is based on adopted HIPAA standards. A major purpose of the Privacy Rule is to define and limit the circumstances in which an individual's protected health information may be used or disclosed by the entities listed above. Information is disclosed only if allowed by the Privacy Rule.

Under this act, the client can request copies of his/her medical record and request that corrections be made if he or she identifies errors. The act specifies that personal healthcare information may not be used for any purpose not related to health care. The act also provides for client information to be given only to the client, or his/her representative, unless directed to do otherwise.

Compliance with HIPPA regulations is mandatory. Noncompliance can lead to civil penalties up to $25,000 per calendar year for multiple violations of a single standard. There are also penalties from $50,000 to $250,000 and/or imprisonment up to 10 years for other violations of the act.

Medicare Prescription Act

The **Medicare Prescription Drug Improvement and Modernization Act of 2003** was signed into law on December 8, 2003, although it was not enacted until 2005. This law brings affordable health care and prescription drug coverage to all Medicare recipients, seniors, and individuals with disabilities; expanded health plan options; improved healthcare access to rural Americans; and preventative care services such as mammograms. This is the first innovative change to the Medicare program since its inception in 1965. There are still proposed changes regarding the legislative healthcare tax credits and expansion of tax-free medical savings accounts.

CLIENTS' RIGHTS AND RESPONSIBILITIES

State and federal regulations governing healthcare facilities mandate that certain rights be afforded clients receiving health care. Hospitals and healthcare facilities must have established policies that discuss client rights and how staff are to adhere to them. The American Hospital Association (AHA) distributes "The Patient Care Partnership" brochure to all clients. This brochure describes what to expect during the hospital stay, the client's rights and privacy, and a short definition of a living will and advance directives. The AHA directs clients to the individual healthcare facility for further information.

Because clients' rights may conflict with nursing functions, you should be familiar with the key elements of these rights. It is important to remember that within a healthcare system, all clients retain their basic constitutional rights, such as freedom of expression, due process of law, freedom from cruel and inhumane punishment, equal protection, and so forth. Clients also have the right to know the identity of all healthcare providers and others involved in their care, which includes student nurses. All healthcare workers must wear a name badge indicating their title (e.g., Jane Doe, Student Nurse). The name of the nursing program is also included on the name badge. Most badges include a photo ID in addition to the name.

Under the Patient's Bill of Rights, hospitals must provide a foundation for understanding and respecting the rights and responsibilities of clients, their families, physicians, and other caregivers. The hospital must ensure and respect the role of clients in decision making about treatment choices and other aspects of their care. There must be a sensitivity to cultural, racial, linguistic, religious, age, and gender differences. In addition, the needs of persons with disabilities must be considered when providing healthcare services. Each hospital is encouraged to tailor its bill of rights to its particular community and client population. Individualization to the community ensures that the families and their specific rights are considered when the bill of rights is written.

Clients have a responsibility for their role in utilizing healthcare facilities. Their responsibilities include providing the physician with a complete history, relevant clinical manifestations, current medications, and herbal remedies. The client is responsible for asking questions and informing the physician of changes in clinical manifestations or general medical situations. Clients also need to respect the hospital personnel and treat hospital property and equipment with respect.

Consent to Receive Health Services

There are two major forms of consent signed by clients in a healthcare facility. The first consent is completed at the time of admission; the client signs the form in the admissions office or in the emergency department, wherever the admission is initiated. This agreement usually indicates that the client has agreed to such things as medical treatment, x-ray examinations, blood transfusions, and injections. The second type of consent is for invasive testing procedures, such as a liver biopsy, surgery, special studies involving contrast media, or other treatments in which there are risks associated with the procedure.

Consent is the client's approval to have his or her body touched by specific individuals, such as doctors, nurses, and laboratory technicians. Informed consent refers to the process of informing the client before granting a consent regarding treatment, such as tests and surgery, and must be understood by the client in terms of the intended outcome and the potential harmful results. The client may rescind a prior consent verbally or in writing.

The authority to sign a consent must be given by a mentally competent adult. Court-authorized persons may give consent for mentally incompetent adults. In emergency situations, if the client is in immediate danger of serious harm or death, action may be taken to preserve life without the client's consent.

The practitioner who will perform the procedure is legally responsible for obtaining the client's informed consent. The nurse's liability in terms of consent is to ensure that the client is fully informed before being asked to sign a consent form. The physician, nurse, or other health personnel must inform the client of any potentially harmful effects of the treatment. If this is not done, it may result in the nurse being held personally liable. The nurse must respect the right of a mentally competent adult client to refuse health care; however, a life-threatening situation may alter the client's right to refuse treatment.

In life-threatening emergencies, informed consent may not be required, because the law assumes a client will want treatment to save his or her life. The practitioner therefore

The Client's Bill of Rights

1. The client has the right to considerate and respectful care.
2. The client has the right to and is encouraged to obtain from physicians and other direct caregivers relevant, current, and understandable information concerning diagnosis, treatment, and prognosis. In emergencies, the client is entitled to the opportunity to discuss and request information related to specific procedures and/or treatments, the risk involved, and the financial implications of the treatment choices, etc. Clients also have the right to know the identity of healthcare professionals caring for them, including students, residents, or other trainees. The client has the right to know the immediate and long-term financial implications of treatment choices insofar as they are known.
3. The client has the right to make decisions about the plan of care prior to and during the course of treatment and to refuse a recommended treatment or plan of care to the extent permitted by law and hospital policy and be informed of medical consequences of this action.
4. The client has the right to have an advance directive and have the hospital honor the intent of the directive to the extent permitted by law and hospital policy. The institution must advise clients of their rights under state law and hospital policy to make informed medical choices. Hospitals must identify if a client has an advance directive and place it in the client records.
5. The client has the right to every consideration of privacy including examination, treatment, consultation, and case discussion.
6. The client has the right to expect all communications and records pertaining to his/her care be treated as confidential by the hospital, except in cases of suspected abuse and public health hazards when reporting is permitted or required by law.
7. The client has the right to review the records pertaining to his/her medical care and have the information explained or interpreted as necessary, except when restricted by law.
8. The client has the right to expect that, within its capacity and policies, a hospital will make reasonable response to the request of a client for appropriate and medically indicated care and services. Clients have the right to request a transfer to another facility. After the facility accepts the client, complete information must be provided.
9. The client has the right to ask and be informed of the existence of business relationships among the hospital, educational institutions, other healthcare providers, or payers that may influence the client's treatment and care.
10. The client has the right to consent to or decline to participate in proposed research studies or human experimentation affecting care and treatment or requiring direct client involvement and to have those studies fully explained prior to consent.
11. The client has the right to expect reasonable continuity of care when appropriate and to be informed by physician and other caregivers of available and realistic client care options when hospital care is no longer appropriate.
12. The client has the right to be informed of hospital policies and practices that relate to client care, treatment, and responsibilities, including grievances and conflicts. Clients have the right to be informed of available resources for resolving disputes, grievances, and conflicts.

Source: American Hospital Association, revision October 21, 1992.

intervenes appropriately to save the client's life regardless of whether informed consent was obtained.

Confidentiality

As stated earlier, clients are protected by law (invasion of privacy) against unauthorized release of personal clinical data, such as symptoms, diagnoses, and treatments. Nurses, as well as other healthcare personnel, may be held personally liable for invasion of privacy, should litigation arise from the unauthorized release of client data. Advances in technology, including computerized medical databases, the Internet, and telehealth, pose potential (unintentional) breaches of confidentiality and privacy. Changes in technology have changed not only the delivery of health care, but also the system used to record and retrieve health information.

The computer, fax machine, and phone calls between facilities and agencies leave the client at risk for information dissemination to unintended sources. Information is readily available to anyone walking by a fax machine or a computer. Confidential information, however, may be released with the client's consent. Information release is mandatory when ordered by a court or when state statutes require reporting child abuse, communicable diseases, or other incidents. Nurses have a legal and ethical responsibility to become familiar with their employer's policies and procedures regarding protection of clients' information.

Medical records are the key written account of such client information as signs and symptoms, diagnosis, treatment, and responses to treatment. Not only do these records document care given to clients, but they also provide effective means of communication among healthcare personnel. These records contain important data for insurance and other expense claims and are used in court in the event of litigation.

Healthcare professionals are becoming more aware of the implications of clients' rights as society in general becomes more aware of every human being's basic rights. Although there are still gaps in the legal process, many states are beginning to grapple with the status of laws applicable to clients who are hospitalized. It is essential that nurses be aware of the particular state's laws and statutes affecting clients and themselves. Nurses as well as physicians are accountable for their actions, and the threat of civil and criminal prosecution is becoming more prevalent. The American Nurses Association has developed a position statement supporting the principles of client privacy and confidentiality as a commitment to client advocacy. This statement is part of the Code of Ethics for Nurses (Privacy and Confidentiality Interpretive Statements 3.1 and 3.2).

Patient Self-Determination Act

Patient Self-Determination Act of 1991 (PSDA) is a federal law that applies to all healthcare institutions receiving Medicaid funds. It imposes on the state and providers of health care, such as hospitals, nursing homes, hospices, home health agencies, and prepaid health care organizations, certain requirements concerning advance directives and an individual's rights under state law to make decisions concerning medical care; this includes the right to accept or refuse medical or surgical care. This act informs clients about existing rights, but does not create new rights or change existing state law. The act did serve as an incentive for many states to pass durable power of attorney for healthcare statutes. It does not require clients to execute advance directives, but it does require that they be apprised and educated about advance directives. It also requires that assistance be offered in the execution of the advance directives if the client elects to do so. The PSDA defines an *advance directive* as a written instruction, such as a living will or durable power of attorney, for health care. A competent adult can communicate preferences about future medical treatment through the advance directive. Clients must be provided written documentation regarding their rights to formulate advance directives. Clients must be made aware of their rights to make decisions about these issues on admission to all healthcare facilities and health maintenance organizations (HMOs); however, they are not required to sign an advance directive if they do not choose to do so. Client education regarding advance directives should be accomplished outside the acute care setting. The directives allow clients to control their own healthcare decisions, even if they become incapacitated in the future.

Classifications of Law Related to Nursing

Classification	Example
Constitutional	Clients' rights to equal treatment
Administrative	Licensure and the state BRN
Labor relations	Union negotiations
Contract	Relationship with employer
Criminal	Handling of narcotics
Tort	
Medical malpractice	Reasonable and prudent client care
Product liability	Warranty on medical equipment

Advance Medical Directives

Advance medical directives are of two types: treatment directives, such as living wills, and appointment directives, such as durable power of attorney for health care. An advance medical directive is a document that allows clients to make legal decisions about how they wish to receive future medical treatment. It is written and signed before any such care becomes necessary. The document becomes effective only when the client becomes incapacitated. The directives may be in the form of a living will or durable power of attorney. Within this document, the client may indicate the person or persons he or she wishes to make medical decisions in situations in which the client is unable to do so. An advance directive does not need to be written, reviewed, or signed by an attorney. It must, however, be signed and witnessed by two individuals, and the witnesses should not be hospital employees, relatives, or heirs to the estate. Copies of the document should be kept on file in the physician's office and the hospital. Advance directives vary among states, and therefore the nurse must be knowledgeable about the use and type of directives in the state in which he or she practices.

> **Advance Directives**
>
> An advance directive allows the client to participate in the following decisions:
>
> - Choosing healthcare providers such as physicians and nurses.
> - Deciding who may have access to medical records.
> - Choosing the type of medical treatments the client desires.
> - Consenting to or refusing certain types of medical treatments.
> - Choosing the agent who will make decisions about the client's health care when the client is unable to do so.

Living Will A living will is a type of advance directive that indicates the client's wishes regarding prolonging life using life support measures, refusing or stopping medical interventions, or making decisions about his or her medical care when the client is diagnosed as having a terminal or permanent unconscious condition. It does not apply to any other healthcare decisions. Living wills are executed while the client is competent and able to make sound decisions. As conditions change, a living will needs to be evaluated for relevance. (States differ in their acceptance of living wills as legal documents.)

Durable Power of Attorney for Health Care This legal document must be prepared and signed while the client is competent. The document gives power to make healthcare decisions to a designated individual (agent) in the event the client is unable to make competent decisions for himself or herself. The designated person is obligated to follow the directives outlined in the document. The document gives the client's agent specific healthcare decisions or the authority to make any and all healthcare decisions the client would make if able. Decisions regarding withdrawing or using life support, organ donation, or consent to treatment or procedures are included in the directive. As long as the client is competent, the agent does not have the authority to make treatment decisions.

The major difference between living wills and the durable power of attorney is that the durable power of attorney is more flexible. A living will is used only if the client's condition is terminal or they are in a permanently unconscious state. A living will only allows the client to direct that life-sustaining treatments be withheld or withdrawn. The durable power of attorney is not limited to terminal or permanent unconscious conditions. It also addresses all types of healthcare decisions, including life-sustaining treatments.

Clients should be encouraged to carry a card in their wallet indicating that they have a living will and/or durable power of attorney on file. The name of their agent should be listed.

Do Not Resuscitate

Health care facilities must provide written information to clients concerning their right to make decisions regarding their care.

A "Do Not Resuscitate" (DNR; sometimes called "Do Not Attempt to Resuscitate" [DNAR]) order is another type of advance directive. A DNR is a request to not have cardiopulmonary resuscitation (CPR) if the client ceases to breathe or is unable to sustain a heartbeat. An advance directive form can be signed at any time before or during hospitalization. When signed, the physician places a DNR notation in the client's medical chart. (See Chapter 34.) In some facilities these orders are reviewed every 48 to 72 hours.

If a terminally ill client without a DNR order tells you orally that he/she does not want to be resuscitated in a crisis, document this information and state the client's level of orientation. Notify the physician and administration, legal services, or social services of the client's wishes.

CLINICAL PRACTICE

Legal Issues

As a student nurse, you need to maintain a high standard of practice and protect yourself against legal problems. Most legal actions against nurses result from a claim that the nurse breached a standard of care that results in injury to the client. In order to prevent legal problems, the nurse must always follow the five steps of the nursing process; administer medications following the seven rights of medication administration; continually assess the client, clearly communicate changes in the client's condition to the appropriate individual, and then document findings on proper forms or computer screens (the medical record is a legal document); follow hospital policies and procedures; and understand and use equipment safely and appropriately. Constantly refer to these guidelines to protect the client from harm and to protect yourself from potential lawsuits.

Before your first clinical experience, you should review the most essential components of client care to enable you to practice safe and efficient nursing care. Laws in each state vary in relationship to how the law applies to your practice and the medical record; therefore, check that you are familiar with your individual state laws.

Guidelines for clinical practice, the parts of a client chart or computer printout, communication techniques, principles of medical asepsis, a basic nursing assessment, and protocols for nursing care procedures are presented to give you confidence and background information in providing nursing care.

Guidelines for Safe Clinical Practice

Before attempting to provide client care, you need to familiarize yourself with all aspects of the care the client requires. The following guidelines will assist you in this preparation. Usually, the preparation is completed the night before you go to the clinical setting. If this is not possible, you need to identify those aspects of preparation that will render you a safe practitioner.

- Obtain the clinical assignment in sufficient time to be able to prepare for safe practice.
- Read the client's chart or computer data and obtain information necessary to assist you in client care. This usually encompasses the following items: history and physical,

physician's progress notes, graphic sheet, medication record, laboratory findings, nurses' notes or flow sheets or both, admissions database, client care plan, Kardex card or computer plan of care, and physician's orders. Each of these documents is illustrated later in this chapter.

- Review all procedures that you will provide for the client. Use your skills and fundamentals books for your review.
- Research the medical diagnosis so that you are more aware of signs and symptoms the client may exhibit. Identify alterations from normal such as altered laboratory values, vital signs, and so forth.
- Research nursing diagnoses identified on the chart or potential diagnoses you identify from review of the chart. Your client care will focus on the nursing diagnoses and interventions associated with collaborative care.
- Research all medications you will administer to the client. Many instructors require that medication cards or documents be completed on all medications before administration.
- Plan your day's schedule by developing a time management plan to help keep you organized and to enable you to complete client care in a timely manner.
- Practice charting the procedures you will be administering so that you can identify appropriate vocabulary and include necessary information. Pertinent charting information is included with each procedure described in this text.
- Complete a clinical prep sheet as required by the instructor. The sheet usually has a section for all pertinent data.

Military Time The use of "military time" is becoming more common in healthcare facilities today. One advantage of using this time frame is that the confusion of whether something is ordered or documented in the AM or PM is avoided. Military time describes time as a 24-hour clock rather than the standard 12-hour clock like your watch. Midnight is identified as 2400, 1:00 AM is 0100, 3:00 PM is 1500, and so on. Review both the 24-hour clock and the chart below to acquaint yourself with this method of keeping time.

Use of PDAs in Clinical Setting

A PDA is a personal digital assistant or handheld computer. Students are becoming more adept in the use of these aids, especially as they have pocket drug guides, diagnostic test guides, and clinical calculators contained within the PDA.

24-HOUR CLOCK

12-hour clock	24-hour clock
12 midnight	2400
1:30 AM	0130
1:59 AM	0159
12 noon	1200
2:18 PM	1418
7:30 PM	1930
9:00 PM	2100

3:30 PM standard time or 1530 military time.

HIPAA requires that you recognize and protect oral, written, and electronic information that could reveal a client's identity and health-related information. This information is referred to as the PHI (protected health information).

HIPAA has developed guidelines for using a PDA safely. HIPAA recommends that the client's name or any identifying data not be input into the PDA. Personal demographics or client identifiers such as history and physical findings, lab data, physical data, and phone numbers must be input using passwords only. If identifying data must be input into the PDA, the nurse needs to utilize the "Security" feature, which requires a password to enter the system. Most nursing students will not use this type of data entry. It is more usual for a home health nurse to need the personal identifiers.

Providing Client Care

You have prepared for clinical practice before coming to the nursing unit. Information regarding client needs and care is provided through shift report and an individualized, in-depth client report by the team leader or preceptor. Each hospital has a method for presenting the report. Some facilities tape a report from the off-going shift that is listened to by the on-coming staff. Other nursing units give a verbal report in which they review the information obtained by the previous shift. Facilities where primary nursing is practiced have a one-to-one report between the on-coming nurse and the off-going nurse for a specific group of clients. At this time a worksheet is completed that lists times for treatments and medications. Following the report, the team leader or your preceptor nurse goes over all aspects of the care you will deliver for the client. This is the time to ask any questions you may have regarding policy or procedure for the nursing unit or the client.

The following outline of client care will assist you in planning your nursing care for the day. Before you begin client care, you need to review the client's profile or computer plan of care and check that all medications are available in the computer on wheels (COW), Pyxis, or medication care.

1. Perform hand hygiene.
2. Gather equipment, such as a stethoscope, sphygmomanometer, thermometer, and linen.
3. Check two forms of client identification (other than room number). Introduce yourself to the client and explain the nursing care you will be giving.
4. Check if the client has any preference for the order in which the care is to be given when possible.
5. Complete a nursing assessment. You may use the basic nursing assessment outlined in this chapter as a guide if your instructor does not have one she or he prefers you to use.
6. Document your findings as you are completing the physical assessment, and enter it in the nurses' notes section of the chart or on the flow sheet or in the computerized documentation system.
7. Take vital signs if it is the policy of the unit. In some facilities, nursing assistants take vital signs, while nursing staff receives report.

8. If using a PDA to enter client data, follow HIPAA guidelines specific to such devices.
9. Don gloves (if appropriate) and complete all nursing interventions, and document the findings immediately after completion.
10. Administer all medications, including checking two identifiers, according to policies and procedures in the healthcare facility. If gloves were used, remove and wash hands.
11. Document medication administration in the appropriate place, and observe for signs of side effects or unusual findings.
12. During your nursing care, practice good communication techniques.
13. Complete all charting.
14. Terminate the relationship with the client.
15. Report off to the appropriate person.
16. Perform hand hygiene after providing nursing care and before leaving the nursing unit.

Client's Forms

Become familiar with each form or computer screen, its placement in the chart or computer, and the information that it contains. Brief examples of some computer screens are included in this chapter, and examples of these forms are included in Chapter 3.

Kardex/Client Profile The Kardex card or Client Profile represents the "hub" for all client activities. Physician's orders are transcribed on the card. Laboratory tests, medications, and activity levels are just a few items documented in designated areas of the Kardex or profile.

The computerized plan of care is replacing the Kardex card in many facilities today. The same information is contained in the electronic version, but in many cases, the information is more up to date.

Care Plan Client care plans vary among healthcare facilities. The older individualized handwritten care plan is being replaced by preprinted standardized care plans, computerized care plans, or critical pathways. Regardless of the type of care plan used, the purpose does not change. Care plans are written guidelines for client care that all healthcare workers use to deliver individualized care. Most care plans today are termed *Multidisciplinary Care Plans* because all health team providers document treatments and observations on one form. Pertinent data regarding client care needs can be communicated to all providers using the multidisciplinary care plan. Client teaching is frequently detailed on the same form.

Critical or Clinical Pathway You may see either of these terms used to describe an approach to deliver collaborative, outcome-driven health care to clients. These documents are another approach to providing individualized care to clients. Interventions and outcomes are progressively outlined within the pathway as illustrated.

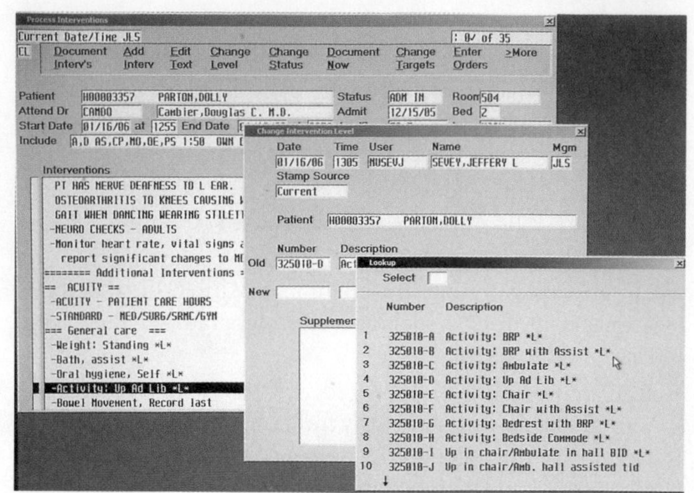

▲ Computer-generated client profile.

Client's Chart

Client information is contained on several forms or computer screens, depending on documentation systems used in the healthcare facility. These forms or computer screens are important to your preparation and administration of nursing care. Be sure to familiarize yourself with the specific forms or screens in the healthcare facility where you have your clinical experience. The following forms are intended to be just examples. Refer to Chapter 3 for complete description of forms or screens.

Nurses' Notes *Nurses' notes* are documents that contain clinical observations and nursing interventions. Many facilities have limited the narrative charting format and increased the use of flow sheets and checklists, termed *Patient Care Records* or *Multidisciplinary Team Records*. This type of charting decreases the time it takes nurses to document and promotes comprehensive documentation. Each hospital has developed its own documentation system; therefore, it is important to

COMMUNITY HOSPITAL

CLIENT CARE PLAN
Individualized

Client Information

Discharge Criteria
1) *Wound healing progressing satisfactorily*
2) *Verbalizes ability to care for wound at home*
3) *Verbalizes understanding of discharge instructions*
4)

Admitting Diagnosis

Relevant Info:

Date	Problem/Need	Expected Outcome/Goal	CP	DL	Nursing Interventions	Update/DC	Initial
3/22/12	*Impaired skin integrity*	*Wound healing s̄*	*q4h*	*Prior*	*4a. Place on Lt side c̄ chux under hips & abd.*		
	related to prolonged	*s̄ complications*		*to dis-*	*Gently move into this position. Do not rush c̄ move.*		
	immobility			*charge*	*b. Note drainage location, quantity color & odor.*		
					c. Irrig. wound c̄ 50 ml. saline solution. Use		
					asepto syringe. Catch solution in emesis basin.		
					d. Cover wound with ABD dressings. Use		
					Montgomery straps.		

▲ Individualized client care plan.

Day 3 POD 2	Day 4 POD 3	Day 5 POD 4
• **q 8 hr. ✓** Basic assessment, CMS, Drsg, I&O, SPO_2, VS, IV site, skin assessment. • ✓ Homan sign. HV dc'd. • Oxygen protocol.	• **q 8 hr. ✓** Basic assessment, CMS, Drsg, I&O, past or present IV site healing, skin assessment, Homan sign. • Oxygen protocol.	• **q 8 hr. ✓** Basic assessment, skin, assessment, CMS, Drsg, I&O, Homan sign. • Oxygen protocol. • ✓ past or present IV site healing.
• ↑ gait training. • Ambulate BID if able.	• Ambulate BID. • PT/Nursing.	• Ambulate BID. • PT/Nursing.
• TED/SCD, I.S., TCDB. Foley remains if needed or until Epidural dc'd. • *Hip Precaution for hemiathroplasty only*	• TED/SCD • DC Foley. • TCDB, especially prior to SpO_2✓. • *Hip Precaution for hemiathroplasty only*	• TED/SCD. • TCDB. • *Hip Precaution for hemiathroplasty only*
• Stool softener, Iron supp. BID (hold if GI upset). Cathartic if no BM. • Anticoagulant.	• Stool softener, Iron supp. BID (hold if GI upset). • Anticoagulant.	• Stool softener, Iron supp. BID (hold if GI upset). • Anticoagulant.
• IV TKO, IVL, or DC if not needed (leave IVL until Epidural dc'd).	• IV dc'd.	
• Diet as tolerated.	• DAT.	• DAT.
• If PCA or Epidural taper dose & give PO pain meds.	• Taper and DC PCA; give PO pain meds. ✓ SpO_2 × 1. SpO_2 reading.	• PO pain meds, reassessing pain level.
• Analgesia method.	• Analgesia method, Pharmaceutical & non-pharmaceutical pain control. • Discharge plan reinforced.	• Understands Ortho inst, risk of DVT/PE, Hip precautions. • Reinforce any instruction given. • Answer any questions patient may have.
• BCP CN or RN to notify MD if platelet count shows 100,000 drop in past 24 hr.	• BCP CN or RN notify MD if platelet count shows 100,000 drop in past 24 hr.	• As indicated.
• PT BID. • Chaplain Services & Dietary consult PRN.	• PT. Chaplain Services & Dietary consult PRN.	• PT. Chaplain Services & Dietary consult PRN.
• SS assess if needed for SNF transfer (notify SS if min. assist needed).	• Discharge decision, S.S. assess if needed and not done.	• Arrange equipment needed for home. • Complete transfer sheet or discharge instructions.
Shift: 7-3 | 3-11 | 11-7 — Circle Yes (Y) or No (N) Y N | Y N | Y N Ambulation started (PT).	Shift: 7-3 | 3-11 | 11-7 — Circle Yes (Y) or No (N) Y N | Y N | Y N Voiding without Foley. Y N | Y N | Y N SS note re. discharge plan (SS).* Y N | Y N | Y N BM passed (RN). Y N | Y N | Y N Pain managed with PO medicine (RN).*	Shift: 7-3 | 3-11 | 11-7 — Circle Yes (Y) or No (N) Y N | Y N | Y N Discharge plan reinforced (RN). Y N | Y N | Y N Discharged to appropriate care level (RN).

11-7		11-7		11-7	
11-7		11-7		11-7	
7-3		7-3		7-3	
7-3		7-3		7-3	
7-3		7-3		7-3	
3-11		3-11		3-11	
3-11		3-11		3-11	
3-11		3-11		3-11	

▲ Clinical pathway.

become familiar with the system before beginning to document. Many facilities have gone to computerized charting systems that facilitate a more thorough mechanism for data input. In-service education programs on use of the computer for charting and data retrieval need to be completed before clinical experience is begun to ensure that you can obtain all the necessary information to provide safe care for the client.

Medication Records Medication records are usually similar to those illustrated. All medications should be documented on a medication record. Some facilities chart routine medications on one medication sheet, and PRN and one-time only medications are charted on another sheet. Check the institution's policy for each record's use. Electronic health records also have medication screens.

Graphic Records Vital signs are recorded on the graphic sheet; see also Chapter 3, including blood pressure, pulse, respirations, temperature, and pain level. Most facilities have included the pain scale on the graphic record as it is referred to as the fifth vital sign. Weight is also included on this form. Intake and output results may be recorded on this record or on a separate form, depending on the facility.

Physician's Orders Physician's orders may be written on forms with carbon copies attached, preprinted, or computerized, depending on the facility. If the orders are carbon copied, copies can be sent to the pharmacy and to the lab, with the original retained in the client's chart. Computerized orders can be easily utilized by all hospital departments.

Physician's Progress Notes Physician's progress notes contain daily observations and thoughts regarding treatments, signs, and symptoms experienced by the client, operative risks explained to the client, and the client's responses to therapy.

History and Physical The physician's report of his/her assessment is written on a special form. Most hospitals type the history and physical from notes dictated by the physician. When this occurs, it may be several days before this information is available.

Laboratory Forms Laboratory results are sent back to the unit on the original laboratory order form. The information from each form may be transcribed to a laboratory data flow sheet. This sheet provides a valuable overview of all laboratory results. Computerized reports of laboratory findings may be used in some facilities.

Basic Nursing Assessment

Each nurse develops her or his own routine for completing a basic nursing assessment. There is no right or wrong way, although it should be consistent and complete. The following outline for basic assessment is a simple approach to the assessment and one you may wish to adopt until you have established a good system for yourself.

The basic assessment is completed at the beginning of each shift (usually a complete assessment is done once per day and focus assessments at the beginning and end of the other shifts). You should focus on the specific physiologic system that correlates with the client's diagnosis. For a more in-depth discussion of each system in the assessment, see Chapter 11, Physical Assessment.

The following outline will assist you in completing a basic physical assessment.

1. Vital signs:
    a. Temperature (method dictated by condition)
    b. Radial or apical pulse (depending on condition)
    c. Respirations: rate, depth, and rhythm
    d. Blood pressure: Korotkoff's sounds
    e. Pain: location and intensity of pain; use pain scale to determine pain level.
2. Response to medications if given.

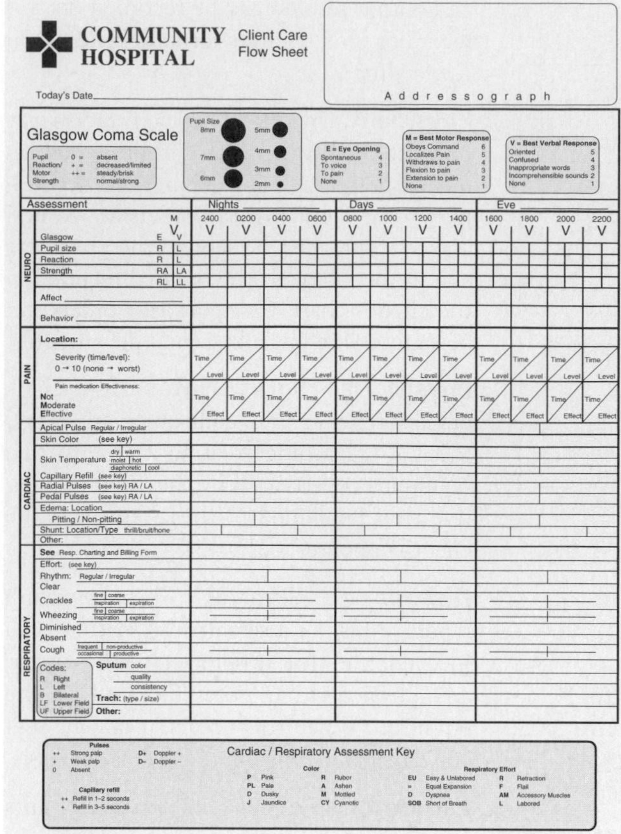

COMMUNITY HOSPITAL
Client Care Flow Sheet

Today's Date________ Addressograph

Glasgow Coma Scale

Pupil Reaction/Motor Strength: 0 = absent; + = decreased/limited; ++ = steady/brisk, normal/strong

Pupil Size: 8mm, 7mm, 6mm, 5mm, 4mm, 3mm, 2mm

E = Eye Opening	
Spontaneous	4
To voice	3
To pain	2
None	1

M = Best Motor Response	
Obeys Command	6
Localizes Pain	5
Withdraws to pain	4
Flexion to pain	3
Extension to pain	2
None	1

V = Best Verbal Response	
Oriented	5
Confused	4
Inappropriate words	3
Incomprehensible sounds	2
None	1

Assessment	Nights 2400	0200	0400	0600	Days 0800	1000	1200	1400	Eve 1600	1800	2000	2200
NEURO: Glasgow (M, E, V)												
Pupil size R L												
Reaction R L												
Strength RA LA, RL LL												
Affect												
Behavior												
PAIN: Location; Severity (time/level): 0 → 10 (none → worst)	Time/Level	Time/Level	Time/Level	Time/Level	Time/Level	Time/Level	Time/Level	Time/Level	Time/Level	Time/Level	Time/Level	Time/Level
Pain medication Effectiveness: Not, Moderate, Effective	Time/Effect	Time/Effect	Time/Effect	Time/Effect	Time/Effect	Time/Effect	Time/Effect	Time/Effect	Time/Effect	Time/Effect	Time/Effect	Time/Effect
CARDIAC: Apical Pulse Regular / Irregular												
Skin Color (see key)												
Skin Temperature dry/warm, moist/hot, diaphoretic/cool												
Capillary Refill (see key)												
Radial Pulses (see key) RA / LA												
Pedal Pulses (see key) RA / LA												
Edema: Location												
Pitting / Non-pitting												
Shunt: Location/Type thrill/bruit/none												
Other:												
RESPIRATORY: See Resp. Charting and Billing Form												
Effort: (see key)												
Rhythm: Regular / Irregular												
Clear												
Crackles fine/coarse, inspiration/expiration												
Wheezing fine/coarse, inspiration/expiration												
Diminished												
Absent												
Cough frequent/non-productive, occasional/productive												
Sputum color, quality, consistency												
Trach: (type / size)												
Other:												

Codes: R Right; L Left; B Bilateral; LF Lower Field; UF Upper Field

Cardiac / Respiratory Assessment Key

Pulses: ++ Strong palp; + Weak palp; 0 Absent; D+ Doppler +; D− Doppler −

Capillary refill: ++ Refill in 1–2 seconds; + Refill in 3–5 seconds

Color: P Pink; PL Pale; D Dusky; J Jaundice; R Rubor; A Ashen; M Mottled; CY Cyanotic

Respiratory Effort: EU Easy & Unlabored; = Equal Expansion; D Dyspnea; SOB Short of Breath; R Retraction; F Flail; AM Accessory Muscles; L Labored

▲ Flow sheet.

FROM UNIVERSITY MEDICAL CENTER TO MEDICATION ADMINISTRATION RECORD

INTRAMUSCULAR/SUBCUTANEOUS SITE CODES		PAIN SCALE	SEDATION SCALE
A-Right Arm	F-Right Thigh	0-No Pain	1-Wide Awake
B-Left Arm	F-Left Thigh	1-Mild Pain	2-Drowsy
C-Right Hip	G-Right Abdomen	2-Discomforting	3-Dozing Intermittently
D-Left Hip	H-Left Abdomen	3-Distressing	4-Mostly Sleeping
		4-Horrible	5-Awakens Only When Aroused
		5-Excruciating	

	MEDICATIONS AND DIRECTIONS	RT	2301-0700	0701-1500	1501-2300
03/11	Dilantin 2 caps PO Every Morning (Phenytoin Sodium Cap 100 Mg)				
03/11	Phenobarbital 1 Tab PO Bedtime (Phenobarbital Tab 30 Mg)				
03/11	Folvite Generic 1 Tab PO Once Daily (Folic Acid Tab 1 Mg)				
03/11	A-Methylpred 40 Mg IV Every 12 HR from 9 AM (Methylprednisolone Sod Sul)				
03/11	Prilosec 1 Cap PO Every 24 Hours (Omperazole Cap 20 Mg)				
03/11	Xylocaine Viscous 5-10 mL PO Every 4 Hours-PRN (Lidocaine Viscous Soln 3%) To wash mouth				

MESSAGE — MAR CHECKED

Time
Pain Rating
Sedation Level
Respiration Rate

NURSE INITIALS AND SIGNATURE | NURSE INITIALS AND SIGNATURE | NURSE INITIALS AND SIGNATURE

CONFIDENTIAL INFORMATION

Rm & Bed # Name CHART COPY Med Rec # Page____ of____

▲ Medication administration record (MAR).

COMMUNITY HOSPITAL ROUTINE

PRESS HARD

MEDICATION DOSAGE ROUTE	SHIFT	/ /19	/ /19	/ /19	/ /19
	2300-0700				
	0700-1500				
	1500-2300				

SITE CODE: Ⓐ - RUOQ; Ⓑ - LUOQ; Ⓒ - R THIGH; Ⓓ - L THIGH; Ⓔ - R LOWER ABD; Ⓕ - L LOWER ABD; Ⓖ - R DELTOID; Ⓗ - L DELTOID

CHART COPY

▲ Medication record.

COMMUNITY HOSPITAL

CLINICAL RECORD

DATE
HOSP. DAY/POSTOP DAY
TIME: 0200 0600 1000 1400 1800 2200 | 0200 0600 1000 1400 1800 2200 | 0200 0600 1000 1400 1800 2200

KEY	PULSE	TEMP. C	F
	140	40.6	105
	130	40.0	104
	120	39.4	103
	110	38.8	102
	100	38.3	101
	90	37.7	100
	80	37.2	99
	70	36.6	98
	60	36.1	97
	50	35.5	96

BLACK – PULSE & RESPIRATIONS; RED – TEMPERATURE

RESPIRATIONS
BLOOD PRESSURE
HEIGHT — WEIGHT
BREAKFAST LUNCH DINNER
DIET – TYPE
% CONSUMED
INTAKE & OUTPUT HOURS: 0600-1400, 1400-2200, 2200-0600
INTAKE: Oral, IV, Blood Plasma, Other
8 Hr. Total
Output: Urine, Emesis, Stools, GI Suction
8 Hr. Total
24 Hr. Intake
24 Hr. Output
SIGNATURE
DATE: CLINICAL RECORD

▲ Graphic record.

COMMUNITY HOSPITAL

COMMUNITY HOSPITAL
HISTORY and PHYSICAL EXAMINATION

Record all positive and all important negative findings in the following order:

Client Complaint
History of P.I.
Past History
Illness
Operations
Injuries
Family History
System Review
Physical Examination
General
Skin
EENT
Lungs
Breasts
Heart
Abdomen
Rectal
Pelvic
Vascular/system
Extremities
Locomotor
Neurological
Provisional Diagnosis

Name — Last — First — Initial — Adm. No. — Date

M.D.
HISTORY AND PHYSICAL EXAMINATION

▲ Physician's history and physical record.

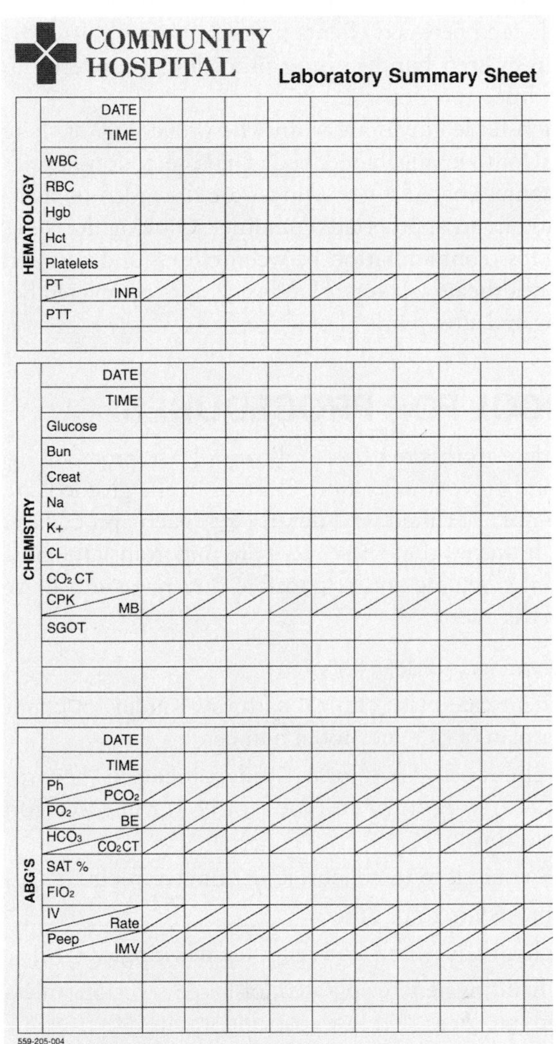

COMMUNITY HOSPITAL Laboratory Summary Sheet

HEMATOLOGY: DATE, TIME, WBC, RBC, Hgb, Hct, Platelets, PT / INR, PTT

CHEMISTRY: DATE, TIME, Glucose, Bun, Creat, Na, K+, CL, CO_2 CT, CPK / MB, SGOT

ABG'S: DATE, TIME, Ph / PCO_2, PO_2 / BE, HCO_3 / CO_2CT, SAT %, FIO_2, IV / Rate, Peep / IMV

559-205-004

▲ Laboratory results flow sheet.

THE JOINT COMMISSION REQUIRES COMPLETE COLLECTION INFORMATION!

COMMUNITY HOSPITAL Laboratory Request - Form #5

NURSING — Ordered By: Date / / Time — Collected By: Date / / Time

COLLECTION PRIORITY:
ROUTINE COLLECTION - AM PICK UP
DRAW TODAY - PROCESS ROUTINELY
TIMED - DRAW @
DRAW STAT - PROCESS ROUTINELY
STAT - LIFE THREATENING
PRE - OP - SURGERY @
FASTING
RANDOM

ORDER PHYSICIAN:
IN:

IMMUNOLOGY
INFLUENZA ANTIBODY T — INFLUENZA 90-32060
CHLAMYDIA ANTIBODY T — CHLMY IGG 90-01475
LEGIONELLA ANTIBODY T — LEGION IFA 90-32010
MYCOPLASMA ANTIBODY T — MYCOPLASMA 90-32030
RUBEOLA ANTIBODY T — RUBEOLA 90-01230
HERPES SIMPLEX I T — HERPES I 50-20040
HERPES SIMPLEX II T — HERPES II 50-20050
CYTOMEGALOVIRUS T — CMV SERO 90-32130

THYROID
Hypothyroid panel - Order T — THY PNL & TSH2
Hyperthyroid panel - Order T — THY PNL & T3
T3 UPTAKE T — T3 U 10-01761
T4 T — T42 10-01781
FREE T4 T — FT4 10-03460
T3 Uptake, T4 and FTI T — THY PNL
TOTAL T3 T — T3 10-03440
FREE T3 T — FT3 10-03400
TSH, HIGHLY SENSITIVE T — TSH2 10-03480
OTHER

IRON STUDIES
FERRITIN T — FERRITIN3 10-01110
TRANSFERRIN T — TRNSFERRIN 90-01240

KIDNEY STONE
KIDNEY STONES-CHEM QUANT — KIDS 90-30001

URINE TESTS
VMA, 24 HOURS — VMA URINE 90-01120
5-HIAA — 5-HIAA URINE 90-01360
TOTAL PROTEIN, 24 HOURS — UT PROT 10-00830
CALCIUM, 24 HOURS — UCA 24 HR 90-03100

TOM / TOXICOLOGY
NORPACE R — DISOPYRAMI 90 00200
VANCOMYCIN T
Random: Next Dose @ — VANCO R 70-01100
PRE 1/2 Hour Before Dose @ — VANCO T 70-01120
POST 1/2 Hour After Dose @ — VANCO P 70-01140
NAPA AND PROCAINAMIDE T — LGNAPA 70-01050
LITHIUM T — LI 10-02600
STAT QUALITATIVE URINE DRUG SCREEN 5 ml — U TRIAGE 70-10000
COMPREHENSIVE TOX SCREEN T, L&U — COMP TOX2 90-04040
RAPID URINE DRUG SCREEN 50 ml — RPD URDRG 90-04060

HEPATITIS TESTS
HEP B SURFACE ANTIGEN T — HEP BS AG 50-00460
HEP B SURFACE ANTIBODY T — HEP BS AB 50-10010
HEP B CORE ANTIBODY T — HEP BC AB 50-10020
HEPATITIS EVALUATION T (HBsAG, HBsAB, HBcAB, HAIgM HAAB TOTAL, HEP C AB) — HEP4 50-11104
HEPATITIS B PANEL T (HBsAG, HBsAB, HBcAB, HBeAG, HBeAB) — HEP BMPNL 50-11001
HEPATITIS C ANTIBODY T — HEP C AB 90-01960

MISCELLANEOUS
NEWBORN SCREEN CARD — NB SCRN 90-33030
AFP-TUMOR MARKER T — AFP TMR 90-00160
PSA T — PSA2 10-03420
CEA T — CEA2 10-10160
FSH T — FSH 90-00330
PAP Prostatic Acid Phosphate T — PAP 90-00290
GLU-6-PTASE DEHYDROGENASE L — G6PD SCRN 90-02220
RESPIRATORY SYNCYTIAL VIRUS T — RSV 90-32000
QUANTITATIVE HCG T — HCG 10-10104
ACTH T — ACTH 90-00040
HAPTOGLOBIN T — HAPTOGLOB 10-01040
ANTI-NUCLEAR ANTIBODY (ANA) T — ANA2 90-02800
VITAMIN B12 T — B12 10-05050
FOLATE T — FOLATE3 10-05022
OTHER:
OTHER:

T = Tiger Top
R = Red Top
L = Lavender Top
U = Urine
# ml = Volume Requested

559-410-020 (8/95) Rev. 10/98 LG4613/302168

▲ Laboratory order form.

3. Emotional responses: client behavior, reactions, and demeanor; general mood (crying, depression)
4. Skin, hair, and nails: Skin: presence or absence of abrasions, contusions, tears, erythema, pressure ulcers, incision line, color, turgor, temperature, edema. Inspect hair distribution, thickness or thinness, texture, and amount. Inspect nails for curvature and angle, texture, color, and surrounding tissue.
5. Musculoskeletal: activity level, general mobility, gait, range of motion
6. Neurologic: pupils (size, response, equality); hand grips; strength and sensation of all extremities; ability to follow commands; level of consciousness
7. Respiratory: breath sounds; sputum color and consistency; cough (productive or nonproductive)
8. Cardiovascular: heart sounds; presence of pulses; edema; observe presence of hair on extremities (lack of indicates poor circulation)
9. Gastrointestinal: bowel pattern and sounds; presence of nausea or vomiting; abdominal distention; consumption of diet
10. Genitourinary: voiding; color, odor, and consistency of urine; dysuria; vaginal drainage or discomfort; penile discharge

If any unusual findings are assessed, complete a more in-depth assessment of the particular system affected. Throughout the day, continue to assess changes in the client's condition by paying particular attention to the alterations from normal that you identified in the initial assessment. At the end of the shift, make a notation of any changes in the client's condition.

MEDICAL ASEPSIS PRINCIPLES

Microorganisms are found everywhere in nature. Pathogenic microorganisms, or pathogens, cause disease; nonpathogenic microorganisms, or nonpathogens, do not cause disease. Some microorganisms are nonpathogens in their normal body environment. An example of this is *Escherichia coli*, which is normally present in the intestinal tract and does not cause a problem until it inhabits another environment such as the urinary tract.

The spread of microorganisms is prevented by the use of two forms of asepsis: medical asepsis and surgical asepsis. Medical asepsis occurs when there is an absence of pathogens. Surgical asepsis occurs when there is an absence of all organisms. Medical asepsis is often referred to as "clean technique," whereas surgical asepsis is termed "sterile technique." A discussion of surgical asepsis can be found later in this book. This chapter discusses medical asepsis as it affects nursing care.

Principles of medical asepsis are used in all aspects of client care. In fact, the use of medical asepsis begins before you report to the nursing unit. To ensure protection for the client, you begin practicing medical asepsis by limiting jewelry to only a wedding band and perhaps small earrings for pierced ears when administering client care. Fingernails are short and in good repair. Your hair is off your collar and under control to prevent contaminating sterile fields and falling into client's food or wounds. While providing client care, the following principles should be kept in mind:

- Linen rooms or carts are considered clean; therefore linen not used for client care cannot be returned.
- Utility rooms are designated as areas for clean and dirty supplies. Cross-contamination must be avoided by not placing articles in the wrong area.
- Linen and articles are carried away from your uniform and are not held close to your body.
- Articles dropped on the floor are considered contaminated and must be discarded appropriately. If linen is accidentally dropped on the floor, it is placed in a soiled linen hamper.
- Clients are to wear slippers or shoes when out of bed.
- Paper tissue is used for removing client's secretions. Discard the tissue in the trash basket.
- Each client has his or her own supplies and equipment, which are not used by other clients. Sterilization or disinfection of equipment is carried out between use.
- Equipment is cleaned and rinsed with cold water to remove secretions or substances before being returned to the central supply area. Heat coagulates the substances and makes them more difficult to remove.
- Soap and water are considered the best cleansers because they help break down soil so it can be more readily removed. Detergents may be more effective in hard or cold water; however, tissue damage can result from their use. Germicides, when added to soap or detergent, increase the effectiveness of the cleansing agent.
- Friction is used to facilitate soil removal. A brush, sponge, or cloth may be used to produce the friction.
- When aseptic technique is used, cleaning is conducted from the cleanest to the least clean area. For example, always clean the incision area from the center of the incision to the periphery of the skin.
- If you are not feeling well, you should not report for clinical experience. If you are running a temperature or have a cold and a runny nose, call the appropriate person and report that you are ill.

Hand Hygiene

The single most effective medical aseptic practice is handwashing. When you first arrive at the nursing unit and before beginning nursing practice, you should complete a medical handwashing procedure. The important concept to remember is that you thoroughly soap and rinse your hands twice before providing any nursing care to the client. Hands are washed before all procedures and between clients. Alcohol-based hand rub is usually used between clients if hands are not dirty. The specific step-by-step handwashing procedure is covered in Chapter 14, Infection Control.

Clean, nonsterile gloves are worn when touching, or there is a potential for touching, blood, body fluids, secretions, excretions, and contaminated items. Gloves are discarded immediately after use in an appropriate container. Gloving decreases the risk of cross-contamination between clients and between clients and healthcare workers. Handwashing is completed before donning and after removal of gloves.

PROTOCOL FOR PROCEDURES

Each procedure in this textbook follows a basic protocol. To save space and prevent repetition, all steps in the protocol are frequently not outlined in detail for each procedure. Remember, however, that these steps are important and must be followed if complete and responsible nursing care is to be delivered to the client.

- Check physician's orders.
- Check client care plan, clinical pathway, Kardex, or client computer plan of care, not room number.
- Identify client using two forms of identification (according to facility policy, and not only for medication administration).
- Introduce yourself to the client, if first time in room.
- Explain procedure to be done.
- Answer client's questions and reinforce teaching.
- Perform hand hygiene using alcohol-based solution unless your hands are dirty; then use soap and water.
- Gather equipment and fill out charge slips.
- Take all of the required equipment and linens to the room.
- Provide privacy for the client by drawing curtain or screen around bed.
- Raise bed to HIGH position.
- Lower side rail nearest you.
- Drape client (if appropriate).
- Don gloves (if appropriate).

- Perform procedure according to protocol.
- Clean client as necessary.
- Remove drape and position client for comfort.
- Remove gloves.
- Raise side rail to UP position.
- Lower bed.
- Replace call bell.
- Pull back curtain or remove screen.
- Remove equipment and clean, dispose of, and disperse used equipment.
- Perform hand hygiene using alcohol-based solution unless your hands are dirty; then use soap and water.
- Document or chart findings.

MANAGEMENT Guidelines

Each state legislates a Nurse Practice Act for RNs and LVN/LPNs. Healthcare facilities are responsible for establishing and implementing policies and procedures that conform to their state's regulations. Verify the regulations and role parameters for each healthcare worker in your facility.

Delegation

- As an RN you will be held accountable and responsible for your actions. When delegating client care, you must know the healthcare worker's level of client care tasks that can be assigned to each category of worker. The Nurse Practice Act for both RN and LVN/PN must be adhered to when assigning client care. The skill level and scope of practice of unassisted licensed personnel must be evaluated before assigning client care.
- The RN must abide by and function within the American Nurses Association Code of Ethics for Nurses. The RN is responsible for the appropriate delegation of nursing tasks to others in order to provide safe, competent client care.
- Legal issues and regulations must be followed in order to establish appropriate client care standards when delegating to other healthcare workers. The RN has a responsibility for a level of performance that must be carried out and cannot be delegated, including healthcare teaching, initial assessment, and the administration of IV medications.
- The signing of a consent form for surgery or an invasive procedure may be delegated to the LVN/LPN, and in some facilities a ward clerk may obtain the consent. Informed consent is the responsibility of the physician; however, most facilities allow nurses and other healthcare workers to witness the client's signature on the consent form after an explanation has been provided by the physician. Some facilities require that a physician obtain the signed consent form. The signature of the witness indicates only that he or she obtained the client's signature on the form. The RN is still responsible for ensuring that the client understands what the procedure is, including potential complications. If the client is unsure of the procedure, the physician needs to be notified to re-explain the procedure until the client understands.

Communication Matrix

- Each member of the nursing unit should be given appropriate directions on the tasks to be completed, keeping in mind the legal issues surrounding delegation. Assign only those tasks the healthcare worker is legally responsible to carry out.
- The RN must ensure that proper consent forms are signed by the client prior to invasive procedures or surgery. Even when the task of witnessing a consent form signing is delegated, the RN is responsible for ensuring it is completed and placed in the client's chart. Ask the witness to inform you when all paperwork is completed for the procedure in order for you to check the forms.
- Ensure that all healthcare workers are aware of DNR orders. Make sure the Kardex or plan of care adequately states the DNR order, and provide that information during report.
- Give specific directions to healthcare workers regarding the client information you wish reported and how you wish to receive it (i.e., written or verbal).
- Provide current information to healthcare workers in a timely manner as it impacts their care of the client (i.e., changes in activity or diet orders).
- Ensure that all forms of documentation are completed in a timely manner; if computerized charting is utilized in the facility, all healthcare workers have responsibility to complete particular forms.

CRITICAL THINKING Strategies

Scenario 1

As a new student you are going into the hospital to prepare for the clinical experience tomorrow morning. There are two stages of preparation. The first stage is obtaining all the necessary information you will need to provide safe care. The second stage is reviewing your textbooks and lecture notes to gain an understanding of the client's diagnosis, medications, lab values, and diagnostic tests that will be done during his/her hospitalization.

- If you have only a limited time to review the client's chart, what sections of the chart will provide you with sufficient information to render you safe to care for the client?

- In preparing for clinical practice, what information is essential to review in addition to the data you have obtained from the clinical record? Where is the most appropriate place to find this information?
- List the priority interventions you will carry out within the first hour of the clinical experience. Explain the rationale for your answers.

Scenario 2

As a student nurse you have been assigned to complete an activity where you compare and contrast legal/ethical issues related to nursing practice. You are assigned to research the ANA Standards of Clinical Nursing Practice, The Nurse Practice Act in your state, and the Code of Academic and Clinical Conduct from the National Student Nurses' Association, Inc.

- Briefly describe the primary purpose/function of each of these nursing regulations or guidelines.
- Select one of the above nursing regulations/guidelines and describe how the regulation/guideline will impact your role as a professional nurse.
- The National Student Nurses' Association developed the Code of Academic and Clinical Conduct. How do you plan to incorporate the code into your practice as a student nurse? How will this practice prepare you for the Registered Nurse profession?

NCLEX® Review Questions

Unless otherwise specified, choose only one (1) answer.

1. According to the American Nurses Association, nursing is best defined as a profession that
   1. Cares for clients in all types of settings.
   2. Protects, promotes, and optimizes health and abilities of clients.
   3. Provides client care as ordered by the physician.
   4. Assists clients in activities of daily living and prepares them for home care.
2. The National Student Association has formulated a code for nursing students. The most important rationale for adhering to this code is it
   1. Encompasses ethical principles that guide professional behavior.
   2. Governs nursing behavior in the clinical setting.
   3. Lets the student know what is acceptable behavior.
   4. Gives guidelines for administering medications.
3. Guidelines for clinical preparation include which of the following activities?
   1. Ensure your uniform is similar to the staff nurse uniform.
   2. Begin the nurse–client relationship using a more social communication to place the client at ease.
   3. Address the client by first name to make him or her feel comfortable.
   4. Listen to client's statements and feelings regarding their clinical manifestations because they are more familiar with their bodily functions.
4. The Nurse Practice Act regulates the practice of nursing in each state. Which skills and functions are included?

   Select all that apply.
   1. Delegate registered nursing responsibilities to an LVN/LPN who has many years of practice.
   2. Instruct the CNA to obtain the vital signs and health history on a newly admitted client.
   3. Complete a client care plan on a newly admitted client.
   4. Refer a client to the discharge planning nurse.
   5. Administer IV medications ordered by the physician.
   6. Observe and document client's responses to medications and treatments.
5. The best statement regarding the Standards of Clinical Nursing Practice is that the standards
   1. Apply only to nurses in specialty practice or who function under a physician.
   2. Do not apply to nurses who are advance practice nurses as they are not accountable for maintaining the basic standards of clinical practice.
   3. Describe a competent level of professional nursing care and professional performance common to all categories of nurses.
   4. Apply to nurses employed in acute care and long-term care settings only.
6. The penalties for professional misconduct could include which of the following?

   Select all that apply.
   1. Probation.
   2. Revocation of license.
   3. Imprisonment for practicing without a license.
   4. Compensation to facility for costs accrued from criminal act.
   5. Reprimand.
7. The nurse can be charged with gross negligence when
   1. There is an act that causes death of a client.
   2. The nurse demonstrates a reckless disregard for client safety.
   3. There is an improper use of restraints.
   4. The nurse refuses a client assignment before the shift begins.

8. Before providing client care, the nurse will
   1. Gather appropriate equipment.
   2. Ask the RN what order of care the client usually likes.
   3. Check the Kardex or computerized plan of care record to determine the order of care for the client.
   4. Identify the client by calling his/her name.

9. When performing a basic nursing assessment, the nurse will
   1. Perform the assessment following morning care, after the client is more relaxed.
   2. Complete an assessment of the physiologic system most affected by the client's condition.
   3. Perform a brief overall system assessment, with a focus on the system most affected by the client's diagnosis.
   4. Complete an in-depth assessment at the end of each shift to provide client-centered information to the on-coming shift.

10. Principles of medical asepsis include
    1. Placing soiled linen only on the bottom of the linen cart.
    2. Cleaning (with alcohol) equipment that has been dropped on the floor.
    3. Using equipment from another client providing it is cleaned with 2% chlorhexidine before and after use.
    4. Cleaning equipment with cold water before returning it to central supply according to facility policies.

2

Nursing Process and Critical Thinking

LEARNING OBJECTIVES

1. Define the term *critical thinking*.
2. Explain how critical thinking is used in each step of the nursing process.
3. Define the term *nursing process*.
4. Describe how the nursing process relates to nursing.
5. Discuss the term *assessment*, and describe how it influences the nursing process.
6. List the components of the assessment step.
7. Describe the primary purpose of the analysis phase of the nursing process.
8. Define outcome identification and planning, and give an example of this step in the nursing process.
9. Define what is meant by the implementation phase of the nursing process.
10. Explain evaluation and include your understanding of why it is an important step in the nursing process.
11. Define the term *nursing diagnosis*.
12. Differentiate nursing diagnosis from medical diagnosis.
13. Define NIC and NOC and their role in standardizing nursing language.
14. Compare and contrast the two-part and three-part Nursing Diagnosis Statement.
15. Define evidence-based nursing practice.
16. State two examples of nursing diagnoses.

CHAPTER OUTLINE

NURSING PROCESS

Nursing process is a familiar term in nursing and is used as a way of organizing nursing actions in healthcare delivery. It is a systematic, problem-solving approach to client care. It is considered a critical thinking competency that assists the nurse to intervene in client care. The nurse's actions are based on reasoning and scientific knowledge. By definition, the term *process* refers to a series of actions that lead toward a particular result. When attached to nursing, the term *nursing process* becomes a general description of nursing: assessment, analysis/nursing diagnosis, planning, implementation, and evaluation. The nursing process is used to diagnose and treat human responses to health and illness (American Nurses Association, 1980). The nursing process provides an organized structure and framework for the delivery of nursing care in all settings. It provides the basis for critical thinking in nursing. Although the five steps can be described separately and in logical order, in practice the steps overlap and events may not always occur in the order listed here. For purposes of understanding this process, however, it is appropriate to work through each phase in logical progression.

The five steps of the nursing process are presented, defined, and illustrated to assist you in understanding the importance of integrating this framework in your beginning mastery of nursing content. A model of each step will enable you to visualize how the individual components can be translated into direct nursing actions or behaviors.

Assessment

Assessment, the first step in the nursing process, refers to the establishment of a database for a specific client. Assessment requires skilled observation, reasoning, and a theoretical

Assessment

Gather data
- Objective data
- Subjective data

Verify data
Confirm observations
Organize data
Make inferences from data
Communicate data

Observe—Interview—Examine

Identify client needs
Be aware of staff reactions to client
Assess sources of data
- Client history
- Data from family
- Client status—physical/emotional
- Signs and symptoms
- Test results and findings

Recall stored knowledge

knowledge base to gather and differentiate, verify and organize data, and document the findings. The nurse gathers information relevant to the client from a variety of sources and then assigns meaning to this data. Assessment is a critical phase because all the other steps in the process depend on the accuracy and reliability of the assessment. Assessment is based on concepts of physiology, pathophysiology, psychology, and social adjustment.

Assessment is also the initial step in critical thinking that leads to the appropriate nursing diagnosis.

Nursing Diagnosis

Nursing diagnosis is an integral component of the nursing process. Following the assessment step of the nursing process, a nursing diagnosis is formulated. Nursing diagnosis is the statement of a client problem derived from the systematic collection of data and its analysis. It is a clinical judgment about a designated client, family, or community that provides the basis for completion of the nursing process. Nursing diagnosis includes the etiology, when known, and relates directly to the defining characteristics. Nursing diagnosis provides the foundation for each individual client's therapeutic plan of care, and once it is established, the nurse is accountable for actions that occur within the scope of this nursing diagnosis framework.

Nursing diagnosis is a clinical judgment about individual, family, or community responses to actual or potential health problems/life processes. Nursing diagnoses provide the basis for selection of nursing interventions to achieve outcomes for which the nurse is accountable (North American Nursing Diagnosis Association, 1997). The nurse must use critical thinking and decision-making skills when determining nursing diagnoses.

Nursing Diagnosis

Analyze and synthesize collected data
Examine defining characteristics, both major and minor
Determine clusters of clues
Identify related factors
Identify potential nursing diagnoses
Develop nursing diagnosis appropriate to client problem

Planning

Identify short- and long-term goals and outcomes
Prioritize nursing diagnoses
Develop a plan based on goals and outcomes, including a teaching plan
Anticipate needs of client and family based on priorities
Select nursing behaviors needed to accomplish goals
Specify deadlines for completion of plan
Coordinate care and community resources
Consider contingencies for modifying plan
Record relevant information

Outcome Identification and Planning

This phase refers to the identification of nursing actions that are strategies for achieving the goals or the desired outcome of nursing care. The planning and outcome phases are directly related to solving or alleviating the problems identified in the nursing diagnosis. The plan includes short- and long-term client-centered goals, strategies for goal outcome, and nursing measures for the delivery of care. During this phase, the nursing diagnoses are prioritized to meet the client's immediate needs.

Clients should be involved in the planning phase to ensure that the client's and the healthcare team members' goals are congruent. If they are not, goal achievement can be impaired. Planning focuses on the development of a plan of care individualized for a specific client.

Planning is based on the client's healthcare needs, selected goals, and strategies directed toward goal achievement. It is a plan of care in which the appropriate nursing actions and the client's desires are considered and chosen to achieve a goal.

Implementation

The fourth phase in the nursing process is the implementation, or intervention, phase. This phase refers to the priority nursing actions or interventions performed to accomplish a specified goal. It explicitly describes the action component of the nursing process. This phase involves initiating and completing those nursing actions necessary to accomplish the identified client goals and outcomes. Nursing actions must be appropriate, individualized for the client, and based on safe nursing practice; they should be formulated on scientific principles and derived from the problem-solving process. Finally, the

Implementation

Implement client care plan by giving direct care based on goals and outcomes

Perform actions and procedures in accordance with client needs

Counsel and teach client, family, or both

Use preventive, palliative, or emergency measures for client's welfare

Encourage independence and self-care

Motivate and maintain optimum wellness

Communicate appropriately to client and client's family

Record data

Continue assessment process

interventions must be congruent with the total medical as well as nursing treatment plan. Implementation of the plan involves giving direct care to the client to accomplish the specified goal.

Implementation is based on accurate and complete assessment, interpretation of data, identified client needs, goals and outcomes, analysis, nursing diagnosis, and strategies to achieve goals.

Evaluation

The final phase of the nursing process is evaluation. Evaluation is the examination of the outcome of nursing actions or the extent to which the expected outcomes or goals were achieved. Was the goal achieved? What parts of the goal were not achieved? Was client behavior modified? Evaluation is a necessary phase to complete the nursing process. It allows the nurse to continue to identify goals in the overall treatment plan and to alter the current plan to the client's needs.

Evaluation is based on the previous phases of the nursing process (assessment, analysis, outcomes and planning, and implementation). The evaluation phase completes the process and examines the outcome.

The nursing process has provided the framework for the immense amount of nursing content that is contained in this textbook. The rationale for choosing this framework is that it provides a way to organize and present nursing knowledge as well as being an essential component of providing quality client care.

Evaluation

Determine effects of nursing actions

Determine extent to which goals and outcomes were achieved

Examine appropriateness of nursing actions

Investigate effect and degree of compliance for client and family

Reassess care plan—judge if goal modification is necessary

Consider alternative nursing actions

Record client responses

CRITICAL THINKING

All nurses are required to use critical thinking skills as they provide nursing care for clients. Nurses are expected not only to master nursing content from many disciplines, but to think creatively, solve problems, communicate, and use reflective judgment in the practice of nursing. Though critical thinking involves problem solving and decision making, it is a more complex process involving higher-level thinking. It employs interpretation, analysis, evaluation, and inference. Critical thinking requires understanding abstract ideas, consideration of the context in which a situation exists, and openness to new ideas.

There is no single accepted definition, but many authors have defined critical thinking in terms that are relevant to nursing. The word *critical* is derived from the Greek word *kritikos*, meaning "critic." To be critical means to ask questions, to analyze, to examine your own thinking and the thinking of others (Chaffee, 1994). Critical thinking focuses on judgment, and nurses must use reflective judgment because each clinical situation they encounter is different and unique. Effective critical thinking and problem solving actually depend on relevant knowledge and previous experience (Facione 1998; McKeachie, 1999). The definition of critical thinking by Scriven and Paul (1996) for the National Council for Excellence in Critical Thinking Instruction is widely accepted today by many in the field of education. "Critical thinking is an intellectually disciplined process of actively and skillfully conceptualizing, applying, analyzing, synthesizing, and/or evaluating information gathered from, or generated by observation, experience, reflection, reasoning, or communication, as a guide to belief and action." To expand on this statement, critical thinking requires cognitive skills, the ability to ask pertinent questions, knowledge, and the ability to think clearly. As stated, an important aspect of critical thinking is also the ability to use reflection and language properly. Reflection is the action of thinking back or recalling an earlier clinical situation, remembering nursing actions that worked or didn't work, and determining whether this information is helpful in the current situation. The ability to use language is associated with the ability to think meaningfully. Thinking and language are closely related processes (Miller & Babcock, 1996). To become a critical thinker, the nurse must use language accurately. If nurses are unable to use appropriate terminology, communication with the client and other healthcare workers may be impaired. In addition to these skills, nurses need to be creative thinkers in order to develop appropriate plans of care for clients.

Critical thinking competencies are the cognitive processes a nurse uses to make judgments. Specific critical thinking competencies in clinical situations include diagnostic reasoning, clinical inferences, and clinical decision making. These competencies are used by many healthcare professionals. The nursing process is considered the specific critical thinking competency in nursing. Diagnostic reasoning is a series of clinical judgments made during and after data collection, resulting in an informal judgment or formal diagnosis (Carnevali & Thomas, 1993). The clinical decision-making process uses reasoning to ensure that after evaluating all options available, the best are chosen to improve the client's health status.

Critical thinking skills assist the nurse to look at all aspects of a situation and then arrive at a conclusion. Critical thinkers identify and question assumptions, determine what is important in each situation, and examine each alternative before making an informed decision. When critical thinking is employed in a clinical situation, you would expect that one would examine ideas, beliefs, principles, assumptions, conclusions, statements, and inferences before coming to a conclusion and then making a decision. The conclusions and decisions made by nurses affect clients' lives; therefore, they must be guided by precise, disciplined thinking, which leads to accurate and complete data collection. While examining the situation, using these concepts, the nurse would also be using scientific reasoning, the nursing process, and decision-making processes.

NURSES ARE CRITICAL THINKERS

Nurses are required to be problem solvers and decision makers, to acquire nursing judgment skills, and to think critically in order to practice in today's nursing climate. Decision-making and problem-solving skills are necessary for managing and delivering client care. Both of these skills require critical thinking.

Watson and Glaser have described critical thinking as a process that defines a problem, selects pertinent information for a solution, recognizes stated and unstated assumptions, formulates and selects relevant hypotheses, draws conclusions, and judges the validity of inferences. The outcome of critical thinking is forming a conclusion and stating the justification for that conclusion. This is what differentiates critical thinking from usual thinking.

Nurses who are considered critical thinkers are those who use logic, creativity, and good communication and are flexible and competent in delivering client care. Additional attitudes attributed to nurses who are considered critical thinkers include open-mindedness, empathy, realism, and being a team player.

Nurses use critical thinking skills as they relate theory to practice, apply the nursing process in client care, and make critical clinical decisions. The ability to use critical thinking skills assists the nurse to recognize and analyze problems and to solve them using a systematic approach.

To acquire critical thinking skills, the nurse must first develop a sound theoretical knowledge base. This means studying the concepts appropriate to each clinical discipline (e.g., the pathophysiology related to the medical diagnosis or disease state; knowledge of pharmacology, growth and development, nutrition, and psychology; and client problem in each area of nursing practice). This knowledge is transferred to clinical situations by determining the appropriate nursing diagnosis in order to provide safe client care and make independent judgments. In addition to reflecting on previous knowledge, the nurse gains immeasurable experience in the identification of clients' problems with each clinical experience. Over time, the nurse is able to select the best solution for assisting clients to resume a healthy state.

Critical thinking is a process as well as a cognitive skill that is used to identify and define problems, assess clients, and evaluate their responses to treatment and care. Nurses select and classify data and organize it into clusters or patterns to formulate nursing diagnoses. Critical thinking is used when multiple nursing actions are considered and the most appropriate action is selected for each client problem. After the client intervention is carried out, the effectiveness of the intervention and client outcome is evaluated using critical thinking. It is easy to see from this statement that critical thinking is used throughout the steps of the nursing process.

You have used problem-solving methodologies throughout your education as you have faced everyday situations. The nursing process provides the basis for critical thinking in nursing when problem solving is required in client care. The following examples demonstrate how critical thinking is used throughout the five steps of the nursing process. When the steps are followed consistently and accuracy of the data is maintained, habits that promote critical thinking in nursing are developed.

Assessment in Critical Thinking

Identifying essential assessment data and where the data can be found requires critical thinking. Obtaining, classifying, and organizing data is a principal function of critical thinking.

A leading cause of error in making clinical judgments or decisions is the collection of inaccurate or incomplete data during the assessment phase. The data collection or assessment step of the nursing process assists the nurse to predict, detect, prevent, and control client problems. A nurse with good critical thinking skills develops a systematic approach to obtaining and validating data. This includes using all sources for data collection (i.e., reviewing the client's chart, asking pertinent questions, and completing the assessment in a systematic manner). If an assessment tool is used, ensure that thought goes into the way the data is recorded; don't just write information down in a rote manner. Review the assessment form to determine whether additional or more in-depth information is required based on the initial findings—this action involves critical thinking. Ask yourself, "Is this information relevant?" and "Do I need to assess anything else?" Listen to the client. Clients provide important subjective data to add to objective information. Once all of the data are collected, information should be validated to ensure that data are not missing and that existing data are correct. Data also need to be organized or categorized in a usable system. Clustering of similar information assists the nurse in forming a picture of the client's problems and strengths. Critical thinking is necessary to determine the significance of reported data, and clustering identifies whether patterns of behavior or responses exist. Clustering data helps determine relevant from irrelevant data as well as gaps in information. It also pinpoints cause-and-effect relationships. Once the clustering is completed, inferences may be formulated.

Nursing Diagnosis in Critical Thinking

A nursing diagnosis is the identification of a client problem. Before a nursing diagnosis is made, the nurse has critically analyzed, synthesized, clustered, and interpreted all the collected data. Use of critical thinking skills is essential in this step of the nursing process. As you cluster data, you are applying the scientific principle of classifying information in order to determine whether relationships exist among the data and whether data are relevant or irrelevant in this situation. As information is clustered, inconsistencies among the collected data may prompt the nurse to look for additional assessment findings. Determining when additional information is needed for an accurate diagnosis prevents the nurse from making a very common critical thinking error—making a judgment based on incomplete information. It is important to recheck the client's records, asking additional questions of the client in order to obtain the necessary information needed to complete the appropriate nursing diagnosis. After the data are clustered, the nurse begins to organize defining characteristics into meaningful patterns. This is a major step toward identifying the client's problems. Usually, the presence of two to three defining characteristics validates the nursing diagnosis. The identification of this information assists the nurse in determining the appropriate nursing diagnosis. Identifying patterns requires critical thinking skills associated with a sound scientific knowledge base. The nurse must differentiate the normal from the abnormal findings, as well as the risk factors for abnormal patterns of functioning. Using a nursing diagnosis reference book will assist the nurse in clarifying data relevant to defining characteristics or risk factors related to the client's clinical manifestations.

During this step of the nursing process, actual client problems are identified, potential problems are predicted, and priorities are established. Establishing nursing diagnoses is an important independent action of the nurse; however, medical diagnoses must be considered as well. Nursing diagnoses cannot be treated in isolation. Collaborative problem identification and treatment with other healthcare workers form the basis of client care and contribute to a holistic approach to client care. Priorities of care are determined by the severity of the client's problems. These priorities are identified within the planning and intervention steps of the nursing process.

Planning in Critical Thinking and Outcome Identification

Long- and short-term goals are formulated after deliberating with the client, family, and other healthcare team members. Defining realistic goals that are acceptable to the client requires critical thinking. A prioritized plan of care is developed during this phase of the nursing process.

Determining outcomes (goals) and strategies for achieving goals are paramount to providing effective client care. Outcomes are time-specific as well as setting-specific. Long-term outcomes or goals are usually based on what is expected by the time of discharge from a nursing unit or a facility. In acute care facilities, short-term outcomes are based on time frames as short as by the end of the shift, within 24 hours, etc. The long-term goal or discharge expected outcome should be determined before other outcomes and interventions are initiated. When setting priorities for client problems, keep in mind that treating these problems must be addressed on the plan of care in order to achieve the client's discharge goal or outcome. There are two critical thinking skills inherent in this step. One is listing the client problems and determining whether there are relationships between the problems, and the other is assigning the problems by highest priority. These critical thinking skills require sound scientific principles and scientific method, clinical judgment, reasoning skills, and goal-directed thinking.

When listing the actual and potential problems identified by the assessment data, identify which problems need immediate intervention and those that are underlying causes of the problems. Those situations identified as causing the problem must be assigned the highest priority. After listing the problems, determine whether there are relationships among the problems. If relationships exist, explore how one problem affects another. Maslow's Hierarchy of Human Needs is employed by many nurses to determine prioritization of problems. Maslow lists problems with survival needs (food, fluids, oxygen) as the highest priority. These needs must be addressed first in the plan of care for the client's well-being.

To write specific, realistic, client-centered outcomes, the problems must be stated clearly. Outcomes are derived directly from the problem statement, and the subject of the problem statement is the client. An example of a clear, client-centered outcome is "The client will ambulate the length of the hall before discharge." Remember, problem statements are written as nursing diagnoses. An example of a client outcome utilizing a nursing diagnosis is "The client will demonstrate accurate administration of insulin according to the guidelines established by the diabetic educator within 24 hours of admission." This outcome is directly related to a "Knowledge Deficit: Insulin Administration" nursing diagnosis. You will also notice there is a time-specific statement included within the outcome statement. This time frame assists the nurse to evaluate outcome achievement and the need to re-evaluate the plan of care.

Implementation in Critical Thinking

Nursing interventions are specific strategies developed to achieve positive client outcomes. These interventions are determined by using the critical thinking skills of generalizing, explaining, and predicting outcomes. After consideration of all identified possible actions, nursing interventions are implemented.

Identifying appropriate nursing actions is critical to the outcome of client care. Determining these actions requires critical thinking skills. These skills include the ability to identify specific actions, predict and monitor the client's response to the actions, and weigh risks and consequences of each action. Examining the risks and consequences of an action, a nurse is determining the most beneficial and least harmful approach to client care. When interventions are clearly delineated on the plan of care, the likelihood of the actions being carried out is enhanced. The more specific the intervention, the greater chance of outcome success. If increasing fluid intake is the intervention, specifics regarding fluid likes and dislikes of the client should be addressed. For example, "Client prefers noncarbonated beverages at room temperature." Another example of a specific intervention is "Ambulate the client after his bath, before lunch, and before dinner." This would be appropriate for the goal to ambulate the length of the hall by discharge. Putting times for interventions or distances for ambulation increases the likelihood of compliance with the intervention by all healthcare workers.

Evaluation in Critical Thinking

During the final phase of the nursing process, the nurse critically analyzes each of the client outcomes. If the client need (goal/objective) was not met, the plan is revised. Clearly documenting a comprehensive plan provides the basis for evaluation. Evaluating progress toward outcome achievement assists the nurse in evaluating the effectiveness of the plan. A critical thinking question during this phase of the nursing process is "How well did the client accomplish the goal?" The nurse might also ask "What could have been done differently?"

NURSING DIAGNOSIS

An important implication of nursing diagnosis is that it refers to a health problem or condition that nurses are legally licensed to treat. Establishment and acceptance of using nursing diagnoses will demonstrate recognition and legal sanction of nursing as a profession with its own body of knowledge, education, and experience.

Nursing diagnoses provide the basis for selection of nursing interventions to achieve outcomes for which the nurse is accountable. In 1987, the Center for Nursing Classification at the University of Iowa College of Nursing introduced the Nursing Interventions Classification (NIC) system and in 1991 the Nursing Outcomes Classification (NOC) system. These classification systems and NANDA were merged and formed the NNN Alliance International in 2001. NIC is a comprehensive list of nursing interventions that are grouped according to nursing activities. The NIC includes physiological and psychosocial interventions to treat and prevent illness and promote health for clients, families, and the community. NOC has developed a taxonomy of standardized outcomes to measure the effects of nursing interventions. These outcomes can be used in all settings and with all client populations. Nursing diagnosis textbooks are now integrating the three components. Each nursing diagnosis statement includes domains, classes, diagnosis, outcomes, and interventions. The nursing diagnoses are continually changing as the NANDA research continues. New diagnoses are introduced at each biennial meeting.

Nursing diagnosis will play a pivotal role when evidence-based, professionally led nursing care is more universally implemented in client care. Using standardized terminology, such as Nursing Diagnosis, Nursing Interventions Classifications (NIC), and Nursing Outcomes Classifications (NOC) as electronic client health records become a requirement, will allow for systematic collection of nursing data across all healthcare organizations. Collecting data in this manner provides for analysis and audit of a large volume of information at minimal cost. Standardized terminology more effectively meets client needs while ensuring client safety.

The term *nursing diagnosis* is not comparable to or the same as a medical diagnosis. The major difference between medical and nursing diagnoses is the focus on illness, injury, or disease by the physician. The nursing diagnosis focuses on the response to actual or potential health problems or life processes and the client's responses to illness, change in lifestyle, etc. Medical diagnoses do not vary until treatment is completed, whereas the nursing diagnosis is fluid and changes as the client's condition or response to treatment changes. Nursing diagnosis highlights critical thinking and decision making and provides a universal terminology that all nurses, irrespective of work site, can understand. Nursing diagnosis is derived from the assessment phase of the nursing process and is based on both subjective and objective data. As the database evolves, patterns of health problems emerge, and alterations from normal health states are identified. A nursing diagnosis is a concise label that describes the observed behavior of the client. The nursing diagnosis can be an actual or potential problem. The specific problem identified implies that the nurse is qualified and prepared to intervene and treat that condition. The nurse is not legally able to intervene and treat a medical diagnosis without specific physician's orders. Thus the nurse is not able to intervene if the client has a diagnosis of, for example, *potential atelectasis* or *pneumonia*. This is a medical diagnosis, whereas *breathing pattern, ineffective*, is a nursing diagnosis, and nursing interventions can be instituted to assist the client.

Comparison of Diagnoses

Medical	Nursing
Cancer of liver	Pain, acute
Heart failure	Fluid volume, excess
Chronic obstructive pulmonary disease	Breathing patterns, ineffective

Nursing diagnoses provide a written communication to all healthcare workers regarding the client's status. The use of nursing diagnoses provides a vocabulary that is used to describe specific nursing practice, research, and education. It provides a method to synthesize and communicate nurses' observations and judgments to all members of the healthcare team.

Types of Nursing Diagnoses

The North American Nursing Diagnosis Association (NANDA International) states that a nursing diagnosis can be written as an "actual" or as a "risk for" statement, "possible," "syndrome," or "wellness."

Actual: The nurse has validated an actual nursing diagnosis using clinical judgment, and the client has presented with specific defining characteristics.

Risk for: Based on clinical judgment, the client is more vulnerable to develop the problem than others in similar circumstances. This may also be referred to as a "potential problem." Risk diagnoses include risk factors.

The term *possible diagnosis* is not considered a type of diagnosis. It is an option indicating some data are present to confirm the diagnosis, but the data are incomplete or insufficient. Writing a nursing diagnosis as "possible" alerts other nurses of your concern but there is insufficient data to support a specific diagnosis as yet. Further data collection is needed to confirm or deny the diagnosis.

The term *syndrome* is used when a cluster of specific nursing diagnoses is seen together. A *wellness* diagnosis describes a client at a low level of wellness. Many diagnoses are further qualified by terms such as effective, ineffective, impaired, imbalanced, readiness for, disturbed, and decreased.

Diagnostic Statement

The diagnostic statement describes the health status of the client and the factors that have contributed to the status. These statements have been developed through research by NANDA and are termed *nursing diagnoses*. One hundred eighty-eight nursing diagnoses were endorsed by NANDA International. For 2009 to 2011, there were 21 new diagnoses, 9 revisions, and 6 retired diagnoses, for a total of 203 nursing diagnoses. Because of the increased use of computers for documentation, a standardized language for describing client problems is mandatory. Nursing diagnosis provides the necessary terminology for use in a variety of clinical settings. NIC can be used both with a paper-based documentation system and electronic documentation system.

TABLE 2-1 Nursing Diagnosis: Impaired Skin Integrity

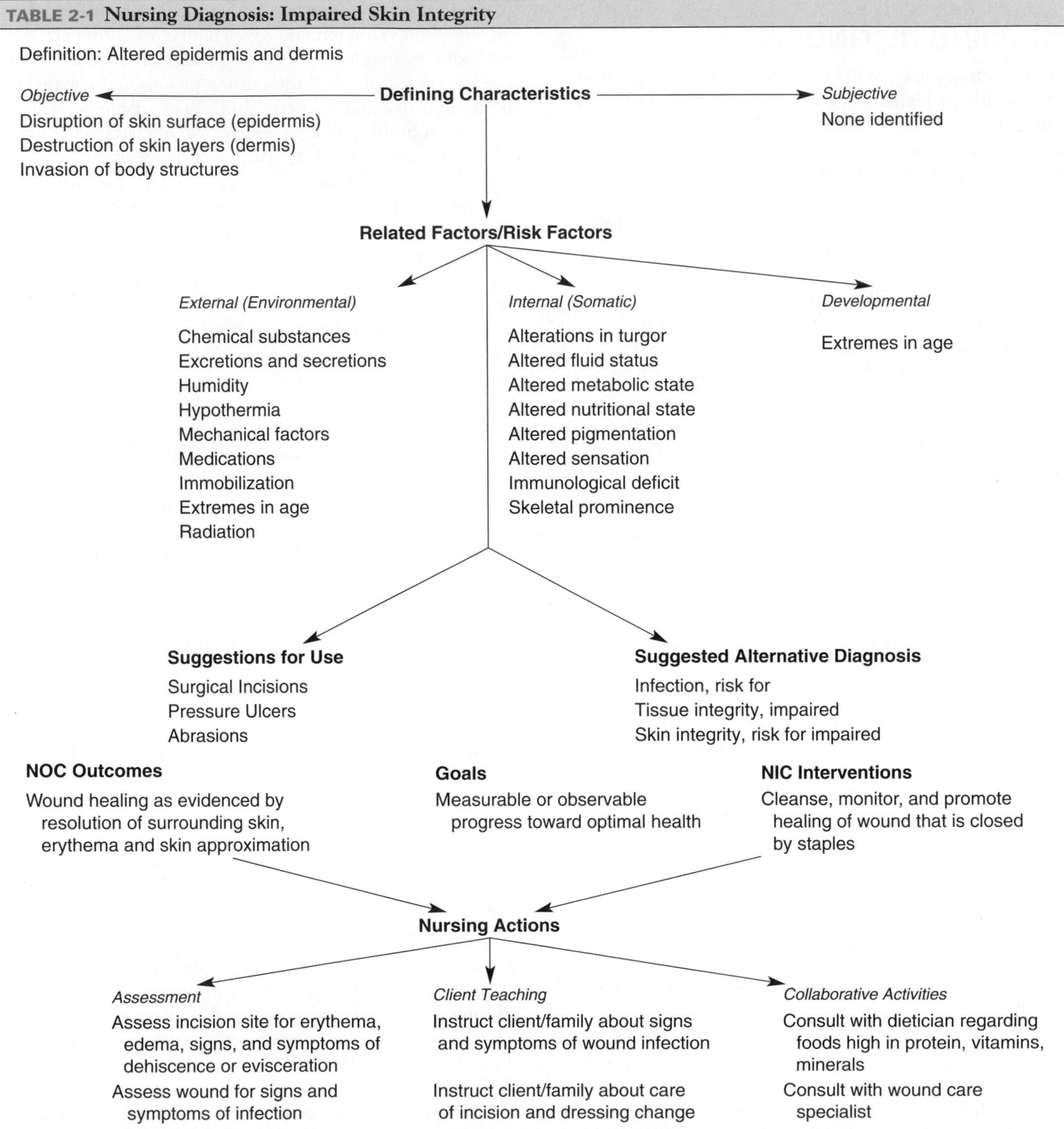

Definition: Altered epidermis and dermis
Objective
Defining Characteristics
Subjective
Disruption of skin surface (epidermis)
Destruction of skin layers (dermis)
Invasion of body structures
None identified
Related Factors/Risk Factors
External (Environmental)
Chemical substances
Excretions and secretions
Humidity
Hypothermia
Mechanical factors
Medications
Immobilization
Extremes in age
Radiation
Internal (Somatic)
Alterations in turgor
Altered fluid status
Altered metabolic state
Altered nutritional state
Altered pigmentation
Altered sensation
Immunological deficit
Skeletal prominence
Developmental
Extremes in age
Suggestions for Use
Surgical Incisions
Pressure Ulcers
Abrasions
Suggested Alternative Diagnosis
Infection, risk for
Tissue integrity, impaired
Skin integrity, risk for impaired
NOC Outcomes
Wound healing as evidenced by resolution of surrounding skin, erythema and skin approximation
Goals
Measurable or observable progress toward optimal health
NIC Interventions
Cleanse, monitor, and promote healing of wound that is closed by staples
Nursing Actions
Assessment
Assess incision site for erythema, edema, signs, and symptoms of dehiscence or evisceration
Assess wound for signs and symptoms of infection
Client Teaching
Instruct client/family about signs and symptoms of wound infection
Instruct client/family about care of incision and dressing change
Collaborative Activities
Consult with dietician regarding foods high in protein, vitamins, minerals
Consult with wound care specialist

Source: NANDA International. (2008, November 10). *Nursing Diagnoses; Definitions and Classifications, 2009-2011*, 2nd ed. Oxford, United Kingdom: Wiley Blackwell.

TABLE 2-2 Nursing Diagnosis Care Plan Data

Each nursing diagnosis care plan includes the following data:

- Definition of the individual nursing diagnosis
- Defining characteristics as cues describing client behavior
  a. Objective data, observed or gathered through other sources such as assessment findings by the nurse
  b. Subjective data, verbalized by the client
  c. Meaningful patterns that identify potential client problems
  d. Two to three defining characteristics that verify an actual or potential nursing diagnosis
- Related factors or risk factors
  a. "Related to" indicates what should change for the client to return to optimal health
  b. Related factors are stated as: "related to," "associated with," or "contributing to" the diagnosis. They are classified as:
    1. Environmental (external) (e.g., hypothermia, moisture, physical immobilization)
    2. Somatic (internal) (e.g., alterations in fluid status, altered circulation)
    3. Developmental factors (e.g., extremes in age)
  c. Risk factors lead to potential nursing diagnoses
- Suggestions for use: how to use the diagnosis appropriately or differentiating it from similar diagnosis
- Suggested alternative diagnosis
  a. Similar diagnosis that can be considered when identifying client's problems
  b. Diagnosis that can be substituted for one that only partially matches client data
- NOC outcomes
  a. Client outcomes that reflect client states or behaviors that nursing care can affect
  b. Outcomes are not goals but can be used to set goals
- Goals and evaluation criteria
  a. Goals represent measurable or observable criteria that represent whether the client problems have been resolved
  b. Use NOC outcomes, indicators, and measuring scales to establish goals
  c. Documented times and dates for meeting goals are stated
  d. Documentation of progress toward meeting goals is set according to client's condition and standards set by facility for documentation
- NIC Interventions
  a. Guide for selecting appropriate interventions
  b. Each intervention has a label name and a set of activities that are identified as steps to carry out the intervention
- Nursing activities are actions taken by the nurse related to the nursing diagnosis
  a. Assessments
  b. Nursing interventions
  c. Client/family teaching
  d. Collaborative activities with other healthcare team members

By 2010, the plan is that all healthcare events will be electronically recorded, and healthcare agencies will be required to submit the data to regional and national data banks according to the Department of Health and Human Services (DHHS). With the implementation of the electronic health records (EHRs), standardized nursing languages such as NANDA International (NANDA-I) will be used to provide a broad base of nursing knowledge at the point of care.

The 2009–2011 Taxonomy of Nursing Diagnosis, now Taxonomy II, is a classification in which the diagnostic data are grouped within the following concepts:

Health promotion
Nutrition
Elimination and exchange
Activity/rest
Perception/cognition
Self-perception
Role relationship
Sexuality
Coping/stress tolerance
Life principles
Safety/protection
Comfort
Growth/development

Components of Nursing Diagnosis

There are basically two formats used to write the nursing diagnosis: the two-part statement and the three-part statement.

The two-part statement is the most common type of format used in practice. The first component is the *Diagnostic Label* or problem statement. This describes the client's response to an actual or risk health problem. The second component,

An *Actual Nursing Diagnosis*, written as a three-part statement:

DIAGNOSTIC LABEL (Problem)	Transfer ability, impaired
CONTRIBUTING FACTORS (Etiology or Cause)	Related to inability to move left side
CLINICAL MANIFESTATIONS (Defining Characteristics)	Evidenced by flaccid paralysis of left side

A Risk for Diagnosis, written as a two-part statement, when there are no defining characteristics:

DIAGNOSTIC Label (Problem)	Walking, impaired
RISK FACTORS	Related to long leg cast secondary to fractured femur

Etiology, is the cause or contributing factor to the problem. The two components are linked by the "*related to (r/t)*" term.

The three-part statement includes the *Diagnostic Label*, *Etiology*, and the *Defining Characteristics*. Defining Characteristics are defined as signs and symptoms or clinical manifestations and subjective and objective data. The characteristics are linked to the other two components by the "*as evidenced by*" statement.

The accompanying box is an example of nursing diagnoses written in a two-part and three-part statement.

The PES framework is a commonly used approach or organizing framework developed by Marjory Gordon that uses the three-part diagnostic statement.

P refers to the *problem*, or state of health, of the individual, family, or community. This problem is expressed as clearly as possible; for example, Skin Integrity, Impaired.

E describes the *etiology*, or probable cause, of the health problem. This may refer to many factors that include client behaviors, environmental components, or the interaction of both. The etiology is combined with the problem statement by using the words "related to," for example, prolonged bed rest.

S signifies the relevant *signs and symptoms*—usually a summary of the objective assessment findings (signs) and subjective data reported by the client (symptoms). The phrase that connects this part of the statement is "as evidenced by"; for example, Impaired Skin Integrity, related to prolonged bed rest, as evidenced by a 2×2 cm circular red lesion or erythematous macules with moderate serosanguineous drainage.

Although there are several approaches to formulating a statement of nursing diagnosis, the PES system is used by many schools of nursing throughout the United States.

EVIDENCE-BASED PRACTICE

This term and use of evidence-based practice (EBP) is relatively new to the practice of nursing, even though nursing has recognized the importance of research as an essential basis for its development. Nurses should make clinical decisions using the best available research and other evidence that is reflected in approved policies, procedures, and clinical guidelines in a particular healthcare agency. Using evidence-based data is critical in nursing to promote a consistent approach to client care that results in less care-quality variability. This is significant as nurses provide care in settings where a group of nurses provides the care to groups of clients. Other health-related disciplines have long relied on this type of empirical data when making clinical decisions.

Evidence-based nursing practice is defined as the application of the best available empirical evidence that applies recent research findings to clinical practice in order to aid clinical decision making.

Evidence-based nursing practice (EBNP) or evidence-based practice (EBP) is differentiated from research in several key ways. Basing nursing practice on evidence entails locating the latest research and other evidence, such as synthesizing results, and translating the evidence into a protocol or guideline that can be used to guide practice. Research is systematic investigation aimed at

Evidence-Based Research Project

When completing an evidence-based research project you need to complete the following steps:

Step 1: State the question you wish to study. It may be a simple question related to a standard nursing procedure that has been done a certain way for many years, or it may be a totally new way of completing a procedure.

Step 2: Gather the evidence (information). Do a literature search, use the Internet, and review medical and nursing studies reported in journals that relate to your subject of interest.

Step 3: Analyze and assess the evidence. Did it come from a valid source? Who did the study, and how was the study actually conducted?

Step 4: Based on research findings, conduct a pilot study to validate your hypothesis. Individuals can make changes in a pilot study, but for an institution to make changes, a plan must be developed, it must be based on research findings, and it must be formally implemented.

Step 5: Obtain feedback from individuals involved in the research. Monitor the research and identify the specific response(s) and alterations that have occurred in the practice setting as a result of the research findings.

Step 6: Analyze and report the outcome resulting from the research project. Reporting a change in practice that improves nursing procedures will encourage others to make changes in practice settings as well.

Source: Domrose, C. (2001, November 19). Information based on interviews with nurse researchers and clinicians including Lisa Sams, Carolyn K. Davis, Kathleen Stevens, Brigitte Failner. *NurseWeek*.

generating new knowledge or refining existing knowledge. EBNP and research involve some of the same tasks, but the purposes of the tasks differ in the way they achieve their goals. Research generates new knowledge, whereas EBNP applies the knowledge to practice.

The levels of evidence vary among researchers. Some researchers believe that the synthesis and use of scientific information comes from randomized clinical trials. Others look at the process more broadly and include information gleaned from case reports and expert opinion to guide healthcare decisions.

The University of Minnesota Evidence-Based Health Care Project concludes that evidence-based practice solves problems by carrying out four steps:

1. Identify issues or problems based on analysis of current nursing knowledge and practice.
2. Identify relevant research through literature search.
3. Evaluate research by using criteria that has scientific merit.
4. Select interventions by using the most valid evidence.

Nurses must recognize the importance of using research findings in clinical practice. It is paramount that nurses begin to not just read research articles but critically examine the content of the article and question current practice. Once research data are available, nursing must consider making changes in clinical practice based on the findings. In many facilities, this involves research teams that review current literature and then make appropriate recommendations for clinical practice. Unfortunately, very little is known about the best methods for implementing research evidence into nursing practice. Evidence-based nursing will strengthen client outcomes, improve client safety, provide effective nursing practice, and increase nursing's credibility among other healthcare professionals and the general public. This should be considered another step in developing nursing's theory base.

One note of caution when you are reading about evidence-based practice: Do not confuse it with best practices. These terms are sometimes used interchangeably, but they do not mean the same thing. *Best practices* is a term used to describe nursing interventions that have proven effective in promoting positive client outcomes or in reducing overall costs to the client or facility. Best practices refers to nursing practices that are based on the "best evidence" available from nursing research. The goal of best practices is to apply the most recent, relevant, and helpful nursing interventions, based on research, in real-life practice. Although the two terms, best practices and EBP, are used interchangeably, the two are different in some respects. Best practice is a generic or general phrase for a process of infusing nursing practice with research-based knowledge. EBP emerges from evidence-based medicine (EBM). EBM is more rigorous and integrates individual clinical expertise with evidence from systematic research. Systematic reviews are more comprehensive in scope and quality of research, and they use mostly randomized clinical trials as the gold standard by which evidence is judged.

EBP highlights can be found throughout the book. EBP will provide you with a framework for determining the effectiveness of selected nursing skills and practice issues. As you proceed through your nursing program, you will be exposed to additional EBP research and its effect on clinical practice.

MANAGEMENT Guidelines

Each state legislates a Nurse Practice Act for RNs, LVN/LPNs, and advanced nurse practitioners. Healthcare facilities are responsible for establishing and implementing policies and procedures that conform to their state's regulations. Verify the regulations and role parameters for each healthcare worker in your facility.

Delegation

- The RN's responsibility when delegating client care tasks is to ensure that the care plan is followed for each client. Information contained on the care plan is reported to each healthcare worker assigned to client care.
- The RN is responsible for implementing the nursing process in all aspects of client care. LVN/LPNs may be assigned to carry out tasks within the nursing process, such as assessing clients after the initial assessment and executing interventions based on the client care plan. The RN, however, is ultimately responsible for client care, developing the plan of care, and ensuring that the plan is followed.
- The LVN/LPN may assist the RN in planning and updating the plan of care, but may not be responsible for this action.
- Assistive personnel, such as unlicensed assistive personnel (UAP) and CNAs, are delegated client tasks, but do participate in the actual development of the plan of care. Their input is valuable and should be considered when changes in the plan of care are necessary.
- Critical thinking processes are used by all team members as they provide client care. The RN has a more expanded scientific knowledge base and experience in utilizing these skills to provide the leadership necessary for effective and safe client care. The RN must use these skills when assigning client care and delegating activities.

Communication Matrix

- The RN synthesizes client data and determines the most appropriate healthcare worker to provide care to each client in her/his assignment.
- Each healthcare worker is given a report on activities to be completed during the shift.
- Dissemination of client care information is based on the client's plan of care.
- Directions are given to all healthcare workers indicating the type of client information the nurse needs immediately and information that can be given during report times. For example, if a client has a fever, the RN may want to know the temperature as soon as it is obtained.

CRITICAL THINKING Strategies

Scenario 1

You have been assigned to care for Mr. Peters, a 76-year-old widower who was admitted with the diagnosis of heart failure. He has lived alone for the last 2 years since his wife died. His children live about 1 hour away and visit him once a month. The children ordered Meals on Wheels for him, but he refused to eat the food that was delivered. "I can do my own cooking, I am not an invalid," was the answer when the nurse asked why he didn't like the Meals on Wheels program. He had not seen the physician for at least 6 months. At the last visit, the physician prescribed a moderately low-sodium diet, Lasix 40 mg daily, Calan, and multiple vitamins. His admitting vital signs were BP 180/90, P 98, R 22. His weight indicated a gain of 10 pounds since the last visit. His physical assessment indicated rales in the lung bases, 3+ edema of the ankles, and difficulty breathing in the supine position, and with the least amount of exertion.

- How will you use the nursing process to determine an accurate assessment database?
- What information is missing that might be important to the nurse to assist in planning care for this client? What is the best approach for obtaining the information?
- Identify at least four nursing diagnoses that are relevant for this client's plan of care. Write a two-part and a three-part diagnostic statement for each nursing diagnosis.
- Using a nursing diagnosis book, identify NIC and NOC statements for the four nursing diagnoses listed in question 3.
- Identify the priority nursing diagnosis, and provide the rationale for your decision.
- Develop a very brief nursing care plan using the nursing process format as outlined in the text.

Scenario 2

8 AM. You are assigned to a 22-year-old male client who was in a motorcycle accident yesterday. He sustained a compound fracture of the right fibula and tibia. He states his pain is 9/10 and it is throbbing. He is nauseated all the time. He is scheduled for surgery later in the day. You assess his wound area and notice there is a large amount of serosanguineous drainage in the dressing. You reinforce the dressing.

- Based on the information provided in the scenario, identify two nursing interventions.
- Determine priority nursing diagnoses and provide rationale for your decision.
- Using a nursing diagnosis textbook, develop a client care plan incorporating NIC and NOC data.

NCLEX® Review Questions

Unless otherwise specified, choose only one (1) answer.

1. Place the steps of the nursing process in sequence.
   1. Evaluation
   2. Planning
   3. Implementation
   4. Assessment
   5. Nursing diagnosis
2. Nurses who are considered critical thinkers exhibit which of the following attributes?
   Select all that apply.
   1. Possess good communication skills and are flexible.
   2. Use logic and creativity.
   3. Are structured in their delivery of nursing care.
   4. Use a systematic method for providing care in the same order for each client.
3. Which one of the following examples accurately describes a properly stated nursing diagnosis?
   1. Poor airway exchange r/t mucus accumulation in the alveoli.
   2. Client exhibits pain as a result of coughing as evidenced by grimacing.
   3. Knowledge deficit r/t inadequate understanding of diabetes as evidenced by lack of regular blood glucose testing.
   4. Pneumonia r/t inadequate ventilation during surgery.
4. Select all of the following diagnoses that are considered a nursing, not a medical diagnosis.
   1. Acute pain
   2. Heart failure
   3. Cancer of the liver
   4. Ineffective breathing patterns
   5. Pulmonary edema
   6. Excess fluid volume
5. Evidence-based nursing practice research is used to
   1. Aid in clinical decision making.
   2. Determine the most often used method to provide nursing care.
   3. Develop new techniques for providing nursing care.
   4. Differentiate nursing diagnosis from medical diagnosis.

6. The major role of assessment, the first step of the nursing process, is to
   1. Develop a nursing diagnosis after collecting client health data.
   2. Assess client and establish a database.
   3. Identify short- and long-term goals based on client's verbal statements regarding health needs.
   4. Assess sources of client data to determine whether accurate and before implementing client care.
7. Client care planning effectively promotes compliance by:
   1. Ensuring all healthcare needs are identified.
   2. Developing the plan within 1 hour of admission.
   3. Involving the client and family with the healthcare team to develop congruent healthcare goals.
   4. Including a teaching plan as part of the overall short-term goals.
8. During the implementation phase of the nursing process, the nurse
   1. Gathers all data and prioritizes client needs.
   2. Determines clusters of clues from collected data.
   3. Collects data and then provides education to client and/or family.
   4. Considers contingencies for modifying care plan.
9. The implementation of Nursing Interventions Classification (NIC) with nursing diagnosis is primarily because
   1. The diagnosis is stated more clearly in nursing terminology.
   2. It is not easily confused with a medical diagnosis.
   3. It can only be used as a paper-based documentation system.
   4. It can be sent to national and regional databases.
10. Delegation of responsibilities to other healthcare members can be completed in which one of the following situations?
    1. Ask the unlicensed assistive personnel to assist in the development of the client's plan of care.
    2. Assign the certified nursing assistants to clients who require completion of care plan goals before discharge.
    3. Ask the LVN (LPN) to assist in revising the care plan.
    4. Request that the LVN (LPN) complete the initial care plan after admitting the client.

3

Managing Client Care: Documentation and Delegation

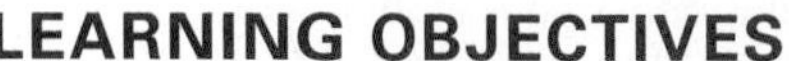

LEARNING OBJECTIVES

1. Describe the components of the client care plan.
2. State the two types of client care plan.
3. Explain the method for individualizing the care plan when a standard care plan is used.
4. Define the term "client problem or need."
5. State the most important reason for using nursing diagnosis in care planning.
6. Define the use of deadlines and checkpoints in the client care plan.
7. Compare and contrast a clinical pathway and a client care plan.
8. Explain at least three purposes of charting.
9. Describe at least three major components of accurate charting.
10. Complete a charting exercise in any of the charting systems using a simulated situation.
11. List the four items that should be charted for every client.
12. Define the terms "subjective data" and "objective data."
13. Describe the legal ramifications for completing unusual occurrence reports.
14. Discuss specific client activities requiring consent forms.
15. Discuss the legal risks of computer charting.
16. Discuss the RN's role in delegating client care.
17. Complete a data collection tool based on a clinical situation.
18. Develop a time-management worksheet for client care.

CHAPTER OUTLINE

Cross Reference: At the end of each chapter, see Delegation as it applies to that chapter's skills.

TERMINOLOGY

Acuity system a method for determining staffing requirements based on the assessment of client needs.

Care plan, client a plan of care, usually written, that meets the special needs of each client.

Charting process of recording information about a client concerning the progress of his or her disease and treatment.

Charting by exception documenting only exceptions to predetermined nursing standards in a narrative format.

Clinical pathways interdisciplinary client care plans using specific assessments, interventions, and outcomes for specified health-related conditions.

Computer-assisted charting client information is entered into the computer for storage and retrieval at a later time.

Delegation transferring to a competent individual the authority to perform a selected task in a selected situation.

EHR electronic health records.

Flow sheets client data are recorded or graphed to show patterns or alterations in findings.

Focus charting charting on one "focus" area. Using DAR format (data, action, response).

HIPAA health insurance portability and accountability act.

HITs health information technologies.

Kardex a convenient and readily accessible file of cards containing current client information.

Nursing process a set of actions that includes assessment, planning, intervention, and evaluation.

Problem-oriented medical record (POMR) a client record that is organized according to the person's specific health problems.

Report to give an account of something that has been seen, heard, done, or considered.

SBAR a tool that standardizes a "hand-off communication" when one nurse turns a client over to another nurse; situation, background, assessment, and recommendations.

SOAP notes nursing notes organized consistently by what the client feels "subjectively," what the nurse observes "objectively," how the nurse "assesses" the situation, and what the nurse "plans."

SOAPIE nursing notes similar to SOAP with additional data; implementation (i) and evaluation (e).

Source-oriented charting information in the chart is organized according to its source; for example, physician's progress notes, nurses' notes.

Systems charting charting or documentation relative to the assessment data obtained during the physical assessment of the client.

Unusual occurrence recording of an unusual happening or event that could affect client or staff safety; also commonly referred to as variance or incident report.

CLIENT CARE PLANS

Documentation is a major component of the nurse's role. Importance is based on several factors: evaluation of planned client care, communication to other healthcare professionals, The Joint Commission and client safety regulations, reimbursement from the federal government, and legal implications. If a treatment, medication, or activity has not been documented in the chart, legally it is very difficult to prove that the client actually received the care. Contact with the client and care delivered to the client must be documented. One of the most useful tools to provide this care is the client care plan.

Client care plans are an integral part of providing nursing care. Without them, quality and consistency of client care may not be obtained. Client care plans provide a means of communication among nurses and other healthcare providers. The plan should serve as a focal point for client care assignments and reporting.

In earlier years, The Joint Commission required an individualized care plan be developed for each client. According to the guidelines from The Joint Commission, the client or family must be involved in the development of the care plan and it must be interdisciplinary. One reason the critical or clinical pathway (see explanation on page 36) is becoming more popular is the interdisciplinary approach involved in this system. Some facilities still use the standardized or individualized care plan. The only modification they need to make is to ensure that multidisciplinary planning and intervention are included in the care of each client. Documentation of client care must also be interdisciplinary.

Regardless of the type of care plan used, the following information should be included: client's needs or problems, both actual and potential, expected outcomes or short-term goals; nursing interventions or actions; and discharge criteria or long-term goals.

Once the goals of client care are established, they are included in a multidisciplinary care plan. Each step in meeting these goals is detailed, including specific observations and how often the observations are made. Step-by-step directions are included for difficult problems, such as lengthy and involved dressing changes. Individualized client teaching programs are described on the care plan. As is evident, all of this information is essential in providing continuity of client care.

Types of Plans

Client care plans consist of two types: an individualized care plan, completely written by the nurse and other health team members for each specific client, and a standard client care plan (Form 3-A). Because of the time required to write individualized care plans, hospital nursing departments have developed preprinted standard care plans. These plans, based on the facility's standards of nursing practice, are guidelines that outline the usual problems or needs. They contain a list of usual nursing actions or interventions and the standard expected outcomes for each problem. Advantages include standards of care; continuity of care, with all nurses providing the same level of care; decreased documentation time; and more accurate documentation. The major disadvantage is the risk that individualized client care may not be provided. The care plan becomes a part of the permanent client record.

Components of a Care Plan

Individualizing Care Plans All clients must have an individualized plan of care even though the standard care plan is used. To individualize the care plan, space is generally provided at the end of the preprinted form to allow the nurse to identify unusual problems or needs. Standard care plans are individualized by activating only those problems that pertain

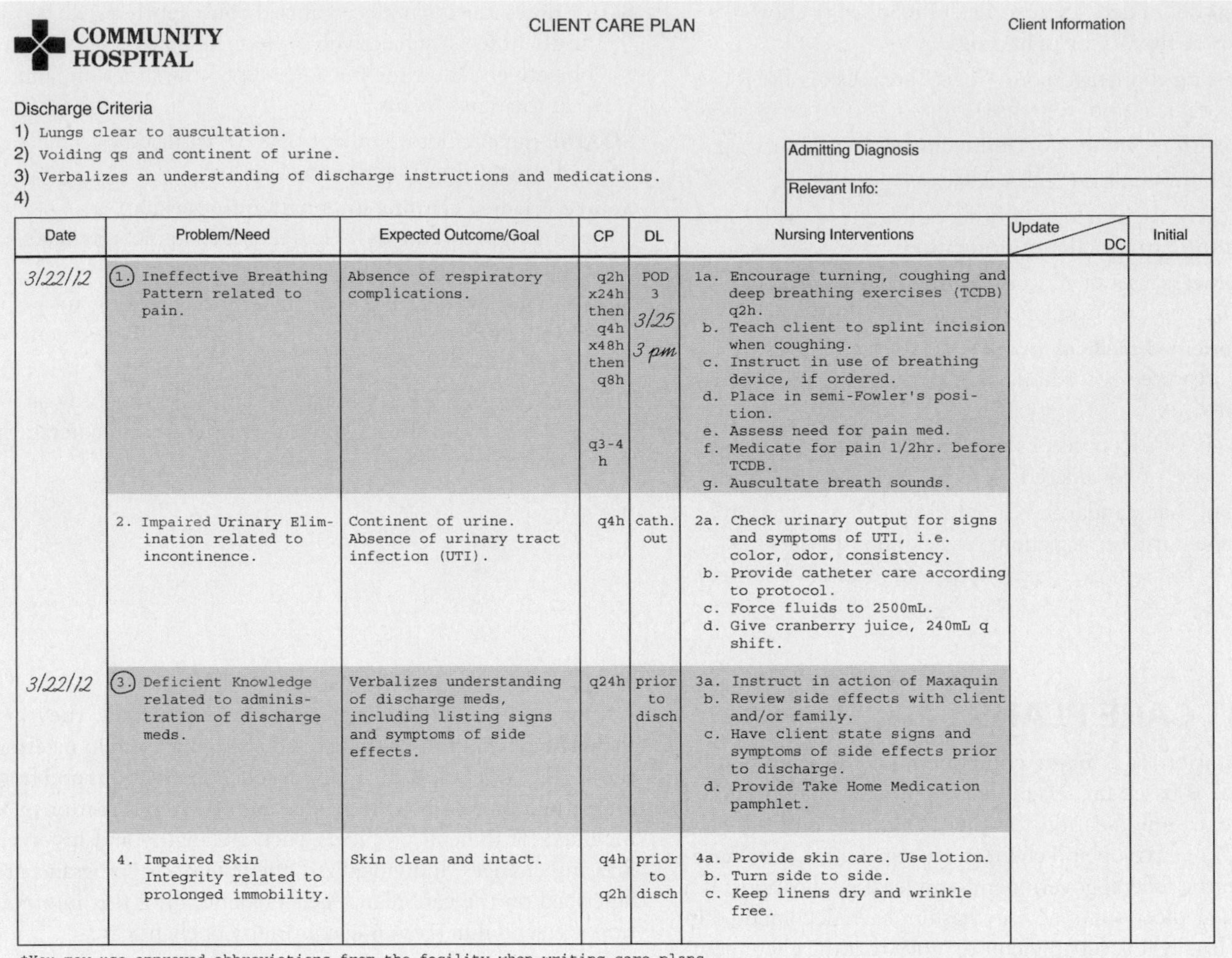

COMMUNITY HOSPITAL

CLIENT CARE PLAN

Client Information

Discharge Criteria
1) Lungs clear to auscultation.
2) Voiding qs and continent of urine.
3) Verbalizes an understanding of discharge instructions and medications.
4)

Admitting Diagnosis

Relevant Info:

Date	Problem/Need	Expected Outcome/Goal	CP	DL	Nursing Interventions	Update / DC	Initial
3/22/12	(1.) Ineffective Breathing Pattern related to pain.	Absence of respiratory complications.	q2h x24h then q4h x48h then q8h q3-4 h	POD 3 3/25 3 pm	1a. Encourage turning, coughing and deep breathing exercises (TCDB) q2h. b. Teach client to splint incision when coughing. c. Instruct in use of breathing device, if ordered. d. Place in semi-Fowler's position. e. Assess need for pain med. f. Medicate for pain 1/2hr. before TCDB. g. Auscultate breath sounds.		
	2. Impaired Urinary Elimination related to incontinence.	Continent of urine. Absence of urinary tract infection (UTI).	q4h	cath. out	2a. Check urinary output for signs and symptoms of UTI, i.e. color, odor, consistency. b. Provide catheter care according to protocol. c. Force fluids to 2500mL. d. Give cranberry juice, 240mL q shift.		
3/22/12	(3.) Deficient Knowledge related to administration of discharge meds.	Verbalizes understanding of discharge meds, including listing signs and symptoms of side effects.	q24h	prior to disch	3a. Instruct in action of Maxaquin b. Review side effects with client and/or family. c. Have client state signs and symptoms of side effects prior to discharge. d. Provide Take Home Medication pamphlet.		
	4. Impaired Skin Integrity related to prolonged immobility.	Skin clean and intact.	q4h q2h	prior to disch	4a. Provide skin care. Use lotion. b. Turn side to side. c. Keep linens dry and wrinkle free.		

*You may use approved abbreviations from the facility when writing care plans.

▲ Form 3-A. Preprinted standardized client care plan.

to a particular client. The nurse may add another problem to the bottom of the form to further individualize the care plan.

Initiating the Plan The client care plan is formulated after the assessment phase of the nursing process. The nurse, after completing the nursing history and assessment, determines whether a standard care plan is available for the client's medical diagnosis or if an individualized care plan must be written. If a standard care plan is available, the nurse need only circle, date, and initial the needs that are relevant for that client. When an individualized care plan is being written, the nurse translates the client's needs or problems into nursing diagnoses and enters the data into the computer or writes them on the care plan. Nursing diagnoses are the acceptable terminology for use on client care plans throughout the country. The terminology was established by the National Conference on Classification of Nursing Diagnosis, published for the first time in 1973.

Identifying Client Problems or Needs A client problem or need is a condition that requires assistance or intervention from a healthcare team member to return the client to a healthy state. The client problem is identified as any unmet need. It can be as basic as the need for adequate comfort or nourishment to the more complex psychosocial needs.

On many care plans, problems are identified as either actual or potential. An actual problem is one that exists at that time. Interventions are planned to resolve or alter the problem. A potential problem describes a condition that frequently occurs with the client's diagnosis or health problem. An actual problem, for example, is a reddened coccyx related to urinary incontinence. Interventions are developed to treat the reddened area to prevent further breakdown or pressure ulcer formation. A potential problem, such as "ineffective breathing patterns related to acute pain" after gallbladder surgery, could affect any client with that condition. Interventions are planned to prevent the problem. Some potential problems are identified to assess more carefully for them. For example, a debilitated client with poor nutrition is assessed for possible wound infection.

Formulating Nursing Diagnoses Using a nursing diagnosis to state the client's real or potential problems takes the problem out of the realm of medical diagnosis. Nursing diagnosis does not focus on a problem or disease state but rather on a physical, psychological, or behavioral response.

Nursing diagnosis can change frequently as the client's health status changes and potential health problems become actual health problems. The nursing diagnosis approach, unlike the medical model or systems approach to care planning, allows for this flexibility in focus.

The use of nursing diagnosis in care planning is a universal method of communication to all health team members. When the diagnosis "Impaired Skin Integrity" is written, the entire health team knows that the client has a broken area on the skin with destruction of skin layers. The relationship of skin impairment to cause is usually stated as "Impaired Skin Integrity, *related to* prolonged immobility."

Expected Outcomes or Goals After the problems have been identified, the nurse sets goals or expected outcomes for client care that are congruent with the goals of the client or significant other. Client-centered goals should be clear, concise, realistic, and should identify specific observable and measurable behaviors. Expected outcomes or goals should indicate what is to be expected when the goal is achieved, by whom, when, to what degree of accuracy, and should be time-limited. The client care plan on page 34 shows several examples of a client-centered goal and the nursing interventions necessary to attain each goal.

Client care plans must include both short- and long-term goals. Long-term goals are frequently stated as discharge criteria and as such should be met before discharge, if possible. Short-term goals usually appear in the form of expected outcomes for each problem. They are designed as stepping stones to assist the client to meet discharge criteria or long-term goals. Some hospitals, particularly rehabilitation facilities, use short-term goals differently. They frequently set weekly steps or phases in the rehabilitative process that clients meet before the final expected outcome is achieved. For example, to meet the long-term goal of ambulation without use of devices, a short-term goal is to ambulate with a walker without assistance. These types of goals are prioritized and updated regularly.

Interventions After problems and expected outcomes are written on the care plan, the nurse determines appropriate nursing interventions that meet the goals of care. Interventions, if written properly, specify the exact nursing actions to be carried out or provide explicit instructions on how care is to be delivered. Time and frequency of the intervention should also be provided.

Checkpoints and Deadlines The standard care plan illustrated in this text includes checkpoint (CP) and deadline (DL) columns. The checkpoint indicates how often the action or intervention should be checked, observed, or carried out and therefore how often it should be charted. The deadline column indicates the time when the goal should be met or the action is no longer necessary. It is important to document the exact time and date when the nursing action should be completed to communicate this information to the entire nursing staff. On the sample client care plan on page 34, notice that item 1—Ineffective breathing pattern—should be alleviated by the third postoperative day, in this case, March 25 at 3:00 PM. The checkpoints are listed in sequence to meet the goal. For the first 24 hours, the nursing interventions (la through 1d) should be completed every 2 hours and then advanced to every 4 hours for the next 48 hours.

Updating Care Plans To ensure that client care plans are current and relevant, they should be reviewed on a daily basis and updated at least every 24 to 48 hours. There are several ways to update a care plan. Some facilities have spaces designated on the nursing Kardex or nurses' notes. In the figure, the update column is used when the original deadline is reached but the problem persists. A new deadline must then be established. If the ineffective breathing pattern exists beyond the third postoperative day, a new time frame for goal achievement is determined and documented in the update column.

Activating Care Plans When standard care plans are used, a systematic approach to activation and deactivation must be understood by all nursing personnel. As already stated, a common approach is to circle, date, and initial problems that are relevant for the individual client. Any problem that is not circled remains inactivated and should not be assessed, treated, or documented. From the example, you can see that the client has two of the problems listed, an ineffective breathing pattern and a knowledge deficit regarding discharge medication. Items 1 and 3 are circled. In the date column, date, time, and initials of the nurse activating the problem are entered. The second problem is not activated; therefore, a circle is not placed around the number.

Inactivating Care Plans To inactivate the problem, a single line through the problem or intervention with a black pen can be made. In the update/DC column, the date, time, and nurse's initials should be placed next to the crossed out, inactivated information. If only one of the interventions is not necessary, a line is drawn through that intervention and initials placed next to it in the initial column. The other interventions are left current and active.

Evaluating Care Plans The evaluation of how well the client care plan was individualized to meet the needs of the client is tested at discharge. If the care plan was appropriate, the discharge criteria are met. The nursing interventions and problems are then inactivated or discontinued. Frequently, there are clients who, on discharge, have not met the discharge criteria for various reasons. The documentation in the chart should reflect those problems that still exist, the extent to which the problem is being resolved, and additional information to indicate which plans were formulated for goal achievement.

Changing Care Plan Formats As computers are being used more commonly to document nursing care and workplace redesign is transforming how we deliver nursing care, the type and method of using the nursing care plan is changing. The Joint Commission's requirements are becoming more flexible and are allowing new ways to document client care. Critical paths, protocols, and standardized nursing care plans are used with or are replacing the more traditional care plans.

Computerized Client Care Plans The format used in computer software packages individualizes client care plans according to each health care facility's specifications. This type of format is very popular now that computerized documentation systems have been implemented in many facilities. Preparation time for writing individualized care plans is decreased and standardized plans are developed and written by clinical experts. One disadvantage of this software is that nurses must carefully determine the relevance and appropriateness of the care plan for each individual client. The care plan for each client is generated by the computer each shift. Changes must be entered into the computer frequently to ensure the accuracy of the plan.

Critical Paths or Clinical Pathways

This type of documentation is used primarily with managed care delivery systems. In this system, traditional nursing care plans do not exist. A critical path or clinical pathway is a standardized multidisciplinary plan of care developed for clients with common or prevalent conditions (Form 3-B). It is a tool developed collaboratively by all health team members to facilitate achievement of client outcomes in a predictable and established time frame. The clinical pathways are used on each shift to direct and monitor client care. The plan indicates the actions and interventions achieved at designated times in order to meet the criteria for reimbursable length of stay. For example, a client with a total hip replacement has a critical path that states time frames for out of bed, gait training, and ambulation listed under the physical activity section of the form. On the second postoperative day the client should move from bed to chair with assistance. Nursing diagnoses are not always incorporated in the critical path. Documentation of nursing activities completed in response to the critical path varies according to facility policies and guidelines. Some facilities initial each day's completed tasks on the critical path document, whereas others use flow charts and narrative charting.

If the client does not achieve the expected outcome in the specified time, a "variance" occurs, and an individual plan of care is developed that may then incorporate nursing diagnosis. For example, if a client is unable to ambulate by Day 3, a nursing diagnosis can be used to individualize the client's variance from the critical path expectations. An individualized care plan is initiated, and charting continues on the variance until it is resolved. The individualized section of the care path is usually found on the back of the form. In the sample "clinical pathway for operative hip," the form used to chart the variance is termed "multidisciplinary problem record." The problem is identified and listed as Problem 1. In the space provided

CLINICAL PATHWAY FOR OPERATIVE HIP

Use Ortho Admit Orders	**Day 1** **Admit/ to OR in 24–36 hrs.** **Date** ____________	**Day 2** **Post Operative Day (POD) 1**
Assessment A *If mechanical fall with no medical hx of problems, then surgery immediately. If hx of medical problems eval. suggested.*	• **Adm. assessment, q 8 hr.** ✓ Basic assessment, CMS, HV Drsg, I&O, IV, skin assess, B/S, flatus. **q 4 hr. Post-op** ✓ VS, O_2 protocol. SpO_2 reading (see graphic)	• **q 8 hr.** ✓ Basic assessment, CMS, HV Drsg, I&O, SpO_2, VS, IV site, skin assess. sign. • BID ✓ Homan sign. Oxygen protocol.
Physical Activity P • Ambulate BID if able.	• Bedrest, move in bed with assistance. • Pre admit activity level:	• OOB chair. • Commode with help. • Transfer & gait training.
Treatment T *Hip Precautions for hemiarthroplasty only*	• Incentive Spirometry (IS), TCDB, TED/ Sequential Compression Device (SCD). • Foley cath. insert	• TED/SCD, I.S., TCDB. • Foley cath. remains if needed. • *Hip Precaution for hemiathroplasty only*
Medications IV, PO, IM, SQ, etc. M	• Ancef pre operative. • Ancef 8 hr. × 24 hr. (after Surgery). Antiemetic PRN, Anticoagulant.	• Stool softener • Iron supp. BID (hold if GI upset). • Anticoagulant.
IV Fluids/Blood Products I	• Transfuse blood if needed. • IV at 75–100cc till tol. P.O. then switch to IVL.	• IV at TKO or IVL.
Nutrition N	• Advance diet as tolerated.	• Diet as tolerated.
Comfort/Pain C	• PCA or other pain medication as ordered by Surgeon or Anesthesia.	• PCA or other pain medication as ordered by Surgeon or Anesthesia.
Education E	• Pre & Post op. Patient Clinical pathway, TED/SCD, Analgesia method. • Discharge plan reinforced.	• Reinforce Post op. & Clinical pathway, TED/SCD, Analgesia method.

▲ Form 3-B. Clinical pathway for operative hip care.

MULTIDISCIPLINARY PROBLEM RECORD

When a particular problem no longer exists the caregiver should yellow out the problem and date when it was resolved. • Review and update problem list q shift. •

Date/Time		Problem #	PROBLEM State the problem with description of findings	INTERVENTION Refer to Pathways, Flow Sheets, Standards of Care as appropriate	EVALUATION Reassessment of problem or results of interventions	Initial

▲ Form 3-C. Sample of variance charting.

for the PROBLEM—a nursing diagnosis is used or a client problem is listed. Interventions are developed, and an evaluation section is added. All other documentation continues on the care path.

In addition to the pathway and multidisciplinary problem record, the more sophisticated clinical pathways also include an admitting assessment, nursing history including risk factors for falls and skin, nutrition risk evaluation, and social or cultural variables. An ongoing admission database is included in the packet. Also, this section contains a discharge planning risk assessment and multidisciplinary team conference section. Routine Assessment and Care Record frequently are included in this system of documentation.

There are several advantages for using critical or clinical pathways including continuity of care among all health care workers—discharge planning is begun on admission, and teaching plans are initiated early in the hospitalization. Clinical or critical pathways have been proven to reduce length of hospital stay, complications, and costs. Client satisfaction has also increased with the use of pathways.

Not all clients can be placed on pathways. For more complex clients, those requiring specialized care or clients experiencing complications, individualized care plans are more appropriate.

Protocols There are several uses for protocols within the various healthcare settings. Protocols can be used when specific equipment, such as a Roto Bed, is used in client care. They are also useful for specific nursing interventions such as administration of IV antifibrinolytic agents. In both of these situations, specific actions must be taken to ensure accurate and safe care of clients requiring these treatments. Using protocols in these situations promotes safety.

Protocols can be used in conjunction with standard care plans, individualized care plans, and critical paths. The use of protocols decreases the amount of documentation required on the care plan as actions and interventions are described in detail on the protocol.

In some areas of the hospital, protocols are used in place of care plans. This is particularly true in emergency departments, outpatient surgery, labor and delivery, postanesthesia departments, and operating rooms. Protocols for client care in each of these areas are practical because clients have common needs. For example, clients in the postanesthesia area must have their respiratory status monitored, fluid balance maintained, and level of consciousness assessed. These clients must also meet certain criteria for discharge from the unit. There is no real requirement for an individualized plan of care for the clients in these settings. The time spent in these specialty areas is usually very limited and the service very specific.

CHARTING/DOCUMENTATION

Next to direct client care, charting is one of the nurse's most important functions. Charting, the process of recording vital information, serves many important purposes:

- Charting communicates information, such as facts, figures, and observations, to other members of the client's healthcare team.
- Charting assists supervisory personnel to evaluate the staff's performance on a day-by-day basis for specific clients.
- Charting provides a permanent record for future reference that may become a legal document in the event of litigation or prosecution.

Documentation—A Method of Communication

Complete and accurate documentation is essential to protect both the client and the nurse. In communicating your observations and actions, charting helps to ensure both quality and continuity of health care for your clients. Information recorded by you becomes a valuable database for nurses on subsequent shifts. Then, when you reassume responsibility for the client, you can determine what events occurred during prior time periods. Frequently, a client's reaction time is nearly as important as the reaction itself; therefore, accuracy of time observations becomes an integral part of the charting process. In addition to the client's attending physician, other personnel interested in the chart may include the infection control nurse, discharge coordinator, utilization review personnel, or other hospital staff specialists who are checking on the client's progress or lack of positive reaction to treatment.

The client, as an individual, should receive individualized attention that focuses on his or her specific needs. As these needs are identified by each member of the healthcare team, they can be communicated to the others. Since nurses have the greatest amount of direct client contact, it is appropriate for the nurse to coordinate the important function of charting.

Charting provides one means for assessing the quality and effectiveness of nursing care. Nurse managers, team leaders, and supervisors use nurses' notes as a basis for staff evaluations. Because charts are documented descriptions of nursing actions, the quality of nursing care may be evaluated on the basis of the quality of charting notes.

Since charting describes nursing interventions and their outcomes, other healthcare personnel can determine whether subsequent treatment should be changed.

A client's record includes all charting and becomes part of a legal document. Should a client's hospital record be introduced in court, the notes become a legal record of the care provided by each healthcare provider. Legally, care that is not recorded is considered to be care that was not provided. It is necessary therefore to chart all care that you *do* provide, as well as any care that you *do not* provide.

The legal requirement for charting is found in state laws and professional requirements. For example, Title 22 of the California Code of Regulation states:

> Nurses' notes which shall include but not be limited to the following: concise and accurate record of nursing care administered; record of pertinent observations including psychosocial and physical manifestations as well as incidents and unusual occurrences, and relevant nursing interpretation of such observations; name, dosage and time of administration of medications and treatment. Route of administration and site of injection shall be recorded if other than by oral administration; record of type of restraint and time of application and removal. The time of application and removal shall not be required for soft tie restraints used for support and protection of the patient.

In addition to the nurses' notes, Title 22 requires that a written client care plan must be a permanent part of the medical record.

> There shall be a written patient care plan developed for each patient in coordination with the total health team. This plan shall include goals, problems/needs, and approach and shall be available to all members of the health team.

The Joint Commission also states its requirements for documentation in its nursing care standards. Examples of the documentation standards include an admission assessment performed and documented by a registered nurse that includes consideration of biophysical, psychosocial, environmental, self-care, educational, and discharge planning; nursing care based on identified nursing diagnoses or client care needs and client care standards; needs that are consistent with the therapies of other disciplines; interventions identified to meet the client's needs; the actual client care provided while hospitalized; educational information provided; and the ability of the client or family to manage the continuing care on discharge.

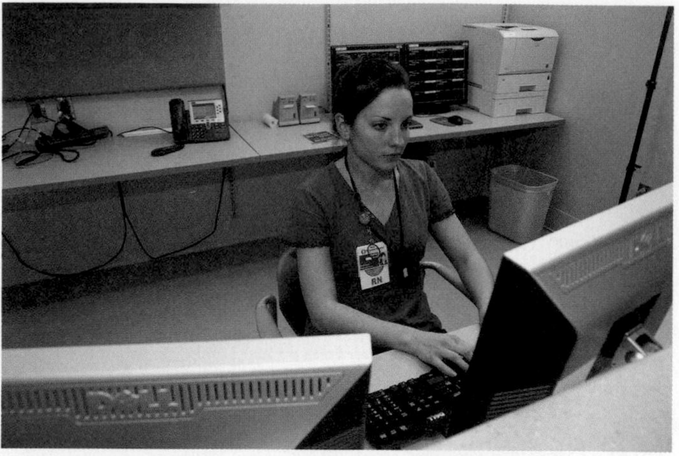

▲ Charting is completed immediately following client care, either at the bedside or nurses' station.

Charting Format

The format of the chart, whether in the computer or on paper, varies from hospital to hospital. Most important is the content of the notes. First, your notes should describe the assessment that you completed at the beginning of your shift. This information provides a baseline for changes that may occur later in the client's condition. If there are no such changes, this fact should be entered as the final note. Some hospitals require that all parts of the assessment be documented; others require that only abnormalities be documented.

As your shift progresses, you should always include certain items in your notes, including changes in the client's medical, mental, or emotional condition. Nurses are well attuned to medical changes, such as shock, hemorrhage, or a change in level of consciousness; however, the nurse may overlook subtle emotional changes. Anger, depression, or joy should also be documented because these emotions often are indications of the client's response to the illness. Recording these changes is absolutely necessary if other nurses are to act appropriately during subsequent shifts. You should also chart if *no* changes occurred in the client's condition so that treatments can be modified as necessary. Normal aspects of the client's condition should be noted also.

New Trends

Meditech's Software Improves Quality of Care

Meditech's fully integrated Health Care Information System displays real-time client information so that all healthcare professionals, including ancillary departments, may access data at any time. Communication between providers appears instantly on the computer; for example, new physician's orders. This system also provides for sending alerts or messages throughout the organization.

Source: http://meditech.com/Industrynews/pages/jcaho.htm

Why Documentation Is So Important

It is the communication mode that nurses and other healthcare providers use to provide continuity of care and to deliver safe care.

It assists in maintaining The Joint Commission accreditation and reimbursement from Medicare.

It protects nurses legally when it verifies the care that has been delivered, demonstrating that the care has met professional standards.

Reactions to any unscheduled or PRN medications must be recorded. Because each medication is given to meet a specified need, the client's response or lack of response must be recorded to document whether the need was met. To complete this part of the entry, note the time the medication was given, the problem for which the medication was given, and the expected solution. For example: "7 AM. c/o moderate RUOQ abdominal incisional pain, '7' on pain scale. Roxanol, 30 mg, PO for pain." When the effects of the medication are known, write another note: "8 AM. States pain relieved."

Finally, it is important to record the client's response to teaching. These notes may describe return demonstrations, verbalization of learning, or resistance to instruction. Because most teaching takes place over a period of days, record both what you taught and how the client responded. Then other nurses will know whether to repeat the previous instructions, reinforce them, or start a new topic.

Frequently, repetitive aspects of nursing care, such as vital signs and intake and output, are recorded on flow sheets. If flow sheets are used, you need not repeat the same information in your notes. An exception is an abnormal measurement that is a part of a larger assessment. For example: "c/o sharp abd. pain. BP 78/50. P 136. Skin cold & diaphoretic. NG tube draining bright red bloody fluid with small clots. Reported to Dr. Jones."

Avoiding Legal Problems in Documentation

- Use facts. If you chart "physician notified," include time called, facts you gave, and his or her response.
- Do not use pat phrases. Be specific and use individual assessment parameters. Do not chart global assessments such as "IV running."
- Be professional when you chart. Do not make interpretations; state what happened; for instance, "suggested to physician that client requires heart monitor" and physician responded "case does not warrant a monitor." If this client were later to be involved in a lawsuit, these notes indicate that the nurse was observant, alert, and aware that the client might be in danger.
- Do not use words such as *mistake* or *accident*; write specifically what incident occurred and what actions were taken.
- Do not use tentative or vague statements such as *appears* or *apparently*.
- Use correct language and medical terms. Do not use slang, pat phrases, or abbreviations that are not generally accepted.
- Use correct grammar and spelling.
- Do not chart for someone else.
- Do not chart ahead of time. Chart after the care is complete, but do not wait until the end of the shift.
- Do not alter a medical record. Draw a single line through an incorrect entry and initial and date the error.
- Write in late entries when you think about them; do not try to go back into earlier charting and insert the information. Label the information as "late entry" and put the time it actually happened in the entry.
- Countersign care given by assistive staff only if the facility allows you to countersign, and then do so only after you review the entry and are familiar with the care provided to the client.
- Chart potentially serious situations; include observations, reports to the physician and supervisor, and whether any action was taken. Be precise; add quotes or specific communication. This is the only kind of charting that holds up in court.
- Report problems to appropriate authorities, such as suspected child abuse to social services.
- Provide the best care you are capable of giving; then precisely chart your observations, interventions, and communications. This is the best deterrent to later legal problems.

Poor Documentation May Lead to Legal Problems

The client was admitted with a fractured right femur. Physician's orders were to turn the client every 2 hours. While hospitalized, the client developed several pressure ulcers, one severe enough to cause her right leg to be amputated. Examining the records, the court determined the client was turned 18 times and should have been turned 117 times. Most cases will be judged on the basis of "if it was not documented, it was not done." Good documentation is critical for the nurse's defense.

Source: Hurlock v. Parklane Medical Center (1985)

Forensic Charting

The content of nurse's notes may affect the outcome of criminal investigations; when charting, especially in the ER, OR, or suspected assault cases, nurses must document exactly and carefully. Forensics is not only linked to criminal investigations; it is the connection between medical data and the legal process. Nurses must be aware that their documentation may be involved in a future legal case.

Charting Systems

The three main charting systems are *source-oriented, problem-oriented,* and *computer-assisted* charting. Two additional systems used are *focus charting* and *charting by exception. Source-oriented charting* is so named because the information is organized and presented according to its source. For example, there are separate sections for doctors' progress notes, nurses' notes, and respiratory therapy notes. To obtain a complete "picture" of the client, one must read through all sections and piece together the separate bits of data. This may be a time-consuming process, and the result may not produce an accurate or complete assessment of the client. Narrative charting is found within this charting system.

A second system for chart organization is the *problem-oriented medical record.* In this system the chart is based on the problem list—all problems, present or potential, identified with that client. Using the problems as reference points, each person giving care charts progress notes on the same sheets. In this way assessment of a specific incident by everyone concerned (e.g., physician, RN, dietitian, enterostomal therapist) is in the same location, and the client's overall picture can be easily seen.

The third method of organizing data is *computer-assisted charting* (see Electronic Charting, page 42). This type of charting constantly updates information from many sources. For example, physiologic measurements are recorded and updated on the computer terminal at least hourly. The information is easily retrievable by the nursing personnel as questions arise. Reference material for common nursing problems ensures quick reference and easily retrieved information to provide safe nursing care.

Focus Charting As the name implies, *focus charting* makes client needs or problems the focus of care in the progress notes. This method moves away from labeling client status a problem because it includes the client's condition, nursing diagnosis, signs or symptoms, or a significant client event or change in status (need for surgical intervention). The focus is not necessarily written as a nursing diagnosis. The progress notes are organized using the DAR format: data, action, and response. Data includes the information that supports the focus, action is the nursing intervention used to treat the problem, and response is how the client responds to the intervention and the outcome. The following is an example:

D: Client found grimacing, hands clenched, and body rigid. Verbalized pain at 9 on pain scale.

A: Administered 15 mg MS IV push. Called physician to request PCA for client.

R: Pain moderately relieved after 35 minutes. Able to understand instruction in use of PCA.

Charting by Exception (CBE) is a system that focuses on significant findings or deviations from the norm. It reduces time spent documenting and reduces multiple data entries in the record. It uses flow sheets, protocols and standards of practice, nursing diagnosis, care plans, SOAP progress notes, and a nursing database. A nursing and physician order flow sheet is used to document physical assessments and implementation of physician and nursing orders as well as completion of nursing and physician orders. The form also contains the teaching record and discharge notes. Only changes or findings significantly different from the norm are documented. Nurses chart only when the client does not meet the predetermined standard or norm. All exceptions to the standards must be documented narratively. When nurses see entries in the chart, it alerts them that something unusual has occurred with the client. An additional advantage in CBE charting is that all flow sheets are kept at the bedside, which eliminates the need to transcribe information from a work sheet to the permanent record.

Some legal or reimbursement issues, such as admissibility in court, may be related to charting by exception. At this time, the rule "if it wasn't charted, it wasn't done" is still the prevailing attitude in legal issues.

Narrative Charting Another system of charting, now infrequently used, is source-oriented narrative charting. This form is based on chronology rather than systems.

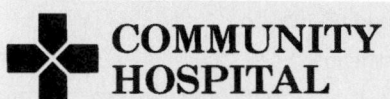

ICU NEURO/SPINAL FLOW CHART

Date: 3/22/12	Time:	8 am		
Pupils	Right: size	4 mm		
	Reaction	S		
	Left: Size	4 mm		
	Reaction	S		
	Visual Acuity	C		
Mental Status				
COMA SCALE — Eyes Open	Spontaneously			
	To Speech			
	To Pain	+		
	Never			
Verbal Response	Clear			
	Confused			
	Inappropriate	+		
	Incomprehensible			
	None			
MOVEMENT — Arms	Normal Power			
	Weakness	+		
	Flexion			
	Extension			
	No Response			
Legs	Normal Power			
	Weakness	+		
	Flexion			
	Extension			
	No Response			
Reflexes	Gag/Cough	0		
	Corneal	+		
	Babinski R/L	+/+		
	Oculocephalic	0		
Respiratory	Pattern	Reg.		
	Rate	28		
Seizures	Type	0		
	Duration			
Fluid Drainage from Ears or		0		
Nose		0		

Signature D. Jones RN

▲ Form 3-D. Neurologic flow sheet.

When using narrative charting, an assessment should be performed at the beginning of the shift and as needed thereafter. When assessment is the initial entry in narrative charting, subsequent entries are more relevant and understandable. This combination of assessment and narrative charting is the best technique to ensure that adequate information about the client is recorded for all personnel who use nurses' notes.

There is a tendency for hospitals to move away from traditional narrative charting to focus on charting by exception. Because the client's chart is considered a legal document, it is important that nurses chart relevant, accurate, and appropriate information in a timely manner. The following rules involve the issues that become problematic if they are not done and may result in litigation.

Rules for Documenting Client Care

1. Document from first-hand knowledge—if you chart for other caregivers, you may have errors or inaccurate data. An exception to this rule is when you are responsible for charting for nonprofessional personnel.
2. Document clearly and legibly in black or blue ink, not felt pen or pencil.
3. Give clear, concise, and unambiguous information. Go back to the client to clarify or validate if information is incomplete. Avoid vague expressions or clichés in charting (i.e., slept well).
4. Select neutral terms or describe observed behaviors, rather than value judgments or generalizations. For example, rather than "client was drunk," use "noted alcohol odor on breath and speech was slurred."
5. Correct errors by drawing a single line through the error, write the words mistaken entry (ME) above it, and then initial the error. The error must be readable. Ink eradication, erasures, or use of occlusive materials is not acceptable. The word error is no longer advised because juries tend to associate the word error with an actual nursing care mistake.
6. Sign each entry with your first initial, last name, and status; for example, SN for student nurse, LVN for licensed vocational nurse, or RN for registered nurse. Script, not printing, is used for the signature. Each signature should appear at the right-hand margin of the nurses' notes.
7. Notes should appear on each succeeding line. Lines should not be omitted in the nurses' notes. A horizontal line is drawn to "fill up" a partial line. Continuous charting is done for each entry unless a time change occurs. You may or may not need a new line for each new idea or statement, depending on agency protocol.
8. The date is entered in the data column on the first line of every page of nurses' notes and whenever the date changes. Time is entered in the time column whenever a new time entry occurs. Do not put time changes in the text of the nurses' notes. If only one time is entered for block charting, enter the last time you were with the client.
9. Chart objective facts, not your interpretations. For example, chart "ate 100%," not "good appetite." If the client complains, place the complaint in quotation marks to indicate that it is his or her statement. For example, "c/o chest pain radiating down left arm."
10. Refusal of medications and treatments must be documented. A circle is placed around the time the medication or treatment is to be given in the appropriate area of the chart. An explanation regarding the reason the medication was not given is entered in the nurses' notes.
11. Sign each entry before it is replaced in the chart rack. An entry is not to be left unsigned. If all the charting is completed for the shift at one time, a single signature is placed at the end of the charting.
12. Accuracy is important. Describe behaviors rather than feelings. This allows other health team members to determine the client's actual problems.
13. Chart only those abbreviations and symbols approved by the facility. Information can be misinterpreted or misleading when unfamiliar abbreviations are used. (*See* the listing at the end of Chapter 18 for examples of commonly used abbreviations.)
14. Spell correctly, using proper terminology and grammar.
15. Write legibly. If your writing is not legible, then print.
16. Do not use the word "client" in the chart. The chart belongs to that client.
17. Do not double chart. If something appears on a flow sheet, it does not need to appear on the nurses' narrative record unless there is an alteration from normal.
18. Do not squeeze information into a space because you forgot to chart it earlier. Add the information on the first available line. Write in the time the event occurred, not the time you entered the information. The words *late entry* can be inserted before the charting.
19. The following information should be charted.
    a. Physician's visits.
    b. Times the client leaves and returns to the unit, mode of transportation, and destination.
    c. Medications (chart immediately after given). Include dosage, route of administration (if parenteral, where given), whether pain was relieved (if pain medication), and side effects.
    d. Treatments (chart immediately after given).

A form of narrative charting is assessment–intervention–response (AIR). In the assessment (A) section of the chart, the nurse summarizes data and impressions of problems found via assessment. The intervention (I) section is for summaries

The Air Format

A Respirations 30 and labored. Rales bilateral in the bases.

I Deep breathing and coughing, incentive spirometer with Mucomyst. Up in chair.

R Respiration 24, decreased intensity of rales but still present.

Narrative Charting

Advantages

- Can be used in conjunction with flow sheets and other documentation systems
- Quick method of charting chronologic data
- Familiar method of charting
- Easy to use
- Used in all types of clinical settings

Disadvantages

- Lack of systematic structure leading to difficulty in determining data relationships
- Time-consuming
- Frequently lacks information on client care outcomes
- Difficult to monitor data for quality assurance
- Relevant information found in several areas in chart

about interventions based on assessment findings. The summary may include a condensed nursing care plan or plans for additional monitoring. The response (R) section focuses on the client's response to nursing interventions. Each assessment and intervention is labeled so that other nurses can chart pertinent responses. With appropriate flow sheets and the AIR method of narrative charting, client care is more clearly and concisely documented.

Informatics

The American Nurses Association in 2001 defined nursing informatics as "a specialty that integrates nursing science, computer science and information science to manage and communicate data, information and knowledge in nursing practice." This new paradigm emphasizes content, structure, context, and the flow of information and technology. Research in the next decade will be based on an understanding of nursing informatics, intervention, and solution. In fact, the National League for Nursing (NLN) has stated that without curriculum reform, nurses will not be able to function in three critical areas: computer literacy, information literacy, and informatics.

Research in 2009 indicates that only 8% of the nation's 5,000 hospitals are currently using computer charting, although many are beginning to incorporate bar coding for medication administration. Approximately 25% of United States hospitals give their nurses hand-held devices for scanning bar codes for medication labels and client's wristbands to prevent medication mistakes. These numbers will increase, as there is a more determined effort to adhere to safety regulations.

Nurses are at the hub of client health information, so it is becoming more and more important for nurses to master technology. Nursing informatics is a specialty area in which nurses develop, customize, and evaluate various information technologies for adaptation to their particular facilities needs. Nurse informaticists' major responsibilities are to develop systems and act as communication liaisons for their care facility.

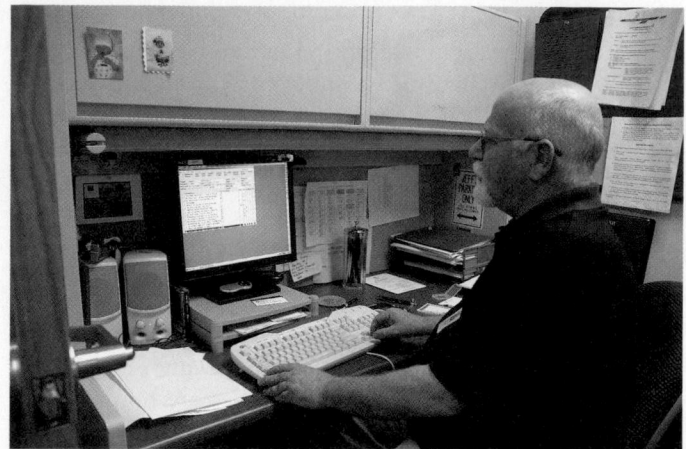

▲ RN informatics tech specialist helps to update and maintain the electronic database.

Electronic Charting

Many hospitals are integrating computer information systems as a way of improving client care and utilizing nurses' time more efficiently. Electronic information systems are moving documentation of client care from handwritten charting into the computer. With these systems, client data can be input and retrieved with the click of a mouse. Data can be input and a new assessment generated within minutes. These information computer systems not only improve client care, but also save nurses' time. Nursing organizations and accrediting agencies are placing more and more emphasis on electronic documentation.

Computer-assisted charting can be implemented by itself, or, as in most cases, it is a component of a facility medical information system. There are so many constraints on time and resources that this type of system is becoming a necessity for healthcare agencies today. Inaccurate documentation has a significant impact on quality of client care, costs, and revenues. Redundant information input wastes valuable nursing time. Missing or incomplete documentation is costly and frustrating. If supplies or treatments are not documented, payment cannot be obtained.

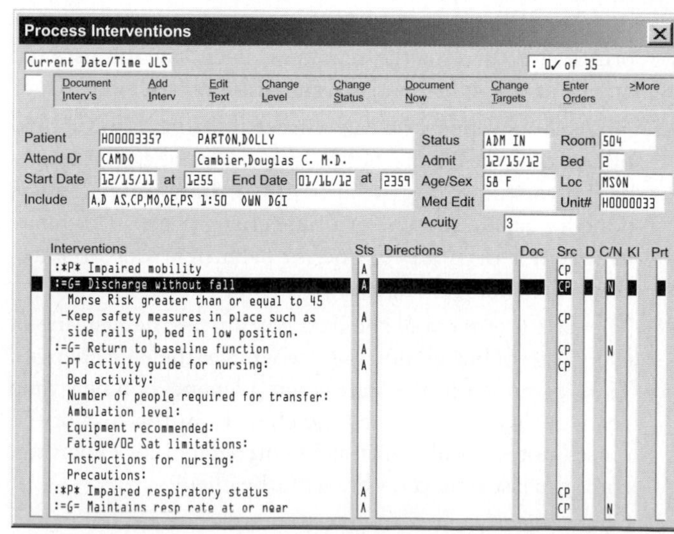

▲ Example of computer charting.

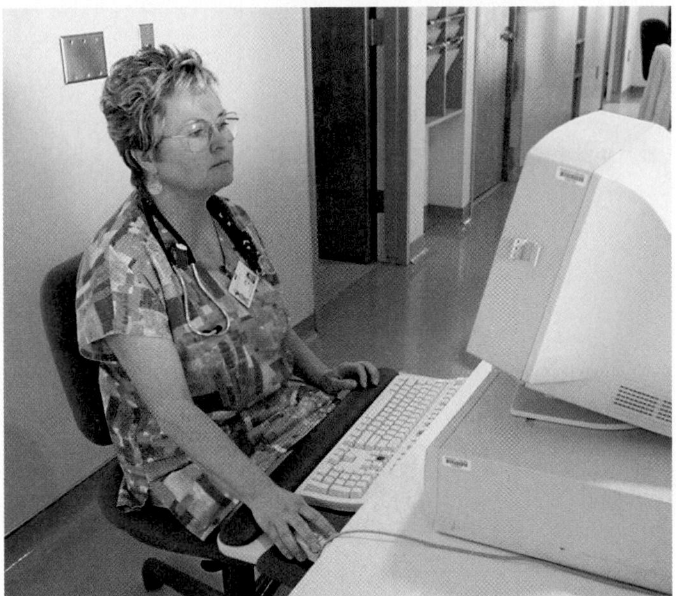

▲ Each nursing unit has several computer terminals for documentation.

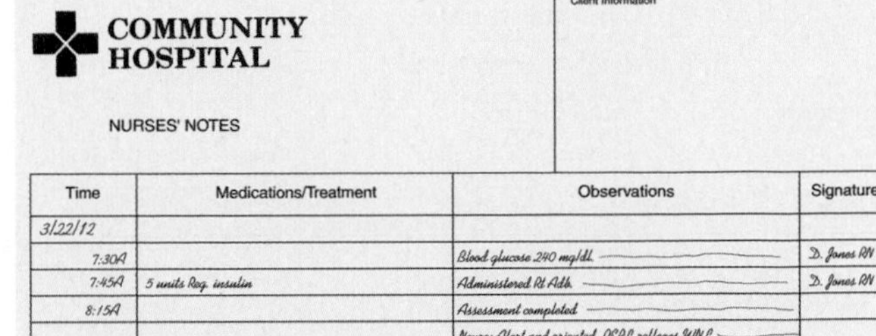

COMMUNITY HOSPITAL

NURSES' NOTES

Client Information

Time	Medications/Treatment	Observations	Signature
3/22/12			
7:30A		Blood glucose 240 mg/dl.	D. Jones RN
7:45A	5 units Reg. insulin	Administered Rt Abd.	D. Jones RN
8:15A		Assessment completed	
		Neuro: Alert and oriented. PERL reflexes WNL	
		Cardio: p. 102 irregular ō pericardial friction rub	
		present.	
		Resp. Rales present bilaterally in bases. Non-productive	
		cough.	
		GI: Bowel sounds present. Abd. soft and non-tender.	
		GU: Voided lge. amts. light straw-colored urine ō sediment	
		M/S: No c/o pain or limitation of movement.	
		Skin clean and moist. No reddened areas or breakdown	D. Jones RN

▲ Form 3-E. Example of data entry options.

Nursing information systems can manage clinical data in a variety of healthcare settings. These systems allow nurses to provide and access accurate and timely information. This type of charting allows the nurse to select content phrases on a screen that automatically builds a comprehensive record without inputting all the individual pieces of information.

Computer-assisted charting can be accomplished in a nurses' station or at the bedside. Most of the necessary documentation can be done at the bedside if the equipment is available. This includes vital signs, admission assessment, nursing assessment, intake and output records, client education records, and client care plans. Once the information is entered into the computer, it can be disseminated to different reports without the nurse's intervention. Some of the documentation systems offer packages, such as customized flow sheets for each nursing unit in the hospital, and individualized critical pathways for each service area in the facility. Laboratory results, respiratory therapy notes, and client care documentation are fully integrated into the electronic chart. Management reports can also be generated through this type of system. Shift reports, client acuity, and client care plan variance can be generated in some systems.

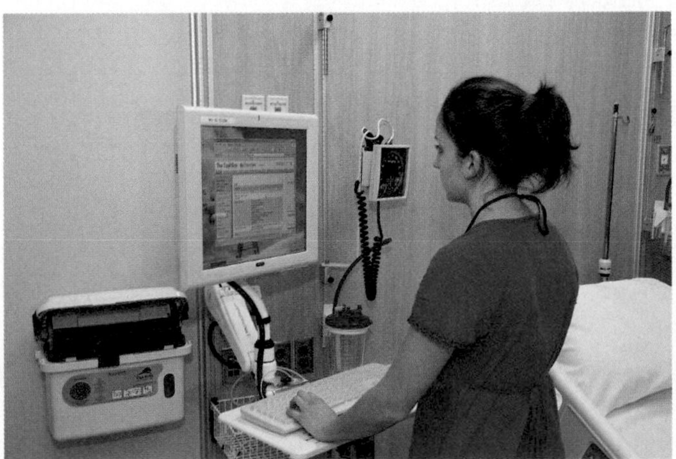

▲ Bedside E-documentation is becoming more accessible to nurses in hospital settings.

Computer systems record, store, and retrieve many pieces of data about the client that must be communicated throughout the hospital for the client to receive optimal care. For example, when a client is admitted and the physician enters orders into the computer, many things automatically happen. The dietary department is notified of the diet needs, pharmacy is notified of medications and IVs that are ordered, CSR is notified of special equipment needs, and the laboratory is notified of required tests. It is no longer necessary for the nurse to make out and deliver requests to all these departments and then arrange for delivery or pick up of the desired items. Each nursing unit has

Electronic Health Records (EHRS) Being Implemented

The president, in 2005, announced that we were to have electronic health care records (EHRs) available by 2010. The initiative states that the United States should have a record interoperable database, while ensuring privacy and security. Interoperable EHRs would benefit both the clients and healthcare providers by eliminating redundancies, enabling access of medical records when clients are away from home, allowing biosurveillance of disease or tracking of disease movement (pandemic flu), and improving quality of care.

Despite this commitment, progress has been slow. One study showed only 17% to 24% of physicians in ambulatory facilities use EHRs to some extent. As benefits are becoming more and more obvious (improved safety, quality, and overall efficiency of care), more facilities are adopting EHRs.

Source: Saunders, K. (April, 2006). Bridging digital gaps. *Advance for Nurses*, 8(9), 38. Nelson, R. (March, 2007). Electronic health records: useful tools or high-tech headache? *American Journal of Nursing*, *107*(3), 25–26.

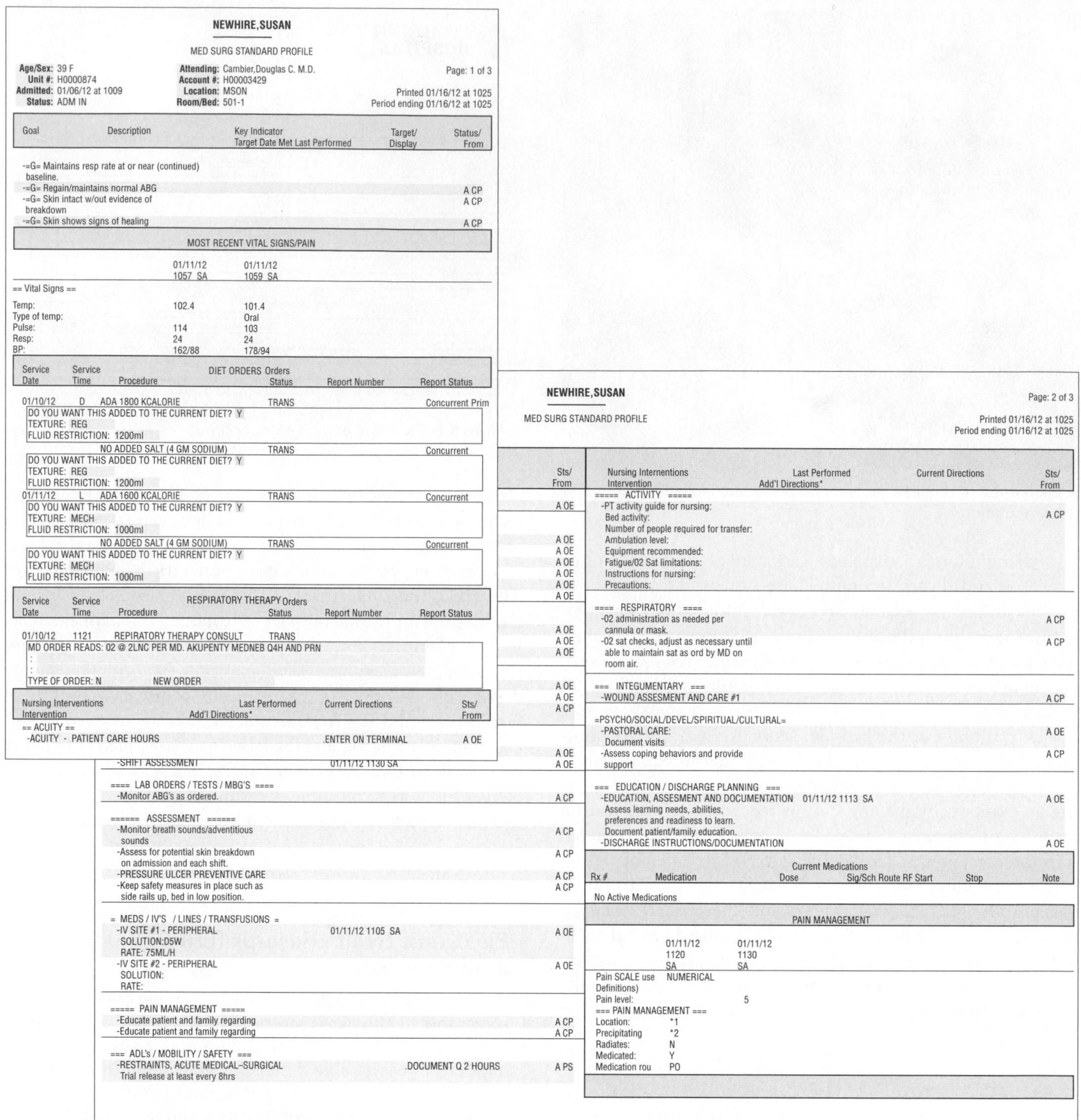

NEWHIRE,SUSAN

MED SURG STANDARD PROFILE

Age/Sex: 39 F
Unit #: H0000874
Admitted: 01/06/12 at 1009
Status: ADM IN

Attending: Cambier,Douglas C. M.D.
Account #: H00003429
Location: MSON
Room/Bed: 501-1

Page: 1 of 3
Printed 01/16/12 at 1025
Period ending 01/16/12 at 1025

Goal	Description	Key Indicator Target Date Met Last Performed	Target/ Display	Status/ From
-=G= Maintains resp rate at or near (continued) baseline.				
-=G= Regain/maintains normal ABG				A CP
-=G= Skin intact w/out evidence of breakdown				A CP
-=G= Skin shows signs of healing				A CP

MOST RECENT VITAL SIGNS/PAIN

	01/11/12 1057 SA	01/11/12 1059 SA
== Vital Signs ==		
Temp:	102.4	101.4
Type of temp:		Oral
Pulse:	114	103
Resp:	24	24
BP:	162/88	178/94

DIET ORDERS Orders

Service Date	Service Time	Procedure	Status	Report Number	Report Status
01/10/12	D	ADA 1800 KCALORIE	TRANS		Concurrent Prim
DO YOU WANT THIS ADDED TO THE CURRENT DIET? Y TEXTURE: REG FLUID RESTRICTION: 1200ml					
		NO ADDED SALT (4 GM SODIUM)	TRANS		Concurrent
DO YOU WANT THIS ADDED TO THE CURRENT DIET? Y TEXTURE: REG FLUID RESTRICTION: 1200ml					
01/11/12	L	ADA 1600 KCALORIE	TRANS		Concurrent
DO YOU WANT THIS ADDED TO THE CURRENT DIET? Y TEXTURE: MECH FLUID RESTRICTION: 1000ml					
		NO ADDED SALT (4 GM SODIUM)	TRANS		Concurrent
DO YOU WANT THIS ADDED TO THE CURRENT DIET? Y TEXTURE: MECH FLUID RESTRICTION: 1000ml					

RESPIRATORY THERAPY Orders

Service Date	Service Time	Procedure	Status	Report Number	Report Status
01/10/12	1121	REPIRATORY THERAPY CONSULT	TRANS		
MD ORDER READS: 02 @ 2LNC PER MD. AKUPENTY MEDNEB Q4H AND PRN : : TYPE OF ORDER: N NEW ORDER					

Nursing Interventions Intervention	Last Performed Add'l Directions*	Current Directions	Sts/ From
== ACUITY ==			
-ACUITY - PATIENT CARE HOURS		.ENTER ON TERMINAL	A OE
-SHIFT ASSESSMENT	01/11/12 1130 SA		A OE
==== LAB ORDERS / TESTS / MBG'S ====			
-Monitor ABG's as ordered.			A CP
====== ASSESSMENT ======			
-Monitor breath sounds/adventitious sounds			A CP
-Assess for potential skin breakdown on admission and each shift.			A CP
-PRESSURE ULCER PREVENTIVE CARE			A CP
-Keep safety measures in place such as side rails up, bed in low position.			A CP
= MEDS / IV'S / LINES / TRANSFUSIONS =			
-IV SITE #1 - PERIPHERAL SOLUTION:D5W RATE: 75ML/H	01/11/12 1105 SA		A OE
-IV SITE #2 - PERIPHERAL SOLUTION: RATE:			A OE
===== PAIN MANAGEMENT =====			
-Educate patient and family regarding			A CP
-Educate patient and family regarding			A CP
=== ADL's / MOBILITY / SAFETY ===			
-RESTRAINTS, ACUTE MEDICAL-SURGICAL Trial release at least every 8hrs		.DOCUMENT Q 2 HOURS	A PS

NEWHIRE,SUSAN

MED SURG STANDARD PROFILE

Page: 2 of 3
Printed 01/16/12 at 1025
Period ending 01/16/12 at 1025

Sts/ From	Nursing Internentions Intervention	Last Performed Add'l Directions*	Current Directions	Sts/ From
A OE	===== ACTIVITY =====			
	-PT activity guide for nursing:			
	Bed activity:			A CP
	Number of people required for transfer:			
A OE	Ambulation level:			
A OE	Equipment recommended:			
A OE	Fatigue/02 Sat limitations:			
A OE	Instructions for nursing:			
A OE	Precautions:			
A OE	==== RESPIRATORY ====			
A OE	-02 administration as needed per cannula or mask.			A CP
A OE	-02 sat checks, adjust as necessary until able to maintain sat as ord by MD on room air.			A CP
A OE	=== INTEGUMENTARY ===			
A OE	-WOUND ASSESMENT AND CARE #1			A CP
A CP	=PSYCHO/SOCIAL/DEVEL/SPIRITUAL/CULTURAL=			
	-PASTORAL CARE: Document visits			A OE
A OE	-Assess coping behaviors and provide support			A CP
A OE				
	=== EDUCATION / DISCHARGE PLANNING ===			
	-EDUCATION, ASSESMENT AND DOCUMENTATION Assess learning needs, abilities, preferences and readiness to learn. Document patient/family education.	01/11/12 1113 SA		A OE
	-DISCHARGE INSTRUCTIONS/DOCUMENTATION			A OE

Current Medications

Rx #	Medication	Dose	Sig/Sch	Route	RF	Start	Stop	Note
No Active Medications								

PAIN MANAGEMENT

	01/11/12 1120 SA	01/11/12 1130 SA
Pain SCALE use Definitions)	NUMERICAL	
Pain level:		5
=== PAIN MANAGEMENT ===		
Location:	*1	
Precipitating	*2	
Radiates:	N	
Medicated:	Y	
Medication rou	PO	

▲ Sample—computer-generated client data.

several computer terminals, or the terminals may be at the bedside. Before accessing the terminal, the sign-on code must be entered. Each person accessing information must have their own sign-on code. This prevents unauthorized persons from accessing confidential information. After sending the code by pressing a SEND button, the nurse can select the section of the record needed. The cursor is pointed at the data category and after clicking, the selection comes up on the screen. The most common category selections are nurses' notes, physician orders, laboratory or x-ray reports, and client care plans.

Hospitals usually have programs that contain special matrices of "Nursing Retrieval Guide(s)." Once the retrieval guide appears on the screen, the nurse can choose the specific category of data needed. Much of the routine ordering and care a nurse gives can be charted rapidly and completely in a matter of seconds using this system.

When the nurse has completed the charting, the information is displayed. At this time the nurse can make corrections, additions, or deletions. If the data displayed are correct, the nurse enters the data and it becomes a permanent part of the

Innovation in Transcription Orders

El Camino Hospital in Mountain View, CA, was the first hospital in the world to use computerized physician order entry (CPOE). They began this innovative approach to transcription orders in 1971. Now, their 400 physicians prescribe everything electronically—from treatment orders to medications—using the windows system. A physician can enter orders from any computer and nurses view electronic orders in real time, regardless of when they were updated. The clinical nurse manager at El Camino says, "We don't have transcription errors. Ever. It's just something that doesn't happen." Because one of the major causes of errors in health care is transcription orders, this is a goal most hospitals would like to emulate.

Source: McPeck, P. (May, 2006). Beyond illegible scrawl: Computerized order entry. *Nurse Week*, California Edition, San Jose, CA.

computer record for that client, and a hard copy is printed out to be put in the chart.

When the client is to be discharged, the nursing discharge summary is completed. This shows not only the client's physical condition, but also the status of client teaching and follow-up plans. Again, it is simply punched or tapped on the terminal and the data are displayed. This information and the client instruction sheet generated by the computer are sent home with the client.

In addition to making the charting of client care and the communication between departments much simpler and less time-consuming, the computer provides reference material for common nursing problems. For example, a matrix may show the signs and symptoms associated with diabetes mellitus. If the nurse is unsure of the signs and symptoms of the different forms of this disease, he or she can easily find them in the computer, and, if needed, this information can be printed out and put in the chart. In this way the nurse can be quickly updated about the client's condition and thereby provide optimal care.

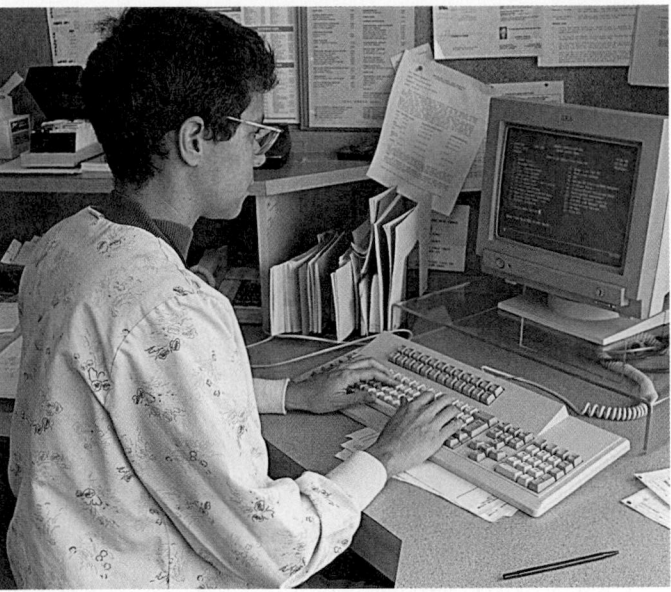

▲ Entry data becomes part of permanent record.

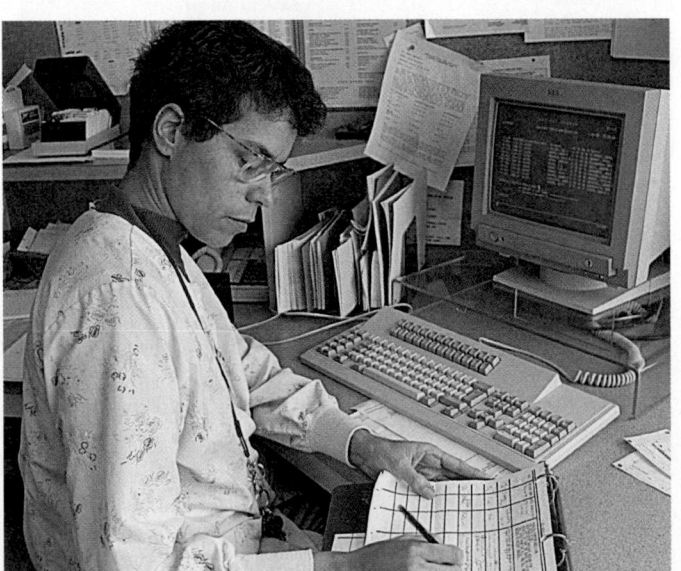

▲ Client data is entered into computer at nurse's station.

As in many professions, use of the computer in nursing and medicine has become more common, and its possible uses are rapidly expanding. In the very near future, automated speech recognition will allow nurses to document into the computer by just speaking. Also, handwriting recognition programs are being tested and will soon be available. This will allow nurses to write, rather than type, information into a book-sized computer. If learning the skills of computer use is viewed as a challenge and the reward is more efficient nursing care and less time spent on paperwork, the learning time will have been well spent.

New software and high-tech equipment are also beginning to change client care. One example is the linking of ICU point-of-care to board-certified intensivist physicians and experienced critical care nurses. By providing remote care from a central location to several hospital ICUs, the level of care for critically ill clients will be substantially upgraded. For example, a study completed in 2004 in Norfolk, VA, noted a 27% reduction in mortality for ICU clients, a 17% reduction in length of stay, and savings of more than $2,000 per client. This use of limited manpower can result in saving lives.

Health Information Technologies

Information technology is being integrated into the healthcare system. As evidence of this trend, President Bush in 2004 created a new position called the National Health Information Technology coordinator.

Bedside E-documentation Electronic charting is becoming more familiar in hospitals and clinics. Portable bedside and handheld computers have the following advantages:

- Data are entered into the client's chart immediately.
- This method saves nurses' time.
- Entry may be more accurate, because it is entered immediately after the intervention.
- Charges to the client are automatic.

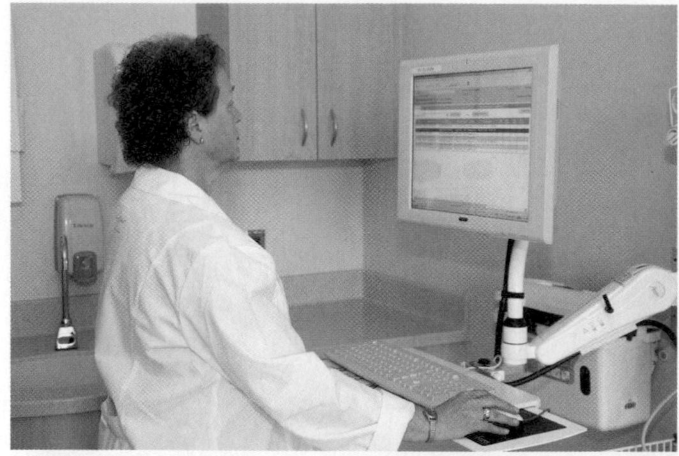

▲ When the computer is at the bedside, charting can be completed immediately after client care.

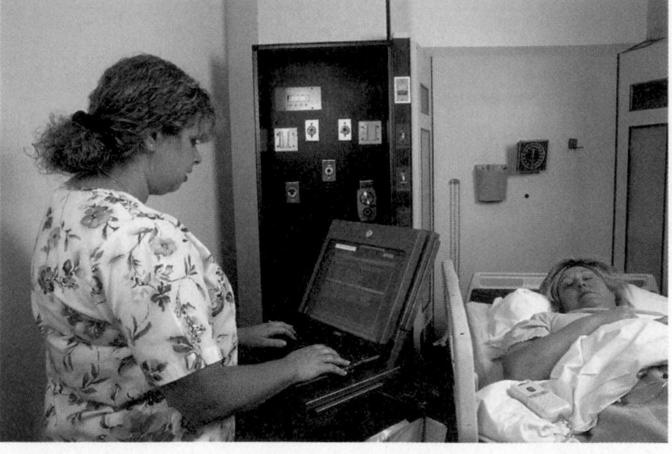

▲ Portable bedside computer unit facilitates client charting.

There are disadvantages to using E-documentation. The computer may not be equipped for narrative charting, and if there is a central data bank, a computer problem could affect obtaining important client information.

At this time there are many issues with E-documentation, but for expediency (especially with the shortage of nurses), it will probably become a primary mode of client charting.

Technology at the Bedside The PDA (personal digital assistant) has the ability to share information with a host or central computer. Nurses can use the PDA as a clinical resource for medication doses and calculations, as well as drug side effects. This device can also be used to access diagnostic test results, evaluate lab tests, and review treatments and interventions. It may also assist the nurse to review medical

Electronic Charting

Advantages

- Minimizes errors when physicians enter orders into the computer
- Allows nurses to document more client details quickly and error correction is easier
- Provides more time to spend on direct client care
- Gives supporting healthcare providers more details about the client
- Provides templates for most conditions, problems, and associated outcomes; standardization is increased
- Protects against human error (i.e., IV pumps feed directly into the computer to monitor the medication rate)
- Provides interdisciplinary plans of care online and is upgraded each shift
- Compensates for messy, incomplete handwritten nurses' notes; quality of notes improves
- Offers instant information results from tests, lab work, x-rays, etc., and allows for instant data retrieval and access ability
- Gives new caregivers a quick and complete total picture of the client; medical management improves

Disadvantages

- Computer system is expensive to purchase and update
- "Downtime" or computer "crashes" can create problems of not receiving information or it is not charted on time

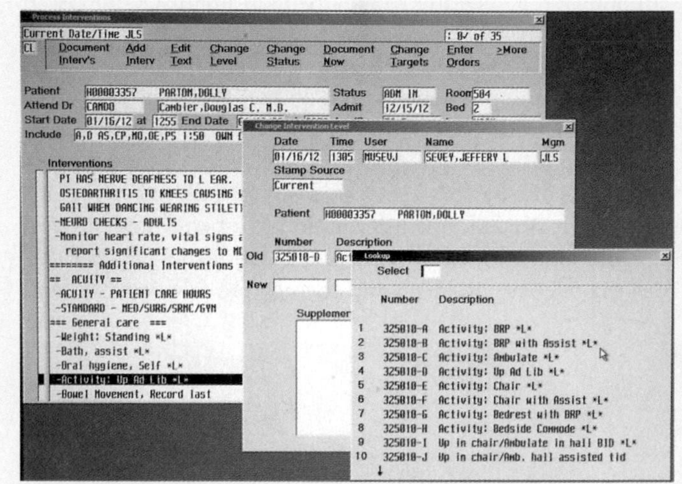

▲ Nurses may access specific categories of data for each client.

- Computer may increase charting time if number of terminals is insufficient
- Nurses rely on computers and don't question information when it may be wrong
- Unfamiliarity with computers (not enough experience in nursing school) may increase errors
- Health Insurance Portability and Accountability Act (HIPAA) and client confidentiality may be compromised; potential for unauthorized persons to access confidential records

EVIDENCE-BASED PRACTICE

Value of Using Computer Information Systems

A study conducted by David Wong, MD, at Long Beach VA Hospital showed that implementing information systems saved nurses an average of 1 hour per 12-hour shift in documentation time, thus freeing up more time for client care.

Source: Wong, D, M.D. (September 2004). *Nurse Week*, California Edition, San Jose, CA (nurseweek.com/news/archives (Sept. 2005).

diagnoses and the steps of procedures. In addition, certified nurse assistants are using the PDA to record point-of-care at the bedside (for example, vital signs), which will be instantly transmitted to the RN. With all of these attributes, the PDA has the potential to improve nursing care, save nurses' time, and promote client safety.

HIPAA Guidelines for Using a PDA The HIPAA Privacy Rule establishes standards to protect the confidentiality of individually identifiable health information maintained or transmitted electronically. The security rule adopts standards for the security of electronic protected health information. This rule is comprehensive in that it includes 19 standards and 42 specifications. Healthcare providers must check with their employers to be sure that they are compliant in adhering to the electronic standards for security.

Protected Health Information (PHI) is a component of the HIPAA guidelines. It is recommended that the client's name or any identifying data not be input into the PDA. Personal demographics or client identifiers such as history, physical findings, data, and phone numbers must be input using passwords only. If identifying data must be input, the healthcare provider should use the "security" feature, which requires a password to enter the system.

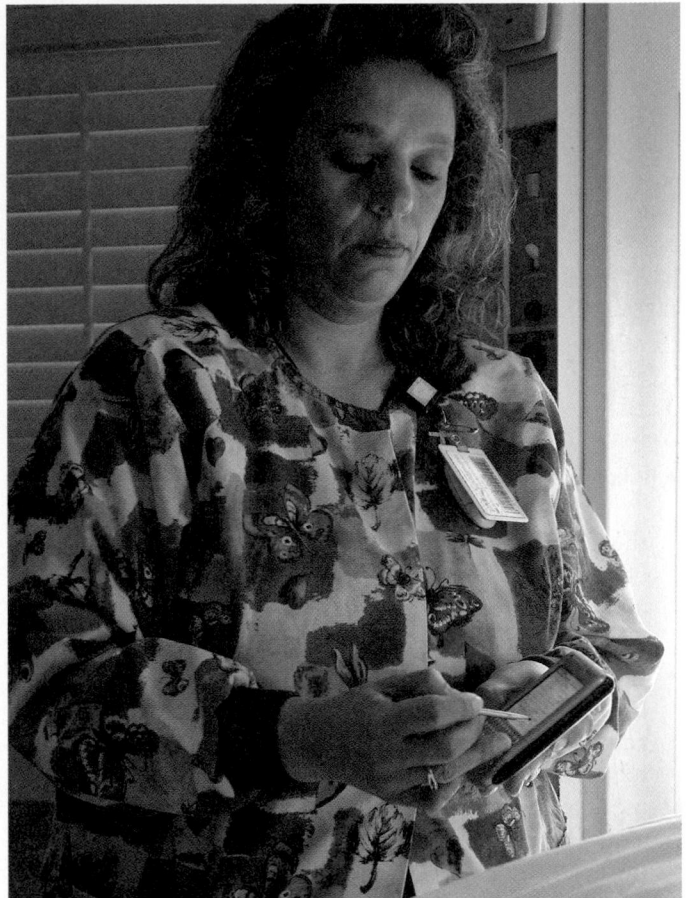

▲ PDA at bedside.

High-Tech Innovations Improve Health Care

- The Vocera B2000 communication system is a small device worn around a nurse's neck that allows for two-way voice communication. This device enables nurses at the bedside to communicate instantly with each other and physicians. Because it is hands-free, the nurse can communicate without stopping a procedure such as changing a sterile dressing. This device also saves time in locating another staff member or asking for assistance, as well as alerting the nurse to a client call or alarm.

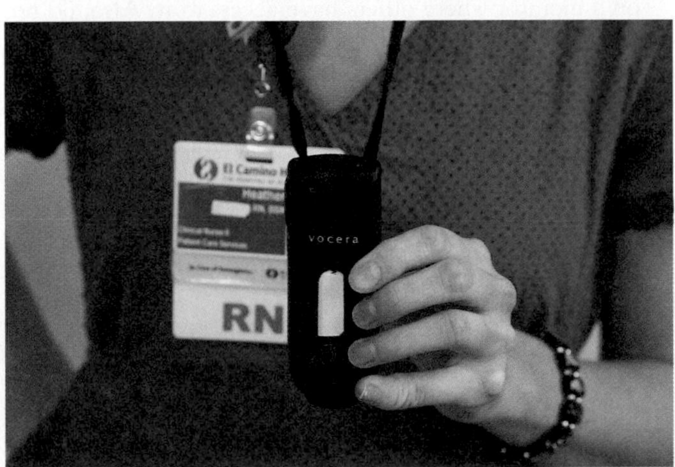

▲ Vocera communication system.

- The AccuNurse is a wearable computer headset and speech recognition system. This system prioritizes interventions and enables nurses to dictate documentation into the electronic medical record. The software is a voice-activated system and can alert the nurse about a new order. Butler Memorial Hospital in Pennsylvania developed the system.
- A specialized PDA device for use at the client's bedside allows the nurse to scan the client's bar-coded identification and medications. The PDA displays all of the critical information, including the five rights of medication administration. This device also documents the medications given and alerts the nurse to adjunct information such as vital signs, pain level, and lab results. It includes a PDA reference based on McGraw-Hill Medical's *Pharmacotherapy Handbook* and is available as an electronic database that provides information on 82 topics and 140 diseases.
- Multimedia phones or iPhones are also being considered to assist nurses working at the bedside. Information and software can be downloaded to these devices to include such information as procedures, lab values, medication information, calculations, medical terminology, physician's preferences, and much more, including a rhythm strip comparing

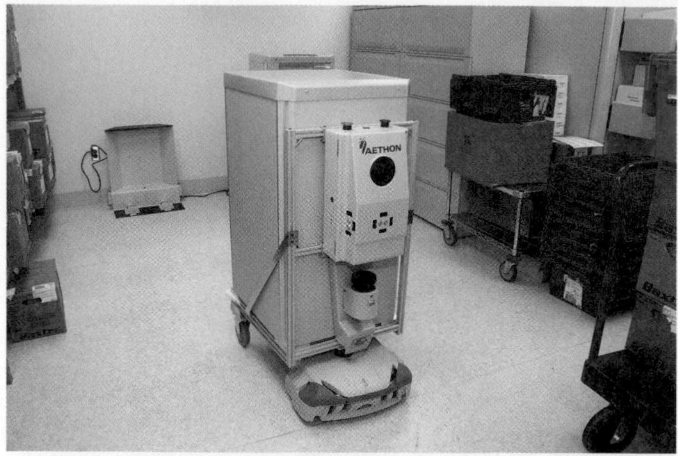

▲ Robot delivering medication to a nurse assigned to the client.

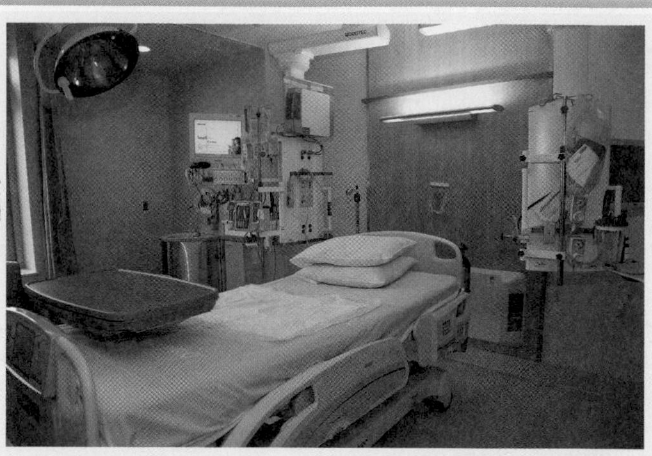

Check out this "smart" room at El Camino Hospital in Mountain View, CA, which opened in November 2009. This high-tech room brings EHRs to the client's bedside and incorporates advanced technology for client care. For example, the nurse enters the client's room and sensors detect a presence. The client's health data are instantly displayed on a wall-mounted monitor listing allergies, risk factors, medications, tests or procedures scheduled, and any information that the nurse requires to care effectively for the client.

the client's strip with a normal one. In fact, the application of the iPhone may be preferable to a computer because it allows the nurse to access information any time, any place, whereas the computer is at the client's bedside.

- Robots are another technological device becoming more and more available. Designed to take over certain clinical activities, they can save precious time, allowing the nurses to spend more time with the client. One example of robot use at a California hospital is as follows: A physician orders a new medication, and the robot in the pharmacy takes the medication directly to the specific nurse assigned to the client. The nurse then uses an ID smart card to access the drug. No other staff member can access the drug. Certain robots (e.g., the RD-7) are very versatile. They have telescopic vision and the technology to transfer vital information, such as a live image, a client's ECG tracings, urine output, heart sounds, etc. This aspect allows nurses off-site to teach, mentor, or help with client monitoring.
- PDAs, robots, telehealth devices, tablet computers, subnotebook computers, wireless networks, and related software represent the current technology and will be the healthcare technology of the future.

Minimizing Legal Risks of Computer Charting

The American Nurses' Association, the American Medical Record Association, and the Canadian Nurses' Association offer guidelines and strategies for computer safety in charting.

- Your personal password or computer signature should not be given to anyone: neither another nurse on the unit, a float nurse, nor a physician. The hospital issues a short-term password with access to certain records for infrequent users.
- Do not leave a computer terminal unattended after you have logged on. Most computers do have a timing device that shuts down a terminal when it has not been used for a certain time.
- Computer entries are part of the client's permanent record and, as such, cannot be deleted. It is possible, however, to correct an error before the material has been stored. If the entry has already been moved to storage, handle the error by marking the entry "mistaken entry," add correct information, and date and initial the entry. If you record information in the wrong chart, write "mistaken entry," add "wrong chart," and sign off.
- Once information about a client is stored, it is difficult to delete accidentally. Do check that stored records have backup files. This is an important safety check. If you inadvertently delete a part of the permanent record (this is difficult to do, since the computer always asks if you are sure), type an explanation into the computer file with date, time, and your initials. Submit an explanation in writing to your supervisor.
- Do not leave computer information about a client displayed on a monitor where others have access to it. Also, do not leave printed files unattended. Keep a log that accounts for every copy of a computerized file that you have generated from the system.
- A positive diagnosis of human immunodeficiency virus (HIV) or hepatitis B virus (HBV) is part of the client's confidential record. Disclosure of this information to unauthorized people may have legal implications. If the diagnosis is entered as any other diagnosis, take steps to follow your hospital's confidentiality procedures. Check your state's special protocols for treatment of a client's HBV or HIV status.
- Computer entry errors are most common when using electronic documentation. In 2003, 15% of the errors reported involved the use of a computer system. Many of these (45%) occurred in the transcribing phase and involved the wrong dose/wrong quantity of a medication.

LEGAL FORMS OF DOCUMENTATION

Unusual Occurrence, Variance, or Incident Report

Unusual occurrence, also called incident report (IR), or unexpected occurrence, serves three main purposes: to help document quality of care, to identify areas where in-service education is needed, and to record the details of an incident for possible legal reference.

With some staff nurses, unusual occurrence forms have a poor reputation and, perhaps, with some justification. When something goes wrong and a nurse is told to "make out a report," it is interpreted as a form of punishment.

Although these forms should be completed regularly with any unusual occurrence and may, on occasion, be used as a form of reprimand, they are no more nor less than what their title suggests: a report of an incident.

As a tool for documenting quality of care, unusual occurrences inform the quality assurance coordinator and the head nurse of areas of practice on the unit that need improvement. For example, there may be an increase in the number of clients who fell out of bed. Further research may show that because the census is up, the staff is very busy and is forgetting to reposition clients' overbed tables. In their attempts to get water or tissues, for example, more clients are falling out of bed. The solution to the problem may be to speak with the staff regarding the consequences of this action, and as a group find a mutually acceptable way of preventing this type of incident from recurring.

Unusual occurrences also suggest and document the need for in-service education. For example, when an unusual number is written regarding a new piece of equipment, the head nurse may conclude that the staff, especially those on evening and night shifts, needs instruction on operating this equipment properly and effectively. Another example is IVs that are behind or ahead of schedule. This might indicate that the nurses do not know how to regulate the IV pump correctly. A solution to this problem is to conduct a series of classes for all shifts in which the operation of the IV pump is discussed and hands-on practice is given. Such classes could be given by someone in the hospital's in-service education department or by a representative of the manufacturer of the IV pumps.

Unusual occurrences may also record the details of an occurrence for possible legal use. In some hospitals, unusual occurrences cover any situation that prevented the client from having a normal recovery. These incidents could include non-nursing actions such as returning to surgery for control of bleeding or having chest tubes inserted for a pneumothorax.

When completing an unusual occurrence with possible legal implications, it is doubly important to record all details of the incident. It is not easy to recall details of the care you gave a client 1 or 2 months ago. Frequently lawsuits are not filed for months or even years after an incident, so it is essential that you record important details promptly.

Information to record on the unusual occurrence includes general details of the incident, the client's response, your action or reaction to the incident, and a list of other personnel who were aware of the details of the incident. Often there is space on the form to record the physician's report of the client's condition after the incident. To fill in the section regarding the physician's report, the nurse later copies the doctor's progress notes from the chart onto the form. At no time is the unusual occurrences given to the physician. This is a written document between the hospital and its insurance carrier, not the physician.

On completion, unusual occurrences are forwarded to the unit manager or head nurse and then to nursing administration. Information from the report of interest to in-service education or quality assurance departments can be obtained at this time. Ultimately, the unusual occurrence is passed along to the hospital's legal department to be retained indefinitely in the event that legal action is later initiated on behalf of the client.

Consent Forms

When an individual enters a hospital, some of his or her basic legal rights are affected. So that these rights are not violated, the client must give permission (consent) for all treatment. If consent is not obtained, the hospital, physician, or nurse may be charged with committing "battery" against the client. *Battery*, as defined by law, is an "offensive touching" of the client. This could include an injection or any breaking of the skin's surface, use of x-rays, or insertion of tubes, for example.

Before you panic and attempt to get a consent signed for such a routine procedure as taking the client's next blood pressure, you should know that routine nursing care is "consented to" when the client signs the "conditions of admissions" form. Also, certain procedures, such as injections, intubations, and dressings, are treatments ordered by the physician and agreed to by the client. If the client has listened to the explanation of a specific procedure and has agreed to allow the procedure to be carried out, he or she is giving implied consent; however, the client has the right to refuse any treatment, including changing his or her mind about a procedure previously agreed to. In that case the physician must be contacted regarding alternative actions.

When discussing the formal written or explicit consents, the two key nursing activities are obtaining and witnessing consent. Initiating consent is not a nursing function because it includes the explanation of what is to be done, the risks of the procedure to that client, alternative procedures, and probable outcomes. This information should be given by the doctor. The nurse may clarify the information to be sure the client understands.

The nurse's role is to witness the signing of the consent. When the consent form is presented to the client, it should be explained, and the client should be encouraged to read it thoroughly before signing. Occasionally a nurse is asked to explain or expand the physician's presentation. Acceptable practice is for the nurse to clarify, define a medical term, or add more details to the physician's initial information. If the nurse feels that the client does not really understand what is going to occur, it is the nurse's responsibility to notify the doctor to give further explanation before the client signs the consent. An easy way to determine what the client understands is to ask him or her to repeat the physician's explanation. Under ordinary circumstances, only one witness to signing the consent is necessary. The witness does not have to be an RN, just someone over the age of 18 years.

UNUSUAL OCCURRENCE

COMPLETE IMMEDIATELY FOR EVERY INCIDENT AND SEND TO ADMINISTRATOR

______ HOSPITAL NAME

ADMINISTRATOR: Please forward to Hospital Attorney

______ CITY

______ FOR ADDRESSOGRAPH PLATE

CONFIDENTIAL REPORT OF INCIDENT (NOT A PART OF MEDICAL RECORD)

CLIENT ______ (LAST NAME) ______ (FIRST NAME) AGE ______ SEX ______ (M OR F) ROOM ______

ADMITTING DIAGNOSIS ______ DATE OF ADMISSION ______

ATTENDING PHYSICIAN ______ DATE OF INCIDENT ______ TIME ______ M

WERE BED RAILS UP? ______ WAS SAFETY BELT IN USE? ______

WAS CLIENT RATIONAL? ______ HI LO BED POSITION ______

SEDATIVES ______ DOSE ______ T ______ IME ______

NARCOTICS ______ DOSE ______ T ______ IME ______

GIVEN WITHIN 12 HOURS PREVIOUS TO INCIDENT

TIME DOCTOR WAS CALLED ______ A.M. ______ P.M. TIME RESPONDED ______ A.M. ______ P.M.

(I.E., HOUSE PHYSICIAN-RESIDENT-INTERN-ETC.)

I NOTIFIED DR. ______ TIME ______ M BY ______

NURSE'S ACCOUNT OF THE INCIDENT (INCLUDE EXACT LOCATION)

______

LIST PERSONS FAMILIAR WITH DETAILS OF INCIDENT - AND OTHER CLIENTS IN THE SAME ROOM

NAME ______ ADDRESS ______

NAME ______ ADDRESS ______

NAME ______ ADDRESS ______

HISTORY OF INCIDENT AS RELATED BY CLIENT ______

DATE OF REPORT ______

▲ Form 3-F. Example of unusual occurrence.

COMMUNITY HOSPITAL

Client Information

AUTHORIZATION FOR AND CONSENT TO SURGERY, ADMINISTRATION OF ANESTHETICS, SPECIAL DIAGNOSTIC OR THERAPEUTIC PROCEDURES

Date ______ Time ______

Your admitting physician is ______, M.D.

Your surgeon is ______, M.D.

1. The hospital staff and facilities assist your physicians and surgeons in the performance of various surgical operations and other diagnostic and therapeutic procedures. These surgical operations and special diagnostic or therapeutic procedures all may involve calculated risks of complications, injury or even death, from both known and unknown causes and no warranty or guarantee has been made as to result or cure. Except in a case of emergency or exceptional circumstances, these operations and procedures are not performed upon clients unless and until the client has had an opportunity to discuss them with his/her physician. Each client has the right to consent to or to refuse any proposed operation or special procedure (based upon the description or explanation received).
2. Your physicians and surgeons have determined that the operations or special procedures listed below may be beneficial in the diagnosis or treatment of your condition. Upon your authorization and consent, the operations or special procedures will be performed by your physicians and surgeons and their staff. The persons in attendance for the purpose of administering anesthesia or performing other specialized professional services, such as radiology, pathology and the like, are not the agents, servants or employees of the hospital or your physician or surgeon, but are independent contractors performing specialized services on your behalf and, as such, are your agents, servants, or employees. Any tissue or member severed in any operation will be disposed of in the discretion of the pathologist, except ______ and those body parts specified as donor organs.
3. Your signature opposite the operations or special procedures listed below constitutes your acknowledgement (a) that you have read and agreed to the foregoing, (b) that the operations or special procedures have been adequately explained to you by your attending physicians or surgeons and that you have all of the information that you desire, and (c) that you authorize and consent to the performance of the operations or special procedures.

Operation or Procedure

______

Signature ______ Client Signature ______ Witness

(If client is a minor or unable to sign, complete the following): Client is a minor, is unable to sign because

______

______ Father ______ Guardian

______ Mother ______ Other person and relationship

▲ Form 3-G. Example of consent form.

There are many rules and regulations governing consents. If you have questions about them, consult the consent manual for your hospital, or a supervisory person. There are several important situations in which more information may be needed. One relates to the client's mental competency. Generally, the client must sign personally, and spouses are unable to sign for the client. Permanent incompetence usually involves legal action to assign someone else as conservator. Temporary incompetence may be the result of hospital treatments, such as drugs or anesthetics. When a narcotic or sedative has been given, at least 4 hours' elapsed time is recommended before the client is considered competent to sign a consent. A second situation concerns the client who is a minor. The age of consent varies by state and also according to specific situations, such as emancipation (being away from the family and self-supporting) and the type of medical problem (reportable diseases or pregnancy). An associated problem may arise when deciding who can legally sign for a minor.

REPORTING

A shift-to-shift report should be given not only from the Kardex but from the client care plan. There is no need to review particular procedures for such activities as dressing changes, when they are outlined on the care plan. A simple statement to the effect that the procedure is listed on the care plan is all that is necessary. This decreases both time and repetition of information.

To avoid confusion from shift to shift, specific times for treatments and for activities of daily living (ADLs) are indicated. For example, it is noted on the care plan that the client prefers his bath before 8 AM to avoid having to ask him every day when he wants his bath. This consistency promotes a feeling of confidence in the nursing staff and alleviates fear.

Intrashift Reports

Reporting your observations and interventions to other health team members is as essential as documenting them on the client's chart. Intrashift reports are usually verbal reports relayed to team members, team leaders, or charge nurses to keep them informed of changes in the client's conditions. Examples of findings that need to be communicated to other health team members include significant changes in vital signs, unusual responses to treatments, medications, or changes in the client's physical or emotional condition.

EVIDENCE-BASED PRACTICE

Interdisciplinary Collaboration

A 2004 study of the literature found positive outcomes from interdisciplinary collaboration. The most significant were coordination of care amongst clinical team members; improved efficiency and client outcomes; interdisciplinary communication, particularly with pharmacists; and reduced medication errors and adverse drug events.

Source: National Association for Healthcare Quality (2004, March-April). Patient safety: A case study in team building and interdisciplinary collaboration. www.nahq.org/Journal/ce/article_ID=171

Intershift Reports

Intershift reports disseminate client information between shifts. It may be accomplished through a verbal report or by tape recording the information. The intershift report should include the following data: client's name, room number, physician's name, diagnosis, and date of surgery when appropriate. In addition, report unusual findings based on the nursing assessment, response to treatments or medications, unusual occurrences, laboratory results, laboratory studies, tests to be completed on the next shift, and any physical or psychosocial problems that exist.

SBAR is a relatively new technique that nurses are using to focus communication relative to the client's condition. When the nurse is making an inter- or intrashift report, this technique includes the critical elements that must be transferred from one healthcare team to another: situation, background, assessment, and recommendations.

Physician/Advanced Practitioner Notification

Physicians should be notified whenever treatment or nursing care parameters are exceeded, significant alterations occur in physical assessment findings, or abnormal laboratory findings and test results are obtained.

Before calling the physician, have all data available to allow you to answer questions: current vital signs, laboratory results, when medications were given last, and so on. It is a good idea to have the entire chart with you.

When calling the physician, identify yourself by name, your status (RN or SN), nursing unit, and the client's name. State the exact reason you are calling. Give pertinent and succinct information.

Nurse Manager

Written or verbal reports are given to nurse managers, nursing supervisors, or clinical coordinators during each shift. The report includes information on all critically ill clients, those with unusual occurrences or complications, and clients with conditions that are difficult to manage. It is also a good idea to alert the supervisor to problems with families, physicians, or other health disciplines so she or he can assist you in the problem solving.

Client Care Conferences

Client care conferences and care plans play an integral role in planning and delivering health care for difficult or unusual problems. The client care conference can focus on developing the care plan or on identifying difficult problems. A conference can be scheduled to plan appropriate interventions and to inform all health team members of the goals for that client's care.

HEALTHCARE DELIVERY

Client Acuity Systems

State law, such as Title 22 of the California Code of Regulation, provides information on how staffing is determined in hospitals within that state. Title 22 states the following regulations regarding staffing.

There shall be a method for determining staffing requirements based on assessment of client needs. This assessment shall take into consideration at least the following:

1. The ability of the client to do self-care
2. Degree of illness
3. Requirements for special nursing activities
4. Skill level of personnel required in delivery care
5. Placement of the client in the nursing unit

There shall be documentation of the methodology used in making staffing determinations. Such documentation shall be part of the records of the nursing service and be available for review.

Various systems to determine staffing patterns have been used for many years. With the advent of diagnosis-related groups (DRGs), acuity systems for planning staffing needs are being used in many hospitals. This system forms the basis for client care delivery. Categories of nursing care are identified, and a numerical value is assigned to each category. These categories of care include areas such as ADLs, ambulation, client teaching, and medication administration. The numerical values assigned to each category are based on a point scale. For example, using a scale of 1 to 5, a score of 1 indicates the client can function independently in certain tasks; a score of 5 indicates complete dependency on a caregiver for that category.

The scores from all categories are totaled; this score is divided by the number of categories in the acuity system. The final score is designated as the client's acuity level, which is determined for each 8-hour shift. Every nursing unit has a predetermined number of client care hours assigned for each acuity level. For example, a client acuity level of 4.0 on the day shift is allotted 2.8 hours of nursing care for that shift.

After all clients in the nursing unit are assigned an acuity level, the total client care acuity number is used to determine the number of nursing staff required for the next shift. Then, the acuity level of individual clients is used to plan care assignments for the staff. A nurse may be able to safely care for a total acuity of 16. This method seems equitable, since each staff member is assigned to clients based on acuity. Thus instead of assigning the nursing staff to clients based on room location or number of clients, the acuity level is used to allocate staff resources. Staffing patterns based on the acuity system have been found to be the most practical, equitable, and manageable.

Disease Management

A current trend in delivering health care specifies a goal of reducing complications associated with chronic diseases. Designed to incorporate healthcare interventions based on standard practice guidelines, this system is a cost-saving, empowering approach for clients.

It is a process that begins when the group paying for the health care identifies a client with a targeted chronic disease, including such diseases as cancer, chronic obstructive pulmonary disease (COPD), asthma, diabetes, or depression.

A nurse contacts the client, asks his permission to enter him in the program, and does an initial assessment. Following this, the nurse discusses recommended medical care to the client. The nurse then discusses lifestyle behaviors proven to improve the chronic conditions. All are based on evidence-backed practice guidelines. Self-care efforts have proved to be significant in altering the course of the disease.

Most programs involve telephone communications from a registered nurse, although home visits may be arranged.

Clinical Alert

Studies show that 90 million U.S. citizens live with chronic diseases which are responsible for 7 out of 10 deaths in the United States.

DELEGATING CLIENT CARE

Client care assignments should be based on careful analysis of each client's needs and goals of care. The care plan may be consulted for an effective use of healthcare team members to their best advantage, as well as for the client's welfare. A client requiring extensive sterile dressing changes, frequent assessments, and IV medications is more appropriately assigned to a professional nurse. A client who is convalescing after a stroke and requires mainly bathing and ambulation assistance can usually be assigned to another member of the health team such as a nursing assistant.

In most healthcare facilities, delegating client care to healthcare workers has become a financially driven reality. RNs have less responsibility for actual direct care activities such as hygienic care, ambulation, and feeding. However, delegation of these tasks is under the jurisdiction of the RN. To delegate appropriate tasks, the nurse must be familiar with the Nurse Practice Act for RNs and Licensed Vocational Nurses (LVNs) in their state and with the hospital's job descriptions for each level of healthcare worker. More unlicensed assistive personnel (UAP) are being employed by facilities as a method of cost containment. The goal is still to deliver service to the clients. This classification of healthcare worker includes many titles, such as patient-focused care technician, patient care technician, UAP, and nurse assistant. This level of healthcare worker provides basic care functions and can be a help to the overburdened nurse. UAPs must receive training in the skills

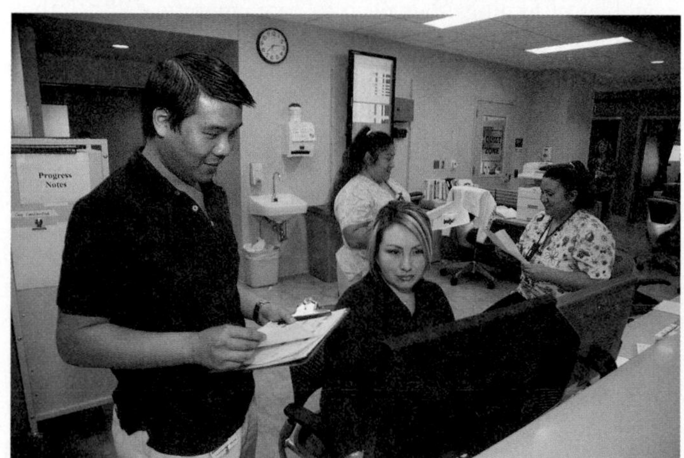

▲ Client care assignments are delegated based on client acuity and competence of the healthcare worker.

they are to perform before client care is assigned. The usual tasks assigned to these workers are similar to those of certified nurse assistants (CNAs), with added responsibilities such as changing clean dressings or suctioning long-standing tracheostomies using clean technique. The RN is still responsible for the care that is provided by this category of healthcare worker. Because of this, many state boards of nursing have developed position statements and guidelines to help RNs delegate activities safely. Guidelines vary among states, so you need to check your state's guidelines. Also, there are general guidelines that should be followed regardless of the state in which you practice. According to the National Council of State Boards of Nursing (NCSBN), tasks that involve nursing judgment and the need to assess the client's responses to the care plan must not be delegated to any other level of worker than an RN. Any nursing intervention that requires independent, specialized nursing knowledge, skill, or judgment can only be delegated to an RN, according to the American Nurses Association. The hospital cannot expand the duties of healthcare workers beyond those legally allowed by the state. The hospital may, however, decrease their task levels and require certification or credentials for some tasks.

RN Delegation

Delegation is defined as "transferring to a competent individual the authority to perform a selected nursing task in a selected situation" (National Council of State Boards of Nursing). State licensing laws designate that nurses are legally accountable for quality of care and for direct client care. For example:

- RNs decide which tasks to delegate and under what circumstances.
- RNs must know what is safe delegation of nursing care tasks.
- RNs must supervise (monitor and evaluate) outcomes for all delegated tasks. The RN retains accountability for the delegation.

RNs must know the legal scope of practice of other licensed providers. They must also know competency of licensed and unlicensed personnel as well as the tasks which may be delegated.

- Some states identify tasks that may *not ever* be delegated (such as a sterile dressing to unlicensed personnel).
- RNs may *not* delegate assessment, evaluation, or nursing judgment functions.

RNs and LVNs must check with their own states' laws and regulations to determine which activities may *not* be performed by unlicensed assistive personnel (UAP).

Examples are as follows:

- Administration of medications or IV drugs.
- Venipuncture or intravenous therapy.
- Parenteral or tube feedings.
- Any invasive procedures such as NG tube insertion, catheters, or suctioning.
- Assessment of the client's condition.
- Educating client or family concerning healthcare problems.
- Reporting on laboratory tests.

RN Responsibilities That Cannot Be Delegated

- Data entry into client's charts for all unlicensed personnel to whom tasks are delegated.
- Initial health assessments (only by RN).
- Care plan objectives—checked by RN if completed by LVN.
- Review data obtained by other healthcare workers.
- Complete referral form for additional client services.
- Receive reports of client conditions and any unexpected findings from delegated activities.
- Identify parameters for which worker is to notify nurse.
- Carry out pain management activities (epidural narcotic analgesia done only by RN).
- Check advanced directives in client's chart.
- Organ donation—RN or LVN responsible for carrying out hospital policies.
- Complete discharge teaching plan.

Activities That May Be Delegated to LVN/PN The RN is legally responsible for client care. As such, the nurse must determine which task may be delegated. These decisions are based on the client's diagnosis, what the state allows the LVN to do, the amount of judgment and experience needed to complete the task, and whether the assistant is capable of performing and completing the task. Following are guidelines for delegation:

- While the RN initiates the care plan, the LVN may update the plan.
- After the RN completes the initial assessment, the LVN records assessment changes.
- The LVN may reinforce client teaching, but the RN must initiate the teaching and evaluate the results.
- LVNs, depending on the individual state standards, may or may not add medications to the IV. They may add vitamins and minerals in most states. After completing an IV course, LVNs may initiate IV therapy.

Delegation Regulations of Unlicensed Assistive Personnel (UAPs) and Certified Nurse Assistants (CNAs)

These terms refer to a group of workers who are trained and/or certified, but not licensed. These workers cannot be assigned tasks in lieu of a registered nurse. The nurse must determine which tasks may be performed by a UAP or CNA.

How to delegate to a UAP or CNA:

- The assistant's areas of competence must be judged against the specific needs of the client.
- The nurse must give specific instructions and do active monitoring during the assignment.
- Progress in client care through feedback and evaluation of outcomes should occur frequently.
- The nurse must be sure that the appropriate delegation is made: Can the assistant legally do this task, has the worker

been trained to perform this task, has the worker demonstrated that they can complete the task, and is the client response predictable?

- When performing the task, can the worker obtain the same result as the RN?

Duties Most Often Delegated to Unlicensed Assistive Personnel

- Taking vital signs and charting results
- Obtaining height and weight
- Repositioning a client or assisting a client to bed
- Bathing a client and making the bed
- Transferring a client between units
- Escorting a client out of the hospital
- Recording drainage from an NG tube
- Serving food trays and feeding a client
- Obtaining a specimen that is nonsterile and noninvasive
- Performing range-of-motion activities after instruction
- Initiating CPR after certification
- Working with a dying client
- Completing postmortem care

Standards of Competent Performance

- A registered nurse shall be considered competent when he/she consistently demonstrates the ability to transfer scientific knowledge from social, biological, and physical sciences in applying the nursing process.
- *Incompetence* means lacking possession of or failure to exercise that degree of learning, skill, care, and experience ordinarily possessed and exercised by a competent registered nurse.

Professional Functions of the RN (Denoted by State)

- Formulates a nursing diagnosis through observation of the client's physical condition and behavior, and through interpretation of information obtained from the client and others, including the health team.
- Formulates a care plan, in collaboration with the client, which ensures that nursing care services provide for the client's safety, comfort, hygiene, and protection, and for disease prevention and restorative measures.
- Performs skill essential to the kind of nursing action to be taken, explains the health treatment to the client and family, and teaches the client and family how to care for the client's health needs.
- Delegates tasks to subordinates based on the legal scope of practice of the subordinate and on the preparation and capability needed in the tasks to be delegated and effectively supervises nursing care being given by subordinates.
- Evaluates the effectiveness of the care plan through observation of the client's physical condition and behavior, signs, and symptoms through communication with the client and health team members and modifies the plan as needed.
- Acts as the client's advocate, as circumstances require, by initiating action to improve health care or change decisions or activities that are against the interests or wishes of the client and by giving the client the opportunity to make informed decisions about health care before it is provided.

Parameters of Delegation

Many state boards of nursing have identified the parameters of delegation. Examples of these "Rights of Delegation" are:

Right Task—a task that can be legally delegated to an LVN/LPN, PCT, or UAP. Check the state nurse practice act to determine whether the caregiver is trained to perform the task. Judge whether the UAP or LVN is competent to perform the task.

Right Circumstances—the LVN, PCT, or UAP understands the elements of the procedure and the RN is assured that the UAP can perform the procedure safely in an appropriate setting. Caregiver is able to collect the right supplies to perform the procedure.

Right Person—the right person (RN or LVN) delegates the right task (legally can be delegated to a UAP) to the right person (legally can perform the task) on the right client (stable with predictable outcomes).

Right Communication—person delegating the task (RN or LVN) has described the task clearly, including directions, special steps of the task, and the expected outcomes. Then, the delegator must trust those they are delegating to, supporting the right to make certain decisions.

Right Supervisor—the RN or LVN delegating the activity answers the UAP's questions and is available to problem solve, if necessary.

Source: Smith, S. F. (2006). *Sandra Smith's Review of Nursing for NCLEX-RN*. Los Altos, CA: National Nursing Review.

STUDENT CLINICAL PLANNING

Preclinical Planning

To assist students with client care planning prior to clinical experience, many nursing programs have developed a Student Clinical Prep Form. This form helps focus the student's attention on the information necessary to ensure safe nursing practice. Most forms of this type, such as the example provided, include information related to the client's biographical data, history and physical assessment findings, medical diagnosis, nursing diagnosis, medications including IVs, and nursing interventions.

Time Management

Implementing time management techniques during your student clinical experience will assist you not only in organizing client care management, but also in completing your assignment efficiently. Some techniques you may find helpful are listed below.

- Design a time management work sheet you can follow.
- Collect the appropriate information you will require to identify client care tasks (e.g., RN report, care plan, Kardex, medication record).

STUDENT CLINICAL PREP FORM

IDENTIFYING DATA

Client Initials ______ Room # ______ Age ______ M ___ F ___ Date of Admission ______ Allergies ______

Cultural/Ethnic Background ______ Primary Language Spoken ______ Religious Preference ______

Occupation ______ Retired ______ Family/Living Arrangements ______

Admitting Diagnosis ______ Diagnostic Procedures (dates): ______

Brief History of Present Illness ______ Surgical Procedures (dates): ______

Pertinent Lab Data: ______

PHYSICAL Assessment Findings ______

PATHOPHYSIOLOGY of Primary & Secondary Diagnoses ______

Medications (Routine & PRNs currently taking)

Drug	Dosage	Route	Classification	Expected Effects	Usual Side Effects	Critical Assessment Data

IV Solutions	Additives	Drip rate	Site Assess.	**Special Equipment/Considerations**

Interventions	Time	Outcome		Drains/Tubes

▲ Form 3-H. Clinical prep form.

CLINICAL TIME MANAGEMENT WORK SHEET

Client #1 ______	7 AM	8 9	10 11	12 1	2 3	Assessment Data
Room number ______				VS BP TPR Meds	I&O I O	Neuro
Med Diag: ______						Resp
______						GU
______						GI
Nsg Diag: ______						M/S
______						Psy/Soc
Diet ______						
Activity level ______						
IV Solution ______						
IV# ______						
Credit ______						
Rate ______						
IV to follow ______						
IV# ______	Lab: ______					
Rate ______	X-ray: ______					
	Special Procedures: ______					

▲ Form 3-I. Time management work sheet.

- Identify specific tasks of client care and the time frame needed for completion.
- Prioritize tasks included in the client care plan.
- Make an initial visit to assess your client's status.
- Revise priorities based on your assessment.
- Plan nursing interventions in sequence.
- Group and sequence client care activities for completion in the same time frame. Allocate sufficient time to complete client assignment.
- Consider client's wishes for completing nonpriority tasks, such as bathing and grooming.
- Identify tasks for which you will require assistance.
- Notify the appropriate colleague to assist you (e.g., ambulating your client).
- Identify and collect necessary equipment for task completion.
- Complete client care, implementing the prioritized plan of action (POA) using your time management work sheet.
- Allocate appropriate time to interact with your client.
- Mark off tasks on the time management sheet as you complete them, leaving a record for giving verbal report to the nurse when leaving the unit.
- Document client care as soon as feasible, or at least every 2 hours, on the appropriate records.

Word Roots, Prefixes, and Suffixes

a, an: without, not
ab: away from
abd: abdominal
ac: before meals
acro: extreme, top, extremity
acu: sharp
ad, al: to, toward
adeno: gland
adip: fat
ad lib: freely, as desired
-aemia: blood
aero: air, gas
-aesthesia: sensation
-al: action, process
alg: pain
-algesia, algia: suffering pain
amb: ambulatory, walking
amput: cut away, cut off
amt: amount
ante: before
anti: against, opposed to
ap, apo: away from
arteri: artery
arthro: joint
-ase: enzyme
aur: ear
auto: self
bacill: rod
bacter: rod
bi: double, two
bid: twice each day
bile: bile
bio: life
blephar: eyelid
BM: bowel movement
brachi: arm
brady: slow
BRP: bathroom privileges
bucc: check
c̄: with
cale: stone
capit: head
cardi, cardio: heart
cathart: cleansing
caud: tail
cav: hollow
cec: blind
cent: hundred
-chem, -chemo: chemical
chole: bile
chron: time
cid: kill
-cide: causing death
cili: eyelid
circum: ring, circle
C/O: complains of
cogni: know
colo: colon
com, con: with, together
crani: skull
cry: cold
cut: skin
cyan: blue
cyst: bladder
cyt: cell
-cyte: cell
DC: discontinue
demi: half
dent: tooth
derm: skin
di, dis: double, separation, reversal
dors: back
dur: hard
dy: two
-dynia: pain
dys: abnormal, different
e, ec: out from
-ectomy: cutting out
em, en: in, within
embol: inserted a wedge
-emesis: vomiting
-emia: blood
emulsi: milk out, exhaust
endo: within
entero: intestinal
epi: upon
erythro: red
eso: inside
-esthesia: sensation
et: and
eu: normal
ex: out of
exo: the outside, beyond
fore: before, in front of
gastro: stomach
genito: genital
-gens, -gent: clan, tribe
glosso: relating to the tongue
glyco: sugar
-gram: tracing, a mark
-graphy: a writing, a record
grav: heavy
gyn: woman
H_2O: water
hemi: half
hemo: blood
hepar, hepatio: liver
hisc: open
homeo: same, similar
homo: same, similar
HS: bedtime
hydro: related to water
hyper: above, beyond
hypo: under, below
I&O: intake and output
-iasis: condition, pathologic state
ile, ilo: intestine
in: not, within, into
in: inch
incont: incontinent
infra: below
inter: between
intra: inside
is: equal
isch, ischo: hold, suppress
-ism: condition, theory
itis: inflammation
juxta: next to
latero: side
lb or #: pound
leuko: white
lip: fat
lith: stone
ly: loose, dissolve
-lysis: dissolving, decomposition
macro: large, big
mal: bad, poor
mamm: breast
man: hand
mani: mental alterations
megaly: large
meta: beyond
metra, metro: uterus
micro: small
ne: young, new
nebul: cloud, mist
necr, necro: dead
neo: new
neuro: nerve
noct: night
-nos, -noso: disease
npo: nothing by mouth
nucleo: nucleus
nutri: nourish
ob: against
oc: occlude
olig: few, small
oob: out of bed
opisth: backward
-opsy: examination
opthalm: eye
-orrhaphy: repair of
ortho: straight, normal
-osis: process, condition
oss, ost: bone
-ostomy: creation of an opening
-otomy: opening into
palp: touch, feel
pan: all, entire
para: beside, beyond
paten, patent: spreading open
path: disease, sickness
pc: after meals
ped, pedi, pedo: foot
ped, pedo: child
pen: lack of
per: by, through
peri: around
pet: tend toward
pha: speak
phag: eat
phleb: vein
phon: sound
phot: light
phthi: waste away
-phylaxis: protection
-plasm: to mold
-plasty: formed or repaired by plastic surgery
platy: broad, flat
-plegia: paralysis
pleur: rib
plur: more
pne: breathing
-pnea: respiration, respiratory condition

Word Roots, Prefixes, and Suffixes (*Continued*)

pneumo: air, gas, lung
post: after, behind
pre: before
PRN: whenever necessary
pro: before
pruri: itch
pseud, pseudo: false
psych: the soul, mind
-ptosis: a lowered position of an organ
pulmo: lung
pur: pus
pyo: pus
pyro: fire
qd: every day
qh: every hour
qid: four times each day
qs: as much as required
q2h: every 2 hours
q3h: every 3 hours
q4h: every 4 hours
ren: kidneys
retro: backwards
-rhage, -rhagia: hemorrhage, excessive flow or discharge
s̄: without
-sclerosis: dryness, hardness
-scopy: to see
sedat: soothed, calm
semi: half
sens: sense
sept: wall off
socio: social
som: sleep
spiro: breathe
stasis: stoppage, slowing
stat: immediately
steat: fat
sub, sup: under, below
super: over, above, higher
syn: with, together
tach: fast
therapeu: serve, treatment
therm: heat
thromb: clot
tid: three times each day
-tomy: cut
top: place
toxic: poisonous
troch: wheel
trop: turn, change
-trophy: nutrition, nourishment
ultra: beyond, excessively
un: one
-uria: a specific condition of, or related to urine
vaso: vessel
veno: vein
ventro: abdomen
°: degree

MANAGEMENT Guidelines

Each state legislates a Nurse Practice Act for RNs and LVN/LPNs. Healthcare facilities are responsible for establishing and implementing policies and procedures that conform to their state's regulations. Verify the regulations and role parameters for each healthcare worker in your facility.

Delegation

- The RN must complete the initial assessment, develop the client care plan, and develop the teaching plan. These activities cannot be delegated to any other healthcare team worker.
- Tasks that require judgment or the need to assess outcomes of the task may not be delegated to other healthcare team workers.
- Before delegating any client care to an LVN/LPN, review the Nurse Practice Act and the facility policies to determine which tasks may be delegated and which may not be delegated.
- Before delegating client care to Unlicensed Assistive Personnel (UAP), review the board of nursing (BRN) guidelines in your state as well as the facility policy governing their skill level. Remember the facility may decrease the level of responsibility for healthcare workers, but they cannot exceed the skill level outlined in Practice Acts or the BRN guidelines.
- When delegating client care, refer to the Kardex as well as the client care plan or critical pathway to determine the level of care required in order to appropriately assign the healthcare workers. Assign clients according to care needs, not location of rooms.
- Charting basic care modalities such as hygienic care can be assigned to CNAs and UAPs when flow sheets are used. These caregivers cannot be assigned to complete narrative charting.
- LVNs/LPNs are responsible for charting using all formats: narrative, flow sheets, problem-oriented, and computer-assisted charting.
- RNs are responsible for the data entry in charts for all unlicensed healthcare workers.

Communication Matrix

- Information relative to client care is provided both in written and verbal communication. Written information is found on the Kardex card, client care plan, or critical pathway. Verbal communication consists of the shift and team report and directions provided to the workers throughout the shift. When assigning client care to healthcare workers, the RN uses both communication processes. When directions are given to healthcare workers, the Kardex card and care plan or pathway is the foundation for client information. This information is provided in a verbal report at the beginning of the shift. Two-way communication is encouraged throughout the shift, as client's needs change or new orders are written for client care.
- Verbal reports can be given individually or to a group of healthcare workers. It depends on the type of healthcare delivery system that is employed in the facility.
- Specific information regarding client care must be provided to each healthcare worker. This information includes activity level, vital sign times, diet, ability to perform

ADLs, procedures or treatments that will be conducted during the shift and the approximate time this will occur, specimens needing collection as well as any safety precautions necessary, visual and hearing deficits, dentures, and specific tasks to be completed by the healthcare worker.

- Communicate with all members of the healthcare team through the multidisciplinary care plan. Ensure they follow the plan of care and document to the care plan.
- After receiving report from unlicensed health care workers, the RN must complete the charting except where flow sheets are used.
- The RN is responsible for the accuracy of all documentation, including information contained in the flow sheet; therefore, it should be checked each shift.
- Licensed nursing staff should review the documentation for the past 24 hours before beginning nursing care. The chart will provide details on the client's status, including assessment findings, response to pain medication, and client's response to treatments. Continuity of care can be provided when client information is known.
- The RN should review necessary data, obtained by reading the chart, with the unlicensed personnel to provide for continuity of care.
- RNs should review principles of charting with personnel if guidelines for charting are not being followed. The records are permanent and reflect the care provided the client while hospitalized. The chart can be subpoenaed if a lawsuit is filed.

CRITICAL THINKING Strategies

Scenario 1

Determine appropriate delegation of client activities for a staff team on a unit. This scenario does not take into consideration the acuity of the client, only the nursing tasks needed for the day shift. Each facility and state have differing policies regarding personnel; therefore, these policies need to be reviewed before this activity is completed.

The team consists of one RN, one LVN/LPN, and one UAP. There are 10 clients and 2 unoccupied beds. There is a charge nurse and ward clerk assigned to the nursing unit. There are two other teams, and these three teams make up the medical–surgical nursing unit.

RM 601A	Mr. Rodrigues, 98, admitted 24 hours earlier Diagnosis: congestive heart failure Bed rest, bed bath and assistance with oral hygiene, daily weight, I&O Vital signs q 4 hrs., low sodium diet, restricted fluids to 1500mL IV #2 1000mL D5/.2NS with 20mEq KCL at 50mL/hr—800mL remaining IV medications: lasix 40mEq BID Oral medications: Digoxin 0.25mg daily, vitamin supplement
RM 601B	Mr. Jamisen, 69, admitted this AM Diagnosis: coronary artery disease Surgery at 10 AM: triple bypass—will go to ICU following surgery Preop checklist and client teaching has been completed Preop meds on call to OR IV medications IV #1 1000mL D5/.2NS at 75mL/hr
RM 602A	Mrs. Jones, 59, admitted 2 days ago Diagnosis: cholelithiasis Surgery 2 days ago: Laparoscopic cholecystectomy Ambulate ad lib, self-care Oral medications for pain IV discontinued at 8 AM To be discharged today with discharge teaching
RM 602B	Not occupied
RM 603A	Mrs. Henderson, 38, admitted yesterday Diagnosis: metastatic cancer to the brain CAT scan scheduled for 12 noon IV #2 1000mL D5W with 20 mEq KCL at 50mL/hr Assist with ADLs Vital signs and neuro checks q 4 hrs, I&O Oral medications for pain
RM 603B	Miss Johnson, 70, admitted 3 days ago Diagnosis: pancreatic cancer with metastasis to the lungs Chair TID, and ambulate to bathroom Vital signs q 4 hrs Spirometry q 4 hrs with RT Deep breathing and coughing exercises q 4 hrs Nasotracheal suction PRN IV #5 1000mL D5W at 50 mL/hr PCA pump for pain medication Chemotherapy IV daily
RM 604A	Mr. Scott, 64, admitted this AM Diagnosis: benign prostatic hypertrophy Surgery for TURP at 1 PM—to return to the nursing unit Needs preop teaching and a surgical checklist completed
RM 604B	Mr. Jackson, 37, admitted last night Diagnosis: torn ACL Surgery this AM at 7:30—will return to unit by 10:30 AM CPM ordered postop

RM 605A	Mrs. Price, 89, admitted 1 week ago Diagnosis: terminal heart failure, semi-comatose Complete ADLs, keep comfortable, turn q 2 hrs Vital signs q 8 hrs, I&O Foley catheter to drainage IV #8 D5/.45 NS with 40mEq KCL at KO rate
RM 605B	Not occupied
RM 606A	Mrs. Fellipe, 28, admitted last evening Diagnosis: gastroenteritis for past 4 days Ambulate to bathroom, chair as tolerated Independent in ADLs Vital signs q 4 hrs, NPO, I&O IV #3 1000mL NS with 40mEq KCL at 125mL/hr
RM 606B	Mrs. Blake, 48, admitted yesterday Diagnosis: sickle cell crisis Bed rest until pain subsides Vital signs q 4 hrs, I&O, diet as tolerated Oral medications: folic acid, nonsteroidal antiinflammatory drug Narcotic analgesic medication for pain IV #3 1000mL D5/.2NS with 40mEq KCL at 125mL/hr

- Determine the appropriate staff assignment for this client roster. What information do you need to complete this assignment?
- How would you as team leader make client assignments for each individual staff member?
- How do the theory of delegation and the facility/state policies of delegation impact on your assignment?
- What additional factors would you need to consider in making these assignments?

Scenario 2

You are assigned to provide nursing care for Mr. Fred Smith, 39 years of age. He is admitted to the hospital for severe dehydration due to the effects of chemotherapy. On your initial rounds at 7:30 AM, you find him sleeping. His respirations are labored and stertorous. His color is ashen, eyes sunken, and skin dry. At 8 AM you enter the room and find him awake. He complains of being very thirsty and wants a glass of water. He cannot tolerate oral fluids and is receiving IV fluids with KCl added because of his nausea and vomiting on admission the day before. After taking his vital signs (T: 100.6; P: 100; R: 32) you give him his bath and make his bed. You notice he has reddened areas over his coccyx and on his elbows and heels, each area about the size of a quarter. His skin is dry and peeling. Drainage from his Foley catheter is a dark amber color with a very strong odor. You measure the urine at 8 AM. The total is 75 mL. The last output was measured at 6 AM.

- How would you chart the information obtained from the simulated situation? What would be appropriate forms to use?
- What assessment information (that you just charted) would require nursing interventions?
- If you were assigning this client to a team member, who would be most appropriate—RN, LVN/LPN, or CNA?

Scenario 3

As a new student, you are going into the hospital to prepare for the clinical experience tomorrow morning. There are two stages of preparation. The first stage is obtaining all the necessary information you will need to provide safe care. The second stage is reviewing your textbooks and lecture notes to gain an understanding of the client's diagnosis, medications, lab values, and diagnostic tests that will be done during his/her hospitalization.

- If you have only a limited time to review the client's chart, what sections of the chart will provide you with sufficient information to render you safe to care for the client?
- In preparing for clinical practice, what information is essential to review in addition to the data you have obtained from the clinical record? Where is the most appropriate place to find this information?
- List the priority interventions you will carry out within the first hour of the clinical experience. Explain the rationale for your answers.

NCLEX® Review Questions

Unless otherwise specified, choose only one (1) answer.

1. Charting is an important nursing activity. The following is a list of functions that client charting fulfills.

   Select all those that apply.

   1. Communicates information to members of the health team.
   2. Is a legal document.
   3. Reminds nurse of the treatments to be performed for the client.
   4. Assists supervisors to evaluate staff performance.
   5. Provides a permanent client record.
   6. Protects both client and nurse in terms of quality and continuity of health care.

2. Hospitals are rapidly adopting electronic charting programs that have many advantages. One of the disadvantages of using this system is it

   1. Allows nurse to document more client details quickly.

2. Encourages nurses to rely on the computer data without questioning the information.
3. Gives the nurse more time to spend on client care.
4. Offers instant test results and information.

3. The nurse finishes documenting a client's chart and notices that the information has been written in the wrong chart. The next action is to
   1. Notify the team leader to correct it.
   2. Completely cross out the writing so it is not visible.
   3. Line out the entry with a single line, write "mistaken entry" above it, and initial the entry.
   4. Draw a red line through the incorrect entry, write "wrong entry" and initial.

4. When completing an unusual occurrence (incident report), it is necessary to record
   1. Major details of the incident.
   2. Only the actual nursing interventions made.
   3. All of the details of the incident.
   4. General details with focus on client's reactions.

5. Your hospital has implemented the use of standard clinical pathways as the major type of documentation. One of the advantages of this type of documentation is
   1. It allows for individual plans of care.
   2. There is continuity of care among all healthcare workers.
   3. It includes history, assessment, and risk factors.
   4. It allows for complex clients to receive specialized care.

6. A bedridden Islamic client asks the nurse to bring a basin of water every morning and evening. The unit is understaffed and extremely busy. You will resolve this issue by
   1. Explaining to the client that you are too busy to bring him water today.
   2. Bringing him the water regardless of the busy schedule.
   3. Asking an unlicensed helper to explain the situation to him.
   4. Telling him that you will try to do it, but it may be late.

7. When planning client care assignments in team nursing, the action that could lead to instability and inadequate care is
   1. Changing assignments frequently.
   2. Considering the job description of the team members.
   3. Considering the geographical location of the clients.
   4. Considering the acuity level of the clients.

8. Which of the following actions will help a nurse manager to increase leadership skills through the process of delegation?
   1. Close supervision, thereby not allowing any errors.
   2. Clearly making all decisions about how a task is to be completed.
   3. Delegating responsibility in such a way that the worker is capable of handling responsibility.
   4. Delegating those tasks that are distasteful to the nurse manager.

9. Witnessing a client sign a surgical consent form implies that the nurse
   1. Saw the client sign the consent form.
   2. Knows the client understands the proposed procedure.
   3. Believes the client to be competent.
   4. Believes the client is able to tolerate the procedure.

10. Delegation is an important nursing function. Of the following statements, which one is incorrect?
    1. RNs decide which tasks to delegate.
    2. RNs must supervise outcomes for all delegated tasks,
    3. All nursing tasks may be delegated if an RN takes responsibility.
    4. RNs must know the legal scope of practice of other licensed providers.

4

Communication and Nurse–Client Relationship

LEARNING OBJECTIVES

1. Define the term *communication*.
2. Explain why communication is an important concept in nursing.
3. Describe what is meant by the term *confidentiality*.
4. Discuss four factors that affect communication.
5. List five examples of therapeutic communication.
6. List five examples of blocks to communication.
7. Explain why multicultural health care is important and discuss the term *cultural diversity*.
8. List three components of a cultural sensitivity assessment.
9. List two questions that would elicit information about the client's spiritual issues.
10. Demonstrate the steps for beginning a client interaction.
11. Explain why it is therapeutic to encourage the client to express feelings and thoughts.
12. Describe the phases of a nurse–client relationship.
13. List three components for maintaining a nurse–client relationship.
14. Describe the rationale for discussing termination at the beginning of the relationship.
15. Practice assisting a client to communicate with his/her physician.
16. List at least three cues you would observe if a client were depressed, anxious, or angry.
17. Discuss two interventions you would make if one of your assigned clients was depressed, anxious, or angry.

CHAPTER OUTLINE

TERMINOLOGY

Acceptance favorable reception; basic acknowledgment.

Agitation excessive restlessness and increased mental and especially physical activity.

Anxiety a state of uneasiness and distress; diffuse apprehension.

Apprehension a fearful or uneasy anticipation of the future; dread.

Assistance aiding, helping, or giving support.

Attitude a state of mind or feeling with regard to some matter; disposition.

Behavior the actions or reactions of persons under specified circumstances.

Clarify to make clear or easier to understand.

Cliché stereotyped response; a trite or overused expression or idea.

Cognition the mental process or faculty by which knowledge is acquired.

Communication the exchange of thoughts, information, or messages.

Confusion disorder; jumble; distraction; bewilderment.

Congruence agreement; conformity.

Consent to agree; to be of the same mind.

Convey to communicate or make known; to impart.

Coping mechanism a means by which to adjust or adapt to disequilibrium; defense mechanism against anxiety.

Counseling to give support or to provide guidance.

Cultural diversity differences among people with respect to their values, beliefs, language, customs, and general patterns of behavior.

Cultural sensitivity being aware of and accepting diversity among people.

Depression a mental state characterized by dejection, lack of hope, and absence of cheerfulness.

Emotion any strong feeling, as of joy, hate, sorrow, love.

Empathy ability to readily comprehend the feelings, thoughts, and motives of another person.

Esteem to consider as of a certain value; regard; respect.

Ethnocentrism belief in the superiority of one's own ethnic group.

Evaluate to examine and judge; appraise.

Expression to manifest or communicate; make known.

Feedback the return of information to the place of origin.

"Hand-Off" Communication *See* SBAR definition.

Helping relationship an interaction of individuals that sets the climate for movement of the participants toward common goals.

HIPAA Health Insurance Portability and Accountability Act, enacted into law in 1996 to improve Medicare and Medicaid programs and efficiency of healthcare system.

Maladaptive inability to, or faulty adjustment or adaptation.

Multicultural health care a consideration of client's varying cultures (including beliefs, values, customs, traditions, language, etc.) when delivering health care.

Noncompliance failure or refusal to go along with a plan or program.

Nonverbal communication aspects of communication that are not content (such as body language or gestures) but still convey meaning.

Overdependence the state of needing or relying on someone or something too much.

Perception the process of receiving and interrupting sensory impressions.

Rapport a feeling of mutual trust experienced by persons in a satisfactory relationship.

Refer to send or direct someone for action or help.

Relationship an interaction of individuals over a period of time.

SBAR a tool that standardizes a "hand-off communication" when one nurse turns a client over to another nurse; situation, background, assessment, and recommendations.

Self-esteem a sense of pride in oneself; self-love.

Social involvement with communities and other persons.

Spiritual assessment assessing a client's religious or spiritual beliefs and values.

Support to lend strength or give assistance to.

Termination the end of something; a limit or boundary; conclusion or cessation.

Therapeutic having medicinal or healing properties; a healing agent.

Understanding to perceive and comprehend the nature and significance of; to know.

Validate to substantiate or verify.

Verbal communication the words, content, or information conveyed in the message.

COMMUNICATION

Communication is the process of sending and receiving messages by means of symbols, words, signs, gestures, or other actions. It is a multilevel process consisting of the content, or information, part of the message and the part that defines the meaning of the message. Messages sent and received define the relationship between people. From the point of view of a learned skill, communication is intended to accomplish a defined goal. It is the transmission of facts, feelings, and meaning through the communication process.

The communication process forms one of the primary bases for administering all skills. Without clear communication, the nurse cannot assess, administer, or evaluate his or her actions in performing the skill. The principles of therapeutic communication also form a basis for interviewing and counseling skills.

Communication is a vital element in nursing. Everything that occurs within the nurse–client interaction involves some form or mode of communication, whether it includes listening to an upset family member, assisting a client in health teaching, or performing a nursing procedure. Without communication, the nurse could not give nursing care.

The communication process includes both verbal and nonverbal expressions and is affected by the intrapersonal framework of the person, the relationship between the participants, and the purpose of the sender. The content of the message and the context also influence the communication process. The manner in which the message is sent and the effect on the receiver also play a role in the eventual outcome of the communication process. As you can see, the communication process can be very complex. As a beginning practitioner, however, the most important factor to remember is that *what* you say and *how* you say it have a very great influence on your client.

One of the most important skills you must master is to be able to talk therapeutically to clients and to be able to listen to them. Nurse–client communication is an intimate process of providing nursing care. In fact, the initial step in the nursing process—assessment—comprises observation, interview, and examination. The interview involves talking and listening to the client. Initially, it may be difficult for you to concentrate on both talking and listening, since you have not yet mastered the basic skills, such as a bed bath or taking vital signs. As you gain experience, however, these skills will become more familiar and you can focus on the communication-interaction process with the client.

Confidentiality (Client's Right to Privacy)

Clients are protected by law (invasion of privacy) against unauthorized release of personal clinical data such as symptoms, diagnoses, and treatments. Confidential information may be released with the consent of the client. Information release is mandatory when ordered by the court or when a state statute requires reporting child abuse, communicable diseases, or other specific incidents.

Nurses, as well as other healthcare providers and their employers, may be held personally liable for invasion of privacy (as well as other torts) should litigation arise from the unauthorized release of client information. Nurses have a legal and ethical responsibility to become familiar with their employers' policies and procedures, as well as the new aspects of HIPAA, regarding production of client information.

Health Insurance Portability and Accountability Act (HIPAA)

This act, enacted into law in 1996 and phased in gradually, requires the Secretary of Health and Human Services to devise certain standards. This act improves the efficiency and effectiveness of Medicare and Medicaid programs, ensures continuing healthcare insurance if the client has had existing group insurance, and ensures the privacy of individual health information. One of the most important components of HIPAA is the privacy rule, which became effective in April 2003.

This act requires healthcare providers to protect clients against unauthorized disclosures of personal medical information. HIPAA requires client consent for any information dispersed to others. It states that clients must receive written notice of privacy practices and their rights. Clients may access personal medical records more freely than previously.

Guidelines That Influence Effective Communication

- A person cannot *not* communicate. This idea is basic to communication. We have an inherent need to communicate, whether it be verbal or nonverbal. Even silence is a form of communication.
- There is a content, or informational, value to messages sent and received that explains what the message is about and expresses how the sender regards the receiver.
- The message sent is not necessarily the meaning received.
- Messages contain overt and covert meanings. The sender is aware of the overt, or direct, meaning and may or may not be aware of the hidden, or covert, meaning.
- Communication becomes dysfunctional when a person does not assume responsibility for his or her communication. Dysfunctional communications result from failing to learn to communicate properly and leaving the responsibility for communicating to others.

Learning to talk with clients and listening to them is the beginning of a nurse–client relationship. Some of you come to nursing with many of these basic communication skills already mastered. Others experience shyness, hesitancy, and awkwardness in relating to clients. Try to keep in mind that you are being educated to be a professional person—a nurse—and as such you have a great deal to give to your clients. They will learn to respect your skill, value your presence, and depend on you when they are ill. One of the most rewarding aspects to nursing is experiencing a communication between you and your client. If you do feel shy or hesitant, remember that communication skills can be learned. Begin by practicing or role-playing with your classmates until you feel comfortable in the initial phases of a relationship.

All communication between nurse and client should be therapeutic, whether it involves obtaining information for an assessment, interacting with the client during a bed bath, or doing client teaching. The difference between therapeutic communication and a therapeutic relationship is that a relationship has a beginning, middle, and end with specified goals for each phase. Therapeutic communication techniques should be used in all forms of communication.

Guidelines for Communicating With Clients

In establishing nurse–client communication, some basic guidelines should be remembered.

- Accept the client as a valued and worthwhile individual, for this acceptance is a prerequisite for a nurse–client relationship.
- Be aware of the total client, not just his or her physical needs. The client's social, emotional, and spiritual needs are also important.
- Understand your own needs, feelings, and reactions so that they do not interfere with the therapeutic process with the client.
- Be prepared to feel some degree of emotional involvement with your client, evidencing caring and concern for his or her welfare. At the same time, however, it is necessary to maintain objectivity.
- Remember that the nurse–client interaction is a professional one. As such, you as the nurse possess the skills, abilities, and resources to relieve the other person's pain and discomfort, and your client seeks comfort and assistance for alleviation of some existing problem.
- A nurse–client relationship does not require a long-term agreement or formal meetings between nurse and client to be effective. You may still meet the objectives of such a relationship in a short clinical experience.
- Take an active role and guide the conversation if the client is overly hesitant. For example, "I'm here to listen to any concerns you might have, Mr. Smith. You were mentioning having trouble understanding. …"
- Give broad opening statements and ask open-ended questions to help the client describe what is happening to him or her. Pick up cues and follow through with the subject that the client introduces to provide continuity.
- Use body language to convey empathy, interest, and encouragement to facilitate communication.
- Use silence as a therapeutic tool, as it allows the client to pace and direct his or her own communications. Long periods of silence, however, may increase the client's anxiety level, so use this technique wisely.

New Trends in Communication

Text messaging nurse to nurse or nurse to physician allows the person receiving the text to instantly learn the critical nature of the text. For example, texting "please review these critical lab values," or "please call back STAT referencing client X." This service enables a nurse to use only a name and web browser to locate the person who is receiving the text rather than taking time to look up a phone or pager number. A problem with this system is that the nurse must document separately that a message was sent so that it goes into the client's record.

A growing service called "pagerbox" is a Web site launched at Johns Hopkins University that allows a person to page a colleague using only the name and web browser and then confirm the page has been sent via a computer that is available. This system may well be adopted by other hospitals because it is so easy to use. (For more information, visit www.pagerbox.com.)

The Joint Commission Safety Goal 2: Improve Effectiveness of Caregiver Communication

The National Patient Safety Goals identified in 2003 by The Joint Commission (formerly JCAHO) are updated every year. One important safety goal targets good communication because poor communication between caregivers can cause errors and risk client safety. The Joint Commission, to improve the effectiveness of this goal, has identified four requirements that apply to nurses:

1. "Read back" or take three steps to verify a verbal telephone order or if the nurse is notified of a critical test result. In these situations, the nurse should write down the information, enter it into the computer, read it back to the person with whom the nurse is speaking, and then confirm what was read back.
2. Develop a list of abbreviations, acronyms, symbols, or dose designations that cannot be used in the facility because they are often misread or confused. (See list on page XX.)
3. Critical test results must be reported immediately. These are test results that are abnormal and for client safety may require an immediate intervention.
4. "Hand-off" communication means that a nurse must pass off crucial information about a client—status, their condition, recent changes, or ongoing treatment—to the next clinical caregiver. A tool available that standardizes hand-off is the SBAR technique. This is a technique that covers situation, background, assessment, and recommendations for the client that is being handed off.

"Hand-Off" Communication

"Hand-off" communication is a system or process that includes all relevant (especially critical elements) information about a client when one member of a healthcare team is "handing off" a client to another member. Using this technique increases client safety and implements a continuum of care.

SBAR is particularly important when you are handing off a client between preoperative and intraoperative areas. The transition of care must summarize critical client data, and SBAR provides a framework to accomplish this goal. Further, TJC's universal protocol is now included in the 2009 Hospital National Patient Safety Goals, which state that there must be three aspects of this protocol:

- Active communication among all members of the surgical team.
- Involvement of the client or the client's legal representative.
- Requirement for site marking and prevention of the wrong site, wrong procedure, and wrong person.

SBAR

The SBAR mnemonic communication technique is a standardized, focused method of communicating essential client information when members of the health team are transitioning from one member or team to another. This technique consists of four parts.

1. Situation—Identify yourself and the client and state the primary problem.
2. Background—Give the background of the client and be ready to answer any questions the other care provider may have.
3. Assessment—Give the essential assessment parameters of the client's current state (for example, BP, P, R).
4. Recommendations—Make suggestions for continued care of the client in a priority framework.

Adhering to this format when one nurse is handing off a client to another caregiver will help to minimize safety risks for the client as well as assist the new health team members to give the best care possible. This method also provides a framework that directs a focus on a critical situation, if present, so that an immediate intervention may be made.

Source: Amato-Vealey, E. J., Barba, M. P., & Vealey, R. J. (2008, November). Hand-off communication: A requisite for perioperative patient safety. *AORN Journal*, 88(5), 763–770.

THERAPEUTIC COMMUNICATION TECHNIQUES

Communication includes the totality of the human person and reflects what is happening within and outside of us. Body sensations, thoughts, feelings, emotions, ideas, perceptions, judgments, previous experiences, and memories are all part of how and what we communicate. Effective, functional communication only occurs when what is happening within is congruent with what we share with the outside. It is important to be a therapeutic as well as a functional communicator and not to disturb the communication process by using nontherapeutic techniques or blocks to communication.

Therapeutic communication techniques assist the flow of communication and always focus on the client. Nontherapeutic communication techniques block or hinder communication and generally focus on the nurse and meet the nurse's needs. The major therapeutic and nontherapeutic techniques are listed below.

Acknowledgment Acknowledging the client without inserting your own values or judgments. Acknowledgment may be simple and with or without understanding, verbal or nonverbal.

EVIDENCE-BASED PRACTICE

Results of the Harvard Medical Practice study revealed that poor communication is the most frequently cited cause of sentinel or adverse events. Using the SBAR technique will reduce errors and increase client safety.

Source: Brennan, T. A., Leape, L. L., Laird, N. M., Hebert, L., Localio, A. R., Lawthers, A. G., . . . Hiatt, H. H. (2004). Incidence of adverse events and negligence in hospitalized patients: Results of the Harvard Medical Practice Study I. 1991. *Quality & Safety in Health Care*, 13(2), 145–151.

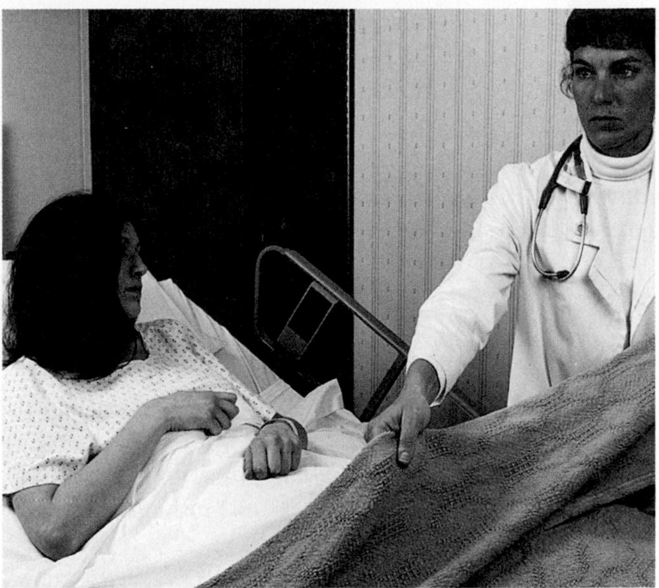

▲ Therapeutic communication implies the nurse is focusing on the client. Here we see an example of nontherapeutic communication.

Example: In the response "I hear what you're saying," the nurse acknowledges a statement without agreeing with it.

Example: "Yes, go on." "Uh huh."

Clarification Clarifying the client's message. Check out or make clear either the intent or hidden meaning of the message, or determine if the message sent was the message received.

Example: "I don't understand. Can you say it in a different way?"

Example: "Are you saying ..." (Repeat meaning of client's message as understood by you.)

Feedback Using feedback to relay to the client the effect of his or her words. This method helps keep the client on course or alters the course. It involves acknowledging, validating, clarifying, extending, and altering.

Example: "You changed the bag on your colostomy very well."

Example: "When you say that, it makes me feel uncomfortable." (If the client is making personal comments about the nurse.)

Focus Focusing or refocusing on the client's statement. Pick up on central topics or "cues" given by the client.

Example: "You were telling me how hard it is to talk to your doctor."

Example: "You said the Doppler test tomorrow is frightening."

Incomplete Sentences Encouraging the client to continue.

Example: "Then your life is . . ."

Listening Consciously receiving the client's message.

Example: Listening eagerly, actively, responsively, and seriously.

Minimum Verbal Activity Keeping your own verbalization minimal and letting the client lead the conversation.

Example: "You feel . . . ?" "Go on."

Mutual Fit or Congruence Creating harmony of verbal and nonverbal messages.

Example: A client is crying, and the nurse says, "I'll sit with you awhile," and puts his or her hand on the client's shoulder.

Example: A client tells the nurse he or she feels fine, but the client's body language indicates that he or she is in pain. "You say you feel fine, but you look like you are in pain."

Nonverbal Encouragement Using body language to communicate interest, attention, understanding, support, caring, and listening to promote data gathering.

Example: The nurse nods appropriately as the client talks.

Example: The nurse leans forward.

Open-Ended Questions Asking questions that cannot be answered with a simple "yes" or "no" or "maybe." Generally ask questions requiring an answer of several words to broaden conversational opportunities and to help the client communicate.

Example: "How is your PCA working?" rather than "Is the pain gone?"

Reflection Identifying and sending back a message acknowledging the feeling or repeating the last few words the client said. (Conveys acceptance and great understanding.)

Example: ". . . distrust your diagnosis?"

Restatement Repeating the client's statement as encouragement for him or her to continue.

Example: "You said that you can't bear to look at your stoma."

Validation Verifying the accuracy of the sender's message.

Example: "Yes, it is confusing when so many staff are in the room."

BLOCKS TO COMMUNICATION

Changing the Subject Introducing new topics inappropriately, a pattern that may indicate anxiety.

Example: The client is crying and discussing his or her fear of surgery when the nurse asks, "How many children do you have?"

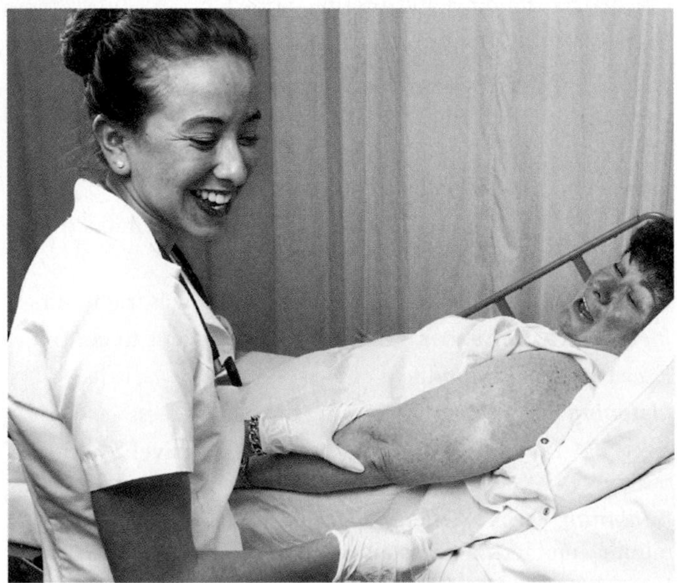

▲ Within the interpersonal framework, nurses share part of who they are with the client.

False Reassurance Using clichés, pat answers, "cheery" words, advice, and "comforting" statements in an attempt to reassure the client. Most of what is called "reassurance" is really false reassurance.

Example: "It's going to be all right."

Example: "Don't worry. This pain medication always works."

Giving Advice Telling the client what to do. Giving your opinion or making decisions for the client implies he or she cannot handle his or her own life decisions and that you are accepting responsibility for him or her.

Example: "If I were you. . . ."

Example: "You should try some alternative treatments."

Incongruence Sending verbal and nonverbal messages that contradict one another; two or more messages, sent via different levels, seriously contradicting one another. The contradiction may be between the verbal/nonverbal content or time/space content.

Example: "I'd like to talk to you" (but I'm just too busy), said while nurse is turning away from the client.

Assumptions Making an assumption about the meaning of someone else's behavior that is not validated by the other person.

Example: The nurse finds the suicidal patient smiling and tells the staff he's in a cheerful mood and much better.

Invalidation Ignoring or denying another person's presence, thoughts, or feelings.

Example: Client: "Hi, how are you?" Nurse: "I can't talk now, I'm on my way to lunch."

Overloading Talking rapidly, changing subjects, and giving more information than can be absorbed at one time.

Example: "I see you're 48 years old and were admitted yesterday. Have you had a physical assessment? Where do you come from?"

Social Response Responding in a way that focuses attention on the nurse instead of the client.

Example: "This sunshine is good for my roses. I have a beautiful rose garden."

Underloading Remaining silent and unresponsive, not picking up cues, and failing to give feedback.

Example: Nurse asking, "I hope your pain is better" as he or she smiles and walks away.

Value Judgments Giving one's own opinion, moralizing, or implying one's own values by using words such as *nice*, *good*, *bad*, *right*, *wrong*, *should*, and *ought*.

Example: "I think he's a very good doctor."

Example: "I think it's good that you decided to have the blood transfusion."

MULTICULTURAL HEALTH CARE

As we move into the 21st century, there are demographic shifts occurring that will change the direction of health care. The last census showed that over 29% of the population is comprised of people of color, and 12% are of Hispanic or

Spanish origin. The total foreign-born population in 2000 was over 20 million, or over 12% of the total population, and 14 million Americans did not speak English. This trend can be expected to increase as the new census statistics are tallied. In fact, those groups that were minority may now be classified as majority.

Because of this change in the United States population demographics, there are emerging barriers to health care for many groups of people. Perhaps the greatest barrier is language, and since communication is an essential component of providing nursing care, it is important to consider language under the topic of communication. Other barriers may be living in urban, poor neighborhoods; poor prevention practices such as poor nutrition; and beliefs that affect how certain cultural groups understand illness and respond to treatment. Perhaps the greatest barrier for many ethnic groups is poverty. Those in the lower socioeconomic group have reduced access to health care, including health insurance, availability and location of health facilities, transportation, and so on.

Cultural Awareness

It is important for nurses to understand the impact of various cultures on healthcare practices if they are to become culturally competent. As more and more people immigrate to this country, nurses will be faced with cultural diversity problems in administering health care. Cultural diversity implies the range of differences in values, beliefs, customs, folklore, traditions, language, and patterns of behavior for the various cultural groups. For example, people from different cultures define personal space differently. Some may prefer closer personal contact, while others are offended by a person moving into their personal space. The nurse needs to be aware that personal space is related to culture, gender, and group behavior. Because all of these aspects potentially affect how an individual experiences, copes with, and responds to illness, nurses must be aware of these cultural differences.

Cultural Sensitivity

Nurses must become sensitive to people from cultures other than their own if they are to meet the needs of their clients. People from different cultures may have different beliefs and values about illness and treatment and different health practices and patterns of behavior. In order to treat the client holistically, the nurse should be aware of these differences and be able to incorporate them into the individual client's plan of care. For example, if a client is Native American and this person believes in and values shamanic healers, the nurse could formulate a plan that includes a healer visiting the client. This addition to the care plan could occur without interfering with the Western approach, in which the primary provider would be a physician.

Diversity in Health Care

Diversity is a key to delivering competent and safe nursing care because U.S. population projections beyond 2007 show that Hispanics, Asian Americans, and African Americans will outnumber whites. These diverse cultural groups will present all healthcare workers with a challenge: a challenge to make appropriate ethical decisions based on the unique cultural values, beliefs, and practices of each group.

Diversity awareness can be viewed in three parts: how people are different, recognizing the unique needs of others, and sensitivity (recognizing personal biases) so that they do not interfere with giving professional and safe nursing care.

Cultural Assessment

When completing a total assessment on a client, the individual cultural components that are important to include are:

- Cultural background and orientation
- Communication patterns (based on culture)
- Nutritional practices
- Family relationships
- Beliefs and perceptions relating to health, illness, and treatment modalities
- Values relating to health practices
- Education
- Issues affecting the delivery of health care

Spiritual Assessment

When you are completing a total client assessment, it is important to include a spiritual assessment. This need not be invasive or intrusive. The purpose of such an assessment is to open the channels of communication so that the client will feel comfortable in discussing spiritual issues. If the client experiences no opening from the nurse, he or she may conclude that the nurse does not wish to discuss spirituality; therefore, just asking a few pertinent questions during a general assessment may accomplish the goal of opening communication.

RELATIONSHIP THERAPY

Nurses are given the unique opportunity to share part of who they are with others who have asked directly or indirectly for assistance. It is within this interpersonal framework that the nurse–client relationship begins to develop and take on its individual characteristics.

Both individuals bring into the relationship their thoughts, feelings, sense of self or self-worth, behavior patterns, abilities to adapt and cope, belief systems, and points of view about life and how they interact with it. Within all these complex variables, there is a commonly shared point at which the nurse–client relationship begins.

This relationship may be defined as the interaction between the nurse and a client with shared therapeutic goals and objectives. Characteristics of the relationship include acceptance, honesty, understanding, and empathy of the nurse

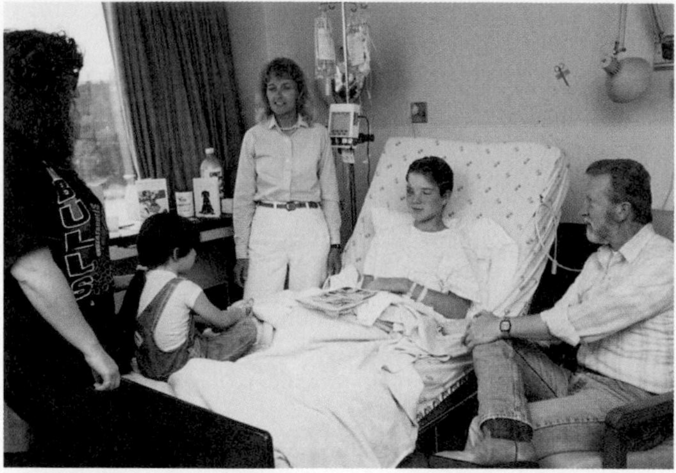

▲ Relationship therapy includes bringing the family together to discuss client care needs.

toward the client who is willingly or unwillingly seeking help. Generally, it is important for the nurse to view the client as a unique individual who is responsible for his or her own feelings, actions, and behaviors and who is an active participant in a healthcare program. The relationship is more effective if the client shows a willingness to accept responsibility and actively participates in the therapeutic relationship. This is not always possible, and the nurse must begin the relationship by accepting the level at which the client is able to participate. This, at times, is a difficult and frustrating process. The goal of relationship therapy is to assist the client to identify and meet his or her own needs. The nurse may assist the client in reaching the goals by demonstrating acceptance so that the client may experience the feeling of being accepted as an individual; by developing mutual trust through consistent, congruent nursing behaviors; by providing corrective emotional experiences to increase self-esteem; and finally by creating a safe, supportive environment. Some degree of emotional involvement and honest, open communication is essential throughout the relationship. The nurse must encourage the client to express his or her feelings, concerns, expectations, fears, and the like within safe limits.

Relationship Principles

Principles underlying a helping relationship include:

- Awareness of the total client, including emotional, physical, cultural, and spiritual needs.
- Some degree of emotional involvement while maintaining objectivity.
- The setting of appropriate limits and consistency in behavior while caring for the client.
- Open, honest, clear communication.
- Encouragement of the expression of feelings.
- Focus on "here and now."

Dangers to the relationship include overemotional involvment and judgmental attitudes on the part of the nurse and the staff.

Phases in Nurse–Client Relationship Therapy

There are three phases in a traditional nurse–client relationship.

Initiation, or Orientation, Phase In the initial interaction with the client, you introduce yourself and establish the boundaries of the relationship. It is also the phase in which you identify problems, expectations, and relevant issues (cultural and spiritual) that need to be addressed during the relationship. It is at this stage in the relationship that you would identify any impairments, such as hearing, speaking, developmental, or psychological, that must be taken into account so that adjustments in the relationship may be made.

Continuation, or Active Working, Phase This is the phase in which you would develop a working relationship, and in conjunction with meeting the client's needs, begin resolving the client's problems: for example, working with the client to handle his pain; teaching the client to care for a new device, such as a colostomy; or implementing a plan to increase the client's independent functioning.

Termination Phase At this final phase, when the client is soon to be discharged; you would follow the plan that you began when the client was admitted: for example, anticipate problems the client will face when he goes home; complete discharge planning and teaching; deal with client's fears about being on his own after leaving the hospital.

CULTURAL AWARENESS

One way to become culturally competent is to learn the language that a majority of your clients speak—this will give you insight into the culture and help you recognize individual cultural impediments to the client's receiving health care.

Source: Gaskill, M. (2002, May 6). Just say the words. *NurseWeek:* Santa Clara, CA.

Reference for Hispanics Because Hispanics are now the largest minority group in the United States, nurses should be aware of references that help to facilitate communication with this group. One such reference is *Procedures of Critical Care* by Judith Ann Lewis, Spanish edition. Physical examination is one topic covered in this text. Using this book will assist the nurse to help the client understand the procedures and treatments he or she receives while hospitalized.

Source: Kleinpell, R. M., Vazquez, M. G., Gailani, K. (2000, April). Translating Spanish: A brief guide for intensive care and acute care nurses. *Critical Care Nurse,* 20(2), 100–104.

TABLE 4-1 Religious Diversity Considerations for Client Care

Religious Orientation	Baptism	Death Rituals	Health Crisis	Diet
Adventist	Opposed to infant baptism	No last rites	Communion or baptism may be desirable	No alcohol, coffee, tea, or any narcotic
Baptist	Opposed to infant baptism	Clergy supports and counsels	Some believe in healing and laying on of hands. Some sects resist medical help	Condemn alcohol. Some do not allow coffee and tea
Islam	No baptism	Prescribed procedures by family for washing body and shrouding after death	No faith healing Ritual washing after prayers every day	Prohibit alcohol and pork
Buddhist	Rites are given after child is mature	Send for Buddhist priest Last rite chanting	Family should request priest to be notified	Alcohol and drugs discouraged; some are vegetarian
Christian Scientist	No baptism	No last rites No autopsy	Deny the existence of health crises Many refuse all medical help, blood transfusions, or drugs	Alcohol, coffee, and tobacco viewed as drugs and not allowed
Episcopalian	Infant baptism mandatory	Last rites not essential for all members	Medical treatment acceptable	Some do not eat meat on Fridays
Jehovah's Witness	No infant baptism	No last rites	Opposed to blood transfusions	Do not eat anything to which blood has been added
Judaism	No baptism but ritual circumcision on eighth day after birth	Ritual washing of body of death	All ill people seek medical care Treatment supersedes dietary restrictions	Orthodox observe kosher dietary laws, which prohibit pork, shellfish, and the eating of meat and milk products at the same time
Methodist	Baptism encouraged	No last rites	Medical treatment acceptable	No restrictions
Mormon	Baptism eight years or older	Baptism for the dead can be done by proxy	Do not prohibit medical treatment, although they believe in divine healing	Do not allow alcohol, caffeine, tobacco, tea, and coffee
Roman Catholic	Infant baptism mandatory	Last rites required	Sacrament of the sick	Most ill people are exempt from fasting

Note: There may exist circumstances that require a court order to supervene religious practices (e.g., a blood transfusion to save the life of a child).

NURSING DIAGNOSES

The following nursing diagnoses may be appropriate to include in a client care plan when the components are related to establishing and maintaining a nurse–client relationship.

NURSING DIAGNOSIS	RELATED FACTORS
Impaired Communication Verbal	Psychologic barrier, inability to speak dominant language, impaired cognitive function, lack of privacy
Powerlessness	Perceived lack of control resulting in dissatisfaction
Impaired Social Interaction	Lack of motivation, anxiety, depression, lack of self-esteem, disorganized thinking, delusions, hallucinations
Social Isolation	Hospitalization, terminal illness
Disturbed Thought Processess	Depression, anxiety, fear of unknown, emotional trauma, unclear communication, negative response from others

CLEANSE HANDS The single most important nursing action to decrease the incidence of hospital-based infections is hand hygiene. Remember to wash your hands or use antibacterial gel before and after each and every client contact.

IDENTIFY CLIENT Before every procedure, introduce yourself and check two forms of client identification, not including room number. These actions prevent errors and conform to TJC standards.

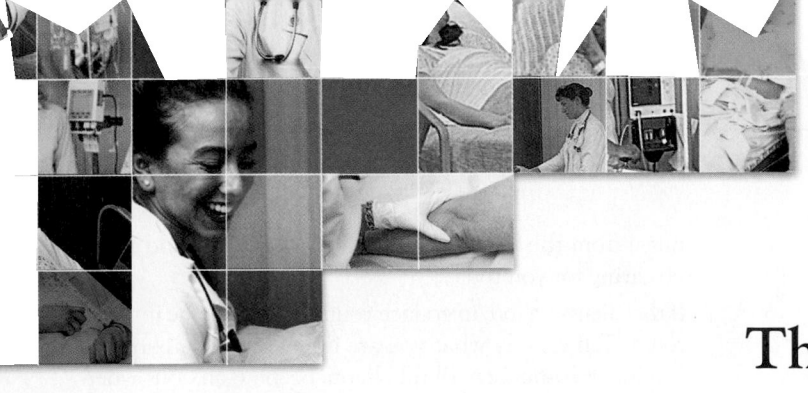

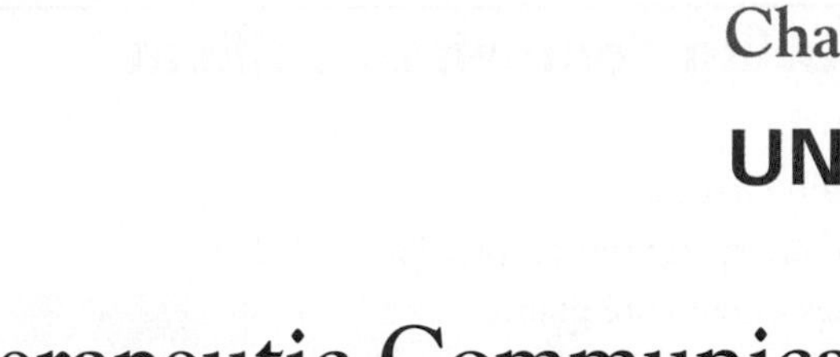

Chapter 4

UNIT 1

Therapeutic Communication

Nursing Process Data

ASSESSMENT Data Base

- Determine client's ability to process information at the cognitive level.
- Assess mental status data to establish baseline for intervention.
- Assess client's ability to communicate on a verbal level.
- Observe what is happening with the client here and now.
- Identify client's developmental level so interaction expectations will be realistic.
- Assess client's anxiety level because anxiety interferes with communication.
- Assess client's cultural background.
- Teaching Clients to Communicate With Their Physicians
- Assessing Cultural Preferences
- Assessing Spiritual Issues
- Assisting a Client to Describe Personal Experiences
- Encouraging a Client to Express Needs, Feelings, and Thoughts
- Using Communication to Increase a Client's Sense of Self-Worth

PLANNING Objectives

- To assist client to meet his or her own needs
- To assist client to experience the feeling of being accepted
- To increase client's self-esteem
- To provide a supportive environment for change
- To institute therapeutic rather than casual or non–goal-oriented communication
- To affect or influence the client's physical, emotional, and social environment
- To be sensitive to client's cultural orientation

IMPLEMENTATION Procedures

EVALUATION Expected Outcomes

- Client develops the ability to assess and meet his or her own needs.
- Communication becomes clearer, more explicit, and centered on problem areas.
- A supportive environment is created so that the client can reduce the level of anxiety and experience change.
- Cultural diversity is accepted by the healthcare team.
- Cultural preferences and spiritual issues are addressed.
- Clients are able to communicate effectively with their physicians.

Pearson Nursing Student Resources

Find additional review materials at **nursing.pearsonhighered.com**

Prepare for success with NCLEX®-style practice questions and Skill Checklists

Introducing Yourself to a Client

Procedure

1. Obtain client assignment.
2. Read chart and review physician's orders.
3. Check client care plan.
4. Clarify any questions about client assignment.
5. Proceed to client's room and check client ID.
6. Introduce yourself to the client. (Example: "Good morning, Mr. Jones. My name is Miss Barnes. I am a student nurse from the Bellington School of Nursing, and I will be caring for you today.")
7. If the client is blind, introduce yourself as you come into the room: Tell exactly what you are doing and when you are leaving. ▸ ***Rationale:*** Blind clients become anxious when they hear someone enter the room who does not speak.
8. Begin to establish a nurse–client relationship using clear, open communication.

Beginning a Client Interaction

Procedure

1. Following introduction (at which time you call the client by name and tell the client your name), relate purpose of interaction.
2. Tell client specifically what you will be doing in terms of his or her care.
3. Ask if the client understands or has any questions.
4. Encourage client to describe how he or she is feeling at the time (especially focusing on the pain level).
5. Encourage client to participate in his or her care—both verbally and nonverbally.
6. Pay attention to communication as well as the procedure you are administering. ▸ ***Rationale:*** Often, your best data base is drawn from observation.
7. Assess nonverbal behavior and determine if it fits (is congruent) with verbal communication, especially when you are evaluating pain level.
8. Complete communication by asking client for feedback.

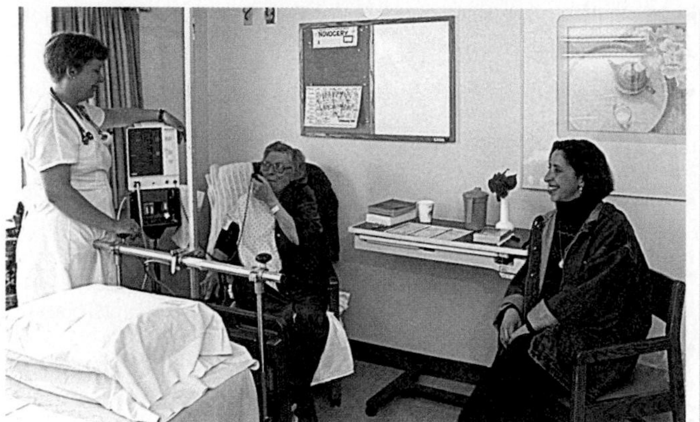

▲ When interacting with a client, the nurse includes friends as an important element in client's support system.

9. Complete interaction by telling client when you will return.
10. Follow through on agreed-upon meeting time to build client trust.

Teaching Clients to Communicate With Their Physicians

Procedure

1. Practice with client how to formulate and verbalize direct (vs. indirect) questions.
2. Role-play with client how to extract the specific information they wish to receive from the physician. ▸ ***Rationale:*** Receiving the information will increase client satisfaction and lower anxiety.
3. Verify directly (clarify) the information the client receives from the physician. ▸ ***Rationale:*** This will decrease client's anger and anxiety.
4. Assist client to ask about functional status of the disease and symptoms. ▸ ***Rationale:*** Increases client's sense of control over their condition.
5. Assist client to ask the physician purpose and expected outcomes of treatments. ▸ ***Rationale:*** Increases adherence and compliance to treatment.

Beginning in 2006, The Joint Commission requires hospitals to document client's language and communication needs in the medical record. The Joint Commission is implementing this because research shows that differences in language and culture can have a major impact on quality and safety in client care.

EVIDENCE-BASED PRACTICE

Teaching Clients to Communicate With Physicians

This study reviewed communication training interventions for 1,665 clients to determine the effectiveness of teaching clients how to communicate with doctors. The results indicated that clients who received this training asked more questions, had a significant increase in direct (vs. indirect) questions to the physician, and received more information. The author's conclusions were that training clients to communicate with their doctors showed improvements in a variety of outcomes.

Source: Cegala, D. J., Miser, W. F. (2002). The other half of the whole: Teaching patients to communicate with physicians. *Family Medicine, 34*(15), 344–352.

Assessing Cultural Preferences

Procedure

1. Review client history related to cultural orientation to determine if adequate information pertaining to cultural preferences is included. ▸ ***Rationale:*** A complete history will detail cultural diversity patterns.
   a. Ethnic heritage and language.
   b. Family organization and role of members.
   c. Dietary practices and knowledge about nutrition.
   d. Education, formal and informal.
   e. Healthcare practices and beliefs.
2. Introduce self to client and identify client.
3. Determine client's perception of illness based on cultural beliefs.
4. Validate verbal and nonverbal communication from client based on cultural understanding. ▸ ***Rationale:*** When the client's cultural background is different from the nurse's, communication problems may result.
5. Consider using an interpreter if communication seems unclear. ▸ ***Rationale:*** An interpreter will facilitate communication and reduce stress on the client.
6. Examine expectations of health care based on the client's cultural influences. ▸ ***Rationale:*** Health care should be congruent with the client's expectations or a positive outcome of treatment may be in jeopardy.

Assessing Spiritual Issues

Procedure

1. Ask the client relevant questions concerning spiritual issues. ▸ ***Rationale:*** If the nurse never opens this subject, the client will not feel free to discuss spiritual issues.
   a. Do you have a spiritual component in your life?
   b. If so, how will this help you during your illness?
   c. Is there any particular person or spiritual advisor that you would like me to contact for you?
   d. Is there anything that I (as your nurse) can do to support your spiritual beliefs?
2. "Are there any spiritual issues that you would like to discuss? If so, let's arrange a time to talk about these issues." ▸ ***Rationale:*** This approach will open communication and notify the client that you are willing to discuss these issues.

Communicating With the Hearing Impaired

If your client is hearing impaired, it is very important to establish a method of communication (pen and pencil, sign language, speaking loudly and clearly). Other factors to take into consideration when communicating with the hearing impaired are to pay attention to the client's nonverbal cues, decrease background noise such as television, and always face the client when speaking. It is also important to check with the family regarding how they communicate with the client. Finally, it may be necessary to contact the appropriate department resource person for this type of disability.

Assisting a Client to Describe Personal Experiences

Procedure

1. Encourage client to describe his or her perceptions and feelings.
2. Focus on communication as well as body reactions.
3. Don't dominate the conversation. ▸ ***Rationale:*** The less you say, the more you encourage spontaneity and verbalization from the client.
4. Assist client to clarify feelings.
5. Maintain an accepting, nonjudgmental attitude. ▸ ***Rationale:*** Making value judgments, even nonverbal ones, negatively affects the nurse–client relationship.
6. Give broad opening statements, and ask open-ended questions. ▸ ***Rationale:*** This open approach enables the client to describe what is happening.

Encouraging a Client to Express Needs, Feelings, and Thoughts

Procedure

1. Focus on feelings rather than superficial topics during interactions.
2. Assist client to identify thoughts and feelings.
3. Pick up on verbal cues, leads, and signals from the client.
4. Convey attitude of acceptance and empathy toward the client. ▸ ***Rationale:*** Being aware of your own feelings and attitudes and separating them from the client's contributes to acceptance.
5. Note what is said as well as what is not said.
6. Assist the client to become aware of differences between behavior, feelings, and thoughts.
7. Give honest, nonjudgmental feedback to the client.

Using Communication to Increase a Client's Sense of Self-Worth

Procedure

1. Use body language as well as verbal communication to convey empathy. ▸ ***Rationale:*** Sitting down at the client's bedside or not acting as if you are in a hurry encourages communication.
2. Respect the client's need for emotional privacy, but be available to the client.
3. Encourage the client to apply the problem-solving approach to different situations.
4. Be nonjudgmental (see example of making judgmental responses).
5. Mutually identify goals to meet the client's individual needs.
6. Keep all agreements with the client.
7. Become the client's advocate.
8. Give the client positive feedback when appropriate.

DOCUMENTATION for Therapeutic Communication

- Identification of client needs
- Explicit goals of interaction
- Communication patterns of client
- Emotional state of client
- Expressed feelings and thoughts if relevant
- Cultural issues if relevant
- Spiritual issues if relevant

TABLE 4-2 Communication Deficits and Interventions

Deficit	Intervention
Language/Culture	Determine client's level of fluency in English and understanding
	Use an interpreter or translator
	Pay attention to nonverbal communication
	Learn client's cultural values
	Be aware of client's cultural preferences that may affect etiquette (personal space, use of touch, eye contact)
	Avoid jargon or slang—select words you use carefully
Sensory—Hearing, Seeing	Speak slowly, clearly, and directly to the client; do not use a loud voice
	Use gestures to clarify or drawings to illustrate
	Describe carefully the care you are giving to the client
	Provide alternate means of communication: writing pad, gestures, etc.
	Work out a code with client for answers to basic questions; for example, "Are you in pain? For yes, blink once."

TABLE 4-2 Communication Deficits and Interventions (Continued)

Deficit	Intervention
Cognitive	Orient to reality frequently (day, year, etc.) Use the same staff as much as possible Introduce self repeatedly, explain simply aspects of care Speak in clear, simple sentences
Verbal Communication	Speak directly to clients and treat them with dignity and respect even if they are nonverbal Ask specific questions that require a yes or no, not an open-ended question Recognize a client's facial expressions as well as their gestures If a client's behavior changes drastically, look for an acute illness, such as an infection Try flash cards or a chalkboard for a response Use nonverbal techniques yourself, such as touch Include client in the conversation even though there is no response

Legal Considerations

A neonate receiving an IV in his right foot showed discoloration and edema at the injection site. The infiltration was noted on a transfer sheet as the baby was being transferred to another unit. It was not noted in the medical record. When the parents questioned the injury, they were told that it was just a "blister." In time, the infiltration led to scarring and loss of motion. The nurse who originally noted the infiltration was sued.

This is an example of poor or inadequate communication when "handing-off" a client.

CRITICAL THINKING Application

Expected Outcomes

- Client develops the ability to assess and meet his or her own needs.
- Communication becomes clearer, more explicit, and centered on problem areas.
- A supportive environment is created so that the client can reduce the level of anxiety and experience change.
- Cultural diversity is accepted by the healthcare team.
- Cultural preferences and spiritual issues are addressed.
- Clients are able to communicate effectively with their physicians.

Unexpected Outcomes	Alternative Actions
Therapeutic communication is not achieved.	• Eliminate blocks to communication from interaction style. If a block does occur, recognize it. Move to correct communication by using therapeutic modes of communication. • Evaluate your own process of communication during and after interaction. • If client needs to verbalize and you cannot help him or her do so, contact another nurse or the social worker.
Client's demanding behavior interferes with the therapeutic communication process.	• Do not ignore demands; they will only increase in intensity. • Attempt to determine causal factors of behavior, such as high anxiety level. • Set limits to response patterns when client is demanding. Control own feelings of anger and irritation. • Teach alternative means to getting needs met.
Cultural preferences/issues were not recognized, so communication was hindered.	• Complete a cultural assessment before revising a plan of care. • Bring in a translator to converse with the client to establish baseline communication. • Evaluate values, beliefs, preferences, and expectations related to health care.
Spiritual issues were not discussed until the client asked for a priest or minister.	• At this time, assess the client's spiritual beliefs and ask if there is any way you can assist him/her in this area.
Client remains uncomfortable in talking to physician.	• Continue to work with client by role-playing with nurse taking role of physician. • Be present when client is questioning physician and give support.

Chapter 4

UNIT 2

Nurse–Client Relationship

Nursing Process Data

ASSESSMENT Data Base

- Determine the purpose of establishing a nurse–client relationship.
- Consider the overall condition of client to determine if he or she can benefit from a nurse–client relationship.
  - A specific relationship could feed into secondary gains of attention.
  - An individual with chronic organic brain disorder cannot benefit from a relationship per se.
- Identify client expectations of a therapeutic relationship to determine if you can meet these needs.
- Examine your own feelings and expectations to evaluate potential effect on such a relationship.

PLANNING Objectives

- To provide an environment in which client can feel secure enough to alter behavior patterns
- To allow a client to experience a positive, satisfying relationship
- To enable client to test more adaptive ways to handle anxiety
- To provide a climate conducive to raising the client's self-esteem
- To allocate enough time to complete planned process of interaction
- To terminate relationship successfully

IMPLEMENTATION Procedures

EVALUATION Expected Outcomes

- Principles of therapeutic communication are used.
- Boundaries of professional relationship are maintained.
- The appropriate environment for interaction is established.
- Termination of the relationship is completed successfully.

Initiating a Nurse–Client Relationship

Procedure

1. Read client's chart and be familiar with history, medications, etc.
2. Identify client with at least one form of client ID.
3. Perform hand hygiene.
4. Approach client and introduce self.
5. Assess client's symptoms and problems, and communicate a willingness to help alleviate these discomforts.
6. Establish a beginning relationship. ▶ ***Rationale:*** Open, honest, congruent communication and consistent behavior help lay the groundwork for trust in a relationship.
7. Establish mutual goals as a basis for the relationship. ▶ ***Rationale:*** Goals mutually set and agreed on are more easily accepted by both parties in the relationship.
8. Be consistent in your behavior; do what you say you will do, and only make promises you are willing to keep. ▶ ***Rationale:*** The most important element is the beginning of trust. Without trust the nurse–client relationship is ineffective.
9. Encourage client's participation in his or her care. ▶ ***Rationale:*** This focus enhances compliance to treatment.
10. Approach client in a warm, accepting manner during interactions. ▶ ***Rationale:*** The client may interpret a cool, aloof manner as lack of interest.

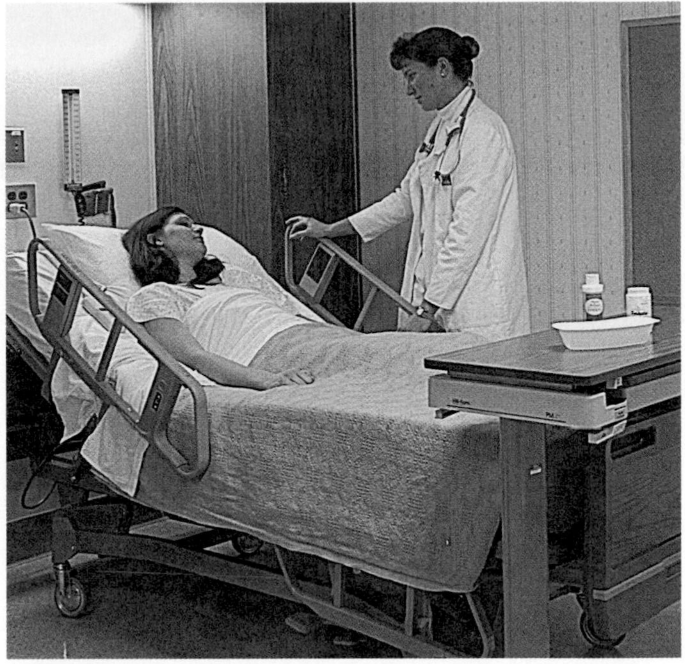

▲ Initiating a relationship is an important component of client care.

Facilitating a Nurse–Client Relationship

Procedure

1. Assume the role of facilitator in the relationship.
2. Accept client as having value and worth as an individual. ▶ ***Rationale:*** Basic acceptance is a fundamental prerequisite of a relationship.
3. Provide a safe environment conducive to client's willingness to share.
4. Maintain the relationship on a professional level. ▶ ***Rationale:*** Responding on a professional rather than a social level defines the relationship.
5. Keep interaction reality-oriented, that is, in the here and now. ▶ ***Rationale:*** Discussion of past or future experiences does not contribute to a change in behavior now.
6. Listen actively; that is, respond to the client's cues.
7. Use nonverbal communication to support and encourage client.
   a. Recognize meaning and purpose of nonverbal communication, especially in assessing pain.
   b. Keep verbal and nonverbal communication congruent.
8. Focus content and direction of conversation on client's cues, not on social or superficial topics.
9. Interact on client's intellectual, developmental, and emotional level.

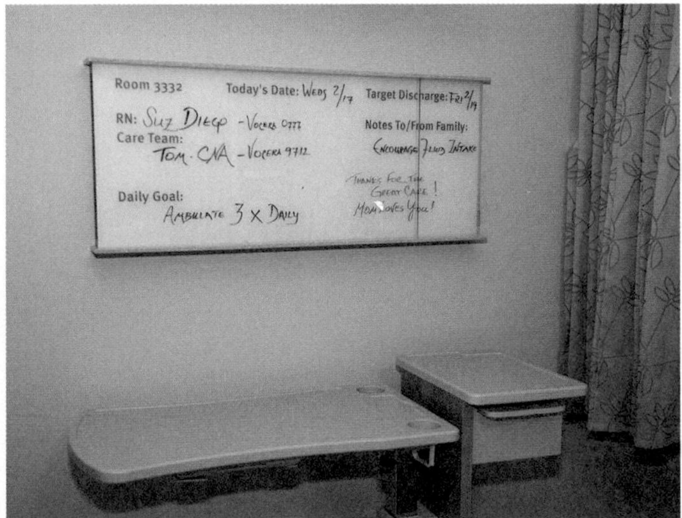

▲ Communication to and from the client can be verbal as well as written.

10. Focus on "how," "what," "when," "where," and "who" rather than "why." ▶ ***Rationale:*** Asking "why" places the client on the defensive because it requires justification of behavior.

11. Teach client problem solving to correct maladaptive patterns.
12. Assist client to identify, express, and cope with feelings.
13. Help client develop alternative coping mechanisms that are more adaptive.
14. Recognize a high level of anxiety, and assist client to deal with it.

Terminating a Nurse–Client Relationship

Procedure

1. Work closely with the client in discharge planning and in planning the termination of the relationship from its beginning. ▶ ***Rationale:*** This approach promotes the client's independence and increases his or her sense of self-esteem.
2. Anticipate problems of termination and plan for their resolution. • *Rationale:* Saying goodbye is often uncomfortable and difficult for both the client and the nurse.
3. Be aware that the client's behavior may reflect fear that he or she can't cope at home, overdependence, depression, and withdrawal. ▶ ***Rationale:*** Allowing this behavior to be expressed helps the client to work it through.
4. Do not terminate the relationship too abruptly or allow it to persist beyond the client's needs.
5. Complete a satisfactory termination of the relationship. ▶ ***Rationale:*** This enables the client to move on.

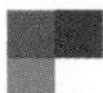

DOCUMENTATION for Nurse–Client Relationship

- Primary goals of nurse–client relationship and identified client needs
- Ongoing process of relationship therapy, including client's expressed feelings, thoughts, and so forth
- Client's behavior and changes in behavior, both positive and negative
- Cues to other team members on how best to relate to this particular client
- Elements of discharge planning

CRITICAL THINKING Application

Expected Outcomes

- Principles of therapeutic communication are used.
- Boundaries of professional relationship are maintained.
- The appropriate environment for interaction is established.
- Termination of the relationship is completed successfully.

Unexpected Outcomes	Alternative Actions
Client refuses to participate in a nurse–client relationship.	• Comply with client's request, and do not force or impose relationship therapy. • Continue to offer relationship therapy at intervals. • Suggest that another team member attempt to establish a relationship.
Nurse–client relationship frequently degenerates into a social conversation.	• Reevaluate the goals for the relationship, and remind client of terms originally established. • Set firm limits, and continually reexamine progress.
Termination of the nurse–client relationship is not successful.	• Reexamine the process of termination (termination should begin at the beginning of the relationship). • Devote more interaction time to this aspect of the relationship. • Attempt to elicit feelings about termination from the client as well as examining your own feelings.
Nurse–client relationship cannot be established due to cultural differences.	• Allow the client's behavior to be expressed without making value judgments, and assist the client to discuss his or her feelings. • The nurse may make a special effort to understand the cultural preferences of the client. • Consider finding another nurse to establish the relationship—one with a similar background.

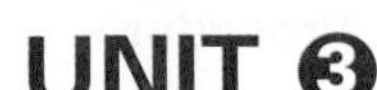

Chapter 4

UNIT ❸

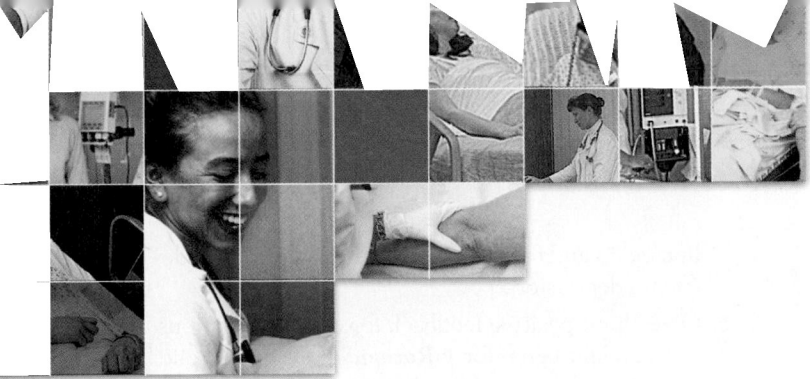

Communication in Special Situations: Depression, Anxiety, Anger, and Denial

Nursing Process Data

ASSESSMENT Data Base

- Observe for behaviors that do not fit expected reactions to illness or hospitalization.

  Depression: *verbal cues* (expressing feelings of sadness, hopelessness, helplessness); *physical cues* (loss of motivation, vegetative, frequent crying episodes, bodily complaints, psychomotor retardation, weight loss); *emotional cues* (low self-esteem, preoccupation with inner thoughts, thoughts of suicide).

  Anxiety: *psychological symptoms* (confusion, dread, agitation, difficulty making decisions, rumination); *physical symptoms* (tremors, dyspnea, palpitations, tachycardia, sweating, sleep disturbance); stages of anxiety (mild, moderate to severe).

  Aggression/anger: *verbal expressions* (voicing anger in loud voice, yelling, cursing); *physically acting out* (clenching fists, throwing objects, refusing treatments, threatening actions).

  Denial: *Verbal expressions* (expressing denial of the client's condition or diagnosis).

PLANNING Objectives

- To recognize client's behavior that fits special situations of depression, anxiety, anger, or denial
- To intervene therapeutically when special circumstances exist
- To provide a supportive climate for the client to work through feelings of depression, anxiety, or anger
- To assist client to develop more adaptive ways of handling feelings

IMPLEMENTATION Procures

EVALUATION Expected Outcomes

- Client's unhealthy responses were recognized and identified, and planned interventions were made.
- Verbal, physical, and emotional cues indicating depression, anxiety, anger, or denial decreased.
- Nurse's therapeutic interventions resulted in more adaptive behaviors. Clients developed new coping mechanisms to handle feelings.

Communicating With a Depressed Client

Procedure

1. Identify cues that client is depressed (see assessment cues).
2. Establish a nurse–client relationship. ▸ ***Rationale:*** A relationship provides the framework for therapeutic intervention.
3. Ask if client is feeling "down," sad, or upset. ▸ ***Rationale:*** The answer will validate nurse's perceptions or behavioral cues.
4. Remain with client, but it is not useful to encourage client to talk at length about feeling depressed; he/she will become even more depressed as conversation progresses. ▸ ***Rationale:*** Depression is best handled by mobilizing client, not talking.
5. Respond to client by suggesting activity, exercise, involvement with another client. ▸ ***Rationale:*** Activity lifts mood and focus outside client's feelings and decreases depression.
6. Give client positive feedback for decisions, actions, and independent behavior. ▸ ***Rationale:*** Depressed clients have difficulty in making decisions.
7. Convey to client you care by spending time talking or participating in activities. ▸ ***Rationale:*** Knowing someone cares helps to lift depression.
8. Focus away from somatic complaints. ▸ ***Rationale:*** Depressed people often focus on somatic problems, but discussing them only increases depression.
9. Assess if client is considering suicide and intervene appropriately.

Communicating With an Anxious Client

Procedure

1. Identify cues that client is anxious (see assessment) and degree of anxiety manifested.
2. Establish nurse–client relationship. ▸ ***Rationale:*** Anxious clients may have difficulty relating to others.
3. Identify anxiety in self and maintain a calm, quiet approach. ▸ ***Rationale:*** Anxiety in the nurse will be transmitted to the client.
4. Assist client to identify anxiety and describe feelings and reactions. ▸ ***Rationale:*** Identifying presence and/or source will help to relieve anxiety.
5. Provide physical outlet for anxiety if possible (i.e., pacing).
6. Remain with anxious client, answering questions, supporting, etc. ▸ ***Rationale:*** This will help to prevent anxiety escalating, especially if client is in critical condition.
7. Provide structured, nonstimulating environment. Give clear, firm directions and information.

Communicating With an Aggressive or Angry Client

Procedure

1. Observe client for cues of anger or aggression getting out of control (see assessment).
2. Intervene immediately when loss of control is imminent.
3. Use a nonthreatening approach to client. ▸ ***Rationale:*** This approach will help to defuse situation.
4. Set firm limits and give specific expectations concerning behavior.
5. Avoid engaging in arguments or provoking client.
6. Calm client so that he/she may regain control.
7. Use problem-solving focus. ▸ ***Rationale:*** Discussion of feelings, examining causal factors and client's response will help to defuse situation.
8. Responses to verbally abusive behavior: do not respond in kind; do not take abuse personally; do not reject client; help client calm down by remaining calm, give feedback concerning your response to comments, and teach alternative ways for client to express feelings.

Communicating With a Client in Denial

Procedure

1. Establish a relationship with the client while determining that the client is using the coping mechanism of denial—that is, denying the diagnosis or condition.
2. Do NOT confront client that he/she is in denial. ▸ ***Rationale:*** This is a protective defense mechanism the client needs at this time.

3. Be aware that denial may be a phase the client will pass through and eventually be able to cope with reality of the condition.
4. Discuss client's condition honestly and the options for treatment. ▸ ***Rationale:*** This focus may enable client to move more rapidly through the denial phase.
5. Offer to spend time with the client and respond to cues that he/she is ready to discuss feelings, but do not force client to confront issues before he/she is ready.

Denial is a defense mechanism whereby the ego protects itself from pain or conflict by denying reality. Elisabeth Kübler-Ross first identified denial as the first stage of the dying process, when the client is stunned at the knowledge, and handles it by denying the reality.

DOCUMENTATION for Communication in Special Situations

- Description of specific cues of client's behavior evidencing depression, anxiety, or anger
- Interventions completed and client's response
- Instructions for other team members on how best to relate to client

CRITICAL THINKING Application

Expected Outcomes

- Client's unhealthy responses were recognized and identified, and planned interventions were made.
- Verbal, physical, and emotional cues indicating depression, anxiety, or anger decreased.
- Nurse's therapeutic interventions resulted in more adaptive behavior.
- Client developed new coping mechanisms to handle feelings.

Unexpected Outcomes	Alternative Actions
Client remains depressed, anxious or angry; interventions do not bring about change in behavior.	• Transfer to another nurse to work with client or request mental health consultant.
Client has thoughts of suicide and is identified as a suicide risk.	• Place client on suicide precautions.
Client remains angry and abusive to staff and others.	• Try to change source of anger or aggressive behavior by identifying source, changing staff, relocating client to another room or private room.

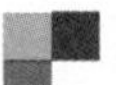

GERONTOLOGIC Considerations

Physical Changes That Affect Communication

- Hearing changes (e.g., presbycusis, tympanic membrane atrophy, and distorted sounds) may make communication difficult. The nurse must speak clearly, loudly, and in view of the client. Use simple sentences and request feedback to validate understanding.
- Visual changes, such as presbyopia, and pupil, cornea, and lens impairment may diminish visualization. The nurse should be aware of eye changes and check that client sees clearly enough to perform required activities.

Psychosocial Changes That Affect Communication

- Relationships change with age. There is a loss of nurturing functions within the family. The nurse may need to perform this function with the elderly.
- Role changes within and outside the family occur—loss of spouse and loss of support systems. Elderly may require more support from caregivers.
- Elderly have fears of physical dependency, chronic illness, and loneliness. Caregiver may need to address these fears and work with client through communication and relationship to reduce them.

MANAGEMENT Guidelines

Each state legislates a Nurse Practice Act for RNs and LVN/LPNs. Healthcare facilities are responsible for establishing and implementing policies and procedures that conform to their state's regulations. Verify the regulations and role parameters for each healthcare worker in your facility.

Delegation

- Evaluation of cultural diversity and spiritual issues should be completed by either the RN or LVN, not by a nursing assistant (NA).
- A full history should be completed by the RN or LVN.
- Care plan objectives relating to communication, spiritual issues, and cultural differences should be completed by the RN or checked by the RN if completed by the LVN.

Communication Matrix

- All staff caring for the client from a different cultural heritage should be informed of special needs of the client based on cultural diversity theory.
- The unit manager should include special needs of the client based on communication patterns and cultural background when making staff assignments. (For example, is there a nurse from the same cultural background or who speaks the same language as the client who can be assigned to that client's care?)
- Assign a nurse who is comfortable dealing with spiritual issues if the initial assessment indicates the client wishes to discuss these issues.

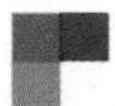

CRITICAL THINKING Strategies

Scenario 1

A 25-year-old male comes to the emergency department. He has a bleeding wound on his arm, and he refuses surgical intervention when told he must remove his clothes and jewelry.

1. What effect would this client response have on the initial nursing plan of care?
2. What is your understanding of this client response? What are some questions you might ask the client?
3. Describe the strategies and goals you would devise to solve this problem.
4. Describe the measures you would implement to resolve this situation.

Scenario 2

A client has just been admitted with a diagnosis of rectal cancer. He is scheduled for surgery the next day. When you are completing an assessment and you ask about spiritual beliefs, the client says, "I'm a washed-out Catholic and I don't think I'm going to live, so what's the sense in talking about it?"

1. What would be the consequence of not responding to the client's comments about spiritual beliefs?
2. How would the goals of establishing a nurse–client relationship and assessing spiritual beliefs overlap in this situation?
3. Describe the actions you would take to engage this client in a discussion about these issues.

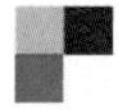

NCLEX® Review Questions

Unless otherwise specified, choose only one (1) answer.

1. Which intervention is most useful when communicating with an aphasic client?
   1. Use correct medical terminology when teaching or explaining.
   2. Ask open-ended questions to obtain information.
   3. Repeat the same word until the client understands.
   4. Provide frequent praise and encouragement.
2. A psychiatric client rapidly improves and is scheduled to be discharged tomorrow. Which of the following responses demonstrates that the nurse has a good understanding of termination of a relationship?
   1. "You have worked really hard the last three weeks. Good-bye and good luck."
   2. "Stop by and let us know how things are going."
   3. "You've done some good work here. I hope you are able follow through with it."
   4. "Good bye and good luck. Hopefully, we won't be seeing you here again."

3. One characteristic of a nurse–client relationship is that it is a professional one. This implies that the nurse
   1. Should be primarily concerned with implementing the policies of the hospital.
   2. Views the client's needs as her/his primary concern.
   3. Maintains a distance between self and client.
   4. Establishes boundaries, formulates goals, and maintains the boundaries of a professional relationship.
4. One day a client with terminal cancer says to the nurse, "Well, I've given up all hope. I know I'm going to die soon." The most therapeutic response is to say
   1. "Now, one should never give up hope. We are finding new cures all the time."
   2. "We should talk about dying."
   3. "You've given up all hope?"
   4. "Your doctor will be here soon. Why don't you talk to him about your feelings?"
5. Which of the following statements would be best to stimulate conversation with a client about his or her social history?
   1. "Are you married?"
   2. "Do you have any children?"
   3. "Tell me about your family."
   4. "Is your role in the family important?"
6. A client is admitted to CCU with a diagnosis of anterior myocardial infarction. Shortly after admission, he states: "I might as well have died because now I won't be able to do anything." The most appropriate response by the nurse is
   1. "Don't worry, everything will turn out all right."
   2. "What do you mean, not able to do anything?"
   3. "Take one day at a time and it will all work out."
   4. "You shouldn't be thinking like this because you are doing well now."
7. A male client is becoming increasingly angry and verbally abusive. The appropriate intervention is to
   1. Send the client back to his room.
   2. Ask the physician for an order for restraints.
   3. Summon assistance from a male staff member.
   4. Set firm limits on the abusive behavior.
8. Which of the following components would you include in a cultural assessment?

   Select all that apply.
   1. Cultural background.
   2. Nutritional practices.
   3. Beliefs and perceptions of health.
   4. Age of the client.
   5. Belief in God.
   6. Communication patterns.
   7. Health practices including alternative.
9. A client you are assigned to care for has impaired hearing. The most effective way to communicate with this client is to
   1. Use a writing pad and gestures.
   2. Speak clearly and slowly.
   3. Use nonverbal communication.
   4. Describe loudly and carefully what you are doing.
10. The highest priority in a nursing intervention when caring for a client who is depressed is to
    1. Form a good nurse–client relationship.
    2. Encourage the client to talk about his feelings of depression.
    3. Suggest that the client do an activity.
    4. Assess the client frequently for potential suicide.

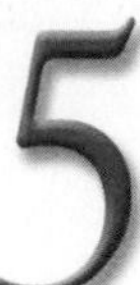

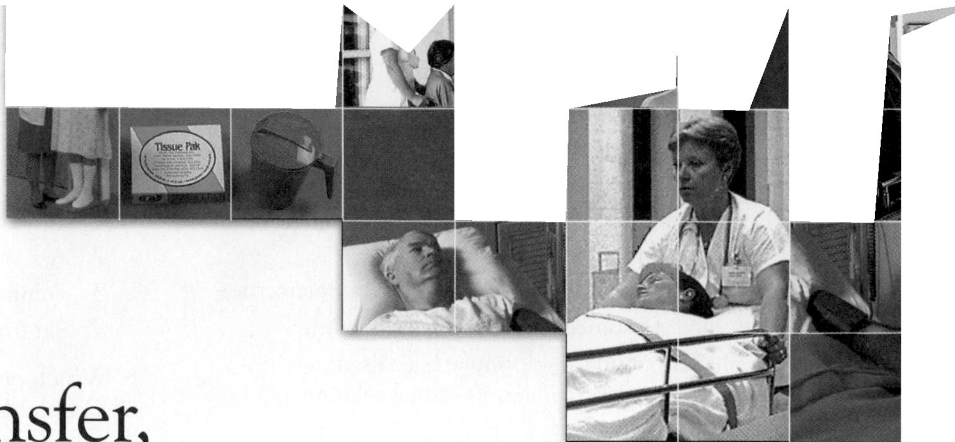

Admission, Transfer, and Discharge

LEARNING OBJECTIVES

1. Explain the steps of admitting a client to the hospital.
2. List client data that are included in documentation when admitting a client to the hospital, including the plan of care, goals, and outcome criteria.
3. Describe the disposition process for safeguarding client's valuables.
4. State what is meant by advance directives.
5. List documents that may be included in the client's admission record (Patient's Bill of Rights, Advance Directives, DNAR, etc.).
6. Propose two solutions for clients who are unable to adapt to the hospital environment.
7. Identify essential "hand-off" information to be communicated when client care is transferred to another caregiver, setting, or home.
8. Describe the process and rationale for medication reconciliation across the continuum of care.
9. Outline steps for transferring a client to another unit within the hospital or to the home.
10. Discuss discharge procedures when a client leaves the hospital.
11. Describe expected outcomes for clients being discharged from the hospital, including meeting criteria in the initial plan of care.
12. Complete discharge documentation including client's achievement of criteria established in the initial plan of care.
13. Describe three solutions for clients leaving the hospital against medical advice.
14. Outline discharge procedures that must be completed when a client leaves the hospital against medical advice.

CHAPTER OUTLINE

TERMINOLOGY

Adaptation ability to adjust to a change in environment.

Admit the process of signing a client into the hospital.

Ambulatory able to walk, or not confined to bed.

Assessment critical evaluation of information; the first step in the nursing process.

Behavior a person's total activity—actions or reactions, especially conduct that can be observed.

Caring thoughtful attentiveness accompanied by responsibility.

Client Care Plan a plan for care of a specific client or one designed especially for one client.

Comfort to ease physically; relieve, as of pain.

Communication transmission of knowledge, information, or messages to another person.

Diagnostic test a test used to determine a diagnosis or to determine the cause and nature of a pathological condition.

Disability a disabled state or condition; incapacity.

Discharge to let go, as in discharging a client from the hospital.

DMEe durable medical equipment.

DRG diagnosis-related group. A system to classify all types of clients to determine how much Medicare pays the hospital, since clients within each category are similar clinically and are expected to use the same level of hospital resources.

Empathy the vicarious experience of another's situation.

Home care assistance nursing care given in the client's home.

Ident-A-Band a band, usually worn on a client's wrist, with the client's name and medical record number.

Limitation the state of being limited or restricted.

Maladaptation inability to adjust to a change in environment.

Potential possible but not yet realized.

Procedure a particular way of accomplishing a desired result.

Reconcile to resolve discrepancies.

Stress a state of agitation that renders the body out of balance.

Supervise to direct or inspect performance; to oversee.

Termination the spatial or temporal end of something; a limit or boundary.

Therapeutic having healing or curative powers.

Transfer to convey or shift from one person or place to another.

Transition the process or an instance of changing from one form, state, activity, or place to another.

Verbalize to express in words (written or spoken).

Volunteer a person who performs or gives his or her services of his or her own free will.

ADMISSION, TRANSFER, AND DISCHARGE

Admission to the hospital can be a positive event if handled with attention and empathy. On the other hand, it can be a negative experience if it is impersonal or mechanized.

Impressions formed by clients during the admission process can affect their attitude toward and ability to adapt to their total hospital experience, so the nurse should consider this an important aspect of client care.

Admission to the Hospital

The process of admitting a client to a healthcare facility varies among institutions, such as nursing homes, clinics, and hospitals. Regardless of the size or type of facility, the admission process assists in the provision of safe, effective care. Because the nurse–client relationship begins with admission, the nurse should have a thorough understanding of the standard admission process for the particular facility.

Clients who present to the emergency department (ED) are stabilized, then discharged, or admitted to the hospital by a general practitioner or specialist who writes, faxes, or telephones admitting orders. In some cases, the nurse calls the admitting physician for these orders.

Admission Protocol

- Advance directives are made available to clients.
- The *Client's Bill of Rights* is presented to each client.
- The admission assessment is completed by a registered nurse within a specified time after admission.
- All clients must be clearly identified by a legible identification band.
- When consent forms are required (for invasive procedures), they must be signed by an adult or guardian who is mentally competent. The adult must give voluntary consent, understand the risks and benefits of the treatment, and have the opportunity to ask questions.

Initial laboratory procedures and x-rays (according to client's DRG admitting diagnosis, surgeon, or anesthesiologist's orders) are usually completed before admission. The client may be provided a copy and/or explanation of an admission plan outlining the client's projected clinical course. Preadmission instructions discourage the client from bringing valuables to the hospital.

If a client enters the hospital in an emergency situation, he or she may feel insecure or fearful because there has been little time to make plans concerning family, travel, finances, or employment. When a client enters the hospital for elective treatment or surgery, both the nurse and client have more time for orientation and preparation for the hospital experience. The initial contact with the nurse leaves a lasting impression, so it should be conducted in an unrushed, organized, and respectful manner.

When the elective client arrives at the hospital, the first contact is usually with the admitting receptionist, who assigns a hospital number and interviews the client. If preadmission forms were mailed to the client, the information is verified by the receptionist at this time; otherwise, the client must answer questions about age, address, financial or insurance status, next of kin, religion, employment, and consent for treatment. If the client cannot answer these questions because of age or condition, a relative usually gives the information. A parent or guardian must do this for a child. At this time, the client receives an identification bracelet or Ident-A-Band. This bracelet includes the client's name, hospital number, and admitting physician's name.

Admission to the Nursing Unit

When admission to the hospital is complete, the client is either directed to the nursing unit or escorted by a volunteer. The client may be met by a staff nurse assigned to admission for that day or by a delegate who will orient the client to the unit and obtain baseline assessment data. Within a specific time, a professional nurse performs a more thorough history and physical assessment, determines a priority of needs, and initiates an individualized plan of care.

The client is informed about telephone use, clergy availability, recreational area and lounge use, mealtimes, visiting hours, and other hospital schedules. Some hospitals have printed booklets describing this information. The client is also familiarized with the immediate environment, including the space for belongings, the bathroom, and operation of the nurse call system inside the bathroom. The nurse also demonstrates operation of the bedside nurse call system, television, radio, and bed controls. The more information the client receives, the more control he or she has over the environment.

Clients are discouraged from bringing items of monetary or sentimental value to the hospital (e.g., money, credit cards, jewelry, photographs, documents). If they are brought, the client may send them home with a family member or friend or place them in the agency vault per security personnel, or the client may retain them, assuming total responsibility and signing a "Release from Responsibility" form. Valuables retained in the agency vault are inventoried and witnessed, and the client is given a receipt. Safeguarded items may be withdrawn from the vault upon presentation of the receipt and completion of the "Request for Release of Valuables" form. Prosthetic devices such as hearing aids, dentures, and glasses are also considered to be valuables, but these are retained by the client.

Upon admission, a comprehensive list of the client's home medications is obtained (prescribed, OTC medications, and supplements), including route, dose, and frequency of use. A list of allergies to foods, drugs, devices, and materials is also obtained. The physician then orders continuation or discontinuation of

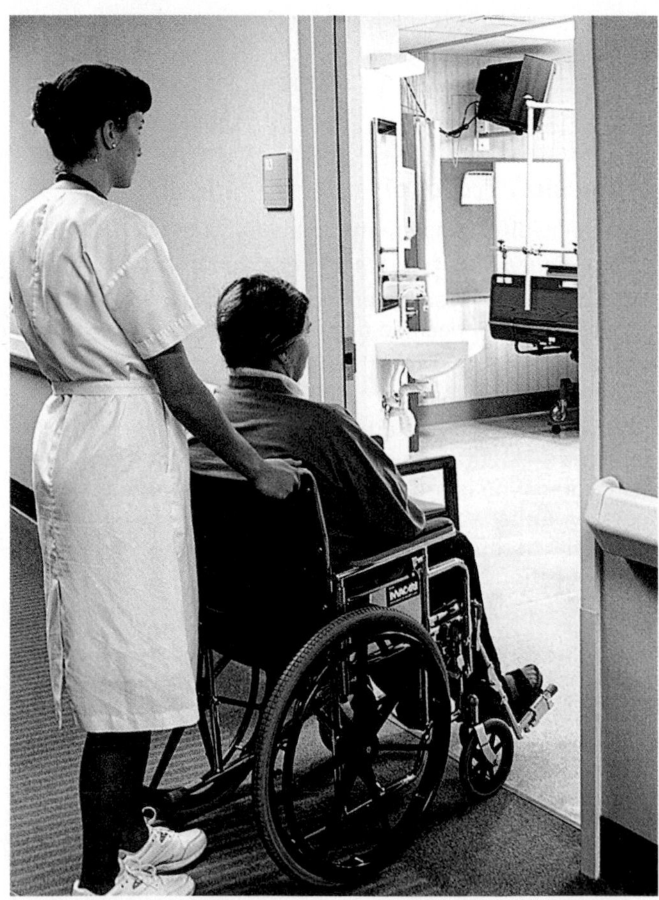

▲ Client may be admitted to the hospital in a wheelchair.

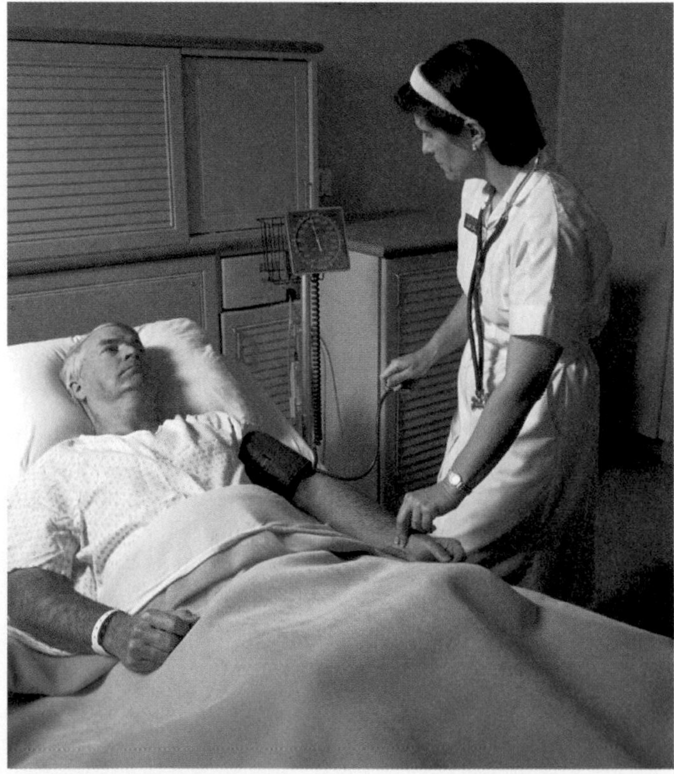

▲ Vital signs are obtained during the admission procedure.

home medications during hospitalization. If the client brings medications or supplements to the hospital, they should be verified by the hospital pharmacist, then placed in the client's medication drawer or sent home (according to agency policy). No medication should be kept at the client's bedside unless there is a specific physician's order that it be placed there.

In some circumstances, upon a physician's order, a client's labeled and pharmacist-verified home medication may be stored in the client's medication drawer and then administered by nursing staff in lieu of a hospital-dispensed preparation. In this case, the medication administration record (MAR) reflects that the client supplies the particular medication and the hospital does not charge for dispensing it.

Because clients may not be sure of their role while in the hospital, many hospitals have adopted versions of the American Hospital Association's *Client's Bill of Rights* (see The Client's Bill of Rights, Chapter 1, page 8). This bill includes the client's rights to obtain information about the client's illness or injury, to refuse medication or treatment, to participate in his or her own care, to know the rationale and risks of the treatment, and to receive courteous care.

The *Patient Self-Determination Act* requires all Medicare and Medicaid recipient hospitals to provide clients with information regarding their rights to reject medical treatment and to complete advance directives. An advance directive is a document the client creates that reflects goals, values, and preferences for health care. A "Living Will" specifies medical treatments the client wants or does not want at the end of life (e.g., feeding tube, mechanical ventilation). Another form of advance directive is the "Durable Power of Attorney," which designates an individual to make decisions for the client when the client is unable to make them for himself or herself. These documents vary from state to state. Copies of advance directives are placed in the client's chart. Additionally, many states mandate that an agency inquire about a client's requests concerning resuscitation. Competent clients who have been informed about their diagnosis and prognosis may be asked to execute a "Do Not Attempt Resuscitation" directive at the time of admission. Following such a request, the physician attaches an order to the client's record, and the order is then reevaluated according to agency policy. (See Chapter 1 for more information about advance directives, living wills, and durable power of attorney.)

Transfer to Another Unit

When a client is admitted through the ED, the nurse must carefully review the ED record for any treatment or diagnostic test the client has received, as these may indicate the need for follow-up assessment or intervention. Similarly, when the client returns from x-ray or other procedures, the nurse considers intervening events (e.g., medications administered) that may influence care decisions. This information, as well as any special instructions for client care, is included on the "hand-off" communication form.

Clients are frequently transferred from one unit to another within the same facility as their condition fluctuates. When a client is moved, all records, charts, medications, MAR, belongings, and personal hygiene and special equipment are transferred with him or her. A complete hand-off report is given to the receiving unit's nursing staff. The new unit's receiving nurse has an obligation to validate all information relayed about the client, to perform an independent client history and physical assessment, and to handle the client's transfer as a "new admission" to the receiving unit. The client also has a right to receive an orientation to the new setting just like that provided in the previous setting. Sometimes clients are transferred within the same unit (e.g., from a semiprivate to a private room or vice versa) for various reasons. While these transfers are readily accomplished within a short time frame, communication about such transactions may be delayed, and confusion about a client's identification or location may result in the client's injury. Always ensure that the client's chart reflects the client's current room number and that all departments participating in the client's care are informed about the client's transfer to a new room number.

A client's transfer to another facility, and sometimes to another unit within the same facility, closes the current hospital record just as if it were a "discharge." A new record is established when the client arrives at the new receiving unit (equivalent to a new hospital admission). In these circumstances, a copy of the client's records may or may not accompany the client; therefore, a thorough report of the client's pretransfer hospital course and current health status must be thoroughly communicated to receiving personnel in order to facilitate continuity of care.

"Hand-Off" Process

Each healthcare facility must define and implement a consistent process by which relevant details about client care are communicated among hospital personnel throughout the continuum of care. This process must allow opportunity for clarifying information in a time frame that is consistent with safe care for the patient

Source: The Joint Commission National Patient Safety Goals. NPSG. 02-05-10 (www.jointcommission.org).

Discharge From the Hospital

From the time of admission, healthcare team conferences help to identify ongoing needs and to make arrangements for the client's reintegration into the community setting. This discharge planning process takes into consideration the physical, emotional, and psychosocial needs of the client, family, and caregiver. Sometimes hospitalization introduces the client to a lifelong need to chronically adapt to declining physical health and to chronically affiliate with the healthcare system. The nurse must be empathetic to the client's response at discharge and approach the client with all possible options for continued care, educational and financial resources, and any other services to assist the client to adapt to a chronic situation. The final responsibilities of the discharge process are to terminate the nurse–client relationship and evaluate the discharge process.

Discharge Against Medical Advice (AMA)

If, for a variety of reasons, a client decides to leave the hospital against medical advice (AMA), it is imperative that the nurse notify the physician, especially if the client is still undergoing diagnosis and ongoing treatment. Most hospitals have AMA protocols that include a mental status evaluation and possible psychiatric consult or detention proceedings.

A competent client, of course, has the right to refuse treatment, but the nurse must still advocate for the client by attempting to determine the reason for the client's decision to leave and explaining that diagnosis and/or treatment have not been completed. An AMA discharge form should be signed by the client and witnessed. This form usually includes follow-up instructions, prescriptions, and documentation that there may be negative consequences of premature discharge.

See Chapter 6 (Client Education and Discharge Planning) for further information on discharging clients to home or another healthcare facility.

ADAPTATION TO HOME CARE

The home healthcare industry has experienced drastically reduced payments and fewer reimbursable visits as a result of the Balanced Budget Act of 1997. Now home healthcare agencies are required to complete data collection information forms. The Outcome and Assessment Information Set (OASIS) was instituted in February 1999, and the newest form, OASIS C, was implemented in January 2010. (See Chapter 6, page 116, for additional information on OASIS C).

The OASIS items were designed to enable systematic measurement of client home healthcare outcomes, with appropriate adjustment for client risk factors affecting those outcomes. The items have specific definitions used to measure changes in client's health status between two or more time points.

OASIS addresses sociodemographic, environmental, support system, health status, functional status, and health service utilization characteristics of the client. Data are collected at the start of care, 60 days after initial care, and at discharge. Additional data are collected if the client has a significant change in condition that requires emergent hospitalization.

In addition to measuring client outcomes, OASIS data have the following uses:

- Client assessment and care planning for individual adult clients
- Agency reports on various client characteristics such as demographic, health, or functional status at the start of care
- Internal Home Health Agency (HHA) performance improvement

The information collected through OASIS is much more comprehensive, particularly in the area of the client's health history.

Legal Issues in Home Care

Home health nurses are at risk for potential legal liability. Nurses work alone in the home care setting and do not have the advantage of calling on a colleague to collaborate on a client situation. This situation leaves the nurse vulnerable to legal risks. Home health nurses must be extremely skilled in handling equipment of all types, as well as performing specialized procedures without the assistance of another nurse. It is critical that these nurses attend workshops, keep abreast of new equipment and procedures, and continue to read nursing journals on a regular basis. If home equipment is not functioning properly, the nurse should inform the client, call the medical equipment provider, fill out an incident report, and not use the equipment.

Home health nurses are also responsible for care provided by unlicensed personnel and LVN/LPNs. It is the responsibility of the nurse to know the competence level of the staff, evaluate their skill level, provide in-service instruction on new equipment or skills, and instruct them only within their specific scope of practice.

It is extremely important to maintain open communication with physicians and professionals in other disciplines providing care to clients in the caseload. Cell phones and e-mail allow for quick response time and improved communication.

Another legal issue is the need for appropriate client documentation that supports the need for home care services. If documentation is not accurate, timely, and complete, the client's reimbursement may be denied. This can lead to hours of time attempting to recover the costs of service, or it could lead to legal repercussions. Maintaining appropriate client records protects the nurse, client, and agency in cases under investigation. Writing legibly, using correct grammar and English, and being succinct and descriptive provide a good legal stance if necessary. Writing notes at the time care is delivered is essential so that information is not forgotten. Many agencies have documentation forms on a computer, so the nurse can enter data as he or she provides care.

The purpose of the unit "Admission to Home Care" in this chapter is to present clinical skills appropriate for the home setting. Many of these skills are exactly the same as those presented in other sections of this book. Some skills require minor change for adaptation to the home environment.

The use of the nursing process is just as important in home care as it is in the hospital. Nursing care plans are required by Medicare regulations and are also used as a justification for skilled nursing services by private insurers. Information regarding admission to home care is presented in the nursing process format to assist in organizing nursing actions and evaluating health care.

Plan of Treatment

A plan of care for home health care based on previous hospitalization admission findings. Centers for Medicare and Medicaid Services (the federal office that administers the Medicare program) requires that all agencies certified to provide home health care to Medicare clients complete the OASIS forms and the home health certification and plan of treatment form (form CMS-485) within 7 days. These forms must be completed on admission to home health care and signed by a physician. The plan of treatment is effective for 60 days. If the client's condition changes, an updated plan must be signed and submitted to the Medicare office every 60 days.

In addition to form CMS-485 and the OASIS forms, the documentation includes the home care agency's admission worksheet, nursing care plan, medication profile, plan of treatment, and consent for admission and service.

Documentation

Charting must follow the nursing care plan and cover the areas listed in the OASIS C docmentation system. OASIS C is an assessment instrument used to collect specific information when a person is receiving Medicaid or Medicare and requires the services of a home health agency. OASIS C is a key component of Medicare's partnership with the home care industry to foster and monitor client outcomes and assist with quality improvement. Oasis C data items include sociodemographic, environmental, support system, health status, and functional status attributes of adult clients. Information gathered in the OASIS C form is forwarded to the state, where it goes to the Centers for Medicare and Medicaid Services. There, the information is used for reimbursement purposes for the specific home health agency. This prospective payment system went into effect in October 2000. Several forms must be completed for each client.

An in-depth assessment identifies areas in which client status differs from optimal health or functional status and is used as the basis of client care planning. Many agencies use standardized care plans and individualize them for each client.

Since interventions are implemented by the client, family, and part-time caregivers, all are involved in the treatment plan. The nurse or the case manager is responsible to coordinate and evaluate the care. The physical therapist can assume the role of case manager when the client is receiving rehabilitation services only.

Because home health aides provide care without direct daily supervision of a nurse, agencies usually hire only experienced nursing assistants (in most states, those who have worked in a hospital or nursing home). Home health aide certification is voluntary in some states and required in others. In many states, the training is completed after nursing assistants have obtained a CNA certificate.

Medicare requires the nurse to make a home visit at least every 14 days to reassess client and family needs and to revise the care plan. One visit each month is to discuss the treatment plan with the family. The nurse also accompanies the home health aide once a month for a supervised visit.

Home health nurses must meet the national standards of care as published by the American Nurses Association. The best preparation for home health nursing continues to be a sound base of nursing skills coupled with a broad knowledge of agency procedures and protocols.

CULTURAL AWARENESS

With the increasing number of clients from culturally diverse backgrounds, it is imperative that nurses be culturally sensitive. Cultural generalizations should only be utilized as a starting point, since differences exist within each culture and among individuals.

Several areas where cultural diversity is common include handshakes, use of eye contact, violation of personal space, facial expressions, and gestures.

The American healthcare system emphasizes medical science and care, informed consent, self-care, advance directives, and risk management. In contrast, clients of other cultures may prefer to rely on faith in God, beliefs, hope, and acceptance of fate as their primary coping mechanisms. A medical interpreter's assistance may be sought to help bridge these two sets of values and to help the client understand the hospitalization experience. The nurse should be aware of different cultural responses to Western protocols (e.g., Chinese-Americans believe the number 4 is unlucky because it sounds like the Chinese word for death; if possible, do not assign 4 as a room number).

Source: Pagana, KD (2009, July). Mind your manners multiculturally. *Nurseweek: Mountain West*, 18–22.

NURSING DIAGNOSES

The following nursing diagnoses may be appropriate to include in a client care plan when the components are related to admission, transfer, and discharge of a client.

NURSING DIAGNOSIS	RELATED FACTORS
Anxiety	Actual or perceived threat to self-concept, threat to biologic integrity, unfamiliar environment and treatments, change in socioeconomic status
Fear	Known or unknown outcome of hospitalization, medical or surgical diagnosis, and treatments
Grieving	Loss of function, change in lifestyle, lack of social support system, change in social role or economic status
Ineffective Health Maintenance	System impairment, surgery, musculoskeletal impairment, visual disorders, external devices
Powerlessness	Actual or perceived lack of control over situation, imposed regimens, lack of privacy
Social Isolation	Hospitalization, chemical dependency, altered appearance

CLEANSE HANDS The single most important nursing action to decrease the incidence of hospital-based infections is hand hygiene. *Remember to wash your hands or use antibacterial gel before and after each and every client contact.*

IDENTIFY CLIENT Before every procedure, introduce yourself and check two forms of client identification, not including room number. These actions prevent errors and conform to The Joint Commission standards.

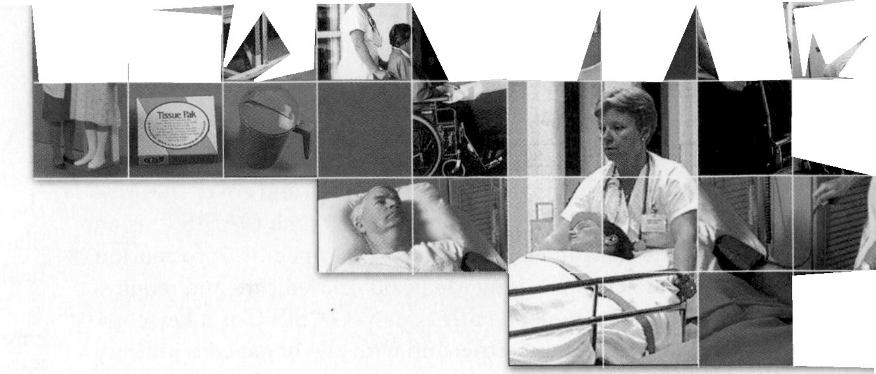

Chapter 5

UNIT ❶

Admission and Transfer

Nursing Process Data

ASSESSMENT Data Base

- Determine client's understanding of reason for hospitalization
- Observe and record client's physical, emotional, and mental status.
- Observe and record client's ability to adapt to the hospital environment.
- Observe for disabilities or limitations.
- Obtain a list of medications client is currently taking (prescribed, OTC, and supplemental), including dose, route, and frequency of use.
- Identify any food, drug, device, or device material allergies.
- Assess the client's level of comfort.
- Assess client for potential discharge needs.
- Assess condition prior to transfer.
- Obtain a thorough "hand off" report of client's progress and status at shift report, when receiving from another unit, or when returning from any test or procedure.

PLANNING Objectives

- To obtain a preliminary nursing history/assessment
- To assist client to adapt to hospital environment with minimal distress
- To encourage the client to participate in his or her own plan of care
- To provide a comfortable and aesthetically pleasing environment for the client
- To provide the client with some control over his or her immediate environment
- To provide the client with an opportunity to verbalize his or her feelings about hospitalization
- To facilitate safe and individualized continuity of care at all transition points throughout the continuum of care.

IMPLEMENTATION Procedures

EVALUATION Expected Outcomes

- Client adapts to hospital environment.
- Client participates in the individualized plan of care.
- Client understands rationale for and accepts transfer to a new care unit.
- Client is transferred to new unit without complication.

Pearson Nursing Student Resources

Find additional review materials at **nursing.pearsonhighered.com**

Prepare for success with NCLEX®-style practice questions and Skill Checklists

Admitting a Client

Equipment

Admission kit with personal hygiene articles (if indicated)
Hospital gown
Thermometer
Blood pressure cuff and stethoscope (or automated unit)
Hospital Nursing History and Assessment form
Client's chart or access to electronic documentation
Labeled containers for client's dentures, etc.

Clinical Alert

The Joint Commission Performance Measurement Initiative requires that all clients admitted with a diagnosis of myocardial infarction, community-acquired pneumonia, or heart failure be assessed for tobacco dependence and that smoking cessation advice/counseling be provided.

Source: www.jointcommission.org

Procedure

1. Refer to client's chart to determine reason for hospitalization and note any orders to be initiated immediately (e.g., oxygen administration). ▶ ***Rationale:*** Timely initiation of tests or treatments reduces hospitalization time and costs.
2. Notify physician of client's admission and obtain orders if not already done.
3. Check client's Ident-A-Band and have client state name and date of birth (according to agency policy).
4. Introduce yourself to the client and begin to establish a therapeutic nurse–client relationship.
5. Orient client to hospital room, various controls, and routines. ▶ ***Rationale:*** Reduces anxiety about hospitalization.
6. Provide labeled container for client's prosthetic items (e.g., dentures).
7. Assist client to don hospital gown.
8. Perform preliminary nursing assessment (may be obtained by a delegate).
9. Obtain client's health history and complete the physical assessment (performed by the professional nurse).
10. Complete score assessments for fall and pressure ulcer risk status.
11. Obtain a complete list of medications client is currently taking (prescribed, OTC, and supplements) including dose, route, and frequency. ▶ ***Rationale:*** The physician reconciles this list by continuing or discontinuing each medication and by ordering new ones.
12. Place allergy and other alert bands on client's wrist if indicated.
13. Initiate client's care plan: Identify individual client's problem areas and needs.
14. Reassess client's level of comfort and ability to adapt to hospitalization.
15. Complete client teaching for all unfamiliar procedures or interventions.
16. Document information on appropriate forms in chart.

Obtaining a Health History

- Past medical history or health problems, including those for which client was not hospitalized
- Signs and symptoms of current problems according to client's perceptions
- Client's knowledge of illness (understanding of present illness) and expectations of care
- Lifestyle patterns: diet, elimination pattern, exercise, habits (i.e., smoking, alcohol intake), sleep patterns
- Relationships and social support systems; emergency contacts
- Values, beliefs, religious or spiritual practices
- History of food, drug, device, or device materials allergies and nature of reaction
- Medications (prescribed and OTC) and supplemental products including dose, route, and frequency used
- Risk analysis for discharge (anticipated needs)
- Special data base for elderly client: level of independence, ability to complete activities of daily living (ADLs), side effects of medications, history of recent loss of loved one, management of chronic conditions

COMMUNITY HOSPITAL

NURSING HISTORY / ASSESSMENT

White areas may be completed by patient / family.
Shaded areas must be completed by nurse / N.A.

CONFIDENTIAL INFORMATION

PATIENT'S NAME

INFORMATION PROVIDED BY
☐ Patient ☐ Family ☐ Friend ☐ Unable to Obtain

DATE OF ADMISSION | TIME OF ADMISSION

ROUTE OF ADMISSION
☐ Ambulatory ☐ Wheelchair ☐ Stretcher

ORIENTATION TO UNIT ☐ Floor Brochure ☐ Channel 50 / 52 ☐ Call Light ☐ Bed Control ☐ Emergency Light ☐ Telephone ☐ Visiting hr ☐ Mealtime

DISBURSEMENT OF VALUABLES ☐ Patient ☐ Home ☐ Security | VALUABLES KEPT BY PATIENT

HEALTH PERCEPTION / HEALTH MANAGEMENT PATTERN

DESCRIBE YOUR USUAL STATE OF HEALTH
☐ Excellent ☐ Good ☐ Fair ☐ Poor

WHY ARE YOU BEING ADMITTED TO THE HOSPITAL?

VITAL SIGNS

STATED WEIGHT Kg.	ACTUAL WEIGHT Kg.	STATED HEIGHT cm	ACTUAL HEIGHT cm
BP	Temp. °C	PULSE	RESPIRATION

ADVANCE DIRECTIVE INFORMATION

Do you have an Advance Directive? (Also may be called a Living Will) ☐ Yes ☐ No
If so, is it on file at this facility. ☐ Yes ☐ No
If not, will you bring / send a copy? ☐ Yes ☐ No
If you do not have an Advance Directive, do you want one? ☐ Yes ☐ No ☐ Not Sure
Do you want help with this? ☐ Yes ☐ No
☐ See Progress Note for additional comments. Date & Time:

Please list any medical problems or previous surgeries below. Include pacemakers, artificial joints, or diabetes.

PROBLEM / SURGERY	DATE

IMMUNIZATIONS ☐ Influenza ☐ Pneumonia

☐ Pacemaker ☐ Artificial Joint ☐ Diabetes

Are you an Organ Donor? ☐ Yes ☐ No
If necessary, would you consent to a blood transfusion? ☐ Yes ☐ No

MEDICATIONS – List medications, including aspirin, laxatives, birth control pills, cough medicines, vitamins, herbal supplements, non-prescriptions, all prescriptions.

NAME	DOSE	FREQUENCY	LAST DOSE

ALLERGIES

NAME (Drug or Other)	DESCRIBE REACTION

Latex Rubber ☐ Yes ☐ No ☐ Unknown
Shellfish ☐ Yes ☐ No ☐ Unknown
X-Ray Dye ☐ Yes ☐ No ☐ Unknown

WHAT DO

DO YOU W ILLNESS, T

WHAT INF

DO YOU U BEEN TOL

IS THERE ☐ No

Interpre

Phone #

DISCHARGE PLANNING NEEDS

COMMUNITY AGENCIES CURRENTLY USED
☐ Home Health ☐ Meals on Wheels ☐ Assistance Program
☐ Other

WHO IS AVAILABLE TO HELP YOU WHEN YOU RETURN HOME?

DO YOU ANTICIPATE ANY PROBLEM CARING FOR YOURSELF WHEN YOU RETURN HOME?
☐ No ☐ Yes Explain:

EMERGENCY CONTACTS

NAME	RELATIONSHIP	TELEPHONE #

Areas within BOLD lines may contain information written elsewhere on th please indicate where the information may be found (Example: "S

1229-1 (1/01)

CONFIDENTIAL INFORMATION

▲ Sample nursing history/assessment form (a).

COMMUNITY HOSPITAL

NURSING HISTORY / ASSESSMENT

White areas may be completed by patient / family.
Shaded areas must be completed by nurse / N.A.

CONFIDENTIAL INFORMATION

ACTIVITY / EXERCISE PATTERN

PHYSICAL LIMITATIONS
Hearing ☐ Yes ☐ No
Sight ☐ Yes ☐ No
Speech ☐ Yes ☐ No
Mobility ☐ Yes ☐ No

FUNCTIONAL ABILITY LEVEL
0 = Self Care
1 = Requires equipment
2 = Requires supervision or assistance
3 = Requires equipment & supervision / assistance
4 = Total care required

___ Feeding ___ Dressing
___ Bathing ___ Bed Mobility
___ Ambulating ___ Toileting

PHYSICAL AIDS

	HOSPITAL	HOME	N/A
Glasses	☐	☐	☐
Contacts	☐	☐	☐
Hearing Aid	☐	☐	☐
Dentures	☐	☐	☐
Partial	☐	☐	☐
Complete	☐	☐	☐
Cane	☐	☐	☐
Walker	☐	☐	☐
Wheelchair	☐	☐	☐
Prosthesis	☐	☐	☐
______	☐	☐	☐
______	☐	☐	☐

GENERAL SAFETY
High Risk for Fall (HRFF)
Any one indicator checked indicates HRFF
History of Falls ☐
Impaired Mobility ☐
Impaired Cognition ☐
Sensory Deficit ☐
Incontinence or Urgency ☐
Age over 75 ☐
Any other reason for which the health card team judges the patient to be at risk ☐

Central Line ☐ Yes ☐ No Type ______ Dialysis Access ______

PAIN MANAGEMENT (Cognitive—Perceptual Pattern)

Have you experienced any discomfort / pain in the past 24 hours? ☐ Yes ☐ No
If yes, how did you treat this pain? ______
Was the treatment of pain / discomfort effective? ☐ Yes ☐ No

ELIMINATION PATTERN

Last Bowel Movement ______
Normal Bowel Pattern ☐ Yes ☐ No
Regular ☐ Yes ☐ No
Laxatives / Enemas ☐ Yes ☐ No
Problems Urinating ☐ Yes ☐ No

ROLE / RELATIONSHIP-SEXUALITY / REPRODUCTIVE PATTERN

Do you have any emotional, family, or home concerns that need to be addressed during this hospitalization? ☐ Yes ☐ No
Possibly pregnant? ☐ Yes ☐ No Last Period ______ Do you feel safe in home? ☐ Yes ☐ No
Comments:

VALUE / BELIEF PATTERN

Do you have any special request with regard to your religious beliefs while you are in the hospital? ☐ Yes ☐ No
Comments:

NUTRITION / METABOLIC PATTERN

Special Diet at Home ☐ Yes ☐ No Specify ______
Food Allergies ☐ Yes ☐ No Specify ______

NUTRITION SCREEN

READ THE QUESTIONS BELOW. CIRCLE THE NUMBER IN THE YES COLUMN FOR THOSE THAT APPLY TO YOU.	NO	YES
Without wanting to, have you lost 10 pounds or more within the last 6 months?	0	1
Do you have a pressure sore or non-healing / infected wound?	0	1
Have you had daily nausea, vomiting, or diarrhea lasting more than 5 days?	0	1
Has your food intake declined within the past 3 months due to chewing / swallowing problems?	0	1
Have you been hospitalized for an illness or a surgery for more than 7 consecutive days within the past 3 months?	0	1

Total the nutritional score (all "yes" answers) and enter in the computer. **At nutrition risk** = any "yes" answer. (Score 1–5) TOTAL:

Do you have any concerns that have not been discussed? ☐ No ☐ Yes Please explain below:

RN SIGNATURE	DATE	TIME

1229-2 (1/01)

CONFIDENTIAL INFORMATION

Sample nursing history assessment form (b). ▶

Transferring a Client

Equipment

Wheelchair or gurney
Covering for client
Client's records, chart MAR, and care plan
Client's valuables receipt
Special equipment (e.g., walker)
Personal belongings

Procedure

1. Verify physician's order if needed. ▸ ***Rationale:*** Physicians order client transfers from and to hospital units. They do not always order transfers within a unit.
2. Contact admitting office to arrange for transfer.
3. Communicate with transfer unit to determine the best time for transferring client.
4. Identify client and inform client of impending transfer. ▸ ***Rationale:*** Discussing the rationale for transfer facilitates adjustment to the new unit.
5. Gather equipment, belongings, and records.
6. Obtain necessary staff assistance for transfer.
7. Transfer client to wheelchair or gurney unless client is remaining in bed for the transfer. Use protective belts and rails as indicated.
8. Cover client to provide warmth and to avoid exposure during transfer.
9. Notify receiving nurse when you arrive on the unit.
10. Introduce client to new staff who will be caring for the client that day.
11. Give complete report to staff, using the client care plan medication reconciliation list, MAR and Kardex. Give information concerning client's current status, individualized care needs (e.g., bed alarm), client problems/alerts, and when next medications or treatments are due. Note any completed or pending test results. If necessary, give phone report to receiving nurse. ▸ ***Rationale:*** Complete "Hand-Off" communication maintains continuity of care after transfer and promotes client safety.
12. Notify physician when client's transfer is completed.

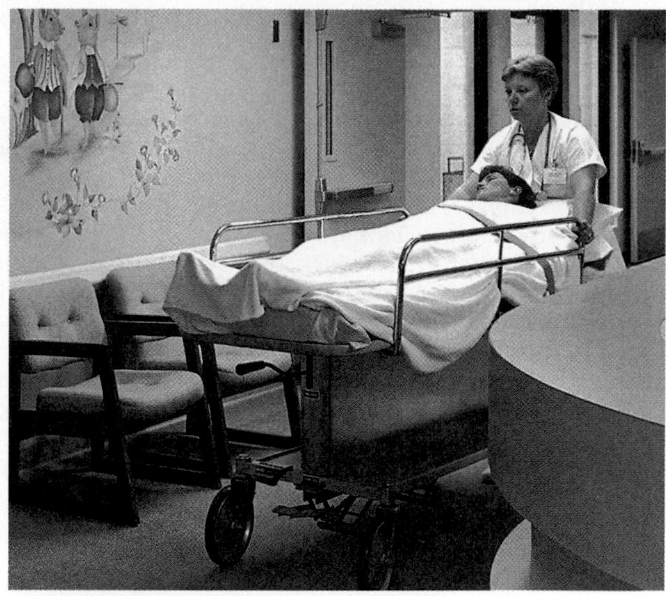

▲ Clients may be admitted or transferred on a gurney.

13. Notify appropriate departments (dietary, pharmacy) as required by hospital protocol when transfer is completed.
14. Notify x-ray and laboratory if tests were scheduled or results are pending.

Clinical Alert

Healthcare facilities must accurately and completely reconcile medications and other treatments at every transition of care: change in setting, service, practitioner, or level of care (National Patient Safety Goal # 8). Reconciliation at every transition point helps avoid medication errors such as omissions, duplications, dosing errors, or drug interactions.

Source: www.jointcommission.org

Clinical Alert

When a client is moved to another bed or room within the same unit, make certain the room/bed number is changed on the client's chart, MAR, and all other documents at the time the client is transferred. All appropriate departments must receive transfer notification.

DOCUMENTATION for Admitting and Transferring

- Admission procedures/orientation provided
- Adaptation to hospitalization
- Client's health history and physical assessment including risk assessment scores
- Individualized care plan and progress toward goal achievement.
- Client-signed documents added to the chart (e.g., advance directive)
- Inventory and dispensation of client's valuables and home medications
- Transfer time, destination, mode of transfer, transporter's name, and client's status
- Name of receiving unit's staff to whom report was given

Legal Considerations

Misidentification of Clients Does Not Ordinarily Occur in Absence of Negligence

This client underwent an apparently uncomplicated hysterectomy. She was placed in Bed B of a semiprivate room to recover.

Several hours later, the client occupying Bed A in the same room was moved elsewhere in the facility, but hospital staff failed to note the move in its records. Two shifts of nurses also failed to note the move.

The next day, the nurses on the unit directed the orderly to the room to find the woman who had previously been in Bed A to transport her to the lab for an ultrasound.

The hysterectomy client in Bed B, who wore a traditional hospital ID bracelet and whose name was posted on her bed, protested that she had just come from surgery, had been instructed not to move without direction, and that she knew of no scheduled test. Nevertheless, the orderly persisted without checking the client's identity.

The client testified that she felt excruciating pain and nearly passed out, but the orderly proceeded to take her to the lab. The lab commenced the procedure, and after client complaints, finally determined her true identity and returned her to her room, but failed to notify the attending nurse of the mistake.

The client suffered an incisional dehiscence and hernia, necessitating further surgery. Based on evidence at trial, the jury found the hospital had a "lackadaisical attitude" toward client identification procedures, evincing a "reckless and wanton disregard of the rights of the client." Potentially, this would allow an award of punitive damages in excess of actual damages determined.

Source: Scribner v. Hillcrest Medical Center (1992).

CRITICAL THINKING Application

Expected Outcomes

- Client adapts to hospital environment.
- Client participates in the individualized plan of care.
- Client understands rationale for and accepts transfer to a new care unit.
- Client is transferred to new unit without complication.

Unexpected Outcomes	Alternative Actions
Client has difficulty adapting to hospital environment.	• Assess physiologic, emotional, or cultural basis for difficulty. • Consult case manager, interpreter, clergy, or other assistant to facilitate client's adaptation.
Foreign client appears depressed, refuses to participate in the plan of care.	• Understand client's cultural acceptance of fate and fear that the diagnosis actually caused the disease process. • Explore client's concept of hot/cold balance; assist in meal planning accordingly. • Emphasize essentials of care and discharge planning as many feel the hospital is a place to die. • Be flexible regarding timing of meals and other aspects of care as much as feasible.
Client is anxious about transfer.	• Orient client to new setting and elicit client's perception of reason for transfer. • Correct misperceptions regarding transfer and continuity of care. • Explain that transfer decision is based on client's clinical progress and that new unit will be appropriate to provide client's current care needs.
Upon transfer, client's personal belongings are lost.	• Check with transferring unit for retained items. • Check with security personnel for client's registered items. • File a variance report if belongings are not located.

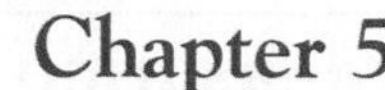

Chapter 5

UNIT 2

Height and Weight

Nursing Process Data

ASSESSMENT Data Base

- Check the need for daily or weekly body weight measurements.
- Determine appropriate method for obtaining client's weight (standing scale, bed scale).
- Determine client's ability to stand for height measurement.
- Obtain previous height and weight measurements to compare with expected norms or to establish a base for identifying trends.

PLANNING Objectives

- To identify excess or deficit of fluid balance
- To establish baseline data to monitor response to drug therapy (e.g., diuretic)
- To determine weight-based drug dosages
- To determine nutritional status in relation to body requirements (see Chapter 19)

IMPLEMENTATION Procedures

EVALUATION Expected Outcomes

- Height and weight are obtained and recorded.
- Client's weight, depending on disease state and therapy, shows expected losses, gains, or stabilization.

Pearson Nursing Student Resources

Find additional review materials at
nursing.pearsonhighered.com

Prepare for success with NCLEX®-style practice questions and Skill Checklists

Measuring Height and Weight

Equipment

Balance beam scale (for clients who are able to stand without assistance)

Bed scale (for clients who are confined to bed or who are unable to stand) or

Bed scale (built into the bed)

Floor scale (for clients in wheelchairs)

Paper towel

Preparation

1. Perform hand hygiene and check client ID.
2. Weigh client in the morning before breakfast. Ask client to void before weighing.
3. Use the same scale each time you weigh the client.
   ▸ ***Rationale:*** For consistency in weight from day to day, keep variables the same as possible.
4. Make sure the client wears the same type of clothing (e.g., gown or robe) for each weighing.
5. If bedscale is used, account for weight of linens, etc.
   ▸ ***Rationale:*** Extraneous variables, such as linens, extra pillows, etc., result in inaccurate client measurements.
6. Change wet gown or heavily saturated dressings before weighing the client.

Procedure

1. Transport client to scale or bring scale to bedside.
2. Balance scale so that weight is accurate. (See Table 5-1 for desirable weight based on sex and height.)
3. Place a clean paper towel on scale and ask client to remove shoes.
4. Assist client to stand on scale.
5. Move weights until the weight bar is level or balanced.
6. Record weight on appropriate record.
7. Ask client to face front so back is toward scale's balancing bar.
8. Instruct client to stand erect.

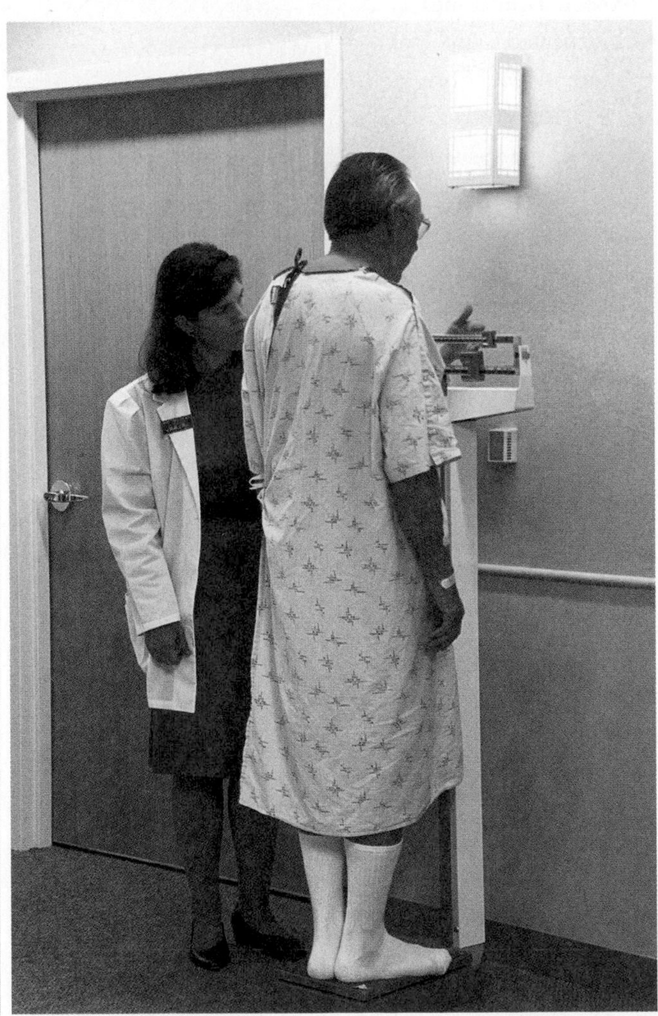

▲ Weigh client in the morning, before eating or drinking, using the same scale each time.

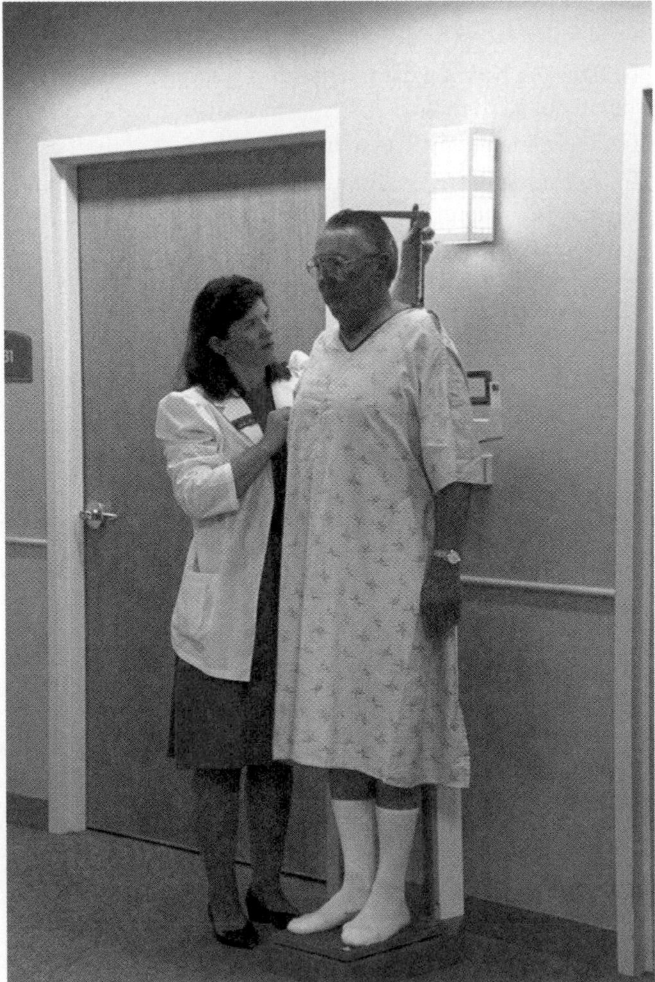

▲ Instruct client to stand erect to measure height.

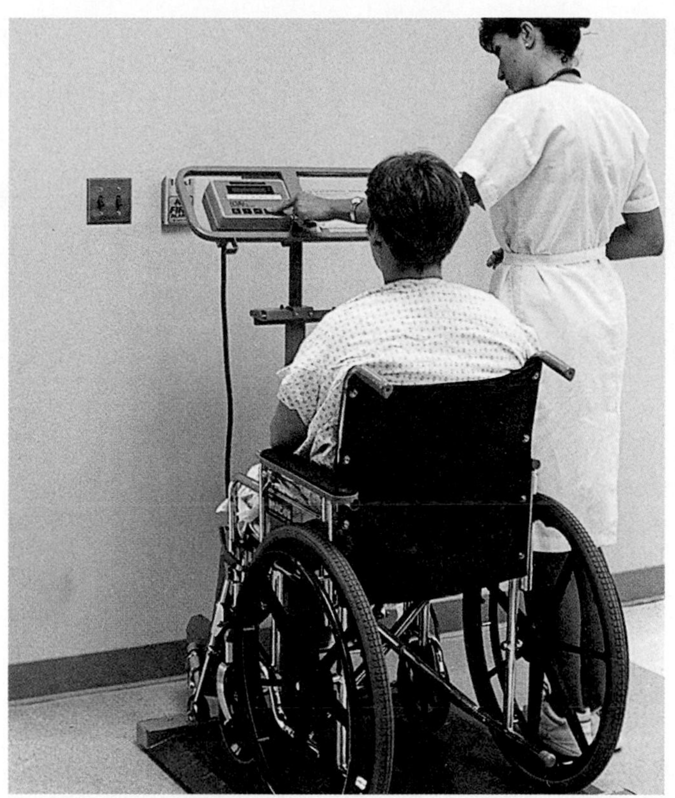

▲ Scales accommodate wheelchairs for weighing clients.

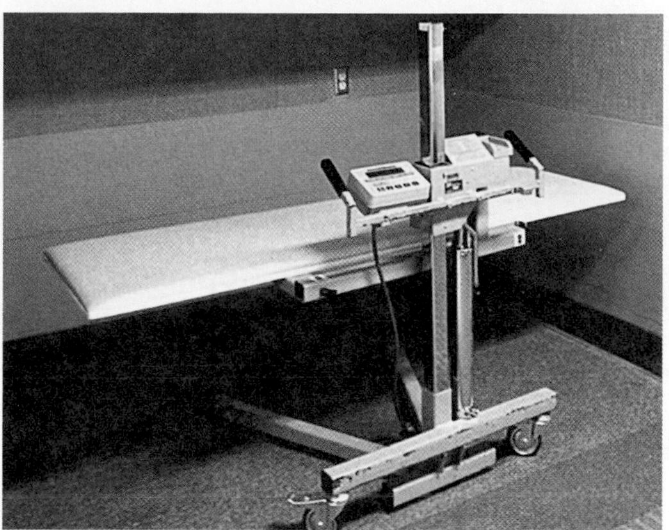

▲ Bed scale is used to weigh clients who are on complete bed rest. *Note: See Chapter 6 for specialty beds that include scale capability.*

9. Place L-shaped sliding height bar on top of client's head.
10. Read client's height as measured.
11. Record height on appropriate record.
12. Discard paper towel (if used) and assist client back to room.
13. Perform hand hygiene.

TABLE 5-1 Weight Chart (Desirable Weights in Pounds, According to Frame—in Indoor Clothing)

WOMEN Height		Small Frame	Medium Frame	Large Frame	MEN Height		Small Frame	Medium Frame	Large Frame
Feet	Inches	Pounds	Pounds	Pounds	Feet	Inches	Pounds	Pounds	Pounds
4	10	92–98	96–107	104–119	N/A		N/A	N/A	N/A
4	11	94–101	98–110	106–122	N/A		N/A	N/A	N/A
5	0	96–104	101–113	109–125	N/A		N/A	N/A	N/A
5	1	99–107	104–116	112–128	N/A		N/A	N/A	N/A
5	2	102–110	107–119	115–131	5	2	112–120	118–129	124–141
5	3	105–113	110–122	118–134	5	3	115–123	121–133	129–144
5	4	108–116	113–126	121–138	5	4	118–126	124–136	132–148
5	5	111–119	116–130	125–142	5	5	121–129	127–139	135–142
5	6	114–123	120–135	129–146	5	6	124–133	130–143	138–156
5	7	118–127	124–139	133–150	5	7	128–137	134–147	142–161
5	8	122–131	128–143	137–154	5	8	132–141	138–152	147–162
5	9	126–135	132–147	141–158	5	9	136–145	142–156	151–170
5	10	130–140	136–151	145–163	5	10	140–150	146–160	155–174
5	11	134–144	140–155	149–168	5	11	144–154	150–165	159–179
6	0	138–148	144–159	153–173	6	0	148–158	154–170	164–184
6	1	N/A	N/A	N/A	6	1	152–162	158–175	168–189
6	2	N/A	N/A	N/A	6	2	156–167	162–180	173–194
6	3	N/A	N/A	N/A	6	3	160–171	167–185	178–199
6	4	N/A	N/A	N/A	6	4	164–175	172–190	182–204

Height is in feet and inches, including shoes. Weight is in pounds, including indoor clothing. Assumption: Male indoor clothing with shoes weighed seven pounds. Female clothing with shoes weighed four pounds. Identify clothes client wore for accurate weight.
For girls between 18 and 25, subtract 1 pound for each year under 25.
Source: Blue Cross/Blue Shield of Delaware, 1997; American Heart Association.
NOTE: See Chapter 19, Nutritional Management, for body mass index table.

DOCUMENTATION for Height and Weight

- Time of day height and weight were measured
- Client's height and weight measurement recorded on client's chart and MAR
- Type and identifying number of scale used for weighing
- Weight of any attached equipment shoes or clothing that adds to client's actual weight

CRITICAL THINKING Application

Expected Outcomes

- Height and weight are obtained and recorded.
- Client's weight shows expected losses, gains, or stabilization.

Unexpected Outcomes	Alternative Actions
Client cannot be weighed accurately because of attached mechanical devices.	• Analyze unexpected weight loss or gain by assessing other factors, such as fluid intake and urinary output, presence of edema, lung sounds. • Remove attached device momentarily to obtain accurate weight.
Client's weight varies more than expected from one day to the next.	• Check time of day weight was measured. • Check if same scale was used for both weighings. • For equipment reliability, check client's weight with another scale and compare findings. • Check what clothing or linen was on the client when weighed on both days. • Check MAR for medications that alter fluid balance (e.g., diuretics). • Check I & O record for sources of fluid loss or gain.

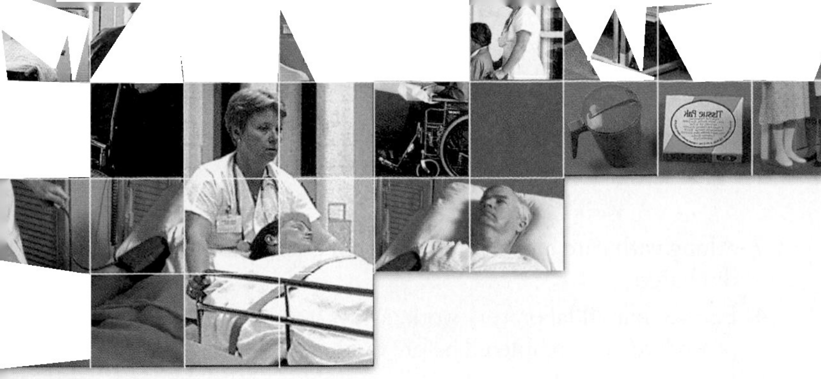

Chapter 5

UNIT 3

Discharge

Nursing Process Data

ASSESSMENT Data Base

- Verify order for client's discharge.
- Identify discharge destination (home, rehabilitation unit, etc.).
- Assess client's feelings about discharge.
- Review care plan to determine client's progress toward goal achievement during hospitalization.
- Identify client's teaching needs for discharge and report findings to multidisciplinary team.
- Assess for any unaddressed need for healthcare assistance in the home.
- Determine that discharge needs have been addressed by case manager, dietitian, occupational or physical therapist, social worker, or other specialist.
- Verify that client is ready for discharge.
- Try to determine reason for client's intent to leave the hospital against medical advice.

PLANNING Objectives

- To collaborate with the multidisciplinary team
- To prepare client for discharge and complete discharge planning
- To assist in the discharge of a client whose condition necessitates lifestyle changes or care at another facility
- To allow the client to verbalize feelings about discharge and to identify the client's strengths and needs
- To inform client of risks involved in leaving the hospital against medical advice (AMA)

IMPLEMENTATION Procedures

EVALUATION Expected Outcomes

- Client understands discharge process and is not exhibiting anxiety.
- Client remains in the hospital until discharged by the physician.

Pearson Nursing Student Resources

Find additional review materials at **nursing.pearsonhighered.com**

Prepare for success with NCLEX®-style practice questions and Skill Checklists

Discharging a Client

Equipment

Client's record

Hospital Discharge Instructions form

Copy of discharge medication order list and any new physician's written prescription

Educational pamphlets/instructions

Telephone numbers and information regarding follow-up appointments or special referrals

Adaptive aids (e.g., walker, toilet seat extender) needed on discharge (may be dispensed by the hospital)

Client's home medications retained, hospital dispensed liquids, MDIs (metered dose inhalers), if continuation is prescribed.

Materials for dressing changes (if indicated), antiembolic stockings, or any additional items previously dispensed for individual client use

Transport vehicle for discharge

Preparation

1. Determine that physician's discharge orders have been written.
2. Notify client's interdisciplinary team of discharge order.

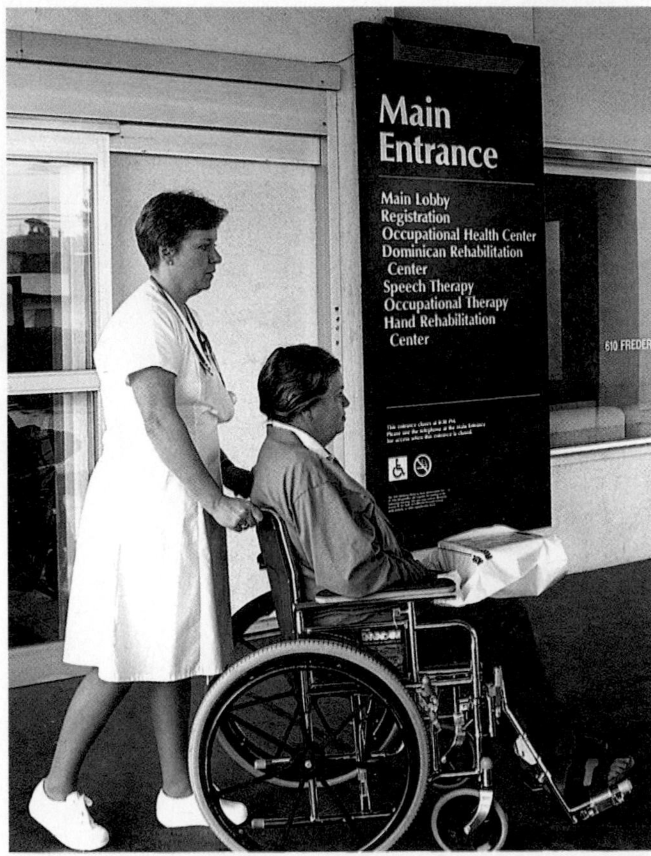

▲ Clients are discharged in a wheelchair for their safety.

3. Along with care team, determine that client is ready for discharge.
4. Ensure that all laboratory work, x-rays, treatments, and procedures are completed before discharge.
5. Determine that client understands instructions for self-care, including medications and follow-up arrangements.
6. Complete client teaching if applicable. (See Chapter 6.)
7. Notify client's caregiver to arrange transportation.
8. Obtain adaptive aids or other supplies that can be dispensed by the hospital (e.g., dressings, potty extender).
9. Provide opportunities for client to discuss impending discharge.

Procedure

1. Identify client.
2. Review details of discharge with client (see Discharge Planning unit in Chapter 6).
3. At discharge, the client's list of medications received during hospitalization is reconciled by the physician and prescriptions are written for new medications to be taken if indicated. The physician should document reasons for discontinuing or omitting certain medications upon discharge from the hospital, such as a beta-blocker and aspirin for the post–myocardial infarction client.
4. Review any teaching and answer questions about medications, diet, bathing, any activity restrictions (e.g., lifting, sexual activity, driving), physical/wound care, use of special equipment or supplies, and follow-up appointments.
5. Explain how to recognize complications and what to do if they occur.
6. Complete written instructions on Discharge Instructions form using lay terminology that client can understand.
7. Have client sign Discharge Instructions form and provide the client with a copy.
8. Place copy of client's signed Discharge Instructions form and discharge medication order list on client's chart.
9. Assist client to retrieve safeguarded valuables per hospital policy.
10. Terminate relationship with client. ▶ ***Rationale:*** Providing an opportunity for the client to express feelings and impressions contributes to a positive termination.
11. Follow hospital procedure for client discharge, including time and method of leaving hospital unit.
12. Document time and method of client's discharge, destination, individual accompanying, and any supplies, prescriptions, and forms sent with client.
13. Notify appropriate departments of client's discharge.

Discharging a Client Against Medical Advice (AMA)

Equipment

Client's record

Form for discharge against medical advice (AMA)

Procedure

1. Immediately notify physician and nurse manager if client insists on leaving the hospital prematurely. ▸ ***Rationale:*** If the nurse judges that the client is endangered by leaving AMA, the physician should be notified immediately.
2. Ascertain why the client wants to leave the hospital prematurely.
3. Explain reasons that continued hospital care is necessary (e.g., diagnosis, treatment).
4. Explain risks of leaving hospital AMA (e.g., incomplete testing or treatment).
5. Inform client that some insurance companies may not pay for hospitalization if the client leaves AMA. Refer client to his or her insurance plan.
6. Request client to sign the AMA form if he/she still insists on leaving AMA. The nurse witnesses and cosigns the document. ▸ ***Rationale:*** This form states that the hospital is relieved from responsibility for any ill effects which may result from AMA discharge.
7. Place signed AMA form in client's record and provide a copy to the client along with prescriptions, self-care and follow-up instructions, etc.
8. *If the client refuses to sign the AMA form,* note this on the form, have it witnessed, notify appropriate hospital personnel, and file a variance report. ▸ ***Rationale:*** This fulfills legal requirements if the client insists on discharge AMA without signing form.
9. Document client's verbatim statement in nurses' notes indicating reason for leaving.
10. The client is not escorted by hospital personnel, but leaves the hospital on his own or with family or friends whose names should be documented on the client's chart.
11. Notify client's caregiver and hospital security if there is concern for the client's welfare or safety.
12. Notify appropriate people when the client leaves (physician, case manager, nursing supervisor, risk management personnel).

Clinical Alert

Refer to agency standard operating procedures (SOPs) for specific instructions related to client admission, transfer, or discharge.

DOCUMENTATION for Discharging a Client

- Day-to-day preparatory activities for discharge such as teaching, return demonstrations
- List Copy of Discharge Instructions form, discharge medication order list, and client teaching/instructions provided
- Discharge data (time, destination, how discharged, and accompanied by whom)
- Client's own medications, physician-written prescriptions, special equipment taken home by client
- Discharge criteria not met and reason criteria were not met as identified on client's care plan
- Client's signed Release from Responsibility for Discharge (AMA) form, instructions provided, name of individual accompanying client out of the hospital, and client's telephone number and address for follow-up call or visit by social worker
- Individuals notified of client's discharge AMA

CRITICAL THINKING Application

Exected Outcomes

- Client understands discharge process and is not exhibiting anxiety.
- Client remains in the hospital until discharged by the physician.

Unexpected Outcomes	Alternative Actions
Client is anxious about discharge to an extended care unit.	• Reinforce physician/hospital's recommendation for extended care. • Provide time for client and caregiver to recognize that the goal is to increase client's strength and independence.
Client wants to leave the hospital AMA.	• Attempt to identify client's reasons for wanting to leave AMA. • Notify client's physician.

(Continued)

Unexpected Outcomes	Alternative Actions
	• Consult hospital policy and procedures regarding AMA before releasing client. • Negotiate possible alternative to leaving hospital (e.g., child care arrangements, employment concerns). • Encourage discussion about risk of leaving/benefits of remaining hospitalized. • Notify charge nurse, or supervisor, case manager and social worker, or clergy to discuss situation with client. • In case of a minor or mentally incompetent client, contact hospital attorney ASAP. • Have client sign hospital AMA form. • If client will not sign AMA form, have another nurse witness refusal, and chart details of discharge.

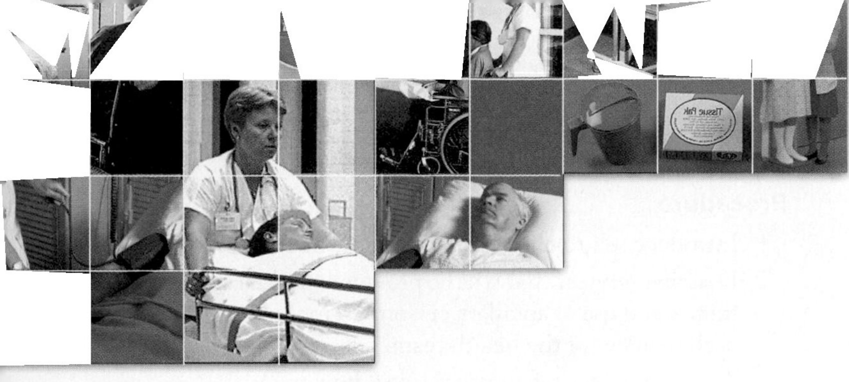

Chapter 5

UNIT 4

Admission to Home Care

Nursing Process Data

ASSESSMENT Data Base

- Assess client's financial eligibility for home care service.
- Observe client's physical, emotional, and intellectual status.
- Observe client's ability to adapt to the home setting.
- Assess the client's level of comfort.
- Determine client's understanding of the health status and any limitations.
- Assess home condition and safety factors prior to client returning home.
- Examine equipment for safety features.
- Assess nurse's safety for making home visits.

PLANNING Objectives

- To assist client to adapt to home care with minimal distress
- To encourage client and family to participate in the plan of care
- To provide a comfortable and safe environment for the client
- To maximize client's outcomes after discharge from hospital
- To provide the necessary and appropriate home care treatment modalities
- To provide a safe environment for the nurse

IMPLEMENTATION Procedures

Note: See Chapter 7 for Safety Interventions for Home Care

EVALUATION Expected Outcomes

- Client adapts to home setting with minimal difficulties.
- Client and family participate in the plan of care.
- Safe environment is provided for client.
- Nurse's safety is maintained during home visits.

Pearson Nursing Student Resources

Find additional review materials at **nursing.pearsonhighered.com**

Prepare for success with NCLEX®-style practice questions and Skill Checklists

Nurse's Role in Home Care

Equipment

Discharge Planning Records
OASIS C Forms
H485 Forms
Consent Forms
Agency Forms

Preparation

1. Obtain appropriate documents from healthcare facility.
   a. History and physical examination
   b. Diagnosis
   c. Treatments
   d. Medications
   e. Subjective and objective discharge notes.
   f. Physical or occupational therapy during home care.
   g. Hospital follow-up care appointments.
   h. Caregiver status (i.e., family member or home health aide).
2. Obtain all OASIS C documents to be completed during initial visit.
3. Contact discharge planner at facility to determine date, time of discharge, method of transfer to home, and availability of health caregiver when client reaches home.
4. Contact client, health caregiver, or family to arrange time for initial visit.

Procedure

1. Introduce self to client, family, and health caregiver.
2. Describe services that will be provided, including time frames and use of ancillary personnel, including role of each member of the health team.
3. Assess home for safety issues (see Chapter 7).
4. Determine client's eligibility for services.
5. Complete OASIS C forms and CMS-485 forms, in addition to relevant forms based on assessment (pressure ulcer forms, mental status, sensory status, etc.). Develop client care plan.
6. Review client's or caregiver's responsibility for care during absence of agency staff.
7. Provide telephone numbers for agency, emergency services, and, if appropriate, the RN (will vary among agencies).
8. Review medication names, doses, and time of administration and side effects that should be reported to the physician.
9. Review and have client or caregiver demonstrate any treatments that will be completed when agency personnel are not in home.
10. Develop a nurses' worksheet and care plan to be reviewed each visit. ▸ ***Rationale:*** To ensure all activities have been completed and documented.
    NOTE: Worksheet to include assessment findings, flow sheets (ADLs, pain assessment, medications, etc.), vital signs, education provided, IVs. Care plan update.

Identifying Eligibility for Medicare Reimbursement

Procedure

1. Complete OASIS C forms.
   a. Integrate information with CMS-485 data.
   b. Complete all sections of document. ▸ ***Rationale:*** Denial of service can result if documentation incomplete.
   c. Complete forms within 7 days.
   d. Ensure information from forms is transcribed accurately onto CMS-485 forms. ▸ ***Rationale:*** To prevent denial of service.
2. Check required criteria for Medicare coverage eligibility. ▸ ***Rationale:*** This prevents administering care for which reimbursement will not be received.
3. Identify client as homebound.
   a. Client's condition severely restricts leaving the home.
   b. Leaving the home requires considerable effort and assistance of another person.
   c. Special transportation is necessary.
   d. Absences from the home are infrequent and short.
4. Check that home service is considered skilled. To be skilled, service must be under the supervision of a registered nurse or a physical therapist.
   a. Registered nurse performs specific functions:
      Client teaching
      Dressings or irrigations
      Catheterization
      Parenteral therapies
      Medication administration and teaching
   b. Physical therapist performs certain functions:
      Gait training
      Therapeutic exercises
      Ultrasound, diathermy, TENS
      Restorative therapy
   c. Speech therapist performs certain functions:
      Therapy for clients with certain diagnoses (e.g., cerebrovascular accident, laryngectomy)
      Selected diagnostic and evaluative services
5. Provide supplemental services from home health aide, social worker, or occupational therapist; care is reimbursed by Medicare only when one of the three skilled services is required.
   a. Supplemental services may be obtained even if one of the skilled services is not needed; however, Medicare does not reimburse, and client is responsible for payment.

Clinical Alert

The Outcome and Assessment Information Set (OASIS-B1) and the Discharge Form in the OASIS paperwork is more extensive than previously gathered information on documentation forms. Be careful to complete all sections of the form.

b. Home health aide services are reimbursable only if plan of care is established and supervised by registered nurse.
   Personal care (activities of daily living [ADLs])
   Light housekeeping (e.g., food preparation, client's laundry)
   Selected semiskilled care (e.g., passive range-of-motion exercises)
c. Social worker.
   Interventions must contribute significantly to the improvement of the client's medical condition.
   Indication that social, environmental, or family conditions inhibit progress of recovery from medical condition.
d. Occupational therapy.
   Design maintenance program.
   Teach compensatory techniques and ADLs.
   Design self-help devices to assist with ADLs.
   Provide restorative therapy.

6. Provide care that is part-time and intermittent.
   a. Care must be episodic or acute and not chronic.
   b. Medically predictable recurring need for care must be present.
   c. Knowledge that condition will improve in a limited time frame.
   d. Frequency of service ranges from daily to every 90 days, depending on individual client's need.
7. Check that plan of treatment is authorized by physician and recertified every 60 days.
   a. Centers for Medicare and Medicaid Services form (CMS-485) is standardized for plan of treatment.
      This form is used by all home health agencies for Medicare clients.
   b. Form must include:
      Identifying data
      Diagnosis (ICD-9CM)
      Start of care
      Types of services required and frequency
      Functional limitations
      Activities permitted
      Safety measures
      Treatments
      Medications
      Mental status
      Nutritional status and diet orders
      Medical supplies and DME
      Goals and discharge plans
      Significant clinical findings
      Prognosis
      Physician's name, address, signature
      Certification of homebound status
8. Assess that care is medically reasonable and necessary.
   a. Entire plan of care must correlate with client's medical problems and client's clinical status.
   b. Each service's goals (client outcomes) must be clearly stated and realistic for the client.

Guidelines for Home Care

- Take as little with you into the home as possible.
- Use appropriate nursing protocols in home setting.
- Perform hand hygiene on entering and leaving home.
- Maintain clean technique in the home.
- Know CDC infection control guidelines.
- Review state and federal guidelines and protocol for reimbursement.

Completing Admission Documentation

Procedure

1. Complete all sections of the OASIS C document.
   a. Demographic data: address, referring physician, payment source, etc.
   b. Present history.
   c. Present illness.
   d. Living arrangements.
   e. Supportive assistance.
   f. Physical assessment/review of systems.
   g. ADLs.
   h. Medications.
   i. Equipment management.
   j. Homebound status.
   k. Therapy modalities required.
   l. Unmet needs.
   m. Lack of Knowledge section.
   n. Treatment/Procedures Performed.
   o. Response to Teaching/Training Performed.
   p. Patient Rights and Responsibilities.
   q. Coordination of Patient Services.
   r. Discharge Planning.
2. Signed consent forms.
   a. IV therapy.
   b. Consent for treatment.
   c. Consent for service
3. Signed HIPAA form.
4. Signed Advance Directive document.
5. Signed Patient's Bill of Rights document.

6. Billing Data Base.
7. Discipline Specific Evaluation, if therapy was instituted.
8. Plan of Care.
9. CMS-485 Worksheet.
10. Aide Assignment and Duties, if appropriate.
11. Physician Plan of Care.
12. Home Health Plan of Care.
13. Nurses' Notes as necessary.
14. Identify if prehospital "Do Not Resuscitate" form has been signed.

Maintaining Nurse's Safety

Procedure

1. Evaluate safety of nurse before the visit.
   a. Call the client before the visit to determine convenient time.
   b. Confirm directions to home.
   c. Determine whether household pets are present; if so, ask that they be secured during visit.
   d. Check neighborhood to determine need for assistance from police to make home visit.
2. Wear identifying name badge. Most agencies request that the nurse wear a lab coat.
3. Wear flat shoes to allow you to walk quickly or to run if necessary.
4. Maintain personal safety while traveling in the car.
   a. Keep car in good working order and stocked with necessary equipment.
   b. Keep gas tank at least half full at all times.
   c. Obtain automobile club membership for emergency use. ▸ ***Rationale:*** To call for assistance with car problems.
   d. Keep a windshield cover with CALL POLICE sign available. ▸ ***Rationale:*** To alert neighbors you need immediate assistance.
   e. Have car phone available and charged at all times.
   f. Keep blanket in car. ▸ ***Rationale:*** To keep warm in the winter if you need to wait for assistance.
   g. Keep thermos of water in car at all times. ▸ ***Rationale:*** In case you need to wait for assistance in hot weather.
   h. Keep doors locked and windows up at all times.
   i. Park in full view of neighbors, preferably directly in front of home.
   j. Lock all personal items in the car trunk before leaving home or office.
   k. Keep all equipment in the car trunk.
   l. Restock the nurses' bag before the visits for the day. Keep nurses' bag on front seat.
   m. Keep change in car for phone calls if necessary.
   n. Place all valuable objects out of direct sight in car (i.e., laptop computers, phone). Place these under the seat if possible. ▸ ***Rationale:*** To prevent car break-in and theft.
5. Maintain personal safety while walking on the street.
   a. Keep one arm and hand free when walking from car to house.
   b. Walk directly to client's residence.
   c. When approaching a group of strangers, cross the street or walkway, if appropriate.
   d. When leaving a residence, keep keys in your hand with the pointed end of the key facing outward. ▸ ***Rationale:*** The keys can be used as a weapon if necessary.
   e. Carry a chemical spray and whistle within easy reach.

Clinical Alert

If your safety is in jeopardy, use one of the following defensive strategies: Scream or yell *FIRE* or *STRANGER.* Kick the person in the shin or groin. Bite or scratch the person. Use chemical spray or blow a whistle. If you feel your personal safety is in question, do not make a visit or stay in the residence.

NOTE: Attendance at a class is necessary before it is legal to carry a chemical spray such as Mace.

6. Maintain personal safety when making home visit.
   a. Use common walkways or hallways. Do not park behind a building or in a dark area.
   b. Knock on the door and wait for permission to enter.
   c. Keep a clear pathway to the door if the situation is potentially unsafe.
   d. Observe home environment for safety hazards (i.e., weapons).
   e. Make a joint visit with another agency staff member or ask for an escort if there is a potentially unsafe situation.
   f. Call for police support if the visit is essential and the situation is unsafe. ▸ ***Rationale:*** There may be times when a visit is essential, but it is unsafe for one individual to make a visit.
   g. Make a visit in the morning when good visual support exists if neighborhood is unsafe.
   h. Close the case if the nurse feels the situation is unsafe and there are no alternative actions that can guarantee nurse's safety.

Assessing for Elder Abuse

Procedure

1. Assess client for indications of neglect: failure to provide adequate food, clothing, medical assistance, or assistance with ADLs. Check body for signs of cleanliness. Determine whether emotional abuse is present. Ask about threats, intimidation, or isolation.
2. Identify whether financial abuse has occurred, such as misuse of finances or property.
3. Assess for signs of physical abuse: signs of restraining; hitting, biting, burning; black and blue marks on trunk, abdomen, buttocks, upper thighs; scars; and abrasions. Bilateral bruises or parallel injuries may indicate forceful restraining; shaking may cause parallel injuries of upper arms. Accidental injuries affect knees, back of hands, forehead, and elbows.
4. Assess for signs of malnourishment or dehydration.
5. Check skin for pressure ulcers.
6. Assess for signs of sprains or dislocations from pulling or pushing the client.
7. Ask about visits to the hospital ER. Ask why client sought medical care, how much time elapsed between injury and visit to ER.
8. Assess for signs of emotional abuse. Observe if client is fearful of strangers, becomes quiet when caregiver enters room, craves attention and socialization.

Questions to Ask If Suspicion of Abuse

- Who cares for you at home?
- Did someone hurt you?
- Are you happy with where you live?
- Tell me about your daily routine.
- Who assists you with ADLs?
- Do you feel safe living here?
- Who manages your money?
- How did the injury (or bruises) occur?
- Did you receive medical attention?
- Has this type of injury happened before?

DOCUMENTATION for Admission to Home Care

- Complete all required forms, i.e., OASIS C, CMS-485, agency-specific forms
- Safety issues occurring within house
- Mental status of client and ability to care for self
- Teaching activities for client or caregiver
- Nursing care plan update
- Medication side effects and referral to physician
- Changes in client status
- Notification of physician

CRITICAL THINKING Applications

Expected Outcomes

- Client is acclimated to home environment and is able to provide care after a period of support from agency staff.
- Client is provided appropriate home care modalities.
- Safe environment provides for client safety in home.
- Nurse's safety is maintained during home visit.

Unexpected Outcomes	Alternative Actions
Client is noncompliant with treatments, safety procedures, and taking medications at home.	• Explain rationale for following home care plan. • Discuss reason with client, caregiver, and family members to determine whether change in plan would increase compliance. • Remind client that if he or she refuses to follow plan, he or she will be taken off services. • Document appropriately on all forms indicating noncompliance issues. • Notify physician.

GERONTOLOGIC Considerations

U.S. Demographics Affect Hospital Admissions

- The average life expectancy has increased.
- The number of elderly will double by 2020.
- Healthcare services are used by the elderly more than any other age group.
- Three of four elderly people die of heart disease, cancer, or stroke.

Elderly Clients Admitted to the Hospital Require Special Consideration

- Fatigue and pain may be pronounced; admission procedures may need to be altered.
- Repeated orientation may be indicated due to short-term memory deficit, confusion, sensory impairment.
- Special problems associated with age must be anticipated and nursing care planned appropriately (e.g., risk for falls).

Elderly Clients Admitted to Home Care Require Special Consideration

MANAGEMENT Guidelines

Each state legislates a Nurse Practice Act for RNs and LVN/LPNs. Healthcare facilities are responsible for establishing and implementing policies and procedures that conform to their state's regulations. Verify the regulations and role parameters for each healthcare worker in your facility.

Delegation

- Delegation for the admission of a new client may be divided into three task areas:
  1. A CNA may assist the client into bed, place client's personal items in a designated area, describe the room environment including the use of telephone, television, and nurse summon controls, visiting hours, mealtimes, and other hospital routines. The CNA may also take vital signs and obtain height and weight measurements.
  2. The LVN/LPN may complete a health history form, obtain admission data required by the hospital, witness consent forms, and complete the same tasks identified above.
  3. The RN is responsible for the complete health history and reviewing the data obtained by other health care workers, initiating the client care plan (nursing diagnosis, goals, and interventions), and beginning the discharge plan in collaboration with the healthcare team.
- An LVN/LPN may complete discharge teaching following the established discharge teaching plan.
- Escorting a client out of the hospital can be delegated to a volunteer, CNA, or LVN/LPN. Many facilities have escort services that utilize volunteers.

Communication Matrix

- Clients being admitted to the hospital are usually frightened and unsure of the events that will take place. It is important to communicate their needs to and collaborate with all staff members involved in the client's care. This will provide a team approach for comprehensive care.
- A complete report on the newly admitted client must be given to all team members. If an LVN/LPN or CNA assisted in the admission process, he or she must provide immediate feedback to the RN manager regarding their findings.
- The client Kardex and Medication Reconciliation List must be completed in a timely manner to facilitate safe and effective care. It is often the responsibility of the unit secretary to process orders and initiate the documentation; however, it is the responsibility of the RN to check the processing and documents for accuracy and completeness.
- A client care plan must be established within a designated time frame. The time is determined by the facility in accordance with The Joint Commission guidelines.
- "Hand-Off" shift report must contain a brief history: reason for admission, overview of the client's assessment, current status, and any special needs. Diet, specific treatments, procedures, test results or those pending, and any alerts (e.g., DNAR, isolation) should be included. The hand-off process (including audio-taped reports) must allow opportunity for asking and receiving answers to questions relevant to safe client care.

CRITICAL THINKING Strategies

Scenario 1

Mr. Moore has been told by his cardiologist that his coronary arteriogram indicates he has three-vessel disease and he is a candidate for coronary artery bypass surgery. The surgery is scheduled and Mr. Moore is welcomed at the facility's preadmission testing unit 1 week before admission for preliminary blood work and preoperative instructions. At this time he receives information about his expected clinical course, which includes a multidisciplinary Plan of Care.

1. What is the advantage of providing the client with information this far in advance of surgery?
2. What is included in the Plan of Care?
3. Who participates in the development of the Plan of Care?
4. How does the Plan of Care facilitate the client's admission, transfer, and discharge processes? Are there drawbacks?

Scenario 2

Marilyn James, age 45, has been admitted to the hospital for incision and drainage of a wound infection following knee surgery she had 3 weeks ago. Her therapy now requires 2 more weeks of hospitalization for twice-daily intravenous antibiotic therapy.

After the first day of antibiotic therapy, she says she's going to leave the hospital AMA without completing the recommended course of treatment. She "wasn't prepared for prolonged hospitalization" and has to go home to care for her 3-year-old granddaughter and elderly mother who live with her.

1. What right does a client have to leave the agency prematurely, AMA?
2. What should the nurse's initial response to this client be?
3. How can the nurse advocate for this client?
4. What are the usual procedures involved in discharging a client AMA?
5. How is this process documented in the client's record?

NCLEX® Review Questions

Unless otherwise specified, choose only one (1) answer.

1. DNR decisions are made by the
   1. Client's family.
   2. Advance Directive counselor.
   3. Client.
   4. Client's physician.
2. Who is responsible for inquiring if the client has an Advance Directive?
   1. The hospital chaplain.
   2. The admitting nurse.
   3. The hospital attorney.
   4. The client's physician.
3. During the admission process, the client receives an identification bracelet (Ident-A-Band)
   1. Before arriving on the nursing unit.
   2. Upon arrival to the nursing unit.
   3. After the initial assessment has been completed.
   4. Upon receipt of admitting physician's orders.
4. The Ident-A-Band contains the client's name as well as this information

   Select all that apply.
   1. Client's room number.
   2. Admitting physician's name.
   3. Client's date of birth.
   4. Client's hospital number.
5. During the admission process, the client is oriented to the hospital unit, including use of various control systems. The purpose of this orientation is to
   1. Save time for the nursing staff.
   2. Provide client control over the environment.
   3. Release the hospital from liability in case the client falls.
   4. Prevent the client's abuse of expensive equipment.
6. This information should be included in the client's orientation to the hospital environment

   Select all that apply.
   1. Meal times.
   2. Use of emergency call system.
   3. Roommate's name.
   4. Use of nurse call system.
   5. Physician visit times.
7. Mr. Jones has been admitted to your unit with a diagnosis of "Rule Out MI" (myocardial infarction). The Joint Commission requires that this client be assessed for and counseled about
   1. Smoking.
   2. Diet.
   3. Exercise.
   4. Stress.
8. The client's body mass index (BMI) is calculated using the client's
   1. Age and waist measurement.
   2. Age and weight.
   3. Height and weight.
   4. Sex and waist measurement.
9. Serious injuries can occur when clients are transferred from one hospital unit or one bed to another because of
   1. Client misidentification.
   2. Loss of personal items.
   3. Delays in medication administration.
   4. Falls during transport.
10. When a client intends to leave the hospital prematurely, against medical advice, the nurse should first
    1. Have the client sign the hospital AMA form.
    2. Try to identify the reasons why the client wants to leave AMA.
    3. Notify the client's physician.
    4. Inform the client about risks of leaving AMA.

6

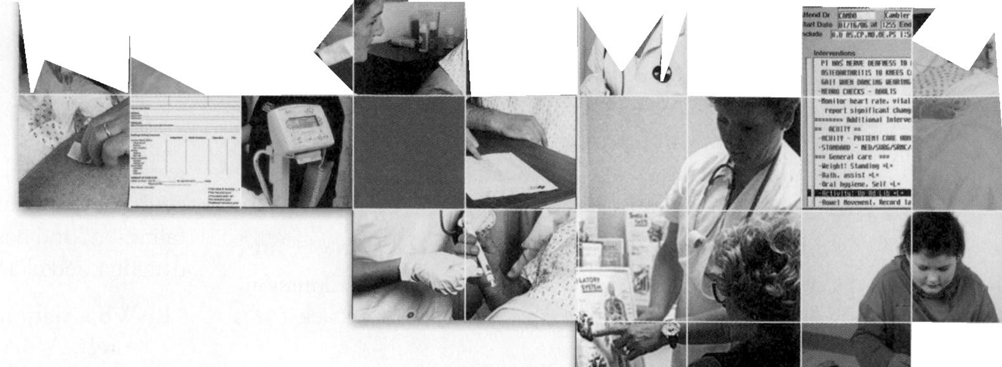

Client Education and Discharge Planning

LEARNING OBJECTIVES

1. Define the process of client education.
2. Discuss the meaning of the term *learning theory*.
3. Outline the process of collecting client data to determine learning needs.
4. Explain the application of the nursing process to client education.
5. List two factors to consider when determining an appropriate teaching strategy.
6. List and describe two specific teaching strategies appropriate for clients and families.
7. Define cultural competence.
8. Identify assessments to determine readiness to learn.
9. Discuss the application of Adult Learning Principles (Knowles) to client education.
10. Identify one strategy to determine readability level of written material.
11. Describe how to develop an evaluation tool.
12. Discuss the meaning of the term *discharge planning*.
13. List three risk factors that require discharge planning.
14. Identify the steps necessary to complete a discharge summary.
15. Describe documents required to accompany client to home.
16. Identify appropriate referral for Home Health Team.

CHAPTER OUTLINE

UNIT ❶ Client Education

UNIT ❷ Discharge Planning

TERMINOLOGY

Assessment the first step in identifying client's knowledge base is to set meaningful learning goals and strategies.

Client education the process of influencing behavior and teaching the client self-care techniques so that he or she can resume responsibility for certain aspects of health care following discharge from the health facility.

Compliance follow-through on advice and direction by medical personnel to promote wellness and rehabilitation.

Comprehensive health care a total system of health care that takes the whole person into account.

Counseling giving support or providing guidance.

Culture a way of living, thinking, and behaving. It is learned within the family and guides the way we solve problems in our daily lives.

Cultural competence a set of congruent behaviors, attitudes, and policies that enables nurses and other healthcare workers to work effectively in a cross-cultural situation.

Diagnosis-related groups (DRGs) categorization of disease diagnoses that standardizes the reimbursement of government funds for number of days in the hospital.

Discharge to release from care; done by a physician, nurse, or medical care facility.

Discharge planning systematic process of planning for client care following discharge; includes client needs, goals of care, and strategies for implementation.

Evaluation tool a test, questionnaire, or direct observation that evaluates the effectiveness of the teaching.

Helping relationship an interaction of individuals that sets the climate for movement of the participants toward common goals.

Home care assistance nursing care provided by licensed and unlicensed personnel in the client's home setting.

Learning The process of conceptual change, within the framework of the client's perceptions, that leads to modifications in behavior.

Maladaptive inability to, or faulty adjustment or adaptation.

Readiness to learn a component of the learning process; referring to the psychologic state of being open and accepting of new information and the learning process.

Relationship an interaction of individuals over time.

Resistance inability to listen and participate in discussion of health behavioral changes.

Support to lend strength or give assistance to.

Termination the end of something; a limit or boundary; conclusion or cessation.

Therapeutic having medicinal or healing properties; a healing agent.

Transfer to convey or shift from one person or place to another.

Transition the process or an instance of changing from one form, state, activity, or place to another.

Transitional care the process of facilitating the transition or move between hospital and home to maintain continuity of health care.

Understanding to perceive and comprehend the nature and significance of, to know.

Validate to substantiate or verify.

CLIENT EDUCATION

Historically, client education has been one of the most important responsibilities of the professional nurse. With advances in medical science and an increasing number of clients with progressive chronic illness, the role of client education can directly affect the client's health, adaptation to illness, and recovery. While a segment of healthcare consumers are more informed and active in making healthcare decisions, there still remain those who lack "health literacy," or lack the ability to read, comprehend, and act on medical information. These factors contribute to the increasingly difficult task of providing appropriate and comprehensive client education. In addition, the influx of clients from various diverse cultures, different languages, availability of educational materials written at appropriate readability levels and/or languages, lack of time, and shorter hospital stays present challenges for nursing.

The purpose of client and family education is for them to gain knowledge, skills, and behavior changes necessary to meet the client's healthcare needs. Client education should be individualized, specific, and understandable. Clients have a right to know about their illness, medications, and any procedures being performed. Client education is an expected standard for nursing practice.

The Joint Commission (formerly JCAHO) has mandated that client and family education be part of comprehensive care and devised Patient and Family Education (PFE) Standards for accredited agencies.

Challenges to Providing Client Education

- Various cultures
- Various languages
- Lack of time
- Lack of reimbursement
- Lack of appropriate readable materials
- Lack of literacy appropriate materials
- Lack of training in providing client education and/or the development of materials

The Joint Commission set the following goals for client and family teaching:

- Client participation and decision making about health care options
- Increased potential to follow the healthcare plans
- Development of self-care skills
- Improved client/family coping
- Increased participation in continuing care
- Adopting a healthy lifestyle

The Joint Commission reviews for evidence of three major processes involved in client education: the hospital's internal focus on education, direct education of the client and family, and evaluation of how well the education program achieves the identified goals. The Joint Commission stresses the need for a multidisciplinary approach to planning and implementing client education. Because nurses are the principal providers of care and have legal responsibility for client education, as outlined in each state's Nurse Practice Act and emphasized in documents published by the American Nurses Association and many specialty associations, they usually provide the leadership role in directing the educational plan for the client and family. Nurses provide the communication link between the multidisciplinary team members to ensure the client's goals are met in a timely manner.

The cultural beliefs and practices of the client have a major influence on healthcare behaviors, beliefs, and willingness to learn. Client education must be sensitive to these beliefs. For example, if teaching a Chinese diabetic, the nurse must consider the food the client likes to eat, as well as the social values. Eating may not be merely for nutrients, but also a gesture of politeness and social interaction. It is important that nurses gain an awareness of the various cultures in order to provide *culturally competent* care.

The goal of client and family education is to promote optimal client health. To achieve this goal, clients and families must learn in a way that is meaningful and acceptable to their concept of self and in relationship to the illness. Thus learning is a process of conceptual change within the framework of the client's perceptions that leads to behavioral change.

To be effective and facilitate the teaching/learning process, the nurse must utilize excellent listening and communication skills to establish rapport. Determining learning needs, preferred learning style, and learning readiness are all requirements included in the The Joint Commission's Standards for Patient & Family Education. Once a client has received a new diagnosis or new information about his/her condition, the nurse must assess three areas: (1) what they already know, (2) what they need to know and, (3) how best to assist with learning. Clients need to be able to identify and understand what the illness is, effects of the treatment, whether it is acute or chronic, and short- and long-term care needs and outcomes. Discussing possible outcomes of the illness will help the client accept the condition, be open for new ideas or teaching, and be motivated to learn and make appropriate health behavior changes. The client must recognize any gaps in knowledge and misconceptions and then assimilate new information for possible actions. When the client and family assist in goal setting and the information is presented based on their preferences, learning becomes more meaningful.

The client education plan is a component of the total nursing care plan, which is part of the nursing process. Thus the same principles of the nursing process apply to client education: assess the learning needs, and plan appropriate teaching, implementation, and evaluation. Client education, when viewed as a process rather than the simple action of imparting information, helps the client to actively participate in his or her health plan for wellness. Individualized to the specific client needs and included as part of a total care plan, client education contributes to continuity of care following discharge.

Principles of Client Education

Malcolm Knowles, author of *The Modern Practice of Adult Education*, discusses strategies for adult learning. He suggests that adult learning and readiness to learn are influenced by developmental tasks. Knowles formulated what he called the "Adult Learning Principles," which include the following:

- Adults learn best when there is a perceived need. In order for learning to occur, the client must understand why they need to know about a subject. Therefore, the nurse must ensure that the client understands the underlying health issue that is to be prevented or the illness that is to be resolved before teaching.
- Teaching plan is considered part of client care plan.
- Teaching of adults should progress from the known to the unknown. Assess what they already know; don't reteach the things they already know.
- Teaching of adults should progress from the simpler concepts to more complex topics.
- Adults learn best using active participation. Asking the client to restate what has been discussed will encourage learning and provide for clarification.
- Adults require opportunities to practice new skills. When acquiring new manual skills, such as drawing up or injecting insulin, it is essential that the client be allowed to practice the skill. It is important to observe a return demonstration in order to evaluate the effectiveness of the teaching.
- Adults need behavior reinforced. An example of reinforcing behavior would be to allow the client to draw up and give their insulin each time it is required.
- Immediate feedback and correction of misconceptions increases learning.

Similar to Knowles's principles of adult learning, simplicity and reinforcement are essential in providing client education. An understanding of these principles is essential for individuals who teach adults in the healthcare setting.

Resistance to Change

Most nurses recognize that the client may resist learning and cannot be forced to learn; the nurse can only assist the client, encourage him or her, and facilitate learning. To master information, the client must have internalized some form of motivation to learn; for example, the client realizes that to adequately control diabetes and feel better, he or she must understand the relationship of insulin and food to body needs.

Tips to Facilitate Client-Focused Education

- Get to know the client, his/her knowledge level, perception, current practices, and preferences.
- Determine client's goals and readiness to learn, and individualize ways to achieve goals.
- Take into account client's goals, learning style, special skills, cultural beliefs, and developmental level.
- Utilize simple language and interact at client's level with empathy and concern.
- Utilize a variety of materials and methods that encourage active learning and participation.
- Plan for right time and right place to maximize client and family learning.
- Follow up at another time to clarify information and reassess learning.

Many clients appear to resist change, even when changing would result in a positive outcome. When this occurs, the process of learning is blocked. As a nurse educator, you are functioning as an agent of change, and dealing with resistance to change is a necessary task. There are several reasons underlying resistance; one of the most common is that change is frightening, even when a person consciously wishes to alter his or her behavior. If a person perceives change as a possible threat, he or she may resist. Another cause of resistance is inaccurately perceiving the reason for or effect of change. Other sources of resistance include psychologic inflexibility, cultural practices, inability to tolerate change, and not believing that change will have a positive effect.

The nurse is both an educator and an agent of change. If the client resists change (the teaching process), attempting to identify the reason for that resistance and altering the teaching approach accordingly may assist the nurse to accomplish the goals of client education.

Barriers to Change	Nursing Approaches
Perceived threat or fear of change	Identify specific fears or threats and impart accurate information that may reduce fears. Focus on the positive outcome of change.
Inaccurate perceptions of effect of change	Clarify client perceptions. Impart accurate information, and discuss results of behavior change.
Disagreement that change is positive	Work to agree on mutual goals and demonstrate positive outcomes so client views change as positive rather than negative.
Psychologic resistance or perceived loss of freedoms or behaviors	Focus on discussion of client's perceived loss of freedom and demonstrate willingness to alter plan or adapt to client's needs.
Inability to tolerate change	Recognize that low tolerance is often caused by fear—allaying fear through developing trust, being supportive when client attempts to change, and giving positive feedback decreases fear of change.

Client education is more than imparting information to a client; it is the process of influencing behavior. As such, it needs to be directed toward the client's thinking to facilitate meaningful behavioral changes. When goals are mutually agreed on and clearly stated, the learner understands what is expected, the nurse understands his or her role and can evaluate it, and the results can more easily be measured. Because of the need to control costs and the current practice of discharging clients earlier, a more extensive teaching plan must be developed and implemented.

Readiness to Learn

Assessing the client's readiness to learn is an essential component of client education. Readiness to learn can be limited by physical and psychosocial demands caused by illness, such as pain and fatigue. For many clients, the post-acute or recovery phase and desire to return to normalcy act as an incentive to learning.

Methods of Teaching

The methods of client teaching may include:

- One-to-one education: most common methodology used in hospitals, clinics, and physician offices.
- Group teaching: most often utilizes videotapes or similar technology, such as CDs or DVDs.
- Computer-aided instruction: used in clinics, hospitals, and physician offices or for client to learn at home.
- Internet: can increase client's understanding of symptoms, conditions, and treatments—key to Internet use is choosing appropriate health Web sites.

Regardless of the methodology chosen, selection of educational materials and resources should be appropriate for age, developmental level, cognitive level, culture, and language.

DISCHARGE PLANNING

Recent changes in healthcare delivery systems, as an attempt to contain rapidly rising costs, have altered client care. The number of hospital days for clients in acute care hospitals has decreased; frequently, these clients are discharged still requiring care; and this care is frequently delivered in the home setting. Most clients, especially those who are high risk, benefit from the process of discharge planning. Discharge planning is defined as the systematic process of planning for client care after discharge from the hospital. The emphasis and goal of discharge planning are to meet client needs through continuity of care—from an acute care setting to a discharge facility.

To comply with The Joint Commission requirements related to discharge planning, initial assessment at admission, ongoing assessments, and referrals must be documented.

When the client is admitted and the care plan formulated, discharge planning should be initiated. The process includes an assessment of the client and family's anticipated needs; physical, emotional, and psychosocial status; home environment; and family and community resources. Two common assessment instruments measuring physical and cognitive function are frequently given to at-risk clients at the time of admission. The Lawton IADL and Katz ADL scales provide information useful when developing the discharge plans.

Comparison of the two scales:

Activities of Daily Living	Instrumental Activities of Daily Living
(Katz ADL)	(Lawton IADL)
Feeding	Using the telephone
Continence	Shopping
Transferring	Preparing food
Toileting	Housekeeping
Dressing	Doing laundry
Bathing	Using transportation
	Handling medications
	Handling finances

Source: Graf, C. (2008, April). The Lawton instrumental activities of daily living scale. *American Journal of Nursing, 108*(4), 52–62.

Discharge planning requires a multidisciplinary approach with participation by all members of the healthcare team, including the client and family. Many of the larger hospitals have discharge planners or coordinators, who orchestrate the discharge planning. This is especially important when the client is considered high risk. The nursing staff still play a major role in assessing discharge needs and preparing the client and caregivers to assume responsibility for care after hospital discharge. With the assistance of social workers or community-based nurses, the nurse identifies and anticipates client needs and formulates a plan for meeting these needs after discharge from the hospital.

Discharge Planning: High-Risk Clients

- Elderly
- Multisystem disease process
- Major surgical procedure
- Chronic or terminal illness
- Emotional or mental instability
- Inadequate or inappropriate living arrangement
- Lack of transportation
- Financial insecurity
- Unsafe features in the home

Successful discharge planning includes:

1. A transitional plan of care from the acute care setting to home or another healthcare facility.
2. Appropriate teaching for family and client in self-care.
3. Knowledge and skills necessary for self-care and emergency procedures.
4. Appropriate agencies involved in transition to the home care setting.

A new approach to discharge planning is transitional care using transition specialists. This category of practitioner was implemented to facilitate the transition from hospital (where discharge planning is initiated) to recovery (in the home). The transition specialist meets with the family and client in the acute setting, begins discharge planning, and usually makes a home visit before the client is discharged. After discharge to the home, this specialist is available to the client and family.

The Joint Commission Standards for Client Education

- Hospital plans for and supports the provision and coordination of client education activities.
- Hospital identifies and provides the resources necessary for achieving educational objectives.
- Education process is coordinated among appropriate staff or disciplines who are providing care or services.
- Client receives education and training specific to the client's assessed needs, abilities, learning preferences, and readiness to learn as appropriate to the care and services provided by the hospital.
- Client is educated, based on assessed needs, about how to safely and effectively use medications according to law and regulation and the hospital's scope of services, as appropriate.
- Client is educated about nutrition interventions, modified diets, or oral health, when applicable.
- Hospital ensures client is educated about how to safely and effectively use medical equipment or supplies, as appropriate.
- Client is educated about pain and managing pain as part of treatment, as appropriate.
- Client is educated about habilitation or rehabilitation techniques to help him or her become more functionally independent, as appropriate.
- Client is educated about other available resources, and when necessary, how to obtain further care, services, or treatment to meet his or her identified needs.
- Education includes information about client's responsibilities in his or her care.
- Education includes self-care activities, as appropriate.
- Discharge instructions are given to client and those responsible for providing continuing care.
- Academic education is provided for a hospitalized child or adolescent, either directly by the hospital or through other arrangements, when appropriate.

Source: Adapted from Joint Commission on Accreditation of Healthcare Organizations (JCAHO). *Comprehensive Accreditation Manual for Hospital: The Official Handbook.* JCAHO Patient and Family Education (PFE 2001) Standards. Oakbrook Terrace, IL.

Federal Requirements for Discharge Planning Process

- Hospitals must identify at an early stage of hospitalization all Medicare clients who are likely to suffer adverse health consequences on discharge if there is no planning.
- The hospital must provide a discharge planning evaluation.
- A registered nurse, social worker, or other qualified person must develop or supervise development of the evaluation.
- Discharge planning must include an evaluation of the likelihood of needing posthospital services and of the availability of the services.
- The evaluation must include the client's capacity for self-care or the possibility of the client being cared for in the environment from which the client entered the hospital.
- The evaluation must be completed on a timely basis so that appropriate arrangements for posthospital care are made before discharge.
- The discharge planning evaluation must be in the client's medical record.

This type of transitional care and coordination has proven to be cost-effective and has improved the quality of client care.

Communication between the client, family, and healthcare agencies is essential for effective discharge planning. According to HIPAA, discussing client information with the family members or friends is only permitted if it directly affects them and the client agrees. The information reflecting client approval needs to be documented in the client's record. Family members involved in discharge planning are helpful, as they can inform the healthcare team about cultural traditions, financial issues, unsafe living conditions, and support for the client at home. The nurse establishes a dialogue between these various people and coordinates the discharge plan before the client leaves the hospital. When referrals to other agencies are necessary, these are initiated before the client is discharged. The nurse, if there is no discharge planner available, is responsible for coordinating such referrals—including signed physician's orders for specific care, treatments, or medications.

ADAPTATION TO HOME CARE

Home Care Definition

The term *home health care* refers to all services that promote, maintain, or restore physical, social, or emotional health to clients in the home setting. Home care is provided in the individual's residence. For a smooth transition from hospital to home, the home care coordinator communicates with the family members and the home health nurse. Home care is also provided to clients in long-term care or residential care facilities in which there are no or limited staff members.

A variety of health workers are needed to provide comprehensive home care services to clients and families. Table 6-1 presents an overview of healthcare providers and their major responsibilities. The list and responsibilities are not inclusive; consult an additional home care reference for more detailed information.

TABLE 6-1 Home Health Team

Healthcare Provider	Major Responsibilities
Registered Nurse	Performs as a case manager. Initiates physician-ordered plan of care; performs assessment, planning, and interventions for needed home care skills and teaching. Assists in evaluating treatment regimens for all services.
Home Care Aide	Performs hygienic care, skin care, exercise, ambulation, dressing, and elimination skills. Some may prepare and serve meals. Assists in maintaining a clean, safe, client environment (e.g., client's bedroom).
Homemaker	Maintains the home environment, shops for and prepares meals, transports client, and runs errands.
Social Worker	Assists in planning for home care needs, instructs in use of social and community services and resources. Provides information relative to long-term planning and respite care in the home.
Physical Therapist	Evaluates environment in preparation for client's return home. Assists with safety adaptations for the home, instructs in exercise program, gait training, and use of special adaptive equipment.
Occupational Therapist	Instructs in activities of daily living, grooming, upper extremity strengthening, function activities, and use of adaptive equipment.
Speech Therapist	Evaluates swallowing and chewing ability; memory; assists with increasing communication techniques for client, family, and healthcare provider; and provides speech reeducation program.
Registered Dietician	Evaluates and provides for nutritional needs of client. Plans and instructs in appropriate diet.
Physician	Prescribes medical plan of treatment. Writes specific prescriptions for medications, diet, supplies, nursing interventions, and therapist parameters.
Licensed Vocational Nurse	Provides skilled nursing care similar to a Home Care Aide under RN supervision. They are not used by all agencies because of limited independent activities allowed.

Referral to Home Care

It is necessary for nurses in all settings to be aware of the referral process and the type of client who should be referred for home care services. Although most home care clients have been hospitalized, it is not a prerequisite for service. Physicians, individual clients, families, residential care administrators, and friends may refer a client by calling a home health agency and requesting service. A physician's approval is needed for reimbursement. An evaluation visit is made by the RN or PT, who act as case managers, to determine if service is needed, and if so, an appropriate plan of care is established. Speech therapists are not allowed to do initial evaluations in California and in most other states.

Most hospitals have a designated protocol for making referrals, which is described in the hospital policy manual. In most hospitals it is the discharge planner, case manager, or social worker who makes the referral. The nurse may alert the appropriate person to the client's need for home care. It is essential that the nurse provide complete and thorough information about the client's condition, including physical and psychosocial needs. This information is documented on a standard referral form or on an official form from the Department of Health and Human Services and sent to the home health agency. Accurate information and orders are needed to facilitate a smooth transition from hospital to home. Incomplete or inadequate communication could mean a lapse in service and inadequate care for the client.

All age groups use home health services. The criteria for referral depends on various factors, such as client need, agency protocol, and insurance criteria. Since the elderly on Medicare represent the largest segment of the population using home care services, it is important that all nurses know Medicare eligibility criteria for home visits. This ensures that accurate information is given to the client and family. In addition to eligibility criteria, many regulations govern the type and frequency of care. Since these regulations are subject to change and interpretation by the fiscal intermediaries who administer Medicare insurance, frequent review of Medicare regulations should be done. Eligibility for another funding agency, Medicaid, differs from state to state. It is the nurse's responsibility to be familiar with these policies. Each individual insurance company reimburses for services at different rates and for different levels of service. Each insurance plan needs to be reviewed to determine reimbursement.

Transition From Hospital to Home

A smooth transition from hospital to home depends on an appropriate discharge plan. The shorter duration in hospital stay requires a thorough, efficient discharge plan that must be initiated at the time of hospital admission. Identifying the client's needs and resources before planning for discharge results in a realistic plan. Since any illness causes additional stress in the family and necessitates an adaptive coping response, the needs of the family or significant other must be included in the teaching and discharge plan. Discharge planning is completed during meetings of the interdisciplinary healthcare team. A representative member of each discipline discusses the client's progress and individual needs for discharge. In addition, accurate and comprehensive documentation must accompany the physician's plan of treatment to ensure a smooth transition. A description of the client at discharge should be provided; include physical assessment findings, ability to assist in ADLs, adaptive devices needed for care, and a brief summary of hospitalization. These data greatly assist in the transition from hospital to home.

Home Health Care Changes

Home health care, a rapidly growing field of health care, has developed in response to recent changes in political and social forces in the United States. These changes have demanded that nurses expand their knowledge about home care and acquire skills needed to provide safe, competent care to clients in the home setting.

Several factors have contributed to the emergence of home health care as a primary delivery system. The fastest growing segment of the American population is 85 years of age or older. The elderly constitute the largest proportion of population currently using home healthcare services. Nine percent of those 65 to 74 years of age and 25% of those 75 years and older require some type of home care service. Many younger clients are receiving home care visits as a direct result of early discharge from hospitals. Home care visits are funded by private insurance companies and are a cost-effective measure for providing nursing care.

Another factor is the changing structure and role of the American family. Traditionally, women have provided health care for the family members at home. With more women working outside the home, the demand for home health services has increased.

Political factors have had an effect on healthcare delivery patterns. A cost-containment measure initiated by the federal government in 1983 to curb rising costs of hospitalized Medicare clients drastically altered the extent of care administered in the hospital setting. A prospective payment system (DRGs), rather than a retrospective payment system, was implemented. This resulted in shorter hospital stays for Medicare clients. With the shorter stays came a dramatic increase in the need for professional services to care for high-acuity clients in the home. Additional types of services have also had to be added to the home care system to meet the needs of these clients. Even more changes occurred with healthcare reform in the 1990s. Health maintenance organizations (HMOs) and reimbursement policies directly affected the home healthcare agencies.

Documentation using Outcome and Assessment Information Set (OASIS) is regulated by the Health Care Financing Administration. The OASIS system was developed by The Center for Health Policy Research in Denver, Colorado. Oasis C has added 30 process meaures that will affect outcomes. The new client assessment information was also used to develop a prospective payment system for home health agencies, which went into effect October 2000. Home visits for maternity clients and children under 18 do not require completion of these forms.

Client Teaching

Client teaching is an essential component of both hospital and home care. Since clients are discharged earlier and with a higher acuity level, the client and his or her family are expected to accept more responsibility for follow-up care. It is essential for client teaching to begin in the hospital and provide a description of the disease or condition and the treatment regimen. The client and family should be instructed in skills and treatments necessary to restore health and prevent other illness or complications. The home health nurse builds on the teaching plan, with the main emphasis on adapting care in the home environment. Continuity of care depends on comprehensive communication between the discharging and home care agencies.

Adapting Care to the Home Setting

The client is often a passive recipient of care in the hospital. In the home setting, on the other hand, the client is in control—it is his or her environment. That is, the environment is determined by the client and family according to their needs, desires, values, and resources. The nurse is a guest in this environment, which requires flexibility in adapting to a variety of situations.

In the hospital, equipment is readily available. Nurses perform procedures or treatments and provide 24-hour-a-day coverage of nursing care. In the home, equipment must be ordered or improvised, and the emphasis is on teaching the client or caregiver self-care activities. The home care nurse must become very creative in adapting and improvising equipment and techniques.

When a client referral is received by a home health agency, a nurse or physical therapist makes an initial admission visit. This visit includes a thorough assessment of the client, family, and home environment. The home environment is evaluated for safety, and the client and family are assessed for knowledge of safety and emergency procedures. Assessment of the client includes physical, emotional, psychologic, and economic status. The home is assessed for any adaptations that must be made to enable the client to function optimally in his or her environment. Family members are assessed for understanding of the client's illness or needs; cultural, ethnic, and health beliefs and values; ability to cope with the current situation; the physical, emotional, and spiritual needs of family members; financial resources; and knowledge of how to use community resources. A complete list of assessment parameters for each of these areas is included on the initial assessment form.

CULTURAL AWARENESS

The Developmental Disabilities and Bill of Rights Act of 2000 defined culturally competent services as services that are (a) provided in a manner responsive to the beliefs, interpersonal styles, attitudes, language, and behaviors of individuals; and (b) provided in a manner that demonstrates respect for individual dignity, personal preference, and cultural differences.

It is essential to remember that all client teaching plans and strategies must consider cultural aspects in the planning phase. Cultural differences affect client's open-mindedness to client education and their willingness to listen to the teaching and then be compliant with the changes that need to occur. Cultural differences affect client's attitudes about illness, healthcare workers, and treatment modalities. The Joint Commission has mandated that there must be greater awareness of diversity, attention to the needs of special populations, and staff training to meet their needs.

When taking cultural competence into account, nurses should consider the following to make client teaching more effective:

- Be aware of own cultural biases and prejudices.
- Become familiar with the core cultural values of client groups.
- Whenever possible, use a translator to convey information.

All cultures have health beliefs about illness: what causes it and what cures it, as well as who they will allow to treat them. It is important for nurses to understand each culture's differences, as it will impact the client teaching process. Table 6-2 summarizes cultural beliefs that may have an effect on health care and client teaching.

Included in the discharge plan is a discharge summary. This summary includes an overall review of hospitalization activities and the client's learning needs. There is a statement indicating how well the learning needs have been met, the client teaching completed, short- and long-term goals of care, referrals made, and coordinated care plan to be implemented after discharge.

Since 1988, hospitals have been mandated by federal requirements to provide a discharge planning process for all Medicare clients. These same requirements now apply to all clients within hospitals in the United States.

TABLE 6-2 Cultural Beliefs Affecting Client Teaching

Ethnic Group	Cultural Beliefs
Asian/Pacific Islander	Extended family has large influence on client.
	Older family members are honored and respected, and their authority is unquestioned.
	Oldest male is decision maker and spokesman.
	Strong emphasis on avoiding conflict and direct confrontation.
	Respect authority and do not disagree with healthcare recommendations—but they may not follow recommendations.
Chinese	Chinese clients will not discuss symptoms of mental illness or depression because they believe this behavior reflects on family; therefore, it may produce shame and guilt.
	Use herbalists, spiritual healers, and physicians for care.
Japanese	Believe physical contact with blood, skin diseases, and corpses will cause illness.
	Believe improper care of the body, including poor diet and lack of sleep, causes illness.

(Continued)

TABLE 6-2 Cultural Beliefs Affecting Client Teaching (*Continued*)

Ethnic Group	Cultural Beliefs
	Believe in healers, herbalists, and physicians for healing, and energy can be restored with acupuncture and acupressure.
	Use group decision making for health concerns.
Hindu and Muslim	Indians and Pakistanis do not acknowledge a diagnosis of severe emotional illness or mental retardation because it reduces the chance of other family members getting married.
Vietnamese	Vietnamese accept mental health counseling and interventions, particularly when they have established trust with the healthcare worker.
Hispanic	Older family members are consulted on issues involving health and illness.
	Patriarchal family—men make decisions for family.
	Illness is viewed as God's will or divine punishment resulting from sinful behavior.
	Prefer to use home remedies and consult folk healers known as *curanderos* rather than traditional Western healthcare providers.
African American	Family and church oriented.
	Extensive extended family bonds.
	Key family member is consulted for important health-related decisions.
	Illness is a punishment from God for wrongdoing, or is due to voodoo, spirits, or demons.
	Health prevention is through good diet, herbs, rest, cleanliness, and laxatives to clean the system.
	Wear copper and silver bracelets to prevent illness.
Native American	Oriented to the present.
	Value cooperation.
	Value family and spiritual beliefs.
	Strong ties to family and tribe.
	Believe state of health exists when client lives in total harmony with nature.
	Illness is viewed as an imbalance between the ill person and natural or supernatural forces.
	Use medicine man or woman known as a shaman.
	Illness is prevented through elaborate religious rituals.

NURSING DIAGNOSES

The following nursing diagnoses are appropriate to include in a client care plan when the components are related to establishing and maintaining a client teaching and discharge planning.

NURSING DIAGNOSIS	RELATED FACTORS
Impaired Communication Verbal	Cognitive impairment, auditory impairment, language barrier
Denial	Attempt to disavow need to alter lifestyle by avoiding client teaching
Ineffective Health Maintenance	Cultural and religious beliefs, information misinterpretation, lack of education, lack of motivation, inadequate healthcare services
Deficient Knowledge	Inadequate understanding of condition, misinformation, language differences
Noncompliance	Impaired ability to perform tasks, poor self-esteem, lack of motivation
Relocation Stress Syndrome	Changes associated with transfer between facilities or facility and home, effects of losses associated with moving, stress in family members
Ineffective Role Performance	Change in self-perception of role; change in others' perception of role as a result of an altered health status, which leads to denial of learning need

CLEANSE HANDS The single most important nursing action to decrease the incidence of hospital-based infections is hand hygiene. *Remember to wash your hands or use antibacterial gel before and after each and every client contact.*

IDENTIFY CLIENT Before every procedure, check two forms of client identification, not including room number. These actions prevent errors and conform to The Joint Commission standards.

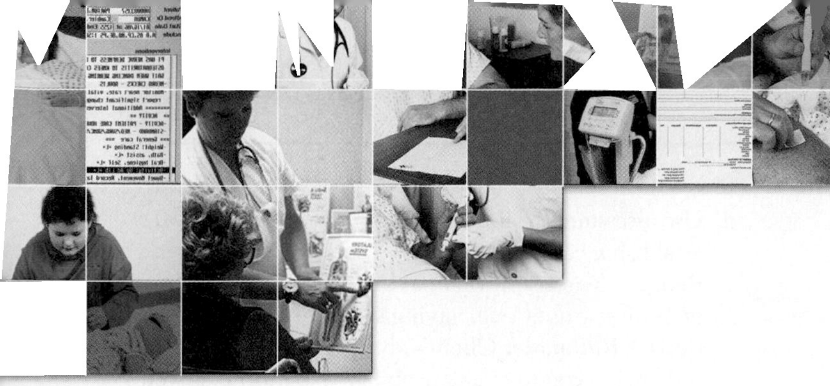

Chapter 6

UNIT 1

Client Education

Nursing Process Data

ASSESSMENT Data Base

- Assess high-risk criteria for client education.
- Determine the need for client teaching program.
- Identify client learning style and preferences.
- Assess knowledge and skill level of client.
- Assess motivation to learn.
- Assess readiness to learn.
- Identify physical or emotional barriers that may affect client's ability to participate in teaching plan.
- Identify health beliefs and practices.
- Assess developmental and educational level of client.
- Determine appropriate methodology for client teaching sessions.
- Identify appropriate adjunctive materials, such as audiovisual aids, to enhance learning process.
- Assess appropriate setting for the individual client.
- Determine family members or significant others who will be involved in client education.

PLANNING Objectives

- To develop a plan using the nursing process framework and adult learning principles
- To determine learning needs and establish learning objectives
- To select appropriate teaching strategies
- To increase client's knowledge to promote compliance with health regimen
- To encourage client participation in goal selection and implementation program
- To encourage client to acknowledge individual responsibility for health behaviors and health status
- To improve client's ability to make informed decisions affecting health status
- To facilitate behavioral changes that are conducive to optimum health status
- To provide continuity of care when the client is moving from one healthcare setting to another

IMPLEMENTATION Procedures

EVALUATION Expected Outcomes

- Client's knowledge regarding his or her health status has increased.
- Client's ability to make informed and effective health-related decisions, based on accurate information and awareness of self, has improved.
- Effective use of the healthcare delivery system has been promoted.
- Continuity of care and information exchange has occurred between health agencies or between the hospital and client's home and family.
- The nurse has evaluated his or her teaching effectiveness and revised the plan, teaching style, and content as necessary.
- Increased compliance to medical regimen as demonstrated by client's ability to manage condition/disease process.

Pearson Nursing Student Resources

Find additional review materials at
nursing.pearsonhighered.com

Prepare for success with NCLEX®-style practice questions and Skill Checklists

Collecting Data and Establishing Rapport

Equipment

Client teaching plan

Room or suitable setting to complete assessment

Adjunct materials, such as audiovisual equipment, charts, and illustrations

Written materials, such as outlines or other handouts

Equipment for demonstration and return demonstration

Documentation forms: Kardex, client's chart, electronic forms

Preparation

1. Develop a client teaching plan utilizing the following information: assessment findings, expected learning outcomes, teaching strategies, teaching materials, education methods.
   a. Use adult (and/or age-appropriate) learning principles.
   b. Use communication and interpersonal relationship skills. ▶ ***Rationale:*** To encourage client's participation in the plan.
   c. Use a nonjudgmental approach. ▶ ***Rationale:*** A nonjudgmental attitude assists client to be honest with feelings.
      1. Use "how" questions to facilitate communication. ▶ ***Rationale:*** "How" is more effective than "why" in a question, as "why" tends to set up a defensive reaction to the question.
      2. Use verbal and nonverbal behavior and congruency of behavior to build relationship with the client.
   d. Use assessment (observation) skills. ▶ ***Rationale:*** To establish a baseline for client teaching.
   e. Request demonstration of a skill previously learned or currently used (e.g., giving self an insulin injection). ▶ ***Rationale:*** Client's ability to demonstrate skill assists you to evaluate ability to perform, as well as mastery of previous teaching principles.
2. Develop an evaluation plan that determines extent of client learning goals.

Procedure

1. Identify personal characteristics.
   a. Age, sex, developmental level.
   b. Educational level.
   c. Marital status.
   d. Family composition and living situation.
   e. Ethnic group and cultural practices pertinent to language skill and preference.
2. Identify resources available; both personal and community.
3. Identify values and attitudes toward self and others having his or her particular disease or condition.
4. Assess baseline knowledge—anatomy and physiology (normal and disease-related) and the disease process—by asking specific questions.
5. Assess current knowledge and ability to perform specific skills.
6. Assess patterns of coping.
   a. Past experiences of self and others in relation to the disease.
   b. Perception by client of how ill he or she is at this time.
   c. Reactions to stress and ways of managing anxiety.
   d. Current level of self-management.
   e. Willingness of client to change behavior.

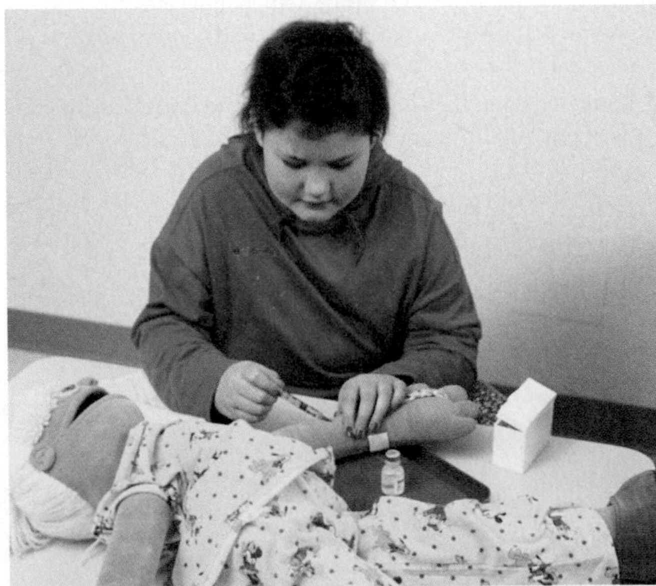

▲ When collecting data to determine learning needs and strategies, use age-appropriate materials.

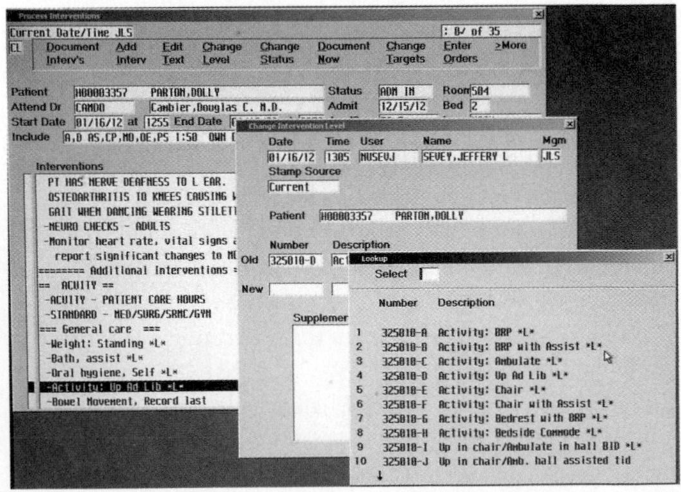

▲ Obtain data from Client Profile to prepare teaching plan.

Determining Readiness to Learn

Procedure

1. Determine client's physiologic readiness.
   a. Degree of physical comfort of client (level of pain), level of alertness, ability to concentrate, degree of interest.
   b. Acuteness of the illness and its influence on client's ability to learn.
   c. Environmental factors that may affect client's degree of readiness.
   d. Safety issues and need for supervision.
2. Evaluate client's psychologic readiness.
   a. State of client's feelings and their influence on receptivity to learning. ▸ ***Rationale:*** An angry and hostile client is not going to absorb information until his or her anger is acknowledged or worked through.
   b. Psychologic barriers (for example, the presence of denial) and their influence on the learning process.
   c. Client's intellectual capacity and level of comprehension.
3. Assess client's willingness to make changes and be compliant with the teaching plan.
4. Assess family's ability and willingness to participate in teaching.
   a. Determine willingness to participate in actual hospital instruction.
   b. Determine cognitive ability to understand instruction.
   c. Evaluate the extent of time and active participation of the family during instruction.
   d. Assess the interaction of the client and family during client teaching. ▸ ***Rationale:*** This will provide data on potential compliance and noncompliance issues related to the teaching plan.
5. Assess the extent of support and actual care the family members will provide for the client at home. ▸ ***Rationale:*** This will determine the extent of the instruction necessary for the family.

Clinical Alert

The Joint Commission's Standards for Patient and Family Education require that client's learning needs, preferred learning styles, literacy level, educational level, language spoken and understood, and learning readiness are assessed.

Assessing Learning Needs

Procedure

1. Assess if client has learning needs related to diagnosis, hospitalization, surgical procedures, or treatments.
   a. Ask specific questions relative to what physician has told client related to specific learning need(s).
   b. Ask client what he/she is most interested in learning about specific learning need(s).
   c. Ask client to tell you in his/her own words what they know about specific learning need(s).

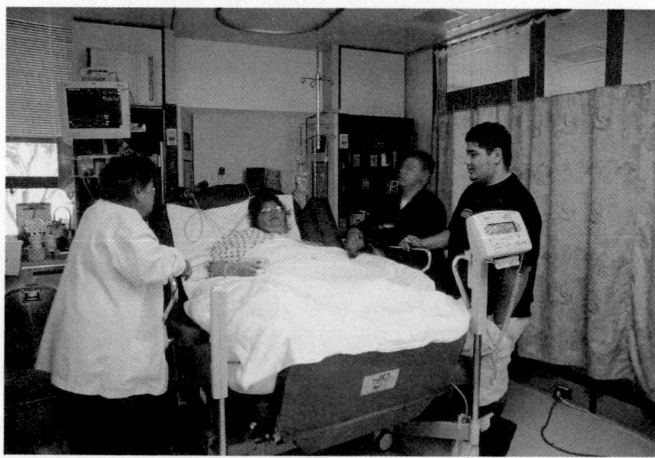

▲ Include family in teaching, particularly if they will play a role in caring for client.

2. Interview client to determine what his/her daily life is like. ▸ ***Rationale:*** The information will assist you in determining impact of changes in client's lifestyle brought on by illness or condition. This will help you determine how to approach the teaching plan.
   a. Ask client to describe his/her usual daily routine.
   b. Determine whether anything has changed with this pattern since illness began.
   c. Describe hobbies or sports activities in which client participates.
   d. Describe normal workday and what activities are involved with employment, if still working.
   e. Discuss usual family responsibilities. Will the family be involved with his/her care?
3. Determine client's age and developmental level. ▸ ***Rationale:*** Knowing client's developmental level is necessary to provide the most effective teaching strategies.
4. Determine client's learning style. ▸ ***Rationale:*** This will assist in matching the most appropriate teaching strategy for client education.
   a. Ask questions related to what time of day he/she learns best.
   b. Determine whether he/she learns best by reading, listening, hands-on learning, or a combination of styles.
   c. Use a commercial learning style inventory, if available.

5. Complete a cultural assessment. ▸ ***Rationale:*** To develop a culturally responsive teaching plan based on client's beliefs.
   a. Determine client's belief about illness.
   b. Determine how strong the client's belief system is relative to his/her traditional culture.
   c. Determine whether he/she uses folk medicine practices and uses a traditional healer. Clients from Asia, Africa, and South America are more likely to maintain this cultural component of their former country.
   d. Identify whether traditional dietary habits are practiced in the home. If so, these should be included in the teaching plan, particularly nutritional counseling.
6. Determine client's educational and literacy levels. ▸ ***Rationale:*** Clients may seem disinterested in learning when in fact they do not understand what is being said and are embarrassed to ask. This can lead to missed physician appointments, noncompliance with treatment or medication usage, and even disability.
   a. Determine client's reading level by measuring his/her reading and comprehension skills.
   b. Use a test of reading and comprehension to obtain a client profile before beginning teaching process. ▸ ***Rationale:*** To determine most appropriate written material for client.
7. Assess client's ability to speak and read English.
   a. Determine whether client requires an interpreter during assessment of learning needs and teaching process.
   b. Ensure that words you use in client's language are correct for the situation.
   c. Do not use slang that could be misunderstood.
   d. Use simple words and phrases to allow interpreter to relate the intent of your statement.

Family Assessment is an integral part of planning an effective teaching plan if family members will be affected by, or part of, the care of the client. Include the following information in the assessment:

- Which family members will be involved with care of client?
- Has client approved that family members be given confidential medical information?
- Can family members provide necessary care or will additional support be necessary?
- Does home environment support client's care needs?
- Are any changes to home necessary to provide a safe environment?
- Do family members speak English and have basic literacy skills?
- Are there any cultural belief conflicts that could inhibit adequate care in home?
- Do family members interact in a supportive manner with the client?
- What do family members know about the client's condition? Do they need additional teaching?

8. Use assessment data and assessment instrument to jointly determine client's learning needs: educational, physical, psychosocial, and financial needs.
9. Formulate needs as goals.
10. Prioritize learning needs or goals.
11. Review with client alternative resources available to accomplish goals.
12. Determine ability of facility, family, staff, or multidisciplinary team to meet goals or learning needs.
13. Identify potential barriers to learning.
    a. Physical: visual or auditory, pain level, literacy level, reading level.
    b. Emotional barriers: stress or anxiety, inability to focus on information.
    c. Language or culture: ability to understand and speak English, beliefs about health, folk practices, or communication style differences.
14. Obtain verbal or written contract with client for educational program.
15. Refer client to other resources or agencies when appropriate.

Clinical Alert

Agencies contract with telephone language lines to provide interpreter services. These services are available through AT&T Language Line Services and Pacific Interpreters Inc. on a 24-hour basis and in over 140 languages.

Determining Reading Grade Level

Readability Formulas

The Fry Formula assesses three samples of 100 words from different parts of a written handout and is useful to determine client's reading grade level. The Simplified Measure of Gobbledygook (SMOG) formula is very similar. The Fry Formula plots the average number of syllables and average number of sentences on a graph that then shows grade level. The SMOG formula also measures the number of syllables in a particular sample of written material, which is then converted by a chart that determines reading grade level.

The Rapid Estimation of Adult Literacy in Medicine (REALM) reading test can be easily administered in a few minutes. This test provides the reading grade level for clients who read below ninth-grade level. Words the client reads are all common health terms. The client reads as many words as he/she can correctly pronounce. A chart is used to convert raw scores obtained from word reading into a reading grade estimate.

Source: REALM, Department of Internal Medicine, Louisiana State University, Baton Rouge, LA.

Determining Appropriate Teaching Strategy

Procedure

1. Consider the following factors when determining appropriate strategy:
   a. Input from client about how he or she learns best.
   b. Specific task or nature of the content to be transmitted and how it is best learned.
   c. Client attention span and retention ability.
   d. Reading level of client.
   e. Teaching materials and resources available. Electronic material is available for client education; it is used particularly for medications, diagnostic tests, and diagnoses.
   f. Time, availability, skills, and abilities of staff; appropriate use of paraprofessional and professional staff.
   g. Participation by members of other healthcare disciplines as part of a team.
   h. Determination of most appropriate time for teaching.
2. Use appropriate reading material for individual client.
   a. Determine reading level of written material.
   b. Use a readability formula to determine most appropriate written information for client.
   c. Use brochures, handouts, and written material written at a sixth-grade level if client has low literacy skills.
   ▸ ***Rationale:*** Seventy-five percent of the adults in the United States should be able to read the material.
   d. Use short, common words in written material.
   ▸ ***Rationale:*** Medical terminology may be misunderstood.

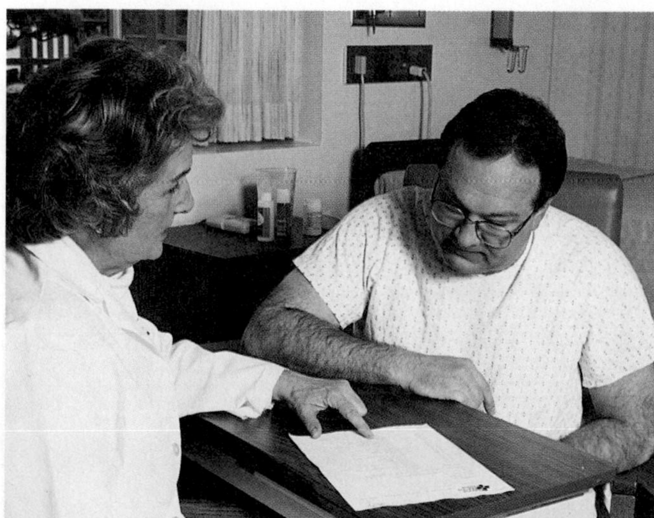

▲ Determine which teaching strategy will be most effective for client.

   e. Make sentences 10 words or less and written in active voice.
   f. Make paragraphs short with one focus.
   g. Use large type (fonts) and lowercase letters.
   ▸ ***Rationale:*** Large font size is easier for clients with visual impairments or elderly clients, and lowercase letters are easier to read.
   h. Use diagrams and photos whenever possible to make a point.
   i. Set realistic goals and only one or two objectives for each teaching session. ▸ ***Rationale:*** Overloading client with information will not allow him/her to master information necessary for compliance.
   j. Ensure client completes a return demonstration, if appropriate. ▸ ***Rationale:*** This assists you to determine the extent to which client understands information presented. The greater the understanding and ability to perform a particular skill, the greater the compliance to treatment.
3. Determine which type of teaching strategy will be effective in a given situation.
   a. Group process: use of principles from group dynamics, mental health, or other related fields to enhance learning or behavior changes in a small group setting.
   b. Lecture–discussion: presentation of content in a didactic fashion with opportunity for questions and interaction during or at the conclusion of the presentation.
   c. Demonstration–return demonstration: demonstration (videotape) by the instructor with practice by the learner and return demonstration of mastery of the skill.
   d. Role playing: assumption of roles by various participants or learners for the purpose of clarifying various aspects of a situation.
   e. Games: structured (age-appropriate) game situation with rules designed for the learner to accomplish specific educational objectives.

Components of a Teaching Plan

- Client learning needs
- Expected learning outcomes
- Teaching content organized from simple to complex
- Teaching methods and tools
- Barriers to learning and readiness to learn
- Evaluation tools

EVIDENCE-BASED PRACTICE

Silent Clients

A qualitative study in Finland (N = 38 patients, N = 19 nurses) found that 18 clients who were identified as aloof or silent spoke little about themselves and followed the lead of the nurse. The nurse often used communication techniques that did not facilitate communication and were nontherapeutic. The study concluded that client's quietness or silence in client education settings "was complex, supported by the hospital's institutional standard, nurses' lack of expertise, and client's restrictive and face-saving speech." This underscores the necessity that client education be client focused, based on client's knowledge, experience, and preferences, rather than comply to a preset standardized, structured format.

Source: Kettunen, T., Poskiparta, M., Liimatainen, L., Sjögren, A., & Karhila, P. (2001, May). Taciturn patients in health counseling at a hospital: passive recipients or active participators? *Qualitative Health Research, 11*(3), 399–422. From Mynatt, S. (2002, January). Patient taciturnity in health counselling was understood in terms of 4 participation frames. *Evidence-Based Nursing,* 5(1), 30.

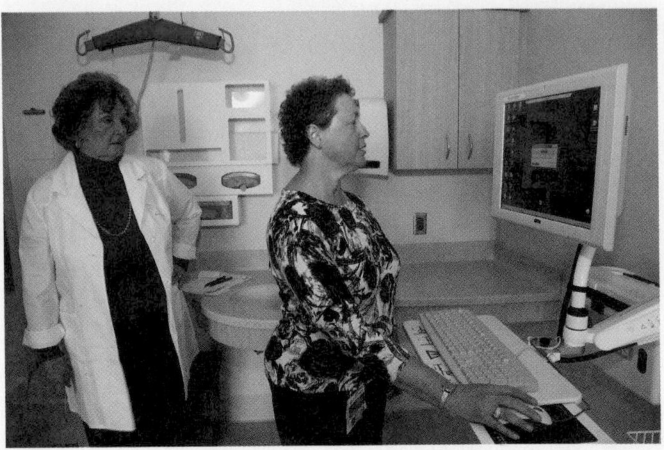

▲ Client education using computerized program assists nurse in providing information that is relevant to client's needs.

4. Select appropriate teaching adjuncts based on developmental level, learning style, and reading literacy.

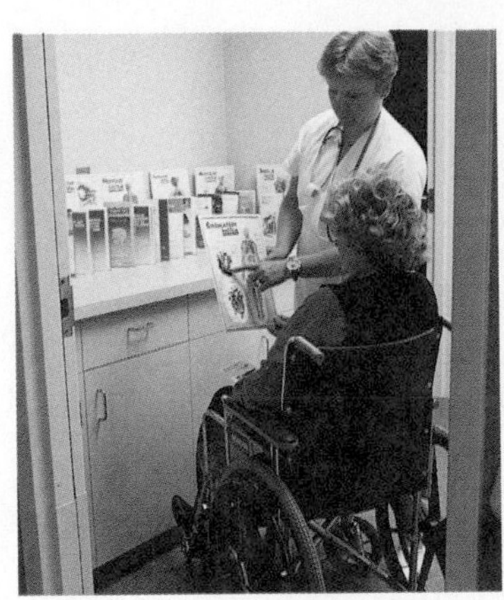

◀ After selecting the appropriate setting, choose the teaching adjuncts.

   a. Videotape or videocassette programs.
   b. Films; slide and tape presentations.
   c. Diagrams, charts, and illustrations.
   d. Programmed instruction materials, i.e., computer/Internet.
   e. Books.
   f. Pamphlets and other written handouts.
5. Provide language-specific material for non–English-speaking clients.
   a. Photos.
   b. Models of specific body parts.
   c. Audio tapes in specific language.

Selecting the Educational Setting

Procedure

1. Choose an appropriate setting based on selected teaching strategy and available facility space.
2. Evaluate types of setting most appropriate to individual client and family learning needs.
3. Consider an informal setting.
   a. Spontaneous teaching interactions between nurse and client can occur at any time in any setting.
   b. Usually no formal plan or evaluation tool is used.
4. Consider a formal setting.
   a. Teaching is carried out in a specified area of the facility such as an in-service classroom.
   b. Teaching can occur independently, such as with audiovisual programmed instruction modules, or in a group setting.
   c. Formal plan for the teaching program includes written goals, objectives, teaching strategies, content, and evaluation method.

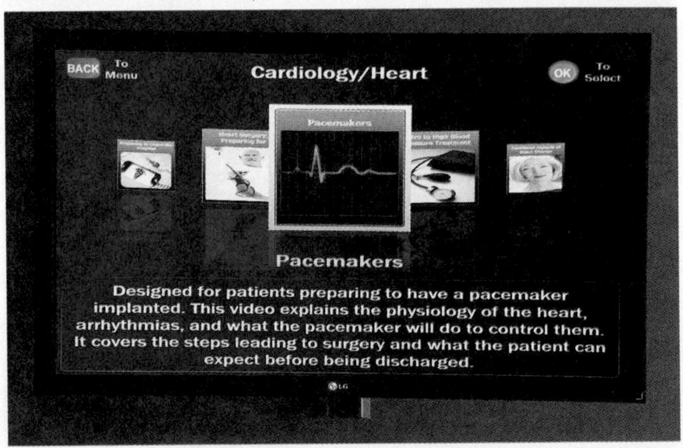

▲ Preoperative teaching using computerized module.

Implementing the Teaching Strategy

Procedure

1. Gather teaching materials appropriate for client's learning needs and teaching strategy.
2. Sit with client in designated setting, and establish a warm and accepting relationship. ▶ ***Rationale:*** This is conducive to teaching and assists client in learning.
3. Specify previously established mutual goals and behavioral objectives of the program. ▶ ***Rationale:*** Mutually agreed-on goals promote acceptance of teaching strategy by the client.
4. Clarify or reclarify contract, agreements, or expected outcomes with individual or group. ▶ ***Rationale:*** Beginning at the level of understanding of person or group facilitates the process.
5. Assess teaching situation for any modifications needed and adjust plans accordingly.
6. Teach content or components of the plan to client. ▶ ***Rationale:*** Sticking to the plan and not deviating or going off on a tangent reinforces your commitment to help client master the content.
7. Use appropriate communication skills throughout session. ***Rationale:*** Therapeutic communication techniques enhance learning environment.
8. Request feedback (evaluation interchange) during teaching process. ***Rationale:*** Feedback lets you know how client is understanding content and allows for modification as indicated.
9. Plan for short teaching sessions on a frequent basis.
10. Adhere to agreed-upon starting and ending times; negotiate any changes. ▶ ***Rationale:*** This encourages client to trust you.
11. Provide closure to teaching situation by summarizing and reiterating agreements made, actions to be taken, or subsequent events to follow.
12. Provide positive reinforcement if not done previously. ▶ ***Rationale:*** This approach increases self-esteem and encourages learning in client.
13. Terminate teaching session by establishing time for next client contact.
14. Do post-assessment of your own participation, and plan for corrections and improvements in presentation. ▶ ***Rationale:*** Ongoing evaluation assists in final step of nursing process evaluation.
15. Reinforce teaching throughout hospitalization.
    a. Use return demonstration of skills frequently throughout hospital stay.
    b. Review teaching content through use of videotapes and reading material.
    c. Provide positive reinforcement for changes in behavior.
    d. Discuss teaching content and written information by asking pertinent questions and providing answers to client's questions.
16. Send teaching plan and written materials home with client and family. Computer-generated written material (medications, tests, diagnosis, etc.) should be discussed verbally, in addition to providing written material.
17. Place copy of written instructions in chart for documentation. Instructions must be signed by client. This stays in chart.
18. Provide copy of teaching plan and written material to home health agency if referral has been made for visiting nurse. ▶ ***Rationale:*** This promotes consistency in information dissemination and reinforces teaching provided to client while hospitalized.
19. Document your teaching on specific client teaching forms, or electronic forms.

    Documentation should include:
    a. Educational assessment/comprehension level.
    b. Knowledge and skill level of learning need(s).
    c. Motivational level (interaction during teaching session).
    d. Learning barriers (language, speech, vision, hearing).
    e. Overall goal achievement.

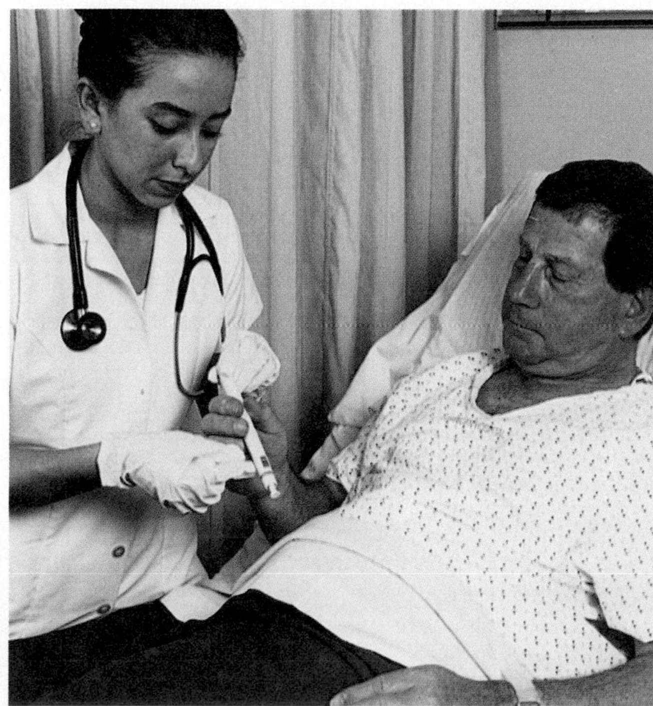

▲ Demonstration is an important component of teaching strategy.

EVIDENCE-BASED PRACTICE

Computer-Generated Client Education

Computer-generated client education has been studied several times. Leaffer and Gonda found that clients taught how to use the Internet to retrieve health information were still using it 90 days later, and 66% of them were taking the information they found on the Internet to their healthcare providers when they had a scheduled visit. More than 50% of the clients stated that using the Internet made them feel more knowledgeable, and thus they were more satisfied with the treatment they received.

Source: Leaffer, T., & Gonda, B. (2000). The Internet: An underutilized tool in patient education. *Computer Nursing, 18,* 47–52. http:///www.medscape.com/viewarticle/478283_print

Baker et al. surveyed 4,764 individuals, and the results indicated that 40% stated they had used the Internet for information or advice about health or health care during the last year. Sixty-seven percent stated that using the Internet improved their understanding of symptoms, conditions, or treatments.

Source: Baker, L., Wagner, T. H., Singer, S., & Bundorf, M. K. (2003). Use of the Internet and e-mail for health care information: results from a national survey. *JAMA, 289*(18), 2400–2406.

Evaluating Teaching/Learning Outcomes

Procedure

1. After demonstrating skill(s), ask client to complete a return demonstration. Evaluate client's ability to perform tasks.
2. Ask client and/or family to explain demonstration using own words.
3. Ask client and/or family specific questions regarding information provided. ▶***Rationale:*** To determine necessity of reinforcing or reteaching information.
4. Develop a simple pre- and posttest to determine client's knowledge base.
5. Develop hypothetical situations for client to problem solve. ▶***Rationale:*** This will help determine client's understanding of disease or condition.
6. Use an evaluation tool, if appropriate. ▶***Rationale:*** Evaluating with a specific tool focuses the evaluation phase better.

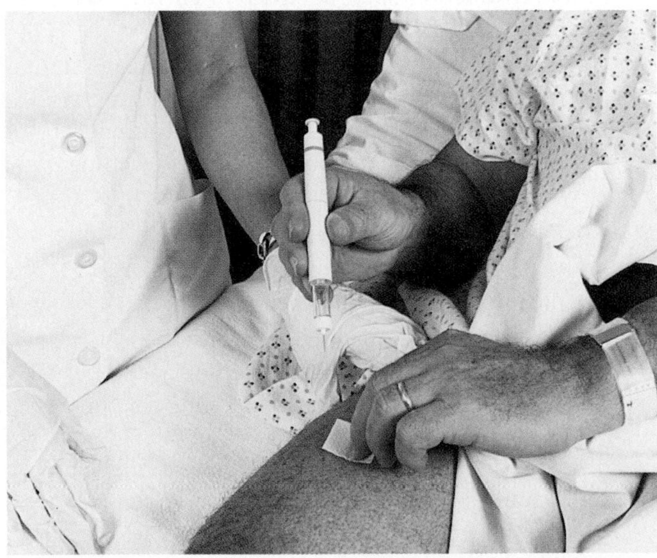

▲ Request a return demonstration to evaluate client understanding.

COMMUNITY HOSPITAL — Client Information

MULTIDISCIPLINARY TEACHING RECORD

INITIAL ASSESSMENT: Interested in health instruction? ___Yes ___No Can patient read? ___Yes ___No

Language used: English___ Other ______ Glasses: Y / N Blind: Y / N Hearing Aid: Y / N Deaf: Y / N

Other______ Signature ______ Date ______

BARRIERS TO LEARNING CODES	NEEDS CODES	TEACHING METHOD CODES	EVALUATION CODES
N = None	1 = Knows well	A = Audiovisual	Patient/Significant Other
C = Cognitive Limitations	2 = Needs review	D = Demonstration	1 = Able to repeat information in own words and/or perform return demonstration. (Education Completed)
E = Emotional	3 = New material	P = Printed Materials	2 = Needs further instructions (Requires entry in Comments)
F = Financial	* = See Comments	MIS = Medication Information Sheet	3 = Unable to retain information or perform return demonstration (Requires entry in Comments)
L = Language		MM = Material Mailed	4 = Not ready to learn (Requires entry in Comments)
M = Motivation/desire		T = Telephone Call	* = See Comments
P = Physical Limitations		V = Verbal Instructions	
R = Religious/Cultural		* = See Comments	
* = See Comments			

TOPIC	*ASSESSMENT*		*PATIENT EDUCATION / EVALUATION*				
DISEASE PROCESS (Specify)	Barrier Code	Needs Code	Person Taught Pt/Other	Teaching Method Codes	**INSTRUCTION**	Evalution Code	**DATE/ INITIALS**
					☐ Cause/effect of Disease Process ☐ Methods of Control ☐ Common Signs/Symptoms to Report ☐ Risk Factors to Modify:______ ☐ Smoking Cessation ☐ ______		
ABILITY TO COPE WITH ILLNESS					☐ Coping Methods and Relaxation Techniques ☐ Spiritual and Emotional Support Provided ☐ Referral If Indicated ______		
DISCHARGE PLANNING/CONTINUING CARE NEEDS					☐ Community Resources ☐ Home Health / SNF Referral ☐ See UM/Social Service Section ☐ ______		
MEDICATIONS					☐ Indications, Dosage, Route, Precautions ☐ Drug/Food Interactions ☐ Adverse Drug Effects ☐ Insulin Injection Technique ☐ MDI Inhaler		
WOUND CARE					☐ Wound Care ☐ Dressing Change ☐ Signs/Symptoms of Infection ☐ Importance of Hand Washing		
ACTIVITY LEVEL					☐ Activity Level ☐ Restrictions/Limitations ☐ ______		
NUTRITION/DIET					☐ Prescribed diet ______ ☐ Hospital Phone # Given for Dietician Referral		
OTHER EDUCATION					☐ ☐		

Comments (Include Date/Time and Initials):

INITIALS	SIGNATURE/TITLE	DEPT.	INITIALS	SIGNATURE/TITLE	DEPT.

▲ Multidisciplinary teaching record.

a. Evaluate forms, format, and types of tools available for evaluation.
   1. Pretest–posttest: measures changes in areas such as knowledge level, attitudes, and values.
   2. Questionnaire: completed by client to report attitudes, certain behaviors, and, most frequently, level of satisfaction with the teaching program.
   3. Physiologic tracers: determined before teaching episode to be the criterion of measurement of success

(e.g., changes in blood pressure values after teaching program for hypertensive clients).

4. Direct observation of behavior changes: report of level of performance during return demonstrations.

b. Choose an evaluative tool based on goals and objectives of the teaching program. ▶ ***Rationale:*** The purpose is to achieve goals, thus evaluative tool should be based on goals.

DOCUMENTATION for Client Education

- Client's learning needs
- Client's learning objectives and goals set by client and staff
- Topics or subjects covered as a part of client education process, such as medications, procedures, dietary plan, activity restrictions, or follow-up care
- Teaching strategies used
- Degree of client's participation in the teaching activity
- Client's reading level
- Client's learning style preference
- Progress in meeting the expected outcomes of teaching
- Client's emotional response to the learning process
- Information or equipment sent home with client
- Client's developmental level

CRITICAL THINKING Application

Expected Outcomes

- Client's knowledge regarding his or her health status has increased.
- Client's ability to make informed and effective health-related decisions, based on accurate information and awareness of self, has improved.
- Effective use of the healthcare delivery system has been promoted.
- Continuity of care and information exchange has occurred between health agencies or between the hospital and client's home and family.
- The nurse has evaluated his or her teaching effectiveness and revised the plan, teaching style, and content as necessary.
- Increased compliance to medical regimen as demonstrated by client's ability to manage condition/disease process.

Unexpected Outcomes	Alternative Actions
Client's health status or treatment compliance has not improved as a result of the teaching program.	• Reevaluate nursing care plan according to the nursing process. • Reassess client for barriers to learning. • Assess client's reading and developmental levels. • Reevaluate testing tool. • Review client's learning style preference. • Determine readability level of written material. • Problem solve with client as to next step to take. • Request assistance from in-service consultant for determining which aspects of the teaching program were not successful and why. • Assist in revising parts of the program and restructure for individual client needs.
Client is hostile to teaching program.	• Attempt to determine underlying reason for hostility. • Terminate this session of teaching program, but tell client you will return tomorrow or at a later time. • Bring another nurse along to assist you in teaching as well as to help you evaluate reason for hostility.
Client's ability to make informed and effective health-related decisions, based on accurate information and awareness of self, has not improved.	• Assist client to take realistic responsibility for ineffective decisions without guilt and shame attached. • Assist client to identify those areas in which he or she is willing to make changes and support development of a plan of action. • Refer to other resources such as groups with like conditions (e.g., cancer, diabetes).

(Continued)

Unexpected Outcomes	Alternative Actions
Client is unable to understand client teaching due to language barrier.	• Identify a volunteer or family member who can be used as an interpreter. • Use the AT&T Language Line. • Obtain teaching material in client's native language. • Use photos or models, or make drawings that depict task to be performed.

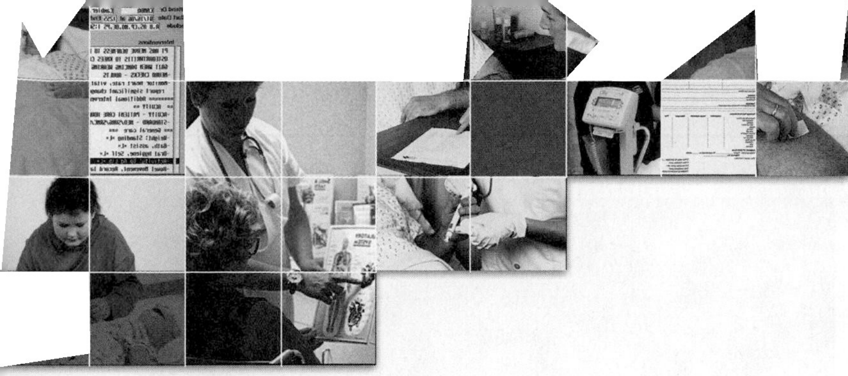

Chapter 6

UNIT 2

Discharge Planning

Nursing Process Data

ASSESSMENT Data Base

- Determine client discharge planning needs.
- Determine if client is in a high-risk category.
- Assess special needs of client for individualized planning.
- Assess need for multidisciplinary healthcare workers.
- Determine information needed for compiling discharge summary.

PLANNING Objectives

- To complete a discharge risk factor assessment when admitting a client
- To determine healthcare workers needed for discharge planning
- To make appropriate referrals for client discharge
- To complete discharge teaching
- To develop a discharge plan
- To complete a discharge summary

IMPLEMENTATION Procedures

EVALUATION Expected Outcomes

- Client's discharge plan is initiated upon admission.
- Client's discharge teaching is completed before discharge.
- Client's plan for discharge is based on identified long-term goals.

Pearson Nursing Student Resources

Find additional review materials at **nursing.pearsonhighered.com**

Prepare for success with NCLEX®-style practice questions and Skill Checklists

Preparing a Client for Discharge

Procedure

1. Obtain admission history, physical, and hospital progress notes.
2. Determine risk factors for discharge planning at time of admission.
3. Refer high-risk clients to discharge coordinator or social service department, if appropriate.
4. Develop discharge plan (if not already completed) including short- and long-term goals in conjunction with physician and client. Plan components should include:
   a. Diet.
   b. Medications.
   c. Treatmnts.
   d. Physical activity limitations.
   e. Signs and symptoms to report.
   f. Follow-up medical care.
   g. Equipment.
   h. Appropriate community resources.
5. Evaluate degree to which client education plan was implemented; reinforce aspects that were incomplete or refer to home agency.
6. Identify need for follow-up care after discharge in conjunction with physician.
7. Make appropriate agency referrals.
8. Complete a discharge referral form, and communicate directly with referral agency about client.

NOTE: Healthcare agency may prefer their own discharge form to be completed rather than documentation in the nurses' notes.

9. Develop written discharge instructions for client and family, including medication administration times, dose, and side effects; treatments to be carried out at home for in a facility, potential side effects or complications from treatments or surgery; when to notify physician regarding symptoms; etc.
10. Update client care plan, and send copy to referral agency.
11. Send client teaching plan and materials to referral agency. ▸ ***Rationale:*** To maintain consistency in client teaching.
12. Document discharge summary.

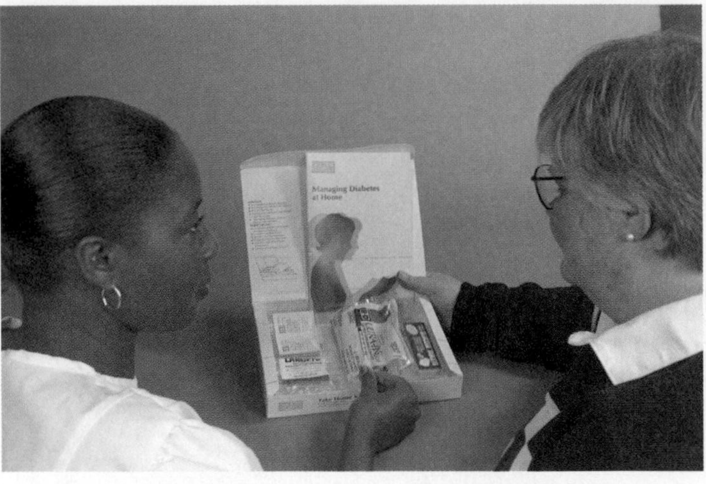

▲ Discharge teaching is an important component of the discharge plan.

DISCHARGE PLAN

Medicare No. ______
MediCal No. ______

Name ______
Admission Date ______ Discharge Date ______

1. Living arrangement: Alone ______ With ______
2. Residence after discharge: ______
   Name and address of nearest relative or friend:
3. Financial situation: Needs assistance ______ Covered ______
4. Agency Referrals: Discharge Coordinator ______
   Home Health: ______

DISCHARGE INSTRUCTIONS

Medications

Name/Dose	Time	Special Instructions

Potential Side Effects ______

Nutrition
Special Diet ______
Restrictions ______

Treatments
Special Equipment Resources and Instructions ______

Discharge Nursing Evaluation

	Independent	Needs Assistance	Dependent	Plan
Personal Needs (ADLs)				
Dressing self				
Bathing				
Skin condition				
Mobility				
Walking				
Bed rest				
Sensory capability				
Glasses				
Hearing aid				
Mental State				
Confused				
Alert				
Oriented				

SUMMARY OF CARE PLAN
Follow-up Care: Call Dr. ______ for appointment in ______ weeks
Telephone No.: ______

Other relevant information

- ❒ Pain rating @ discharge ___/10
- ❒ Pain Pamphlet given
- ❒ Prescription given **–or–**
- ❒ No medication given
- ❒ Additional instructions given

▲ Sample discharge plan form.

Completing a Discharge Summary

Procedure

1. Document a complete physical and psychosocial assessment at time of discharge.
2. Review vital sign ranges, and state latest vital signs.
3. Identify activity level of client.
4. Describe use of adaptive devices or equipment needs.
5. Review client teaching plan. Provide explanation of areas where teaching was adequate and where additional reinforcement is required.
6. Identify prescribed medications, dosage, and administration times. Provide information on client's knowledge of medication.
7. Describe goal achievement based on client care plan. Describe action taken if goal not achieved.
8. Identify referral agencies contacted.
9. Provide information regarding instructions on physician office visits, appointments to healthcare agencies, or support services.
10. Describe client's condition at time of discharge.
11. Document discharge instructions provided to client and family.

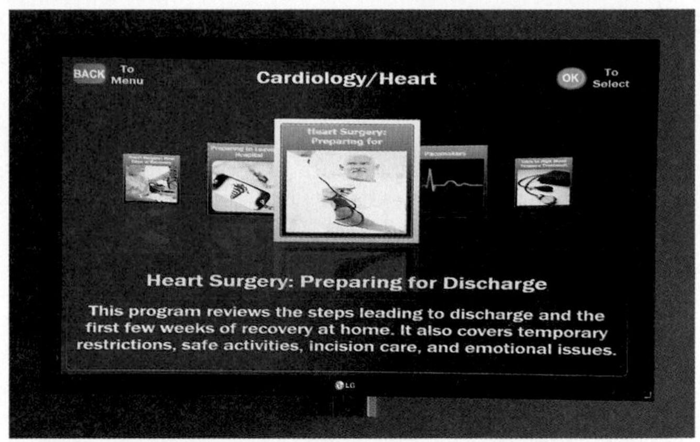

▲ Computer programs provide discharge teaching that is accurate and inclusive.

12. Describe method of discharge (e.g., wheelchair) and person accompanying client at discharge.
13. State means of discharge transportation (e.g., private car, ambulance).
14. Specify discharge facility where client is going.

NOTE: Many facilities have developed forms that combine discharge summaries and client instructions.

DOCUMENTATION for Discharge Planning

- Discharge teaching completed, and additional teaching need(s) necessary after discharge
- Discharge plan completed, including risk factors, short- and long-term goals, and degree to which plan was implemented
- Summary of client care during hospitalization, client interventions provided
- Need for follow-up after discharge
- Referral agencies contacted
- Discharge summary form completed; discharge instructions including medications, treatments, etc.
- Client's condition at time of discharge
- Date, time, location, and mode of discharge

Legal Considerations

Lawsuit Regarding Follow-Up Discharge Teaching: Roberts v. Sisters of St. Francis Health Services (1990)

A 3-year-old presented to the emergency room with an upper respiratory infection. The child was discharged home in the care of her mother. The nurse gave both verbal and written instructions, including a pretyped instruction, for treating a fever. The child's condition worsened a few days later and the mother brought the child to another hospital, where the child subsequently died from meningitis.

The mother brought a lawsuit against the first hospital for failure to provide adequate instructions upon discharge. The suit contended the nurse was negligent for not providing written follow-up instructions to see another physician and not warning the mother to observe for symptoms of meningitis. The court found in favor of the nurse stating she was not negligent and that she provided written instructions for fever treatment and other instructions. The court held that the mother was negligent for not seeking help when the child needed additional care.

Based on this court ruling, remember to give both written instructions and verbal explanations. Written client teaching sheets should be used to reinforce, not replace, discharge teaching. It is recommended that this type of information (teaching sheets) should be written at the sixth-grade reading level. Non–English-speaking clients should have instructions translated into the client's primary language.

CRITICAL THINKING Application

Expected Outcomes	
• Client's discharge plan is initiated upon admission. • Client's discharge teaching is completed before discharge.	• Client's plan for discharge is based on identified long-term goals.
Unexpected Outcomes	**Alternative Actions**
Client is discharged before discharge plan is completed.	• Continue to complete discharge plan, and send to referral agency. • Verbally communicate to referral agency and discuss discharge needs of client.
Discharge plan does not contain adequate data.	• Reassess parameters of a discharge plan, and revise accordingly. • Elicit assistance from another nurse or supervisor to revise discharge plan.
Goals of discharge plan were not accomplished.	• Attempt to assess reason goals were not met. • Reformulate or revise goals so that they are mutually agreed on and more realistic. • Request assistance from expert healthcare workers or in-service consultant.
Discharge referral plan is not implemented and client receives no referral notice before discharge.	• Attempt to contact other referral agencies to provide continuity of care for client. • Notify physician and discharge coordinator (if available) of necessity of providing follow-through care after discharge.

GERONTOLOGIC Considerations

Teaching Strategies

Memory changes occur with the elderly population.

- There is better short-term memory with auditory rather than visual presentation of information.
- Structure should be brief and simple.
- Repetition is important.
- Older clients learn better by doing, using multiple senses, than by reading instructions.
- Memory is better for things considered important.
- Clients remember best what is told *first*.
- Declining mentation is not inevitable with aging, but some memory loss is usual.

Retention facts that underlie teaching strategies. People remember:

- 5% to 10% of what they read.
- 10% to 20% of what they hear.
- 30% to 50% of what they hear and verbalize.
- 70% of what they verbalize and write.
- 90% of what they say as they perform a task.

Interventions for teaching the elderly

- Speak distinctly and sit close to learner.
- Face the learner so that lip reading can supplement hearing.
- Use visual aids and verbal teaching.
- Decrease extraneous noise.
- Use printed materials with large type and high contrast.
- Limit use of blue, green, and violet illustrations. Use red.
- Avoid totally dark room for audiovisual presentations.
- Increase time allowed for psychomotor skills, and allow time for repetition.
- Slow the pace of presentation.
- Give small amounts of information at one time.
- Use analogies and examples to explain information. Mnemonic devices are helpful to compensate for imperfect memory.
- Establish attainable short-term goals.
- Encourage participation in goal setting and planning.
- Integrate new behaviors with previously learned ones.
- Focus on problem solving, not just delivery of facts.
- Apply teaching to present situation.
- Bolster self-esteem and self-confidence in self-care.
- Stress the "why" of what is presented.
- Recognize that the elderly client may prefer to be alone when learning.
- Make follow-up phone calls, if indicated, to check on the client, reinforce teaching, or to clarify any misunderstanding.

Discharge Planning

A discharge plan for the elderly contains some of the same components as a plan for a younger adult; at every step in the plan, however, the coordinator must remember that this is an elderly person and he or she must be evaluated for the ability and resources to manage at home. Include family and/or caregiver in discharge planning. This is especially so if the elderly person lives alone or with another elderly person. Following are several issues that the discharge planner must consider when formulating the plan:

- Was the person functioning independently at home before hospitalization, and is it realistic to expect him/her to do so again?
- Does this person have capable family or friend resources to assist with functioning in the home (in addition to the necessary professional resources)?
- What is the baseline health status of the person (assuming he/she recovers from the current hospitalization), and does this status allow for independent functioning after hospitalization?
- What are the long-term financial resources of the elderly person and do special measures need to be initiated for coverage?
- If the elderly person cannot return to the facility he or she was in before hospitalization, what special arrangements need to be made?
- Special considerations the discharge planner must take into account when coordinating a plan for an elderly individual. For example:
    1. Does the person have a hearing or visual impairment that interferes with learning?
    2. Does the teaching need to be done in written form (not just verbal)?
    3. Would a return demonstration of care procedures by the home health nurse be beneficial after the client has returned home?
    4. Will the anxiety level of the client to be discharged interfere with understanding and learning?
    5. Is the health status of the client a way of gaining attention? If so, this need should be separated from the needs of self-care after discharge. It is important to convey this need to the follow-up caregiver.

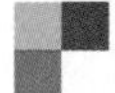

MANAGEMENT Guidelines

Each state legislates a Nurse Practice Act for RNs and LVN/LPNs. Healthcare facilities are responsible for establishing and implementing policies and procedures that conform to their state's regulations. Verify the regulations and role parameters for each healthcare worker in your facility.

Delegation

- RNs must develop the teaching and discharge plans based on the assessment of client needs. The Nurse Practice Act sets the standards for who assesses and plans client care. Multidisciplinary team input is critical and a major component of both plans. The nurse is usually the coordinator of most client care plans and teaching plans.
- Once the teaching and discharge plans have been developed, other members of the healthcare team may participate in implementing them.
- LVN/LPNs follow the guidelines established in the teaching plans. They can assist with the discharge plans; however, an RN must write the discharge referral summary and communicate with the referring agency.

Communication Matrix

- The teaching plan should be developed in concert with the client and family. Mutually acceptable goals should be established with realistic time frames.
- The teaching plan is initiated early in the hospitalization. It must be written because it is a permanent part of the client record. It is updated as goals are achieved.
- Team members are kept apprised of the progress toward meeting the teaching goals by updates during shift report.
- Client information is disseminated between referral agencies and the hospital through a written discharge summary and/or referral sheet. The data in the summary includes pertinent information on the hospitalization and the condition at discharge, the medications and treatments the client is to continue to take, and specific equipment required for client care.

CRITICAL THINKING Strategies

Scenario 1

Mr. John Johanson, age 58, was admitted to the medical unit with a diagnosis of heart failure. He is African American, 5'7", and weighs 260 pounds. He is a cross-country truck driver. He lives alone when not working. He usually watches TV and eats fast foods or frozen dinners. This is his second hospital admission in the last month. His vital signs are BP 230/108, P 108 and irregular, R 36. He has bibasilar rales and a 3+ pitting edema of the lower extremities. His point of maximal impulse (PMI) is at the sixth intercostal space (ICS), midaxillary line. He states he is short of breath and has had difficulty ambulating the last few days. He states he has tried to lose weight but even after dieting he gains more weight back. When asked about his smoking habits, he states he knows he is not supposed to smoke and he has tried to stop, but with his work it is too difficult because he is alone so much. He states he is on blood pressure drugs, but unsure of the name.

1. Identify the current nursing diagnoses by priority and provide rationale for answers.
2. From these data, identify the teaching needs by priority and develop a teaching plan for Mr. Johanson.
3. Are there any cultural considerations that need to be taken into account when considering his teaching plan? If so, identify actions you will take relative to the cultural considerations.
4. Briefly outline how you will determine when it is appropriate to initiate the teaching plan.
5. Describe the discharge plan you might develop for Mr. Johanson.

Scenario 2

A very young mother brings a 6-month-old child to the emergency room and tells the triage nurse that she doesn't know what is wrong her child, but she doesn't seem to be "normal." The child is assessed by the pediatrician and the child is admitted for further testing. The pediatrician's admitting diagnosis is *failure to thrive*. The child's weight is only 5 pounds over what it was at birth (7lb 2 oz), and the child is still not turning over from back to front. As the admitting nurse, you need to begin the discharge plan and the teaching plan. Based on the limited information from the physician and the admitting diagnosis, complete the following scenario.

1. What information will you need to obtain before you can plan for discharge?
2. What information is necessary to obtain before you can develop a teaching plan?
3. What approach will you take with the mother in order to obtain the necessary information for both the discharge and teaching plan?
4. Describe the nurse's role in client teaching for this mother.

NCLEX® Review Questions

Unless otherwise specified, choose only one (1) answer.

1. The healthcare team member (HCT) who assumes the leadership role in directing the educational plan for the client and/or family is usually the
    1. Physician.
    2. HCT member whose role represents the greatest teaching need requiring education.
    3. Discharge planner.
    4. Nurse.
2. Clients at high risk for discharge, usually requiring specific instructions, include those who are/have
    1. Living alone.
    2. Multisystem issues.
    3. Small children.
    4. A job requiring them to return to work immediately.
3. Data for which one of the personal characteristics below is least necessary to obtain when planning for client teaching?
    1. Educational level.
    2. Family composition and living situations.
    3. Ethnic group.
    4. Employment/occupation.
4. It is imperative the client's family participate in teaching activities. What actions would *not be* used to determine their ability and willingness to participate?
    1. Assess cognitive ability to understand instruction.
    2. Assess how attentive they are to the client and how often they visit.
    3. Evaluate extent of time and active participation of family during instruction.
    4. Evaluate interactions between client and family.
5. You have been assigned to develop a teaching plan for a client being discharged after a laparoscopic procedure for gallbladder removal. Your priority intervention is to
    1. Assess the home environment for specialized equipment needs.
    2. Determine when the client plans to return to work.
    3. Determine who will be at home with the client after discharge.
    4. Assess the client's usual lifestyle and daily activities.
6. You are developing the strategy for an initial teaching plan for a 24-year-old client admitted with newly diagnosed acute leukemia. Which one of the factors would *not* be taken into consideration as you develop the initial teaching plan?
    1. Attention span and retention ability.
    2. Reading level.
    3. Input from client on how he/she learns best.
    4. Support for client at home.
7. Nurses evaluate the effectiveness of the teaching strategies by

    Select all that apply.
    1. Asking the client to do a return demonstration of the skill being discussed.
    2. Having the client take a posttest of the teaching content.

3. Asking pertinent questions relative to the teaching content.
4. Summarizing the teaching content they presented.
5. Clarifying misinformation after each teaching session.

8. A client becomes very agitated and hostile when you approach him to begin client teaching for discharge. Which one of the actions would *not* be an appropriate action by the nurse?
   1. Begin the teaching and explain you are required to complete the teaching.
   2. Attempt to determine the reason for the agitation and hostility.
   3. Do not begin the teaching program but explain that you will return later.
   4. Ask another nurse to assist you in assessing the reason why the client is refusing the teaching.

9. Documentation for discharge includes which of the following statements?

   Select all that apply.
   1. Summarize vital signs during hospitalization and include latest vital signs.
   2. Describe the activity level of the client during hospitalization.
   3. Summarize the teaching plan and client's response to teaching.
   4. Summarize nursing interventions provided during hospitalization.
   5. Provide intake and output findings during hospitalization.

10. Gerontologic considerations for client education should include which one of the following concepts for older clients? They
    1. Learn best through reading material.
    2. Remember 30% to 50% of what they read.
    3. Need extraneous noises decreased while teaching is being presented.
    4. Learn best in group settings.

7

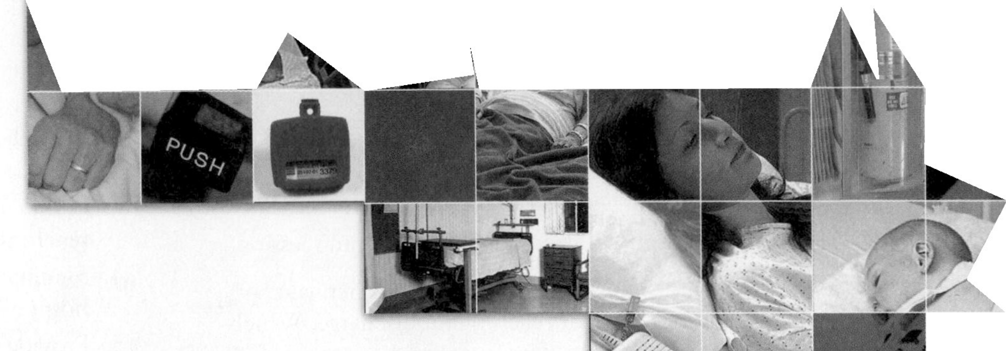

Safe Client Environment and Restraints

LEARNING OBJECTIVES

1. Define the term *adaptation*.
2. Describe three characteristics that influence adaptation.
3. Outline four sociocultural dimensions of environmental adaptation.
4. State two nursing diagnoses relevant to maintaining a safe environment.
5. Outline the objectives for providing a safe environment.
6. Identify clients who are at high risk for falls.
7. List and briefly describe at least four guidelines for using restraints to prevent mechanical injuries.
8. Describe nursing actions for clients with seizure activity.
9. List the guidelines for providing safety when clients are receiving radioactive materials.
10. Demonstrate two methods of client evacuation when a fire occurs in a nursing unit.
11. Demonstrate the application of wrist restraints.
12. Demonstrate the application of a torso/belt restraint.
13. List the components that should be included when charting for application of restraints.
14. Describe The Joint Commission Standards for restraint use.
15. Describe the Home Assessment Checklist.

CHAPTER OUTLINE

TERMINOLOGY

Adaptation ability of an organism to adjust to a change in environment.

Ambiance the pervading atmosphere of the surrounding environment.

Ambulation to move from place to place by walking.

Aseptic sterile; a condition free from bacteria and infection.

Assessment critical evaluation of information; the first step in the nursing process.

Behavior a person's total activity—actions or reactions; especially conduct that can be observed.

Centers for Medicare and Medical Services (CMS) previously named Health Care Financing Administration (HCFA).

Chemical restraint use of a sedating psychotropic drug to manage or control behavior.

Comprehensive health care a total system of health care that takes the whole person into account.

Contaminated waste radioactive waste, which, if improperly disposed of, may be harmful or cause a radiation hazard.

Decibel a unit for measuring difference in acoustic signals; a unit of intensity and volume of sound.

Ecosystem the biologic and physical dimensions of the environment that refers to all living and nonliving elements.

Epidemiologist one who studies the causes, distribution, and frequency of disease outbreaks in a human community.

Homeostasis a state of equilibrium of the internal environment.

Hospital acquired infection (HAI) (formerly termed nosocomial) infection or disease originating in a hospital.

Hygiene pertinent to a state of health and its preservation.

Limitation the state of being limited or restricted.

Licensed independent practitioner (LIP) an individual licensed by the state or institution who is permitted to provide and monitor conscious sedation to clients and order restraints or seclusion. This practitioner is either a physician, dentist, advanced nurse practitioner, or physician's assistant.

Maladaptation inability of an organism to adjust to a change in environment.

Mechanical restraint containment of a person in a chair or bed to provide safety.

Nosocomial formerly used term for infection or disease originating in a hospital (now called hospital acquired infection).

Physical restraint any manual method or physical or mechanical device that restricts freedom of movement or normal access to one's body, material, or equipment, attached to or adjacent to the client's body that he/she cannot easily remove. Holding a client in a manner that restricts his/her movement.

Physiologic in accord with or characteristic of the normal functioning of a living organism.

Psycho prefix referring to the mind or mental processes of an individual.

Psychosocial a term that refers both to psychologic and social factors.

Restraint any involuntary method (chemical or physical) of restricting an individual's freedom or movement, physical activity, or normal access to the body.

Seclusion the isolation of a client in a special room to decrease stimuli that might be causing or exacerbating the client's emotional distress, free from objects that could cause the client harm.

Sentinel event any unexpected occurrence involving death or serious physical or psychological injury or the risk thereof.

Sociocultural a term that refers both to society and culture.

Stress any emotional, physical, social, economic, or other factor that requires a response or change.

Supervise to direct or inspect performance; to oversee.

Therapeutic having healing or curative powers.

Thermal pertaining to using, producing, or caused by heat.

ORIENTATION TO THE CLIENT ENVIRONMENT

Maintaining Homeostasis

As a nurse, one of your primary responsibilities is to make sure your clients have a safe and comfortable healthcare environment. It is your responsibility to help clients adapt to this environment as well as to their health care in general.

From a holistic view, the term *environment* can generally be explained as the total of all conditions and influences, both external and internal, that affect the life and development of an organism. As human beings we are constantly exposed to changing physical, biologic, and social conditions. To survive, we continually assess our relationship to our changing surroundings. We also learn how to make adjustments that help us control and improve our environment. This complex process is called *adaptation*.

Adaptation includes psychologic and physiologic adjustments. People in most situations are able to control or adapt to their immediate surroundings. Although no two people respond to the environment in exactly the same way, common principles related to adaptation can be found in all human beings:

- All adaptations are attempts to maintain optimum physical and chemical states, or homeostasis.
- Individuals retain their own identity and uniqueness regardless of the degree of adaptation required.
- Adaptation affects all aspects of human existence.

- Human beings have limits in the process and degree of their adaptation.
- Adaptation is measured in relationship to time.
- Adaptive responses to the environment may or may not be adequate or appropriate.
- Adaptive attempts may be stressful.
- The degree and process of adaptation varies from individual to individual.
- Adaptation is an ongoing process about which the individual may be consciously or unconsciously aware.

Each of us adjusts to our immediate environment in a way that is unique to us. When this environment changes suddenly, for instance when we are hospitalized, we may not be able to adapt independently to our immediate surroundings safely and comfortably. It is at this point that assistance must be provided.

CHARACTERISTICS THAT INFLUENCE ADAPTATION

The characteristics that make all people unique also provide information about the process of adaptation to the environment. These factors must be considered when assessing clients' needs and abilities to safely adjust to their immediate surroundings.

Age

A client's age is a critical factor in the assessment process. Because terms such as *elderly* and *young* can be interpreted in many different ways, the nurse may need to look at the client's developmental stage (physical and mental growth) rather than at the client's chronologic age.

As people develop, sensory receptors help process day-to-day events. Human beings learn how to protect themselves and how to adjust to changing needs through experiencing these events. During the learning process, young children may require entirely different protection than teenagers. Even a 30-year-old man who has learned through experience how to protect himself in a routine environment may not have adequate skills in an unfamiliar atmosphere.

The older adult often requires special assistance. Sensory and motor changes, such as slowness of movement, postural instability, decreased vision or hearing, and even diminished acuity for taste and touch, are not uncommon. These changes can result in an altered ability to sense and adapt to harmful environmental stimuli. The older person may not see or hear an approaching car, detect the taste of spoiling food, or move quickly enough to avoid falling.

Mental Status

The ability to perceive and react to environmental stimuli is closely related to mental status. Adapting to a new or different environment requires learning through experience and possessing a cognitive awareness of the immediate surroundings. Making adjustments to the environment requires stimuli to travel over the sensory pathways of nerves to the central nervous system. To respond to stimuli, such as avoiding a burn from a hot object, motor neurons carry impulses to muscles to cause an involuntary reflex action, such as withdrawing the hand from hot water. Sensory impulses traveling to the cerebral cortex of the brain inform the person that this stimulus is potentially harmful. Voluntary movement then provides additional adaptation.

Consciousness is the state in which individuals are aware of themselves and their relationship to their surroundings. Unconsciousness indicates a lack of awareness and inability to cognitively respond to the environment. Levels of consciousness range from fully conscious to nonresponsive. Difficulty in adapting to the immediate environment due to alterations in mental status can manifest itself in a variety of ways:

- Confused clients often view their environment in a distorted way. This condition can lead to extreme behavioral changes, injury, or combativeness.
- Neurologically injured clients may have decreased perception of stimuli such as heat, cold, pain, or friction. In extreme cases, they may have no perception of any stimuli.
- Paralysis inhibits movement and is accompanied by a loss of position sense (dangling limbs or poor body alignment).
- Alterations in communication, sight, or hearing are barriers to identifying hazards and sharing fears or concerns with others.
- Fluctuating levels of consciousness create difficulty in promoting self-care and self-image.

Continuous assessment of changes in the client's ability to relate and adapt to the environment is essential. Ability to adapt influences the type and amount of assistance the client needs, especially while in less than familiar surroundings.

States of Illness

Illness or injury causes a person to focus more intensely on himself or herself. The very nature of disease or trauma requires the individual to use physical and mental energy to adapt to the situation and to become more egocentric. A client often cannot perform even the simplest daily activity. Fatigue or pain may render clients helpless. Assistance with activities, such as bathing, eating, skin care, and elimination, may be necessary.

Some medications produce such side effects as drowsiness, which prevent the individual from adequately assessing the environment. Perceptions may be distorted, and the client is more vulnerable to hazards.

Emotional stress and anxiety can occur in mild to acute degrees. Although mild anxiety very often increases perceptual awareness, acute anxiety reduces perceptual awareness.

Because an individual is able to focus only on a specific amount of stimuli at one time, additional stimuli that may be equally important are not perceived. Potential environmental dangers are not processed. The client whose energy is focused on pain may not even hear instructions from the nurse. Depressed clients also require assistance. Depression often results in slower than normal responses to stimuli. Alcohol, a central nervous system depressant, also causes dull, slow reactions to stimuli.

When pain, anxiety, illness, injury, weakness, medications, or even lack of sleep cause a decrease in sensory acuity, awareness of potential hazards is altered. The client may not be able to make the necessary biologic, physical, or emotional adjustments to adapt to the immediate environment. Any of these conditions necessitates immediate assessment and action.

PHYSICAL AND BIOLOGICAL DIMENSIONS

The influences that make up an environment include the basic categories of biological and physical conditions, and the third dimension termed sociocultural. The biological dimensions of our environment covered in this section include all living things, such as plants, animals, and microorganisms. Water, oxygen, sunlight, organic compounds, and other components in which living things exist and develop make up the physical dimensions of an environment.

As the nurse becomes more aware of the factors that affect environmental adaptation, a safe and comfortable atmosphere for the clients becomes a greater challenge. As you assess your clients and help them adapt to the environment of a healthcare facility, you should consider the following essential elements: space, lighting, humidity, temperature, ventilation, sound levels, surfaces and equipment, safety, food and water, and waste disposal.

Adequate Space

Everyone needs space in which to grow and develop. This space may consist of a room or an area as small as a shelf or corner. No matter what form space takes, individuals need to feel they have control over it—that they can arrange it or decorate it to their liking.

Providing space for clients encourages stimulation and experimentation. Toddlers need the space of an area like a recreation room for discovery and motor skills, since playtime is their primary source of development. Adults often enjoy the social activities of a lounge but may also require well-defined personal areas, even if these areas are as simple as a bedside table or a bulletin board.

Natural and Artificial Light

Light, like space, is necessary for growth and development. The production of vitamin D, a critical component of bone metabolism, occurs from ultraviolet radiation on the skin. Natural light also assists in wound healing. In a hospital setting, natural light can be used to decrease feelings of isolation and to encourage clients to continue their normal routine.

Whether natural or artificial, adequate light is essential for the preservation of sight, for safety, and for accurate assessments and nursing care. Because eye strain, as well as nervousness and fatigue, can result from improper lighting, care should be taken to avoid glare, sharp contrast, and flickering lights. Night lights promote safety and orientation for the elderly.

Humidity and Temperature

The ability to adapt to changes in humidity or temperature is directly related to comfort. Most people in this country are comfortable at a room temperature of between 18.3° and 25°C (65°– 77°F) with the humidity at 30% to 60%. People in other cultures function equally well at lower or higher readings.

Conditions that may inhibit a person's ability to adjust to high temperatures include excessive physical work, dehydration, extremes in age (the very young and very old), decreased physical fitness, and inappropriate clothing. An individual who has difficulty adapting to high temperatures may experience a rapid rise in pulse rate, cramps, nausea, and vomiting. Severe inability to adapt to heat can result in heat stroke and death.

An individual who has difficulty adapting to lower temperatures may experience a change in behavior, depressed vital signs, and eventual unconsciousness. Hypothermia, or abnormally low body temperature, occurs when there is an imbalance between heat loss and heat production.

Extremes of heat or cold increase the incidence of infection and add to discomfort. Temperatures in healthcare institutions can be regulated with air conditioners and dehumidifiers, although care should be taken to avoid drafts and excessive dryness.

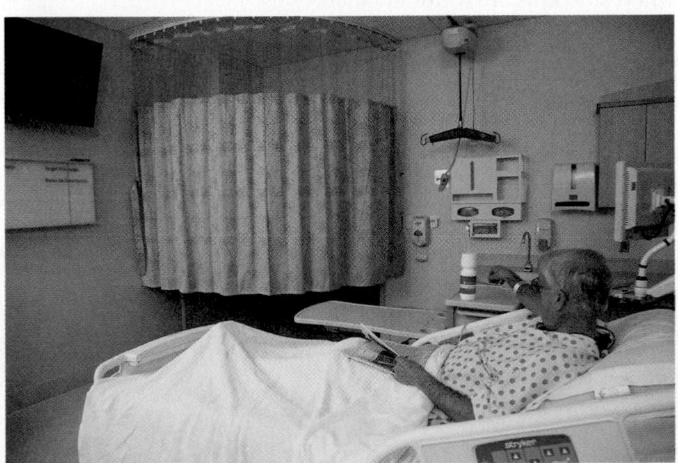

▲ Provide a comfortable environment with space for personal effects.

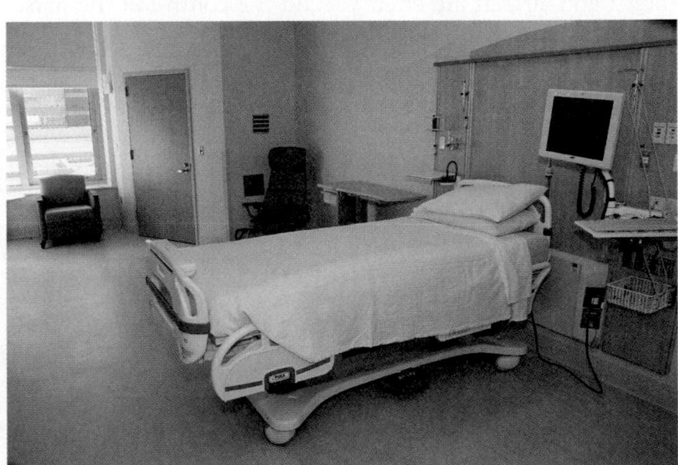

▲ A pleasant environment promotes a sense of well-being.

Ventilation

Particular attention should be given to assessing the movement of air within a client's immediate environment. An adequately ventilated room should contain a comfortable amount of moisture; be free of irritating pollutants, odors, or noxious fumes; and be at a tolerable temperature.

Adequate ventilation is especially important when more than one client is in a room. Other areas requiring optimum ventilation are operating rooms, delivery rooms, nurseries, isolation rooms, and sterile supply rooms.

A properly functioning ventilation system reduces airborne contaminants by regulating the amount of air movement within an enclosed area. When ventilation cannot be maintained by using doors and windows, mechanical devices, such as fans or air conditioners, may be used.

Clients requiring airborne isolation are placed in private rooms where the ventilation system is a directional air flow negative-pressure ventilation system. Six to 12 air exchanges per hour occur with this system.

Comfortable Sound Levels

Noise can be defined as any undesirable sound. The intensity and kind of noise that is comfortable is highly individual and related to past experiences. A businessman who lives on a busy street in a city may not adjust well to the quiet he may experience at night in a hospital room. On the other hand, a farmer from a rural community may be disturbed by the slightest sound. Infants often sleep peacefully in an atmosphere of loud noise and activity.

Decibel is the unit for measuring the intensity of noise. At close range, noise produced from heavy traffic, for example, has a decibel measure of 90, whereas a whisper at 3 feet has an intensity of 20 decibels.

At certain levels noise is considered hazardous. Temporary or permanent hearing loss or damage can occur when noise is present for a prolonged time at intensities over 90 decibels. Other effects of sustained loud noise are muscle tension, increased blood pressure, blood vessel constriction, pallor, increased secretion of the adrenal hormone, and nervous tension.

The pitch, quality, and duration of noise may also affect the client's environment. Unwanted sounds produced by sirens, traffic, and aircraft are often beyond the control of the nurse. But noise within a hospital setting, such as television, call systems, careless handling of dishes and other equipment, visitors, excessive conversation at the nurses' station, and some care-related sounds (e.g., beeping monitors), can be controlled.

Nursing personnel should always be aware of the noise level and its effects on the clients' well-being. Very ill individuals are often more sensitive to excessive or meaningless stimuli. Certain sounds can be reassuring because they represent activity or assistance to the client.

Furniture: Bed Safety

Today, most healthcare facilities are designed to be attractive, orderly, efficient, and clean. Since a person's outlook is strongly influenced by the surroundings, careful attention to appearance and cleanliness can assist with adjustment to the healthcare environment. Although it is essential to assess the routines and standards of cleanliness of each client, the nurse may also have to teach the client how to organize and clean up. In some cases, instruction to the client may be critical to maintaining or improving a healthcare condition.

The standards and routine cleaning procedures of the hospital are generally not a nursing function now because hospital housekeeping has become a specialized occupation. Maintaining an organized, clean environment, however, requires coordination by all healthcare providers.

Furnishings should be arranged to be physically safe, comfortable, aesthetically appealing for the client, and easily cleaned. Adequate cleaning of the room should be done at a time of day that is coordinated with the client's needs so that the resulting sense of security adds to the client's ability to adapt adequately to the surroundings. The ambiance of the room and a sense of order contribute to the client's sense of well-being.

Hospital beds are adjustable in height from the floor; when the bed is in LOW position, the client can more easily and safely get in or out of it; when it is in HIGH position, the nursing staff can more efficiently render care. The head and sometimes the knee areas of the bed can be elevated; this is accomplished by electric controls. The electric controls are found on the foot, the side of the bed, or on the side rails. When placed at the side, the client can more easily control bed positions. Bed wheels are equipped with locks and kept in locked position.

For many years, side rails have provided what everyone thought was safe nursing care, protecting clients from injury as a result of falling out of bed. Changes have occurred in both long-term care and acute-care settings regarding the use of side rails. The Center for Medicare and Medicaid Services (CMS, formerly called Health Care Financing Administration, HCFA) and the Food and Drug Administration (FDA) have established guidelines that decrease the routine use of side rails. There is still controversy over the safety of side rails. Appropriately placed half-rails function as assistive devices, helping clients transfer from bed to chair or wheelchair. The HCFA believed that regardless of whether side rails were used as restrictive or assistive devices, risk of client entrapment in the side rails overshadows the potential benefit. Elderly clients and those with altered mental status are at high risk for injury when side rails are routinely used.

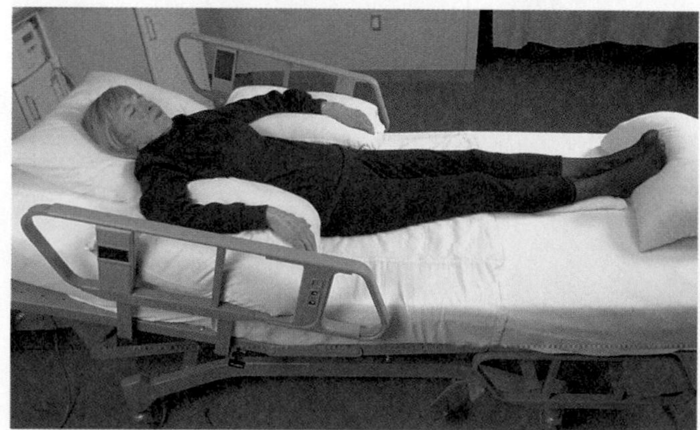

▲ Half-length side rails can be requested by clients to use as an assistive device.

The HCFA stated that a half- or quarter-length upper side rail is not considered a restraint if the client uses it as an aid for moving in and out of bed. A full-length or four half-length rails are not considered restraints if the client requests them in order to feel more secure and if he is able to lower them by himself before getting into or out of bed.

Nurses must assess appropriateness for side rail use for each client and inform both client and family of benefits and risks for their use. These assessments must be completed according to hospital policies and procedures to ensure that client is not at risk for injury if they are in use.

The overbed table is adjustable in height and slides over the bed to provide space for self-care activities or additional working surface for the nurse. The overbed table may also be used when the client sits in a chair. Small bed trays are sometimes convenient when the overbed table cannot be used.

The bedside table, similar to a nightstand, holds the client's personal possessions in drawers. A cabinet section in the table can be used to store bathing or toiletry equipment, and the top provides space for the client's familiar items, such as pictures or books.

A chair with firm back and arm supports should always be a part of the client's furnishings. Chairs should be made of durable, easily cleanable materials, such as plastic or Naugahyde. The client should be instructed to avoid contact between skin surfaces and the chair when sitting in a chair. A small towel or blanket can be placed under the client for this purpose.

A signaling system is also essential for the client to call for assistance. A signaling system may be an intercom, buzzer, electric light, or handbell. Whatever device is available must be within the client's reach and ability to use.

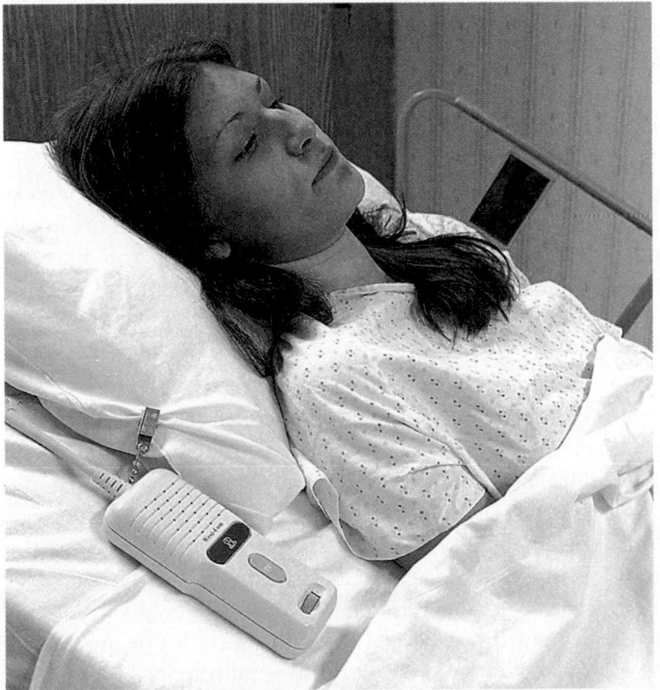

▲ Ensure that call light or other summoning device is within easy reach of client to provide access to nursing staff.

Food and Water

Fresh, nourishing food and clean water are vital to recovering and maintaining health and must be planned for and provided in appropriate amounts in healthcare facilities. A client's well-being can be positively affected by the ingestion of the correct number of calories, fat, proteins, carbohydrates, minerals, vitamins, and water, but it is well known that many people have nutritional habits that can negatively affect their well-being. A careful nutritional assessment is a critical step in helping the client adjust to the environment.

Hazardous Products and Waste Management

All waste products, whether contaminated equipment, blood or body fluid, waste, garbage, soiled dressings, refuse, or hazardous products, must be handled and disposed of in a way that prevents risk for injury or illness.

Nurses must be aware of potential dangers to themselves as well as to their clients when handling and disposing of hazardous materials. Just a few of the hazardous chemicals that nurses and other healthcare workers may be exposed to include disinfectants, such as isopropyl alcohol and iodine; sterilizing agents, such as formaldehyde and ethylene oxide; and anesthetic waste gases, such as nitrous oxide and Fluothane. Antineoplastic agents used in cancer treatment may also pose a hazard even when proper prevention policies and procedures are in place. All healthcare agencies have specific guidelines regarding the handling and disposal of such materials. For example, unit Material Safety Data Sheets provide information about area-specific chemical hazards and precautionary measures. Each toxic agent sheet (Material Safety Data Sheet) in the facility details information on the chemical's makeup, its health effects, exposure information, and emergency care procedures. These are available and accessible to the staff.

The U.S. Public Health Service, Centers for Disease Control and Prevention, the Environmental Protection Agency, the Occupational Health and Safety Administration (OSHA), the American Hospital Association, and state departments of health are some of the agencies that prepare guidelines for the handling and disposal of biohazards and dangerous products. Familiarity with general and unit-specific hazards and adherence to recommended standards for their control is essential for safe nursing practice. OSHA requires hospitals to educate employees about chemical hazards and to train them in safety precautions before they work in an area where toxic agents are used. Most hospitals require annual hazardous chemical training as part of their required staff development and training updates. (Refer to Chapter 14, Infection Control, for more details in handling hazardous material.)

In many healthcare facilities, a position of infection control nurse has been created to gather data on the type and frequency of various infections found in the hospital. These data help the infection control nurse to locate the source of the problem, predict its spread, and identify the best method of preventing its recurrence. Many of the hospital-acquired infections (HAIs, formerly called nosocomial) can be traced to inadvertent transmission by care providers. Each nurse plays a significant role in establishing a safe environment for the client by using standard precautions in client care and by handling and disposing of biohazards appropriately. The infection control nurse plays a major role in identifying the "no pay" adverse events in the hospital acquired conditions. The 10 identified events listed by Centers for Medicare and Medicaid Services (CMS) will not be reimbursed by Medicare-Medicaid. (See Chapter 14, Infection Control.)

SOCIOCULTURAL DIMENSIONS

The first two dimensions of the environment, the biologic and physical, or ecosystem, refer to all living and nonliving elements. The third dimension of an environment is sociocultural, which includes both past and present influences from the people and the culture surrounding the individual. Customs, religious and legal systems, and economic and political beliefs are all part of this environment. This dimension also involves responses and adjustments to the ideals, concepts, beliefs, activities, and pressure of various groups, such as social clubs, peer groups, or colleagues.

Organization of Time

How clients perceive and deal with time and the passing of time depends on their age, immediate situation, culture, and past experiences, as well as their present physical and emotional condition. To a mother waiting for her child to return from surgery, hours seem like days. Small children generally do not have a well-developed sense of time. A 3-year-old may act out feelings of abandonment when separated from a parent for just a few minutes. In an intensive care unit, time can be severely disrupted, since healthcare activities continue around the clock. The ability to organize time is a critical element in adaptation. Helping clients assess and plan their time is one of the most important ways you can help them cope with their new surroundings.

Privacy

Many people who enter a healthcare facility fear exposure and loss of identity. Providing privacy for a client is more than a luxury or a mere courtesy. It is necessary and vitally important to the individual's attitude toward health care.

Clients should be given as much privacy as possible. Most individuals give clues to the nurse about the degree of privacy they need. The client's culture, past experience, values, and age should all be considered when planning for privacy.

Hospital routines should be planned to promote privacy. If an embarrassing or upsetting situation occurs, the feelings of the client must be protected. People require time and space to think, organize, and reflect. Privacy is necessary for human development, even at home. In the hospital, privacy is critical to the client's attitude and well-being.

Privacy can be promoted by drawing curtains or screens. Doors and window shades may also be used. Signs stating "Do Not Enter Without Checking at Desk" posted on room entrances give the client a sense of security from disturbances. This is especially important during physical examinations, personal care, or emotional upset. Knocking or asking for permission to enter the client's room or area promotes mutual respect and enhances a sense of emotional space.

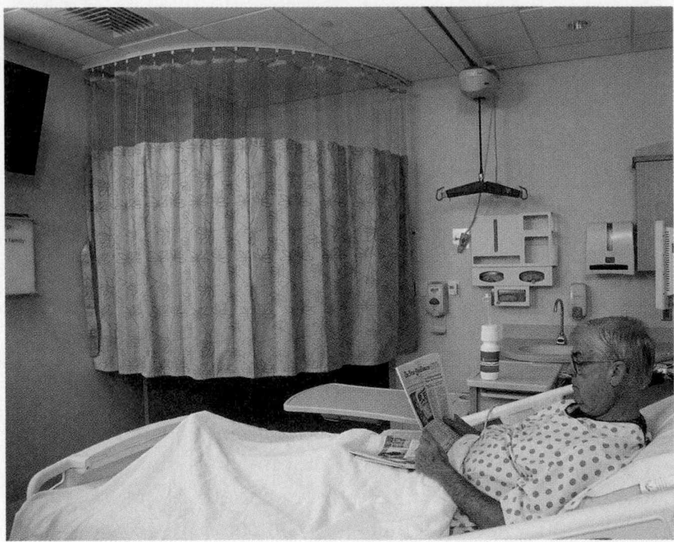

▲ Clients should be given as much privacy as possible by drawing curtains or using screens.

Privacy also extends beyond the physical need of the individual. Health status, conversation, and records are privileged information. Since the privacy rule, a part of HIPAA, went into effect on April 2003, this has greatly increased the confidentiality of client's information. A more trusting, therapeutic relationship evolves if the client understands that confidences shared with nurses are used appropriately.

Individualized Care

Providing an environment that is comfortable, safe, and individualized to meet the specific needs of a client is a challenging task. The client's ability to adapt to the immediate environment can either improve or interfere with his or her well-being. To assist the client in adjusting to the environment, a careful assessment of the situation should always include the person's usual routines, self-care abilities, cultural beliefs, current perceptions, and past experiences. To promote the best adaptation to a different environment, encourage as much independence as possible with each client. You may be required to use your resourcefulness, imagination, and ingenuity to assist the client through difficult periods. Ongoing assessment and open communication between client and staff is essential if positive adaptation is to occur.

Hospitalized clients also need emotional space. This form of space is that psychological area where the person can experience a sense of self. This is particularly difficult to achieve in a hospital setting when caregivers exercise control over many of the activities of daily living. It is important that the staff be aware of this psychological need so that they can provide adequate privacy, quiet, and freedom of choice over all of the areas that the client can control. The staff must also be aware that the client rarely needs to relinquish total responsibility for his or her care.

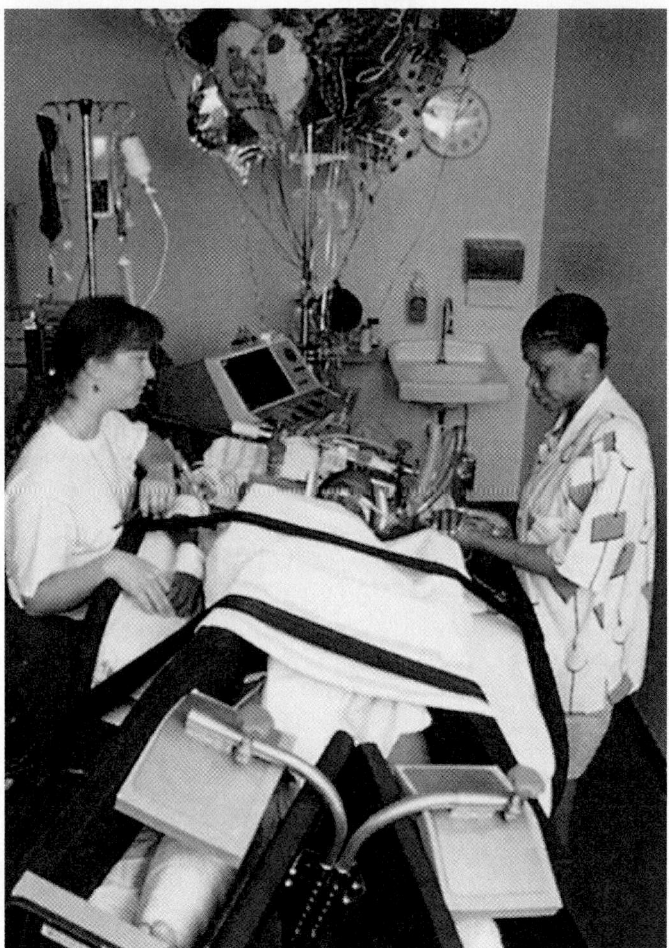

▲ Providing an environment that is both safe and individualized is a challenging task for the nursing staff.

Information and Teaching

The amount of information the client has about the environment and immediate situation directly affects his or her ability to adjust safely and comfortably. When the individual is given information and explanation about strange equipment, diagnostic procedures, or unfamiliar healthcare personnel, fears and feelings of helplessness can be reduced and a shared sense of responsibility enhanced. The client becomes more capable of asking questions and expressing concerns if prepared for unfamiliar occurrences.

Providing the client and his or her family, if appropriate, with information about the client's environment is the responsibility of the nurse. As more people assume the role of consumers of health care, there is more demand for knowledge about aspects of health care. Including the client in planning and caring for himself or herself promotes a sense of responsibility, independence, and self-respect.

Teaching the client about various aspects of health care is one method of information sharing. Over the years, the focus has changed from the professional staff doing everything for the client to helping the client be more independent. This change enables the client to adapt to the environment with guided assistance from nurses. As the client learns about his or her own health care and becomes involved in meeting his or her particular needs, a sense of trust, responsibility, and usefulness develops.

A SAFE ENVIRONMENT

The Joint Commission and CMS are taking the lead in attempting to ensure that Americans are better protected from unsafe health care. Nurses are expected to carry a major responsibility in preventing medical errors, as they are the managers of client care. The Joint Commission is committed to improving safety for clients and residents in healthcare organizations. About 50% of The Joint Commission standards are directly related to safety. The Joint Commission has standards that address restraints and seclusion, environment of care (fire drills, medical equipment monitoring), physical environment, and infection control policies, to name only a few.

The mission statement indicates it is continuously trying to improve the safety and quality of care provided to the public through its accreditation standards. In 2009 the new National Patient Safety Goals (NPSGs) were published by TJC. Among the goals are using at least two client identifiers (not the room number) when administering medications; implementation of a Universal Protocol for Preventing Wrong Site, Wrong Procedure, Wrong Person Surgery; standardizing a list of abbreviations, acronyms, and symbols used for medication administration and physician orders; and reducing the risk of client falls by implementing a fall reduction program and then evaluating the program. In 2010 the National Patient Standards have decreased from the 2009 NPSGs of 20. The missing goals have now become "Standards of Care" (see Table 7-1, NPSGs). Table 7-1 outlines the client/patient safety goals that directly affect hospitals.

SENTINEL EVENTS

One of the policies implemented by The Joint Commission in 1996 addressed sentinel events. This policy ensured that healthcare organizations identified sentinel events and took action to prevent their recurrence. These events include an unexpected death or serious physical or psychological injury. Serious injuries such as the loss of limb or function were included in this policy. All sentinel events are to be documented, and this documentation is forwarded to TJC. A total of 6,780 (4,590 in hospital) events have been reported to TJC since the initiation of data collection through the first quarter of 2010. Of these, 67% resulted in client death, 9% resulted in loss of function, and 24% resulted from other causes. These figures include sentinel events in hospitals, home care, emergency rooms, psychiatric care setting, etc.

It is assumed that 50% of more than 5,000 to 6,000 hospitals in the United States have experienced a sentinel event in the past 10 years. Unfortunately, not all sentinel events are reported. Approximately 67.7% of all reported events occur in general hospitals. When a sentinel event occurs, the facility must conduct what is termed a root cause analysis and must develop an action plan within 45 days of the facility becoming aware of the event. A root cause analysis examines the reasons the error occurred and suggests changes to the

TABLE 7-1 National Patient Safety Goals 2010

Goal 1—Improve the accuracy of patient identification.
- Use of Two Patient Identifiers When Administering Medications, Blood and Blood Products (NPSG.01.01.01)
- Eliminating Transfusion Errors (NPSG.01.03.01)

Goal 2—Improve the effectiveness of communication among caregivers.
- Timely Reporting of Critical Tests and Critical Results (NPSG.02.03.01)

Goal 3—Improve the safety of using medications.
- Labeling Medications (NPSG.03.04.01)
- Reducing Harm from Anticoagulation Therapy (NPSG.03.05.01)

Goal 7—Reduce the risk of healthcare-associated infections.
- Meeting Hand Hygiene Guidelines (NPSG.07.01.01)
- Preventing Multidrug-Resistant Organism Infections (NPSG.07.03.01)
- Preventing Central Line–Associated Blood Stream Infections (NPSG.07.04.01)
- Preventing Surgical Site Infections (NPSG.07.05.01)

Goal 8—Accurately and completely reconcile medications across the continuum of care.

Note: *All requirements for Goal 8 are not in effect at this time.*
- Comparing Current and Newly Ordered Medications (NPSG.08.01.01)
- Communicating Medications to the Next Provider (NPSG.08.02.01)
- Providing a Reconciled Medication List to the Patient (NPSG.08.03.01)
- Settings in Which Medications Are Minimally Used (NPSG.08.04.01)

Goal 9—Reduce the risk of patient harm resulting from falls. (NPSG.09.02.01)

Goal 14—Prevent health care-associated pressure ulcers (decubitus ulcers). (NPSG.14.01.01)

Goal 15—The organization identifies safety risks inherent in its patient population. Identifying Individuals at Risk for Suicide (NPSG.15.01.01)

NPSG goal numbers are current for 2010. Other goals not listed here (4, 5, 6, 10, 11, 12, 13, and 16) are not applicable for hospitals. Refer to www.jointcommission.org/PatientSafety/National Patient Safety Goals for additional information.

In addition to the above goals, the Universal Protocol for Preventing Wrong Site, Wrong Procedure, and Wrong Person Surgery has been implemented to prevent surgical patient errors.

system that can prevent the incident from happening again in the future. Root causes of sentinel events indicate that communication is the primary reason leading to the sentinel event (66%). Client assessment errors are responsible for 42% of the events, and staffing issues account for 22% of the events.

"NEVER EVENTS"

The use of the term "Never Events" was first discussed in 2001 by the National Quality Forum (NQF). Since the inception, the term has expanded to include 28 events grouped into six categories (Surgical, Product or Device, Client Protection,

The Joint Commission Sentinel Events

According to TJC, the following events are considered sentinel events.

- Incidents that involve unexpected death or serious injury or the risk of death and serious injury that is not related to the natural course of the client's condition.
- Any of the following incidents, even if the outcome was not death or serious injury:
  1. Suicide of a client receiving around-the-clock care.
  2. Unanticipated death of a full-term infant, weighing more than 2,500 g, unrelated to congenital conditions.
  3. Infant abduction or discharge to the wrong family.
  4. Intrapartum maternal death.
  5. Medication error resulting in major permanent loss of function or death.
  6. Client fall resulting in permanent loss of function or death.
  7. Rape.
  8. Hemolytic transfusion reaction involving administration of blood or blood products having major blood group incompatibilities.
  9. Surgery on the wrong client or body part.
  10. Assault, homicide, or other crime resulting in permanent loss of function or death.
  11. Any unauthorized departure of client from an around-the-clock care setting resulting in temporally related death or major permanent loss of function.

Source: The Joint Commission. (2009). Oakbrook Terrace, IL.

TABLE 7-2 Root Causes of Sentinel Events

Communication	66%
Orientation/training	57%
Client assessment	42%
Staffing	22%
Availability of information	20%
Competency/credentialing	20%
Procedural compliance	19%
Environmental safety/security	17%
Leadership	13%
Continuum of care	13%
Care planning	12%
Organization culture	10%

All categories 1995–2005; 3,548 total reported events.
Source: http://www.jointcommission.org/.

Care Management, Environmental, and Criminal) that can lead to serious error, indicating a problem with the safety of a health facility. It has been estimated that medical errors cost from $17 million to $29 million annually and account for 2.4 million additional hospital days (Haberly, 2009).

As of October 2008, the CMS has ceased reimbursing hospitals for costs associated with specific events, such as serious hospital-acquired pressure ulcers it considers preventable. In fall 2009, 20 states had plans to deny payment for some of the "Never Events." Studies have indicated that 30% to 40% of clients receive care inconsistent with scientific evidence. It is estimated that implementation of evidence-based practice will result in increased client outcomes during hospitalization.

Providing a safe environment involves a number of people, including the client, visitors, and healthcare providers. Providing protection from hazardous situations and education about safety precautions is one of your most important responsibilities as a nurse.

TABLE 7-3 "Never Events"

1. Artificial insemination with the wrong donor sperm or donor egg
2. Unintended retention of a foreign object in a patient after surgery or other procedure
3. Surgery performed on the wrong patient
4. Wrong surgical procedure performed on a patient
5. Intraoperative or immediately postoperative death in an ASA class I patient (ASA is a physical status classification system; ASA I indicates the client is considered normal and healthy)
6. Infant discharged to the wrong person
7. Patient suicide, or attempted suicide resulting in serious disability, while being cared for in a healthcare facility
8. Maternal death or serious disability associated with labor or delivery in a low-risk pregnancy while being cared for in a healthcare facility
9. Stage 3 or 4 pressure ulcers acquired after admission to a healthcare facility
10. Any incident in which a line designated for oxygen or other gas to be delivered to a patient contains the wrong gas or is contaminated by toxic substances
11. Any instance of care ordered by or provided by someone impersonating a physician, nurse, pharmacist, or other licensed healthcare provider
12. Abduction of a patient of any age
13. Sexual assault on a patient within or on the grounds of the healthcare facility
14. Death or significant injury of a patient or staff member resulting from a physical assault (i.e., battery) that occurs within or on the grounds of the healthcare facility
15. Patient death, or serious disability associated with:
    - Patient elopement (disappearance)
    - Medication error
    - Hemolytic reaction due to the administration of ABO/HLA-incompatible blood or blood products
    - Electric shock or elective cardioversion while being cared for in a healthcare facility
    - A fall
    - Use of contaminated drugs, devices, or biologics provided by the healthcare facility
    - Use or function of a device in patient care in which the device is used or functions other than as intended
    - Intravascular air embolism that occurs while being cared for in a healthcare facility
    - Hypoglycemia, the onset of which occurs while the patient is being cared for in a healthcare facility
    - Kernicterus associated with failure to identify and treat hyperbilirubinemia in neonates
    - Spinal manipulative therapy
    - Burn incurred from any source while being cared for in a healthcare facility
    - Use of restraints or bedrails while being cared for in a healthcare facility

Source: The Joint Commission. (2006). Oakbrook Terrace, IL.

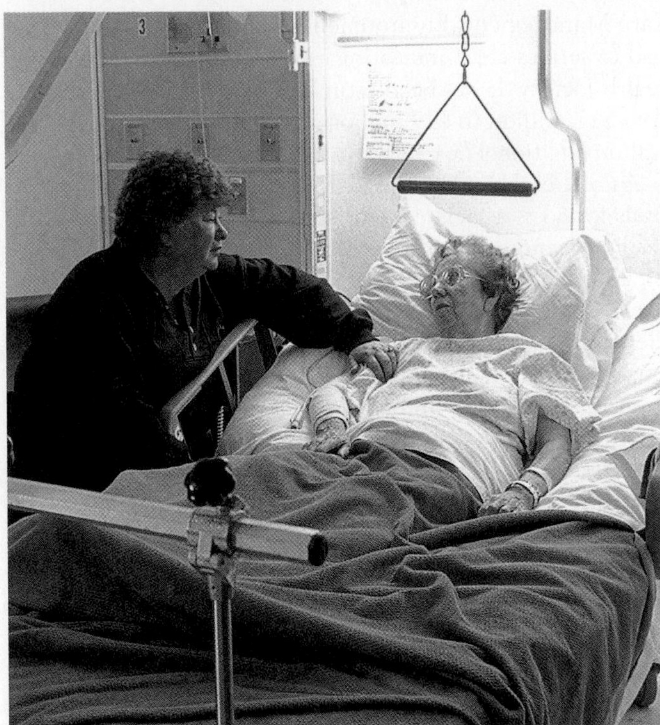

▲ Providing a safe environment involves instructing the client, family, and visitors in safety measures.

Clients who are moved from their usual environment into one that is unfamiliar and often frightening may act in ways that are very different from their usual behavior. A threatening situation can interfere with the individual's adaptation to the immediate surroundings.

The design and decor of the client's room must satisfy two needs: comfort and safety. Tasteful, unobtrusive colors help to normalize the hospital room. Interesting color combinations and patterns generally appeal more to the senses than do the traditional white or green choices. Pictures, flowers, cards, colorful linens, and curtains can add variety and familiarity to a room.

Safety Precautions

The client's age and health status influence the specific safety precautions that need to be taken to provide a safe environment. For example, infants require constant supervision, since they may attempt to put anything in their mouths or noses.

Preschool-aged children can be taught more detailed aspects of safety. Fire precautions and guidelines for bathing should be stressed.

Elementary school-aged children can usually protect themselves from hazards. They do, however, require instruction on how to operate mechanical equipment as well as information about fires and emergency exits.

All hospitals in the United States are required to be smoke-free facilities. Teenagers, adolescents, and adults should be given instruction about nonsmoking, the use of special equipment, and emergency exits. In addition, general information regarding their safety during hospitalization should be explained.

Smoking Policies

The Joint Commission standards require hospital smoking policies be disseminated and enforced throughout hospital buildings.

- Directives on smoking policy should be conveyed to each client on admission.
- Smoking is prohibited throughout the hospital.
- A physician may write orders for an exception to this policy for an individual client.
- A designated smoking area may be made available for family or visitors. (See Chapter 30 for safety measures for clients receiving oxygen therapy.)

Client Falls

Falling is a common cause of morbidity and the leading cause of nonfatal injuries and trauma-related hospitalization. Falls account for 70% of accidental deaths among individuals 75 or older. Complications that occur from falls include soft tissue injury, bone fractures, and the fear of falling again. More than 90% of hip fractures result from falls, most occurring in individuals over 70 years of age.

It is estimated that one-third of individuals over 65 years of age and more than half of individuals over 80 years of age will fall at least one time per year. Nearly 70% of all emergency room visits by individuals older than 75 years are directly related to falls. More than 60% of the falls occur in the home. Fall-related injuries account for 6% of all medical expenditures for persons 65 years and older. It has been shown that most of the falls in the hospital have occurred from or near the client's bed. Other common areas where falls occur include the bathroom and corridor. Even though much research has been done on falls and fall prevention, it is still a major problem for healthcare organizations. Clients at risk for falls include those with impaired mental status due to confusion, disorientation,

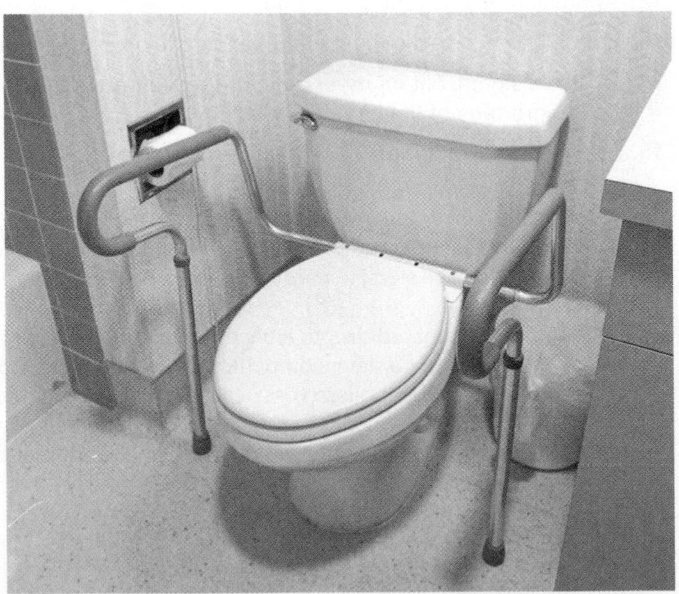

▲ Rails next to the toilet assist in preventing client falls.

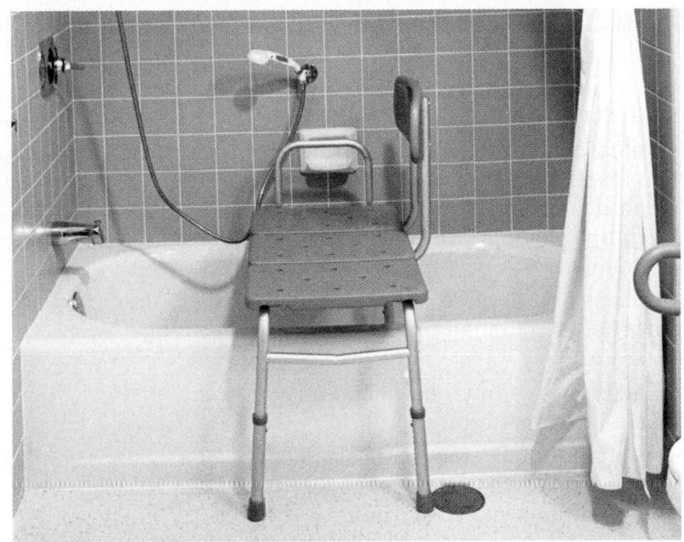

▲ Shower chairs provide for client safety.

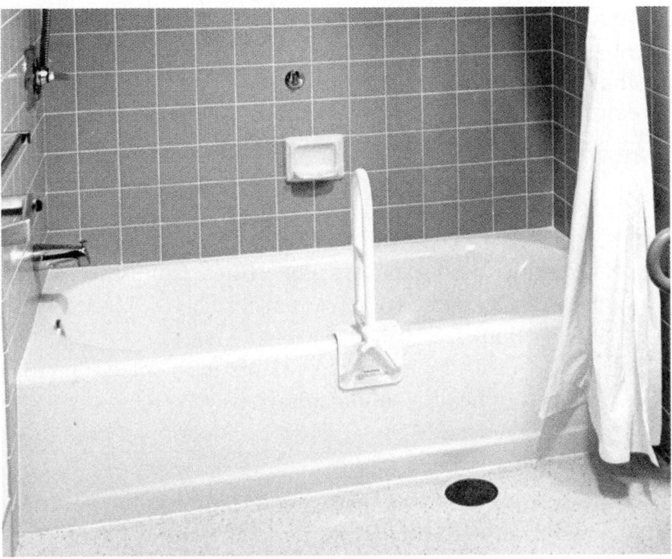

▲ Safety features such as handrail on bathtubs assist in preventing client falls.

impaired memory, and inability to understand and those taking medications such as sedatives, tranquilizers, antihypertensives, and beta-blockers. In addition to physical injury, falls result in substantial psychological and social consequences, such as anxiety, loss of independence, and increased rate of nursing home placements.

A fall risk assessment is now part of the admission assessment of all clients. If the client is at high risk for falling, appropriate interventions are implemented immediately. (See Fall Risk Assessment Form, page 153.)

Elderly adults are especially at risk for injury from falls. Decreased sensory acuity, decreased balance and postural instability, acute confusion, or chronic physical problems such as arthritis contribute to the high risk for falls among the elderly. Specialized safety equipment, such as toilet and bathtub railing and modified seats, are often used in geriatric units to decrease risk of injury during bathroom use.

It is sometimes difficult to balance the need for client safety with that for autonomy. Surveillance by agency personnel or family members, use of alarm systems, or special monitoring devices provide alternatives to use of restraints in promoting client safety.

Use of Restraints

Restraints are defined as any physical or chemical means used to restrict a client's movement or activity or access to their body.

For many years, restraining a client or placing a client in seclusion was considered a method to protect the client or the staff from injury. After much research into the subject, it has been determined that use of restraints is very problematic and actually leads to severe client injury and even death.

Because of client injury or potential injury from use of restraints or seclusion, both The Joint Commission and the CMS, formerly Health Care Financing Administration (HCFA), have developed regulations regarding use of restraints in acute care, long-term care, and psychiatric settings. The standards require that the facility exhaust all reasonable alternatives before a client is placed in restraints or seclusion. CMS standards used in long-term and psychiatric settings are more stringent than those of The Joint Commission. A licensed independent practitioner (LIP) is permitted by the state and hospital to order a restraint or seclusion. CMS requires that restraints can only be implemented with an order from a physician or LIP. An LIP must evaluate the client in person as soon as possible after implementation of restraints. In long-term care facilities, restraints may be used only to ensure physical safety of the resident or other residents and can only be applied after a written order by the physician. Orders for restraints can be written for up to 4 hours for an adult. The order can be renewed every 4 hours, up to a total of 24 hours. The Joint Commission allows that after an assessment by an RN, restraints may be implemented, and then the physician must be contacted within a specified time frame. Each facility determines the time frame for rewriting restraint orders. Continued use of restraints must be reevaluated every 4 hours for clients over 18 years of age, every 2 hours for clients 9 to 17 years of age, and every hour for children under 9 years. No standing orders or PRN orders are allowed for restraints. Facilities may choose to be more restrictive, but they cannot be less restrictive in the time frame for renewal of orders.

Documentation of the client's symptoms that lead to the implementation of restraints must be both subjective and objective and derived from a clinical evaluation. All less restrictive interventions utilized must be documented as well. Before caring for a client requiring behavioral seclusion or restraints, review facility policies, as they do vary from policies in an acute hospital.

When restraints are employed, they must be an appropriate method of restraint and be used in the least restrictive manner. The family, significant other, or guardian must be informed immediately when restraints are required. Many hospitals use "sitters" in place of restraints for clients whenever possible. Family members may be called on to sit with the client as well.

Devices and immobilization that are considered protective interventions but not "restraint" interventions include arm boards for IV stabilization, procedural immobilization such as the temporary use of soft restraints to prevent a client from interfering with a related treatment, or soft restraints and tabletop chairs that are used as a temporary preventative measure.

Restraint Guidelines

Review hospital policy for the use of restraints. Requires a physician's order.

Use restraints for the client's protection and to prevent injury only if all other less restrictive measures are not effective.

- Use the least amount of restraint possible. A torso belt is least restrictive, limb restraint is more restrictive, and chemical (medication) is most restrictive.
- Allow clients as much freedom of movement as possible. Use slip knots for quick release. Do not use square knots or bows.
- Always explain the purpose of the restraint to the client and family. Afford as much dignity to the client as possible.
- Remember that restraints can cause emotional, mental, and physical deterioration and increase the risk of injury if falls occur.
- Remember that circulation and skin integrity can be affected by restraints.
- Special precautions should be taken for adult females in restraints to protect breast tissue.
- Clients must be observed every 15 minutes.
- Release restraints every 2 hours for at least 5 minutes to inspect tissues and provide joint range of motion and position change to prevent circulatory impairment. When a client is combative, release only one restraint at a time.
- Assess and provide for client's fluid and elimination needs, pain management, and position change every 2 hours.
- Pad bony prominences, such as wrists and ankles, beneath a restraint.
- Attempt to make restraints as inconspicuous as possible for the sake of the client's relatives and friends, who may be upset by seeing restraints.
- Clearly document rationale and precautions taken for client safety.
- Notify family, significant other, or guardian if restraints are necessary.
- Enlist support of family members or significant other to sit with client rather than implement restraints.

ADAPTATION TO HOME CARE

The home environment should be evaluated for safety issues before the client is discharged from the hospital. The National Home Care Patient Safety Goals should be followed at home in order to improve the client's safety while recuperating. The following eight safety goals should be discussed with the client, family, and healthcare provider.

1. Identify patients correctly.

   Use at least two ways to identify patients. Use the patient's name and date of birth. Ask the patient and staff questions to make sure that the treatment being done is the correct one. Make sure that the treatment will be done at the correct place on the patient's body.
2. Improve staff communication.
   - Read back spoken or phone orders to the person who gave the order.
   - Create a list of abbreviations and symbols that are not to be used.
   - Quickly get important test results to the right staff person. Create steps for staff to follow when sending patients to the next caregiver. Make sure there is time to ask and answer questions.
3. Use medicines safely.
   - Create a list of medicines with names that look alike or sound alike. Update the list every year.
   - Take extra care with patients who take medicines to thin their blood.
4. Prevent infection.
   - Use the hand-cleaning guidelines from the World Health Organization or Centers for Disease Control and Prevention.
   - Report death or injury to patients from infections that happen in healthcare organizations.
   - Use proven guidelines to prevent infection of the blood.
5. Check patient medicines.
   - Ensure that it is OK for the patient to take any new medicines with their current medicines.
   - Provide a list of patient's medicines to their next caregiver. Give the list to the patient's regular doctor before the patient goes home.
   - Give a list of the patient's medicines to the patient and their family before they go home. Explain the list. Some patients may get medicine in small amounts for a short time. Make sure that it is OK for those patients to take those medicines with their current medicines.
6. Prevent patients from falling.
   - Determine which patients are most likely to fall. Take action to prevent falls in these patients.
7. Help patients to be involved in their care.
   - Tell each patient and their family how to report their complaints about safety.
8. Identify safety risks.
   - Find out if there are any risks for patients who are getting oxygen; for example, fires in the patient's home.

NOTE: For complete description of Home Care National Patient Safety Goals, refer to list available on The Joint Commission Web site (http://www.jointcommission.org/PatientSafety/NationalPatientSafetyGoals/08_ome_npsgs.htm).

NURSING DIAGNOSES

The following nursing diagnoses may be appropriate to include in a client care plan when the components are related to maintaining a safe environment.

NURSING DIAGNOSIS	RELATED FACTORS
Injury, Risk for	Motor, sensory, or cognitive alterations; elimination urgency; bleeding tendency; physiologic instability due to medications, aging, illness, environmental hazards
Disturbed Sensory Perception (Specify)	Medications, decreased sensory acuity, altered level of consciousness, mental status changes, environmental conditions
Impaired Tissue Integrity	Chemical, thermal, or mechanical factors, decreased mobility, nutritional deficiency
Self-Mutilation, Risk for	Labile behavior, depression, guilt, inadequate coping, loss of control over problem-solving situations

CLEANSE HANDS The single most important nursing action to decrease the incidence of hospital-based infections is hand hygiene. ***Remember to wash your hands or use antibacterial gel before and after each and every client contact.***

IDENTIFY CLIENT Before every procedure, introduce yourself and check two forms of client identification, not including room number. These actions prevent errors and conform to The Joint Commission standards.

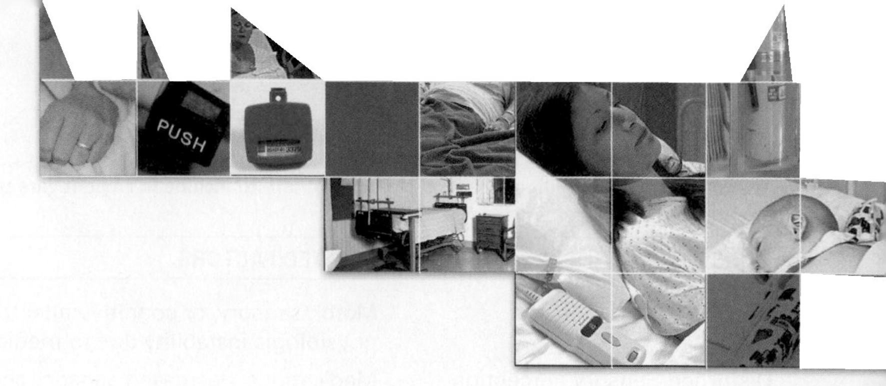

Chapter 7

UNIT 1

A Safe Environment

Nursing Process Data

ASSESSMENT Data Base

- Identify client's age, previous or chronic sensory impairments, previous level of mobility, ambulatory aids used, and general health history.
- Assess the client's reliability as an accurate health historian.
- Identify any alteration of sensory or motor abilities or emotional adaptation due to illness, injury, or hospitalization.
- Observe and record client's present level of consciousness, orientation, mobility, and any sensory or motor restrictions.
- Evaluate client's ability to comprehend instruction about how to use potentially dangerous equipment.
- Evaluate client's ability to make judgments.
- Assess need for specific precautions to promote a safe environment.
- Assess type of fire extinguisher needed for specific types of fires or use ABC extinguisher.
- Assess the need for protection while administering care to clients with radioactive implant.
- Assess prodromal signs and symptoms (aura) for potential seizure activity.
- Assess home for environmental safety.

PLANNING Objectives

- To provide protection when states of illness decrease the individual's ability to receive and interpret environmental stimuli
- To assist client to interpret environmental stimuli relevant to his or her safety
- To determine safety equipment necessary to promote a safe environment
- To place all personal articles and call light within easy reach of client
- To enhance degrees of mobility in a safe environment
- To determine that all electrical equipment is intact and operated safely
- To determine the protective devices needed when caring for clients receiving radioactive material
- To provide a safe environment for a client with seizure activity
- To determine that home environment is safe

IMPLEMENTATION Procedures

EVALUATION Expected Outcomes

- Client's environment is safe from potential mechanical, chemical, and fire or electrical hazards.
- All personal articles and call light are within easy reach of the client.
- All electrical equipment is intact and operated safely.
- If oxygen is used, appropriate safety measures are in effect.
- Personnel are protected from radioactive material.
- Client is free of injury after seizure.
- Client does not experience sequelae from seizure activity.

Pearson Nursing Student Resources

Find additional review materials at **nursing.pearsonhighered.com**

Prepare for success with NCLEX®-style practice questions and Skill Checklists

Preventing Client Falls

Equipment

Side rails, handrails
Alarm systems
Restraints
Locks for movable equipment, such as beds, wheelchairs, and gurneys

Procedure

1. Assess all clients for risk factors for falls.
2. Complete a comprehensive interview to determine potential for falls. Determine how many falls the client experienced in the last 6 months. Ask how they fall, backward or forward? Determine if medications are taken correctly and any dietary supplements the client is taking. Discuss client's diet: What foods and fluids do they eat and drink?
3. Determine psychosocial status. ▸ ***Rationale:*** To gain insight into how the client will react to necessary changes in their daily routine or changes in their house necessary to prevent falls.
4. Orient new clients to their surroundings, including use of call light.
5. Instruct ambulatory client in use of toilet and shower controls and emergency signals in bathroom.
6. Determine client's ability to safely use mobility aids.
7. Place bed in low position when you are not providing direct client care.
8. Determine appropriateness for side rail use.
9. Keep half side rails up for all heavily sedated, elderly, confused, and immediate postsurgical clients according to hospital policy.
10. Place articles such as call light, cups, and water within the client's reach.
11. Pad bed rails for client with high risk for seizures.
12. Remind client and hospital personnel to lock beds, wheelchairs, and gurneys and to release the lock only after client is secure for transport.
13. Tell clients who are weak, sedated, in pain, or who have had surgery to ask for assistance before getting out of bed.
14. Use two staff to transport client on gurney or wheelchair when nonattached equipment, such as chest-tube system or IV poles, must accompany client in transport.
15. Respond to client's summons as soon as possible.
16. Make sure floors are free of debris that might cause clients to slip and fall. Spilled liquids should be wiped up immediately. Encourage housekeepers to use signs for slippery areas.

Assess Clients for Risk Factors for Falls

- Adverse reaction to medications
- Alterations in vision
- Weakness and decreased physical functioning
- Altered mental acuity or confusion
- Neurological conditions (i.e., paralysis, stroke)
- Agitation
- Environmental hazards
- Difficulties with elimination
- Unsafe footwear and/or foot problems
- Orthostatic hypotension
- Reaching for articles out of the way
- Elderly clients
- Chronic health problems
- Alcohol consumption
- Pain
- Cardiovascular alterations

Source: Gustafson, S. (2007, December). Assess for fall risk, intervene—and bump up patient safety. *Nursing, 37,* 24–25.

17. Check to see that client's unit and hallway are neat and free of hazardous obstacles, such as foot stools, electrical cords, or shoes.

For the High-Risk Client

Clinical Alert

Risk Factors for Falls

There is a tendency for multiple fallers to repeat the type and location of the fall on successive falls (e.g., use of commode). Studies have identified a variety of fall risk factors that have led to the development of a number of fall risk assessment tools. Clients at high risk for fall generally demonstrate more than one of the following:

- History of falls
- Advanced age
- Sensory or motor impairment
- Urgent need for elimination
- Postural blood pressure instability

18. Attend to acute changes in client's behavior (e.g., hallucinations, abrupt disorientation, or altered responses or cognitive impairment). Monitor client frequently.

19. Continuously orient the disoriented client.
20. Assess and respond to fluid and elimination needs every 2 hours.
21. Employ bed, chair, and wander alarms. Bed alarms involve placing a sensor on the client's bed. When a change in position or loss of contact with the sensor occurs, an alarm alerts the nurse. Ambualarm devices are placed on the client's leg and signal an alarm when the legs are in a dependent position, indicating the client is trying to get out of bed.
22. Apply hip protectors on clients at risk for a fractured hip if they fall (i.e., clients with osteoporosis). Soft foam pads are held in place at the hips with specially designed removable briefs.
23. Assign aides or elicit the assistance of sitters or family to monitor the high-risk client; make certain they inform you when they leave the client's side.
24. Relocate high-risk client to room near nurses' station.
25. Utilize a recliner chair for client safety.
26. Place absorbent pad next to bed. ▶ ***Rationale:*** Prevents severe injury if client falls out of bed.
27. Keep intercom open between client's room and nurses' station.
28. Obtain physician's specific orders if restraints are deemed absolutely necessary.

EVIDENCE-BASED PRACTICE

Do Side Rails Prevent Falls?

A New Zealand study of almost 2,000 clients tested a new policy of restricting side rails. The results revealed that even though the use of side rails decreased (from 29% to 7%), the mean fall rate remained the same (36.6 falls/100 admissions). However, the falls that did occur were less severe.

Source: Hanger, H. C., Ball, M. C., & Wood, L. A. (1999). An analysis of falls in the hospital: Can we do without bedrails? *Journal of the American Geriatric Society*, 47(5):529–531.

Clinical Alert

Methods to Prevent Falls

To prevent at-risk clients from falling out of bed, consider using one of the following interventions:

- Use a mattress with raised edges; use body-length pillows, rolled blankets, or "swimming noodles" (foam flotation aids) under mattress edges.
- Place mat on floor next to bed.
- Place client in a very low to ground bed (7 to 13 inches above floor).
- Use bed alert alarms.
- Use half or three-fourth length side rails.
- Identify high-risk clients and implement a plan of action to prevent falls.
- Place high-risk client near nurses' station.
- Monitor high-risk client frequently, make rounds every 1 to 2 hours.
- Educate staff in fall prevention programs.
- Decrease environmental risks, obstacles, and clutter.
- Implement grab bars in bathroom and stabilize beds.
- Support client's elimination needs.
- Monitor client's reaction to medications.
- Assist clients with mobility.
- Ensure client wears nonskid slippers.
- Monitor client's mental status.
- Institute interventions to prevent falls from bed.
- Use safety straps or seat belts when in wheelchairs or geri-chairs.
- Involve family members in client prevention program.

Risk Assessment Tools for Falls

- Falls Efficacy Scale—measures how confident the individual is when performing ADLs
- Balance Self-Perception Test
- Berg Balance Scale
- Tinetti Mobility Assessment
- The Mini Mental State Examination—for assessing cognition

Exit Alarms

Posture indicator:	Adhesive transmitter patch is applied to thigh and to a receiver alarm box. When client attempts to get up, alarm goes off.
Pressure release:	Pads, mats, or other devices are placed on the floor or chair. They sense changes in weight and pressure.
Pressure-sensitive:	Pad or mat placed on floor by bed or chair sounds when stepped on.
Clip-on alarms:	Alarms activated by pulling detachable tab from the unit, a small box attached to the bed, chair, or wheelchair. A clip is attached to client's clothes. When client gets up, tab detaches from box and sounds an alarm.

TABLE 7-4 Fall Risk Assessment Form (Required Form)

Fall Risk Assessment Form (REQUIRED FORM)				
Name________		Date________	Examiner________	
PARAMETER		**SCORE**	**RESIDENT STATUS/CONDITION**	
A.	Level of Consciousness/Mental Status	0	ALERT (oriented X 3) OR COMATOSE	
		2	DISORIENTED X 3 at all times	
		4	INTERMITTENT CONFUSION	
B.	History of Falls (past 3 months)	0	NO FALLS in past 3 months	
		2	1 - 2 FALLS in past 3 months	
		4	3 OR MORE FALLS in past 3 months	
C.	Ambulation/Elimination Status	0	AMBULATORY/CONTINENT	
		2	CHAIR BOUND - requires restraints and assist with elimination	
		4	AMBULATORY/INCONTINENT	
D.	Vision Status	0	ADEQUATE (with or without glasses)	
		2	POOR (with or without glasses)	
		4	LEGALLY BLIND	
E.	Gait/Balance	To assess the resident's Gait/Balance, have him/her stand on both feet without holding onto anything; walk straight forward; walk through a doorway, and make a turn.		
		0	Gait/Balance normal	
		1	Balance problem while standing	
		1	Balance problem while walking	
		1	Decreased muscular coordination	
		1	Change in gait pattern when walking through doorway	
		1	Jerking or unstable when making turns	
		1	Requires use of assistive devices (i.e., cane, w/c, walker, furniture)	
F.	Systolic Blood Pressure	0	NO NOTED DROP between lying and standing	
		2	Drop LESS THAN 20 mm Hg between lying and standing	
		4	Drop MORE THAN 20 mm Hg between lying and standing	
G.	Medications	Respond below based on the following types of medications: Anesthetics, Antihistamines, Antihypertensives, Antiseizure, Benzodiazepines, Cathartics, Diuretics, Hypoglycemics, Narcotics, Psychotropics, Sedatives/Hypnotics.		
		0	NONE of these medications taken currently or within last 7 days	
		2	TAKES 1 - 2 of these medications currently and/or within last 7 days	
		4	TAKES 3 - 4 of these medications currently and/or within last 7 days	
		1	If resident has had a change in medications and/or change in dosage in past 5 days = score 1 additional point	
H.	Predisposing Diseases	Respond below based on the following predisposing conditions: Hypotension, Vertigo, CVA, Parkinson's disease, Loss of limb(s), Seizures, Arthritis, Osteoporosis, Fractures.		
		0	NONE PRESENT	
		2	1 - 2 PRESENT	
		4	3 OR MORE PRESENT	
Total score of 10 or above represents HIGH RISK			**TOTAL SCORE:________**	

Source: http://classes.Kume.edu/som/amed900/ExposureSkills/long_term_care_fall_risk_assessm (from LTCS Books.com)

TABLE 7-5 Clinical Guidelines for the Prevention of Falls and Injuries in the Older Adult

- Brief assessment of all clients will identify those who should be referred for a comprehensive fall evaluation.
- Assessments may be done by all healthcare professionals.
- Because of the many factors associated with falls, one test cannot identify individuals at risk for falls. Several tests assessing for risk factors should be utilized.
- **Clients at risk for falls include older clients with:**
  Medical needs who have experienced one or more falls
  Reported recurrent falls
  Abnormalities in gait and/or balance
- **Comprehensive clinical risk assessment usually consists of:**
  A review of falls, history, and circumstances
  Assessing home for hazards
  Identifying medications routinely taken
  Assessing gait, balance, mobility, and muscle weakness
  Identifying risk for osteoporosis
  Evaluating perceived functional ability and fear of falling
  Assessing visual impairment and effects of corrective eyewear
  Presence of urinary incontinence
  Assessing acute and chronic health problems, joint function, and basic neurological function
- **Fall prevention:**
  Utilize exercise programs
  Implement behavior changes
  Review medications
  Treat contributing health conditions
  Use assistive and protective devices
  Modify house to prevent injury
  Educate client and family in ways to prevent falls

Source: American Geriatrics Society. (2004). Guideline for the Prevention of Falls in Older Persons.

Preventing Thermal/Electrical Injuries

Equipment

Fire extinguishers

Procedure

1. Make sure that all electrical apparatuses are routinely checked and maintained. Look for safety inspection expiration dates on biomedical equipment.
2. Have all electrical appliances brought to the hospital by client (radios, electric razors, hair dryers, etc.) inspected by hospital maintenance staff. It is best to discourage use of nonhospital equipment.
3. Make sure water in the tub or shower is not more than 110°F (95°F for those with circulatory insufficiency).
4. When heating pads, sitz bath, or hot compresses are used, check the client frequently for redness. Maximum temperature should not exceed 105°F (95°F for those with circulatory insufficiency).
5. Hospitals do not allow smoking in the facility. There may be designated smoking areas outside the building. Inform clients and visitors about the hospital's smoking regulations. Do not allow confused, sedated, or severely incapacitated clients to smoke without direct supervision.
6. Store all combustible materials securely to prevent spontaneous combustion.
7. Make sure that all staff and employees participate in and understand fire safety measures, such as extinguishing fires and plan for evacuating clients.
8. Report and do not use any apparatus that produces a shock, has a broken plug or ground pin, or has a frayed cord.
9. Never apply direct heat (e.g., heating pad) to ischemic tissue—doing so increases the tissue's need for oxygen.
10. Turn equipment off before unplugging it. ▶ ***Rationale:*** This prevents sparks that can cause a fire.
11. Plug devices that require a high current (i.e., ventilators or radiant warmers) into separate outlets. ▶ ***Rationale:*** This prevents overloading the circuit that could lead to a fire.
12. Use only three-pronged grounded plugs.

Clinical Alert

The elderly, diabetic, or comatose client is especially vulnerable to thermal injuries.

Providing Safety for Clients During a Fire

Equipment

Appropriate extinguisher for fire:

Water type
Soda-acid type
Foam type
Dry chemical type
ABC extinguisher

Procedure

1. Follow hospital policy and procedure for type of fire safety program and for ringing the fire alarm to summon help.
2. Remove all clients from the immediate area to a safe place. Be familiar with fire exits and agency evacuation plan.
3. To remove a client safely from the fire, use carrying method that is most comfortable for you and safe for client.
   a. Place blanket (or bedspread) on floor. Lower client onto blanket. Lift up head end of blanket and drag client out of danger.
   b. Use two-person swing method. Place client in sitting position. Form a seat by having two people clasp forearms or shoulders. Lift client into "seat" and carry out of danger.
   c. Carry client using "back-strap" carry method. Step in front of client. Place client's arms around your neck. Grasp client's wrists and hold tight against your chest. Pull client onto your back and carry to safety.
4. Activate fire alarm.
5. Secure the burning area by closing all doors and windows.
6. Shut off all possible oxygen sources and electrical appliances in the fire area.
7. If possible, employ the appropriate extinguishing method without endangering yourself. Fire extinguishers should not be used directly on a person.
8. Be familiar with the different types of fire extinguishers and their location.

Class A

a. Water-under-pressure type or soda-acid type.
b. Use on cloth, wood, paper, plastic, rubber or leather.
c. Never use on electrical or chemical fires due to danger of shock.

Class B

a. Foam, dry chemical, carbon dioxide types.
b. Use on fires such as gasoline, alcohol, acetone, oil, grease, or paint thinner and remover.
c. Class A extinguisher is never used on class B fires.

Class C

a. Dry chemical or carbon dioxide types.
b. Use on electrical wiring, electrical equipment, or motors.
c. Class A or class B extinguishers are never used on class C fires.

Class ABC combination

a. Contains graphite.
b. Use on any type of fire.
c. Most common extinguisher in use.

9. Keep fire exits clear at all times.

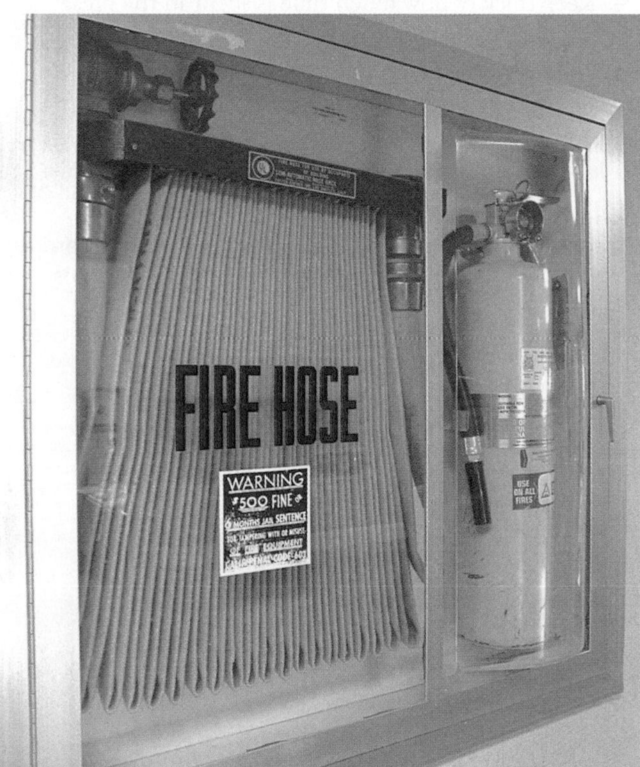

▲ Become familiar with the location and use of fire extinguishers in the hospital.

Priorities for Fire Safety

R Rescue and remove all clients in immediate danger
A Activate fire alarm
C Confine the fire; close doors, windows; turn off oxygen supplies and electrical equipment
E Extinguish fire when possible

Providing Safety for Clients Receiving Radioactive Materials

Equipment

Protective shields for x-ray
Lead-shielded container if required
Film badge if required
Sign for client's door: "Caution, Radioactive Material"

General Guidelines for Radiation Precautions*

Radioactive Implant

- Care time not to exceed 15 minutes per employee per day.
- No pregnant woman or anyone under age 18 should enter room.
- No special handling of excreta other than standard precautions
- Bath usually omitted, client movement restricted.
- Visitors limited to 1 hour/day, keeping distance from client.
- All linens, gloves, trash, and dressings kept in room until cleared by radiation safety officer.

Systemic Radioactive Material

- No lab specimens to be taken without consent of radiation safety officer.
- Use disposable dietary tray.
- Handle all excreta and secretions with gloves.
- Have client use toilet—flushing twice.
- Shielding not needed.
- Visitors require special instructions.
- Keep gloves, dressings, linens, and trash in contaminated container.

***NOTE:** See Institutional Policy for Specifics.

Procedure

1. Review these guidelines:
   a. Determine type and amount of radiation used and its side effects and hazards.
   b. Rotate care providers because increased time in the presence of a radioactive source increases exposure to radiation.
   c. Use shields, such as lead walls or lead aprons, to protect from radioactive source.
   d. Inform staff that exposure is greater the closer the person is to the radioactive source.
   e. Store radioactive material in lead-shielded containers when not in use.
   f. Issue monitoring badge to all who enter room to record exposure.
2. If nurse or family member is assisting with a radioactive procedure, they must put on a shield.
3. If a radioactive implant is used in a client, all nurses and visitors must be protected with a shield. Limit exposure with the client.
4. Keep track of how much time is spent in the presence of radioactive material. Check film badge frequently.
5. Constantly assess and support clients who are undergoing radiation therapy. Bed rest, isolation, and unpleasant side effects are sometimes common.

Clinical Alert

Pregnant nurses should check hospital policy regarding working with clients receiving radioactive materials.

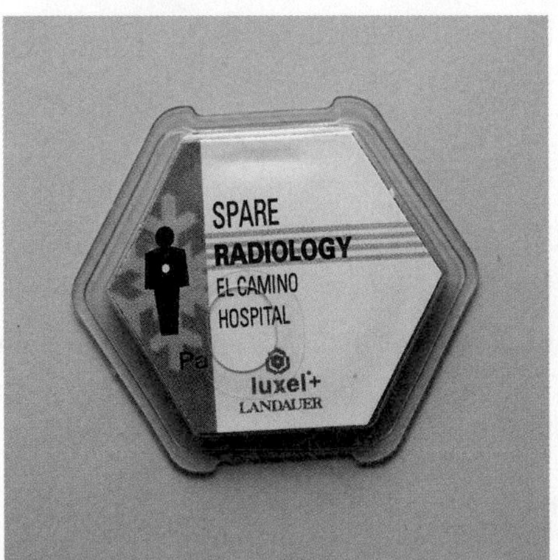

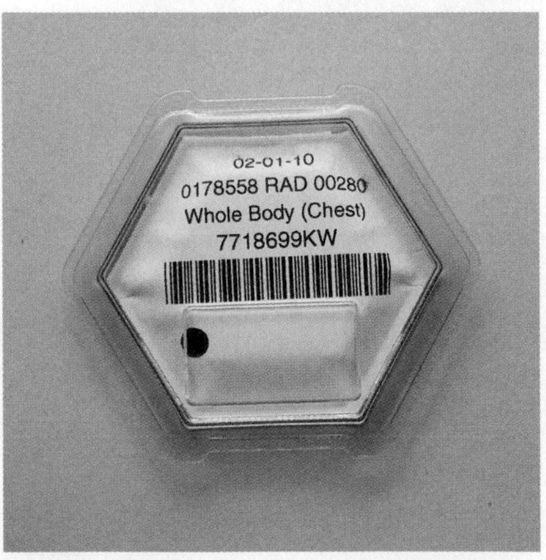

▲ Badge worn when working with clients receiving radioactive material.

6. Follow guidelines for working with clients with unsealed sources of iodine-131.
   a. Wear rubber gloves at all times when providing care.
   b. Wash gloves before removing, and place in designated waste container.
   c. Wash hands with soap and water after removing gloves.
   d. Dispose of all bed linen in contaminated linen bag.
   e. Wrap all nondisposable items that have come in contact with client's blood, saliva, or gastric juices in plastic bag. Send to appropriate hospital department for decontamination (usually nuclear medicine department).
   f. Notify radiation safety officer (usually in radiology department) if clothes or shoes have been contaminated.
   g. Instruct visitors and family member of no visitations for 24 hours.

Clinical Alert

Client Education After Receiving Radioactive Iodine

- Check with physician regarding guidelines
- Follow these guidelines, if approved by physician

7. If client is discharged immediately after radioactive iodine, provide client instructions.
   a. Minimize contact (less than 3 feet or 0.6 meter for more than 1 hour each day) with everyone for the first 5 days, and with small children or pregnant women for 8 days.
   b. Do not sit next to someone in an automobile for more than 1 hour.
   c. Sleep in a separate room and use separate bath linen and launder these and underclothing separately for 1 week.
   d. Wash hands with soap and water every time the toilet is used.
   e. Rinse the sink and tub thoroughly after using them.
   f. Use separate eating utensils or disposable eating utensils. Wash eating utensils separately for 1 week. Do not prepare food for others.
   g. Flush toilet 2 to 3 times after use for 2 weeks after discharge.
   h. Males should sit when urinating to avoid splashing for 1 week.

Providing Safety for Clients With Seizure Activity

Equipment

Oral airway

Padding material for side rails

Suction equipment and catheters

Clean gloves

Preparation

1. Identify client at risk for seizure activity (e.g., clients with closed head injury, neurosurgical clients, meningitis, history of seizures).
2. Place suction equipment and catheters on bedside stand.
3. Tape oral airway to head of bed or place on wall.
4. Pad side rails with blankets or other heavy material.

Procedure

1. Determine type of seizure activity, if client has a previous history of seizures. ▸ ***Rationale:*** Assists in determining potential type of seizure activity, client response, and presence of an aura.
2. Place client in side-lying position, with pillow at head of bed and side rails in raised position, if seizure activity is anticipated. ▸ ***Rationale:*** To protect client from injury.
3. When seizure activity begins, provide privacy; ensure bed is in low position and side rails are raised.
4. Maintain client in side-lying position with head flexed slightly forward. Do not restrain client or place anything in client's mouth. ▸ ***Rationale:*** To prevent injury to jaw or teeth. Flexed head will prevent tongue from occluding airway.
5. Remain with client during seizure to ensure airway is not occluded and client does not require suctioning.
6. Explain that client had a seizure when he/she is alert.
7. Remain with client after seizure to ensure he/she has an uneventful postictal period. Client usually sleeps for a period of time after seizure.
8. Document findings and notify physician of seizure.

Assessing Home for Safe Environment

Equipment

Home Assessment Checklist

Outcome and Assessment Information Act (OASIS-B1)

Procedure

1. Identify type of dwelling (i.e., client-owned, boarding home, rental, mobile home).
2. Identify water source.

3. Identify sewer source.
4. Identify type of plumbing available.
5. Determine if any pollutants are present in the environment.
6. Assess exterior of the home for:
   a. Condition of sidewalks and steps.
   b. Presence of railings on steps.
   c. Barriers that prevent easy access to the home.
   d. Adequacy of lighting.
   e. Adequacy of roof and windows.
7. Assess interior of the home for:
   a. Presence of scatter rugs or worn carpeting.
   b. Uncluttered pathways throughout the house.
   c. Adequacy of lighting.
   d. Doorways wide enough to permit assistive devices.
   e. Cleanliness of house.
   f. Presence of insects, rodents, or infective agents.
   g. Presence of functioning smoke detectors.
   h. Adequate heating and cooling systems.
   i. Presence of running water.
8. Determine whether hazardous materials are safely stored.
9. Assess for presence of lead-based paint.
10. Determine whether medications can be adequately stored out of reach of children and impaired individuals.
11. Assess stairway and halls for:
    a. Adequacy of light.
    b. Handrails that are securely fastened to wall.
    c. Flooring in good repair.
    d. Rugs or carpeting in good repair.
    e. Light switches in easy reach and accessible at both ends of stairs or hallway.
12. Assess kitchen for:
    a. Properly functioning stove.
    b. Adequacy of light surrounding stove and sink.
    c. Condition of small appliances.
    d. Accessibility of appliances to clients in wheelchairs.
    e. Adequacy of sewage disposal.
13. Assess bathroom for:
    a. Skidproof strips or mat in tub or shower.
    b. Handrails around toilet and tub or shower.
    c. Accessibility of medicine cabinet.
    d. Adequate space if wheelchairs or walkers are used.
    e. Temperature of hot water from faucets in sink, tub, or shower.
14. Assess bedroom for:
    a. Accessibility of closets and cabinets.
    b. Ease in getting into and out of bed.
    c. Adequate space, if commode or wheelchair is required.
    d. Night light availability.
    e. Accessibility of medications, water on night stand.
    f. Calling system to alert healthcare provider.
    g. Flooring in good repair and nonslippery surface.

DOCUMENTATION for Providing a Safe Environment

- Assessment notes
- Actual incidents involving mechanical, chemical, or thermal trauma
- Client education provided
- Safety devices used
- Behaviors occurring before, during, and after seizure activity
- Safety issues instituted for client receiving radioactive iodine
- Completion of home environment forms

Legal Considerations

Using Bed Alarms to Prevent Falls

Several small studies, with low numbers of clients, were conducted to determine whether use of bed alarms prevents falls. The conclusion indicated insufficient evidence regarding the effectiveness of bed alarms in preventing falls in elderly clients. Additional studies will need to be conducted to determine the usefulness of these devices in fall prevention.

Source: http://www.injuryboard.com, Using Bed Alarms to Prevent Falls.

Client Falls

Even though client falls are second only to medication errors in untoward events that happen to clients in hospitals, it does not mean that fault will be assessed against healthcare providers.

If it can be proven that the nursing staff used poor judgment in preventing client falls, liability will be assessed against the staff. A client was noted to be at high risk for falls but even with this data, was not placed on fall prevention interventions.*

In a second case, *Sullivan v. Edward Hospital,* 2004, the court found that the institution had taken appropriate measures to safeguard a client who fell and developed a subdural hematoma.**

Source: **Williams v. Covenant Medical Center*, 2000. **Guido, G.W. (2006). *Legal and Ethical Issues in Nursing*, 4th ed. Upper Saddle River, NJ: Prentice Hall, 2006, p. 395.

CRITICAL THINKING Application

Expected Outcomes

- Client's environment is safe from potential mechanical, chemical, and fire or electrical hazards.
- All personal articles and call light are within easy reach of the client.
- All electrical equipment is intact and operated safely.
- If oxygen is used, appropriate safety measures are in effect.
- Personnel are protected from radioactive material.
- Client is free of injury after seizure.
- Client does not experience sequelae from seizure activity.

Unexpected Outcomes	Alternative Actions
The client, nurse, or visitor experiences an accident or injury related to mechanical, chemical, or thermal trauma.	• Provide immediate first aid or care. • Assess vital signs and notify physician. • Report the incident according to hospital procedure. Unusual occurrence forms are used to protect the injured individual, the nurse, and the hospital. • Review safety procedures to ensure a safe environment. • Report all malfunctioning equipment immediately to the proper department.
Unfamiliarity with hospital fire and disaster protocol results in poor performance.	• Review protocols frequently to update knowledge base. • Participate in fire and disaster drills to become familiar with protocols.
Radium implant becomes dislodged and falls out.	• Put on lead gloves, pick up radium with forceps, and place in lead-shielded container in client's room. • Notify physician and hospital radiation safety officer immediately. • Never touch radioactive source directly.
Spillage of excreta from client with systemic radioactive therapy.	• Cover spillage with absorbent material and notify radiation safety officer. • Wash with soap and water if skin is contaminated.

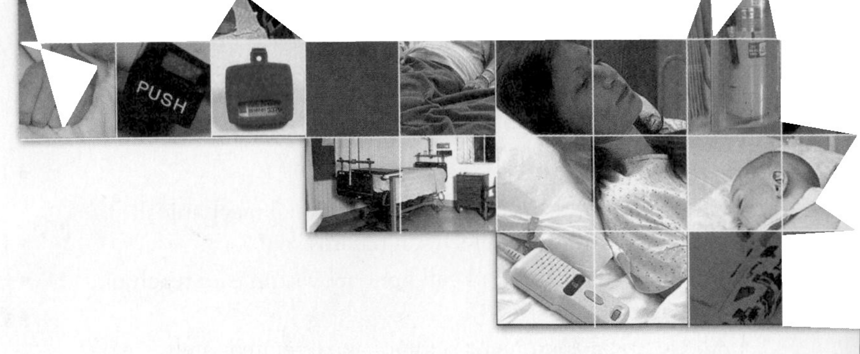

Chapter 7

UNIT 2

Restraints

Nursing Process Data

ASSESSMENT Data Base

- Assess client's risk for falls on an ongoing basis.
- Assess need for fall prevention measures.
- Assess area under and surrounding a restraint to ensure it is not restrictive.
- Evaluate client's response to restraint use.

PLANNING Objectives

- To identify clients who are at risk for injury
- To prevent a client from injuring himself/herself or others
- To employ fall prevention measures
- To obtain physician's order for restraints if deemed absolutely necessary
- To apply restraints safely and effectively
- To restrain a child's elbow to prevent the child from reaching an incision
- To promote client safety when ambulating or sitting in a chair

IMPLEMENTATION Procedures

EVALUATION Expected Outcomes

- Client is prevented from injuring himself (herself) or others.
- Restraints are applied appropriately.
- Client does not develop complications due to restraint use (e.g., agitation, pressure ulcers, circulatory disturbance).
- Child is prevented from reaching the incision site, IVs, or tubes.
- Client remains in restraints for a limited amount of time.
- Client does not experience complications as a result of restraint placement.
- Client does not endure undue psychological stress while being placed in restraints.

Pearson Nursing Student Resources

Find additional review materials at **nursing.pearsonhighered.com**

Prepare for success with NCLEX®-style practice questions and Skill Checklists

Managing Clients in Restraints

Equipment

Appropriate restraint, limb, torso, and vest

Preparation

1. Identify and evaluate if less restrictive measures have been explored before the client is placed in restraints.
2. Call physician or licensed independent practitioners (LIP) for restraint order before applying restraints. If restraints must be placed before the order is obtained, ensure the order is obtained within 1 hour for either a nonbehavioral health client or a behavioral health client. ▸ ***Rationale:*** Physician's order is required to apply restraints.

NOTE: Follow guidelines for obtaining restraint orders and updating orders according to hospital policy.

3. Ensure that a face-to-face assessment is completed on the client within 8 hours for a nonbehavioral health client and 1 hour for a behavioral (psychiatric) health client. ▸ ***Rationale:*** Frequent assessments prevent complications.
4. Ensure that restraint orders are renewed every 24 hours or sooner according to facility policy for nonbehavioral health clients or every 2 to 4 hours for behavioral health clients. Children from 12 to 17 must have orders renewed every 2 hours, for a maximum of 24 hours. ▸ ***Rationale:*** Restraints should be discontinued as soon as possible.
5. Establish and implement a plan of care for the client to eliminate the need for restraints.
6. Discuss the use of restraints with the client and family members. If possible, elicit the support of the family or use sitters to stay with the client rather than place the client in restraints.

Clinical Alert

Restraints are indicated only if there is no other viable option available to protect the client, and then they are implemented only when the client is assessed and evaluated by an appropriate licensed independent practitioner (LIP).

There are three types of restraints used in clinical practice:

1. *Chemical:* Sedating psychotropic drugs to manage or control behavior. Psychoactive medication used in this manner is an inappropriate use of medication.
2. *Physical:* Direct application of physical force to a client, without the client's permission, to restrict his or her freedom of movement.
3. *Seclusion:* Involuntary confinement of a client in a locked room. Physical force may be applied by individuals, mechanical devices, or a combination of any of them.

Source: The Joint Commission. (2000). www.thejointcommission.org.

Procedure

1. Gather appropriate restraint and perform hand hygiene.
2. Identify client using two identifiers and seek client's cooperation with restraint procedure, if possible.
3. Apply restraint according to manufacturer's specific directions.
4. Monitor and assess the client every 15 minutes, or according to facility policy.
5. Release restraint at least every 2 hours or sooner (The Joint Commission). ▸ ***Rationale:*** Releasing restraints allows the client to be provided with the following:
   a. Toileting.
   b. Fluids and food.
   c. Hygiene care such as brushing teeth or washing face and hands.
   d. Circulation checked; skin care provided.
   e. Body alignment checked.
   f. Range of motion to all joints, particularly those in restraints.

Clinical Alert

In acute medical and postsurgical care, a restraint may be necessary to ensure that an IV or tube feeding is not removed, or the client cannot be allowed out of bed after surgery. This type of medical restraint may be used temporarily to limit mobility or prevent injury to the client.

Additional types of activities that may constitute a restraint include:

- Tucking a client's sheet so tight that he/she cannot move.
- Using a side rail to prevent a client from voluntarily getting out of bed.
- Placing the client in a geri-chair with a table.
- Placing a wheelchair-bound client so close to the wall that it prevents them from moving.

6. Avoid application of force on long bone joints and pad bony prominences beneath restraint. ▸ ***Rationale:*** Reduces pressure on skin.
7. Take vital signs every 8 hours unless indicated more frequently.
8. Bathe client every 24 hours or more often as needed.
9. Do not interrupt the client's sleep unless indicated by his/her medical condition.
10. Ensure that a new order and the physician or LIP completes a medical assessment every 24 hours.
11. Obtain a physician's order and discontinue restraints as soon as it is clinically indicated.
12. Document all assessments and findings on appropriate forms.

EVIDENCE-BASED PRACTICE

Effects of Restraints on Reducing Falls

Studies have indicated that restraints do not reduce falls, prevent the removal of medical devices such as tracheostomy tubes or IVs, or increase client safety. Forty-seven percent of clients who fall are restrained, and 81% who remove their endotracheal tubes are restrained with wrist restraints. Restrained clients are eight times more likely to die during hospitalization. This is directly related not only to the use of restraints but to the fact they usually have IVs, dementia, or surgical intervention. The use of restraints or seclusion has led to more than 140 deaths in the past decade in behavioral health care facilities. Asphyxiation is the most common cause of restraint-related death when clients are trapped between the side rail and the mattress or bed frame.

Source: http://www2.nursingspectrum.com (Geriatic Anthology, 2005 Edition. Avelene Orhon. JECH.

TABLE 7-6 Methods to Decrease Use of Physical or Chemical Restraints

Environmental Alterations	Physiological Approaches
• Use alternatives such as wedge or roll cushions for positional support	• Potential complication assessment (i.e., increased temperature or hypoxia)
• Adjust lighting at night to decrease fear of unknown and facilitate vision of where bed is in room	• Pain relief
• Use rolled edge mattresses	• Comfort measures
• Use low-level beds (7 to 13 in. from floor)	• Physical therapy/exercises
• Place mats on floor in case of client fall	**Psychosocial Interventions**
• Use special beds	• Identify and alter factors that are causing client anxiety, if possible
• Place in special unit where client can be watched more carefully	• Talk with client
• Use sitters or family members	• Involve client in activities that take his or her mind off what is happening
• Use upper side rails only for aid in turning and moving	• Encourage interaction with family members by phone if necessary

Applying Torso/Belt Restraint

Equipment

Safety belt restraint (usually 2-in. soft webbing material) with waist and side belts (for bed)

Procedure

1. Check physician's order and client care plan for torso/belt restraint. Perform hand hygiene.
2. Obtain belt. Belts usually have a key-locked buckle.
   ▸ ***Rationale:*** To prevent slipping and to provide a snug fit.
3. Identify client using two identifiers and explain necessity for safety belt to client and family.
4. Apply torso restraint as follows:
   a. Slip waist belt through flat buckle, adjusting to client's size.
   b. Snap hinged plate shut by hooking plain end of key over cross bar and lifting upward.
   c. Attach side belts to bed frame in similar manner.
   d. Release restraint by hooking green end of key over cross bar from below and pulling downward.
5. Document time, rationale, and type of safety belt used in nurses' notes, along with client monitoring, client response, frequency of care measures, and time and rationale for discontinuing restraint. Documentation must be done every 15 minutes.

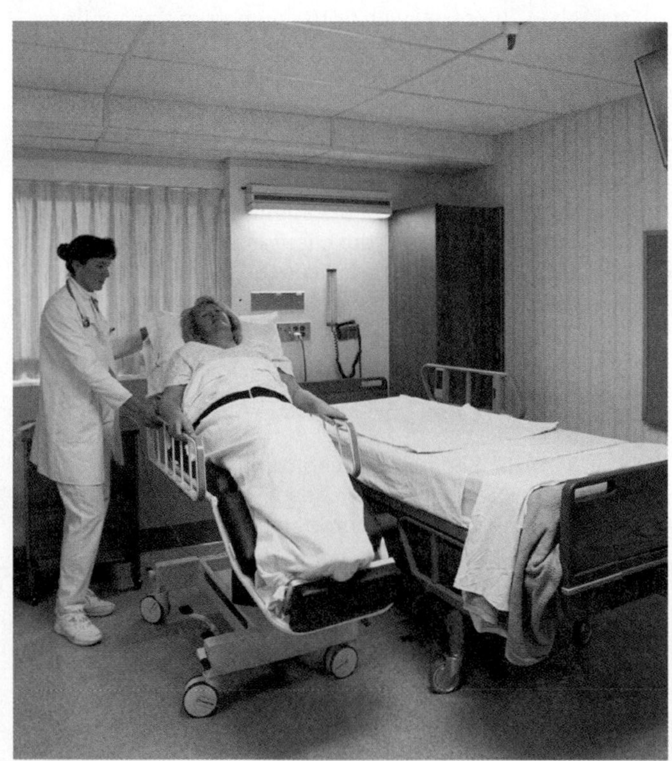

▲ Some belts have a key-locked buckle to prevent slipping and to provide a snug fit.

EVIDENCE-BASED PRACTICE

Deaths Due to Use of Physical Restraint or Seclusion

A 50-state survey by the *Hartford Courant* in 1998 identified at least 142 deaths related to the use of physical restraint or seclusion since 1988. The true number of deaths is much higher since data regarding this type of information is not public information. According to statistical projections commissioned by the *Courant* and conducted by the Harvard Center for Risk Analysis, between 50 and 150 deaths occur every year across the country due to improper restraint procedures. Based on this data, it was felt there is a critical need for mandated monitoring of the use of restraints and seclusion.

Source: American Nurses Association. (2001). Position Statements: Reduction of Patient Restraint and Seclusion in Health Care Settings. www.nursingworld.org/EthicsHumanRights.

Using Wrist Restraints

Equipment

Commercial cloth restraints with flannel padding
Ace bandages of appropriate size for area to be immobilized
Call bell for communication

Procedure

1. Attempt all other methods of client protection or less restrictive measures before applying restraints.
2. Check physician's order for wrist or ankle soft restraint. If necessary, place restraint on client, then phone physician or LIP for orders within 1 hour of application of restraint.

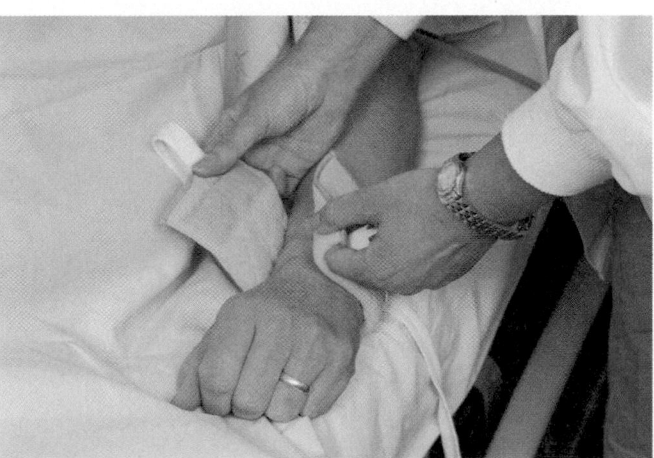

▲ First, apply padded portion of restraint around wrist or ankle.

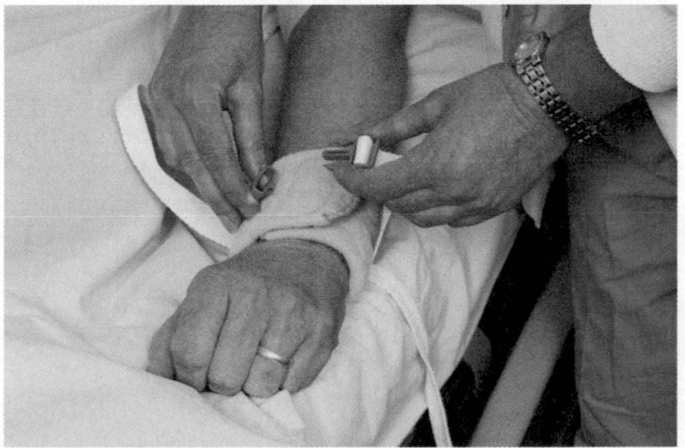

▲ Secure restraint by pinching long-pronged adapter and inserting into buckle end of restraint.

3. Obtain soft restraints. Check correct size of restraints.
4. When applying restraint, place padded section over the wrist or ankle. Ensure restraint will not interfere with IVs or tubes.
5. Secure restraint by pinching long-pronged adapter and inserting into buckle end of restraint, or follow manufacturer's directions.
6. Slip two fingers under restraint. ▸ ***Rationale:*** This ensures it is not too tight and will not constrict blood flow.
7. Attach other end of restraint under movable portion of bed frame by using a half-bow knot. ▸ ***Rationale:*** This is a quick release knot and will untie quickly in an emergency.

Clinical Alert

Always keep scissors in easy access to facilitate cutting restraints in case of an emergency.

8. Release restraints every 2 hours. ▸ ***Rationale:*** Release is necessary to:
   a. Check limb circulation and skin condition.
   b. Provide extremity range of motion.
   c. Change client's position.
   d. Attend to elimination, fluid, or other needs.
9. Document use of and rationale for wrist restraints in nurses' notes. Identify all less restrictive actions tried before restraints.
10. Monitor client every 15 minutes. ▸ ***Rationale:*** Frequent monitoring prevents complications.

Clinical Alert

Limb, vest, and mitt restraints are considered a type II restraint. A type I restraint is a four-point locked restraint. Type I restraints are used primarily in psychiatric or emergency room settings.

If using any locked restraint, keep the key in client's room taped to the top of bed or near "stat" call button. It must be in sight and easily accessible in case of emergency.

Alternate Type of Soft Restraint

- Slide strap through slit in restraint.
- Tighten strap, leaving fingerbreadth space between restraint and client's limb.

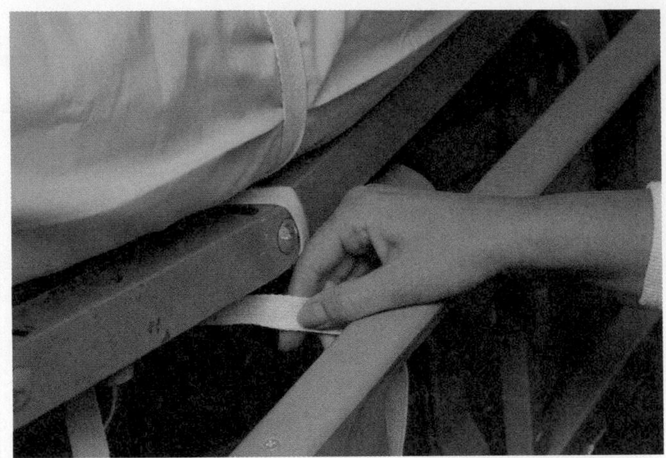

▲ Secure restraint under moveable part of bed, using slipknot.

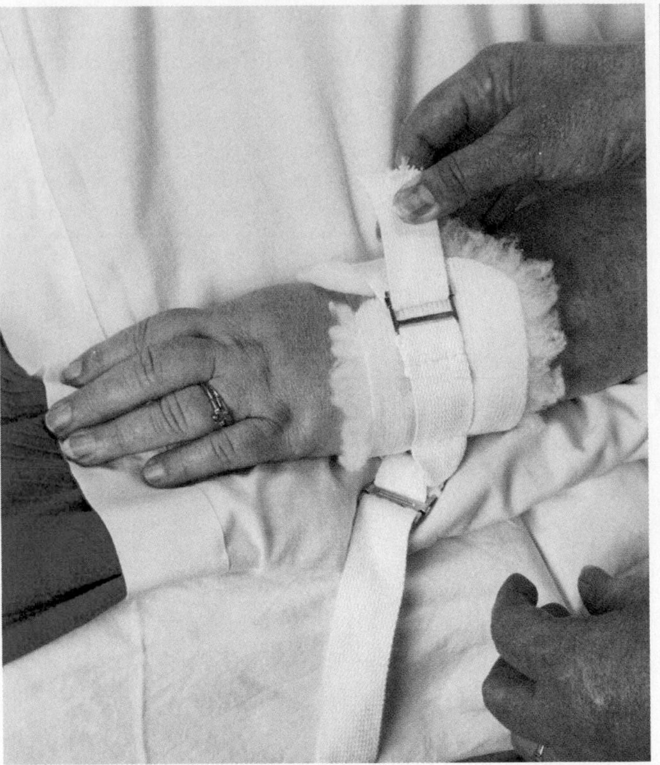

Using Mitt Restraints

Equipment

Mitt restraint
Gauze padding
Call bell for communication

Procedure

1. Check physician's order, or after placing mitt restraint, phone physician or LIP for orders.
2. Determine whether less restrictive actions could be used.
3. Perform hand hygiene.
4. Obtain appropriate size mitt restraint and gauze padding, if needed.
5. Identify the client by checking two forms of identification.
6. Explain steps and purpose of procedure to family and client (to gain his or her cooperation) if client is able to understand.
7. Raise bed to high position.
8. Lower side rail as needed.
9. Check condition of skin and circulation in involved extremity.
10. Wrap fingers with gauze to absorb moisture and prevent abrasion, if necessary.
11. Apply mitt; secure wrist ties snugly, but maintain circulation by ensuring that two fingers can be slipped under the restraint.
12. For hand control, use slip knot to tie restraints to immovable part of bed frame, not to side rail.
13. Place call bell within access and monitor client every 15 minutes.
14. Remove mitt every 2 hours. ► ***Rationale:*** This is necessary to:
    a. Check adequacy of circulation and skin condition.
    b. Provide extremity range of motion.
    c. Change client's position.
    d. Provide for fluid.
15. Reapply mitt.
16. Raise bedrail and lower bed, according to facility policy.
17. Perform hand hygiene.
18. Chart on nurses' notes: client behavior necessitating restraint, all less restrictive actions taken, condition of skin, adequacy of circulation of involved extremity, time of mitt application, times of release and observed responses, and care needs met. Documentation must be done every 15 minutes.

Clinical Alert

Restraints are never used as a substitute for surveillance.

NOTE: In confused ambulatory clients, restraint use has been associated with increased falls.

Using Elbow Restraints

Equipment

Elbow restraint
Soft padding

Procedure

1. Check physician's order. This type of restraint, if used for medical procedures or to protect IVs, does not require specific restraint orders.
2. Obtain elbow restraints (many types are available).
3. Explain necessity of restraints to child's parents.
4. Place restraints over elbow of both arms. You may need to insert tongue blades into pockets of restraint.
5. Wrap restraints snugly around the arm. Secure by tying the restraints at the top. Many restraints have ties long enough to cross under the child's back and tie under the opposite arm.
6. For small infants and children, tie or pin restraints to their shirts.

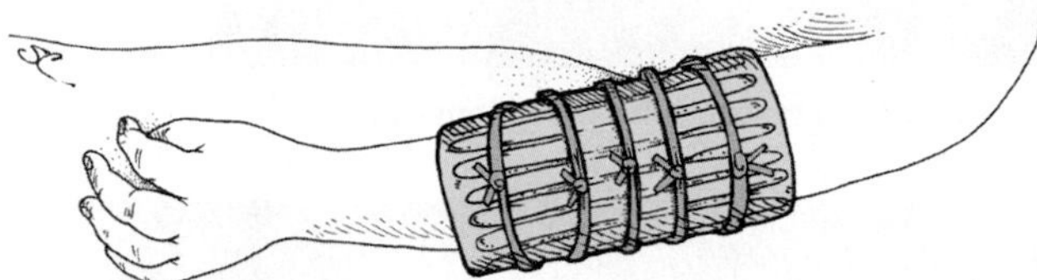

▲ Elbow restraints prevent children from reaching equipment.

7. Release the restraints every 2 hours. ▶ ***Rationale:*** This allows for joint mobility.
8. Assess position of restraints, circulation, skin condition, and sensation every hour.
9. Provide diversionary activity for small child.
10. Encourage parents or hospital personnel to hold child to promote a feeling of security.
11. Document use of restraints in nurses' notes. Document release of restraints, skin, and circulatory condition. Documentation must be done every 15 minutes.

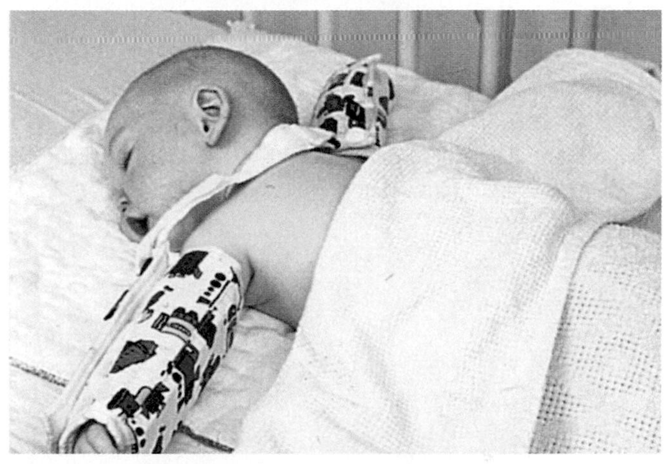

▲ Elbow restraints may be used to prevent child from reaching his or her face or head.

Applying a Vest Restraint

Equipment

Safety vest
Call bell for communication

Procedure

For Client in Bed

1. Check physician's order or apply vest and call physician or LIP within 1 hour for order.
2. Determine whether less restrictive actions could be used.
3. Explain necessity for jacket or vest restraint to client and family.
4. Place vest over gown.
5. Place safety vest on client so that closed side of vest is in back and front side of vest crosses over chest or according to manufacturer's directions. ▶ ***Rationale:*** This prevents choking if client slumps forward.
6. Bring strap through slit in front of the vest. ▶ ***Rationale:*** Criss-crossing vest in the back may cause serious injury.

Clinical Alert

The use of vest restraint has been associated with serious injury, including client suffocation. If your facility still uses this restraint, exercise extreme caution in applying restraint and monitor frequently.

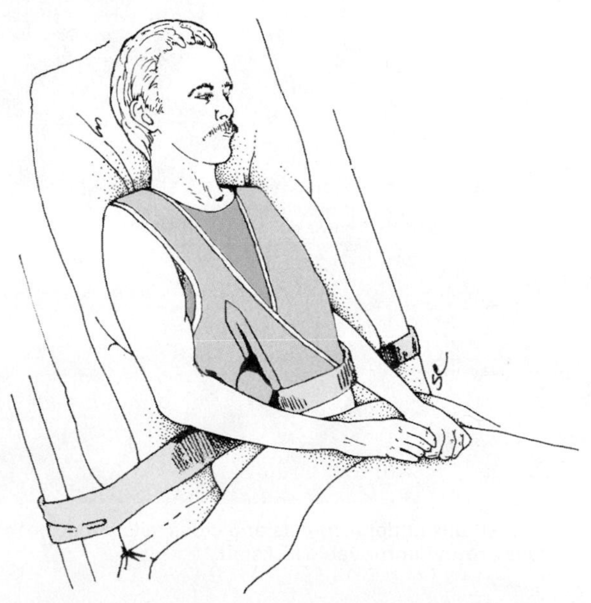

▲ Vest restraint can be used for client on bed rest.

7. Tie straps to nonmovable upper section of bed frame using slipknot. ▶ ***Rationale:*** This position minimizes risk of inadvertent release, which may cause subsequent injury.
8. Observe client every 15 minutes to ensure proper fit of jacket.
9. Release vest restraint every 2 hours. Follow interventions for releasing restraints of all types.
10. Document use and rationale for restraint in nurses' notes every 15 minutes.
11. Document client assessment and attendance to fluid and elimination needs regularly.

For Client in Wheelchair

1. Place client in wheelchair with buttocks against chair back.
2. Place vest on client (zipper vest is best) place zipper to back of client. Zip vest from bottom to top. Ensure that there is adequate space between vest and client.

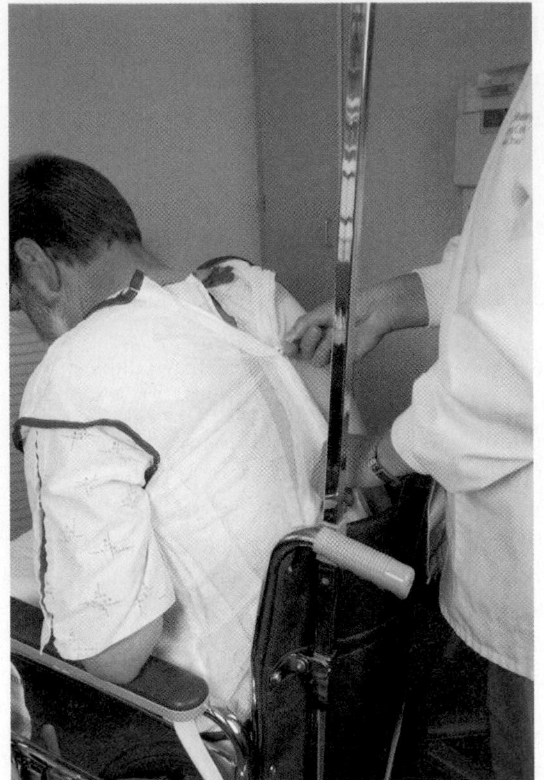

▲ Zip vest from bottom to top at client's back.

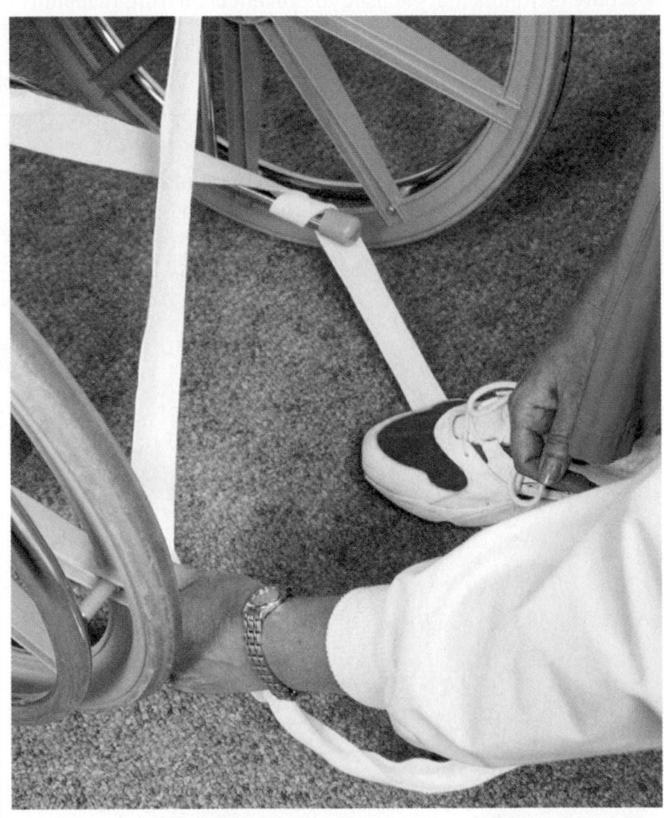

▲ Pull vest tails under armrests and cross tails in back of chair. Wrap tails around immovable kickspur.

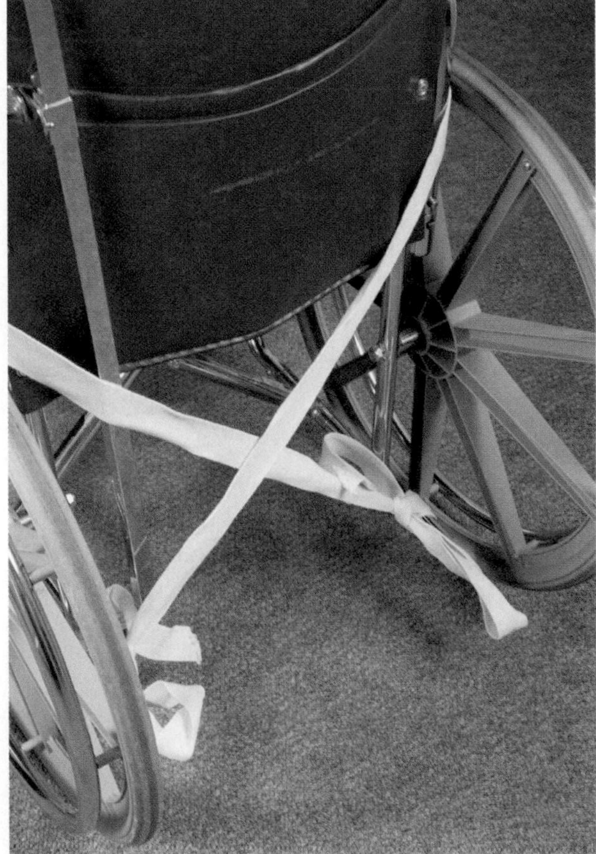

▲ Tie each tail to kickspur using half-bow knot.

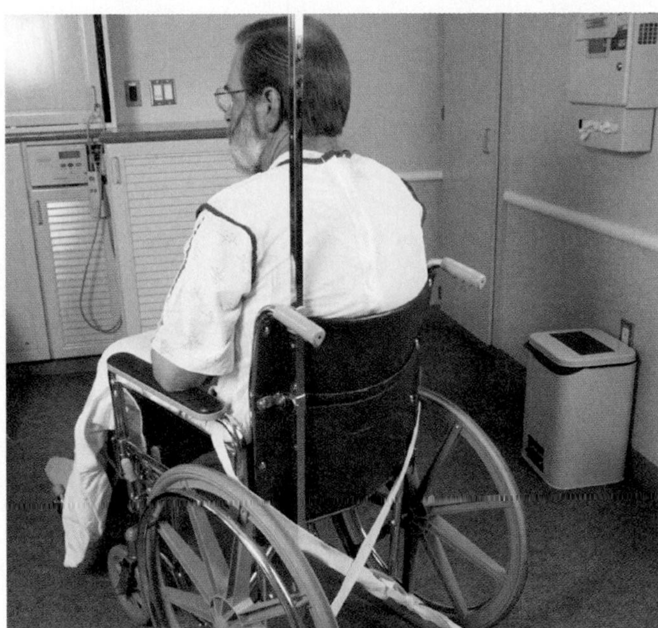
3 Check client every 15 minutes while in restraint.

▸ ***Rationale:*** To prevent constriction from vest that is too tight.

3. Pull straps at 45-degree angle to rear of seat and pull vest tails under armrests and cross tails in back of chair. ▸ ***Rationale:*** Tying vest tails in back of chair prevents client from reaching the tails and untying the vest.
4. Wrap tails around immovable kickspur. ▸ ***Rationale:*** This anchors the tails and prevents client from slipping out of restraints.
5. Tie each tail to kickspur using half-bow knot. ▸ ***Rationale:*** This type of knot is used because it can be quickly released if necessary.
6. Check client every 15 minutes to ensure vest is on correctly and client is not in compromising situation.
7. Document every 15 minutes according to policy.

Source: Health Resources Unlimited, LLC (2006, January).

Tying a Half-Bow Knot

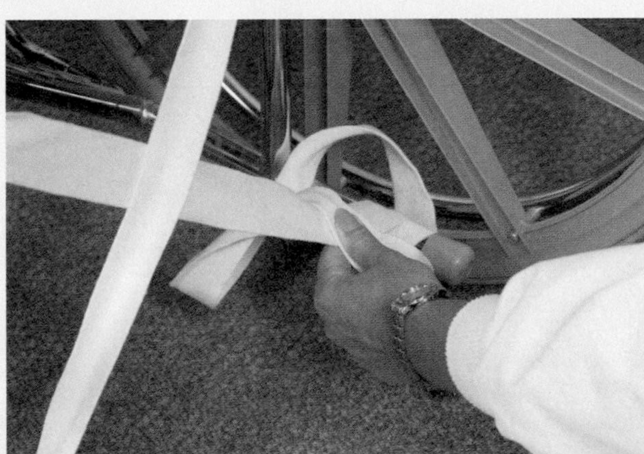
1 Place restraint tie around wheelchair kickspur. Bring free end up, around, under, and over attached end of tie and pull tight.

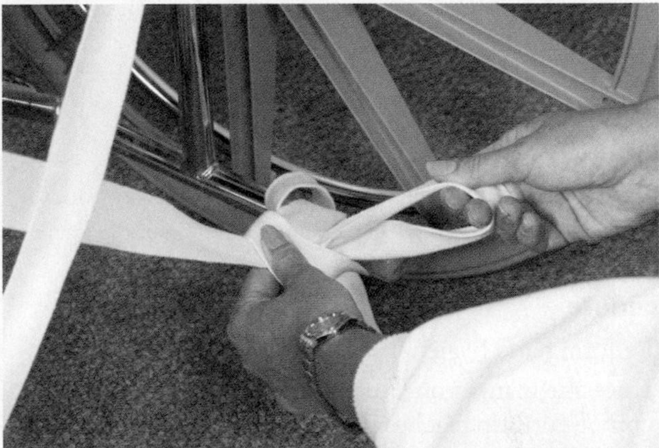
2 Take free end over and under attached end of tie, but this time make half-bow loop.

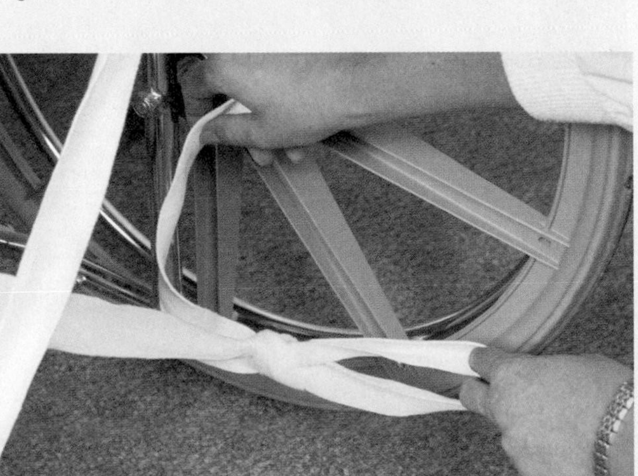
3 Tighten free end of tie and bow until knot is secure.

Clinical Alert

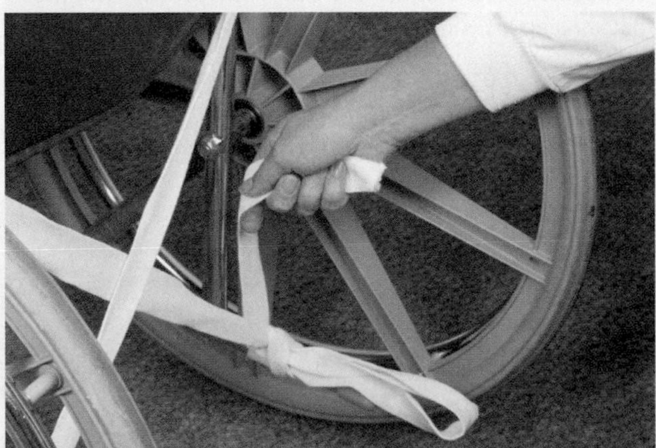
▲ Pull end of tie and loosen first crossover tie in an emergency.

Alternate Method

Daisy chain tie is used as an alternate method to prevent tie from dangling to floor or to prevent client from releasing tie.

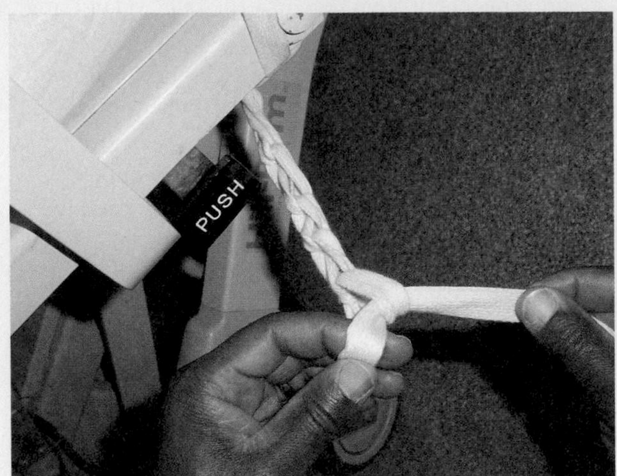

1 Complete daisy chain.

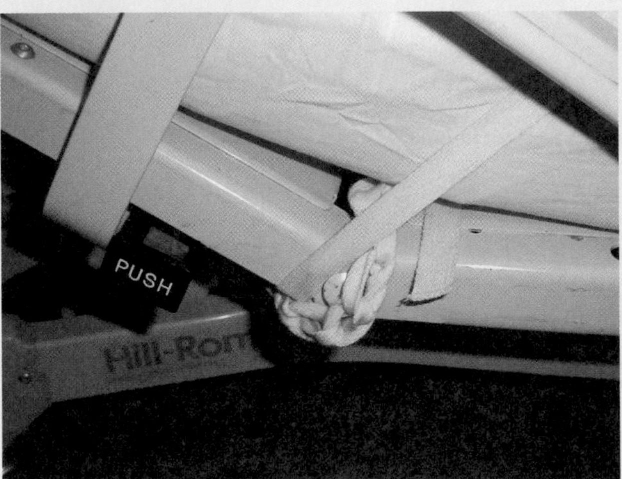

2 Tuck chain under mattress.

Applying Mummy Restraints

Equipment

Blanket large enough to fit child, or sheet, if blanket not large enough for infant.

Procedure

1. Perform hand hygiene.
2. Place the blanket on a secure surface and fold down one corner until tip reaches the middle of the blanket.
3. Place the baby in a diagonal position with the head halfway off the folded edge of the blanket.
4. Bring one side of the blanket over the infant's arm and trunk, and tuck it under the other arm and around the back. Keep arms in natural position to the side.
5. Tuck the bottom part of the blanket up onto the infant's abdomen.
6. Fold the second side over the infant, and tuck it snugly around the body.
7. Use the restraint only until procedure is completed.

Mummy boards with Velcro straps are used more often in the hospital setting. A diaper or Chux is placed on the board, and the infant is placed on the board and secured with the Velcro straps.

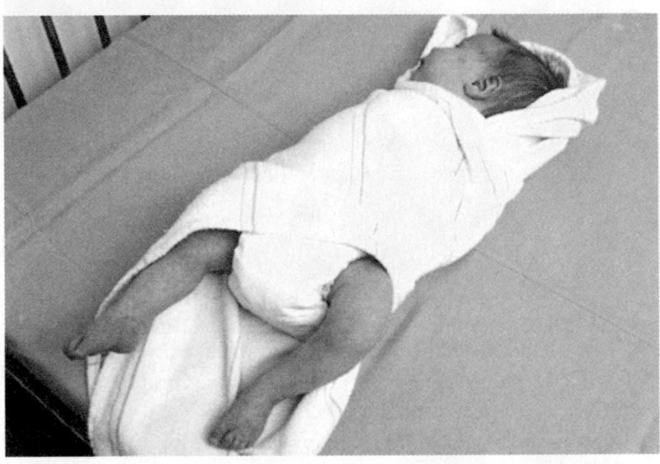

▲ A mummy restraint is used when certain procedures are to be done.

Clinical Alert

Generally, restraint policies do not apply to:

- Restriction for security purposes.
- Procedure-related immobilization (e.g., for medical, surgical, or diagnostic procedure).
- Use of adaptive support devices (e.g., brace, orthopedic appliances).
- Use of medical protective devices (e.g., tabletop chairs, bed rails).
- Voluntary restraint (client consent).

DOCUMENTATION for Applying Restraints

- Description of specific behaviors leading to restraint.
- Note all less restrictive techniques used. If less restrictive techniques were not used, provide rationale.
- Extent to which client is able to cooperate with restraint procedure.
- Any injury to client or others.
- All observation data for entire time restraint is applied. Include skin integrity, neurovascular changes, etc.
- Client's behavior after and during time restraint is applied.
- Justification and reassessment for continued use of restraints.
- Document review of care plan for effectiveness or rationale for ineffectiveness of care plan.

DATE: ______________ UNIT: ______________ REASON FOR RESTRAINT: ______________________________

SUGGESTED ALTERNATIVES TO RESTRAINT USE CONSIDERED DURING THE RE-ASSESSMENT PROCESS:

TIME

____ ____ ____ Met patient's comfort needs

____ ____ ____ Changed or elimin ated bothersome treatments

____ ____ ____ Modified the environment

____ ____ ____ Reality orientation and psychosocial interventions

____ ____ ____ Provided companionship and supervision

____ ____ ____ Offered diversion and physical activities

____ ____ ____ Designed creative alternatives

CODES:

DESCRIPTION
2P = 2 POINT
3P = 3 POINT
4P = 4 POINT
G = GERICHAIR
M = MITTENS
4S = 4 SIDERAILS WITH PROTECTIVE PADS

LEVEL OF CONSCIOUSNESS
A = ALERT
D = DROWSY
C = CONFUSED

RESPONSE
C = CALM
A = AGITATED
S = SLEEPING

RESTRAINT RESOLUTION
A = APPLIED
R = RELEASED
A/R = APPLIED & RELEASED

EFFECT
A = ADEQUATE
I = INADEQUATE

SIGN/CIRCULATION
I = INTACT
B = BROKEN
R = REDDENED
M = MOTTLED
P = PULSES PALPABLE

RANGE OF MOTION
Y = YES
N = NO
S = SLEEPING

POSITION
R = RIGHT SIDE
L = LEFT SIDE
S = SUPINE
P = PRONE

FLUIDS/NOURISHMENT/TOILETING
Y = YES
N = NO
R = REFUSED
*SEE OBSERVATIONS

TIME	0800	1000	1200	1400	1600	1800	2000	2200	2400	0200	0400	0600
NOTE: PATIENT IS MONITORED EVERY 15 MINUTES. DOCUMENT EVERY 2 HOURS.												
DESCRIPTION												
LEVEL OF CONSCIOUSNESS												
RESPONSE to RESTRAINT												
RESTRAINT RESOLUTION												
EFFECT of RESTRAINT												
SKIN/CIRCULATION												
NOTE: PATIENT IS MONITORED AND DOCUMENTED ON EVERY 2 HOURS.												
RANGE OF MOTION												
POSITION												
FLUIDS/ NOURISHMENT												
TOILETING												
INITIALS												

SIGNATURE/TITLE	INITIALS	SIGNATURE/TITLE	INITIALS	SIGNATURE/TITLE	INITIALS
SIGNATURE/TITLE	INITIALS	SIGNATURE/TITLE	INITIALS	SIGNATURE/TITLE	INITIALS
SIGNATURE/TITLE	INITIALS	SIGNATURE/TITLE	INITIALS	SIGNATURE/TITLE	INITIALS

COMMUNITY HOSPITAL

PATIENT I.D. #
NAME
SEX AGE SS #
BIRTH DATE MED. REC. # FIN. CLASS
DOCTOR ADMIT. DATE

▲ Restraint/Seclusion flow sheet.

Legal Considerations

Restraints: Swann v. Len-Care Rest Home Inc. (1997)

Family members requested the confused grandmother be restrained when they were not in attendance. The physician ordered the restraints and wrote a letter indicating he wanted the restraints placed when the client was alone. The client was left unattended and unrestrained, fell, and sustained a head injury. The family brought suit against the facility. During the trial, it was noted this was the client's third fall while she was unrestrained. The court found for the plaintiff. To avoid liability, always follow hospital policies related to use of restraints.

Source: Health Resources Unlimited, LLC. January 2006.

CRITICAL THINKING Application

Expected Outcomes

- Client is prevented from injuring himself/herself or others.
- Restraints are applied appropriately.
- Client does not develop complications due to restraint use (e.g., agitation, pressure ulcers, circulatory disturbance).
- Child is prevented from reaching the incision site, IVs, or tubes.
- Client remains in restraints for a limited amount of time.
- Client does not experience complications as a result of restraint placement.
- Client does not endure undue psychological stress while being placed in restraints.

Unexpected Outcomes	Alternative Actions
Skin abrasion, maceration, or rash occurs after application of restraints.	• Reassess absolute need for restraint. • Reassess application method. • Increase padding of soft restraints before application. • Keep restraints off as much as possible and have staff or family member stay with client.
Impaired circulation or edema evidenced by change in color, sensation, movement, and blanching of nail beds.	• On observation of signs of neurovascular changes, immediately release restraints. • Massage area gently to increase circulation. • If extremity is edematous, elevate extremity above level of heart. Encourage range of motion. • Request order for different type of restraint
Client unties restraints.	• Camouflage restraint to decrease client's awareness. • Reassess need for restraint. • Exhaust alternative measures to promote safety. • Anticipate and attend to client's needs.
Client with history of falling has developed acute cognitive changes.	• Alert all personnel that client is high risk for fall. • Review medication regimen (e.g., Demerol and psychoactive drugs can cause acute confusion). • Assess for physiologic causes (e.g., hypoxemia, infection, pain) and address alterations. • Place bedside commode away from bed and remove all obstacles; provide good lighting as well as night light. • Reduce environmental stimuli (e.g., television). • Reorient client with each encounter. • Move client for better surveillance. • Employ monitoring alarm/device or engage family attendance. • Request floor mattress or recliner chair.
Child is able to reach incision site even with elbow restraints in place.	• Make sure the elbow restraints are tight enough and extend over the elbow. • Tie the one elbow restraint to the opposite elbow restraint by placing the tie under the child's back and securing the tie with the upper tie on the opposite restraint. • Check that the restraint is large enough to completely immobilize the elbow. If not, obtain a larger size or use two restraints and tie them together securely.

GERONTOLOGIC Considerations

Safety Precautions for the Elderly

- Ensure sensory adaptive devices are used (glasses, hearing aid).
- Use one-half to three-quarter rails rather than full rails.
- Provide adequate lighting.
- Provide and encourage use of call bell/summons device.
- Assess fluid and elimination needs regularly.
- Promote activities of daily living and exercise to maintain muscle strength and flexibility.
- Assist client in ambulation if unsteady on feet.
- Heed client's summons promptly.

- Put necessary articles for personal hygiene and activities of daily living within easy reach.
- Provide nonslip mats and grab bars in bathtubs, showers, and near toilets.
- Use shower chair.
- Mop up spills promptly.
- Keep hallways clear of obstacles.
- Lock all equipment when not moving client.
- Provide handrails in hallways.
- Instruct in use of assistive devices when in use.
- Maintain a consistent environment: keep furniture in established places.

Preventing Thermal Injury

- Skin is fragile and prone to injury as client's age increases. Use thermal treatments with caution. Do not apply *direct* heat to areas with ischemic tissue.
- Check skin frequently when any type of heat therapy (e.g., Aqua K pad) is used.
- Check water temperature before placing client in bathtub (95°F for the elderly and those with peripheral circulation impairment).

Wandering-Client Management Plan

- Clients who are identified as potential wanderers from a facility or at risk for falls should wear a monitor device.
- Monitors come in various models, each one designed to identify clients who move away from a designated monitor zone.
- Clients need to be checked regularly to ensure the monitor is appropriately positioned and the alarm functions properly.

MANAGEMENT Guidelines

Each state legislates a Nurse Practice Act for RNs and LVN/LPNs. Healthcare facilities are responsible for establishing and implementing policies and procedures that conform to their state's regulations. Verify the regulations and role parameters for each healthcare worker in your facility.

Delegation

- Before nursing staff is assigned to care for clients requiring restraints, the team leader and/or charge nurse must ensure they have been properly educated in the legal requirements as well as in the application of restraints.
- All personnel must be aware of environmental and client risks for injury. Remind staff to notify RN of risks.
- Nurses must help identify clients at high risk for injury and must be familiar with agency plan/protocol for the prevention of injury.
- Nurses must individualize restraint implementation.

Communication Matrix

- Clients at high risk for injury: Report client risk behaviors, attempts to determine underlying cause, attempted alternative protective measures, and rationale for choice of restraint.
- Document type and time restraint initiated, regular monitoring, and client response. According to the FDA, approximately 20 clients die every year from protective restraints. It is critical to instruct all personnel (including CNAs and UAPs who may not administer the restraints, but give client care and therefore, observe restraint use) in the proper use of restraints.

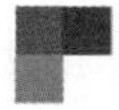

CRITICAL THINKING Strategies

Scenario 1

As you enter Mrs. Lake's room, you find her with one leg over the side rail, making attempts to get out of bed unassisted. Mrs. Lake is an 82-year-old client with a history of heart failure (HF). When you question what she is doing, she tells you, "I need to go to the bathroom." She also tells you she is sure her dog needs to be let out because she hasn't been able to get out of the bed all morning. This is your second day caring for Mrs. Lake. Your initial assessment on admission 2 days ago included her being oriented to person, place, time, and thing. The night shift reported off saying she was disoriented all night.

1. What is your first nursing action? Provide rationale for your response.

2. What additional priority nursing actions are justified for Mrs. Lake?
3. What additional information do you need to gather to determine the next step in her plan of care?
4. If, in the assessment completed by the RN, it is determined she needs to be closely monitored for possible falls, what interventions, by priority, will you implement?
5. Identify the legal requirements that must be implemented when a client is placed in restraints.
6. Identify other least restrictive measures that can be utilized before restraints are applied.

Scenario 2

A 75-year-old female was admitted to the hospital after sustaining a fractured hip after a fall on the sidewalk in front of her house. The admission nurse calls the unit to apprise them of the new admission. The nurse explains that the client is not sure what day it is nor where she is at the moment. She did sustain a cut on her forehead in the fall, requiring five stitches. You have been assigned to admit the client when she arrives on the unit.

1. Identify the priority assessment you will complete at the time of admission.
2. Describe the environmental alterations that can be initiated to prevent injury to the client.
3. Considering the fall, determine what assessment findings you will evaluate in the initial assessment.
4. Describe two priority nursing interventions that will be included in the client care plan for this client.
5. The client has surgery the next day and returns to the nursing unit. The client comes back with two IVs, hip dressings with a drain, and O2 per nasal cannula. The client responds to painful stimuli but is not fully awake. Determine the appropriate safety interventions that will be employed to prevent injury to the client as she awakens.

NCLEX® Review Questions

Unless otherwise specified, choose only one (1) answer.

1. Which one of the following factors is not considered a characteristic that promotes adaptation to the environment?
   1. Environmental influences.
   2. Age.
   3. Mental status.
   4. State of illness.
2. The primary root cause of a sentinel event is:
   1. Poor staffing ratio.
   2. Errors in procedure.
   3. Inaccurate client assessment.
   4. Communication.
3. A client has an order for application of wrist restraints as a result of exhibiting confusion. How often in hours must a renewal order be written?
   1. 2.
   2. 4.
   3. 8.
   4. 24.
4. Restraint guidelines include which of the following?
   1. Client must be observed every 2 hours while in restraints.
   2. Wrist restraints must be the first type of restraints used before proceeding to other types of restraints.
   3. Slip knots or the daisy chain is used for securing restraints to the bed frame.
   4. Use of restraints is encouraged to replace sitters for clients at risk for falls.
5. You are preparing to care for a client with a radioactive implant. The most important client care principle is to
   1. Keep soiled dressings, gloves, and linens in contaminated container in the room.
   2. Assist client to sit at edge of bed to participate in bathing.
   3. Increase time available for client care; provide care by standing at head or foot of bed.
   4. Instruct visitors to limit visits to no more than 4 hours each day.
6. The priority nursing intervention when a client has a seizure is to
   1. Turn client on abdomen to prevent tongue from occluding airway.
   2. Insert tongue blade to side of mouth to prevent tongue from falling back.
   3. Place vest restraint on client after initial seizure activity to prevent client from falling out of bed.
   4. Stay with client during postictal state to ensure client has an uneventful recovery.
7. In case of fire in the nursing unit, the priority intervention is to
   1. Extinguish fire, if possible.
   2. Close doors and windows of clients' rooms.
   3. Remove clients from immediate danger.
   4. Activate the fire alarm.

8. The client teaching plan for an 88-year-old female client who is being discharged to home includes all but which one of the following safety precautions?
   1. Explain to client that he/she needs to be on bedrest until lower extremity strength and flexibility returns.
   2. Place essential articles for personal hygiene near the bed.
   3. Install grab bars in tubs and near the toilet.
   4. Use a shower chair when bathing the client in the shower.

9. You assess a client for potential falls and determine that an environmental alteration could be used to prevent the need for restraints. This type of alteration would include
   1. Placing a rolled-edge mattress on the bed.
   2. Placing client in a room near nurses' desk for easy observation.
   3. Using a geri-chair and placing client near the nurses' desk.
   4. Placing bed in low position, with two upper side rails in the "up" position.

10. The client is being positioned in a wheelchair with an order for a Posey vest to prevent him from falling out of the chair. Which actions should be taken by the nurses to secure the vest on the client?
    Select all that apply.
    1. Place vest on client with the zipper in front.
    2. Place vest tails under arm rests and cross tails in back of chair.
    3. Tie vest tails using a daisy chain and anchoring on kickspur of the wheelchair.
    4. Tie each tail to the kickspur using a half-knot.

8

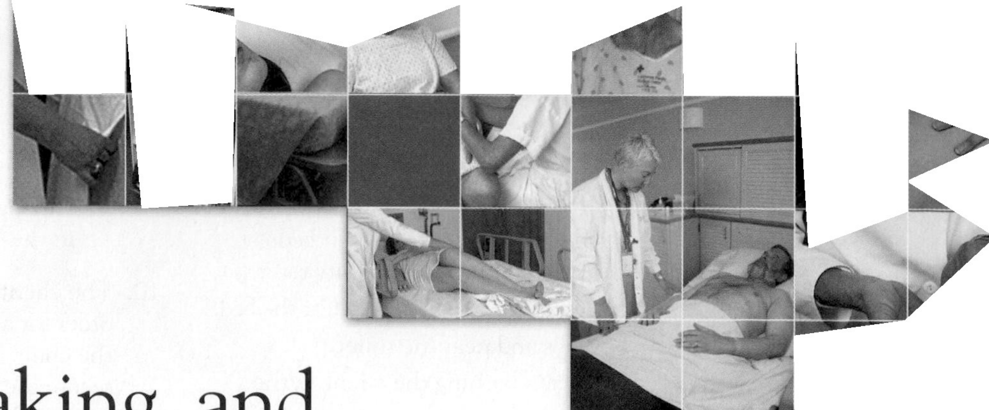

Bathing, Bedmaking, and Maintaining Skin Integrity

LEARNING OBJECTIVES

1. Compare and contrast the steps in making an occupied and unoccupied bed.
2. Demonstrate the skill of folding a mitered corner.
3. Outline the steps in bathing a bedridden adult client.
4. Differentiate between bathing a bedridden client and a critically ill client.
5. Compare and contrast the differences in bathing an infant, a child, and an adult client.
6. State the advantages of using a commercial bathing system.
7. Describe the assessment modalities completed while bathing a client.
8. Outline the steps in providing morning care.
9. Describe the skin assessment steps that must be completed on a daily basis.
10. Outline the steps in providing foot care.
11. Describe the changes in skin that occur with aging and appropriate nursing interventions to prevent a skin tear.
12. Describe briefly the components of evening care.
13. Define the three back care strokes and their use in back care.
14. Complete client charting for evening care on nurses' notes.
15. Write three nursing diagnoses appropriate for providing basic hygienic care to clients.

CHAPTER OUTLINE

TERMINOLOGY

Bedmaking

Closed bed a bed not being used by a client; the linens are left to cover the bed.

Occupied bed the client remains in the bed while it is being made.

Open bed a bed being used by a client; the linens are fan-folded down.

Unoccupied bed the client is out of the bed while it is being made.

Equipment Used With Beds

Aside from the standard types of equipment used on the basic hospital bed, specialized equipment can be added to meet the client's healthcare needs.

Balkan overbed frame an overhead bar used to support a trapeze, or a series of pulleys and weights used for traction equipment.

Footboard usually a solid support placed on the bed where the soles of the feet touch. It is secured to the mattress or bed frame. Footboards are used to prevent permanent plantar flexion (footdrop) and to exercise leg muscles. The footboard may also have side supports to help maintain proper alignment of feet.

Sheets for Bedmaking

Fitted sheets sheets that have elastic at each corner.

Drawsheets sheets made of fabric or waterproof material that are placed across the shoulder-to-knee area of the bed and tucked in on the sides.

Full sheets regular full-length flat sheets that can be used as the top and/or bottom sheet.

Incontinent pads large cloth or disposable pads that can be placed under the buttocks area, head, drains, or any place where excess moisture or fluid may collect on the bed.

Pull sheets sheets placed across the shoulder-to-knee area of the bed. The sides are not tucked under the mattress. The sheet is kept wrinkle-free and folded under the client. Pull sheets are used to lift the client in the bed.

Levels of Personal Care

Complete or total care the client requires total assistance from the nurse because he or she is able to do little or nothing for him or herself. Complete bathing, skin care, oral care, nail and hair care, care of the feet, eyes, ears, and nose, and a total bed linen change are usually provided.

Early morning care or AM care given by the night shift or day shift nurses and may include bathing the hands and face, use of the bedpan, urinal, or bedside commode, oral care, and other preparations before breakfast.

Evening care (H.S. care, hour of sleep care) evening care is usually provided to prepare the client for a relaxing, uninterrupted period of sleep. Activities may include oral care, partial bathing, skin care, a soothing back massage, straightening or changing the bed linen, and offering the bedpan or urinal. The client should also be assessed for the need of food, drink, or medication before sleep.

Preoperative care clients who will be undergoing surgery or diagnostic tests may be required to bathe the evening before. Partial bathing is sometimes allowed in the morning if time permits. If the client is not allowed to have anything by mouth, care must be taken not to allow swallowing of water or dentifrice while providing oral care. The client is usually given a clean gown. All dentures, hairpins, makeup, nail polish, contact lenses, and jewelry are removed. Valuables are locked up. The client is encouraged to void before leaving for the operating room.

Partial care the client performs as much of his or her own care as possible. The nurse completes the remaining care.

Independent care the client is able to complete his or her own care. The nurse provides the client with any needed equipment.

Skin Care

Acne skin condition due to irritation and infection of the sebaceous glands.

Blanching a whitish hue to an area of the skin when pressure is applied.

Ecchymosis collection of blood underneath skin surface; bruise.

Emollient soothing, softening agent applied to body surfaces.

Epidermis superficial, or top, layer of skin.

Erythema redness of skin associated with rashes, inflammation, infections, allergic responses, or congestion of the capillaries.

Hyperemia influx of blood into an area causing redness to the skin.

Ischemia decreased, insufficient blood supply to body area.

Lesion an area of broken skin as a result of trauma or a pathologic interruption of tissue.

Necrosis cellular death resulting from decreased blood flow to tissue.

Pediculosis infestation of lice.

Pediculus capitis head lice.

Pediculus corporis body lice.

Pediculus pubis crab lice or pubic lice.

Petechiae pinpoint reddish spots.

Pressure ulcer an area of cellular necrosis due to decreased circulation.

Purpura reddish purple area.

Shearing force layers of skin moving on each other.

Skin tear traumatic wound resulting from separation of the epidermis from the dermis.

Turgor the degree of elasticity of the skin.

Back Care

Effleurage long stroking motions of the hands up and down the back. Hands do not leave the skin surface. Pressure is light.

Petrissage pinching of the skin, subcutaneous tissue, and muscle as you move up and down the client's back.

Tapotement alternate striking of fleshy part of hands on client's back as you move up and down the back.

Foot Care

Athlete's foot irritation characterized by itching, burning skin; caused by an easily transmitted fungus.

Calluses thickened epidermis over area of pressure.

Corns high calluses caused by pressure on toes, joints, or bony prominences.

Cracks and fissures between toes this problem can occur anyplace on feet, often on heels; often occurs as a result of excessively dry skin.

Decreased circulation to the feet a problem that is often caused by diabetes, vascular diseases, or the constriction of major vessels to the lower extremities.

Incurvated or ingrown toenails the corners of the nail tend to press into skin, causing pain, ulceration, and infection.

Plantar warts virus manifested as a deep, often painful wart on the soles of the feet.

GENERAL TERMINOLOGY

Assessment the collection, verification, organization, interpretation, and documentation of client data; the first step in the nursing process.

Complete bath all areas of the body are bathed. This bath can be done completely by the nurse or by the client.

Cyanosis blueness of the skin related to decreased oxygenation of the blood.

Dermis layer of skin below the epidermis containing blood and lymphatic vessels, nerves, nerve endings, glands, and hair follicles.

Epidermis superficial, avascular layer of skin primarily used for protection.

Excreta waste matter; materials cast out by the body.

Fissure a groove, slit, or natural division; ulcer or crack-like sore.

Flush a redness of the face and neck due to dilation of the capillaries.

Hypoallergenic against allergy, as hypoallergenic tape.

Incurvate curved, especially inward.

Inflammation swelling, pain, heat, and redness of tissue.

Intervention the act of coming between, so as to hinder or modify.

Jaundice yellowish appearance caused by deposition of bile pigment in the skin.

Mucosa mucous membrane lining passages and cavities communicating with the air.

Pallor paleness; absence of skin coloration.

Partial bath certain parts of the body are bathed such as the face, hands, underarms, back, and perineal area. Another definition of a partial bath is a bath that occurs when the nurse bathes areas which the client cannot reach and the client washes all other areas.

Pigment any normal or abnormal coloring of the skin.

Plaque a patch on the skin or on a mucous surface.

Pressure point area for exerting pressure to control bleeding; an area of skin that can become injured with pressure, especially over bony prominences.

Sensory deprivation enforced absence of usual and accustomed sensory stimuli.

Sensory overload too much stimuli for the senses to adjust to at once.

Therapeutic bath baths requiring a physician's order used for specific conditions. The order should include type of bath, water temperature, solution to be used, and frequency.

Ulcer an open sore or lesion of the skin or mucous membrane of the body.

BASIC HEALTH CARE

Clients enter the hospital environment for a variety of reasons requiring immediate care, or because the physician has recommended diagnostic procedures or surgery. The latter is commonly referred to as an *elective admission*. Whatever the reason, the client must rapidly alter everyday routines and activities of daily living. The client may be concerned about his or her health and well-being and may experience varying degrees of anxiety as a reaction to unfamiliar procedures, hospital personnel, or the hospital environment itself.

After the client has been admitted to the healthcare unit, many independent actions, such as bathing, personal hygiene, and general care, may be curtailed by the nature of the illness and confinement. The client may require assistance with even the simplest of actions. Without therapeutic intervention, the total adaptation process may be put in jeopardy as additional physical problems occur. Knowing when and how to intervene and performing such skills as bedmaking, bathing, and personal hygiene facilitate the client's process of adapting to the healthcare environment.

When the client is confined to bed even for a short time, comfort is essential in order to promote rest and sleep. To prevent skin irritation and breakdown, beds must be kept clean and free of debris and wrinkles. The bed needs to be straightened frequently throughout the day to accomplish this. If the client is to remain in bed for an extended time, all care and daily routines are directed from bed. It becomes the center of activity.

Types of Beds

There are many different types of beds and related equipment available to meet the special healthcare needs of individual clients.

The hospital bed is a standard twin-size bed in a frame that allows for different positions to facilitate care and comfort for the client. The height, head, and foot positions in most beds are electrically operated to assist both the client and the nursing staff. The nurse instructs the client in the proper use of bed controls and in bed positions that could be helpful or dangerous for the client.

Support Surfaces

Support surfaces such as mattress overlays filled with foam, gel, or water are commonly used as the first line of defense against skin breakdown. These surfaces prevent pressure on bony prominences, thus reducing pressure ulcer incidence. They are cost-effective surfaces that prevent pressure ulcers in clients who are classified as low risk. These surfaces can also be used to treat those clients who already have pressure ulcers. (See Chapter 25 for pressure ulcer care.)

Foam overlay (Care-Gard, Geo-Matt) support surfaces are used for prevention in low-risk clients. The foam pads are ventilated for moisture control and have an antishearing surface. Foam mattresses (Comfortline Ultimate, basic PRIMA, and SimpliMATT) can be placed on top of existing mattresses. An alternating therapy system mattress can also be used as a replacement for the mattress (DUO DETEQ, TRINOVA®). A third type of support system, the continuous airflow system (ACUCAIR), is also placed over an existing mattress. It keeps skin dry with the continuous airflow and moisture control feature. It also reduces friction and shear. This system is portable and easily transported and placed on the existing mattress.

Specialty Beds

New types of specialty beds are used to provide care to clients at risk for developing skin breakdown and pressure ulcers. Clients most susceptible to these conditions (where a specialty bed is critical) include spinal cord injury clients or those who need frequent turning and are difficult to move, such as CVA clients.

Specialty beds replace the entire hospital bed and are classified as air fluidized, low air-loss, kinetic therapy, and critical care therapy. High air-loss beds are used for clients with stage III and IV pressure ulcers. These beds have antifriction/shear surfaces and built-in scales. Low air-loss beds are used for clients who are difficult to reposition or when moving is contraindicated. Air-filled beds are used for clients who require minimal movement. It makes turning easy and facilitates drainage.

There are two additional types of specialty beds used as preventative or treatment measures for clients having special needs. The first type, the kinetic bed (TotalCare, SpO_2RT, and RotoRest®) is used to provide continuous passive motion or oscillation for clients with unstable spines. The second type of bed, the bariatric bed (Magnum II®, Burke®, BariMaxx II®), is used with obese clients. These beds have a special feature that allows clients to be weighed in the bed, and it can also be converted into a chair.

Bathing

Routine bathing is an essential component of daily care. It is essential to prevent body odor, because excessive perspiration interacts with bacteria to cause odor. Dead skin cells can lead to infection if impaired skin integrity occurs. Excessive bathing, on the other hand, can increase the risk for impaired skin integrity in elderly clients. In the elderly, the skin may become dry and cracked due to a natural decrease in the production of moisturizing oils, which can lead to infection.

Bathing promotes a feeling of self-worth by improving the person's appearance. Relaxation and improved circulation are benefits of bathing and play a therapeutic role in the care of clients on bedrest. The apocrine glands, found in the axillae and pubic areas, produce sweat, which leads to odor. Therefore, thorough bathing should be provided to these areas.

In addition to the therapeutic effects, the bath affords the nurse time to communicate with and assess the client. Assessment of skin conditions, mobility, and self-care deficits can be detected while bathing the client.

In addition to the basin, wash cloth and soap bathing procedure, there are several types of commercial body cleansing systems currently used in hospitals and other healthcare facilities. The systems are a body bath, shampoo, and a perineal care package. The bath system uses disposable washcloths to cleanse the client. This type of system cleans, moisturizes, conditions, and protects the skin; therefore, it is a good alternative for elderly clients or clients with sensitive skin. The system contains ingredients that are hypoallergenic and bactericidal.

Bathing is accomplished in a variety of ways, according to the client's needs, condition, and personal habits. Bathing is necessary to cleanse the skin and to promote circulation. Baths may also be used as a treatment to promote healing for a client with burns. Various types of bathing include:

- **Complete bed bath:** The client, who is usually totally dependent, is bathed in bed by the nurse due to physical or mental incapacity. The client is encouraged to complete as much of his or her bath as possible.
- **Partial bath:** Face, axilla, hands, back, and genital area are bathed. Partial bath may be completed by client or nurse.
- **Therapeutic bath:** This bath is used as part of a treatment regimen for specific conditions, such as skin disorders, burns, high body temperature, and muscular injuries. Medicinal substances, such as oatmeal, Aveeno, and cornstarch, may be included in the bath water. Therapeutic baths require physician's orders.
- **Shower:** Preferred method of bathing if client is ambulatory or can be transported to use a shower chair.

- **Tub bath:** Used by ambulatory clients as well as those who must be assisted by a device such as the Hoyer lift.
- **Cooling bath:** The client is placed in a tub of tepid water to reduce body temperature.

Skin Conditions

The skin is the largest organ of the body. Skin is exposed to environmental risks as well as physical and mechanical injury. Skin is composed of the epidermis (outer layer) and the dermis (inner layer). The skin provides protection, thermoregulation, excretion, metabolism, sensation, and communication for the body.

Skin types, colors, textures, and condition are as different and unique as each person. The condition of a client's skin is determined by his or her health status, age, activity level, and environmental exposure. For example, the skin of an infant is often more sensitive and delicate than that of an adult because it has not been exposed to many environmental elements. Most infants cannot tolerate strong soaps and lotions and must be handled gently to avoid trauma. Adolescents are affected by acne and have areas of increased oil secretion. Adults may have drier skin, especially as they age. Older adults cannot always tolerate harsh soaps because their skin is more delicate. They require less frequent bathing and more lubrication with oil-rich creams and lotions.

According to Payne and Martin (1998), the classification of skin tears is a traumatic wound usually occuring on the extremities of elderly clients as a result of friction, or shearing and friction forces, resulting in separation of the epidermis from the dermis. This occurs more frequently with elderly clients as a result of changes in their skin with aging. The epidermis gradually thins as a result of loss in dermal thickness and becomes more susceptible to mild mechanical trauma. In addition, the skin loses its elasticity as elastin fibers decrease. This leads to a less effective barrier against fluid loss, bruising, and infection. Impaired thermoregulation leads to decreased tactile sensitivity and pain perception. Blood vessels become thin and fragile, which presents as purpura or the appearance of little hemorrhages under the skin. Skin tears often occur at the site where purpura is present. Skin tears are more prevalent on the arms and hands, but can occur anywhere on the body. A skin tear on the back or buttocks is often mistaken for a pressure ulcer; however, the etiology of a skin tear is different.

Maintaining skin integrity is an integral part of providing nursing care; being aware of the client's skin condition and alterations in the integrity is a critical aspect of providing total client care. The feet are especially susceptible to discomfort, trauma, and infection due to the amount of stress they must endure as well as to their distance from main blood supplies. Many conditions can be avoided if proper foot care is taken.

CULTURAL AWARENESS

When providing hygienic care for clients, the nurse needs to assess the client's usual pattern of bathing, hygienic products usually used, and cultural rituals and beliefs.

Modesty and bathing rituals and beliefs must be considered in caring for clients. For example, some cultures and religions do not allow members of the opposite sex to see them from the waist to the knees (Gypsy culture, Southeast Asian cultures). Hispanic women have a strong sense of modesty and do not want healthcare workers to see them unclothed.

NURSING DIAGNOSES

The following nursing diagnoses may be appropriate to include in a client care plan when the components are related to basic care of the client.

NURSING DIAGNOSIS	RELATED FACTORS
Activity Intolerance	Prolonged bed rest, surgery, pain, treatment schedule, weakness, fatigue
Ineffective Health Maintenance	Ineffective coping, lack of motivation, motor impairment, lack of financial resources
Impaired Bed Mobility	Unable to ambulate, difficulty moving into or out of bed. Lack of coordination, motor impairment, visual disorders, surgery, muscle weakness, pain
Impaired Skin Integrity	Surgery, immobility, prolonged bed rest, mechanical factors (shearing force, pressure)

CLEANSE HANDS The single most important nursing action to decrease the incidence of hospital-based infections is hand hygiene. *Remember to wash your hands or use antibacterial gel before and after each and every client contact.*

IDENTIFY CLIENT Before every procedure, introduce yourself and check two forms of client identification, not including room number. *These actions prevent errors and conform to The Joint Commission standards.*

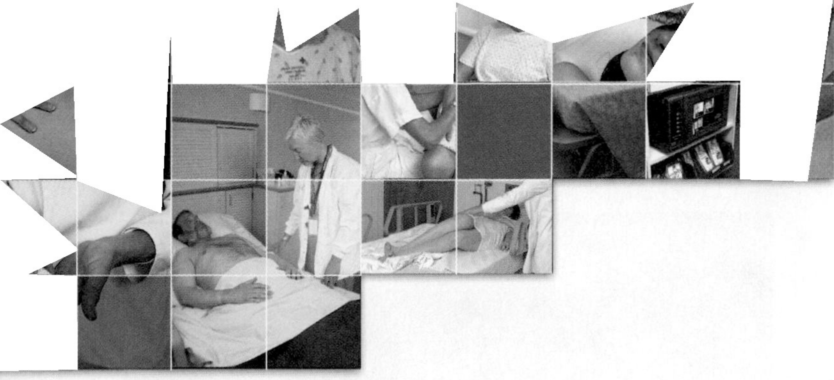

Chapter 8

UNIT 1

Bedmaking

Nursing Process Data

ASSESSMENT Data Base

- Assess the client's need to have linen changed.
- Determine whether the client's present condition permits a change of bed linen.
- Determine how many and what type of linens are required.
- Check client's unit for available linens.
- Determine client's prescribed level of activity and any special precautions in movement.
- Assess client's ability to get out of bed during linen change.

PLANNING Objectives

- To provide a clean, comfortable sleeping and resting environment for the client
- To eliminate irritants to skin by providing wrinkle-free sheets and blankets
- To avoid client exertion, do not move client more than necessary when making an occupied bed (Do not move client more than necessary)
- To enhance client's self-image by providing a clean, neat, and comfortable bed
- To properly dispose of soiled linens and prevent cross-contamination
- To correctly align clients to assist in promoting a physically and emotionally safe and comfortable position
- To prevent stress to the nurse's back or limbs during procedure

IMPLEMENTATION Procedures

EVALUATION Expected Outcomes

- Bed remains clean, dry, and free of wrinkles.
- Client's skin is intact, and free of irritation.
- Nurse does not experience stress on back or joints during bathing and bedmaking.

Folding a Mitered Corner

Equipment

Same as for an unoccupied bed

Procedure

1. Tuck sheet tightly and smoothly under mattress at top or bottom of the bed depending on where mitered corner is needed.
2. Grasp edge of sheet with hand and bring sheet onto mattress so that edge forms a right angle.
3. Tuck lower edge of sheet under mattress.
4. Place finger on sheet where it meets mattress and lower top of sheet over finger. ▶ ***Rationale:*** This action makes the mitered corner neat, tight, and secure.
5. Remove finger without disturbing folds.
6. Tuck sheet securely under mattress.

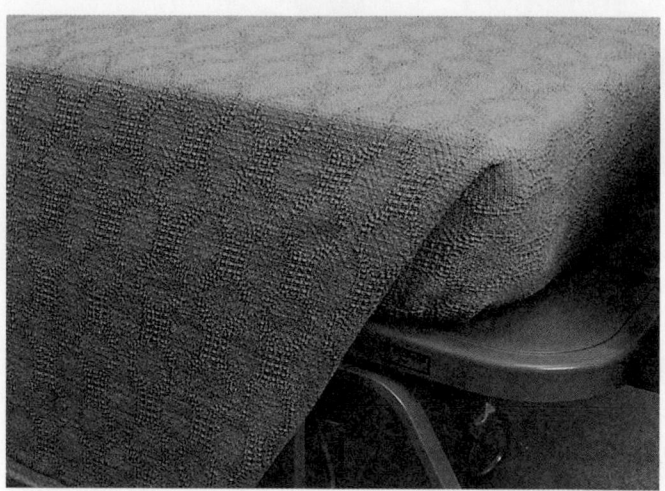

▲ Mitered corners keep bed linens tight and wrinkle-free.

Changing a Pillowcase

Equipment

Clean pillowcase

Procedure

1. Perform hand hygiene.
2. Pick up center of closed end of pillowcase.
3. Continue to firmly grip end of pillowcase; then with other hand, gather pillowcase from open end and fold back (inside-out) over closed end.
4. Pick up center of one end of pillow with the hand holding the gathered pillowcase.
5. Invert pillow so pillowcase drapes down over pillow.
6. Pull pillowcase over pillow with other hand. Do not place pillow or case under arm, chin, or in teeth. ▶ ***Rationale:*** Contamination occurs from using these methods.
7. Adjust pillow corners in pillowcase by placing hand between case and pillow. Do not shake the pillow to position it in its case.

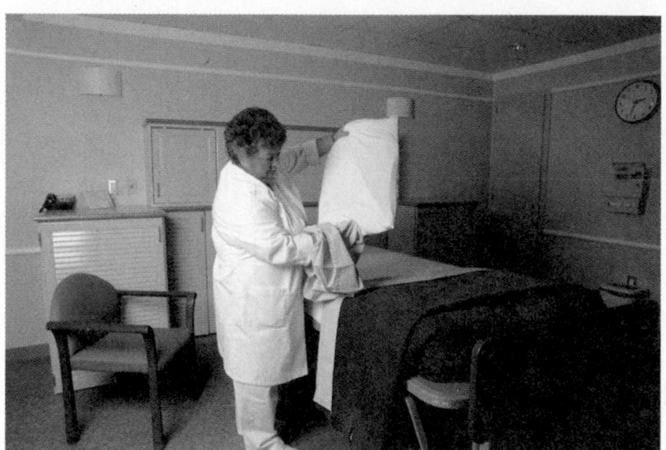

▲ Pick up center of one end of pillow with the hand holding the gathered pillowcase and pull case over pillow with the other hand.

Making an Unoccupied/Surgical Bed

Equipment

- Chair or table
- Linen hamper
- Linens (in order of use):
  - Top sheet
  - Mattress pad, optional
  - Bottom sheet
  - Drawsheet
  - Incontinent pad, if needed
  - Top sheet
  - Blanket
  - Bedspread
  - Pillowcase
- Clean gloves, as needed

NOTE: Whenever possible, make an unoccupied bed rather than occupied. This is physically less stressful for both the client and the nurse.

Preparation

1. Gather clean linen and hamper and bring to room.
2. Explain need for client to be out of bed during procedure.
3. Perform hand hygiene. Don gloves if needed. ▶ ***Rationale:*** Linens may be contaminated from urine, stool, or drainage.
4. Assist client out of bed and into chair.
5. Arrange second chair and hamper conveniently for use.
6. Place linen on chair; ensure chair is clean. ▶ ***Rationale:*** This action provides a clean surface and promotes infection control.
7. Place clean linen on chair in order of use; pillow case at bottom.
8. Detach call signal from bed linen.
9. Adjust bed to a comfortable working height and use body mechanics principles.

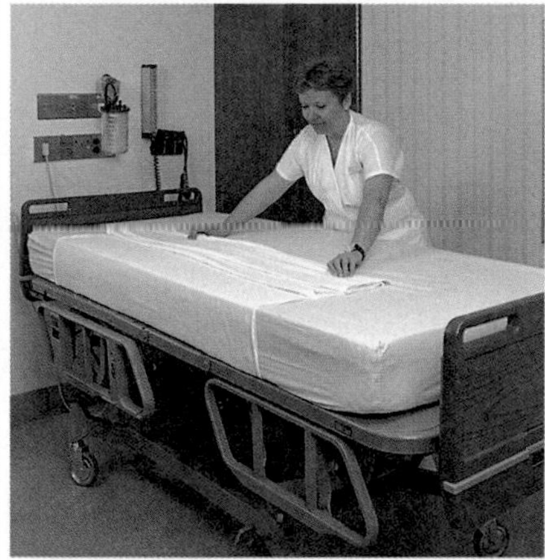

▲ Tuck drawsheet in tightly over bottom sheet.

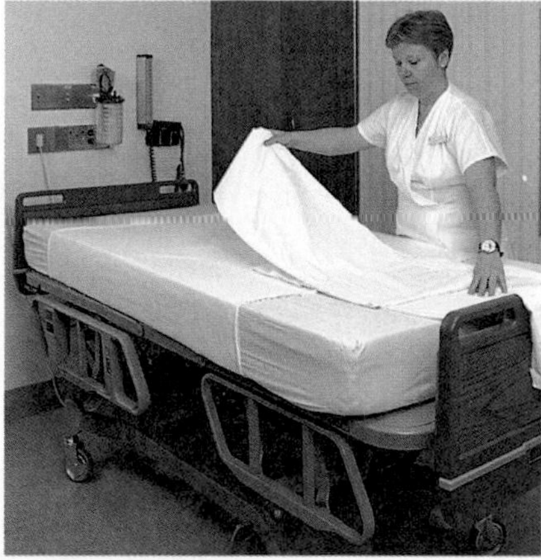

▲ Unfold top sheet to cover mattress.

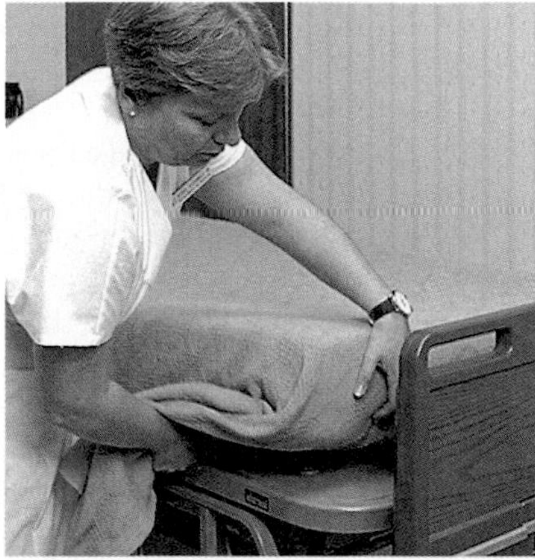

▲ Smooth linen before mitering corners.

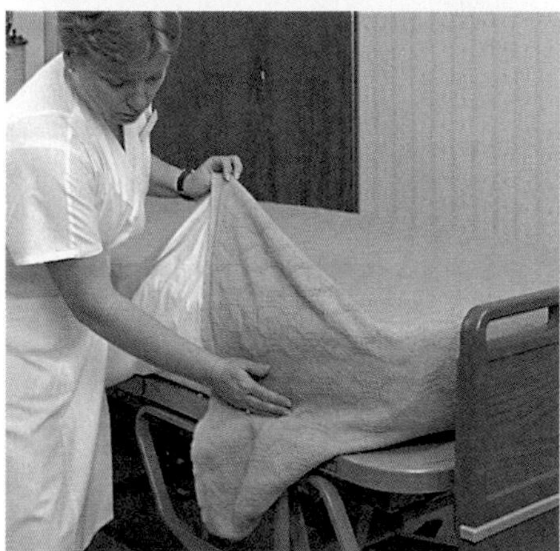

▲ Form triangle and tuck in linen.

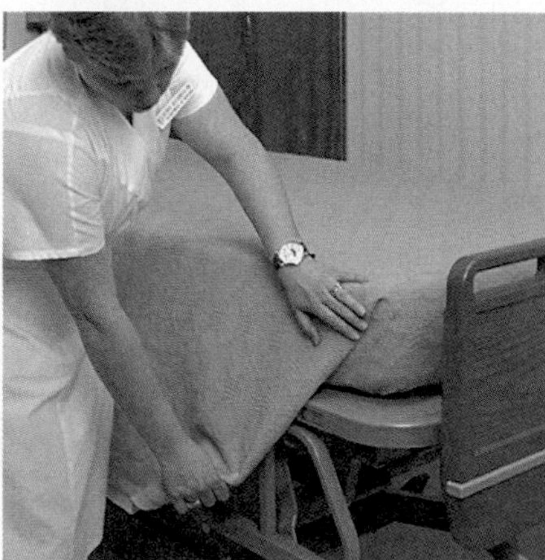

▲ Pull down top linen while holding corner.

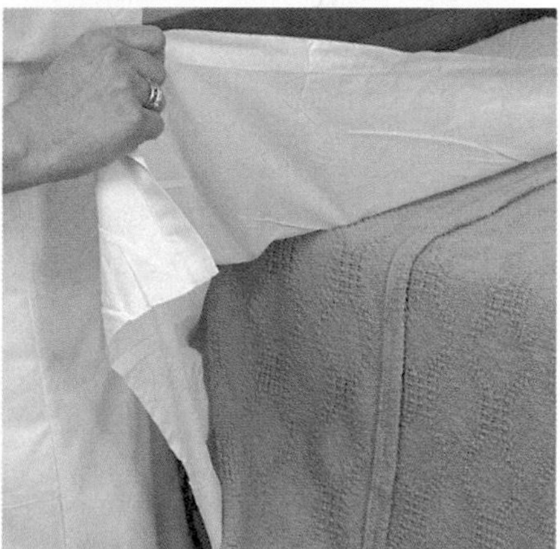

▲ Fold cuff of sheet over spread.

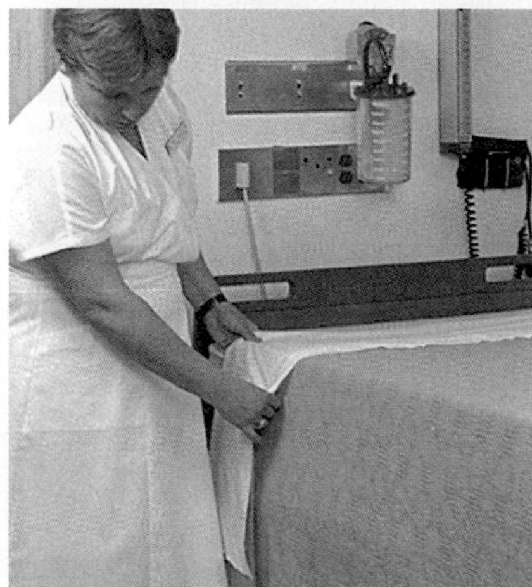

▲ Fold sheet over spread and leave cuff.

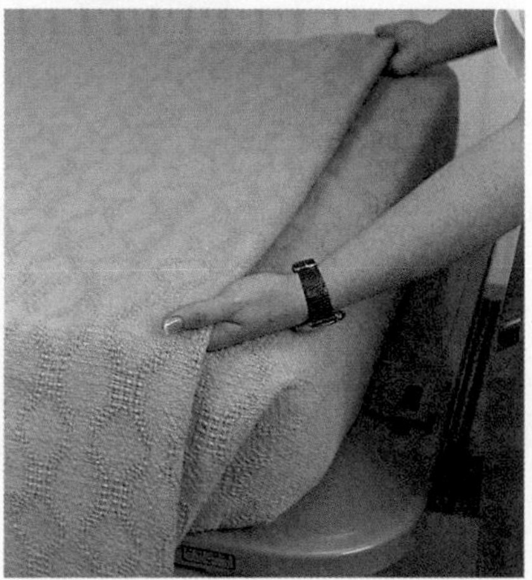

▲ Pleat top linen to allow space for feet.

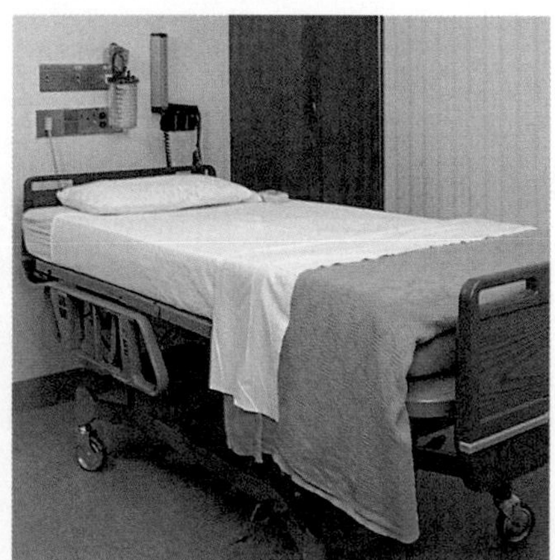

▲ Fanfold linen to foot of bed.

Procedure

1. Lower both side rails and place bed in flat position.
2. Remove spread and blanket. If they are to be reused, fold them and place on the chair.
3. Loosen linen on all sides, including head and foot of the bed.
4. Remove top, draw, and bottom sheet, and place in soiled linen hamper. ▸ ***Rationale:*** Never place dirty linen on the floor as cross-contamination occurs from this action.
5. Push mattress to head of bed. Center the mattress if necessary.
6. If mattress pad is not changed, smooth out wrinkles and recenter pad on the bed surface. ▸ ***Rationale:*** Wrinkles can cause skin abrasions if skin is compromised by age, disease, or malnutrition.
7. Make up one side of the bed, then move to the other side of bed and make it. ▸ ***Rationale:*** This step saves time and expenditure of nurse's energy.
8. Place fitted bottom sheet on mattress, and continue making bed at Step 13. If using a flat bottom sheet, place the center fold of the sheet in the middle of the mattress with the end of the sheet even with the end of the mattress.
9. Unfold the bottom sheet, and cover the mattress.
10. Tuck the top of the sheet under the head of the bed.
11. Miter the corner of the bottom sheet at the head of the bed. (See procedure for mitered corner.) ▸ ***Rationale:*** A mitered corner is tighter and less likely to come apart.
12. Tuck the remaining side of the bottom sheet well under the mattress.
13. If the client needs a drawsheet, place the drawsheet on the bed and open drawsheet. Tuck the sheet under the mattress. Smooth out wrinkles.
    a. If a pull sheet is needed, fold drawsheet in half or quarters. Position sheet in middle of bed. ▸ ***Rationale:*** Pull sheets are used with heavy or difficult-to-move clients.
    b. If absorbent pad is needed, center it on bed over draw or pull sheet.
14. Move to the other side of the bed. Pull linen toward you and straighten out linen.
15. Tuck the top of the sheet under the head of the bed if using a flat sheet.
16. Miter the corner of the bottom sheet at the head of the bed if not using a fitted sheet.
17. Tuck remaining bottom sheet well under the mattress. Gather sheet into your hand, lean away from the bed, and pull sheet downward. Tuck sheet under mattress.
18. If drawsheet is used, tighten and tuck the same as bottom sheet.
19. Straighten out absorbent pad and pull sheet if used.
20. Place top sheet, blanket, and spread full length on top of bed.
21. Leave a cuff of top sheet and spread at the head of the bed. Fold back top sheet and spread to form 5 inch cuff. ▸ ***Rationale:*** This prevents client's face from rubbing against blanket.
22. Tuck sheet, spread, and blanket well under foot of mattress, one side at a time.
23. Miter corners at the foot of the bed, one side at a time.
24. Make a small pleat or slightly loosen linen to allow room for client's feet. ▸ ***Rationale:*** To prevents friction and pressure on feet and toes.
25. Fanfold linen to foot of bed. ▸ ***Rationale:*** To facilitate client getting into bed.
26. Change pillowcase. See skill "Changing a Pillowcase."
27. Return bed to lowest position. Reattach call signal to linens.

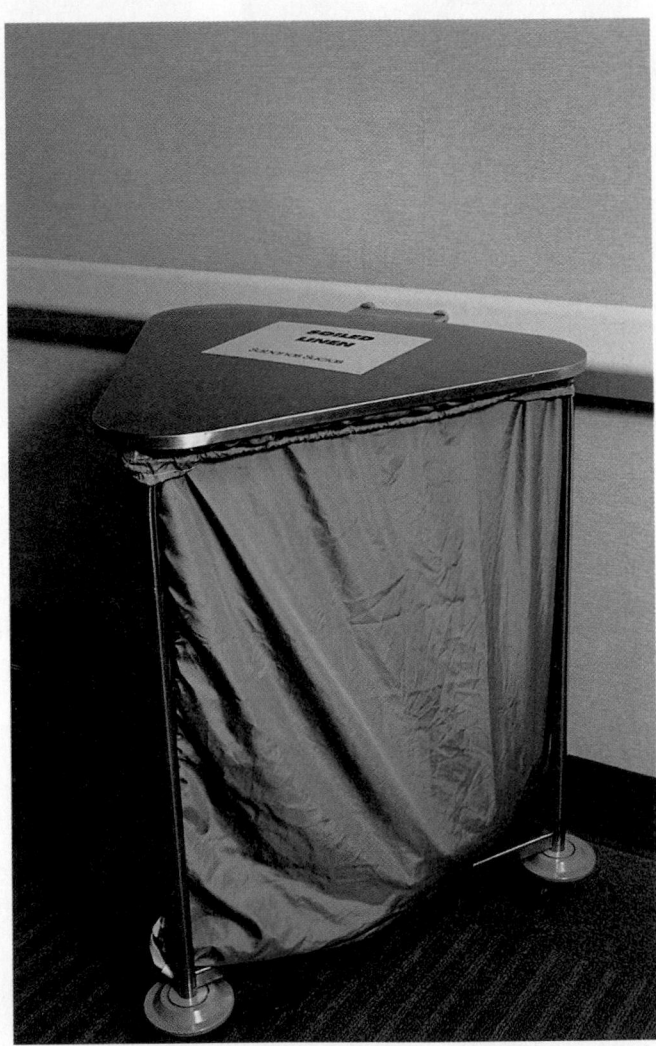

▲ Keep linen hamper covered to prevent spread of microorganisms. Position hamper outside client's room for easy access.

28. Pull side rail up on side farthest from client.
   ▸ ***Rationale:*** To allow client to position self in bed.
29. If the bed is unassigned, leave top linen pulled up, covering the bed.
30. Dispose of soiled linen in dirty utility room or hamper.
31. Perform hand hygiene.

NOTE: Some facilities use individualized plastic bags to transfer linens to dirty utility room.

Principles of Medical Asepsis

- Place dirty linen in hamper.
- Do not place dirty linen on floor.
- Discard all unused linen from client area.
- Do not transfer linen from one client area to another.
- Do not allow dirty linen to touch uniform.
- Perform hand hygiene.

Changing an Occupied Bed

Equipment

Chair or table
Soiled linen hamper
Linens (in order of use):
- Bath blanket or top sheet
- Mattress pad, optional
- Bottom sheet
- Cloth drawsheet

Incontinent pad, if needed
Top sheet
Blanket
Bedspread
Pillowcase
Clean gloves, if indicated

Preparation

1. Talk with the client and explain how he or she can be involved in the procedure.
2. Explain the sequence for the procedure.
3. Arrange furniture and equipment (e.g., soiled linen hamper and chair) for convenience of use.
4. Perform hand hygiene and then collect the clean linen.
5. Place linen on chair; ensure that chair is clean.
6. Detach call signal from linens.
7. Provide for privacy for the client.
8. Adjust the bed to a comfortable working height with side rails up. Help client into a supine position.
9. Don gloves if bed linen is soiled with body fluids.

Procedure

1. Lower side rail on your side of the bed, but make sure side rail on opposite side is in UP position. ▸ ***Rationale:*** This ensures client safety as client rolls to edge of bed.
2. Loosen top linens.
3. Remove spread, sheet, and blanket at the same time the bath blanket is pulled over client. Top sheet may be used in place of bath blankets in some facilities. ▸ ***Rationale:*** Blanket keeps client warm during bed change. If they are to be reused, fold them and place on the chair.
4. Place top sheet in soiled linen hamper, unless being used to cover client during bedmaking.
5. Push mattress to head of bed. Center the mattress if necessary.
6. Assist client to the side of the bed, place in side-lying position facing away from you as near the far side rail as possible.

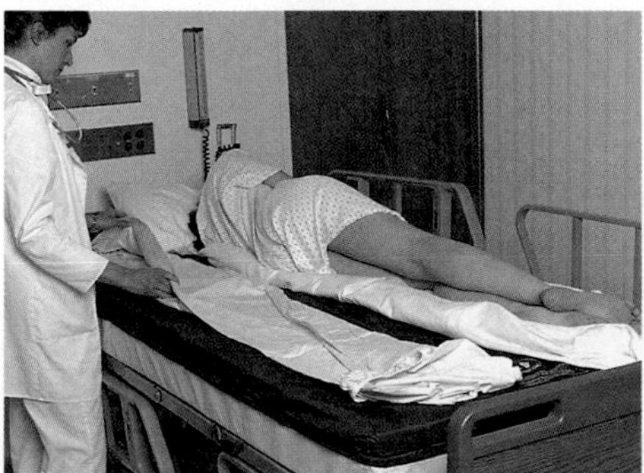
▲ Place center of sheet in middle of bed.

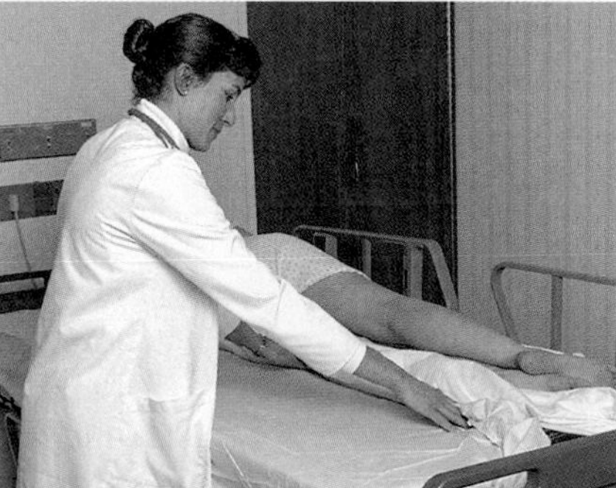
▲ Tighten bottom sheet under mattress.

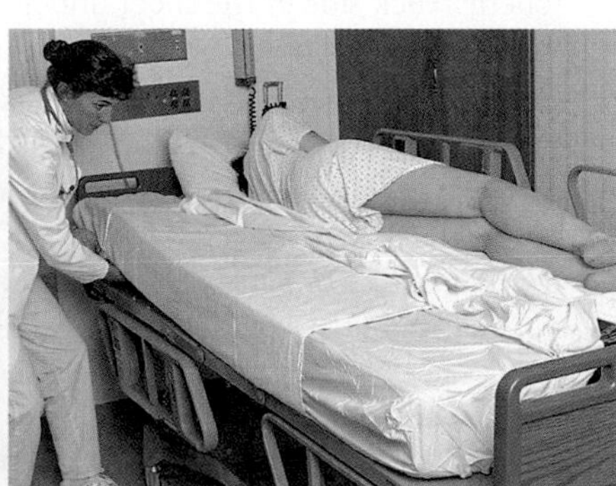
▲ Place drawsheet in middle of bed.

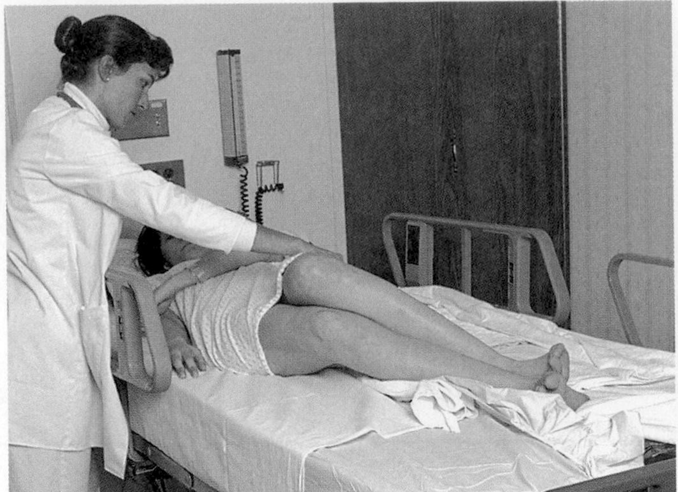

▲ Assist client to roll over to side of bed toward you.

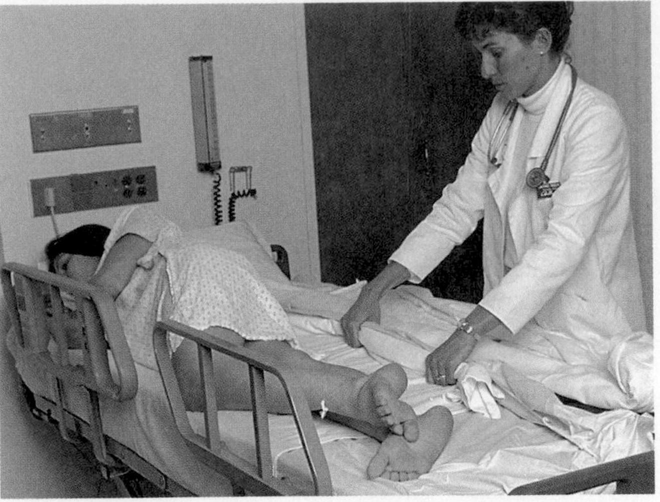

▲ Move to other side of bed, and pull linen toward you.

7. Loosen bottom linens on your side of the bed.
8. Fold or roll dirty linen under or as close as possible to client. ▸ ***Rationale:*** To keep soiled linen contained and away from client's skin.
9. Smooth out wrinkles and recenter pad on the bed surface if mattress pad is used but not changed. ▸ ***Rationale:*** Wrinkles may cause skin irritation.
10. Place clean bottom sheet on mattress with client on the opposite side of the bed. Place the center fold of the sheet in the middle of the mattress with the end of the sheet even with the end of the mattress.
11. Unfold the bottom sheet and cover the mattress. Make sure the clean bottom sheet is underneath any used linen. ▸ ***Rationale:*** This keeps the clean linen uncontaminated.
12. Tuck the top of the sheet under the head of the bed, or position fitted sheet around corner of mattress.
13. Miter the corner of the bottom sheet at the head of the bed if flat sheet is used.
14. Tuck the remaining bottom sheet well under the mattress from head to foot.
15. Center drawsheet on the bed, if the client requires a drawsheet, and fanfold half of the sheet under the client. Tuck side of the sheet under the mattress. Smooth out wrinkles.
    a. Fold drawsheet in half or quarters if a pull sheet is needed. Position sheet in middle of bed. Fanfold half of the pull sheet under client, from client's shoulders to knees.
    b. Fanfold absorbent pad and center it on bed under client's buttocks. Place the pad, absorbent side up and plastic side down, close to the client. ▸ ***Rationale:*** This position makes it easy to pull through to the other side of the bed.
16. Help the client roll over to the other side of the bed.
17. Tell the client why there is a hump of linen in the center of the bed. Ensure client comfort (i.e., reposition pillows).
18. Raise the side rail. Move to other side of bed.
19. Move linens to the other side of the bed, by gently pulling linens toward you.
20. Lower side rail, and loosen bottom sheets.
21. Pull dirty linen to side of bed and roll into a bundle at the foot of the bed or place linen in linen hamper. ▸ ***Rationale:*** This reduces the spread of microorganisms.
22. Never place dirty linen on the floor. ▸ ***Rationale:*** Cross-contamination occurs from this action.
23. Pull clean linen across mattress and straighten under client.
24. Miter the top corner of the flat bottom sheet or tuck fitted sheet over mattress edge.
25. Gather bottom sheet into your hand, lean away from the bed, and pull linens downward at an angle. Tuck remaining bottom sheet well under the mattress. If drawsheet is used, tighten and tuck it in the same way.
26. Help the client into a supine position and adjust the pillow.
27. Place top sheet, blanket, and spread over the client. Leave at least a 6-inch cuff of top sheet at the head of the bed.
28. Remove bath blanket, and straighten top sheet and blanket.
29. Miter corners at foot of bed.
30. Pull up all layers of linen at client's toes. Make a small pleat. ▸ ***Rationale:*** This allows room for client's feet and prevents sheets from rubbing on client's toes.
31. Raise side rail.
32. Remove pillow from bed, and change pillowcase.
33. Return bed to lowest position. Reattach call signal to linens.
34. Position client for comfort.
35. Dispose of soiled laundry.
36. Remove gloves, if used, and perform hand hygiene.

EVIDENCE-BASED PRACTICE

To reduce or eliminate the risk for pressure ulcers, research recommends limiting the layers of linen on which a client lies. Use only the minimum amount of bed linens needed for the specific client's needs or condition.

Source: Gibbons, W., Shanks, H. T., Kleinhelter, P., Jones, P. (2006). Eliminating facility-acquired pressure ulcers at Ascension Health. *The Joint Commission Journal on Quality and Patient Safety, 32*(9), 488–496.

DOCUMENTATION for Bedmaking

- Specific linens or equipment that cause discomfort for the client
- Special requirements for linens (e.g., certain detergents or elimination of starch)
- Use of pull sheets, incontinent pads, or specified ways to keep bed dry
- Addition or removal of linen to adjust for accurate client weight, if using bed scale

CRITICAL THINKING Application

Expected Outcomes

- Bed remains clean, dry, and free of wrinkles.
- Client's skin is intact and free of irritation.
- Nurse does not experience stress on back during bathing and bedmaking.

Unexpected Outcomes	Alternative Actions
Client refuses to have bed made.	• Assess reason for refusal. Client may be in pain or does not want to be disturbed. • Offer to make the bed at a later time. • Change only the pillowcase and drawsheet, if client allows. • Beds do not need to be changed unless soiled or damp, so allow client's independence if possible.
Cross-contamination occurs from improper linen disposal.	• Provide adequate linen hampers for the nursing personnel. • Attend in-service education programs on infection control.
Client's skin becomes irritated from linen or begins to break down.	• Obtain hypoallergenic linen. • Place therapeutic mattress under client. • Provide skin care with appropriate lotion.
The nurse feels stress on back during bedmaking.	• Make sure bed is positioned for comfort of the nurse. High position is generally used. • If client is heavy, ask for assistance with bedmaking, especially in moving side to side. • Use full sheet or Booster Lift for turning. • Attend in-service classes on preventing back strain. • Use body mechanics principles during bedmaking procedure. • Use assistive devices for large clients, as available.

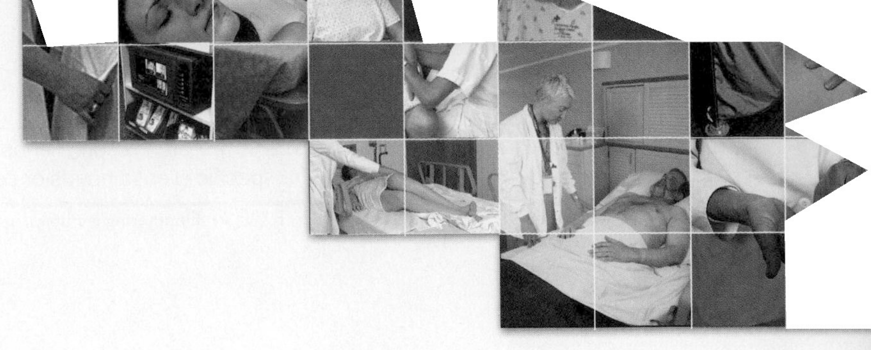

Chapter 8

UNIT 2

Bath Care

Nursing Process Data

ASSESSMENT Data Base

- Assess client's need for bathing and other personal hygiene activities.
- Check client's activity order. Note special precautions related to movement or exercise.
- Assess client's ability to perform his or her own care and determine how much assistance he or she needs.
- Discuss client's preferences for the bathing procedure, bath, and personal articles.
- Check client's room for availability of bathing articles and linens.
- Assess client's skin (see Unit 3 on Skin Integrity).

PLANNING Objectives

- To decrease the possibility of infection by removing transient bacteria, excessive debris, secretions, and perspiration from the skin
- To eliminate odors and rid body of microorganisms
- To promote circulation
- To maintain muscle tone through active or passive movement during bathing
- To alternate points of pressure on the body by changing client's position during the bath
- To provide comfort for the client
- To assess the client's overall status, skin condition, level of mobility, comfort

IMPLEMENTATION Procedures

EVALUATION Expected Outcomes

- Client's skin is free of excessive perspiration, secretions, and offensive odors.
- Client feels comfortable and does not experience itching or irritation.
- Client's skin is moist and free of itching sensation.
- Client is able to take bath or shower without excessive fatigue or anxiety.
- Client is able to bathe self using disposable cleansing system.

Providing Morning Care

Equipment

Basin of warm water
Soap
Towel and washcloth
Emesis basin
Toothbrush and paste
Bedpan or urinal
Toilet tissue
Clean gloves

Preparation

1. Determine whether client wishes morning care. ▸ ***Rationale:*** Morning care is provided to "freshen" the client in preparation for breakfast, physicians' visits, and procedures occurring before bathing.
2. Perform hand hygiene. ▸ ***Rationale:*** When providing morning care to several clients, it is important to perform hand hygiene between clients so that microorganisms are not transmitted from one client to another.
3. Gather equipment and take it to client's room.
4. Identify client using two indicators.
5. Explain that early morning care is available while client remains in bed. If client is able, assist him or her to the bathroom.
6. Provide privacy.

Procedure

1. Perform hand hygiene.
2. Offer bedpan or urinal and assist client as needed. Don gloves when giving client bedpan or urinal.
3. Move bed to comfortable working height and lower side rail.
4. Put equipment on over-bed table within reach. Place towel under client's chin. ▸ ***Rationale:*** To keep gown and linens dry.
5. Wash client's face and hands or assist as needed. Dry face and hands.
6. Offer oral hygiene. Assist as needed. Gloves should be worn if client needs assistance with oral hygiene.
7. Hold emesis basin so client can rinse after brushing teeth.
8. Assist client to comfortable position.
9. Reposition bed, and replace side rails.
10. Remove equipment and draw curtains.
11. Remove gloves, if used.
12. Perform hand hygiene.

Bathing an Adult Client

Equipment

Basin or sink with warm water (110°–115°F)
Soap and soap dish
Personal articles (i.e., deodorant, powder, lotions)
Laundry hamper
Two to three towels and several washcloths
Gloves if appropriate
Bath blanket
Pajamas or hospital gown
Table for bathing equipment
Shaving equipment for male clients

NOTE: Use a new cloth for each section of the body to prevent cross-contamination.

Preparation

1. Provide a comfortable room environment (i.e., comfortable temperature, lighting).
2. Identify client; talk with client about plan for bathing to meet personal care needs.
3. Encourage client to bathe himself or herself. ▸ ***Rationale:*** To increase independence, promote exercise and a sense of self-worth.
4. Explain any unfamiliar methods or procedures regarding bathing.
5. Perform hand hygiene.
6. Collect necessary equipment, and place articles within reach on over-bed table.
7. Ask the client if he or she needs to void or defecate before starting the bath. ▸ ***Rationale:*** Warm water of the bath and movement can stimulate the client to void.
8. Position the bed at a comfortable working height.
9. Ensure privacy.

Procedure

1. Place bath blanket over client and over top linen. Loosen top linen at edges and foot of bed.
   a. Ask client to grasp and hold top edge of bath blanket to keep it in place while you pull linen to foot of bed.
   b. Remove dirty top linen from under bath blanket, starting at client's shoulders and rolling linen down

EVIDENCE-BASED PRACTICE

Bed Bath or Disposable Bed Bath

Very few studies have been published on the effect that bed baths or tub baths have on client comfort or healing. One study by Dunn et al. (2002) stated that there was a high level of stress for clients receiving tub baths with the diagnosis of dementia. A study by Collins and Hampton (2003) indicated only that the bed bath was more costly than the disposable bed bath. There is a school of thought that indicates bed baths should be eliminated as part of nursing care, particularly since the average length of hospital stay is so short; however, there is insufficient evidence-based data to support this decision.

Source: Dunn, J. C., Thiru-Chelvam, B., & Beck, C. H. (2002). Bathing, pleasure or pain? *Journal of Gerontologic Nursing, 28*, 6.
Collins, F., & Hampton, S. (2003). The cost-effective use of BagBath: a new concept in patient hygiene. *The British Journal of Nursing, 12*, 984.
Moore, K. (2005). Does "arriving" mean we give up the bed bath? *Journal of Wound, Ostomy and Continence Nursing, 32*(5), 285–286.

toward the client's feet. If bath blanket is not available, use top sheet.

c. Place dirty linen in laundry hamper.

2. Help client to the side of the bed closest to you. Keep the side rail on the far side of the bed in the UP position.
3. Remove client's gown. Most gowns have snaps and can be taken off without disturbing IVs or other tubes. Place gown in laundry bag. Keep client covered with bath blanket. ▸ ***Rationale:*** To protect client's modesty and keep client warm during bathing.
4. Remove pillow if client can tolerate.
5. Place towel under client's head.
6. Don clean gloves if risk of exposure to body fluids when bathing client. ▸ ***Rationale:*** To maintain Standard Precautions.
7. Make a mitt with a washcloth. Fold washcloth around your hand as illustrated. ▸ ***Rationale:*** This prevents wet ends of cloth from annoying client.
8. Bathe client's face. ▸ ***Rationale:*** Begin bath at cleanest area and work downward toward feet.
   a. Wash around client's eyes, using clear water. With one edge of washcloth, wipe from the inner canthus toward the outer canthus. ▸ ***Rationale:*** This prevents secretions from entering the lacrimal duct. Using a different section of the washcloth, repeat procedure on other eye. Dry thoroughly.
   b. Wash, rinse, and dry client's forehead, cheeks, nose, and area around lips. Use soap with client's permission.
   c. Wash, rinse, and dry area behind and around the client's ears.
   d. Wash, rinse, and dry client's neck.
9. Remove towel from under client's head.
10. Use a clean washcloth for each section of the body. Bathe client's upper body and extremities. Place towel under area to be bathed.
    a. Wash both arms by elevating client's arm and holding client's wrist. Use long, firm strokes from the wrist toward the shoulder, including the axillary area. ▸ ***Rationale:*** Movement distal to proximal increases venous return and promotes circulation.
    b. Wash, rinse, and dry client's axillae. Apply deodorant and powder if desired.
    c. Wash client's hands by soaking them in the basin or with a washcloth. Nails can be cleaned now or after the bath.
    d. Keeping chest covered with the towel, wash, rinse, and thoroughly dry client's chest, especially under breasts. (Apply powder or cornstarch under breasts if desired.)
11. Bathe client's abdomen. Using a towel over chest area and bath blanket, cover areas you are not bathing. Wash, rinse, and dry abdomen and umbilicus. Replace bath blanket over client's upper body and abdomen.
12. Bathe client's legs and feet. Place towel under leg to be bathed. Drape other leg, hip, and genital area with the bath blanket.
    a. Carefully place bath basin on the towel near the client's foot, with knee bent.
    b. With one arm under the client's leg, grasp the client's foot and bend knee. Place foot in basin of water.
    c. Bathe client's leg, moving toward hip with long, firm strokes. Rinse and dry client's leg. ▸ ***Rationale:*** This promotes circulation.

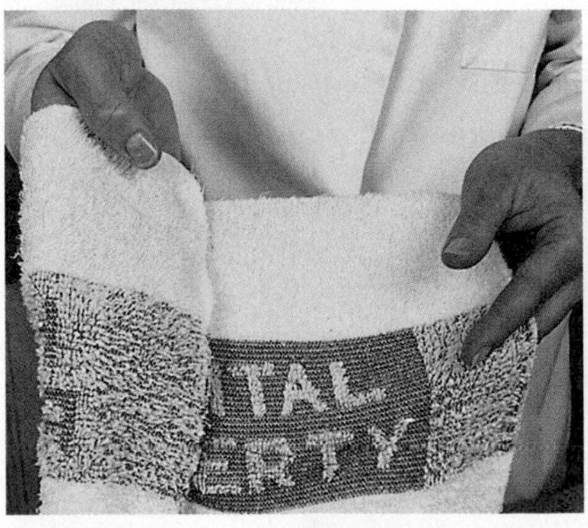
▲ Wrap one edge of cloth around palm and fingers.

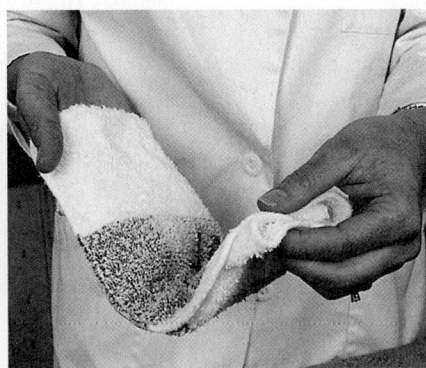
▲ Wrap cloth around hand and anchor with thumb.

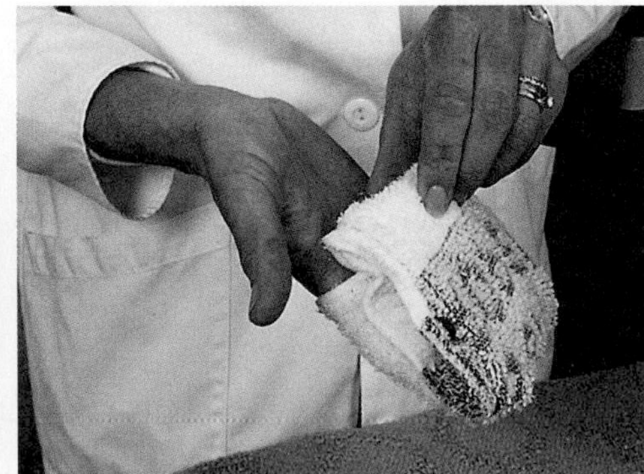
▲ Tuck far edge of cloth under edge in palm of hand.

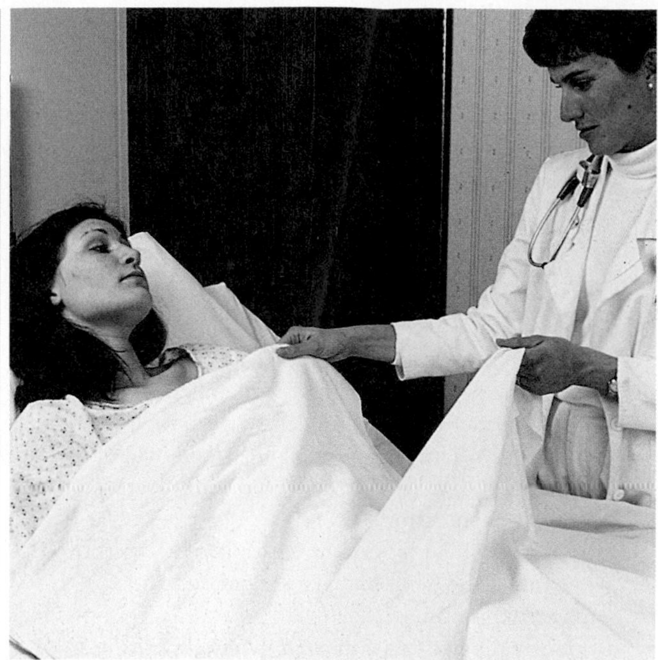

▲ Remove top linen and replace with bath blanket.

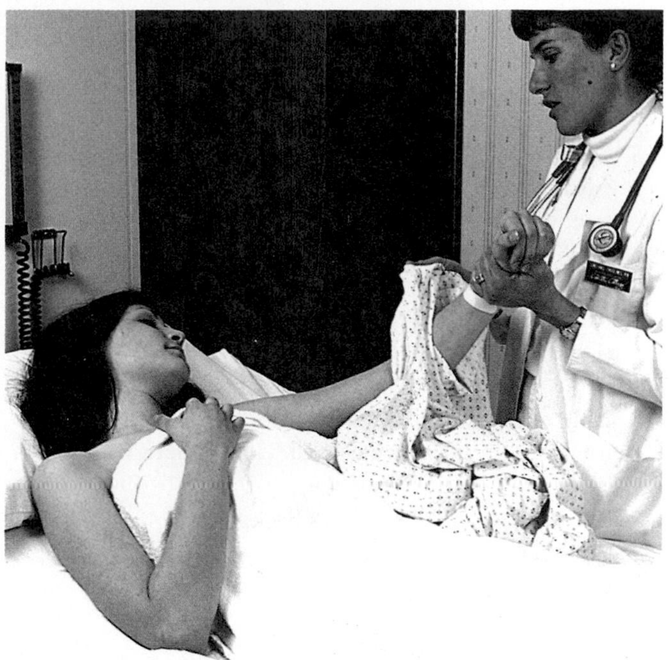

▲ Remove gown while covering client with bath blanket.

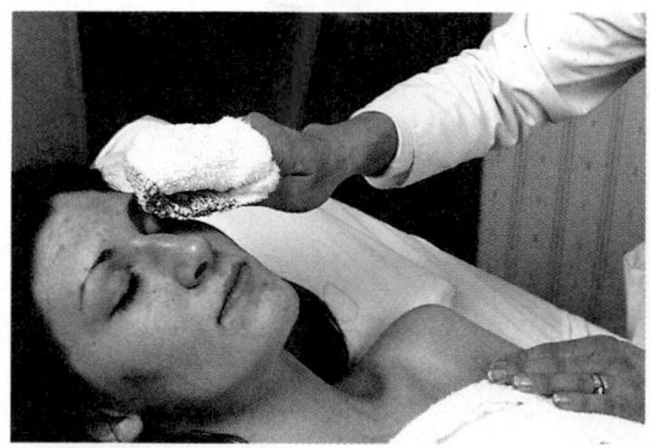

▲ Wash eyes first, from inner to outer canthus.

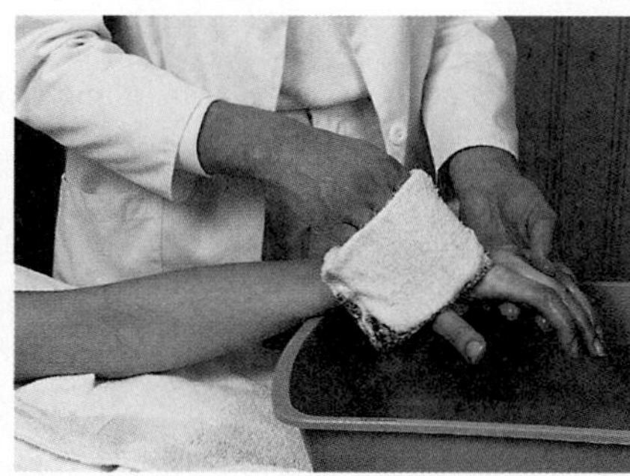

▲ Wash hands by soaking them in a basin.

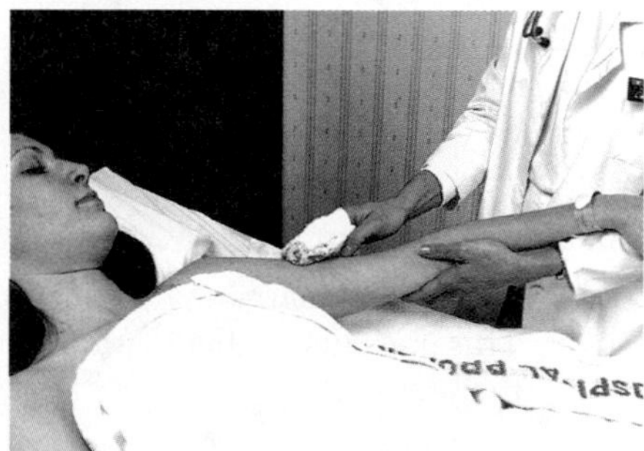

▲ Support wrist when washing client's arm.

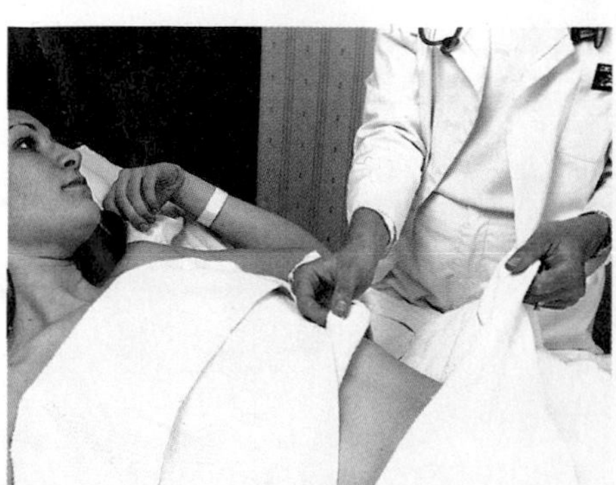

▲ Keep client covered with towel during bath.

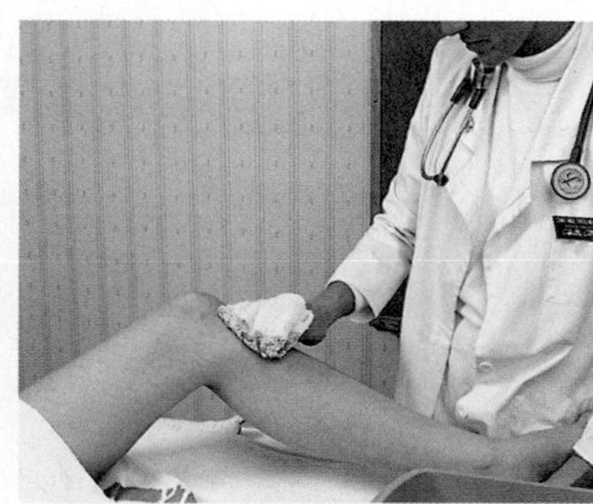

▲ Wash client's legs and feet for a total bed bath.

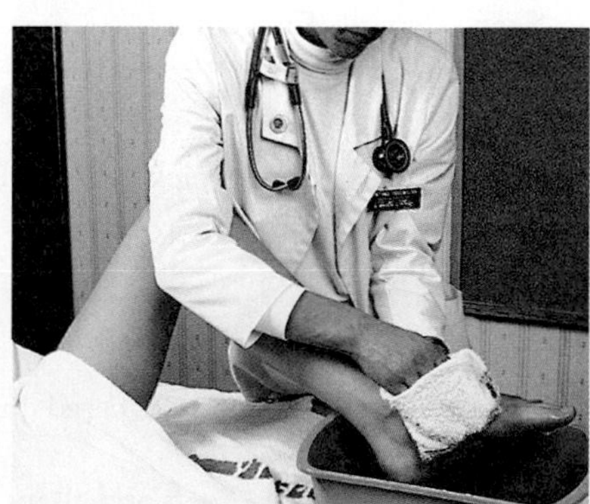

▲ Place client's feet in basin while bathing.

d. Wash client's foot with washcloth. Rinse and dry foot and area between toes thoroughly.
e. Carefully move basin to other side of bed, and repeat procedure for client's other leg and foot.

13. Change bath water. Raise side rails when refilling basin. ▸ ***Rationale:*** This ensures client safety. Check the water temperature before continuing with the bath.
14. During the bath, continuously assess the client's skin and musculoskeletal system. Careful attention should be paid to the verbal statements and nonverbal expressions. ▸ ***Rationale:*** This data yields information about client's overall condition.
15. Help client turn to a side-lying or prone position. Place towel under area to be bathed. Cover client with a bath blanket.
16. Wash, rinse, and dry client's back, moving from the shoulders to the buttocks. ▸ ***Rationale:*** Move from clean to dirty area on body.

Clinical Alert

Bathe lower extremities gently if client is at high risk for deep vein thrombosis. DO NOT rub legs. This action could dislodge a clot.

17. Provide back massage now or after completion of bath. (For procedure, see Providing Back Care.)
18. Bathe client's genital area if client is unable to do this by self. Cover all body parts except area to be bathed. Place towel under client's hips.

For Female Client

a. Bathe perineum from pubis to rectum. ▸ ***Rationale:*** This prevents contamination from the rectal area to the urethra.
b. Use separate areas of the washcloth for each stroke.
c. Discard soiled washcloths as needed.
d. Clean the labia majora by separating the labia and clean between the majora and labia minora.
e. Wash, rinse, and dry the clitoris, urethral meatus, and vaginal orifice.
f. Ensure all folds of skin are thoroughly dry.

For Male Client

a. Place a towel under the penis.
b. Hold the penis by the shaft. If the client is uncircumcised, retract the foreskin before washing if it retracts easily. ▸ ***Rationale:*** This will allow removal of smegma that may have collected, thus decreasing chance of infection.
c. Using a circular motion, wash, rinse, and dry the meatus of the penis and glans in an outward direction.
d. Gently replace foreskin to its original position.
e. Cleanse the shaft of the penis moving from the tip to the base of the penis.
f. Wash, rinse, and pat the scrotum dry, especially the posterior rugae.

19. Remove gloves and place in receptacle.
20. Assist client to dress in a clean hospital gown or pajamas.
21. Clean and store bath equipment. Dispose of dirty linen.
22. Proceed with any other personal hygiene activities as needed.
23. Replace call light, lower bed, and place side rails in UP position before leaving client.
24. Remove gloves, if used, and perform hand hygiene.

Providing Foot Care

Equipment

Basin of warm water
Soap or emollient agent
Washcloth
Two towels
Nail file, emery board, pick, or orangewood stick
Skin care lotion or lanolin
Clean gloves (use if risk of contacting body fluids)

Preparation

1. Determine foot care needs based on client's condition and assessment data.
2. Check physician's orders and client care plan.
3. Collect necessary equipment.
4. Help client into a chair in a comfortable sitting position if possible.

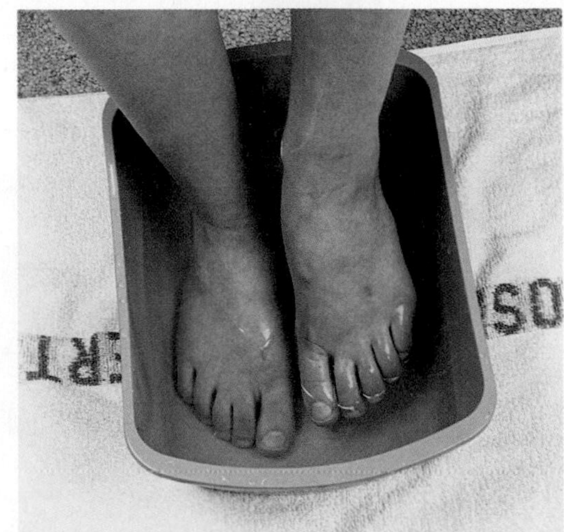

▲ Place towel on floor in front of client and place feet in basin for soaking.

5. Discuss procedure with client.
6. Perform hand hygiene.

Procedure

1. Place towel or bath mat on floor in front of client.
2. Place basin of warm water on towel.
3. Help client place feet in basin.
4. Add emollient agent to water, if desired.
5. Assist client with other personal hygiene activities while feet are soaking. Let feet soak for 10 minutes.
6. Using a washcloth, gently wash client's feet with soap and water.
7. Dry each foot thoroughly with a second towel. Dry between each toe.
8. Using nail clippers, cut straight across the nails. ▸ ***Rationale:*** Prevents trauma to surrounding tissue.
9. Clean underneath and on sides of nails using a file or orangewood stick.
10. If necessary, push back cuticles using an orangewood stick. Smooth rough edges with an emery board.
11. Apply lotion to entire foot focusing on callused or dry areas. If client's feet are cracking or excessively dry, instruct client to use a deep-penetrating moisturizer like shea butter.
12. Assist client in putting on clean socks and shoes or slippers.
13. Replace equipment.
14. Assist client to bed or position for comfort in chair.
15. Perform hand hygiene.

Bathing a Client in Tub or Shower

Equipment

Two towels and washcloth
Soap
Clean gown, robe, and slippers

Preparation

1. Identify client; perform hand hygiene.
2. Assess client's ability to tolerate tub or shower.
3. Cover all tubings and dressings with plastic covering and instruct client to minimize getting these areas wet.
4. Ensure that tub or shower and equipment is cleansed per agency policy. ▸ ***Rationale:*** To prevent spread of microorganisms.
5. Place a rubber mat or towel on floor. Use shower chair if indicated. ▸ ***Rationale:*** To prevent client slipping and ensure safety.
6. Fill tub or adjust shower with warm water (temperature if tested 105°–110°F).

Procedure

1. Assist client into tub or shower. Use hydraulic bathtub chair if necessary (see procedure for Bathing in a Hydraulic Bathtub Chair).
2. Show client how to call for help when needed.
3. Provide client privacy. Assist client with washing back, lower legs, or feet, as needed.
4. Assist client with putting on clean gown, robe, and transporting back to room.
5. Clean shower or tub area and dispose of dirty linen.
6. Perform hand hygiene.

Bathing Using Disposable System

Equipment

Commercial cleansing system
Bath blanket
Clean gown
Disposable bag
Clean gloves, if appropriate

Preparation

1. Obtain package with cleansing cloths. Cloths are premoistened with an aloe and vitamin E formula. ▸ ***Rationale:*** The cleansing cloths are less drying as they maintain the skin at pH of 4.7–4.9.
2. Heat package in microwave for no more than 45 seconds. Check temperature before applying to skin. ▸ ***Rationale:*** Increased time could lead to excessive heat and burning of the skin. The commercial system can be used at room temperature.
3. Explain procedure to client. ▸ ***Rationale:*** This procedure may be new to the client and an explanation is needed to ensure client understands the difference between a bed bath and a bath using a cleansing system. The client may not think he has had a complete bath but only "a sponge bath."
4. Perform hand hygiene.
5. Don gloves if there is a risk of contact with body secretions.
6. Replace top linen and gown with bath blanket or top sheet if bath blanket not available.

Procedure

1. Open package and remove one cloth at a time.
2. Remove bath blanket at each site when cleansing with cloth.
3. Replace bath blanket when cloth removed. ▸ ***Rationale:*** To prevent client chilling.

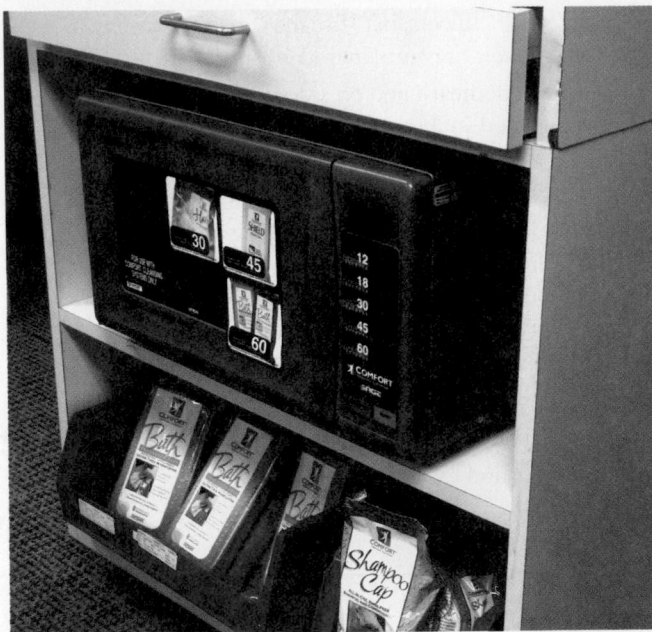
▲ Place package containing cleansing cloths in microwave to warm, according to directions (usually no more than 45 seconds).

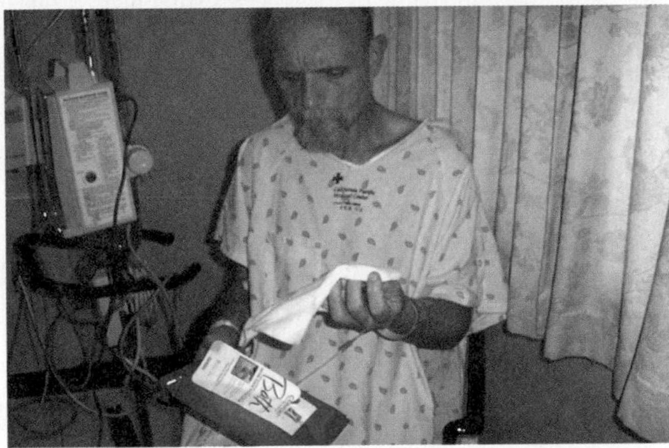
▲ Each towel is used once and discarded.

4. Use a new cloth for each section of the body as follows:
   a. Face, neck, and chest
   b. Right arm and axilla
   c. Left arm and axilla
   d. Perineum
   e. Right leg
   f. Left leg
   g. Back
   h. Buttocks
5. Discard cloth after cleansing each area. Do not flush down toilet. Rinsing is not required with this system. Replace bath blanket or sheet over each part of the body after it has been cleaned. ▸ ***Rationale:*** To prevent the client from becoming chilled.
6. Place clean gown on client.
7. Place client in comfortable position.
8. Discard cloths in appropriate receptacle.
9. Perform hand hygiene.
10. Document bath on flow sheet or nurses' notes.

EVIDENCE-BASED PRACTICE

Bath Basins as Potential Sources of Infection

A recent study (2009) conducted at three acute care hospitals examined 92 bath basins from three intensive care units. Sterile culture sponges were used to obtain samples from the basins. Some form of bacteria grew in 98% of the samples. The organisms with the highest positive rates of growth were enterococci (54%), gram-negative organisms (32%), *staphylococcus aureus* (23%), vancomycin-resistant enterococci (13%), and methicillin-resistant *staphylococcus aureus* (8%). The conclusion of the study indicated that bath basins are a reservoir for bacteria and may be a source of transmission of hospital-acquired infections.

Using a prepackaged bath indicated that microbial counts were significantly lower than basin baths. The study concluded that using a disposable bath is more efficacious for bathing, particularly for high-risk clients.

Source: Johnson, D., Lineweaver, L., & Maze, L. M. (2009). Patient's bath basins as potential sources of infection: a multcenter sampling study. *American Journal of Critical Care*, *18*(1), 31–40.

Bathing an Infant

Equipment

Tub or basin filled with warm water (100°F)
Two towels
Washcloth
Suction bulb
Mild soap
Cotton balls
Blanket
Clean clothing
Clean gloves, if indicated

Preparation

1. Provide a comfortable room environment (i.e., comfortable temperature, lighting).
2. Check client ID.
3. Perform hand hygiene.
4. Collect necessary equipment, and place articles within reach.
5. Position the bed at a comfortable working height.
6. Place towel, laid out in diamond fashion, on bed next to basin.
7. Don gloves if there is a risk of exposure to body secretions.

Procedure

1. Test water temperature with your wrist or elbow.
2. Lift infant using football hold.

Some facilities use disposable cleansing systems to bathe neonates and infants. There are four infant-size washcloths for infants up to 25 pounds. The bathing procedure is the same for infants and adults.

3. Remove all clothing except shirt and diaper.
4. Cover infant with towel or blanket. Never let go of the infant during the bath. ▶ ***Rationale:*** This is a safety intervention to prevent falls or other injury.
5. Clean infant's eyes using a cotton ball moistened with water. Wipe from inner to outer canthus, using a new cotton ball for each eye. ▶ ***Rationale:*** This procedure prevents water and particles from entering the lacrimal duct.

Clinical Alert
Discharge from the eyes may be present for 2 to 3 days due to prophylactic eyedrops administered at birth.

6. Make a mitt with the washcloth.
7. Wash infant's face with water.
8. Suction nose, if necessary, by compressing suction bulb before placing it in nostril. ▶ ***Rationale:*** This prevents aspiration of moisture. Gently release bulb after it is placed in nostril.
9. Wash infant's ears and neck, paying attention to folds; dry all areas thoroughly. Use mild soap and rinse.
10. Remove shirt or gown.
11. Remove diaper by picking up infant's ankles in your hand.
12. Pick up infant and place feet first into basin or tub. Immerse infant in tub of water only after umbilical cord has healed. Pick up infant by placing your hand and arm around infant, cradling the infant's head and neck in your elbow. Grasp the infant's thigh with your hand. ▶ ***Rationale:*** The umbilical cord is kept dry to prevent infection.
13. Wash and rinse the infant's body, especially the skin folds.
14. Wash infant's genitalia.
    a. For a female infant: Separate labia and with a cotton ball moistened with soap and water, cleanse downward once on each side. Use a new piece of cotton on each side.
    b. For an uncircumcised male infant: Do not force foreskin back. Gently cleanse the exposed surface with a cotton ball moistened with soap and water.
    c. For a circumcised male infant: Gently cleanse with plain water.
15. Wrap the infant in a towel and use a football hold when washing an infant's head. Soap your own hands and wash infant's hair and scalp, paying attention to the nape of the neck and using a circular motion. Rinse hair and scalp thoroughly. ▶ ***Rationale:*** Football hold is the most secure for active infants.
16. Place infant on a clean, dry towel with head facing the top corner and wrap infant.
17. Use the corner of the towel to dry infant's head with gentle, yet firm, circular movements.
18. Replace infant's diaper and redress in a new gown or shirt.
19. Provide comfort by holding the infant for a time after the bath procedure.
20. Perform hand hygiene.

Bathing in a Hydraulic Bathtub Chair

Equipment

Two towels and washcloth
Soap
Clean gown, robe, and slippers

Procedure

1. Check client's ID using two identifiers; perform hand hygiene.
2. Bring client to tub room in wheelchair.

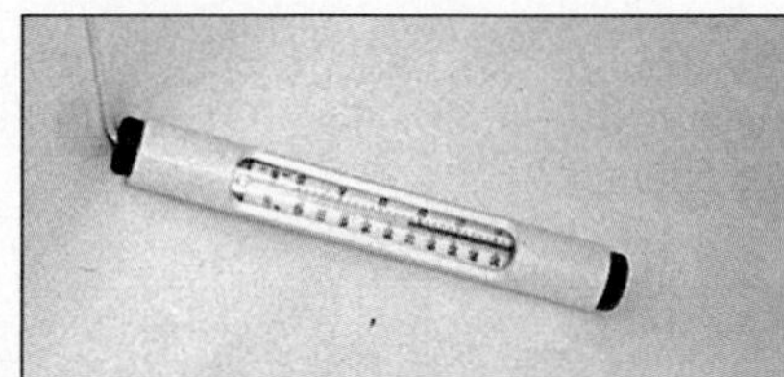

▲ Check that water temperature is not above 105° For safety.

3. Fill tub with water and check temperature. ▶ ***Rationale:*** Temperature must not be more than 105°F or client may burn skin.
4. Release chair to lowest point beside tub, and place towel on floor under chair.
5. Move client into bathtub chair, and attach seat belt.
6. Swing chair into position over tub.
7. Direct client to move legs down, then lower chair into low position in the tub filled with water.
8. When client is finished bathing, reverse chair out of tub.
9. Assist client to towel dry.
10. Put clean gown, robe, and slippers on client and transport to room.
11. Transfer client to wheelchair.
12. Assist client to settle comfortably in bed.
13. Perform hand hygiene.

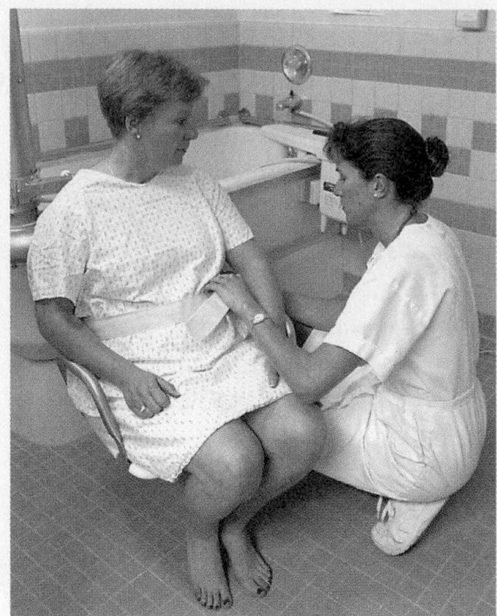
▲ Attach seat belt before swinging chair over the tub.

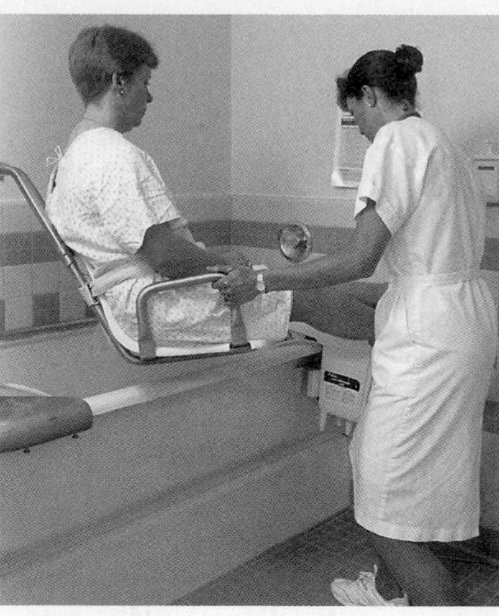
▲ Support client in chair as chair is swung over tub.

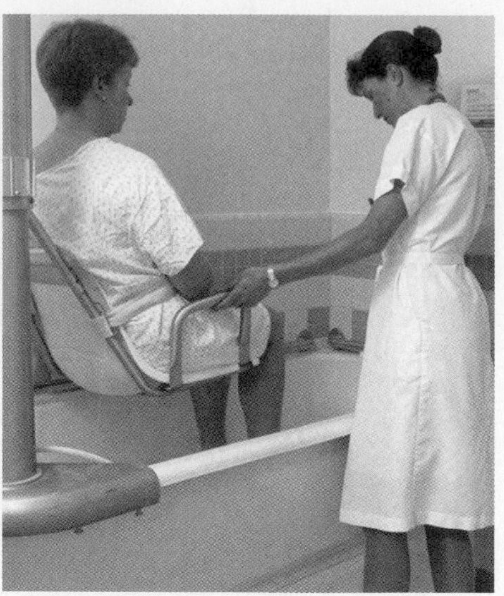
▲ Lower chair into tub filled with water.

DOCUMENTATION for Bath Care

- Client's overall ability to participate in own care
- Type of bath given (i.e., complete or partial) and by whom (e.g., client, nurse, family member)
- Condition of client's skin and any interventions provided for the skin (e.g., lotion, massage)
- Client's educational needs regarding hygienic care
- Information shared with client or family
- Infant bath demonstration to parents with return demonstration

CRITICAL THINKING Application

Expected Outcomes

- Client's skin is free of excessive perspiration, secretions, and offensive odors.
- Client feels comfortable and does not experience itching or irritation.
- Client's skin is moist and free of itching sensation.
- Client is able to take bath or shower without excessive fatigue or anxiety.
- Client is able to bathe self using disposable cleansing system.

Unexpected Outcomes	Alternative Actions
Client is unwilling to accept a complete bed bath.	• Respect client's wishes and take other opportunities for assessment. • Have client wash hands, face, and genitals. You should wash back and give back care. Re-explain the purpose of the bath to the client and request client participation.
Client is too shy to allow bath.	• Respect client's privacy and only wash areas client wishes you to do. • Give assistance so client can bathe himself or herself. • Allow spouse or parent to give bath if this is more acceptable to client.
Client complains of dry, itching skin after the bath.	• Assess for cause of itching. • Ask physician for an order for special lotion. • Do not use soap for the bath.

Chapter 8

UNIT 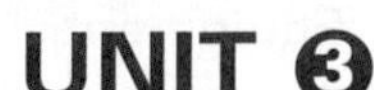

Skin Integrity

Nursing Process Data

ASSESSMENT Data Base

- Assess for signs of skin breakdown or the eruption of lesions.
- Assess color of skin.
- Assess color of mucous membranes.
- Check for alterations in skin turgor.
- Assess for complaints of itching, tingling, or numbness.
- Assess texture of skin.
- Assess general hygienic state.
- Observe skin for increased or decreased pigmentation and discoloration.
- Assess client's condition to determine appropriate support surface or specialty bed.

PLANNING Objectives

- To maintain intact skin
- To recognize a break in skin integrity
- To avoid introduction of pathogens through break in skin
- To prevent skin breakdown from pressure points or strain
- To prevent excessive dryness, flaking, itching, or burning
- To use support surface or specialty bed to prevent or treat altered skin integrity

IMPLEMENTATION Procedures

EVALUATION Expected Outcomes

- Client's skin is intact.
- Client's skin does not show evidence of dryness, flaking, itching, or burning.
- Client is comfortable with no complaints of pain or discomfort.

Pearson Nursing Student Resources

Find additional review materials at **nursing.pearsonhighered.com**

Prepare for success with NCLEX®-style practice questions and Skill Checklists

Monitoring Skin Condition

Equipment

Artificial light for observation if natural light is not available

Bath blanket

Gown

Clean gloves, if indicated

Procedure

1. Perform hand hygiene.
2. Check two client identifiers and explain monitoring process to client.
3. Provide privacy for client.
4. Remove linens and gown if necessary. Cover client with bath blanket.
5. Compare color of client's skin with normal range of color within the individual's race. Observe for pallor (white color), flushing (red color), jaundice (yellow color), ashen (gray color), or cyanosis (blue color).
6. Place the back of your fingers or hand on client's skin to check temperature. Consider the temperature of the room and of your hands. ▶ ***Rationale:*** The back of the hand is more sensitive to changes in temperature than the palm.
7. Correlate abnormalities in skin color with changes in skin temperature. ▶ ***Rationale:*** Skin temperature reflects blood circulation in the dermis layer.
8. Observe for areas of excessive dryness, moisture, wrinkling, flaking, and general texture of skin.
9. Gently pick up a small section of the skin with your thumb and finger. Observe for ease of movement and speed of return to original position to check for skin turgor. ▶ ***Rationale:*** Degree of hydration is reflected in the skin turgor or elasticity of the skin.
10. Press your finger firmly against client's skin for several seconds (especially ankle area). After removing your finger, observe for lasting impression or indentation. ▶ ***Rationale:*** This identifies the severity of pitting edema. It is based on a 4-point scale: +1 (slight) to +4 (very marked).
11. When checking skin temperature and texture, note the client's response to heat, cold, gentle touch, and pressure.
12. Observe the amount of oil, moisture, and dirt on the skin surface. ▶ ***Rationale:*** Degree of moisture or dryness may indicate disease states or hydration status.
13. Note presence of strong body odor or odor in the skin folds.
14. Observe for areas of broken skin (lesions) or ulcers. If present, wear gloves. Check if lesions are present over entire body or if they are localized to a specific area.
15. Check for skin discolorations (e.g., ecchymosis, petechiae, purpura, erythema, and altered pigmentation). ▶ ***Rationale:*** These signs may indicate generalized disease states, such as leukemia, vitamin deficiency, or hemophilia.
16. Ensure client is resettled comfortably.
17. Perform hand hygiene.
18. Document findings in chart.

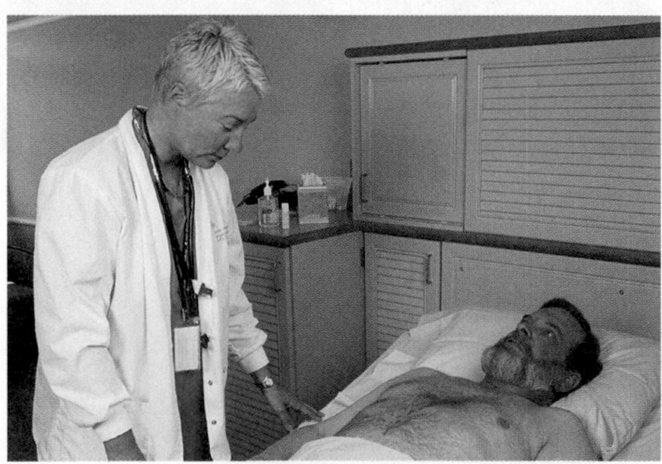

▲ Compare color of client's skin with normal range of color within the individual's race.

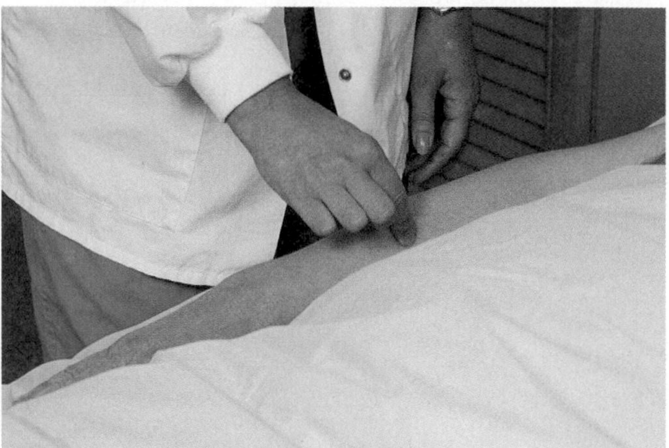

▲ Gently pick up a small section of skin with your thumb and finger to check for skin turgor.

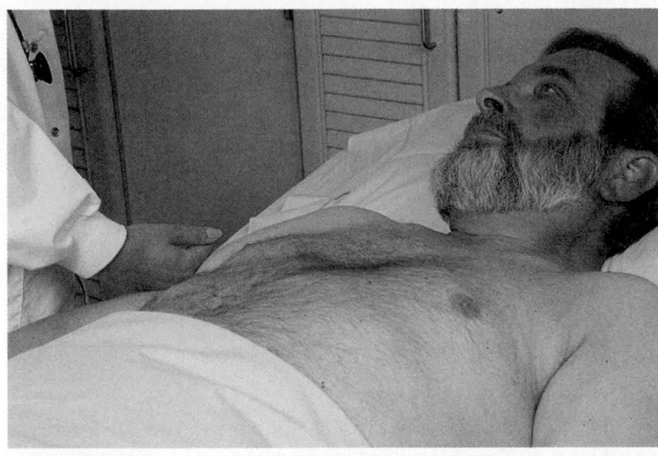

▲ Place back of your fingers or hand on client's skin to check temperature.

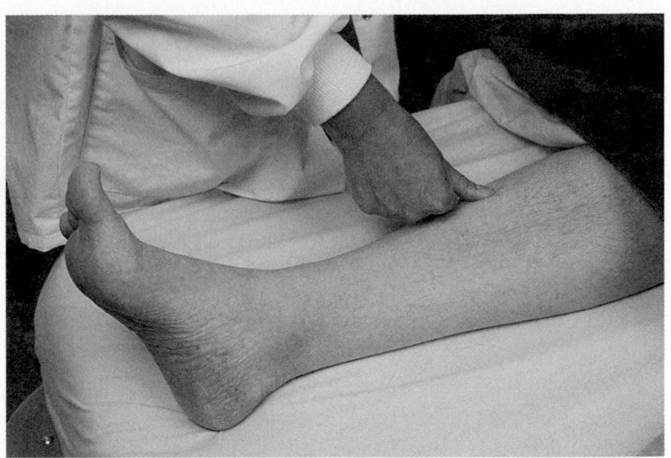

▲ Press your finger firmly against client's skin for several seconds to check for pitting edema.

TABLE 8-1 Potential Skin Problems

Skin Condition	Problem	Nursing Responsibility
Xeroderma, or dry skin	If skin is extremely dry, it could crack and become infected. May cause pruritus.	Maintain skin integrity. Bathe less frequently. Relieve discomfort. Use emollient or moisturizing lotion after bathing. Encourage nutritious diet. Increase fluid intake. Maintain cool, humid environment.
Skin rash or contact dermatitis. May be allergic or nonallergic reaction; may have exudate.	Erythema, flat or raised eruptions, and inflammation. Could cause pruritus, discomfort, and infection if scratched.	Avoid soap and heat, and rubbing area. Bathe area: may use antiseptic soap with orders. Apply ordered lotion or spray (steroids) to prevent itching. Use cool, wet dressing. If exudate present, check bed linens and client's gown, change if moist.
Abrasions	Break in skin integrity could result in infection. Healing may be prolonged due to age (poor circulation, etc.).	Wash abrasions with soap and water. Apply lotion as ordered.
Fungal skin infection	Fungal skin infection: common in diabetics, those on antibiotics or immunosuppressive therapy, those who are incontinent.	Apply topical antifungal medication as ordered. Dry skin folds well before applying antifungal medication. Apply medication sparingly to prevent skin from becoming too moist. Keep incontinent clients dry and provide good perineal care. Avoid using plastic pants or liners next to client's skin. Use nonocclusive dressings if needed.
Yeast skin infection	Seen with prolonged antibiotic use and in skin folds.	Cleanse and dry skin folds, apply medicated lotion or cream as ordered.

Preventing Skin Breakdown

Equipment

Skin lotion
Pressure-relieving mattress
Clean gloves if open lesions are present

Procedure

1. Perform hand hygiene.
2. Check two client identifiers.
3. Provide for client privacy.
4. Inspect skin daily; observe the client's most vulnerable body surfaces for ischemia, hyperemia, or broken areas.
5. Change the client's body position at least once every 2 hours to rotate weight-bearing areas. Use turning techniques. ▶ ***Rationale:*** To minimize skin injury caused by friction and shear forces. Observe all vulnerable areas at this time. Include right and left lateral, prone, supine, and swimming-type positioning if possible.

6. Massage client's skin and pressure-prone areas, if skin is not reddened, when client changes position. ▸ ***Rationale:*** Massage increases risk of breakdown in clients with reddened areas over bony prominences.
7. Lubricate dry, unbroken skin to prevent breakdown.

NOTE: Products used to prevent skin breakdown and treat impaired skin integrity are selected based on client's skin type, product application, cost, and desired outcome.

8. Apply lotion to bedridden client's sacrum, elbows, and heels several times during the day.
9. Cleanse skin with warm water and a mild pH-balanced cleansing agent, then apply moisturizers and a barrier cream as ordered.
10. Protect healthy skin from drainage secretions.
11. Use protective padding on heels and elbows if needed.
12. Keep linens clean, dry, and wrinkle-free.
13. Minimize the layers between the client and mattress. ▸ ***Rationale:*** Allows for proper functioning of pressure relief mattresses.
14. Encourage active exercise or range-of-motion exercise.
15. Encourage client to eat a well-balanced diet with protein-rich foods and adequate fluids.
16. Teach client and family how to prevent pressure areas and pressure ulcer formation.
17. Perform hand hygiene.
18. Document findings in chart.

Clinical Alert

Current guidelines from the U.S. Department of Health and Human Services advocate no skin massage on reddened skin or skin that has a potential for breakdown because massage causes friction and shearing.

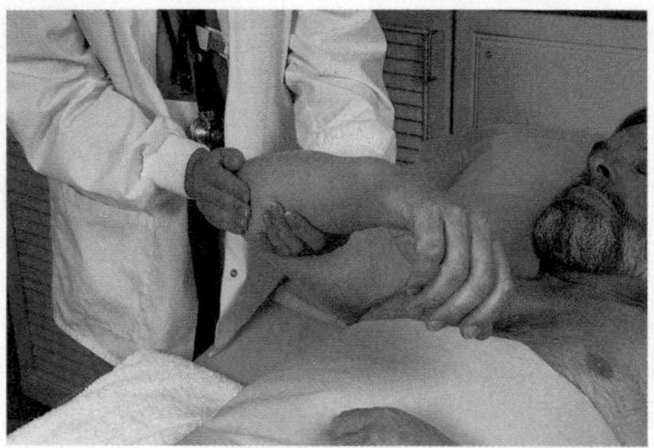

▲ Observe client's most vulnerable body surfaces for ischemia, hyperemia, or broken skin.

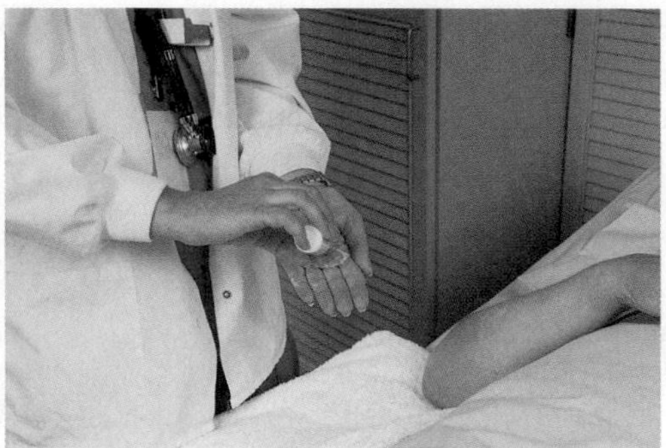

▲ Lubricate dry, unbroken skin to prevent breakdown.

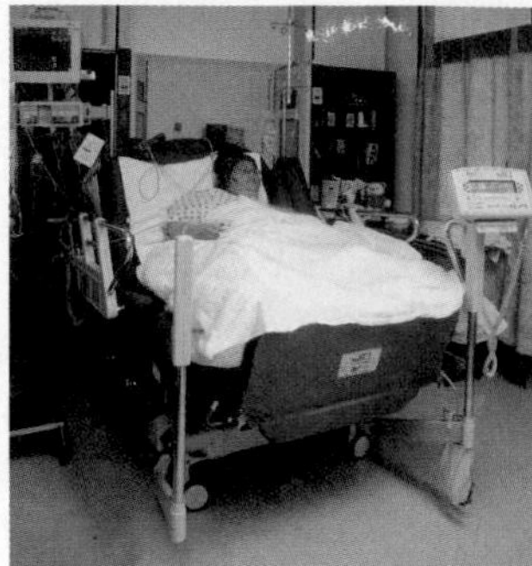

▲ High-risk, obese clients should be placed on a bariatric bed such as the BariMaxx II® or Magnum®.

Preventing Skin Tears

Equipment

Lift or turning sheet or booster lift device
Padding for bedrails, or other equipment
Pillows and blankets
Paper tape
Moisturizing agent for skin
Clean gloves as needed

Preparation

1. Identify clients at risk for developing skin tears. ▸ ***Rationale:*** To identify clients at risk and then determine appropriate preventative measures. Clients at risk include those on bedrest, those with purpura or ecchymosis, paper-thin skin such as geriatric clients, those on long-term steroid use, or those with poor vision resulting in accidental bumping into objects.
2. Identify the category of skin tear, if present. ▸ ***Rationale:*** To determine correct nursing action to be completed.
3. Perform hand hygiene before providing client care.

Procedure

1. Check two client identifiers.
2. Use lift sheet or the Booster lift device when moving clients at risk for developing skin tears. ▸ ***Rationale:*** This will assist in preventing tears resulting from friction or shearing.
3. Remove tape from dressings carefully; use only paper or nonadherent dressing for at-risk clients, if possible.

Clinical Alert

Ensure that all healthcare workers are aware of proper handling of elderly clients with fragile skin. Slight friction and shearing can create a skin tear when turning or lifting these clients.

4. Assist clients with ambulation if unsteady gait. Remove objects in pathway. ▸ ***Rationale:*** To prevent client from bumping into objects, causing bruises, cuts or skin tears, from falling.
5. Ensure clients use glasses, if necessary, when ambulating or transferring into chair. ▸ ***Rationale:*** To prevent falling or unsteady gait due to impaired vision leading to potential skin tears from falls.
6. Place padding on beds, wheelchairs, or equipment. ▸ ***Rationale:*** To prevent client from rubbing on hard surfaces and causing bruising.
7. Don gloves and apply moisturizing agent to dry skin to keep moist.
8. Remove gloves and place in appropriate receptacle.
9. Perform hand hygiene.
10. Document findings in chart.

Payne–Martin Classification System for Skin Tears

Category I: skin tears without tissue loss
- Linear type: epidermis and dermis pulled apart
- Flap type: epidermal flap completely covers dermis to within 1 mm of the wound margin

Category II: skin tears with partial tissue loss
- Scant tissue loss type: 25% or less of epidermal flap lost
- Moderate to large tissue loss type: more than 25% epidermal flap lost

Category III: skin tears with complete tissue loss, no epidermal flap

Source: Fleck, C. (2007). Preventing and treating skin tears. *Advances in Skin and Wound Care: The Journal for Preventing and Healing*, 20(6), 315–321. Payne, R. L., & Martin, M. L. (1993). Defining and classifying skin tears: need for a common language. *Ostomy Wound Management*, 39(5), 16–26.

Managing Skin Tears

Equipment

Saline
Nontoxic wound cleanser
Moist wound dressing (e.g., Hydrogel, foam, petrolatum ointment)
Nonadherent dressings
Tegaderm
Gauze
Clean gloves

Procedure

1. Perform hand hygiene.
2. Check two client identifiers.
3. Don clean gloves.
4. Remove old dressing, being careful to not cause additional skin damage. Moisten dressing with saline before removing if dressing sticks to skin.
5. Assess for signs of infection.
6. Cleanse skin tear with saline or nontoxic wound cleanser. Be careful not to put pressure on skin as you are cleaning. ▸ ***Rationale:*** To prevent additional pain and trauma to skin.
7. Place Tegaderm or clear adherent dressing over tear site.
8. Change dressings according to hospital policy.
9. Remove gloves and place in appropriate receptacle.
10. Perform hand hygiene.
11. Document findings in chart.

DOCUMENTATION for Skin Integrity

- Client's skin condition: odor, temperature, turgor, sensation, cleanliness, integrity
- Client's mobility
- Turning frequency and client positioning
- Type of care given (e.g., massage, bathing)
- Client's complaints about skin or pressure ulcer
- Time and method used to obtain wound specimen
- Type of lesion, rashes and bruises; state location, size, shape, color
- Alterations in sensation in skin lesion area
- Skin or body odor
- Presence of skin tear and assessment findings
- Treatment given for skin tear

Support Surfaces and Specialty Beds

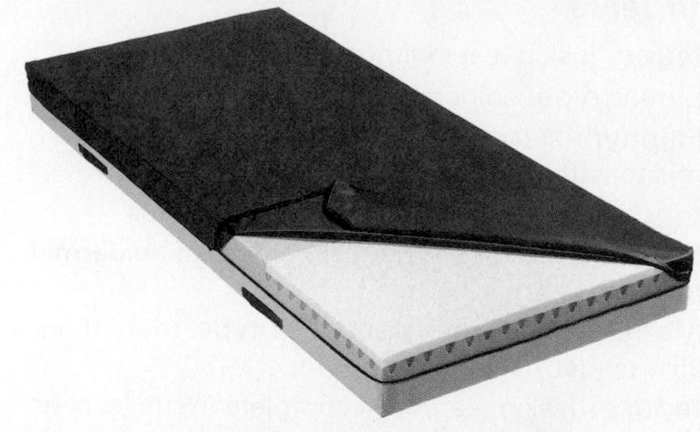

▲ First Step Plus, an overlay mattress from KCI.

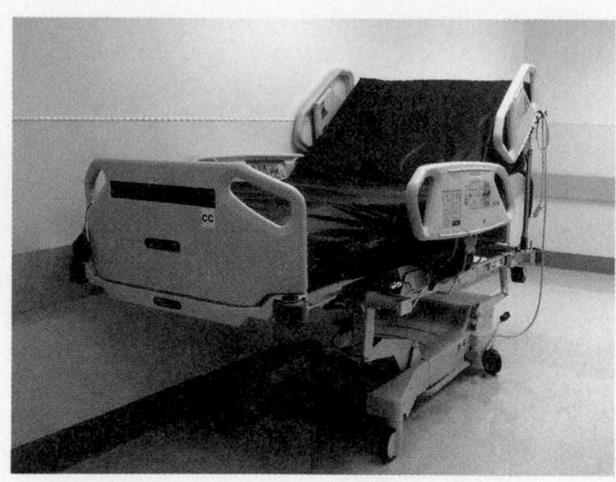

▲ Total Care $SpO_2RT^{®}$ Pulmonary Therapy System (Hill-Rom).

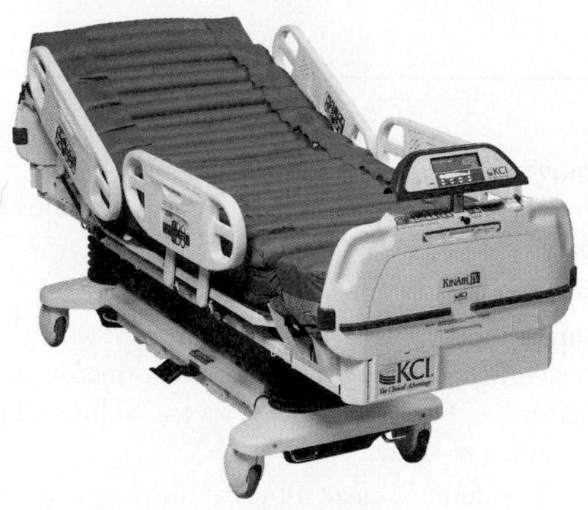

▲ KinAir IV®, a low air-pressure bed from KCI.

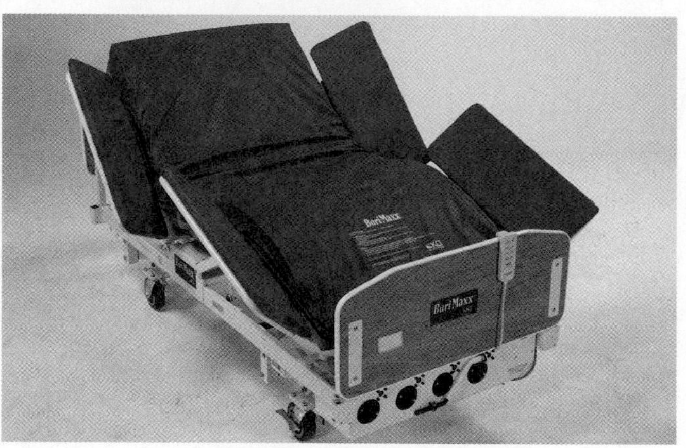

▲ BariMaxx II®, a bariatric pressure bed from KCI.

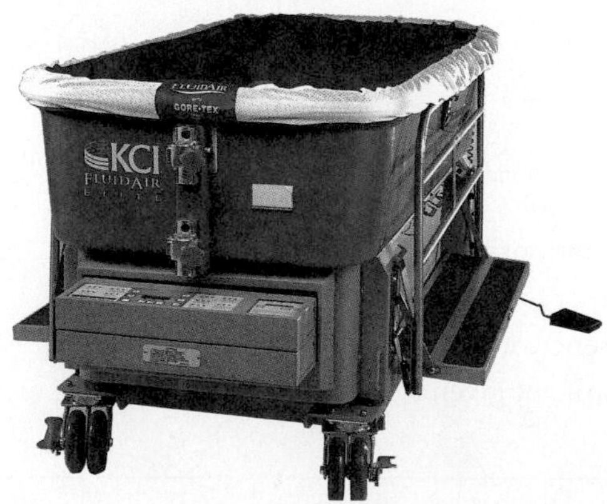

▲ FluidAir Elite®, air-fluidized therapy from KCI.

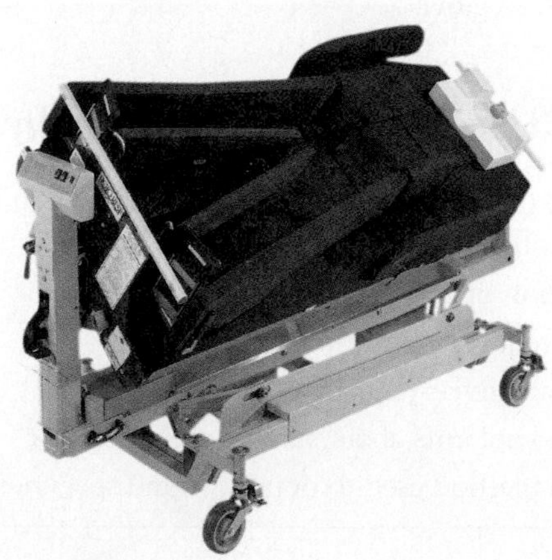

▲ RotoRest® Delta Kinetic®, a kinetic bed from KCI.

TABLE 8-2 Therapeutic Beds

Type of Bed	Client Recommendations
Air fluidized and low air-loss	High risk for skin breakdown
KinAir IV® (KCI)	Obese clients
Clinitron Rite Hite® (Hill-Rom)	Skin grafts, flaps
	All four stages of pressure ulcers
	Wound healing
Air-fluidized	Severe skin disorders
Clinitron II® (Hill-Rom)	Pressure ulcers
Fluid Air Elite® (KCI)	Burns
Low air-loss	Massive edema
KinAir Med Surg®(KCI)	Critical care
Flexicair Eclipse ® (Hill-Rom)	Pneumonia or other pulmonary problems with compromised skin integrity
Kinetic therapy	Obese—850–1,000 lbs.
Bariatric Client Care Systems	Difficult to move out of bed
MAGNUM II® (Hill Rom)	Assistance to place in a sitting position
BariAir®(KCI)	Difficult to move due to obesity
BariMaxx® II(KCI)	Difficult to move due to obesity
Critical care therapy	Pulmonary condition related to immobility (pneumonia), COPD
TriaDyne Proventa® (KCL)	Skin complications related to bed rest
SpO_2RT® (Hill Rom)	Spinal cord–injured, requiring skeletal traction
RotoRest Delta® (KCI) Kinetic	Spinal cord-injured, at risk for respiratory complications

CRITICAL THINKING Application

Expected Outcomes

- Client's skin is intact.
- Client's skin does not show evidence of dryness, flaking, itching, or burning.
- Client is comfortable with no complaints of pain or discomfort.

Unexpected Outcomes	Alternative Actions
Skin is erythematous but remains intact.	• Monitor fluid balance and nutritional status. • Obtain pressure-relieving mattress. • Turn client every 2 hours. • Ambulate if able.
Client cannot be positioned in a manner to avoid erythematous areas entirely.	• Turn at least every hour. • Do not turn on erythematous site. • Use protocol for stage 1 ulcer treatment on affected area. • Place support mattress on bed.
Skin integrity is interrupted, even with skin care.	• Use aseptic technique in treating area to prevent spread of bacteria and promote wound healing. • Use appropriate skin care products. • Place support mattress on bed.
Skin tear occurs.	• If skin is sensitive and breakdown occurs over large area, the use of a Clinitron unit or air-fluidized bed might be indicated (Table 8-2).

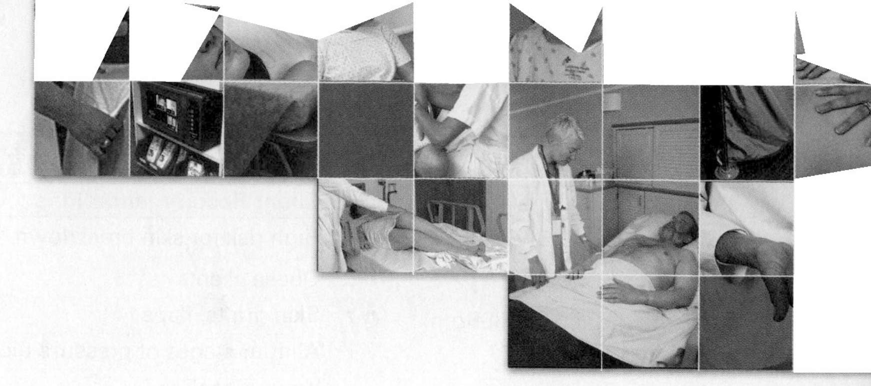

Chapter 8

UNIT 4

Evening Care

Nursing Process Data

ASSESSMENT Data Base

- Review client's usual routines before sleep.
  - Usual time of sleep and length of sleeping period
  - Personal hygiene routines
  - Temperature of room and number of blankets
  - Anticipated elimination needs
  - Religious or meditation needs
- Assess client's understanding and acceptance of safety precautions, such as use of side rails.
- Assess client's needs for comfort and security.
  - Dressings
  - Medication
  - Linen change or adjustment
  - Positioning
  - Television, radio, light
  - Communication needs
- Assess physical and emotional status during evening care.
- Assess condition of back, especially bony prominences.

PLANNING Objectives

- To encourage a period of comfortable, uninterrupted rest
- To evaluate the client's present health status
- To make observations about the client's physical and emotional status
- To provide time for the client and nurse to review the day's events
- To provide time for the client to communicate needs and questions regarding health care
- To provide the client with a clean, secure environment in which to sleep

IMPLEMENTATION Procedures

EVALUATION Expected Outcomes

- Client states he/she is comfortable and ready for sleep after evening care.
- Client states that back care has decreased muscle tension and improved comfort level.

Providing Evening Care

Equipment

Disposable cleansing cloth system or towels, washcloth, basin with water and soap
Clean linens if needed
Dental care items (i.e., toothbrush, dentifrice, denture cup)
Emesis basin, cup
Fresh pitcher of water if allowed
Skin care lotion if desired
Personal care items (e.g., deodorant, skin moisturizers)
Bedpan, urinal, toilet paper
Miscellaneous supplies as needed (e.g., dressing, special equipment)
Clean gloves, if indicated

Preparation

1. Perform hand hygiene.
2. Check two client identifiers.
3. Explain the needs and benefits of evening care; discuss how the client can be involved.
4. Collect and arrange equipment.
5. Adjust the bed to a comfortable working height, and assist the client into a comfortable position.
6. Ensure privacy.
7. Don gloves if indicated.

Procedure

1. Assess for pain. Medicate as necessary.
2. Offer bedpan or urinal if client is unable to use bathroom. Assist with handwashing.
3. If client needs or requests a bath, provide assistance as needed.
4. Assist with mouth and dental care as needed.
5. Remove equipment, extra linens, and pillows if possible. Remove sequential compression devices, ace wraps, and binders.
6. Change dressings, if necessary. Perform any required procedural techniques.
7. Wash face, hands, and back. Provide back massage.
8. Assist with combing or brushing hair if desired.
9. Replace sequential compression devices, stockings, and binders.
10. Replace soiled linen, or straighten and tuck remaining linen. Fluff pillow and turn cool side next to client.
11. Straighten top linens. Provide additional blankets if desired.
12. Remove any unnecessary equipment. Place call signal and water (if allowed) within client's reach.
13. Administer sleeping medication if ordered and client requests.
14. Assist client into a comfortable position.
15. Ensure that the client's environment is safe and comfortable.
16. Remove gloves, if used.
17. Raise upper side rails, place bed in LOW position, and turn lighting to low.

NOTE: Side rails are now considered restraints by the Centers for Medicare and Medicaid Services and the Food and Drug Administration. Check with your facility about agency policies on use of side rails.

18. Perform hand hygiene.
19. Document evening care provided.

Providing Back Care

Equipment

Disposable cleansing cloth system or
Basin of warm water, washcloth, towel, soap
Skin care lotion
Clean gloves if indicated

Procedure

1. Perform hand hygiene.
2. Check two client identifiers.
3. Explain the purpose of a back rub, and ask client if he or she would like one.
4. Provide privacy.
5. Assess for pain.
6. Warm lotion by holding bottle under water.
7. Raise bed to comfortable height for you, and assist the client into a comfortable prone or semiprone position. Keep farthest side rail in UP position. Placing pillow below breasts may increase comfort for female clients.
8. Don gloves if necessary.
9. Drape bed clothes for warmth, and untie the client's gown. Cleanse back with disposable cleansing cloth or washcloth with soap.
10. Place lotion on your hands and rub hands together to warm lotion.
11. Once you place your hands on a client's back to begin a back rub, your hands should remain in constant skin contact with the client until back rub is complete. ▸ ***Rationale:*** To prevent "tickling" sensation.
12. Repeatedly move your hands up on either side of the client's spine, across shoulders, and down the lateral aspects of the back using the effleurage stroke, applying firm and steady pressure.

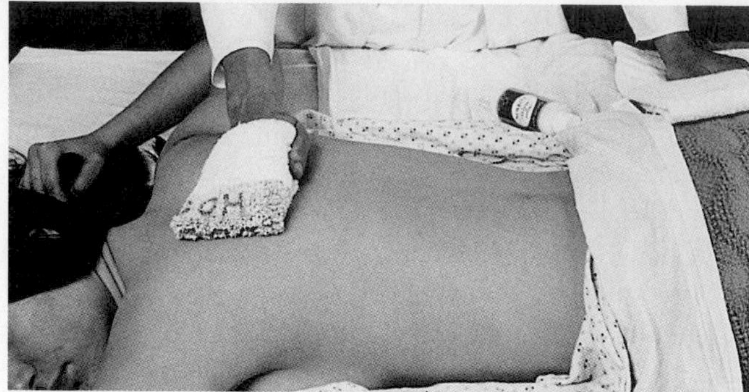

▲ Cleanse back using a disposable cleansing cloth before begining back rub.

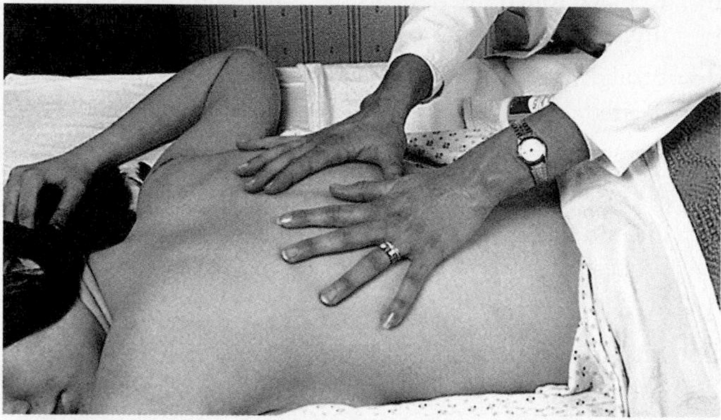

▲ Without lifting hands from skin surface, massage in continuous motion.

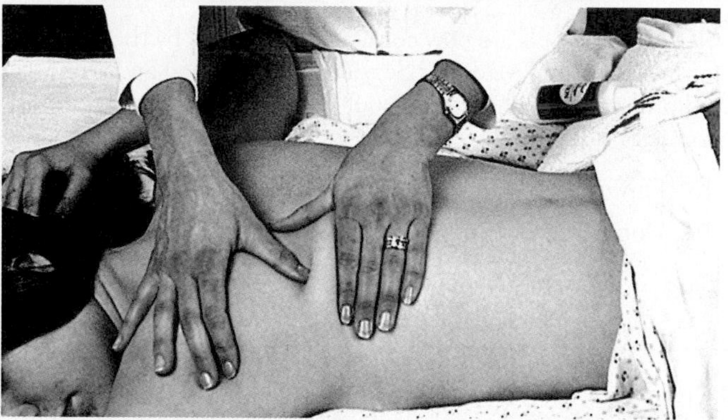

▲ The petrissage, or kneading stroke, is issued over the shoulders and along back.

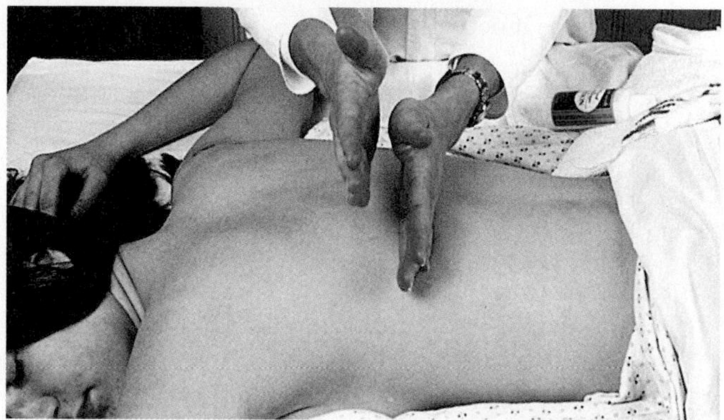

▲ The tapotement stroke stimulates the skin as the hands move up and down the back. The kidneys area should be avoided.

13. Move your hands down the center of the client's back to sacral area.
14. Massage with a figure-eight motion from the sacrum out over each buttock.
15. Finally, rub lightly up and down the back a few strokes before lifting hands from client's back.
16. Throughout back rub, assess skin for color, turgor, skin breakdown.
17. When percussion is desired, the back and buttocks can be lightly struck with the fleshy sides of your hands, called tapotement. Using an alternating rhythm, move up and down the back several times, avoiding the kidney area. In addition, kneading can be accomplished by picking up the skin between the thumb and fingers as you move up the back. This movement is called petrissage.
18. Close client's gown, pull up bedcovers, and assist client to change position if desired. Place top half of side rails in UP position. (See Chapter 7 regarding use of side rails.) Place bed in LOW position.
19. Remove gloves, if used.
20. Return lotion to the proper area.
21. Perform hand hygiene.
22. Document care provided.

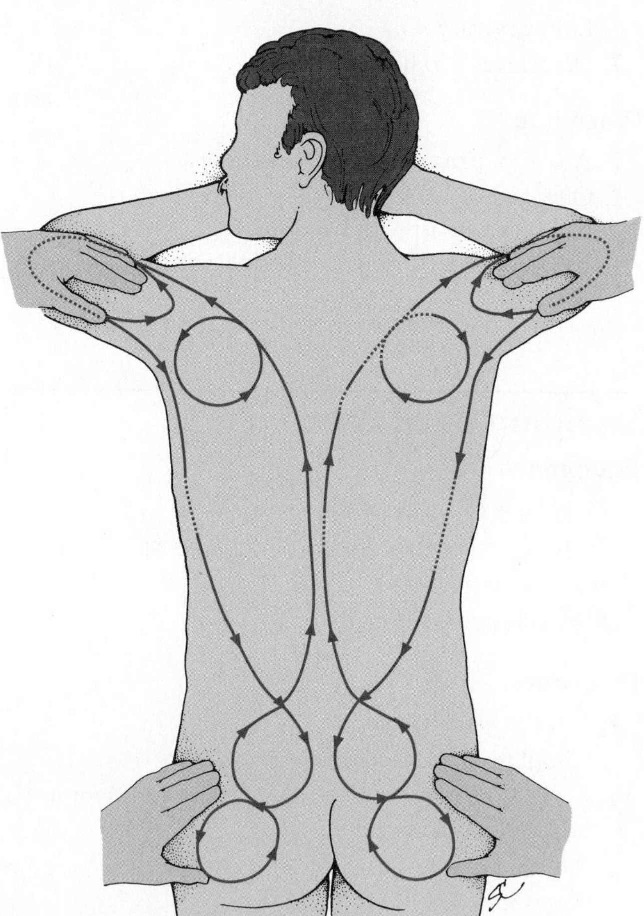

▲ Maintain constant skin contact during care by moving hands in figure-eight motion from shoulder to buttocks and back.

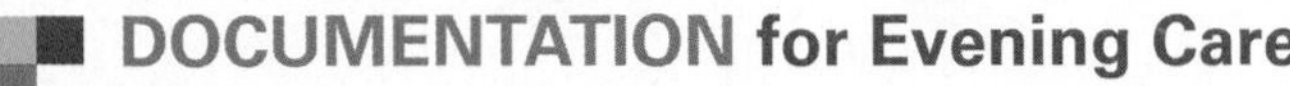

DOCUMENTATION for Evening Care

- Client's level of comfort or discomfort
- Type of care given (i.e., back care, evening care)
- Any significant complaints
- Nature of client teaching if done
- Medication required for discomfort or sleep
- Client's physical and emotional status after evening care completed

CRITICAL THINKING Application

Expected Outcomes

- Client states he/she is comfortable and ready for sleep after evening care.
- Client states that back care has decreased muscle tension, improved comfort level, and increased feelings of relaxation.

Unexpected Outcomes	Alternative Actions
Client refuses back care because he/she does not want to be touched.	• Tell client that if he or she cannot accept back care as part of the therapeutic regimen, you will stop.
Client refuses back care because he or she thinks you are too busy or disinterested.	• Make sure you offer the back care in an unhurried and meaningful manner. Do not allow the client to misinterpret your offer for care. • Return to client and offer back care later in the evening.
Client is unable to sleep even after evening care is given.	• Encourage verbalization of feelings, fears, etc. • Check to see if sleeping medication can be given. • Provide additional back care.

GERONTOLOGIC Considerations

Factors That Can Increase Risk of Skin Breakdown and Delay Wound Healing

- Inadequate nutritional intake.
- Compromised immune system.
- Compromised circulatory and respiratory systems.
- Poor hydration.
- Decreased mobility and activity.

Skin Changes With Age

- Delayed cellular migration and proliferation.
- Skin is less effective as barrier and slow to heal.
- There is increased vulnerability to trauma.
- There is less ability to retain water.
- Geriatric skin is dry (osteotosis) due to decreased endocrine secretion and loss of elastin. This can cause pruritus, which could lead to skin ulceration.
- Increased skin susceptibility to shearing stress leading to blister formation and skin tears.
- There is increased vascular fragility.

The Skin of the Elderly Should Be Assessed

- Decreased temperature, degree of moisture, dryness resulting from decreased dermal vascularity.
- Skin not intact, open lesions, tears, pressure ulcers as a result of increased skin fragility.
- Decreased turgor, dehydration as a result of decreased oil and sweat glands.
- Pigmentation alterations, potential cancer.
- Pruritus—dry skin most common cause because of decreased oil and sweat glands.
- Bruises, tears, scars from increased skin fragility.

Bathing Adaptations to Minimize Dryness

- Have client take complete bath only twice a week.
- Use superfatted or mild soap or lotions to aid in moisturizing.
- Use tepid, not hot, water.
- Apply emollient (lanolin) to skin after bathing.

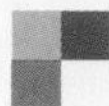

MANAGEMENT Guidelines

Each state legislates a Nurse Practice Act for RNs and LVN/LPNs. Healthcare facilities are responsible for establishing and implementing policies and procedures that conform to their state's regulations. Verify the regulations and role parameters for each healthcare worker in your facility.

Delegation

- All personnel interacting with clients must report any client risk behaviors or signs or symptoms that are unusual or new. Since activities of bathing or bedmaking have predictable outcomes and do not require nursing judgment, they are usually delegated to CNAs or UAPs. When these activities of daily living are delegated to a CNA or unlicensed personnel, the professional nurse remains responsible for total client care and should receive a complete report from the staff member assigned to the client.
- Even though unlicensed personnel are qualified to complete many tasks that involve activities of daily living, if the client is critically ill or unstable, the RN or LVN/LPN should be assigned to such a client. The professional nurse is responsible for assessing the client's total condition, thereby avoiding complications caused by missed assessment parameters.

Communication Matrix

- CNAs and UAPs must report any unusual or unanticipated signs or symptoms or risk behaviors to the RN or LVN/LPN responsible for the client's care. This report should include mental status as well as previously unreported physical signs and symptoms observed during the interaction period.
- Clients with alterations in skin integrity may be referred to the wound care specialist if the facility has one on staff.

CRITICAL THINKING Strategies

Scenario 1

An 89-year-old male was admitted earlier today, and you were assigned to admit him and provide nursing care for the remainder of the shift (4 hours). His admitting diagnosis is dehydration due to prolonged nausea and vomiting. He lives with his 88-year-old wife. They have some home health care twice a week, and a nursing assistant assists them with bathing and personal hygienic care. He is usually very active, walking, gardening, and attending church every week.

Your nursing history indicates he has not been out of bed for 3 days. He was unable to get to the bathroom and used a urinal, which proved to be difficult for him to manage and he spilled some urine each time he used it. He has not had a bath for 4 days and has also not brushed or cleaned his dentures.

1. Considering the client's issues related to bathing and bedmaking, what is your priority assessment after completing the initial assessment? Provide the rationale for your answer.
2. What information would you place on his plan of care to prevent skin breakdown? List the risk factors the client most likely exhibited.
3. Outline the nursing interventions that will be incorporated in his plan of care for the pressure ulcer.
4. What would you consider priority for his bathing needs? Provide the rationale for your answer.
5. Identify the major preventative measures to prevent skin breakdown or tears that will need to be discussed with the nursing assistant who will continue to care for him when he returns home.

Scenario 2

The client develops a skin tear on the greater trochanter the second day after admission. Refer to Scenario 1 for data.

1. In addition to risk factors identified in Scenario 1, describe additional risk factors that can cause skin tears.
2. Describe nursing interventions that can be used to treat the skin tear.
3. Describe nursing actions you will use when applying a dressing for the skin tear.
4. Explain how skin changes with age and how that leads to skin tears.
5. Are there any bathing changes that will need to be carried out during the time the treatment for the skin tear is being carried out?

NCLEX® Review Questions

Unless otherwise specified, choose only one (1) answer.

1. Which one of the following statements is correct relative to making an occupied bed?
   1. The bed is made by tucking the sheet under the mattress starting at the head of the bed, then pulling the sheet down to the foot of the bed.
   2. One side of the bed is completed first, then the client is moved to that side of the bed while the second side is completed.
   3. Making a bed with the client in the bed consists of changing the drawsheet and pillowcase.
   4. Unoccupied bed changes are completed only when the bed is soiled; then the bed is changed by rolling up

the soiled part of the sheet and having the client move to the opposite side of the bed.

2. You are preparing to complete a bed bath for an elderly client who is experiencing difficulty when moving in and out of bed. Place in order the sequence you will use for bathing the client.
   1. Legs
   2. Arms
   3. Abdomen
   4. Back
   5. Face

3. While assessing the skin of an elderly client, you notice the skin is very dry. The most appropriate intervention is to
   1. Use any fragrant soap when washing the skin.
   2. Bathe the client daily using only lukewarm water and mild soap.
   3. Apply generous amounts of oil-rich cream to the skin.
   4. Have the client only take showers to prevent build-up of soap on the skin.

4. A physician's order must be obtained before you perform which one of the following nursing interventions?
   1. Cooling bath using tepid water.
   2. Tub bath requiring the use of a hydraulic bathtub chair.
   3. Bath using Aveeno or cornstarch.
   4. Partial bath including washing the genitalia.

5. A client's diagnosis is heart failure. He has difficulty breathing when he experiences too much activity. The most appropriate intervention for bathing the client is
   1. The nurse gives him a bed bath.
   2. He is placed in a shower chair, wheeled to the shower, and the nurse showers him.
   3. He is assisted to the side of the bed and instructed to complete a partial bath.
   4. He assists with washing his face and hands if he is able to tolerate the activity.

6. The protocol for client care on the unit where you are gaining clinical practice includes providing morning care to all bedridden clients. This activity includes

   Select all that apply.
   1. Offering oral hygiene.
   2. Providing a wash cloth and assisting the client with washing his/her face and hands.
   3. Changing the drawsheet and pillowcase.
   4. Providing back care.

7. A major advantage of using a disposable bathing system for bathing a client that it
   1. Is less expensive than using regular linen.
   2. Is warmed to provide a soothing effect for the skin.
   3. Maintains a pH of 4.7 to 4.9 and is less drying.
   4. Prevents the spread of infection among clients.

8. The first step in bathing an infant is to
   1. Wash the infant's hair and scalp.
   2. Place the baby into the bathtub and wash the face, neck, and ears.
   3. Cleanse the eyes using a moistened cotton ball.
   4. Lower the baby into the bathtub and wash the abdomen, arms, and legs before washing the genitalia.

9. As part of your morning assessment, you are going to check the client's skin condition for signs of hydration. The most appropriate method to check for hydration is to:
   1. Place the back of your fingers or hand on the client's skin to check for resilience.
   2. Gently pick up a small section of the skin with your thumb and forefinger and observe for speed of return to original position.
   3. Firmly press your finger against the client's skin for several seconds and observe for blanching of skin.
   4. Observe for color change in skin of hands.

10. You are working the afternoon shift and the day nurse asks you to carefully assess an elderly client because she thinks she may have the beginning of a skin tear. You complete the assessment as soon as you are out of report. Your findings are a Category I flap type skin tear on the right arm. The most appropriate nursing action is to
    1. Cleanse the tear with a Betadine swab, and press the tear back onto the skin.
    2. Place Tegaderm or adherent dressing over tear.
    3. Place dry 4" × 4" dressing over tear and tape securely.
    4. Apply a moist dressing over the tear and immobilize the arm to prevent excess movement.

9

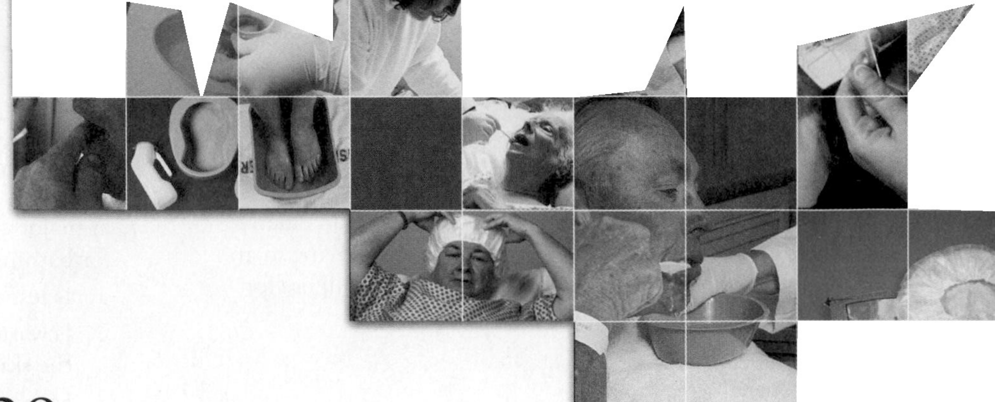

Personal Hygiene

LEARNING OBJECTIVES

1. Discuss oral hygiene needs of clients.
2. Outline the procedure for flossing teeth.
3. Compare and contrast oral hygiene for clients with natural teeth and dentures.
4. Demonstrate safety awareness when providing oral care for unconscious clients.
5. Identify the appropriate method of hair care according to client's condition.
6. Outline the steps for shaving a male client.
7. Describe procedure for removing lice and nits from hair and other body areas.
8. State the rationale for preventing prolonged scalp contact with solutions used to treat pediculosis.
9. Demonstrate proper draping technique for female clients.
10. Demonstrate the skill of placing a bedpan for a bedridden client.
11. Describe the steps in providing perineal care for male and female clients.
12. Describe nursing actions necessary to care for clients with contact lenses.
13. State two suggested solutions when hearing is not improved after cleaning a hearing aid.
14. State at least two nursing diagnoses pertinent to clients requiring assistance with personal hygiene.

CHAPTER OUTLINE

TERMINOLOGY

Abrasion the scraping away of a portion of skin or of a mucous membrane as a result of injury.
Adaptation an alteration or adjustment by which an individual can improve his or her relationship to the environment.
Antibacterial any substance that fights against or suppresses the growth of bacteria.
Anticoagulant any substance that suppresses or counteracts coagulation of blood.
Aspiration to withdraw fluid that has collected in an area to obtain a specimen.
Canthus the angle at either end of the slit between the eyelids.
Capillary minute blood vessel joining arterioles and venules; carries blood, forming the capillary system.
Congenital present at birth, as a congenital anomaly or defect.
Cornea the clear, transparent anterior portion of the fibrous coat of the eye.
Debilitated to become feeble; tired; loss of strength.
Decalcification the act of removing calcium, the basic component of bones and teeth.
Decubitus old term for pressure ulcer.
Dental plaque a thin film on the teeth made up of mucin and colloidal material found in saliva.
Edema a local or generalized condition in which there is excess fluid in the tissues.
Emesis vomiting.
Epidermis the outer layer of skin.
Eversion a turning outwards.
Excoriation an injury to a surface of the body cavity caused by trauma.
Expectoration expulsion of mucus or phlegm from the throat or lungs.
Fissure a groove, slit, or natural division; ulcer or crack-like sore.
Floss a waxed or unwaxed tape or thread used to clean between teeth.
Fungus a vegetable cellular organism that subsists on organic matter.
Genitals organs of generation; reproductive organs.
Hemorrhage abnormal internal or external discharge of blood.
Holistic the philosophy that an individual must be looked at as a whole rather than a sum of the parts.
Hygiene the study and observance of health rules.
Hypoallergenic having a lowered potential for producing an allergic reaction.
Impetigo inflammatory skin disease marked by isolated pustules that rupture and become crusted.
Incontinent inability to retain urine or feces through loss of sphincter control.
Intervention the act of coming between, so as to hinder or modify.
Irritation a source of annoyance; incipient inflammation, soreness or roughness, or irritability of a body part.
Labia the lips of the vulva.
Lesion an injury or wound; a single infected patch in a skin disease.
Metabolism the sum of all physical and chemical changes that take place within an organism; all energy and material transformations that occur within living cells.
Microorganism a minute living body such as a bacterium or protozoon not perceptible to the naked eye.
Mucosa mucous membrane lining passages and cavities communicating with the air.
Nasolacrimal pertaining to the nose and lacrimal apparatus.
Nits lice eggs.
Ophthalmic solution solution designed especially for the eyes.
Oral concerning the mouth.
Palate the roof of the mouth.
Parotid gland either of the largest of the paired salivary glands, located below and in front of each ear.
Pediculosis infestation with lice.
Periodontal disease chronic bacterial infection of the tissues surrounding the teeth.
Perineum the external region between the vulva and anus in a female or between the scrotum and anus in a male.
Plaque a patch on the skin or on a mucous surface; a blood platelet.
Pressure point area for exerting pressure to control bleeding; an area of skin that can become irritated with pressure, especially over bony prominences.
Sclera the tough, white, fibrous outer envelope of tissue covering all of the eyeball except the cornea.
Semi-Fowler's position semisitting position.
Systemic pertaining to the whole body rather than to one of its parts.
Thrush fungus infection of mouth or throat, especially in infants and young children and in clients with AIDS.
Ulcer an open sore or lesion of the skin or mucous membrane of the body.
Urethra canal for the discharge of urine extending from the bladder to the outside.
Vascular pertinent to or composed of blood vessels.

HYGIENIC CARE

Unfamiliar or life-threatening conditions affect the client's adaptation to the healthcare system. A holistic approach on the part of the nurse provides individualized care and assists the client to adapt. Basic hygiene care is an integral part of the total treatment program. Together with its role in enhancing the client's adaptation to the hospital environment and sense of self-worth, it provides an opportunity for the nurse to do a total assessment and evaluation. This time also allows for establishing a working relationship with the client and offers an opportunity to reduce stress by discussing fears and concerns about being in the hospital or the care being received.

The manner in which hygienic care is provided by nursing staff influences the client's perception of the staff. If care is administered in a professional and efficient manner, the client's confidence in the healthcare system is increased. The need to provide personal hygiene depends on each client's physical state and ability to care effectively for himself or herself. Your first responsibility is to assess the client's level of ability. After gathering this data, you should assist the client as necessary, providing any assistance or teaching he or she may require.

Oral Hygiene

The condition of the oral cavity has a direct influence on an individual's overall state of health. Dental diseases require a "host" (the tooth and gum), an "agent" (plaque), and an "environment" (e.g., the presence of saliva and food). When plaque comes in contact with bacterial enzymes, carbohydrates, and acids, cavitation begins as the enamel of the tooth is decalcified. As long as food and plaque remain in the oral cavity, the possibility of dental decay increases. In the hospital the incidence of caries (cavities) can be decreased by using a dentifrice containing fluoride, proper brushing and flossing, and adequate nutrition. Clients at risk for poor oral hygiene include those who are NPO, mouth breathers, and those with oral surgery.

Oral hygiene is a challenge for clients in long-term care settings. It is one of the most important interventions that nurses need to provide for these clients. Evidence links poor oral hygiene to serious systemic illnesses, including diabetes, stroke, hypertension, myocardial infarction, and aspiration pneumonia.

Hair Care

The appearance and condition of a client's hair may reflect his or her general physical and emotional status, individuality and feelings of worth, and the ability to care for him or herself. When complex medical care is required during illness or trauma, hair care is often neglected.

Hair care is an important aspect of regular hygiene. To prevent damage to the hair, scalp, and surrounding skin, and to promote the client's sense of well-being, you should assess the condition of a client's hair. Based on the assessment, provide hair and scalp care, shampooing, and shaving, and intervene to correct special problems.

Pediculosis

Pediculosis is one of the major health problems in school-age children and easily spreads to family members and friends. The use of terminology varies related to the life cycle of the louse. According to biologists, the life cycle of the head louse includes:

Adult Louse: wingless, flat insect about the size of a sesame seed, parasitic on warm blood.

Eggs: head louse eggs are also called nits: cemented firmly to hair shaft and take 6 to 9 days to hatch; nit shells remain on hair shaft.

Nymphs: immature louse released when egg hatches; looks like an adult head louse, but the size of a pinhead; takes 7 to 8 days to become an adult.

Perineal and Genital Care

The perineum consists of the area between the thighs and from the anterior pelvis to the anus. This area contains organs and structures related to sexual functioning, reproduction, and elimination.

Hygienic care involves cleaning the perineum and genitalia to prevent bacterial growth, which can rapidly increase in this warm, dark, moist environment. Perineal care is often provided as a routine part of bathing but may be required more frequently to prevent skin irritation, infection, discomfort, or odor.

All clients are susceptible to perineal irritation or infection. Clients who are especially vulnerable are those who are immobilized, incontinent, debilitated, postsurgical, or comatose; those who have indwelling catheters; those who have metabolic and fluid balance disorders; or those who require systemic medications.

Eye Care

The usual eye care provided for hospitalized clients is for the comatose client and the client with contact lenses. Several types of contact lenses are used by clients. The older, hard lenses were the first on the market and were made of solid plastic. They were easy to keep clean because they did not absorb proteins from the eye. They do inhibit oxygenation of the cornea; therefore, they must not be worn for long periods of time.

Soft lenses, the most popular of the lenses, allow more oxygenation of the cornea, but require care because they are less durable and carry a risk of contamination from collection of bacteria, dirt, and chemicals. Extended-wear lenses, another type of soft contact lenses, are worn for a number of days (usually up to 7) without being removed. The Food and Drug Administration (FDA) has approved the use of continuous 30-day lenses. It is recommended that the lenses be removed every 30 days, cleaned, disinfected, and replaced or discarded. Lenses should not be replaced for 24 hours to allow the eye to rest. There are reported side effects with these lenses, including conjunctivitis, dry eyes, and mild burning or stinging. Some clients use disposable extended-wear lenses. These are considered one-time-only contacts and are discarded, not cleaned, after they are removed.

Individuals who wear contact lenses must be aware of environmental contaminants such as dust, smoke, and sprays because they can irritate the eyes. Certain drugs cause a decrease in the eye fluid on which the contact lens floats and can lead to irritation of the eye. Common drugs that can lead to this problem include antihistamines, birth control pills, and alcohol. Clients who use eye cosmetics must apply the makeup before they insert the contact lenses so makeup will not adhere on the lenses.

CULTURAL AWARENESS

- Cultures define cleanliness in different ways. Western cultures, because of the abundance of detergents and washing machines, value clean clothes. Some underdeveloped countries have limited access to fresh water and therefore may not wash clothes as frequently.
- Anglo-Americans are fastidious about body cleanliness and the absence of body odor. The use of perfumes, deodorants, and aftershave lotions is a major part of their hygienic care. In some cultures, natural body odor is thought to have sex appeal.
- Some cultures incorporate the participation of family members to provide personal care, particularly assistance with using a bedpan or bedside commode, to maintain modesty. Puerto Ricans, African-Americans, and clients of Arab descent should be questioned regarding their preferences for assistance with personal care.

NURSING DIAGNOSES

The following nursing diagnoses may be appropriate to include in a client care plan when a client is admitted and requires basic hygiene care.

NURSING DIAGNOSIS	RELATED FACTORS
Deficient Knowledge	Misinformation or lack of information, impaired cognitive function, lack of motivation
Noncompliance	Inability to perform tasks, disability, impaired memory
Impaired Oral Mucous Membrane	Inadequate oral hygiene, chemotherapy, malnutrition, dehydration, infection, mechanical trauma
Bathing Self-Care Deficit	Impaired motor or cognitive function, pain, disease condition, surgery
Situational Low Self-Esteem	Impaired motor or cognitive function, chronic illness, chronic pain

CLEANSE HANDS The single most important nursing action to decrease the incidence of hospital-based infections is hand hygiene. *Remember to wash your hands or use antibacterial gel before and after each and every client contact.*

IDENTIFY CLIENT Before every procedure, check two forms of client identification, not including room number. *These actions prevent errors and conform to The Joint Commission standards.*

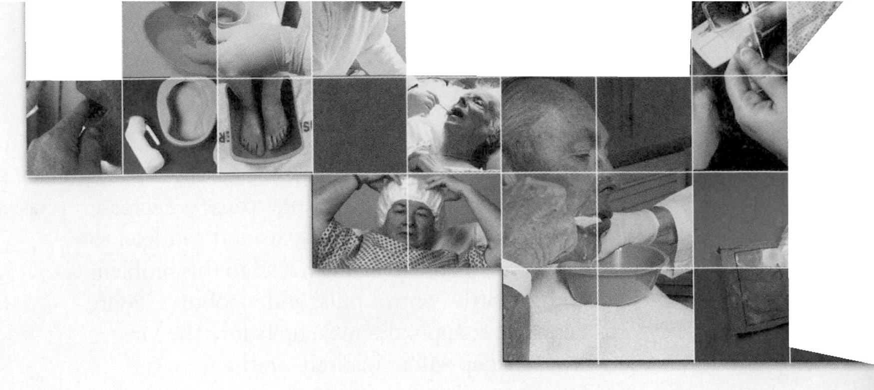

Chapter 9

UNIT 1

Oral Hygiene

Nursing Process Data

ASSESSMENT Data Base

- Assess whether client wears dentures.
- Evaluate client's knowledge of oral hygiene techniques.
- Assess condition of client's oral cavity, teeth, gums, and mouth.
- Assess for color, lesions, tenderness, inflammation, intactness of teeth, and degree of moisture or dryness of the oral cavity.
- Observe external and internal lips.
- Assess palate (roof and floor of mouth), and inspect under tongue.
- Assess entire oral mucosa, noting inside of the cheek.
- Observe tongue. Note tip, sides, back position, and underside.
- Evaluate condition of gums and teeth.
- Assess condition of throat as client says "Ah."
- If dentures or orthodontic appliances are used, observe relationship of the appliances to client's oral cavity (i.e., fit, irritation, condition of dentures).

PLANNING Objectives

- To remove plaque and bacteria-producing agents from oral cavity
- To allow nurse to assess client's oral health status, knowledge, and routines of oral care
- To decrease possibility of irritation or infection of oral cavity
- To remove unpleasant tastes and odors from oral cavity
- To provide comfort for client
- To provide client teaching when appropriate
- To assess hydration status

IMPLEMENTATION Procedures

EVALUATION Expected Outcomes

- The oral health status of client has been assessed and documented by nurse.
- Oral hygiene care is provided without complications.
- Plaque and bacteria-producing agents are removed.

Pearson Nursing Student Resources

Find additional review materials at **nursing.pearsonhighered.com**

Prepare for success with NCLEX®-style practice questions and Skill Checklists

Providing Oral Hygiene

Equipment

Toothbrush: small enough to reach back teeth; soft and rounded with nonfrayed rows of nylon bristles

Dentifrice: client's choice, preferably one containing fluoride; special paste for dentures

Cup of water

Emesis basin or sink

Dental floss: regular or fine, waxed or unwaxed, depending on client's needs

Tissues or towel

Mouthwash if desired

Clean gloves

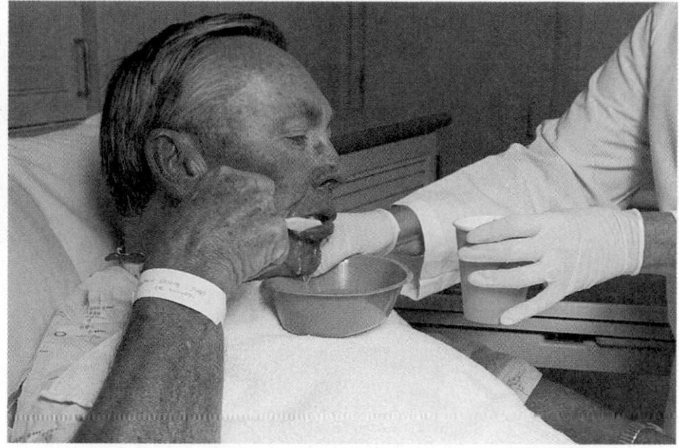

▲ Providing oral hygiene is an essential component of client care.

Preparation

1. Perform hand hygiene.
2. Collect necessary equipment.
3. Check two forms of client ID and introduce yourself.
4. Assist client to sink or provide privacy if care is to be given in bed.
5. Help client into a comfortable semi-Fowler's position or a sitting position. Assist client with the arrangement of equipment if necessary.
6. Don clean gloves.
7. Inspect surface of mouth for any abnormalities.
   a. Inspect surface of mouth, especially buccal mucosa (it should be pink, smooth, and moist), for any abnormalities. ▸ ***Rationale:*** Alterations from normal may indicate presence of disease states such as measles, mumps, or Addison's disease.
   b. Examine condition of teeth and gums. Be alert to changes in gums. ▸ ***Rationale:*** Gingival hypertrophy, crevices between teeth and gums, pockets of debris, and bleeding with slight pressure are indicative of gingivitis.
   c. Ask client about usual oral care routines.
8. Elicit any concerns, comments, or questions client may have about his or her oral health status.
9. Determine oral hygiene needs based on findings.
10. Assess client's need for teaching. Consider educational level, physical, emotional and mental state, previous experiences, and cultural differences.
11. Assess client's physical condition. Consider diagnoses, lab reports, treatments, fluid status, drugs, diet, and level of comfort or pain.
12. Assess client's ability to care for himself or herself.

Procedure

1. Perform hand hygiene and don clean gloves.
2. Request that client open mouth wide and hold emesis basin under chin.
3. Instruct client to complete following steps or provide the care yourself. Direct the bristles of the toothbrush toward the gum line for all areas to be brushed. ▸ ***Rationale:*** Action removes food particles from gum line and stimulates the gums.

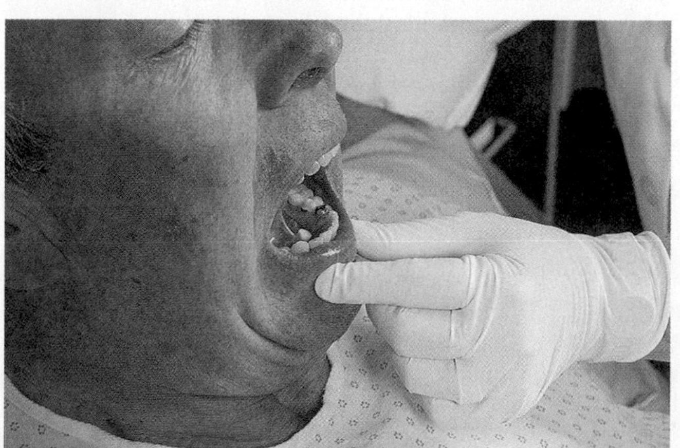

▲ Inspect surface of mouth abnormalities.

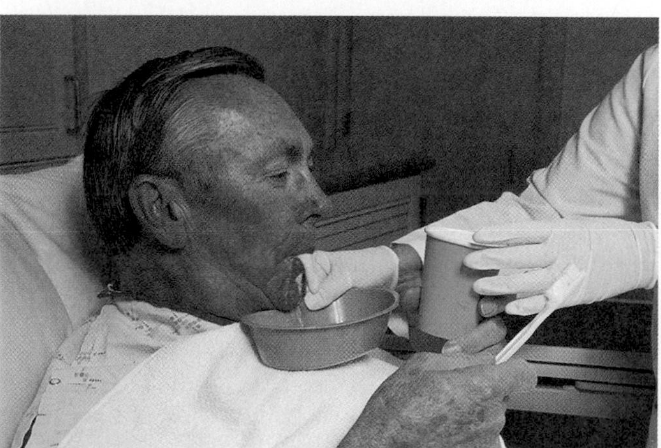

▲ Assist client to rinse mouth with water.

The American Academy of Periodontology estimates that at least half of noninstitutional individuals age 55 and older have periodontitis and that almost 25% ages 65 and older have lost all of their teeth. Periodontal disease affects glycemic controls in diabetic clients. There is also a significantly higher incidence of cardiovascular complications as a result of periodontal disease.

4. Keep the brush positioned over only two or three teeth at a time. Use small rotating movements to cover the outside surfaces of all teeth.
5. Clean the inner surfaces of all back teeth, using the brushing method described above.
6. Use a firm back-and-forth motion to clean the flat chewing surfaces.
7. Use the bristles on the end of the toothbrush and rotate the brush back and forth across the teeth to clean the inner surfaces of the front teeth.
8. Lightly brush all areas of the tongue—this improves the breath. Be careful not to stimulate gag reflex.
9. Rinse the client's mouth thoroughly with water.
10. Inspect oral cavity, and repeat brushing if necessary.
11. Floss thoroughly, using approximately 12 inches of floss loosely wrapped around one finger of each of your hands. Flossing removes plaque from between teeth.
12. Instruct or assist client to complete the following steps.
    a. Wrap one length of floss loosely around index fingers of both hands.
    b. Hold floss taut between two hands, and gently pull back and forth between each tooth.
    c. Move floss up and down sides of teeth to clean plaque. Go as near gum line as possible without injury to gum. Pull floss back and forth gently, working back toward the biting surface of each tooth. Repeat other edge of each tooth, using a new section of floss.
    ▶ ***Rationale:*** Overly vigorous flossing can damage gums.
    d. Floss each tooth several times until all particles of food are removed.
13. Assist client to rinse mouth and expectorate into emesis basin.

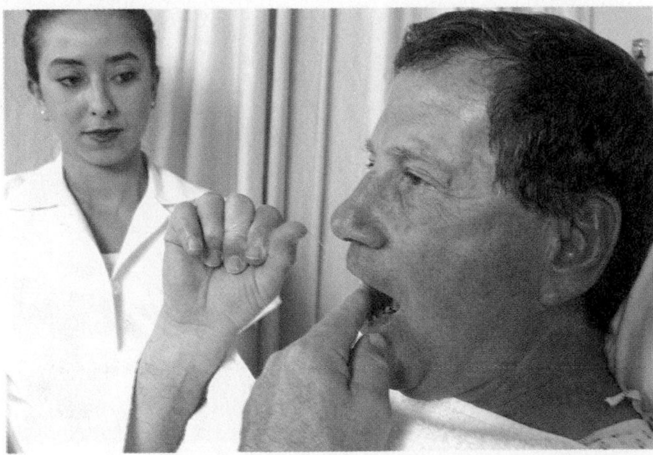

▲ Instruct client to floss to prevent build-up of plaque and food particles between the teeth.

EVIDENCE-BASED PRACTICE

In a longitudinal study of more than 600 individuals with type 2 diabetes, those with severe periodontal disease had 3.2 times the risk of death from ischemic heart disease and diabetic nephropathy than those with little or no periodontal disease.

Source: Saremi, A., Nelson, R. G., Tulloch-Reid, M., Hanson, R. L., Sievers, M. L., Taylor, G. W., ... Knowler, W. C. (2005). Periodontal disease and mortality in type 2 diabetes. *Diabetic Care*, *28*(1), 27–32.

Client Teaching

Begin teaching client about oral care during your initial assessment. Focus teaching on oral health needs and care. You may want to incorporate the following techniques:

- **A demonstration and return demonstration to illustrate correct dental care techniques.**
- **Disclosure tablets or solution that temporarily stains dental plaque pink. This technique helps the client to see where plaque appears on the teeth. After applying tablets or solution, ask the client to brush and floss until plaque is removed.**

14. Wipe off client's mouth and chin.
15. Wash client's toothbrush, rinse, and put the toothbrush and paste away and return additional equipment to the appropriate area.
16. Remove gloves and place in appropriate receptacle.
17. Perform hand hygiene.
18. Check to see that client is comfortable.

Sonic Toothbrush

Many dentists and dental hygienists recommend the use of a sonic toothbrush, especially for clients with plaque formation, stains, and periodontal pockets. The usual recommended time for brushing is 2 minutes twice a day. The toothbrush is charged by plugging the charger into the electrical outlet; therefore, electrical safety procedures must be followed. Do not store or place the charger where it can come in contact with water. Client instructions for using the toothbrush are printed on the owner's manual and must be clearly understood before attempting to use the toothbrush.

NOTE: If the client brings the toothbrush to the hospital, it is not necessary to charge it if hospitalization is less than 2 weeks. If hospitalization is beyond 2 weeks or the toothbrush needs charging, instruct the client's relatives to take the brush home and charge it. It is required by most hospitals that any electrical appliance brought into the hospital must be checked for safety by the hospital engineering department.

Providing Denture Care

Equipment

Denture toothbrush
Denture cup, labeled with client's name
Emesis basin
Cleanser or effervescent tablets for dentures
Clean gloves
Mouthwash, if desired
Adhesive dental liner, optional

Procedure

1. Encourage client to use dentures. ▸ ***Rationale:*** Dentures improve speech, make eating easier, and improve the shape of the mouth, appearance, and self-image.
2. Perform hand hygiene and don gloves.
3. Help client remove dentures. If client is unable to do this, carefully place your finger on the edge of the upper denture. ▸ ***Rationale:*** This action breaks the seal at the roof of the mouth and allows the denture to easily slide out. Lower denture generally lifts out easily.
4. If client is unable to clean own dentures, place them in an unbreakable container. Either wash dentures over a basin or carry them to the sink. Place a towel or washcloth on the bottom of the sink. ▸ ***Rationale:*** To cushion the surface in case you accidentally drop a denture.
5. Hold one denture in your hand. With your other hand, use a toothbrush or special denture brush and a cleaning agent, such as a commercially prepared paste or solution, to brush the denture. Use the same brushing motion as with natural teeth.
6. Rinse denture thoroughly in cold water. ▸ ***Rationale:*** Hot water can damage dentures.
7. If dentures are to remain out of the mouth for a period of time, as at night, store them in a clearly labeled, unbreakable container of cold water.
8. If dentures are to be worn immediately, help client to rinse oral cavity with warm water or mouthwash.
9. You may also gently brush client's gums and tongue. ▸ ***Rationale:*** To remove bacteria and freshen breath.
10. Apply adhesive dental liner if client requests. ▸ ***Rationale:*** Holds dentures in place and provides cushion for more security and comfort.

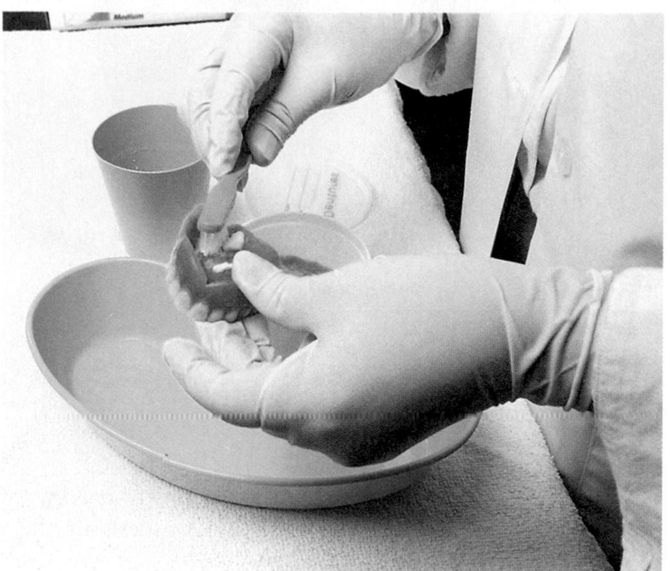

▲ Hold dentures securely while brushing.

11. Moisten dentures according to client's desire.
12. Help client replace dentures.
13. Clean denture cup and emesis basin and replace in client's bedside stand.
14. Remove gloves, and place in appropriate receptacle.
15. Perform hand hygiene.

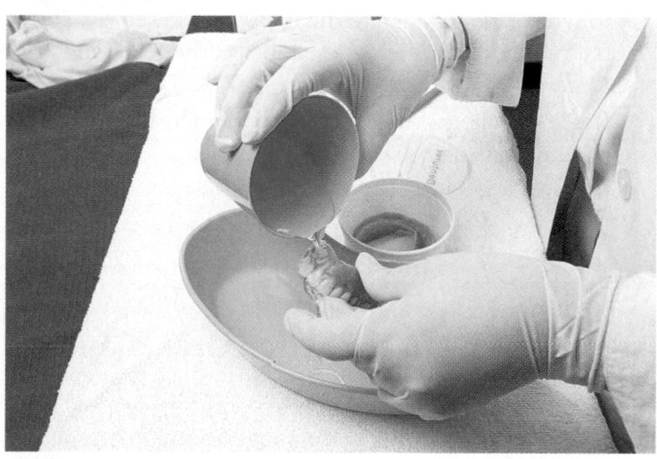

▲ Rinse dentures in cold water.

Providing Oral Care for Unconscious Clients

Equipment

Foam toothette oral swabs
Lubricant for lips
Waterpik devices or brush
Bulb syringe or suction equipment
Tongue blades or bite block
Clean gloves

Procedure

1. Gather equipment.
2. Perform hand hygiene and don gloves.
3. If possible, position client on side in a semi-Fowler's position. If this is not possible, turn client's head to the side. ▸ ***Rationale:*** Allows fluid to drain or be suctioned out of mouth and thus prevents aspiration.

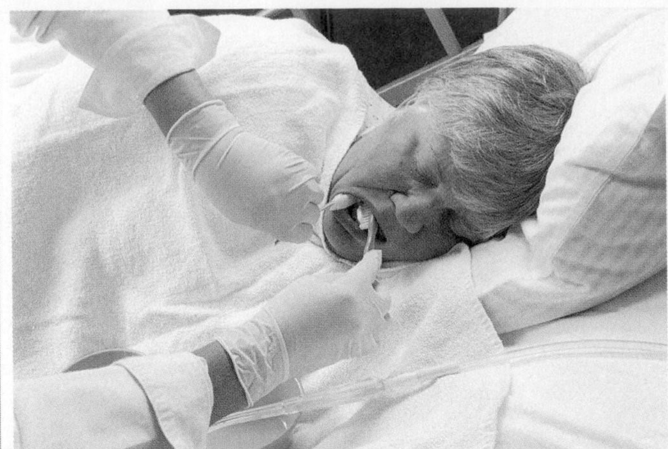
▲ Use padded tongue blade when brushing teeth.

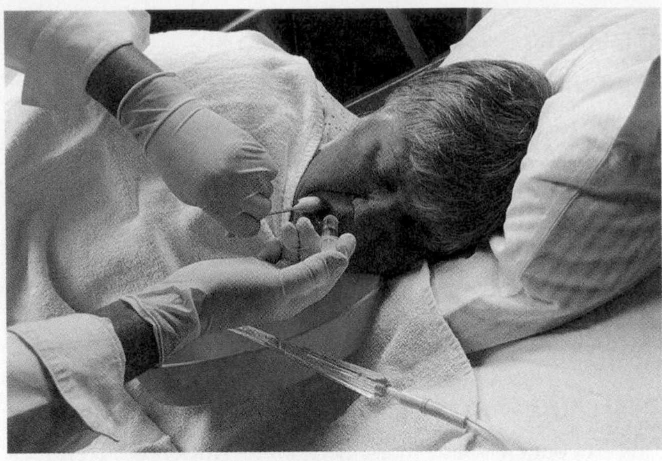
▲ Rinse mouth using water-filled syringe.

4. Place a bulb syringe or suctioning equipment nearby. ▸ ***Rationale:*** Safety precaution to use for suctioning oral cavity as needed.
5. Insert bite block if necessary to keep mouth open while brushing.
6. Place a small amount of toothpaste on brush. Brush the external surfaces of the teeth in the routine manner, using less water on the brush. You may use a tongue blade to move the cheeks and lips. Do not put your fingers in the client's mouth. ▸ ***Rationale:*** This prevents accidental closing down on toothbrush and biting your finger.
7. To clean the inner surfaces of the teeth, use a padded tongue blade to separate the upper and lower sets of teeth, if bite block is not used. Brush the teeth and tongue in the usual manner.
8. Rinse the client's mouth carefully, using very small amounts of water that can be suctioned.
9. Remove bite block.
10. Lubricate client's lips with petroleum jelly.
11. Provide oral care frequently—as often as every 4 hours if necessary. ▸ ***Rationale:*** Oral care maintains adequate oral health.
12. Remove gloves and place in appropriate receptacle.
13. Perform hand hygiene.

NOTE: Foam toothettes can be moistened with water and used as a toothbrush.

Toothette swabs are indicated for the following client conditions: radiation therapy, chemotherapy, bone marrow transplant, immunosuppressed, on a ventilator, nutritionally depleted, or elderly. Toothettes improve the appearance of oral tissue (tongue, palate, lips). Toothbrushes are more effective in stimulating gingival tissue and removing debris from the teeth.

Source: DeWalt, E. M. (2003, January). Effect of timed hygiene measures on oral mucosa in a group of elderly subjects. Journal of American Dental Association, 134(1), 109–110.

DOCUMENTATION for Oral Hygiene

- Findings from assessment of mouth; condition of gums, mucous membranes, and teeth
- Assessment of client's oral hygiene needs
- Planning steps taken to meet client's oral hygiene needs
- Oral care provided or observed
- Effectiveness of oral care on client's teeth, gums, mucosa
- Client's reaction and level of comfort
- Client's level of participation in oral care
- Client's participation in nurse–client teaching

CRITICAL THINKING Application

Expected Outcomes

- The oral health status of client has been assessed and documented by nurse.
- Oral hygiene care is provided without complications.
- Plaque and bacteria-producing agents are removed.

Unexpected Outcomes	Alternative Actions
Even with increased oral hygiene, client still has odorous breath.	• Use antiseptic mouthwash between oral hygiene care. • Notify the physician, as this could be a symptom of systemic disease. • Obtain dental consultation to check for presence of dental caries or gum disease. • Examine client's nutritional intake. Absent nutrients or imbalanced intake of fats, protein, or carbohydrates can result in bad breath.
Client complains of extreme oral mucosal irritation or sensitivity.	• Request physician's order for one of the following solutions: Saline solutions: for soothing, cleansing rinses Anesthetic solutions: to dull extreme pain in the oral cavity Effervescent solutions (e.g., hydrogen peroxide or ginger ale) to loosen and remove debris from the mouth Coating solutions (e.g., Maalox) to protect irritated surfaces Antibacterial—antifungal rinses (e.g., nystatin [Mycostatin]) to prevent the spread of organisms that cause thrush
Vigorous flossing results in bleeding and sore gums.	• Give client warm antiseptic mouthwash to relieve soreness. • Investigate gum condition and refer for consultation.
Client needs care after oral surgery or oral trauma.	• Oral care after surgery or trauma is always ordered by physician. No oral hygiene care should be attempted until physician has clearly defined the specific care. • Suctioning equipment should always be present. • Assessment of client's head, face, neck, and general status is critical at this time.
Normal stimulation and cleaning is not sufficient to remove debris and plaque for the unconscious client.	• Try flossing teeth to dislodge debris. • Provide mouth care with toothbrush and dentifrice at least twice daily. • Check with physician and order sonic toothbrush.
Parotid gland inflammation can occur with improper oral hygiene.	• Rinse mouth with mouthwash. • Use swab to reach back in oral cavity along mandible to temporomandibular area. • Floss teeth at least daily.

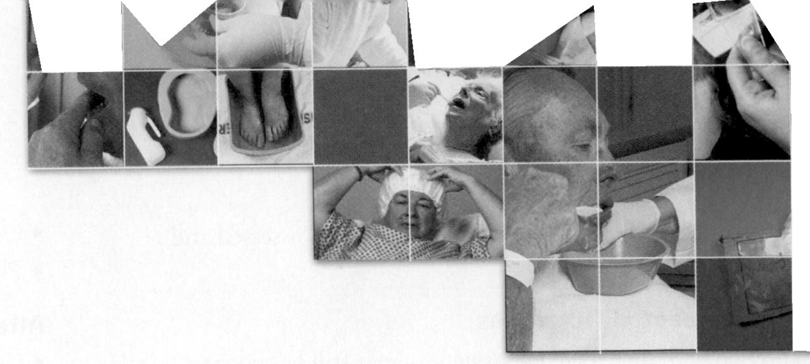

Chapter 9

UNIT 2

Hair Care

Nursing Process Data

ASSESSMENT Data Base

- Review general physical assessment findings.
- Elicit information regarding loss of hair, tenderness of scalp, or itching.
- Determine client's ability to perform own hair care.
- If unable to care for own hair find out who usually assists client.
- Observe client's hair and scalp, noting the following:
  - Texture
  - Color
  - Degree of thickness and hair distribution
  - Degree of gloss or shine
  - Dryness or oiliness
  - Areas of irritation, rash, or scaliness on the scalp or surrounding skin
  - Matting or snarls
  - Pediculosis (lice)
- Assess usual hair care routines, products, and appliances.
- Assess method for providing hair care (e.g., in bed, on gurney, in wheelchair).
- Determine client teaching needs regarding hair care.
- Assess need for frequency of shaving facial hair for male clients.

PLANNING Objectives

- To prevent irritation to the scalp and damage to the hair
- To help maintain or improve client's existing condition of hair and scalp
- To promote circulation to the hair follicle and growth of new hair
- To distribute oils along the hair shaft
- To remove facial hair for client comfort and self-esteem
- To promote self-esteem

IMPLEMENTATION Procedures

EVALUATION Expected Outcomes

- Hair and scalp assessment are performed without complications.
- Appropriate method of hair care provided for client.
- Client's hair and scalp are clean, comfortable, and styled according to client's preference.
- Client is comfortable and rested after shampooing.
- Shaving is accomplished without skin nicks or discomfort.

Pearson Nursing Student Resources

Find additional review materials at **nursing.pearsonhighered.com**

Prepare for success with NCLEX®-style practice questions and Skill Checklists

Providing Hair Care

Equipment

Blunt-ended comb or pick
Brush
Towel
Mirror
Hair care products and ornaments

Preparation

1. Determine client's hair care needs.
2. Perform hand hygiene.
3. Help client into a comfortable position to perform hair care.
4. Collect and assemble equipment.

Procedure

For Routine Hair Care

1. Place all hair care items within reach.
2. Place towel over client's shoulders.
3. Brush or comb client's hair from scalp to hair ends, using gentle, even strokes.
   a. Tangled Hair: Use short gentle strokes. Work from end of hair shaft toward scalp. May use conditioner to make combing easier.
   b. Curly hair: Use wet comb on wet hair (water or oil) for ease of combing.
4. Style hair in a manner suitable to client.
5. Replace hair care items in appropriate place and clean items as needed.
6. Perform hand hygiene.

Shampooing Hair

Equipment

Two bath towels
Washcloth
Large container for water
Shampoo
Conditioner, if desired
Hair dryer, if allowed by hospital
For Disposable System
Package containing shampoo cap
Face or bath towel
Hair care products, as requested by client
Comb and/or brush

NOTE: Ensure that electrical equipment is checked by maintenance department before using. ▶ ***Rationale:*** This confirms that equipment is grounded and mechanically safe.

Preparation

1. Determine client's hair care needs.
2. Perform hand hygiene.
3. Collect and assemble equipment.
4. Help client into a comfortable position to perform hair care.
5. Shampooing the hair can be accomplished in a variety of ways depending on the client's usual routine and physical condition. In many institutions, a physician's order is necessary before shampooing a client's hair.
6. If possible, the easiest way to shampoo is to assist the client while he or she is in the shower. Caution should be taken to prevent the client from becoming overly tired or weak while in the shower. (Use shower chair if necessary.)

Procedure

For Client on a Gurney

1. Have shampoo items readily available.
2. Position gurney with head end at sink.
3. Lock wheels on gurney. ▶ ***Rationale:*** This prevents the gurney from moving away from the sink.
4. Pad the edge of the sink with a towel or bath blanket.
5. Move the client's head just beyond the edge of the gurney. ▶ ***Rationale:*** To allow water to run off more easily.
6. Put a pillow or a rolled blanket under the client's shoulders. ▶ ***Rationale:*** To help elevate and extend the head.
7. Drape one towel over client's shoulders and around neck. Place another towel within reach.
8. Use a washcloth to protect client's eyes. Wet hair and gently make a lather with shampoo.
9. Rinse thoroughly and repeat if necessary.
10. Towel dry, add conditioner if desired, and rinse again.
11. Using a dry towel, pat hair dry, and wrap turban style to transport back to room.
12. Use hair dryer if available.
13. Style as desired.
14. Replace equipment.
15. Perform hand hygiene.

Clinical Alert

If the client is elderly, do not press the neck down on the edge of the sink—this position can diminish circulation to the brain and has been reported to be a possible cause of strokes.

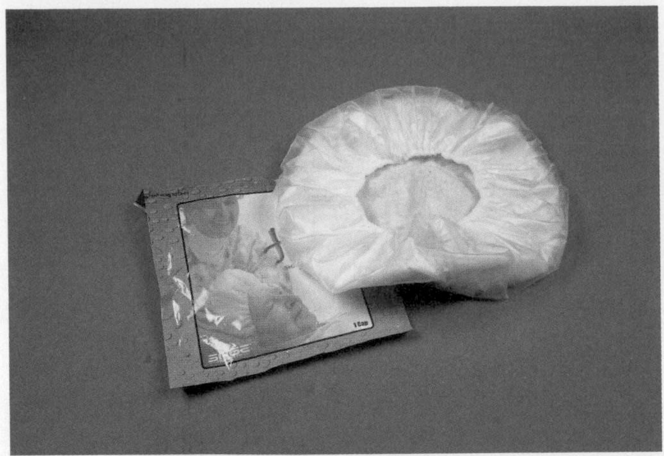

▲ Shampoo system activated by microwave.

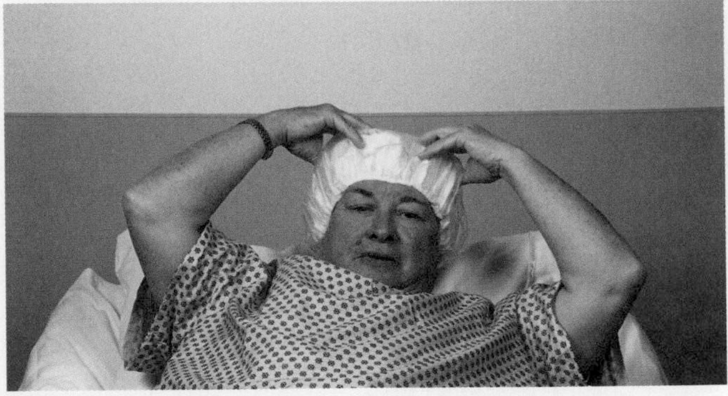

▲ Disposable cap can be used for clients on bed rest.

For Client Using Disposable System

1. Heat shampoo package in microwave for no more than 30 seconds.
2. Perform hand hygiene.
3. Open package and check temperature. ▶ ***Rationale:*** Clients react to heat at different temperatures; therefore, check the cap temperature with client before placing on client's head.
4. Place cap on head. Ensure that all hair is contained within the cap. For longer hair, place cap on top of head and then tuck all hair up inside cap.
5. Gently massage cap with hands, 1–2 minutes for short hair and 2–3 minutes for longer hair. ▶ ***Rationale:*** This will assist in saturating the hair with the solution. There is no need to rinse hair after using solution.
6. Remove cap and place in appropriate receptacle.
7. Towel dry hair.
8. Complete hair care according to client's needs and desires.
9. Perform hand hygiene.

NOTE: Disposable hair care systems provide a quick and easy way to freshen client's hair with minimal client movement

Clinical Alert

If hair is tangled, the cap may need to stay on for longer period of time in order to saturate hair. If blood or other secretions are present on hair, they may need to be removed using the washcloths from the disposable bath system before attempting to shampoo the hair.

Shaving a Client

Equipment

Safety or electric razor, specific to client's needs or wishes
Shaving cream
Aftershave lotion (optional)
Two towels
Basin of warm water

Preparation

1. Place client in sitting position.
2. Perform hand hygiene.
3. Place towel over chest and under chin.
4. Put up mirror on overbed table.
5. Determine how the client usually shaves (i.e., use of safety edge or electric razor; special products).
6. Check to see if the client has excessive bleeding tendencies due to pathologic conditions (hemophilia) or the use of specific medications (anticoagulants or large doses of aspirin). ▶ ***Rationale:*** If client is accidentally cut, it could lead to some loss of blood.

Clinical Alert

Only electric razors can be used to shave clients with excessive bleeding tendencies.

Procedure

1. If using a safety edge razor:
   a. Don gloves and apply a warm, moist towel to soften the hair.
   b. Apply a thick layer of soap or shaving cream to the shaving area.
   c. Holding skin taut, use firm but small strokes in the direction of hair growth.
   d. Gently remove soap or lather with a warm, damp towel. Inspect for areas you may have missed.
2. If using electric razor:
   a. Use rotating motion of razor and start from lateral aspect of face and move toward chin and upper lip area.
   b. Clean razor with brush or remove razor head and clean facial hair from head of razor.

3. Apply aftershave lotion or powder as desired.
4. Reposition client for comfort if needed.
5. Remove gloves and replace equipment.
6. Perform hand hygiene.

Clinical Alert

According to the hospital policy, be sure to have the electric razor checked for safety aspects. Some hospitals do not allow clients to use their own electric razors.

DOCUMENTATION for Hair Care

- Documentation of hair care assessment and needs
- Shampooing method, outcomes, problems encountered
- Client's tolerance to hair care
- Shaving completed; note specific type of razor
- Unusual bleeding from shaving

CRITICAL THINKING Application

Expected Outcomes

- Hair and scalp assessment performed without complications.
- Appropriate method of hair care was provided for client.
- Client's hair and scalp are clean, comfortable, and styled according to client's preference.
- Client is comfortable and rested after shampooing.
- Shaving is accomplished without skin nicks or discomfort.

Unexpected Outcomes	Alternative Actions
Extreme matting, snarling, blood, or nonremovable substances appear in client's hair.	• Never cut a client's hair unless it is absolutely necessary. • Check hospital policy regarding hair cutting. It may not be allowed in some facilities. • Apply alcohol to tangled hair or blood-soaked hair. Keep in place 5 minutes. Wash hair with shampoo to remove alcohol and blood. • Secure permission of family or physician (if order required).
Client is cut during shaving procedure.	• Assess extent of cut, and place a clean towel on the area with pressure to stop bleeding. • If cut appears to be more than a nick, report to physician and fill out unusual occurrence report.
Shaving is difficult and painful for the client.	• Place warm towels on area to be shaved for 15 minutes. • Apply more shaving cream. • Ensure that razor is sharp.

Chapter 9

UNIT ❸

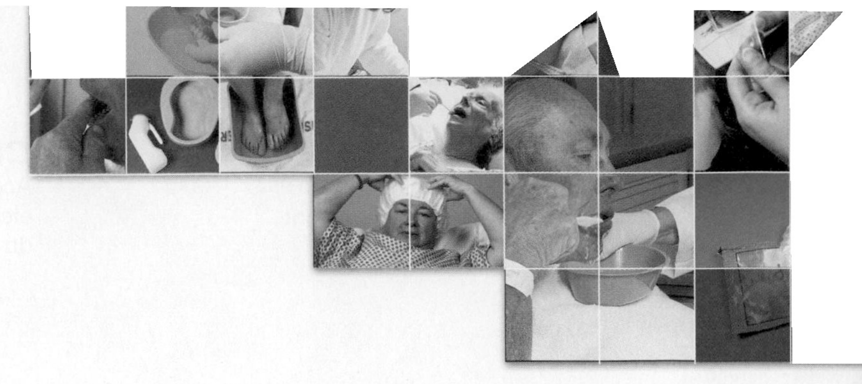

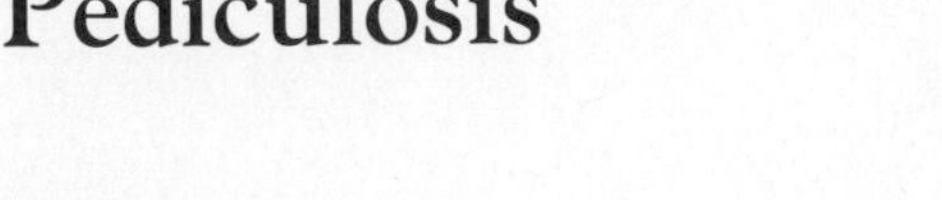

Pediculosis

Nursing Process Data

ASSESSMENT Data Base

- Observe head (scalp), body (nape of neck, behind ears, beard, eyebrows, arms, legs), and pubic areas for the following signs:
  - Small, hemorrhagic areas on the skin
  - Scratches on the skin
  - Habitual itching and scratching, feeling something crawling in hair
  - Insect-type bites or pustular eruptions behind the ears or hairline
  - Small, white dandruff-like particles
  - Gritty feel when running fingers through hair
- Assess client's personal hygiene, living conditions, contact or exposure to others with lice (e.g., school-aged children, sexual partners, siblings).

PLANNING Objectives

- To remove lice from client's hair and prevent further skin problems such as impetigo or infection
- To remove cause of itching and intense need to scratch scalp
- To control spread of lice to others

IMPLEMENTATION Procedures

EVALUATION Expected Outcomes

- Lice removed after treatment.
- Client verbalizes cause of problem and preventive measures.
- Client repeats back to nurse instructions for preventing lice infestation and indicates understanding of process.
- Client and family members remain free of lice infestation.

Pearson Nursing Student Resources

Find additional review materials at **nursing.pearsonhighered.com**

Prepare for success with NCLEX®-style practice questions and Skill Checklists

Identifying the Presence of Lice and Nits (Lice Eggs)

Equipment

Bright lamp/light
Magnifying glass
Clean gloves
Isolation bag
Nit comb or tongue blade (2)

Procedure

NOTE: Louse becomes adult in 7 to 8 days. Each louse lays 4 to 8 eggs/day for the next 18 days, then dies (each louse lays 100–400 eggs). The nits/eggs hatch in 8 days. Adult lice can survive up to 55 hours without a host.

1. Perform hand hygiene. Don clean gloves.
2. Check two forms of client identifiers, introduce yourself, and explain procedure to client.
3. Position client so head or affected body area is well lighted by lamp.
4. Use fine-tooth louse comb after removing tangles and comb from roots to end. After each stroke, examine comb for live louse or a viable egg. Use magnifying glass to observe scalp and hair.
   a. For live lice:
      Gray-white to reddish brown in color
      2–4 mm long; 1 mm wide
      Flat body with 6 clawed legs
      Live lice crawl, but do not fly, jump, or hop
      Feed on blood 3–4 times/day
   b. For viable eggs or nymph:
      Tiny and hard
      Yellow to white oval, tear-drop–shaped capsules
      Attached firmly to base of hair shaft (dandruff will fall from hair shaft when touched)
      Nits hatch after 7–10 days
      Nits within 6 mm of scalp are usually viable and indicate an active infestation
      Easier to detect close behind the ears or at the nape of the neck
5. Identify lice or nits:
   a. Fine-toothed louse comb: after removing tangles, comb from roots to end with the nit comb. After each stroke, examine comb carefully for signs of lice.
   b. Nits present without lice does not indicate there is an active infestation. Assess further: previous treatment, timing, and distance from scalp.
   c. Put hair strands between two tongue blades and scrape white specks. Determine whether they come off the shaft easily. Observe base of scalp carefully for tiny lice.

Removing Lice and Nits

Equipment

Isolation bags (optional)
Topical insecticide/pediculicides:
   Permethrin (Nix®, RID)
   Pyrethrin® (A-200, Pronto, Tisit)
   Malathion (Ovice, by prescription)
   Benzyl Alcohol (Ulesfia, by prescription)
Clean linen
Fine-tooth "nit" comb
Disinfectant for comb
Clean gloves
Towels

Procedure

1. Determine whether client is allergic to ragweed or chrysanthemums. ▶ ***Rationale:*** Pyrethrin is obtained from these plants and cannot be used to treat lice if client has allergic reaction to them.

> **Clinical Alert**
> **When using any of the lice treatment products, the nurse needs to check for allergies to ragweed or chrysanthemum flowers. Allergies to ragweed can cause breathing difficulties or an asthmatic attack. Allergies to chrysanthemums can cause pneumonia, muscle paralysis, or death due to respiratory failure.**

2. Perform hand hygiene.
3. Don clean gloves. Gloves are used even when completing treatment at home.
4. Remove and bag client's clothing and linens. Client's clothes do not need to be bagged separately and placed in isolation bags if standard precautions are used.
5. Notify physician and other healthcare providers of lice infestation. Begin treatment as ordered by physician.
6. Follow manufacturer's directions for product ordered.

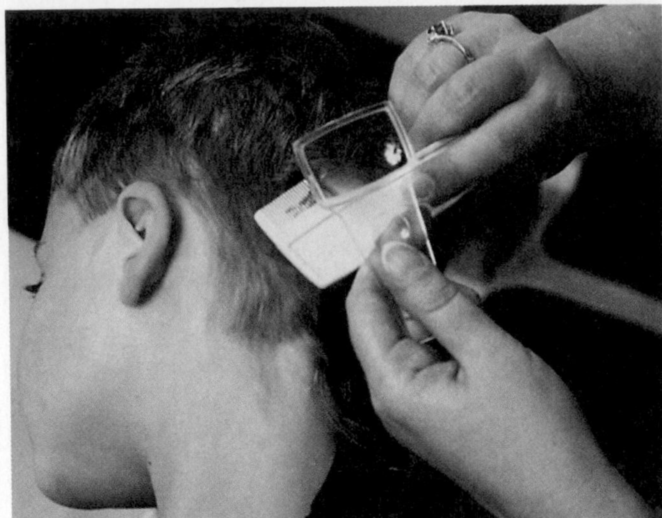
▲ Use magnifying glass when inspecting for head lice.

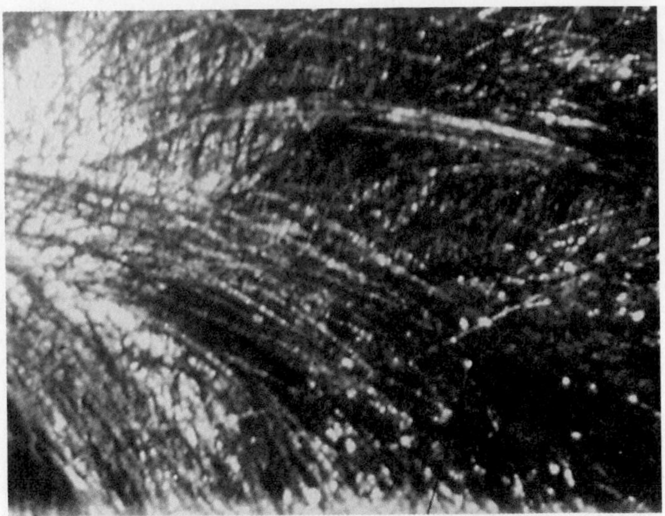
▲ Examine hair closely for white nits on hair shaft.

7. Apply lotion, mousse, or gel to scalp and dry hair, beginning at the roots, and extend to the end of the hair shaft. If using shampoo before treatment, be sure to towel dry hair.
8. Leave product on hair for 10 minutes (leave Malathion longer, according to directions).
9. Rinse hair thoroughly.
10. Give client a towel to protect eyes and face while applying product and rinsing hair.
11. Comb out nits using a fine-tooth or lice/nit comb. Hair should remain slightly damp while removing nits. If hair dries during combing, dampen slightly with water. ▶ ***Rationale:*** Combing is the most important step in the process of lice removal, as eggs can be left behind and hatch at a later time.
12. Disinfect combs and brushes with the shampoo.
13. Remove gloves.
14. Perform hand hygiene.
15. Instruct client, parent, or significant other to check hair and use "nit comb" every 2 to 3 days until lice are gone and to check skin for removal of scabies. (Pruritus may last for 2 weeks after treatment.)
16. Wash clothes and linens that person has used within 48 hours before treatment. ▶ ***Rationale:*** head lice rarely survive more than 48 hours off the body.
17. Place stuffed toys in hot dryer or place in a plastic bag and seal for 2 to 4 weeks.
18. Instruct client or family to vacuum furniture and floors to rid house of lice. ▶ ***Rationale:*** Head lice need a human host and therefore do not survive long after falling off head.
19. Administer Bactrim if ordered (usually used with resistant cases). ▶ ***Rationale:*** used if multiple treatments have tried to rid hair of lice.
20. Inspect all family members using wet louse comb or magnifying glass in bright light for lice/nits (eggs). Look for tiny nits near scalp, beginning at back of neck and behind ears. Examine small section of hair one at a time. Treat each member infested with lice using the same treatment plan.
21. Discuss the cause, treatment, and preventive measures regarding lice infestation with client and family.
22. Reinspect hair every 1 to 3 days for signs of reinfestation.
23. Apply second treatment within 7 to 10 days to kill any newly hatched lice.

NOTE: Nix is treatment of choice and is over-the-counter. Recommended by the American Academy of Pediatrics because of its efficacy and lack of toxicity.

Clinical Alert

- Do not use more than three applications in 2 weeks.
- Do not use cream rinse or conditioner shampoo before applying pediculicide treatment as it will interfere with the medication.

Clinical Alert

- Do not use near eyes, eyebrows, eyelids, inside nose, mouth, or vagina.
- If product gets into eyes, immediately flush eyes with water. If child swallows product, immediately contact a Poison Control Center for directions on care.
- Stop treatment immediately if client complains of breathing difficulties, eye irritation, or skin or scalp irritation.
- Adverse reactions and side effects may be more frequent and severe in younger clients. Consult with physician about treatment dose. Pediculicides are not effective on some resistant strains of lice.

Removing Nits From Hair

- Part hair into sections; start at top of head and do one section at a time.
- Lift a 1- to 2-inch–wide strand of hair. Place comb as close to scalp as possible and comb with a firm, even motion away from scalp.
- Pin back each strand of hair after combing.
- Clean comb often. Wipe nits away with tissue and discard into a plastic bag. Seal bag and discard to prevent lice from spreading.
- After combing, thoroughly recheck for lice/nits. Recomb as needed.
- Check every 1 to 3 days for missed lice.

Guidelines for Diagnosis and Treatment of Pediculosis Capitis in Children and Adults

Diagnosis:

- A live louse or nymph on the scalp or a viable egg is usually found within 1 cm of the scalp.
- Using a fine-tooth louse comb is four times more efficient that direct visualization and two times faster.

Treatment:

- Permethrin is the treatment of choice because of efficacy and lack of toxicity.
- Pyrethrin and Piperonyl butoxide are not ovicidal and application should be repeated in 7 days.
- Malathion lotion.
- Combing wet hair using a conditioner of choice and a louse comb is an alternative regiment and the treatment of choice for children younger than 2 years of age. When using this method, repeat combing needs to be done for the next 2 weeks on days 1, 5, 9, and 13 to break the life cycle.
- A combination of Permethrin and Bactrim should be reserved for cases not responsive to traditional pediculicides and those suspected to have lice-related resistance.

Source: Prepared by University of Texas, Austin (2008), and posted in the National Guideline Clearinghouse; reviewed 19 references, in addition to the 41 previously reviewed to formulate the 2002 guidelines.

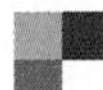

DOCUMENTATION for Removing Lice

- Location of lice infestation
- Notification of physician and healthcare providers
- Medicated shampoo applied
- Side effects of medicated shampoo, if any
- Nursing interventions and the results obtained
- Client teaching activities

CRITICAL THINKING Application

Expected Outcomes

- Lice removed after treatment.
- Client verbalizes cause of problem and preventive measures.
- Client repeats back to nurse instructions for preventing lice infestation and indicates understanding of process.
- Client and family members remain free of lice infestation.

Unexpected Outcomes	Alternative Actions
Special shampoo is left on hair/scalp too long.	• Observe for irritation or burning after rinsing out the shampoo. • If scalp is burned, notify physician for a medication order. • Do not repeat treatment unless specifically ordered by physician.
Other clients or staff become infested with lice.	• Isolate the client's linen and personal hair grooming equipment to prevent spread of lice. • Instruct client or staff on use of medicated lotion, shampoo, or combination therapy.
Lice are not eliminated with treatment.	• Repeat treatment using combination therapy as ordered by physician. • Do not repeat treatment for 7 days. • Utilize another type of insecticide or wet-combing method.

Chapter 9

UNIT ❹

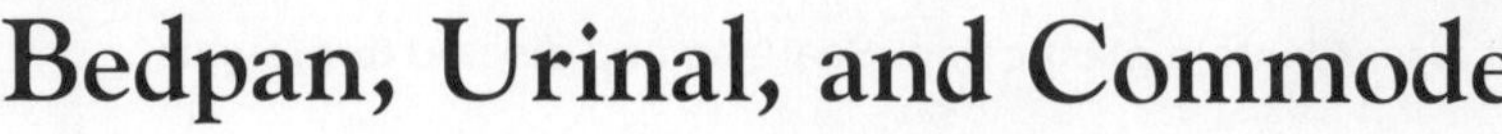

Bedpan, Urinal, and Commode

Nursing Process Data

ASSESSMENT Data Base

- Determine client's usual voiding pattern.
- Assess client's ability to assist with the procedure.

PLANNING Objectives

- To assist the client to void when on bed rest or unable to urinate
- To help client void 200 to 500 mL of urine without discomfort or difficulty

IMPLEMENTATION Procedures

EVALUATION Expected Outcomes

- Client voids 200 to 500 mL of urine without discomfort or difficulty.
- Bladder does not become distended.
- Genitourinary system is free of infection.
- Client transferred to commode for voiding.

Pearson Nursing Student Resources

Find additional review materials at **nursing.pearsonhighered.com**

Prepare for success with NCLEX®-style practice questions and Skill Checklists

Using a Bedpan and Urinal

Equipment

Bedpan or urinal
Toilet tissues
Absorbent pad, if needed
Clean gloves

Procedure

1. Perform hand hygiene and don gloves.
2. Obtain bedpan or urinal and warm pan or urinal by running warm water around the edges of the receptacle if cold. Fracture pan is used for clients in traction, body cast, or with casted extremities.
3. Provide privacy.
4. Place client in a supine position, if possible, or position on edge of bed or in a chair.
5. Instruct the client to sit on bedpan or place penis into urinal. If the client needs assistance, follow these steps:

For Using a Bedpan

a. Place absorbent pad under hips, if needed.
b. Raise the client's hips and slip your arm under the client or turn the client on his or her side. Roll the client onto the pan.
c. Place a rolled towel or blanket under the client's sacrum. ▸ ***Rationale:*** This provides comfort by padding the bony area.
d. Elevate the head of the bed.

For Using a Urinal

a. Place the base of the urinal flat on the bed between the client's thighs.
b. Position the client's penis into opening of the urinal.

NOTE: It may be easier for clients to use a urinal if they sit on the edge of the bed.

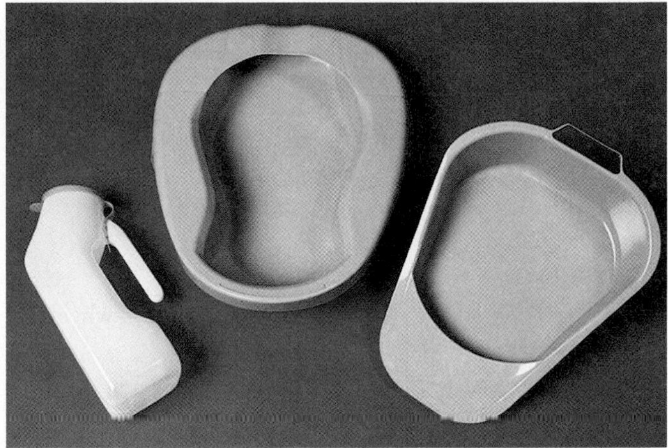

▲ Urinal, bedpan, and fracture pan used for clients on bed rest.

6. Place the signal light or call bell and toilet tissue within easy reach.
7. When the client has voided, remove the bedpan or urinal and assist with wiping as necessary.
   a. Remove bedpan by placing hand under small of back.
   b. Assist client to lift buttocks off pan.
   c. Remove pan by pulling toward edge of bed. Keep bedpan flat when moving. ▸ ***Rationale:*** To prevent spilling urine out of bedpan.
8. Provide an opportunity for the client to perform hand hygiene.
9. Reposition the client for comfort, pull back curtains.
10. Measure intake and output if required.
11. Empty bedpan or urinal, clean equipment, and return to proper area in client's room.
12. Remove gloves and perform hand hygiene.

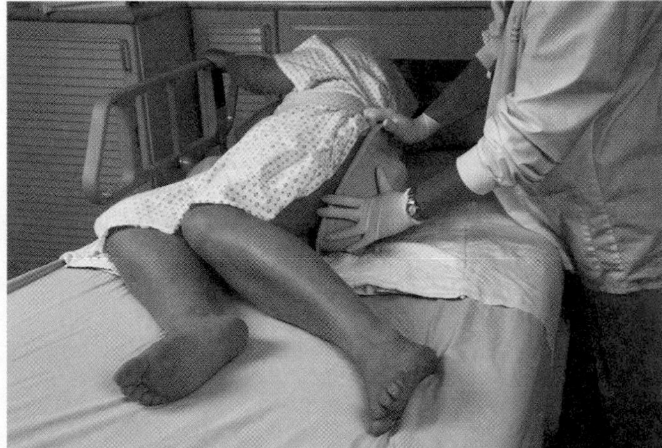

▲ Turn client to side to position on bedpan.

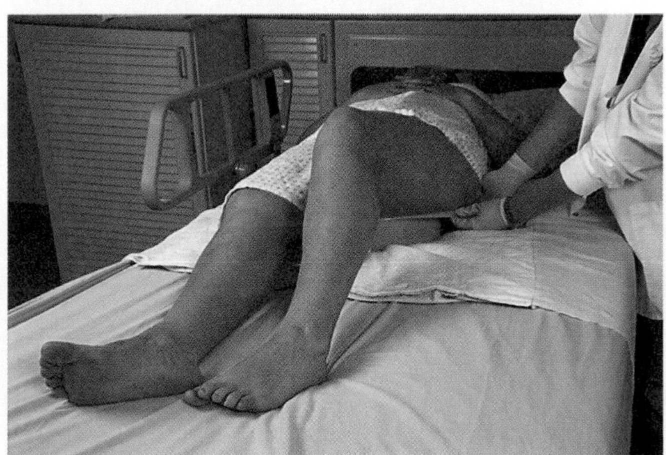

▲ Roll client onto pan and make comfortable.

Assisting Client to Commode

Equipment

Commode with locking wheels or rubber-tipped legs
Toilet tissue
Nurse's call bell
Slippers
Bath blanket

Procedure

1. Place commode at foot of bed. Be sure to lock wheels on commode if needed.
2. Place slippers on client.
3. Raise head of bed to facilitate moving client to edge of bed.
4. Move client to edge of bed and assist to a sitting position at edge of bed. Instruct client to place feet flat on floor.
5. Stand directly in front of client, blocking client's toes with your feet and client's knees with your knees. ▸ ***Rationale:*** Prevents client from buckling knees.
6. Flex your knees.
7. Place your arms securely around client's waist. ▸ ***Rationale:*** Stabilizes client for transfer.
8. When starting to transfer, avoid bending at the waist. ▸ ***Rationale:*** Prevents back strain.
9. Instruct client to push self off bed and support his/her own weight.
10. Straighten your knees and hips as you raise client to standing position.
11. Pivot client in front of commode. Instruct client to grasp arm rest on farthest side.
12. Lower client onto commode, using correct body mechanics (flexing your hip and knees but not your back) to ensure client is securely positioned on commode.
13. Place toilet tissue within easy reach.
14. Cover client with bath blanket for warmth and privacy.
15. Place call bell within easy access of client.
16. Provide privacy by closing curtains and shutting door.
17. Assist client to wipe self as necessary.

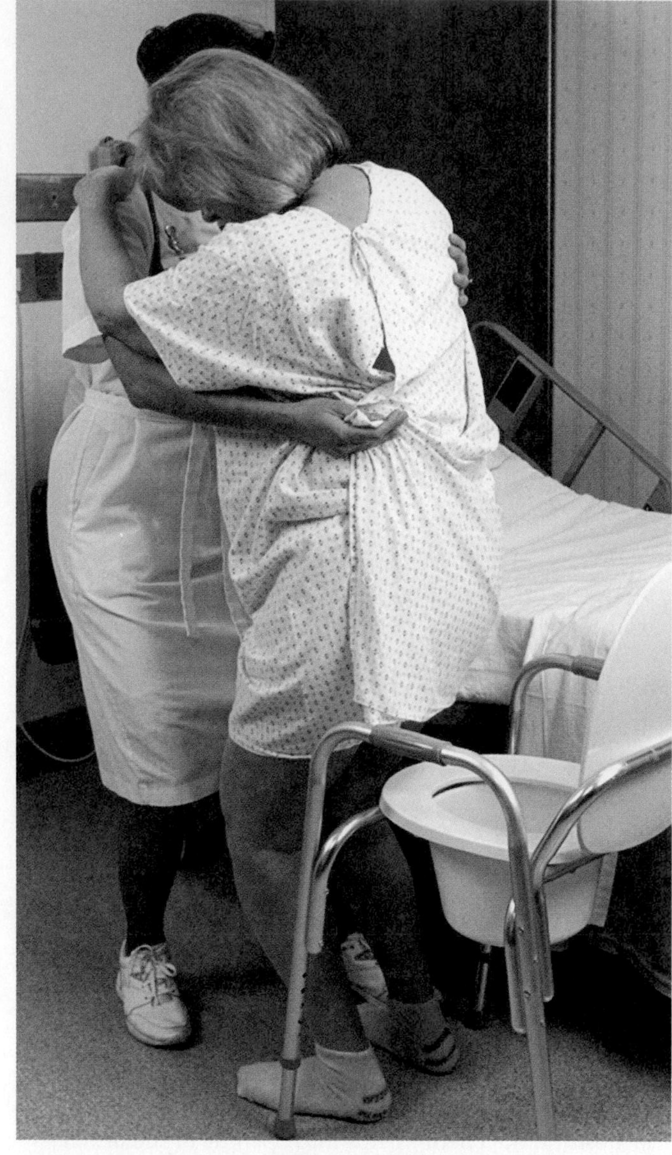

▲ Pivot with client and bend knees when seating client.

18. Assist client back to bed.
19. Empty and clean commode.
20. Perform hand hygiene.

DOCUMENTATION for Bedpan, Urinal, and Commode

- Amount, color, appearance, and odor of urine and feces
- Techniques effective in stimulating voiding
- Equipment used (e.g., commode, bedpan)
- Type of support needed for transfer to commode

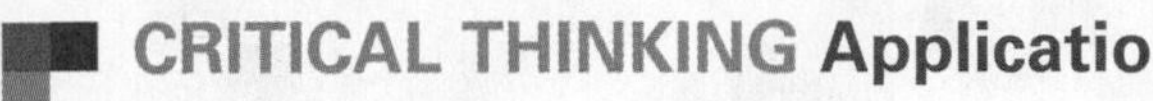

CRITICAL THINKING Application

Expected Outcomes

- Client voids 200 to 500 mL of urine without discomfort or difficulty.
- Bladder does not become distended.
- Genitourinary system is free of infection.
- Client transferred to commode for voiding as soon as able.

Unexpected Outcomes	Critical Thinking Options
Unable to turn and has difficulty raising hips	• Use a fracture pan rather than a bedpan. Powder the fracture pan. • Insert the fracture pan with the flat side toward the head, under the client's thighs. • Assess reason for difficulty. • Maintain complete privacy.
Unable to void on bedpan.	• Run water in sink. • Massage the lower abdomen. • Place a hot washcloth on the abdomen. • Pour warm water over the perineum with client positioned on toilet or bedpan. • Give client a sitz bath after obtaining an order.

Chapter 9

UNIT 5

Perineal and Genital Care

Nursing Process Data

ASSESSMENT Data Base

- Review client's general assessment data.
- Observe for signs of perineal itching, burning on urination, or skin irritation. Ask client if he or she experiences any of these problems.
- Assess client's ability to bathe himself or herself and to perform perineal care.
- While providing privacy, observe the perineal–genital area for abnormal secretions, ulcerations, skin excoriations and sensitivity, drainage (amount, consistency, odor, color), swelling, enlarged lymph glands, catheter patency, and comfort.
- Assess client's learning needs related to perineal and genital care.

PLANNING Objectives

- To decrease the growth of bacteria
- To remove excessive secretions
- To promote healing after surgery and vaginal deliveries
- To prevent the spread of microorganisms for clients with indwelling catheters
- To increase client comfort

IMPLEMENTATION Procedures

EVALUATION Expected Outcomes

- Perineal care has been comfortably and effectively provided.
- Perineal area is clean, odor-free, and without irritation or discharge.
- Skin remains intact after perineal care.

Draping a Female Client

Equipment

Bath blanket

Procedure

1. Bring bath blanket to bedside.
2. Identify client and explain procedure.
3. Provide privacy.
4. Perform hand hygiene.
5. Assess bladder for distention. ▸ ***Rationale:*** Offer bedpan before providing perineal care to prevent urge to urinate during perineal care.
6. Place bed in HIGH position, and lower side rail nearest you.
7. Place bath blanket over client's top linen so that one corner of the blanket is pointed toward the client's head to form a diamond shape over the client.
8. Instruct client to hold onto bath blanket. Fanfold linen to foot of bed.
9. Request that client flex knees and keep them apart with feet firmly on bed.
10. Wrap lateral corners of bath blanket around feet in a spiral fashion until they are completely covered.
11. The corner of the blanket between knees and extending over perineum can later be folded back over the abdomen.

Providing Female Perineal Care

Equipment

Bath blanket or sheet
Two to three bath towels or perineal cloths
Protective pad
Three washclothes
Clean gloves

Preparation

1. Check to see if specific physician orders are to be followed.
2. Talk with client about how she can perform care or assist with procedure. ▸ ***Rationale:*** This gives client a sense of control.
3. Collect and arrange necessary equipment. Warm disposable cloth package if using disposable system. ▸ ***Rationale:*** Warm cloth is more comfortable for client.
4. Provide privacy by closing door and pulling drapes.
5. Perform hand hygiene.
6. Position client in a comfortable position in bed. Head of bed can be elevated to low-Fowler's position. Drape according to procedure described above.
7. If possible, encourage the client to bend her knees and separate her legs. ▸ ***Rationale:*** The perineal area can be cleansed more efficiently in this position.

Procedure

1. Place a protective pad or towel under the client's hips. ▸ ***Rationale:*** Keeps the linen clean and dry.
2. Don gloves.
3. Lift corner of drape away from perineal area.
4. Place first washcloth into basin. Rub cloth with soap, wring out excess water or open disposable cloth package.
5. Fold washcloth into mitt or gather into palm of hand.
6. Separate labia with one hand to expose urethral and vaginal openings.

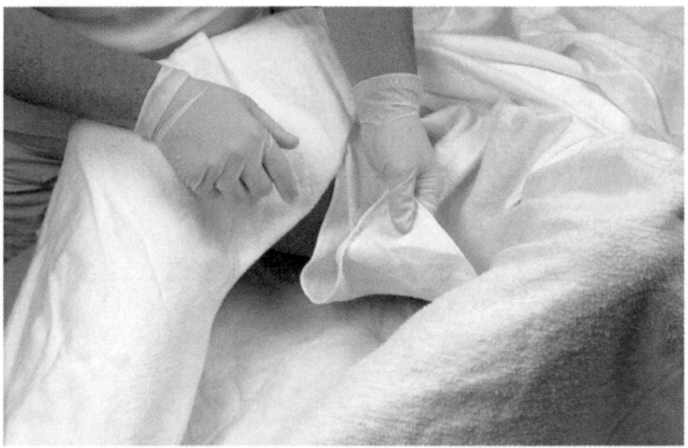

▲ Draping protects client's privacy when performing perineal care.

7. Wash labia minora, from front to back, in a downward motion on one side. ▸ ***Rationale:*** This promotes the principle of washing from a clean to a dirty area to prevent a urinary tract infection.

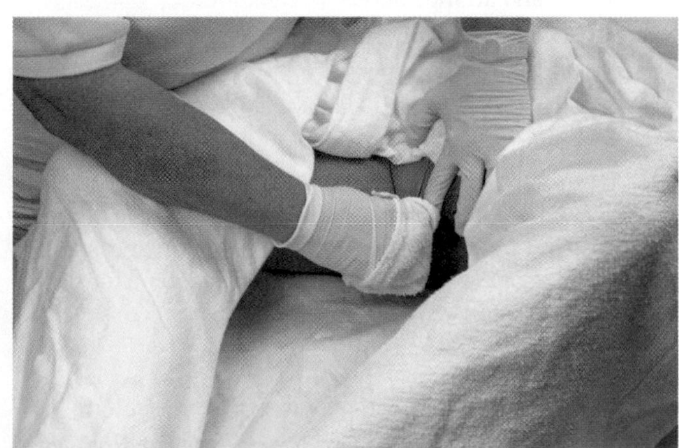

▲ Separate labia and expose urethral and vaginal areas.

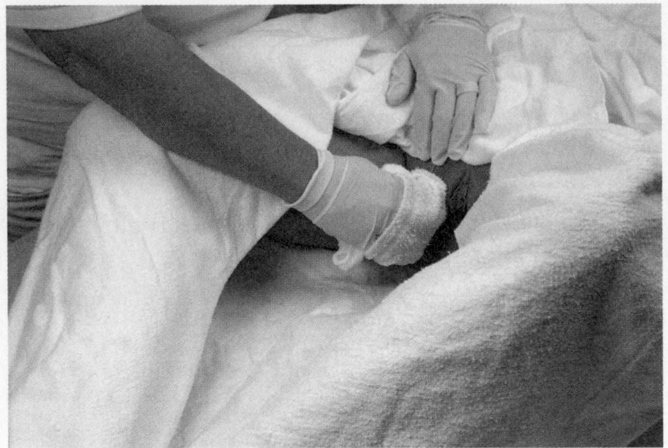

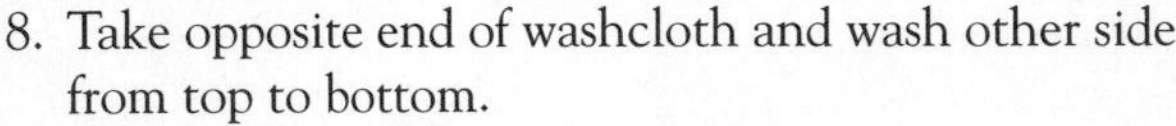

▲ Use different section of washcloth for each area of perineum.

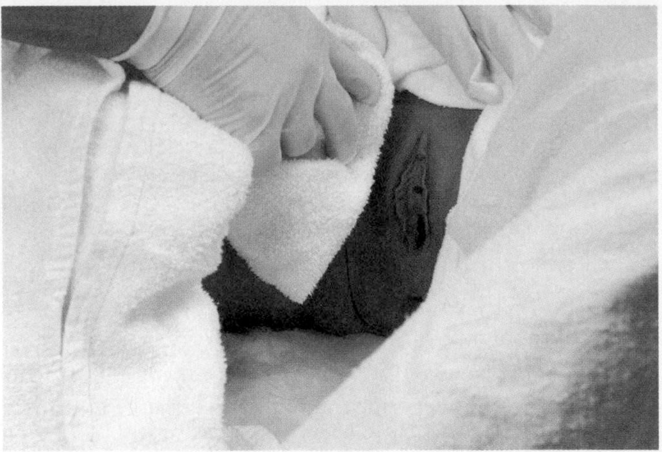

▲ Thoroughly pat dry perineal area.

8. Take opposite end of washcloth and wash other side from top to bottom.
9. Do not replace washcloth in basin.
10. Place second washcloth in water and soap washcloth, wash labia majora from top to bottom. ▸ ***Rationale:*** Prevents contamination from previous cleansing area.
11. Take opposite side of washcloth and clean external labia (labia majora) and perineal area from front to back.
12. Wring out new washcloth and rinse perineum.
13. Thoroughly pat dry perineal area. ▸ ***Rationale:*** Prevents moisture accumulation and potential fungal infections.
14. Use washcloth used for rinsing and clean around anal area. ▸ ***Rationale:*** Anal area is last to be washed to prevent cross-contamination.
15. Discard washcloths in appropriate receptacle.
16. Remove gloves.
17. Position client for comfort.
18. Perform hand hygiene.

Providing Male Perineal Care

Equipment

Bath blanket or sheet
Two bath towels
Protective pad or plastic sheet
Three washcloths
Basin of warm water
Clean gloves

Preparation

1. Collect and arrange necessary equipment.
2. Talk with client about how he can perform care or assist with procedure.
3. Ask client to attempt to empty bladder.
4. Provide privacy by closing door and pulling drapes.
5. Perform hand hygiene and don gloves.
6. Cover client with bath blanket or towel over abdomen and cover client's legs with sheet or towel, exposing genital area as little as possible. ▸ ***Rationale:*** This contributes to client's comfort and privacy.

Procedure

1. Place washcloth in basin. Apply soap to washcloth.
2. Wring washcloth out to remove excess water. ▸ ***Rationale:*** This will prevent the protective pad from getting too wet.
3. If the client has not been circumcised, retract his foreskin carefully to expose the glans penis.
4. Gently but securely hold the shaft of the penis in one hand.
5. Using a circular motion, start at the tip of the penis and wash downwards toward the shaft with soap and water. Do not repeat washing over an area without using a new washcloth. ▸ ***Rationale:*** This procedure prevents cross-contamination.

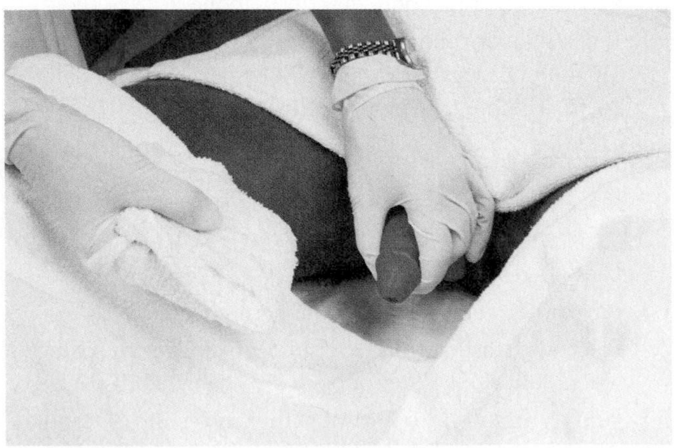

▲ Hold shaft of penis in one hand.

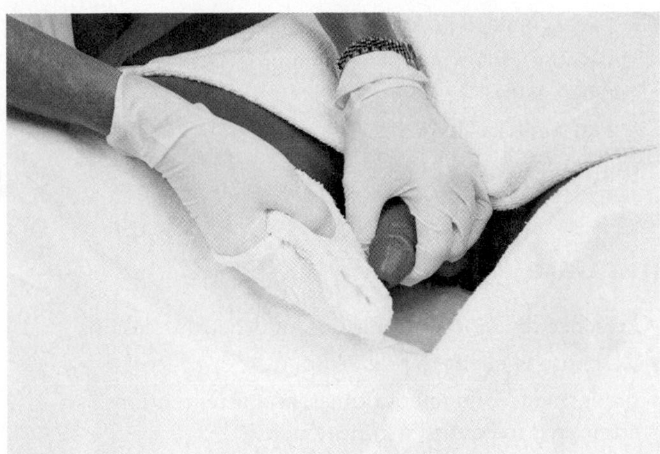

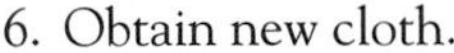

▲ Use circular motion, starting at tip of penis and wash toward shaft.

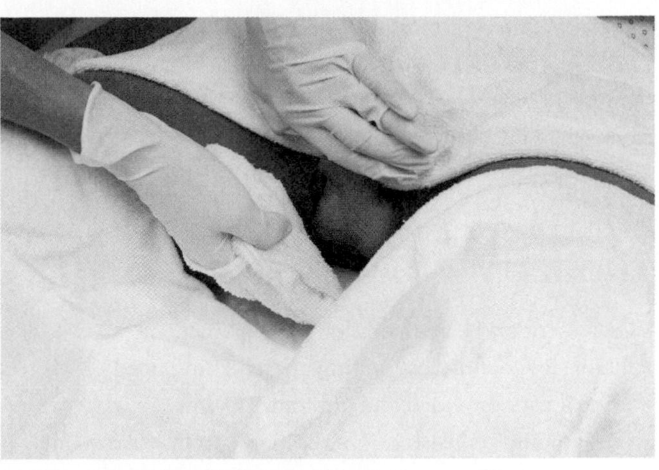

▲ Wash around scrotum using new washcloth.

6. Obtain new cloth.
7. Replace the foreskin over the glans penis and cleanse area.
8. Obtain new washcloth and wash around the scrotum using new washcloth.
9. Wash the anus last.
10. Use new washcloth and rinse the perineal area.
11. Dry all areas.
12. Remove articles and cover client.
13. Reposition client for comfort.
14. Place disposable cloth in garbage or washcloth in linen hamper.
15. Remove gloves, and place in appropriate receptacle.
16. Perform hand hygiene.

Commercial Perineal Care Washcloths for Incontinent Client

- Used for clients with urinary or fecal incontinence.
- Remove soiled gown and place in appropriate receptacle.
- Remove washcloth from tub and wash perineal area.
- Use new washcloth for each swipe: Wash from front (pubis) to back (anus), starting at middle of perineum and working outward.
- Discard washcloth into appropriate receptacle. Several washcloths can be used to clean client.
- Place tub cover over remaining cloths for use at a later time.
- Change bed if needed.
- Place new gown on client.

Providing Incontinence Care

Equipment

Commercially prepared package with premoistened perineal washcloths
Cleansing agent if needed
Clean linen, gown as needed
Clean gloves

Preparation

1. Provide privacy for client and explain what you will be doing.
2. Obtain package of three washcloths premoistened with 3% dimethicone, a transparent barrier that remains on the skin to protect it. ▸ ***Rationale:*** This protective barrier is less messy than zinc oxide or other petroleum-based barriers, and it seals out wetness on the perineum.
3. Place in microwave for 12 seconds. ▸ ***Rationale:*** Warming for a longer time can potentially burn the client's perineum. Washcloths may be used at room temperature.
4. Take warmed package to room.
5. Don clean gloves.

Procedure

1. Remove client's soiled gown and place in linen hamper. (Change gloves if they become contaiminated.)
2. Open package.
3. Clean soiled area by cleansing from front to back for females and tip of penis down shaft for males. ▸ ***Rationale:*** Prevents contamination. The cloths provide moisturizing, deodorizing, and a barrier protection.

4. Use a different cloth for each area of the perineum.
5. Discard soiled washcloths and package in appropriate receptacle.
6. Place new gown on client and change linen as needed.
7. Place client in position of comfort.
8. Remove gloves and place in appropriate receptacle.
9. Perform hand hygiene.

DOCUMENTATION for Perineal and Genital Care

- Assessment and care needs for perineal hygiene
- Client's level of understanding and teaching needs
- Perineal care provided and outcomes of care
- Type, amount, consistency of discharge from perineal area
- Presence of lesions, ulcerations, or other skin lesions
- Response of client to procedure
- Incontinence, number of times, and interventions attempted to control incontinence

CRITICAL THINKING Application

Expected Outcomes

- Perineal care has been comfortably and effectively provided.
- Perineal area is clean and odor-free, and without irritation or discharge.
- Skin remains intact after perineal care.

Unexpected Outcomes	Alternative Actions
Client has foul odor even after perineal care.	• Obtain order for sitz bath. • Request order for medicated solution. • Request culture of discharge so the appropriate treatment can be instituted.
Client develops urinary tract infection.	• Instruct client on proper technique for perineal care. • Instruct female clients to wash from anterior to posterior aspects of perineum, using different sections of cloth for each wipe. • Instruct male clients to wash from urethral opening down the shaft of the penis.

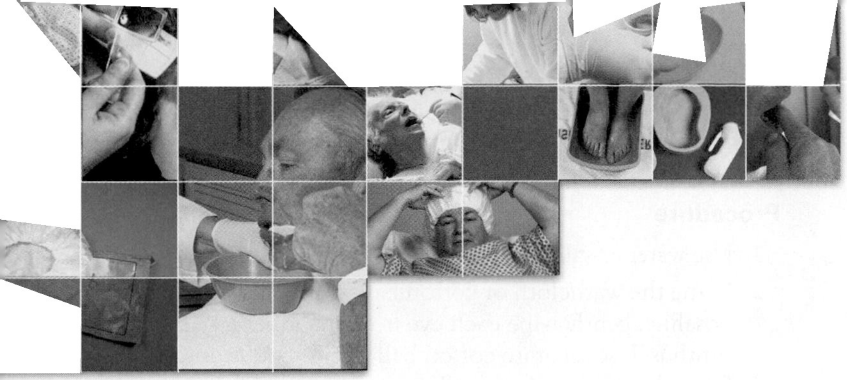

Chapter 9

UNIT 6

Eye and Ear Care

Nursing Process Data

ASSESSMENT Data Base

- Assess whether client is using eyeglasses or contact lenses or is experiencing any eye problems.
- Observe client's eyes for symmetry and clarity.
- Assess skin surrounding client's eyes for excessive dryness, scaling, and irritation.
- Assess eyes for discomfort, irritation, edema, crustation, sties, and lesions.
- Assess client's knowledge related to care of contact lenses.
- Observe client's tear duct areas and sclera for inflammation and excessive tearing.
- Assess client's pupils for response to light.
- Observe client's eye movements or muscle action.
- Evaluate ability to hear and effectiveness of hearing aid.

PLANNING Objectives

- To ensure that eyes and surrounding skin areas are clear, comfortable, and free of crustation
- To improve or maintain the client's vision
- To prevent irritation and infection
- To maintain or improve the client's appearance and self-esteem
- To increase ability to hear

IMPLEMENTATION Procedures

EVALUATION Expected Outcomes

- Eyes and surrounding area are clear and free of crustation.
- Vision is maintained or improved.
- Contact lenses are cleaned and replaced without difficulty.
- Hearing is improved after cleaning of hearing aid.

Providing Routine Eye Care

Equipment

Small basin

Water or normal saline solution

Washcloth or cotton balls

Clean gloves

Preparation

1. Determine client's eye care needs, and obtain physician's order if needed.
2. Explain necessity for and method of eye care to client. Discuss how client can assist you.
3. Collect necessary equipment.
4. Perform hand hygiene and don gloves.

Procedure

1. Use water or saline solution at room temperature.
2. Using the washcloth or cotton balls moistened in water or saline, gently wipe each eye from the inner to outer canthus. Use separate cotton ball or corner of washcloth for each eye. ▸ ***Rationale:*** To prevent cross-contamination from one eye to the other.
3. If crusting is present, gently place a warm, wet compress over eye(s) until crusting is loosened.
4. Dispose of used supplies and return basin to appropriate area.
5. Remove and discard gloves.
6. Perform hand hygiene.

Providing Eye Care for Comatose Client

Equipment

Water or normal saline solution

Washcloth, cotton balls, tissues

Sterile lubricant or eye preparations if ordered by the physician

Eye dropper or Asepto bulb syringe

Eye pads or patches

Clean gloves

Procedure

1. Perform hand hygiene and don clean gloves.
2. Cleanse the eyes using a moistened washcloth or cotton balls moistened in water or saline. Gently wipe each eye from inner to outer canthus. Use separate cotton ball or corner of washcloth for each eye. ▸ ***Rationale:*** Wiping from inner canthus to outer prevents particles and fluid from entering nasolacrimal duct.
3. Use a dropper to instill a sterile ophthalmic solution (liquid tears, saline, methylcellulose) every 3 to 4 hours as ordered by physician. (See procedure for *Instilling Eyedrops* in Chapter 18, Medication Administration.) ▸ ***Rationale:*** To prevent corneal drying and ulceration.
4. Keep client's eyes closed if blink reflex is absent. If eye pads or patches are used, explain their purpose to client's family. Do not tape eyes shut. ▸ ***Rationale:*** Corneal abrasions and drying occur when eyes lose blink reflex.
5. Remove gloves and perform hand hygiene.
6. Remove patch and evaluate condition of eye every 4 hours.

Removing and Cleaning Contact Lenses

Equipment

Towel

Contact lens container

Commercially prepared cleaning solution

Commercially prepared disinfecting solution

Commercially prepared rinsing and storing solution

Enzymatic agent (protein remover)

Clean gloves

Procedure

1. Place client in semi-Fowler's position and place a towel under the client's chin.
2. Perform hand hygiene and don gloves.
3. Place the tip of your thumb across the lower lid below its margin.
4. Place the tip of the forefinger of the same hand on the upper lid above its margin.
5. Spread eyelids apart as wide as possible and locate outer edges of soft lens which should appear as a rim around outer edge of iris.
6. Place thumb and forefinger directly on soft lens.
7. Gently remove soft lens from surface of eyeball by squeezing lens between thumb and fingertip. To remove rigid lens, place thumb on lower eyelid and index finger on upper lid. Press gently against eyeball to release suction; lens is released as eyelids meet lens edge. Catch lens in your hand. ▸ ***Rationale:*** Cornea is avascular and

Clinical Alert

- Extended-wear (overnight) contacts, rigid or soft, increase the risk of corneal ulcers, infection-caused eruptions on the cornea that can lead to blindness. Symptoms include visual changes, eye redness, eye discomfort or pain, and excessive tearing.
- Clean, rinse, and disinfect reusable lenses each time they are removed regardless of number of times each day. Always store lenses in storage solution, not water. Microorganisms from water can feed on corneal tissue.

use of contact lenses interrupts flow of oxygen into cornea. Removing lenses for a period of time allows oxygen to reach cornea and thus prevent corneal complications.

8. Release eyelids.
9. Place lens in palm of hand or place disposable lenses in trash. Some types of disposable lenses are cleaned and reused. Follow eye care specialist directions.
10. Place 2 to 3 drops of cleaning solution on lens.
11. Clean lens thoroughly by rubbing between fingertip and palm of hand for 20 to 30 seconds.
12. Rinse lens thoroughly with sterile saline solution or rinsing solution. Use only lens cleaning system recommended by ophthalmologist. Do not interchange cleaning solution systems.
13. Place lens in disinfecting solution according to physician directions. Time varies from hours to 1 full day. ▶ ***Rationale:*** This destroys microorganisms on lenses.
14. Rinse lens thoroughly with rinsing solution.
15. Repeat procedure on second lens.
16. Use enzyme tablet or solution according to physician orders, usually weekly. ▶ ***Rationale:*** This removes stubborn protein and lipids.
17. Clean lens container daily and leave open to dry. Replace as directed by physician, either weekly or monthly.
18. Remove gloves and perform hand hygiene.

NOTE: A suction cup can be placed gently against lens for easy removal of lens. Squeeze suction cup with dominant hand, place on lens, open finger slightly to create suction between lens and cup. Rock lens gently to remove it.

Client Teaching for Contact Lens Care

Instruct the client in the following safety issues:

- Notify physician immediately if eyes are red, not comfortable, or you can't see clearly.
- Use only rinsing solution, not saliva, to wet lenses.
- Use only commercially prepared saline solution or rinsing solution to cleanse lenses.
- Do not interchange types of lens cleaning systems.
- Maintain lens-care regimen prescribed by physician.
- Put on makeup before inserting lenses.
- Use appropriate type of lenses for their intended use. Do not use daily-wear lenses at night or disposable lenses more than once.
- Do not allow soft lenses to dry out.
- Contact lens wearers should be instructed to carry appropriate identification on type and care for specific lens he/she wears.

Cleaning and Checking a Hearing Aid

Equipment

Soap
Water
Petroleum jelly
Pipe cleaner
Cotton-tipped applicator
Hearing aid batteries
Clean gloves

Procedure

1. Determine ability of client to perform all or part of cleaning procedure, and teach procedure when necessary. Have client remove hearing aid if able to do so.
2. Perform hand hygiene and don gloves.
3. Wipe casing with dry cloth.

Types of Hearing Aids

- **Analog:** Two types, conventional and programmed. Programmed aids adjust amplifier more precisely to match hearing loss and provide greater fitting flexibility.
- **Digital:** Continuous sound waves are broken into small, discrete bits of information, digitalizing the signal. Computer programs are written for each client's hearing loss.

NOTE: 75% of all hearing aids sold are digital.

4. Check batteries if hearing aid has not been functioning. Insert new batteries, matching positive (+) and negative (−) signs.
5. Before inserting ear mold, cleanse outer ear gently with cotton-tipped applicator.

6. Turn receiver switch to ON. Assist client to adjust volume control to desired level. If whistling or feedback noises occur, check for tightness of fit as ear mold probably has not been inserted properly or there is a buildup of ear wax.
7. Place hearing aid in labeled container when not in use and place in bedside stand.
8. Remove gloves.
9. Perform hand hygiene.

Client Teaching for Hearing Aids

- Replace batteries when needed.
- Turn hearing aid off when not in use.
- Clean hearing aids according to manufacturers directions.
- Refrain from using hairspray or other hair products.
- Keep hearing aids away from moisture and heat.

Source: National Institute on Deafness and Other Communication Disorders (NIDCD), http://www.nidcd.nih.gov/health/hearingaid.asp.

DOCUMENTATION for Eye and Ear Care

- Documentation of eye assessment and eye care needs
- Method and outcome of eye care provided
- Condition of eye and surrounding structure
- Client's response to client teaching regarding contact lenses
- Response to using hearing aid
- Improved hearing after cleaning hearing aid
- Client's ability to insert, remove, and clean hearing aid

CRITICAL THINKING Application

Expected Outcomes

- Eyes and surrounding area are clear and free of crustation.
- Vision is maintained or improved.
- Contact lenses are cleaned and replaced without difficulty.
- Hearing is improved after cleaning of hearing aid.

Unexpected Outcomes	Alternative Actions
Eyelids become crusted from exudate.	• Place warm, moist washcloth across eyes and leave in place for several minutes. • Moisten cotton applicator stick with sterile saline and gently twist the applicator stick over crusted surface to assist in removing crust.
Wrong solution used on contact lens causes excessive tearing and burning sensation when lens is placed in eye.	• Immediately remove lens from eye and place in proper storage container. • Immediately rinse client's eye with copious amounts of sterile water. • Have client checked immediately by ophthalmologist for emergency care of potentially burned cornea.
Hearing did not improve with cleaning of hearing aid.	• Check if receiver switch is ON. • Check if batteries are properly in place and that the poles match: positive (+) and negative (−). • Recheck hearing aid with expert.

GERONTOLOGIC Considerations

Clients With Dentures Require Special Nursing Care

- Check for proper fit when replacing dentures. Ill-fitting dentures interfere with chewing and can lead to altered nutrition. Loss of teeth may limit meal planning and the nurse should assist the client to choose a balanced diet taking into account tooth loss.
- Monitor denture cleaning to ensure client has fresh-tasting mouth to encourage eating. Elderly clients have decreased

sensitivity to sweet, sour, salty, and bitter tastes; thus they may compensate by using extra salt. The nurse can counsel the client on alternative seasonings and request dietary consultation.

Fear of the unknown

- Any treatment or activity may be unfamiliar and frightening to the elderly.
- Explain each procedure before attempting it. Ask client to help when appropriate.

Self-Perception/Self-Concept

- Poor self-concept, depression, and negative feelings are common among elderly.
- Encourage personal hygiene activities to promote a more positive self-image.
- A positive body image is enhanced with good personal hygiene. Nursing care should focus on assisting the client to maintain good personal hygiene.
- Encourage elderly clients to have hair and nail care done frequently to increase self-esteem.

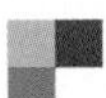

MANAGEMENT Guidelines

Each state legislates a Nurse Practice Act for RNs and LVN/LPNs. Healthcare facilities are responsible for establishing and implementing policies and procedures that conform to their state's regulations. Verify the regulations and role parameters for each healthcare worker in your facility.

Delegation

- The staffing patterns today often require that Certified Nursing Assistants (CNAs) or Unlicensed Assistive Personnel (UAPs) complete personal hygiene activities for most clients because these activities have a predictable outcome and do not require nursing judgment. However, performing these tasks for the client provides an excellent forum for client assessment. When the tasks are delegated to other personnel, the RN and LPN/LVNs responsible for client care must receive specific reports of the client's condition and any unexpected findings. The CNAs and UAPs should receive specific instructions regarding the condition of each client and what to observe for.
- The RN is responsible for assessing all clients because assessment responsibilities cannot be delegated.
- The team member delegating staff assignments should try to implement a staffing pattern that allows professional nurses to be assigned to complete general care, including personal hygiene activities, at least every other day so that important assessment parameters are not missed.
- Check facilities procedure manual for appropriate healthcare worker to remove and replace contact lenses.

Communication Matrix

- CNAs and UAPs should be educated, encouraged, and rewarded with positive feedback when they give excellent reports on the client for whom they have performed the tasks of personal hygiene. When the unit is extremely busy, this may be the major source of information the professional nurse receives about the client for whom he or she is legally responsible.

CRITICAL THINKING Strategies

Scenario 1

You have been assigned to two clients for the 7 AM to 12 noon clinical experience.

Client 1:

A 68-year-old female with a total hip replacement 2 days ago. Her past history indicates she had a cataract removed 2 months ago and had a lens fitted a week ago. She has developed a very uncomfortable incision site. It is red and tender to touch. Her dressings are somewhat moist without observable drainage on the dressings. Her vital signs indicate a temperature of 101°F, P 90, R 28 and unlabored. She tells you she doesn't feel like doing anything today.

Client 2:

An 80-year-old female with a fractured hip, unrepaired, admitted this morning from a local long-term care facility. She is in severe pain and requires pain medications every 4 hours. She is unable to use the patient-controlled analgesia (PCA) because she forgets how it works. Her physical assessment indicates her skin is reddened around the coccyx and very dry. She appears to be unkempt, and her hair is matted.

1. Based on the scenario, what is your first action after you hear report? Provide rationale for your answer.
2. Identify the assessment you will complete on each client. What information will you be gathering in order to make a decision on nursing care for the shift?
3. List, in priority, the nursing care you will provide for each client and provide rationale for your decision.
4. Which client will you assess first and why?
5. Which of the personal hygiene skills will you provide or can be delegated for each client? Will any adjustments need to be made in the skill in order to provide care for

the client? Please state the changes that will need to be made.

Scenario 2

You are working in a pediatric clinic when a mother brings her two preschool children into the clinic. She tells you she is not sure why her children keep scratching their scalps and have something that looks like dandruff. After examining the children's hair you determine they have lice. When the mother receives this information she starts crying and states, "I just knew that preschool was dirty. I should not have sent the children there."

1. What response will be appropriate to this statement?
2. After calming the mother down, how will you approach her to explain the treatment for lice?
3. You begin the explanation with a discussion of potential side effects. What will you tell her about the side effects?
4. Describe the skill of applying a treatment for lice.
5. While shampooing the hair, if the child starts crying and says her eyes are burning, what will you tell the mother to do?
6. Explain the most effective method for removing nits from the child's hair after the treatment.
7. The mother asks you if she needs to do the treatment once and then the lice will be gone. What is your response to her?
8. The mother wants to know if she and her husband can get the lice also. What is your response to her?
9. What is your best response to the mother's question on whether she needs to burn the sheets and children's clothes?

NCLEX® Review Questions

Unless otherwise specified, choose only one (1) answer.

1. You are assigned to provide hygienic care to an unconscious client. Your assessment indicates she needs good oral hygiene. The major safety action for this procedure is to
   1. Turn the client's head to the side.
   2. Keep a suction bulb or equipment at bedside.
   3. Use a tongue blade to keep the mouth open.
   4. Don clean gloves to prevent spread of bacteria.
2. A client has severely tangled hair. The best description on how to provide hair care for this client is to
   1. Brush or comb her hair from the scalp to hair ends.
   2. Apply small amount of oil to tangled areas of scalp before combing.
   3. Use a hair pick to untangle hair and then brush hair.
   4. Use short gentle strokes with a wide-toothed comb, starting at the end of hair shaft.
3. Which of the following statements is true regarding lice eggs? Lice eggs
   1. Are light brown, crawl, and feed on blood.
   2. Are yellow to white and attach to hair shaft.
   3. Hatch in 17 days after louse lays eggs.
   4. Have clawed legs that assist in jumping and hopping.
4. Identifying a live louse or nymph on the scalp is evidenced by nits/eggs located on the hair shaft
   1. Less than 1 cm from the scalp are usually not viable.
   2. Within 10 mm from the scalp are usually not viable.
   3. Within 6 mm are usually viable.
   4. Easily seen on the hair shaft are viable.
5. The primary intervention to prevent spread of lice or nits is to
   1. Discard all clothing and bedding used by client.
   2. Use one of the products to prevent lice on all family members at same time client is being treated.
   3. Launder all clothing and bedding in hot water, followed by drying using hot cycle of dryer.
   4. Observe family members for signs of nits near scalp; if present, use same treatment plan as client.
6. The client requires denture care but is unable to remove his dentures. When removing the dentures, the nurse will place his/her finger
   1. To the side of the lower denture and move it sideways to remove it.
   2. On the middle of the upper denture and ask the client to move it with his tongue.
   3. On the edge of the upper denture and gently break the suction.
   4. In the middle of the teeth on the lower denture and gently pull the denture upward to remove it.
7. When moving a client from the bed to the commode, the most appropriate movement to prevent client or nurse injury is to
   1. Instruct client to place hands around nurse's neck to stabilize stance when standing.
   2. Ensure the nurse bends back and squats when moving client out of bed.
   3. Stand in front of client, block client's toes with your feet and client's knees with your knees before starting to transfer.
   4. Maintain your hips and knees flexed when pivoting client to commode.

8. When providing male perineal care, it is important to remember
   1. That if the client is not circumcised, wash the penis carefully to prevent retraction of the foreskin.
   2. To wash the penis using a circular motion, starting at the base of the shaft and moving toward the tip.
   3. When washing the penis, do not wash over the same area without using a new cloth.
   4. To always wash the scrotum first before washing the perineum.

9. Client teaching for individuals who wear contact lenses should include explaining that
   1. Daily wear lenses can be worn overnight; however, they need to be disposed of once they are removed.
   2. You can use tap water or rinsing solution to wet reusable contact lenses.
   3. You can use interchangeable types of lens cleaning solutions regardless of type of contact lenses.
   4. Soft contact lenses should not be allowed to dry out.

10. A client asks you about caring for a hearing aid. Your response includes
    Select all that apply.
    1. You need to turn off the hearing aids when not in use.
    2. Keep hearing aids away from moisture and heat.
    3. Newer hearing aids do not have batteries that require changing.
    4. Hairspray should not be used when wearing hearing aids.

10

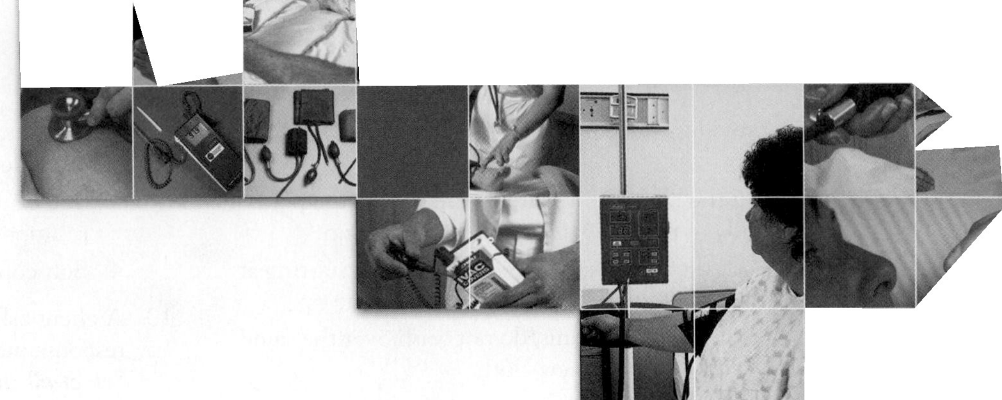

Vital Signs

LEARNING OBJECTIVES

1. Identify the cardinal signs that reflect the body's physiologic status.
2. List three mechanisms that increase heat production.
3. Explain how disease alters the "set point" of the temperature-regulating center.
4. Define hypothermia and list the symptoms of this condition.
5. Differentiate between the oral, rectal, axillary, and tympanic methods of taking temperature.
6. Describe two nursing actions that can be performed when temperature is not within normal range.
7. Describe at least three different types of pulse characteristics.
8. Discuss the pulse, and indicate how it is an index of heart rate and rhythm.
9. Compare normal heart rate range for adults and children.
10. Identify the characteristics of peripheral pulses.
11. Explain why the blood pressure cuff should be the appropriate size for the client.
12. Define Korotkoff's sounds in terms of phases.
13. Identify four of the seven factors that affect blood pressure.
14. Demonstrate the method of palpating systolic arterial blood pressure.
15. Discuss conditions when vital signs may be delegated and when they would not be delegated.
16. Demonstrate the proper techniques for obtaining peripheral pulses.
17. Describe the most effective method of obtaining a respiratory rate.

CHAPTER OUTLINE

TERMINOLOGY

General Terminology

Antipyretic an agent that reduces febrile temperatures.

Apex the pointed end of a cone-shaped part or organ (e.g., lower heart, upper lung).

Arteriosclerosis an arterial disease characterized by inelasticity and thickening of the vessel walls with lessened blood flow.

Atherosclerosis a form of arteriosclerosis in which there are localized accumulations of lipid-containing material within the internal surfaces of blood vessels.

Atrial pertaining to the atrium, the upper cardiac chamber that receives blood from the lungs and systemic circulation.

Autoregulation the intrinsic ability of an organ or tissue to maintain blood flow despite changes in arterial pressure.

Axilla armpit.

Cardiac output the amount of blood ejected by the heart or the stroke volume (SV) times the heart rate (CO = SV × HR).

Cardio pertaining to the heart.

Cardiogenic having origin in the heart itself.

Chemoreceptor a sense organ or sensory nerve ending that is stimulated by and reacts to chemical stimuli.

Contractility having the ability to contract or shorten muscle tissue or cells.

Core temperature the body's interior deep tissue temperature (e.g., the abdominal cavity).

Diastole the period in which the heart dilates and fills with blood; the period of relaxation.

Doppler a type of ultrasound stethoscope or probe that uses an ultrasound beam to detect blood flow.

Febrile feverish, increased body temperature.

Fibrillation quivering, involuntary contraction of individual muscle fibers.

Hypertension blood pressure that is considered to be higher than the normal range.

Hyperthermia unusually high body temperature.

Hypervolemia abnormal increase in the volume of circulating body fluid.

Hypotension blood pressure that is lower than the normal range.

Hypothalamus the part of the brain that lies below the thalamus; it maintains or regulates body temperature, certain metabolic processes, and other autonomic activities.

Hypothermia a body temperature below the average normal range.

Hypovolemia diminished blood volume.

Infarction an area of tissue in an organ or part that undergoes necrosis after cessation of blood supply.

Infrared scanner thermometer a noncontact digital thermometer that measures a client's temperature without physical contact by using infrared technology.

Ischemia local and temporary hypoxia due to obstruction of the circulation to a part.

Korotkoff's sounds low-frequency sounds that are regarded by the American Heart Association as the best index of blood pressure in an adult—sounds are produced as a result of changes in blood flow through a compressed artery.

mmHg millimeters of mercury, used for measuring blood pressure.

Myocardium the middle muscle layer of the walls of the heart.

Normotensive a normal tone, tension or pressure, as in normal blood pressure.

Palpate to examine by touch; feel.

Peripheral pertinent to the periphery, away from the central structure.

Peripheral vascular disease indicates diseases of the arteries and veins of the extremities, especially those conditions that interfere with adequate flow of blood.

Piloerection hair standing on end when heat production is stimulated through vasoconstriction.

Pyrogen any substance that produces fever.

Set point the constant temperature that the hypothalamus (the body's thermostat) strives to maintain.

Shock state of inadequate tissue perfusion resulting from circulatory failure, precipitated by many factors and identified by various signs and symptoms.

Sonorous loud breathing.

Sphygmomanometer instrument for indirectly determining arterial blood pressure.

Stertorous loud, noisy breathing.

Thermoregulation the body's physiological function of heat regulation to maintain a constant internal body temperature.

Valsalva's maneuver attempt to forcibly exhale with the glottis, nose, and mouth closed, producing an increased intrathoracic pressure.

Vasoconstriction constriction of the blood vessels and stimulation of heat production.

Vasodilation dilation of blood vessels and the inhibition of heat production.

Pulse Terminology

Atrial fibrillation atrial arrhythmia characterized by rapid, random contractions of the atrial myocardium causing a rapid, irregular ventricular rate.

Bigeminal pulse a regularly irregular pulse where every second beat has a decreased amplitude.

Bradycardia a pulse rate below 60 BPM.

Bounding pulse pulse pressure is increased. It is felt as a slapping against the fingers because of the rapid upstroke and quick downstroke. It is seen in conditions of increased cardiac output, such as exercise, anxiety, alcoholic intake, and pregnancy. It is also noted in pathology with fever, anemia, hyperthyroidism, liver failure, complete heart block with bradycardia, and hypertension.

Normal pulse pulse is smooth and rounded and is felt as a sharp upstroke and gradual downstroke. Provides information about cardiac status and blood volume. Correlates with cardiac contraction.

PMI apical pulse or point of maximum impulse; palpated at fifth intercostal space, left midclavicular line. Pulse occurs with contraction of left ventricle.

Premature beats a pacemaker outside the sinus node fires earlier than the sinus node, the normal pacemaker of the heart. Since the beat is early, the stroke volume is less because the ventricles do not have time to fill. This condition causes a pause in rhythm, which may result in a pulse deficit.

Pulse deficit occurs when the heart rate counted at the apex by auscultation is greater than the heart rate counted by palpation of the radial pulse. The pulse wave is not transmitted to the periphery to produce a palpable radial pulse.

Pulsus alternans rhythm is regular but the amplitude alternates from beat to beat. May be related to left ventricular failure.

Pulsus paradoxus detected by blood pressure measurement. The disappearance of Korotkoff's sounds during inspiration phase of breathing, with sounds appearing throughout the respiratory cycle (during inspiration and exhalation) at a pressure 10 mmHg lower than heard during exhalation alone. This phenomenon occurs in COPD and with cardiac tamponade and should be further evaluated.

Pulse pressure the difference between systolic and diastolic pressure (about 30 to 40 points).

Sinus arrhythmia common in children and young adults. The rate accelerates with inspiration and slows with expiration.

Tachycardia heart rate greater than 100 beats/min.

Weak or thready pulse pulse pressure is diminished. It is smooth and rounded, but is felt as a gradual upstroke and prolonged downstroke. It is commonly seen in conditions resulting in decreased cardiac output, such as heart failure and shock, and with obstruction to left ventricular ejection, such as aortic stenosis.

VITAL SIGNS

Vital signs, also termed cardinal signs, reflect the body's physiologic status and provide information critical to evaluating homeostatic balance. Vital signs include four critical assessment areas: temperature, pulse, respiration, and blood pressure. The term *vital* is used because the information gathered is the clearest indicator of overall health status. These four signs form baseline assessment data necessary for ongoing evaluation of a client's condition. If the nurse has established the normal range for a client, deviations can be more easily recognized. Although not a cardinal sign, pain is considered the fifth vital sign and must be assessed at the same time as all other vital signs.

Routine vital signs (including pain assessment) are important to assess on every client. These parameters should be assessed by a staff member who is familiar with the client's health history so results can be evaluated against previous data. Vital signs should be taken at regular intervals, and serial readings are important with all vital signs. In fact, trends yield more information than singular readings. The more critical the client's condition, the more often these assessments need to be taken and evaluated. They are not only indicators of a client's present condition, but are also cues to a positive or negative change in status.

Obtaining the total picture of a client's health status is a major objective of client care. Although vital signs yield important information in themselves, they gain even more relevance when compared with the client's diagnosis, laboratory tests, history, and records. The five vital signs are as follows:

1. *Temperature* represents the balance between heat gain and heat loss and is regulated in the hypothalamus of the brain. Variations in temperature indicate the health status of the body; thermostatic function may be altered by pyrogens, nervous system disease, or injury.
2. The *pulse* is an index of the heart's action; by evaluating its rate, rhythm, and volume, one can gain an overall impression of the heart's action.
3. *Respiration*, the act of bringing oxygen into the body and removing carbon dioxide, yields data on the client's entire breathing process. When the pattern of respiration is

altered, ongoing evaluation yields important clues to a client's changing condition.

4. *Blood pressure* readings provide information about the condition of the heart, the arteries and arterioles, vessel resistance, and the cardiac output. Serial readings provide the best indication of a client's cardiovascular status.
5. *Pain assessment* that is ongoing and constant is essential to maintain the client's homeostasis and quality of life. Pain assessment provides information on location, quality, and intensity, as well as outcomes of relief measures. (See Vital Sign Assessment Record.)

Factors Influencing Vital Signs

Factors that cause alterations in vital signs include age, gender, race, heredity, medications, lifestyle, environment, pain, exercise, anxiety, stress, metabolism, circadian rhythms, and hormones. The normal variations in vital signs may be caused by age, disease, trauma, etc. The most common alterations are listed below.

Age Age influences body temperature. Body temperature varies from 96.0° to 99.5°F in newborns and 96.8° to 98.3°F in elderly clients due to thermoregulation deficiencies in both age groups. Newborns have an immature thermoregulation mechanism that causes temperature fluctuations in response to the environment. Elderly clients have an ineffective thermoregulating system due to physiological changes of aging. These changes are related to loss of subcutaneous fat, decreased sweat glands, reduced metabolism, and poor vasomotor control. Environmental conditions may also play a role in an elderly person's ability to effectively adapt body heat and cooling to changes in external temperature. Respirations vary according to age as well. Newborns have a respiratory range of 30 to 80 breaths/minute with an average rate of 32 breaths/minute. As age increases, respirations decrease; adults average 16 breaths/minute. The pulse rate also decreases with age. Newborns average 140 beats/min and adults average 80 beats/min. On the other hand, blood pressure may increase with age. The newborn's mean blood pressure is 65/42, while the normal adult client's blood pressure ranges from 120/80 to 100/60.

VITAL SIGN ASSESSMENT RECORD

*SCALE 0 – Absent 1 – Markedly impaired 2 – Moderately impaired 3 – Slightly impaired 4 – Normal

KEY: Black/Blue – Heart Rate & Respirations RED – Temperature

	DATE
	TIME
HEART RATE	TEMP.
140	106°
130	105°
120	104°
110	103°
100	102°
90	101°
80	100°
70	99°
60	NORMAL 98°
50	97°
	RESPIRATIONS
	BLOOD PRESSURE
	WEIGHT
PERIPHERAL	(R/L)*
PULSES	SITE
PAIN SCALE (0–10) **	10
	5
	0
	INITIALS

Assessment Strategies applicable to all patients

Hierarchy of importance of Basic Measures of Pain Intensity

a. Patient's self report using a pain rating scale
b. Pathologic conditions or procedures that usually cause pain
c. Behaviors such as crying, facial expressions, body movements
d. Report of pain from parent, family or others close outpatient
e. Physiologic measures recognized as the least sensitive

Persistent pain

The RN shall communicate with the physician to coordinate an alternative treatment plan when pain is above the identified comfort goal in 2 consecutive assessments.

****Analgesic Rating Scale: 0–10**

0 = no pain 10 = worst pain

Pain Assessment Scales

Mild Pain Moderate Pain Severe Pain

No Pain Distressing Pain Unbearable Pain

0 1 2 3 4 5 6 7 8 9 10

Modified Wong-Baker FACES Pain Rating Scale

0 No Hurt 2 Hurts Little Bit 4 Hurts Little More 6 Hurts Even More 8 Hurts Whole Lot 10 Hurts Worst

Initials	Signature/Title	Initials	Signature/Title	Initials	Signature/Title	Initials	Signature/Title

COMMUNITY HOSPITAL

PATIENT I.D.#

NAME

SEX AGE SS#

▲ Vital signs assessment record.

Gender Women experience greater temperature fluctuations than men, probably due to hormonal changes. Temperature variations occur during the menstrual cycle. During menopause, the instability of the vasomotor controls leads to periods of intense body heat and sweating.

Race and Heredity Studies have been mostly inconclusive as to race and heredity being related factors in vital signs alteration. Blood pressure alterations appear to be the main difference in vital signs, usually as a result of particular groups being more susceptible to hemodynamic alterations. African Americans are more prone to high blood pressure resulting from increased salt sensitivity or increased blood cholesterol levels.

Medications Some medications can directly or indirectly alter temperature, pulse, respirations, and blood pressure. For example, narcotic analgesics can depress the rate and depth of respirations and lower blood pressure.

Pain Acute pain leads to sympathetic stimulation, which in turn increases the heart rate, respiratory rate, and blood pressure. Chronic pain decreases the pulse rate as a response to parasympathetic stimulation and may decrease heart rate and respirations.

Circadian Rhythms Biologic rhythms, or biorhythms, control certain physiological patterns in conjunction with environmental factors. The most familiar biorhythm is the circadian rhythm that controls sleep patterns. These rhythms influence blood pressure (pressure is lowest in the morning and peaks in late afternoon and evening) and temperature (highest in the evening—8 PM to 12 midnight—and lowest in the early morning—4 to 6 AM).

TEMPERATURE

Temperature control of the body is a homeostatic function, regulated by a complex mechanism involving the hypothalamus. The temperature of the body's interior (core temperature) is maintained within ±1°F except in the case of febrile illness. The surface temperature of the skin and tissues immediately underlying the skin rises and falls with a change in temperature of the surrounding environment. Core temperature is maintained when heat production equals heat loss. The temperature regulating center in the hypothalamus keeps the core temperature constant. Temperature receptors, which determine whether the body is too hot or too cold, relay signals to the hypothalamus.

Regulatory Mechanisms

When the body becomes overheated, heat-sensitive neurons stimulate sweat glands to secrete fluid. This enhances heat loss through evaporation. The vasoconstrictor mechanism of the skin vessels is reduced, thereby conducting heat from the core of the body to the body surface. Heat loss occurs through radiation, evaporation, and conduction.

When the body core is cooled below 98.6°F (37°C), heat conservation is affected. Intense vasoconstriction of the skin vessels results. There is also piloerection and a decrease in sweating to conserve heat. Heat production is stimulated by shivering and increased cellular metabolism.

The "set point" is the critical temperature level to which the regulatory mechanisms attempt to maintain the body's core temperature. Above the set point, heat-losing mechanisms are brought into play, and below that level, heat-conserving and heat-producing mechanisms are set into action.

Disease can alter the set point of the temperature-regulating center to cause fever, a body temperature above normal. Inflammation, brain lesions, pyrogens from bacteria or viruses, or degenerating tissue (i.e., gangrenous areas or myocardial infarction) also increase the set point. Dehydration can cause fever due to lack of available fluid for perspiration and by increasing the set point, which brings more heat-conserving and heat-producing mechanisms into play. When the "thermostat" is suddenly set higher, the client complains of feeling cold, has cool extremities, shivers, and has piloerection. Hypoxia can occur due to increased oxygen use with the increased metabolism of heat production. When the thermostat returns to normal, heat-losing mechanisms again are activated. The client feels hot and starts perspiring. Other symptoms of fever the client may experience are perspiration over the body surface, body warm to touch, flushed face, feeling cold alternately with feeling hot, increased pulse and respirations, malaise and fatigue, parched lips and dry skin, and convulsions, especially with rapid temperature increase in children.

When the body temperature falls below the normal range, the client experiences hypothermia and complains of being cold, shivers, and has cool extremities. Hypothermia may be caused by accidental cold exposure, frostbite, or GI hemorrhage. Medically induced hypothermia is used for some cardiovascular and neurosurgical interventions. The ability of the hypothalamus to regulate body temperature is greatly impaired when the body temperature falls below 94°F (34.4°C) and is lost below 85°F (29.4°C). Cellular metabolism and heat production are also depressed by a low temperature.

Fever Signs

Fever is considered to be any abnormal elevation of body temperature (over 100.8°F). The most common signs and symptoms are:

- Perspiration over the body surface
- Body warm to the touch
- Chills and shivers
- Flushed face
- Client complaints of feeling alternately cold and hot
- Increased pulse and respirations
- Complaints of malaise and fatigue
- Parched lips and dry skin
- Convulsions, especially in children

Measuring Body Temperature

Oral or rectal temperatures reflect the body's core temperature. Tympanic and axillary temperatures are somewhat variable but are clinically acceptable for tracking important changes. The normal range of an oral temperature is 97° to 99.5°F, or 36° to 37.5°C. Rectal temperatures are approximately 1°F higher, ear canal 0.5° higher, and axillary temperatures are 1°F lower than oral readings. Body temperature may vary according to age (lower for the aged), time of day (lower in the morning and higher in the afternoon and evening), amount of exercise, or extremes in the environmental temperature.

The thermometer is the instrument used to measure body heat. Oral and rectal (also used for axillary temperature) thermometers in hospitals are commonly, as of 2002, digital, disposable, and electronic. Before 1998, when the American Hospital Association agreed to eliminate mercury from the healthcare environment, mercury thermometers were used in hospitals. The thermometer is marked in degrees and tenths of degrees with either a Fahrenheit or Celsius (centigrade) scale and a range of 93° to 108°F (34°–42.2°C).

Electronic thermometers are now widely used in hospitals. They have disposable covers, which promote infection control, and therefore should always be used. The electronic thermometer plugs into a receptacle and has a heat sensor that records the client's core temperature in seconds. The ear canal provides another noninvasive site for temperature measurement using infrared thermometers.

Heat-sensitive tapes are also used to record temperature. A chemical strip tape is applied to the skin, and color changes indicate the temperature level. A continuous-reading wearable tape can be used for 2 days; the temperature is also read by a change in color. These tapes are both disposable and nonbreakable. They are most appropriate for use with small children and in situations when proper cleaning of the thermometer is difficult.

A new type of thermometer, the temporal artery (sensor touch by Exergen), is now being used in hospitals. It is more cost effective and more accurate than the ear thermometer. It takes 0.1 second to respond and automatically self-calibrates. This device is configured to give either oral or arterial temperatures.

PULSE

The pulse is an index of the heart's rate and rhythm. The apical pulse rate is the number of heart beats per minute. With each beat, the heart's left ventricle contracts and forces blood into the aorta. Closure of the heart valves creates the sounds heard. The forceful ejection of blood by the left ventricle produces a wave that is transmitted through the arteries to the periphery of the body. The pulse is a transient expansion of peripheral arteries resulting from internal pressure changes. If cardiac output is reduced (such as with a premature or irregular heartbeat), the peripheral pulse is weak; if the radial pulse rate is less than the apical rate, the difference is called a *pulse deficit*. The pulse wave is influenced by the elasticity of the larger vessels, blood volume, blood viscosity, and arteriolar and capillary resistance.

Circulatory System Control

The circulatory system is under the dual control of the autonomic nervous system and autoregulation (at the microcirculation level). This dual control allows the circulatory system to vary blood flow to meet the body's requirements. Local control of blood flow is called autoregulation. Blood flow is adjusted according to oxygen need based on changing metabolic activity of different tissues.

The autonomic nervous system regulates circulation through the vasomotor center in the medulla oblongata. Stimulation of the sympathetic nervous system causes vasoconstriction, increased heart rate and cardiac contractility, and a resulting increase in blood pressure. On the other hand, sympathetic inhibition causes vasodilation, reduced heart rate, and a reduction in blood pressure.

Pressure receptors, called baroreceptors, located in the walls of the carotid sinus and arch of the aorta also influence the vasomotor center. Decreased circulating volume (as in hemorrhage) stimulates these receptors, which then transmit signals to the vasomotor center to stimulate the sympathetic nervous system. Resulting cardiovascular responses divert blood flow to vital organs.

Heart Rate and Rhythm

A normal adult heart rate is from 60 to 100 beats/min; the average rate is 72 beats/min. Rates are slightly faster in women and more rapid in children and infants (90–140 beats/min; Table 10-1). The resting heart rate usually does not change with age. Tachycardia is a pulse rate over 100 beats/min. Bradycardia is a pulse rate below 60 beats/min.

When taking a client's pulse, be aware that many pathologic conditions produce bradycardia. Among the most common causes are decreased thyroid activity, hyperkalemia, cardiac conduction blocks, and increased intracranial pressure.

Tachycardia is associated with stressful conditions, hypoxia, exercise, and fever. Client conditions, such as congestive heart failure, hemorrhage and shock, dehydration, and anemia produce tachycardia as a compensatory response to poor tissue oxygenation.

Heart rhythm is the time interval between each heartbeat. Normally, the heart rhythm is regular, although slight irregularities do not necessarily indicate cardiac malfunction. An irregular cardiac rhythm, especially if sustained, requires cardiac evaluation because it may be indicative of cardiac disease.

Variance in heart rate, either increased or decreased, may be attributed to many factors, such as drug intake, lack of oxygen, loss of blood, exercise, and body temperature. When evaluating a pulse rate, it is important to ascertain the normal baseline for each client and then to determine variances from the normal for that particular client. The heart normally pumps about 5 L of blood through the body each minute. This cardiac output is calculated by multiplying the heart rate per minute by the stroke volume, the amount of blood ejected with one contraction. Increasing the heart rate is one of the first compensatory mechanisms the body employs to maintain cardiac output.

Evaluating Pulse Quality

The quality of the pulse is determined by the amount of blood pumped through the peripheral arteries. Normally, the amount of pumped blood remains fairly constant; when it varies, it is also indicative of cardiac malfunction. A so-called bounding pulse occurs when the nurse is able to feel the pulse by exerting only a slight pressure over the artery. If, by exerting pressure, the nurse cannot clearly determine the flow, the pulse is called weak or thready.

The arterial pulse can be felt over arteries that lie close to the body surface and over a bone or firm surface that can support the artery when pressure is applied. In adults and children older than age 3, the radial artery is palpated most frequently because it is the most accessible. The femoral and carotid arteries are used in cases of cardiac arrest to determine the adequacy of perfusion.

Peripheral pulses may be absent or weak. The amplitude of a pulse depends on the degree of filling in the artery during systole (ventricular contraction) and emptying during diastole

TABLE 10-1 Vital Sign Chart for Children

Age	Normal Pulse Range	Normal Pulse Average	Blood Pressure Average	Respiration Average
Newborn	110–180	140	90/55	30–50
1 year	80–150	120	90/60	20–40
2 years	80–130	110	95/60	20–30
4 years	80–120	100	99/65	20–25
6 years	75–115	100	100/56	20–25
8 years	70–110	90	105/56	15–20
10 years	70–110	90	110/58	15–20

(ventricular relaxation). It is important to note characteristics of peripheral pulses: 0 = absent; 1+ = weak; 2+ = diminished; 3+ = strong; and 4+ = full and bounding. (Use the system described in your hospital procedure manual.)

When peripheral pulses cannot be palpated, a Doppler ultrasound stethoscope is used by the nurse to confirm the presence or absence of the pulse. Even though the peripheral pulse is an indicator of cardiac function, it is not always an accurate indication of the force of cardiac contractions. If cardiac contractions are weak or ventricular filling is incomplete, the pulse is weak; however, in the case of aortic stenosis, the pulse may be weak in spite of forceful cardiac contraction.

The pulse should be taken frequently (every 15 minutes to 1–2 hours) on an acutely ill hospitalized client and less frequently (every 4–8 hours) on more stable hospitalized clients. Once a week or even once a month is adequate for clients in long-term care facilities. Do not wait until the next routinely scheduled time if the client develops unexpected symptoms or has experienced trauma.

RESPIRATION

Respiration is the process of bringing oxygen to body tissues and removing carbon dioxide. The lungs play a major role in this process. Another respiratory function is to maintain arterial blood homeostasis by maintaining the pH of the blood. The lungs accomplish this by the process of breathing.

Breathing consists of two phases, inspiration and expiration. Inspiration is an active process in which the diaphragm descends, the external intercostal muscles contract, and the chest expands to allow air to move into the tracheobronchial tree. Expiration is a passive process in which air flows out of the respiratory tree.

The respiratory center in the medulla of the brain and the level of carbon dioxide in the blood both control the rate and depth of breathing. Peripheral receptors in the carotid body and the aortic arch also respond to the level of oxygen in the blood. To some extent, respiration can be voluntarily controlled by holding the breath and hyperventilation. Talking, laughing, and crying also affect respiration.

The diaphragm and the intercostal muscles are the main muscles used for breathing. Other accessory muscles, such as the abdominal muscles, the sternocleidomastoid, the trapezius, and the scalene, can be used to assist with respiration if necessary.

Evaluating Respirations

The quality of breathing is important baseline information. Normal breathing, termed eupnea, is almost invisible, effortless, quiet, automatic, and regular. When the breathing pattern varies from normal, it needs to be evaluated thoroughly. For example, bronchial sounds heard over the large airways are fairly loud. There is normally a pause between inspiration and expiration. Softer sounds are heard over peripheral lung areas, and there are no pauses between inspiration, which is a long sound, and expiration, which is a short sound. If breathing is noisy, labored, or strained, an obstruction may be affecting the breathing pattern that could lead to major alterations in homeostasis.

In addition to evaluating the breathing pattern, it is also necessary to evaluate the rate and depth of breathing. The normal rate for a resting adult is 12 to 18 breaths per minute. A rate of 24 or above is considered tachypnea, and a rate of 10 or less is considered bradypnea. The rate for infants ranges from 20 to 30 breaths per minute and is often irregular. Older children average about 20 to 26. The ratio of pulse to breathing is usually 5:1 and remains fairly constant.

The depth of a person's breathing (tidal volume) is the amount of air that moves in and out with each breath. The tidal volume is 500 mL in the healthy adult. Alveolar air is only partially replenished by atmospheric air with each inspiratory phase. Approximately 350 mL (tidal volume minus dead space) of new air is exchanged with the functional residual capacity volume during each respiratory cycle. Accurate tidal volume can be measured by a spirometer, but an experienced nurse can judge the approximate depth by placing the back of the hand next to the client's nose and mouth and feeling the expired air. Another method of estimating volume capacity is to observe chest expansion and to check both sides of the thorax for symmetrical movement.

After assessing the pattern, rate, and depth of breathing, it is important to observe the physical characteristics of chest expansion. The chest normally expands symmetrically without rib flaring or retractions. In addition, observation of chest deformities should also be made, as all of these signs yield information about the respiratory process and overall health status of the client.

BLOOD PRESSURE

The heart generates pressure during the cardiac cycle to perfuse the organs of the body with blood. Blood flows from the heart to the arteries, into the capillaries and veins, and then flows back to the heart. Blood pressure in the arterial system varies with the cardiac cycle, reaching the highest level at the peak of systole and the lowest level at the end of diastole. The difference between the systolic and diastolic blood pressure is the pulse pressure, which is normally 30 to 50 points (mmHg).

There are seven major factors that affect blood pressure:

Cardiac Output The force of heart contractions (the amount of blood ejected by the heart) influences blood pressure, especially systolic pressure.

Peripheral Vascular Resistance Resistance to the flow of blood is due to resistant vessels under the influence of the autonomic nervous system. Peripheral vascular resistance is the most important determinant of diastolic pressure.

Elasticity and Distensibility of Arteries Elasticity refers to the action of the blood vessel walls to spring back after blood is ejected into them. When blood is ejected into the aorta and large arteries, the arterial vessel walls distend. Recoil during diastole propels blood through the arterial tree and maintains diastolic pressure. Both elasticity and distensibility decrease with age, resulting in increased systolic pressure and slightly increased diastolic pressure.

Blood Volume Increased blood volume causes an increase in both systolic and diastolic blood pressure, whereas decreased blood volume causes the reverse effect. Hemorrhage decreases blood pressure, whereas overhydration from excessive blood transfusions may cause an increase in blood pressure.

Blood Viscosity Blood viscosity (thickness) influences blood flow velocity through the arterial tree. For example, increased viscosity, which occurs with polycythemia, increases resistance to blood flow, whereas decreased viscosity, resulting from anemia, decreases resistance.

Hormones and Enzymes These substances have an important influence on blood pressure. For example, epinephrine and norepinephrine produce a profound vasoconstrictor effect on peripheral blood vessels (mediators of the sympathetic nervous system). Aldosterone (released by the adrenal cortex), renin (released by the juxtaglomerular apparatus of the kidney), and angiotensin (activated by the renin response) also produce effects that raise blood pressure. Histamine and acetylcholine (a parasympathetic mediator) cause vasodilation, therefore lowering blood pressure.

Chemoreceptors Chemoreceptors in the aortic arch and carotid sinus also exert control over the blood pressure. They are sensitive to changes in PaO_2, $PaCO_2$, and pH. Decreased PaO_2 stimulates the chemoreceptors, which stimulate the vasomotor center. Increased $PaCO_2$ and decreased pH directly stimulate the vasomotor center, causing increased peripheral vascular resistance.

Measuring Blood Pressure

Measuring arterial blood pressure provides important information about the overall health status of the client. For example, the systolic pressure provides a database about the condition of the heart and great arteries. The diastolic pressure indicates arteriolar or peripheral vascular resistance. The pulse pressure, or difference between the systolic and diastolic pressure, provides information about cardiac function and blood volume. A single blood pressure reading, however, does not provide adequate data from which conclusions can be drawn about all of these factors. Rather, a series of blood pressure readings should be taken to establish a baseline for further evaluation.

The *indirect method* of taking a blood pressure using a recently calibrated aneroid manometer and a stethoscope is accurate for most clients. New electronic blood pressure devices constantly monitor systolic, diastolic, and mean readings at preset time intervals and are helpful to measure blood pressure trends in clients who are at risk for hyper- or hypotension. These devices also provide a printout if needed for documentation. If a stethoscope is unavailable or the brachial artery amplitude is decreased, the brachial or radial artery can be palpated as the blood pressure cuff is inflated to determine the systolic blood pressure (palpated pulse disappears at this point). Alternatively, an inflated blood pressure cuff may be slowly deflated and the point at which distal pulsation is first palpated reflects systolic blood pressure. Those who are severely hypotensive or hypertensive (hemodynamically unstable), have low blood volume, or are on rapid-acting intravenous vasoconstricting or vasodilating drugs should have blood pressure measured by direct (intraarterial) method. The *direct method* is continuous and measures mean arterial pressures. A needle or catheter is inserted into the brachial, radial, or femoral artery. An oscilloscope displays arterial pressure waveforms.

Normal blood pressure in an adult varies between 100 and 120 systolic and 60 and 80 diastolic (See box on Blood Pressure Classification on page 273.) As blood moves toward smaller arteries and into arterioles, where it enters the capillaries, pressure falls to 35. It continues to fall as blood goes through the capillaries, where the flow is steady and not pulsatile. As blood moves into the venous system, pressure falls until it is the lowest in the venae cavae.

Blood pressures vary widely. A blood pressure of 100/60 may be normal for one person but may be hypotensive for another. Hypotension (90–100 systolic) in a healthy adult without other clinical symptoms is little reason for concern.

Blood pressure readings are recorded in association with Korotkoff's sounds. These sounds are described as "K" phases. The systolic, or first, pressure reading occurs with the advent of the first Korotkoff's sound. The systolic reading represents the maximal pressure in the aorta after contraction of the left ventricle and is heard as a faint tapping sound.

According to American Heart Association standards, the diastolic, or second, reading should be taken at the time of the last Korotkoff's sound (phase V) for adults. The diastolic reading represents the minimal pressure exerted against the arterial walls at all times. In children under age 13, pregnant women, and clients with high cardiac output or peripheral vasodilation, sounds are often heard to a level far below muffling and sometimes to levels near 0. In these individuals, muffling (phase IV) should be used to indicate diastolic pressure, but both muffling (phase IV) and disappearance (phase V) should be recorded (e.g., 110/80/20).

Frequency of blood pressure assessment should be individualized or as ordered. Blood pressure for an acutely ill client should be taken every 15 minutes to 1 to 2 hours and the blood pressure of more stabilized clients should be taken every 4 to 8 hours to once a day. Clients with severe hypotension or hypertension, with low blood volume, or those on vasoconstrictor or vasodilator drugs require checking every 5 to 15 minutes.

There are approximately 58 million Americans with hypertension, and only 25% are controlled to normotensive. Another 30% were not even aware they had the disease. High blood pressure is one of the leading risk factors for cardiovascular disease.

Currently there are five methods of lifestyle modification suggested for management of hypertension:

1. Weight reduction
2. Diet modification (one rich in fruits and vegetables, with a reduced amount of saturated and total fat)
3. Sodium reduction
4. Physical activity—regular aerobic exercise
5. Moderate alcohol intake

The other important method of reducing blood pressure is prescriptive medications, monitored by a physician.

PAIN

According to The Joint Commission, pain should be considered the fifth vital sign. Pain must be evaluated every time vital signs are taken, and it should be documented on the vital sign record. Refer to Chapter 16, Pain Management, for a more in-depth explanation of pain and the options available for pain management.

CULTURAL AWARENESS

Many cultures believe that certain substances protect one's health. For example, Italians, Greeks, and Native Americans believe that garlic or onions eaten raw or worn on the body will prevent an illness such as high blood pressure. If a client wishes to include these items in his or her diet or wear them, the nursing staff should respect this practice, since it is an important cultural tradition for many groups.

NURSING DIAGNOSES

The following nursing diagnoses are appropriate to use on client care plans when the components are related to vital signs.

NURSING DIAGNOSIS	RELATED FACTORS
Ineffective Airway Clearance	Obstruction of airway, increased secretions, fatigue
Ineffective Breathing Pattern	Change in rate, depth, or pattern of breathing that alters normal gas exchange
Decreased Cardiac Output	Hypovolemia, rapid pulse, changes in breathing patterns, alteration in heart rhythm or rate, or vascular tone
Deficient Fluid Volume	Excessive urinary output, abnormal fluid loss, infection, fever
Excess Fluid Volume	Decreased cardiac output, fluid retention, inflammatory process, low protein diet, increased fluid intake
Chronic Pain	Chronic disease conditions, tissue trauma, injury
Ineffective Thermoregulation	Disease, infection, drug reactions, or damage to the hypothalamic temperature regulating center; possibly dehydration
Ineffective Peripheral Tissue Perfusion	Vascular disorders, hypovolemia, medications, hypoxemia
Impaired Spontaneous Ventilation	Metabolic factors; respiratory muscle fatigue

CLEANSE HANDS The single most important nursing action to decrease the incidence of hospital-based infections is hand hygiene. *Remember to wash your hands or use antibacterial gel before and after each and every client contact.*

IDENTIFY CLIENT Before every procedure, introduce yourself and check two forms of client identification, not including room number. These actions prevent errors and conform to The Joint Commission standards.

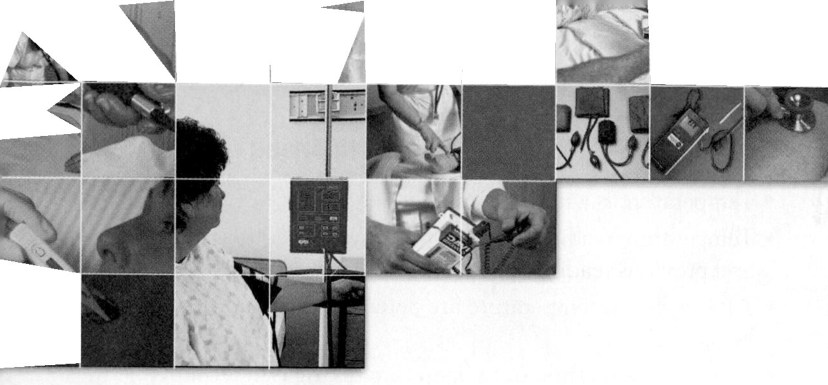

Chapter 10

UNIT 1

Temperature

Nursing Process Data

ASSESSMENT Data Base

- Determine number of times temperature needs to be taken daily.
- Assess temperature in relationship to time of day and age of client.
- Compare temperature with other vital signs to establish baseline data.
- Determine the method most appropriate for obtaining temperature.

Oral Method

- Accurate method of determining body temperature
- Used only for alert and cooperative clients; not unconscious clients or those with active signs
- Not appropriate for use with tachypneic or mouth-breathing clients
- Not appropriate for clients with oral inflammatory processes or oral surgery
- Delivery of oxygen by nasal cannula does not affect oral temperature readings
- Determine client has not taken hot or cold liquids or smoked for 15 to 30 minutes before taking temperature orally

Rectal Method

- Appropriate for tachypneic, uncooperative, confused, or comatose clients or for clients on seizure precautions
- Used for clients with open-mouth breathing, such as those with nasal or oral intubation
- Appropriate for clients with wired jaws, facial fractures, or other abnormalities, or for clients with nasogastric tubes who cannot breathe easily with mouth closed
- Contraindicated for infants or clients who have had surgery involving the rectum

Axillary Method

- Least accurate, but safe
- Often used for infants and young children
- Used in recovery rooms to avoid turning clients
- Time-consuming

Electronic Thermometer

- Accurate for oral or rectal temperature measurement, but inaccurate for axillary temperature measurement
- Prevents infection between clients
- Time-efficient and easy to read

Infrared Ear Thermometer

- Measures body heat radiating from the tympanic membrane
- Noninvasive, safe, efficient
- Less sensitive in detecting fever in the very young child and infant

Infrared Scanner Thermometer

- Measures temperature without physical contact via infrared technology.
- Used for children or unconscious clients.

Heat Sensitive Tape

- Disposable and nonbreakable
- Appropriate for children when proper cleaning of thermometer is difficult

PLANNING Objectives

- To determine whether core temperature is within normal range
- To provide baseline data for further evaluation
- To determine alterations in disease conditions

IMPLEMENTATION Procedures

EVALUATION Expected Outcomes

- Temperature is within normal range.
- Temperature readings are compared with age, time of day, and previous readings.
- Alterations in temperature are detected early and treatment begun.
- Appropriate method of temperature taking is determined for each client.
- Correct length of time is used for thermometer insertion to obtain an accurate reading.

Pearson Nursing Student Resources

Find additional review materials at **nursing.pearsonhighered.com**

Prepare for success with NCLEX®-style practice questions and Skill Checklists

Using a Digital Thermometer

Equipment

Client's individual digital thermometer or if multiple client use, thermometer with disposable sheaths

Gloves, if necessary

Procedure

1. Perform hand hygiene.
2. Don gloves if risk of contact with saliva.
3. Identify client with two forms of ID.

For Oral Temperature

a. Wait 20 to 30 minutes to take oral temperature if client has been eating, drinking, chewing gum, smoking, or exercising. ▸ ***Rationale:*** These activities may alter the temperature.

b. Place thermometer in client's mouth under front of tongue and along gum line. ▸ ***Rationale:*** Location ensures contact with large vessels under tongue.

c. Have client hold lips closed and leave thermometer in place for 45 to 90 seconds. The alert sound will indicate time. ▸ ***Rationale:*** Open-mouth breathing produces abnormally low readings.

d. Remove thermometer and read temperature displayed in digital window.

For Axillary Temperature

a. Assist client to comfortable position and expose axilla area.

b. Dry axilla if necessary. ▸ ***Rationale:*** A false low reading may result if axilla is moist.

c. Place thermometer in center of axilla and lower arm down across chest. ▸ ***Rationale:*** This position allows thermometer to be in contact with large vessels.

d. Leave in place 1 to 2 minutes. ▸ ***Rationale:*** Axilla temperature recordings take a longer time to register.

4. Record temperature noting route and return thermometer to its case at client's bedside stand.
5. Perform hand hygiene.

TABLE 10-2 Comparing Centigrade and Fahrenheit Temperatures

Centigrade (C)	Fahrenheit (F)
36.0	96.8
36.5	97.7
37.0	**98.6**
37.5	99.5
38.0	100.4
38.3	101.0
39.0	102.2
39.5	103.1
40.0	104.0

To convert degrees F to degrees C, subtract 32, then divide by 1.8. To convert degrees C to degrees F, multiply by 1.8, then add 32.

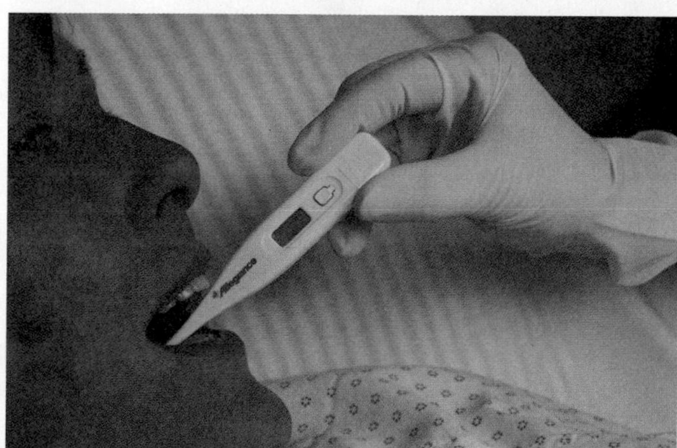

▲ Place thermometer in client's mouth under tongue.

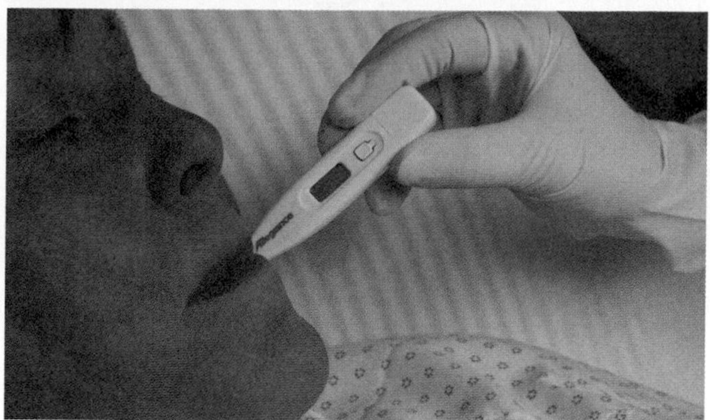

▲ Ask client to hold lips closed and leave thermometer in place 45–90 seconds.

EVIDENCE-BASED PRACTICE

Reducing Mercury in Hospitals

A survey of American hospitals released in late September 2005 indicated that 97% of hospitals have taken steps to reduce or eliminate mercury. Seventy-two percent of hospitals have inventoried and replaced mercury-containing devices or labeled them for proper handling.

Source: Survey conducted by American Hospital Association, Health Care Without Harm, and U.S. Environmental Protection Agency.

Clinical Alert

Temperature varies with time of day: It is highest between 5 and 7 PM and lowest between 2 and 6 AM. This variation is termed *circadian thermal rhythm.* A consistent method of body temperature measurement should be used so that readings are comparable.

Mercury Thermometers

Mercury thermometers are no longer used in hospitals. In 2001, a U.S. senator introduced a comprehensive bill to totally eliminate and retire mercury because of its toxic effects on people and the environment.

Using an Electronic Thermometer

Equipment

Electronic thermometer unit with digital readout and probe
Disposable cover for thermometer
Lubricant on tissue (for rectal temperature)
Clean gloves

Procedure

1. Perform hand hygiene and don gloves, if necessary.
2. Remove thermometer from charger unit.
3. Place carrying strap around your neck or remove thermometer from rolling stand.
4. Grasp probe at top of stem using your thumb and forefinger. ▸ ***Rationale:*** Pressure on top releases the ejection button.
5. Firmly insert probe in disposable probe cover.
6. Identify client with two forms of ID.
7. Provide privacy for rectal temperature.

Clinical Alert

Temperature assessment is the single most important infection control monitoring criterion for HAIs (nosocomial infections) and fever of unknown origin.

For Oral Temperature

a. Instruct client to open mouth. Slide probe under front of client's tongue and along the gum line in the sublingual pocket. ▸ ***Rationale:*** The larger blood vessels in the pocket more accurately reflect the core temperature.
b. Instruct client to close lips (not teeth). Lips should close at the ridge on the probe cover.

For Rectal Temperature

a. Don clean gloves. ▸ ***Rationale:*** Prevents exposure to feces.
b. Position client on side facing away from you, separate buttocks, instruct client to take in a deep breath, and insert covered and lubricated probe ¼ to 1 ½ in. (depending on client's age) through anal sphincter. ▸ ***Rationale:*** Taking in a deep breath relaxes the sphincter and the lubrication prevents tissue trauma.
c. Position probe to side of rectum to ensure contact with tissue wall. ▸ ***Rationale:*** This ensures probe is in contact with large vessels of rectal wall.

8. Remove probe when audible signal occurs. Client's temperature is now registered on the dial.
9. Discard oral probe cover into trash by pushing ejection button.
   a. Discard rectal probe cover, tissue, and gloves. ▸ ***Rationale:*** Proper disposal prevents transmission of microorganisms.
   b. Wipe anal area to remove lubricant and stool.
10. Assist client to comfortable position.
11. Perform hand hygiene.
12. Record temperature, and then return probe to storage well. ▸ ***Rationale:*** This ensures that system is ready for next use.
13. Return thermometer unit to charging base. Ensure charging base is plugged into electric outlet.

Clinical Alert

The temperature of an unconscious client is never taken by mouth. The rectal, tympanic, or scanner method is preferred.

Clinical Alert

Only use client's own dedicated electronic thermometer (including rectal and oral) if diagnosis includes *Clostridium difficile*-associated diarrhea because of the potential for spreading the bacteria and increasing the risk of transmitting an HAI (nosocomial) to other clients.

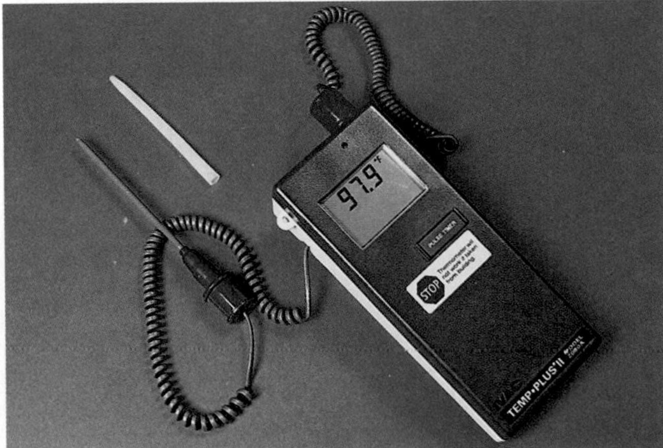

▲ Electronic thermometer unit with digital probe.

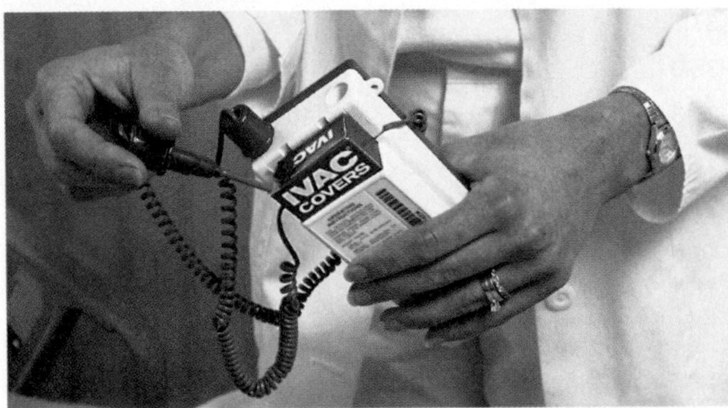

▲ Cover probe of thermometer before taking temperature.

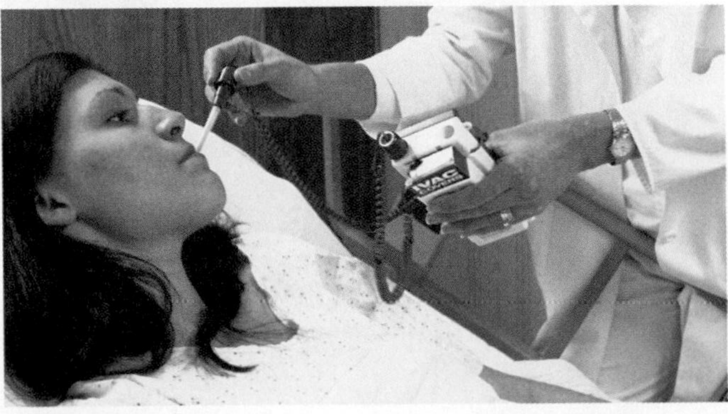
▲ Slide probe under front of tongue to sublingual pocket.

Measuring an Infant or Child's Temperature

Equipment

Digital or electronic thermometer with disposable probe cover
Water-soluble lubricant
Gloves, if necessary

Procedure

1. Determine appropriate thermometer and route for child. ▸ ***Rationale:*** Oral route is appropriate only for child over 3 years of age. Electronic, nonbreakable thermometer or scanner is preferred.
2. Perform hand hygiene and identify client with two forms of ID.
3. Explain procedure at child's level of understanding.
4. Remove probe from cover or attach probe tip to electronic thermometer.

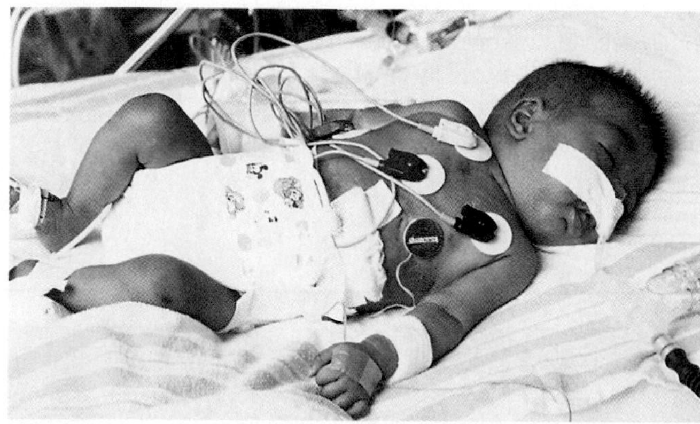

▲ The new scanner method is often used for children who are unconscious, have seizures, or have a structural abnormality.

For Oral Route (only for child 3 years or older)

a. Place probe under child's tongue, one side or the other.
b. Have child close mouth and either hold thermometer in place or monitor while taking temperature.
c. Leave digital thermometer in place for 45 to 90 seconds or remove electronic thermometer when audible signal occurs.

For Rectal Route

a. Place infant or child in prone or side-lying position.
b. Lubricate probe.
c. Insert thermometer ¼ to ½ in. into rectum for infant or ½ to 1 in. for child and hold in place.
d. Turn on scanner and follow directions.
e. Remove probe when tone or beep is heard.

For Axillary Route

a. Assist infant or child to a comfortable position and expose axilla.
b. Dry axilla if necessary. ▸ ***Rationale:*** A moist axillary area can produce a false low reading.
c. Place thermometer in center of axilla. Lower child's arm down and across the chest. ▸ ***Rationale:*** This position ensures that thermometer remains in contact with large vessels of axilla.
d. Leave in place 1-2 minutes or until tone is heard. ▸ ***Rationale:*** Axillary temperature recordings take longer to register than oral or rectal.

5. Read and record temperature; indicate method.
6. Discard probe cover into trash by pushing ejection button, or return digital thermometer into its case.

Using an Infrared Thermometer for Tympanic Temperature

Equipment

Infrared thermometer unit
Disposable probe cover

NOTE: A tympanic thermometer measures the infrared energy that naturally radiates from the tympanic membrane and surrounding tissues.

Procedure

1. Perform hand hygiene and identify client with two forms of ID.
2. Attach disposable cover centering probe on film and press firmly until backing frame of probe cover engages base of probe. ▸ ***Rationale:*** Cover protects client from transmission of microorganisms.
3. Turn the client's head to one side and stabilize the client's head.
4. Pull pinna upward and backward for an adult or down and backward for a child. ▸ ***Rationale:*** This procedure provides better access to the ear canal.
5. Center probe and gently advance into ear canal to make a firm seal, directing probe toward tympanic membrane. ▸ ***Rationale:*** Pressure close to the tympanic membrane seals ear canal and allows for accurate reading.
6. Press and hold temperature switch until green light flashes and temperature reading displays (approximately 3 seconds). ▸ ***Rationale:*** Method records core body temperature.
7. Remove thermometer. Discard probe cover.
8. Return thermometer to home base or storage unit for recharge.

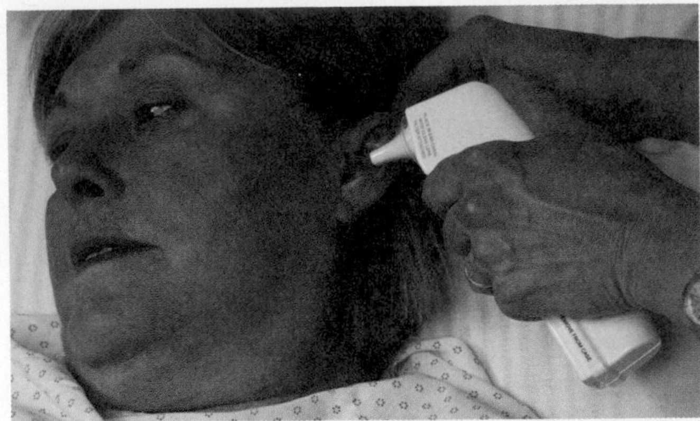

▲ Position client so ear canal is easily seen and pull pinna back and up.

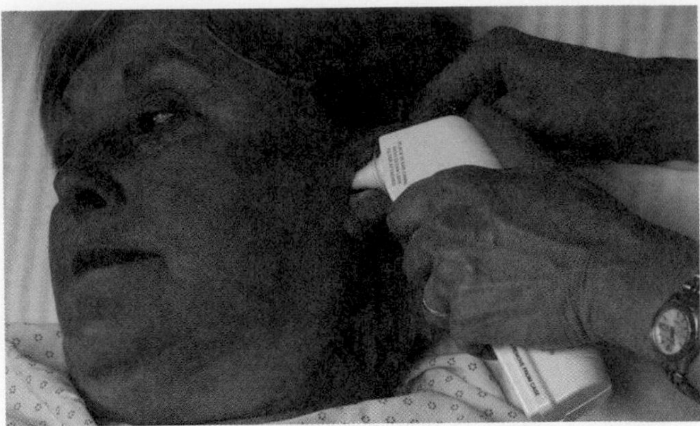

▲ Place probe in client's ear and advance into ear canal to make a firm seal.

9. Keep lens clean using lint-free wipe or alcohol swab, then wipe dry. Do not use povidone-iodine (Betadine).
10. Perform hand hygiene.
11. May be used for clients over 3 months of age.

Clinical Alert
Do not use ear thermometer in infected or draining ear or if adjacent lesion or incision exists.

EVIDENCE-BASED PRACTICE

Correct Technique for Taking a Tympanic Temperature

Studies on the correct technique for taking a tympanic temperature indicate that the ear tug (pulling the pinna upward and backward for an adult and down and backward for a child) is essential for an accurate reading. Eliminating this step will not allow the thermometer to be directly at the tympanic membrane.

Source: The Joanna Briggs Institute. (1999). Vital signs. *Best Practice*, 3(3), 5. http://www.joannabriggs.edu.au/pdf/BPISEng_3_3.pdf.

Using an Infrared Scanner Thermometer

Equipment

Scanner temperature thermometer

Procedure

1. Check orders for scanner device (may be used with children to check temperature without waking).
2. Press power button to turn device on. Check to see thermometer is in person mode (see symbol in window).
3. Press and hold scan button. "00" will be displayed.
4. Aim infrared lens at client's forehead, holding thermometer 2 to 3 in. away.
5. Release scan button and note reading that is displayed.
6. Clean device with antiseptic wipe.
7. Record temperature in record.

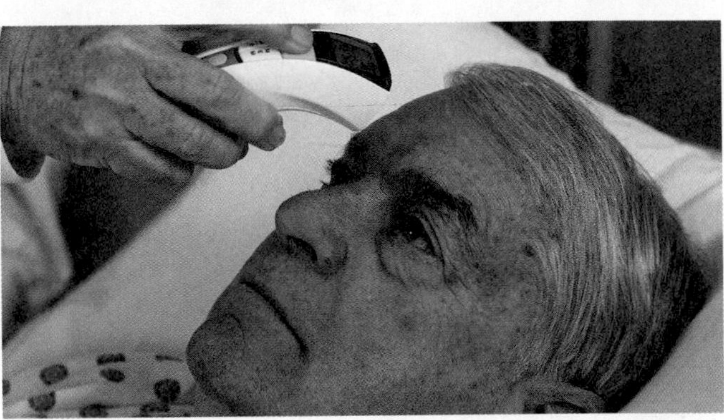

▲ Follow manufacturer's directions for scanner device.

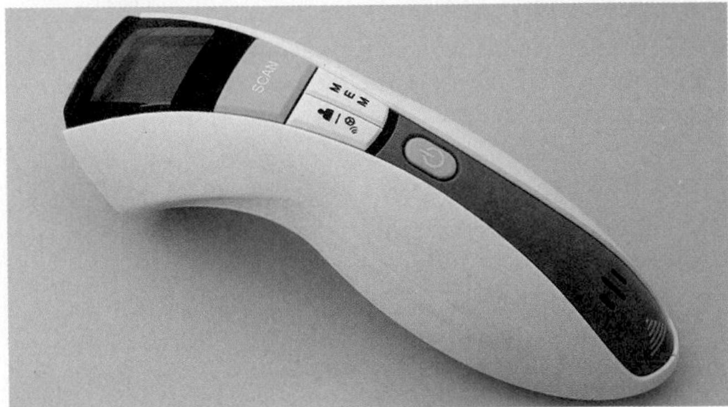

▲ After releasing scan button, note reading in window.

Using a Heat-Sensitive Wearable Thermometer

Equipment

Wearable thermometer (TraxIt), chemical strip tape or liquid crystal thermometer

Procedure

1. Check orders for continuous-reading thermometer and identify client with two forms of identification.
2. Dry forehead or axilla area, if necessary.
3. Please strip on forehead or deep in client's axilla—may stay in place for two days.
4. Read correct temperature by checking color changes or dots that turn from green to black.
5. Record temperature on appropriate form or record.

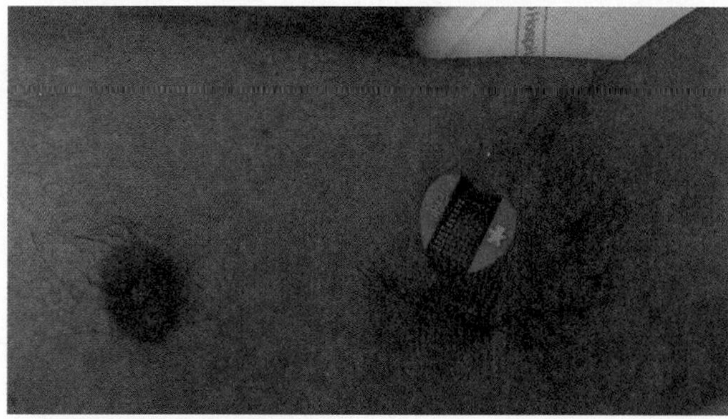

▲ Place Traxit®, a continuous-reading wearable thermometer, deep in the client's axilla.

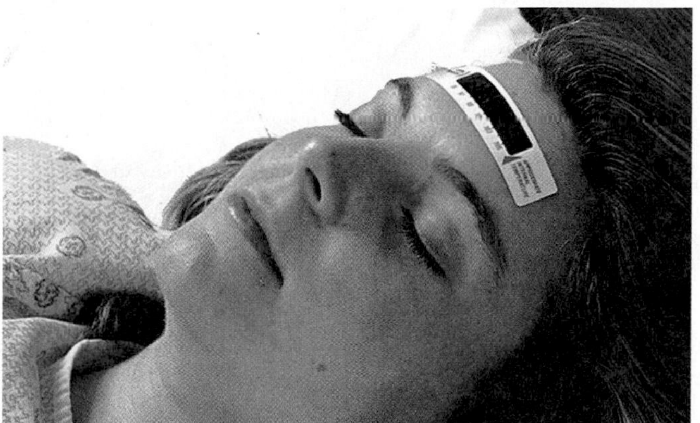

▲ Liquid crystal thermometer is placed against lower forehead for 15 seconds.

DOCUMENTATION for Temperature

- Site designated: "O" (oral), "R" (rectal), "A" (axillary), or "T" (tympanic)
- Temperature recorded on temp sheet and graph
- Nursing interventions used for alterations in temperature
- Condition of skin related to alterations from normothermia (e.g., diaphoresis)
- Signs and symptoms associated with alterations in temperature (e.g., shivering, dehydration)

Legal Considerations

Nurse's Negligence

The client had transthoracic vagotomy after which the doctor ordered vital signs every 15 minutes × 1 hour and every hour for 10 hours. Vital signs were recorded 4 times for 1 day. The next day the client's temperature was 102°F and it remained there until the next day when it was 105°F. The nurse administered aspirin when it rose to 106°F. The nurse then contacted the doctor who found signs of serious wound infection. The client suffered organic brain syndrome as a direct result of the continued high temperature. The court found that the nurses breached standard of care when they failed to notify the doctor of the client's high temperature.

CRITICAL THINKING Application

Expected Outcomes

- Temperature is within normal range.
- Temperature readings are compared with age, time of day, and previous readings.
- Alterations in temperature are detected early and treatment begun.
- Appropriate method of temperature taking is determined for each client.
- Correct length of time is used for thermometer insertion to obtain an accurate reading.

Unexpected Outcomes	Alternative Actions
Fever develops.	• Check possible sources of infection and take preventative measures. • Notify physician. • Employ cooling methods if temperature is dangerously high, such as tepid sponge bath, cool oral fluids, ice packs, or antipyretic drugs. • Assess all vital signs.
Despite initial cooling measure, temperature remains elevated due to hypothalamus damage from brain disease or injury.	• Notify physician and request cooling blanket. • Monitor temperature every 15 to 30 minutes and record. • Continue to administer antipyretic drugs as ordered.
Temperature remains elevated because of bacterial-produced pyrogens.	• Check for order to obtain culture of possible sources of infection. • Give antipyretic drugs as ordered. • Decrease room temperature and remove excess covers. • Give tepid sponge bath.
Temperature remains subnormal.	• Extreme low temperature can cause vasoconstriction; assess for blood clots. • Institute measures to promote vasodilation (application of warmth). • If extremity is ischemic, monitor that heat source does not exceed body temperature.
Using a tympanic thermometer, client's temperature reading seems too low.	• Be sure client has been indoors for at least 10 minutes. • Replace probe cover and retake temperature. • Check that probe cover and lens are clean and intact.

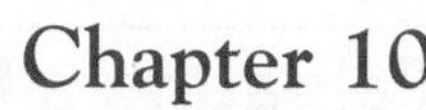

Chapter 10

UNIT 2

Pulse Rate

Nursing Process Data

ASSESSMENT Data Base

- Assess appropriate site to obtain pulse.
- Check pulse with health status changes, as ordered by physician, or before administering certain medications.
- Assess for rate, rhythm, volume, and quality.
- Assess an apical pulse on clients with irregular rhythms or those on cardiac medications.
- Obtain baseline peripheral pulses with initial assessment or in any client going for cardiac or vascular surgery. Also obtain pulse for medical clients with diabetes, arterial occlusive diseases, atherosclerosis, or aneurysm, or any color or temperature changes in the periphery.
- Obtain an apical–radial pulse when deficits occur between apical and radial measurements.
- Assess the need to monitor pulses with an ultrasound or electronic device.

PLANNING Objectives

- To determine whether the pulse rate is within normal range and if the rhythm is regular
- To evaluate the quality (amount of blood pumped through peripheral arteries) of arterial pulses
- To determine whether peripheral pulses are equal in amplitude when compared with corresponding pulses
- To determine presence of peripheral pulses with ultrasound device when palpation is ineffective
- To monitor and evaluate changes in the client's health status
- To determine apical pulse rate before heart medications are administered

IMPLEMENTATION Procedures

EVALUATION Expected Outcomes

- Pulse is palpated without difficulty.
- Pulse rate is within normal range and rhythm is regular.
- All peripheral pulses are equal in amplitude when compared with the corresponding pulse on the other side and when compared with the next proximal site.
- Apical pulse is easily detected and counted.

Palpating a Radial Pulse

Equipment

Watch with sweep second hand or digital watch that indicates seconds.

NOTE: To assess a pulse correctly, the nurse's watch must have second-hand capability.

Procedure

1. Perform hand hygiene.
2. Check client identity with two forms of ID and place client in comfortable position.
3. Ask about activity level within last 15 minutes. ▸ ***Rationale:*** Pulse rate increases with activity, then returns to preactivity rate.
4. Palpate arteries by using pads of the middle three fingers of your hand. ▸ ***Rationale:*** The nurse may feel own pulse if palpating with the thumb.
   a. Radial artery is usually used because it lies close to the skin surface and is easily accessible at the wrist.
   b. Press the artery against the bone or underlying firm surface to occlude vessel and then gradually release pressure. ▸ ***Rationale:*** Too much pressure obliterates the pulse.
   c. Note pulse characteristics, i.e., quality (strength) of pulse. ▸ ***Rationale:*** Strength of the pulse is an indication of stroke volume or amplitude.
   d. If pulse is difficult to palpate, try exerting more pressure on the most distal palpating finger. ▸ ***Rationale:*** This amplifies the pulse wave against the two more proximal palpating fingers.
5. Count pulse for 30 seconds, and multiply by two to obtain pulse rate. ▸ ***Rationale:*** This is sufficient time for rate determination if pulse rhythm is regular.

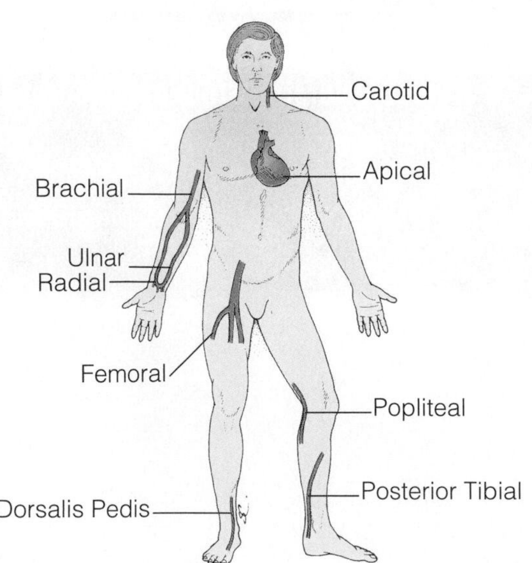

▲ Radial artery is the most commonly used site for determining pulse rate.

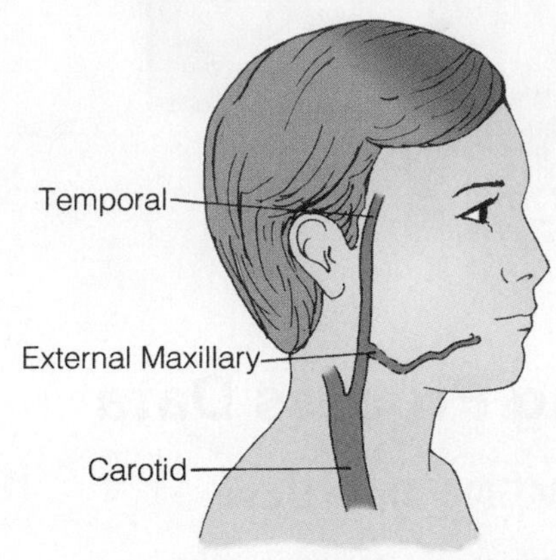

▲ Carotid artery is used when other sites are inaccessible or when there is a cardiac arrest to determine the adequacy of perfusion during CPR.

6. Count radial pulse for at least 1 minute if rhythm is irregular or difficult to count. ▸ ***Rationale:*** It may take a minute or so to detect the irregularity. This method assists you to count the pulse more accurately.
7. Check to see that client is comfortable.
8. Perform hand hygiene.
9. Record pulse rate, rhythm, and strength (volume).

TABLE 10-3 Pulse Quality

Pulse quality is determined by the amount of blood pumped through the peripheral arteries. The amount of pumped blood usually remains fairly constant; when it varies, it is also indicative of cardiac malfunction.

- *Bounding pulse:* Occurs when the nurse is able to feel the pulse by exerting only a slight pressure over the artery. May occur with increased stroke volume.
- *Weak or thready pulse:* Occurs if, by exerting firm pressure, the nurse cannot clearly determine the flow. May be associated with decreased stroke volume.
- *Pulsus alternans:* A regular pulse that the nurse feels as strong alternating with weak beats. May be related to left ventricular failure.
- *Bigeminal pulse:* Every second beat has a decreased amplitude. May be due to premature contractions.

Normal pulse

Hypokinetic (weak) pulse

Pulsus alternans

Hyperkinetic (bounding) pulse

Bigeminal pulse

Source: LeMone, P., & Burke, K. M. (2008). *Medical–Surgical Nursing: Critical Thinking in Clinical Care* (4th ed.). Upper Saddle River, NJ: Prentice Hall Health.

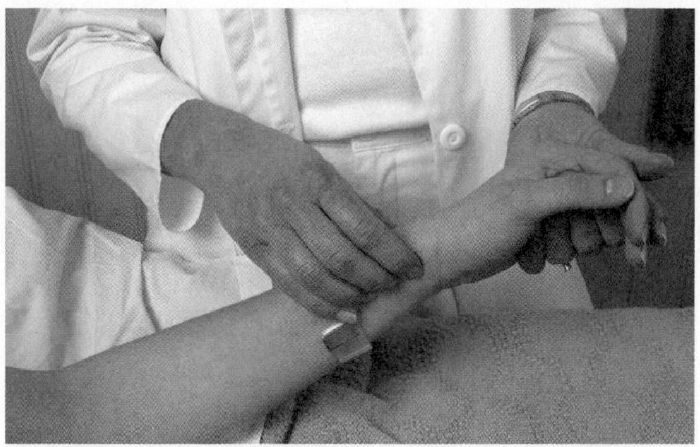
▲ Palpate radial pulse by using pads of middle three fingers, not thumb, for accurate results.

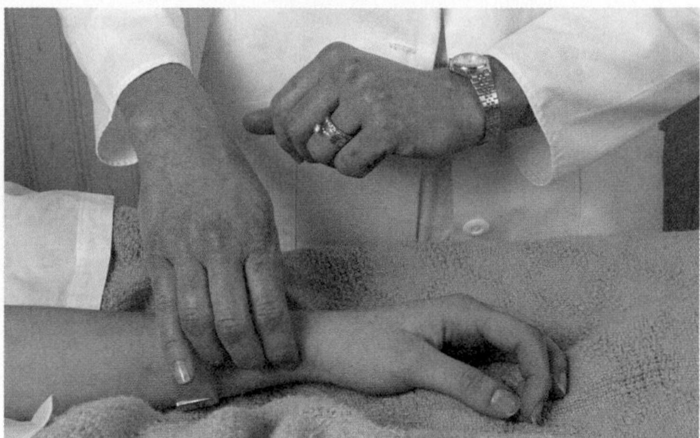
▲ Count pulse for at least 30 seconds and multiply by two to obtain pulse rate.

Pulse Characteristics

When counting the pulse rate, pay attention to:

- Rate: Average is 72 beats/min. The normal adult heart rate range is 60 to 100 beats/min. If pulse rate is below 60 or above 100 beats/min (outside the normal parameters), notify the physician.
- Rhythm: The pattern of beats, either regular or irregular.
- Volume or amplitude: The force of blood with each beat; can range from absent to bounding.
- Symmetry: Bilateral uniformity of pulse.

Palpate a Child's Pulse or Listen to the Heart

The best practice for taking a pulse for infants or children is to listen to the heart itself, rather than palpating the pulse—too much pressure may obliterate it and inadequate pressure may not detect it.

EVIDENCE-BASED PRACTICE

Pulse Rate Measurement

Studies have indicated that the accuracy of pulse rate measurement is influenced by the number of counted seconds (counting the pulse for 60 seconds is more accurate than 15 or 30 seconds). However, clinical significance of the result is not clear because in one study using a 15- or 30-second count was just as accurate as a 60-second count.

Source: The Joanna Briggs Institute. (1999). Vital signs. *Best Practice*, 3(3), 2. http://www.joannabriggs.edu.au/pdf/BPISEng_3_3.pdf Craven, R.F., Hinnle, C.J. (2006) *Fundamentals of Nursing Human Health and Function*, 5th ed. Philadelphia: Lippincott Williams and Wilkins.

Taking an Apical Pulse

Equipment

Watch with sweep second hand

Stethoscope

Procedure

1. Gather equipment.
2. Perform hand hygiene.
3. Check two forms of client's ID. Provide privacy.
4. Explain procedure to client.
5. Place client in a supine position and expose chest area. If possible, stand at client's right side. ▸ ***Rationale:*** Auscultation of heart sounds is often enhanced when examiner is at client's right side.
6. Locate the apical impulse, termed the point of maximal impulse (PMI), by palpating the angle of Louis just below the suprasternal notch. This is the angle between the manubrium, top of the sternum, and the body of the sternum.

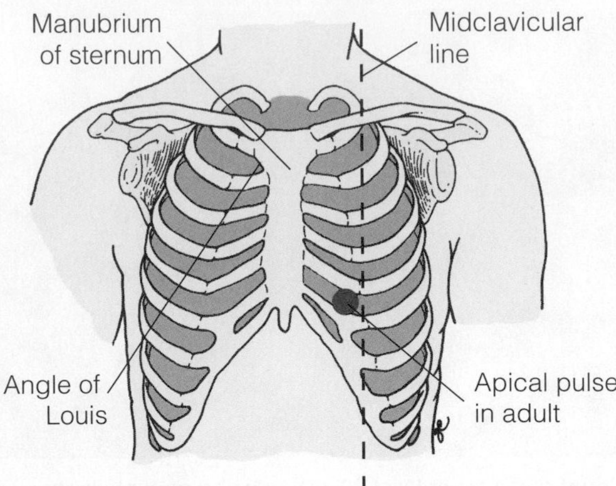

▲ Apical pulse site in adult.

a. Place your index finger just to the left of the client's sternum and palpate the second intercostal space.
b. Place your middle finger in the third intercostal space and continue palpating downward until you locate the apical impulse at the fifth intercostal space.
c. Move your index finger laterally along the fifth intercostal space to the midclavicular line (MCL).

7. Warm the stethoscope in the palm of your hand for 5 to 10 seconds. ▸ ***Rationale:*** Warming the stethoscope prevents startling the client.
8. Count client's apical pulse.
   a. Place diaphragm of stethoscope firmly over apical impulse site. ▸ ***Rationale:*** Heart sounds are high-pitched and most clearly heard with diaphragm of stethoscope.
   b. Count the rate for 1 minute when taking an apical pulse. Count *lub-dub* sound as one beat. ▸ ***Rationale:*** More accurate readings are obtained over 1 minute, especially if pulse is irregular.

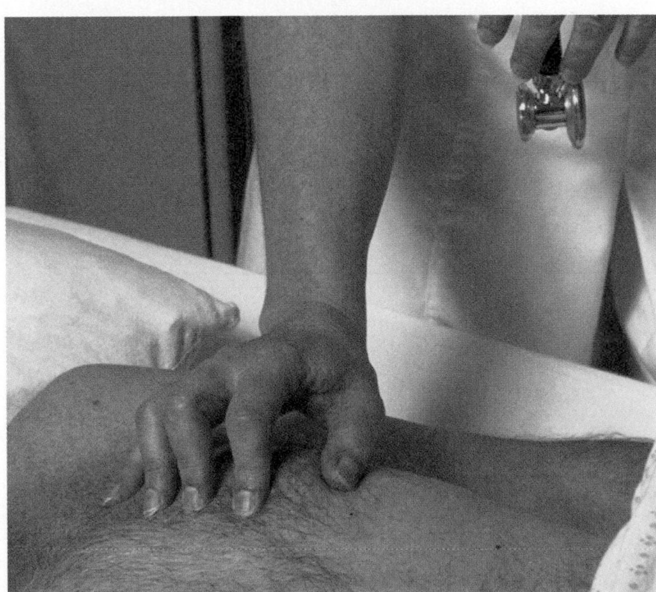

▲ Place middle finger in third intercostal space and continue to move downward to the fifth intercostal space.

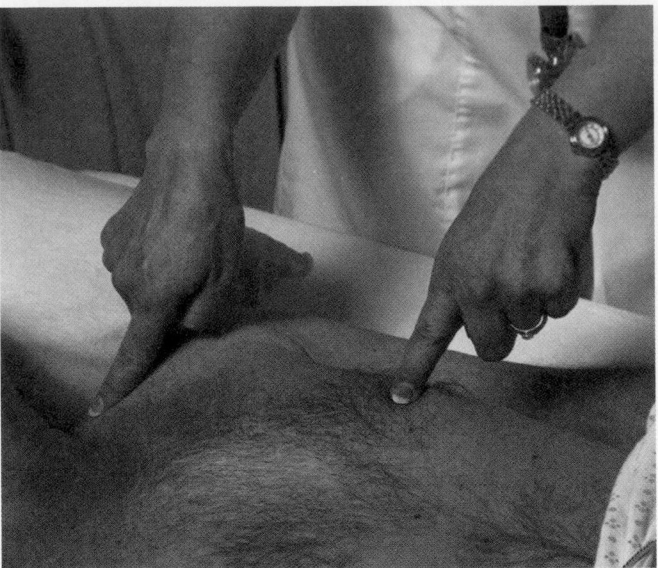

▲ Move index finger along fifth intercostal space to midclavicular line.

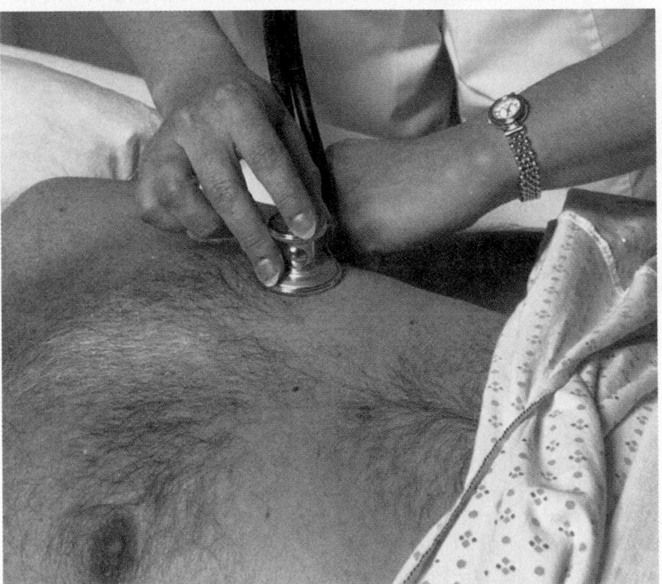

▲ Accurate apical pulse is found in fifth intercostal space, left of sternum at midclavicular line, or at Erb's point.

   c. Determine if there is a regular pattern to any irregularity or if it is chaotically irregular. ▸ ***Rationale:*** This finding helps describe the rhythm disturbance.
9. Check to see that client is comfortable.
10. Perform hand hygiene and clean stethoscope, if necessary.
11. Record apical pulse rate, rhythm, and intensity.

EVIDENCED-BASED PRACTICE

Effect of Music on Vital Signs

The impact of music (Mendelson's classical violin) on vital signs was studied on a pulmonary medical unit. The results showed a trend toward a decrease in systolic and diastolic blood pressure as well as a decrease in heart rate.

Source: Burgner, K. (2005, June 27). Musical intervention. *Advance for Nurses, 2,* 21–23.

Taking an Apical–Radial Pulse

Equipment

Watch with sweep second hand
Stethoscope
Another nurse to assist with procedure

NOTE: An experienced nurse may be able to assess apical and radial rates simultaneously without an assistant.

Procedure

1. Gather equipment.
2. Perform hand hygiene.
3. Check two forms of client's ID.
4. Provide privacy.
5. Explain procedure to client, especially if two nurses are taking the pulse. ▸ ***Rationale:*** Clients may be apprehensive when two nurses are at the bedside, so a full explanation helps allay fears.
6. Assist client to a supine position and expose chest area.

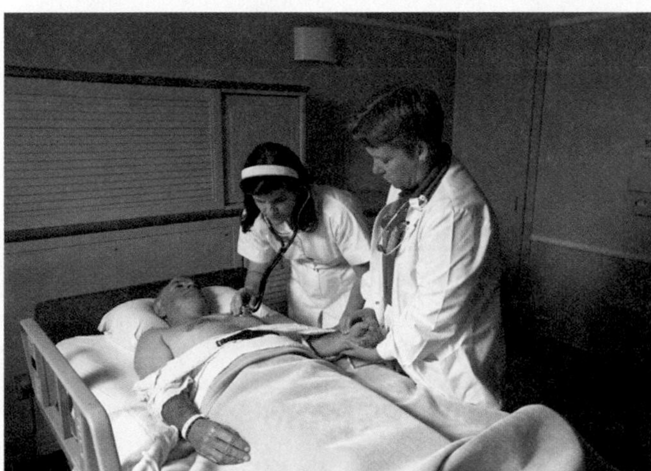

▲ Auscultate apical pulse and palpate radial pulse simultaneously, preferable using two nurses.

7. Place watch where clearly visible to both nurses. ▸ ***Rationale:*** Both nurses count pulse rates within the same time span, preferably using one watch.
8. Warm stethoscope in palm of your hand. ▸ ***Rationale:*** Prevents startling the client with cold stethoscope.
9. Locate radial pulse. The second nurse locates apical pulse at the fifth intercostal space left of sternum at the midclavicular line and firmly places diaphragm of stethoscope on the site. ▸ ***Rationale:*** Firm application helps transmit high-pitched heart sounds.
10. With assistant, select number on watch to start counting pulse (e.g., 12:00).
11. Signal to the other nurse with your hand when to start taking the pulse and when to stop. Both nurses simultaneously count pulse for 1 full minute.
12. Auscultate the apical pulse and palpate the radial pulse simultaneously (preferably using two nurses, one at each site).
    a. Note a pulse deficit between apical and radial pulses when rhythm is irregular. ▸ ***Rationale:*** Atrial dysrhythmias and premature ventricular beats generally produce pulse deficits (apical greater than radial rate). A pulse deficit results from the ejection of a volume of blood that is too small to initiate a peripheral pulse wave.
    b. If a significant pulse deficit is found, assess for other abnormal signs (BP).
    c. Assess pulse volume by feeling the pressure of the beat. The quality is described as normal, weak, strong, or bounding.
13. Subtract radial rate from apical rate to obtain pulse deficit. ▸ ***Rationale:*** The pulse deficit represents the number of ineffective or nonperfused heartbeats.
14. Position client for comfort.
15. Perform hand hygiene.
16. Chart apical and radial rate and pulse deficit.

Palpating a Peripheral Pulse

Equipment

Felt-tipped pen
Watch with second hand

Procedure

1. Gather equipment.
2. Perform hand hygiene.
3. Check two forms of client ID.
4. Provide privacy. Explain procedure.
5. Place client in a supine position with relaxed legs.
6. Palpate peripheral pulses: radial, carotid (when other sites are inaccessible), brachial, femoral, popliteal, dorsalis pedis, posterior tibial. (For special cases, after carotid surgery, palpate temporal pulse also.)
7. Compare pulse sites bilaterally by palpating with pads of the middle three fingers of your hand.
8. Press artery against the bone or underlying firm structure to occlude vessel and then gradually release pressure.
9. Palpate weak pulses gently. ▸ ***Rationale:*** Too much pressure obliterates a weak pulse.
10. Assess if bilateral pulses are equal in amplitude (strength).

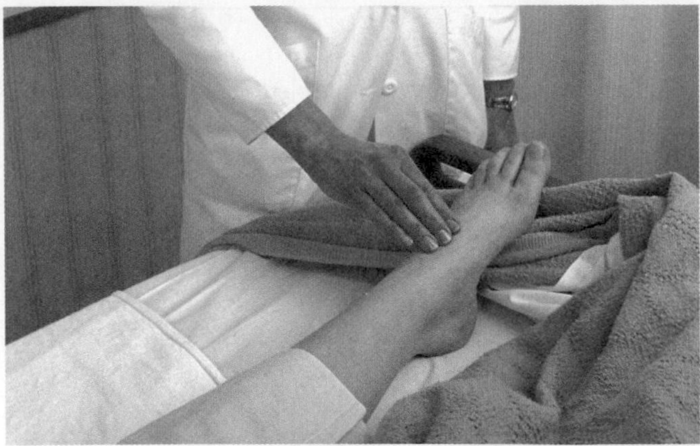

▲ Apply firm pressure against underlying structure, then release to find peripheral pulse.

a. If pulse is not immediately palpable, examine adjacent area. ▸ ***Rationale:*** This action identifies where interruption or alteration in circulation occurs in an extremity.

b. Since pulse locations differ, mark pulse locations with felt-tipped pen, especially when they are difficult to palpate. ▸ ***Rationale:*** Marking site allows the next nurse to find location without spending extra time.

c. Compare presence and characteristic of peripheral pulses with previous findings. ▸ ***Rationale:*** This action allows early identification of alterations in peripheral circulation.

11. Check to see that client is comfortable.
12. Wash your hands.
13. Record pulse rate, rhythm, pattern, and volume.

Characteristics of Peripheral Pulses

Peripheral pulses may be absent or weak. The size (amplitude) of a pulse depends on the degree of filling of the artery during systole (ventricular contraction) and emptying during diastole (ventricular relaxation). The amplitude of a pulse is described as being large or small and determines the pulse pressure (the difference between systolic and diastolic pressure).

0 = Absent
1+ = Weak
2+ = Diminished
3+ = Strong
4+ = Full and bounding

Clinical Alert

If palpating the carotid pulse, avoid pressing on the carotid sinus in the upper neck area near the jaw. *Do not* palpate both carotids simultaneously because this decreases blood flow to the brain.

EVIDENCED-BASED PRACTICE

Determining Pulse Rate With a Doppler Device

Determining a pulse rate with a Doppler device is more accurate than palpation, which detects arterial wall expansion and retraction. The Doppler detects the motion of red blood cells and thus is more sensitive.

Source: Thomas, J., Feliciano, C. (July, 2003). Measuring blood pressure with a doppler device. *Nursing* 33(7): 52–53.

Monitoring Peripheral Pulses With a Doppler Ultrasound Stethoscope

Equipment

Doppler ultrasound stethoscope or probe
Conductive jelly (not K-Y)

Procedure

1. Gather equipment.
2. Perform hand hygiene.
3. Check two forms of client ID; explain procedure.
4. Provide privacy.
5. Uncover extremity to be assessed.
6. Place extremity in a comfortable position.
7. Plug headset (stethoscope) into one of the two outlet

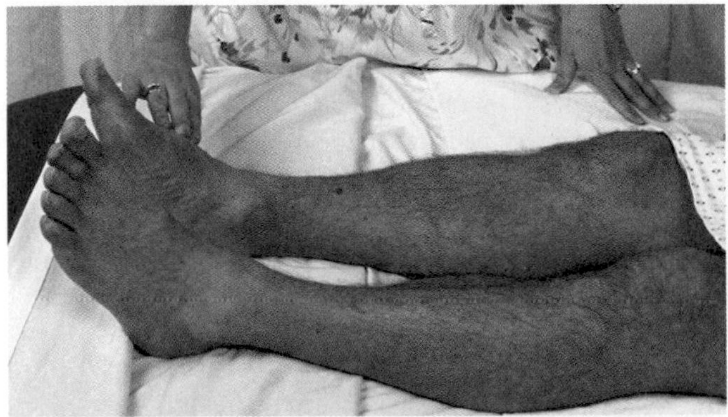

▲ Locate peripheral pulse with fingers before applying gel.

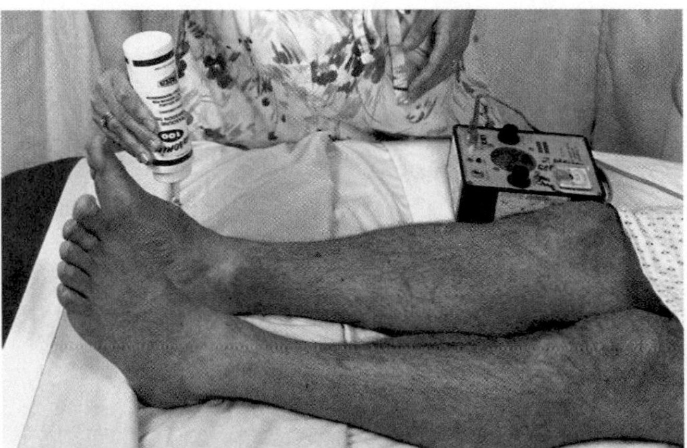

▲ Apply gel to skin to facilitate beam transmission.

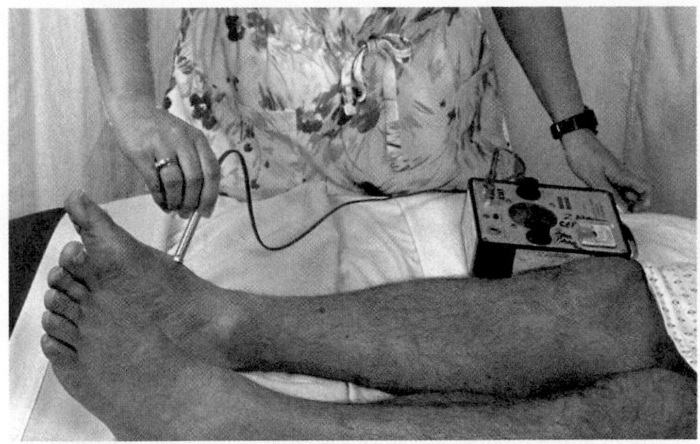

▲ Hold probe against skin at 90° angle.

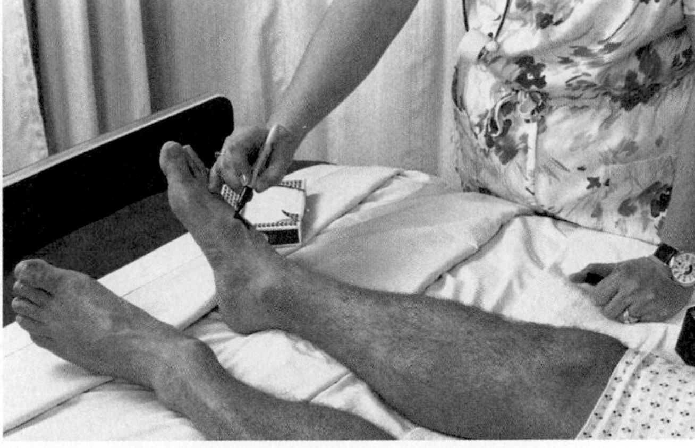

▲ Mark site where pulsations were heard.

jacks located next to the volume control. If not using stethoscope, plug probe into monitor.

8. Apply conductive gel to client's skin. ▸ ***Rationale:*** The ultrasound beam travels best through gel and requires an airtight seal between the probe and the skin.
9. Hold probe (at tapered end of plastic core) against skin at a 90° angle to the blood vessel being examined.
10. Turn on Doppler by pressing down the "ON" switch.
11. Move probe over site if pulse is not detected. Keep it in direct contact with skin, and adjust volume to detect blood flow. ▸ ***Rationale:*** This action should facilitate detection of whooshing pulse sounds.
12. Reapply new gel if pulse is still not detected and, with light pressure, place probe over site and turn switch ON. Increase volume control, or check if batteries are weak.
13. Mark site where pulsations were heard. ▸ ***Rationale:*** This facilitates future assessments.
14. Clean gel from skin and Doppler probe. Replace cover over extremity.
15. Position client for comfort.
16. Replace Doppler equipment to appropriate location.
17. Perform hand hygiene.

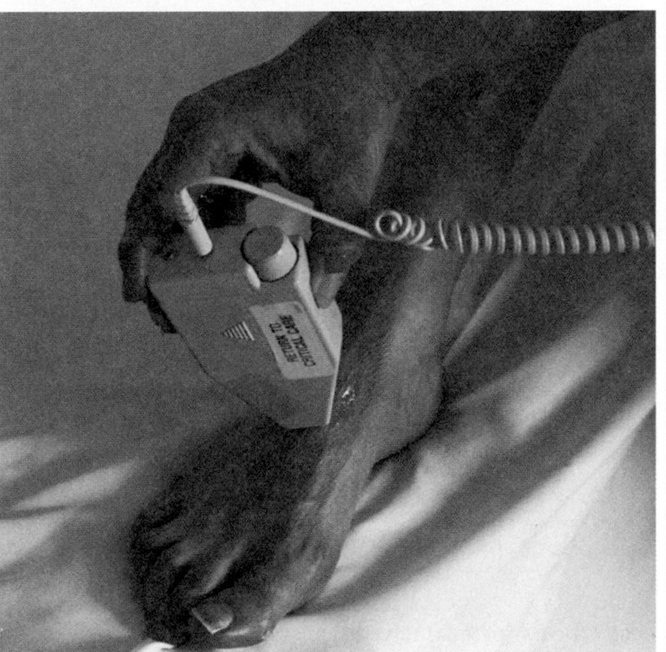

▲ Alternate equipment for Doppler probe. Skill steps are the same.

Monitoring Pulse Oximetry

NOTE: See Procedure in Chapter 30, Respiratory Care.

DOCUMENTATION for Taking a Pulse

- Type of pulse taken
- Rate, rhythm, intensity, and quality of pulse
- Pulse deficit, if any, present
- Characteristics of all peripheral pulses—use rating scale
- Use of Doppler stethoscope if needed
- Effects of nursing interventions or medical treatments on abnormal pulse rates or rhythms

CRITICAL THINKING Application

Expected Outcomes	
• Pulse is palpated without difficulty. • Pulse rate is within normal range and rhythm is regular.	• All peripheral pulses are equal in amplitude when compared with the corresponding pulse on the other side and when compared with the next proximal site. • Apical pulse is easily detected and counted.

Unexpected Outcomes	Alternative Actions
Apical, femoral, and carotid pulse is absent.	• *Note:* For all unexpected outcomes, assess all vital signs and status of the client. • Immediately call a Code. • Initiate CPR immediately, and continue to assess the femoral or carotid pulse during resuscitation. • For absent femoral pulse, assess for systemic circulation and presence of disorders affecting circulation to extremities. • Use Doppler stethoscope to assess for presence of pulse.
Abnormal heartbeats are present.	• Relieve anxiety, fear, or stress through communication and pertinent information. • If client has pain, relieve with change of position, back rub, and analgesic.
Tachycardia (pulse rate over 100 beats/min in adults or 140 in children)	• Decrease heart rate by reducing an elevated temperature to normal. • Take vital signs every 15 minutes to 2 hours until condition stabilizes and pulse rate is within normal limits. • Determine significance of pulse rate as it affects blood pressure, sensorium, and client comfort. • Reassess client for shock because a rise in pulse rate is one of the earliest signs of shock. • Notify physician if persistent tachycardia continues or if there is a change in blood pressure. • Determine whether tachycardia is normal for this client.
Bradycardia (pulse rate less than 60 in adults or less than70 in children)	• Notify physician for electrocardiogram request to determine if heart block is present. • If client is on digitalis, hold the drug, or on beta-blockers or other medications, notify physician. • Have atropine and temporary pacemaker available for physician if pulse is consistently slow (less than 50) and client is not an athlete (who may well have a pulse less than 50). • Continue monitoring pulse rate every 15 minutes to 2 hours until pulse is within normal limits.
Ectopic Beats (premature ventricular or atrial contractions)	• Relieve pain if irregularity is due to premature beats associated with pain. • Administer oxygen if client has an order to do so. • If associated with stimuli from noise, visitors, caffeinated beverages, or smoking, eliminate the cause of the stimulation. • Notify physician to request a medical order for an electrocardiogram since premature beats in a client with myocardial infarction may be potentially harmful. • Obtain order from physician to draw serum electrolytes, especially magnesium or potassium. Low levels can cause ectopic beats. • Continue monitoring pulse rate every 15 minutes to 2 hours until irregularity is controlled.
Peripheral pulse is absent.	• Assess for other signs and symptoms of circulatory impairment.
Loss of peripheral pulse.	• Use a Doppler ultrasound and stethoscope to find pulse and report to physician.
Doppler stethoscope unable to detect sounds.	• Check that conductive jelly is used because salt from K-Y Jelly can damage the probe. • Check that batteries are less than 6 months old. The date should be indicated on all batteries. • Use alkaline batteries; they last longer. • Check that abnormal pressure is not applied, as this obliterates pulse.
Client is in isolation and requires vascular assessment.	• Clean with gas sterilization after discontinuing use of Doppler stethoscope. • Do not clean with alcohol or autoclave.

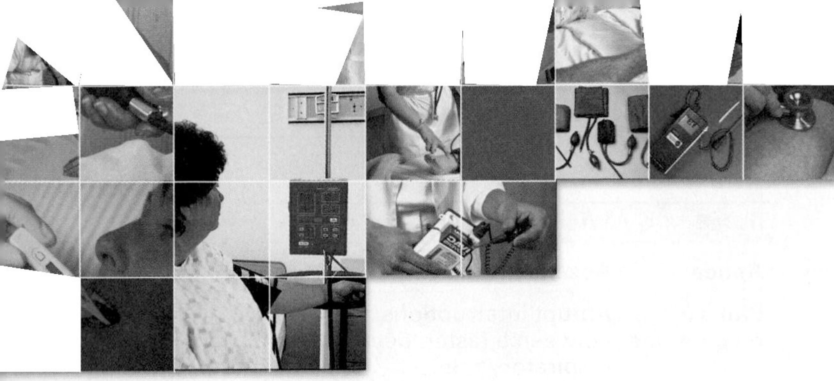

Chapter 10

UNIT 3

Respirations

Nursing Process Data

ASSESSMENT Data Base

- Assess client's respiratory rate, depth, and rhythm.
- Note any abnormalities noted during inspection and palpation or by percussion and auscultation.
- Assess presence of dyspnea or cyanosis.
- Assess for presence of abnormal sounds, such as stertorous or sonorous breathing.
- Assess if accessory muscles are used for breathing.

PLANNING Objectives

- To note respiratory rate, rhythm, and depth
- To establish baseline information on admission to the unit
- To note labored, difficult, or noisy respirations or cyanosis
- To identify alterations in respiratory pattern resulting from disease condition
- To determine whether respiratory rate is within normal range compared with pulse and blood pressure readings

IMPLEMENTATION Procedures

EVALUATION Expected Outcomes

- Respiratory rate, rhythm, and depth are within normal limits.
- Baseline information upon admission is documented.
- Labored, difficult, or noisy respirations are evaluated.
- Alterations in respiratory patterns resulting from disease conditions are identified.

Pearson Nursing Student Resources

Find additional review materials at **nursing.pearsonhighered.com**

Prepare for success with NCLEX®-style practice questions and Skill Checklists

Obtaining the Respiratory Rate

Equipment

Watch with a second hand

Procedure

1. Perform hand hygiene.
2. Check two forms of client ID and explain procedure to client.
3. Check lighting to ensure it is adequate for procedure.
4. Maintain client's privacy.
5. Place hand on chest or observe chest rise and fall and count respirations.
6. Note relationship of inspiration to expiration. Note also depth and effort of breathing.
7. Count respirations for preferably 1 minute, or for 30 seconds and multiply by 2. ▶ ***Rationale:*** One full minute is more accurate for abnormal breathing patterns.
8. Perform hand hygiene.
9. Compare respiratory rate with previous recordings.
10. Record respiratory rate. Record if rhythm or depth altered from normal.

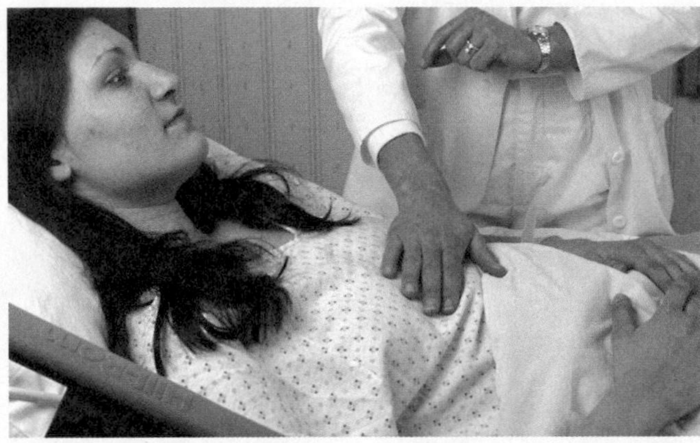

▲ Place hand on chest when respirations are difficult to count.

TABLE 10-4 Abnormal Breathing Patterns

Apnea	Absence of breathing.	
Biot's respirations	Abrupt interruptions between a faster, deeper respiratory rate.	
Bradypnea	Slow, regular respirations. Rate is below 10 per minute.	
Cheyne–Stokes	Periods of apnea appear throughout cycle. Respirations become deeper and faster than normal followed by a slower rate and progressing to periods of apnea lasting from 15 to 60 seconds.	
Hyperpnea	Abnormal increase in depth and rate.	
Kussmaul's respirations	Deep, gasping breathing. Attempt to blow off carbon dioxide as respiratory compensation for metabolic acidosis (e.g., diabetic ketoacidosis).	
Tachypnea	Respiratory rate increased above 24 breaths per minute. Rate remains regular but shallow in pattern.	

Normal Respiratory Rate

Adults: 12–20 per minute

Young children: 20–25 per minute

Infants: Up to 40 per minute

NOTE: One study found that counting respirations for 15 seconds versus a full minute produced a significant difference in the rate; thus the conclusion is respirations should be counted for a full minute.

DOCUMENTATION for Respiration

- Rate, depth, and rhythm of respirations
- Abnormal sounds associated with breathing
- Effectiveness of therapy if needed to correct respiratory problems
- Ratio of inspiration and expiration
- Alterations from baseline respiratory patterns

Legal Considerations

Failure to Assess and Monitor Vital Signs

A client entered the hospital with pain from a kidney stone. From 4:35 PM to 10:30 PM, he received three 5-mg doses of morphine, 1 mg of Dilaudid, and an additional 15 mg of morphine with 50 mg of Phenergan IV. At 1:05 AM, the night shift found the client in respiratory and cardiac arrest. He died shortly thereafter. After being transferred from the emergency department to a unit at 8:15 PM, the client did not have his vital signs taken, even though hospital policy stated that after IV narcotic administration, the client must be monitored every hour for respiratory depression for 24 hours. The court found a breach of standard of care by the nurse's failure to assess, monitor, and document care of a client receiving narcotics.

Source: McMinn *v.* Mount Carmel Health, 1998.

CRITICAL THINKING Application

Expected Outcomes

- Respiratory rate, rhythm, and depth are within normal limits.
- Baseline information upon admission is documented.
- Labored, difficult, or noisy respirations are evaluated.
- Alterations in respiratory patterns resulting from disease conditions are identified.

Unexpected Outcomes	Alternative Actions
Apnea (absence of breathing) occurs, may be intermittent.	• *Note:* For all unexpected outcomes, assess client for all vital signs and comfort/condition. • Begin artificial ventilation by mouth-to-mask, mouth-to-nose, or other airway adjunct method at the rate of 12 per minute for an adult or 20 per minute for a child. • Summon help immediately; call a Code.
Tachypnea (rate faster than normal and more shallow >24) occurs.	• Relieve anxiety, fear, and stress through communication and pertinent information. • Relieve fever if that is the cause. • Correct respiratory insufficiency with low-flow oxygen administration, good pulmonary toilet, and deep breathing and coughing exercises.
Bradypnea (rate slower than normal <10) occurs.	• A sleeping adult's respirations can be less than 10 per minute; if so, use other vital signs to check condition. • If due to respiratory depressant drugs, such as opiates, barbiturates, and tranquilizers, be prepared to assist respirations or administer mouth-to-mask resuscitation. • Administer oxygen at 4 to 6 L/min via nasal cannulae as ordered. If client has COPD use 2 L/min. • Stimulate client to take breaths at least 10 times per minute.
Hyperpnea (increased depth of respiration) occurs.	• Rest after period of exertion. • Relieve fear, anxiety, or stress. • May be indicative of respiratory compensation for metabolic acidotic state (Kussmaul's pattern).
Cheyne–Stokes respirations (respiratory cycle in which respirations increase in rate and depth, then decrease, followed by a period of apnea) occur.	• Follow physician's orders to treat underlying disease state (e.g., heart failure, increased intracranial pressure). • Monitor respirations every 15 minutes to hourly, depending on client's status. • Be prepared to administer CPR if apnea occurs. • Evaluate cause—one of the indicators that death is approaching.
Biot's (irregular pattern—slow and deep or rapid and shallow, followed by apnea) respirations occur.	• Assess for central nervous system (CNS) abnormalities (increased intracranial pressure, meningitis).
Kussmaul's (deep and gasping breaths—more than 20 breaths/minute) respirations occur.	• Follow orders to treat for renal failure, septic shock, or diabetic ketoacidosis.

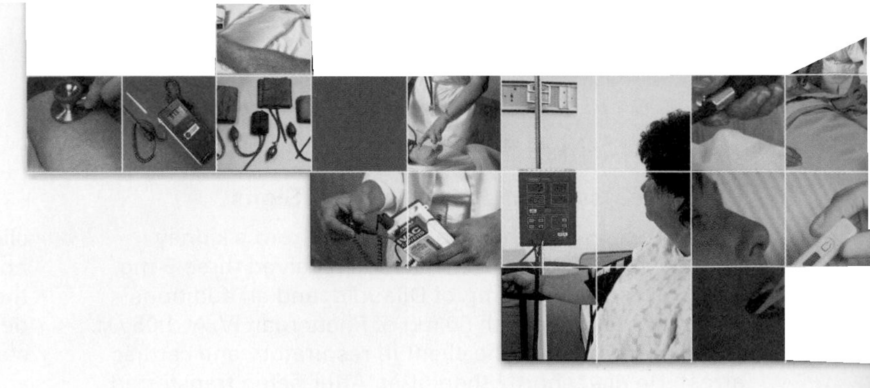

Chapter 10

UNIT 4

Blood Pressure

Nursing Process Data

ASSESSMENT Data Base

- Assess blood pressure initially and whenever client's status changes.
- Assess size of cuff needed for accurate reading.
- Assess the beginning and disappearance of Korotkoff's sounds during a blood pressure reading.
- Assess presence of factors that can alter blood pressure readings.
- Note any changes from prior assessments.

PLANNING Objectives

- To determine whether arterial blood pressure reading is within normal range for the individual client
- To assess condition of heart, arteries, blood vessel resistance, and stroke volume
- To establish a baseline for further evaluation
- To identify alterations in blood pressure resulting from a change in disease condition
- To correlate blood pressure readings with pulse and respirations

IMPLEMENTATION Procedures

EVALUATION Expected Outcomes

- Blood pressure readings provide information regarding the overall health status of client.
- Major changes from prior assessments are documented.
- Accurate readings are taken by using correct cuff size and procedure.
- Beginning and disappearance of Korotkoff's sounds during a blood pressure reading are evaluated and documented.
- The presence of factors that can alter blood pressure readings is identified.

Measuring a Blood Pressure

Equipment

Sphygmomanometer with proper size cuff
Stethoscope
Alcohol wipe

Procedure

1. Gather equipment. Clean stethoscope before use. Be sure the cuff is an appropriate size for the client. ▸ ***Rationale:*** A cuff that is too narrow results in erroneously high readings; a cuff too large may result in false low readings.
2. Provide quiet environment.
3. Perform hand hygiene.
4. Check two forms of client ID.
5. Explain procedure to client. If client is a child, take blood pressure after the other vital signs. ▸ ***Rationale:*** This intervention may upset the child and affect pulse and respirations.
6. Place client in relaxed reclining or sitting position. (Sitting position with feet on the floor is the preferred position.) ▸ ***Rationale:*** Blood pressure can vary by position in certain persons.
7. Prepare client for blood pressure reading.
   a. Assess whether client has smoked or exercised within last 15 minutes. Prepare client for blood pressure reading.
   b. Allow client to rest several minutes before beginning a reading.
   c. Client should be instructed not to cross legs or talk during the procedure. ▸ ***Rationale:*** Client activities and a slouched position yield false high readings.
8. Expose upper part of client's arm and position it with palm upward, arm slightly flexed with the whole arm supported at heart level. ▸ ***Rationale:*** If arm is below level of heart, the blood pressure reading is higher than normal, and if above the heart, is lower than normal.
9. Choose appropriate size cuff and wrap totally deflated cuff snugly and smoothly around upper part of arm (lower border of cuff 1 in. above antecubital space) with center of cuff bladder over brachial artery (pressure dial at zero).

Stethoscopes—Carriers of Bacterial Infection

A study conducted at the emergency department, Michigan State University, found that 89% of the stethoscopes grew staphylococci and 29% yielded *staphylococcus aureus.* When the stethoscope diaphragms were cleaned (using alcohol swabs), it resulted in immediate reduction in the bacterial count by 94%.

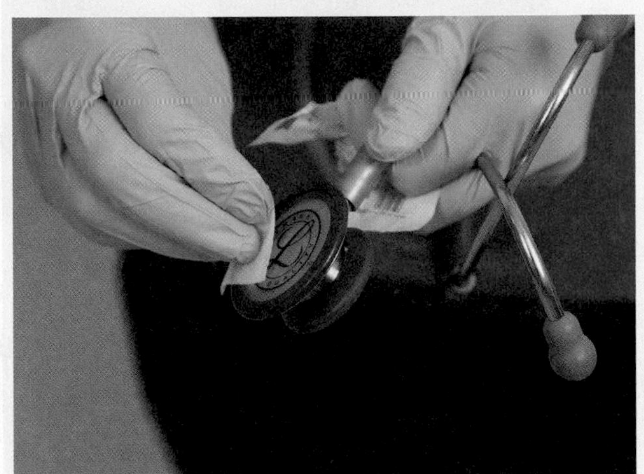

▲ Clean the bell/diaphragm of the stethoscope after taking client's blood pressure.

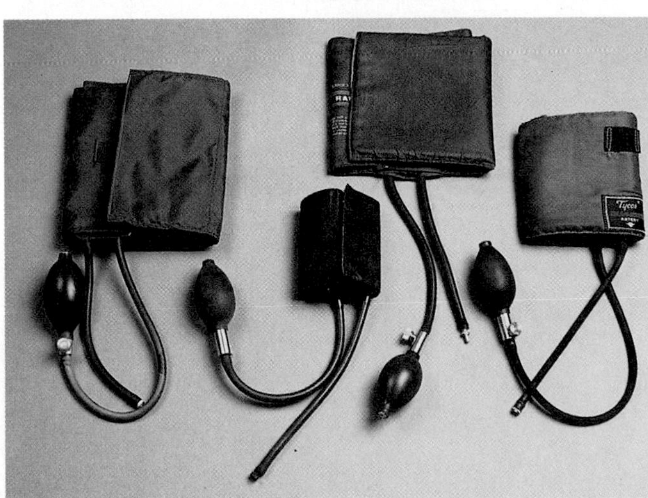

▲ Blood pressure cuffs are available in various sizes.

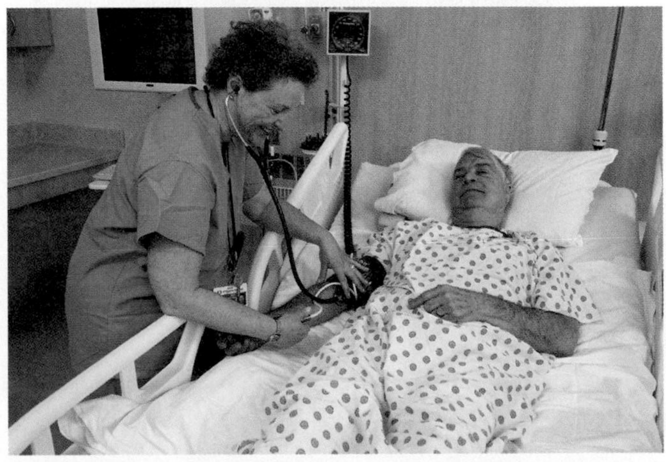

▲ Before starting procedure, explain steps to the client.

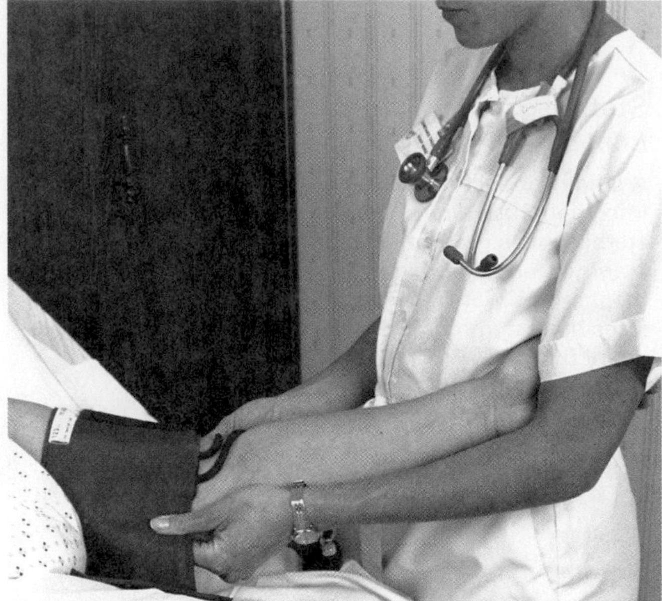

▲ Wrap blood pressure cuff snugly around upper arm.

10. Locate and palpate brachial artery with fingertips (medial aspect of antecubital fossa).
11. Position stethoscope ear pieces in ears. The ear pieces should tilt slightly forward. ▸ ***Rationale:*** Sounds are heard more clearly.
12. Ensure stethoscope hangs freely from ears. ▸ ***Rationale:*** Rubbing of stethoscope against an object can cause artifact and inaccurate readings.
13. Close valve on sphygmomanometer pump.
14. Inflate cuff rapidly (while palpating radial artery) to a level 30 mmHg above level at which radial pulsations are no longer felt. ▸ ***Rationale:*** This level ensures that cuff is inflated to a pressure exceeding the client's systolic pressure. Slow inflation can yield gaps in pressure readings.

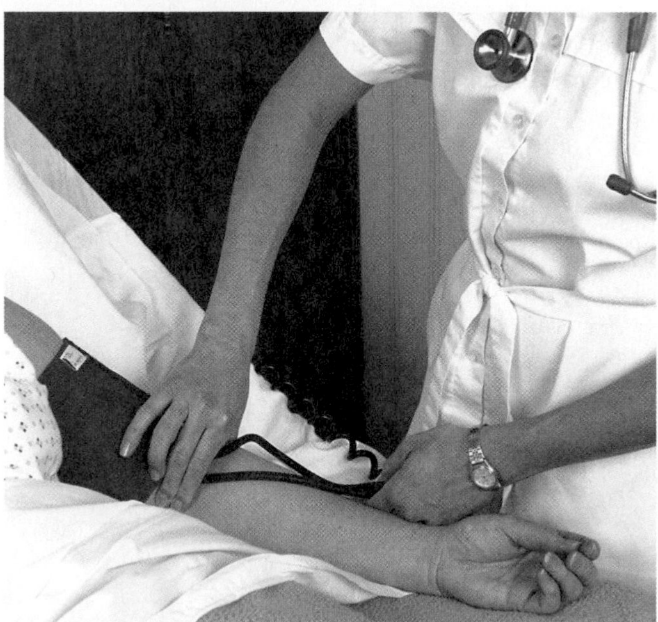

▲ Palpate brachial artery on medial antecubital fossa.

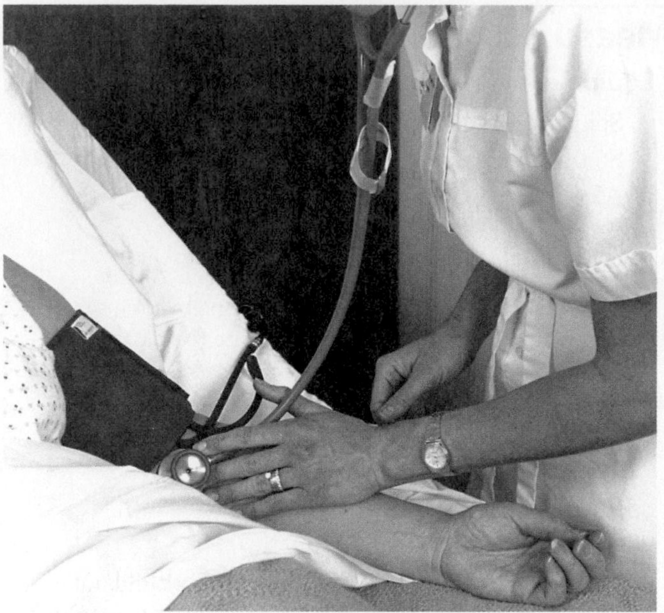

▲ Place stethoscope on medial antecubital fossa.

15. Note level and rapidly deflate, waiting 60 seconds. ▸ ***Rationale:*** This is enough time for venous congestion to decrease.
16. Place bell (or diaphragm) of stethoscope lightly on the medial antecubital fossa where brachial artery pulsations are located and rapidly inflate cuff to 30 mmHg above point where radial pulse disappeared. ▸ ***Rationale:*** This pressure ensures that cuff is inflated to exceed client's systolic pressure.
17. Deflate cuff gradually at a constant rate by opening valve on pump (2–4 mmHg/sec) until the first Korotkoff's sound is heard. This is the systolic pressure, or phase I, of Korotkoff's sounds. ▸ ***Rationale:*** Slower or faster deflation yields false readings.
18. Read pressure on manometer at eye level. ▸ ***Rationale:*** This ensures accurate reading.
19. Continue to deflate cuff at a rate of 2 to 4 mmHg/sec. Do not reinflate without letting cuff totally deflate. ▸ ***Rationale:*** Reinflating cuff results in erroneously high readings.

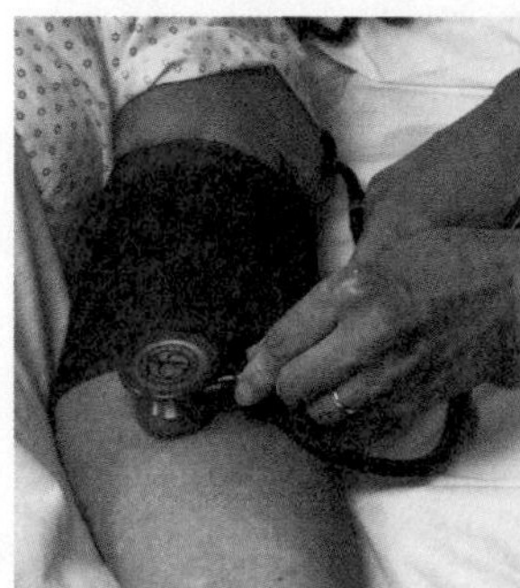

▲ Bell of stethoscope

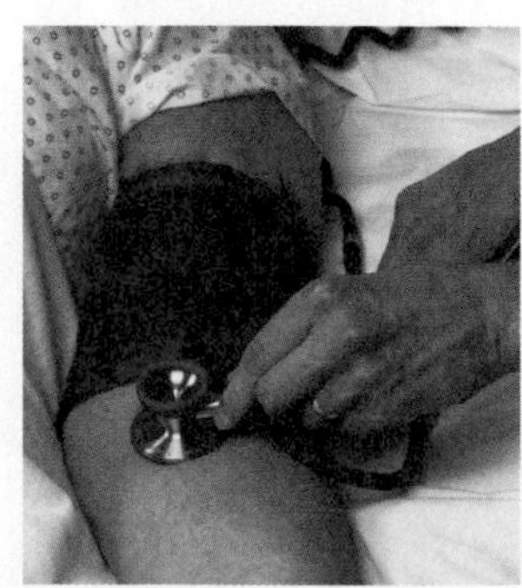

▲ Diaphragm of stethoscope.

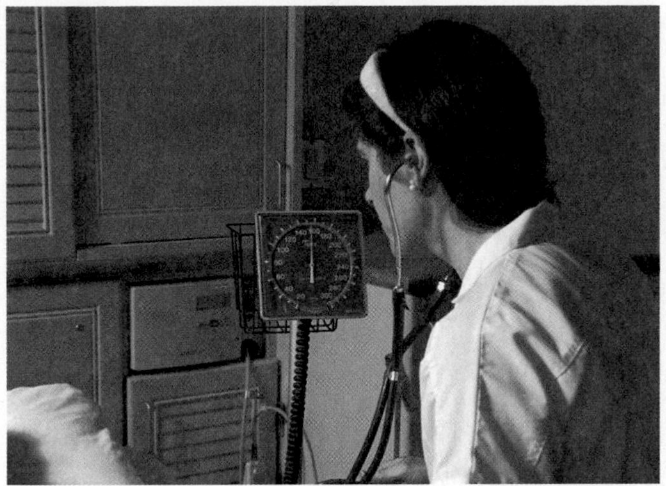

▲ Read manometer at eye level.

20. Note point at which Korotkoff's sounds begin (phase I) and when they disappear completely (phase V). Disappearance of sounds (phase V) is regarded by the American Heart Association as the best index of diastolic blood pressure in individuals over age 13. If the child is younger than 12 years, the best indication of diastolic pressure is the distinct muffling of sounds at phase IV.

NOTE: Some facilities require that all five phases be recorded.

21. Do not leave cuff inflated for a prolonged period. ▸ ***Rationale:*** Leaving cuff inflated produces client discomfort.
22. Deflate cuff completely and wait at least 1 to 2 minutes before rechecking the blood pressure. ▸ ***Rationale:*** This allows time for blood vessels to return to normal.

NOTE: Check level of comfort of client and level of consciousness (as well as other vital signs) when evaluating blood pressure reading. If all signs and symptoms don't correlate, reevaluate blood pressure.

EVIDENCE-BASED PRACTICE

Forearm Blood Pressure

Statistical analysis has shown that blood pressure taken in the upper arm versus the forearm varies by 14 to 20 mmHg. The two pressures are therefore not interchangeable. If the appropriate size cuff is not available and the forearm has to be used, document the site used.

Source: Schell, K., Bradley, E., Bucher, L., Seckel, M., Lyons, D., Wakai, S., . . . Simpson, K. (2005). Clinical comparison of automatic, noninvasive blood pressure in the forearm and upper arm. *American Journal of Critical Care, 14*(3), 232–241.

Body Positioning Affects Blood Pressure

A study in an ambulatory cardiac clinic found that clients seated in proper position (in a chair with back support, feet on the floor and arms at heart level) had readings 12 to 14 percent lower than those who were seated on exam tables.

Source: Turner, M. (2008). University of Virginia Health System reported by the Academy of Medical-Surgical Nurses.

23. Remove cuff from client's arm.
24. Clean the diaphragm/bell and cuff with an approved antiseptic. If possible, each client should have a disposable blood pressure cuff. ▸ ***Rationale:*** Studies have shown that cuffs (as well as stethoscopes) can become contaminated.
25. Check that client is comfortable.
26. Compare blood pressure reading with previous recordings.
27. Perform hand hygiene.
28. Record blood pressure readings using two phases: 120/80 where 120 is the systolic (phase I) and 80 is the diastolic (phase V) pressure; or three phases: 130/110/80 where 130 is the systolic (phase I), 110 is the first diastolic (phase IV), and 80 is the second diastolic (phase V) pressure.
29. Repeat this procedure on the opposite arm if this is an initial reading. ▸ ***Rationale:*** Clients may have a difference of 10 points between the two arms. For ongoing monitoring, note that BP should be taken on the arm with the higher blood pressure.

NOTE: If there is more than 20 points difference, report to physician.

Clinical Alert

When a client moves from recumbent to standing position, systolic pressure can fall 10 to 15 mmHg and diastolic may rise by 5 mmHg.

Blood Pressure Cuff Sizes

- Standard (12–14 cm wide) for the average adult arm.
- Narrower cuff for infant, child, or adult with thin arms.
- For children (younger than 13 years) the bladder should be large enough to encircle the arm completely (100%).
- Wider cuff (18–22 cm) for client with obese arms or thigh pressure readings.

The cuff's inflatable bladder width should be 40% of the circumference of the limb on which it is used. The length of the bladder should be twice its width.

Blood Pressure Classification

Blood Pressure	Systolic	Diastolic
Normal	<120	
Pre high blood pressure	120–139	80–89
Stage I high blood pressure	140–159	90–99
Stage II high blood pressure	160 and higher	100 and higher

Source: National Heart, Lung, and Blood Institute, 2003.

Korotkoff's Sound Phases

Phase I: The pressure level at which the first faint, clear tapping sounds are heard. The sounds gradually increase in intensity as the cuff is deflated. This phase coincides with the reappearance of a palpable pulse (systolic sound).

Phase II: That time during cuff deflation when a murmur or swishing sounds are heard.

Phase III: The period during which sounds are crisper and increase in intensity.

Phase IV: That time when a distinct, abrupt, muffling of sound (usually of a soft, blowing quality) is heard (diastolic sound in children or physically active adults).

Phase V: That pressure level when the last sound is heard and after which all sound disappears (second diastolic sound).

In person with hypertension, an auscultatory gap may be present. This gap is an absence of sounds after the first Korotkoff's sounds appear and then the reappearance of the sounds at a lower level. This condition can be avoided if the brachial artery is palpated first and the cuff is inflated above the level where the pulsations disappear.

Source: American Heart Association.

Clinical Alert

The American Heart Association recommends routine use of the *bell* of the stethoscope for blood pressure (Korotkoff's sounds) auscultation. Studies indicate that when measuring the blood pressure, accuracy is much higher when using the bell (rather than the diaphragm) of the stethoscope.

Source: The Joanna Briggs Institute. (1999). Vital signs. *Best Practice*, 3(3), 3. http://www.joannabriggs.edu.au/pdf/BPISEng_3_3.pdf

Routinely, blood pressure for an acutely ill client should be taken every 1 to 2 hours, and blood pressure for more stabilized clients should be taken every 4 to 8 hours. Clients with severe hypotension or hypertension, with low blood volume, or on vasoconstrictor or vasodilator drugs may require checking every 15 minutes.

EVIDENCE-BASED PRACTICE

Body Position Influence on Blood Pressure

When the client's arm was placed above or below the level of the heart, BP changed by as much as 20 mmHg. Therefore, it is recommended that clients sit with their arm supported horizontally at heart level.

Studies showed that when hypertensive clients crossed their legs while having their BP taken, the systolic readings rose by 9.45 mmHg and the diastolic rose by 3.7 mmHg. Clients should have their feet on the floor during a BP measurement.

Sources: The Joanna Briggs Institute. (1999). Vital signs. *Best Practice*, 3(3), 3. http://www.joannabriggs.edu.au/pdf/BPISEng_3_3.pdf. Foster-Fitzpatrick, L., Ortiz, A., Sibilano, H., Marcantonio, R., & Braun, L. T. (1999). The effects of crossed leg on blood pressure measurement. *Nursing Research*, 48(2), 105–108.

Children's Blood Pressure

Children as young as 3 should have their blood pressure checked to identify possible heart disease. Children under age 3 can have their BP checked by palpation method. The normal systolic BP can be determined by using the formula 80 + 2× the child's age. A newborn's systolic BP ranges between 50 and 80 mmHg and diastolic between 25 and 55 mmHg.

Palpating Systolic Arterial Blood Pressure

Equipment

Sphygmomanometer with proper size cuff

Procedure

1. Gather equipment. Check that cuff is appropriate size for client. ▶ ***Rationale:*** A cuff that is too narrow results in erroneously high readings.
2. Perform hand hygiene.
3. Check two forms of client ID.
4. Explain procedure to client.
5. Place client in relaxed position and support arm at heart level.
6. Wrap cuff snugly and smoothly around the upper part of the arm (1 in. above antecubital space) with center of bladder over brachial artery.
7. Keep pressure level in cuff at zero.

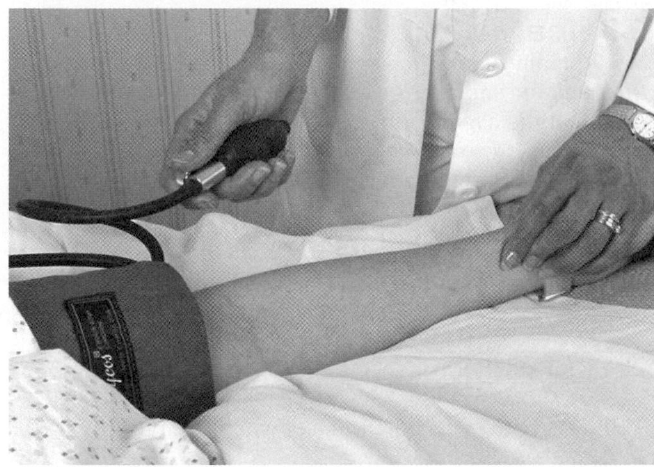
▲ Palpate radial artery while inflating cuff and releasing pressure.

8. Locate radial artery pulsations on cuffed arm.
9. Inflate cuff rapidly (while palpating radial artery), to a level 30 mmHg above level at which radial artery pulsations are no longer felt. ▸ ***Rationale:*** This level ensures that cuff is inflated to a pressure exceeding client's systolic pressure.
10. Continue to palpate artery and release pressure from cuff slowly (2–3 mmHg/sec). The first palpated beat is the systolic pressure. This should be the same point at which the last pulsation was felt during inflation of cuff.
11. Remove cuff and return equipment.
12. Perform hand hygiene.
13. Record systolic blood pressure reading as "palpated systolic pressure."

Clinical Alert

- Avoid measuring blood pressure in an arm with extensive axillary node dissection (e.g., radical mastectomy) or an arteriovenous fistula (e.g., for dialysis).
- Ultrasound techniques such as using a Doppler stethoscope can be used to measure systolic blood pressure when auscultatory sounds are too faint to be heard.

Measuring Lower-Extremity Blood Pressure

Equipment

Stethoscope
Sphygmomanometer with standard or large-size cuff

Procedure

1. Gather equipment.
2. Perform hand hygiene.
3. Check two forms of client ID.
4. Explain procedure to client.
5. Wrap cuff snugly and smoothly around lower leg with cuff's distal edge at the malleolus.
6. Locate either the dorsalis pedis or posterior tibial artery pulsations.
7. Inflate cuff rapidly while palpating foot artery, to a level 30 mmHg above level at which artery pulsations are no longer felt.
8. Place bell (or diaphragm) of stethoscope quickly on pulse site.
9. Deflate cuff slowly (2–4 mmHg/sec) while auscultating sounds over the selected artery.
10. Remove cuff and return equipment.
11. Check to see that client is comfortable.
12. Record readings for first (systolic) and last (diastolic) sounds, noting site and client position.

For Alternative Methods

13. Measure blood pressure in thigh by using a large cuff with bladder placed over posterior mid-thigh and bottom edge above knee. ▸ ***Rationale:*** The cuff bladder must be directly over the posterior popliteal artery for accurate reading. Listen with stethoscope at popliteal fossa with client in prone position, or supine with knee flexed enough for stethoscope placement.

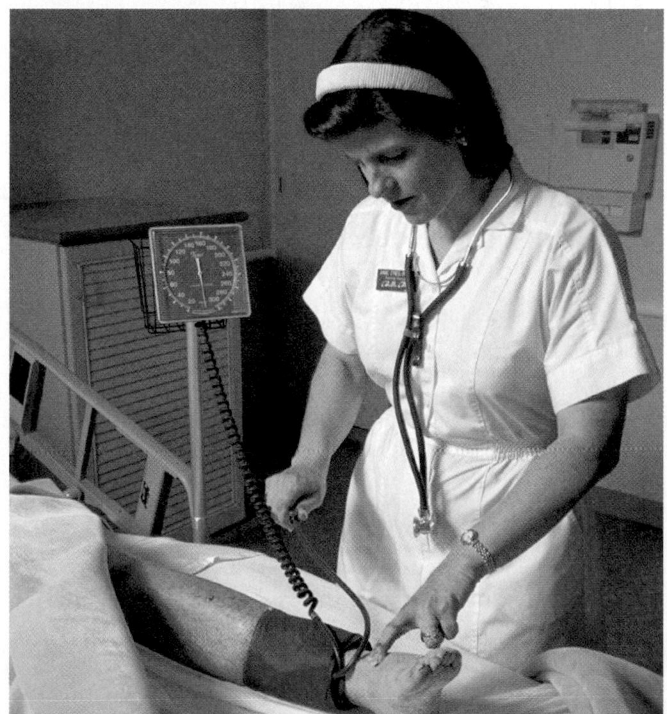
▲ Wrap cuff snugly around lower leg and locate dorsalis pedis.

NOTE: The systolic pressure is 20 to 30 mmHg higher than in the brachial artery. The diastolic pressure is the same.

14. Measure blood pressure in forearm by placing appropriate size cuff around forearm 13 cm from elbow; listen for Korotkoff's sounds over radial artery at wrist.
15. Compare blood pressures measured indirectly in the arm, leg, and thigh to reveal similar values. Measurements may be difficult to obtain in clients with peripheral vascular disease.

Clinical Alert

Traditionally, vital signs provided the basis for assessing the need for and adequacy of sedation in critically ill clients. If the client is on drug therapy, vital signs may not always be a reliable indicator of sedation, because they do not directly reflect the level of consciousness.

Measuring Blood Pressure by Flush Method in Small Infant

Equipment

Sphygmomanometer with appropriate cuff
Elastic bandage
Assistant for observing flush
Well-lighted room

Procedure

1. Gather equipment.
2. Perform hand hygiene.
3. Check two forms of client ID.
4. Wrap blood pressure cuff snugly and smoothly just above wrist or ankle.
5. Elevate extremity above heart level.
6. Wrap elastic bandage firmly around exposed hand or foot. ▶ ***Rationale:*** Bandage compression empties the veins.
7. Lower extremity to heart level when compression is complete.
8. Inflate cuff rapidly to 200 mmHg.
9. Remove elastic bandage.
10. Deflate cuff slowly (not exceeding 5 mmHg/sec).
11. Instruct assistant to watch for appearance of flush in the extremity distal to cuff. ▶ ***Rationale:*** An assistant is necessary so that pressure at which flush appears can be precisely noted. This reading more clearly reflects the *mean* blood pressure than the systolic pressure.
12. Document that blood pressure was taken by flush method.

Clinical Alert

Flush pressures are taken on small infants or on adults when unable to auscultate or palpate blood pressure readings.

Using a Continuous Noninvasive Monitoring Device

Equipment

Blood pressure cuff
Display monitor
Readout paper for monitor

Procedure

1. Check two forms of client ID and perform hand hygiene.
2. Gather equipment. Select proper size blood pressure cuff. (Size should be two-thirds the size of upper arm.) Attach the cuff to the air hose by firmly pushing the valve from the cuff into the air hose and twisting to secure fit.
3. Squeeze the air from the cuff.
4. Wrap the cuff securely around the extremity (usually the arm).
    a. Place cuff over brachial artery with lower edge 1 in. above antecubital fossa.
    b. If skin is fragile, place single layer of cotton under cuff.
5. Turn power switch ON.

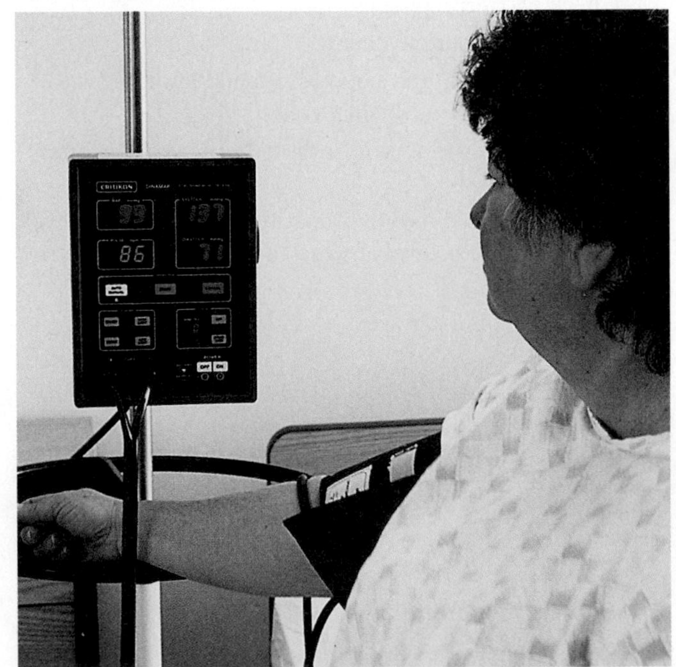

▲ Continuous monitoring of blood pressure is done by attaching cuff to display monitor.

6. Position the extremity at the level of the heart. ▸ ***Rationale:*** If arm is below heart level, reading will be higher than normal.
7. Set arterial pressure alarm limits by pushing *Alarm* to ON and set both HIGH and LOW parameters by depressing the *Alarm* button until the parameters read out on the digital display. ▸ ***Rationale:*** The alarm parameters provide a safety factor by alerting the nurse when the readings exceed the parameters.
8. Test time cycles by turning wheel (found above alarm button) to 1 minute and check for cycling effects. Then, to set automatic cycle time, move the wheel to desired time increments.
9. Press START button for approximately 4 seconds to activate printer for readout of blood pressure; press again to begin reading. Systolic, diastolic, mean arterial pressures, and heart rates can be monitored with this system.
10. Alternate extremities if device is used for a prolonged period of time.
11. Check position of cuff and skin under cuff frequently. ▸ ***Rationale:*** It is important to note bruises or skin trauma and to check if position of cuff has changed.
12. Perform hand hygiene.

New Trends—Electronic Stethoscope

A new electronic stethoscope is now available. It measures a client's blood pressure via Bluetooth-Enabled Cardioscan and sends the results directly into the client's computer record for immediate evaluation.

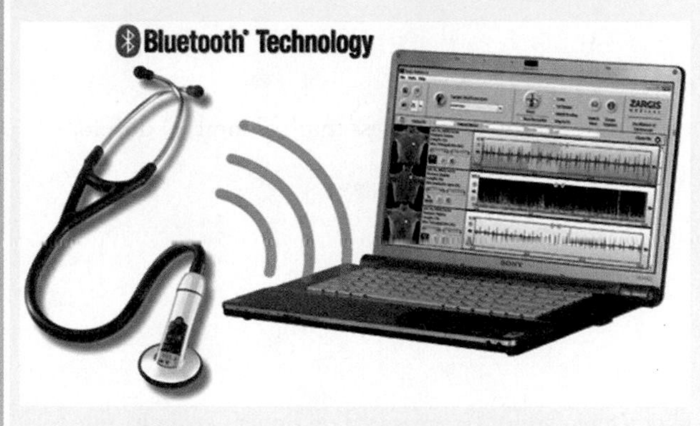

Source: Courtesy 3M® Littman®.

DOCUMENTATION for Blood Pressure

- Two phases of Korotkoff's sounds (e.g., 120/80) and site
- Three phases of Korotkoff's sounds (e.g., 130/110/80) and site
- Response to alternative nursing actions
- Response to position changes
- Document vital signs in chart, in addition to attaching digital read-outs

CRITICAL THINKING Application

Expected Outcomes

- Blood pressure readings provide information regarding the overall health status of the client.
- Major changes from prior assessments are documented.
- Accurate readings are taken by using the correct cuff size and procedure.
- Beginning and disappearance of Korotkoff's sounds during a blood pressure reading are evaluated and documented.
- The presence of factors that can alter blood pressure readings is identified.

Unexpected Outcomes

Blood pressure reading is abnormally high without apparent physiologic cause.

Alternative Actions

- Check if arm was unsupported.
- Check if cuff was too narrow.
- Check if cuff was not snug.
- Check if cuff was deflated too slowly or reinflated during deflation, causing venous engorgement and abnormally high diastolic readings.
- Ask if client has pain, was anxious (white coat syndrome), or had just exercised, eaten, or smoked. Recheck pressure as indicated.
- Check blood pressure on both arms. The normal difference from arm to arm is usually no more than 5 mmHg.
- Check if insufficient rest before assessment.

(continued)

CRITICAL THINKING Application *(Continued)*

Unexpected Outcomes	Alternative Actions
Blood pressure reading is very low and there are no significant clinical indicators.	• Assess if cuff is too wide. • Check if client's arm was above heart level. • Check if inflation was too slow. This reduces intensity of Korotkoff's sounds. • Assess if Korotkoff's sounds were barely audible. Raise client's arm, and then recheck. Sounds should be louder. • Identify if stethoscope was misplaced and was not on brachial artery. • Take blood pressure 3 minutes after client rises from supine to standing if postural hypotension is suspected.
Hypotension (systolic pressure less than 90 mmHg) develops.	• Take all vital signs more frequently (every 15 minutes to 2 hours) until condition has stabilized. • Place client in supine position with lower extremities elevated 45° and head on pillow. • Assess cause of hypotension, and notify physician. • Increase or administer fluids as ordered by physician. • Observe postoperative clients for signs of bleeding. • Administer oxygen.
Blood pressure cannot be measured on upper extremity due to casts or other causes of inaccessibility	• Use lower extremity to obtain blood pressures. Systolic pressure in thigh is usually 20 to 30 mmHg higher than in arms, but diastolic pressure is equivalent to arm readings.
Korotkoff's sounds cannot be heard due to hypotension.	• Use the palpation method or ultrasound technique. Client may be candidate for intraarterial (direct method) pressure monitoring.
Hypertension (blood pressure consistently over 140/90 mmHg) develops.	• For clients with severe, acute hypertension, take vital signs more frequently (every 15 minutes to 2 hours) until condition has stabilized. • Notify physician. • If client is anxious or excited, institute relaxation techniques to lower blood pressure. • Allow client to rest after strenuous exercise. • Relieve pain with reassurance, change of position, and analgesia as ordered by physician. • For clients with essential hypertension, administer antihypertensive and diuretic drugs as ordered by the physician. Evaluate response by checking blood pressure in reclining, sitting, and standing position. Instruct client in diet therapy, such as low salt, low fat, and inclusion of vitamins and garlic.
Continuous BP monitoring system displays 00 instead of blood pressure reading. (00 indicates the unit is unable to determine parameters.)	• Check cuff placement and size to determine if appropriately placed.
Client's blood pressure continues to be high with a diagnosis of hypertension.	• Evaluate any medication client is taking, including antihypertensive agents. • Teach client about lifestyle modifications as a cornerstone for managing hypertension. 1. Lose excess weight. 2. Maintain a low-fat diet with many fruits and vegetables. 3. Limit alcohol intake. 4. Stop smoking. 5. Exercise regularly. 6. Include extra minerals in diet: potassium, calcium, and magnesium. 7. Reduce sodium intake and switch to sea salt. 8. Practice stress-reducing exercises such as meditation, yoga, tai chi.

GERONTOLOGIC Considerations

Cardiac Status—Changes

- Changes in cardiovascular status with aging are often insidious and may become apparent when system is stressed and there is increased demand for cardiac output (which may occur with illness and hospitalization). Nursing care assessment should focus on client's cardiovascular status, even when diagnosis does not include a cardiac condition.
- Blood pressure measurement should take age into account. If client has severe joint stiffness, pseudohypertension may be present. If this is suspected, raise the cuff pressure above the systolic blood pressure and, if the radial pulse remains palpable, the reading may show 10 to 15 mmHg in error.
- Postural hypotension is common in the elderly (positional drop of less than 20 mmHg); nurses should take note when helping a client out of bed. Hypertension is also common in this age group.
- A rise in blood pressure may be associated with reduced cardiac output, vasoconstriction, increased blood volume, or fluid overload.
- Pulse changes, particularly an irregular pulse, can be related to hypoxia, airway obstruction, or electrolyte imbalance.
- The arteries in elderly clients may feel stiff and knotty due to decreased elasticity. Excessive pressure to site when taking pulse may obliterate it. The normal rate is 60 to 90 beats/min.
- If pulses are not palpated, the Doppler may need to be used.

Respiratory Status—Changes

- Changes in the respiratory system may be subtle and gradual with the elderly: oxygen saturation is decreased to 93% to 94%; there is often poor cough response and incomplete lung expansion—all of which leads to increased risk of pulmonary infection when the elderly client is hospitalized.
- Slightly irregular breathing patterns are not unusual in the elderly.

Temperature—Changes

- With the elderly, temperature may be as low as 95°F. Because they may be easily dehydrated with increased temperature, nursing assessment should include baseline temperature at admission and continued monitoring during hospitalization.
- Elderly who have acute infections may have a subnormal temperature.
- Increased temperatures can lead to increased metabolism, thus increasing the body's demand for oxygen. This causes the heart to work harder.
- Oral temperatures are the preferred method for obtaining the elderly client's temperature.

MANAGEMENT Guidelines

Each state legislates a Nurse Practice Act for RNs and LPN/LVNs. Healthcare facilities are responsible for establishing and implementing policies and procedures that conform to their state's regulations. Verify the regulations and role parameters for each healthcare worker in your facility.

Delegation

- Taking vital signs for clients may be assigned to any healthcare worker provided they have been assessed for competency in the procedure. This includes LPN/LVN, CNA, UAP, and EMT.
- The registered nurse must identify parameters for which the healthcare worker is to notify the nurse (i.e., blood pressure above or below a certain reading, pulse rate, or irregular pulse).
- The nurse must provide detailed explanations and/or demonstrate alterations in the procedure or specific methods of obtaining the vital signs to CNA, UAP, or EMTs.
- Obtaining peripheral pulses by use of the Doppler is the responsibility of the RN or LPN/LVN. A CNA or UAP is not responsible for using the Doppler.
- The CNA or UAP may monitor blood pressure using the noninvasive monitoring device; however, the CNA or UAP is not responsible for initiating the procedure or setting the alarms.

Communication Matrix

- Directions must be given to healthcare workers on documentation procedures. Do they complete the graphic record, write the findings on a vital sign sheet at the nurses' desk, or give the results to the nurse?
- The registered nurse must evaluate all abnormal or changed vital signs identified by the healthcare workers. The nurse maintains total responsibility for client care even though someone else performs the task of taking the vital signs.
- The registered nurse must ensure that the healthcare workers know the parameters for reporting unusual vital signs. Periodic checks with the workers may be necessary.

CRITICAL THINKING Strategies

Scenario 1

Mr. Trager (age 92) has been admitted to your unit with a temperature of 103°F, BP 140/90, P 114, and R 30 and labored. He reports a history of 3 days of diarrhea and fever and asks you for something to drink.

1. From your analysis of the admission data, determine the following:
   a. Appropriate nursing diagnosis in priority for this client.
   b. The metabolic effects of fever on pulse and respiration.
   c. Age factors that contribute to the existing problem.
2. What are the other assessment findings indicative of the diagnosis established from primary admitting data?
3. Develop a plan of care for this client.
4. Describe the evaluative outcomes for problem resolution.

Scenario 2

Mr. Sondheim is admitted to the hospital with unstable hypertension for evaluation. He has a family history of hypertension and heart disease. The nurse will complete a physical exam and a history.

1. What information is missing in the family history that the nurse will want to elicit from the client?
2. Which questions regarding lifestyle would be appropriate to ask?
3. Which aspects of client teaching would the nurse want to cover before Mr. Sondheim is discharged?

Scenario 3

You are caring for a client, and when checking his vital signs, you are unable to palpate his radial pulse.

1. What would be your follow-up intervention?
2. When you still cannot find a pulse clear enough to document, what would be your next intervention?
3. What parameters of the pulse will you pay attention to when assessing and recording a client's pulse?

NCLEX® Review Questions

Unless otherwise specified, choose only one (1) answer.

1. During a shift assessment, the nurse notes that the client's peripheral pulses are absent. The next intervention would be to
   1. Palpate the peripheral pulse.
   2. Assess for other signs of circulatory impairment.
   3. Notify the physician.
   4. Administer O_2 as ordered.
2. When a pulse deficit is detected in a client, the nurse would expect that the client is experiencing
   1. Premature ventricular beats.
   2. Bradycardia.
   3. Tachycardia.
   4. Heart block.
3. A client's temperature remains elevated despite the administration of antipyretic drugs. The first intervention after determining this is to
   1. Administer a cool bath.
   2. Assess all remaining signs.
   3. Request orders for a cooling blanket.
   4. Obtain an order for a blood culture.
4. Taking a client's blood pressure that has been within normal limits, the nurse gets a reading that is very low without any significant clinical indicators. The appropriate intervention is to
   1. Assess if the BP cuff is too narrow.
   2. Assess if the BP cuff is too wide.
   3. Assess if the client's arm was positioned below heart level.
   4. Notify the physician.
5. Taking a client's blood pressure, the reading is very altered from previous readings recorded on his chart. The first intervention is to
   1. Recheck the blood pressure with different equipment.
   2. Notify the physician.
   3. Validate the reading with another nurse.
   4. Check the client's circulatory status.
6. Which of the following breathing patterns of adults are abnormal?
   Select all those that apply.
   1. Apnea.
   2. Rate of 12 to 20 per minute.

3. Hyperpnea.
4. Biot's.
5. Bradypnea.

7. Assessing a client newly admitted to the ER, an early sign of shock would be a
   1. Pulse rate of 120.
   2. Blood pressure of 110/70.
   3. Respiratory rate of 24.
   4. Fever of 101 degrees F.

8. An accurate graph of blood pressure readings is very important for evaluation. For taking a blood pressure reading, the nurse should apply the cuff to the
   1. Same arm, while the client is in the same position each time.
   2. Right arm, while the client is in a sitting position.
   3. Left arm, while the client is in a left lateral recumbent position.
   4. Left arm, while the client is in a supine position.

9. When using the tympanic route for taking a temperature, what is the rationale for directing the probe toward the tympanic membrane?
   1. Pressure seals the ear canal.
   2. The probe will not record unless it is near the tympanic membrane.
   3. This method records the core temperature.
   4. This method provides better access to the ear canal.

10. The RN is in charge of the team assigned to care for six clients for morning shift. The staffing includes the RN, an LVN, and two Nursing Assistants. All clients need to have vital signs taken as part of their shift assessment. How will the RN best assign these duties?
    1. The LVN should do all of the vital signs.
    2. The RN and LVN should split the vital signs.
    3. The RN should assign vital signs to the two Nursing Assistants.
    4. The RN should do all of the vital signs.

11

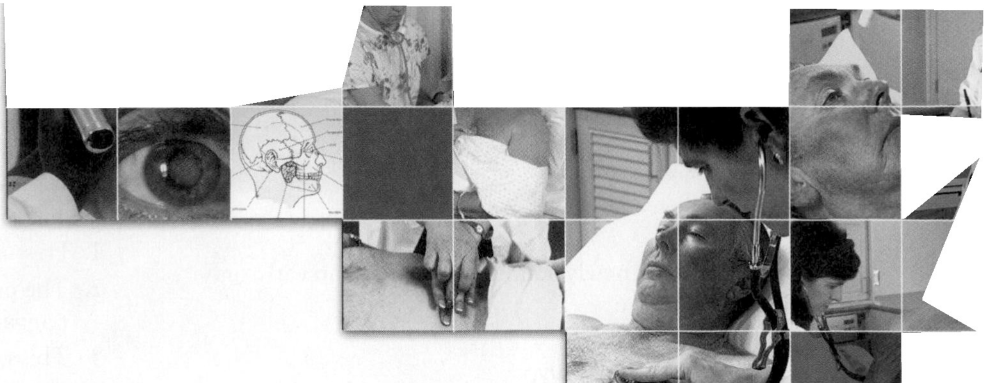

Physical Assessment

LEARNING OBJECTIVES

1. Outline the essential elements obtained from a health history.
2. List the four techniques of physical assessment.
3. Demonstrate six steps of the focus assessment.
4. Describe the abnormal manifestations associated with each specific body system for one client with whom you are familiar.
5. List four normal responses that determine the client's level of consciousness.
6. Describe four abnormal responses in pupil assessment.
7. State three assessment components of the skin.
8. Describe normal and abnormal lung sounds.
9. Describe the assessment techniques use in an abdominal assessment in sequential order.
10. Outline the steps of breast assessment.
11. Identify the four areas for heart sound auscultation.
12. List at least five essential elements included in a mental status assessment.
13. Compare and contrast three elements of the antepartum obstetrical assessment.
14. Relate the elements of a "9" score on the Apgar test.
15. Describe basic components of a pediatric physical assessment.

CHAPTER OUTLINE

ASSESSMENT

Basic assessment discussed in this chapter can be performed in less than 10 minutes using a stethoscope, penlight, reflex hammer, your hands, and observational skills. Although you may not be able to perform assessment rapidly at first, you will have many opportunities to practice your skills, because every client should be assessed at least once a shift.

While interviewing the client, note such characteristics as hair, skin, posture, facial expression, and body language—in other words, the general appearance of the client. Then proceed with a head-to-toe systems assessment using the four techniques of assessment: inspection, palpation, percussion, and auscultation. This IPPA sequence is used for all systems except for the abdominal assessment, which requires auscultation *before* palpation and percussion. Palpation and percussion are performed using fingers and hands to assess abnormalities of sound, such as vocal fremitus, enlarged organs, organ displacement, and chest expansion. Auscultation is accomplished by using a stethoscope to listen to breath, heart, and bowel sounds. Observe the client's response as each system is assessed.

Equipment

The stethoscope is the primary instrument used for assessment. Remember that any movement of the tubing or chest piece by clothing or hands can cause extraneous noise that obliterates the sounds you want to hear. The diaphragm piece should be applied firmly to the skin. It enhances high-pitched sounds (breath sounds, normal heart sounds, bowel sounds). The bell piece should be placed very lightly to pick up low-pitched sounds, such as vascular sounds and abnormal heart sounds. If the bell is pressed firmly, it stretches the skin and acts as a diaphragm. Other instruments used include the penlight, reflex hammer, ophthalmoscope, otoscope, and tuning fork.

HEALTH HISTORY

A total client assessment begins with a nursing health history. Using open-ended questions such as "Tell me about . . .," collect data about past health conditions, current problems, and present needs. The information is obtained through objective (observed) and subjective (stated by client) data collection.

Information obtained from the interview and the physical assessment constitutes the basis for identifying nursing diagnoses and establishing the individualized client care plan. A complete health history includes the following elements:

- *Biographic information:* age, sex, educational level, marital status, living arrangements.
- *Chief complaint:* condition that brought client to healthcare facility; reason for visit; any recent changes.
- *Present health status or illness:* onset of the problem; clinical manifestations, including severity of symptoms; pain characteristics if present.
- *Health history:* general state of health, past illnesses, surgeries, hospitalizations, allergies, over the counter (OTC) medications, herbal supplements, current medications, and general habits such as smoking, alcohol consumption, or recreational drug use.
- *Family history:* age and health status of parents, siblings, and children; cause of death for immediate family members.
- *Psychosocial factors, lifestyles:* cultural beliefs that influence health management; religious or spiritual beliefs.
- *Nutrition:* dietary habits, preferences, or restrictions.
- *Domestic violence:* (The Joint Commission requirement).

NURSES' ROLE

The nurses' role in obtaining a health history and completing a physical assessment has expanded dramatically over the last 40 years. Today nurses must be adequately instructed to perform a total assessment, as well as a focus assessment, including the use of equipment, formerly the domain of physicians only. The skill of performing a physical assessment must be practiced repeatedly to acquire expertise.

EXAMINATION TECHNIQUES

Inspection

Observe the client while facing him or her in the bed or chair. Observe the client's skin color and texture; check for lesions and hair distribution. Look at overall body structure. If the client can be out of bed, observe gait and stance. Note all parts of the body as the examination proceeds. Inspection also evaluates verbal and behavioral responses and mental status.

Palpation

Obtain information by using the hands and fingers to palpate. A light or deep palpation depends on the area being palpated. The palmar surface of fingers and finger pads are used to determine position of the organs, size and consistency, fluid accumulation, pain, and masses. The ulnar surface of the hand is used to distinguish vibration and temperature. The moisture and warmth of the skin can also be determined during palpation.

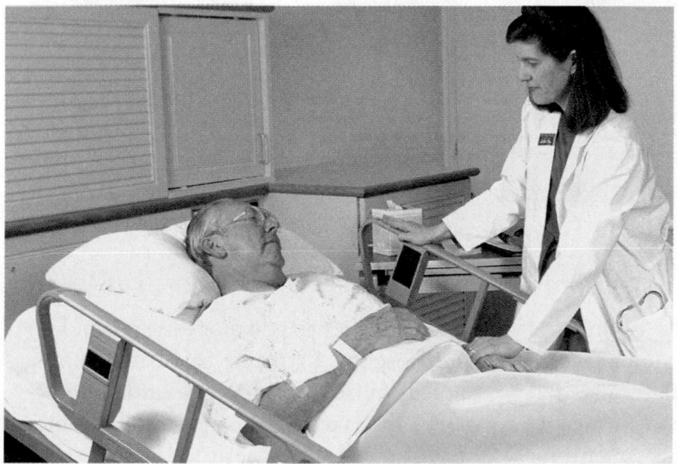

▲ Inspection.

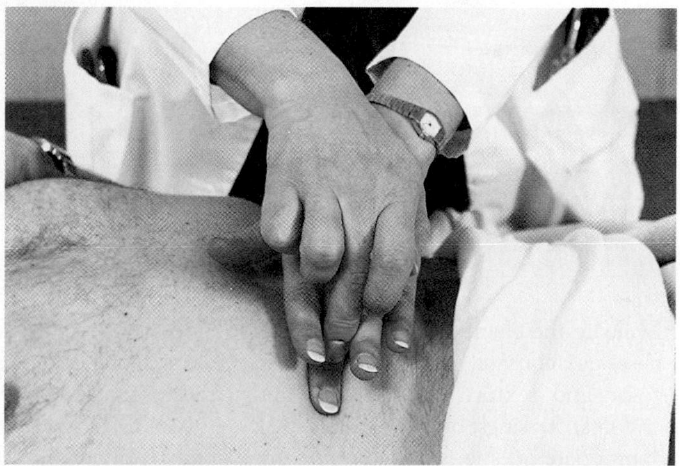

▲ Percussion.

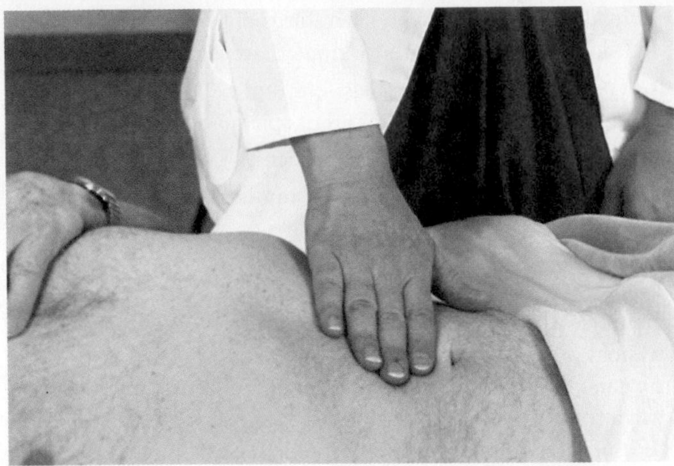
▲ Palpation.

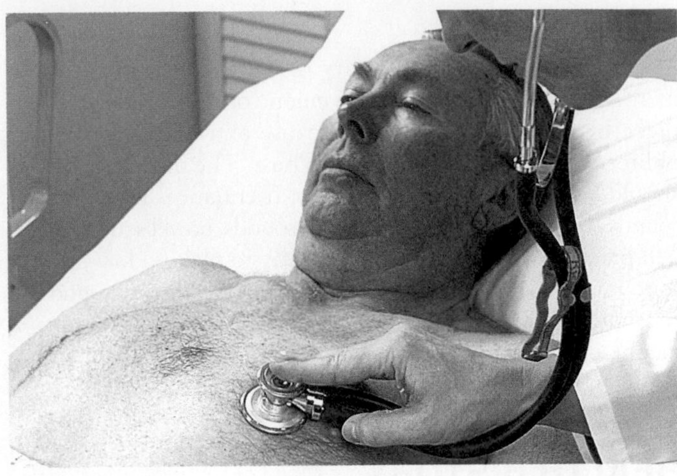
▲ Auscultation.

Percussion

With percussion, sound waves are produced by using the fingers as a hammer. Place the interphalangeal joint of the middle finger on the skin surface of the nondominant hand. Using the tip of the middle finger of the dominant hand, strike the placed finger. Vibration is produced by the impact of the fingers striking against underlying tissue. Sound or tone of the vibration is determined by body area or organ percussed. Normal lung areas produce a resonance sound; liver sounds are dull, and a flat sound is heard over muscle.

Auscultation

Place the stethoscope on the client's bare skin to listen for the presence and characteristics of sound waves. The bell of the stethoscope is used to detect low-pitched sounds; the diaphragm detects high-pitched sounds. Note variations in intensity, pitch, duration, and quality.

Assessment: Focus (Shift)

A full, comprehensive physical assessment is completed upon admission. A focus assessment, also called a bedside or shift assessment, is performed at the beginning and ending of the shift and concentrates on vital assessment parameters; it tracks changes or problem-oriented assessments from shift-to-shift and should take no more than 5 minutes to complete. Several activities in the assessment can be completed at the same time. Usually, it is individualized to fit the client's condition, diagnosis, and level of acuity.

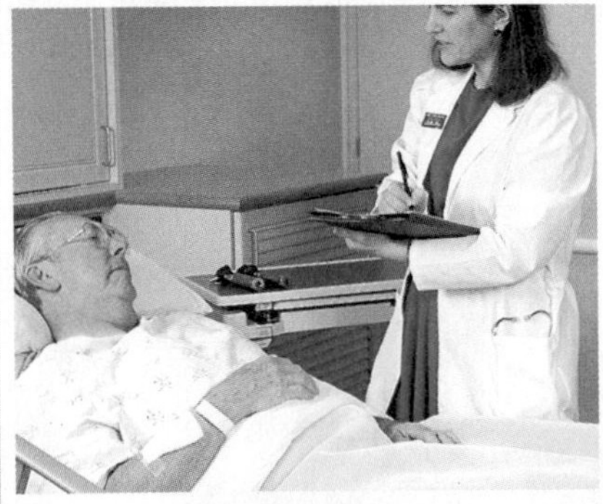
▲ **Step 1**

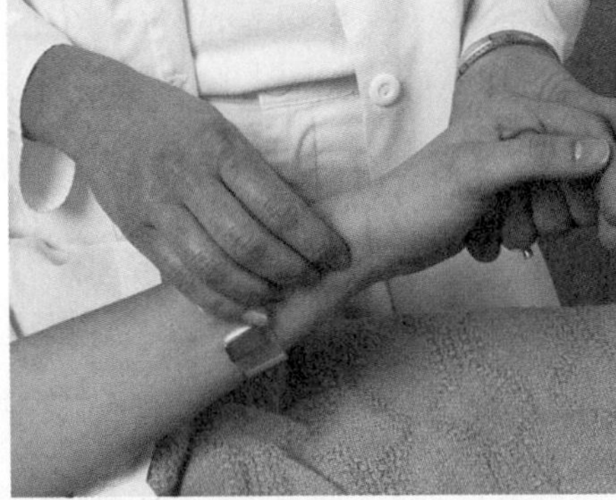
▲ **Step 2**

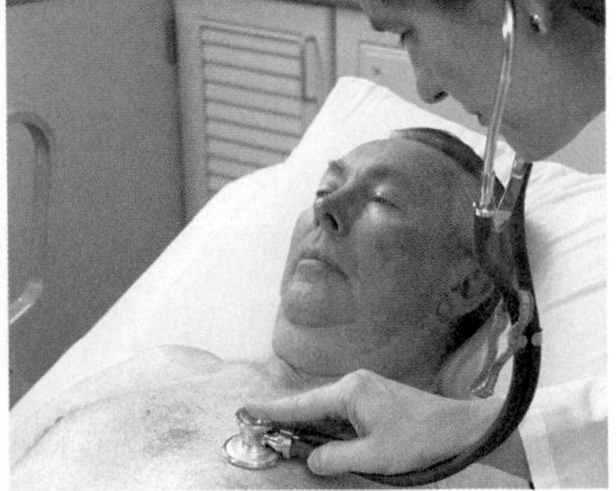
▲ **Step 3**

Step 1
Evaluate the client's level of consciousness, eye contact and responsiveness, color and texture of the skin, and any IVs, dressings, or tubes visible. Ask appropriate questions to determine orientation to time and place. Establish the nurse–client relationship at this time.

Step 2
Assess vital signs. While taking the client's pulse, feel skin temperature and moisture. Check bilateral radial pulses. Observe for edema in face or neck. Individualize the assessment; for example, with a neurologic condition, check pupils.

Step 3
Remove client's gown or raise gown. Use stethoscope to listen to heart sounds, apical pulse and breath sounds bilaterally. Observe breathing patterns, symmetry of chest movement, shape of chest, and depth of respirations. Check for skin turgor.

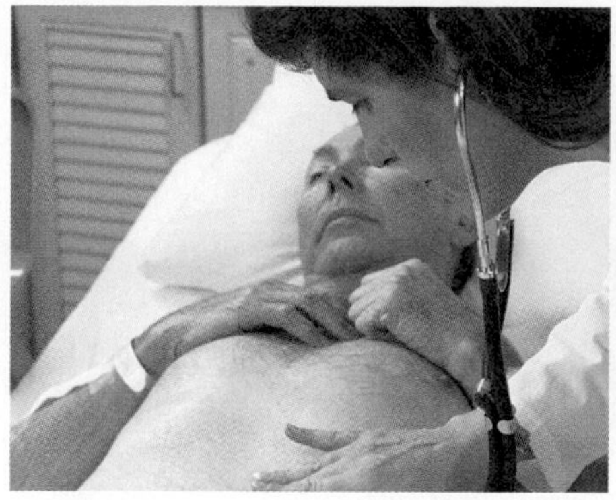

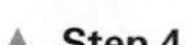 Step 4

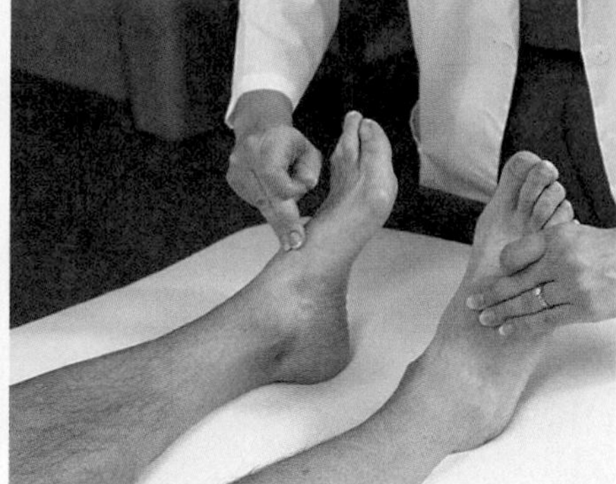

▲ Step 5

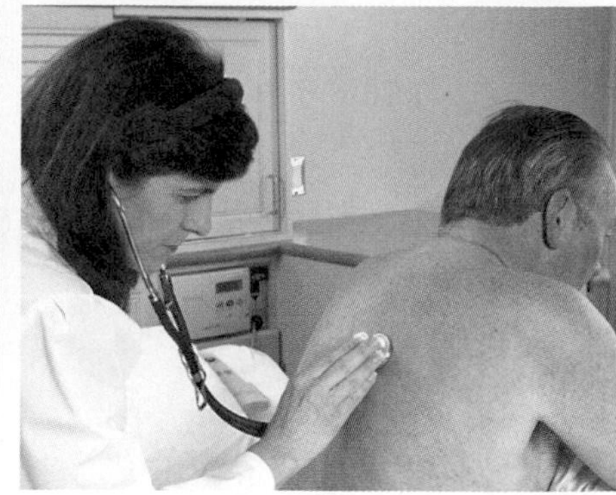

▲ Step 6

Step 4
Auscultate abdomen for bowel sounds. Use palpation and percussion techniques only if appropriate to diagnosis. Palpate bladder if necessary (based on output). If catheter is in place, observe urinary output for color, odor, consistency, and amount.

Step 5
Assess lower extremities for warmth, color, moisture, presence of pedal or popliteal pulses, muscle tone, and sensation. Assess for pedal edema or general edema in the lower extremities. Check traction or casted areas for skin breakdown, alignment, and placement.

Step 6
Have client turn onto side or sit at edge of bed. Assess posterior lung fields and symmetry of chest movement with inspiration. Assess skin for pressure areas, particularly coccyx and heels when client returns to side-lying position. Evaluate client's ability to move in bed.

ASSESSMENT OF THE NERVOUS SYSTEM

- Level of Consciousness
  - Glasgow Coma Scale
  - Respiratory Assessment
  - Cranial Nerves
  - Spinal Nerves
- Pupil Assessment
- Motor Function Assessment
- Coordination Assessment
- Reflex Assessment
- Sensory Function
- Vital Signs

An understanding of the function of each lobe of the brain allows the nurse to be able to identify potential client problems when an injury occurs to that portion of the brain.

The brain comprises three segments: the brainstem, cerebrum, and the cerebellum. There are 12 cranial nerves, which are discussed later in this chapter, and 31 pairs of spinal nerves with dorsal and ventral roots.

The brainstem is divided into four sections: The *diencephalon* comprises the thalamus, which screens and relays sensory impulses to the cortex, and the hypothalamus, which regulates the autonomic nervous system, stress response, sleep, appetite, body temperature, water balance, and emotions. The *midbrain* is responsible for motor coordination and conjugate eye movements. The *pons* controls involuntary respiratory reflexes and contains projection tracts between the spinal cord, medulla, and brain. The *medulla* contains cardiac, respiratory, vomiting, and vasomotor centers. In addition, all afferent and efferent nerve tracts must pass between the spinal cord and brain through the medulla.

The cerebral hemispheres have an outer layer formed by cellular gray matter, called the cerebral cortex. The two cerebral hemispheres are divided into four major lobes. The frontal lobe controls emotions, judgments, motor function, and the motor speech area. The parietal lobe integrates general sensations; interprets pain, touch, and temperature; and governs discrimination. The temporal lobe contains the auditory center and sensory speech center. The occipital lobe controls the visual area. The cerebellum coordinates muscle movement, posture, equilibrium, and muscle tone.

The 12 cranial nerves are summarized in Table 11-2. The 2nd through 12th nerves arise from the brainstem. The cranial nerves are 12 pairs of parasympathetic nerves with their nuclei along the brainstem.

The neurologic examination begins with the initial contact with the client. Evaluation of verbal responses, movement, and sensation is carried out throughout the examination. In addition, functions of the cerebrum, cerebellum, cranial nerves, spinal cord, and peripheral nerves are assessed. The level of consciousness is the most sensitive and reliable index of cerebral function.

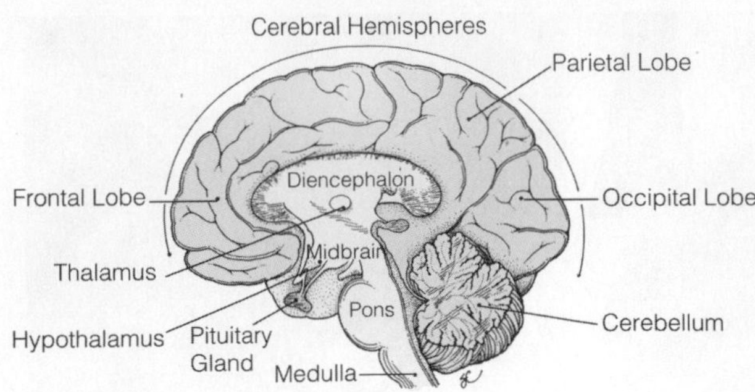

▲ Lobes of the brain.

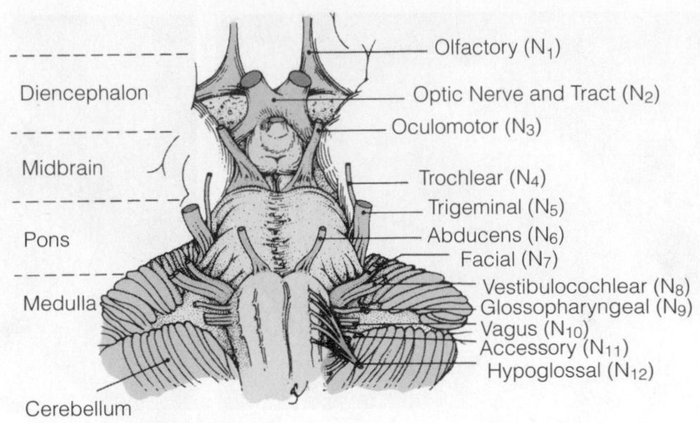

▲ Brain segments and cranial nerves.

TABLE 11-1 Glasgow Coma Scale

A. Motor response.	Points
1. Obeys a simple command	6
2. Localizes painful stimuli; attempts to remove offending stimulus; lack of obedience	5
3. Withdrawn—moves purposelessly in response to pain	4
4. Abnormal flexion—decorticate posturing	3
5. Extensor response—decerebrate posturing	2
6. No motor response to pain	1
B. Verbal response.	**Points**
1. Oriented—to time, place, and person	5
2. Confused conversation; disorientation in *one* or more spheres	4
3. Inappropriate or disorganized use of words (cursing); lack of sustained conversion	3
4. Responds with incomprehensible sounds	2
5. No verbal response (Record T if an endotracheal or tracheostomy tube is in place)	1
C. Eye opening.	**Points**
1. Spontaneous when a person approaches	4
2. In response to speech	3
3. Only in response to pain	2
4. Eyes do not open, even to painful stimuli (Record C if eyes are closed by swelling)	1

NOTE: This scale is a tool for assessing a client's response to stimuli. Scores range from 3 (deep coma) to 15 (normal). Add numbers to get a total score.

TABLE 11-2 Cranial Nerves and Their Function

Cranial Nerve	Function	Testing Cranial Nerves
I Olfactory	Sensory nerve	Recognizes odor in each nostril separately (e.g., coffee)
II Optio	Sensory nerve: conducts sensory information from the retina	Demonstrates visual acuity: can read newsprint
III Oculomotor	Motor nerve: controls four of the six extraocular muscles; raises eyelid and controls the constrictor pupillae and ciliary muscles of the eyeball	Responds to light: pupils constrict; moves eyes medially; elevates upper eyelid

TABLE 11-2 Cranial Nerves and Their Function *(Continued)*

Cranial Nerve	Function	Testing Cranial Nerves
IV Trochlear	Motor nerve: controls the superior oblique eye muscle	Move eyes to the right, up then down, and to the left
V Trigeminal	Mixed nerve with three sensory branches and one motor branch: the ophthalmic branch supplies the corneal reflex	Demonstrates normal facial sensation; clenches teeth with no lateral jaw deviation; blinks as wisp touched to cornea
VI Abducens	Motor nerve: controls the lateral rectus muscle of the eye	Moves eyes laterally
VII Facial	Mixed nerve: anterior tongue receives sensory supply, motor supply to glands of nose, palate lacrimal submaxillary, and sublingual; motor branch supplies hyoid elevators and muscles of expression and closes eyelid	Elevates eyebrows; puffs cheeks; recognizes tastes (sugar, salt)
VIII Acoustic	Sensory nerve with two divisions: hearing and semicircular canals	Hears whisper separately with each ear
IX Glossopharyngeal	Mixed nerve: motor innervates parotid gland; sensory innervates auditory tube and posterior portion of taste buds	Demonstrates gag reflex to tongue blade when touched to back of tongue
X Vagus	Mixed nerve: motor branches to the pharyngeal and laryngeal muscles and to the viscera of the thorax and abdomen; sensory portion supplies the pinna of the ear, thoracic, and abdominal viscera	Same as IX
XI Accessory	Motor nerve: innervates the sternocleidomastoid and trapezius muscles	Shrugs shoulders
XII Hypoglossal	Motor nerve: controls tongue muscles	Sticks tongue out in midline without deviation

Assessment: Neurologic

Assessment	Normal Responses	Abnormal Responses
Level of Consciousness		
Apply **Glasgow Coma Scale** Evaluate **verbal responses and orientation** If client seems awake and alert but does not respond properly, check to see if client is blind, deaf, or speaks another language	A score of 15 is evaluated as normal Alert Mood appropriate to situation Responds to verbal command Answers questions appropriately Speaks clearly Oriented to time, person, place, and purpose Recent and remote memory intact	A score under 15 is not normal; a comatose client is 7 or less Drowsy Difficult to awaken Unable to give date, month, place Irritable Memory defect Difficulty finding words Does not recognize family Does not respond to own name
Observe and test symmetry of **motor responses** on both sides of body	Eyes open Follows command to stick out tongue, squeeze fingers, move extremities	Eyes closed Does not follow directions to stick out tongue, squeeze fingers, or move extremities
Exert pressure on nailbed with pen Apply pressure to supraorbital ridge Pinch Achilles tendon Test each side independently	Responds to painful stimuli by reaching out or trying to stop pressure	Does not localize or withdraw from painful stimuli or withdraws abnormally Assumes *decorticate posturing* (legs extended; feet extended with plantar flexion; arms internally rotated and flexed on chest): may

(continued)

Assessment: Neurologic *(Continued)*

Assessment	Abnormal Responses
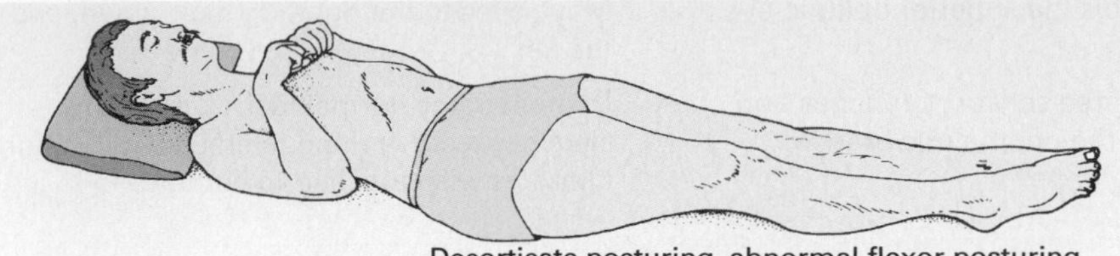 Decorticate posturing–abnormal flexor posturing 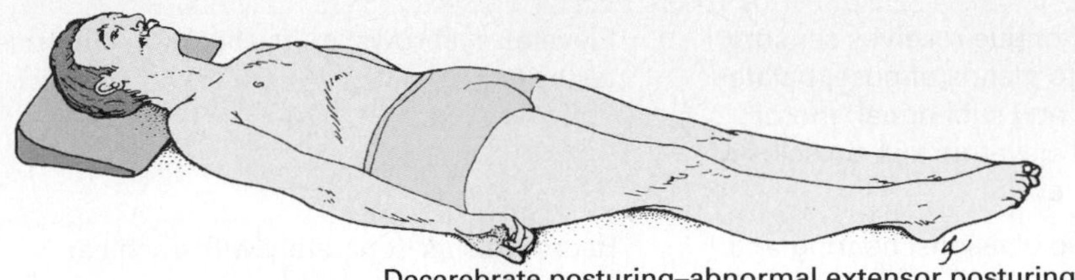 Decerebrate posturing–abnormal extensor posturing	be due to lesion of corticospinal tract near cerebral hemisphere Assumes *decerebrate posturing* (arms stiffly extended and hands turned outward and flexed; legs extended with plantar flexion): may be due to lesion in diencephalon, pons, or midbrain Assumes *flaccid posturing* (no motor response): may be due to extreme brain injury to motor area of brain *Involuntary movements* *Choreiform* (jerky and quick): present in Sydenham's chorea *Athetoid* (twisting and slow): present in cerebral palsy *Tremors:* hyperthyroidism, cerebellar ataxia, parkinsonism *Spasms:* cord-injured clients *Seizures:* brain injury, heat stroke, electrolyte imbalance

Respiratory Assessment

Clients with neurologic damage are at risk for respiratory complications

Respirations are normal
Oxygen levels are normal

Asterixis: metabolic encephalopathy due to liver or kidney failure
Respiratory complications may include traumatic or spinal cord injury

Cranial Nerves

See Table 11-2 for specific functions and testing.

Spinal Nerves

Thirty-one pairs of peripheral nerves that originate on the spinal cord from anterior roots. Each pair of spinal nerves is related to a specific region of the body.

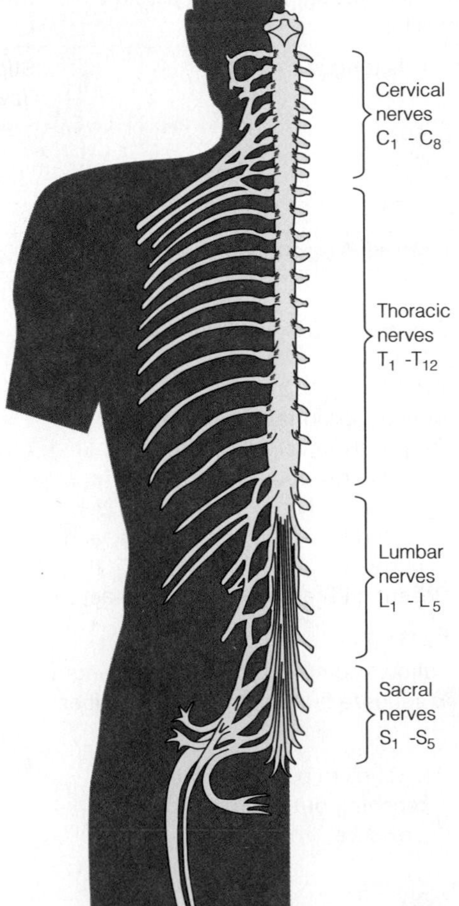

▲ Spinal nerves.

Assessment	Normal Responses	Abnormal Responses
Pupil Assessment Observe **pupils** using penlight and pupil gauge or an automated pupillometer		
Size of pupils	Diameter: 1.5–6 mm	Unilateral dilation: sign of third cranial nerve involvement Bilateral dilation: sign of upper brainstem damage Unilateral dilation and nonreactive: sign of increased intracranial pressure (ICP) or ipsilateral oculomotor nerve (III) compression from tumor or injury
Shape of pupils	Round and midposition	Midposition and fixed: sign of midbrain involvement Pinpoint and fixed: sign of pontine involvement or opiate effect
Equality of pupils	Equal	Unequal: sign that parasympathetic and sympathetic nervous systems are not in synchronization
Observe **reaction to light** by using penlight in darkened room	Pupil constricts promptly	Sluggish reaction or failure to react to light: early warning of deteriorating condition or elevated ICP 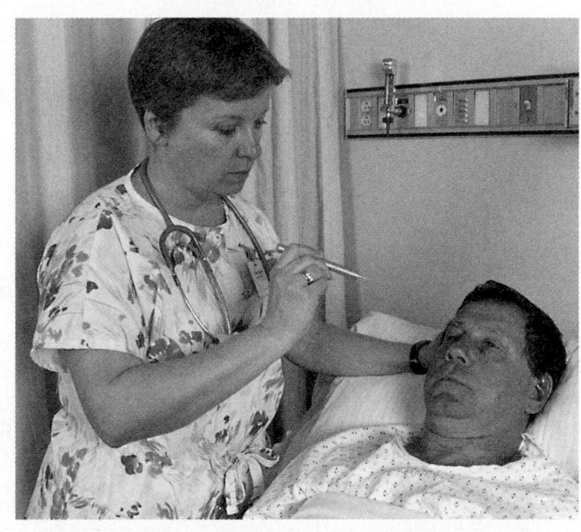 ▲ Move light toward client's eye from side position.
Open eyelid being tested; cover opposite eye		Light reflex is the most important sign differentiating structural (cranial involvement) from metabolic coma due to extracranial cause (e.g., diabetic coma), which does not alter light reflex
Observe consensual **light reflex** Hold both eyelids open Shine light into one eye only Observe opposite eye	Both pupils constrict	Pupil does not constrict: sign that connection between brainstem and pupils is not intact
Check **accommodation** (ability of lens to adjust to objects at varying distances)	Lens can adjust	When the lens thickens (often in the fifth decade of life) accommodation can be limited

(continued)

Assessment: Neurologic *(Continued)*

Assessment	Normal Responses	Abnormal Responses
Motor Function Assessment Assess bilateral **muscle strength** Test hand grip by asking client to squeeze your fingers Rate muscle strength from 0 to 5, with 0 indicating no muscle contraction and 5 (normal) indicating full range of motion against gravity with full resistance	Muscle strength is equal bilaterally	Absent or weak muscle function on one side may be sign of hemiplegia (paralysis of one side of the body); or hemiparesis (weakness on one side); paraplegia (paralysis of the legs or lower part of the body); tetraplegia or quadriplegia (paralysis of arms and legs)
Test arm strength by asking client to close eyes and hold arms out in front with palms up	Maintains position for 20–30 seconds	Cannot maintain position—downdrifts one extremity

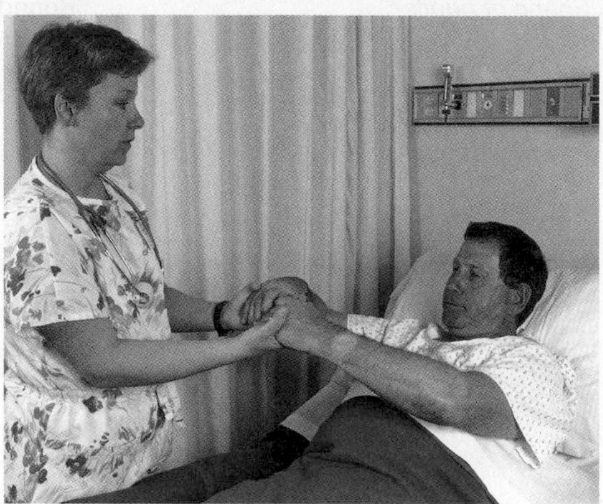

▲ Test client's hand grip.

Muscle Grading Scale

Muscle Graduations	***Description***
5 – Normal	*Complete range of motion against gravity with full resistance*
4 – Good	*Complete range of motion against gravity with some resistance*
3 – Fair	*Complete range of motion against gravity*
2 – Poor	*Complete range of motion with gravity eliminated*
1 – Trace	*Evidence of slight contractility, no joint motion*
0 – Zero	*No evidence of contractility*

Assessment	Normal Responses	Abnormal Responses
Assess **flexion** and **extension** strength in extremities Stand in front of client, place your hand in front of client, and ask client to push your hand away	Equal response in both arms	Unequal response in arms Asymmetrical response Inability to perform movements
Place your hand on client's forearm and ask client to pull arm upward		

Assessment	Normal Responses	Abnormal Responses
Position client's leg with knee flexed and foot resting on bed; as you try to extend leg, ask client to keep foot down Place one hand on client's knee and one hand on client's ankle; ask client to straighten leg as you apply resistant force to knee and ankle	Equal response in both legs	Unequal response in legs
Assess **muscle tone** Flex and extend client's upper extremities to assess how well client resists your movements	Client resistance is apparent	Increased resistance: sign of increased muscle tone from muscle rigidity or spasticity in upper motor neuron (UMN) lesions; for example, as with cerebrovascular accident (CVA) and parkinsonism Decreased resistance to leg extension and arm flexion in UMN lesion (CVA)
Flex and extend client's lower extremities to assess resistance		Weakness in lower motor neuron (LMN) and cerebellar lesion
Coordination Assessment		
Hand coordination		
Ask client to pat both thighs as rapidly as possible Ask client to turn hands over and back in quick succession Ask client to touch thumb with each finger in rapid succession—repeat with other hand	Client able to perform coordinated movements on request: hand, foot, hand and leg positioning	Uncoordinated movements: may be due to cerebellum or basal ganglia involvement Clumsy movement with cerebellar involvement
Foot coordination Place your hands close to client's feet Ask client to tap your hands alternately with the balls of feet		
Hand positioning coordination With client's eyes open, extend your hand in front of client's face Ask client to touch nose with index finger several times in rapid succession Repeat test with client's eyes closed		Tremor as nose is approached indicates cerebellar involvement Inability to perform task with eyes closed: may be due to loss of positioning sense
Leg positioning coordination Ask client to put heel on opposite knee and to slide heel down leg to foot		
Reflex Assessment		
Blink reflex Hold client's eyelid open Approach client's eye unexpectedly from side of head Complete corneal touch	Eyes close immediately	Absence of blink response; eyelid continuously in open position: due to fifth or seventh cranial nerve (pons) involvement; blindness
Gag and swallow reflex Open client's mouth and hold tongue down with tongue blade Touch back of pharynx on each side with applicator stick	Gag and swallow reflex present	Absence of gag and swallow reflex; inability to swallow food or liquid: due to ninth or 10th cranial nerve (medulla) involvement

(continued)

Assessment: Neurologic *(Continued)*

Assessment	Normal Responses	Abnormal Responses
Plantar reflex		
Run top of pen along outer lateral aspect from heel to little toe of client's foot Continue tracing a line across ball of foot toward great toe	Toes are pointed down	Babinski response: great toe dorsiflexes; other toes fan on foot of paralyzed side in CVA, and bilaterally in spinal cord injury (SCI)
▲ Testing plantar reflex.	▲ Normal plantar reflex.	▲ Babinski response (abnormal).
Deep tendon reflex Ask client to relax Position limb to be assessed so that muscle is somewhat stretched Using reflex hammer, strike tendon quickly Assess according to scale	Biceps reflex: flexion at elbow and contracting of biceps muscle Triceps reflex: extension at elbow and contraction of triceps muscle Patellar reflex: extension of knee and contraction of quadriceps	Absent or diminished: sign of cervical cord (C–5 or C–6) involvement Absent or diminished: C–7 or C–8 cord involvement Absent or diminished: L2–3 or L3–4 cord involvement
Grading Scale 4+ Hyperactive or exaggerated 3+ More brisk than usual but not indicative of disease state 2+ Average or normal 1+ Slightly diminished, low normal 0 No response		Indicates upper motor neuron (UMN) lesion or SCI Seen with lower motor neuron (LMN) lesion
Sensory Function Assess **superficial sensations** *Pain* Ask client to close eyes Stroke or touch skin with cotton-tipped applicator, alternating cotton tip with wooden end Ask client to distinguish sharp and dull pain	Ability to distinguish between sharp and dull sensations	Alterations in pain or temperature sensations: indicate lesion in posterior horn of spinal cord or spinothalamic tract of cord
Temperature Fill two test tubes with water, one hot, one cold Ask client to close eyes and touch client's skin with test tubes	Ability to distinguish between hot and cold	
Touch Ask client to close eyes Stroke cotton wisp over client's skin	Ability to identify light touch— equal bilaterally	Anesthesia = loss of light touch Analgesia = absence of sense of pain Hypalgesia = decreased pain sensation Hyperalgesia = exaggerated sensitivity to pin prick (pain)

Assessment	Normal Responses	Abnormal Responses
Positioning Ask client to close eyes Grasp client's finger with your thumb and index finger Move client's finger up and down Ask client to identify direction finger is moving. Repeat with great toe.	Ability to identify position or mimic position with other hand	Inability to determine direction of movement: may be due to posterior column or peripheral nerve disease
Vital Signs Temperature Apical/radial pulses Respiration Blood pressure Assess **temperature** If client is semiresponsive or nonresponsive, take rectal, axillary, or tympanic temperature If rectal temperature is contraindicated or there are signs of increased ICP, use alternate method.	Ability to maintain normal body temperature (approximately 98.6°F, or 37°C)	Inability to maintain normal temperature: may be due to damage to hypothalamus No sweating below level of injury; due to spinal cord injury Hypothermia
Assess **apical** and **radial pulses** Note character of pulses Count heart rate Count radial pulse rate	Regular rhythm Rate 60–100 beats/min Apical and radial rates are equal	Fast heart rate due to decreased blood volume, arrhythmia, heart failure, fever, medulla dysfunction Irregular rhythm with premature beats due to hypoxia, cardiac irritability, or electrolyte imbalance Pulse deficit due to premature beats or ineffectual cardiac contraction.
Assess **respiration** Assess rate and pattern of breathing	Regular rate: 12–20 breaths per minute	Cheyne–Stokes (rhythmic increase in depth of breathing followed by period of apnea) may be due to deep cerebral or cerebellar lesion or condition altering cerebral perfusion Central neurogenic (sustained) hyperventilation due to upper brainstem involvement Ataxic (Biot's) breathing unpredictably irregular, due to lower brainstem involvement
Monitor arterial blood gases if signs of respiratory imbalances occur	pH: 7.35–7.45 PCO_2: 35–45 mmHg HCO_3: 22–26 mEq/L	Alterations in pH and PCO_2 values indicate respiratory imbalances: pH below 7.35 and PCO_2 above 45: sign of respiratory acidosis (hypoventilation) pH above 7.45 and PCO_2 below 35: sign of respiratory alkalosis (hyperventilation) HCO_3 above 26 indicates metabolic compensation for chronic respiratory acidosis (hypoventilation)

▲ Assess client's apical pulse.

(continued)

Assessment: Neurologic *(Continued)*

Assessment	Normal Responses	Abnormal Responses
Assess **blood pressure** Position neurologic clients in low- to semi-Fowler's position	Normal pressure (range <120/<80)	Systolic blood pressure rises with diastolic pressure remaining same (widening pulse pressure): sign of increased intracranial pressure Blood pressure over 140/90 is a sign of stage 1 hypertension Blood pressure below 90/60 is a sign of hypotension

Korotkoff's Sound Phases for Blood Pressure

Phase I: The pressure level at which the first faint, clear tapping sounds are heard. The sounds gradually increase in intensity as the cuff is deflated. This phase coincides with the reappearance of a palpable pulse (systolic sound).

Phase II: That time during cuff deflation when a murmur or swishing sounds are heard.

Phases III: The period during which sounds are crisper and increase in intensity.

Phase IV: That time when a distinct, abrupt, muffling of sound (usually of a soft, blowing quality) is heard (diastolic sound in children or physically active adults).

Phase V: That pressure level when the last sound is heard and after which all sound disappears (second diastolic sound).

Source: American Heart Association, 1996.

Blood Pressure Classification

Blood Pressure	Systolic	Diastolic
Normal	<120	<80
Pre high blood pressure	120–139	80–89
Stage I high blood pressure	140–159	90–99
Stage II high blood pressure	160 and higher	100 and higher

Source: National Heart, Lung, and Blood Institute, 2003.

ASSESSMENT OF THE HEAD AND NECK

Eye Assessment
Ear Assessment
Nose Assessment
Mouth and Lips Assessment
Neck Assessment

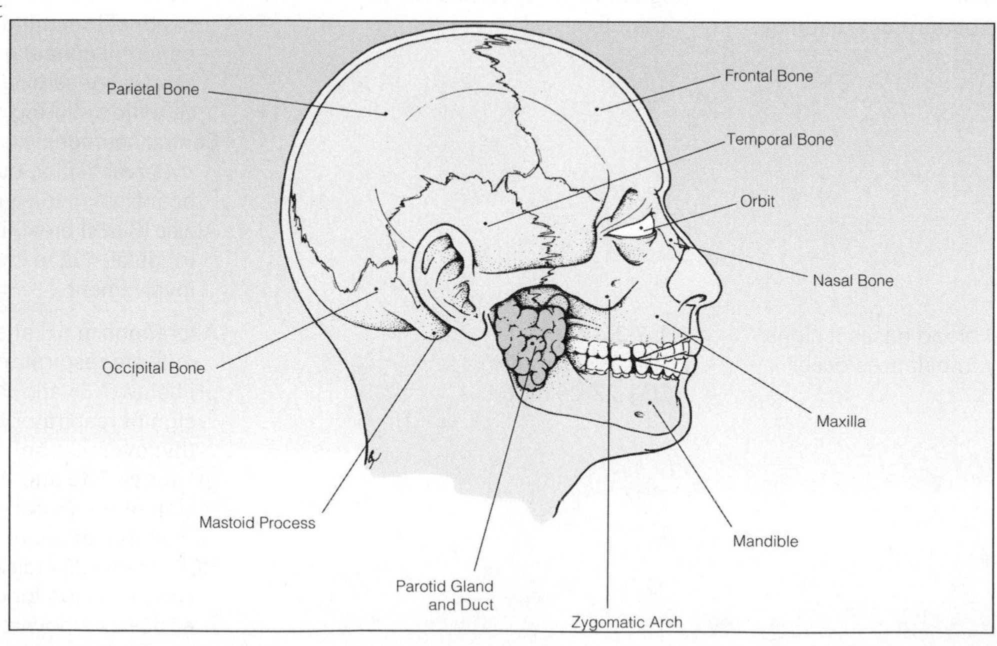

▲ Bones that form the skull.

The names of the regions of the head are derived from the bones that form the skull. Knowing the names of the bones and regions of the skull can assist in describing the location of the physical findings.

The size and shape of the head should be noted, as well as the placement of the eyes and facial structures. Note any lesions or discharge from the ears; if there are any lesions of the lips or mouth, assess further.

When palpating the neck, note the head position and neck muscles. Using your fingers, palpate the lymph nodes in the neck to determine swelling. Check the thyroid gland in the front of the neck, and if enlarged, note that this condition requires further assessment.

Assessment: Head and Neck

Assessment	Normal	Abnormal
Eye Assessment		
Note **visual acuity** by observing client performance of activities of daily living Factors influencing visual acuity include client's previous status and age Note exact location, size, and color of any **external lesions** Palpate for mobility and firmness	Adequate performance of activities of daily living Appropriate responses to environment No external lesions	Age-related macular degeneration (AMD) Hyperopia (farsightedness) Myopia (nearsightedness) Cataract (opacification of the lens) Enucleation (loss of an eye): may have prosthesis in place Circumocular ecchymosis: may be sign of basal skull fracture Xanthelasma (small, yellowish, well-circumscribed plaques): may appear on eyelids of clients with lipid disorders. *Example:* atherosclerosis
Note **equality of eyelid movement**	Eyelids are equal in movement	Ptosis (paralytic drooping of the upper eyelid)
Note color, consistency, amount, and origin of **discharge** from eyes	No discharge	Sty or hordeolum Thick white discharge; may be due to conjunctivitis
Note **internal lesions**	No internal lesions	Conjunctival or ciliary injection (dilatation of the blood vessels)
Assess differences between **pupil size and reaction** Note presence of hemorrhage	Both pupils are the same size	Anisocoria (indicates unequal pupil size): may be indicative of neurologic trauma or deficit Corneal edema (very soft, movable mass that looks like raw egg white): frequently occurs in clients who have increased intracranial pressure Arcus senilis (partial or complete whitish circle near the outer edge of the cornea); usually due to aging; does not affect vision

▲ Anatomy of the eye.

(continued)

Assessment: Head and Neck *(Continued)*

Assessment	Normal	Abnormal
▲ Assess pupil size and reaction.		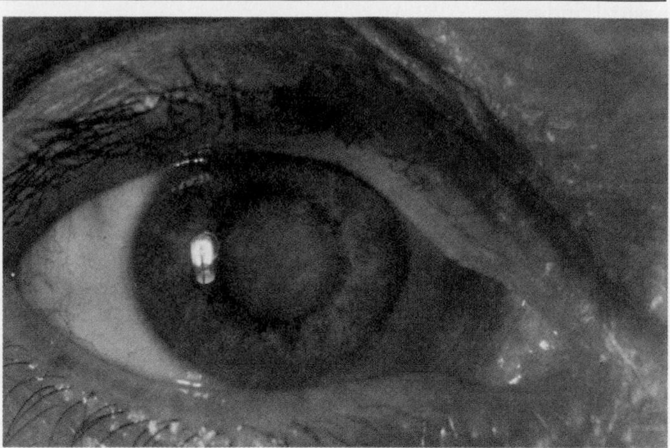 ▲ Cataract: Opacity of the crystalline lens.
Observe for opacity of lens—**cataract**	No opacity noted	Cataract present—one or both eyes
Ear Assessment		
Note **auditory acuity** by asking client to indicate if he or she hears normal sounds as you make them	Adequate responses to normal sounds Auditory changes due to aging	Deafness or impaired hearing; excess cerumen in auditory canal Abnormal sounds in the ears (ringing or buzzing) may be caused by ototoxic drugs
Note exact size, color, and location of any **external** lesions Palpate lesions for mobility and firmness	No external lesions	Battle's sign (ecchymosis behind the ear): may be sign of basilar skull fracture
Examine tympanic membrane using an otoscope Malleus Surface of Eardrum Umbo (Lower Malleus Projection) Cone of Light ▲ Anatomy of the tympanic membrane (ear drum).	Membrane intact, flat, gray, with no scarring	White patches show prior infections: yellow or red patches may be infection of middle ear Bulging membrane may indicate increased pressure in middle ear Depressed membrane may indicate vacuum due to blocked eustachian tube.
Note color, quantity, and consistency of any **discharge** from the ears Test clear fluid for glucose using a Labstix	No discharge Wax buildup Glucose test negative	Redness, swelling, and pain may be signs of otitis externa Cerebrospinal fluid leak: may be due to head injury. If drainage is blood and CSF, it will develop a "halo" with a reddish area in the center surrounded by a whitish circle if placed on white material Perforation of tympanic membrane: serosanguineous or purulent drainage Glucose test of clear drainage is positive if CSF

Assessment	Normal	Abnormal

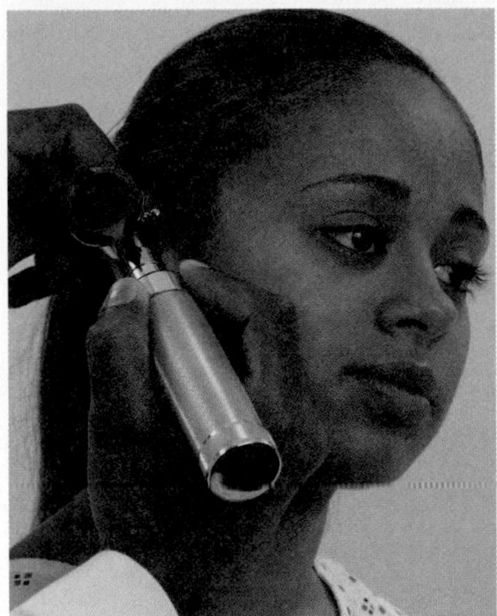

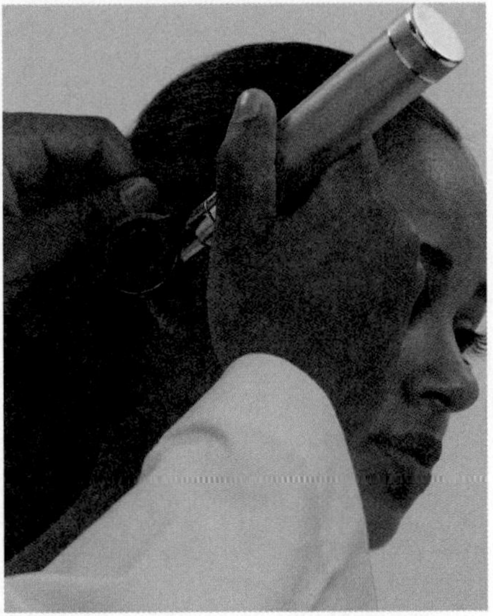

▲ Two techniques for positioning and inserting an otoscope into ear before viewing.

Assessment	Normal	Abnormal
Nose Assessment		
Note any **structural changes** in the nose by observing client breathing Gently occlude one nostril at a time; ask client to breathe through the nonoccluded nostril	Regular breathing with mouth closed Breathing through nonoccluded nostril	Breathing through the mouth only: furuncles may occlude breathing Obstruction in the nose due to deviated nasal septum, swelling of the nasal turbinates, or excessive mucus secretions
Note color, quantity, and consistency of any **discharge** from the nose	Minimal discharge	Cerebrospinal fluid leak (fluid tests positive for glucose with Labstix) Copious, watery-to-thick, mucopurulent discharge: may be due to acute rhinitis Excessive buildup of mucous secretions
Mouth and Lip Assessment		
Note size, color, and location of any **external lesions** Palpate for mobility and firmness	No external lesions	Dehydrated mouth or lips Fissures Pressure sores Necrosis
Note size, color, and location of any **internal lesions** Palpate for mobility and firmness	No internal lesions	Candidiasis (a fungal infection indicated by adherent, white patches)
Neck Assessment		
Note any **lesion or swelling** in the neck Ask client to relax and flex neck slightly Palpate the neck, using the pads of your fingers to move the skin and underlying tissues	Occasional small, mobile, discrete, nontender lymph nodes	Enlarged tender immobile nodes

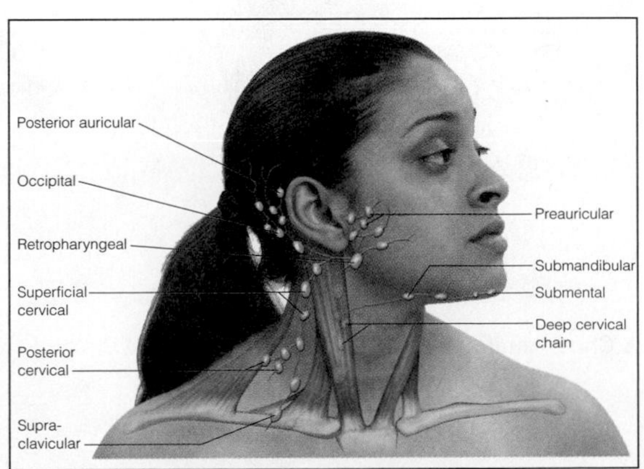

► Lymph notes in the head and neck.

ASSESSMENT OF THE SKIN AND NAILS

Skin Assessment
Nail Assessment

The skin is the body's first line of defense against disease and injury. It is made up of three layers: the epidermis, the dermis, and the subcutaneous tissues.

The epidermis is divided into two avascular, or bloodless, layers: an outer layer that consists of dead keratinized cells and an inner layer that consists of live cells where keratin and melanin are formed. The dermis contains blood vessels, connective tissue, sebaceous glands, and some of the hair follicles. The subcutaneous tissues contain the remainder of the hair follicles, fat, and the sweat glands.

Hair, nails, sweat glands, and sebaceous glands are appendages of the skin. There are two types of sweat glands: eccrine and apocrine. Eccrine glands are distributed over most of the body except for the palms and soles. These glands help control body temperature through their sweat production. The apocrine glands are found mainly in the axillary and genital areas and are stimulated by emotional stress. Bacterial decomposition by apocrine sweat glands causes adult body odor.

The nail body is made up of dead keratinized cells. Nail production occurs at the nail root. Underlying vessels give the nail its pink color.

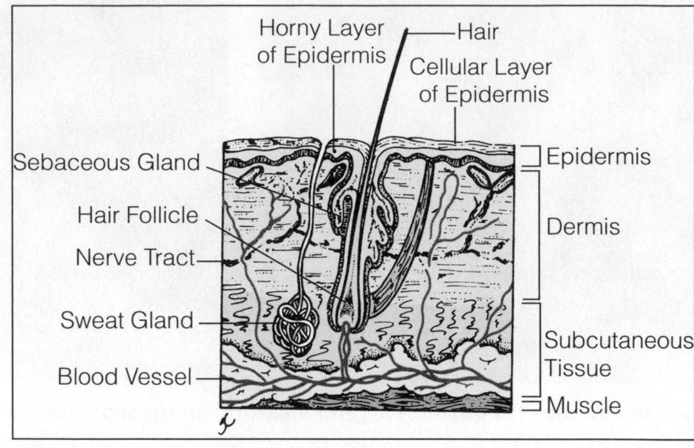

▲ Anatomy of the skin.

Assessment: Skin

Assessment	Normal	Abnormal
Note **color** of the skin by assessing the oral mucous membranes, the conjunctiva, and the nailbeds	Pink, tan, or brown, depending on the client's basic skin color Oral mucous membrane: moist, pink Conjunctiva: moist, pink Nailbeds: pink	Pallor (decrease in color) *Example*: anemia from acute blood loss (hemorrhage), renal failure, dietary deficiencies, or arterial insufficiency Jaundice (icterus): due to the presence of conjugated or unconjugated bilirubin in the blood and tissues; appears most frequently in the face and sclerae; seen best under natural light *Example*: liver disease Cyanosis (blue, blue-gray, or purple discoloration of the skin and mucous membranes): caused by hypoxia, a result of an increased amount of reduced hemoglobin Peripheral: seen in nailbeds and earlobes *Example*: vasoconstriction, venous insufficiency Central: seen in nailbeds, lips (circumoral), and oral mucosa Erythema (redness of the skin): caused by capillary congestion; occurs with inflammation or infection; usually a local finding

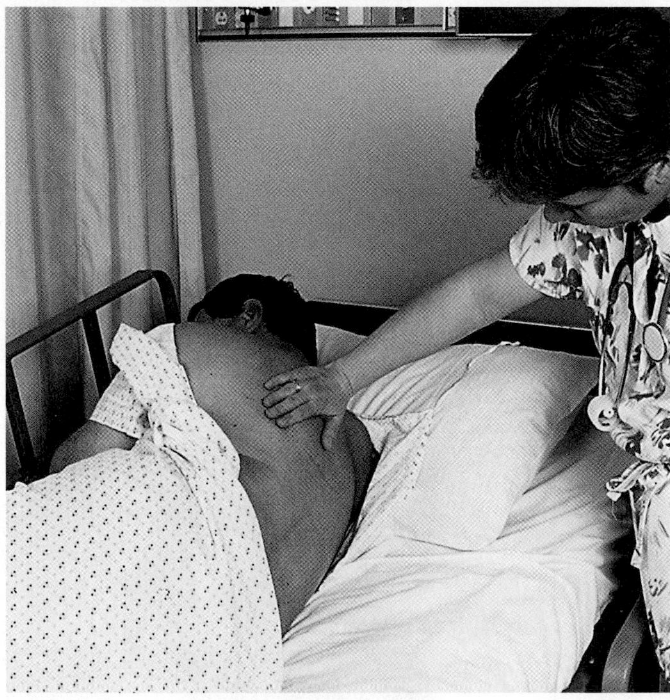

▲ Check quality of the skin.

Assessment	Normal	Abnormal
Note **pigmentation**	Discolored spots may be due to normal aging	Hyperpigmentation (especially in skin creases) *Example*: use of oral contraceptives, pregnancy, Addison's disease, and hyperthyroidism
Note **turgor** and **mobility**	Smooth and elastic	Tight or stretched and difficult to move: due to local or generalized edema Wrinkled: due to dehydration or caused by rapid weight loss
Pinch skin over the sternum If the fold persists, skin turgor is poor	Resilient and supple	Thin and translucent (parchment) *Example*: chronic steroid use. Thin, shiny, and smooth with alopecia on lower extremities *Example*: chronic arterial insufficiency
Assess for **edema** Press finger firmly for 5 seconds into skin on top of foot or inner ankle bone	Resilient and no depression remains after pressure released	Pitting edema: excess interstitial fluid *Example:* congestive heart failure, renal failure, cirrhosis of the liver, venous stasis

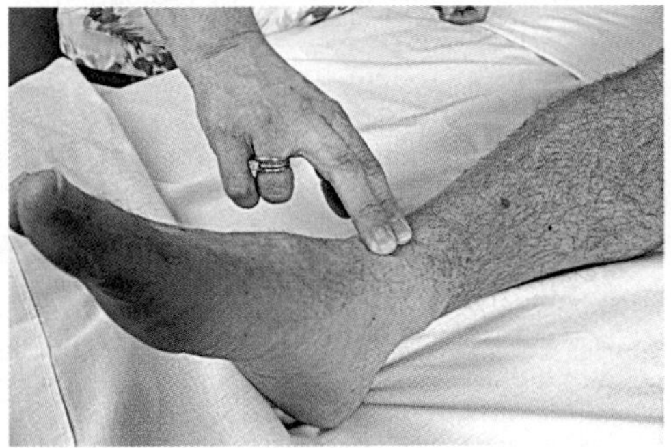

▲ Check client for edema.

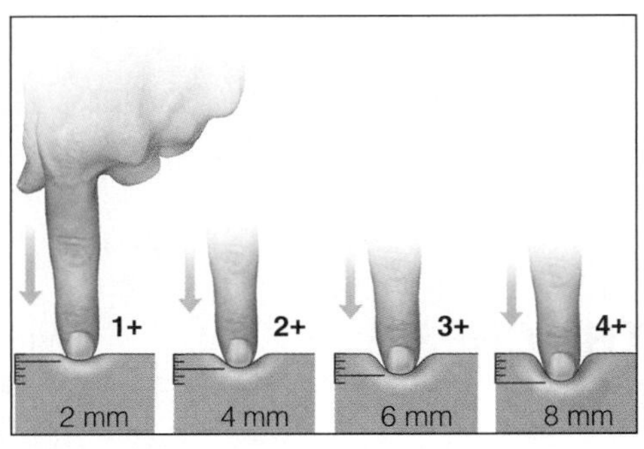

▲ Grading pitting edema.

Assessment	Normal	Abnormal
Note **moistness** and **temperature** of the skin	Warm and dry	Warm (hot) and moist due to temperature elevation Cool and moist (cold and clammy): may be due to shock states Abnormally dry: may be due to dehydration, decreased sebaceous gland secretions, or the excessive use of soap
Assess for **sensation**—response to external stimuli	Feels touch, sensitive to heat and cold and pressure	Absence of touch or pain sensation *Example*: spinal cord injury or nerve damage Diminished heat and cold sensation *Example*: peripheral vascular disease Itching and tingling *Example:* peripheral vascular disease, peripheral neuropathy, allergy
Note **lesions** on the skin Physical characteristics include color, elevation, shape, mobility, and contents	No lesions present	Macules (flat localized changes in color) *Example*: petechiae, first-degree burns, purpura Papules, plaques, nodules (solid, elevated, varying in size) *Example*: psoriasis, xanthomas Cancerous lesions *Examples:* Basal cell epithelioma—small, smooth papule with atrophic center

(continued)

Assessment: Skin *(Continued)*

Assessment	Normal	Abnormal
		Melanoma—pigmented tumor; may arise from a blue-black mole Squamous cell—macules with indistinct margins; surface may be crusted Wheals (elevated, circumscribed, transient) *Example:* urticaria, insect bites Vesicles and bullae (clear, fluid-filled pockets between skin layers) *Example:* second-degree burns Pustules (vesicles or bullae filled with purulent exudate) *Example:* furuncles, acne
Nail Assessment		
Note condition of the nails	Smooth transparent layer with white crescent called a lunula	Clubbing occurs with hypoxia or decreased tissue perfusion, cirrhosis, and other conditions Spoon-shaped nails may indicate iron deficiency Thickened nails may relate to circulatory disorder Cracked, split, or broken nails may result from nutrient deficiencies

ASSESSMENT OF THE CHEST, LUNGS, AND HEART

Chest Assessment

Lung /Respiratory (Breath Sounds) Assessment

Heart Assessment

The chest, or thorax area, extends from the base of the neck to the diaphragm. The overall shape of the thorax should be elliptical, although deformities such as barrel chest, pigeon chest, or funnel chest do occur. Total assessment includes the external aspect: The nurse should observe for movement, posture, shape, and symmetry, especially of the breast and axilla area, and the internal components of the lungs and the heart.

The lungs anteriorly extend from 2 to 4 cm above the inner third of the clavicle to the eighth rib at the midaxillary line and the sixth rib at the midclavicular line.

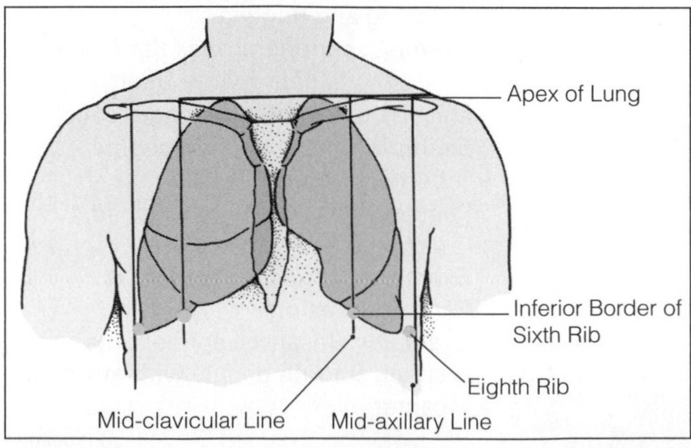

▲ Anterior anatomical relationship of lungs to skeletal structure.

Posteriorly the lungs extend from the third thoracic spinous process and descend to the 10th process or, on deep inspiration, to the 12th process.

Chest assessment begins with inspection, proceeds to palpation, and then to auscultation. Breath sounds of clients differ due to the depth of breathing, underlying disease, or obesity. Because of these differences, it is difficult to compare the breath sounds of one client with another. The basic principle to remember when auscultating the lungs is to do a comparison between the right and left lung. To make these comparisons, begin auscultating at the apices of one lung, alternating sides as you work down through both lungs. By comparing similar areas in both lungs, you can note changes and determine causes for these changes more easily.

Examination of the chest usually proceeds from posterior to anterior. For posterior assessment of the lungs, place the client in an upright sitting position with shoulders pulled forward. For anterior assessment, the client can be sitting or supine (especially if female). If the client is lying on his or her side, the lung closest to the bed is mechanically compressed, and true lung sounds cannot be heard.

Ask the client to breathe a little deeper than usual through the mouth. Breathing through the nose produces extra sounds that mask true lung sounds.

The heart is located directly behind the sternum, with the left ventricle projecting into the left chest. The heart is usually thought to be in the left chest for two reasons: the left ventricle produces the most movement (ventricular contraction), and three of the valve sound areas are located to the left of the sternum.

The action of the heart should be assessed both proximally and distally. Proximal assessment involves evaluating heart sounds, heart rate, and rhythm to obtain information about the mechanical activity of the heart. Distal assessment involves evaluating the peripheral pulses to obtain information about the effectiveness of the heart's pumping action.

One method for assessing heart sounds is to start at the aortic area, moving slowly across to the pulmonic area, down to the tricuspid area, and over to the mitral area. This same general progression can also be used in reverse, starting at the mitral area and progressing up to the aortic area. Most clinicians begin the assessment at the mitral area, which is the point of maximum impulse and where the apical pulse is the loudest.

The most important point to remember in heart assessment is to use the same method every time, repeating the same steps in the same sequence. By using one systematic approach, you learn how to compare the different sounds more easily and not neglect to listen to all areas on the chest.

Breast assessment should include observing for lumps, drainage, dimpling of breast tissue, and presence of asymmetry. The client should also be asked if she has noted any recent changes.

Assessment: Chest

Assessment	Normal	Abnormal
Chest Assessment		
Note respiratory rate—increase may be due to fever, pain, anxiety	A normal or increased rate does not assume a normal tidal volume	Clients may have an increased rate to compensate for decreased tidal volume, but the resultant minute volume is still not sufficient. (Normal minute volume is 6–8 L/min.) Increased depth: due to neurologic disease, intracranial pressure (ICP) from trauma, drug overdose, exertion, fear, or anxiety Decreased depth: due to neurologic disease, ICP from trauma, drug overdose, respiratory disease, pneumothorax, or pain
Note the **general appearance** of the chest and movement when client breathes	Straight spine, level shoulders	Breathes sitting forward with arms on pillows or overbed table (present with emphysema)
	Relaxed breathing; rib cage moves symmetrically with respirations	Uses accessory muscles (i.e., scalene, trapezius, sternocleidomastoid, pectoralis, or intercostal)
Note **shape of chest**	Anterior–posterior dimension is half of lateral dimension	Anterior–posterior dimension increased in emphysema (barrel chest) Deformities such as scoliosis (lateral curvature), kyphosis (forward curvature), or kyphoscoliosis
Note **position of ribs**	Ribs slant downward	Horizontal is common in COPD Bulging of interspaces during exhalation with retraction on inhalation (present with asthma and emphysema) Chest tilted to one side when client sits or stands: may be due to pain in ribs or chest wall or trauma (i.e., fractured ribs or surgery such as a thoracotomy)
Measure **chest excursion** for range and symmetry: place hands parallel to 10th rib (under scapulae) with thumbs beside spine. Bunch up fold of skin pushing thumbs medially. Ask client to inhale. For anterior assessment, place hands over lower thorax, push medially, then have client inhale. Note equidistant lateral movement of hands.	On inhalation, the thumbs move equidistant away from midline indicating equal expansion ▲ Measure chest excursion while client takes deep breath.	Flail chest: occurs when four or more ribs are broken; area collapses inward during inhalations and outward on exhalation Asymmetrical (unequal) chest expansion occurs with pneumothorax, fractured ribs, atelectasis, or when client's chest splints due to pain

(continued)

Assessment: Chest *(Continued)*

Assessment	Normal	Abnormal
Tactile and Vocal Fremitus		
Tactile fremitus (vibrations felt on surface of chest as sound passes through tissue) Palpate upper thorax and ask client to say "ninety-nine"; vibrations detected as hands move down thorax	Varied because it depends on thickness of chest wall 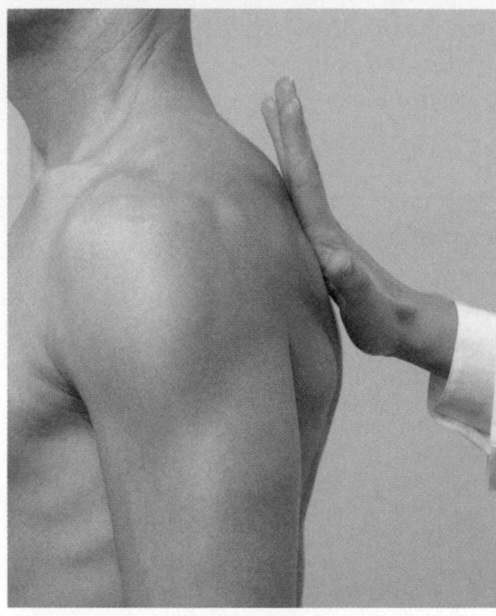 ▲ Palpation for tactile fremitus.	Decreased sounds: obesity, emphysema, pneumothorax, and possible Increased sounds: heard when lung is filled with fluid-consolidation (pneumonia) or tumors Absent sounds: atelectasis or pleural effusion Asymmetric sounds: abnormal Normal sounds: found with bronchitis or pulmonary edema
Lung/Respiratory Assessment		
Complete a **general assessment** of the lungs		
Respiratory rate *Respiratory depth or volume* Auscultation: note location and quality of **lung sounds**	12–20 respirations/minute Normal depth is equal to about 500 mL	Increased respiratory rate: may be due to increased metabolic needs (fever), mechanical injury, surgery, or trauma to chest wall
Note presence of *adventitious (extra) sounds,* such as rales/crackles, wheezes, and rhonchi, or pleural friction rub	No extra sounds heard—symmetrical areas should be the same in quality and intensity	*Discontinuous Sounds: Crackles* (rales) are due to sudden opening of closed airways, indicating hypoventilation; usually heard as soft, high-pitched scratching sounds, like hair strands rubbing together at end of inspiration Heard in dependent areas of bedridden clients or in early congestive heart failure. May be collapsed or fluid-filled alveoli. Simulate by rubbing hair together in front of your ear *Continuous Sounds:* *Wheezes* are produced by air passing through airways narrowed by edema, spasm or mucus; may be heard on inspiration but more often louder on expiration; high-pitched and musical *Rhonchi* are low-pitched rumbling, coarse; sounds heard on inhalation and exhalation. Fluid-blocked airways—may be cleared with coughing. *Sibilant wheezes* are high-pitched, musical sounds; may be caused by asthma, increased secretions, or edema

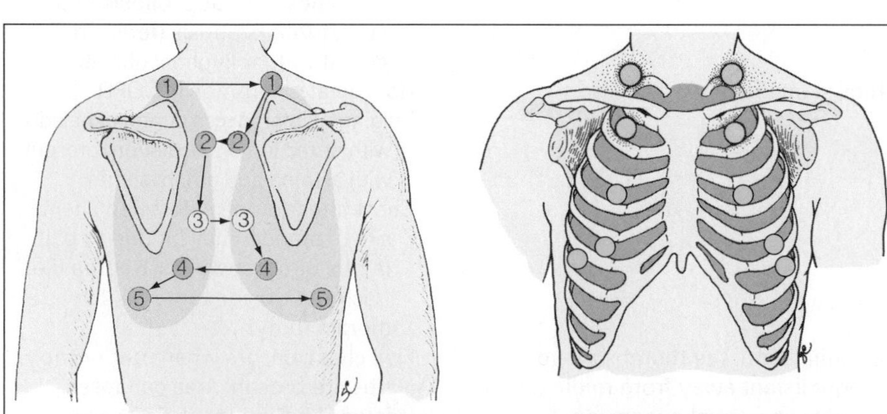

▲ Stethoscope placement sites for posterior (left) and anterior (right) auscultation of breath sounds. Follow arrows for sequence of examination.

Assessment	Normal	Abnormal
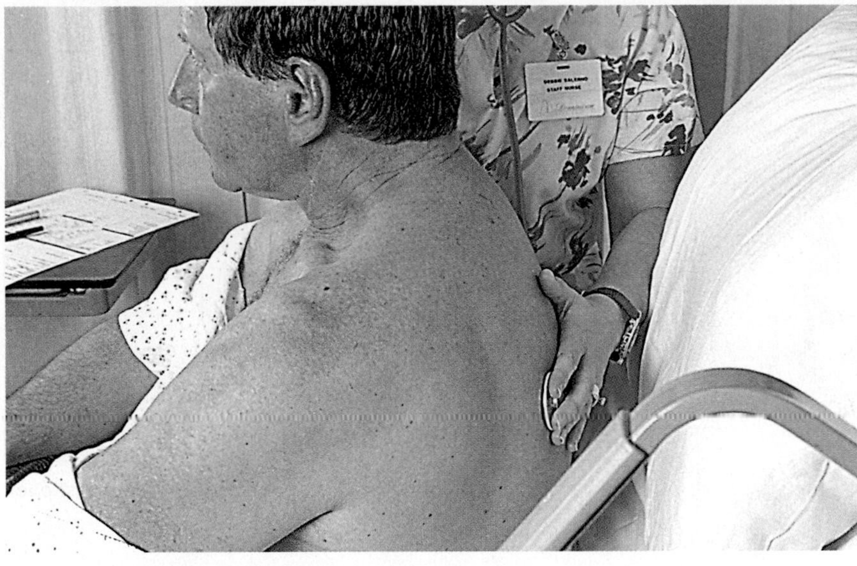 ▲ Listen to posterior breath sounds.		*Pleural friction rub* is produced when inflamed pleurae rub together in the absence of normal pleural fluid; localized, high-pitched, harsh, and scratchy; frequently transient; may be heard on inspiration and expiration *Stridor* is an inspiratory wheeze heard in the neck due to partial obstruction at upper airway—tracheal or laryngeal level
Evaluate ***breath sounds***		
Bronchovesicular breath sounds Heard over the mainstem bronchi below the clavicles and adjacent to the sternum, between scapulae	Moderate to high pitch, with moderate amplitude Hollow, muffled quality Inspiration and expiration equal in duration	Bronchial or bronchovesicular sounds heard in the perimeter where vesicular sounds are expected indicate consolidation such as pneumonia. The client's spoken and whispered words are also clearly heard by the examiner over consolidated lung areas
Vesicular (normal) breath sounds Heard over lung parenchyma (heart will mask breath sounds on the left side)	Low to medium pitch, with low amplitude Soft, whooshing quality	Breath sounds may be absent over areas of atelectasis, pneumothorax, or pleural effusion
Lungs extend anteriorly to the sixth intercostal space	Inspiration two to three times longer than expiration	
Bronchial breath sounds Heard over the trachea above the sternal notch	High pitch and amplitude Harsh, loud, tubular quality Expiration longer than inspiration	
Lungs extend posteriorly to T10 on expiration, to T12 on deep inspiration		Breath sounds are decreased (faint) with hypoventilation, early atelectasis, and COPD
Heart Assessment		
Evaluate **atrioventricular heart sounds** (S_1 heart sound). Use diaphragm of stethoscope—best for picking up high-pitched sounds	S_1 (the first heart sound, a combination of the mitral and tricuspid closure) heard best over the mitral and tricuspid areas. S_1 louder than S_2 in this area	Heart sounds not heard in the area prescribed (e.g., with left ventricular hypertrophy, mitral sound moves laterally)
Mitral value sounds Heard best at left, fifth intercostal space at, or medial to, the midclavicular line		
Tricuspid valve sounds Heard best at fifth intercostal space, left sternal border	S_1 also heard at this area and is louder than S_2	
Evaluate **semilunar heart sounds** (S_2 heart sounds)	S_2 (the second heart sound, a combination of the aortic and pulmonic closure): heard best over the aortic and pulmonic areas	Sounds altered with aortic stenosis (thrill) and hypertension (accentuated sound)

(continued)

Assessment: Chest *(Continued)*

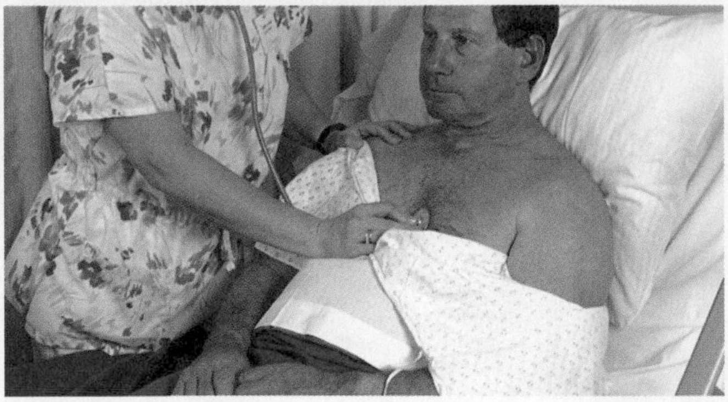

▲ Auscultate heart sounds.

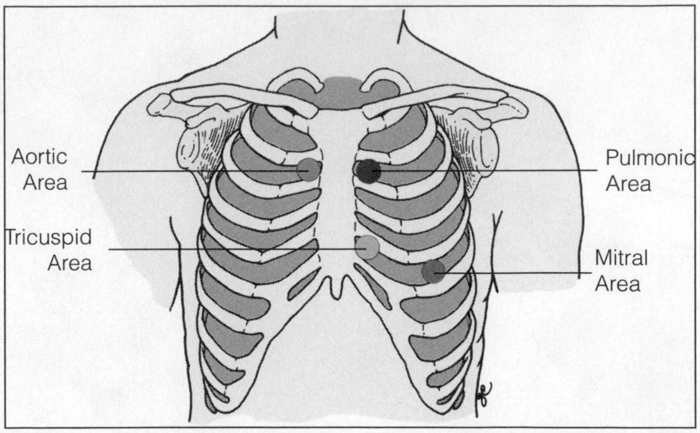

▲ S_1 heard best over mitral and tricuspid areas. S_2 heard best over aortic and pulmonic areas.

Assessment	Normal	Abnormal
Aortic valve sounds		
Heard best at second intercostal space, right sternal border		
Pulmonic valve sounds		
Heard best at second intercostal space, left sternal border	Part of S_2 is louder than S_1 in this area. May be heard separately from aortic closure if client inhales deeply	Accentuated with pulmonary hypertension
Evaluate presence of **diastolic heart sounds**		
Use bell of stethoscope—best for picking up low-pitched sounds and gallops. Place lightly on chest with client in left side lying position.	Quiet and low-pitched	Murmurs originating from stenotic valves
S_3 (ventricular gallop)		
Heard just after S_2, at the apex or at lower, left sternal border	May be a physiologic finding in children and young adults Abnormal finding in older clients	Almost always signifies heart failure in client over age 40
S_4 (atrial gallop)		
Heard just before S_1, at the apex or at lower, left sternal border; occurs when blood flow from atrial contraction meets increased resistance in ventricle	Normal finding in elderly	Heard in older individual with hypertension
Assess for **heart murmurs**, heard between heart sounds Produced by atypical flow of blood through the heart (e.g., irregularity or partial obstruction, increased flow in normal area, flow into dilated chamber, flow through abnormal passage); regurgitant flow Occurs during systole (between S_1 and S_2) or during diastole (between S_2 and S_1)	Faint sound More common during systole Often found in children and young adults	Faint or loud enough to be heard without a stethoscope Occurs during systole or diastole (diastolic murmurs are almost always pathologic)—found in older clients with heart disease or infants and children with congenital heart defects
Evaluate the **apical pulse** when assessing for general heart rate and rhythm of contractions	Regular rhythm Heart rate: 60–100 beats/min	Irregular rhythm (dysrhythmia) may be regularly irregular or irregularly irregular (i.e., atrial fibrillation)
Auscultate at the apex of the heart (left, fifth intercostal space at the midclavicular line)	Moderate bradycardia common in well-trained athletes	Bradycardia (less than 60 beats/min)

Assessment	Normal	Abnormal

Describing a Murmur

Murmurs are classified by timing and are heard between heart sounds:

Timing—When does it occur? Between systolic (S_1 and S_2) sounds or between diastolic (S_2 and S_1) sounds.

Location—Point where murmur is loudest.

Radiation—Where murmur starts (point of maximum intensity) and moves to surrounding areas.

Quality—Blowing, harsh, musical, or rumbling.

Pitch—High, low, medium.

Intensity—Grade 1, barely audible; to grade 6, audible with stethoscope just off client's skin.

Pattern—Intensity over time; soft to loud/loud to soft.

Source: Smith, S. (2009). *Sandra Smith's Review for NCLEX-RN*, 12th ed. Sudbury, MA: Jones & Bartlett Publishers, p. 216.

Assessment	Normal	Abnormal
Palpate and view pulse on chest wall if client's chest wall is thin enough	Mild tachycardia possible with stress, infection, or fever	Tachycardia (more than 100 beats/min)
Assess for **irregular apical pulse** With another nurse, take apical and radial pulses *simultaneously* Compare beats per minute for both pulses	Equal apical and radial pulses = no pulse deficit	Fewer beats at the radial area may indicate an irregular apical pulse, producing ineffective pumping
Auscultate apical pulse and compare to carotid pulse	Two pulses are synchronous	Apical pulse greater than carotid pulse indicates a pulse deficit
Palpate **peripheral pulses***: radial, brachial, femoral, popliteal, dorsalis pedis, posterior tibial (For special cases, after carotid surgery, palpate temporal pulse also) Guidelines for palpating peripheral pulses: If pulse is not immediately palpable, examine adjacent area—pulse locations differ with clients Palpate weak pulses gently so that you do not obliterate pulse with too much pressure If you cannot differentiate your pulse from client's pulse, check your radial or carotid pulse, or observe monitor pattern When peripheral pulses cannot be palpated, use a Doppler ultrasound stethoscope and grade according to scale	Easily palpated Equally strong on both sides Posterior tibial pulse usually weaker than femoral	Difficult to palpate Unequal pulses Weak pulse Absent pulses

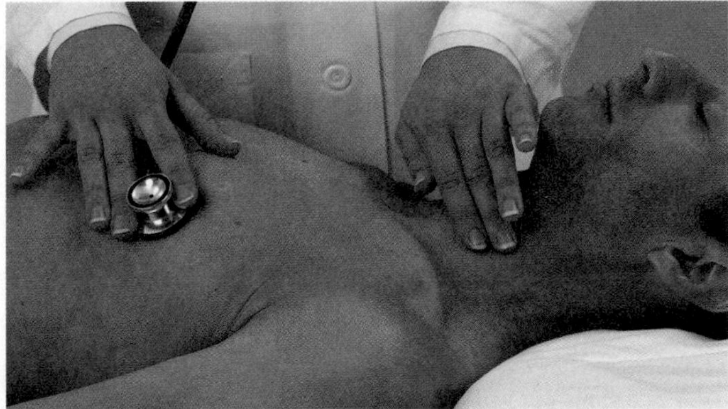

▲ Compare apical and carotid pulse to identify pulse deficit.

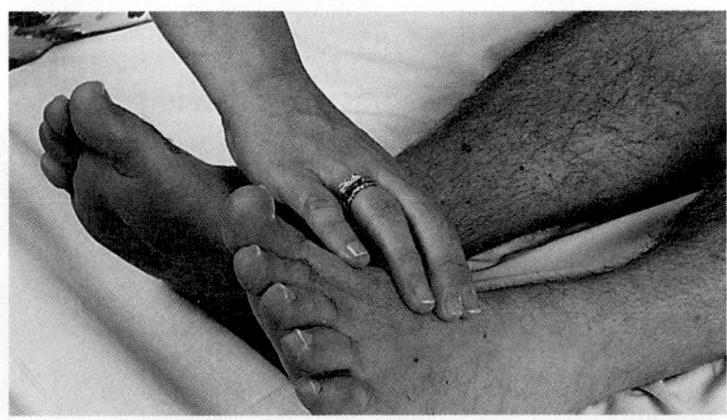

▲ Palpate peripheral pulse, dorsalis pedis.

*See assessing peripheral pulses in Chapter 10, Vital Signs

ASSESSMENT OF THE ABDOMEN, SPLEEN, KIDNEY, LIVER, AND GENITOURINARY TRACT

Abdomen Assessment
Liver Assessment
Spleen Assessment
Urinary Tract Assessment
Genital Assessment
Breast Assessment
Testicular Examination

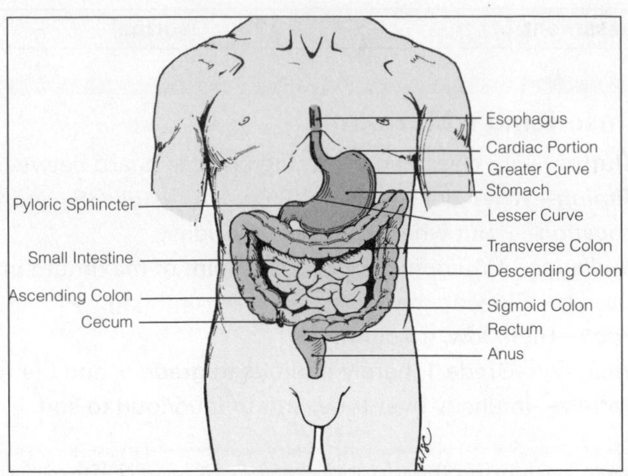

▲ Assessment requires knowledge of abdominal organ anatomy.

The abdomen extends from the diaphragm to the pelvis. Generally speaking, there are two body systems present in this area: the gastrointestinal system and the genitourinary system.

The gastrointestinal system begins at the mouth and consists of the esophagus, stomach, the small and large intestines, and associated organs that include the liver, pancreas, and spleen.

The urinary tract consists of the kidneys, ureters, bladder, and the urethra. The urinary tract should be assessed frequently and accurately because changes in urine production reflect changes in other body systems.

The most common way to assess the urinary tract is to note the quantity and quality of the urinary output. Some medications or foods produce unusual odors and colors in urine (e.g., sulfasalazine [Azulfidine] turns urine a yellow-orange color; asparagus gives urine a musty odor).

External male genitalia include the penis, the scrotum, and the testicles. External female genitalia include the vulva, the urethral orifice, and the vagina.

Assessment: Abdomen, Liver, Spleen, Kidney, and Genitourinary Tract

Assessment	Normal	Abnormal
Abdomen Assessment		
Have client lie flat in bed At the client's abdominal level, inspect the **general contour** of the abdomen	Abdomen flat from chest to pubis with concave indentation at umbilicus	Scaphoid (concave) abdominal contour: due to inadequate nutritional intake to meet caloric need or inadequate food absorption Distended abdomen: caused by gas and fluid accumulation due to lack of peristalsis, hemorrhage, or intestinal leakage after trauma (e.g., auto accident or surgery), or ascitic fluid (e.g., liver or cardiac failure)
Inspect for bruising around umbilicus and over flanks	No change of skin color around umbilicus or flanks	Acute abdomen
Observe for scars, stretch marks, dilated veins, presence of hernia	Correlate with health history	Dilated veins caused by liver disease Bulge seen with defect in abdominal wall
Assess **circumference** for intraabdominal hemorrhage or ascites by placing a tape measure around the largest circumference of the abdomen. Draw two lines around client's entire abdomen, one line at the top of the tape measure, one line at the bottom of the tape measure; perform measurement when client exhales	No increase in abdominal circumference	Abdominal circumference increases steadily within 1–2 hours
Auscultate abdomen to assess presence and quality of **bowel sounds**		

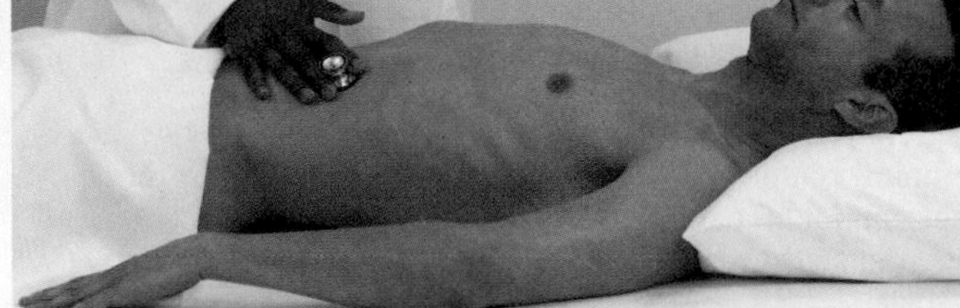

▲ Auscultate abdomen for bowel sounds.

Note: After abdominal surgery, the return of GI function is determined by the (1) return of flatus, (2) bowel movement, (3) hunger, (4) no nausea or tolerance of oral feeding, (5) flat abdomen/nondistension, rather than the return of bowel sounds.

Assessment	Normal	Abnormal
Place diaphragm of stethoscope firmly on right lower quadrant and count sounds for 1 minute	Bowel sounds gurgle, about 5–30 per minute	Hyperactive bowel sounds: due to blood in GI tract, diarrhea, or to partial bowel obstruction (sounds become high-pitched and tinkling or come in "rushes," followed by silence as obstruction progresses)
Listen at all quadrants, near the center, for several minutes if sounds not heard initially	Varying frequency of sounds with clients and time of day (i.e., more sounds right before and after eating) Decreased or absent bowel sounds after surgery After general anesthesia, normal sounds in 1–2 days After abdominal surgery, normal sounds in 3–5 days	Bowel sounds hypoactive, quiet, and infrequent: may be due to peritonitis, paralytic ileus, or no obvious cause Absent bowel sounds: may be due to complete bowel obstruction or systemic illness
Palpate abdomen lightly to determine area of tenderness. Palpate deeper to check **abdominal muscles** and organs beneath muscles. Assist client to relax, lie flat in bed, and flex knees. Have client mouth-breathe.	No tenderness, abdomen is relaxed.	Tenderness is present—hypersensitivity.

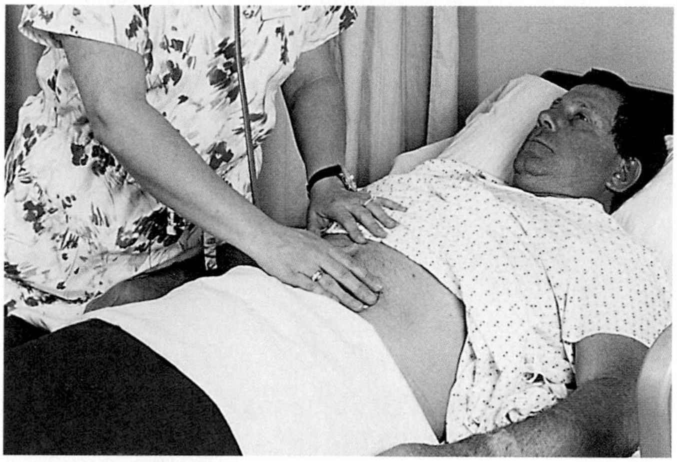

▲ Palpate client's abdomen.

Assessment	Normal	Abnormal
Place your hand flat on client's abdomen, holding your four fingers together and depress ½ in. or 1 cm.	Soft, pliant musculature when relaxed	Rigid, tender muscles/pain produced with cough: may be due to presence of muscle spasm, inflammation, or infection (peritonitis)
Have client cough to determine any areas of abdominal tenderness	Cough does not produce pain in abdomen	
Begin palpation at the pubis, moving upward. Palpate any problem areas last to minimize effects of discomfort. Palpate all quadrants of abdomen to assess organs contained in each quadrant Superficial palpation: use slight pressure only with your fingers extended	No bulges felt No masses felt	Pain or tenderness with quick release of pressure indicates rebound tenderness suggesting peritoneal inflammation If hernia is suspected, have client raise head and shoulders and observe for abdominal bulge
Deep palpation: indent the abdominal wall 4–5 cm—may use one hand over the other to apply pressure	No masses felt	Masses felt with colon disease, vascular aneurysm, dilated bowel, distended bladder, or cancer
Liver Assessment		
Palpate **liver** by placing left hand behind 11th and 12th ribs with right hand on right abdomen lateral to rectus muscle	Normal liver (difficult to palpate) may feel like sharp ridge with smooth surface	Tenderness may be due to inflammation (hepatitis) Enlarged liver with nontender edge may be due to cirrhosis

(continued)

Assessment: Abdomen, Liver, Spleen, Kidney, and Genitourinary Tract *(Continued)*

Assessment	Normal	Abnormal
		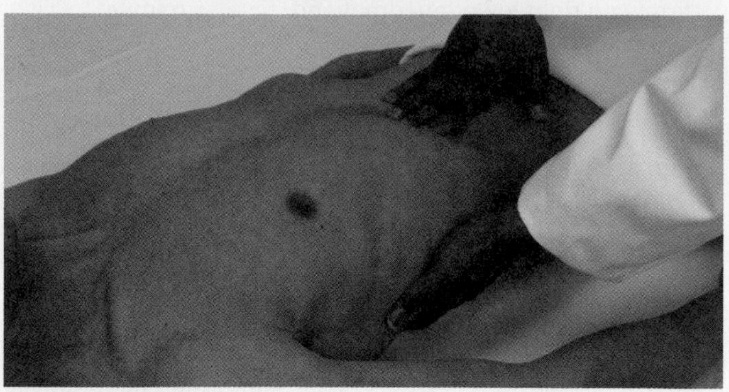 ▲ Palpation of the liver.
Spleen Assessment		
Standing on client's right side, palpate spleen. Place left hand under rib cage on left side and elevate rib cage. Press fingers of right hand into left costal margin area and ask client to take a deep breath. You should feel spleen move forward toward right hand.	A normal spleen is usually not palpable	Enlarged spleen (which can be palpated) occurs in acute infections such as mononucleosis 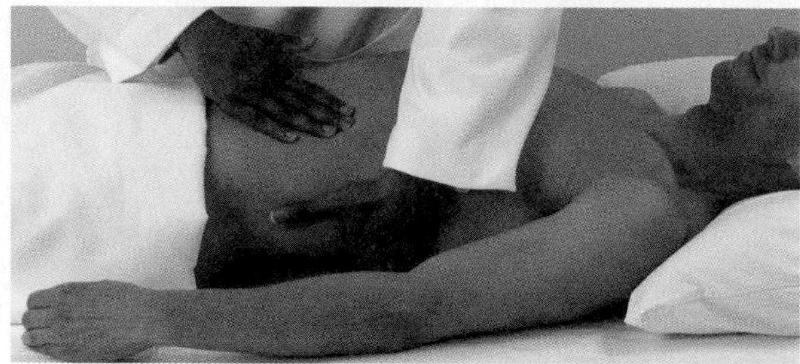 ▲ Palpation of the spleen.
Urinary Tract Assessment		
Assess the **external urethra**	Orifice is pink and moist; clear, minimal discharge	Burning or pain at urethral orifice: may indicate urinary infection

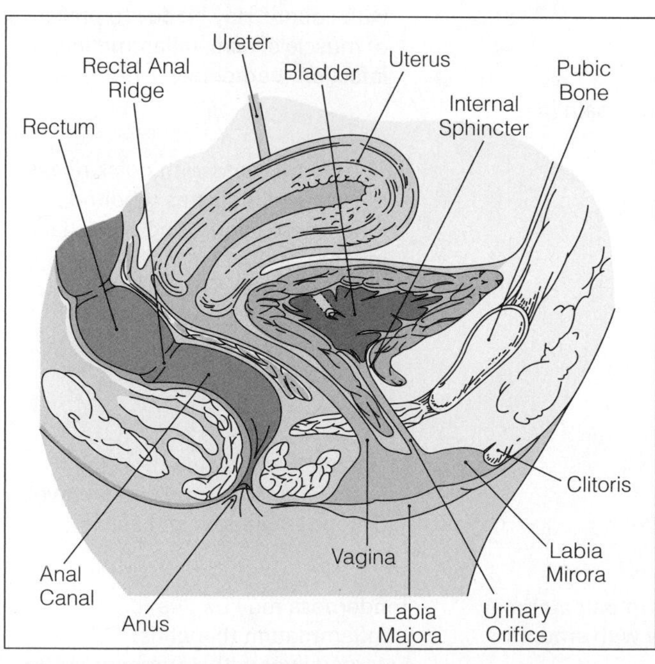

▲ Female genitourinary system.

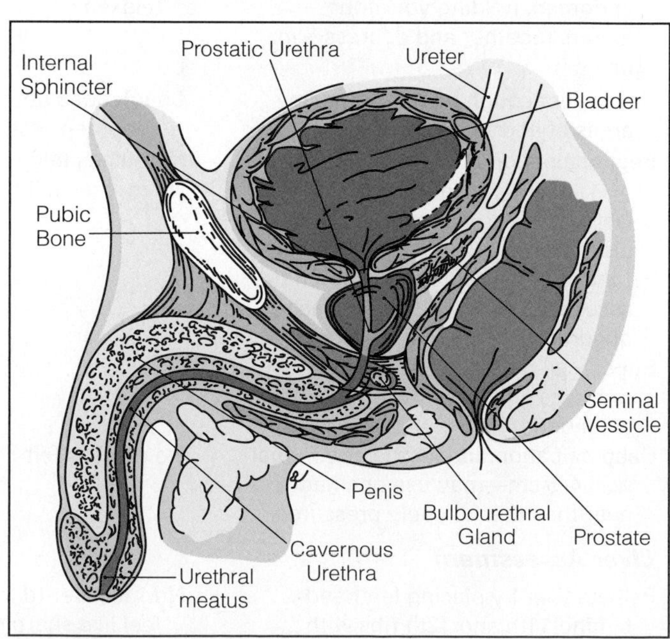

▲ Male genitourinary system.

Assessment	Normal	Abnormal
Assess the quantity, color, odor, specific gravity, and pH of **urine output**	Output: average 1,200–1,500 mL/24 hours, or 30–50 mL/hour—should equal oral and IV intake	Increased output: may indicate increased intake, diuresis, potential diabetes mellitus, or inappropriate antidiuretic hormone (ADH) response (e.g., diabetes insipidus) Frequent small amounts of urine output indicate urinary retention or urinary tract infection Decreased output: may indicate dehydration, acute nephritis, cardiac disease, renal failure, or excess ADH response (e.g., head injury)
	Clear, yellow-amber color (vegetarians may have slightly cloudy urine)	Cloudy *(turbid)*: may indicate possible urinary tract infection Dark amber: may indicate very concentrated urine due to dehydration Dark amber to green: may indicate hepatitis or obstructive jaundice
	Slight odor (ammonia-like odor indicates that specimen has been sitting for some time)	Foul-smelling: may indicate urinary tract infection, drug or specific food ingestion (e.g., asparagus) Sweet odor: may indicate acetone from ketoacidosis (i.e., diabetes mellitus)
	Specific gravity: 1.003–1.030	Specific gravity of more than 1.030: indicates dehydration Constant specific gravity of 1.010, regardless of fluid intake: indicates renal failure
	pH range from 4.5–7.5; average is 6–7	Acidic pH—when below 6.0 may indicate starvation or acidosis Alkaline pH greater than 7.0: indicates metabolic alkalosis or alkaline ash diet (e.g., vegetarian)
Assess for **blood** in urine using Hemastix or Labstix	No blood present	Smokey to mildly pink-tinged to grossly red-colored urine: indicates blood in urine
Palpate for **bladder distention**	Not normally palpated	Distended bladder (firm, round mass) accompanied by discomfort and urge to void: indicates urine retention (common following surgery, where catheter is not used)
Kidney Assessment		
Assess (palpate) for kidney pain on either side of vertebrae column between last thoracic and third lumbar vertebrae Use indirect percussion to further assess the kidneys	When palpated, client feels no pain 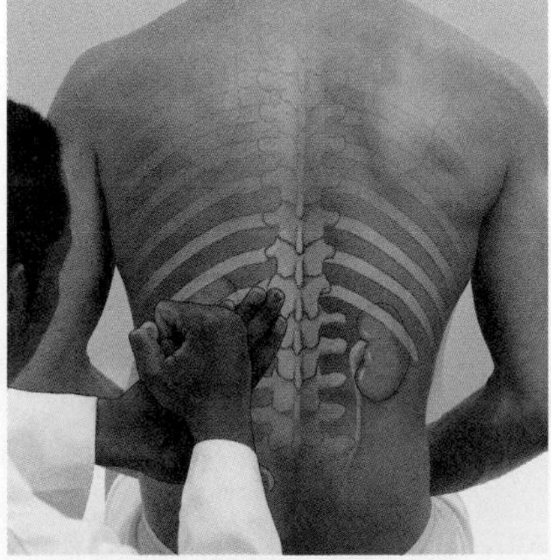 ▲ Use of indirect percussion will identify pain.	Severe pain, discomfort, or tenderness in the flank region (below rib cage posteriorly and lateral to spine): indicates kidney infection, stones, or kidney disease. Kidney enlargement may indicate neoplasm or polycystic disease.

(continued)

Assessment: Abdomen, Liver, Spleen, Kidney, and Genitourinary Tract *(Continued)*

Assessment	Normal	Abnormal
Genital Assessment Male		
Visually examine the **male genitalia** Retract the foreskin of the uncircumcised penis to note cleanliness, any **lesions**, and **discharge**	Clean No odor No lesions	Unclean Odor Lesions and discharge may indicate venereal disease or cancer
Lift scrotum to inspect for rash	No discharge Size of penis and scrotum vary	Oval and round, dark erosion: may indicate syphilitic chancre
Noting groin area, ask client to strain down	Urethra opens midline of the tip of the glans No bulges in groin area	Hypospadias: due to congenital displacement of the urethral meatus Bulge on straining seen with hernias Indurated nodule or ulcer: may indicate carcinoma
Testicular Examination		
Palpate scrotum, testes, and observe shape and contour.	Should be pear-shaped with left side lower than right; no masses; testes nontender, smooth, and solid	Swelling may indicate orchitis or scrotal edema; scrotal hernia or testicular torsion; varicocele
Observe for swelling, redness, and distended veins or lesions inguinal area.	Flat, no evidence of masses	Mass may be related to inguinal hernia or cancer
Using thumb and first two fingers, gently palpate each testicle for size, shape, and consistency	Two testicles in the scrotum No nodules felt, no swelling or tenderness	Mass in scrotum: indicates possible hernia, hydrocele, testicular tumor, or cyst Pain indicates inflammatory disease
Female		
Visually examine **female genitalia**	Clean No odor	Unclean Odor (musty with bacterial infection)
Assess for signs of sexual abuse	No signs	Bruises, welts, burns, unusual swelling
Assess for **lesions** or **discharge** or complaints of itching	Minimal, clear discharge Menstrual flow Lochia (normal discharge after delivery) No lesions No pruritus	Thick; thin, white, yellowish, or green discharge: may indicate trichomoniasis Thick, white, and curdy discharge with pruritus may indicate candidiasis Lesions: could indicate syphilitic chancre, herpes infection, venereal wart, or carcinoma of vulva
Breast Assessment		
Inspect **size, symmetry**, and **contour** of breasts, comparing one side with the other Place client in sitting position Have client remove clothing from waist up Have client raise arms over her head	Size varies with each client Breasts should be fairly equal in size and contour and symmetric in position	Masses, skin thickening, dimpling, or flattened areas: indicate possible cancer
Color, edema, and **venous pattern of skin**	Normal skin color with darker area surrounding nipples No edema or prominent vessels	Erythema: indicates infection or inflammatory carcinoma Edema or increased venous prominence: indicates carcinoma
Inspect **size and shape of nipples** Note direction in which they point, and any **rashes** or **discharge** To palpate breasts, position client supine or on side Place a pillow under the shoulder of the side being examined Using three fingers in a circular motion, compress breast tissue gently against chest wall	Simple inversion of nipples is common	Flattening, nipple retraction, or axis deviation of nipple points: may be due to fibrosis associated with cancer Ulcerations of nipples and areola: may be due to Paget's disease Discharge: may not be malignant but should be observed closely Mobile nodules may indicate cystic disease

Assessment	Normal	Abnormal
Systematically examine entire breast, top to bottom, moving medially to laterally into the axilla	Soft, elastic tissue with mobile nodules 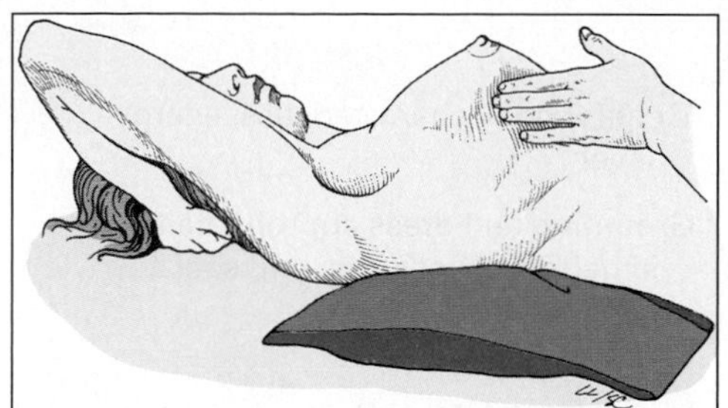 ▲ Examine breast tissue in circular movement.	Hard nodules fixed to skin or underlying tissue may indicate cancer When nodules are present: Describe location and quadrant of breast where found Note size in centimeters Describe consistency and shape Note tenderness and mobility of nodule in relationship to underlying tissue
Palpate nipples		
Compress nipple and areola between thumb and index finger to inspect for discharge	No discharge or small amount of milky discharge in previously nursing mother	Bloody discharge: may indicate papilloma
Note **elasticity**	Elastic, no retraction of nipple	Loss of elasticity: indicates possible cancer
Observe for erection of nipple with palpation		Inversion, flattening, or retraction: may indicate cancer

MENTAL HEALTH ASSESSMENT

The mental assessment is completed throughout the physical assessment during the history taking. It is not generally considered a separate entity. Mood, memory, orientation, and thought processes can be evaluated while obtaining the health history. Nutritional preferences and restrictions can be determined as a part of a client care plan and may or may not be included in the general client assessment.

A spiritual assessment can be obtained as a part of the health history, although specific sociocultural beliefs may need to be ascertained separately. The purpose of a spiritual assessment is to facilitate the client adapting to the hospital environment and to help the staff understand stressors the client may be experiencing as a result of belief systems.*

The purpose of a mental status assessment is to evaluate the present state of psychologic functioning and to monitor safety needs of the client. It is not designed to make a diagnosis; rather it should yield data that contribute to the total picture of the client as he or she is functioning at the time the assessment is made.

The specific rationale for completing a mental status assessment is:

- To collect baseline data to aid in establishing the cause, diagnosis, and prognosis
- To evaluate the present state of psychologic functioning

NOTE: For more information on a spiritual–religious assessment, see Chapter 4.

- To evaluate changes in the individual's emotional, intellectual, motor, and perceptual responses
- To determine the client's ability to cope with the present situation
- To assess the need and availability of support systems
- To ascertain if some seemingly psychopathologic response is, in fact, a disorder of a sensory organ (i.e., a deaf person appearing hostile, depressed, or suspicious)
- To determine the guidelines of the treatment plan
- To document altered mental status for legal records

The initial factors that the nurse must consider in completing a mental status assessment are to correctly identify the client, the reason for admission, record of previous mental illness, present complaint, any personal history that is relevant (living arrangements, role in family, interactional experience, history of alcoholism, domestic violence), family history if appropriate, significant others and available support systems, assets, and interests.

The actual assessment process begins with an initial evaluation of the appropriateness of the client's behavior and orientation to reality. The assessment continues by noting any abnormal behavior and ascertaining the client's chief verbalized complaint. Finally, the evaluation determines if the client is in contact with reality enough to answer particular questions that further assess the client's condition.

Assessment: Mental Status

Assessment	Normal	Abnormal
General Appearance, Manner, and Attitude		
Assess **physical appearance**	General body characteristics, energy level	Inappropriate physical appearance, high or low extremes of energy
Note **grooming**, mode of dress, and **personal hygiene**	Grooming and dress appropriate to situation, client's age, and social circumstance Clean	Poor grooming Inappropriate or bizarre dress or combination of clothes Unclean
Note **posture**	Upright, straight, and appropriate	Slumped, tipped, or stooped
Note speed, pressure, pace, quantity, volume, and diction of **speech**	Moderated speed, volume, and quantity Appropriate diction	Tremors Accelerated or retarded speech and high quantity Poor or inappropriate diction
Note relevance, content, and organization of **responses**	Questions answered directly, accurately, and with relevance	Inappropriate responses, unorganized pattern of speech Tangential, circumstantial, or out of-context replies
Expressive Aspects of Behavior		
Note **general motor activity**	Calm, ordered movement appropriate to situation	Overactive (e.g., restless, agitated, impulsive) Underactive (e.g., slow to initiate or execute actions)
Assess **purposeful movements and gestures**	Reasonably responsive with purposeful movements, appropriate gestures	Repetitious activities (e.g., rituals or compulsions)
Assess style of **gait**		Command automation Parkinsonian movements Ataxic, shuffling, off-balance gait
Consciousness		
Assess **level of consciousness**	Alert, attentive, and responsive Knowledgeable about time, place, and person	Disordered attention; distracted, cloudy consciousness Delirious Stuporous
Thought Processes and Perception		
Assess **coherency, logic,** and **relevance** of thought processes by asking questions about personal history (e.g., "Where were you born?" "What kind of work do you do?")	Clear, understandable responses to questions Attentiveness	Disoriented in time, place, person Disordered thought forms Autistic or dereistic (absorbed with self and withdrawn); abstract (absent-mindedness); concrete thinking (dogmatic, preaching)
Assess **reality orientation**: time, place, and person awareness	Orderly progression of thoughts based in reality Awareness of time, place, and person	Disorders of progression of thought; looseness, circumstantial, incoherent, irrelevant conversation, blocking Delusions of grandeur or persecution: neologisms, use of words whose meaning is known only to the client Echolalia (automatic repeating of questions) No awareness of day, time, place, or person

Assessment	Normal	Abnormal
Assess **perceptions** and reactions to personal experiences by asking questions, such as "How do you see yourself now that you are in the hospital?" "What do you think about when you're in a situation like this?"	Thoughtful, clear responses expressed with understanding of self	Altered, narrowed, or expanded perception illusions Depersonalization
Thought Content and Mental Trend		
Assess degree of anxiety Ask questions to determine general themes that identify **degree of anxiety** (e.g., "How are you feeling right now?" "What kinds of things make you afraid?")	Mild or 1+ level of anxiety in which individual is alert, motivated, and attentive	Moderate to severe (2+ to 4+) levels of anxiety
Assess **ideation** and **concentration**	Ideas based in reality Able to concentrate	Ideas of reference Hypochondria (abnormal concerns about health) Obsessional Phobias (irrational fears) Poor or shortened concentration
Mood or Affect		
Assess prevailing or **variability in mood** by observing behavior and asking questions, such as "How are you feeling right now?" Check for presence of abnormal **euphoria**	Appropriate, even mood without wide variations high to low	Cyclothymic mood swings; euphoria, elation, ecstasy, depressed, withdrawn
If you suspect **depression**, continue questioning to determine depth and significance of mood (e.g., "How badly do you feel?" "Have you ever thought of suicide?")	May be sad or grieving but mood does not persist indefinitely	Flat or dampened responses Inappropriate responses Ambivalence
Memory		
Assess **past and present memory** and **retention** (ability to listen and respond with understanding or knowledge); ask client to repeat a phrase (e.g., an address)	Alert, accurate responses Able to complete digit span Past and present memory appropriate	Hyperamnesia (excessive loss of memory); amnesia; paramnesia (belief in events that never occurred) Preoccupied Unable to follow directions
Assess **recall** (recent and remote) by asking questions, such as "When is your birthday?" "What year were you born?" "How old are you?" "Who is the president of the United States now?"	Good recall of immediate and past events	Poor recall of immediate or past events
Judgment		
Assess **judgment, decision-making ability**, and **interpretations** by asking questions, such as "What should you do if you hear a siren while you're driving?" "If you lost a library book, what would you do?"	Ability to make accurate decisions Realistic interpretation of events	Poor judgment, poor decision-making ability, poor choice Inappropriate interpretation of events or situations

(continued)

Assessment: Mental Status *(Continued)*

Assessment	Normal	Abnormal
Awareness		
Assess **insight**, the ability to understand the inner nature of events or problems, by asking questions, such as "If you saw someone dressed in a fur coat on a hot day, what would you think?"	Thoughtful responses indicating an understanding of the inner nature of an event or problem	Lack of insight or understanding of problems or situations Distorted view of situation
Intelligence		
Assess **intelligence** by asking client to define or use words in sentences (e.g., recede, join, plural)	Correct responses to majority of questions	Incorrect responses to majority of questions indicate possible severe psychiatric disorders
Assess **fund of information** by asking questions, such as "Who is president of the United States?" "Who was the president before him?" "When is Memorial Day?" "What is a thermometer?" (Consider client's cultural and educational background and his or her grasp of English)	Correct responses to majority of questions	Deteriorated or impaired cognitive processes
Sensory Ability		
Assess the **five senses** (i.e., vision, hearing, taste, feeling, and smell)	Able to perceive, hear, feel, touch appropriate to stimulus	Lack of response Suspicious, hostile, depressed Kinesthetic imbalance
Developmental Level		
Assess **developmental level** compared with normal	Behavior and thought processes appropriate to age level	Wide span between chronologic and developmental age Mentally retarded
Lifestyle Patterns		
Identify **addictive patterns** and effect on individual's overall health	Normal amount of alcohol ingested Smoking habits, number of years Prescriptive medications Adequate food intake for physical characteristics	High quantity of alcohol taken frequently Heavy smoker Addicted to illegal drugs Habituative medication; user of over-the-counter or legal medications Anorexic eating patterns Obese or overindulgence of food
Coping Devices		
Identify **defense-coping mechanisms** and their effect on individual	Conscious coping mechanisms used appropriately, such as compensation, fantasy, rationalization, suppression, sublimation, or displacement Mechanisms effective, appropriate, and useful	Unconscious mechanisms used frequently, such as repression, regression, projection, reaction formation, insulation, or denial Mechanisms inappropriate, ineffective, and not useful

Assessment: Obstetrical

Assessment	Normal	Abnormal
Baseline Data		
Assess **breasts** and **nipples**		
Contour and size		
Presence of lumps	No lumps	Lumps
Secretions	Colostrum secretions in late first trimester or early second trimester	Secretions, other than colostrum
Assess **abdomen**		
Contour and size		
Changes in skin color	*Linea nigra* (black line of pregnancy along midline of abdomen) Primiparas: coincidentally with growth of fundus Multiparas: after 13–15 weeks' gestation	
Striae (reddish-purple lines)	On breasts, hips, and thighs during pregnancy After pregnancy, faint silvery-gray	
Scar, rashes, or other skin disturbances	Usually none present	
Fundal height in centimeters (fingerbreadths less accurate): measure from symphysis pubis to top of fundus	Fundus palpable just above symphysis at 8–10 weeks Halfway between symphysis and umbilicus at 16 weeks Umbilicus at 20–22 weeks	Large measurements: Expected date of confinement, or delivery (EDC) is incorrect; tumor; ascites; multiple pregnancy; polyhydramnios, hydatidiform mole Less than normal enlargement: fetal abnormality, oligohydramnios, placental dysmaturity, missed abortion, fetal death
Perineum: assess for scars, lesions, or discharge	None present	Rash, warts, discharge
Evaluate **weight**		
Take **vital signs, blood pressure** (BP), **temperature, pulse,** and **respiration** (TPR)	Vital signs normal	
Evaluate **lab findings**		
Urine: sugar, protein, albumin	Negative for sugar, protein, and albumin throughout pregnancy	Positive for sugar, protein, and/or albumin
Hematocrit (HCT)	38%–47%	
Hemoglobin (Hgb)	12–16 gm/dL	
Blood type and Rh factor		If Rh negative, father's blood should be typed If Rh positive, titers should be followed; possible RhoGAM at termination of pregnancy
Pap smear		
VD smears and screening		
Antepartum Assessment		
Evaluate **weight** to assess maternal health and nutritional status and growth of fetus	Minimum weight gain during pregnancy: 24 lb If underweight: gain 28–42 lb If obese: gain 15 lb or more Normal weight gain: 25–35 to 40 lb	Inadequate weight gain; possible maternal malnutrition Excessive weight gain: if sudden at onset, may indicate preeclampsia; if gradual and continual, may indicate overeating

(continued)

Assessment: Obstetrical *(Continued)*

Assessment	Normal	Abnormal
Evaluate **blood pressure**	Fairly constant with baseline data throughout pregnancy	Increased: possible anxiety (client should rest 20 to 30 minutes before you take BP again) Rise of 30/15 above baseline data: sign of preeclampsia Decreased: sign of supine hypotensive syndrome. If lying on back, turn client on left side and take BP again
Evaluate **fundal height**	Drop around 38th week: sign of fetus engaging in birth canal Primipara: sudden drop Multipara: slower, sometimes not until onset of labor	Large fundal growth: may indicate wrong dates, multiple pregnancy, hydatidiform mole, polyhydramnios, tumors Small fundal growth: may indicate fetal demise, fetal anomaly, retarded fetal growth, abnormal presentation or lie, decreased amniotic fluid
Determine **fetal position,** using **Leopold's maneuvers.** Complete external palpations of the abdomen to determine fetal position, lie, presentation, and engagement		
First maneuver: to determine part of fetus presenting into pelvis	Vertex presentation	Breech presentation or transverse lie
Second maneuver: to locate the back, arms, and legs: fetal heart heard best over fetal back		

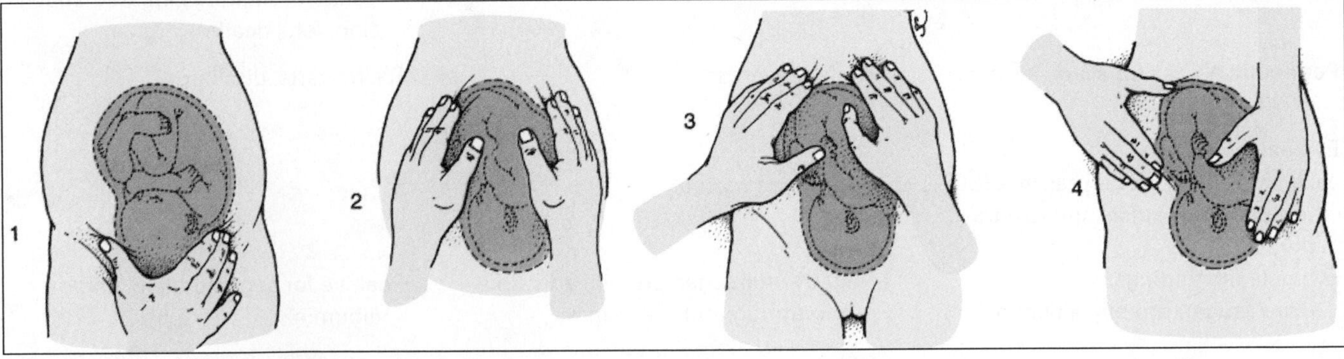

▲ Steps of Leopold's maneuvers.

Assessment	Normal	Abnormal
Third maneuver: to determine part of fetus in fundus		
Fourth maneuver: to determine degree of cephalic flexion and engagement		
Evaluate **fetal heart rate** by quadrant, location, and rate	120–160 beats/min	>160 or <120: may indicate fetal distress. *Notify physician*
Check for presence of **edema**	In lower extremities toward end of pregnancy	In upper extremities and face: may indicate preeclampsia
Evaluate **urine** (clean catch midstream)	Negative for sugar, protein, and albumin	Positive for sugar: may indicate subclinical or gestational diabetes Positive for protein and/or albumin: may indicate preeclampsia
Evaluate **levels of discomfort**		

Assessment	Normal	Abnormal
Intrapartum Assessment		
Assess for **lightening** and **dropping** (the descent of the presenting part into the pelvis)	Several days to 2 weeks before onset of labor Multipara: may not occur until onset of labor Relief of shortness of breath and increase in urinary frequency	No lightening or dropping: may indicate disproportion between fetal presenting part and maternal pelvis
Check if **mucous plug** has been expelled from cervix	Usually expelled from cervix before onset of labor	
Assess for "**bloody show**"	Clear, pinkish, or blood-tinged vaginal discharge that occurs as cervix begins to dilate and efface	
Assess for **ruptured membranes** Time water breaks	Before, during, or after onset of labor	Breech presentation: frank meconium or meconium staining
Color of **amniotic fluid**	Clear, straw color	Greenish-brown: indicates meconium has passed from fetus, possible fetal distress Yellow-stained: fetal hypoxia 36 hours or more before rupture of membrane or hemolytic disease
Quantity of amniotic fluid	Normal is 500–1,000 mL of amniotic fluid, rarely expelled at one time	**Polyhydramnios**—excessive amniotic fluid over 2,000 mL Observe newborn for congenital anomalies: craniospinal malformation, oro-gastrointestinal anomalies. Down's syndrome, and congenital heart defects **Oligohydramnios**—minimal amniotic fluid, less than 500 mL Observe newborn for malformation of ear, genitourinary tract anomalies, and renal agenesis
Odor of fluid	No odor	Odor may indicate infection; deliver within 24 hours
Fetal heart rate	120–160 beats/min	Decreased: indicates fetal distress with possible cord prolapse or cord compression
	Regular rhythm	Accelerated: initial sign of fetal hypoxia Absent: may indicate fetal demise
Labor and Delivery Assessment		
Evaluate Contractions		
Frequency: from start of one contraction to start of next	3–5 minutes between contractions	Irregular contractions with long intervals between: indicates false labor
Duration: from beginning of contraction to time uterus begins to relax	50–90 seconds	>90 seconds: uterine tetany; stop oxytocin if running
Intensity (strength of contraction): measured with monitoring device	Peak 25 mmHg End of labor may reach 50–75 mmHg	>75 mmHg: uterine tetany or uterine rupture
First-Stage		
Latent phase (0–4 cm dilation)	0–3 to 4 cm; average 6.4 hours	Prolonged time in any phase: may indicate poor fetal position, incomplete fetal flexion, cephalopelvic disproportion, or poor uterine contractions

(continued)

Assessment: Obstetrical *(Continued)*

Assessment	Normal	Abnormal
Active phase (4–8 cm) *Transitional phase* (8–10 cm)	Length of time varies—may be 1–2 hours	If total labor <3 hours: indicates precipitous labor, increasing risk of fetal complications, or maternal lacerations and tears
Assess for **bloody show** Observe for presence of **nausea or vomiting** Assess **perineum**	Beginning to bulge	
Evaluate **urge to bear down**		Often uncontrolled Multipara: can cause precipitous delivery "Panting" (can be controlled until safe delivery area established)
Second stage (10 cm to delivery)	Primipara: up to 2 hours Multipara: several minutes to 2 hours	>2 hours: increased risk of fetal brain damage and maternal exhaustion
Assess for **presenting part**	Vertex with ROA or LOA presentation	Occiput posterior, breech, face, or transverse lie
Assess **caput** (infant head) Multipara: move to delivery room when caput size of dime Primipara: move to delivery room when caput size of half dollar	Visible when bearing down during contraction	"Crowns" in room other than delivery room: delivery imminent (do not move client)
Assess **fetal heart rate (FHR)** Bradycardia, drop of 20 beats/min below base line (↓120 beats/min) Tachycardia, increase in FHR over 160 beats/min for 10 min	120–160/min	Decreased: may indicate supine hypotensive syndrome (turn client on side and take again) Hemorrhage (check for other signs of bleeding: notify physician) Increased or decreased: may indicate fetal distress secondary to cord progression or compression (place client in Trendelenburg or knee–chest position; give oxygen if necessary; inform physician)
Evaluate **fetal heart rate tracing**	Short-term variability is present Long-term variability ranges from 3–5 cycles/min	Absence of variability (no short term or long term present) Severe variable decelerations (fetal heart rate <70 for longer than 30–45 seconds with decreasing variability)
Deceleration	Early deceleration (10–20 beat drop) Recovery when acme contraction passes—often not serious	Monitor closely—distinguish from decrease with hypertonic contraction; leads to fetal distress
Variable deceleration; decrease in FHR, below 120/min Loss of beat-to-beat variation	Mild; may be within normal parameters—continue to monitor If continues less than 15 minutes, no problem apparent	Cord compression—may result in fetal difficulty Late deceleration pattern occurs—monitor for hypertonic contraction; leads to total distress.
Evaluate **breathing**	Controlled with contractions	Heavy or excessive: may lead to hyperventilation and/or dehydration

Assessment	Normal	Abnormal
Evaluate **pain** and **anxiety**	Medication required after dilated 4–5 cm unless using natural childbirth methods	Severe pain early in first stage of labor: inadequate prenatal teaching, backache due to position in bed, uterine tetany
Third stage (from delivery of baby to delivery of placenta)	Placental separation occurs within 30 minutes (usually 3–5 min)	Failure of placental separation Abnormality of uterus or cervix, weak, ineffectual uterine contraction, tetanic contractions causing closure of cervix >3 hours: indicates retained placenta
Fourth stage (first hour postpartum)		Mother in unstable condition (hemorrhage usual cause) Highest risk of hemorrhage in first postpartum hour
Temperature	36.5°C–37.5°C	>37.5°C: may indicate infection Slight elevation: due to dehydration from mouth breathing and NPO
Pulse	Pulse: 60–100	Increased: may indicate pain or hemorrhage
Respiration	Respirations: 12–22	
Blood pressure	Blood pressure: 120–140/80	Increased: may indicate anxiety, pain, or post-eclamptic condition Decreased: hemorrhage
Postpartum Assessment		
Assess **vital signs** every 15 minutes for 1 hour, every 30 minutes for 1 hour, every hour for 4 hours, every 8 hours, and as needed	Pulse may be 45–60/min in stage 4 Pulse to normal range about third day	Decreased BP and increased pulse: probably postpartum hemorrhage Elevated temperature >38°C indicates possible infection Temperature elevates when lactation occurs
Assess **fundus** every 15 minutes for 1 hour, every 8 hours for 48 hours, then daily	Firm (like a grapefruit) in midline and at or slightly above umbilicus Return to prepregnant size in 6 weeks: descending at rate of 1 fingerbreadth/day	Boggy fundus: immediately massage gently until firm; report to physician and observe closely; empty bladder; medicate with oxytocin if ordered Fundus misplaced 1–2 fingerbreadths from midline: indicates full bladder (client must void or be catheterized)
Assess **lochia** every 15 minutes for 1 hour, every 8 hours for 48 hours, then daily *Color*	3 days postpartum: dark red (rubra) 4–10 days postpartum: clear pink (serosa) 10–21 days postpartum: white, yellow brown (alba)	Heavy, bright-red: indicates hemorrhage (massage fundus, give medication on order, notify physician) Spurts: may indicate cervical tear No lochia: may indicate clot occluding cervical opening (support fundus; express clot)
Quantity	Moderate amount, steadily decreases	Foul: may indicate infection
Odor	Minimal	
Assess **breasts** and **nipples** daily	Days 1–2: soft, intact, secreting colostrum Days 2–3: engorged, tender, full, tight, painful	Sore or cracked (clean and dry nipples; decrease breast-feeding time; apply breast shield between feeding)

(continued)

Assessment: Obstetrical *(Continued)*

Assessment	Normal	Abnormal
	Day 3+: secreting milk Increased pains as baby sucks: common in multiparas	Milk does not "let down": help client relax and decrease anxiety; give glass of wine or beer if not culturally, religiously, or otherwise contraindicated
Assess **perineum** daily	Episiotomy intact, no swelling, no discoloration	Swelling or bruising: may indicate hematoma
Assess **bladder** every 4 hours	Voiding regularly with no pain	Not voiding: bladder may be full and displaced to one side, leading to increased lochia (catheterization may be necessary)
Assess **bowels**	Spontaneous bowel movement 2–3 days after delivery	Fear associated with pain from hemorrhoids
Assess mother–infant **bonding**	Touching infant, talking to infant, talking about infant	Refuses to touch or hold infant
Evaluate **Rh-negative status**	Client does not require RhoGAM	RhoGAM administered
Maternal History: Definition of Terms *Abortion:* pregnancy loss before fetus is viable (usually <20 weeks or 500 g)	*Multigravida:* refers to second or any subsequent pregnancy	*Nullipara:* refers to female who has never carried pregnancy to viable age for fetus
Gravida: any pregnancy, including present one	*Para:* past pregnancies that continued to viable age (20 weeks); infants may be alive or dead at birth	*Multipara:* refers to female who has given birth to two or more viable infants; either alive or dead
Primigravida: refers to first-time pregnancy	*Primipara:* refers to female who has delivered first viable infant; born either alive or dead	

Assessment: Newborn

Assessment	Normal	Abnormal
Skin Assessment Note skin **color, pigmentation,** and **lesions**	Pink Mongolian spots	Cyanosis, pallor, beefy red Petechiae, ecchymoses, or purpuric spots: signs of possible hematologic disorder
	Capillary hemangiomas on face or neck	Café au lait spots (patches of brown discoloration): possible sign of congenital neurologic disorder Raised capillary hemangiomas on areas other than face or neck
	Localized edema in presenting part Cheesy white vernix Desquamation (peeling off)	Edema of peritoneal wall Poor skin turgor: indicates dehydration Yellow discolored vernix (meconium stained)

Assessment	Normal	Abnormal
	Milia (small white pustules over nose and chin) Jaundice after 24 hours; gone by second week	Impetigo neonatorum (small pustules with surrounding red areas) Jaundice at birth or within 12 hours Dermal sinuses (opening to brain) Holes along spinal column Low hairline posteriorly: possible chromosomal abnormality Sparse or spotty hair: congenital goiter or chromosomal abnormality
Note color of **nails**	Pink	Yellowing of nail beds (meconium stained)
Note **muscle strength/tone**	Strong, tremulous	Flaccid, convulsions Muscular twitching, hypertonicity
Head and Neck Assessment Note **shape of head**	Fontanels: anterior open until 18 months; posterior closed shortly after birth	Depressed fontanels indicate dehydration; closed or bulging indicate congenital anomalies; full or bulging indicate edema or increased ICP Cephalohematoma that crosses the midline Microcephaly and macrocephaly
Assess **eyes**	Slight edema of lids	Purulent discharge Lateral upward slope of eye with an inner epicanthal fold in infants not of Asian descent Exophthalmos (bulging of eyeball): may be congenital anomaly, sign of congenital glaucoma or thyroid abnormality Enophthalmos (recession of eyeball): may indicate damage to brain or cervical spine
	Pupils equal and reactive to light by 3 weeks of age Intermittent strabismus (occasional crossing of eyes) Conjunctival or scleral hemorrhages Symmetrical light reflex (light reflects off each eye in the same quadrant): sign of conjugate gaze	Constricted pupil, unilateral dilated fixed pupil, nystagmus (rhythmic nonpurposeful movement of eyeball): continuous strabismus Haziness of cornea Absence of red reflex; asymmetrical light reflex
Note **placement of ears,** shape and position The top of the ear should be on an imaginary line from the edge of the eye		Low-set ears: may indicate chromosomal or renal system abnormality
Assess **nose**	Discharge, sneezing	Thick, bloody nasal discharge
Assess **mouth**	Sucking, rooting reflexes Retention cysts Occasional vomiting	Cleft lip, palate Flat, white nonremovable spots (thrush) Frequent vomiting: may indicate pyloric stenosis Vomitus with bile: fecal vomiting Profuse salivation: may indicate tracheoesophageal fistula

(continued)

Assessment: Newborn *(Continued)*

Assessment	Normal	Abnormal
Assess **neck**	Tonic neck reflex (Fencer's position)	Distended neck veins Fractured clavicle Unusually short neck Excess posterior cervical skin Resistance to neck flexion
Assess **cry**	Lusty cry	Weak, groaning cry: possible neurologic abnormality High-pitched cry: newborn drug withdrawal (may occur 6–12 months after birth); hoarse or crowing inspirations; catlike cry: possible neurologic or chromosomal abnormality
Chest and Lung Assessment		
Assess **chest**	Circular Enlargement of breasts Milky discharge from breasts	Depressed sternum Retractions, asymmetry of chest movements: indicates respiratory distress and possible pneumothorax
Assess **respirations/lungs**	Abdominal respirations	Thoracic breathing, unequal motion of chest, rapid grasping or grunting respirations, flaring nares
	Respiration rate: 30–50 Respiration movement irregular in rate and depth Resonant chest (hollow sound on percussion)	Deep sighing respirations Grunt on expiration: possible respiratory distress Hyper-resonance of chest or decreased resonance
Heart Assessment		
Assess the **rate, rhythm,** and **murmurs** of the heart	Rate: 100–160 at birth; stabilizes at 120–140 Regular rhythm Murmurs: significance cannot usually be determined in newborn	Heart rate >200 or <100 Irregular rhythm Dextrocardia, enlarged heart
Abdomen and Gastrointestinal Tract Assessment		
Assess the **abdomen**	Prominent	Distention of abdominal veins: possible portal vein obstruction
Assess the **gastrointestinal tract**	Bowel sounds present	Visible peristaltic waves Increased pitch or frequency: intestinal obstruction Decreased sounds: paralytic ileus Distention of abdomen
	Liver 2–3 cm below right costal margin Spleen tip palpable	Enlarged liver or spleen Midline suprapubic mass: may indicate Hirschsprung's disease
	Umbilical cord with one vein and two arteries Soft granulation tissue at umbilicus	One artery present in umbilical cord: may indicate other anomalies Wet umbilical stump or fetid odor from stump
Genitourinary Tract Assessment		
Assess **kidneys and bladder**	May be able to palpate kidneys Bladder percussed 1–4 cm above symphysis pubis	Enlarged kidney Distended bladder; presence of any masses

Assessment	Normal	Abnormal
Assess the **genitalia**	Edema and bruising after delivery Unusually large clitoris in females a short time after birth Vaginal mucoid or bloody discharge may be present in the first week Inguinal hernia	Ambiguous genitalia (chromosomal abnormality)
Urethral orifice	Urethra opens on ventral surface of penile shaft	Hypospadias (urethra opens on the inferior surface of the penis) Epispadias (urethra opens on the dorsal surface of the penis) Ulceration of urethral orifice
Testes	Testes in scrotal sac or inguinal canal	Hydroceles in males
Spine and Extremities Assessment		
Assess the **spine**	Straight spine	Spina bifida, pilonidal sinus; scoliosis
Assess **extremities**	Soft click with thigh rotation	Asymmetry of movement Sharp click with thigh rotation: indicates possible congenital hip Uneven major gluteal folds: indicates possible congenital hip Polydactyly (extra digits on a hand or foot); syndactyly (webbing or fusion of fingers or toes)
Assess **anus and rectum**	Patent anus	Closed anus: no meconium

TABLE 11-3 Apgar Scoring

Sign	0	1	2
Heart rate	Absent	Slow (less than 100)	Over 100
Respiratory effort	Absent	Slow, irregular	Good, crying
Muscle tone	Flaccid	Some flexion of extremities	Active motion
Reflex irritability	No response	Cry	Vigorous cry
Color	Blue, pale	Body pink, extremities blue	Completely pink

APGAR scoring system is a method of evaluating a newborn's condition at 1 and 5 minutes after birth.

- Newborns who score 7–10 are considered free of immediate danger.
- Newborns who score 4–6 are moderately depressed.
- Newborns who score 0–3 are severely depressed.

Scores less than 7 at 5 minutes, repeat every 5 minutes for 20 minutes. Infant may be intubated unless 2 successive scores of 7 or more occur.

Assessment: Pediatric

Assessment	Normal	Abnormal
Measurements		
Measure **height** and **weight** and plot on a standardized growth chart	Height/weight proportional Sequential measurements: pattern follows normal growth curves	Height/weight below fifth percentile Sudden drop in percentile range of height and/or weight: possible sign of disease process or congenital problem Sudden and persistent increase (above 95th percentile)

(continued)

Assessment: Pediatric *(Continued)*

Assessment	Normal	Abnormal
Assess **temperature** (axillary or tympanic until 6 years of age)	Axillary 36.5°–37.5°C (97.7°F) Elevations after eating or playing not unusual Rectal 36.6°–37.2°C (97.8°F)	Temperature of 104°–105°F: corresponds roughly with 101°–102°F in an adult Large daily temperature variations Hypothermia: usually result of chilling
Measure **circumference of head and chest** Examine or check circumferences when child is less than 2 years old Compare measurements with standardized charts	Head at birth: about 2 cm greater than chest During first year: equalization of head and chest After 2 years: rapid growth of chest; slight increase in size of head	Increase in head circumference greater than 2.5 cm per month: sign of hydrocephalus
Assess **pulse** apically	Birth–1 year: 100–180 1 year: 80–150 2 years: 80–130 3 years: 80–120 Over 3 years: 70–110	Pulse over 180 *at rest* after first month of life: cardiac or respiratory condition Inability to palpate or very weak femoral and pedal pulses: possible coarctation of the aorta
Assess **respirations**	Birth: 30–50 6 years: 20–25 Puberty: 14–16 (Young children have abnormally high respiration rate with even slight excitement)	Consistent tachypnea: usually a sign of respiratory distress Respiratory rate over 100; lower respiratory tract obstruction Slow rate: may be sign of CNS depression
Assess **blood pressure**	Birth: 55–60/80–90 1 year: 90–60 Rise in both pressures: 2–3 points per year of age Adult level reached at puberty	Elevated blood pressure in upper extremities *and* decrease in lower extremities: coarctation of aorta Narrowed pulse pressure (normal or elevated diastolic with lowered systolic; less than 30 points difference between systolic and diastolic readings): possible sign of aortic or subaortic stenosis or hypothyroidism Widened pulse pressure: possible sign of hyperthyroidism
Appearance		
Observe **general appearance**	Alert, well-nourished, comfortable, responsive	Lethargic, uncomfortable, malnourished, gross anomalies, dull
Listen to **voice and cry**	Strong, lusty cry	Weak cry, low- or high-pitched cry: may indicate neurologic problem or chromosomal abnormality Stridor: possible upper airway edema or obstruction or hoarse cry
	Facial expression animated No indications of pain	Expressionless, unresponsive Doubling over, rubbing a body part, general fretfulness, irritability
Assess presence of **odor**	No odor	Musty odor: sign of phenylketonuria, diphtheria Odor of maple syrup: may be maple syrup urine disease Odor of sweaty feet: one type of acidemia Fishy odor: may be metabolic disorder Acetone odor: acidosis, particularly diabetic ketoacidosis

Assessment	Normal	Abnormal
Skin Assessment		
Assess **pigmentation**	Usually even Pigmented nevi common Large, flat, black and blue areas over sacrum, buttocks (mongolian spots)	Multiple cafe au lait spots: possible neurofibromatosis Cyanosis Jaundice Pallor
Assess **lesions**	Usually none Adolescence: acne	Erythematous lesions Multiple macules, papules, or vesicles Petechiae and ecchymoses: may indicate coagulation disorder
Assess **signs/symptoms of abuse**	None present	Hives (allergy) Subcutaneous nodules: may indicate juvenile rheumatoid arthritis Any unexplained bruises, welts, scars, burn marks, rope marks, failure to thrive, x-ray findings of multiple bone injuries, passive, noncommunicating child
Note **consistency of skin**	Good turgor Smooth and firm Check fontanel in infant	Poor turgor Dryness Edema Lack or excess of subcutaneous fat: sign of malnutrition or excess nutrition (obesity)
Assess **nails**	Nailbeds: normally pigmented Good nail growth	Cyanosis Pallor Capillary pulsations Pitting of the nails: possible sign of fungal disease or psoriasis Broad nailbeds: possible sign of Down's syndrome or other chromosomal abnormality
Assess **hair** (consistency appropriate to ethnic group)	No excessive breaking Consistent growth pattern	Dry, coarse, brittle hair: possible sign of hypothyroidism Alopecia (loss of hair): may be psychosomatic or due to drug therapy Unusual hairiness in places other than scalp, eyebrows, and lashes: may indicate hypothyroidism, vitamin A poisoning, chronic infections, reaction to Dilantin therapy Tufts of hair over spine or sacrum: may indicate site of spina bifida occulta or spina bifida Absence of the start of pubic hair during adolescence: possible hypothyroidism, hypopituitarism, gonadal deficiency, or Addison's disease
Assess **lymph nodes**	Nontender, movable, discrete nodes up to 3 mm in diameter in occipital, postauricular, parotid, submaxillary, sublingual, axillary, and epitrochlear nodes Up to 1 mm in diameter inguinal and cervical nodes	Tender or enlarged nodes: may be sign of systemic infection

(continued)

Assessment: Pediatric *(Continued)*

Assessment	Normal	Abnormal
Head and Neck Assessment		
Assess **scalp**	Usually without lesions	Ringworm, lice
Assess frontal and maxillary **sinuses**	Nontender	Tenderness: indicative of inflammatory process Seborrheic dermatitis
Assess **face**	Symmetrical movement	Asymmetry: signs of facial paralysis Twitching: could be due to psychosomatic causes; vitamin/mineral deficiency
Evaluate the eyes Gross screening of vision Snellen chart	With younger child, ability to focus and follow movement and to see objects placed a few feet away	Inability to follow movement or to see objects placed a few feet away
Sclerae	Completely white	Yellow sclera: sign of jaundice Blue sclera: may be normal or indicative of osteogenesis imperfecta
Placement in eye socket	Normally placed	Exophthalmos (protrusion of eyeball) Enophthalmos (deeply placed eyeball)
Iris	At rest: upper and lower margins of iris visible between the lids	Setting sun sign (iris appears to be beneath lower lid): if marked, may be sign of increased intracranial pressure or hydrocephalus
Movement	In newborn, intermittent strabismus or nystagmus	Fixed strabismus or intermittent strabismus continuing after 6 months of age: indication of muscle paralysis or weakness Involuntary, repetitive oscillations of one or both eyes: normal with *extreme* lateral gaze Nystagmus: may be cerebellar dysfunction indicative of use of certain drugs (anticonvulsants, barbiturates, alcohol)
Eyelids	Fully covers eye Fully raised on opening	Ptosis of eyelid: may be an early sign of a neurologic disorder Sty
Conjunctiva	Clear	Inflammation (conjunctivitis) Hemorrhage Stimson's lines (small red transverse lines on conjunctiva)
Cornea	Clear	Opacity: sign of ulceration Inflammation Redness
Discharge	Tears	Purulent discharges: note amount, color, consistency (bacterial conjunctivitis)
Pupils	Round, regular Clear, equal Brisk reaction to light Accommodation reflex (ability of lens to adjust to objects at different distances)	Sluggish or asymmetrical reaction to light: indicates intracranial disease Lack of accommodation reflex
Lens	Clear	Opacities (cataracts)

Assessment	Normal	Abnormal
Evaluate the **ears**		
Sinuses	No abnormality	Small holes or pits anterior to ear: may be superficial but could indicate the presence of a sinus leading into brain
Position	Top of ear above level of eye	Top of ear below level of eye: associated with some congenital defects
Discharge	None	Discharge: note color, odor, consistency, and amount
Hearing	In infant: turning to sound In older child: responds to whispered command	Diminished hearing in one or both ears
Assess the **nose**	No secretions	Secretions: note characteristics Any unusual shape or flaring of nostrils
	Breathing through nose	Breathing through mouth
Assess the **mouth**		Circumoral pallor: possible sign of cyanotic heart disease, scarlet fever, rheumatic fever, hypoglycemia; also seen in other febrile diseases Asymmetry of lips: seen in nerve paralysis
	Intact palate Teeth in good condition In older child presence of permanent teeth	Cleft palate Delayed appearance of deciduous teeth: may indicate cretinism, rickets, congenital syphilis, or Down's syndrome; may also be normal Poor tooth formation: may be seen with systemic diseases Green or black teeth: seen after iron ingestion or death of tooth Stained teeth: may be seen after prolonged use of tetracyclines
Assess the **gums**	Retention cysts in newborn	Inflammation, abnormal color, drooling, pus, tenderness Black line along gums: may indicate lead poisoning
Assess the **tongue**	Moves freely	Tremors on protrusion: may indicate chorea, hypothyroidism, cerebral palsy Protruding tongue—Down's syndrome White spots (thrush) Tongue-tie (frenulum)
	Pink, with conical, filiform nontender papillae	Strawberry tongue (scarlet fever)
Assess the **throat**	Tonsils normally enlarged in childhood	White membrane over tonsils (diphtheria) White pus on sacs, erythema (bacterial pharyngitis), tender: vitamin deficiencies, anemia
Assess the **larynx**	Normal vocal tones	Hoarseness or stridor: possible upper respiratory tract obstruction

(continued)

Assessment: Pediatric *(Continued)*

Assessment	Normal	Abnormal
Assess the **neck**	Short in infancy Lengthens at 2–3 years Trachea slightly right of midline	Trachea deviated to left or right: may indicate shift with atelectasis
Thyroid	Not enlarged	Enlarged: may be due to hyperactive thyroid, malignancy, goiter
Movement	Full lateral and upward/downward motion	Limited movement with pain: may indicate meningeal irritation, lymph node enlargement, rheumatoid arthritis, or other diseases
Lungs and Thorax Assessment		
Assess the **lungs**	Normally clear and equal breath sounds bilaterally	Presence of rhonchi, crackles, or wheezes Diminished breath sounds heard over parts of lung
	No retractions	Mild to severe intercostal or sternal retractions indicative of respiratory distress
	Symmetry of diaphragmatic movement	Asymmetry of movement (phrenic nerve damage)
Assess the **sputum**	None or small amount of clear sputum in morning	Thick, tenacious sputum with foul odor Blood-tinged or green sputum
Assess the **breasts**	Slightly enlarged in infancy Generally slightly asymmetrical at puberty	Discharge or growth in male Masses (especially solid, fixed nonmobile) in older adolescent
Heart Assessment		
Assess **heart sounds**	S_1, S_2, S_3	S_4 indicates congestive heart failure
Assess **femoral pulses**	Strong	Weak
Note **edema**	None present	Edema—note location (initially periorbital) and duration, bulging fontanelles
Note **clubbing** of fingers	None present	Clubbing—congenital cyanotic heart defects; note location and duration
Note **murmurs**		Murmur grade 3 or higher is always abnormal No change in quality with positional changes
Note **cyanosis**	None normally present	Circumoral or peripheral cyanosis: indicates respiratory or cardiac disease (hypoxemia); congenital heart defects
Abdomen Assessment		
Assess **skin condition**	Soft	Hard, rigid, tender
Assess for **peristaltic motion**	Not visible	Visible peristalsis—may indicate pyloric stenosis (olive-shaped mass, palpable, in area of pylorus)

Assessment	Normal	Abnormal
Assess **shape**	"Pot-bellied" toddlers Slightly protuberant in standing adolescent	Large protruding abdomen: may indicate pancreatic fibrosis, hypokalemia, rickets, hypothyroidism, bowel obstruction, constipation, inguinal hernias, unilateral or bilateral: observe for reducibility
	Umbilical protrusion	Umbilical hernia
Genitourinary Tract Assessment		
Assess **female genitalia**		
Discharge	Mucoid, no odor	Foul or copious discharge; any bleeding before puberty
Assess **male genitalia** Presence of urethral orifice	Orifice on distal end of penis	Hypospadias or epispadias (urethral orifice along inferior or dorsal surface)
Urethral opening	Normal size	Stenosis of urethral opening
Foreskin	Covers glans completely	Foreskin incompletely formed ventrally when hypospadias present
Placement of testes	Descended testes	Undescended testes Enlarged scrotum
Signs of abuse	No signs	Bruises, welts, swelling, discharge, bleeding
Assess **urine output**	Full, steady stream of urine	Urine with pus, blood, or odor (infection) Excessive urination or nocturia: possible sign of diabetes
Check **anus and rectum**	No masses or fissures present	Hemorrhoids, fissures, prolapse, pinworms Dark ring around rectal mucosa: may be sign of lead poisoning
Musculoskeletal Assessment		
Assess **extremities**	Coloration of fingers and toes consistent with rest of body	Cyanosis—indicates respiratory or cardiac disease, or hypothermia in newborn Clubbing of fingers and toes indicates cardiac or respiratory disease
	Quick capillary refill on blanching	Sluggish blood return on blanching indicates poor circulation
	Temperature same as rest of body	Temperature variation between extremities and rest of body indicates neurologic or vascular anomalies
	Presence of pedal pulses	Absence of pedal pulses indicates circulatory difficulties
	No pain or tenderness	Presence of localized or generalized pain
	Straight legs after 2 years of age	Any bowing after 2 years of age may be hereditary or indicate rickets
	Broad-based gait until 4 years of age; feet straight ahead afterwards	Scissoring gait indicates spastic cerebral palsy Persistence of broad-based gait after 4 years of age indicates possible abnormalities of legs and feet or balance disturbance Any limp or ataxia

(continued)

Assessment: Pediatric *(Continued)*

Assessment	Normal	Abnormal
Assess **spine**	No dimples Flexible	Presence of dimple or tufts of hair indicates possible spina bifida Limited flexion indicates central nervous system infections Hyperextension (opisthotonos) indicates brainstem irritation, hemorrhage, or intracranial infection
Have child bend forward at waist and check level of scapulae (scoliosis screening)	No lateral curvature or excessive anterior posterior curvature Scapulae at same height	Presence of lordosis (after age 2 years), kyphosis, or scoliosis
Assess **hips**		Asymmetrical thigh folds, clicks on adduction—hip dysplasia
Assess **joints**	Full range of motion without pain, edema, or tenderness	Pain, edema, or tenderness indicates tissue injury
Assess **muscles**	Good tone and purposeful movement Ability to perform motor skills approximate to development level	Decreased or increased tone Spasm or tremors may indicate cerebral palsy Atrophy or contractures

GERONTOLOGIC Considerations

Head and Neck and Neurologic System

Physiologic Changes With Age

- Decreased speed of nerve conduction and delay in response and reaction time, especially with stress
- Diminution of sensory faculties; decreased vision, loss of hearing, diminished sense of smell and taste, greater sensitivity to temperature changes with low tolerance to cold
- Tooth loss
- Poor dentition, inadequate chewing, poor swallowing reflex
- Condition of teeth, gums, buccal cavity
- Periodontal disease

Taste sensation decreases.

- Chronic irritation of mucous membranes
- Atrophy of up to 80% of taste buds
- Loss of sensitivity of those on tip of tongue first: sweet and salt
- Loss of sensitivity of those on sides later: salt, sour, bitter

Assessment

- Facial symmetry
- Poor reflex reactions
- Level of alertness—presence of organic brain changes: memory impairment
- Motor function—strength

Skin

Physiologic Changes With Age

Skin less effective as barrier:

- Decreased protection from trauma
- Less ability to retain water
- Decreased temperature regulation

Skin composition changes:

- Dryness (osteotosis) due to decreased endocrine secretion
- Loss of elastin
- Increased vascular fragility
- Thicker and more wrinkled on sun-exposed areas
- Melanocyte cluster pigmentation

Sweat glands:

- Decreased number and size
- Decreased function of sebaceous glands

Hair:

- General hair loss
- Decreased melanin production
- Facial hair increases in women

Nails:

- More brittle and thick

Assessment

Skin:

- Temperature, degree of moisture, dryness
- Intactness, open lesions, tears, decubiti
- Turgor, dehydration
- Pigmentation alterations, potential cancer
- Pruritus—dry skin most common cause
- Bruises, scars

Condition of nails (hard and brittle):

- Presence of fungus
- Overgrown or horny toenails, ingrown

Condition of hair

Infestations (scabies, lice)

Chest

Physiologic Changes With Age

Respiratory muscles lose strength and become rigid.

Ciliary activity decreases.

Lungs lose elasticity:

- Residual capacity increases.
- Larger on inspiration.
- Maximum breathing capacity decreases; depth of respirations decreases.
- Alveoli increase in size, reduce in number.
- Fewer capillaries at alveoli.
- Dilated and less elastic alveoli.

Gas exchange is reduced:

- Arterial blood oxygen PaO_2 decreases to 75 mmHg at age 70.
- Arterial blood carbon dioxide $PaCO_2$ unchanged.

Coughing ability is reduced—less sensitive mechanism.

More dependent on the diaphragm for breathing.

System less responsive to hypoxia and hypercardia.

Assessment

- Shape of chest excursion
- Lung and breath sounds
- Quality of cough, if present; sputum

Rib cage deformity

Dyspnea, hypoxia, and hypercarbia

Breast—size, symmetry, contour:

- Presence of lumps
- Size and shape of nipples

Heart

Physiologic Changes With Age

Mitral and aortic valves thicken and become rigid.

Cardiac output decreases 1% per year after age 20 due to decreased heart rate and stroke volume.

Vessels lose elasticity:

- Less effective peripheral oxygenation
- Position change from lying-to-sitting or sitting-to-standing can cause blood pressure to drop as much as 65 mmHg

Increased peripheral vessel resistance:

- Blood pressure increases: systolic may normally be 170 mmHg, diastolic may normally be 95 mmHg.
- Smooth muscle in arteries is less responsive.

Blood clotting increases.

Assessment

Heart sounds—murmurs

Peripheral circulation, color, warmth:

- Apical pulse
- Jugular vein distention

Orthostatic hypotension:

- Dizziness
- Fainting

Edema

Activity intolerance

Dyspnea

Transient ischemic attacks (TIAs)

Abdomen

Physiologic Changes With Age

Esophagus dilates, decreased motility.

Stomach:

- Hunger sensations decrease.
- Secretion of hydrochloric acid decreases.
- Emptying time decreases.

Peristalsis decreases and constipation is common.

Absorption function is impaired:

- Body absorbs less nutrients due to reduced intestinal blood flow and atrophy of cells on absorbing surfaces.
- Decrease in gastric enzymes affects absorption.

Hiatal hernia common (40%–60% of elderly).

Diverticulitis common (40% over age 70).

Liver:

- Fewer cells, with decreased storage capacity.
- Decreased blood flow.
- Enzymes decrease.
- Increased risk for drug toxicity.

Impaired pancreatic reserve.

Decreased glucose tolerance.

Assessment

- Indications of possible hiatal hernia.
- Bowel distention.
- Bowel sounds.

Genitourinary Tract

Physiologic Changes With Age

Kidneys:

- Smaller due to nephron atrophy.
- Renal blood flow decreases 50%.
- Glomerular filtration rate decreases 50%.
- Tubular function diminishes: less able to concentrate urine; lower specific gravity; proteinuria 1+ is common; blood urea nitrogen (BUN) increases 21 mg%.
- Renal threshold for glucose increases.

Bladder:

- Muscle weakens.
- Capacity decreases to 200 mL or less, causing frequency.
- Emptying is more difficult, causing increased retention.
- Increased risk of incontinence.

Prostate enlarges to some degree in 75% of men over age 65; hypertrophy.

Menopause occurs by mean age of 50.

Perineal muscle weakens.

Vulva atrophies.

Vagina:

- Mucous membrane becomes dryer.
- Elasticity of tissue decreases, so surface is smooth.
- Secretions become reduced, more alkaline.
- Flora changes.

Sexuality:

- Older people continue to be sexual beings with sexual needs.
- No particular age at which a person's sexual functioning ceases.
- Frequency of genital sexual behavior (intercourse) may tend to decline gradually in later years, but capacity for expression and enjoyment continues far into old age.

Assessment

- Condition of skin—dehydration
- Urinary output; blood in urine; color; specific gravity; prothrombin time (PT)
- Incontinence
- Bladder distention
- Genital assessment

Musculoskeletal System

Physiologic Changes With Age

Contractures:

- Muscles atrophy, regenerate slowly, strength diminishes.
- Tendons shrink and sclerose.

Range of motion of joints decreases:

- Lack of adequate joint motion, ankylosis
- Slight flexion of joints

Assessment

Mobility level:

- Ambulate with more difficulty.
- Limitation to movement.
- Muscle strength cramps.
- Gait becomes unsteady.
- Presence of kyphosis.
- Pain in joints.

MANAGEMENT Guidelines

Each state legislates a Nurse Practice Act for RNs and LVN/LPNs. Healthcare facilities are responsible for establishing and implementing policies and procedures that conform to their state's regulations. Verify the regulations and role parameters for each healthcare worker in your facility.

Delegation

- RNs must complete the admission assessment and document the findings. They cannot delegate this activity to anyone else on the team.
- LVN/LPNs may complete focus assessments each shift; however, any changes in assessment findings must be reported and verified with the RN.
- Unlicensed assistive personnel may not perform assessments on clients.

Communication Matrix

- Changes in assessment data identified in report or in the client's chart must be reported to the appropriate nurse assigned to complete the focus assessment.
- LVN/LPNs delegated the responsibility to complete focus assessments on clients must have clear direction on what is essential information to report back. Remind the LVN/LPN they must verify with the RN any changes identified in the assessment.
- Remind LVN/LPNs that if there are any questions on the client status as a result of their assessment, they must notify the RN immediately.

CRITICAL THINKING Strategies

Scenario 1

Mrs. Smiley has had a history of hypertension for several years. She has recently experienced an inability to use her right arm and leg and has lost ability to express herself. She has been admitted to your unit with the diagnosis of R/O left CVA (stroke) and has been placed on a continuous heparin IV drip.

1. Based on admitting data, make a judgment about what deviations from normal you would find in the physical examination.
2. List appropriate nursing diagnoses based on her physical state and immobility status (this affects virtually all systems).
3. In view of all these existing and potential problems, identify *priority* concerns (all are important concerns) for this client.
4. Develop a plan of care addressing these priority concerns.

Scenario 2

You are caring for a woman in labor and monitoring the fetal heart rate. You note that early deceleration has occurred (a 10- to 20-beat drop in the fetal heart rate).

1. From these symptoms, indicate your priority intervention.
2. What would you conclude about the viability of the fetus?
3. What does this change in condition of the fetus imply?

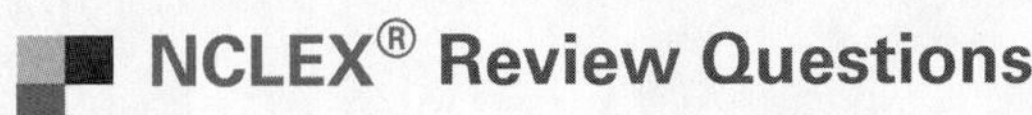

NCLEX® Review Questions

Unless otherwise specified, choose only one (1) answer.

1. The systematic approach the nurse should follow when auscultating a client's lungs is
   1. Anterior to posterior.
   2. Top to bottom.
   3. Posterior to lateral to anterior.
   4. Side to side.
2. The nurse suspects that a client has appendicitis. When assessing for rebound tenderness, the nurse should
   1. Perform this assessment first.
   2. Have the client take a deep breath.
   3. Palpate deeply with quick release of pressure.
   4. Have the client lie flat with legs extended.
3. A client comes into the clinic for evaluation of a burn injury from hot liquid. The lesions are flat and red. The nurse should document the presence of
   1. Macules.
   2. Wheals.
   3. Vesicles.
   4. Papules.
4. The nurse is assessing a client's deep tendon reflexes. When documenting a normal response, the nurse would chart
   1. +1.
   2. 0.
   3. +2.
   4. +4.
5. The cranial nerve that is assessed when testing for the "gag reflex" is the
   1. XI accessory.
   2. VII facial.
   3. IX glossopharyngeal.
   4. XII hypoglossal.
6. During a cardiac assessment, the S_1 heart sound can be heard best
   1. At the second intercostal space.
   2. By using the bell of the stethoscope.
   3. Over the aortic area.
   4. At the apex of the heart.
7. When assessing the lymph nodes in the neck, the nurse should instruct the client to
   1. Raise the chin.
   2. Lie in a supine position.
   3. Swallow a sip of water.
   4. Flex neck slightly.
8. Completing a physical assessment, the nurse is unable to palpate a peripheral pulse, the dorsalis pedis. The next intervention would be to
   1. Notify the physician.
   2. Examine the adjacent area.
   3. Obtain a new Doppler.
   4. Move on to the next area.
9. The urinary tract assessment includes checking the specific gravity of the client's urine to determine if it is within normal limits. The normal range of specific gravity is ______.
10. Suspecting that the client you are assessing may be exhibiting cognitive decline or dementia, which of the following statements would be appropriate?
    1. How do you feel today?
    2. What work did you do 20 years ago?
    3. Who is the president of the United States?
    4. Tell me about why you are in the hospital.

12

Body Mechanics and Positioning

LEARNING OBJECTIVES

1. Discuss the primary function of the skeletal muscles, joints, and bones.
2. Describe nursing measures that assist in preserving joints, bones, and skeletal muscles
3. Describe the ANA Standards that promote safe handling of clients and prevention of injury to healthcare workers.
4. Describe a minimum of two principles of correct body mechanics.
5. State two expected outcomes of using proper body mechanics.
6. Discuss the objectives for moving and turning clients.
7. Compare and contrast the methods used in moving clients up in bed for a single nurse and when assistants are available.
8. Describe the position of the head of the bed in the four Fowler's positions.
9. Describe the correct placement of the canvas pieces when placing a client on the floor-based client lift.
10. Explain the rationale of assisted ambulation for clients.
11. Demonstrate the procedures for moving a client to the side of the bed and dangling a client.
12. Outline the steps in logrolling a client.
13. Describe requirements for lift team members.
14. List the pertinent data that should be charted when moving a client from the bed.
15. Write a client care plan using at least three nursing diagnoses for a client requiring moving and turning interventions.

CHAPTER OUTLINE

TERMINOLOGY

Alignment referring to posture, the relationship of body parts to one another.

Ambulate walking; able to walk.

Appendicular skeleton composed of 126 bones, which include the shoulder girdle, arm bones, pelvic girdle, and leg bones.

Assistive equipment used to move clients without placing pressure on back and trunk.

Atrophy a wasting; decrease in size of an organ or tissue.

Axial skeleton includes the head and trunk, which form the central axis to which the appendicular skeleton is attached.

Balance client's ability to maintain equilibrium.

Base of support surface area on which an object rests (e.g., for a client lying in prone position, the base of support is the entire undersurface of the body).

Body mechanics movement of the body in a coordinated and efficient way so that proper balance, alignment, and conservation of energy is maintained.

Brachial plexus network of spinal nerves supplying arm, forearm, and hand.

Cartilage nonvascular, dense supporting connective tissue. Found in joints, thorax, larynx, trachea, nose, and ear.

Center of gravity midpoint or center of the body weight. In an adult it is the midpelvic cavity between the symphysis pubis and umbilicus.

Dangle to have a client sit on the edge of the bed with feet in a dependent position, flat on floor, if possible.

Dorsiflexion upward or backward flexion of a part of the body, such as the foot at the ankle.

Ergonomics physical stressors involving excessive force; i.e., lifting heavy objects or working in an awkward position.

Flexion the act or condition of being bent.

Footdrop a falling or dragging of the foot from paralysis of the flexors of the ankle.

Fowler's position head of bed is at a 45° angle; client's knees may or may not be flexed.

Gravity the force that pulls objects toward the earth's surface.

High-Fowler's position head of bed is at a 60° angle; often used to achieve maximum chest expansion.

Hoyer lift a mechanical device that enables one person to safely transfer a client from bed to chair.

Joint the portion of the body where two or more bones join together.

Leverage the use of a lever to apply force.

Ligament a band or sheet of strong fibrous connective tissue connecting the articular ends of bones serving to bind them together and to facilitate or limit motion.

Line of gravity an imaginary line that goes from the center of gravity to the base of support.

Manual client handling tasks such as lifting, transferring, and repositioning of clients without use of assistive devices.

Mobility state or quality of being mobile; facility of movement.

Musculo pertaining to muscles.

Musculoskeletal pertaining to the muscles and bones.

Orthosis use of external device or special equipment to stabilize or immobilize a body part, protect against injury, or assist with function.

Paralysis temporary or permanent loss of function, especially loss of sensation or voluntary motion.

Posture attitude or position of body.

Prone lying horizontal with face downward.

Reverse Trendelenburg's position mattress remains unbent, but head of bed is raised and foot is lowered.

Semi-Fowler's position head of bed is at a 30° angle; often used for clients with cardiac and respiratory problems.

Skeletal system system of separate bones (206) bound together by ligaments and responsible for supporting, moving, and giving shape to the body.

Sprain injury caused by wrenching or twisting of a joint that results in tearing or stretching of the associated ligaments.

Stable when the center of gravity is close to the base of support.

Strain injury caused by excessive force or stretching of muscles or tendons around the joint.

Trendelenburg's position mattress remains unbent but the head of the bed is lowered and the foot is raised. "Shock blocks" may be used under the legs of the bed to achieve this position.

Trochanter either of the two bony prominences below the neck of the femur.

MUSCULOSKELETAL SYSTEM

The musculoskeletal system protects the body, provides a structural framework, and allows the body to move. The primary structures in this system are muscles, bones, and joints.

Skeletal Muscles

Skeletal muscles move the bones around the joints by contracting and relaxing so that movement can take place. Each muscle consists of a body, or belly, and tendons, which connect the muscle to another muscle or to bone.

When skeletal muscles contract, they cause two bones to move around the joint between them. One of these bones tends to remain stationary while the other bone moves. The end of the muscle that attaches to the stationary bone is called the origin. The end of the muscle that attaches to the movable bone is called the insertion.

Muscles are designated flexors or extensors according to whether they flex the joint (decrease the angle between the bones) or extend the joint (increase the angle between the bones). For example, when the deltoid muscle contracts, it abducts the arm and raises it laterally to the horizontal position. The anterior fibers aid in flexion of the arm, and the posterior fibers aid in extension of the arm.

Joints

Joints are the places where bones meet. Their primary function is to provide motion and flexibility. Although the internal structure of joints varies, most joints are composed of ligaments, which bind the bones together, and cartilage, or tissue, which covers and cushions the ends of the bones.

Bones

Bones provide the major support for all the body organs. Bone is composed of an organic matrix, deposits of calcium salts, and bone cells. The organic matrix provides the framework and tensile strength for the bone. The calcium salts, which are about 75% of the bone, provide compressional strength by filling in the matrix. As a result, it is very difficult to damage a bone by twisting it or by applying direct pressure.

Bone cells include osteoblasts, osteocytes, and osteoclasts. Osteoblasts deposit the organic matrix; osteocytes and osteoclasts reabsorb this matrix. Because this process is usually in equilibrium, bone is deposited where it is needed in the skeletal system. If increased stress is placed on a bone, such as the stress of continued athletic activity, more bone is deposited. If there is no stress on a bone, as is often the case with clients on prolonged bedrest, part of the bone mass is reabsorbed, or lost.

SYSTEM ALTERATIONS

Alterations in mobility can result from problems in the musculoskeletal system, the nervous system, and the skin. A primary cause for alterations in muscles is inactivity. With forceful activity muscles increase in size. With inactivity muscles decrease in size and strength. When clients are in casts, in traction, on prolonged bedrest, or unable to exercise, their muscles become weak and atrophied.

Alterations in joints result when mobility is limited by changes in the adjacent tissues. When muscle movement decreases, the connective tissue in the joints, tendons, and ligaments becomes thickened and fibrotic.

Chronic flexion and hyperextension can also cause alterations in the joints. Chronic flexion can cause joints to become contracted in one position so that they are unmovable. Hyperextension occurs when joints are extended beyond their normal limits, which is usually 180°. The results of hyperextension are pain and discomfort to the client and abnormal stress on the ligaments and tendons of the joints.

TABLE 12-1 Pathophysiological Effects of Immobility

System Affected	Result
Cardiovascular	• Veins become engorged, leading to valve damage due to lack of muscular activity. • Increased risk of clot formation due to slowing of blood flow and inadequate circulation of blood to cells and tissues.
Heart Effects	• Valsalva maneuver, caused by holding the breath when trying to raise up in bed or when having a bowel movement, leads to increased workload on the heart. • Potential for blood pressure decrease causing orthostatic hypotension when standing; can lead to falls.
Respiratory	• Accumulation of thick secretions pooling in the lower respiratory structures, secondary to spinal positioning. • Prevents lung expansion, decreases movement of secretions in the airways, and decreases expectoration of secretions.
Gastrointestinal	• An indirect effect of immobility on the GI system occurs during the intake of nutrients, both food and water. • Decreased metabolic needs can cause anorexia. • Decreases in food intake lead to protein deficiency. • Constipation or diarrhea may occur due to fecal impaction, weakened muscle tone, and not feeling the urge to defecate.
Urinary	• Immobility causes the kidneys to force urine against gravity. • Sluggish flow leads to pooling of urine in the kidney and increases the risk of renal calculi and infection. • Loss of sphincter muscle tone can lead to urinary incontinence, resulting in losing the urge to void and increased urine dribbling.
Musculoskeletal	• Loss of muscle tone and deterioration of bone leads to weakness and stiffness. • Loss of elasticity and demineralization of bones leads to osteoporosis.

Alterations in bone are caused by disease processes, decalcification, and breaks caused by trauma or twisting. Encouraging clients to stand and to walk is important because the body functions best when it is in a vertical position. Physical activity forces muscles to move and increases blood flow, which improves metabolism and facilitates such body functions as gastrointestinal peristalsis.

Many body systems are affected by immobility. Even a few days of immobility can lead to alterations in many body systems. The following chart indicates a few of the systems affected and what occurs with immobility.

In addition to the system alterations, mental health can be affected. Alterations in mental health can range from depending upon others for care, loss of independence, isolation, and depression.

Nursing Measures

Nursing care measures to preserve the joints, bones, and skeletal muscles should be carried out for all clients who require bedrest. Positions in which clients are placed and methods of moving and turning should all be based on the principles of maintaining the musculoskeletal system in proper alignment. The nurse must also use good body mechanics when moving and turning clients to preserve her or his own musculoskeletal system from injury. These nursing measures are also performed by the home care providers.

In addition to paying attention to the body positioning and moving and turning, it is essential to:

- Perform range-of-motion exercises—maintain blood circulation and muscular activity, as well as promote oxygenation to the cells and tissues.
- Provide frequent turning and proper positioning—essential to prevent skin breakdown.
- Avoid using the Valsalva maneuver when turning or moving the client.
- Increase fluids to maintain blood flow, unless contraindicated by the client's condition.
- Instruct the client in coughing and deep-breathing exercises to prevent and remove secretions from the airways and promote oxygenation.
- Provide nutritious meals, especially high calcium for bone health.

BODY MECHANICS

Knowledge of a client's body and how it moves is important. Knowledge of your own body and what happens to it when you care for clients with altered mobility is also important. Before you lift or move a client, determine the causes and consequences of the client's illness and implement the use of Safe Patient Handling and Management Algorithms to determine the appropriate client moving/transfer protocols. These guidelines also indicate the equipment needed for safe client transfer/moving or the need for the lift team. This knowledge enables you to move the client without causing additional discomfort.

The most common client handling approaches used in the United States in the past included manual client lifting, education related to body mechanics, education in safe lifting techniques, and the use of back belts. There is strong evidence that each of these approaches is not effective in reducing caregiver injuries. Evidence-based practice indicates that use of client handling equipment/devices, client care ergonomic assessment protocols, "No Lift" policies, education of proper use of client handling equipment/devices, and client lift teams reduce injury to both clients and staff.

The physical environment of the healthcare setting and the aging of the nursing workforce also contribute to work-related injuries. The "tight quarters" and configuration of client rooms, nurses' work areas, and equipment can affect use of appropriate body mechanics as well as equipment for moving clients.

A well-designed client care environment assists the staff in using ergonomically sound procedures that improve client handling. The size of the hospital room determines the ability of the staff to use safe handling techniques. It is recommended that 6 feet be left between the door and client's bed to accommodate lifting equipment, such as a floor lift. Leaving 42 in. between the toilet and wall on one side will accommodate a lateral standing transfer. Doorways should be 36 to 43 in. wide to accommodate bariatric equipment.

Trying to lift or move too much weight forces you to use your body incorrectly and frequently causes injuries. The average weight of clients who require lifting is 169 lbs, but with the increasing rates of obesity, it will be changing. The National Institute for Occupational Safety and Health (NIOSH) states that the average worker should not lift more than 51 lb under controlled and limited circumstances. Incorrect lifting puts most of the pressure on the muscles of your lower back. Because these muscles are not strong enough to handle the stress, you can sustain severe injuries. If you do not follow guidelines for promoting proper body mechanics or using equipment, you are putting your own health and safety in jeopardy. It is advisable that healthcare workers do simple exercises to strengthen and stretch the abdominal muscles and muscles that support the back. This will assist in preventing back injuries.

Low back pain is an occupational hazard for many workers. Back injuries account for approximately 20% of all injuries and illnesses in the workplace.

Nursing personnel are among the most at risk for musculoskeletal disorders. Nurses ranked number six among occupations with a high risk of strains and sprains. The ANA research on the impact of musculoskeletal injury indicates 52% of nurses complain of chronic back pain and 30% of nurses who acquired back pain were required to leave work. Twelve percent of all nurses left the profession as a result of back pain. The majority of the injuries occur from manual client handling. Moving or lifting a client in bed precipitated 61% of low back pain episodes and 60% of lost workdays. Other movements, such as forward bending, twisting, and reaching when assisting clients with ADLs are associated factors in musculoskeletal disorders.

The Occupational Safety and Health Administration (OSHA) has developed the following lifting guidelines for healthcare workers to prevent injury to the client and the worker.

- Evaluate need for assistive devices or lift team.
- Never lift clients who have fallen if you are alone. Use team lifts or use mechanical assistance.
- Never transfer clients when off-balance.
- Lift loads close to the body.
- Limit number of allowed lifts per worker per day.
- Avoid heavy lifting, especially, with spine rotated.
- Complete training in "when and how" to use mechanical assistive devices.

Source: Occupational Safety and Health Administration. HealthCare Wide Hazards Module: Ergonomics. http://www.osha.gov/SLTC/etools/hospital/hazards/ergo/ergo.html.

Proper use of body mechanics helps prevent injuries to clients and all members of the health team. Guidelines that underlie the implementation of body mechanics include:

- Assume a proper stance before moving or turning clients.
- Distribute workload evenly before moving or turning clients.
- Establish a comfortable height when working with clients. Keep the client as close to your body as possible when moving.
- Push and pull objects when moving them to conserve energy.
- Use large muscles for lifting and moving, not back muscles. Move the hip and shoulders as one unit.
- Avoid leaning and stretching.
- Request assistance from others or use client-handling equipment/devices when working with heavy clients to avoid strain.
- Avoid twisting your body.
- Maintain low back in neutral position.

In addition to proper use of body mechanics, ergonomic protection and education programs must be implemented in all healthcare facilities to decrease risk factors related to back injuries. Whereas the use of body mechanics, equipment, and devices alone does not prevent back injuries and musculoskeletal disorders among nurses, together, appropriate use of body mechanics and a safe client handling or client care ergonomics program can decrease injuries in both number and severity.

ANA Promotes Safe Handling Legislation

The American Nurses Association (ANA) has been campaigning for the Federal Occupational Safety and Health Administration (OSHA) to develop standards to control ergonomic hazards in the workplace for the prevention of work-related musculoskeletal disorders. This regulation would include stipulations requiring healthcare settings to use assistive lift and transfer equipment for client handling tasks and eliminate total manual client handling. Using assistive equipment and devices prevents injury such as falls and skin tears, especially in geriatric clients. Anxiety reduction and client comfort occurs during lifting, transferring, or repositioning and promotes confidence in the healthcare team. Assistive devices are selected based on the client's ability to assist with moving and thus promotes client autonomy. In the absence of a national standard, the ANA established the Handle With Care national campaign in 2003 (www.NursingWorld.org/handlewithcare/). This proactive plan was developed to promote safe client handling and the prevention of musculoskeletal disorders among nurses.

As part of the campaign, the ANA fostered the development of client care ergonomics, programs that include the use of assistive client handling equipment and devices and the elimination of manual client handling. The ANA Handle With Care Recognition Program rewards and increases visibility of healthcare organizations that have made the commitment to and the investment in safe patient handling programs. The U.S. Senate Bill S1788 was introduced in October 2009 to establish a Safe-Client Handling and Prevention Standard. As of August 2010, the hearings have not yet been completed.

HOME CARE

Knowledge of body mechanics and how to use these principles when giving care is important to both the healthcare provider and the client. Correct use of body mechanics decreases the caregiver's potential for injury and provides safety for the client. Recently, there has been an increase in the number of back injury accident claims among home healthcare providers. One reason for the increase is the improper use of body mechanics while performing skills in the home setting. Also, there may be no one to assist the care provider when lifting and turning clients in the home. The nurse may need to improvise, as the equipment may not be adequate or adjustable. More home care agencies assist clients in obtaining assistive devices. The purpose of this unit is to consider adaptations necessary for providing safe care to the client while using proper body mechanics. In the home setting, much of the care is given by the family; therefore, it is essential that they also be taught good body mechanics.

CULTURAL AWARENESS

Different cultures may have cultural variances regarding distance and space. When clients are being moved or transferred to a bed or gurney, the client is brought close to the nurse's body. It is important to explain the transfer process to client, particularly Americans, Canadians, and British clients. They may be threatened by invasion of personal space and touch. Japanese, Arabs, and Latin Americans may not be as concerned about personal space.

NURSING DIAGNOSES

The following nursing diagnoses are appropriate to use on client care plans when the components are related to body mechanics.

NURSING DIAGNOSIS	RELATED FACTORS
Activity Intolerance	Impaired motor function, weakness, paralysis, or pain
Risk for Injury	Altered mobility, impaired sensory function, prolonged bedrest
Impaired Physical Mobility	Trauma or musculoskeletal impairment, surgical procedure, muscle weakness, pain, decreased strength
Imparied Transfer Ability	Weakness, flaccidity, amputation, decreased strength
Impaired Walking	Muscle weakness, impaired motor function, orthopedic surgery, or dysfunction
Ineffective Breathing Patterns	Musculoskeletal dysfunction; decreased energy
Ineffective Peripheral Tissue Perfusion	Mechanical reduction of venous and/or arterial blood flow

CLEANSE HANDS The single most important nursing action to decrease the incidence of hospital-based infections is hand hygiene. *Remember to wash your hands or use antibacterial gel before and after each and every client contact.*

IDENTIFY CLIENT Before every procedure, check two forms of client identification, not including room number. These actions prevent errors and conform to The Joint Commission standards.

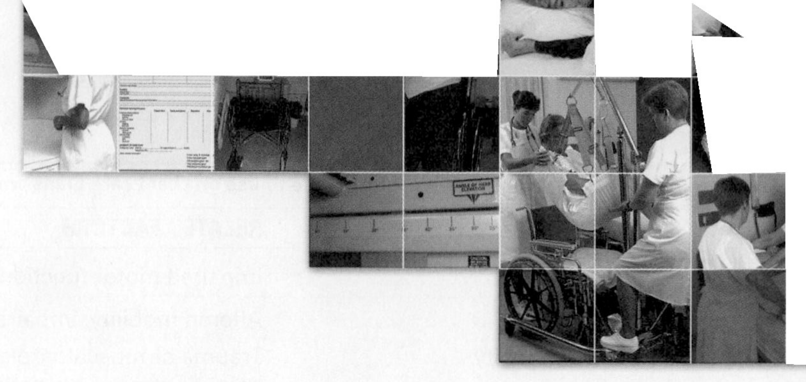

Chapter 12

UNIT 1

Proper Body Mechanics

Nursing Process Data

ASSESSMENT Data Base

- Evaluate personnel's knowledge of the principles of body mechanics.
- Evaluate personnel's knowledge of how to use correct muscle groups for specific activities.
- Assess knowledge and correct any misinformation about body alignment and how to maintain it with each position.
- Assess knowledge of physical science and application to balance and body alignment.
- Assess the competency of spinal cord and associated musculature.
- Assess the muscle mass of the long, thick, and strong muscles of the shoulders and thighs.

PLANNING Objectives

- To promote proper body mechanics while caring for clients
- To maintain good posture, thereby promoting optimum musculoskeletal balance
- To provide knowledge of the musculoskeletal system, body alignment, and balance in order to assist the nurse in caring for clients
- To correct body mechanics, promote health, enhance appearance, and assist body function

IMPLEMENTATION Procedures

EVALUATION Expected Outcomes

- Correct body mechanics are used when preparing for and providing client care.
- Injuries are prevented to both the nurse and the client.
- Proper body mechanics facilitate client care.
- Clients and nurses are not injured when nursing care is provided.
- Center of gravity is maintained when lifting objects.
- Back care exercises promote back health.

Performing Back Exercises

Equipment

Small pillow

NOTE: This skill is for nurses to prevent back strain.

Procedure

1. Complete the four exercises in order, and repeat 10 cycles. ▸ ***Rationale:*** to assist in strengthening stomach, buttocks, and thigh muscles and stretching lower back muscles to prevent back injuries.
2. Complete pelvic tilt exercises.
   a. Lie flat on your back with head on a small pillow or stand against a wall.
   b. Bend knees and hips so feet are flat on the hard surface.
   c. Push lower back onto floor or against wall (back needs to be flat).
   d. Tighten abdominal muscles, then exhale.
   e. Tighten gluteal muscles, then exhale.
   f. Lift hips from floor, or away from wall, and tilt whole pelvis forward while maintaining back flat against hard surface. Hold position for count of 10.
   g. Slowly relax.
3. Complete 10 lumbar stretches to keep natural curves of spine in shape.
   a. Lie flat on floor with head on pillow.
   b. Bend knees and slowly bring them toward your chest. Place hand behind thigh to assist in bending knees.
   c. Keep head on pillow, and elevate buttocks as high as possible off the floor. Keep knees as close to chest as possible.
   d. Hold position, holding onto thighs and keeping knees to chest for count of 10.
4. Complete hamstring stretches for 10 cycles to promote easy bending.
   a. Lie on a hard surface with knees close to the chest in a relaxed position.
   b. Slowly extend one leg toward ceiling, flex foot and push heel upward to feel hamstring muscles stretch. Hold position and count to 10. Bend leg and bring knee back toward chest.
   c. Extend second leg while lowering first leg and complete step b.
   d. Repeat exercise 10 times and then bring both knees toward chest, roll to one side, and take a standing position.
5. Complete reverse sit-ups to strengthen abdominal muscles.
   a. Sit on floor in upright position with knees bent.
   b. Lock hands together behind head and hold arms out to side.
   c. Slowly lean back 15 degrees while tightening stomach muscles. Hold position for count of at least 5.
   d. Slowly lean back about 20 degrees, hold the position, and count to 10.
   e. Slowly return to an upright position, Repeat exercises 10 cycles.

Clinical Alert

Stop exercises if you experience pain or if it gets more difficult with repetitions. Check with your physician before attempting exercises.

Applying Body Mechanics

Procedure

1. Determine need for assistance in moving or turning a client following OSHA Lifting Guidelines. ▸ ***Rationale:*** Half of all back pain is associated with lifting or turning clients. The most common back injury is strain on the lumbar muscle group.
2. Establish a firm base of support by placing both feet flat on the floor, with one foot slightly in front of the other.

Clinical Alert

Proper body mechanics is a myth according to the American Nurses Association "Handle With Care" campaign. "Proper body mechanics" training does not translate well into nursing practice. Body mechanics methods primarily concentrate on the lower back for lifting and do not account for other vulnerable body parts involved in other types of client handling tasks, such as lateral transfers.

3. Distribute weight evenly on both feet.
4. Slightly bend both knees. ▸ ***Rationale:*** Allows strong muscles of legs to do the lifting.
5. Hold abdomen firm and tuck buttocks in so that spine is in alignment. ▸ ***Rationale:*** This position protects the back.
6. Hold head erect and secure firm stance.
7. Use this stance as the basis for all actions in moving, turning, and lifting clients.
8. Maintain weight to be lifted as close to your body as possible. ▸ ***Rationale:*** This position maintains the center of gravity and provides leverage that reduces lower back strain.
9. Align the three natural curves in your back (cervical, thoracic, and lumbar). ▸ ***Rationale:*** Weight of client is evenly distributed throughout spine, lowering risk of back injury.
10. Prevent twisting your body when moving the client. ▸ ***Rationale:*** This prevents injury to the back.

Guidelines on Prevention of Low Back Pain for Workers

- Physical exercise is recommended for prevention of low back pain. There is insufficient evidence to recommend for or against any specific type or intensity of exercises.
- Lumbar supports or back belts are not recommended.
- Shoe inserts/orthoses are not recommended. There is insufficient evidence to recommend for or against insoles, soft shoes, soft flooring, or antifatigue mats.
- Temporary modified work and ergonomic workplace adaptations can be recommended to facilitate early return to work for individuals with low back pain.
- There is insufficient consistent evidence to recommend physical ergonomic interventions alone for prevention of low back pain.
- Further research is necessary to determine appropriate prevention in low back pain. Future studies need to be high quality, using randomized controlled trials.

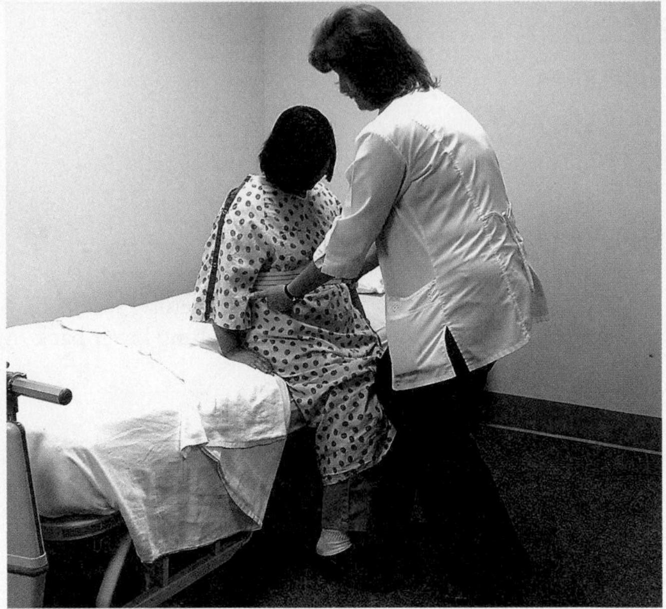

▲ Gait belts are routinely used to assist in manual transfer in most facilities.

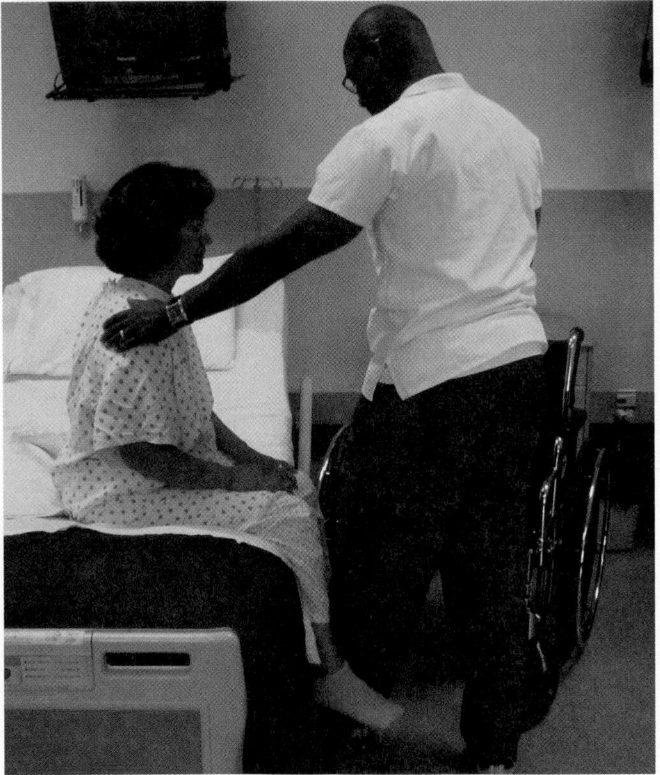

▲ Manual transfers from bed to chair should be done only if client is able to stand.

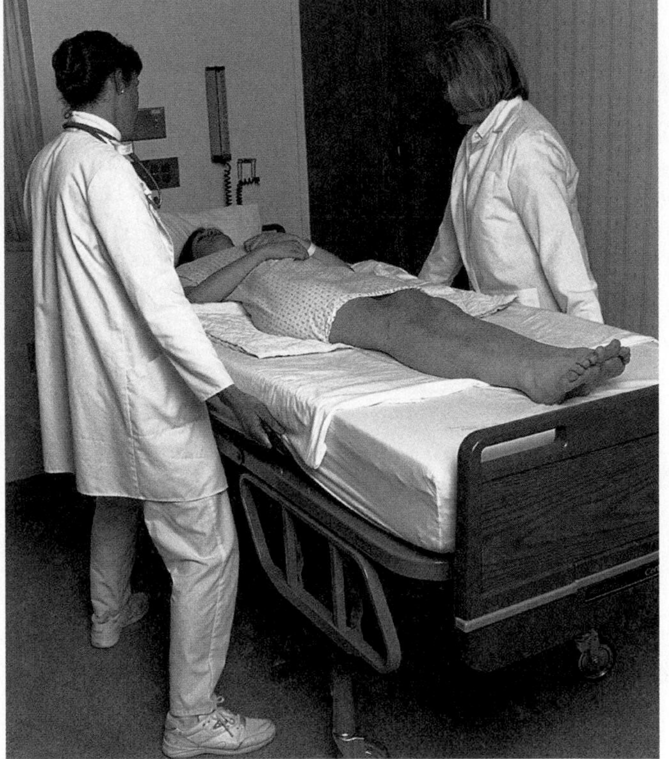

▲ Use proper body mechanics whenever moving clients or objects.

EVIDENCE-BASED PRACTICE

Use of Back Brace to Prevent Back Injury

Two studies on prevention of low back pain using a back support differed in their conclusions. One study, Linton and van Tulder, researched the literature and found 27 investigations that were consistently negative about the use of back braces to prevent low back pain. There is strong evidence not only that they are ineffective in prevention, but that lumbar supports or back belts are no more beneficial than either no intervention or preventative interventions; in fact, they may be detrimental. The results of the Linton and van Tulder study were consistently negative about the use of lumbar supports. The study indicated that exercises, conversely, showed positive results in the randomized controlled trials, providing consistent evidence of their function in prevention.

The second study, conducted at the University of California, Los Angeles (UCLA), by Kraus, McArthur, and Samaniego, found the opposite results. The UCLA study "found compelling evidence that back support can play an important role in helping reduce back injuries among workers who do a lot of lifting." The study, completed in 1994 with 36,000 participants, indicated that low back injuries are reduced by one-third when workers wear a back support. This study recommends worker training and proper workplace ergonomics design and indicates that back supports should be part of an overall back injury prevention program.

The National Institute of Occupational Safety and Health (NIOSH) reviewed the scientific findings in the UCLA study and issued a report in 1994 that concluded the benefit of back supports remained unproven and did not recommend that they be used. A number of preventive measures have been introduced to prevent work-related back injuries. Training, job screening, and ergonomic modification are recommended by NIOSH, but objective evidence of their effectiveness alone or in combination has been elusive and subject to many issues and problems.

These study results have culminated in a recommendation by the European Guidelines for Prevention in Low Back Pain (November 2004) to promote prevention of low back pain using activity/exercise, ergonomics, and orthosis. Physical exercise has a positive effect in prevention of back pain. Various types of activities were reviewed, such as aerobic exercises, physiotherapy, and specific trunk muscle training. The researchers found no specific differences in pain intensity between these interventions. No studies indicated harmful effects of exercise or increased symptoms of pain.

Source: Linton, S. J., & van Tulder, M. W. (2001). Preventive interventions for back and neck problems: What is the evidence? *Spine, 26*(7), 778–787.

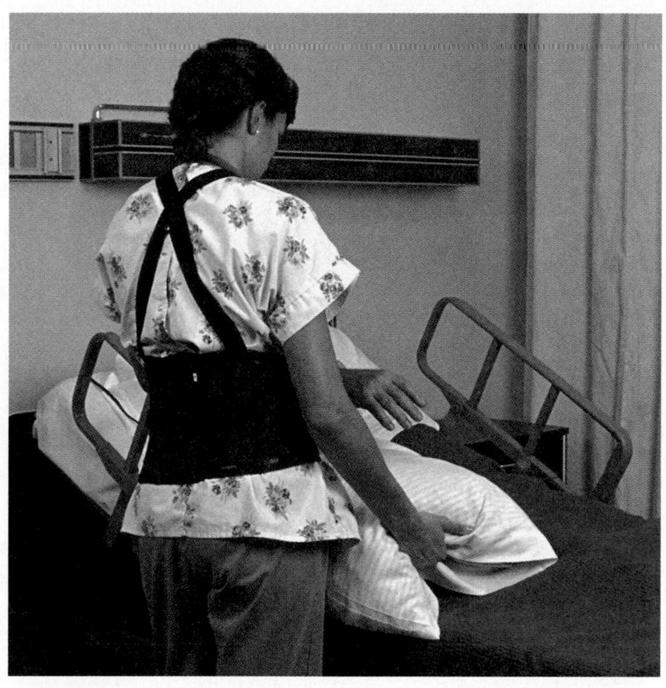

◀ Ensure that height of bed allows you to work without causing injury.

Maintaining Proper Body Alignment

Procedure

1. Begin with the proper stance established in the previous intervention.
2. Evaluate working height necessary to achieve objective.
   a. Test parameters of possible heights (i.e., bed moves within an approximate range of 18 in. from floor).
   b. Establish a comfortable height in which to work; usual height is between waist and lower level of hip joint.
3. Test that this level minimizes muscle strain by extending your arms and checking that your body maintains proper alignment.
4. If you need to work at a lower level, flex your knees. ▸ ***Rationale:*** Bending over at the waist results in back strain.
5. Make accommodations for working at high surface levels. ▸ ***Rationale:*** Reaching up may result in injury to the back through hyperextension of muscles.

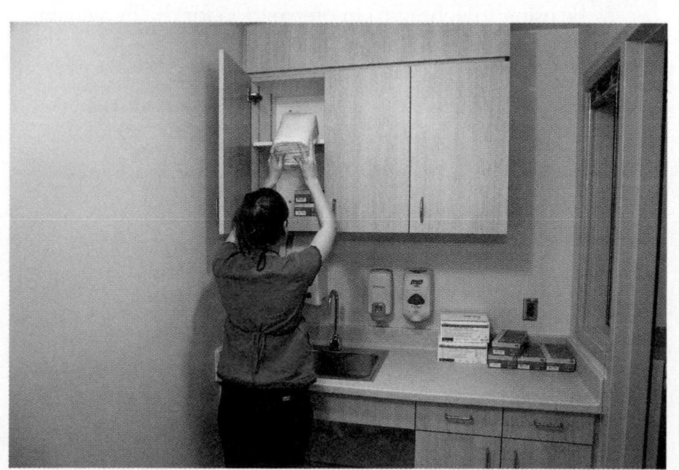

▲ *Correct:* Keep body in correct alignment when turning and reaching for objects to prevent muscle strain or back injury.

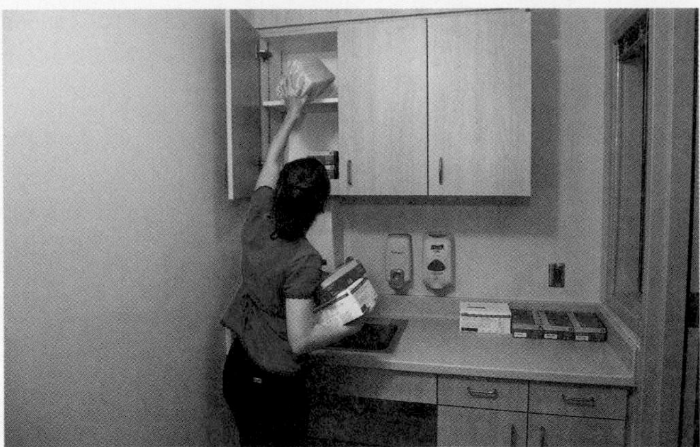

▲ *Incorrect:* Do not use stretching or twisting movements when you reach for objects out of close proximity to your body.

6. Work close to your body so that your center of gravity is not misaligned and your muscles are not hyperextended. ▸ ***Rationale:*** This prevents back strain.
7. Use your longest and strongest muscles (biceps, quadriceps, and gluteal) when moving and turning clients.
8. Whenever possible, roll, push, and pull objects instead of lifting.

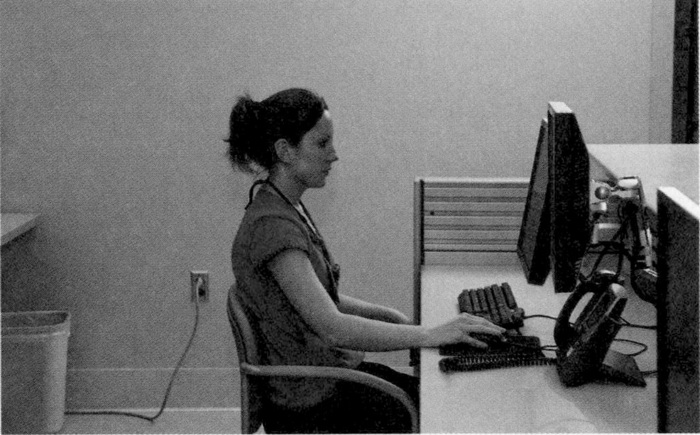

▲ *Correct:* Work close to the body so that center of gravity is not misaligned.

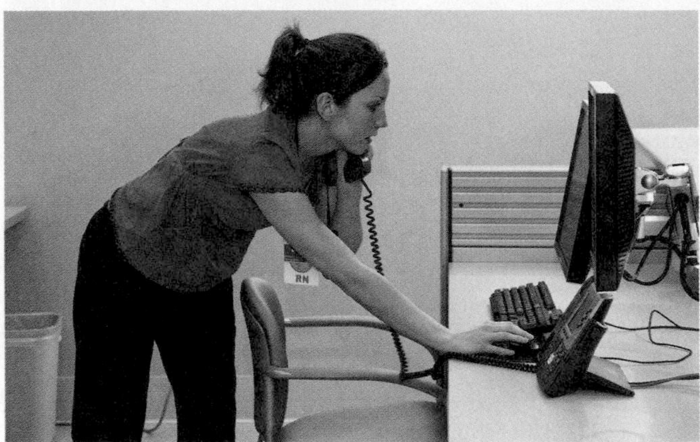

▲ *Incorrect:* Bending over incorrectly could injure back muscles and cause undue strain.

Using Coordinated Movements

Procedure

1. Plan muscle movements to distribute workload before you actually begin turning, moving, or lifting clients.
   a. Establish a clear plan of action before you begin to move.
   b. Take a deep breath so oxygen is available for energy expenditure.
   c. Tense antagonistic muscles (abdomen) to those you will be using (diaphragm) in preparation for the movement.
   d. Release breath and mobilize major muscle groups (abdominal and gluteal) to do the work.
2. Move muscles in a smooth, coordinated manner. ▸ ***Rationale:*** This avoids putting strain on one muscle and is more efficient.
3. Do not make jerky, uncoordinated movements. ▸ ***Rationale:*** This may cause injury or frighten the client.
4. When you are working with another staff member, coordinate plans and movements before implementing them.

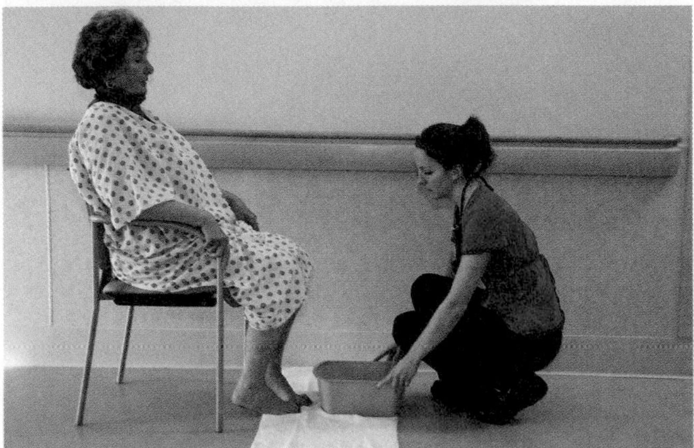

▲ *Correct:* Move muscles as a unit and in alignment rather than twisting.

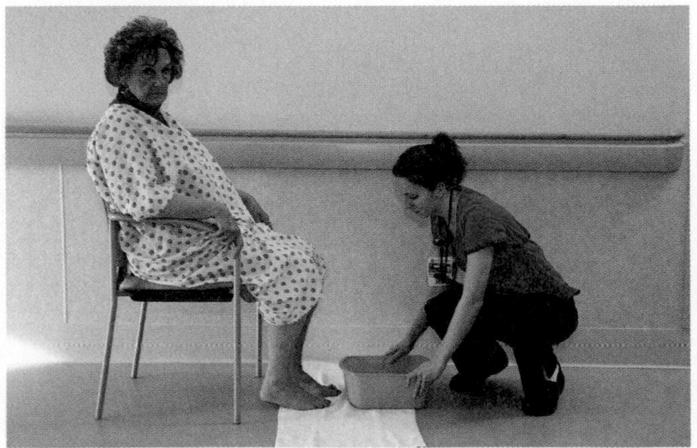

▲ *Incorrect:* Do not twist or rotate upper body when working at lower surface levels.

Using Basic Principles

1. Move an object by pushing and pulling to expend minimal energy.
   a. Stand close to the object.
   b. Place yourself in proper body alignment stance.
   c. Tense muscles, and prepare for movement.
   d. Pull toward you by leaning away from the object and letting arms, hips, and thighs (*not back*) do the work.
   e. Push away from you by leaning toward object, using body weight to add force.

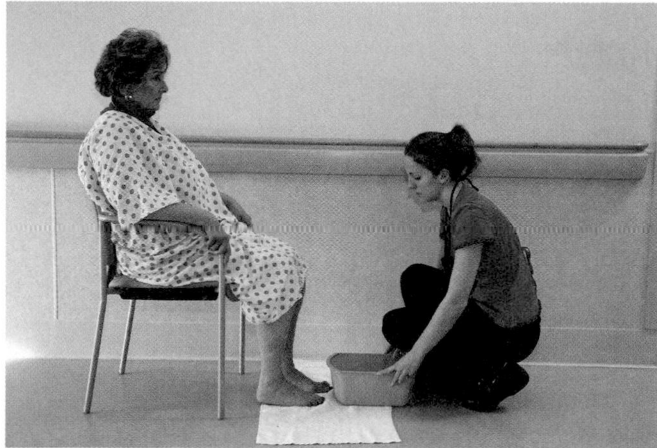

▲ *Correct:* Keep body in proper alignment by bending knees and keeping back straight when lifting objects.

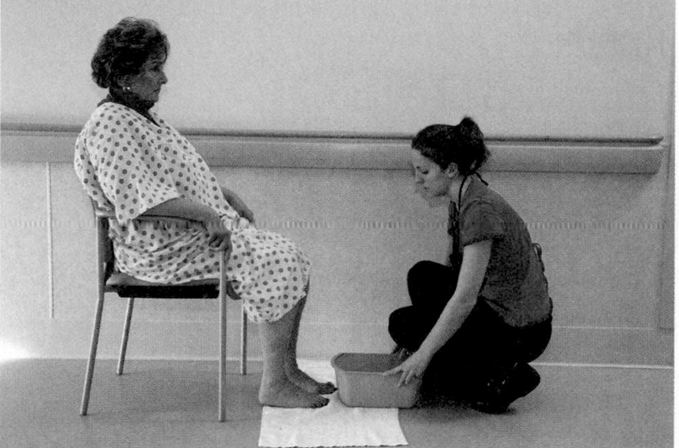

▲ *Incorrect:* Prevent injury to back muscles; for proper alignment, bend at knees and use leg muscles.

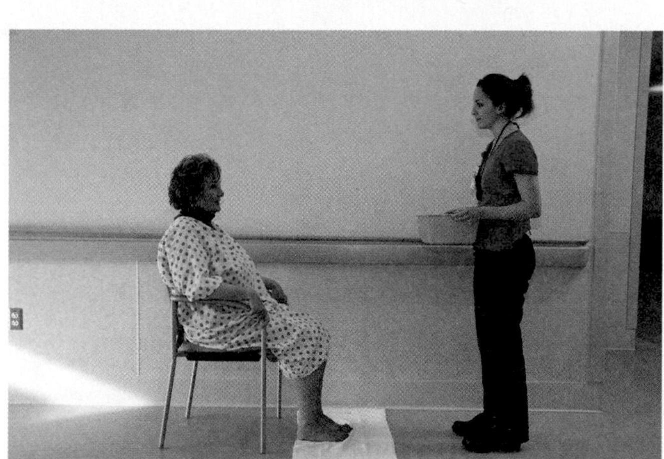

▲ *Correct:* Hold objects close to the body to prevent muscle strain and possible back injury.

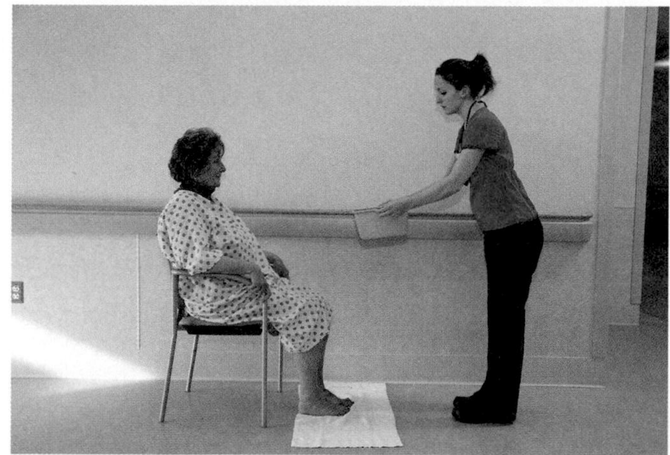

▲ *Incorrect:* Holding objects away from the body may cause back strain or injury.

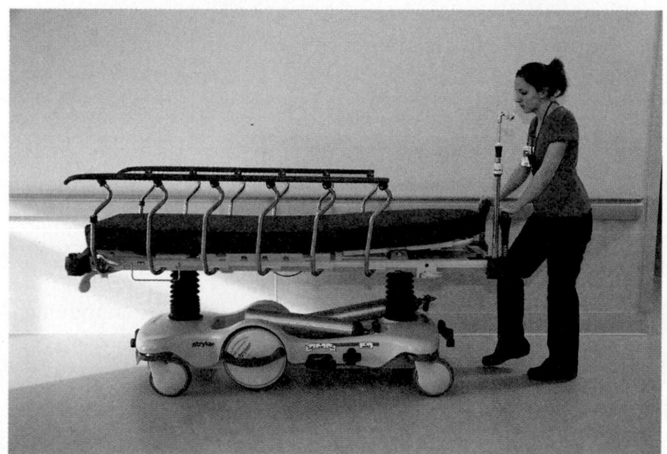

▲ *Correct:* When pushing an object, place yourself in proper body alignment.

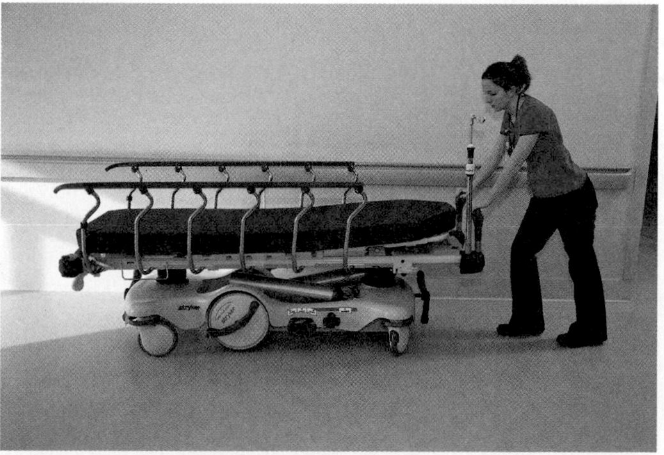

▲ *Incorrect:* Standing away from object puts body out of proper alignment.

2. When changing direction, use pivotal movement—moving muscles as a unit and in alignment, rather than rotating or twisting upper part of body.
3. When working at lower surface levels, do not stoop by bending over. Flex body at knees and, keeping back straight, use thigh and gluteal muscles to accomplish task.
4. Use muscles of arms and upper torso in an extended, coordinated movement parallel to body stance when reaching to prevent twisting or hyperextension of muscles.
5. Lift clients or objects with the maximum use of these body alignment principles:
   a. Determine that the movement is within your capability to perform without injury.
   b. Place yourself in proper body alignment stance.
   c. Stand close to and grasp the object or person near the center of gravity.
   d. Prepare muscles by taking a deep breath, and set muscles.
   e. Lift object with arms or by stooping and using leg and thigh muscles.
   f. Carry object close to your body to prevent strain on your back.
   g. Take frequent rest periods to prevent additional strain.

The Veteran's Health Administration completed a literature review and determined that body mechanics training has proven to be ineffective.

1. Body mechanics training alone is not effective to prevent job-related injuries.
2. There is no evidence that back belts are effective in reducing risks to caregivers.
3. Literature does not support the myth that physically fit nurses are less likely to be injured.
4. The average worker should lift no more than 51 pounds and only under controlled circumstances.
5. The long-term benefits of proper equipment and mechanical lifts far outweigh the costs related to work-related injuries.
6. Staff will use the equipment when they are included in the decision-making process for purchasing new equipment.

Source: American Nurses Association. (2002). http://www.NursingWorld.org.

DOCUMENTATION for Body Mechanics

- Devices needed for turning and moving
- Number of personnel required for turning and moving
- Ways in which client assists in moving
- Special requirements of client for proper body alignment, such as support pillows
- Complete an unusual occurrence report for client or nurse injury during transfer or moving client. (Some facilities refer to this as a Safety Report or Incident Report.)

CRITICAL THINKING Application

Expected Outcomes

- Correct body mechanics are used when preparing for and providing client care.
- Injuries are prevented to both the nurse and the client.
- Proper body mechanics facilitate client care.
- Clients and nurses are not injured when nursing care is provided.
- Center of gravity is maintained when lifting objects.

Unexpected Outcomes

Incorrect body mechanics are used while giving client care.

Alternative Actions

- Identify areas of your body where you feel stress and strain.
- Evaluate the way you use body mechanics.
- Attend an in-service program on using body mechanics appropriately.
- Concentrate on how you are using your body when moving and turning clients.
- Position bed and equipment at a comfortable height and proximity to working area.
- Use your longest and strongest muscles to prevent injury.

Unexpected Outcomes	Alternative Actions
Nurse injures self while giving client care.	• Prevent future episodes of back pain by increasing physical activity and exercises, changing ergonomics, and evaluating use of orthosis. • Report any back strain immediately to supervisor. • Complete unusual occurrence form. • Go to health service or emergency room for evaluation and immediate care. • Evaluate any activities that led to injury to determine incorrect use of body mechanics. • Prevent additional injury by obtaining assistance when needed. • Use devices such as turning sheets or assistive devices to assist in turning difficult clients.
Nurse uses poor body mechanics and injures client.	• Assess the extent of client's injury. • Notify client's physician. • Complete unusual occurrence form. • Carry out physician's orders for follow-up treatment.
Nurse is unable to obtain sufficient assistance with turning and moving clients.	• Place turning sheets on bed for all clients who are difficult to move. • Use principles of leverage in moving clients. • Until adequate staff is available, turn and position client from side to side at least every 2 hr. • Use Hoyer Lift.
Number of client/healthcare worker injuries increases in nursing unit.	• Determine cause of injury and nursing units involved. • Based on causes, compile a survey and walking rounds on all shifts and units to gather data regarding injury status. Look for trends and personnel behaviors. • Form a safety committee made up of direct healthcare providers, nursing staff, management, and risk manager to determine causes and propose changes in patient handling. • Study findings of surveys and unusual occurrence reports to determine appropriate prevention program. • Determine appropriate equipment based on level of injury and dependency. Bring in vendors to demonstrate equipment based on findings. • Complete in-service staff development program on proper use of equipment and safety principles before implementing program. • Continue to keep detailed notes on client and/or staff injury reports after implementation of new protocols. Analyze data and compare with prior injury rates and types.

Source: American Nurses Association. (2006). Based on Preventing Back Injuries: Safe Patient Handling and Movement.

Chapter 12

UNIT 2

Moving and Turning Clients

Nursing Process Data

ASSESSMENT Data Base

- Observe the client and identify ways to improve the client's position and alignment.
- Determine the client's physical ability to assist with positioning.
- Assess appropriate mechanical device for moving clients requiring assistance.
- Note the presence of tubes and incisions that alter the positioning and alignment procedures.
- Assess joint mobility.
- Assess skin condition with each turn.

PLANNING Objectives

- To provide increased comfort
- To provide optimal lung excursion and ventilation
- To prevent contractures due to constant joint flexion
- To promote optimal joint movement
- To help maintain intact skin
- To prevent injury due to improper movement
- To move and transfer clients using mechanical devices

IMPLEMENTATION Procedures

EVALUATION Expected Outcomes

- Client's comfort is increased.
- Skin remains intact without evidence of breakdown as a result of moving and turning.
- Breathing is adequate and unlabored.
- Joint movement is maintained.
- Footdrop is prevented.
- Body alignment is maintained.
- Mechanical equipment and devices are used in client transfers and repositioning as needed.
- Client is moved safely using appropriate device.

Pearson Nursing Student Resources

Find additional review materials at
nursing.pearsonhighered.com

Prepare for success with NCLEX®-style practice questions and Skill Checklists

TABLE 12-2 Bed Positions for Client Care

Positions	Placement	Use
High-Fowler's	Head of bed 60° angle	Thoracic surgery, severe respiratory conditions
Fowler's	Head of bed 45°–60° angle; hips may or may not be flexed	Postoperative, gastrointestinal conditions, promote lung expansion
Semi-Fowler's	Head of bed 30° angle	Cardiac, respiratory, neurosurgical conditions
Low-Fowler's	Head of bed 15° angle	Necessary degree elevation for ease of breathing, promotes skin integrity, client comfort
Knee-gatch	Lower section of bed (under knees) slightly bent	For client comfort; contraindicated for vascular disorders
Trendelenburg's	Head of bed lowered and foot raised	Percussion, vibration, and drainage (PVD) procedure; promotes venous return
Reverse Trendelenburg's	Bed frame is tilted up with foot of bed down	Gastric conditions, prevents esophageal reflux

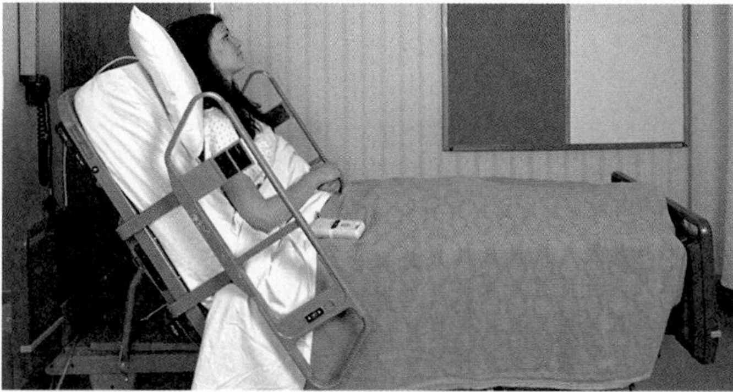

▲ High-Fowler's position at 60° angle.

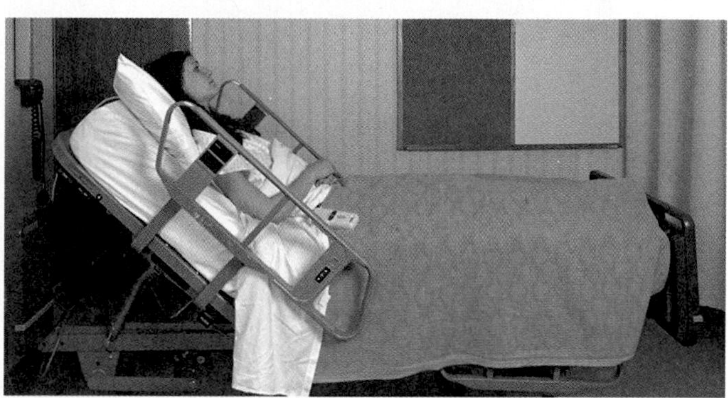

▲ Fowler's position at 45°–60° angle.

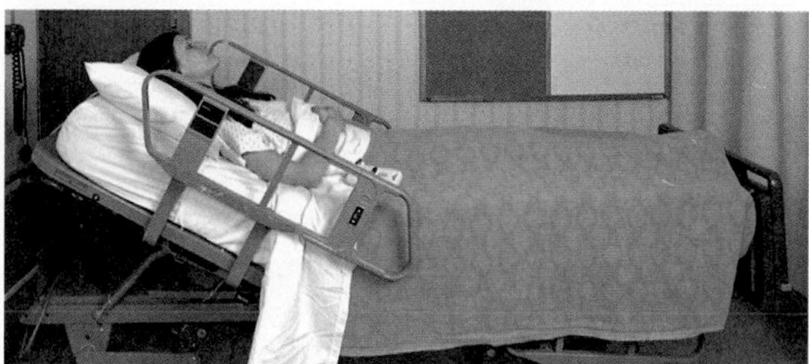

▲ Semi-Fowler's position at 30° angle.

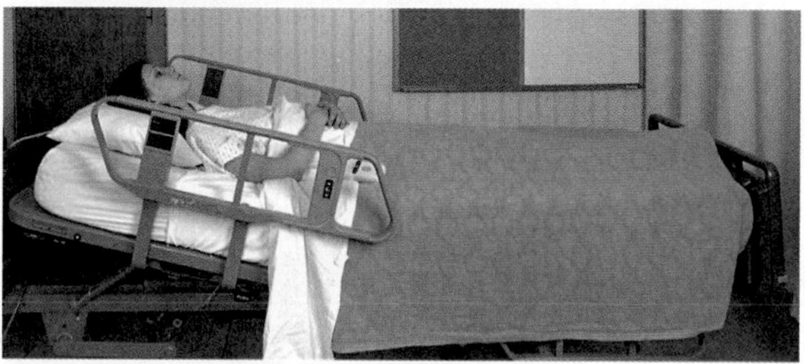

▲ Low-Fowler's position at 15° angle.

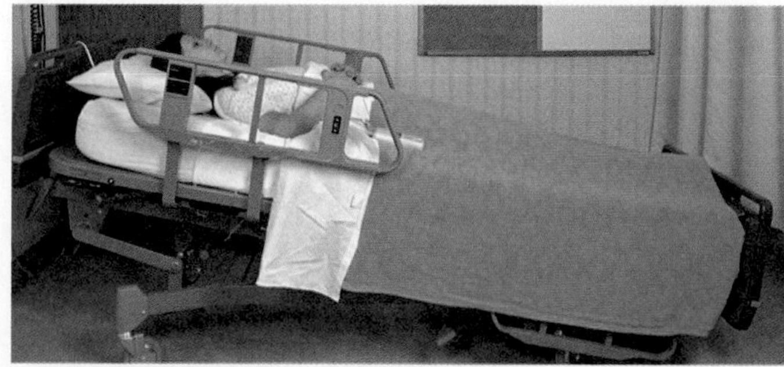

▲ Reverse Trendelenburg position.

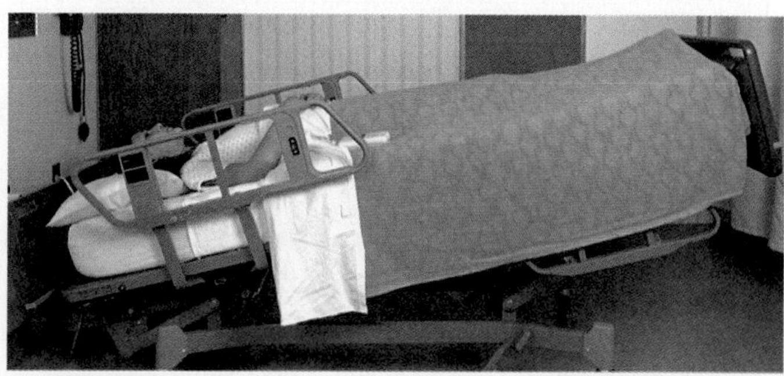

▲ Trendelenburg position.

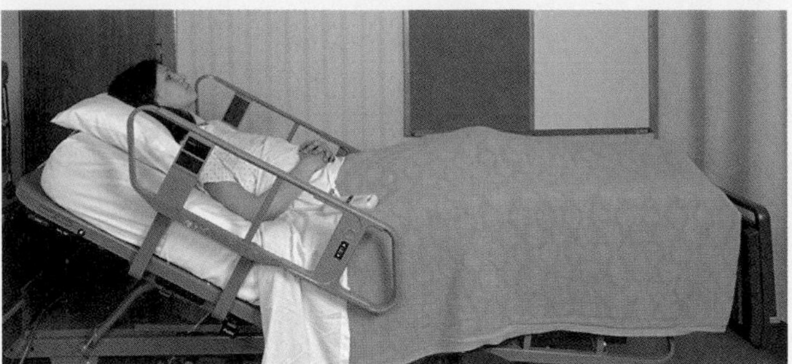

▲ Elevated knee gatch.

Assessing Clients for Safe Moving and Handling

Equipment

Mechanical equipment or devices based on assessment of functional level.

Procedure

1. Perform hand hygiene.
2. Check if physician orders need to be obtained for client transfers or moving (joint replacement, spinal cord injury, or surgical procedure).
3. Use two indicators to identify client and introduce yourself.
4. Explain use of assessment criteria in preparation for safe moving and handling.
5. Complete check list or document findings in nurses' notes.
   a. Identify client's level of assistance.
      (1) Independent: able to perform task safely with or without staff assistance or assistive devices.
      (2) Partial Assist: requires stand-by assistance, cueing, or lifting no more than 35 lb of client's weight by staff.
      (3) Dependent: requires staff to lift more than 35 lb of client's weight or is unpredictable in amount of assistance needed. Assistive devices need to be utilized.

Assessment Criteria and Care Plan for Safe Patient Handling and Movement

A: ASSESSMENT CRITERIA

I. Patient's Level of Assistance:

_____ Independent — Patient performs task safely, with or without staff assistance, with or without assistive devices.

_____ Partial Assist — Patient requires no more help than stand-by, cueing, or coaxing, or caregiver is required to lift no more than 35 lbs. of a patient's weight.

_____ Dependent — Patient requires nurse to lift more than 35 lbs. of the patient's weight, or is unpredictable in the amount of assistance offered. In this case assistive devices should be used.

An assessment should be made prior to each task if the patient has varying level of ability to assist due to medical reasons, fatigue, medications, etc. When in doubt, assume the patient cannot assist with the transfer/repositioning.

II. Weight Bearing Capability

_____ Full
_____ Partial
_____ None

III. Bi-Lateral Upper Extremity Strength

_____ Yes
_____ No

IV. Patient's level of cooperation and comprehension:

_____ Cooperative — may need prompting; able to follow simple commands.

_____ Unpredictable or varies (patient whose behavior changes frequently should be considered as "unpredictable"), not cooperative, or unable to follow simple commands.

V. Weight: _______ Height: _______

Body Mass Index (BMI) [needed if patient's weight is over 300][1]:_______

If BMI exceeds 50, institute Bariatric Algorithms

The presence of the following conditions are likely to affect the transfer/repositioning process and should be considered when identifying equipment and technique needed to move the patient.

VI. Check applicable conditions likely to affect transfer/repositioning techniques.

_____ Hip/Knee Replacements	_____ Postural Hypotension	_____ Amputation
_____ History of Falls	_____ Severe Osteoporosis	_____ Urinary/Fecal Stoma
_____ Paralysis/Paresis	_____ Splints/Traction	_____ Contractures/Spasms
_____ Unstable Spine	_____ Fractures	_____ Tubes (IV, Chest, etc.)
_____ Severe Edema	_____ Respiratory/Cardiac Compromise	_____ Severe Pain, Discomfort
_____ Very Fragile Skin	_____ Wounds Affecting Transfer/Positioning	

Comments: ____________________

B: CARE PLAN

VH. Care Plan:

Algorithm	Task	Equipment/ Assistive Device	# Staff
1	Transfer To and From: Bed to Chair, Chair to Toilet, Chair to Chair, or Car to Chair.		
2	Lateral Transfer To and From: Bed to Stretcher, Trolley.		
3	Transfer To and From: Chair to Stretcher, or Chair to Exam Table.		
4	Reposition in Bed: Side-to-Side, Up in Bed.		
5	Reposition in Chair: Wheelchair and Dependency Chair.		
6	Transfer Patient Up from the Floor		
Bariatric 1	Bariatric Transfer To and From: Bed to Chair, Chair to Toilet, or Chair to Chair		
Bariatric 2	Bariatric Lateral Transfer To and From: Bed to Stretcher or Trolley		
Bariatric 3	Bariatric Reposition in Bed: Side-to-Side, Up in Bed		
Bariatric 4	Bariatric Reposition in Chair: Wheelchair, Chair or Dependency Chair		
Bariatric 5	Patient Handling Tasks Requiring Access to Body Parts (Limb, Abdominal Mass, Gluteal Area)		
Bariatric 6	Bariatric Transporting (Stretcher)		
Bariatric 7	Bariatric Toileting Tasks		

Sling Type (circle choice): Seated____ Seated (Amputation)____ Standing____ Supine____ Ambulation____ Limb Support____

Sling Size: ____________

Signature: ____________________ **Date:** ____________

[1]If patient's weight is over 300 pounds, the BMI is needed. For Online BMI table and calculator see: http://www.nhlbi.nih.gov/guidelines/obesity/bmi_tbl.htm

▲ *Source:* Nelson, A. VISN 8 Patient Safety Center. www.VISN8.med.va.gov/ patientsafetycenter

Sample Algorithm for Client Transfer

Algorithm 1: Transfer to and From: Bed to Chair, Chair to Toilet, Chair to Chair, or Car to Chair

Start Here

rev 4/1/05

Can client bear weight?

Fully

Caregiver assistance not needed; Stand by for safety as needed.

No

Partially

Is the client cooperative?

Yes

Stand and pivot technique using a gait/transfer belt (1 caregiver) or powered standing assist lift (1 caregiver)

No

Is the client cooperative?

No

Use full body sling lift and 2 caregivers.

Yes

Does the client have upper extremity strength?

No

Yes

Seated transfer aid; may use gait/transfer belt until the client is proficient in completing transfer independently.

- For seated transfer aid, must have chair with arms that recess or are removable.
- For full body sling lift, select a lift that was specifically designed to access a client from the car (if the car is the starting or ending destination).
- If client has partial weight bearing capability, transfer toward stronger side.
- Toileting slings are available for toileting.
- Bathing mesh slings are available for bathing.
- During any client transferring task, if any caregiver is required to lift more than 35 lbs of client's weight, then client should be considered to be fully dependent and assistive devices should be used for the transfer.

▲ *Source:* Nelson, A. VISN 8 patient Safety Center. www.VISN8.med.va.gov/ patientsafetycenter

b. Weight-bearing capacity.
   (1) Full.
   (2) Partial.
   (3) None.
c. Evaluate bilateral upper-extremity strength.
d. Determine client's ability to transfer weight, assist with repositioning of body before contractures occur.
e. Client's level of cooperation and comprehension.
   (1) Cooperative: may need prompting, able to follow simple commands.
   (2) Unpredictable or varies: Client's behavior changes frequently, client is not cooperative or is unable to follow simple commands.
f. Record client's:
   (1) Height.
   (2) Weight.
   (3) Client more than 300 lb, must use Bariatric Algorithms for assistance.
g. Identify client's physical condition, which will likely affect transfer/repositioning techniques (i.e., pin sites, surgical incision, fragile skin, fractures, presence of IVs and tubes, etc).

NOTE: See Sample Assessment Criteria and Care Plan for Safe Patient Handling and Movement and Algorithms. (Nelson, A. VISN 8 Patient Safety Center.)

6. Determine appropriate procedure for safe transfer; assistive devices, lift team, number of workers required for procedure for safe transfer.

Bariatric Considerations

Lifting and transferring bariatric clients has become a concern for healthcare providers. Approximately 5% to 10% of the general population is obese. When the body mass index (BMI) is greater than 38, special bariatric equipment is required. If the BMI is over 39, the client is considered morbidly obese.

Equipment may need to be ordered if not available in the facility. To ensure that appropriate equipment is available, the needs assessment should be part of the hospital admission assessment.

Frequently required equipment includes:

- Wider wheelchairs
- Wider beds
- Walkers
- Shower/commode chairs

7. Review algorithms or appropriate use of equipment and devices to determine equipment necessary to meet client's needs.
8. Complete care plan, identifying type of client transfers and specifics to be carried out during transfers.
9. Ensure all staff are properly instructed in techniques and equipment utilized as assistant devices. ▸ ***Rationale:*** promote safe handling of clients during transfer.

Placing a Trochanter Roll

Equipment

Bath blanket

Procedure

1. Perform hand hygiene, use two identifiers to identify client, and place client in supine or prone position.
2. Place folded bath blanket on bed next to client.
3. Extend blanket from greater trochanter to thigh or knee.

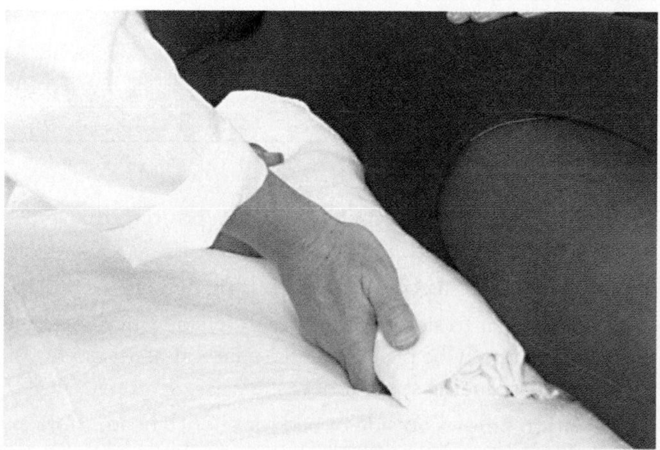

▲ Use trochanter rolls made from bath blankets to align client's hips.

Handroll Positioning

When positioning clients who are on long-term bedrest, all areas of the body must be considered. Handrolls made from folded washcloths rolled into a cone shape (or commercially available) may be used to position and maintain wrist and fingers in a functional position. The purpose is to prevent deformity and contractures.

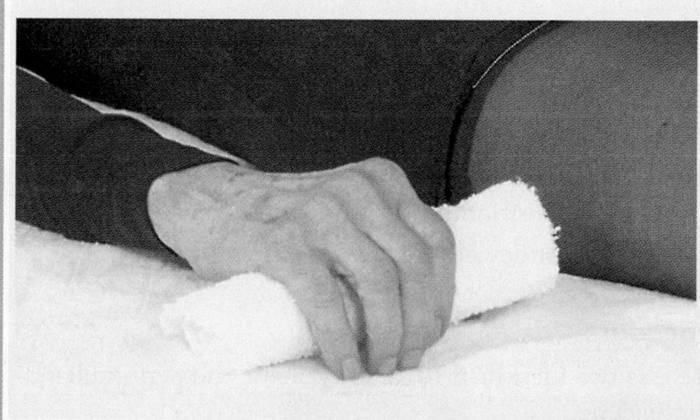

4. Place blanket edge under leg and buttocks to anchor.
5. Roll bath blanket toward client by rolling it under.
6. Rotate affected leg to slight internal hip rotation. ▸ ***Rationale:*** The purpose is to prevent external rotation of the head of the femur in the acetabulum.
7. Tighten the roll by tucking the roll under the hip joint.
8. Allow affected leg to rest against trochanter roll. Hip should be in normal alignment, not internally or externally rotated. Patella should be facing upward if client in supine position. ▸ ***Rationale:*** This is used most commonly for clients who have a muscle weakness or paralysis of that side of the body.

Turning to Lateral Position

Equipment

Pillows for positioning

Lateral-assist device or friction-reducing sheet (see Table 12-3)

Drawsheet for trochanter roll

Procedure

1. Use two identifiers to identify client and perform hand hygiene.
2. Explain rationale for procedure to client.
3. Lower head of the bed completely or to a position as low as client can tolerate.
4. Elevate bed to a comfortable working height.
5. Move client to your side of bed. Put side rails up, and move to other side of bed. Use lateral-assist device or friction-reducing sheet if necessary.
6. Flex client's knees.

Kinetic Bed Therapy

Kinetic bed therapy reduces the odds of developing HAI (nosocomial) pneumonia in mechanically ventilated clients. It has not shown a significant reduction in mortality, duration of mechanical ventilation, or length of ICU or hospital stays.

Source: Delaney, A., Gray, H., Laupland, K. B., & Zuege, D. J. (2006). Kinetic bed therapy to prevent nosocomial pneumonia in mechanically ventilated patients: A systematic review and meta-analysis. *Critical Care, 10*(3), R70.

7. Place one hand on client's hip and one hand on client's shoulder; roll onto side.
8. Position pillow to maintain proper alignment.
9. Be sure to position client's arms so they are not under the body.
10. Perform hand hygiene.

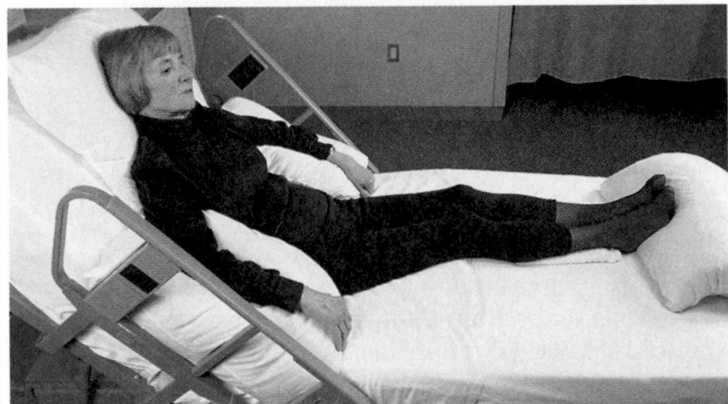

▲ Use pillows to support proper alignment.

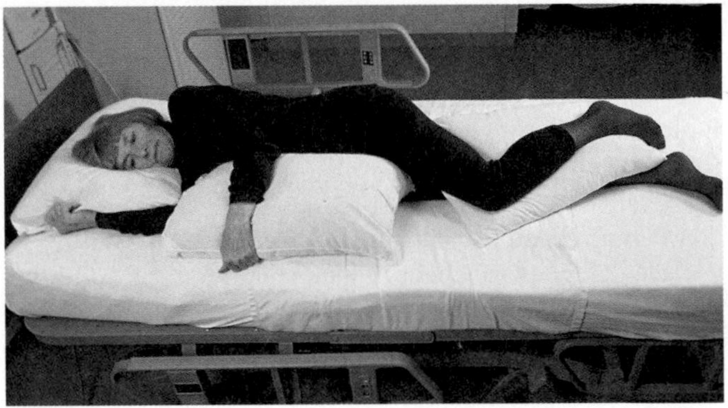

▲ Lateral (side-lying) position.

Turning to a Prone Position

Equipment

Pillows for positioning

Lateral-assist device or friction-reducing sheet

Procedure

1. Use two identifiers to identify client and perform hand hygiene.
2. Explain rationale for procedure to client.
3. Lower head of bed completely or to a position that is as low as client can tolerate.
4. Elevate bed to a comfortable working height.
5. Move client to side of bed away from side where he or she will finally be positioned. Use lateral-assist device or friction-reducing sheet if necessary.
6. Position pillows on side of bed for client's head, thorax, and feet.

7. Roll client onto pillows, making sure that client's arms are not under his or her body.
8. Reposition pillows as necessary for client's comfort.
9. Perform hand hygiene.

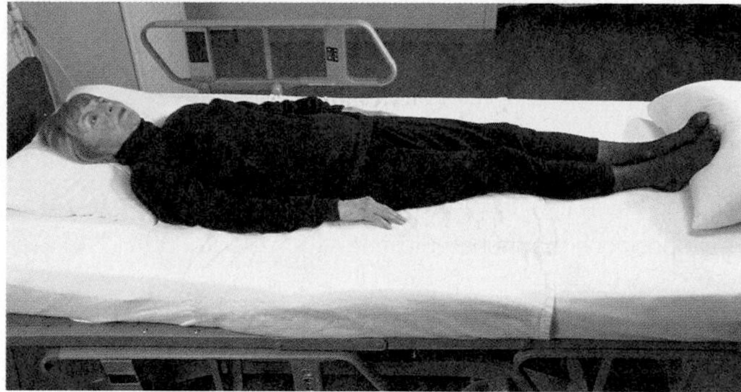

▲ Supino pocition.

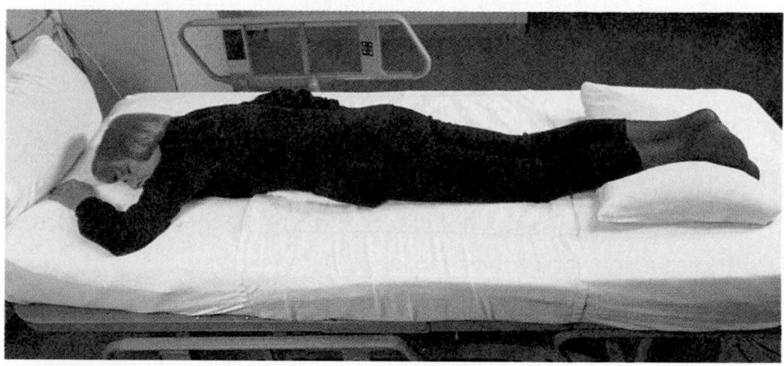

▲ Prone position.

Moving Client Up in Bed

Equipment

Trapeze (optional)
Friction-reducing sheet

Procedure

1. Use two identifiers to identify client and perform hand hygiene.
2. Explain rationale for procedure to client.
3. Lower head of bed so that it is flat or as low as client can tolerate.
4. Raise bed to a comfortable working height. ▸ ***Rationale:*** Allows nurse's center of gravity to assist in turning.
5. Remove pillow and place it at head of bed. ▸ ***Rationale:*** This prevents striking client's head against bed.
6. Place one arm under client's shoulders and other arm under client's thighs. Use this method of moving only if the client can assist with move.
7. Flex your knees and hips. Move feet close to bed.
8. Place your weight on your back foot.
9. Instruct client to put arms across chest, bend legs, and put feet flat on the bed.

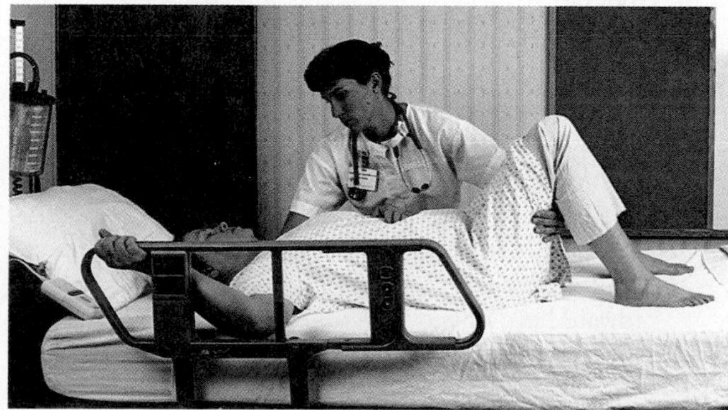

▲1 Place one arm under shoulders and other under thighs.

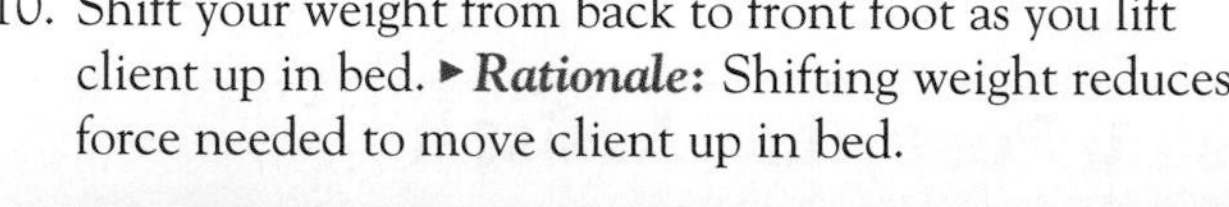

10. Shift your weight from back to front foot as you lift client up in bed. ▸ ***Rationale:*** Shifting weight reduces force needed to move client up in bed.

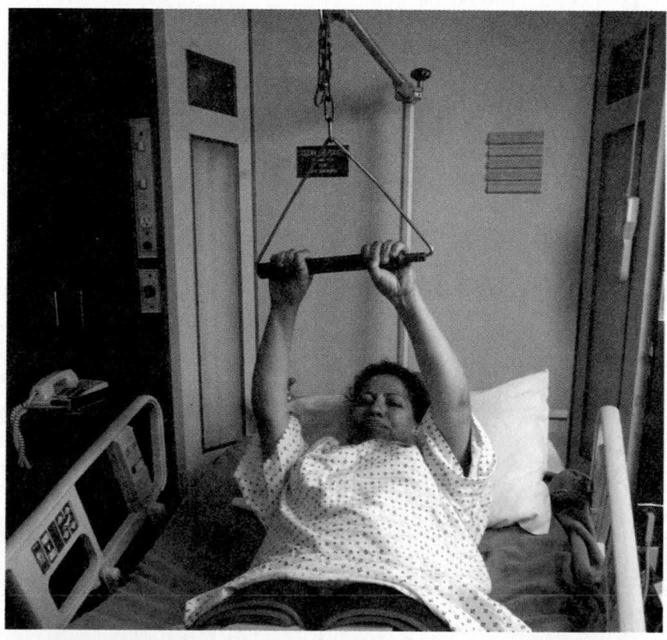

▲ Encourage client to help when repositioning.

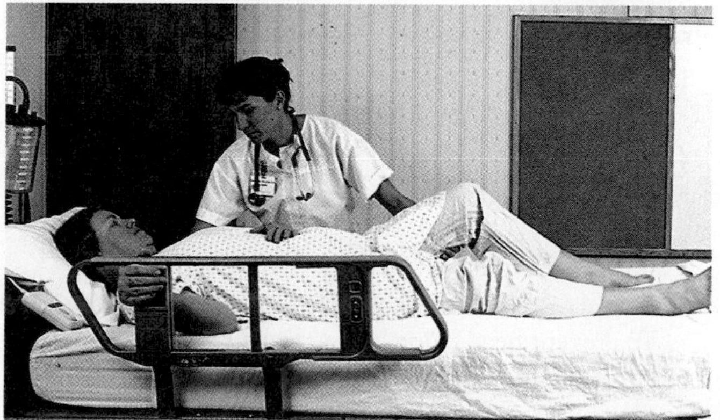

▲2 Maintain proper body alignment when moving client up in bed.

11. Ask client to push with feet as you move him/her.
12. Position client comfortably, replacing pillow and arranging bedding as necessary.
13. Perform hand hygiene.

NOTE: There are several other methods of moving a client up in bed—including using assist devices such as friction-reducing sheet or total lift devices for clients who are unable to assist with moving and turning.

EVIDENCE-BASED PRACTICE

Recommendations for Positioning

- Client experiences consolidated pneumonia in one lung: position good lung down to increase oxygenation.
- Progressive mobilization to dangling legs, standing, and walking are safe positions for intubated clients.
- Clients increase their oxygenation with head of bed elevated.
- Turning every 2 hr is not sufficient to prevent healthcare acquired pneumonia.
- Using kinetic and continuous lateral rotation therapy decreases risk of ventilator-acquired pneumonia (VAP) in clients on ventilators. Eighteen hours of rotation per day and early placement in kinetic bed are necessary to prevent VAP.
- Prone positioning improves oxygenation, but hasn't been shown to affect mortality rates.

Source: Rauen, C. A., Chulay, M., Bridges, E., Vollman, K. M., & Arbour, R. (2008). Seven evidence-based practice habits: Putting some sacred cows out to pasture. *Critical Care Nurse*, *28*(2), 98–124.

Using Posey Lift Assist II

Equipment

Posey Assist II
Chair or wheelchair

NOTE: Posey Lift Assist is used for clients weighing up to 300 lb.

Procedure

1. Use two forms of identification to identify client
2. Introduce self and explain use of Posey Lift.
3. Inspect device for broken stitches; torn, cut, or frayed straps on fabric. ▸ ***Rationale:*** Ensure straps do not break and cause client to fall.
4. Stand in front of client, feet apart with broad base of support, one foot slightly ahead of other.
5. Keep back straight, bend hips and knees.
6. Place lift assist around client's lower back.
7. Firmly grasp handles of lift device.
8. Instruct client to lean forward and upward as you slowly stand upward. If client is weak at the knee, brace your knee against client's weak knee to stabilize as you assist client to standing position.
9. Assist client to pivot into chair. Gently lower client into chair.

Moving Client With Assistance

Equipment

Friction-reducing sheet

Procedure

1. Use two identifiers to identify client and perform hand hygiene.
2. Explain rationale for procedure to client.
3. Lower head of bed so that it is flat or as low as client can tolerate.
4. Raise bed to a comfortable working height.
5. Remove pillow, and place it at head of bed. ▸ ***Rationale:*** To prevent head being bumped when moved.
6. Coordinate the movements of all nurses. ▸ ***Rationale:*** One nurse is responsible for stating when to move client, "on count of three."
7. Position client with two nurses or staff members.
   a. Position one nurse on each side of client. Assume broad base of support; position front foot facing head of bed, body slightly turned toward head of bed.
   b. Assist client to flex knees, if possible.
   c. Each nurse firmly grasps sheet at level of client's upper back with one hand and at level of buttocks with other hand.
   d. Each nurse places weight on back foot.
   e. Then with one firm, coordinated, rocking movement (shifting weight from back to front foot), lift client toward head of bed.
   f. Place client in a comfortable position.
8. Perform hand hygiene.

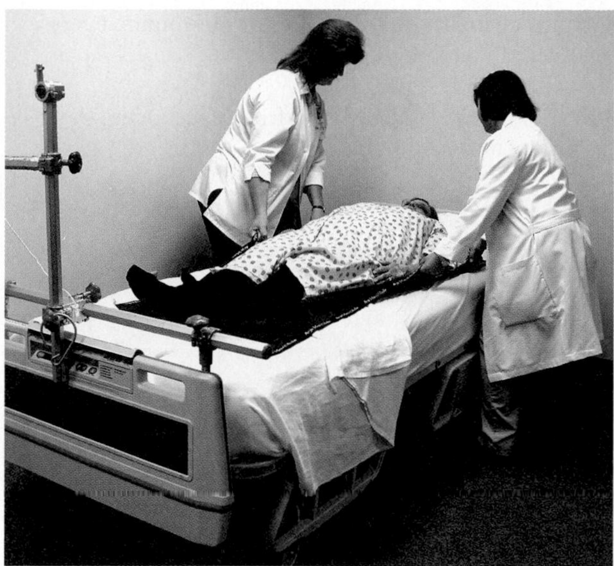

▲ Use friction-reducing sheet and shift weight from back to front leg when moving client up.

Clinical Alert

The ANA reports that an average healthcare worker should lift no more than 51 lb and only under very controlled circumstances. It is advisable to use lifting and transferring devices.

Logrolling the Client

Equipment

Pillows, towels, blankets for positioning

Turning sheet

Procedure

1. Check order for logrolling client and client care plan as to exactly why client needs to be logrolled.
2. Identify the client using two identifiers. Perform hand hygiene.
3. Obtain sufficient assistance to complete procedure with ease. Three nurses are preferable.
4. Place a pillow between the client's knees before moving the client. ▸ ***Rationale:*** To prevent adduction of hip. This will prevent spinal torque.
5. Position two nurses on side of bed to which client will be turned. Position third nurse on opposite side of bed.
6. Designate person at head of bed to be in charge of coordinating move.
7. Assume correct position for client move:
   a. Nurse at head: one arm supports client's head, second arm supports shoulders and neck.
   b. Second nurse: one hand grasps client's other shoulder, the other hand and arm around knee.
   c. Third nurse: on the opposite side of the bed, nurse holds drawsheet firmly to support torso. ▸ ***Rationale:*** This maintains the body in alignment.
8. Instruct client to place arms across chest to keep body straight.
9. Assume broad stance with one foot ahead of the other and knees flexed.
10. Rock onto back foot, and use leg and arm muscles to move client in one coordinated movement when nurse

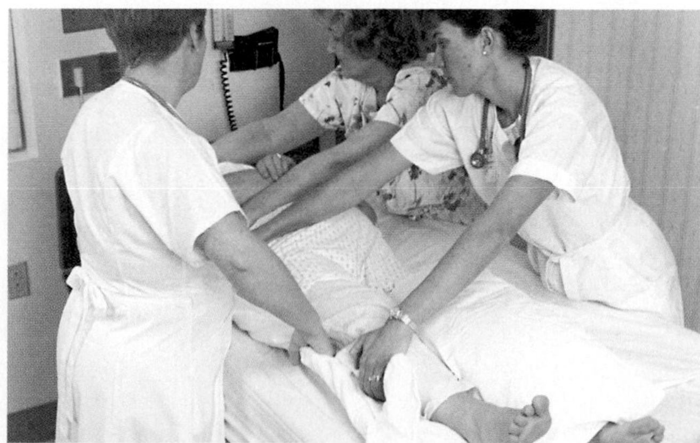

▲ Position nurses on each side of client.

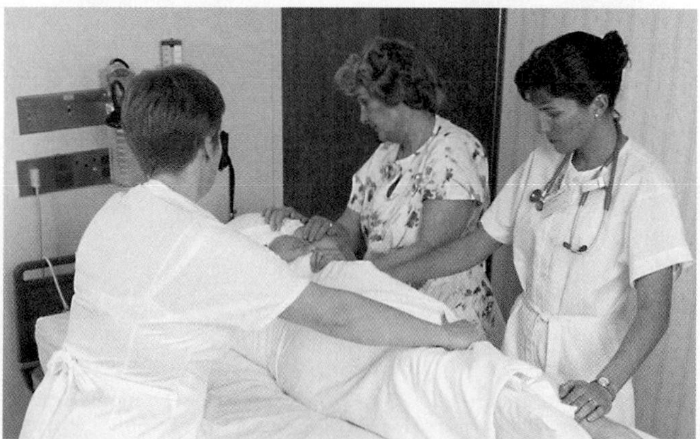

▲ Maintain proper alignment while turning client.

at head of bed signals to move client. ▶ ***Rationale:*** To maintain proper alignment, all of the body parts must be moved at the same time. If not, injury to client's neck and spinal column may occur.

11. Maintain client's position in alignment with pillows, towels, or folded blankets.
12. Change client's position frequently (minimum every 2 hr) according to physician's orders.

NOTE: It is recommended that a friction-reducing sheet be used instead of manual turning.

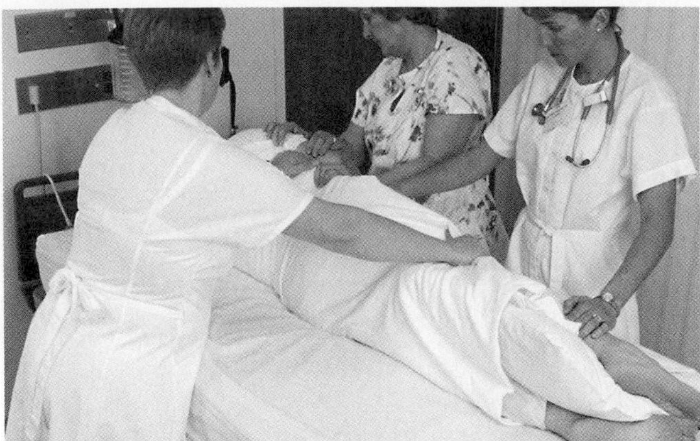

Maintain client's position with pillow support under client's back.

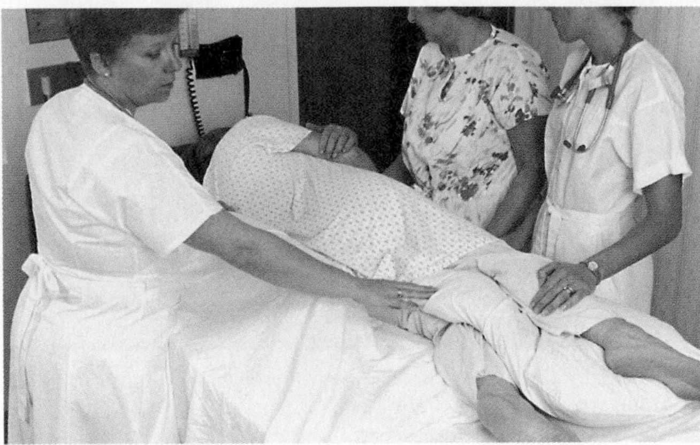

After positioning pillow, allow client to lean back for support.

Client Lift Teams

A lift team consists of two physically fit individuals competent in lifting techniques, who work together to perform high-risk client transfers. The individuals on the team must have no prior history of a musculoskeletal injury and must depend on their physical strength and capabilities. They must have a physical examination and an x-ray of their spine, in addition to not having a history of back injury.

They are trained on the use of mechanical lifting devices. Several clinical trials have been conducted on the use of client lift teams. The outcomes indicated this intervention was effective in decreasing the loss of work days and compensable injury costs.

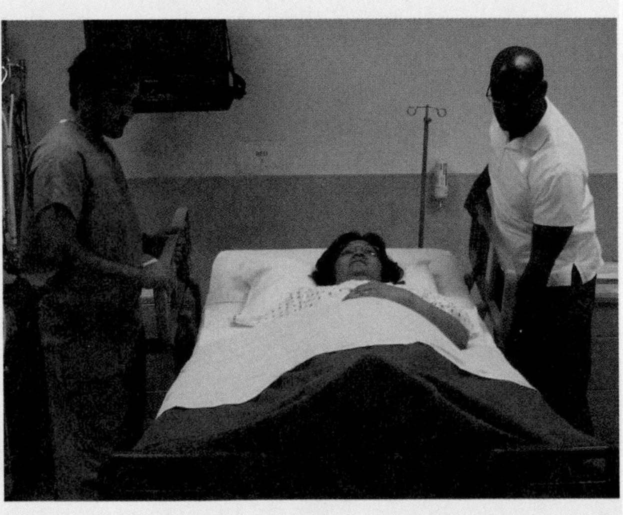

Source: Nelson, A., & Baptiste, A. S. (2004). Evidence-based practices for safe patient handling and movement. *The Online Journal of Issues in Nursing*, 9(3). Available at www.nursingworld.org/ojin. Accessed September 30, 2004.

EVIDENCE-BASED PRACTICE

Use of Draw Sheet for Moving Clients

Few evidence-based studies disagree that the critical task of repositioning a client in bed places caregivers at an increased risk of back injury due to high spinal loads. Although the two-person drawsheet method of repositioning clients has the lowest low-back disorder risk, spinal loads were still high, thus increasing the risk of a back injury.

Most low back injuries are not the result of a single exposure to a high load but repeated small loads (bending) or a sustained load (sitting). Low back pain is shown to result from repetitive motion and excessive loading.

Source: Marras, W. S., Davis, K. G., Kirking, B. C., & Bertsche, P. K. (1999). A comprehensive analysis of low-back disorder risk and spinal loading during transferring and repositioning of patients using different techniques. *Ergonomics*, *42*(7), 904–926.

Transferring Client From Bed to Gurney

Equipment

Transfer board: polyethylene board about 18–22 in. wide by 72 in. long
Sheets to cover board, gurney, and client
Bath blanket (optional)
Gurney, bed, or CT table

Procedure

1. Use two identifiers to identify the client and perform hand hygiene.
2. Introduce self and explain procedure to client and show client transfer board. ▸ ***Rationale:*** To allay client's fears of being dropped from board.
3. Cover client with sheet or bath blanket and cover board and gurney with sheets.
4. Position client on side of bed away from gurney in lateral position.
5. First nurse supports client while second nurse places board as close to client as possible. ▸ ***Rationale:*** This allows client to be positioned on entire board after turn.
6. Instruct client to turn onto back, directly onto board. Client may need assistance to turn.
7. Place both nurses on side of gurney or bed toward which client will be turned.
8. Assume appropriate body mechanics (broad base of support, one foot in front of the other, knees and hips flexed). Place weight on front foot.

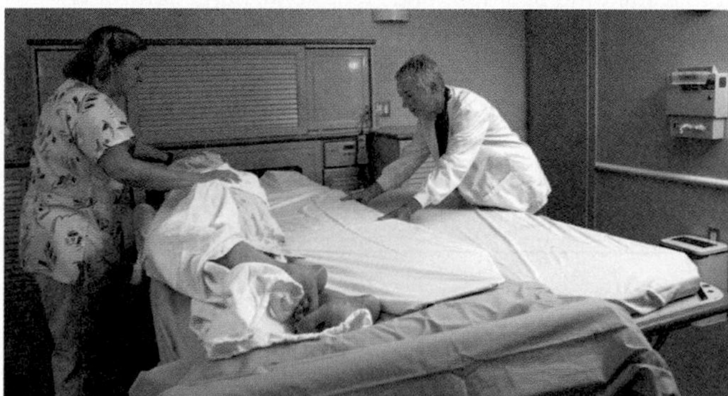

Move client to side of bed in lateral position and position transfer board.

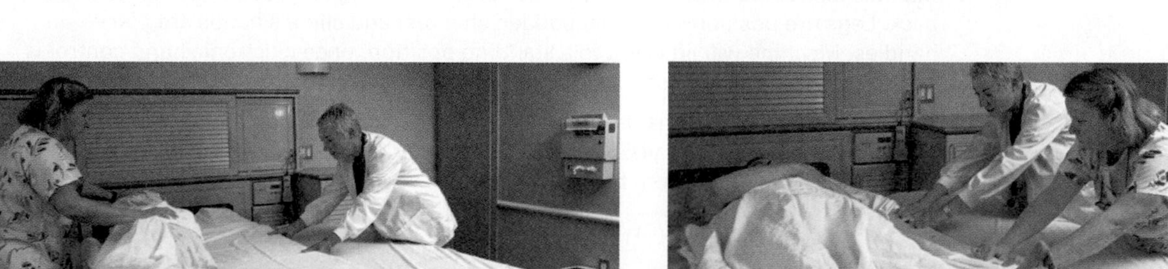

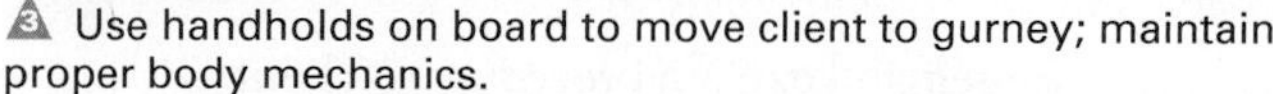

Use handholds on board to move client to gurney; maintain proper body mechanics.

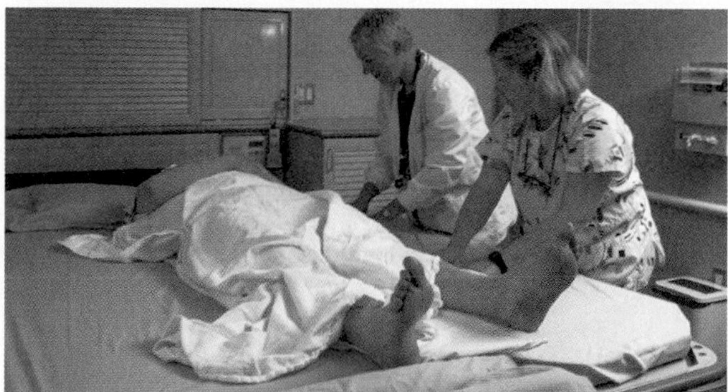

Two nurses move to transfer board side of gurney before moving client.

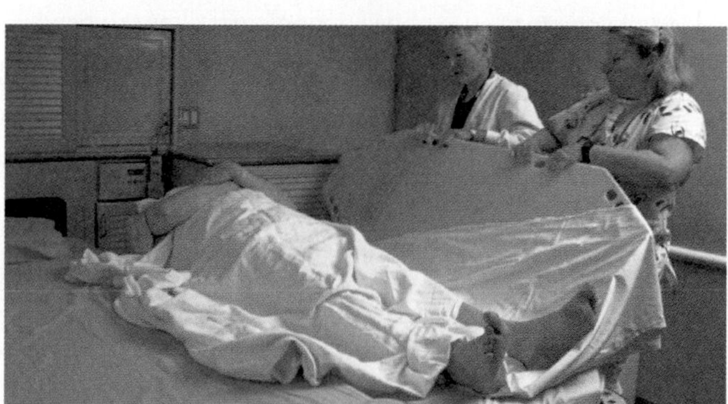

Remove transfer board after centering client on gurney.

9. Transfer weight on count of three from front to back foot as you lift board and pull it toward you.
10. Center client on gurney or bed and remove board by pulling board out and up using handholds along edge of board and using good body mechanics.
11. Place side rails in UP position, or according to facility policy.

NOTE: Lateral-assist devices can be used to transfer clients from bed to gurney.

TABLE 12-3 Assistive Devices for Moving/Turning Clients

Equipment/Device	Use for Client Moving/Handling
Gait belt	Assists client to walk when he/she has leg strength, can cooperate, and requires minimal assistance.
Lateral-assist devices (roller boards, side boards, friction-reducing lateral-assist devices)	Assists clients in lateral transfers, bed-to-gurney, and reduces client-surface friction during transfers, thus preventing skin breakdown and client discomfort. Friction-reducing sheets are used to position clients in bed and in lateral transfers.
Electric beds	Assists clients in lateral transfers. Position the bed so transfer surface (gurney) slightly lower than bed to allow client to move onto new surface. Beds can be placed in high-Fowler's position to assist client into sitting position for easier transfer out of bed.
Nonmechanical sit-to-stand aids	Assists clients with some arm strength and weight-bearing ability and who can follow simple directions to move out of bed. Once client stands, pulling self up by holding onto bars, a seat flap is lowered, and the client can rest on the seat. Transfers to commodes, toilets, showers can be accomplished using this device.
Powered stand-assist device	Assists clients who can bear weight on at least one leg and can follow simple instructions. Client is instructed to place feet on footrest while a sling is placed under arms and around back. Legs are positioned against padded shin rest and client's hands are placed on handles. Machine will lift client to a standing position, once electronic hand control is pushed by nurse. Device can be used to transport client to bathroom or chair.
Powered full-body lifts	Assists clients who are unable to bear any weight. These lifts can also be used to pick clients off the floor after falls. Sling is placed under client, then attached to a positioning bar. Client is then lifted from bed or floor. These lifts are portable or ceiling mounted.

Dangling at the Bedside

Procedure

1. Use two identifiers to identify client and perform hand hygiene.
2. Introduce self and explain procedure to client.
3. Lower bed to lowest position.
4. Move client to edge of bed and instruct client to bend knees. ▶ ***Rationale:*** This allows client to easily move legs and feet over side of bed onto floor.
5. Turn client onto side, keeping knees flexed, or place bed in Fowler's position (head elevated at 45° angle). ▶ ***Rationale:*** This position is sometimes preferred; it may be easier for nurse to pivot client to sitting position.
6. Stand at client's hip level. Assume broad base of support with forward foot closest to client. Flex your knees, hips, and ankles.
7. Place one of your arms under client's shoulders and other arm beneath client's thighs near knees. Instruct client to use arms to push shoulders up from bed. ▶ ***Rationale:*** This prevents client falling backward onto bed.

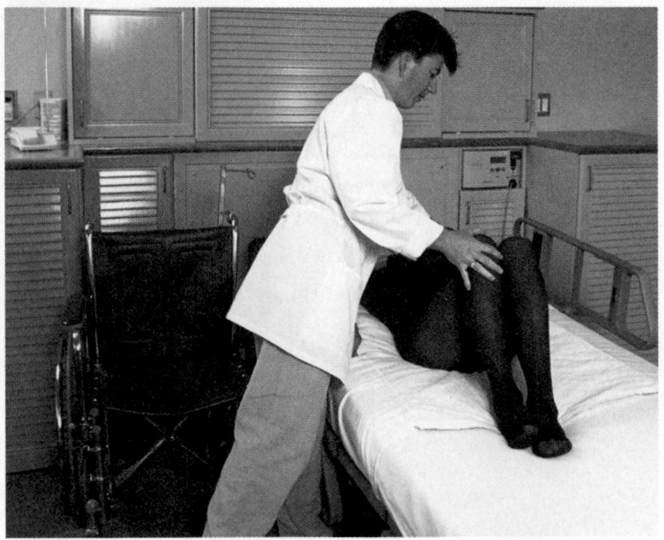

▲ Move client to side of bed and instruct to flex knees.

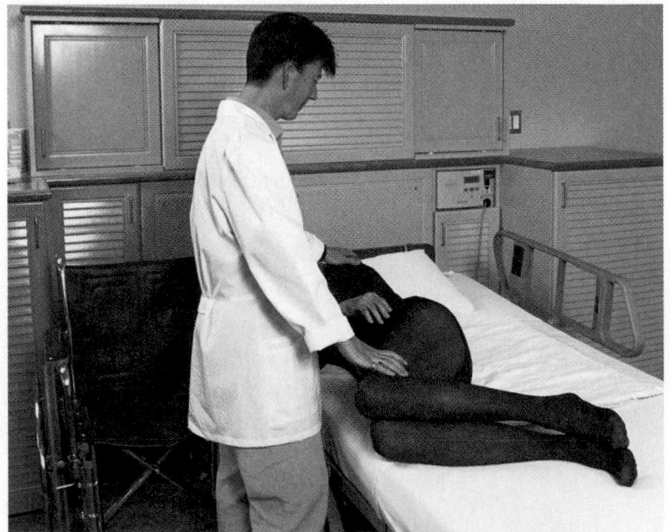

▲ Turn client onto side, maintaining knees in flexed position.

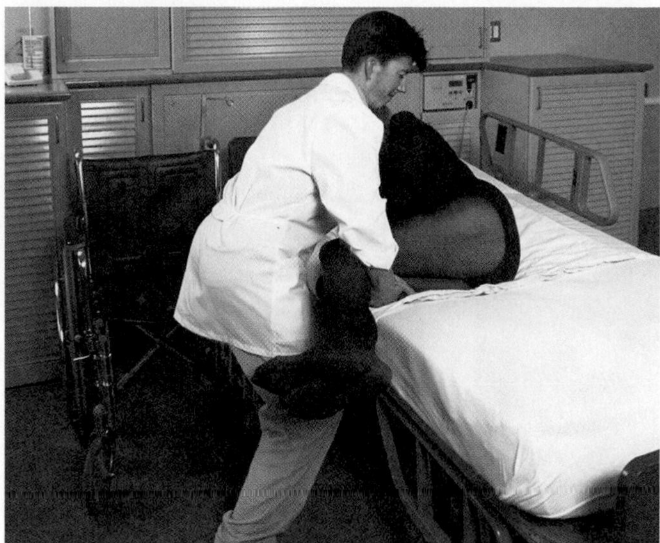
Maintain broad base of support as you pivot client to sitting position.

8. Lift client's thighs slightly and pivot on balls of your feet as you move client into sitting position. Use gluteal, abdominal, leg, and arm muscles to move client.
9. Stand in front of client until client is stable in upright position. ▸ ***Rationale:*** Client may experience orthostatic hypotension if he/she has been on bedrest for a period of time.

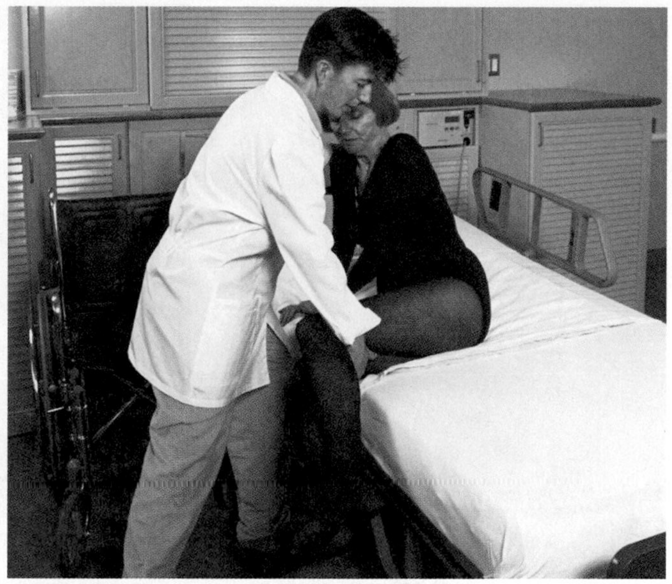
Dangle client with feet flat on floor for several minutes before transferring to chair or ambulating.

10. Take vital signs, especially if this is first time client is dangled. ▸ ***Rationale:*** To determine if orthostatic hypotension is present.
11. Dangle client with feet flat on the floor for a few minutes before transferring to chair or ambulating. ▸ ***Rationale:*** When feet are on floor, it helps to prevent clot formation.

Moving From Bed to Chair

Equipment

Chair
Gait belt

Procedure

1. Use two identifiers to identify the client and perform hand hygiene.
2. Lock bed in place.
3. Place chair at head of bed. If using wheelchair, remove arm and foot closest to bed to facilitate transfer.
4. Lock chair wheels or have someone hold chair as you move client.
5. Follow steps 4–6 in skill *Dangling at the Bedside.*
6. Dangle client until he or she is stable.
7. Give client nonskid shoes or slippers.
8. Place gait belt around client's waist and move client to side of bed using gait belt for support. ▸ ***Rationale:*** Helps stabilize client to prevent falls during transfer to chair.
9. Stand as close to client as possible, place your foot closest to chair between client's feet.

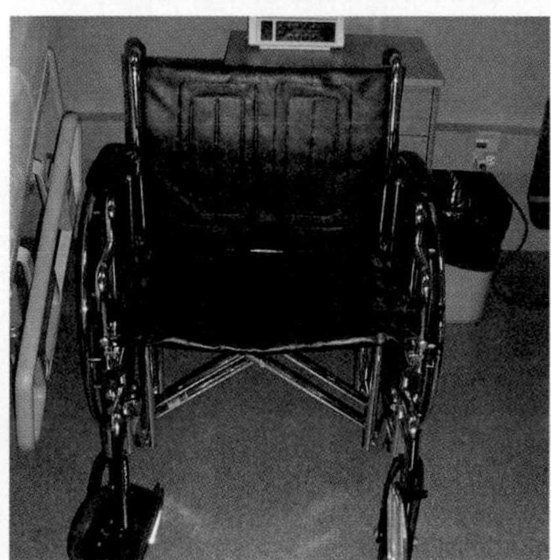
When using wheelchair, remove arm and foot closest to bed for ease of transfer.

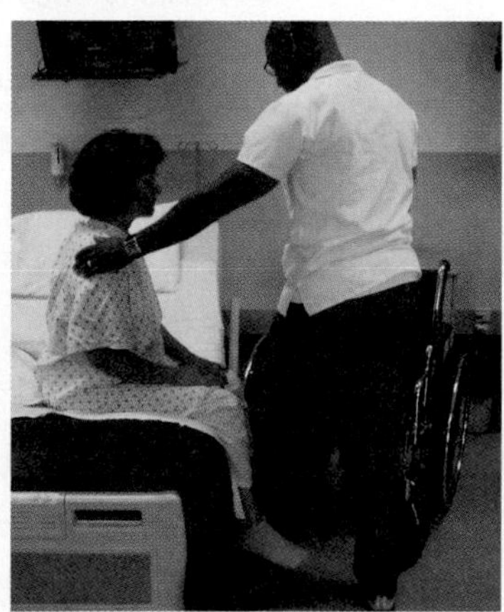
Pivot client to dangling position before placing feet on floor.

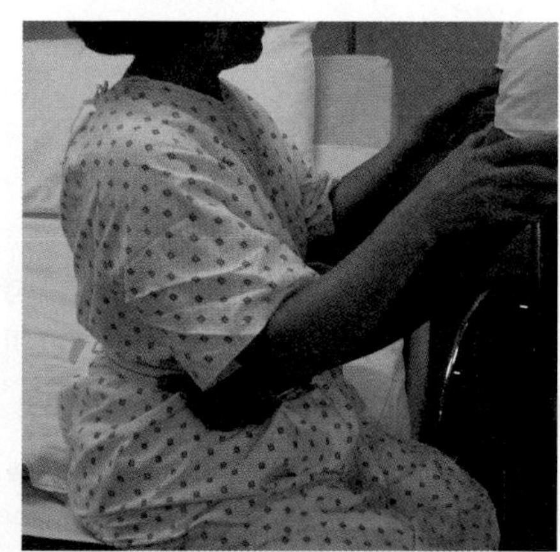
Move client to side of bed using gait belt for support.

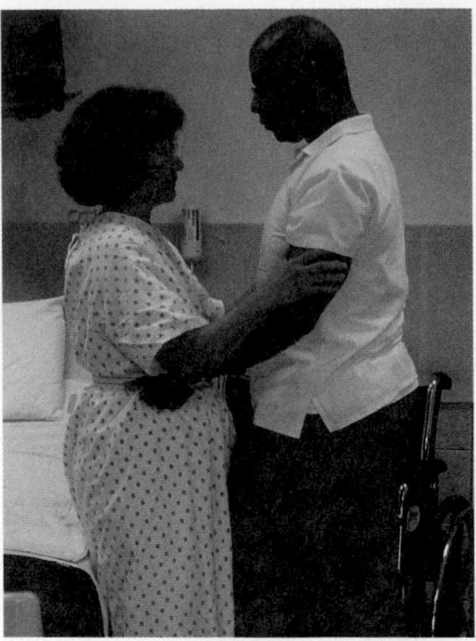

▲ Stand with your foot between client's feet; assist client to standing position.

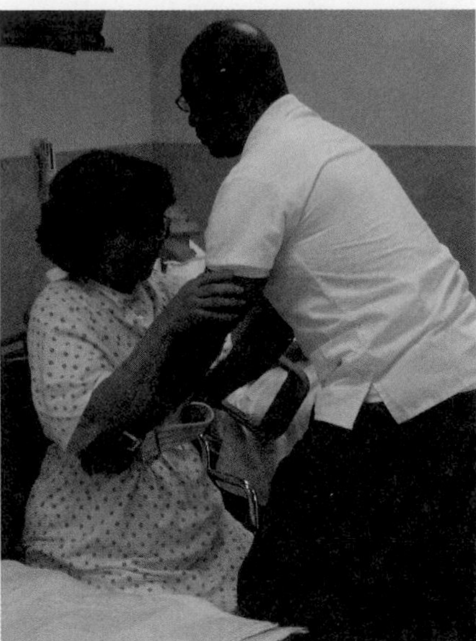

▲ Grasping gait belt for safe transfer, use leg muscles to pivot client into chair.

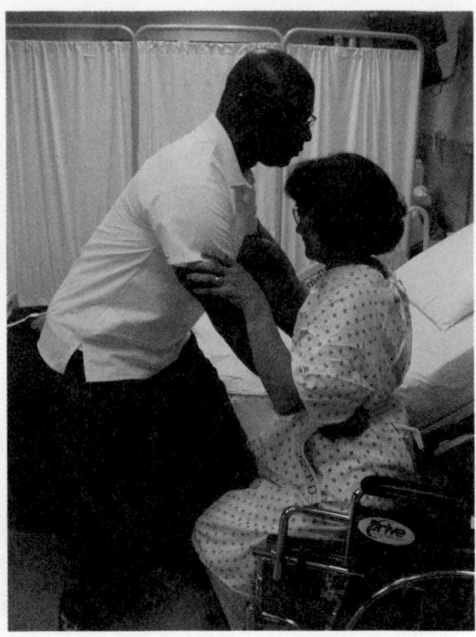

▲ Slowly lower client into chair while holding gait belt securely.

10. Bend your hips and knees, keeping back straight.
11. Rock client and, on count of three, assist client to standing position.
12. Grasp gait belt firmly for safe transfer while using leg muscles to pivot client to chair. Move your body in direction in which transfer is taking place.
13. Slowly lower client into chair.
14. Position client in chair to prevent pressure areas. If client has circulatory impairment, elevate legs while out of bed. ▶ ***Rationale:*** This promotes venous return.

NOTE: It is preferable to use the nonmechanical sit-to-stand aid for transferring clients out of bed unless they require minimal assistance.

Effectiveness of Safe Client Handling Using Assistive Equipment and Devices

Healthcare Staff Benefits

- Use of assistive client handling equipment and devices has made manual client handling unnecessary.
- New assistive devices control the ergonomic hazard associated with lifting and transferring clients, preventing injuries to staff.
- Injuries to nursing staff have decreased dramatically since the advent of the new devices and equipment, leading to cost savings for facilities for workers' compensation benefits.

Client Benefits in Use of Assistive Devices and Equipment

- Reduction in client falls and skin tears as a result of the new equipment and devices.
- Clients feel more secure with transfer and ambulation with new equipment and devices.
- Client is more comfortable in moving and turning using the new devices and equipment.
- Client's dignity is protected by using assistive equipment and devices.
- Assistive devices and equipment are selected to match the client's ability to assist in own movement, allowing client more autonomy.

Criteria for Selection of Lifting and Transfer Devices

- Appropriate for task to be accomplished
- Safe and stable for client's caregiver
- Comfortable for client
- Can be managed with relative ease
- Maneuverable in confined work space
- Efficient use of time
- Minimal maintenance required
- Equipment storage requirements reasonable
- Adequate numbers of device available
- Cost effectiveness

TABLE 12-4 Safe Client Handling Devices

	Device	Use
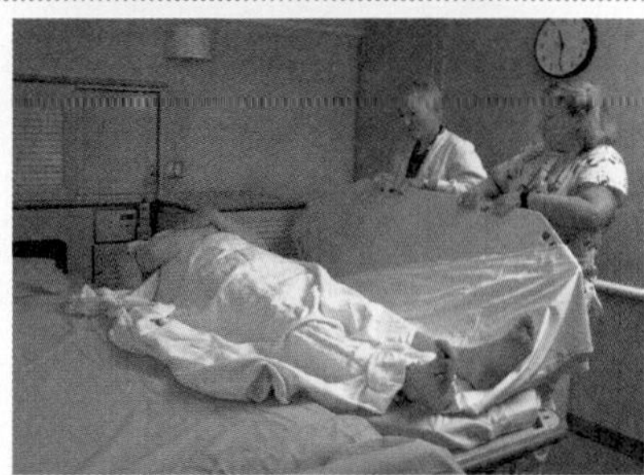	Gait belt	Assist client in walking if he/she has leg strength, can cooperate, and requires minimal assistance.
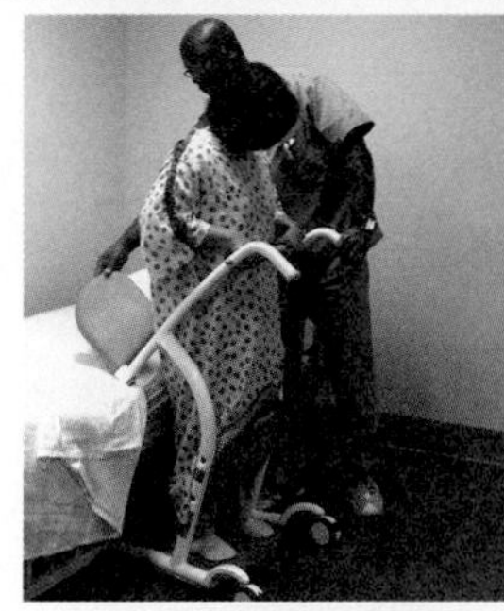	Lateral assist device	Slide boards can be used to transfer clients from bed to gurney.
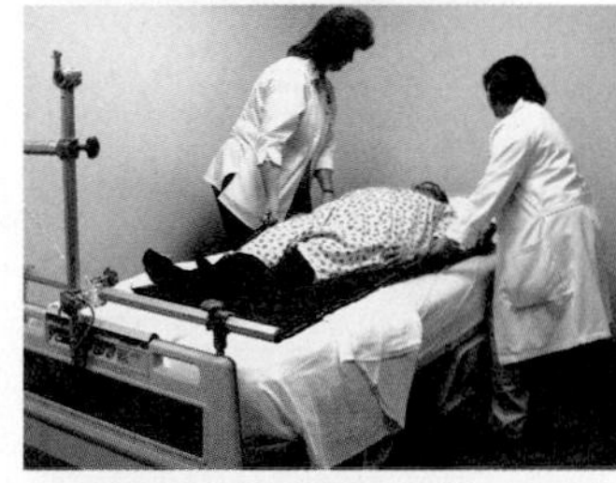	Nonmechanical sit-to-stand aid	Used to assist clients who have some arm strength and some weight-bearing ability out of bed. Client pulls self up by holding onto bar. Unfold a seat flap and have client sit on seat.
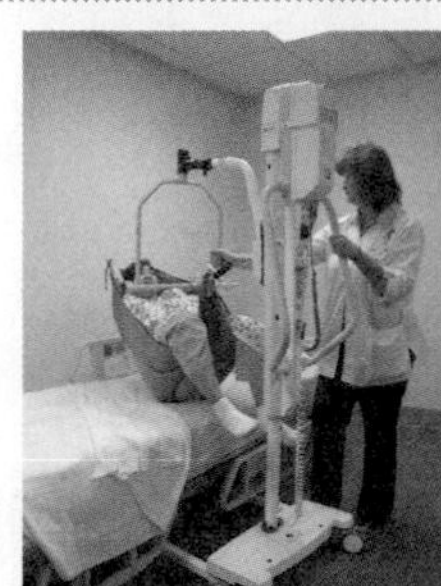	Friction-reducing sheet	Allows clients to be positioned in bed without causing shearing of the skin.
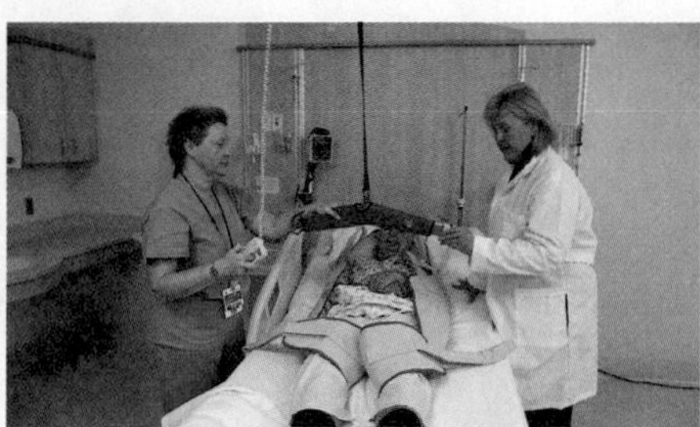	Powered full-body lift	Used for clients unable to bear weight. Clients can be moved out of bed or lifted off the floor after a fall. Ceiling-mounted lifts are also available.

NOTE: Follow manufacturer's directions for use of these assist devices.

Using a Floor-Based (Sling) Lift

Equipment

Floor-based lift (such as a Hoyer)
2 canvas pieces: 1 large, 1 small
2 sets of canvas straps

Procedure

1. Check orders and client care plan. Determine that lift can safely move the weight of the client.
2. Use two identifiers to identify client and explain procedure to client. ▸ ***Rationale:*** Clients may be frightened by use of a mechanical device.
3. Perform hand hygiene.
4. Bring floor-based frame to bedside.
5. Provide privacy for client.
6. Lock wheels of bed.
7. Place client's chair by the bed. Allow adequate space to maneuver the lift.
8. Raise bed to HIGH position and adjust head and knee gatch so that mattress is flat.
9. Keep side rail on opposite side in UP position.
10. Roll client away from you.
11. Place lower edge of wide canvas piece under client's knees.
12. Place upper edge of narrow canvas piece under client's shoulders.
13. Raise side rail on your side of bed.
14. Move to opposite side of bed and lower side rail.
15. Roll client away from you to opposite side and straighten out canvas pieces. Turn client to supine position.
16. Place U base of frame under bed on side where chair is positioned.
17. Lock wheels of frame. Lower side rail.
18. Attach canvas straps from swivel bar to each canvas piece using hooks.
19. Place straps evenly on canvas pieces. Sling extends from shoulders to knees. ▸ ***Rationale:*** This supports client's weight equally.
20. Elevate head of bed.
21. Raise client by turning release knob clockwise to close pressure valve.
22. Pump lift handle until client is lifted clear of the bed.
23. Maneuver client over the chair.
24. Lower client by turning release knob *slowly* counterclockwise.
25. Guide client into chair.
26. Align client into chair.
27. Remove straps from bar and move lift out of the way.
28. Check for client's comfort in chair; place call bell close at hand.
29. Perform hand hygiene.
30. Return client to bed using reverse method.

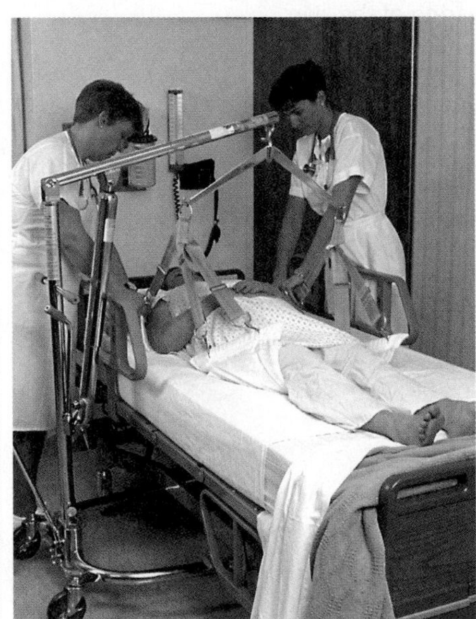

▲ Place canvas piece under client from knees to shoulders.

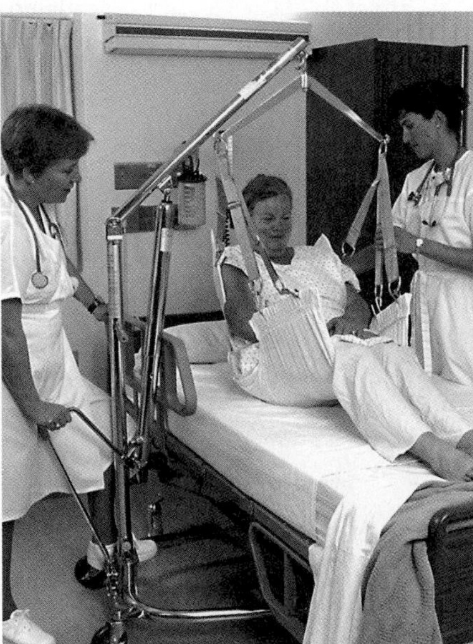

▲ Raise client off bed by turning release knob clockwise.

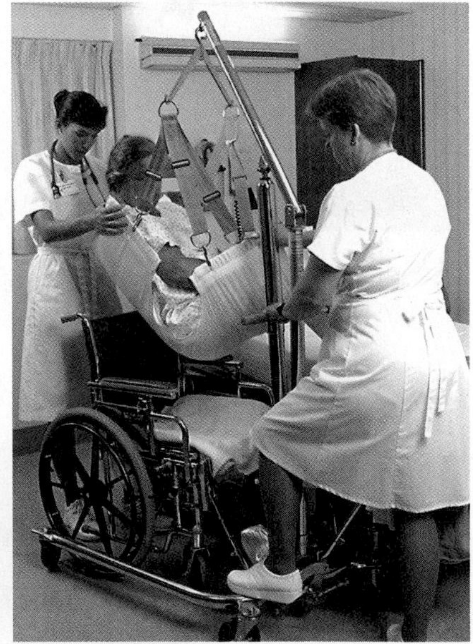

▲ Use one nurse to stabilize client as second nurse guides client into chair.

Using a Hydraulic Lift

Equipment

Sling
Mechanical lift device
Wheelchair

Preparation

1. Check physician's orders for type of assistive device ordered for client (check hospital's policy and procedure for available types of devices in facility).
2. Check equipment to ensure lift sling is intact (no frayed material or weak stitching; straps, hooks, and chains are intact), and mechanical lift devise is functioning appropriately. Check manufacturer's instructions and safety precautions.
3. Use two forms of identifiers to identify client, introduce yourself to client, and explain how the hydraulic lift will transfer the client to the chair or wheelchair.
4. Complete an assessment to determine client's willingness and ability to assist with transfer.
5. Check client's weight. ▶ ***Rationale:*** Some lifts state a weight restriction. If over weight level, a bariatric hydraulic device will need to be ordered.
6. Bring equipment to room.
7. Perform hand hygiene.
8. Provide privacy.

Procedure

1. Place wheelchair close to head of bed, leaving space to maneuver lift between bed and wheelchair.
2. Ensure bed wheels are locked, flat, and in high position.
3. Roll client on side, and with client holding side rail, place sling under client.
4. Roll client to other side and pull sling through and straighten sling flat.

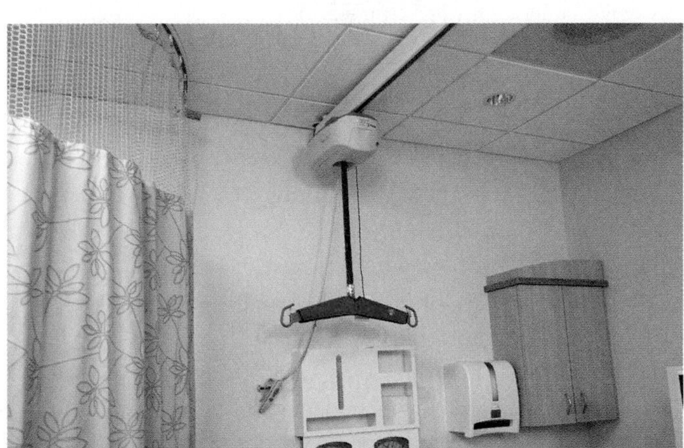

▲ Ceiling mounted lift device for client transfer.

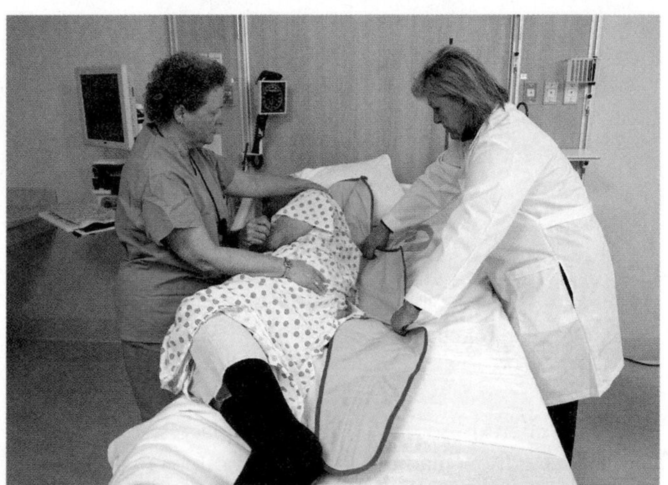

▲ Turn client to side and pull sling under client.

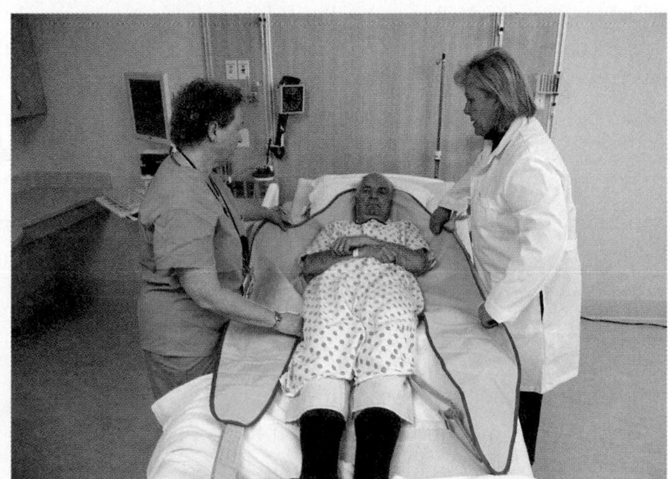

▲ Position client in center of sling.

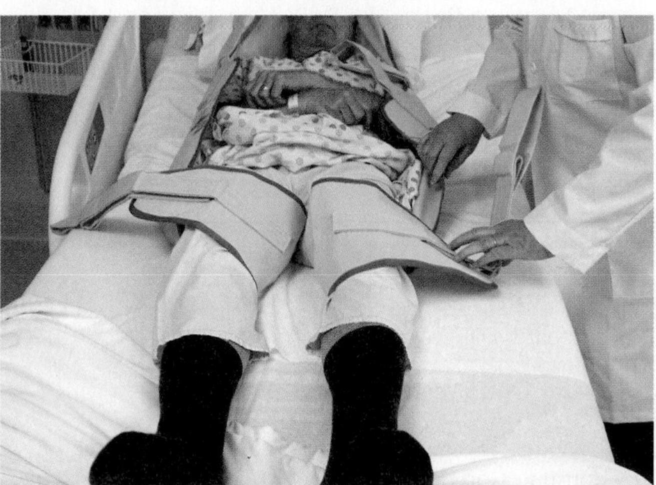

▲ Secure leg straps.

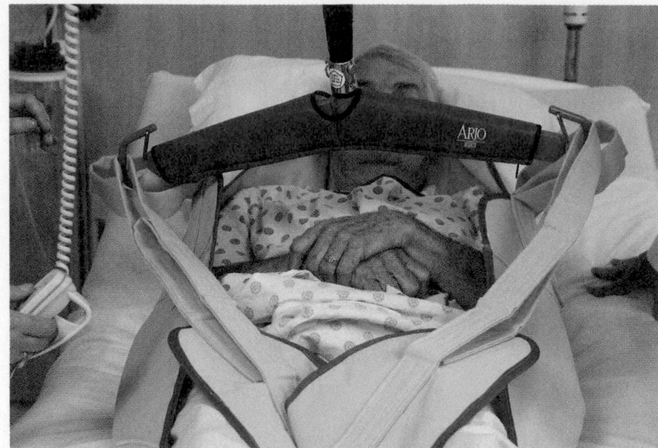

Ensure that sling is securely attached to assist device.

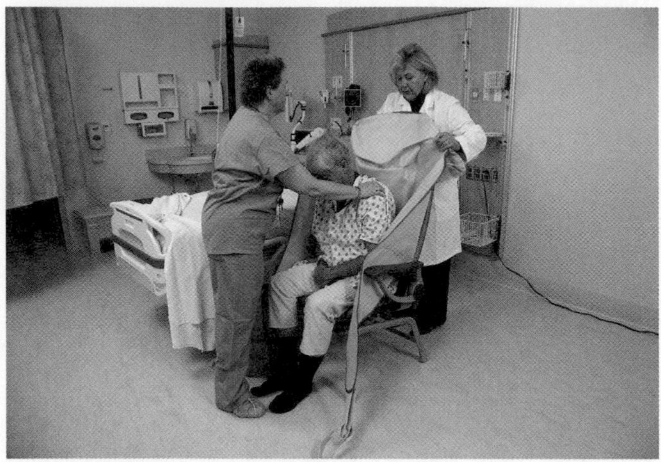

Remove sling for client comfort.

5. Place client in supine position and place leg loops over thighs. Follow manufacturer's instructions to place loops correctly.
6. Roll lift under bed as far as possible. The lift arm should be over client if appropriately placed. Ensure lift base is wide open. ▶ ***Rationale:*** Provides stability for lift.
7. Attach sling straps to lift arm. If using hooks, they should be pointed away from client.

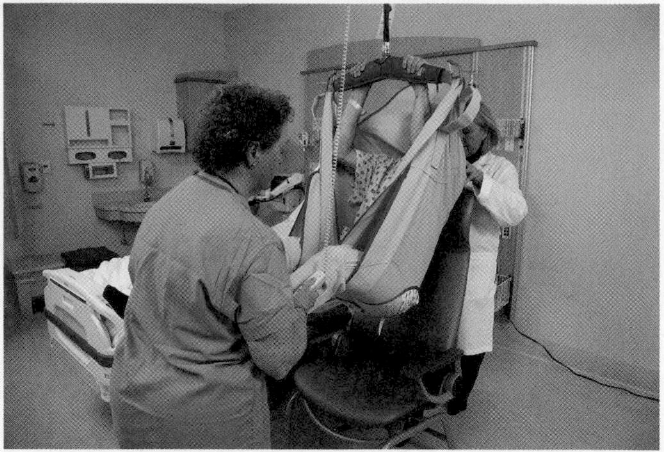

Move client directly over chair.

8. Elevate head of bed to place client in sitting position. Check manufacturer's instruction for client's hand placement.
9. Ensure wheelchair wheels are locked and client is instructed to remain very still during transfer. ▶ ***Rationale:*** Maintain the lift's stability.
10. Slowly raise sling until buttocks is just above mattress. ▶ ***Rationale:*** Self-leveling lift maintains client in sitting position.
11. Turn client to face second nurse who operates the lift. During turning, the client's legs are dangled off bed. Do not pull on client or the lift arm during this step of procedure.
12. Move lift away from bed by grasping steering bar and position client over wheelchair seat.
13. Slowly lower client onto wheelchair until he/she reaches a comfortable position.
14. Unhook sling from lift arm or remove chains or straps from sling. Keep sling in place under client. ▶ ***Rationale:*** Sling will be reattached to lift device to transfer back to bed.
15. Ensure client is positioned maintaining good body alignment.
16. Evaluate client's response to transfer and document findings.
17. Place overbed table near client. Place fluids, tissues, and personal items in easy reach.
18. Perform hand hygiene.

Using a Footboard

Equipment

Footboard

Procedure

1. Provide a footboard if client is unable to place feet in dorsal flexion or plantar flexion.
2. Cover footboard with a bath blanket to protect feet from rough surfaces.
3. Place footboard on bed in a place where client's feet can firmly rest on it without sliding down in bed.
4. Observe legs to ensure that they are not in a flexed position when feet are against the board.
5. Tuck top linen under mattress at foot of bed, and bring linen up over the footboard to the top of the bed. Do not drape top linen over footboard as it can easily be pulled off the bed.

6. Put feet and ankles through range-of-motion exercises every 4 hr for clients on prolonged bedrest.
7. Observe heels and ankles frequently for signs of breakdown.
8. Place pillow under client's calves (not under heels), allowing heels to be off mattress if skin breakdown is assessed.

NOTE: Clients are encouraged to wear high-top sneakers while on bedrest, along with the footboard. ▶ ***Rationale:*** Aids in preventing footdrop. Footboards are used to prevent plantar flexion. Extended periods of plantar flexion can lead to footdrop.

DOCUMENTATION for Moving and Turning Clients

- How often client is turned or moved
- Condition of skin and joint movement
- Unexpected problems with moving or positioning client and solutions to problems
- Client's acceptance of and feelings about the procedure
- Number of staff needed to complete the procedure
- Type of assistive devices needed from bed to chair, if appropriate
- Time client was in chair or dangling at bedside
- Use of a footboard or trochanter roll

Legal Considerations

Back Injuries From Lifting and Transferring

A suit was filed against a large nursing home chain by nursing assistants at five Pennsylvania nursing homes. The complaint with OSHA alleged they had suffered back injuries from lifting and transferring clients. After a 15-month investigation, OSHA issued citations against the nursing home for ergonomics violations under the "general duty" clause of the Occupational Safety and Health Act. The clause states that an employer must provide employees with a workplace free of recognized hazards that are causing or likely to cause death or physical harm. OSHA argued that transferring clients exposed CNAs to serious injury to the upper back and upper extremities. OSHA settled with the nursing home chain. Under the terms of the settlement, the nursing home chain agreed to purchase mechanical lifting equipment at all facilities, nationwide, and to train all workers in the use of the equipment.

Source: Mannix, R. (2002). Health Care Law.

CRITICAL THINKING Application

Expected Outcomes

- Client's comfort is increased.
- Skin remains intact without evidence of breakdown as a result of moving and turning.
- Breathing is adequate and unlabored.
- Joint movement is maintained.
- Footdrop is prevented.
- Body alignment is maintained.
- Mechanical equipment and devices are used in client transfers and repositioning as needed.
- Client is moved safely using appropriate device.

Unexpected Outcomes	Alternative Actions
Client unwilling to move due to fear of pain or discomfort.	• Explain rationale and need for the procedure more thoroughly. • If possible, check if client can be medicated before the procedure. • Obtain additional assistance to decrease client's apprehension.
Client unable to assist with movement.	• Use a friction-reducing sheet to provide more support for client. • Obtain additional assistance to help with moving "dead" weight.
Client unable to maintain any type of position without assistance.	• Use trochanter roll to prevent external rotation of client's hip. • Use foam bolsters to maintain side-lying positions. • Use folded towels, blankets, or small pillows to position client's hands and arms to prevent dependent edema.
Skin begins to break down.	• Change client position every 2 hr. • Request physician's order for therapeutic mattress or dressings for pressure ulcer(s) care.
Client frightened to use assistive device.	• Explain use of equipment (i.e., comfort and safety in transferring). • Demonstrate equipment before using.

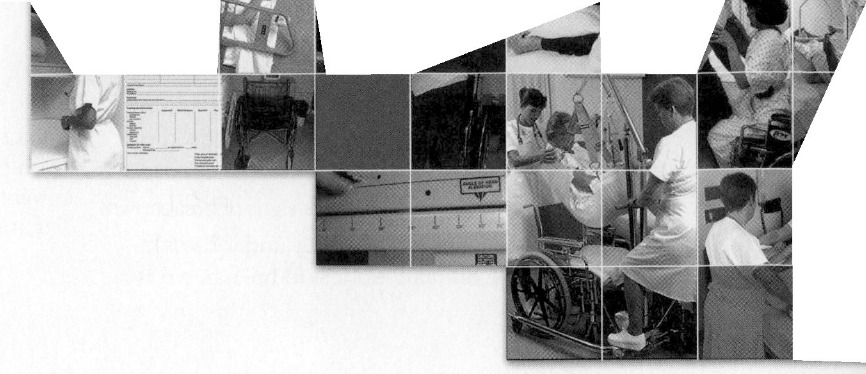

Chapter 12

UNIT 3 Adaptations for Home Care

Nursing Process Data

ASSESSMENT Data Base

- Assess safety factors in home
- Check equipment for safety features
- Determine client's safety in home
- Determine caretaker's ability to provide client care and safety
- Determine need for additional client equipment to promote client and caregiver safety

PLANNING Objectives

- To provide a comfortable and safe client environment
- To ensure caregiver's safety while providing client care
- To provide necessary home care treatments utilizing appropriate safety equipment

IMPLEMENTATION Procedures

EVALUATION Expected Outcomes

- Safe environment is provided for client
- Healthcare worker's safety is maintained during home visit

Pearson Nursing Student Resources

Find additional review materials at **nursing.pearsonhighered.com**

Prepare for success with NCLEX®-style practice questions and Skill Checklists

Evaluating Client's Safety

Procedure

1. Evaluate client's cognitive abilities: level of consciousness, orientation, ability to make appropriate judgments, ability to follow commands and directions.
   a. Knowledge of how to operate appliances (e.g., stoves and heaters).
   b. History of alcohol or drug abuse.
   c. Knowledge of medication times and doses to be taken.
   d. Knowledge of how to call for help: physician, nurse, fire, police.
2. Evaluate client's sensory and motor function.
   a. Hearing and vision acuity
   b. Ability to ambulate with assistance
   c. Need for assistive devices or support in ambulation
3. Determine client's ability to manage self-care.
   a. Bathing, grooming, and dressing
   b. Preparing food and feeding
   c. Toileting
   d. Housekeeping, shopping, transportation to physician and pharmacy
4. Assess if client needs alternatives to physical restraints.
   a. Determine if environment needs to be modified by removing unsafe objects or barriers.
   b. Remove wheels from chairs or bed.
   c. Install bed check system or alarm device.
   d. Decrease auditory and visual stimuli.
   e. Place supplies close to bed or chair (e.g., tissues, water).
   f. Develop routine for client.
5. Evaluate most effective type of restraint, if absolutely necessary.
   a. Determine that less restrictive methods have been attempted.
   b. Assess purpose of restraint to determine most appropriate type.
   c. Obtain physician's order for restraint. Order must include reason, type, and time of restraints.
   d. Obtain informed consent from client or guardian before applying.
   e. Explain purpose of restraints to client and family members.
   f. Ensure caregiver is instructed on use of restraints.
   g. Evaluate effectiveness and continued need for restraints.
6. Determine client's financial support.
   a. Determine healthcare insurance plan, workers' compensation, Medicare, Medicaid.
   b. Determine need for social service intervention.

NOTE: The safety issues in the home are similar to the safety issues of hospitalized clients.

Assessing Caregiver's Safety

Procedure

1. Determine caregiver's cognitive function.
   a. Ability to understand and carry out interventions
   b. Ability to make safe decisions and judgments
   c. Willingness to care for client
2. Determine caregiver's sensory and motor function.
   a. Ability to hear client's needs
   b. Visual acuity to read directions, medication labels
   c. Ability to feel temperature changes (e.g., water for bathing)
3. Determine caregiver's motor function and strength.
   a. Ability to assist client in transfer, moving, turning, and ADLs
   b. Ability to provide treatments and care for client
   c. Ability to prepare food and do housekeeping chores
   d. Ability to do shopping and provide transportation for physician visits
4. Determine need for client care assistance with ADLs
   a. Type of wheelchair, with or without removable arms
   b. Shower chairs that fit over toilet or in shower
   c. Toilet seat risers
5. Determine need for type of transfer assist devices for safe client handling.
   a. Gait belts: provide secure grip without holding onto client's clothes or limbs. ▶ ***Rationale:*** Prevents caregiver strain as client weight is closer to caregiver and he/she can assume upright position.
   b. Small slide/transfer board: used for seated lateral transfers, such as between bed and wheelchair or commode. ▶ ***Rationale:*** Caregiver does not need to manually lift client.
   c. Turning discs: used to pivot seated clients who can bear weight and stand. The client is guided to a standing position without adjusting their feet. The client must be able to stand or the caregiver will have to exert excessive force in an awkward position.
   d. Mechanical lift devices such as the Lean–Stand Assist Lift and Sling–Type Full Lift are used for clients who cannot support their own weight.
   e. Repositioning devices: mechanically pull client up in bed without need for caregiver to assist client.
   f. Trapeze lifts: a bar device suspended above the bed that allows clients to reposition. Client must have upper body muscle strength in order to reposition in bed.

DOCUMENTATION for Home Care

- Client's assessment findings determining ability to care for self and transfer from bed to wheelchair/chair
- Type of assistive devices used in moving and/or transferring client
- Client's ability to assist with transfer and repositioning
- Client's response to moving and repositioning

CRITICAL THINKING Application

Expected Outcomes

- Client is safely repositioned or transferred without injury to client or caregiver.
- Appropriate assistive devices are utilized to transfer client.
- Caregiver is able to manage turning, repositioning, and managing assistive devices.
- Appropriate body mechanisms are utilized by caregiver.

Unexpected Outcomes	Alternative Actions
Unable to transfer client from bed to wheelchair due to excess weight.	• Determine if wheelchair without arms or transfer board can aid in transfer. • Contact social services to obtain bariatric assist devices. • Determine if other family members can assist with transfer. • May need home health aide services to assist with transfer.
Injury occurs to client when caregiver attempts transfer to wheelchair.	• Do not continue to reposition client, place in bed. • Complete sensory, motor, and pain assessment. • Notify physician. • Document findings.

GERONTOLOGIC Considerations

Physiologic Age Changes in the Musculoskeletal System That Affect Nursing Care of the Elderly

- Contractures—muscles atrophy, regenerate slowly; tendons shrink and sclerose.
- Range of motion of joints decreases—lack of adequate joint motion, ankylosis.
- Mobility level is limited—muscle strength lessens and gait may be unsteady.
- Kyphosis occurs—cervical vertebrae may be flexed; intervertebral discs narrow.
- Bodies of thoracic vertebrae compress slowly with aging, leading to the hunchback appearance—loss of overall height results from disk shrinkage and kyphosis.
- Bone changes—loss of trabecular bones and bones become brittle.
- Osteoporosis occurs as a result of calcium loss from the bone and insufficient replacement.
- Osteoarthritis increases with age, equally affecting men and women. This condition results in physical stress on joints as a result of long-term mechanical, horizontal, chemical, and genetic factors.

Psychosocial and Physiological Changes in Elderly Who Are Immobilized

- At risk for confusion, depression, and disorientation—keep clock and calendar in room to help reorient to time and place.
- More susceptible to hazards of immobility—maintain own ADLs as much as possible and change position every 2 hr.

Aging and Changes in Ability to Maintain Activity Levels

- As aging occurs, there is a decrease in the rate or speed of activity.
- Loss of muscle mass interferes with activities that require strength such as bending down, dressing, and reaching for objects.
- Dexterity decreases, leading to a change in performing manipulative skills.

Nursing Care for Positioning Elderly Clients

- Ambulate within limitations of age.
- Alter position every 2 hr; align correctly.
- Prevent osteoporosis of long bones by providing exercises against resistance as ordered.
- Provide active and passive exercises—rest periods necessary and exercise paced throughout the day for the elderly.
- Provide range-of-motion exercises to all joints three times a day.
- Educate family that allowing the client to be sedentary is not helpful.
- Encourage walking, which is the best single exercise for the elderly.

MANAGEMENT Guidelines

Each state legislates a Nurse Practice Act for RNs and LVN/LPNs. Healthcare facilities are responsible for establishing and implementing policies and procedures that conform to their state's regulations. Verify the regulations and role parameters for each healthcare worker in your facility.

Delegation

- All levels of healthcare workers can be assigned to move and turn clients and provide assistance with transfers.
- Positioning clients in bed can be assigned to all levels of healthcare workers.
- Frequently, the physical therapist is assigned to work with postoperative clients or clients requiring special transfer techniques or ambulation until clients are released to nursing.
- Before assigning staff to logroll a client or use assistive devices for moving a client out of bed, ensure they have been properly instructed in the procedures and safety issues associated with these activities.

Communication Matrix

- The RN must give specific directions to the healthcare workers on appropriate positions for clients on bedrest or specifics on how to transfer clients to a chair or gurney.
- Before physical therapy releases clients to nursing for transfer or ambulation activities, the RN must obtain explicit information on the procedures to be used. This information must be written on the Kardex or computer record, as well as reviewed with all staff assigned to the client.
- A team conference may be necessary if special equipment or specific activities are required by a client. This conference ensures all staff will be given a demonstration and provided information necessary for safe client care.
- The RN must ensure that all new personnel are proficient in transfers, logrolling, and use of the assistive devices before assigning them to care for clients requiring these skills.
- It is crucial for safe client care that the RN monitors healthcare workers when they perform logrolling or use mechanical devices for transfer after the initial demonstration.

CRITICAL THINKING Strategies

Scenario 1

You are assigned to a medical unit where many of the clients require assistance moving in and out of bed. The following clients are assigned to you for care on the day shift.

- Onica Jones, 89-year-old (CVA) client who has weakness on the right side and is unable to communicate but seems to understand directions. She has been in the hospital for 4 days and will be transferred to an SNF this afternoon.
- James Metcalf, 60-year-old (MI) client who is about to be discharged. However, you notice he still has not been able to ambulate by himself.
- Madeline Oscar, 70-year-old client with Parkinson's disease and hospitalized for pneumonia. She was admitted last night. She has orders to be up in the chair BID.
- Joseph Nichols, 40-year-old client, hospitalized for possible kidney stones. He is in severe pain and the MD has ordered that he remain on bedrest until further orders.

1. Which client will you assess first? Provide rationale for your answer.
2. How will you determine the client's ability to assist with his or her own care and movement in bed?
3. For each client, identify the type of assistance he or she might need; provide rationale for your answer.
4. Describe the body mechanics you will use when moving clients; this will be based on the type of moving that will need to be performed for each of the four clients.

Scenario 2

You are assigned to care for a client who weighs 300 lb. The client was out of bed for lunch and now insists on getting back into bed. There are insufficient staff members available to help you. The client is able to weight bear but needs maximal assistance to stand.

1. Suggest creative resolutions to this problem.
2. Describe the procedure you will use to transfer the client from chair to bed.
3. If mechanical devices are not available, what action will you take?

NCLEX® Review Questions

Unless otherwise specified choose only one (1) answer.

1. The most effective method for teaching student nurses principles of moving clients is to discuss:
    1. Using a back brace when lifting clients.
    2. Instructions on safe lifting techniques using two to three nurses for heavy clients.
    3. Education related to body mechanics.
    4. Proper use of lift teams for moving clients.

2. According to the National Institute for Occupational Safety and Health (NIOSH), the average client weight that should be lifted by healthcare workers is ________ pounds.
   1. 51.
   2. 75.
   3. 100.
   4. 169.
3. Applying body mechanics includes which of the following principles? Select all that apply.
   1. Establish a base of support by placing the feet close together.
   2. Hold abdomen firm and bend at the waist when lifting client.
   3. Keep weight to be lifted as close to your body as possible when moving clients.
   4. Align three natural curves in your back when moving clients.
4. Maintaining proper body alignment is critical for nurses to prevent injuries when providing client care. Which of the following steps would *not* be included in teaching appropriate body alignment?
   1. The most comfortable height at which to provide client care is above the nurse's waist.
   2. Flex your knees if you need to work at lower than waist level.
   3. Triceps, quadriceps, and gluteal muscles are used when moving and turning clients.
   4. Push, pull, or roll objects instead of lifting whenever possible.
5. If you are injured while providing client care, it is important you immediately
   1. Complete an unusual occurrence (or incident report) form.
   2. Inform charge nurse you need to go home to rest and apply ice.
   3. Report the injury to your supervisor.
   4. Ask for a change in your assignment to prevent reinjury.
6. There is an order for a client to be placed in a low-Fowler's position. You will place the bed in a ________ degree position.
   1. 60.
   2. 45.
   3. 30.
   4. 15
7. During report the team leader stated, "the client needs to be turned to a lateral position every 2 hr." You recall the best way to turn the client is to
   1. Ask a second nurse to assist you in turning the client to his/her side.
   2. Ask the lift team to come every 2 hr to turn the client.
   3. Place a friction-reducing sheet under the client to assist in turning.
   4. Explain to the client that he/she needs to move up in bed before you can assist in turning the client to a lateral position.
8. A client is being moved from the bed to a gurney using a transfer board. The directions given the client include
   1. "You need to move toward the side of the bed nearest the gurney before being placed on the slide board."
   2. "Roll directly onto the transfer board and position yourself on your side."
   3. "The nurse will place the board close to you and you need to roll over the edge of the board onto the gurney while staying in a side-lying position."
   4. "Turn onto your back, directly onto the transfer board."
9. A client assessment indicates the client has some arm strength and weight-bearing ability and can follow simple directions to move out of bed. The most appropriate assistive device to move this client out of bed is the
   1. Powered full-body lift.
   2. Powered stand assist device.
   3. Nonmechanical sit-to-stand aid.
   4. Lateral assist device.
10. As part of a home care admission assessment, you need to determine a client's "Safe Handling and Movement" abilities. This assessment criteria includes: ***Select all that apply.***
    1. Weight-bearing capability.
    2. Client's level of cooperation and comprehension.
    3. Ability to assist in transfer.
    4. Need for assistive device.

13

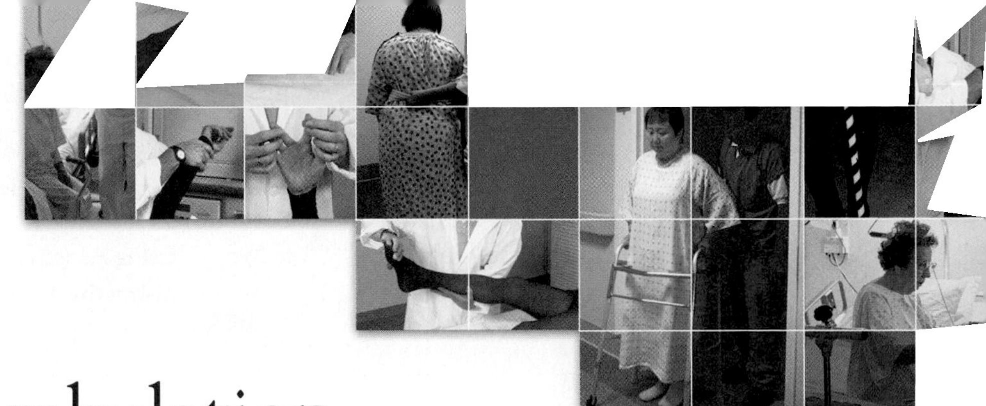

Exercise and Ambulation

LEARNING OBJECTIVES

1. Define rehabilitative nursing.
2. Compare and contrast preservative and restorative methods of care.
3. Identify the joints and the type of movement they accommodate.
4. Compare and contrast passive and active range of motion exercises.
5. Demonstrate passive range-of-motion exercises using all muscle groups.
6. Explain the rationale of assisted ambulation for clients.
7. Complete a client teaching guide for clients requiring muscle-strengthening exercises.
8. Demonstrate the proper method for measuring crutches.
9. Compare and contrast the four crutch-walking gaits.
10. Demonstrate the four crutch-walking gaits.
11. List the components of crutch walking that require documentation.
12. Identify the steps in measuring a client for a cane.
13. Describe client instructions for using a cane.
14. Describe client instructions for using a walker.
15. Write three nursing diagnoses that are appropriate for clients requiring exercise and ambulation activities.
16. Describe safety steps necessary when home care client requests use of assistive devices.

CHAPTER OUTLINE

TERMINOLOGY

Abduction movement of a bone away from the midline of the body or body part, as in raising the arm or spreading the fingers.

Adduction movement of a bone toward the midline of the body or part, as in lowering the arm from a raised position.

Alignment arranged in a straight line; position of body parts in relation to each other.

Ambulate walking; able to walk.

Antagonists muscles that exert an action opposing that of prime mover.

Atrophy a wasting or decrease in size of any organ or body part due to lack of nutrients or oxygen, causing death and reabsorption of cells.

Base of support foundation on which a person's body weight is supported.

Balance a result of body alignment that maintains equilibrium, coordination, and stability of the body in space.

Cardiovascular pertaining to heart and blood vessels.

Circumduction to revolve around an axis in such a way that the proximal end of a limb is fixed and the distal end traces a circle.

Contractility ability of muscle to shorten, tighten, and contract.

Dorsiflexion flexion of the foot at the ankle joint; the act of turning the foot and toes upward, as in standing on the heel.

Elasticity ability of strained muscle to regain original size and shape when applied force is removed.

Eversion turning outward; movement of the foot at the ankle joint so that the sole faces outward.

Excitability capacity of muscle to respond to stimulus without intervention of motor nerves.

Extensibility ability of muscle to stretch in response to applied force.

Extension a movement that increases the angle between two bones, straightening a joint.

Fibrous repair and replacement of inflamed tissues or organs by connective tissue.

Flaccidity decrease in muscle tone.

Flexion a movement that decreases the angle between two bones; the act of bending a joint.

Fracture any break or crack in a bone.

Hyperextension continuation of extension beyond the anatomic position, as in bending the head backward.

Hypertrophy increased muscle fiber leading to increased muscle shape and size.

Inversion turning inward; movement of the foot at the ankle joint so that the sole faces inward.

Ligament a band or sheet of strong fibrous connective tissue connecting the articular ends of bones serving to bind them together and to facilitate or limit motion.

Mobility state or quality of being mobile; facility of movement.

Musculoskeletal pertaining to the muscles and bones.

Paralysis temporary or permanent loss of function, especially loss of sensation or voluntary motion.

Plantar flexion extension of the foot at the ankle joint; the foot and toes are turned downward toward the sole of the foot, as in standing on tiptoe.

Posture attitude or position of body.

Prime movers muscles responsible for the essential movement of contraction.

Pronation rotation of the forearm so that the palm faces backward or downward; movement of the whole body so that the face and abdomen are downward.

Prone lying horizontal with face downward.

Protraction movement of the clavicle (collar bone) or mandible (lower jaw) forward on a plane parallel to the ground.

Proximal nearest the point of attachment or reference point.

Range-of-motion extent to which a joint can move through active or passive exercises.

Retraction movement of the clavicle or mandible backward on a plane parallel to the ground.

Rotation movement of a bone around its own axis, as in moving the head to indicate "no" or turning the palm of the hand up and then down.

Spasticity increase in muscle tension.

Sprain injury caused by wrenching or twisting of a joint that results in tearing or stretching of the associated ligaments.

Strain injury caused by excessive force or stretching of muscles or tendons around the joint.

Supination rotation of forearm so that the palm faces forward or upward; movement of the whole body so that the face and abdomen are upward.

Synergists muscles that enhance action of prime mover.

Tendons fibrous connective tissue serving for the attachment of muscles to bones and other parts.

Tonicity ability of muscle to maintain steady contraction, which determines its firmness.

Ulcer a lesion of the skin marked by inflammation, necrosis, and sloughing of damaged tissue.

REHABILITATION CONCEPTS

Rehabilitative nursing involves the prevention and correction of alterations in the musculoskeletal system. In fact, the definition of rehabilitative nursing is the process of restoring a person's ability to live and work in as normal a manner as possible. To assist clients to achieve and maintain optimal mobility, both preservative and restorative methods are used.

Preservative methods, such as exercises and assisted ambulation, include those interventions that are needed to help clients maintain their normal mobility. Because the changes that occur in the human body when a person is hospitalized are varied and subtle, preservative methods are used with every client. Restorative methods, such as crutch walking and splinting, are used with clients who have decreased mobility caused by such factors as debilitating illness or major surgery. The purpose for applying restorative methods is to assist the client in achieving the level of mobility he or she enjoyed before becoming ill.

The general goals for using these methods are to assist the client to strive for optimal function, to prevent further injury, and to restore the client's mobility to as close to normal function as possible. To achieve these goals of care, it is important for the nurse to accept the philosophy underlying rehabilitative nursing: that every illness is accompanied by the intrinsic threat of disability and that this part of total client care must begin with the initial client contact. Finally, it is important to accept that the principles of rehabilitation are basic to the care of all clients and that rehabilitation must be begun early in the client's hospitalization.

Being hospitalized and immobile seriously affects a person's body image, behavior, and overall adaptation and adjustment. The greater the disability, the more these aspects of a person's life are affected. The nurse's responsibility in providing total client care is to be aware of these responses and to take them into account when developing a client care plan.

MUSCULOSKELETAL SYSTEM

The musculoskeletal system is composed of bones, muscles, joints, cartilage, bursa, tendons, and ligaments. The bones form the infrastructure of the system. The ability of bones to provide weight bearing and mobility is in direct relationship to the size and shape of the bones.

Joints, in conjunction with muscles, provide motion and flexibility. Skeletal muscles are under voluntary control as a result of being innervated by somatic nerves. Muscles, through their ability to contract, convert energy into mechanical work, maintain body alignment, and cause movement.

The muscular system is a system of more than 600 fibers that are attached to bones. The system allows for body movement under the control of the voluntary nervous system. Muscles provide for body movement or locomotion, support the body, and perform several body functions, such as the partial production of heat. The fibers of the voluntary muscles are grouped together in a sheath of connective tissue. Each bundled group of muscle fibers is surrounded by a connective tissue sheath. The sheath tissue may be continuous with fibrous tissue that extends from the muscle as a tendon.

There are several properties of muscle fibers. The first is excitability, or the capacity of a muscle to respond to stimulus without intervention of the motor nerves. Another property is contractility, the ability of a muscle to shorten, tighten, or contract. Muscles are also able to maintain steady contraction (tonicity), stretch in response to applied force (extensibility), and regain their original size and shape when applied force is removed (elasticity).

Muscle Function

Skeletal muscles produce body movements by pulling on the bones. Bones serve as levers, and joints serve as fulcrums of these levers. Each muscle has a point of origin and a point of insertion that are usually attached to the bone. Muscles that move a body part usually do not extend over that part. These muscles usually perform with group action; some contract, and others relax. Prime movers are muscles responsible for the primary movement of contraction. Antagonists are muscles that exert an action opposing that of the prime movers. Synergists are muscles that enhance action of the prime mover. The accessory parts to muscles are the ligaments and the tendons.

JOINTS

A joint of the body is the point at which two or more bones join together. The function of a joint is skeletal flexibility and motion. Joints are classified according to structural variations that allow for different kinds of movements. There are three main types of classification: synarthrotic, amphiarthrotic, and diarthrotic joints.

Synarthrotic joints are immovable and include those areas where tissue grows between articulating surfaces, such as the suture lines of the skull. Amphiarthrotic joints have limited movement. Diarthrotic joints have two freely movable parts. This type of joint is a cavity enclosed by a capsule lined with synovial membrane, which secretes a lubricant. The following types of joint movement allow for structural variations:

- Hinge: allows single directional movement (elbow).
- Ball-and-socket: allows bending (hip).
- Saddle: allows multidirectional shifting (thumb).
- Pivot: allows rotary movement (neck, cervical spine).
- Gliding: allows limited sliding of bones against each other (wrist, ankle, invertebral joints).

Each of these types of joints have specific kinds of movements they can perform. These movements can be described in relationship to the three body planes: sagittal, transverse, and coronal. The sagittal plane divides the body into two portions with a straight vertical line between the two parts. The transverse plane divides the body into upper–lower portions with a horizontal line. The coronal plane divides the body into anterior–posterior portions at right angles to the sagittal plane. The joints accomplish a variety of movements that range from flexion–extension to rotation and circumduction. For definitions of joint movements through the planes of the body, refer to the following.

Joint Movements

Abduction: Movement of a bone away from the midline of the body or body part, as in raising the arm or spreading the fingers.

Adduction: Movement of a bone toward the midline of the body or part.

Circumduction: Movement of a bone in a circular direction so that the distal end scribes a circle while the proximal end remains stationary, as in "winding up" to throw a ball.

Extension: A movement that increases the angle between two bones, straightening a joint.

Eversion: Turning outward; movement of the foot at the ankle joint so that the sole faces outward.

Flexion: A movement that decreases the angle between two bones; the act of bending a joint.

Hyperextension: Continuation of extension beyond the anatomic position, as in bending the head backward.

Inversion: Turning inward; movement of the foot at the ankle joint so that the sole faces inward.

Pronation: Rotation of the forearm so that the palm faces backward or downward; movement of the whole body so that the face and abdomen are downward.

Protraction: Movement of the clavicle (collar bone) or mandible (lower jaw) forward on a plane parallel to the ground.

Retraction: Movement of the clavicle or mandible backward on a plane parallel to the ground.

Rotation: Movement of a bone around its own axis, as in moving the head to indicate "no" or turning the palm of the hand up and then down.

Supination: Rotation of forearm so that the palm faces forward or upward; movement of the whole body so that the face and abdomen are upward.

EXERCISE

Muscles that are not used become weak and shortened. During prolonged bedrest, strength and endurance decrease rapidly. Clients can regain muscle strength and mobility by practicing specific groups of exercises daily. Promoting exercise, both passive and active, is one of the most important nursing functions. The purpose of exercises is to promote proper alignment, prevent contractures, stimulate circulation, and prevent thrombophlebitis and pressure ulcers. Exercise reduces joint pain and stiffness and increases flexibility and endurance. Exercise also prevents edema of the extremities and promotes lung expansion.

The nurse both performs and teaches several types of exercises as a component of providing total client care. Passive exercises are carried out by the therapist or nurse without assistance from the client. These exercises enable the client to retain as much joint range of motion as possible, as well as stimulating circulation. Active exercises, although supervised by the nurse, are performed by the client. These exercises increase muscle strength when the client is partially immobile.

> The 2008 Physical Activity Guidelines for America state that regular physical activity reduces the risk of many adverse health outcomes. Adults should avoid inactivity and participate in physical activity to gain some health benefit. There is a greater increase in health benefits as the amount of physical activity increases. All clients should be instructed to increase their physical activity if they are inactive. Elderly clients need to be encouraged to participate in regular physical activity, including aerobic muscle strengthening and flexibility activities. Balance training for elderly clients will decrease the risk of falls.

Resistive exercises, another rehabilitative measure, provide resistance in order to increase muscle power. These active exercises are performed by the individual working against resistance. Isometric or muscle-setting activities are similar to resistive exercises. These exercises maintain strength in a muscle when the joint is immobilized. They are performed by the individual without assistance.

Range-of-motion (ROM) exercises are the most common form of exercises for maintaining joint mobility and increasing maximal motion of a joint when the client is totally or partially immobilized. These exercises are completed by the nurse or physical therapist. The therapist puts an extremity through its full range so that the joint is moved through all the appropriate planes. Before beginning these exercises, it is important that the therapist and/or nurse assess the client's condition and the baseline ROM capabilities, establish the extent of ROM to be carried out, and ensure that the client is comfortable. Be aware that clients might be fearful of this type of exercise and that a full explanation of what you are going to do is helpful to allay fears. Enlist the cooperation of the client for maximum benefit. Discontinue all range-of-motion exercises if the client complains of pain, for it is at this point that the exercises become counterproductive.

AMBULATION

Ambulation, or walking, is an important function that most of us accomplish automatically; that is, without thinking or conscious effort. When a person has been immobilized, confined to bed after surgery or an injury, or unable to ambulate, this seemingly simple activity can become a major hurdle to overcome. The longer a person is immobilized, the more difficult it is to regain ambulatory ability; likewise, the sooner a person begins to ambulate after being bedridden, the more easily he or she will regain preimmobilization status. Early ambulation decreases hospitalization time and prevents complications, such as paralytic ileus or thrombophlebitis.

The human body functions best when it is frequently placed in a vertical position. Ambulation improves physical and mental well-being. Ambulation increases muscle strength and joint mobility. It also increases respiratory exchange, gastrointestinal muscle tone, and circulation. Without stress on bones, calcium deposits occur anywhere in the body, especially in damaged areas, and renal problems also increase from calcium-based calculi.

Balance, coordination, and good body alignment are aspects important to walking. One must be able to move forward and maintain an upright balance; use muscles, bones, and joints correctly for coordination; and keep the head erect and vertebral column fairly straight with feet and knee caps pointed forward in order to maintain good body alignment.

The major muscle groups used for walking are the thigh and leg muscles. If these muscles have not been used or exercised because the client has been in bed for a long period of time, ambulation must be accomplished step by step. Weak muscles cannot support a human frame for the mechanics of walking. It is important, then, to begin the process of ambulation by administering muscle-strengthening exercises. Several different types of exercises were described previously; however, the most important preambulatory preparation is quadriceps-setting and gluteal-setting exercises. Carried out several times a day, these exercises restore muscle strength and prepare the legs for weight bearing.

Before actually assisting the client to walk, explain precisely what you are going to do, and prepare the client by completing the ambulatory procedure in stages. For example, begin with the muscle-strengthening exercises. Then assist the client to sit up in bed to determine if he or she is experiencing vertigo. Have the client move to the side of the bed with legs down, and only when he or she is ready and feels comfortable in doing so, assist the client to stand beside the bed. You may decide to take the client's vital signs after dangling to determine if they are stable. Allow the client to remain there with the bed as support until he or she feels totally secure. Finally, and with the assistance of one or two nurses (depending on the assessment of the client's ability and readiness to ambulate), have the client walk by taking short steps and walking only as long as he or she can tolerate. Do this several times a day, and it will not be long before the client's legs are strengthened, and he or she can graduate to one assistant, a walker, or cane. Throughout this procedure, do not allow the client to lose confidence in the ability to walk or your ability to support and assist while regaining his or her independence of action.

ASSISTIVE DEVICES

A variety of assistive devices are available to give the client support when ambulating. Assistive devices are used to relieve the client's body weight to enable the client to ambulate. Canes relieve about 40% of the weight mainly attributable to the lower limb. Walkers and crutches allow for complete non–weight-bearing ambulation. Such devices may give the client confidence (especially important with the elderly), stability, support for a weak limb, or reduce the pressure on a limb. These devices may include canes (standard cane, T-handled cane, tripod cane, and quad cane) and walkers (standard, with wheels, or a hemi-walker). Crutches are another type of assistive device used to lessen or remove weight from one or both legs.

Crutches

Crutches are an aid to walking by providing support during ambulating when the lower extremities are unable to support the body weight. It is hoped that this situation is temporary, but even if it is permanent, crutches do allow independence of movement that otherwise could not occur.

There are three main types of crutches: the axillary (most common for short-term use), the Lofstrand, or Canadian (a forearm crutch with a metal band and handle), and the platform, for clients who are unable to use their wrists to bear weight.

Several safety factors should be taken into account before assisting the client to use crutches. The measurement should be 5 cm (2 in.) from the axillary fold to the crutch bar. The handpiece should be adjusted to allow 20° to 30° elbow flexion, and rubber suction tips should be placed on the bottom of the crutches. Finally, the client should be informed that while using crutches, one needs well-fitting shoes with non-slip soles.

The type of crutch used by the client depends on the ability to ambulate, the muscle strength needed for support, and the individual needs of the client.

Walkers

Walkers assist the client with balance and with walking. The client's arms are used to support all or part of the client's body and take weight off the lower limbs as he/she ambulates.

Walkers are a necessary assistive device for postoperative clients requiring help with ambulation. These clients include those with major spinal cord surgery or hip replacement surgery, or those who were/are debilitated from major surgery and are unsteady with ambulation.

Walkers are constructed with or without wheels, or platforms. Wheels are only on the front legs of the walker to prevent falls and possible injury. All walkers have rubber tips that must be observed frequently to ensure they are in good repair.

The height of the walker is adjusted by lowering or raising the legs of the extension piece to properly fit the client's height. The handles of the walker should be at the height of the client's wrist, with elbows slightly bent.

Canes

Canes are used to protect clients from falls. Clients who are unsteady, lose their balance, are weak, or have a leg(s) that cannot hold the client in the upright position are candidates for canes.

Using a cane affords the client the confidence to ambulate and maintain his/her independence. Canes, just like crutches, are measured for a proper fit. The cane is turned upside down with the handle on the floor and the rubber tip is removed. The client is instructed to stand with his/her arms at the sides of the body. The correct measurement is marked with the tip of the cane facing upward and at the level of the wrist. The cane is cut (if a wooden cane) 1/2 in. shorter than the mark. Aluminum canes can be adjusted within 1 in. of the desired height.

ADAPTATION TO HOME CARE

Knowledge of body mechanics and how to use these principles when giving care is important to both the healthcare provider and the client. Correct use of body mechanics decreases the caregiver's potential for injury and provides safety for the client. Recently, there has been an increase in the number of back injury accident claims among home healthcare providers. One reason for the increase is the improper use of body mechanics while performing skills in the home setting. Also, there may be no one to assist the care provider when lifting and turning clients in the home. The nurse may need to improvise, as the equipment may not be adequate or adjustable. The purpose of this unit is to consider adaptations necessary for providing safe care to the client while using proper body mechanics. In the home setting, much of the care is given by the family; therefore, it is essential that they also be taught good body mechanics.

NURSING DIAGNOSES

The following nursing diagnoses are appropriate to use on client care plans when the components are related to exercise and ambulation needs of clients.

NURSING DIAGNOSIS	RELATED FACTORS
Activity Intolerance	Nutritional disorders, surgery, disease states, impaired motor function, pain
Impaired Home Maintenance	Chronic debilitating disease, lack of knowledge, insufficient funds, lack of support or community resources
Impaired Physical Mobility	Neuromuscular impairment, musculoskeletal impairment, surgical procedure, trauma
Acute Pain	Altered body function (muscle spasms or rigidity), musculoskeletal disorders, inflammation, immobility
Self-Care Deficit	Neuromuscular impairment, surgery, musculoskeletal impairment, visual disorders, external devices, decreased strength and endurance

CLEANSE HANDS The single most important nursing action to decrease the incidence of hospital-based infections is hand hygiene. *Remember to wash your hands or use antibacterial gel before and after each and every client contact.*

IDENTIFY CLIENT Before every procedure, check two forms of client identification, not including room number. These actions prevent errors and conform to The Joint Commission standards.

Chapter 13

UNIT ❶

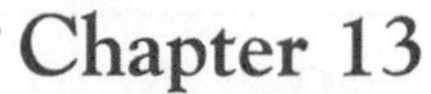

Range of Motion

Nursing Process Data

ASSESSMENT Data Base

- Determine client's physical ability to perform exercises (i.e., level of consciousness, presence of casts, traction).
- Ascertain client's baseline level of joint movement and muscle strength.
- Note amount of spontaneous movement shown by the client.
- Assess client's understanding of ROM exercises.

PLANNING Objectives

- To improve or maintain joint function
- To improve or maintain muscle tone and strength
- To enhance/mainstream soft tissue integrity
- To counteract effects of prolonged bedrest or immobilization
- To facilitate passive range of motion
- To prevent contractures
- To increase client comfort
- To prepare the client for ambulation

IMPLEMENTATION Procedures

EVALUATION Expected Outcomes

- Client improves range of motion and muscle tone after performing range-of-motion exercises.
- Client is able to progress through range-of-motion with minimal to no pain.
- Client is able to ambulate without difficulty following a period of bedrest.

Pearson Nursing Student Resources

Find additional review materials at **nursing.pearsonhighered.com**

Prepare for success with NCLEX®-style practice questions and Skill Checklists

Performing Passive Range of Motion

Equipment

Hospital bed

Procedure

1. Check physician's order to determine if passive range of motion can be performed (according to facility policy).
2. Explain procedure to client and caregiver who may be delivering range of motion at home.
3. Perform hand hygiene.
4. Check two forms of client ID and introduce yourself. Explain rationale for procedure to client.
5. Position client on his or her back with bed as flat as possible. Place bed in high position.
6. Expose limb to be exercised.
7. Put all joints through range of motion slowly and gently (Tables 13-1 and 13-2). Start at head.
8. Protect against gravity and detrimental movement when performing range-of-motion exercises.
9. Provide support above and below joint using a cradling support while performing the exercises.
10. Follow sequence of exercises for upper and lower body according to chart.
11. All joints should be put through five full-range-of-motion exercises to each joint at least twice daily.
12. Encourage client to do active exercises as soon as possible. ▸ ***Rationale:*** Passive exercises only help prevent contractures, but do not maintain muscle.
13. Discontinue exercises if client complains of pain or discomfort. ▸ ***Rationale:*** Range of motion exercises should be performed in prain-free movement.
14. Reassess client's ability to perform ROM exercises and adjust schedule accordingly.

TABLE 13-1 Range of Motion: Upper Body

	Neck	Shoulder	Elbow	Forearm	Wrist	Finger and Thumb
Flexion	Move head forward 90° with chin on chest	Raise arm 180° from side to above head	Bend elbow so arm moves up toward shoulder		Bend hand 90° toward inner arm	Make a fist so fingers are all bent inward
Extension	Move head up from chest 90° to erect position	Move arm to side of body	Straighten elbow and return to position		Move hand straight pointed out	Move fingers 90° to straight position
Hyper-extension	Move head backwards 90°	Move arm to back of body at 50° angle			Bend hand up and back 90° toward arm	Move fingers up toward back of hand
Abduction		Hold arm away from side 180° to above head			Bend wrist out away from arm	Spread fingers as much as possible
Adduction		Move arm from side across chest			Bend wrist inward toward radius	Move fingers and thumb together
External Rotation		Hold arm out to side with elbow bent 45°; move forward so palm faces forward				
Internal Rotation		Move arm to side at shoulder level with elbow bent 45°. Lower arm so palm faces back				
Rotation	Move head in circular motion—90° left, then 90° right					
Circum-duction		Move arm in full circle				
Supination				Rotate forearm 90° so palm is up		
Pronation				Rotate forearm 90° so palm is down		

TABLE 13-2 Range of Motion: Lower Body

	Trunk	Hip	Knee	Ankle	Toes
Flexion	Bend forward 90°	Move leg forward and up 90°	Bend knee 90°; foot moves back and up		Point down 90°
Extension	Stand in straight position	Move leg in straight alignment with trunk	Move foot 90° with knee straight and leg in line with body		Straight out from foot
Hyperextension	Bend backward 30°	Move leg backward 50°			Point up 45°
Lateral Flexion	Bend to both sides 45°				
Internal Rotation		Turn leg and foot inward 90°			
External Rotation		Turn leg and foot outward 90°			
Circumduction		Move leg in circle 360°			
Abduction		Move leg away from body 45°			Spread apart 15°
Adduction		Move leg toward body 45°			Bring together in normal position
Rotation	Move in circle 360° from waist				
Plantar Flexion				Point toes downward	
Dorsiflexion				Point toes upward	
Eversion				Move sole of foot lateral to outside	
Inversion				Move sole of foot medial to inside	

NOTE: ROM exercises should be incorporated into ADL activities whenever possible.

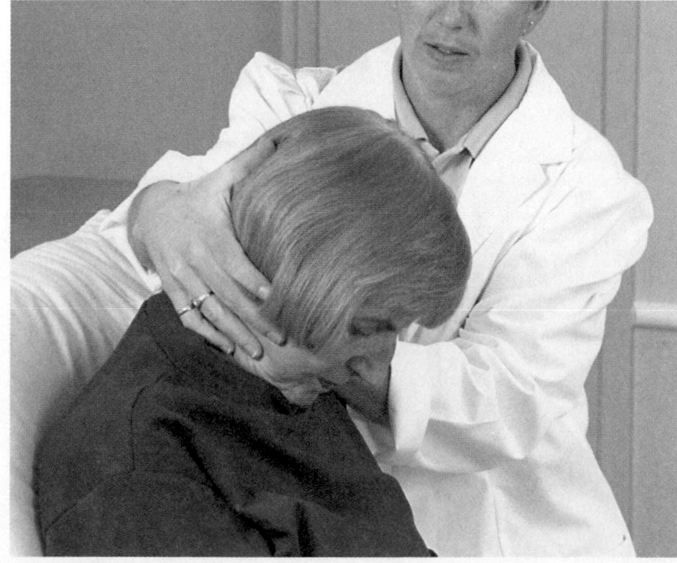
▲ Flexion of neck—move head forward 90° with chin on chest.

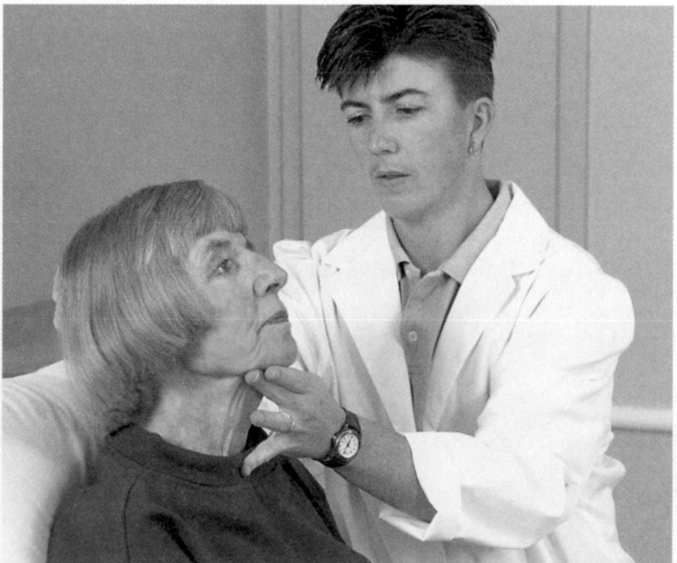
▲ Extension of neck—move head up from chest 90°.

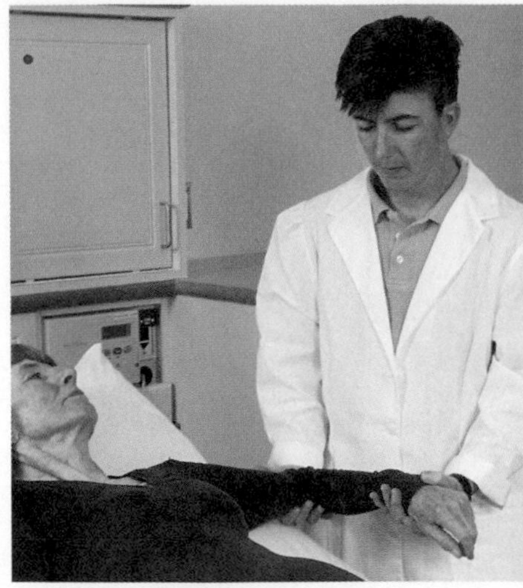
▲ Internal rotation of shoulder.

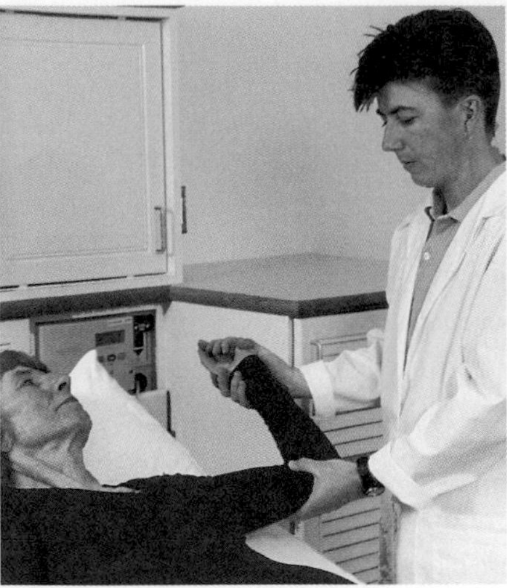
▲ External rotation of shoulder.

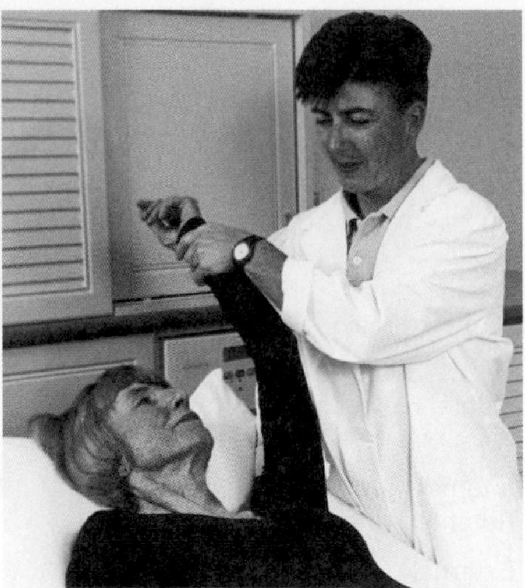
▲ Abduction of shoulder.

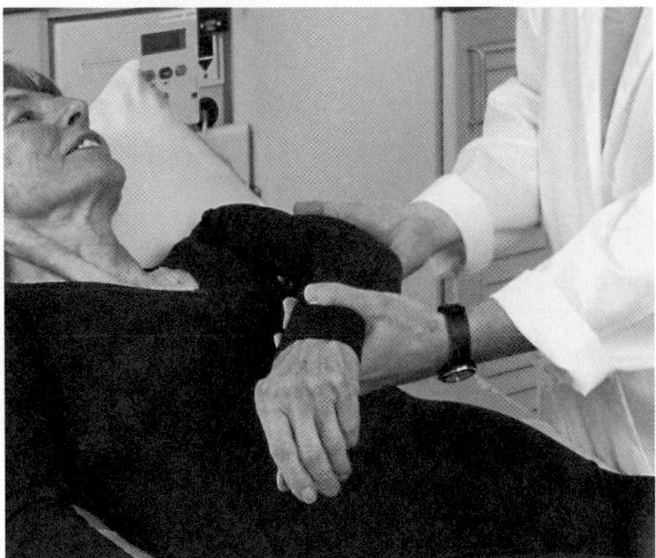
▲ Adduction of shoulder.

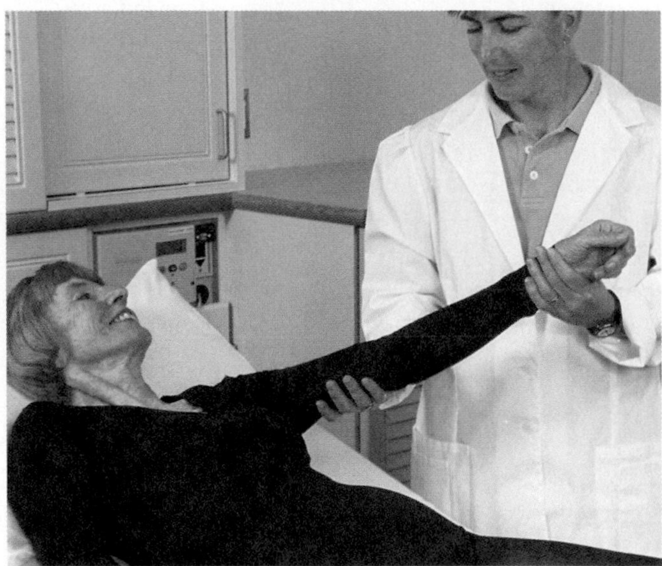
▲ Extension of elbow.

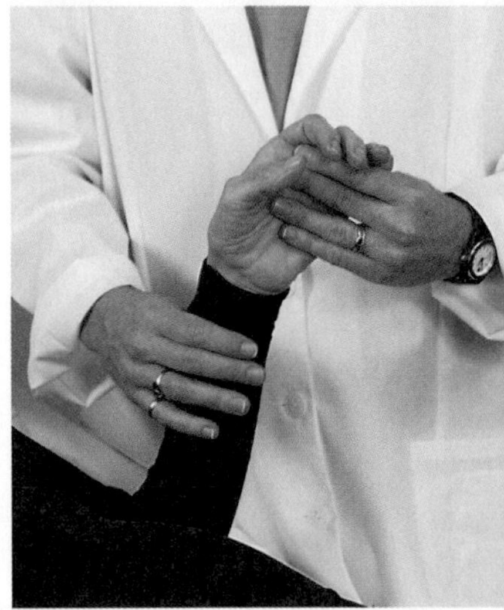
▲ Rotation of the wrist.

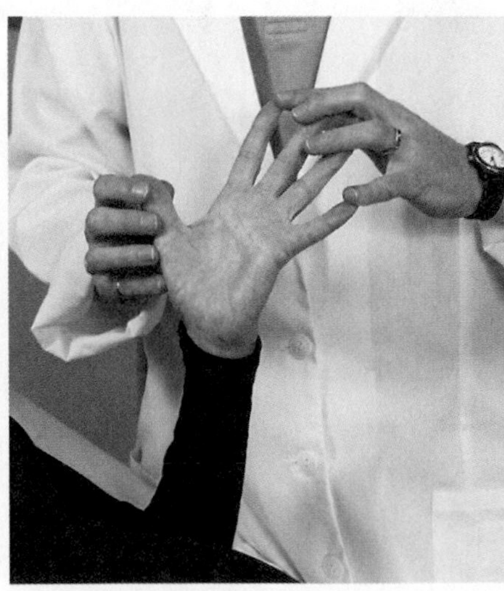
▲ Extension of finger joints.

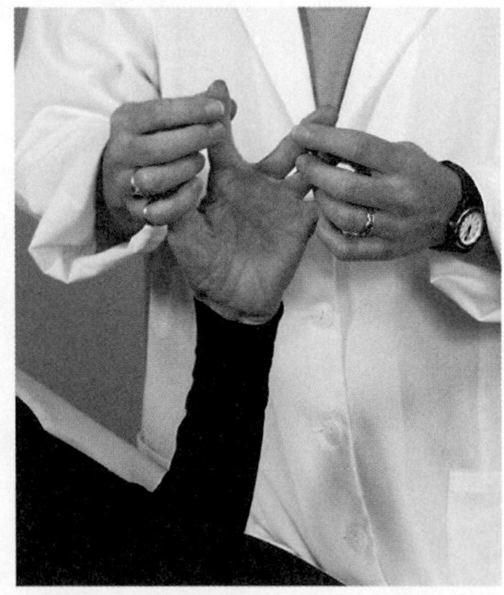
▲ Adduction – abduction finger exercises.

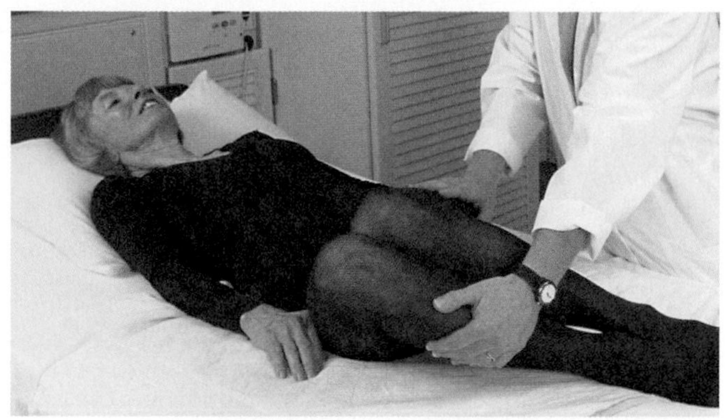

▲ Rotate lower trunk outward 90°.

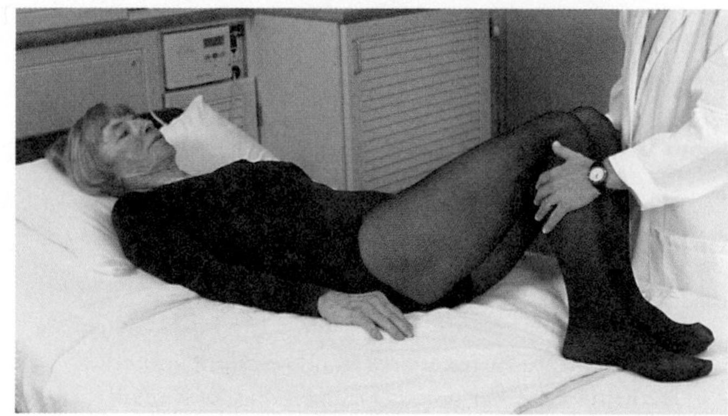

▲ Rotate lower trunk to other side 90°.

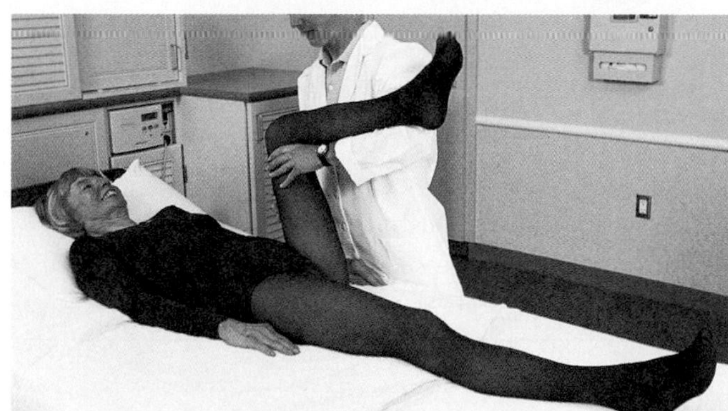

▲ Flex hip and knee.

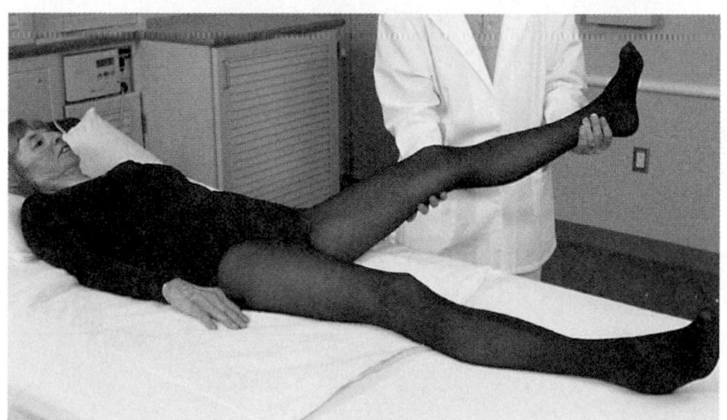

▲ Straight leg raise.

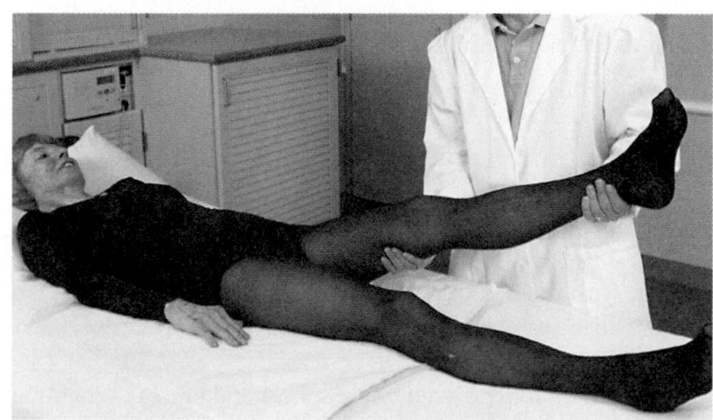

▲ Abduction—Move leg away from the body.

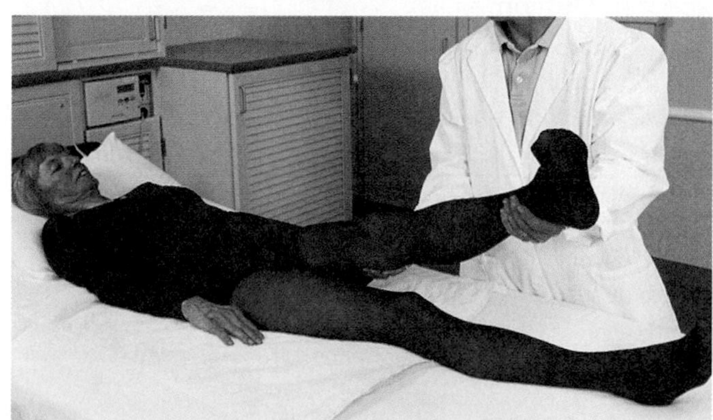

▲ Adduction—Move leg toward midline of body.

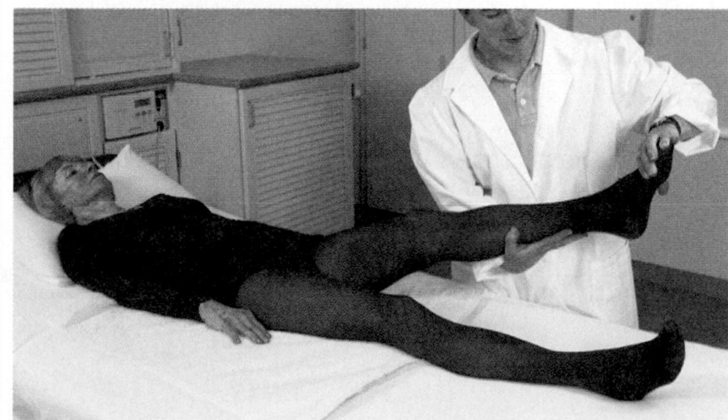

▲ Plantar flexion—Move foot down and away from leg.

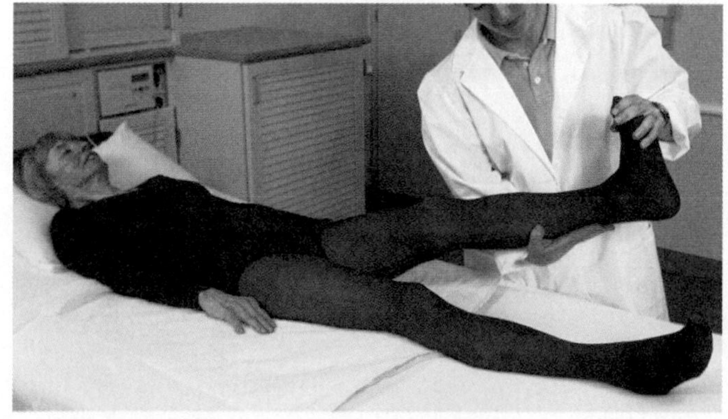

▲ Dorsiflexion—Move foot up and toward leg.

Teaching Active Range of Motion

Equipment

Hospital bed

Sturdy nonslip shoes or slippers

Procedure

1. Explain the rationale for the procedure to the client.
2. Demonstrate the exercises that the client should perform. (See *Performing Passive Range of Motion* for specific steps in exercises.)
3. Observe as the client performs the exercises.
4. Assist with the exercises as needed.
5. Correct any problems you notice in the client's performance.
6. Encourage client to perform as much of the exercises as possible.
7. Instruct client to do range-of-motion exercises every 4 hr, exercising all joints.
8. Move extremities through range of motion five cycles each procedure.

DOCUMENTATION for Range of Motion

ROM Exercises

- Amount of time needed to complete exercises
- Any changes in condition of joint or joint mobility
- Movements that caused unusual pain or discomfort
- Amount of client participation
- Specific joints put through range of motion
- Alterations in usual procedure
- Degree of mobility improvement after exercises

CRITICAL THINKING Application

Expected Outcomes

- Client improves range of motion and muscle tone after performing range-of-motion exercises.
- Client is able to progress through the range-of-motion exercises with minimal to no pain.
- Client is able to ambulate without difficulty after a period of bedrest.

Unexpected Outcomes	Alternative Actions
Client continues to lose mobility and strength despite nursing intervention.	• Discuss the need for additional measures to improve joint range with the health team. • Refer client to physical therapist if range of motion only performed by nursing staff. • Assess client for the need to use splints and braces to maintain the best physiologic position between exercise periods, and discuss your findings with the physician.
Client experiences pain and discomfort during range-of-motion exercises.	• Assess amount and type of pain and report findings to physician. • Reevaluate your technique to ensure you are performing the exercises correctly. • Start exercises with less stress on joints. Do exercises for a shorter period of time and gradually increase time and range of joint mobility.

Chapter 13

UNIT 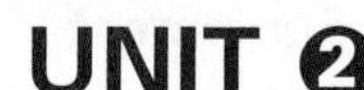

Ambulation

Nursing Process Data

ASSESSMENT Data Base

- Assess client's previous activity level.
- Check physician's orders for activity.
- Assess vital signs and physical ability to ambulate.
- Assess need for safety belt or assistive devices.
- Assess client for vertigo when moved into an upright sitting position.
- Determine if client feels pain from operative site.
- Observe client's balance.
- Assess any sensory deficits (visual, perceptual).

PLANNING Objectives

- To promote increased feelings of physical and mental well-being
- To develop increased tolerance for exercise
- To decrease hospitalization time
- To regain independence by regaining ability to walk
- To prevent paralytic ileus by increasing abdominal wall and gastrointestinal tract muscle tone
- To prevent thrombophlebitis by increasing circulation in the legs
- To promote healing by increasing circulation and muscle contraction

IMPLEMENTATION Procedures

EVALUATION Expected Outcomes

- Feelings of physical and mental well-being increased.
- Balance and muscle tone improve.
- Client progresses from being dependant with ambulation to becoming independent in ambulation.
- Complications of immobility are prevented with ambulation.
- Correct use of assistive devices without supervision.

Pearson Nursing Student Resources

Find additional review materials at
nursing.pearsonhighered.com

Prepare for success with NCLEX®-style practice questions and Skill Checklists

Minimizing Orthostatic Hypotension

Equipment

Elastic stockings, if ordered

Robe and slippers

Stethoscope and sphygmomanometer

Procedure

1. Review client's chart before ambulation to check for a history of orthostatic hypotension. ▶ ***Rationale:*** This condition may occur in any client, but is more common in the elderly or with clients who have been immobilized.
2. Perform hand hygiene.
3. Check two forms of client ID, introduce yourself, and review procedure with client.
4. Place elastic stockings on client's legs if ordered. ▶ ***Rationale:*** Elastic stockings help to reduce blood stasis and promote venous return.
5. Move bed to LOW position. ▶ ***Rationale:*** This position enables client to have feet on the floor and is safer if client experiences vertigo.
6. *Slowly* raise head of bed to Fowler's position. ▶ ***Rationale:*** The more slowly the client's position is changed, the less the effect of postural hypotension.
7. Move client to edge of bed by placing one arm behind client's back and one arm under both thighs. Pivot client to a sitting position and assist to dangle legs over side of bed. ▶ ***Rationale:*** Dangling with feet flat on floor for several minutes with legs in a dependent position will reduce effects of postural hypotension.
8. Take client's blood pressure and pulse and observe for vertigo, fainting, pallor, etc.
9. *Slowly* assist client to stand. Instruct client to take a deep breath and exhale. If there is no evidence of orthostatic hypotensive symptoms, begin ambulation or transfer to a chair.

NOTE: If hypotension continues, client should be returned to flat position in bed.

Clinical Alert

If the client has been on prolonged bedrest or been immobilized, the risk of orthostatic hypotension is increased. Raising and lowering head of bed (HOB) several times to stimulate baroreceptors will help to prevent this condition.

Measuring Orthostatic Hypotension

Postural or orthostatic hypotension is often present after prolonged bedrest or immobilization. It is a sudden drop in blood pressure (25 mmHg systolic or 10 mmHg diastolic) when the client moves from a horizontal to a vertical (lying to sitting or standing) position. Symptoms include dizziness, lightheadedness, fainting, pallor, or nausea.

To measure orthostatic hypotension:

- With client in supine position for 5 minutes, measure pulse and blood pressure. ▶ **Rationale:** This amount of time allows for blood pressure to stabilize.
- Assist client to stand, wait 1 minute, and recheck pulse and blood pressure.
- Reassess blood pressure and pulse after 2 minutes. ▶ **Rationale:** This amount of time will allow for compensatory mechanisms to work.
- Notify physician if blood pressure and/or pulse remain abnormal after 15 minutes.

Ambulating With Two Assistants

Equipment

Robe or second hospital gown (put on backwards so that client is not exposed)

Shoes or slippers that fit well and have nonslip soles

Procedure

1. Perform hand hygiene.
2. Check two forms of client ID, introduce yourself, and explain the rationale for the procedure to the client.
3. Move client to side of bed and assist client to sit on the edge after placing bed in LOW position.
4. Assess the client for vertigo or faintness. Keep client in sitting position until he or she is able to stand without becoming dizzy. ▶ ***Rationale:*** Orthostatic hypotension can occur with prolonged bedrest (see skill *Minimizing Orthostatic Hypotension*).
5. Position one nurse on each side of the client and have each nurse grasp the client's upper arm with the hand that is closest to the client.
6. Have each nurse grasp the client's hand with the other hand and instruct the client to stand.
7. Encourage the client to maintain erect posture and look straight ahead, not down.
8. Ask the client to lift each foot to take a step. The client should not shuffle.
9. Walk the client only as far as he or she is capable of walking and returning without exhaustion.

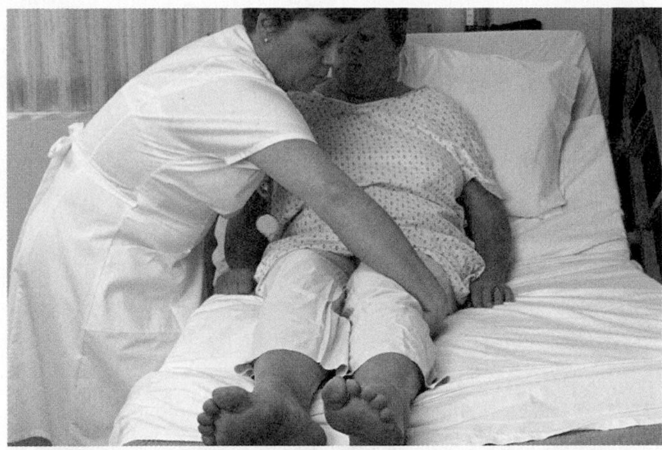
▲ Move client to side of bed.

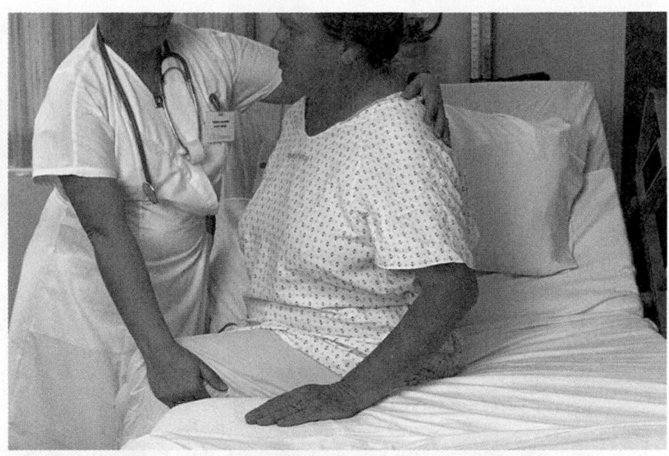
▲ Assist client to sit at edge of bed.

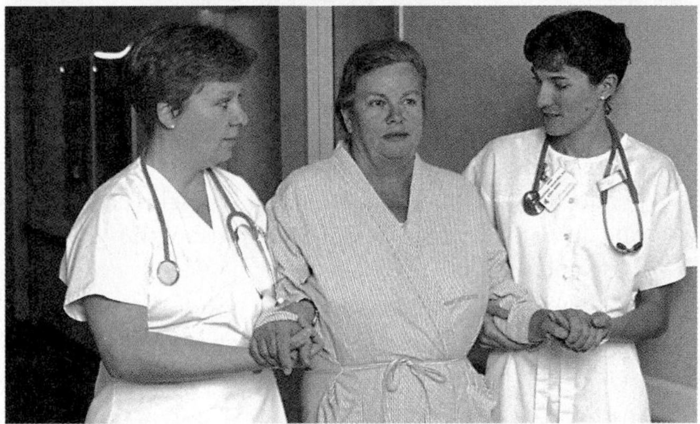
▲ Support is provided by two nurses when client's condition requires.

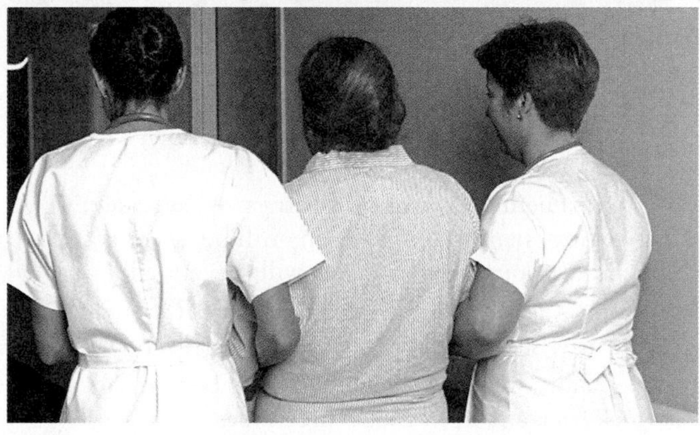
▲ Grasp client's arms firmly on both sides to provide support.

EVIDENCE-BASED PRACTICE

Early Mobilization Promotes Better Outcomes

Clients numbering 5,777 were included in 39 trials. Twenty-four trials evaluated bedrest after a variety of medical procedures. Seventeen trials favored early mobilization. Fifteen trials evaluated bedrest as a primary treatment, and all showed worse outcomes for clients on bedrest. The study provides evidence to support what clinicians have been doing for several decades—mobilizing clients as early as possible. There is evidence that prolonged bedrest is harmful for clients with low-back pain and myocardial infarction. There is a lack of evidence to determine the effects of bedrest for clients with multiple pregnancies, threatened abortion, and impaired fetal growth.

Source: *ACP Journal Club*, May/June 2000, vol. 132, no. 3. Review done on article by Allen, C., Glasziou, P., & Del Mar, C. (1999, October 9). Bed rest: A potentially harmful treatment needing more careful evaluation. *Lancet*, *354*, 1229–1233.

EVIDENCE-BASED PRACTICE

Progressive Mobility Combating Deconditioning

Once a client's hemodynamic status allows forms of mobilization, it is essential to begin progressive mobilization. This decreases severe muscle wasting that occurs particularly in critically ill clients. Start with dangling, standing, and ambulation. Hemodynamic instability is due to prolonged periods in a stationery position.

Source: Rauen, C. A., Chulay, M., Bridges, E., Vollman, K. M., & Arbour, R. (2008). Seven evidence-based practice habits: Putting some sacred cows out to pasture. *Critical Care Nurse*, *28*(2), 98–124.

Ambulating With One Assistant

Equipment

Robe or second hospital gown (put on backward so that client is not exposed)

Shoes or slippers that fit well and have nonslip soles

Safety belt if indicated

Procedure

1. Check client's chart for ambulation problems, orthostatic hypotension, or any specific physician's orders.
2. Perform hand hygiene.
3. Check two forms of client ID, introduce yourself, and explain rationale for procedure to client.

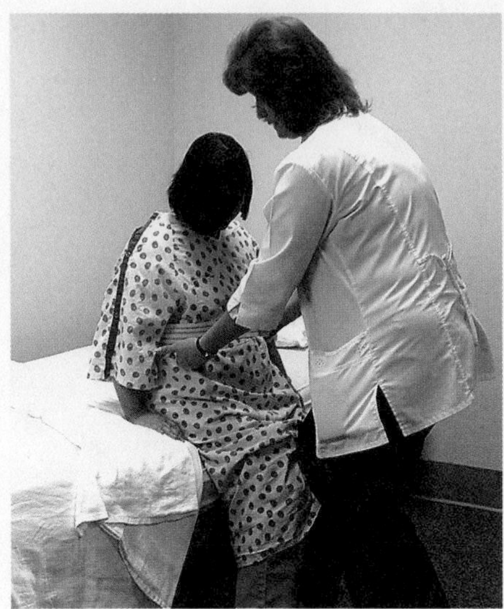

▲ Use gait belt to assist client out of bed.

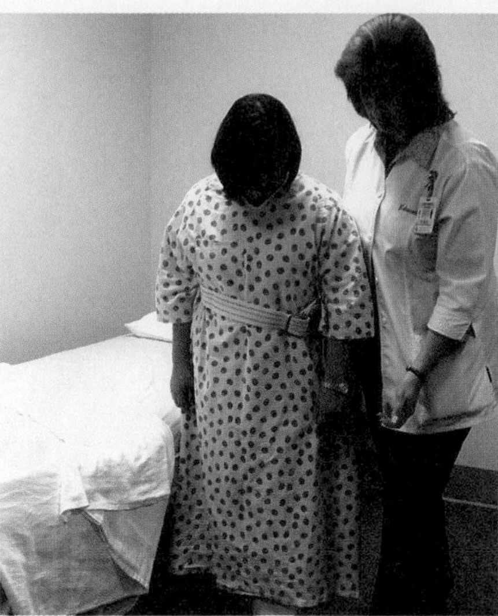

▲ Gait belt provides for stability when ambulating.

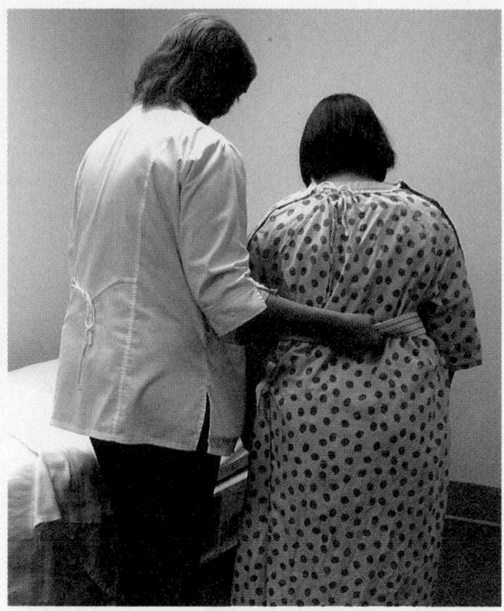

▲ Grasp belt firmly at client's back when ambulating.

4. Help client sit on side of bed after placing bed in LOW position.
5. Assess client for vertigo or faintness. ▸ ***Rationale:*** Keeping client in this position until he or she is able to stand without becoming dizzy will prevent falling.
6. Apply safety belt if client is unsteady. ▸ ***Rationale:*** Provides support if client is weak and prevents injury.
7. Bend forward facing the client, grasp belt, and gently rock back and forth about three times.
8. Instruct the client to assist with standing while pulling client upward with rocking motion, and on the third rocking motion, pull the client to a standing position. Have client take a deep breath and exhale while standing.
9. Stabilize client in a standing position.
10. Stand on weaker side, when client is moderately weak; for cerebrovascular accident (CVA) client, stand on unaffected side. ▸ ***Rationale:*** Flaccid muscles on affected side do not provide sufficient muscle strength for you to grasp and support client.
11. Encourage client to maintain good posture and to look straight ahead. ▸ ***Rationale:*** Tendency is for client to look down, which may increase vertigo.
12. Instruct client to lift each foot to take a step, not to shuffle.
13. Walk client as far as he or she is capable of walking without becoming exhausted. Remember client must walk back to room, so take this into consideration when walking. A wheelchair or walker can be pushed behind client so if he becomes tired he can sit down.

Clinical Alert

If client is collapsing, try to break the fall with your body and guide client to the floor. If client is unsteady or appears to be falling, support his or her body, especially the head and trunk, maintaining your body in good alignment with line of gravity within your base of support. This alignment prevents injury to yourself, while giving client adequate support. If necessary, guide client all the way to the floor.

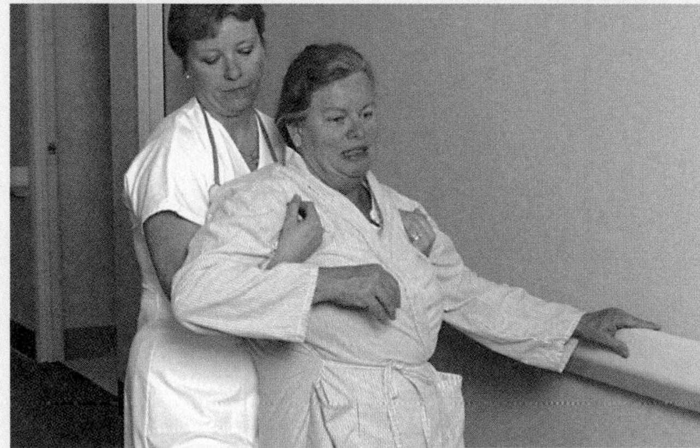

▲ Grasp client under both arms if she begins to fall.

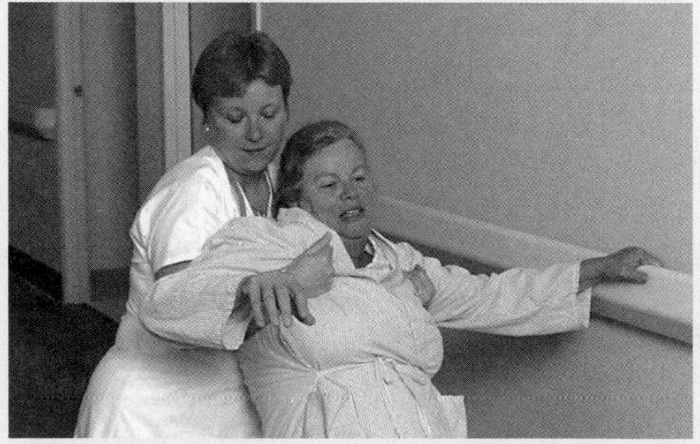

▲ Break client's fall using your body to prevent injury.

Ambulating With a Walker

Equipment

Robe or second hospital gown (put on backward so that client is not exposed)

Shoes or slippers that fit well and have nonslip soles

Walker with safety tips and rubber hand grips (nonrolling walker is used for clients beginning ambulation)

Procedure

1. Perform hand hygiene.
2. Check two forms of client ID, introduce yourself, and explain rationale for procedure to client.

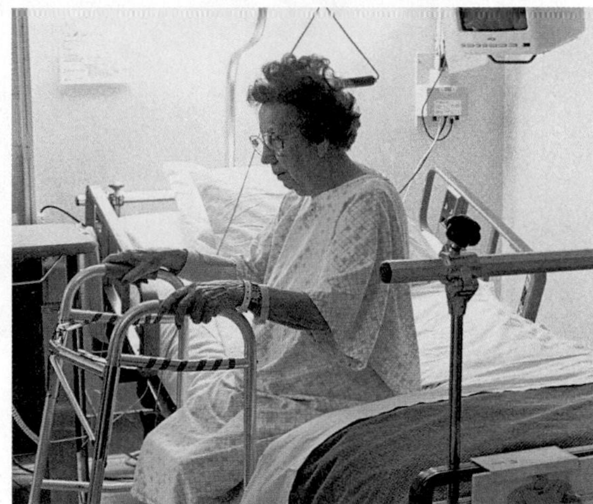

▲ Place walker directly in front of client. Instruct client to hold on to hand grips.

3. Move client to edge of bed and seat client so feet touch floor.
4. Place walker directly in front of client at a comfortable distance. Instruct client to grasp hand grips on walker. ▸ ***Rationale:*** To provide stability when getting up.
5. Ensure legs of walker are level to ground.
6. Instruct client to push self off bed. Client is cautioned to not step completely against front bar of walker. ▸ ***Rationale:*** Client can lose balance.
7. Have client bend elbows slightly and move walker forward 6 to 8 in.; keep all four feet of walker on floor.
8. Instruct client to move weaker side first by supporting body weight on handles and advancing weaker leg into center of walker.
9. Instruct client to balance self and then move unaffected side by placing foot even with first foot.
10. Have client move walker forward and continue same pattern of ambulating.

NOTE: When moving to a chair, instruct client to back all the way to the chair until legs touch the front. Release hands from the walker and grasp the armrests of the chair. Instruct client to slowly lower herself or himself into the chair. Once in the chair, instruct to slide until back touches chair.

Clinical Alert

Adjust walker to client's height. Allow 20° to 30° flexion of the elbows when grasping hand grips of walker.

▲ Instruct client to bend elbows slightly and move walker forward.

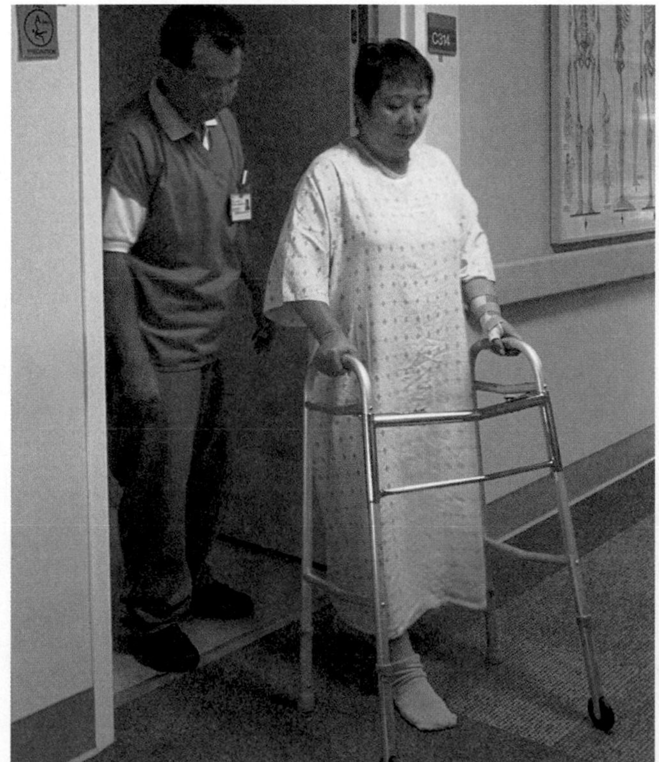

▲ Instruct client to move weaker side first.

Ambulating With a Cane

Equipment

Appropriate type of cane with rubber tips.
- Straight-legged or standard cane
- Tripod or three-pronged cane
- Quad cane

Sturdy shoes with nonskid soles

Safety or gait belt (optional)

Procedure

1. Check physician's orders and client care plan. ▸ ***Rationale:*** To ensure client is ready to use a cane and to ascertain that cane provides sufficient support for client.
2. Perform hand hygiene.
3. Check two forms of client ID, introduce yourself, and explain the purpose of using a cane for ambulation, and answer client questions.
4. Demonstrate use of cane if client is unfamiliar with its use.
5. Assist client to put on appropriate shoes and socks for walking.
6. Assist client to standing position with feet firmly on the floor.
7. Instruct client to hold cane on the stronger side of the body. ▸ ***Rationale:*** This offers the most support.
8. Check that cane extends from greater trochanter to floor with 20° to 30° for elbow flexion. ▸ ***Rationale:*** If cane is too long or too short, client may injure back.

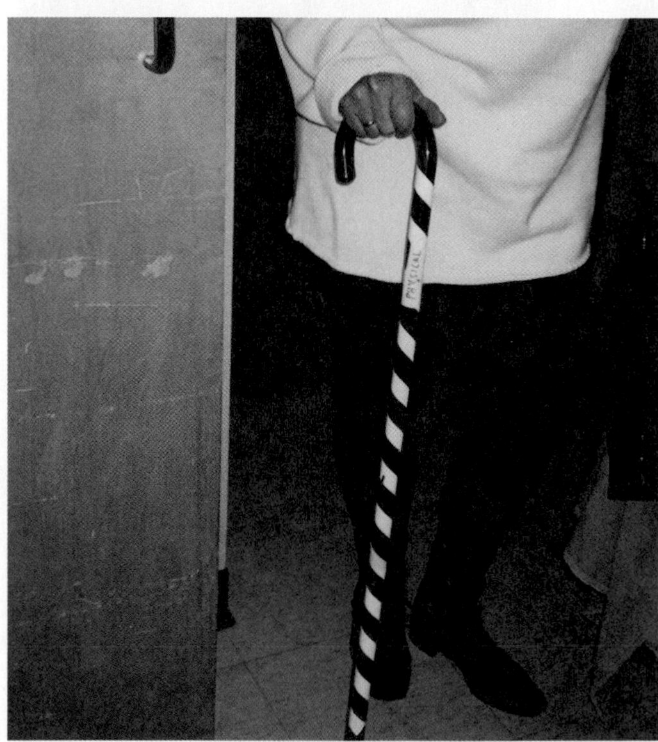

▲ Specially marked cane indicates disability.

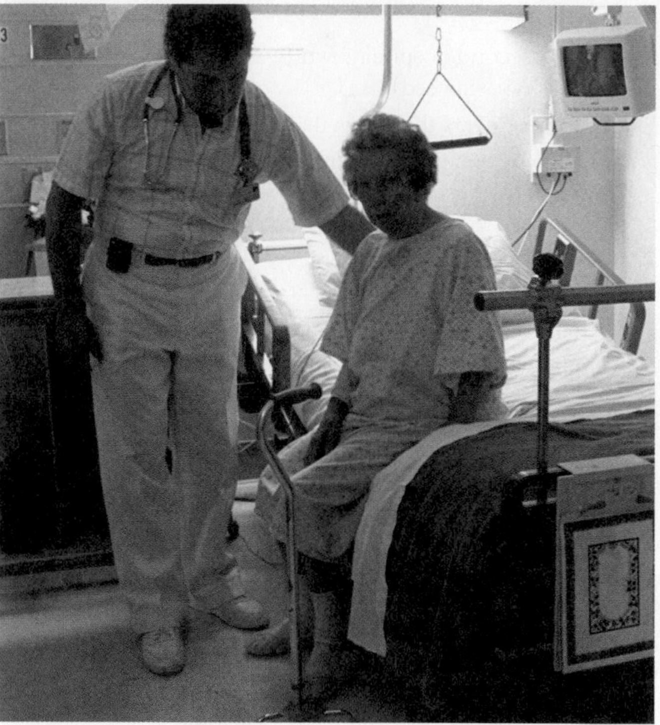

▲ Direct client to hold cane on stronger side of body.

9. Place cane about 12 in. in front of the foot and slightly to the outside. ▸ ***Rationale:*** This position provides the best balance, because the client's center of gravity is within the base of support.
10. Determine that client can maintain balance and does not experience vertigo before taking the first step. Hold cane on unaffected side, keeping the cane close to the body. ▸ ***Rationale:*** To distribute weight away from affected side and prevent the body from leaning forward.
11. Move cane and affected leg 4 in. (10 cm) in front of client.
12. Instruct client to shift his or her weight to affected leg and cane. Then move unaffected leg forward, ahead of cane.
13. Move cane forward, then bring affected leg forward until it is even with cane. Repeat these steps when walking with the cane.
14. Accompany client by walking beside him or her on the unaffected side, or use safety or gait belt if needed. ▸ ***Rationale:*** If the client loses his or her balance, supporting client on unaffected side is most effective. Simply insert your hand and arm underneath the client's axilla and support his or her arm with your other hand.
15. Evaluate client's ability to use the cane, and instruct about its use as needed.
16. Reinforce the client's achievement to assist him or her to gain confidence in ambulating.
17. Continue to accompany client until the time for walking is completed.

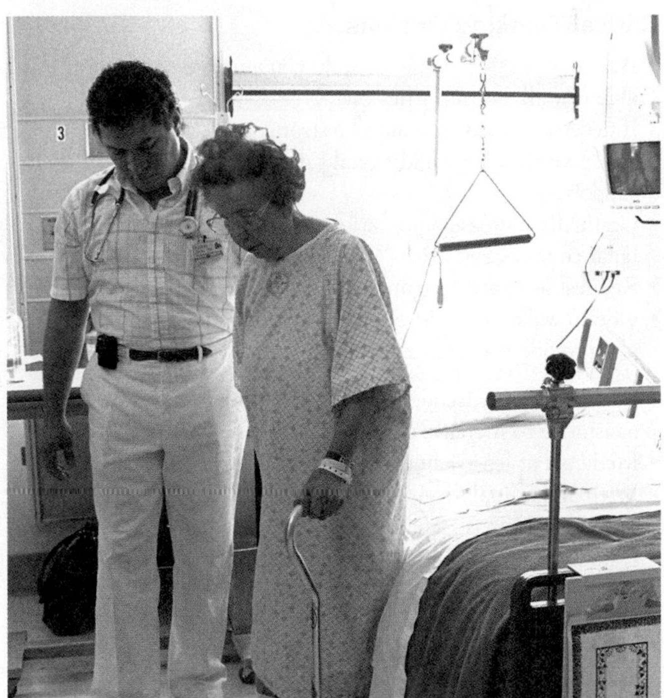

▲ Instruct client to move affected leg forward first, even with cane.

18. Assist client to return to the room and to bed if indicated.
19. Position client for comfort.
20. Assess client's response to ambulation.
21. Perform hand hygiene.
22. Chart client's progress, and evaluate plan for increased periods of ambulation in terms of client's capability.

Managing Steps Using a Cane

Upstairs

- Take first step with strong leg.
- Move cane and affected leg to same step.
- Continue this procedure as client goes up stairs.

Downstairs

- Take first step by placing cane and unaffected leg on step.
- Lower affected leg to same step.
- Continue this procedure as client goes down stairs.

DOCUMENTATION for Ambulation

- Client's ability to balance
- Describe client's posture and gait during ambulation
- Time and distance of ambulation
- Strength and/or weakness of lower extremities
- Use of correct procedure for walker or cane
- Client's perceptions of ambulation

Legal Alert

Whenever the nurse is teaching clients how to use assistive devices, ensure that written instructions are also provided. Document what was taught, results of return demonstrations on use of equipment, and client's understanding of use of equipment. The nurse and hospital can be held liable for negligence if the client falls and suffers an injury if the client does not follow specific instructions on use of assistive devices.

CRITICAL THINKING Application

Expected Outcomes

- Client is able to ambulate independently.
- Client is not experiencing complications of immobility.
- Client is able to prevent orthostatic hypotension by following protocol for moving out of bed.
- Client is able to ambulate using assistive devices without assistance.
- Client is able to ambulate safely with assistance.

Unexpected Outcomes	Alternative Actions
Client experiences vertigo or feels faint.	• If in the client's room, help the client return to the chair or bed. • If in the hall, ease the client down the wall to the floor. Do not attempt to hold the client. • Summon help if possible.
Client is too weak to ambulate.	• Provide active and passive ROM before attempting ambulation. • Begin ambulation protocol as soon as possible using assistive device.

Unexpected Outcomes	Critical Thinking Options
Client is heavy or has poor balance.	• Ask other nurses or staff to help you ambulate the client until able to walk on his or her own. • If necessary, enlist the aid of a stronger assistant whose presence may give the client additional psychologic as well as physical support. • Gradually increase ambulation as muscle tone improves and balance improves. • Request assistance for ambulation from physical therapist. • Obtain walker to assist client with ambulation. The walker will also provide reassurance to client.
Client feels unsafe to ambulate.	• Ambulate more frequently for shorter periods and with more assistance to increase confidence. • Medicate at least 1 hour before ambulation to decrease pain. • With abdominal surgery, check with physician for an order for a binder to decrease fear of dehiscence and pain, if present. • Establish rapport with the client so you can discuss fears about ambulation. • Use assistive devices for client security.

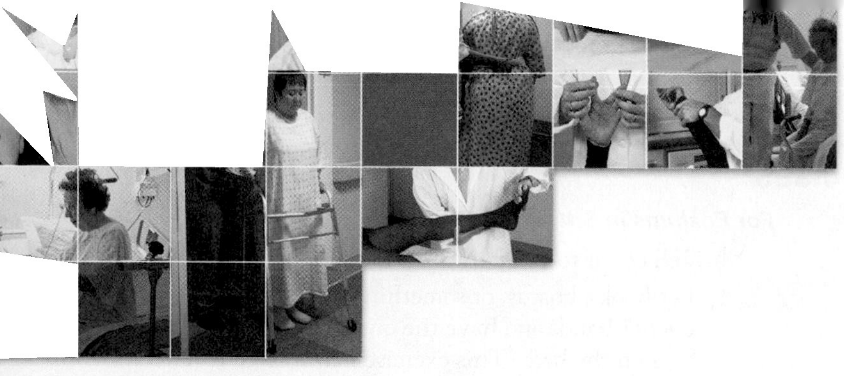

Chapter 13

UNIT 3

Crutch Walking

Nursing Process Data

ASSESSMENT Data Base

- Assess physical ability to use crutches and strength of the client's arm, back, and leg muscles.
- Observe client's ability to balance self.
- Note any unilateral or unusual weakness or vertigo.
- Assess which gait is appropriate for client.
- Assess client's understanding of crutch-walking technique.

PLANNING Objectives

- To improve client's ability to ambulate when he or she has lower extremity injury
- To increase muscle strength, especially in the arms and legs
- To increase feeling of well-being when client can ambulate
- To promote joint mobility
- To resume activities of daily living after injury or surgery

IMPLEMENTATION Procedures

EVALUATION Expected Outcomes

- Client is able to ambulate without assistance.
- Client is able to use crutches to ambulate without fear or anxiety.
- Client is able to move in and out of chair with crutches.
- Crutches are measured appropriately to prevent numbness or tingling in fingers.
- Client is able to resume activities of daily living.

Pearson Nursing Student Resources

Find additional review materials at **nursing.pearsonhighered.com**

Prepare for success with NCLEX®-style practice questions and Skill Checklists

Teaching Muscle-Strengthening Exercises

Equipment

Books, boards, or other firm surface for each hand

Procedure

1. Check the client care plan for physician's orders.
2. Perform hand hygiene.
3. Check two forms of client ID, introduce yourself, and explain rationale for exercises to client.
4. Demonstrate the exercises that client will practice.

For Quadriceps-Setting Exercises

a. Try to hyperextend the client's leg by pushing the popliteal area (the area behind knee) into the bed and lifting heel off the bed.
b. Instruct client to contract muscle for a count of 5, then relax for a count of 5.
c. Have client repeat exercise 2 to 3 times, gradually working up to 10 to 15 times an hour.

For Gluteal-Setting Exercises

a. Tell client to pinch his or her buttocks together for a count of 5 and then to relax for a count of 5.
b. Have client repeat exercise 10 to 15 times an hour.

For Pushups in Sitting Position

a. Tell client to sit up in bed with arms at sides.
b. Put books, boards, or something firm under the client's hands and have the client push down, raising hips off the bed. (This exercise may also be practiced while sitting in a chair.)
c. Have client repeat exercise until he or she can do 10 to 15 pushups an hour.

For Pushups in Prone Position

a. Tell client to lie prone in bed.
b. Ask client to place hands on the bed, close to the shoulders.
c. Tell client to extend arms and to push the upper part of the body into an upright position.
d. Have client repeat exercise until he or she can do 10 to 15 pushups an hour.

5. Monitor as the client performs the exercises and correct any problems that may occur.
6. Assess the client for increasing strength as he or she continues to practice the exercises.
7. Perform hand hygiene.

Measuring Client for Crutches

Equipment

Measuring tape
Hard-soled street shoes
Safety or gait belt

Procedure

1. Perform hand hygiene.
2. Check two forms of client ID, introduce yourself, and explain rationale for procedure to client.
3. Ask client to put on the shoes she or he will be wearing when using the crutches, if possible. Shoes should be low heel and non-skid.
4. Ask client to lie flat in bed with arms at sides.
5. Measure distance from client's axilla (armpit) to a point 15 to 20 cm (6–8 in.) out from heel.
6. Adjust hand bars on the crutches so that client's elbows are always slightly flexed.
7. Instruct client to stand with crutches under arms.
8. Measure the distance between client's axilla and arm pieces on the crutches. You should be able to put two of your fingers in the space between axilla and crutch bar. ▸ ***Rationale:*** Crutches that do not fit client correctly or crutches that are used incorrectly can damage the brachial plexus and cause paralysis of the arms.

NOTE: Use of gait belt can be beneficial when client is beginning to use crutches. ▸ ***Rationale:*** The gait belt provides safety in preventing falls and promotes security for client.

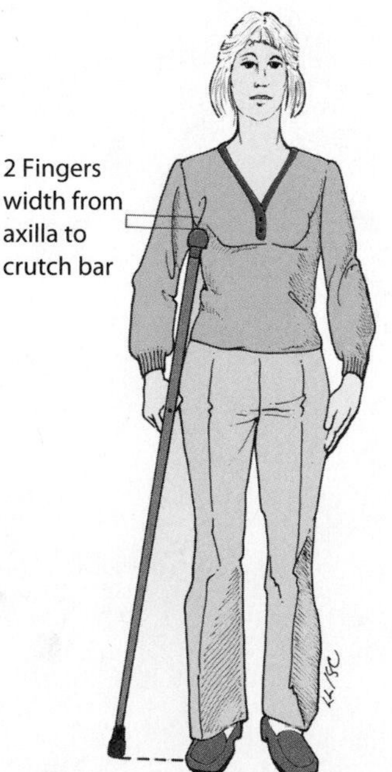

▲ Measure from axilla to heel for crutch height, with crutch tip positioned 6 to 8 inches from foot.

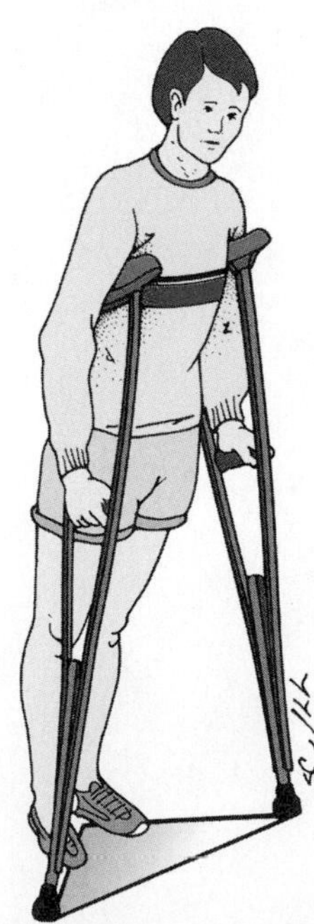
▲ Teach tripod crutch stance for balance in crutch walking.

Teaching Crutch Walking: Four-Point Gait

Equipment

Properly fitted crutches with rubber tips and axillary pads or Lofstrand or Platform crutch.

Regular, hard-soled street shoes

Safety belt, if needed

Procedure

1. Perform hand hygiene.
2. Check two forms of client ID, introduce yourself, and explain the rationale for the procedure to the client.
    a. The gait is rather slow but very stable.
    b. The gait can be performed when the client can move and bear weight on each leg.
3. Demonstrate the crutch-foot sequence to the client.
    a. Move the right crutch.
    b. Move the left foot.
    c. Move the left crutch.
    d. Move the right foot.
4. Help the client practice the gait. Be ready to help with balance if necessary. Use safety belt if necessary.

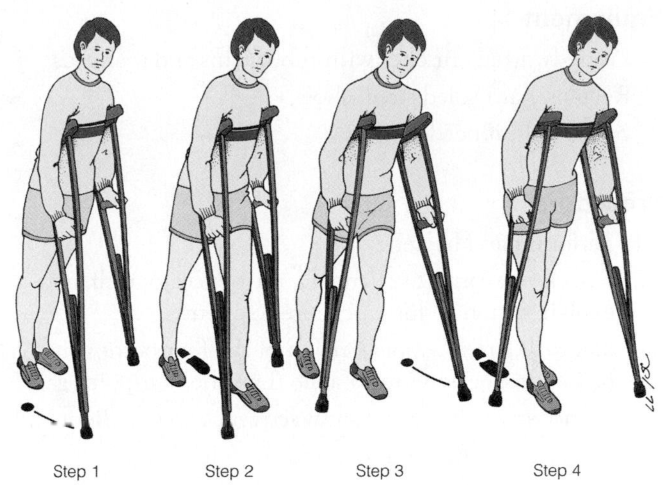

▲ Four-point gait.

5. Assess client's progress and correct mistakes as they occur.
6. Perform hand hygiene.

Teaching Crutch Walking: Three-Point Gait

Equipment

Properly fitted crutches with rubber tips and arm pads

Regular, hard-soled street shoes

Safety belt, if needed

Procedure

1. Perform hand hygiene.
2. Check two forms of client ID, introduce yourself, and explain the rationale for the procedure to the client.
    a. The gait can be performed when the client can bear little or no weight on one leg or when the client has only one leg.
    b. This gait is fairly rapid and requires strong upper extremities and good balance.
3. Demonstrate the crutch-foot sequence to the client.
    a. Two crutches support the weaker extremity.
    b. Balance weight on the crutches.
    c. Move both crutches and affected leg forward.
    d. Move unaffected leg forward.
4. Assess the client's progress, and correct any mistakes as they occur.
5. Remain with client until crutch safety is ensured. Use safety belt if necessary.
6. Perform hand hygiene.

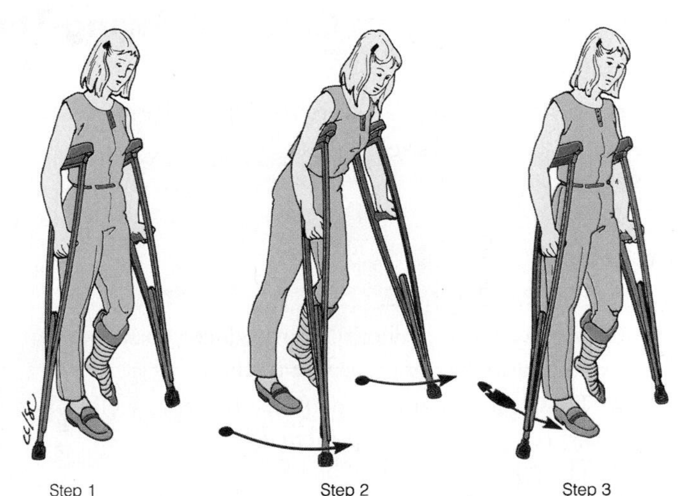

▲ Three-point gait.

Teaching Crutch Walking: Two-Point Gait

Equipment

Properly fitted crutches with rubber tips and arm pads
Regular, hard-soled street shoes
Safety belt, if needed

Procedure

1. Perform hand hygiene.
2. Check two forms of client ID, introduce yourself, and explain rationale for procedure to client.
   a. Procedure is a rapid version of the four-point gait.
   b. Gait requires more balance than the four-point gait.
3. Demonstrate the crutch-foot sequence to the client.
   a. Advance the right foot and the left crutch simultaneously.
   b. Advance the left foot and the right crutch simultaneously.
4. Help the client practice the gait. Use safety belt if necessary.
5. Assess the client's progress and correct any mistakes as they occur.
6. Perform hand hygiene.

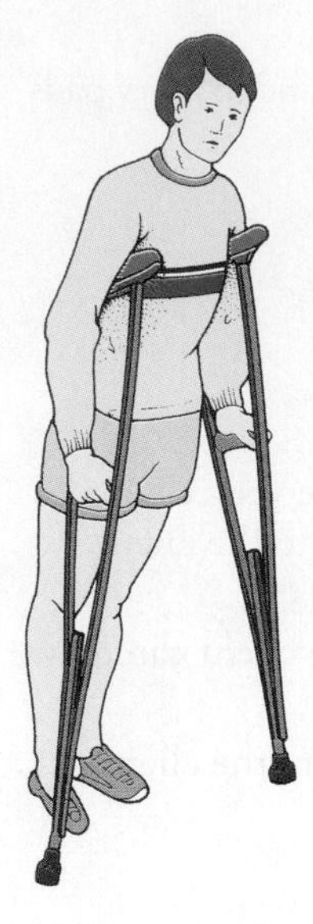
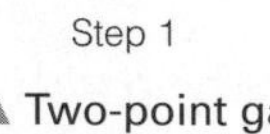
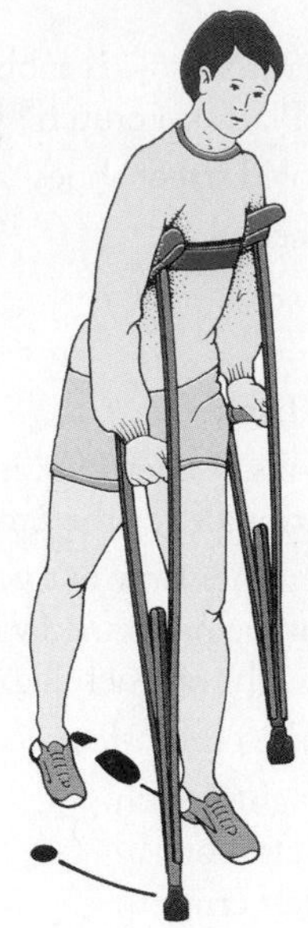

▲ Two-point gait.

Teaching Swing-To Gait and Swing-Through Gait

Equipment

Properly fitted crutches with rubber tips and arm pads
Regular, hard-soled street shoes
Safety belt, if needed

Procedure

1. Perform hand hygiene.
2. Check two forms of client ID, introduce yourself, and explain rationale for procedure to client.
   a. These gaits are usually performed when the client's lower extremities are paralyzed.
   b. The client may require braces.
3. Demonstrate the crutch-foot sequence to the client.
   a. Move both crutches forward.
   b. Swing-to gait: Lift and swing the body to the crutches.
   c. Swing-through gait: Lift and swing the body past the crutches.
   d. Bring crutches in front of the body and repeat.

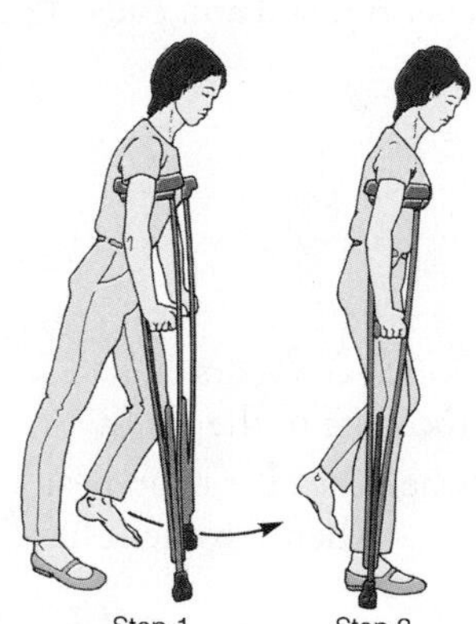
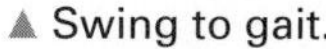

▲ Swing to gait.

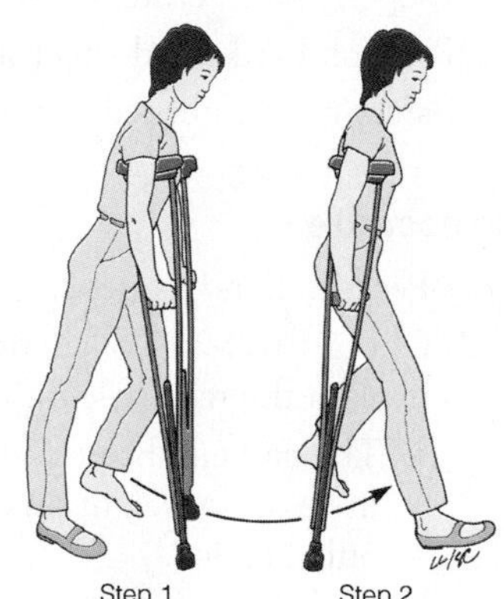

▲ Swing through gait.

4. Help the client practice the gaits. Use safety belt if necessary.
5. Assess the client's progress and correct any mistakes as they occur.
6. Perform hand hygiene.

Teaching Upstairs and Downstairs Ambulation With Crutches

Equipment

Properly fitted crutches with rubber tips and arm pads
Regular, hard-soled street shoes
Safety belt, if needed

Procedure

1. Perform hand hygiene.
2. Check two forms of client ID, introduce yourself, and explain rationale for the procedure to the client.
3. Apply safety belt if client is unsteady or requires support.
4. Demonstrate procedure using a three-point gait.

For Going Downstairs

a. Start with weight on the unaffected leg and crutches on the same level.
b. Put crutches on the first step.
c. Put weight on the crutch handles and transfer unaffected extremity to the step where crutches are placed.
d. Repeat until client understands the procedure.

For Going Upstairs

a. Start with the crutches and unaffected extremity on the same level.
b. Put weight on the crutch handles and lift the unaffected extremity onto the first step of the stairs.
c. Put weight on the unaffected extremity and lift other extremity and the crutches to the step.
d. Repeat until client understands the procedure.

5. Help the client practice.
6. Make sure that the client has adequate balance. Be ready to assist if necessary.
7. Assess the client's progress and correct any mistakes as they occur.
8. Perform hand hygiene.

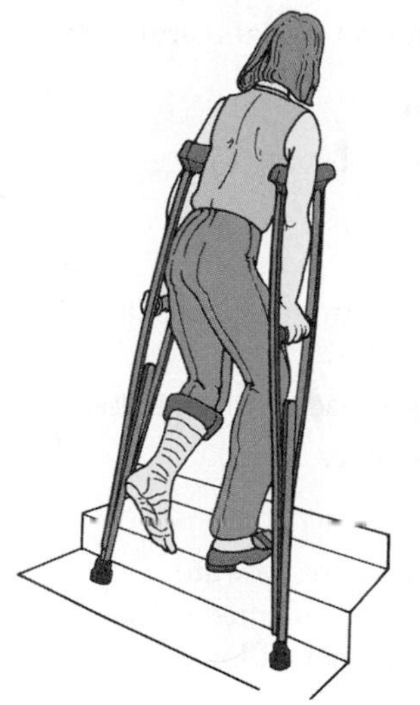
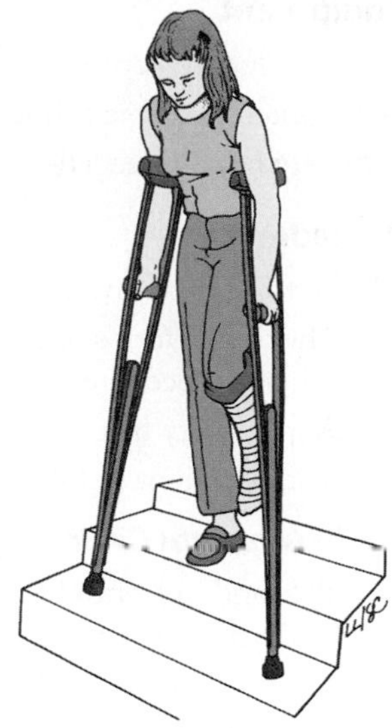

▲ Crutch ambulation—up stairs and down stairs.

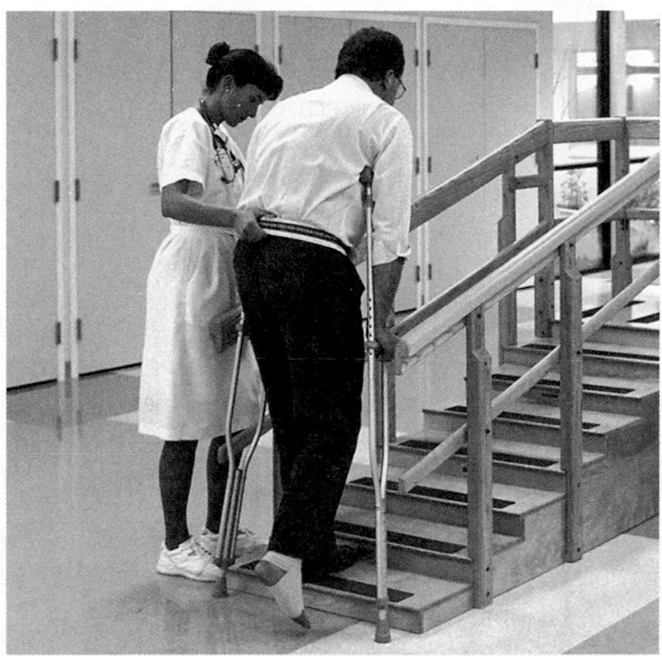

▲ Use safety belt when client is first learning to manipulate stairs.

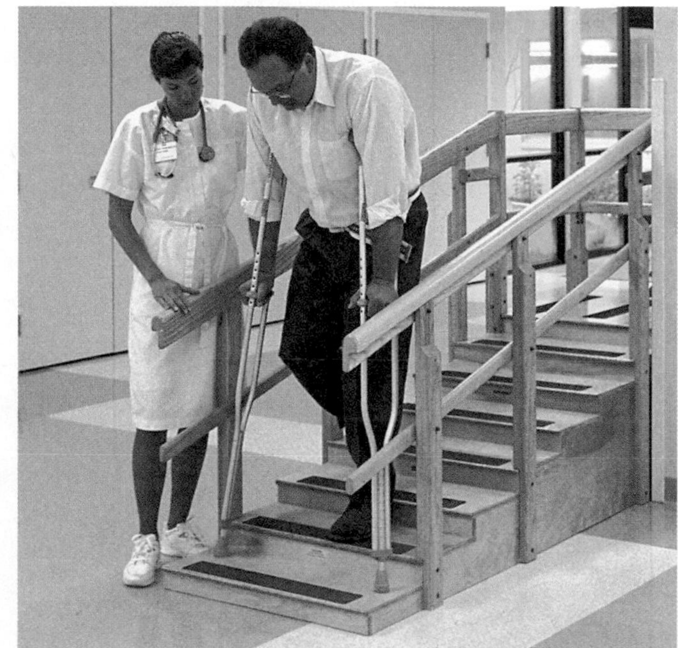

▲ Demonstrate going up or down stairs using a three-point gait.

Teaching Moving in and out of Chair With Crutches

Equipment

Properly fitted crutches with rubber tips and arm pads
Regular, hard-soled shoes
Safety belt, if needed

Procedure

1. Perform hand hygiene.
2. Check two forms of client ID, introduce yourself, and explain procedure to client.
3. Apply safety belt if client is unsteady with crutches.
4. Instruct client to follow these steps.

For Moving Into Chair

a. Stand in front of the chair, facing forward.
b. Place both crutches in hand on affected side.
c. Move backward slowly until back of lower legs touch center of chair.
d. Hold on to chair arm on unaffected side.
e. Lower self into chair by bending knees and hips, keeping back straight.
f. Use crutches and unaffected leg as a support.

For Moving Out of Chair

a. Move forward in chair by using unaffected side to slide body to edge of chair.
b. Hold on to chair arm on unaffected side.
c. Place both crutches in hand on affected side.
d. Lift self out of chair by grasping the chair arm and supporting self with crutches. Put weight on unaffected leg as you lift body out of chair.
e. Stand with back straight, bearing weight on unaffected leg and crutches.
f. Place crutches in front and slightly to side of body and begin crutch walking.

5. Perform hand hygiene.

DOCUMENTATION for Crutch Walking

- Time and distance of ambulation on crutches
- Balance
- Reason for safety belt, if used
- Problems noted with technique
- Remedial teaching
- Client's perceptions of ambulation with crutches
- Ability to move in and out of chair
- Fear of using crutches

CRITICAL THINKING Application

Expected Outcomes

- Client is able to ambulate without assistance.
- Client is able to use crutches to ambulate without fear or anxiety.
- Client is able to move in and out of chair with crutches.
- Crutches are measured appropriately to prevent numbness or tingling in fingers.

Unexpected Outcomes	Alternative Actions
Client states he or she is frightened of the crutches.	• Observe as the client practices the procedures to make sure that he or she is completing the steps correctly for each gait. • Explain that it takes time to become proficient. • Reassure the client that he or she will improve with continued practice. • Assess the client's ability to use the crutches and evaluate level of confidence. • Place safety or gait belt on client until he/she feels confident. • Check with physician about obtaining an order for a walker until the client feels more confident.
Client fears falling while dependent on crutches.	• Slow down crutch protocol until client gains confidence at every level of mastery (e.g., four-point gait to two-point gait). • Remain with client and give verbal reassurance and feedback for improvement.

Unexpected Outcomes	Alternative Actions
Shoulder girdle is too weak to bear client's weight for crutch support.	• Increase exercise of shoulder (biceps and triceps setting) to gain strength. • Request physician to write an order for overhead frame with trapeze for shoulder exercise sets.
Slipping occurs with crutch walking.	• Check crutch tips to ensure they cover all metal or wood. • Observe the client's stance or gait to determine if it is too broad. • Be sure that floor surface is dry and free of scatter rugs.
Client complains of numbness and tingling in fingers when crutch walking.	• Remeasure distance between axilla and crutch bars to determine if two finger breadths can be inserted. • Observe client's gait to determine if he or she is leaning on crutch inappropriately.

Chapter 13

UNIT 4

Adaptation for Home Care

Nursing Process Data

ASSESSMENT Data Base

- Assess family's knowledge of the principles of body mechanics.
- Assess home care provider's knowledge of how to use correct muscle groups for specific activities.
- Assess knowledge of how to improvise for a nonhospital bed.
- Assess knowledge and correct any misinformation about body alignment and ability to move client up in bed without assistance.

PLANNING Objectives

- To promote proper body mechanics while caring for clients
- To move clients without assistance, preventing back injury
- To provide knowledge of the musculoskeletal system, body alignment, and balance in order to prevent back injury when providing care for a client in the home
- To provide methods of improvising for a nonhospital bed
- To discuss four safety tips for home care clients requiring assistive devices

IMPLEMENTATION Procedures

EVALUATION Expected Outcomes

- Correct body mechanics are used in caring for clients.
- Injuries are prevented to both nurse and client.
- Client care is facilitated by proper body mechanics.
- Client is able to move without assistance.
- Center of gravity is maintained when lifting objects.
- Nonhospital bed is easily adapted for home care.

Pearson Nursing Student Resources

Find additional review materials at **nursing.pearsonhighered.com**

Prepare for success with NCLEX®-style practice questions and Skill Checklists

Positioning Nonhospital Bed for Client Care

Procedure

1. Position foam wedges to simulate change in position when head of bed does not move (high-Fowler's/90°; Fowler's/60°; semi-Fowler's/30°).
2. Use correct body mechanics to adjust height.
   a. Flex body at knees and keep back straight if bed is only slightly low.
   b. Kneel on pillow by bed or sit in chair alongside bed if bed is extremely low.
3. Lock each wheel or leg of bed in position by securing with bricks or blocks of wood.
4. Make footboard of lumber or item such as a TV tray; position legs of tray under mattress so that tray becomes footboard.

Correct Body Mechanics

- Place both feet flat on the floor and keep your back straight to prevent back injury.
- Hold objects close to the body to prevent muscle strain and possible back injury.
- Keep body in proper alignment by bending your knees and keeping back straight when lifting objects to prevent injury to back muscles.

Moving a Helpless Client up in Bed Without Assistance

Procedure

1. Lower head of bed and place pillow at head of bed.
2. Stand at side of client's bed.
   a. Face far corner at foot of bed.
   b. Place one foot behind the other, assume a broad stance, and flex knees.
3. Flex arms so forearms are level with bed. Place one arm under client's head and one under small of back.
4. Rock and shift weight from forward to rear foot; hips will move downward.
5. Guide the client as he or she slides diagonally across bed toward head.
6. Repeat for trunk and leg sections.
7. Move to other side of bed and repeat Steps 2 through 5.
8. Repeat until client is satisfactorily positioned in bed.

NOTE: Mechanical lift devices are made for home care clients. See Chapter 12.

Using Assistive Devices in Home

Equipment

Appropriate Device for:
- Assistance with walking
- Cane
- Walker
- Crutches
- Gait belt (optional)

Procedure

For Cane

1. Ensure client was measured appropriately for cane (refer to top of page 375).
2. Review steps in working with a cane. Demonstrate, if necessary.
3. Assist client to use gait belt if unsure of client's balance.
4. Assist client to walk stairs as needed.
5. Review safety issues with cane: observe tips of cane to ensure rubber covers top completely.
6. Instruct caregiver in proper method to walk with cane.

For Crutches

1. Ensure client was measured appropriately for crutches (refer to page 392).
2. Review steps in crutch walking according to type of gait: two point, four point, etc.
3. Demonstrate appropriate gait.
4. Instruct client to demonstrate gait; use gait belt constantly with crutches.
5. Instruct client to walk up and down stairs if needed and have client return demonstration.
6. Instruct client on how to sit down on chair using crutches.
7. Instruct client and caregiver to examine rubber tips and change if they become worn.

For Walker

1. Ensure client was measured appropriately for walker and appropriate type of walker was selected (with wheels, with seat, etc.).
2. Review steps in using walker.
3. Demonstrate moving walker and proper foot.
4. Discuss how to grasp handles on walker with both hands.
5. Instruct client and caregiver to examine rubber tips on walker and change if worn.

Instructing Caregiver on Safety Issues

Procedure

1. Inspect household for general safety issues. Instruct caregiver and client on change necessary to promote safety for clients using assistive devices.
2. Ensure adequate space to allow client to move throughout the house.
   a. Remove small scatter rugs from pathway.
   b. Keep electrical cords out of pathway.
   c. Wipe up spills that can cause slips.
   d. Position furniture to make space for assistive devices.
   e. Keep frequently used household items in easy access in lower shelves to prevent client from falling.
   f. Install nonslip bath mats and grab bars next to toilet and in shower. Install raised toilet seat and shower/tub seats.
   g. Encourage client to use fanny pack or apron to carry items about the house.
   h. Discuss issues related to house pets and safety.
3. Instruct caregiver to watch for warning signs of difficulty. Notify MD if any signs appear.

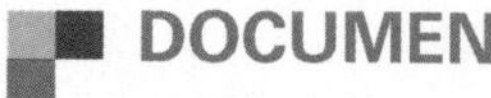

DOCUMENTATION for Home Care

Using appropriate home care forms, document the following:

- Environmental assessment and safety instruction
- Client's ability to use assistive devices safely
- Support needed for assisting client utilizing assistive devices
- Caregiver's ability to move client up in bed

CRITICAL THINKING Application

Expected Outcomes

- Client has safe environment in home for ambulation using assistive devices.
- Client provided appropriate instruction to make ambulation using assistive devices.

Unexpected Outcomes	Alternative Actions
Client not stable ambulating with crutches or cane.	• Place safety belt on client and ambulate with walker. • Increase both upper and lower muscle strength to increase ambulation with cane or crutches.
Unable to lift client up in bed with single healthcare worker.	• If a second person is available, utilize him/her to assist in moving. • Use sliding board if two healthcare workers are available. • Rent a hydraulic lift or Hoyer lift to assist with moving up in bed or getting out of bed.
Client is not ambulating.	• Discuss with caregiver and client reasons why client is not ambulating. • If client is afraid of falling, ensure that a gait belt is worn and the client uses a walker to start with and then moves to a cane, if possible. • Use two individuals to assist with walking, if available.

GERONTOLOGIC Considerations

The Elderly Can Suffer Impaired Mobility and Disability Due to Decreased Physical Function or Accidents

- Nearly 23% of older people living in the community have some degree of disability.
- Persons 85 and older constitute 27% of those who have impaired mobility.
- Impaired mobility can lead to many subsequent problems, including depression, negative self-image, dependent behavior, and loss of independence.
- Effects of disability can influence the individual's body image, physical appearance, and bodily sensations.
- Posture becomes more flexed and center of gravity shifts.

Special Assessment Parameters Are Important for the Elderly

- Specific source of disability or impaired mobility
- Presence of accompanying disease state: arthritis, stroke, dementia, diabetes, heart failure, COPD
- Presence of pain
- Condition of skin
- Drug effects: sedation, incontinence, orthostatic hypotension
- Motivation for rehabilitation
- Nutritional status
- Best assistive aid for client
- Be aware of any vision problems your client may have, especially cataracts, glaucoma, or macular degeneration. Note poorly lighted areas in the home or dark areas in the corridors, throw rugs, uneven or uncarpeted areas adjoining carpeted areas, etc., which may cause the client to stumble or fall.
- Check your client's ability to be mobile—their gait, balance, and posture, and whether the client shuffles or is able to pick up his or her feet. Check if the client leans forward and is therefore off balance. Poor or unsteady mobility is often a direct cause of falling.
- Assess the client's degree of muscle strength on both sides of body and/or loss of flexibility because as age increases, strength declines, resulting in a fall. Check the degree of range of motion to all joints before ambulating. Even a poor hand grip can be dangerous if the client is walking downstairs. If leg muscles are weak, it may be difficult to get off a bed or up from a chair and the client may lose his or her balance.
- Assess for certain medications the client is taking which may cause vertigo, poor balance, blurred vision, weakness, or even drowsiness. Review the medications for elderly clients, keeping in mind the fact that they may require only half the normal dose due to their age and inability to metabolize drugs. The use of alcohol may contribute to falls in the home environment, so if the client uses alcohol there should be client teaching that focuses on the potential danger.
- Chronic diseases such as osteoarthritis, Parkinson's, Alzheimer's, and diabetes with peripheral neuropathy can all contribute to falls. Clients who have these diseases may require special assessment and interventions to prevent falls.
- Most elderly clients are aware of the danger of falling and breaking a hip or a leg, so fear is usually present when they are moving or walking. Proper intervention and instructions with an assistive device (canes, walkers, wheelchairs, etc.) will help to allay these fears, which may become so overpowering that they cause immobilization and depression. Even fear itself, with its concomitant caution, may result in a fall; if the nurse can work with the client to discuss fears about falling and specific behaviors to prevent falling, it would be very therapeutic.

Develop Nursing Care Plan to Meet Elderly Client's Needs

- Focus on disability or impaired mobility.
- Establish supportive relationship.
- Teach activities of daily living. Determine activities that must be accomplished each day for individual to care for own needs and be as independent as possible.
- Use assistive devices until client is stable and able to ambulate independently.
- Increase activities as individual progresses and is able to resume activity.
- Give positive reinforcement for all effort expended.

MANAGEMENT Guidelines

Each state legislates a Nurse Practice Act for RNs and LVN/LPNs. Healthcare facilities are responsible for establishing and implementing policies and procedures that conform to their state's regulations. Verify the regulations and role parameters for each healthcare worker in your facility.

Delegation

- Range of motion is usually performed for the first time by or under the supervision of a licensed physical therapist or RN. If these members are not available, the nurse or healthcare worker must understand the principles of the skill before performing it on the client. Range of motion is important for the client who is immobilized or on long-term bedrest, so if the skill is ordered more than once per day, it will probably be delegated to an LVN/LPN, CNA, or UAP. This staff member should be assigned to observe and be checked by personnel who understand the skill.
- Ambulation may be done by any healthcare worker and is often assigned to a CNA or UAP. However, the first time a

client is ambulated, an assessment is very important for safety reasons, and this should be performed by an RN or LVN/LPN. In some medical–surgical settings, a physical therapist may ambulate specific high-risk clients for the first time. A licensed nurse performing this task will minimize the possibility of orthostatic hypotension occurring, because assessment and vital signs are an important part of the skill.

- Crutch walking is a skill often performed initially with specialized personnel, such as the physical therapist. However, the nurse should understand the principles of crutch walking so that he or she may reinforce the correct steps of the procedure whether the client is in the hospital or in the home setting.

Communication Matrix

- Range-of-motion and muscle-strengthening exercises, ambulation, and crutch walking should all be included in the verbal report at change of shift to all personnel and charted in the client's record.
- Any problems that occur with the exercises or ambulation should also be noted and, if present, the task should be reassigned to licensed personnel. It is especially important to note occurrence of orthostatic hypotension and what actions were effective to minimize the effects on the client.

CRITICAL THINKING Strategies

Scenario 1

You are assigned to care for two clients during the day shift.

Client A: A 65-year-old obese client who had a hysterectomy yesterday. Her orders include ambulation and up-in-chair TID on the first postop day.

Client B: A 70-year-old female client who is to be discharged today after having an inguinal hernia repair yesterday.

1. What is your priority of care of these two clients?
2. What assessment will you focus on for both clients and which assessment will be your priority?
3. Briefly describe the discharge teaching that will be done for Client B.
4. When you approach Client B and tell her you would like to do her discharge teaching, she informs you, "Oh, at my age, I can be a couch potato so I don't need you to tell me anything." What is your best response?
5. Based on the information provided, what generalizations can you make about the general health and projected health of this client?
6. What is the primary danger to the health of this client? Describe how you will explain this to the client.
7. What plan (part of discharge teaching) can you devise to positively affect this situation?
8. You have elicited the help of a nursing assistant to help you ambulate Client A. As you are ambulating the client, she begins to fall. What steps should both you and the nursing assistant take to prevent client injury?
9. After your initial intervention, what other actions should be taken for this client?
10. What preliminary actions should have been taken to prevent this from happening?

Scenario 2

You are a student on an orthopedic unit and are assigned to assist the RN in the care of her clients for the day shift. You obtained the following information during report.

Client A: Client had a right-sided CVA 4 days ago and needs to be instructed on the use of a walker before being discharged to a long-term care facility this morning.

Client B: Client was instructed on the use of a cane yesterday, but no one has seen him practicing with the cane. He had a CVA several years ago and still has some instability when walking. He is 80 years old, wears a hearing aid, and is very independent.

Client C: Client is a 20-year-old who had an arthrotomy last night for injuries from football. He stayed overnight as a result of being nauseated and with low blood pressure. He is to be discharged this morning with crutches.

1. Which client should be assessed first?
2. Provide rationale for your choice.
3. Discuss your priority interventions for each of the clients.
4. Client A: Identify the major nursing action for this client before beginning instruction on the use of a walker.
5. Client B: What hunches do you have regarding why the client may not have been practicing with the cane?

NCLEX® Review Questions

Unless otherwise specified, choose only one (1) answer.

1. The movement of a bone away from the midline is termed:
   1. Flexion.
   2. Eversion.
   3. Adduction.
   4. Abduction.

2. Passive range-of-motion exercises (ROM) were ordered for the client. The nurse has just performed the exercises on the client who is on strict bedrest. The documentation for this skill includes
   Select all that apply.
   1. Total time for exercises.
   2. Specific joints put through ROM.
   3. Specific joints that client was able to exercise independently.
   4. Movements that caused unusual pain.
3. During morning report the nurse states that the client assigned to you experienced orthostatic hypotension when getting out of bed. Your priority intervention before taking the client to the bathroom is to
   1. Move client to side of bed and assist him to transfer to a walker.
   2. Take vital signs before allowing client to stand up.
   3. Raise and lower head of the bed slowly several times before attempting to assist client out of bed.
   4. Obtain assistance from another health team member to assist client to ambulate.
4. Client teaching needs to be completed before the client uses a walker. The correct instructions include
   1. Place walker approximately 2 feet in front of client and instruct client to push self off bed, stand erect, and grasp hand grips on the walker.
   2. Move walker by pulling legs of walker slightly off floor as you move unaffected leg forward.
   3. Move weaker side of body first by supporting body weight on handles of walker and then advancing weaker leg.
   4. Grasp handles of walker and move weaker leg first by moving body toward center of walker.
5. Instructions provided to a client who is using a cane for the first time should include the following information
   1. "You will need to place the cane on the weaker side of your body."
   2. "The cane is placed directly to the side of your weaker leg to help maintain balance."
   3. "The cane and unaffected leg are moved together when walking."
   4. "You need to move the cane forward, then bring the affected leg forward even with the cane."
6. Instructions to the client who is learning to use the cane when walking steps should include
   1. "When going downstairs, the unaffected leg is placed on the step, followed by the cane."
   2. "When going downstairs, the affected leg and cane are moved to the step before moving the unaffected leg to the same step."
   3. "When going upstairs, the first step is placing the affected leg and cane on the step, then the unaffected leg."
   4. "When going upstairs, the unaffected leg is placed on the step, followed by the cane and affected leg."
7. Before the client uses crutches they must be measured to the appropriate length. Which of the following instructions will be given to the client?
   1. Place stocking feet flat on the floor and then measure height of crutches.
   2. With client lying in bed with shoes on, measure distance from axilla to a point 6 to 8 in. out from heel.
   3. Ensure axilla rests on bars of the crutches when measuring for length.
   4. Assist client to standing position with shoes on, keeping crutches tight to body, and measure distance from crutch bar to floor.
8. A client who can move and bear weight on each leg will be taught the __________ gait for crutch walking.
   1. Three-point.
   2. Four-point.
   3. Two-point.
   4. Swing-through.
9. Clients going upstairs with crutches will start with:
   1. Weight on the uninjured leg on the step, and placing crutches on upper step.
   2. Weight on the uninjured leg and crutches at same level.
   3. Crutches on upper step and then bringing injured leg to the step.
   4. Moving injured leg to first step with one crutch, then moving second crutch and uninjured leg to the next step.
10. The client states that when she uses the crutches, she slips. Which of the following critical thinking options should be implemented?
    Select all that apply.
    1. Observe client using the crutches to see if she is leaning on them inappropriately.
    2. Reassure client that this will not occur as she becomes more proficient with the crutches.
    3. Observe client's stance or gait to check if it is too broad, causing her to slip.
    4. Check crutch tips to ensure they cover all the metal or wood from the crutches.

14

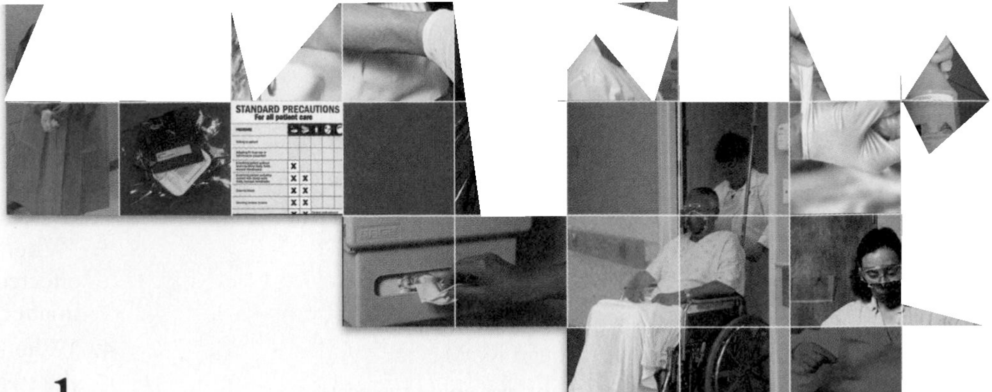

Infection Control

LEARNING OBJECTIVES

1. Describe and draw the six steps in the chain of infection.
2. Explain what is meant by the body's natural defenses.
3. List and describe eight conditions that predispose clients to infection.
4. Describe what is meant by the term healthcare-associated (*nosocomial*) infection and discuss one intervention that will help to prevent it.
5. List the major organisms responsible for healthcare-associated infections.
6. State the main purpose of hand hygiene.
7. Demonstrate donning and removing a gown.
8. Define the terms *surgical asepsis* and *medical asepsis*.
9. Outline the steps in donning isolation clothing before entering an isolation room.
10. Outline the steps in removing isolation clothing before leaving the room.
11. State the isolation procedure for removing specimens and equipment from an isolation room.
12. Describe the modes of transmission of HIV.
13. List three precaution principles and explain their main purpose.
14. List blood and body fluid protection protocol.
15. Describe the difference between the first and second tier of precautions.
16. Compare and contrast infection control practices in the home and hospital.
17. Differentiate assessment modalities to determine potential for infection in home care and hospitalized clients.

CHAPTER OUTLINE

TERMINOLOGY

AIDS acquired immunodeficiency syndrome—a serious condition characterized by a defect in natural immunity against disease. When the immune system is suppressed, the individual is vulnerable to a host of opportunistic infections.

Antibody protein substance developed by the body to fight disease organisms. Not effective against a virus that is inside the cells.

Antimicrobial an agent that prevents the development or pathogenic action of microbes.

Antiseptics agents that are applied to body tissues, such as skin or mucous membrane, to destroy or retard the growth of microorganisms.

Asepsis the absence of disease-producing microorganisms.

Aseptic technique a method to eliminate contamination, germs, or infection.

Autoinfections infections that arise from an individual's own body flora.

AZT an antiviral drug currently being used as an effective drug against HIV.

Bacteriostatic a substance that prevents the growth or multiplication of bacteria.

Barrier nursing any technique that reduces the risk of cross-contamination.

Biohazard waste any solid or liquid waste that may present a threat of infection.

Carrier a person or animal without signs of illness but who carries pathogens on or within his or her body that can be transferred to others.

Cell-mediated immunity reactions to antigens by cells rather than antibody molecules present in body fluids.

Chemotaxis attraction and repulsion of living protoplasm to a chemical stimulus.

Cofactors existing characteristics in the individual that may make them more susceptible to the AIDS virus.

Colonization organisms present in body tissue but not multiplying or invading the tissue.

Contagious disease a disease conveyed easily to others.

Contamination introduction of disease, germs, or infectious materials into or on normally sterile objects.

Detergent compounds (surfactants) that possess a cleaning action, often referred to as soaps. They are composed of a hydrophilic and a lipophilic substance.

Disinfectants chemical agents that are used to destroy or reduce microorganisms on inanimate surfaces and objects.

Disinfection a process that employs physical and chemical means to remove, control, or destroy most of the organisms that may be present on equipment or materials.

Duration of the infectious challenge sustained exposure to even a relatively small number of organisms that poses a significant risk to the client (e.g., intravenous catheters become colonized with microorganisms).

Endogenous organisms natural to an individual's own body.

Enteric precautions isolation practices designed to prevent transmission of pathogens through contact with fecal matter and vomitus.

Exogenous organisms external to an individual's own body.

False negative a negative test in someone who in fact has been infected by a microorganism but for some reason has not developed antibodies.

False positive a positive test for an antibody. Usually the result of an artifact of the laboratory test; the person has not in fact been exposed to the microorganism. All persons who test positive should have the test repeated.

Granulation formation of granules (roughened prominences). Each granulation represents an outgrowth of new capillaries and enriched blood supply.

HAI Healthcare-Associated Infection formerly Hospital-Acquired Infection or nosocomial; an infection not present and without evidence of incubation at the time of admission to a healthcare setting.

HIV human immunodeficiency virus is a blood-borne retrovirus that has a different life cycle from a normal virus.

Host an animal or person on which or within which microorganisms live.

Humoral immunity acquired immunity in which the circulating antibody is predominant.

Hygiene study of health and observance of rules pertinent to health.

Incubation period the time between infection from a microorganism and the onset of symptoms. Seems to range from 6 months to 7 years for AIDS. Not everyone who is exposed to the virus develops the disease.

Infection establishment of a disease process that involves invasion of the body tissue by microorganisms and the reaction of the tissues to their presence and to the toxins generated by them.

Isolation technique practices designed to prevent the transmission of communicable diseases.

Kaposi's sarcoma a type of cancer usually occurring on the surface of the skin or in the mouth. Kaposi's sarcoma may also spread to internal organs of the body and may be responsible for death.

Latex natural rubber used in many gloves and medical equipment. Latex proteins can enter the body and cause latex allergy.

MDR-TB multidrug-resistant tuberculosis is an in vitro resistant strain of TB to antituberculosis drugs.

Medical asepsis all practices that limit the number and growth of microorganisms and their transmission.

Microorganism minute living body, such as a bacterium, protozoan, or virus, not perceptible to the naked eye.

Nosocomial infection see HAI.

Opportunistic infections illness or diseases that would not be a threat to anyone whose immune system is functioning normally, but in a person with AIDS may be responsible for death.

Opsonin a substance in blood serum that acts on microorganisms and other cells and facilitates phagocytosis.

Outbreak a critical incident in which infections occur above an established level and are caused by the same infective agent.

Pathogen a microorganism that can cause infectious disease in the human body.

PEP postexposure prophylaxis; recommendations from the CDC on how to treat a healthcare worker's exposure to HIV.

Pneumocystis carinii pneumonia PCP is a parasitic infection of the lungs. This is one of the two rare diseases that affect 85% of AIDS clients. PCP has symptoms similar to other severe forms of pneumonia.

Primary immune response response that occurs when the B cell recognizes an antigen, becomes activated, and divides into more memory cells.

Protective isolation practices designed to protect a highly susceptible person from contagious diseases, reverse isolation.

Protocol description of steps taken in exact order—may be legally binding.

Resident (normal) flora organisms natural to an individual's own body. Organisms multiply in the environment, not merely survive there.

Retrovirus a virus with a life cycle in which the genetic information is in reverse of that in an ordinary virus: the RNA code is transcribed backward into DNA.

Sepsis condition resulting from the presence of pathogenic bacteria and their products.

Sterile free from any living microorganisms.

Subungual an area beneath a fingernail or toenail.

Surgical asepsis practices which will maintain area free from microorganisms, as by a surgical scrub or sterile technique.

Susceptible sites an area that is sensitive to or can be invaded by a bacterium or other infectious agent.

Virulence recognized pathogenic organisms designated because of their ability to invade and propagate in normal, intact, uncompromised individuals. Some organisms that are avirulent for normal individuals become pathogenic when defense mechanisms are impaired.

Virus minute, parasitic organism that depends on nutrients inside cells for its metabolic and reproductive needs. These organisms cause a variety of infectious diseases and stimulate host antibodies. Unlike a bacteria, viruses are unable to survive long on their own and are not affected by antibodies.

Waterless antiseptic agent an antiseptic agent that does not require use of exogenous water. Agent dries automatically after applying to hands and rubbing hands together.

CHAIN OF INFECTION

For an infection to occur a chain of events must take place. If the chain is broken through the implementation of infection control measures, the infection is less likely to occur. The chain of infection involves six steps.

Infectious Agent (Microorganism) The first step in the chain involves the presence of an infectious agent, or microorganism. Whether the microorganism is capable of producing an infection depends on a number of circumstances: the virulence and number of organisms present, the susceptibility of the host, the existence of a portal of entry, and the affinity of the host to harbor the microorganism.

Reservoir A reservoir must provide a favorable environment for growth and multiplication of the microorganism. These reservoirs include the respiratory, gastrointestinal, reproductive and urinary tract, and blood.

Portal of Exit The third link in the chain must be a portal of exit, which allows the microorganism to move from the reservoir to the host. Without a portal of exit an infection cannot occur. The portal of exit is directly associated with the reservoir. For example, if the reservoir is the respiratory tract, the portal of exit is through sneezing, coughing, breathing, or talking. If the reservoir is blood, the portal of exit is through an open wound, needle puncture site, or nonintact skin surface.

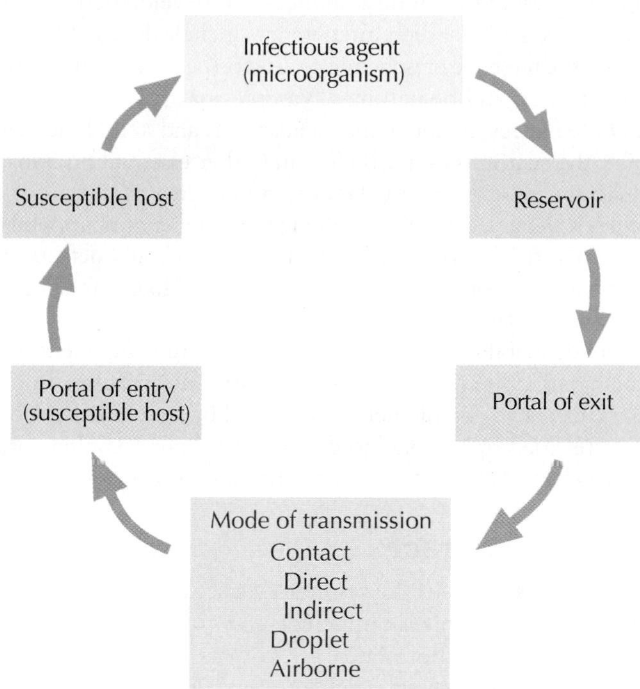

▲ Six steps in the chain of infection.

Mode of Transmission The fourth step is transmission of microorganisms. There are five routes of transmission; the three primary routes are contact, droplet, and airborne. Two lesser routes are common vehicle (transmission by contaminated items such as food, water, devices, or equipment) and vector borne (transmission by vectors such as mosquitoes, fleas, or rats). This last mode of transmission is more significant in other parts of the world than in the United States.

Contact transmission, the most frequent source of nosocomial infection, is transmitted via two modes—direct and indirect contact. Direct contact involves a direct transmission, body-to-body, and the physical transfer of microorganisms from one infected person to another, for example, through sexual contact, kissing, or even touch. It also may occur when a healthcare worker touches a client, gives a client a bath, or performs other care activities. Indirect transmission involves contact with a contaminated intermediate object such as a needle, instrument, or dressing. This also occurs when contaminated hands are not washed, gloves are not changed between clients, and whenever there is a break in technique.

Droplet transmission is a form of contact transmission, but the mechanism of pathogen transfer is so different that it is considered a separate route of transmission. It occurs when droplets from the infected source person are projected a short distance to the host's nasal mucosa, mouth, or conjunctiva. These droplets are not suspended in the air, so it is not considered airborne transmission.

Airborne transmission occurs by dissemination of either small particle nuclei of evaporated droplets or dust particles containing the infectious agent. These agents can be dispersed widely by air currents, as with Legionnaire's disease, and may be inhaled by a susceptible host. These microorganisms include *Mycobacterium tuberculosis*, rubeola, and varicella viruses.

Portal of Entry The most effective barrier to transmission of microorganisms is an intact skin. For an infection to occur it must have a means of entering the body. A disruption in the integrity of the skin provides such a portal of entry for microorganisms. Microorganisms also enter the body the same way they leave the body. The respiratory system provides a viable portal of both exit and entry.

Susceptible Host For an infection to occur a susceptible host is needed—someone who is "at risk." This includes clients who are immunosuppressed, fatigued, stressed, anemic, not immunized, poorly nourished, or those who have underlying diseases. Hospitalized clients with wounds, catheters, and IVs are at high risk for developing infections. Clients who require invasive procedures, blood specimen collections, and surgery are also in the high risk category.

BARRIERS TO INFECTION

An individual's ability to resist infection is determined by the status of the body's defense mechanisms and by the person's general health. Factors that contribute to susceptibility to infection include altered nutritional status, stress, fatigue, disease, drugs, metabolic functions, and age. Clients with severe underlying diseases are most likely to develop nosocomial infections. The body is protected against infection by immunities, by the inflammatory process, and by anatomic barriers that include the skin and mucous membranes.

When the integrity of the skin or mucous membrane is broken, both resident and transient flora or bacteria have a direct route to the internal tissues of the body. To prevent the spread of infection, the body's internal defense mechanisms mobilize and begin clearing and repairing the damaged site. How quickly a wound heals depends on the degree of vascularization in the injured area, the location and cleanliness of the wound, and the degree of tissue damage.

The second way the body resists infections is through immunity, antitoxins, and vaccines. Natural immunity is inherited. Acquired immunity occurs after an individual has been exposed to a disease or infection or has been vaccinated.

The third way the body resists infection is through the inflammatory process. Inflammation involves use of metabolic energy, increased blood flow to the inflamed area, and, in many cases, drainage of inflammatory debris to the external environment.

When an area becomes inflamed, cells at the site activate the plasmin system, the clotting system, and the kinin system. The result of the activation of these systems is the release of histamine, which creates increased vascular permeability around the injured site, and the release of chemotoxic agents, which summon phagocytes into the vascular and tissue spaces. Phagocytes are white blood cells that combat and prevent infection by ingesting harmful microorganisms.

The Body's Natural Defenses

Any alteration in the body's natural defenses increases the probability that an infection will occur. Almost any organism can be the cause of a significant nosocomial infection, given the proper circumstances. Some of the variables that help determine which organism emerges as the pathogen are the virulence and number of organisms, the exposure and attachment of the organism to a susceptible site, and the duration of the client's exposure to the infectious challenge. The following formula illustrates these variables.

$$\frac{\text{Dose} \times \text{Virulence}}{\text{Host Resistance}} = \text{Infection}$$

Using this formula, the client's risk factors can be evaluated. The inherent health and immunologic status of the client are also major factors in determining whether an infection occurs.

Alterations in the skin barrier include any physiologic break in the integrity of the skin. Intentional breaks are caused by the use of percutaneous catheters and needles and by surgical procedures. Unintentional causes of skin breakdown include the development of pressure ulcers and traumatic wounds.

CONDITIONS PREDISPOSING TO INFECTION

Certain conditions and invasive techniques predispose clients to infection because the integrity of the skin is broken or the illness itself establishes a climate favorable for the infectious process to occur. Among the most common are surgical wounds, changes in the antibacterial immune system, or alterations in the respiratory tract or genitourinary tract. Implants such as heart valves, prosthetic grafts, or vascular grafts can lead to nosocomial septicemias. The extensive use of IV therapy and central lines in clients has increased infections dramatically.

Surgical Site Infections

It has been documented that the longer a person is hospitalized before the surgical procedure, the greater the risk of postsurgical infection. Other factors that influence infection rates are duration of time in the operating room, time surgery is done (between midnight and 8:00 AM is period of greatest risk), whether the client has postsurgical drains in place, and if the surgery enters a colonized or infected part of the body.

It is useful for the nurse to be aware of conditions that increase the risk of postoperative infection. Risk reduction measures include preoperative showering with an antiseptic solution, the use of depilatory creams or the clipping of hair in lieu of shaving the surgical site, and keeping the incision site covered with a dry sterile dressing. A wet dressing, through osmosis and diffusion, pulls organisms down into the wound from the surface. This is particularly important during the first 45 hr before the wound becomes "watertight." Research shows that preoperative shaving results in disruption of normal flora on the surface of the skin.

Antibacterial Immune Mechanisms

There are three categories of abnormalities in antibacterial immune mechanisms: those affecting inflammatory responses, those affecting phagocytic functions, and those affecting opsonins (humoral immunity).

Anything that interferes with the migration of phagocytic cells to the area of contamination or with the physical contact of phagocytes and bacteria enhances the development of an infection. Examples of such interferences include deficient blood supplies, the presence of ischemic or dead tissue, sutured material, foreign bodies, and hematomas. Vasopressor agents, radiation injury, uremia, severe nutritional deficiencies, and steroid therapy inhibit the synthesis of antibodies and other essential proteins.

Clients with severe thermal injuries and severe nutritional deficiencies have abnormalities involving the number of neutrophils collected at the site of an inflammatory response and defects of bactericidal chemotoxic capacity. Clients with Hodgkin's disease have a specific defect in cell-mediated immunity.

Genetic inabilities to synthesize complement components or specific antibodies can cause abnormalities in opsonins. Burn clients may have complement inactivated by a circulating substance released by the damaged tissue. Without complement, lysis of cells and destruction of bacteria cannot take place.

Respiratory Tract

Common alterations in the respiratory tract that facilitate the development of an infection include endotracheal intubation, tracheostomy, bronchotracheal suctioning, and stasis due to poor respiratory excursion for clients on bedrest.

The bronchi and trachea are so sensitive to foreign matter that they initiate the cough reflex whenever irritation occurs. Ciliated, mucus-coated epithelium lining the trachea and lungs aids in clearing the respiratory tract of bacteria and mucus by the beating motion of the cilia. Intubation bypasses the cough reflex and compromises the effectiveness of this action. Although the trachea is usually considered sterile, it does not remain sterile after 48 to 72 hr of intubation. Infections associated with endotracheal intubation include pneumonia, tracheitis, and purulent bronchitis.

Catheters placed directly in the trachea can force pathogenic microorganisms into the respiratory system. In addition, catheters may damage the mucous lining of the respiratory tract, further compromising the effectiveness of its clearing mechanisms.

Genitourinary Tract

Instrumentation, including catheterization of the bladder, and complicated obstetric delivery after prolonged confinement in bed are two procedures that introduce potentially pathogenic bacteria into the genitourinary tract. Acute urinary tract infection and pyelonephritis often occur after the use of a catheter or cystoscope.

The most common alteration is the placement of an indwelling urinary catheter. Research has demonstrated that significant bacteriuria develop in only 2% of the clients who have a single "straight" catheterization (in and out) to empty a distended bladder. Although bacteriuria may be considered benign and usually resolves after removal of the catheter, bacteriuria after catheterization may result in symptomatic cystitis and, occasionally, in acute pyelonephritis, chronic pyelonephritis, and persistent asymptomatic bacteriuria. Lack of adequate fluid intake, improper positioning of the catheter and bag, use of an open versus a closed drainage system, and inadequate emptying of the bladder all serve to increase the risk of infection in the catheterized client.

Invasive Devices

Most healthcare-associated (nosocomical) septicemias occur as a result of significant alterations in normal host defenses. These infections may be primary (caused by direct introduction of microorganisms into the bloodstream) or secondary (arising from an infection at another site such as the urinary tract). In fact, the most common site for a healthcare-associated infection (HAI) is the urinary tract.

The use of IV therapy and central line insertions greatly increases the risk of introducing harmful microorganisms. The incidence of septicemia in clients receiving IV therapy varies from 0 to 8%.

Septicemia may also be caused by the introduction of microorganisms from contaminated fluids, infected venipuncture sites, or foci of septic thrombophlebitis as a complication of using an indwelling IV catheter.

Venipuncture Sites

The wounds made by a percutaneous stick at the venipuncture site may become colonized or infected. This opening provides a reservoir for bacteria that could move along the catheter into the bloodstream.

Organisms that travel down the catheter ultimately reside in the thrombus, which is usually present on the catheter tip. Around the thrombus, bacteria are shielded from the immune response and antibiotics. When these microorganisms attain a critical level, they seed the bloodstream and cause bacteremia. Site infections can be reduced by several methods: selecting a catheter appropriate to the size of the vein; avoiding sites near joints; the performance of proper site preparation; maintaining a regimen for site care; and changing the site every 48 to 72 hr as well as maintaining a closed system of therapy. Discontinuing IVs started in emergency situations like codes or "field starts" in which proper site hygiene wasn't carried out also reduces IV-related infections.

Total Parenteral Nutrition Therapy

Total parenteral nutrition therapy (TPN/TNA) is a means of achieving an anabolic state in clients who would otherwise be unable to maintain normal nitrogen balance. Problems with IV-related sepsis in TPN are the same as those seen in conventional IV therapy, only greatly magnified. The hypertonic solution used with these clients supports the growth of a wide variety of organisms, especially fungus, to a greater extent than conventional IV solutions. Clients on TPN are critically ill and malnourished. Peripheral inserted central catheter (PICC) lines are usually inserted for TPN infusions. These lines may not be changed for months. Infection control is of critical importance with TPN. Meticulous site care must be done at least every 3 days to preserve the site, and aseptic technique used when changing solution, tubing, dressings, and filters.

Implanted Prosthetic Devices

Commonly used implanted devices include artificial cardiac valves, synthetic vascular grafts, orthopedic prosthetic joints, neurosurgical shunts, and cerebrospinal fluid pressure monitoring devices. Most infections associated with prosthetic devices require long-term IV antibiotic therapy. If the infection is not controlled, removal and replacement of the prosthesis is indicated.

HEALTHCARE-ASSOCIATED (NOSOCOMIAL) INFECTIONS (HAIs)

HAIs are infections that are acquired while the client is in the hospital—infections that were not present or incubating at the time of admission. The CDC estimates that as many as 2 million infections are acquired in hospitals every year, resulting in 90,000 deaths and an additional $5 billion in healthcare expenses. As of 2006, only six states have adopted laws requiring hospitals to report the incidence of HAIs. Many of these infections are caused by pathogens transmitted from one client to another by healthcare workers. HAIs are usually caused by poor hand hygiene technique or no handwashing between clients. Hand hygiene is the single most important intervention to prevent these infections; various studies have shown that there is very poor compliance with handwashing techniques by healthcare workers. Other interventions important to the prevention of HAIs are the use of sterile technique when indicated, keeping the environment as free as possible of pathogens, and identifying and protecting at-risk clients. The CDC has studied rates of the four "hot spots"—infections of surgical sites, the bloodstream, and urinary tract, and ventilator–associated pneumonia in intensive care units.

The major organisms responsible for the majority of HAIs are *Clostridium difficile*, methicillin-resistant *Staphylococcus aureus* (MRSA), and vancomycin-resistant enterococcus (VRE). The most common organism, C. *difficile* is an anaerobic, gram-positive, spore-forming bacillus associated with infectious diarrhea (CDAD). Twenty to 40% of hospitalized clients become colonized within a few days of entering the hospital. Because it is often resistant to antimicrobial therapy, it is able to proliferate in the hospital setting. *Alert*: The alcohol-based gels do *not* kill c. *difficile*, so soap and water must be used.

MRSA

The second most common infection, affecting 40% of all critically ill or immunosuppressed clients, is pneumonia. The leading cause of this condition is gram-positive *Staphylococcus* that is methicillin resistant, labeled "healthcare-acquired" or "HA-MRSA." This condition often occurs in clients who have invasive procedures such as intravenous or respiratory therapy treatments or surgical procedures. Healthcare personnel easily transmit MRSA to clients because it frequently colonizes skin. Vancomycin, the drug of choice to treat MRSA, is losing its effectiveness as a treatment.

A new and potentially lethal strain of MRSA has developed since the late 1990s (when MRSA was also increasing among hospital-acquired S. *aureus* infections) named the "community-acquired MRSA." This strain is seen among healthy young people with no known exposure. Infections caused by CA-MRSA are easily transmitted through skin-to-skin contact or by contact with contaminated objects or surfaces. Although most clients can be treated successfully, they have the potential of developing necrotizing fasciitis or pneumonia, sepsis, furunculosis, osteomyelitis, etc.

According to the CDC, there are at least three different strains of Staphylococcus that can cause CA-MRSA. This condition can occur without any exposure to HA-MRSA. It is a distinct and separate infection both genetically and epidemiologically from HA-MRSA. This type of MRSA can occur in totally healthy individuals and is not limited to any age group or related to any other diagnosis. This infection usually begins as a skin or soft tissue infection, such as a boil or rash, and can become invasive.

Treatment of CA-MRSA can range from incision and drainage, to hot soaks, to good wound care. Antibiotics are usually the treatment of choice, and it is important that the client continue to take them for the prescribed period (usually 7–10 days). Practicing excellent hand hygiene and proper disposal of contaminated dressings are important to not spreading the infection. Inform the client that if there is blood or body fluids on the hands, they should be washed for 15 seconds, rather than using antibacterial gel. (See Standard Precautions protocol.)

Two-Hour MRSA Test

The first rapid blood test that will detect MRSA and staphylococcus aureus in 2 hr was approved by the U.S. Food and Drug Administration (FDA) in 2008. The manufacturer is BD Diagnostics. This company is developing more rapid assays to quickly identify VRC and C. *difficile*.

VRE

VRE is a gram-positive bacterium normally found in flora of the gastrointestinal tract. When this bacterium mutated and became resistant to common antimicrobial therapies, it became a major cause of HAIs in the hospital setting.

There is a new type of antibiotic available to fight resistant infections. An example of this drug (the first entirely new type of antibiotic in 35 years) is Zyvox. This drug and others of its genre are the drugs of choice for VRE and MRSA.

STANDARD PRECAUTIONS

In 1985, universal precautions were instituted as a result of the human immunodeficiency virus (HIV) epidemic in the United States. Blood and body fluid precautions were practiced on all clients regardless of their potential infectious state.

In 1987, body substance isolation (BSI) was proposed. The intent of this isolation system was to isolate all moist and potentially infectious body substances (blood, feces, urine, sputum, saliva, wound drainage, and other body fluids) from all clients, regardless of their infectious status, primarily through the use of gloves.

In the late fall of 1994, the CDC drafted new guidelines. The revised guidelines contain two tiers of precautions. The first tier, **Standard Precautions**, blends the major features of universal precautions (blood and body fluids precautions) and body substance isolation into a single set of precautions to be used for the care of all clients in hospitals, regardless of their diagnosis or presumed infection status. The new Standard Precautions apply to blood, all body fluids, secretions, and excretions, whether or not they contain visible blood; nonintact skin; and mucous membranes. These precautions are designed to reduce the risk of transmission of both recognized and unrecognized sources of infection in hospitals. As a result of the new category of Standard Precautions, clients with diseases or conditions that previously required category-specific or disease-specific precautions are now covered under this category and do not require additional precautions.

The second tier, **transmission-based precautions**, is designed only for the care of specified clients. (This term and isolation precautions are used interchangeably in much of the literature.) This tier reduces the disease-specific precautions into three sets of precautions based on routes of transmission. These categories are designed for clients documented or suspected to be infected or colonized with highly transmissible or epidemiologically important pathogens for which additional precaution must be used to interrupt transmission to others in the hospital. The three types of transmission-based precautions include airborne, droplet, and contact precautions. Airborne

Innovative Infection Control Approaches

Founded in 1991, the Institute for Healthcare Improvement (IHI) offers healthcare facilities information on how to best control hospital infections. Thus far, 2,700 hospitals have joined together with the goal of saving 100,000 lives by eliminating hospital-acquired infections. Backed by solid evidence-based research, the institute makes recommendations addressing specific risk factors for different infections. There are six "bundles" focused on six separate interventions, three of which include a focus on preventing infections: central-line infections, surgical site infections, and ventilator-associated pneumonia. An example is the central line bundle, which specifies whole-body drapes, masks, and gowns during line insertion.

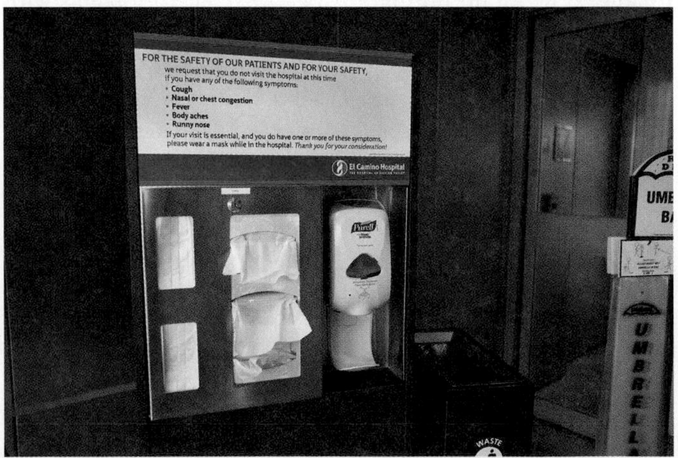
FOR THE SAFETY OF OUR PATIENTS AND FOR YOUR SAFETY,
we request that you do not visit the hospital at this time
if you have any of the following symptoms:
• Cough
• Nasal or chest congestion
• Fever
• Body aches
• Runny nose
If your visit is essential, and you do have one or more of these symptoms,
please wear a mask while in the hospital. Thank you for your consideration!
El Camino Hospital

▲ Many hospitals are adopting measures that support standard precautions. Shown is a Kiosk outside hospital doors that allows visitors to complete hand hygiene both entering and exiting the hospital.

precautions reduce the risk of airborne transmission of infectious agents, such as measles, varicella, and tuberculosis. Droplet precautions are used to prevent the transmission of diseases, such as meningitis, pneumonia, scarlet fever, diphtheria, rubella, and pertussis. Contact precautions are used for clients known or suspected to have serious illnesses easily transmitted by direct contact, such as herpes simplex, staphylococcal infections, hepatitis A, respiratory syncytial virus, and wound or skin infections.

Transmission-based precautions now include educational information to help family members and visitors. They should be taught/informed via fact sheets, pamphlets, and other material about preventing transmission of infections. It is also important to include rationale, risks to household members, and other routine infection prevention strategies, which are a part of respiratory precautions.

All three types of precautions may be used at one time when multiple routes of transmission are suspected in a client. These precautions are always used in conjunction with Standard Precautions. Table 14-1 outlines recommendations for transmission-based precautions. Table 14-2 lists the diseases/conditions in which transmission-based precautions are required or advised.

Hand Hygiene, Hand Antisepsis, and Gloving: CDC Recommendations

- Hands must be washed with antiseptic soap and water or alcohol-based hand rub:
  1. Before and after client contact and between clients.
  2. After contact with a source of microorganisms.
  3. After removing gloves. Before donning gloves.
  4. After touching equipment or surfaces that may be contaminated.
  5. Before handling an invasive device (regardless of glove protocol).
  6. After contact with body fluids, excretions, nonintact skin, wound dressings.
  7. Before handling medication and/or preparing food.
  8. If moving from a contaminated body site to a clean body site during client care.
- Gloves should be used as an adjunct to, not a substitute for, hand hygiene:
  1. Remove gloves and wash hands after any hand contaminating activity.
  2. Change gloves between clients.
  3. Change gloves during care of a single client when moving from one procedure to another. (This is critical when moving from a contaminated to a clean body site.)
  4. Use disposable gloves only once.
  5. Do not touch any body surface that is moist without gloves. (Moisture can be considered potentially contaminated.)
  6. Have latex-free gloves available for personnel with an allergy or sensitivity to latex.
  7. Decontaminate hands before donning sterile gloves.

See CDC Web page for more information: http://www.cdc.gov/hand/hygiene/training.html

Fundamental Principles Certain fundamental principles should be applied to all clients. *The first is hand hygiene.* Hand hygiene is the single most important means of preventing the spread of infection. (People carry between 10,000 and 10 million bacteria on each hand.) A *second fundamental principle involves the use of gloves.* Gloves are worn to provide a protective barrier, prevent gross contamination of the hands when touching body substances or blood, and reduce the risk of exposure to blood pathogens. Gloves also prevent the spread of microorganisms to other clients and to healthcare personnel.

The third fundamental principle is the proper placement of clients in the hospital to prevent the spread of microorganisms to others or to the client. Clients may not always be placed in private rooms when they are infected. They can be placed in a room where the second client has the same infectious process.

The fourth fundamental principle is the appropriate use of isolation equipment to prevent the spread of microorganisms to healthcare workers and other clients. The equipment required is based on the specific transmission route of the microorganism. Specific handling of client care items needs to be considered in preventing the spread of infection.

Hand Hygiene Wash hands with nonantimicrobial soap or use waterless antiseptic agent for routine hand hygiene and after removing gloves. An antimicrobial or antiseptic agent should be used for control of specific outbreaks of infection.

Gloves Clean, nonsterile gloves (or latex-free gloves if latex allergy is present) are worn when touching blood, body fluids, secretions, excretions, and contaminated items. Put gloves on just before touching mucous membranes and nonintact skin. Remove gloves immediately after use and wash hands before touching noncontaminated items and environmental surfaces or giving care to another client. Gloves should be discarded immediately and not reused.

Mask, Eye Protection, Face Shield Wear mask and eye protection during procedures in which splashes or sprays could come in contact with eyes and mucous membranes. Face shields protect the mucous membranes of the eyes, nose, and mouth from splashes of blood, body fluids, secretions, and excretions. Suctioning clients and assisting physicians in insertion of hemodynamic monitoring lines are examples of situations in which this type of protection is required.

Gown Nonsterile disposable gowns are used to protect the skin and clothing from contamination while providing client care. Gowns should be worn whenever there is a risk of contamination from blood, body fluids, secretions, or excretions. Soiled gowns should be removed immediately and hands washed to prevent the spread of microorganisms.

Linen Transport soiled linens in a manner that prevents skin and mucous membrane exposure, contamination of clothing,

TABLE 14-1 HICPAC* Recommendations for Transmission-Based Precautions

	Contact	Droplet	Airborne
Purpose	Prevent transmission of known or suspected infected or colonized microorganisms by direct hand or skin-to-skin contact that occurs when providing direct client care.	Prevent transmission of large-particle droplets, larger than 5 microns (μm).	Prevent transmission of small-particle residue of 5 microns (μm) or smaller droplets.
Client Placement	• Private room • Can be placed in room of client with same microorganism	• Private room • Can be placed in room of client with same diagnosis	• Private room • Can be placed in room of client with same diagnosis • Monitor negative air pressure • Keep door closed • Keep client in room
Respiratory Protection	• Mask not necessary • Family, visitors respiratory hygiene/cough etiquette. *See page 417*	• Use mask when working within 3 feet of client	• Respiratory protective equipment • Do not enter room of clients with rubeola or varicella if susceptible to these infections
Gloves and Gown	• Wear gloves when entering room • Change gloves after contact with infective material, such as wound drainage or fecal material • Wash hands immediately after removing gloves • Wear gown when working with clients with diarrhea, ostomies, or wound drainage not contained in dressing • Wear gown if contact with client or environment will occur	• Follow Standard Precautions	• Follow Standard Precautions
Client Transport	• Transport only if essential • Ensure precautions are maintained to minimize risk of transmission	• Transport only if essential • Place mask on client when outside room	• Transport only if essential • Place mask on client when outside room
Client Care Items	• Client care items and environmental surfaces are cleaned daily • Dedicate equipment to single client use (i.e., stethoscope, thermometer)		

*Hospital Infection Control Practices Advisory Committee.
Source: Adapted from Department of Health and Human Services: CDC, *Federal Register*, "Recommendations for Isolation Precautions in Hospitals" (1997).

and transfer of microorganisms to other clients and environments. This is usually accomplished through double-bagging linen before taking it to the laundry facility.

Occupational Health and Bloodborne Pathogens Take precautions to prevent injuries caused by needles, scalpels, or other sharp instruments or devices. Only use safety needles. Never recap used needles, purposely bend or break needles by hand, remove needles from disposable syringes, or otherwise handle needles directly. All such instruments should be placed in puncture-resistant containers for disposal. The use of needleless systems for IV management has dramatically decreased needle stick injuries.

Mouth pieces, resuscitation bags, or other ventilation devices should be used as an alternative to mouth-to-mouth resuscitation.

Client Placement Clients who are at risk for contaminating the environment or who are unable to maintain appropriate hygiene or environmental control should be placed in a private room. If this is not possible, other arrangements need to be made in consultation with the hospital's infection control department.

In addition to healthcare workers following Standard Precautions, the following guidelines should be considered when providing client care:

- Healthcare workers who have open lesions, upper respiratory infections, or weeping dermatitis should refrain from all direct client contact and from handling client care equipment.
- Because of the risk of transmission of HIV and hepatitis B virus (HBV) from mother to fetus, pregnant healthcare workers

TABLE 14-2 Disease Indications for Transmission-Based Precautions*

Modes of Transmission		
Contact (Direct and Indirect)	**Droplet**	**Airborne**
Clostridium difficile	Diphtheria	Tuberculosis
Diphtheria	Influenza	Chickenpox
Staphylococcus	Pertussis	Herpes zoster
E. coli	*Streptococcal pharyngitis*	Measles
Hepatitis	Pneumonia	
Herpes simplex	Scarlet fever	
Impetigo	Rubella	
Scabies	Mumps	
Major abscesses	Meningitis	
Cellulitis	Sepsis	
Respiratory conditions	Pneumonic plague	
Virus infection–wound/skin	Parvovirus B19	
Rotavirus infection		
Smallpox		
Ebola, Lassa, Marburg		
Rubella–chickenpox		

*Listed above are the diseases/conditions in which transmission-based precautions are required or advised as a part of the treatment protocol.

should be especially familiar with, and strictly adhere to, precautions to minimize risk of these viruses. Currently, pregnant healthcare workers are not known to be at greater risk of contracting HIV or HBV than other workers.

Health Care Worker Protection Act In 1997 the "Health Care Worker Protection Act" was passed to assist in the reduction of incidents in which healthcare workers are accidentally exposed to potentially contaminated, infected blood via a needle stick. This act makes the use of safe needle devices a requirement if the facility receives Medicare funding. The impetus for the bill was a direct result of statistics from the Centers for Disease Control and Prevention (CDC) indicating that more than 800,000 needle sticks and sharps injuries were being reported yearly. This is the most common cause of healthcare worker–related exposure to bloodborne pathogens. Needle stick injuries caused by hollow-bore needles accounted for 86% of all reported occupational HIV exposures. Nurses make up 24% of all the cases of HIV infection among healthcare workers known or thought to have been infected on the job. The use of protective needle devices is estimated to prevent up to 90% of needle sticks. For more information, refer to the PEP protocol (PEP) described later in this chapter.

More than 20 pathogens can be transmitted through small amounts of blood. In addition to HIV and hepatitis B, syphilis, varicella-zoster, and hepatitis C can be transmitted via this route. Hepatitis B is the most common infectious disease transmitted through work-related exposure to blood. About 5,100 healthcare workers become infected with hepatitis B each year.

Principles of Hand Hygiene

Wash hands or use alcohol-based gel:

- At the beginning of the shift before providing client care.
- Before and after providing client care.
- Before and after preparing medications.
- After touching client surroundings (i.e., after handling soiled linen, equipment, or supplies).
- Between contact with different clients.
- After removing gloves.
- After you have sneezed or coughed.
- Before and after eating.
- After body fluid exposure/risk.
- Just before leaving the nursing unit.

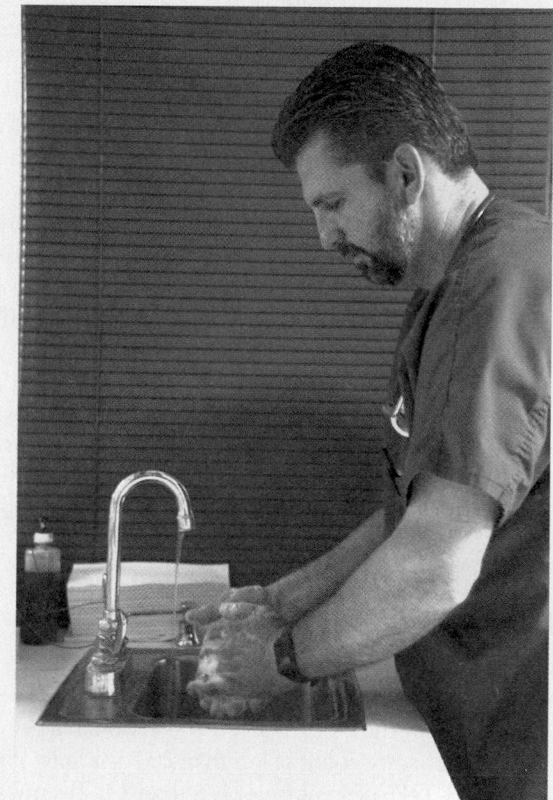

▲ The single most important nursing action to decrease the incidence of hospital-based infection is washing your hands.

ACQUIRED IMMUNODEFICIENCY SYNDROME

Epidemiology and Modes of Transmission

The incidence of acquired immunodeficiency syndrome (AIDS) has grown exponentially since it was first recorded in 1981. The statistics are chilling. Internationally, an estimated 5 million people were infected with HIV in 2005 and, at the end of 2006, 1.1 million persons in the United States were living with HIV/AIDS. The CDC estimates that 56,300 new cases occurred in the United States in 2001. All areas of the world are expected to see increases in HIV (with the exception of the Caribbean), in spite of a massive educational prevention program.

Cumulatively, since AIDS was first identified, the death toll from AIDS in the United States has been 562,793. Data shows that in the number of AIDS cases reported, the highest is African Americans (51%), then Caucasians (29%) and Hispanics (18%).

Estimates for 2007, the most recent year for which data is available, are that the number of AIDS cases have remained stable and the number of deaths decreased.

Now the high-risk groups are male-to-male sexual transmission, accounting for 53% of AIDS cases, and 32% in high-risk heterosexuals. Estimates are that the percentage of AIDS cases will go up in women and in adolescents, who are rapidly becoming the newest high-risk group.

A new (2005) potent strain of HIV has been diagnosed in New York state. The man who received the diagnosis was resistant to three of four antiviral drugs and the HIV status progressed to full-blown AIDS in only 2 months. This situation, coupled with increased resistance to HIV drugs, is very alarming to health professionals.

Definitions

Acquired Immunodeficiency Syndrome AIDS is the most severe form of a continuum of illnesses associated with HIV infection. AIDS is defined by the CDC as an HIV infection in a person with a CD4+ T-lymphocyte count of less than 200 cells/microliter (μL) of blood or a CD4+ percentage of less than 14. Twenty-six clinical conditions are listed in the CDC AIDS surveillance case definition in category C. Once clients have a condition listed in category C, they remain in that surveillance category. Among those 26 conditions listed in the category are cytomegalovirus (CMV) retinitis; Karposi's sarcoma; *Mycobacterium avium* complex (MAC) (which includes the M. *avium* and M. *intracellulare* organisms) or M. *kansasii*; *Mycobacterium tuberculosis*, any site; *Pneumocystis carinii*; and recurrent pneumonia.

Human Immunodeficiency Virus HIV is a bloodborne infective retrovirus that invades the CD4+ T-lymphocyte (immunity) cell, renders it useless, and then duplicates itself by means of that cell. With loss of the client's immune function, the disease becomes clinically manifested. Infection with HIV progresses to AIDS in at least 35% of those infected. Once a client has been diagnosed with HIV, the usual approach to care includes evaluation of the immune system and classification by CDC grouping: (A) asymptomatic, (B) acute symptomatic, and (C) AIDS-indicator conditions. Identification and treatment of infectious and neoplastic complications, initiation of approved antiretroviral therapy, and consideration of experimental measures are also included in the evaluation.

HIV is transmitted through high-risk behaviors or other contact with the virus, including:

- Sexual contact with HIV-infected individuals
- Sharing needles with HIV-infected individuals
- Transfusions of blood or blood products from infected individuals (not common today, but new cases are still reported)
- Babies who become infected from the mother before or during birth, or through breast-feeding
- Contact with contaminated needles, blood, secretions, or excretions from an HIV-infected client

Healthcare Workers' Exposure to HIV

Prospective studies of healthcare workers have estimated that the average risk for HIV transmission after a percutaneous exposure to HIV-infected blood is approximately 0.3%, after a mucous membrane exposure is 0.1% and risk factors for transmission by skin exposure less than 0.1%. The CDC states that approximately 800,000 needle-stick injuries occur each year with potential risk of HIV exposure. The FDA has recently approved a point-of-care HIV test that provides a result in as few as 5 minutes. There are four versions of this test, which identifies the presence of HIV antibodies with 98% accuracy. Since these results are not 100%, a follow-up confirmation test must be done. If a positive Western Blot analysis is found, the healthcare worker would immediately be referred to postexposure prophylaxis (PEP). (See procedure "Obtaining a Gum Swab for HIV Antibodies," Chapter 20, p. 710.) Considerations that influence the use of PEP include the timing of the PEP—how soon after exposure PEP was begun—and the belief that the infection can be improved by the use of the antiretroviral drugs.

In 1997, the Public Health Service updated recommendations for management of healthcare worker exposure to HIV and recommendations for PEP. The decision to recommend HIV PEP takes into account the nature of the exposure, needle stick or mucous membrane contact, and the amount of blood or body fluid involved in the exposure. Other considerations include exposure to a virus known or suspected to be resistant to antiretroviral drugs. Pregnancy is also a consideration. Risk factor assessments are key determinants of PEP. Healthcare facilities should have the protocols available, and prompt reporting and postexposure care should be considered a healthcare emergency and treated as such. This includes access to clinicians who can provide postexposure care during all working hours and the antiretroviral agents for PEP immediately available. Healthcare workers must be educated to report occupational exposures immediately after they occur because PEP is most likely to be effective if implemented as soon after the exposure as possible.

Proper Handling of Biohazard Waste

Speaking for the Florida Department of Health and Rehabilitation Services, an epidemiologist stated that there was an 80% reduction in exposure to biohazard material in seven Florida hospitals after the enactment of the Florida Administrative Code. This code is an example of the principles that additional states are beginning to enact.

What Is Biohazard Waste?

Any solid or liquid waste that may present a threat of infection is considered "biohazard." This could include laboratory waste, blood or blood products, body fluids, absorbent material saturated with blood or body fluids (either wet or dry), discarded sharps, and nonabsorbent disposable devices (such as drains, excretions, gloves, urine specimens, etc.).

Why Separate Biohazard From Other Medical Waste?

It is critical that the biohazard waste be separated at the point of origin or before it leaves the client's room. This reduces the risk of exposure considerably. The principles of separation are:

- Use an impermeable red plastic bag labeled "biohazard"; close bag securely while inside the client's room.
- Use a second red-labeled bag outside the room and place the inside bag in it so that the waste is "double-bagged."
- Do not place red-labeled bag with other waste material, because it could contaminate all waste.
- Sharps should be separated from all other waste and placed in a leak- and puncture-proof container with a biohazard symbol on the outside.
- Fiberboard waste containers should NOT contain scalpels.
- Do not overfill sharps containers, because items could fall out.

Storage of Biohazard Material

Biohazard waste must be appropriately sealed. It may be stored for 30 days; time starts when material is placed in the sharps container or biohazard bag. All biohazard waste must be restricted, locked up, or placed in a separate storage area. Biohazard waste must be in a room with **no** carpeting. Sealed cement is necessary so that a spill can be cleaned up. Biohazard material must be labeled correctly so that there is a tracking method for each bag, container, etc. Labels should say "medical waste" and "biohazard" and be dated when the bag was first placed in the area.

Transporting Biohazard Waste

When transporting biohazard waste within the facility, containers must remain intact. Trash chutes must **not** be used. Outdoor containers should be secured against vandalism and marked or labeled.

A contingency plan for spilled material:

- Spilled or leaked biohazard material must be cleaned with industrial strength detergent and then disinfected.
- Onsite treatment and disposal of waste must be steamed, incinerated, or cleaned with an alternative method (chemical, dry heat, etc.).
- Each facility must post a "Spill Contingency Plan," which includes which substance to be used to disinfect.

If each facility has an administrative code that includes a total plan, policies, and procedures for dealing with biohazard waste, as well as a training program for all employees in how to handle biohazard waste, the incidence of exposure could be dramatically decreased.

Source: Adapted from Department of Health and Human Services.

Recommendations for PEP include a basic 4-week regimen of two drugs (zidovudine and lamivudine, or Combivir, a combination of these two antiretroviral agents) for most HIV exposures. An expanded regimen that includes the addition of a protease inhibitor (indinavir or nelfinavir) is recommended for HIV exposures that pose an increased risk of transmission or when there is a known or suspected resistance to one or more of the antiretroviral agents recommended for PEP. There is now available a boosted protease inhibitor (Kaletra), which helps reduce the viral load in the body, thereby providing greater protection against retroviral activity.

OTHER INFECTIOUS DISEASES

Tuberculosis

Tuberculosis is an infectious disease caused by the tubercle bacillus *Mycobacterium tuberculosis*. The main reservoir for the organism is the human respiratory tract, and transmission occurs between individuals through respiratory contact. The tubercle bacillus enters the respiratory tract on droplets transmitted through productive coughing from the infected individual. Symptoms may occur in 4 to 12 weeks after exposure or may go unnoticed for many years. Active pulmonary tuberculosis has a slow, insidious onset. The progression of the active disease and symptoms of cough, weight loss, and fever usually occur within the first 2 years after the infection. Latent infections, which are asymptomatic, are not infectious and may last a lifetime. Without treatment tuberculosis progresses to other body sites. Disseminated tuberculosis occurs in many of the body areas, not just the lungs. The incidence of tuberculosis cases in this country has increased greatly, due in large part to the AIDS epidemic. Immunosuppressed hosts are very vulnerable to the bacillus. In addition to immunosuppressed individuals, others considered at high risk for infection include alcoholics; IV drug abusers; individuals who share a closed environment with the infected individual; residents of institutions such as long-term care and correctional facilities; foreign-born individuals from countries with a high prevalence of tuberculosis, such as Asia, Latin America, Africa, Mexico, and the former Soviet Union; low-income populations who are medically underserved; and clients who are noncompliant and do not complete the appropriate drug therapy. Healthcare workers who come in contact with any of the high-risk populations are at risk for infection.

A growing number of clients develop MDR-TB, multidrug-resistant tuberculosis. According to the CDC, MDR-TB now accounts for 1.2% of cases for which drug susceptibility data are available (2005). This type of tuberculosis is in vitro resistance of a strain of TBC to antituberculosis drugs. The disease can progress from diagnosis to death in as short a period as 4 to 16 weeks. The increasing incidence of MDR-TB can be attributed to delays in treatment, inadequate isolation and infection control practices, and lack of follow-through after hospital discharge. Clients develop resistance to the standard drug regimen (two first-line therapies, isoniazid and rifampin) as a result of noncompliance and/or inappropriate drug therapy. MDR-TB is also caused by person-to-person contact through sneezing or coughing or from a person with primary drug resistance.

Early recognition and treatment of tuberculosis must be initiated promptly and isolation measures instituted to prevent the spread of the disease. The CDC describes effective tuberculosis control requirements as early identification, isolation, and treatment of persons with active tuberculosis. The purified protein derivative (PPD) skin test is used to quickly identify the infection in the absence of clinical symptoms. Sputum specimens for acid-fast bacillus (AFB) TB culture, and sensitivity and chest x-rays are also ordered to rule out TB. A PPD skin test is read 48 to 72 hr after the injection. A positive skin test is indicated by an induration of 5 to 10 mm at the site of the injection. A two-step method is now being used, particularly with healthcare workers. This procedure involves the first PPD injection to be given and read within 48 to 72 hr. If the PPD is negative or doubtful, the PPD is repeated in 1 week. If the client has a positive reaction, he or she is started on a prophylaxis regimen. A client who is known to be HIV-positive with a 5 mm or larger induration at the site of the PPD injection should be considered positive for tuberculosis.

The CDC recommendation for tuberculosis isolation includes a directional air-flow, negative-pressure ventilation system in the room of tuberculosis clients. Negative-pressure ventilation pulls air away from hallways and exhausts it out of the room to areas away from air intake vents. Six air changes each hour are required to provide microbial dilution within the room. Ultraviolet irradiation lamps can be used to supplement ventilation systems when the risk of tuberculosis transmission is high.

Anyone entering the client's room should wear a mask that forms a tight-fitting seal against particulates 1 to 5 microns (μm). Two examples of tuberculosis masks are the high-efficiency particulate air (HEPA) mask used for suspected or confirmed multidrug-resistant (MDR) tuberculosis and the disposable submicron mask used for confirmed tuberculosis. Disposable particulate respirators are suggested by the CDC when adequate ventilation is not available in the room. All treatments and procedures should be performed in the client's room if at all possible. If the client must leave the room, a valveless particulate respirator must be used.

Viral Hepatitis

There are six forms of hepatitis. Each form differs in regard to incubation period, route of transmission, antigenic properties, and progression to chronicity. All forms of hepatitis produce an inflammatory response to the liver, which is characterized by liver cell necrosis, inflammation, and cell regeneration. The three major forms of hepatitis are hepatitis A virus (HAV), hepatitis B virus (HBV), and hepatitis C virus (HCV). Hepatitis D virus (HDV) is not as common and hepatitis E virus (HEV) is rare in the United States. Hepatitis G virus (HGV) is a recently isolated bloodborne infectious agent transmitted by needle sticks and blood transfusions.

Hepatitis A (HAV) is spread via the fecal–oral route and sexual transmission. Poor sanitation and hand hygiene is a major source of infection. Approximately 152,000 infections occur in the United States each year. Ninety-nine percent of those infected recover without any serious problems. HAVRIX vaccine is available to prevent HAV. Once exposed to the infection or as a preventative therapy, immune serum globulin is administered intramuscularly.

Hepatitis B (HBV) is spread through infected blood or body fluids and through two nonparenteral routes, sexual contact and perinatal transmission. Contaminated needles, syringes, and blood products are the most common mode of transmission, although about 30% of the cases are spread through sexual contact. An estimated 140,000 individuals are infected yearly in the United States. Two to 10% of adults become chronically infected with HBV after an infection. HBV is 100 times more infectious than HIV. HBV vaccine provides active immunity in more than 95% of recipients. The two common vaccines are Engerix-B and Recombivax HB. Hepatitis B immune globulin provides passive immunity to individuals who have had contact with HBV-contaminated material.

Hepatitis C (HCV) is transmitted primarily by contact with contaminated blood and blood products. Eighty-five percent of those infected with HCV will remain chronically infected. Chronic HCV infection is the main causal factor for nearly one-third of all liver transplants. There are three types of interferon used to treat HCV.

The CDC recommends the use of Standard Precautions with clients known to have hepatitis. The precautions should be maintained for 1 week after the onset of symptoms.

EMERGING VIRUSES (POSSIBLE PANDEMIC THREATS)

Severe Acute Respiratory Syndrome (SARS)

In 2003, there was a multi-country outbreak of a virus suspected to be a mutated form of the coronavirus (the common cold). The specific SARS pathogen is not known. There is speculation that this new virus has jumped from animal to human, setting up the possibility for a worldwide pandemic like the 1918 swine or Spanish flu that infected millions of people around the world and killed more than 20 million. Jumping species, from animal to human and being able to

transmit person-to-person, is the worst possible combination of events because it can cause havoc in a nonimmune population. Because of this potential for disaster, the World Health Organization (WHO) issued a global alert when this coronavirus rapidly spread to 26 countries. At this initial juncture, it was critical to employ stringent infection control protocols because both the exact pathogen, as well as the transmission mode, continued to elude scientists.

The primary symptoms of SARS are malaise, aching muscles, a persistent fever >38°C or 100.4°F, dry cough, shortness of breath or breathing difficulties, and an almost normal white blood count. People with these symptoms who have recently traveled to or been in the Far East are advised to see a doctor immediately. The unusual and discriminating characteristic of this illness is that while it appears to be a flulike illness, the symptoms persist and simply do not go away. Administering antiviral drugs (i.e., ribavirin, a drug also used to treat hepatitis C) does not appear to be effective. At this point, there is only supportive treatment, including oxygen and ventilatory assistance, when necessary.

In the initial stages, SARS was transmitted to healthcare personnel because they did not adhere to precise precautions while caring for SARS clients. Also, it was discovered that this particular virus can live for 24 hr or longer on various surfaces, making it even more dangerous.

According to Dr. Steven Garner, NY Methodist Hospital, the SARS virus, as of 2006, has mutated to a weaker virus and is no longer a threat. It could, however, reverse in the future. Even if this particular condition is eliminated, new viruses and bacteria will appear on the world stage and many of them could be mutated forms, not responsive to current antibiotics.

H1N1 (Swine) FLU

Swine influenza, the latest health threat to emerge, is a respiratory disease of pigs caused by type A influenza virus that regularly causes outbreaks of influenza in pigs. Usually, the death rate in pigs is low. This virus, type A H1N1, was first isolated from a pig in 1930. Over the years, variations of this virus have emerged. Now, there appear to be four main subtypes that have been isolated in pigs, but the most recently isolated influenza virus is the H1N1.

While swine flu viruses do not normally infect humans, recently there have been cases that have occurred in persons with direct exposure to pigs. There are now documented cases of one person spreading the swine flu to others, so there is human-to-human transmission. This is thought to occur in the same way other types of flu are transmitted: coughing, sneezing, or touching. In October 2009, President Obama declared swine flu a national emergency, and since June 2009, it was declared an official global pandemic by WHO. However, as of 2010 WHO declared the pandemic over. The downgrade followed recommendations by global influenza experts who reviewed the status.

The symptoms of swine flu are essentially the same as those of seasonal flu: fever, fatigue, coughing, sore throat, body aches, headache, lack of appetite, and sometimes, vomiting and diarrhea. One of the most important teaching tasks of nurses is to teach clients how to protect themselves. People should wash their hands frequently or use antibacterial gel.

Whenever someone is near them and is coughing or sneezing, get out of range, at least 3 feet. Stay home from work or school if you feel symptoms developing. There are two types of flu vaccines: injection and nasal spray. The injection contains dead virus and is approved for healthy people, 6 months old and older. The nasal spray is made from live, attenuated virus, and is approved for healthy persons between 2 and 49 years of age.

There are four different antiviral drugs that are prescribed for the treatment of influenza: amantadine, rimantadine, oseltamivir, and zanamivir. The most recent H1N1 influenza viruses isolated in humans are resistant to amantadine and rimantadine. They currently have developed a swine flu vaccine and have millions of doses on hand. There are several antiviral medications available that prevent infected cells from releasing new viruses. They are known as neuraminidase inhibitors. These medications can prevent and reduce the severity of infection. They include Tamiflu, Relenza, and Peramivir, and the United States has stockpiled 50 million doses over the past few years.

Pandemic Influenza Preparedness and Response

Precautions for Staff	Responses (to Infection)
Modify transmission-based infection control strategies to match organism.	Use airborne infection isolation rooms, including HEPA filter.
Use personal protective equipment: gloves, gown, goggles, face shields, etc.	Use single hospital rooms, or place clients with same organism (H1N1) together.
Modify administrative controls.	Limit number of persons entering area.
Use safe working practices (i.e., stringent hand hygiene).	Limit client transport.
	Use vigorous hand hygiene measures.
	Employ standard practices for used client care equipment.
	Educate clients on hand hygiene and cough etiquette.

The World Health Organization (WHO) maintains a global surveillance system that monitors presence of an influenza pandemic in progress. Pandemic status evolves and is not always accurately assessed or projected.

Avian Influenza

Avian (bird) influenza was a prior health threat to the world's population. Not since the outbreak of SARS in 2003 has the possibility of a worldwide pandemic caused such concern. Avian influenza is an infection caused by avian influenza viruses. These viruses are found in many varieties of wild birds and are carried in the bird's intestines and generally do not cause illness. However, if infection with the virus occurs, the influenza is very contagious among birds.

Infected birds shed influenza virus in their saliva, nasal secretions, and feces. Susceptible birds, including domesticated birds, become infected when they have contact with contaminated excretions or with surfaces that are contaminated with excretions or secretions. During an outbreak of avian influenza among poultry, there is a possible risk to people who have direct or close contact with infected birds, with surfaces that have been contaminated by secretions and excretions from infected birds, or who eat the meat of infected birds that has not been cooked well.

Avian flu viruses do not usually infect humans, but according to WHO, more than 100 confirmed cases of human infection with bird flu viruses have occurred since 1997. Outbreaks of avian influenza, H5N1, occurred among poultry in eight countries in Asia during late 2003 and early 2004. So far, spread of the H5N1 virus from person to person has not continued beyond one person. The concern is that all influenza viruses have the ability to mutate, and there is a 50/50 chance of the avian flu virus mutating. Scientists are concerned that the H5N1 virus one day could be able to infect humans and spread easily from one person to another.

Symptoms of avian influenza in humans have ranged from fever, cough, sore throat, and muscle aches to eye infections, pneumonia, and severe respiratory diseases. The symptoms of avian influenza may depend on which specific virus subtype and strain caused the infection. Because these viruses do not commonly infect humans, there is little or no immune protection against them in the human population. Right now, there is no commercially available vaccine to protect humans against the H5N1 virus. Research studies to test a vaccine that will protect humans against H5N1 virus began in April 2005, and a series of clinical trials is under way. However, if the virus mutates to human-to-human contact, it will take 6 months to produce a vaccine.

Since it is still unknown exactly how avian influenza may first transmit between humans, the CDC has made recommendations for precautions for healthcare workers involved in the care of clients with documented or suspected avian influenza.

Total infection control precautions are essential to prevent transmission for these potential pandemic threats. Isolation precautions should be instituted for clients with a history of travel within 10 days to a country with avian influenza activity and are hospitalized with a severe febrile respiratory illness, or are otherwise under evaluation for severe influenza. In addition, Standard Precautions, especially hand hygiene, should be followed. Use of gloves and gowns for all client contact is necessary. Goggles should be worn if within 3 feet of a client. Equipment such as stethoscopes and blood pressure cuffs should stay in the client's room. Airborne Precautions should also be instituted. Clients should be placed in a HEPA-filtered, negative air pressure isolation room. Healthcare providers should use a respirator mask such as a custom-fitted N-95 face piece when entering the room.

The Secretary of Health and Human Services recommends that citizens begin storing some form of food supply (at least 2 weeks' worth) so that "social distancing," a basic tenet of public health, can be observed. She suggests that any community that fails to prepare will be in danger. Our transient and mobile global society makes it imperative that intervention and containment occur rapidly to prevent a worldwide pandemic when a new or mutated pathogen appears. The other imperative is that healthcare workers protect themselves using infection control protocols so that the spread of a new pathogen is contained in healthcare settings.

HOME CARE ADAPTATIONS

In the home setting, medical asepsis, or clean technique, is often used instead of sterile technique. The major reasons for this protocol change are the nature of the setting and the personnel providing care.

The greatest infection control problem in hospitals is healthcare-associated infections due to the large numbers of antibiotic-resistant organisms present in a hospital setting. When clients are in their own environment, however, they tend to develop fewer infections because they are subjected to fewer organisms. In the home setting, focus is on protecting home care staff and family, not other clients. While there may be transmission of organisms between individuals in the home, there are minimal data on the incidence of home care–acquired infections. Infection-preventing strategies in the home should focus on IV therapy and urinary tract, respiratory, and wound care.

Nevertheless, sterile technique and equipment, such as prepackaged catheter and irrigation kits, parenteral fluid equipment, and dressings, are often purchased for home care. When sterile technique is required, it is the responsibility of the nurse to provide the instruction and evaluate the family's ability to perform the skill accurately. Hospital techniques may need to be modified for the home setting, and ideal environmental working conditions may not be present. Unfortunately, the Division of Healthcare Quality Promotion of the CDC has not developed guidelines for infection control in home care settings at this time. Therefore, adaptations must be made, and the essential infection control measures must be maintained.

Just as in the hospital, effective hand hygiene is the *most* effective means of infection control in the home setting. There is one major difference between hospital and home. Equipment (soap, running water, and paper towels) that is readily available to the nurse in the hospital may not be available in the home. Even if running water is available, there may not be soap or clean towels. Nurses must bring their own handwashing supplies.

A decrease in the duration of hospital stays has dramatically increased the expanded scope of the home care nurse. Unfortunately, infection surveillance, prevention, and control efforts have not kept up. Many home care infection control

practices have been based on ritual and acute care practice, rather than scientific principles. Changes in infection control procedures in the home are currently occurring based on a scientific approach.

Home care assessment for potential infections relies on clinical signs and symptoms and tests, such as the urine dipstick, that can be performed in the home. Routine tests used in hospitals to diagnose infections of the urinary tract, respiratory tract, and wound or skin sites are not routinely done, as the current reimbursement system does not support cultures and laboratory tests. Only cultures that confirm and treat bloodstream infections for clients requiring home infusion therapy are obtained.

If the home care client is suspected of or diagnosed as having an infectious disease or the client is infected or colonized with VRE or MSRA, the nurse should use the same personal protective equipment and protocol used in the hospital setting. The equipment includes gloves, disposable gown or apron, mask, cap, and goggles. Reusable equipment, such as stethoscopes and blood pressure cuffs, should stay in the home and not be used on other home care clients. If possible, these clients should be seen at the end of the day.

CULTURAL AWARENESS

Many cultures believe that certain substances protect one's health. For example, Italians, Greeks, and Native Americans believe that garlic or onions eaten raw or worn on the body will prevent a condition or illness such as infection. If a client wishes to include these items in his or her diet or wear them, the nursing staff should respect this practice, since it is an important cultural tradition for many groups.

NURSING DIAGNOSES

The following nursing diagnoses may be appropriate to use on client care plans when the components are related to clients requiring isolation protocol or sterile procedures.

NURSING DIAGNOSIS	RELATED FACTORS
Ineffective Community Coping	Deficits in social support, disease follow-up protocols, inadequate resources for disease prevention
Deficient Knowledge	Lack of access to healthcare facilities, lack of education, cognitive limitation
Ineffective Health Maintenance	Participation in high-risk activities, substance abuse, infectious states, religious or cultural beliefs detrimental to health
Infection, Risk for	Immunosuppressed hospitalized clients, HIV/AIDS clients, invasive procedures, lack of immunization
	Inadequate defenses (loss of skin integrity, leukopenia, low hemoglobin)
Latex Allergy Response	Allergies to certain foods, allergy to latex, lack of safety procedures for latex allergy
Noncompliance	Lack of motivation, education, or readiness; information misinterpretation; cultural or religious beliefs
	Medical condition (communicable disease, HIV-positive), hospitalization, terminal illness
Ineffective Protection	Poor compliance to protocols, lack of knowledge, lack of resources
Ineffective Family Therapeutic Regimen Management	Choices of daily living precludes maintaining treatment modalities (e.g., drug therapy, hand hygiene)

CLEANSE HANDS The single most important nursing action to decrease the incidence of hospital-based infections is hand hygiene. *Remember to wash your hands or use antibacterial gel before and after each and every client contact.*

IDENTIFY CLIENT Before every procedure, check two forms of client identification, not including room number. These actions prevent errors and conform to The Joint Commission standards.

Chapter 14

UNIT 1

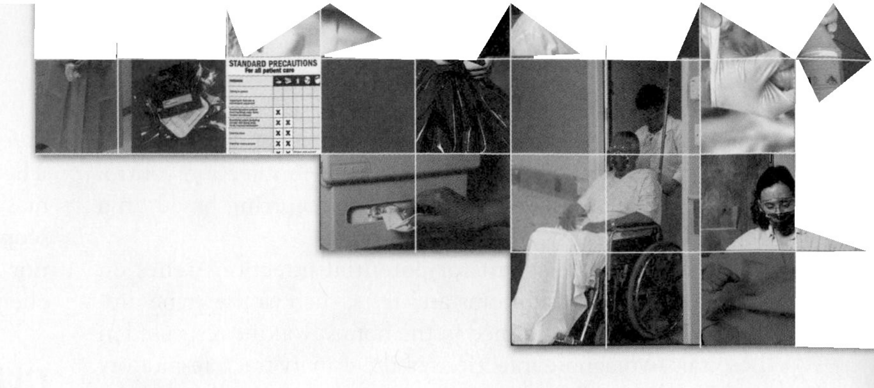

Basic Medical Asepsis

Nursing Process Data

ASSESSMENT Data Base

- Assess method of hand hygiene that is most appropriate for assigned task.
- Identify clients at risk for infection.
- Assess availability of equipment for frequent hand hygiene (soap and water or antiseptic cleansing agent).
- Evaluate health status of the nurse.
- Check agency policy for hand hygiene protocol.
- Assess need for use of nonsterile gloves.
- Assess nurses and clients for latex allergies.
- Assess need for latex-free equipment and/or environment.

PLANNING Objectives

- To deliver client care with pathogen-free hands
- To prevent pathogenic microorganisms from spreading client to client, environment, or healthcare personnel to client
- To protect clients from cross-contamination
- To protect healthcare workers

IMPLEMENTATION Procedures

EVALUATION Expected Outcomes

- Decreased number of bacteria on hands from client to client.
- Delivered care with pathogen-free hands to clients.
- Prevented spread of microorganisms from healthcare workers or environment to clients.
- Prevented cross-contamination between clients.

Pearson Nursing Student Resources

Find additional review materials at **nursing.pearsonhighered.com**

Prepare for success with NCLEX®-style practice questions and Skill Checklists

Hand Hygiene (Medical Asepsis)

Equipment

Nonantimicrobial soap* for routine handwashing
Orangewood stick for cleaning nails
Running warm water
Paper towels
Trash basket

Procedure

1. Stand in front of but away from sink. ▸ ***Rationale:*** Uniform should not touch sink to avoid contamination.
2. Ensure that paper towel is hanging down from dispenser.
3. Turn on water using foot pedal or faucet so that flow is adequate, but not splashing.
4. Adjust temperature to warm. ▸ ***Rationale:*** Cold does not facilitate sudsing and cleaning; hot is damaging to skin.

**According to 1997 HICPAC recommendations.*

5. Wet hands under clean running water, keeping hands below elbow level. ▸ ***Rationale:*** Wet hands facilitate distribution of soap over entire skin surface.

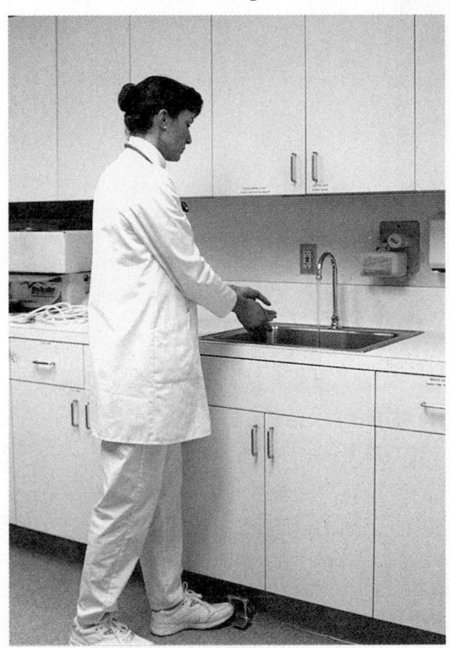

▲ Use foot pedals when available to prevent contamination of hands.

Compliance Studies for Hand Hygiene

- A study of 2,800 opportunities for handwashing showed only a 48% compliance.
- Another study showed hands were washed only 8.5 to 9.5 seconds; a minimum of 15 seconds is necessary to prevent spread of infection.
- Compliance with handwashing technique is higher among nurses than physicians and other healthcare personnel; however, it is estimated to be only 30% to 50%.

Source: Centers for Disease Control and Prevention.

Clinical Alert

Nurses must wash hands for at least 15 seconds before and after each direct contact with a client or each use of client care items to prevent spread of infection (CDC).

EVIDENCE-BASED PRACTICE

Intervention Improves Handwashing Practice

After implementing an educational hand hygiene program, researchers found that before the program, 51% of all health-care workers complied with handwashing guidelines, and after the intervention, 83% did. For nurses, compliance went up from 56% to 89% after the intervention. The program included a handout that specified how important handwashing is and described the proper technique as well as the CDC's hand hygiene guidelines. Five posters were placed around the nurses' station.

Source: Creedon, S. A. (2006). Health care workers' hand decontamination practices: An Irish study. *Clinical Nursing Research, 15*(1), 6.

6. Place a small amount, 1 to 2 teaspoons (3–5 mL) of liquid soap on hands. Thoroughly distribute over hands. Soap should come from a dispenser, not bar soap. ▸ ***Rationale:*** This prevents spread of microorganisms.

Clinical Alert

CDC Alert: The CDC has stated that healthcare workers in contact with clients must remove all fake fingernails because they serve as a reservoir for microorganisms.

7. Rub vigorously, using a firm, circular motion, while keeping your fingers pointed down, lower than wrists. Start with each finger, then between fingers, then palm and back of hand. ▸ ***Rationale:*** This creates friction on all surfaces.
8. Wash your hands for at least 15 to 20 seconds. ▸ ***Rationale:*** Duration of washing is important to produce mechanical action and to allow antimicrobial products time to achieve desired effect.
9. Clean under your fingernails with an orangewood stick. (This should be done at least at start of day and if hands are heavily contaminated.) Move rings up and down fingers to clean if rings are left on.
10. Rinse your hands under running water, keeping fingers pointed downward. ▸ ***Rationale:*** This position prevents contamination of arms.
11. Resoap your hands, rewash, and rerinse if heavily contaminated.
12. Dry hands thoroughly with a paper towel, while keeping hands positioned with fingers pointing up. ▸ ***Rationale:*** Moist hands tend to gather more microorganisms from the environment.

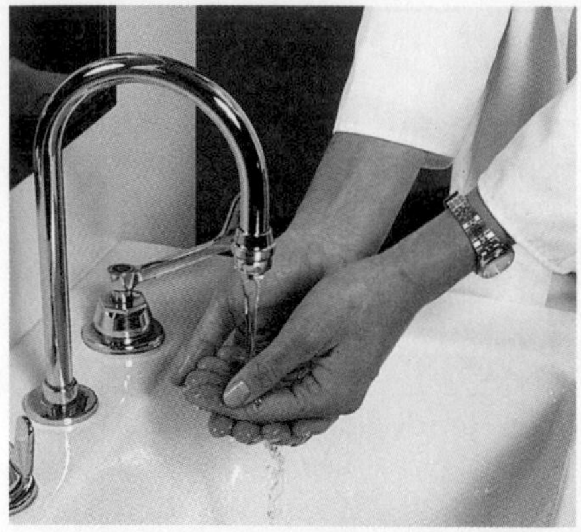

▲ Wet hands thoroughly before applying soap to facilitate removal of pathogens.

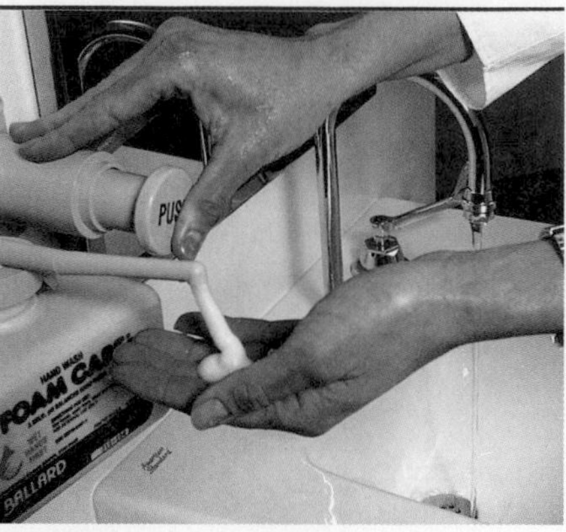

▲ Use a generous amount of soap and friction during handwashing procedure.

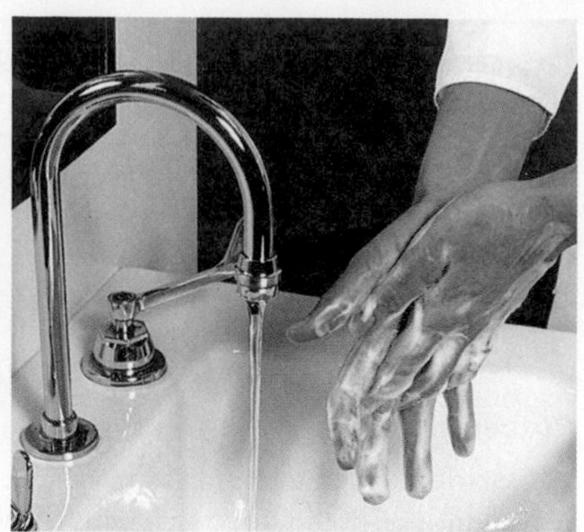

▲ Keep fingers pointed down during handwashing to prevent contaminating arms.

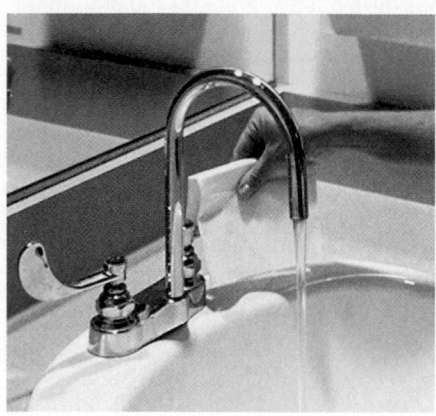

▲ If foot pedal is not available, turn water off using paper towel.

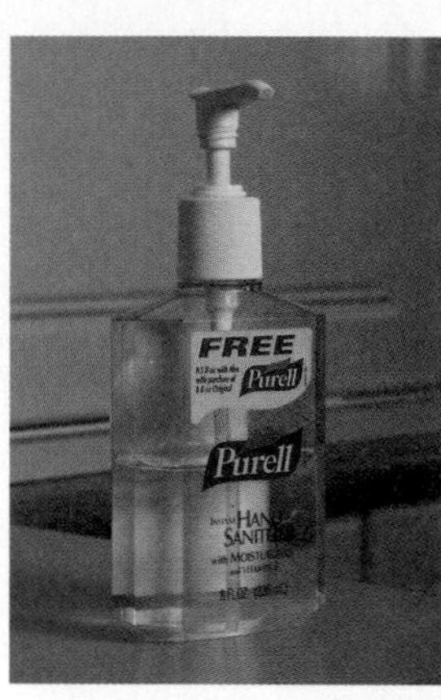

▲ Waterless hand sanitizer kills 99.9% of the most common germs in 15 seconds.

13. Turn off water faucet with dry paper towel, if not using foot pedal. ▸ ***Rationale:*** To avoid recontaminating the hands.
14. Restart procedure at Step 5 if your hands touch the sink anytime between Steps 5 and 13.

For Using Waterless Antiseptic Agents (foam or gels)

1. Check dirt on hands and use waterless agent only if hands are clean. ▸ ***Rationale:*** Hands soiled with dirt or organic matter require soap or detergents that contain antiseptic and water to effectively clean.
2. Apply small amount of alcohol-based rub, foam, or gel (3–5 mL) on palm of hand.

The CDC recommends rubbing hands for 15 to 20 seconds. If you need a timer, imagine singing "Happy Birthday" twice through to a friend.

Centers for Disease Control and Prevention (2009).

How One Hospital Increased Doctors' Compliance in Hand Washing From 65% to 100%

Hospital management first tried self-reporting and nagging doctors to encourage them to wash their hands. This was useless. When they tried a hand hygiene safety posse who would give doctors a small reward (e.g., a $10 Starbuck's gift certificate) for washing their hands, this raised compliance to 80%. What radically worked to increase compliance was when they photographed cultured plates after doctors pressed their palms on the plates and used these disgusting gobs of bacteria (which showed up on the photographs) on every computer screen saver in the hospital. This raised compliance to close to 100%. Perhaps managing the system is preferable to managing the staff.

Dubner, S. J., & Levitt, D. L. (2006, September 24). Selling soap: The Petri dish screen saver. *New York Times Magazine*. Available at: http://www.nytimes.com/2006/09/24/magazine/24wwln_freak.html?ex=1189569600&en=c052a8c2b9420585&ei=5070

EVIDENCE-BASED PRACTICE

Nail Polish and Microbial Threat

Studies show that chipped nail polish or polish worn more than 4 days is linked to higher microbial load than unpolished or freshly polished nails.

Source: Recommended practices for surgical hand antisepsis/hand scrubs. (2004). *AORNJ*, *79*(2), 416.

3. Rub hands together vigorously, covering all surfaces, sides of hands, and fingers. ▶ ***Rationale:*** Failure to cover all surfaces can leave contaminated areas on the hands.
4. Rub hands until dry—waterless agent will dry quickly and automatically without using a towel.

Clinical Alert

OSHA requires that hands be washed with soap and water every third time the hands are cleansed.

5. **NOTE:** *There are now available disposable germicidal wipes that are effective at killing 99.99% of harmful bacteria. These wipes are also effective at removing soil from hands because of natural friction when wiping. The wipes are made from cloth saturated with ethyl alcohol gel solution, free of fragrance and dye. These products are approved by the Environmental Protection Agency (EPA) for both hepatitis B and other viruses.*

Clinical Alert

Antimicrobial soap or waterless agent should be used when there is identified resistant bacteria, colonization outbreaks, or hyperendemic infections with the exception of *C. difficile* and *norovirus,* which are not killed by an alcohol-based gel.

New Health Care Initiative From WHO

Led by WHO in 2009, an initiative to tackle healthcare–associated infection was launched. By focusing on hand hygiene, a major global effort to follow a detailed action plan to save lives has been introduced. This plan is based on global evidence that hand hygiene is integrally linked to transmission of infection by healthcare workers. Some international studies indicate that compliance is as low as 8% and even in developed countries, rates range from 5% to 15%. These rates can affect 10% to 40% of clients admitted to intensive care units. WHO has an improvement strategy that includes "My 5 Moments for Hand Hygiene," which details when hand hygiene needs to be applied:

1. Before touching a client
2. Before clean/aseptic procedures
3. After body fluid exposure/risk
4. After touching a client
5. After touching client surroundings

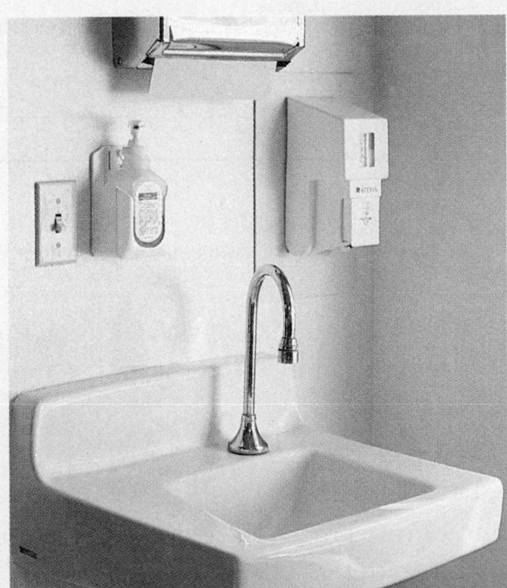

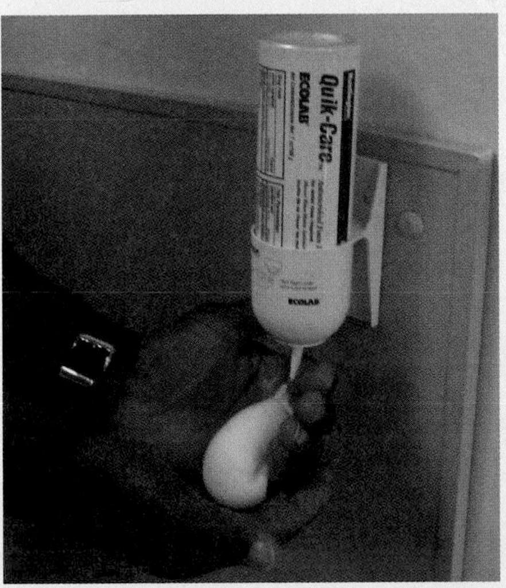

▲ If hands are dirty, wash with soap and water; if clean, use alcohol—gel or foam—as hand hygiene agent.

Source: World Health Organization. (2009). WHO Guidelines on Hand Hygiene in Health Care: Patient Safety.

HyGreen: New Trends

Completing hand hygiene, the staff member passes each hand under a wall-mounted sensor that notes the status of the worker's hands. The device sends a message to the badge the staff member wears. Then, a wireless monitor on the client's bed detects the status, and, if the caregiver's hands are not clean, a wireless message goes to the badge, which vibrates. This reminds the wearer to clean his/her hands before client contact.

The device records all hand hygiene events, allowing the hospital to document events and develop a comprehensive database. During a 5-month test of this device at a Florida medical center, infection rates dropped to zero.

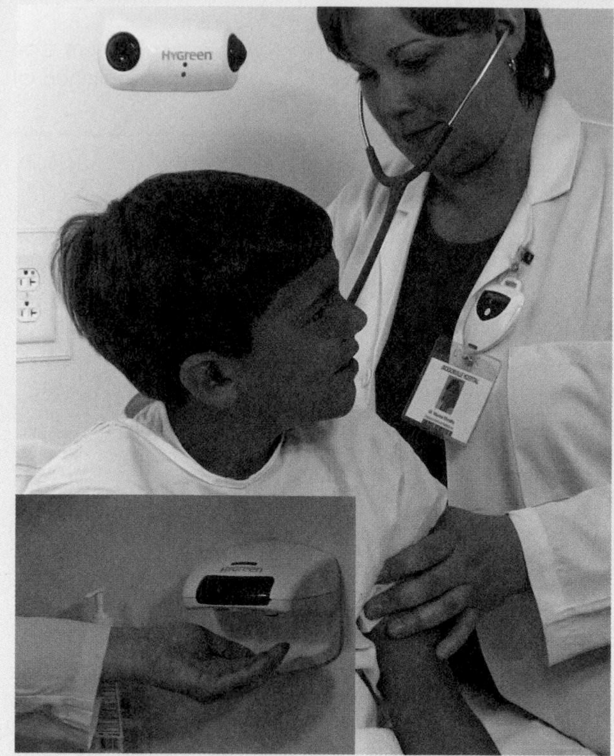

▲ A new screening device from HyGreen could decrease the nearly 2 million in-hospital infections that occur each year.

EVIDENCE-BASED PRACTICE

The Hand Hygiene Resource Center states that 2 million people each year become ill as a result of hospital-acquired infections. Proper hand hygiene is critical to the prevention of these infections, which contribute to the death of nearly 90,000 hospital patients per year and $4.5 billion in medical expenses.

Hand Hygiene Resource Center (www.handhygiene.org)

EVIDENCE-BASED PRACTICE

Bath Basin Contamination

Researchers sampled 92 bath basins at several acute care hospitals and found some form of bacteria in 98%. The conclusion was that bath basins can be reservoirs for bacteria that transmit hospital-acquired infections. Nurses should be aware of this link.

Source: American Association of Critical Care Nurses. (2009, October). www.aacnboldvoicesonLine.org

Cleaning Washable Articles

Equipment

Article to be washed
Antiseptic solution (according to hospital policy)
Running warm water
Paper towels
Trash basket
Clean gloves

Procedure

1. Complete hand hygiene and don clean gloves.
2. Rinse under cold running water. ▸ ***Rationale:*** Cold water removes organic material. Hot water coagulates protein of organic material (pus, blood) and it adheres to a surface.
3. Wash with warm, soapy water using friction or follow hospital protocol for cleaning equipment.
4. Rinse well with clear, hot water.
5. Dry thoroughly.
6. Return to proper place or prepare for sterilization or disinfection if indicated.
7. Remove gloves and complete hand hygiene.

NOTE: If norovirus is identified, use 1 part bleach to 50 parts water for contaminated surfaces. Put washable items in hot water with soap, and dry in hot dryer.

Donning and Removing Clean Gloves

Equipment

Clean gloves
Trash receptacle

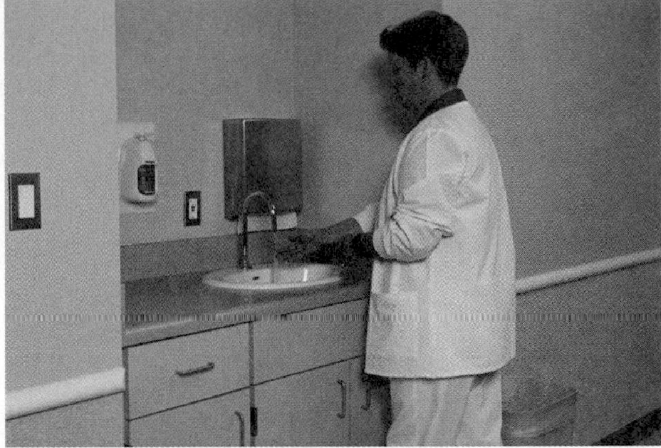

▲ Wash your hands, or complete hand hygiene before donning gloves.

Procedure

1. Complete hand hygiene. ▸ ***Rationale:*** Donning gloves with unclean hands can transfer microorganisms outside gloves.
2. Remove glove from glove receptacle.
3. Hold glove at wrist edge and slip fingers into openings. Pull glove up to wrist.
4. Place gloved hand under wrist edge of second glove and slip fingers into opening.
5. Remove glove by pulling off, touching only outside of glove at cuff, so that glove turns inside out.
6. Place rolled-up glove in palm of second hand.
7. Remove second glove by slipping one finger under glove edge and pulling down and off so that glove turns inside out. Both gloves are removed as a unit.
8. Dispose of gloves in proper container, not at bedside.
9. Complete hand hygiene.

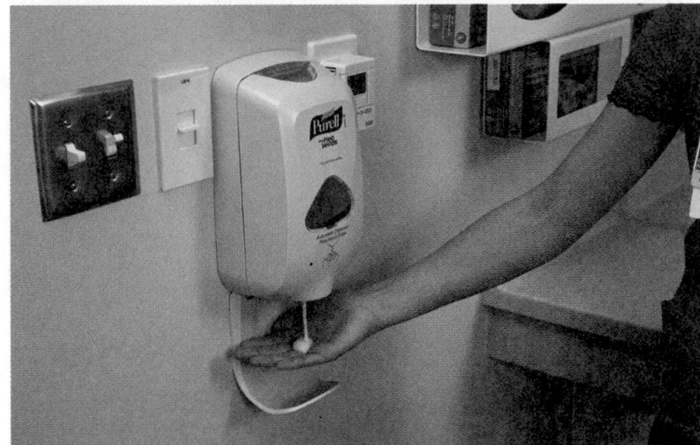

▲1 Complete hand hygiene using anti-bacterial gel or by washing hands.

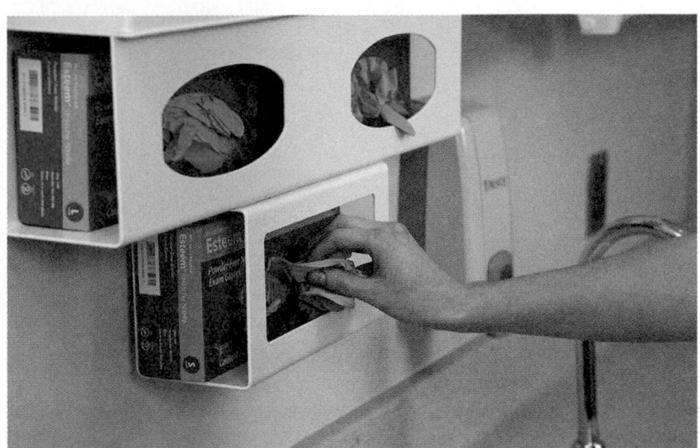

▲2 Remove glove from dispenser.

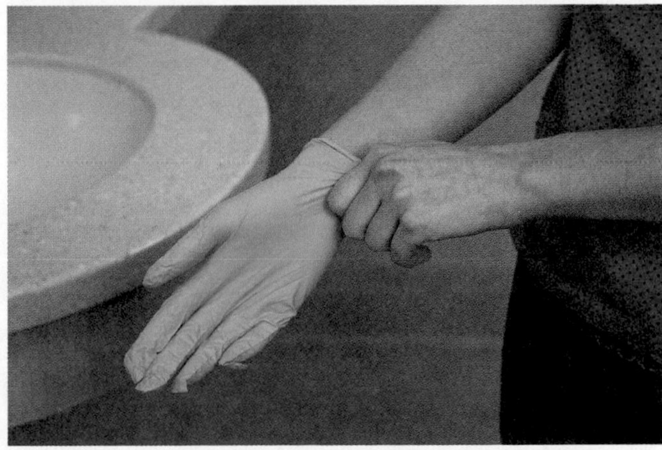

▲3 Hold glove at wrist edge and slip fingers into openings. Pull glove up to wrist.

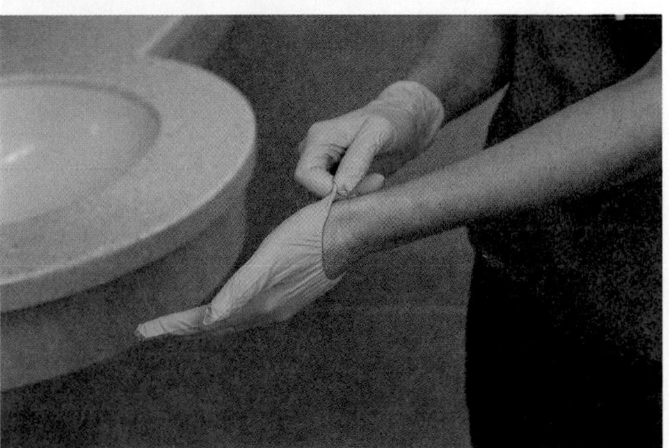

▲4 Place gloved hand under wrist edge of second glove and slip fingers into opening.

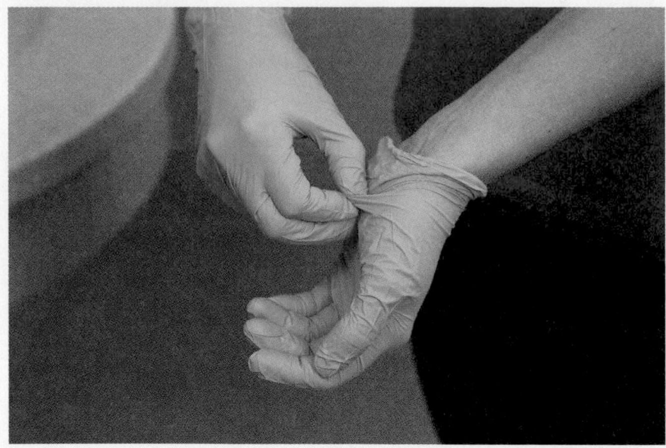

5 Remove glove by pulling off. Touch only outside of glove at cuff, so that glove turns inside out.

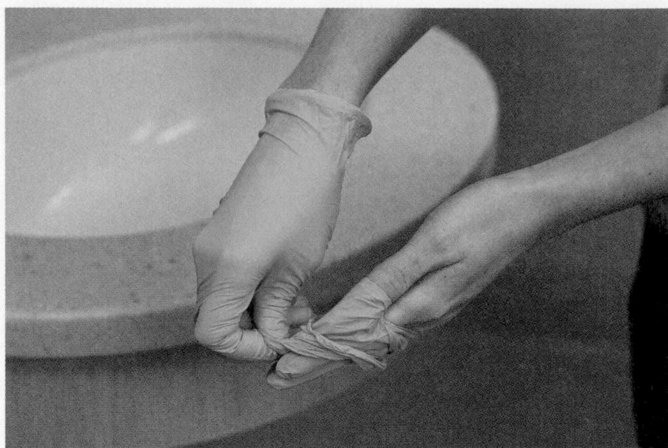

6 Continue pulling off first glove until it is inside out.

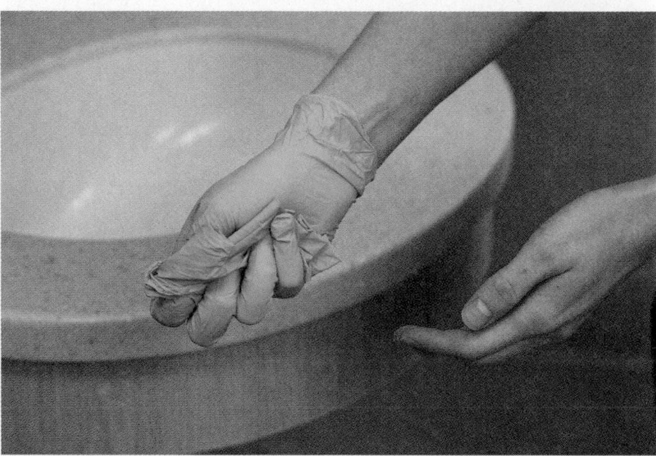

7 Fold rolled-up glove in palm of second hand.

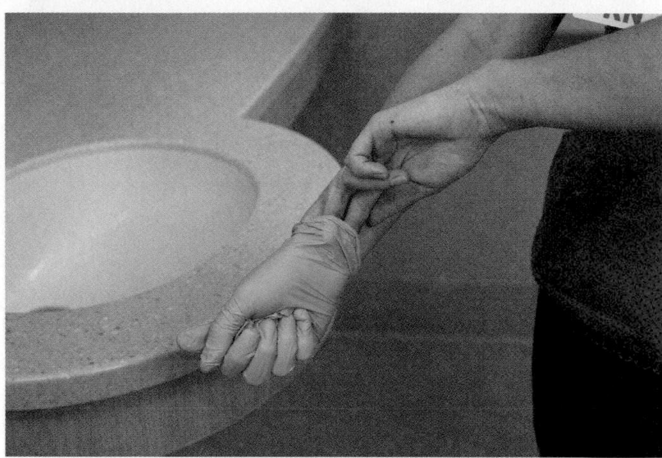

8 Remove second glove by slipping fingers under glove edge.

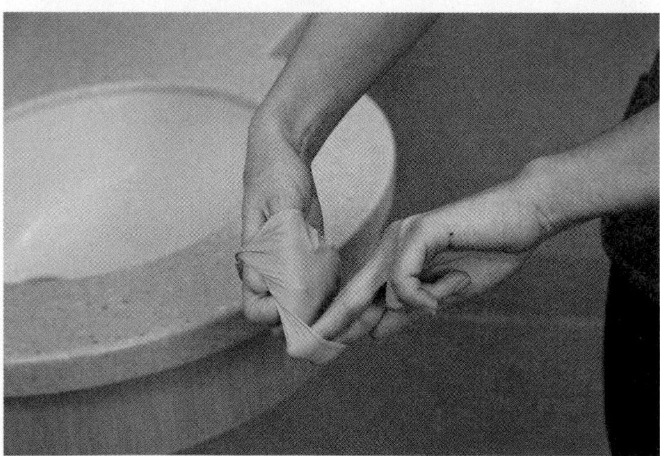

9 Pull glove down and off so that glove turns inside out.

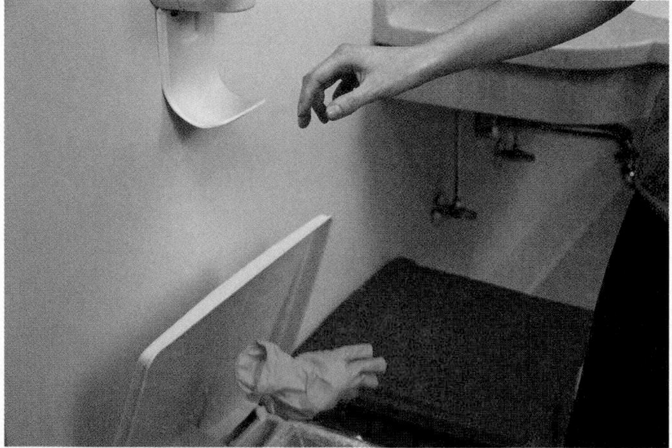

10 Dispose of gloves in proper container, not at bedside. Complete hand hygiene.

Clinical Alert

Ungloved hands should not touch anything that is moist coming from a body surface. The moisture coming from a body surface should be considered potentially contaminated during routine client care.

Source: Pittet, D., Dharan, S., Touveneau, S., Sauvan, V., & Perneger T. V. (1999). Bacterial contamination of the hands of hospital staff during routine patient care. *Archives of Internal Medicine*, 159, 821–826.

EVIDENCE-BASED PRACTICE

C. difficile on the Rise

A study done at 28 community hospitals in North Carolina showed that *C. difficile* infections are on the rise and have surpassed MRSA. The rate of HAI *C. difficile* was 0.28 cases per 1,000 client days and the rate for MRSA was 0.23 cases per 1,000 client days.

Source: Miller, B. (2010). Study presented at International Conference on Health Care Associated Infections.

Glove Selection

- Use sterile gloves for procedures involving contact with normally sterile areas of the body.
- Use examination gloves for procedures involving contact with mucous membranes, unless otherwise indicated, and for client care or procedures that do not require use of sterile gloves.
- Change gloves between clients.
- Do not wash, disinfect, or reuse surgical or examination gloves.
- Use general purpose utility gloves (rubber household gloves) for housekeeping tasks that involve potential blood contact and for instrument cleaning and decontamination procedures.

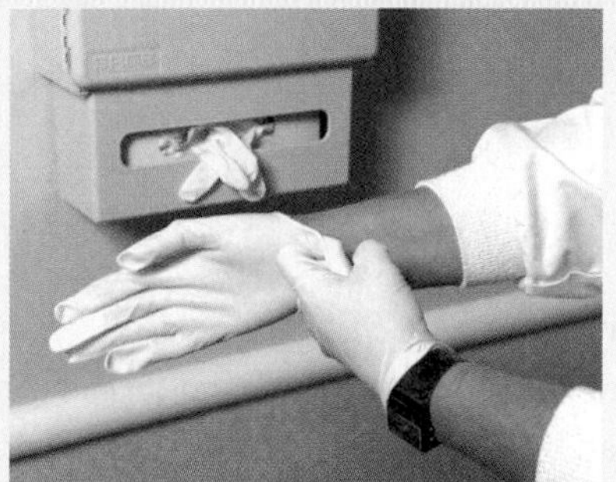

Managing Latex Allergies

Equipment

Latex-free gloves
Latex-free syringes
Latex-free IV tubing and bags of solution
Latex-free cart with supplies for client with latex allergy

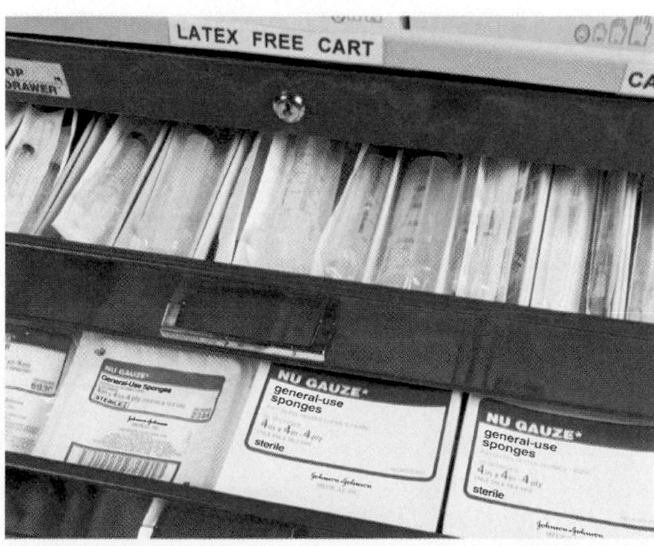

▲ Provide a latex-free cart—supplies for staff and clients with latex allergies.

Procedure

1. Assess clients at high risk or suspected sensitivity to latex (high latex exposure, congenital defects, indwelling catheters, etc.).
2. Assess clients and staff with allergies to cherries, apricots, tomatoes, avocados, bananas, papaya, kiwi, or chestnuts.
   ▸ ***Rationale:*** They may have cross-sensitivity to latex.
3. Recognize symptoms of latex allergy.
   a. Contact dermatitis.
   b. Type IV: facial swelling, itching, hives, rhinitis, eye symptoms.
   c. Type I: potentially dangerous bronchospasms, generalized edema, difficulty breathing, cardiac arrest.
4. Replace latex-containing products (especially gloves) with nonlatex alternatives.
5. Obtain a latex-free cart when a client is identified as having a latex allergy.
   a. Place cart inside client's room.
   b. Check that cart is supplied with latex-free gloves, syringes, IV tubes, suction catheters, etc.
6. Ensure that anaphylaxis medication is available for both clients and staff if latex allergy is suspected.
   ▸ ***Rationale:*** If there is a severe reaction, this medication may be lifesaving.

Ansell Healthcare Company has introduced a new latex-free glove made from synthetic polyisoprene. This glove is safe for use by latex-sensitive nurses, while having the characteristic of a natural rubber latex glove. The Yulex Corporation has introduced a new form of natural rubber latex made from the quayule bush that may prove to be a safer alternative for people with latex sensitivity.

Clinical Alert

Latex allergy or hypersensitivity can be life-threatening, so recognize the primary symptoms in both clients and staff.

DOCUMENTATION for Basic Medical Asepsis

- Infection control measures used
- Clean gloves used for procedure
- Latex allergy identified
- Use of latex-free gloves

CRITICAL THINKING Application

Expected Outcomes

- Decreased number of bacteria on hands from client to client.
- Delivered care with pathogen-free hands to clients.
- Prevented spread of microorganisms from healthcare workers or environment to clients.
- Prevented cross-contamination between clients.

Unexpected Outcomes	Alternative Actions
Infection occurs in client.	• Assess mode of transmission of microorganism. • Administer antibiotics specific to microorganism as ordered. • Review handwashing technique. • Attend in-service program on infection control procedures. • Notify nurse manager of allergy.
Latex allergy identified in healthcare worker or client.	• Institute latex safety procedures for staff and client (if identified). • Educate staff about latex allergy. • Replace latex-containing objects (particularly gloves) with nonlatex alternatives. • Create a latex-free environment in which those who are allergic can work safely.

Chapter 14

UNIT 2

Standard Precautions *(Tier 1)*

Nursing Process Data

ASSESSMENT Data Base

- Assess for skin integrity.
- Assess for presence of drainage from lesions or body cavity.
- Assess for ability to deal with oral secretions.
- Assess for compliance to hygiene measures (i.e., covering mouth when coughing, ability to control body fluids).
- Assess ability to carry out activities of daily living (ADLs).
- Assess extent of barrier techniques needed (i.e., gloves, gown, mask, protective eyewear).
- Assess need for special equipment (i.e., hazardous waste bags, plastic bags for specimens).

PLANNING Objectives

- To prevent the spread of the microorganism to health professionals
- To reduce potential for the transmission of microorganisms
- To protect hospital personnel and others from contamination
- To provide appropriate equipment and techniques for preventive measures
- To prevent clients (especially compromised clients) from acquiring nosocomial infections.

STANDARD PRECAUTIONS
For all patient care

PROCEDURE					
Talking to patient					
Adjusting IV fluid rate or non-invasive equipment					
Examining patient *without* touching blood, body fluids, mucous membranes	X				
Examining patient *including* contact with blood, body fluids, mucous membranes	X	X			
Drawing blood	X	X			
Inserting venous access	X	X			
Suctioning	X	X	*Use gown, mask, eyewear if bloody body fluid splattering is likely*		
Inserting body or face catheters	X	X	*Use gown, mask, eyewear if bloody body fluid splattering is likely*		
Handling soiled waste, linen, other materials	X	X	*Use gown, mask, eyewear only if waste or linen are extensively contaminated and splattering is likely*		
Intubation	X	X	X	X	X
Inserting arterial access	X	X	X	X	X
Endoscopy	X	X	X	X	X
Operative and other procedures which produce extensive splattering of blood or body fluids.	X	X	X	X	X

IMPLEMENTATION Procedures

EVALUATION Expected Outcomes

- Prevented spread of microorganisms between clients and/or healthcare workers.
- Reduced potential for transmission of microorganisms occurs.
- Protected hospital personnel and others from contamination.
- Provided appropriate equipment and techniques for preventive measures.
- Reduced incidence of nosocomial infections.

Pearson Nursing Student Resources

Find additional review materials at **nursing.pearsonhighered.com**

Prepare for success with NCLEX®-style practice questions and Skill Checklists

Donning Protective Gear Utilizing Standard Precautions

Equipment

- Disposable gloves
- Gown
- Mask
- Protective eyewear

Procedure

1. Use alcohol-based antiseptic or wash hands using nonantimicrobial soap and dry.
2. Put on gown by placing one arm at a time through sleeves. Wrap gown around body so it covers clothing completely. ▶ ***Rationale:*** Gowns are worn when it is likely that personal clothing will come in contact with blood, body fluids, secretions, and excretions.
3. Bring waist ties from back to front of gown or tie in back, according to hospital policy. ▶ ***Rationale:*** This will ensure that entire clothing is covered by the gown, preventing accidental contamination.
4. Tie gown at neck or adhere Velcro strap to gown.
5. Don mask. ▶ ***Rationale:*** Masks are worn when there is an anticipated contact with respiratory droplet secretions (e.g., client with suspected or known tuberculosis), the client has a persistent cough and does not cover mouth, or when suction will be performed.
6. Don protective eyewear such as face shield. ▶ ***Rationale:*** Face shields will protect the nurse from splashing of blood or body fluids while caring for clients.
7. Don disposable gloves. ▶ ***Rationale:*** Gloves will prevent contamination of hands when there is contact with blood, body fluids, secretions, or excretions.

New Trends: Software to Improve Quality of Care

Meditech's Health Care Information System provides tools to help organizations increase client safety and assist them to meet The Joint Commission's goals.

Goal 7: Reduce the Risk of Healthcare Associated Infections

The infection control portion of Meditech's Laboratory Information System helps providers to identify and track infections by automatically flagging infections by markers (site of infection, type of infection, and whether sensitive or resistant to certain antibiotics). The infection control group can receive alerts which will assist them in tracking healthcare-associated infections.

See The Joint Commission's goals in Chapter 7.
Source: http://www.meditech.com/IndustryNews/homepage.htm

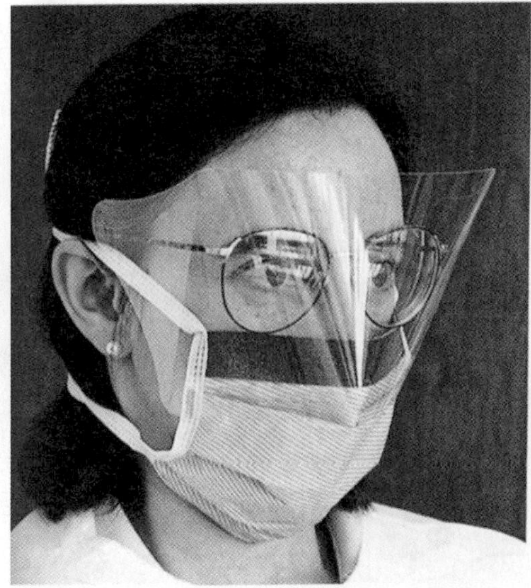

▲ Face shield should be used when there is a risk of splashing from body fluids or blood.

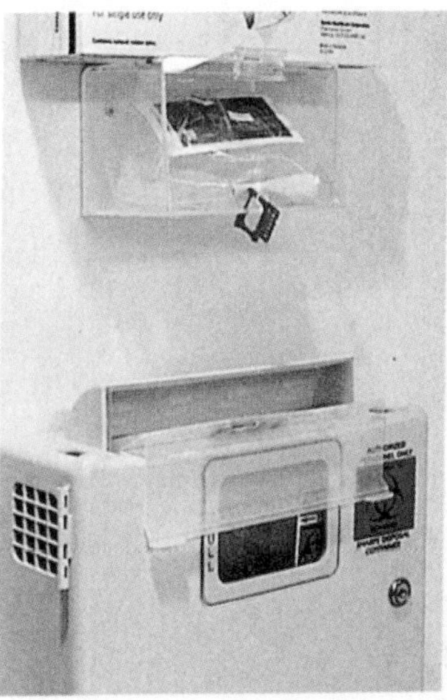

▲ Place sharps container in area for easy access.

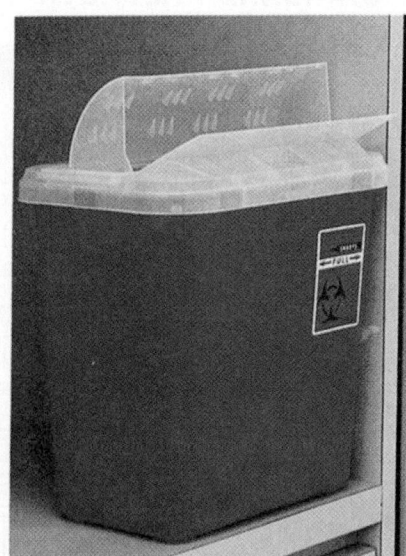

▲ Larger sharps containers are available for areas where usage is greater.

Standard Precaution Guidelines

The following Standard Precautions are recommended for use with clients to prevent transmission of infectious agents. Please follow these guidelines when caring for clients.

- Wash hands thoroughly or use alcohol-based antiseptic after removing gloves and before and after all client contact.
- Wear gloves when there is direct contact with blood, body fluids, secretions, excretions, and contaminated items. This includes a neonate before first bath. Wash as soon as possible if unanticipated contact with these body substances occurs.
- Protect clothing with gowns or plastic aprons if there is a possibility of being splashed or in direct contact with contaminated material.
- Wear masks, goggles, or face shield to avoid being splashed; includes during suctioning, irrigations, and deliveries.
- Do not break or recap needles; discard them intact into puncture-resistant containers.
- Place all contaminated articles and trash in leakproof bags.
- Clean spills quickly with a 1:10 solution of bleach, or according to facility policy, or EPA-approved germicide if spill occurs in an HIV/AIDS client's room.
- Place clients at risk for contaminating the environment in a private room with separate bathroom facilities, or with another client with same infectious organism.
- Transport infected clients using appropriate barriers, i.e., mask and gown.

Exiting a Client's Room Utilizing Standard Precautions

Equipment

Linen hamper
Garbage bag

Procedure

1. Untie string of gown at waist. ▸ ***Rationale:*** Any surface below waist level is considered contaminated; therefore, the strings at the waist are untied before removing gloves.
2. Remove first glove by turning it inside out, place rolled-up glove in second hand, remove second glove by slipping one finger under glove edge and pulling glove off. Dispose of them in garbage bag.
3. Untie gown at neck. ▸ ***Rationale:*** The back of the neck is considered clean and the tie should not be touched with contaminated gloves.
4. Take off gown by pulling down from shoulders, turn gown inside out, and pull arms out of gown. ▸ ***Rationale:*** The inside of the gown is not considered contaminated and therefore, if it accidentally touches your uniform, it will not be contaminated.
5. Dispose of gown in linen hamper. If disposable, place in garbage bag.
6. Remove protective eyewear.

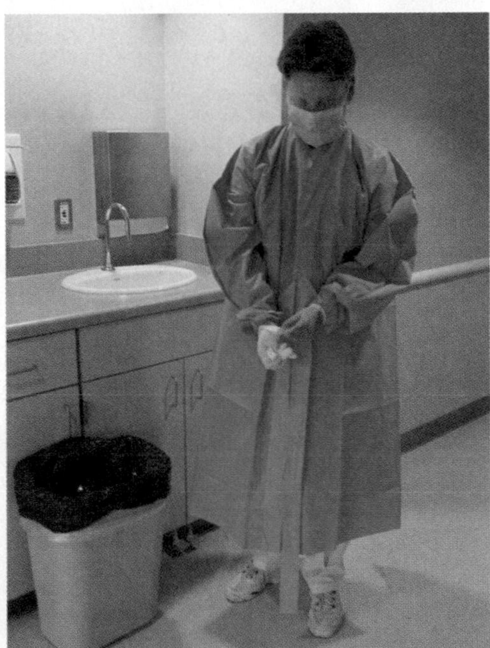

▲ Place rolled-up glove in palm of second hand. Remove second glove by slipping one or two fingers under edge and pulling down and off. Remove second glove by slipping finger under glove edge. Both gloves are removed as a unit.

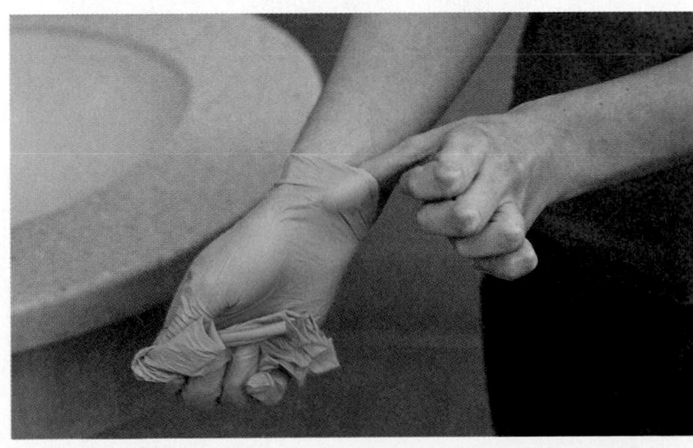

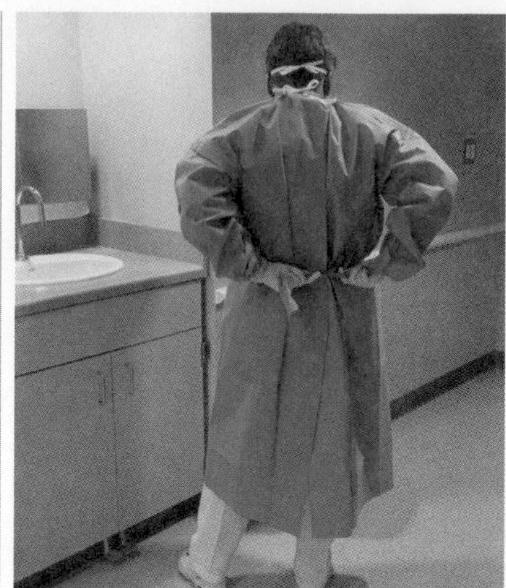

1 Remove gown by first untying string at waist (or in back, as shown in photo).

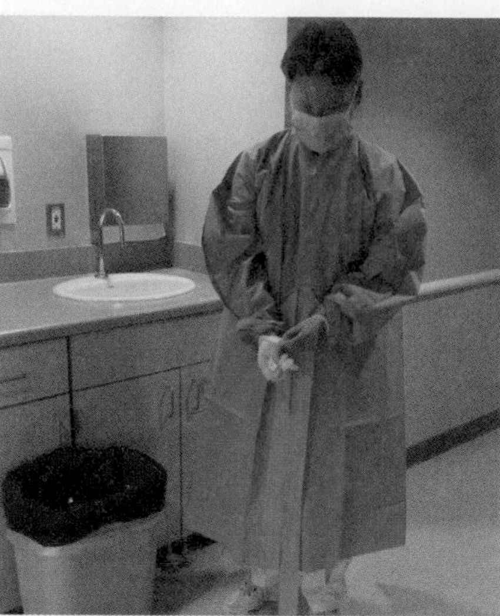

2 Remove first glove by pulling it off so glove turns inside out. Place rolled-up glove in palm of second hand and remove second glove.

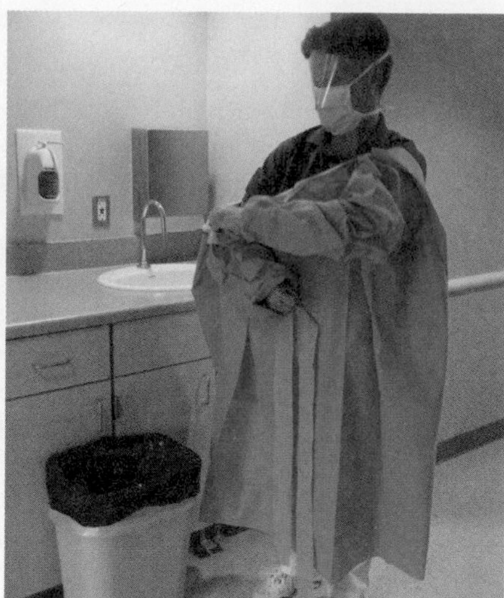

3 Untie gown at neck and take off gown by pulling down from shoulders.

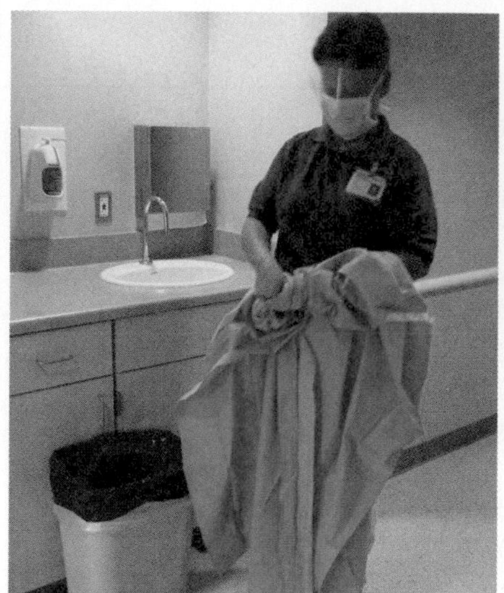

4 Turn gown inside out and pull arms out as you pull gown off.

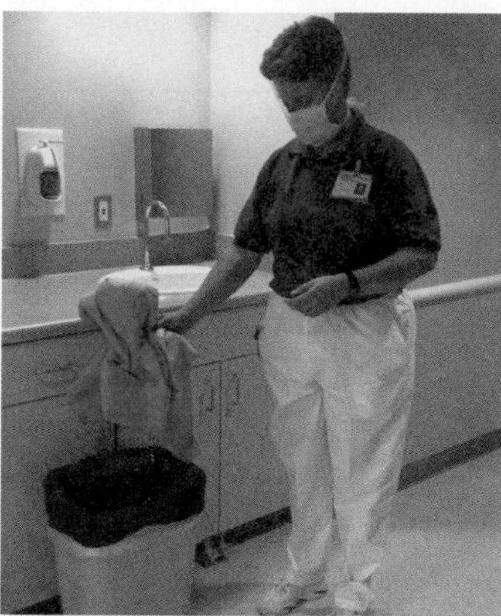

5 Dispose of gown in linen hamper; if disposable, place in garbage bag.

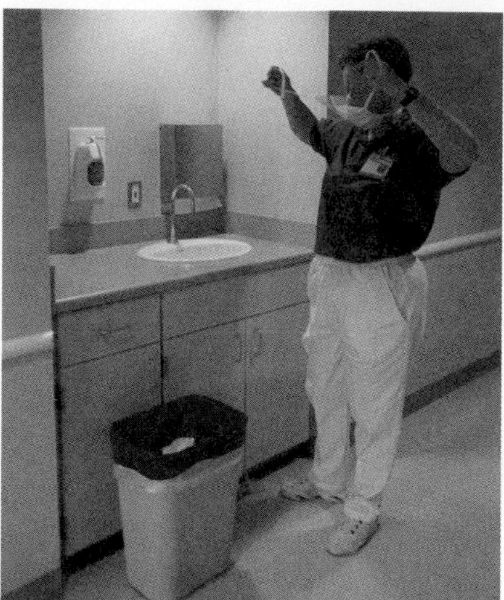

6 Remove protective eyewear, if worn, and mask.

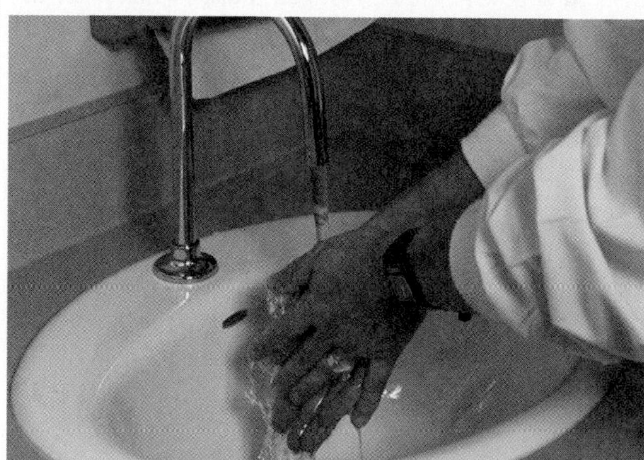

7 Wash hands in room or use antiseptic gel. After exiting room, repeat hand hygiene.

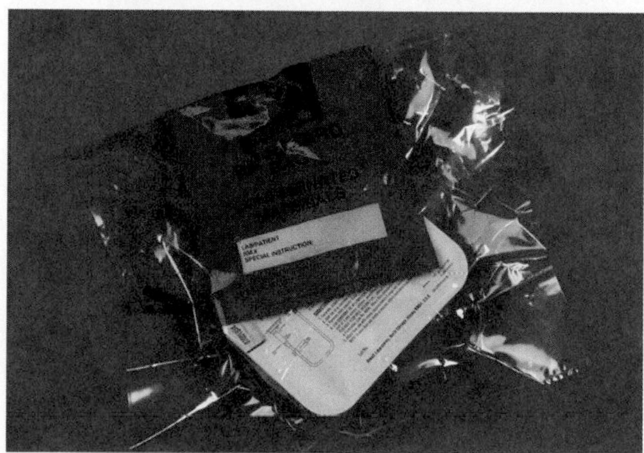

8 Dispose of all soiled equipment or contaminated material in appropriate receptacle.

Clinical Alert

Disposal Precautions

Secretion: Client should be instructed to expectorate into tissue held close to mouth. Suction catheters and gloves should be disposed of in impervious, sealed bags.

Excretion: Excrement should be disposed of by flushing into sewage system. Strict attention should be paid to careful hand hygiene; disease can be spread by oral–fecal route.

Blood: Needles and syringes should be disposable. Used needles should not be recapped. They should be placed in a puncture-resistant container that is prominently labeled "isolation." Specimens should be labeled "blood precaution."

Clinical Alert

HIV–HBV

Sample protocol for accidental contact with blood or body fluids.

1. Any percutaneous or mucocutaneous exposure should receive immediate first aid.
   a. Percutaneous exposure—a break in the skin caused by contaminated needle or sharp instrument, broken glass container holding blood or body fluids, or human bite.
   b. Mucocutaneous exposure—body fluid contact to open wounds, nonintact skin (eczema), or body fluid splash to mucous membranes (mouth, eyes).
2. Apply immediate first aid to site.
   a. Needle stick or puncture wound: Scrub area vigorously with soap and water for 5 minutes.
   b. Oral mucous membrane exposure: Rinse area several times with water.
   c. Ocular exposure: Irrigate immediately with water or normal saline solution.
   d. Human bite: Cleanse wound with povidone–iodine (Betadine) and sterile water.
3. Report unusual occurrence to the charge nurse or supervisor. (See explanation of form and sample in Chapter 3.)
4. Complete an unusual occurrence form and follow reporting requirements mandated by OSHA.
5. Follow facility protocol for emergency care. If risk assessment indicates, follow PEP protocol.
6. Document circumstances of exposure, postexposure management, counseling, and follow-up procedures in healthcare worker's confidential medical file.
7. The CDC has now approved rapid result tests for HIV. Most people exposed to HIV develop antibodies within 2 to 8 weeks, but within 20 minutes will know the results from one of these new diagnostic tests. See Chapter 20 on specimen collection.

NOTE: Use of antiseptics is not contraindicated; however, they have not been proven effective in postexposure care.

7. Remove mask and place in garbage bag.
8. Wash hands or use alcohol-based antiseptic in room.
9. Exit room and complete hand hygiene at nearest sink.
   ▶ ***Rationale:*** To prevent spread of microorganisms.
10. Dispose of all double-bagged equipment by taking to "soiled" utility room. Send specimens to laboratory and deposit linen in appropriate linen hamper.
11. Complete hand hygiene.

TABLE 14-3 Basic and Expanded HIV Postexposure Prophylaxis Regimens

Regimen Category	Application	Drug Regimen
Basic	Occupational HIV exposures for which there is a recognized transmission risk	4 weeks (28 days) of both zidovudine 600 mg every day in 2 or 3 divided doses **and** lamivudine 150 mg twice a day. Now available combined as Combivir, single tablet given 2 × daily.
Expanded	Occupational HIV exposures that pose an increased risk for transmission (e.g., larger volume of blood and/or higher virus titer in blood)	Basic regimen plus **either** indinavir 800 mg every 8 hr on an empty stomach **or** nelfinavir 750 mg 3 × daily with meals or snacks.

Recommendations for the Selection of Drugs for PEP

The selection of a drug regimen for HIV PEP must strive to balance the risk for infection against the potential toxicity of the agent(s) used. Because PEP is potentially toxic, its use is not justified for exposures that pose a negligible risk for transmission. Also, there is insufficient evidence to recommend a highly active regimen for all HIV exposures. Therefore, two regimens for PEP are provided: a "basic" two-drug regimen that should be appropriate for most HIV exposures and an "expanded" three-drug regimen that should be used for exposures that pose an increased risk for transmission or where resistance to one or more antiretroviral agents is known or suspected. When possible, the regimens should be implemented in consultation with persons having expertise in antiretroviral treatment and HIV transmission.

Source: Centers for Disease Control and Prevention. (2001). Appendix C: Basic and expanded HIV postexposure prophylaxis regimens. *Morbidity and Mortality Weekly Report (MMWR)*. Available at: http://cdc.gov/mmwr/preview/mmwrhtml/rr5011a4.htm.

*Indinavir should be taken on an empty stomach (i.e., without food or with a light meal) and with increased fluid consumption (i.e., drinking six 8-oz glasses of water throughout the day); nelfinavir should be taken with meals.

DOCUMENTATION for Standard Precautions

- Standard Precautions maintained
- Client's response to care and protocol used
- Specimens sent to laboratory if appropriate
- Disposal precautions utilized if appropriate

CRITICAL THINKING Application

Expected Outcomes

- Prevented spread of microorganisms between clients and/or healthcare workers.
- Reduced potential for transmission of microorganisms occurs.
- Protected hospital personnel and others from contamination.
- Provided appropriate equipment and techniques for preventive measures.
- Reduced incidence of nosocomial infections.

Unexpected Outcomes	Alternative Actions
Contaminated blood or body fluid comes in contact with your skin or mucous membranes.	• Report incident, and complete unusual occurrence report. (Very important for follow-up legal and medical implications.) • Follow hospital guidelines (they may differ per facility) for postexposure prophylaxis (PEP). • HIV exposure should be immediately reported, as most hospitals offer AZT preventive therapy. This therapy should be administered within 1 hr, not more than 24 hr after exposure. • Obtain AIDS antibody test in ensuing months. • Continue to monitor own health status and carry out specific activities to build immune system. • Do not smoke or drink excessively. • Eat well-balanced meals with reduced fat intake. • Take vitamin supplements designed to boost immune system (vitamin C, beta-carotene, vitamin A, coenzyme Q10, zinc). Check with nutritionist or holistic physician for complete protocol. • Exercise frequently. • Obtain adequate sleep and rest. • Learn and practice stress reduction activities (stress is known to lessen effectiveness of immune system).
Working with AIDS clients becomes extremely stressful, and the nurse experiences burn-out.	• Request consultation therapy to handle feelings and learn new methods of coping with stress. • Leave this type of work temporarily. • Change other aspects of your life to reduce stress. • Follow above-mentioned regimen to enhance immune system.

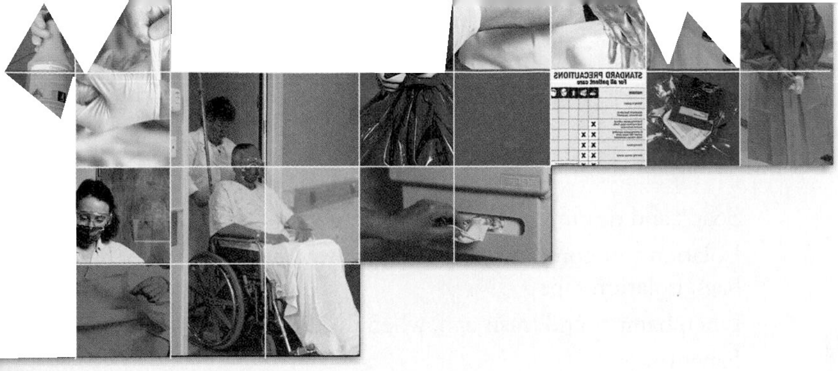

Chapter 14

UNIT 3

Isolation

Nursing Process Data

ASSESSMENT Data Base

- Identify appropriate times for hand hygiene.
- Identify type of protective clothing required for barrier nursing.
- Identify epidemiology of the disease to determine how to prevent infection from spreading.
- Identify equipment needed to prevent spread of organisms.
- Assess method of terminal cleaning and disposing of equipment.

PLANNING Objectives

- To prevent the spread of endogenous and exogenous flora to other clients
- To reduce potential for transferring organisms from the hospital environment to the client
- To protect hospital personnel from becoming infected
- To prevent immunosuppressed clients from acquiring nosocomial infections

IMPLEMENTATION Procedures

EVALUATION Expected Outcomes

- Prevented client-to-client spread of endogenous and exogenous flora.
- Protected hospital personnel from becoming infected.
- Prevented immunosuppressed clients from acquiring nosocomial infections.
- Reduced transferrence of organisms from hospital environment to clients.

Pearson Nursing Student Resources

Find additional review materials at **nursing.pearsonhighered.com**

Prepare for success with NCLEX®-style practice questions and Skill Checklists

Preparing for Isolation

Equipment

Specific equipment depends on isolation precaution system used

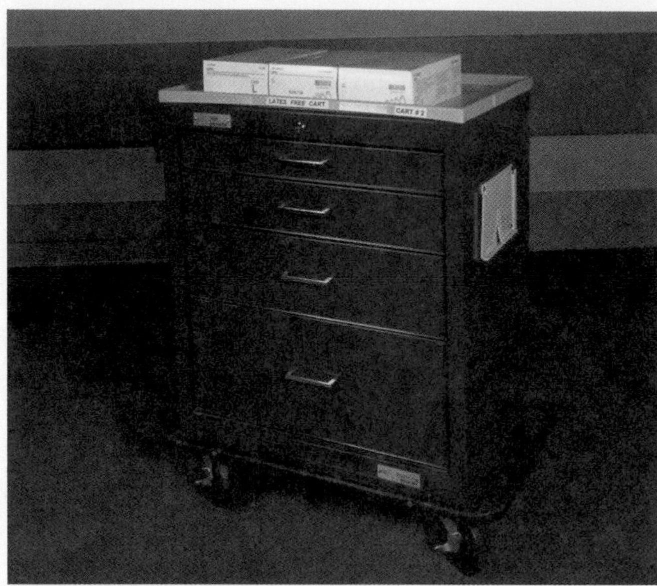

▲ Place isolation cart outside client's door when cart is required.

Soap* and running water

Isolation cart containing masks, gowns, gloves, plastic bags, isolation tape

Linen hamper and trash can, when needed

Paper towels

Door card indicating precautions

Procedure

1. Check physician's order for isolation.
2. Obtain isolation cart from central supply, if needed.
3. Check that all necessary equipment to carry out the isolation order is available.
4. Place isolation card on the client's door.
5. Ensure that linen hamper and trash cans are available, if needed.
6. Explain purpose of isolation to client and family.
7. Instruct family in procedures required.
8. Wash hands with antimicrobial soap* or use alcohol-based gel before and after entering isolation room.

**Type of antimicrobial soap or agent depends on infectious agent and client condition.*

EVIDENCE-BASED PRACTICE

An isolation client with an infection that can be transmitted via airborne route should be admitted to a room that has a directional air-flow negative pressure ventilation system, with a connected anteroom. The door should be kept closed at all times, and the air should undergo 12 air exchanges per hour for rooms developed after 2001. Air should be filtered through a HEPA filter or directly discharged to the outside.

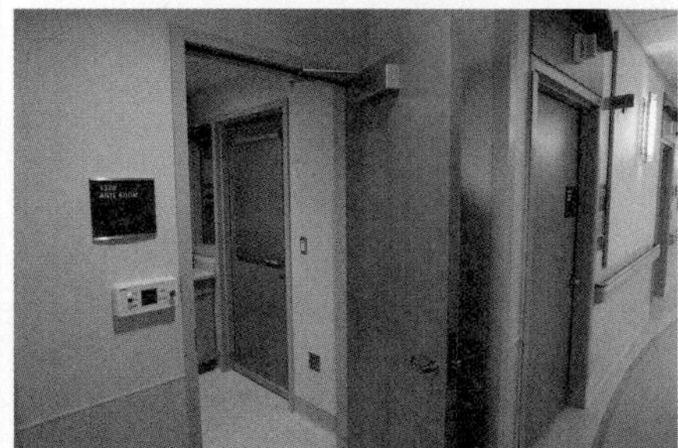

▲ Entrance to Negative Pressure isolation room and the adjoining Anteroom.

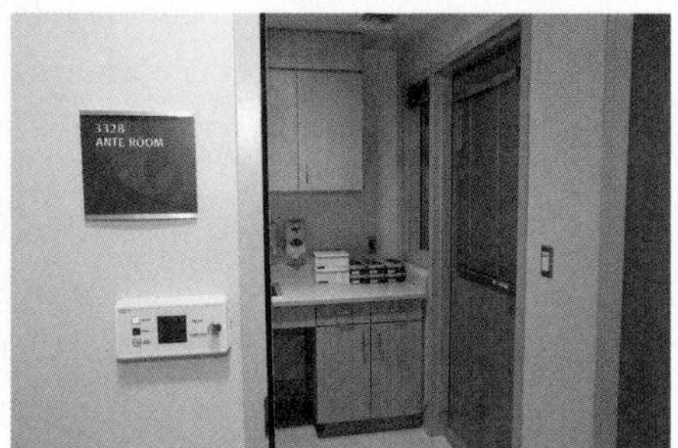

▲ View from anteroom to client's isolation room with directional air-flow negative pressure ventilation system.

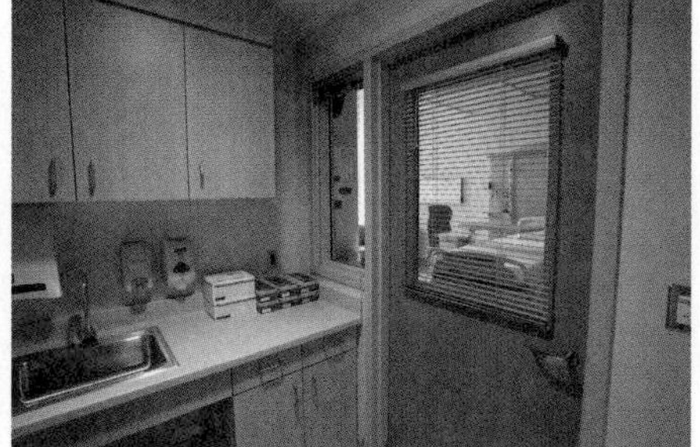

▲ Anteroom connected to isolation room. Staff should use this access to client's room and keep door closed at all times.

Source: Centers for Disease Control and Prevention. (2003, June). Guidelines for Environmental Infection Control in Health Care Facilities. *MMWR Morbidity and Mortality Weekly Report, 52,* 1–4.

EVIDENCE-BASED PRACTICE

Conditions Caused by HAIs

Statistics from the CDC indicate that HAIs (ranging from pneumonia to MRSA) cost hospitals up to $45 billion each year and kill an estimated 100,000 people a year.

Source: TeleTracking Technologies: Fighting hospital-acquired infections with patient flow software. http://.onemedplace.com/blog/archives/5868.

Donning and Removing Isolation Attire

Equipment

Gown
Clean gloves

Procedure

For Donning Attire:

1. Complete hand hygiene.
2. Take gown from isolation cart or cupboard. Put on a new gown each time you enter an isolation room.
3. Hold gown so that opening is in back when you are wearing the gown.
4. Put gown on by placing one arm at a time through sleeves. Pull gown up and over your shoulders.
5. Wrap gown around your back, tying strings at your neck.
6. Wrap gown around your waist, making sure your back is completely covered. Tie strings around your waist.
7. Don eye shield and/or mask, if indicated. ▸ ***Rationale:*** Mask is required if there is a risk of splashing fluids.
8. Don clean gloves and pull gloves over gown wristlets. ▸ ***Rationale:*** Prevents contamination of exposed skin.

For Removing Attire:

1. Untie gown waist strings.
2. Remove gloves and dispose of them in garbage bag.
3. Next, untie neck strings, bringing them around your shoulders so that gown is partially off your shoulders.
4. Using your dominant hand and grasping clean part of wristlet, pull sleeve wristlet over your nondominant hand. Use your nondominant hand to pull sleeve wristlet over your dominant hand.
5. Grasp outside of gown through the sleeves at shoulders. Pull gown down over your arms.
6. Hold both gown shoulders in one hand. Carefully draw your other hand out of gown, turning arm of gown inside out. Repeat this procedure with your other arm.
7. Hold gown away from your body. Fold gown up inside out.
8. Discard gown in appropriate place.
9. Remove eye shield and/or mask and place in receptacle.
10. Complete hand hygiene. ▸ ***Rationale:*** This prevents cross-infection to other clients.

Deadly New Superbug Appears in 2010

A deadly superbug has been detected, surfacing for the first time in India in 2009. Named the New Delhi metallo-beta-lactamose 1, or NDM-I, this bug is an enzyme that can live inside different bacteria. The two types of bacteria that have been host to NDM-I, are *e-coli* (from a human intestine) and *Kebsiella,* found in the lungs. The NDM-I gene alters these bacteria making them resistant to almost all known antibiotics. The young and elderly are the most susceptible to this superbug, which has caused numerous deaths internationally.

Source: Kumarasamy KK, Toleman MA, Walsh TR, et al. (August 2010). Emergence of a new antibiotic resistance mechanism in India, Pakistan, and theUK. *Lancet Infect Dis* 10 (9): 597–602.

Donning Isolation Gear

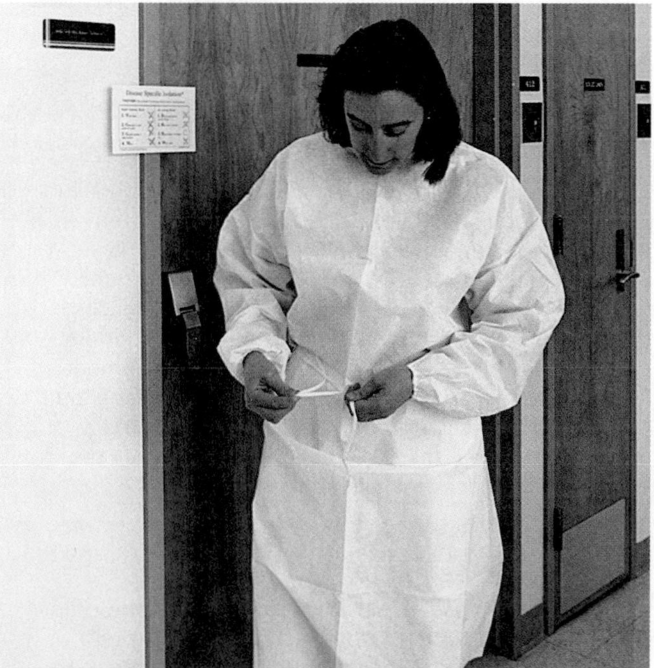

1 Isolation gown is put on before mask, eye shield, or gloves.

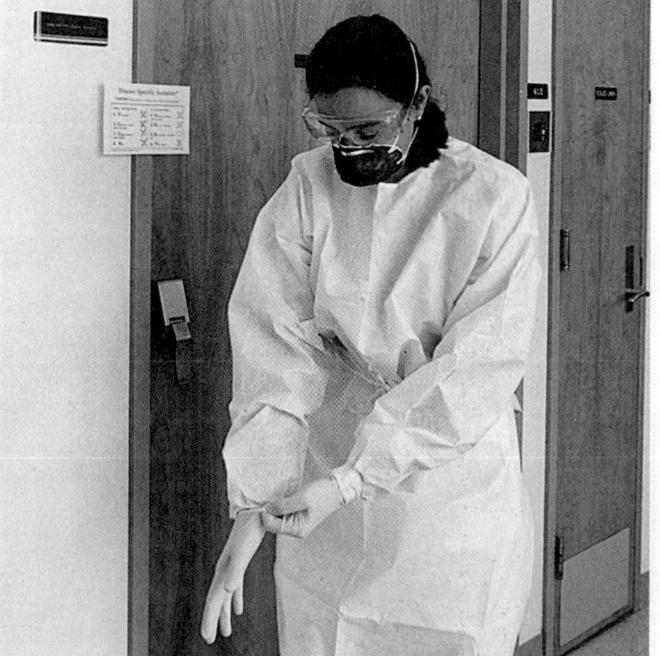

2 Cover wristlets completely to prevent contamination of exposed skin.

Removing Isolation Gear

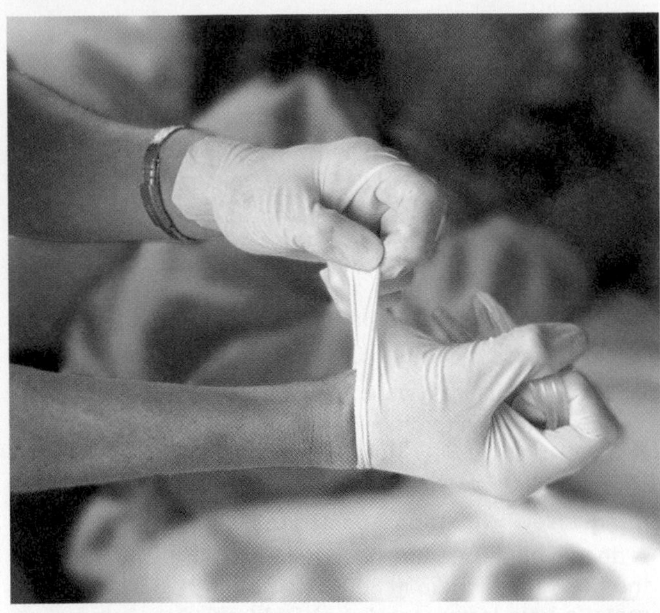

1 Remove gloves before gown, mask or eye shield.

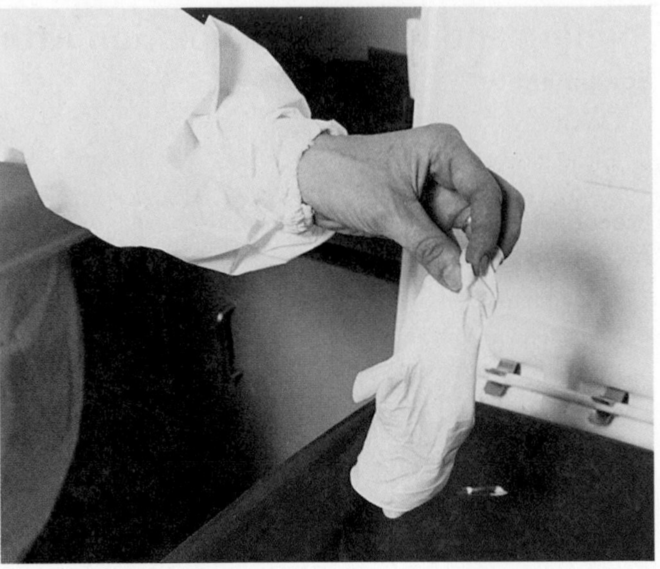

2 Dispose of gloves in appropriate receptacle.

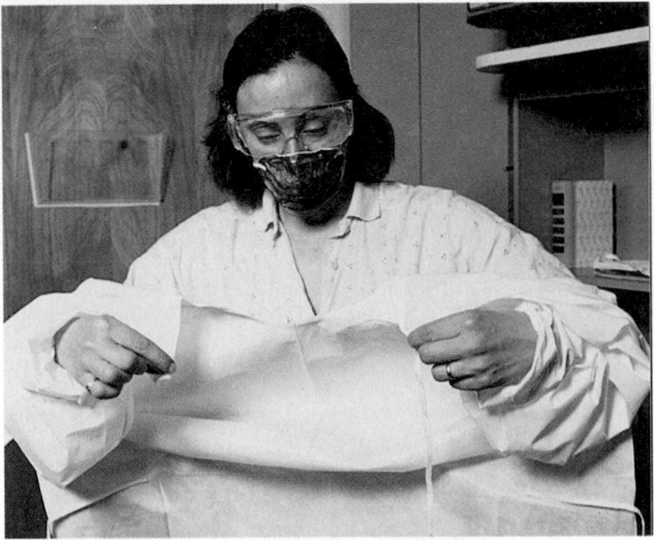

3 Pull gown off shoulders, then down over arms.

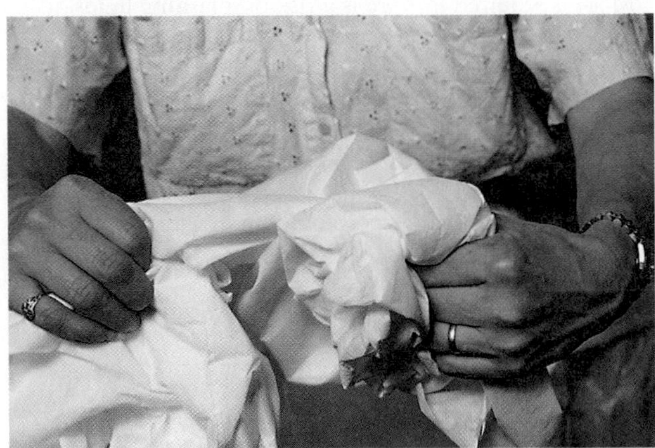

4 Hold gown away from body when rolling inside out.

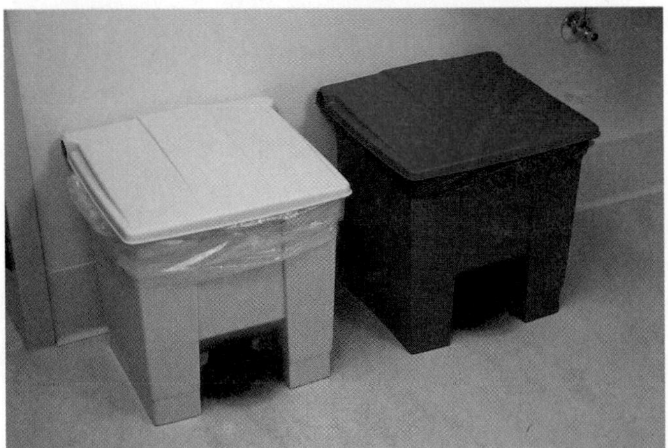

5 Dispose of equipment in appropriate containers that should be in client's room.

Pediatric Considerations

Isolation precautions can increase an already stressful situation for a hospitalized child. Younger children have limited cognitive abilities to understand the implications of isolation. Particularly frightening for them is the presence of people in gowns and masks. To help decrease their fears, preparation is important. Letting the children see and play with the equipment lessens some of the anxiety. Healthcare workers should introduce themselves to the child before donning a mask. Frequent visits to the child can also lessen the fear and loneliness associated with isolation.

Clinical Alert

Some isolation gowns do not tie at the neck; they slip over the head. When removing these gowns, pull shoulders forward to loosen the Velcro at the neck area. Remove gown in the same manner as you would if tied at the neck.

Using a Mask

Equipment

Clean mask

Procedure

1. Obtain mask from box.
2. Position mask to cover your nose and mouth.
3. Bend nose bar so that it conforms over bridge of your nose.
4. If you are using a mask with string ties, tie top strings on top of your head to prevent slipping. If you are using a cone-shaped mask, tie top strings over your ears.
5. Tie bottom strings around your neck to secure mask over your mouth. There should be no gaps between the mask and your face.
6. *Important:* Change mask every 30 minutes or sooner if it becomes damp. ▸ ***Rationale:*** Effectiveness is greatly reduced after 30 minutes or if mask is moist.
7. Complete hand hygiene before removing mask.
8. To remove mask, untie lower strings first, or slip elastic band off without touching mask. ▸ ***Rationale:*** Only strings are considered clean.
9. Discard mask in a trash container.
10. Complete hand hygiene.

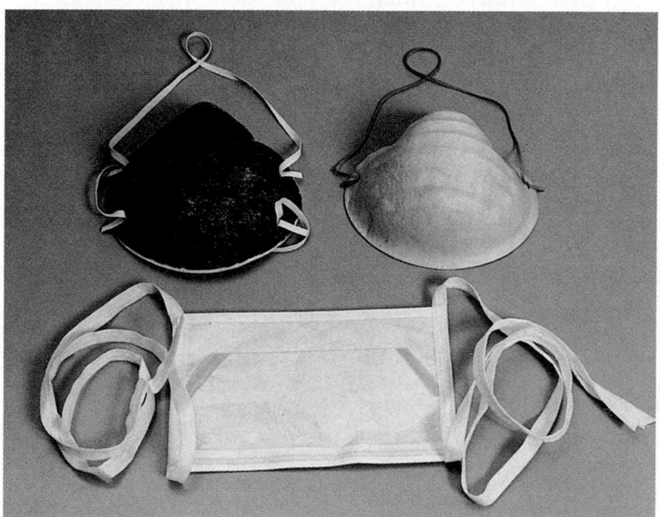

▲ Sample masks used for isolation protocol.

Clinical Alert

Protective eyewear such as goggles and face shield are worn when there is a risk of splashes or sprays from blood, secretions, excretions, or body fluids. Eyewear is removed before taking off mask.

Clinical Alert

Respiratory N95 or HEPA respirators (high-efficiency particulate air) masks are recommended for infectious diseases transmitted by airborne mode; for example, influenza or suspected or confirmed multidrug-resistant tuberculosis.

- Masks are fitted to worker. Mask should have a good sealing surface with no leakage around the edge, providing a tight seal over the nose and mouth.
- Wear mask until it becomes difficult to breathe. This indicates mask is clogged.
- When not in use, store mask in zip-lock bag in safe area.
- Masks are expensive and can be used repeatedly until it is difficult to breathe through them.

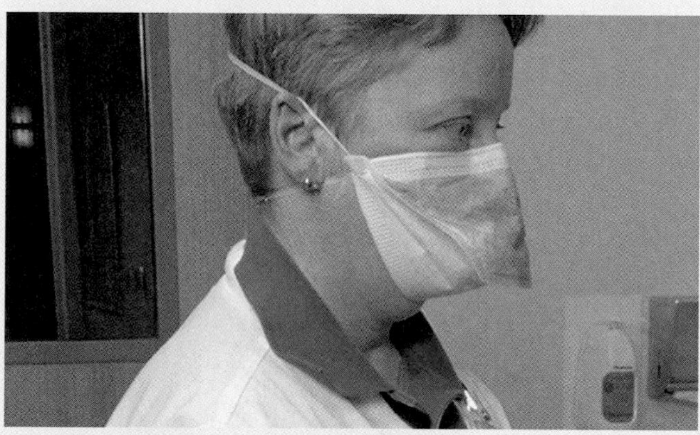

▲ Particulte filter respirator mask must be airtight.

Filligent Limited Biomask

A new flu-killing mask called the Biomask is available in 2010. Made of interwoven cellulose fibers that bind to bacteria and viruses, this mask destroys the cell walls and kills 99.9% of the flu virus. This mask kills germs on contact and can be worn multiple times per day, unlike conventional masks.

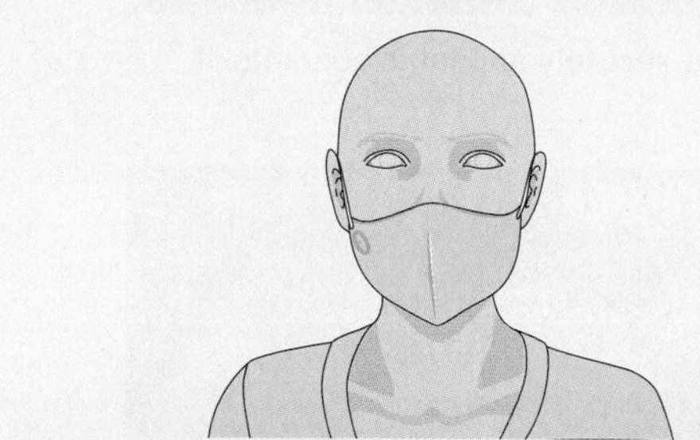

▲ Filligent Limited Biomask.

EVIDENCE-BASED PRACTICE

Using a Mask

A study was done at McMaster University in Canada comparing a surgical mask with the N95 mask for clients with laboratory confirmed influenza. It showed that within a prespecified margin, the surgical mask appeared to be no worse than N95 masks in preventing influenza transmission.

Source: Loeb, M. (2009). McMaster University and Hamilton Science Corp., Ontario, Canada. *Journal of the American Medical Association, 302*(12).

Assessing Vital Signs

Equipment

Thermometer
Stethoscope
Blood pressure cuff and sphygmomanometer
Thermometer stand
Watch with sweep second hand
Isolation clothing

Procedure

1. Complete hand hygiene and use two forms of client ID.
2. Don isolation clothing as required by type of isolation.
3. Proceed to take vital signs as you would for any client.
4. Place equipment in appropriate area if it is to be left in room. Follow appropriate protocol to remove equipment from isolation room.
5. Remove isolation clothing according to protocol.
6. Complete hand hygiene.
7. Wipe watch if accidentally contaminated. Use appropriate solution.

Removing Items From Isolation Room

Equipment

Large red isolation bags
Specimen container
Plastic bag with biohazard label
Laundry bag
Red plastic container for sharps
Cleaning articles

Procedure

1. Place laboratory specimen in biohazard plastic bag.
2. Dispose of all sharps in appropriate red plastic container in room.
3. Place all linen in linen bag.

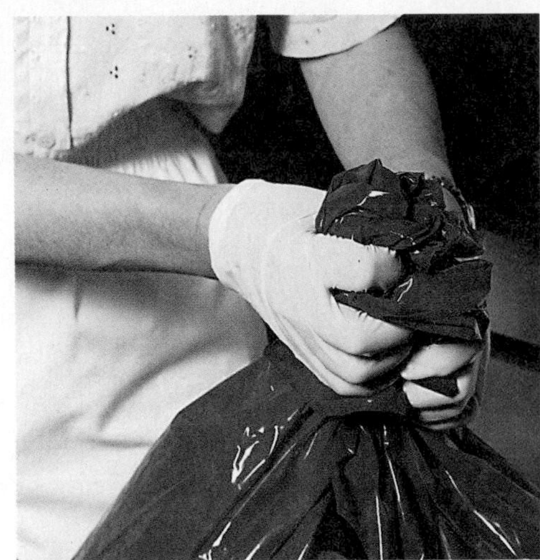

▲ Close bag securely and label contents, if necessary.

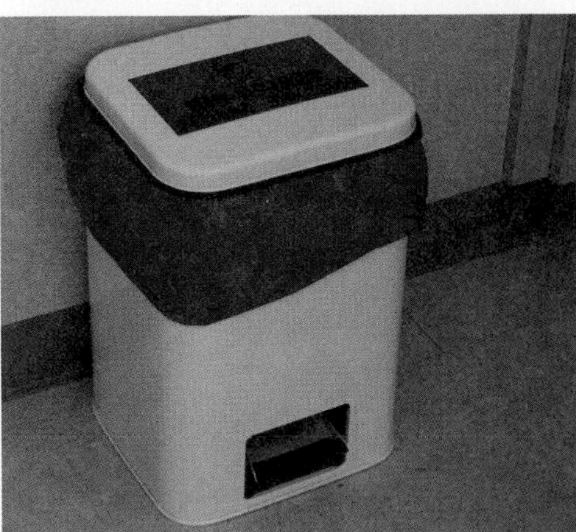

▲ Set up new biohazard bag for continued use in client's room.

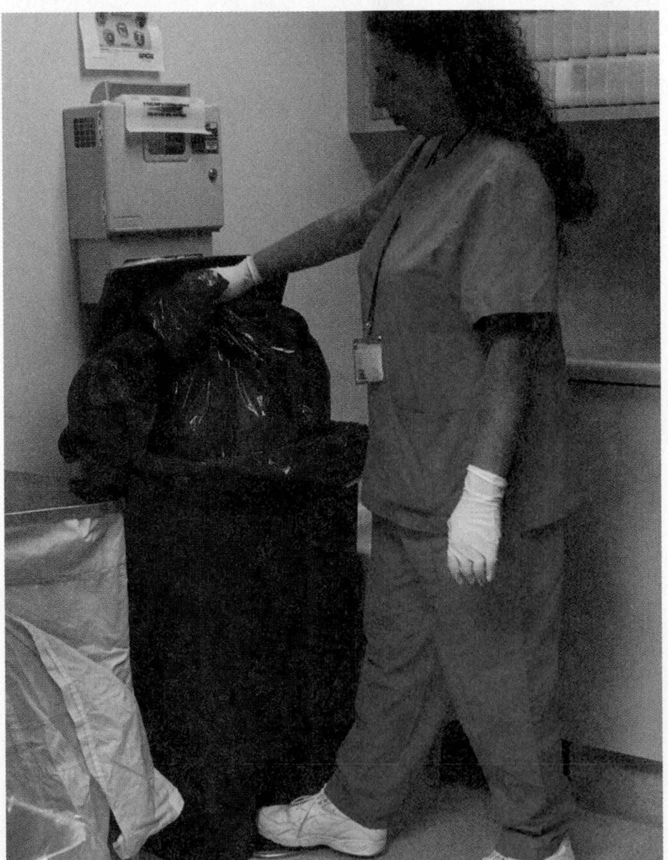

▲ Place red biohazard bag in specified area for disposal.

4. Place reusable equipment such as procedure trays in plastic bags. ▶ ***Rationale:*** Appropriate separation of equipment from isolation room alerts central supply staff that it is contaminated and special handling needs to be carried out.
5. Dispose of all garbage in plastic bags.
6. Place all material to be removed from isolation room in anteroom (if available). ▶ ***Rationale:*** All material removed from an isolation room is potentially contaminated. This will prevent spread of microorganisms.

Clinical Alert

Linen and burnable trash are disposed of in the same manner. Ensure that when placing bags in containers in "dirty" utility room you place in correct container according to bag contents.

7. Replace all bags, such as linen bag and garbage bag, in appropriate container in room.
8. Clean client's room as necessary, using germicidal solution, according to facility protocol.
9. Prepare to leave the client's room.

Removing a Specimen From Isolation Room

Equipment

Specimen container
Clean biohazard bag

Procedure

1. Follow dress protocol for entering isolation room, or, if you are already in the isolation room, continue with Step 2.
2. Mark a specimen container with the client's name, type of specimen, and the word "isolation" before entering an isolation room.
3. Collect specimen, and place container in a clean plastic biohazard bag outside the room. ▶ ***Rationale:*** Use clear bags so that laboratory personnel can see the specimen easily.
4. Complete hand hygiene.
5. Send specimen to laboratory with appropriate laboratory request form.

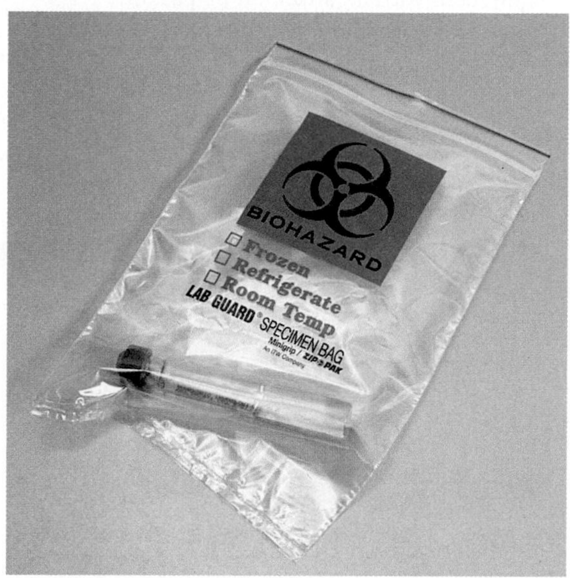

▲ Biohazard bag for transportation of specimens from isolation room.

Transporting Isolation Client Outside the Room

Equipment

Transport vehicle
Bath blanket
Mask for client if needed

Procedure

1. Explain procedure to client.
2. If client is being transported from a respiratory isolation room, instruct him or her to wear a mask for the entire time out of isolation. ▶ ***Rationale:*** This prevents the spread of airborne microbes.
3. Cover the transport vehicle with a bath blanket if there is a chance of soiling when transporting a client who has a draining wound or diarrhea.
4. Help client into transport vehicle. Cover client with a bath blanket.

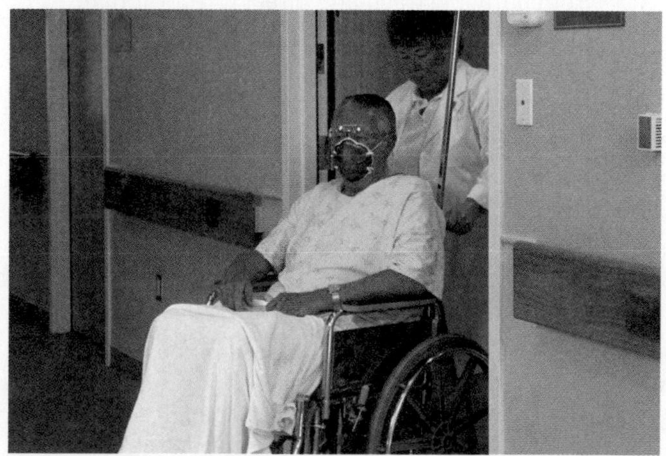

▲ Place surgical mask on client if he needs to be transported outside room.

5. Tell receiving department what type of isolation client needs and what precautions hospital personnel should follow.
6. Remove bath blanket and handle as contaminated linen when client returns to room.
7. Instruct all hospital personnel to complete hand hygiene before they leave the area.
8. Wipe down transportation vehicle with an antimicrobial solution if soiled.

Removing Soiled Large Equipment From Isolation Room

Equipment

Antimicrobial agent and articles needed to wash equipment
Plastic bag

Procedure

1. Don isolation garb as recommended.
2. Wash equipment with an antimicrobial agent. ▸
   Rationale: Washing is preferred to spraying in order to ensure all surfaces are cleaned.
3. Cover equipment with a plastic bag.
4. Remove garb, and complete hand hygiene outside the room. Take equipment to the decontamination area of central supply room (CSR).

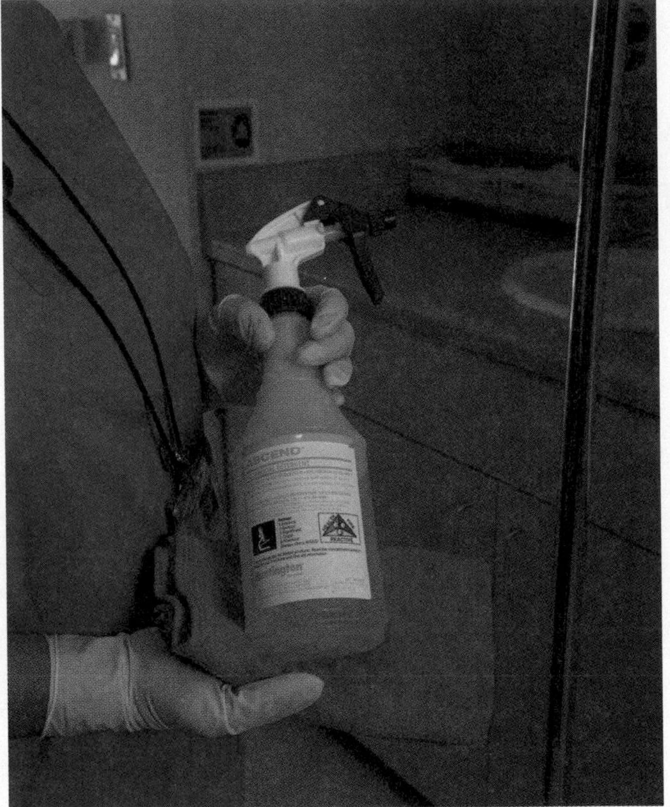

▲ Wash isolation equipment with antimicrobial agent.

Protocol for Leaving Isolation Room

1. Untie gown at waist.
2. Take off gloves.
3. Untie gown at neck.
4. Pull gown off and place in laundry hamper.
5. Take off goggles or face shield.
6. Take off mask.
7. Complete hand hygiene.

Guidelines for Disposing of Contaminated Equipment

- **Disposable glass:** Place in isolation bag separate from burnable trash and direct to appropriate hospital area for disposal.
- **Glass equipment:** Bag separately from metal equipment and return to CSR.
- **Metal equipment:** Bag all equipment together, label, and return to CSR.
- **Rubber and plastic items:** Bag items separately and return to CSR for gas sterilization.
- **Dishes:** Require no special precautions unless contaminated with infected material; then bag, label, and return to kitchen.
- **Plastic or paper dishes:** Dispose of these items in burnable trash.
- **Soiled linens:** Place in laundry bag and send to separate area of laundry room for special care. If possible, place linens in hot-water–soluble bag. This method is safer for handling, as bag may be placed directly into washing machine. (Double-bagging is usually required because these bags are easily punctured or torn. They also dissolve when wet.)
- **Food and liquids:** Dispose of these items by putting them in the toilet—flush thoroughly.
- **Needles and syringes:** Do not recap needles; place in puncture-resistant container.
- **Sphygmomanometer and stethoscope:** Require no special precautions unless they are contaminated. If contaminated, disinfect using the appropriate cleaning protocol based on the infective agent.
- **Thermometers:** Dispose of electronic probe cover with burnable trash. If probe or machine is contaminated, clean with appropriate disinfectant for infective agent. If reusable thermometers are used, disinfect with appropriate solution.

DOCUMENTATION for Isolation

- Type of isolation protocol being practiced
- Specimens sent to laboratory
- Client's reactions to sensory deprivation
- Vital signs if appropriate

Legal Considerations

Every year while in hospitals, 90,000 Americans acquire infections that kill them. In addition, hospital-acquired infections cost an estimated $20 billion each year, according to the CDC.

Source: AARP, March 2009

It may be that while there is no case law relating specifically to noncompliance with infection control practices, current case law could be used to establish whether or not a healthcare professional who had failed to implement acceptable standard infection control practices had acted negligently, and as a result, caused a patient to develop a healthcare-associated infection.

Source: Portsmith, R. (2007). Infection control and the law. *British Journal of Infection Prevention*, 8(2), 14–19.

CRITICAL THINKING Application

Expected Outcomes

- Prevented client-to-client spread of endogenous and exogenous flora.
- Protected hospital personnel from becoming infected.
- Prevented immunosuppressed clients from acquiring healthcare-associated infections.
- Reduced transferrence of organisms from hospital environment to clients.

Unexpected Outcomes

Outbreak of disease occurs in isolation environment.

Alternative Actions

- Identify cause of outbreak, and contact the infection control practitioner for consultation.
- Examine handwashing and infection control practices among staff.
- Attend in-service education program on isolation techniques to increase your awareness of appropriate procedures.

Chapter 14

UNIT 4

Home Care Adaptation

Nursing Process Data

ASSESSMENT Data Base

- Assess need for hand hygiene.
- Identify clients at risk for infection.
- Assess need for cleaning equipment and decontaminating equipment.
- Identify type of waste material requiring special disposal.
- Assess equipment needed to deliver care in the home.
- Assess need for teaching preventive measures in the home of HIV or AIDS clients.

PLANNING Objectives

- To deliver client care with pathogen-free hands
- To clean equipment properly to prevent cross-contamination
- To protect client from cross-contamination
- To protect the nurse
- To properly dispose of contaminated waste material
- To protect client's significant others from contamination of infected material

IMPLEMENTATION Procedures

EVALUATION Expected Outcomes

- Cross-contamination is prevented.
- Nurse is protected from infection.
- Equipment is cleaned appropriately.
- Waste is disposed of in proper manner.

Preparing for Client Care

Equipment

Community health nursing bag
Liquid soap
Antibacterial gel for hand hygiene
Disposable gloves
Disposable apron or gown
Goggles
Masks, air-purifying mask
Thermometers (oral and rectal)
Thermometer sheaths
Nex Temp (disposable thermometer)
Vaseline or lubricant
Cotton balls
Alcohol, one small bottle
Antimicrobial wipes
Cotton-tipped applicators
Tongue depressors
Sterile 4 × 4s
Band-Aids
Bandage scissors
Nonallergic tape
Plastic bags with ties
Keto-Diastix and Chemstrips
Sphygmomanometer
Stethoscope
Paper cups
Bleach, one small bottle

Procedure

1. Arrange equipment in bag before making home visit so that hand hygiene equipment is accessible. Bring only the supplies needed. ▸ ***Rationale:*** This procedure decreases the possibility of cross-contamination.
2. Place bag on flat, dry surface to establish a clean work area during visit. Use of disposable barrier under bag is recommended. ▸ ***Rationale:*** To prevent potential spread of infection between clients' homes. The risk can be high for transmitting undiagnosed infections between home clients.
3. Perform hand hygiene.
   a. Use liquid soap and paper towels from bag and client's water supply. Wash hands with clean running water and apply soap. Rub hands together to make a lather and scrub all surfaces. Rub hands for 10 to 15 seconds. Rinse hands well under running water. Dry hands using paper towel from nurse's bag. Turn off faucet using paper towel.
   b. Use antimicrobial gel as alternative for handwashing when soap and water are not available. Squeeze small amount of germicide onto palm of hand and rub all surfaces of hands, fingers, and nails. Rub until hands and fingers are dry. Germicide evaporates into air, making towels unnecessary.
4. Don disposable gloves when appropriate for infection control, especially when handling blood and body fluids.
5. Take other equipment that will be needed during the visit out of the bag and place on clean work surface.
6. Keep bag closed when not in use to promote cleanliness, safety, and security. Care should be taken not to reenter bag wearing soiled gloves. Washing hands between reentering bag is not necessary unless soiled.
7. Wear disposable apron or gown, goggles, or masks if necessary. ▸ ***Rationale:*** This protects the caregiver from blood or body fluid exposure.
8. Cleanse thoroughly any equipment that left clean area and is to be returned to the bag on completing care.
   a. Rinse equipment (such as bandage scissors, forceps) under *cold* water, wash with soap and water. Use client's personal equipment or disposable equipment whenever possible.
   b. Return stethoscope and blood pressure cuff to nursing bag. ▸ ***Rationale:*** Clean items can be returned to nursing bag if no visible soiling.
9. Ensure nursing bag is monitored regularly for safety.
   a. Keep bag out of reach of children.
   b. Keep bag in trunk of car or keep in your home overnight. ▸ ***Rationale:*** Unattended bags in cars are more often stolen.
   c. Clean bag monthly and PRN.

Clinical Alert

If item is soiled and cannot be returned to the bag, place in separate container for transport to agency. Clean item when it is returned to agency. Most items for home care are disposable.

Assessing Client for Potential Infection

Equipment

Disposable gloves
Disposable impenetrable plastic bag
Disposable gown (if drainage present)
Mask, cap, goggles (if potential respiratory infection)
Blood pressure cuff
Stethoscope
Thermometer
Urine container and dipstick
Blood specimen tubes and Vacutainer with needle
Alcohol swabs
Soap and water and/or germicidal gel

Procedure

1. Wash hands or complete hand hygiene.
2. Don disposable gloves when appropriate for infection control.
3. Take equipment out of bag and place on clean work surface.
4. Don disposable equipment as necessary for infection control.
5. Obtain vital signs; check for elevated temperature and pulse rate.
6. Complete physical assessment; carefully evaluate heart and lung sounds.
7. Observe urine output; color, odor, amount. If catheter in place; observe for purulent drainage around catheter site and consistency of urine in drainage bag. Check for tenderness at insertion site, pain, and swelling. Obtain sample and complete dipstick test if urinary tract infection is suspected.
8. Observe color and consistency of sputum.
9. Observe IV catheter insertion site for erythema tenderness, pain at site, and patency of IV.
10. Observe for inflammation, erythema, warmth of affected soft tissue sites.
11. Evaluate pain; location and severity. Use pain scale.
12. Clean equipment such as stethoscope and blood pressure cuff. Place back into bag.
13. Dispose of any supplies used by placing in appropriate disposal bag (impenetrable plastic) if infection is suspected.
14. Complete hand hygiene and dispose of gloves in plastic bag.
15. Document findings; if symptoms are indicative of potential infection, call physician.

Disposing of Waste Material in the Home Setting

Equipment

Plastic bags, heavy duty
Disposable gloves
Receptacle, rigid and puncture-proof
Bleach
Germicide

Procedure

1. Dispose of wastes contaminated with blood or body fluids.
   a. Place waste products in impenetrable, heavy-duty plastic bag.
   b. Remove plastic gloves by rolling inside out (so contaminated side is on inside) and drop into plastic bag.
   c. Seal plastic bag with tie.
   d. Discard in client's trash.
   e. Perform hand hygiene with soap and water or germicide.
2. Dispose of body wastes, such as urine, feces, respiratory secretions, vomitus, and blood, by flushing them down the toilet. (This is true whether the toilet empties into a septic tank or a sewage system.)
3. Dispose of needles and sharp objects.
   a. Do *not* remove needle from syringe or bend, break, clip, or recap after use.
   b. Drop entire disposable safety syringe intact into rigid, puncture-proof receptacle provided by agency.
   c. Complete hand hygiene.
4. Discard other trash.
   a. Place in plastic bag.
   b. Discard in client's trash.

NOTE: Clothes and bedding do not need to be destroyed. They are laundered separately in hot water with a 10% bleach solution added to the detergent in the washer.

Clinical Alert

All items contaminated with blood, exudates, or other body fluids should be considered to present a risk of transmission of HIV or hepatitis B. These items should be disposed of by incineration if possible. Use mechanisms for disposal of waste into normal trash only when incineration is not available.

Clinical Alert

Do not use glass bottles or plastic bottles that can be returned to store.

Bleach bottle with screw lid can be left in home for use as a sharp container. Tape closed before disposing of bottle. Small biohazard containers can be obtained from drug stores.

Caring for an AIDS or HIV Client in the Home Setting

Equipment

Gloves
Disposable mask, gown, or apron
Protective eyewear
Specimen container if needed
Plastic bag for transport of specimen
Chlorine bleach solution (Clorox)

Procedure

1. Perform hand hygiene before and after client care and after disposing of soiled materials.
2. Don disposable gloves for any procedure.
   a. Don double gloves if tearing is likely during the procedure.
   b. If staff member has any type of open wound or weeping dermatitis, she or he should not administer care (even with gloves) until condition is resolved.
3. Don disposable gown or apron to protect clothing from soilage.
4. Put on mask and protective eyewear if splattering is anticipated during the procedure (e.g., suctioning, wound irrigations).
5. Collect specimens in appropriate containers. Place in plastic sealable biohazard bags.
6. Use extraordinary care to avoid puncture wounds with needles and other sharp objects.
   a. If puncture occurs, bleed wound and wash with soap and water.
   b. Notify supervisor immediately and fill out unusual occurrence report.
7. Transport all specimens in an impermeable container, keeping the container separate from nurse's bag and supplies.
8. Clean spills of blood and body fluids with 10% bleach solution (one part liquid chlorine bleach to nine parts water). Make solution fresh each visit.
9. Wash eating utensils (dishes and silverware) in hot soapy water. Water should be hot enough to need gloves to tolerate the temperature. No other special precautions are required. It is best to use a dishwasher, if available. It is not necessary to wash client's dishes separately.
10. Store linens and laundry soiled with body fluids in a plastic bag and then wash separately with very hot water. Use a detergent and a 10% bleach solution. (Nonchlorine bleaches such as Clorox II are acceptable for colored clothing.)
11. Dispose of gown or apron in plastic bag after completing care.
12. Take off gloves by peeling them down and turning them inside out so that contaminated side is on the inside. Place in plastic bag.
13. Perform hand hygiene.
14. Take off mask and goggles.
15. Perform hand hygiene.

Cleansing Equipment in the Home Setting

Equipment

Article to be cleansed
Soap
Running water
Paper towels
Plastic bags
Disposable gloves

Procedure

1. Don gloves when working with equipment contaminated with any body fluid or blood.
2. First rinse article with cold running water. ▸ ***Rationale:*** Cold water releases organic material from the equipment and warm water may make it adhere to the surface.
3. Second wash with hot, soapy water using friction.
4. Rinse well with clear water.
5. Dry thoroughly.
6. Disinfect equipment or article as indicated: one part chlorine bleach (Clorox) to nine parts water.
7. Dry thoroughly.
8. Remove disposable gloves.
9. Dispose of gloves (inside out) into plastic bag.
10. Perform hand hygiene.

Clinical Alert

If durable medical equipment cannot be sterilized by ethyl oxide or autoclaved, it should be cleaned with 10% chlorine bleach solution after washing with hot soapy water.

Urinary drainage bags can be disinfected in the home. Use soap and water and clean and dry well. Antiseptic solution can be placed in the bag for a few minutes, then bag is rinsed well and dried before attaching to urinary catheter.

Teaching Preventive Measures in the Home Setting

Procedure

1. Discuss the inadvisability of allowing any person who is ill or who has depressed immune function to come in contact with the client.
2. Teach the client these appropriate hygiene principles:
   a. Wash hands after use of toilet or contact with any body fluids.
   b. Do not share thermometers, razors, razor blades, toothbrushes, douche, or enema equipment.
   c. Do not cough without covering mouth.
   d. Be careful to dispose of nasal secretions in tissue, then in plastic bags.
3. Teach these guidelines for sharing kitchens and bathrooms:
   a. Good household cleaning practices prevent spread of infection.
   b. Don't share eating and drinking utensils. After use, they must be cleaned with hot water (hot enough to necessitate use of gloves) and soap. Use of a dishwasher and soap is appropriate.
   c. Kitchen and bathroom surfaces should be cleaned every day with scouring powder or with chlorine bleach solution (10%, one part bleach to nine parts water). Use disposable bathroom cups. Use covered individual toothbrush holders.
   d. Clean refrigerators regularly with soap and water; remove old food to prevent mold.
   e. Mop floors in bathroom and kitchen weekly. Pour dirty water down the toilet and disinfect with bleach solution.
   f. Clean toilet, tub, and shower weekly or as often as necessary with 10% bleach solution. If urine or diarrhea spills on toilet or floor, wipe immediately with the 10% bleach solution.
   g. Sponges used to clean floors or body fluid spills should be soaked for 5 minutes in a 10% bleach solution.
4. Teach the following principles of food preparation:
   a. Discuss the fact that people infected with HIV may prepare food for others. They should follow usual practices for safe food preparation and be especially diligent about handwashing.
   b. Wash hands thoroughly before any food preparation.
   c. Do not lick fingers or taste from the mixing spoon while cooking.
   d. Avoid unpasteurized milk (danger of contact with *Salmonella*); do not eat old or moldy food (danger of food poisoning); and carefully wash and thoroughly cook chicken.
   e. Wash all fresh (raw) fruits and vegetables before eating.
5. Teach how to care for linens and laundry.
   a. When clothing or linen is soiled with blood or body fluids, it should be stored separately in a plastic bag. Wash separately with very hot water, detergent, and bleach. Use Clorox II for colored clothing.
   b. Wear disposable gloves when touching soiled clothes or linen.
   c. Do not share used towels or washcloths, and wash separately. (Towels and washcloths are, however, safe to use after washing.)
   d. Change towels and washcloths daily.
6. Inform client and family of measures for disposing of trash.
   a. Flush body wastes down the toilet.
   b. Discard dressings, diapers, Chux, or any materials soiled with secretions in a plastic bag. Discard into the regular trash.
   c. Sharp items (e.g., razors, needles) should be placed in a rigid, puncture-proof container with a solution of 10% bleach. Incinerate when container is full. Pharmacies collect the used containers in some areas.
7. Discuss procedures for caring for pets.
   a. Clean bird cages wearing gloves. Birds can spread psittacosis (*Chlamydia psittaci*) or *Cryptococcus*.
   b. Clean cat litter boxes wearing gloves to prevent spread of toxoplasmosis.
   c. Tropical fish tanks should not be cleaned by the person with AIDS to prevent spread of *Mycobacterium*.
8. Teach general principles of preventing cross-infection.
   a. Wear gloves when handling body fluids, linens, or other objects contaminated with body fluids.
   b. Disposable gowns or aprons protect clothing from becoming soiled.
   c. Caregivers should not provide care when ill themselves. If this is not possible they should wear a mask when in close contact with the person with AIDS. AIDS clients are very susceptible to infections.
   d. Maintain adequate ventilation in the living quarters.
9. Discuss steps to prevent spread of contagious disease; cold, flu, strep throat.
   a. Clean hands thoroughly before eating or touching food, after using the bathroom, taking out trash, playing with a pet, or being in contact with someone who is ill.
   b. Use tissues when sneezing or coughing, cover mouth and nose, and discard tissue immediately. If tissue is not available, cover mouth and nose with bend in your elbow or your hands. Clean hands immediately.
   c. Avoid contact with others if you are ill.
   d. Maintain up-to-date vaccinations.
10. Medical supplies should be kept in a clean, dry location. If refrigeration is required, place medication in sealed plastic storage bag.

Teaching Safer Practices to IV Drug Users

Procedure

1. Inform persons of risk behaviors and factors associated with IV drug use.
   a. Direct transmission occurs with shared needles and syringes; permits blood-to-blood contact, the most direct method of transmitting the AIDS virus and hepatitis B.
   b. Transmission to sexual partners; permits contact of body fluids.
   c. Transmission to fetus during pregnancy.
   d. Suppression of the immune system caused by alcohol or drug use.
   e. Impaired judgment while under the influence of drugs.
2. Teach IV drug users how to reduce the risk.
   a. Do not share needles or syringes with others.
   b. Clean needles and other equipment vigorously. Wash twice with full-strength bleach or alcohol; rinse twice with water.
   c. Boil needles and other equipment for 15 minutes.
   d. Do not borrow or use needles or equipment from others, even if they appear healthy or say that they do not have AIDS.
3. Teach basic health maintenance measures.
   a. Decrease use of all immunosuppressive drugs (marijuana, speed, cocaine, alcohol).
   b. Maintain an adequate, nutritionally sound diet.
   c. Reduce stress on self through stress-reduction practices or removing self from a stressful situation (living with others who routinely use drugs).
   d. Obtain regular medical and dental care.
   e. Follow lifestyle that provides adequate rest and exercise.
   f. Obtain counseling to assist in living life without dependence on drugs.

DOCUMENTATION for Home Care Adaptations

- Document findings on appropriate home care forms
- Therapies provided and client response
- Follow treatment plan and document goal achievement
- Client status, physical findings, ability to care for self
- Clinically significant observations stated objectively related to potential infection
- Clinically significant observations related to environmental findings related to potential infections

CRITICAL THINKING Application

Expected Outcomes

- Clients do not acquire infections during home care visits.
- Early detection of potential infections is identified through appropriate assessment techniques.
- Infections are treated appropriately and not transmitted to other home care clients or the nurse because effective preventative measures are utilized.

Unexpected Outcomes	Critical Thinking Options
There are potential infection sources in the home environment.	• Explain the necessity of keeping the environment free of potential organisms, by keeping it clean and uncluttered.
	• Instruct the client and family members on proper hand hygiene technique.
	• Explain and develop a plan for family members to discard soiled dressings, diapers, etc., to prevent potentially infecting other household members.

GERONTOLOGIC Considerations

- Social isolation resulting from infection control requirements is more intense with the elderly. They need frequent contact with healthcare workers. Sometimes being ill is the only attention they receive.
- Elderly clients can become confused in the hospital, and when placed in isolation, there is an even greater risk. Frequent monitoring for safety issues is necessary.
- Frequent explanations of why isolation is necessary are important for the elderly. They may have a lapse of memory and forget earlier discussion about isolation.
- Ensure that call lights are easily accessible and the client understands how to call for assistance. They may have impaired hearing and sight, which can interfere with communications.

MANAGEMENT Guidelines

Each state legislates a Nurse Practice Act for RNs and LVN/LPNs. Healthcare facilities are responsible for establishing and implementing policies and procedures that conform to their state's regulations. Verify the regulations and role parameters for each healthcare worker in your facility.

Delegation

- LVN/LPNs and CNAs may be assigned to clients requiring infection control precautions and barriers. Ensure that all healthcare workers have been properly educated in infection control procedures before assigning them to clients requiring these measures.
- It is the RN's responsibility to make assignments that take into account the type of isolation precautions and potential cross-contamination of other clients in the care of the healthcare worker. For example, the same healthcare worker should not take care of a client in contact isolation and an immunosuppressed client.

Communication Matrix

- Ensure that appropriate designations are posted on the door of the room indicating the type of isolation precautions necessary for the client.
- Indicate the type of isolation precautions on the client's chart.
- During shift report and team report, review the type of isolation precautions being maintained for the client.
- Inform and instruct all visitors on the isolation precautions.
- Monitor that all hospital staff practice good hand hygiene technique. Review appropriate technique with those who do not practice these techniques.
- Review isolation precautions, particularly standard precautions, with all new personnel and on a regular basis with all personnel to ensure compliance with hospital policy.
- Monitor healthcare workers for appropriate use of gloves, masks, and gowns when caring for clients in isolation. Instruct healthcare workers in proper use of these items when providing client care.

CRITICAL THINKING Strategies

Scenario 1

You are assigned to care for two clients. One client has just returned from surgery for an abdominal resection. The second client is hospitalized with an acute case of tuberculosis.

1. Is this assignment appropriate, considering the two diagnoses? Provide a rationale for the answer.
2. What special precautions will you take when providing care for these two clients?
3. CDC guidelines are specific for clients with tuberculosis. Identify the differences in providing care for this client versus other clients requiring barrier nursing.
4. Describe the procedure for leaving the tuberculosis client's room. Provide a rationale for the prioritized steps.

Scenario 2

You are assigned to take two clients' vital signs, complete a focus assessment, provide hygienic care, monitor IVs, and complete a dressing change for a client with an abdominal resection.

1. What task will have priority with this assignment?
2. Develop a time management plan and provide a rationale for the time frames and activities.

NCLEX® Review Questions

Unless otherwise specified, choose only one (1) answer.

1. When assessing the following client care situations, which one would require the nurse to wear goggles?
   1. Changing a dressing.
   2. Administering an IM injection.
   3. Catheterizing the urinary bladder.
   4. Emptying a Foley drainage collection bag.
2. A client is hospitalized with complications of AIDS. The best way to clean up a hazardous waste spill is to use
   1. Waterless antiseptic.
   2. 1:10 bleach solution.
   3. Soap and water.
   4. Alcohol solution.
3. Isolation is used for hospitalized children who
   1. Have chicken pox (varicella).
   2. Are immunocompromised.
   3. Are coughing or vomiting.
   4. Have tuberculosis.
4. When working with infants, the most important action for breaking the chain of infection is
   1. Using sterile technique.
   2. Isolation of ill people near the infant.
   3. Treatment with antibiotics.
   4. Proper hand hygiene.
5. When caring for a person with AIDS in the home, the best way to dispose of contaminated needles and syringes is to
   1. Break the needle from the syringe and dispose.
   2. Place them in a puncture-resistant container in the home.
   3. Recap them and bring them to an appropriate disposal area.
   4. Soak them in bleach and then dispose of them in the trash.
6. A nurse is giving an emaciated client an injection. While withdrawing the needle from the site, the needle slips and pierces the nurse's finger. The action most appropriate is to
   1. Recap the needle and save it for laboratory analysis.
   2. Break the needle and discard it in a puncture-proof container.
   3. Obtain an order for the client to receive gamma globulin.
   4. Wash the finger with an antiseptic and water solution.
7. The nurse observes a nursing assistant putting on gloves to deliver a lunch tray to a client with AIDS. The therapeutic intervention would be to
   1. Commend the nursing assistant for the action.
   2. Explain to the nursing assistant that gloves do not need to be worn if there is no client contact.
   3. Ask the nursing assistant to wear a gown, also.
   4. Make sure the nursing assistant does not touch the client.
8. The most frequent mode of transmission of HAI (nosocomial) infections such as vancomycin-resistant enterococcus (VRE) in healthcare facilities is
   1. Soiled linens.
   2. Hands of healthcare workers.
   3. Medical equipment.
   4. Food trays.
9. When leaving an isolation room, prioritize the steps to maintain proper protocol.
   1. Hand hygiene.
   2. Taking off your mask.
   3. Removing your gloves.
   4. Untying waist strings of the gown.
10. To prevent the spread of infection between clients, the home care nurse should:
    1. Use only disposable supplies and equipment in the home and dispose of them in the home before leaving.
    2. Take out necessary supplies from the bag and bring them into the house, leaving the bag in the car.
    3. Take needed supplies from the bag and place on clean work area, then close bag immediately.
    4. Wear clean gloves throughout the visit, and place them in the garbage as you leave the house.

15

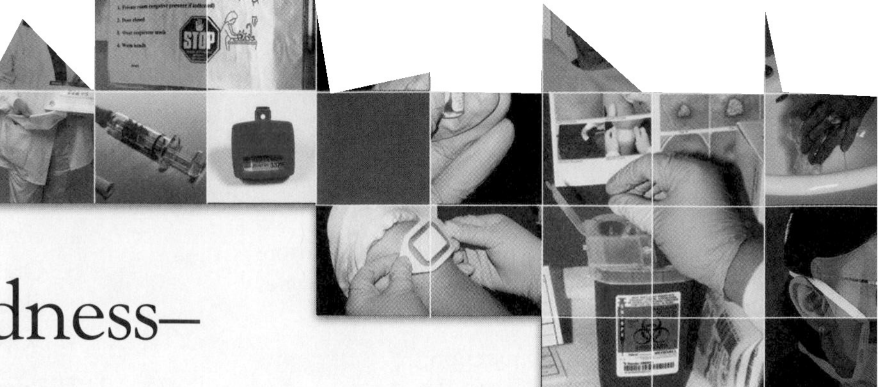

Disaster Preparedness–Bioterrorism

LEARNING OBJECTIVES

1. Discuss the concept of preparedness for a terrorism attack.
2. List the effects on infrastructure that may result from a mass casualty incident.
3. Compare and contrast external and internal communication systems.
4. State the chain of command and reporting requirements when a mass casualty incident occurs.
5. Differentiate between a chemical and a biological attack.
6. Discuss diversity considerations when healthcare workers are responding to a terrorist event.
7. List at least two ethical issues you might encounter during a mass casualty event.
8. List components of a home safety plan.
9. Discuss earthquake safety principles.
10. Identify two diarrhea-related diseases.
11. List signs and symptoms of various biological agents and describe how to distinguish between them.
12. Discuss the clinical features of smallpox.
13. Identify the high-risk groups for smallpox vaccination.
14. Demonstrate the procedure for smallpox vaccination (include reconstituting *vaccinia* vaccine).
15. Describe the steps of collecting and transporting a potentially contaminated clinical specimen.
16. Describe the major agents of a chemical attack.
17. List the primary interventions necessary to care for the psychological needs of disaster victims.
18. Describe how to measure external radiation levels.
19. Review the equipment included in Standard Precautions.
20. List the steps of decontamination via triage.
21. Explain the protective equipment necessary for biological exposure (individualize for anthrax, plague, botulism, and smallpox).
22. Differentiate decontaminating victims after a biological and chemical attack.
23. Demonstrate decontamination procedures for victims of a radiological attack.
24. Discuss establishing public health parameters for triage.
25. Explain the term triage and list the steps of triage.
26. Demonstrate the steps of treating life-threatening conditions.
27. Discuss post-traumatic stress disorder.

CHAPTER OUTLINE

TERMINOLOGY

Aerosol very fine liquid or solid particles suspended in air—small particles in a gaseous medium.

Airborne microorganisms spread by droplets dispersed in the air; a deliberate release of pathogens; could be carried out by using an aerosol delivery system.

Antimicrobial an agent that prevents the development or pathogenic action of microbes.

Antidote a substance that neutralizes a poison or the effects of a poison.

Bioterrorism the planned, deliberate use of a chemical or biological agent (bacteria, virus, fungi, or toxin) with the intent to harm or kill people. Bioterrorism is a general term used to encompass all forms of terrorism.

Centers for Disease Control and Prevention (CDC) a U.S. government agency with the stated purpose of preventing the transmission of communicable diseases. This agency is responsible for identifying and disseminating standards and guidelines for isolation precautions.

Chemical terrorism use of a chemical agent (nerve, blood, blister, volatile) with intent to harm or kill people.

Communicable disease a disease that can be transmitted person-to-person.

Community disaster plan a document that specifies who is in charge, lines of communication, and agencies and resources that will be involved.

Contamination introduction of disease, germs, or infectious materials into or onto normally sterile objects.

Decontamination process of removing contamination from people, equipment, or environment—usually done through a physical (i.e., shower) or chemical process.

Disaster an event of such magnitude that essential services are disrupted and current resources are overwhelmed.

Emergency any event or situation that occurs as an unexpected and sudden incident, demanding immediate action.

EMTALA Emergency Medical Treatment and Labor Act—a federal law to stop hospital EDs from refusing to treat poor or uninsured clients or from transferring clients to other facilities before their medical conditions have stabilized.

Equivalent dose a measure of the effect that radiation has on humans—takes into account the type and absorbed dose of radiation.

Exposure inhalation or contamination by a substance that contains a biological, chemical, or radioactive agent.

Federal Bureau of Investigative (FBI) investigative agency of United States Department of Justice; it has authority and responsibility to investigate specific crimes, such as a bioterrorism event.

Federal Emergency Management Agency (FEMA) primary or lead federal agency that responds to a disaster, such as a terrorism incident.

First responder first trained personnel to arrive at an emergency.

Gray a measurement of the absorbed dose of radiation; used more often than RAD—(1 Gy = 100 RADS).

Hazardous material any substance that is potentially toxic to a biological system.

HAZMAT model hazardous materials; this model is used for situations involving certain toxic or chemical exposures.

Homeland Security the Department of Homeland Security (DHS) coordinates all activities related to a terrorist attack.

Immunization process of rendering a person immune, usually done through vaccination.

Incident Command System (ICS) local and national command structure that organizes emergency responses.

Incubation period time between infection from a microorganism and onset of symptoms.

Infection establishment of a disease process that involves invasion of body tissue by microorganisms, reaction of tissues to their presence, and to toxins generated by them.

Inhalation exposure to a substance through the respiratory tract.

Isolation practices or actions designed to prevent transmission of communicable diseases.

Ionizing radiation radiation that has the energy to cause atoms to lose electrons and become ions—alpha, beta, gamma, and x-rays are examples.

Isotopes elements that have neutrons (they have neither a positive nor negative charge). Not all isotopes are radioactive; those that are, are called radionuclides. Cobalt-69 is an example of a radioactive isotope.

Mass casualty incident (MCI) an incident or emergency event associated with many casualties (airplane crash, terrorism, chemical spill) that has a negative impact on emergency resources.

Microorganism a minute living body, such as a bacterium, protozoan, or virus, not perceptible to the naked eye.

NBC military acronym for nuclear, biological, and chemical weapons.

Nerve agent chemical agent that acts on the body by disrupting normal function of the nervous system.

Occupational Safety and Health Administration (OSHA) section of the Department of Labor that develops and implements regulations requiring employers to have safety policies and to provide training and personal protective equipment to employees who may be exposed to toxic substances.

Outbreak critical incident in which infections occur above an established level and are caused by the same infective agent.

Pandemic denotes a disease that affects the population of a large region, country, or continent.

Pathogen microorganism that can cause disease; may be bacteria, fungi, parasites, or viruses.

Percutaneous agent substance that can be absorbed through the skin.

Personal protective equipment (PPE) equipment for protection of emergency personnel; includes gloves, masks, gowns, eye shields, biohazard bags, and in some cases, head and shoe covers.

Poison any substance that enters the body by absorption, ingestion, inhalation, or infection and interferes with normal physiological functions.

RAD radiation absorbed dose—the unit of measure for radiation exposure.

Radiation energy in the form of waves or particles that is emitted from radioactive material or equipment.

Radioactive contamination radioactive material distributed over some area, equipment, or person; must be decontaminated.

Radiation dose quantity of radiation energy deposited in a material by the radiation to which victim is exposed.

REM roentgen equivalent man—the unit of dose or measure—takes into account type of radiation producing the exposure.

Sodium hypochlorite 0.5% diluted bleach is the active ingredient used for decontamination.

START acronym that stands for "simple treatment and rapid triage," an initial triage system used for triaging large numbers of victims.

Standard (Universal) Precautions a system of disease control; assumes that direct contact with body fluids is infectious and recommends a series of procedures to protect the staff.

Terrorism the use of force or violence against people or property in violation of the criminal laws of the United States for purposes of intimidation, coercion, or ransom (FBI).

Threat assessment an assessment of a community's vulnerability and risk potential.

Toxin poisonous substance produced by a living organism.

Trauma multisystem condition or injury that is potentially life-threatening to the individual.

Vaccine preparation of a killed or weakened microorganism used to induce immunity against disease.

Vesicles blisters on the skin.

Virulence the power of a microorganism to cause disease in a given host.

Virus an infectious microorganism that normally lives within other living cells and cannot reproduce outside the cell.

Weapons of mass destruction (WMD) nuclear, biological, chemical, incendiary, or conventional explosive agents that pose a threat to health, safety, food supply, property, or the environment.

INTRODUCTION

America's world changed on September 11, 2001. From this time, our greatest challenge became to adopt the awareness that we are no longer invulnerable; that biological, chemical, and nuclear terrorism is a future reality; and that we must change our perspective of how to function in the world. Senator Bill Frist stated it clearly: "The United States faces a grave and growing threat from bioterrorism."

Years ago, this chapter would never have been written. Today, a page in history has been turned, and the medical community—indeed, the world—must face terrorism and the probability of disasters caused by terrorism. We cannot predict—we can prepare. In order to steer a course toward a viable future, we must be prepared to cope with such a disaster.

Preparedness for a terrorist-caused disaster is critical for containment and protection of the population. There must be coordinated emergency preparedness plans in place in order that a prompt and effective response to a biological, chemical, or radiation attack is initiated.

Meeting this new challenge will require preparedness in all communities, cities, and states in the United States of America. Nurses are an important part of this response.

NATURAL DISASTERS

Although disasters may be natural or man-made, there are numerous definitions of a disaster. For our purposes, natural disasters will be examined regarding how they affect health and health services. From this standpoint, the type and timing of a disaster event will create the types of injuries and illnesses that occur. Disasters that have a prior warning, such as hurricanes or floods, generally have fewer injuries and deaths than those that occur with little or no warning, such as tsunamis or earthquakes. These disasters tend to have more casualties because the individuals have little time to prepare or to evacuate before the disaster strikes. Of course, there may be a combination of disasters like that which occurred in New Orleans; it started with a hurricane and ended with a severe flood.

Natural disasters have the potential to significantly affect the public health of the people, since access to medical care can be severely limited and resources such as food, water, and medicines become unavailable or depleted.

Natural Disasters

- Earthquakes
- Hurricanes
- Floods
- Tornadoes
- Tsunamis
- Volcano eruptions
- Wildfires
- Landslides and mudslides
- Extreme heat and snow/cold

Disaster Defined

Disaster is defined as an event of such magnitude that essential services are disrupted and current resources are overwhelmed. Disasters may be natural (as listed) or caused by human actions such as civil disturbance, a hazardous material incident, or act of terrorism.

Whatever the cause, disasters have several characteristics in common: They are unexpected and there has been little or no warning; lives, public health, and the environment are endangered; and emergency services and personnel must be called to action if not available during the initial stages of the disaster. The terrorist attack that occurred in Washington, D.C., and New York on September 11, 2001, and the Katrina disaster in 2005 were just such events, events that carried an unforeseen and immediate threat to public health and required the intervention of others to provide outside resources.

PUBLIC POLICY

Mass Casualty Characteristics

- Mass casualty incidents are community-wide incidents—not confined to individual hospitals.
- Event occurs in local community.
- Local government provides "first responders."
- State and federal government will be involved if incident is large enough.
- Hospitals are last link in community response to mass casualty incident.
- Hospitals will receive most seriously injured and ill casualties.

Hospitals are the most comprehensive community health resource. As the last link in the community chain of readiness, the hospital is the organization that will have to, by default, make up for the inadequacies in community preparedness.

Hospitals must follow federal legislation known as EMTALA (the Emergency Medical Treatment and Labor Act), which governs what a hospital must do when clients present themselves. If the emergency department is closed because of client overload or to protect the health of current clients, by federal law the hospital is not allowed to turn away clients. EMTALA ensures that all individuals who appear at an emergency department must be screened, evaluated, and stabilized before being transferred. If the State Survey Agency determines that a violation has occurred, it begins the process to terminate the hospital's Medicare provider agreement. Triage is not equivalent to medical screening, so a hospital could easily be overwhelmed in a disaster, even when victims are processed in the field via triage.

Also, this legislation is still in place even if the community designates some hospitals to receive victims of a disaster and others to remain open to clients not exposed to the contaminant. Authorities are suggesting that an open dialogue with the federal government (officials of the Department of Health and Human Services [HHS]) to revise provisions of EMTALA is necessary, now that the potential for mass casualty disaster is present.

Lessons From Natural Disasters

The implications of natural disasters for nurses and other healthcare providers are profound. For example, throughout a storm-devastated area, nurses were called upon to provide hospital care under extreme conditions caused by the lack of electricity, food, water, and medical supplies, as well as the inability to evacuate patients. Other nurses who assisted at evacuation centers were overwhelmed by the surge of sick and injured.

Potential Threats From Natural Disasters

Certain natural disasters, such as earthquakes and tornadoes, are very unpredictable; others, like Hurricane Katrina in 2005, are carefully tracked. As a major storm approaches, the national weather agencies estimate the potential for major damage and disruption (i.e., wind velocity, snow depth, temperature, tidal surges), which are widely publicized by the media. The lesson is to hope for the best, but prepare for the worst. Soon after Katrina, another hurricane threatened the region. When residents of several Texas cities followed evacuation orders, they experienced traffic delays, gasoline and water shortages, and other obstacles during their disorderly evacuation.

Do Not Assume Government Agencies Will Provide Immediate Relief

The government agencies involved with disaster relief include local police, National Guard, Federal Emergency Management Agency (FEMA), federal troops, the U.S. Coast Guard, and many nongovernmental organizations, such as the Red Cross. The coordination among all these organizations has often failed in a morass of bureaucracy and red tape. Several dire predictions have been made concerning the potential threat to an area from a disaster, with effective response plans either not in place or that have not been tested.

Learn to Cope Without Electricity and Water

Storms involving strong wind, snow, or ice usually disrupt electrical power. So do earthquakes, wildfires, and floods. A severe hurricane's winds can topple trees into power lines and blow down cell phone towers. A storm surge and flood can disable emergency generators and disrupt water and sewer service. Normal communications are crippled as cell phones and cordless phones do not operate, nor do television, air conditioning, refrigeration, hospital equipment, or services that depend upon electricity. The ability to communicate with the "outside world" may be extremely limited, leaving hospitals and evacuation centers unable to adequately communicate their emergency needs or to learn when and in what form they could expect assistance.

Disruption of the water service could result in extreme hardship to many thousands of stranded survivors. Many may have to endure several days without adequate water, ice, or food until they are either rescued or make their way to an emergency center. The implication of the loss of utilities for the individual nurse is that you must keep an emergency supply of water at home, in your automobile, and at work (in case you are stranded at work or in transit) adequate for 3 days. Refer to "Creating a Safety Plan for Disasters," page 470, for a checklist of emergency supplies.

Another lesson learned from natural disasters is that healthcare professionals who may be called upon to assist with disaster relief should be up-to-date with tetanus, hepatitis A, and other preventative injections.

Bioterrorism Response Act

The Public Health Security and Bioterrorism Response Act of 2002, signed into law in June 2002, authorized $4.3 billion to combat terrorism. As of January 2005, the U.S. Department of Homeland Security has provided $2.2 billion in counterterrorism grants to the states. The federal government has focused on three components: detection, treatment, and containment.

One aspect of the law is to allocate funds for the training of healthcare workers, including nurses. The American Nurses Association (ANA), together with HHS, has established the National Nurses Response Team (NNRT). This team, made up of a large number of nurses, is poised to respond to any major disaster, such as an anthrax or smallpox attack.

These nurses, as well as other healthcare professionals, will be "federalized," thus receiving umbrella coverage for licensure, liability, and expenses. Deployments will be limited to 2 weeks. In the law-signing ceremony, President Bush pointed out that biological attacks could occur covertly, and healthcare professionals may well be the first to recognize such an attack. He went on to say, "The speed with which they detect and respond to a threat to public health will make the difference between containment and catastrophe."

To encourage hospitals to be ready to combat bioterrorism, the federal Health Resources and Services Administration is giving millions in grants. The major expenditure is $800,000 to each of 10 hospitals designated as disaster resource centers who will coordinate emergency training and preparedness. These centers will be required to implement procedures that can deal with a "worst case scenario" or a disaster affecting hundreds of thousands of casualties.

The Department of Homeland Security, created in September 2001, coordinates multiple agencies and programs into a single integrated agency focused on protecting the American people and our homeland. This organization directs a comprehensive national strategy to connect agencies at all levels. There are 15 major agencies, including Federal Emergency Management Agency (FEMA), Transportation Security Administration, Customs and Border Protection, U.S. Coast Guard, and the Secret Service.

The Disaster Medical Assistance Team (DMAT) is a regional group under the control of Homeland Security. These groups are trained to activate as a unit that can deploy for any type of disaster; they are trained to provide care for any type of casualty. The three major responsibilities of DMAT are triage, staging, and providing medical care.

Nurses are an essential part of the disaster team and must be prepared to function in the event of either a man-made or natural disaster. To accomplish this effectively, nurses must have a personal and family disaster plan, for it is difficult to care for others if one's own family is not safe.

DISASTER IMPACT ON THE INFRASTRUCTURE

When a disaster occurs, the impact on the infrastructure may be severe. Services and delivery systems, transportation, utilities, fuel, food, water supplies, and communication systems may be affected. Disaster experts point out that when one of the support systems breaks down, it has a domino effect and all elements of the infrastructure could be affected. According to Community Emergency Response Team (CERT) information, some of the ways in which the infrastructure can be affected after a disaster are shown below.

Service	Effect
Transportation	Inability to get emergency service personnel into the affected area
	Inability to transport victims away from the area
Electrical	Increased risk of fire and electrical shock
	Possible disruption to transportation system if downed lines are across roads
Telephone	Lost contact between victims, service providers, and family members
	System overload due to calls from/to friends or relatives
Water	Disruption of service to homes, businesses, and medical providers
	Inadequate water supply for firefighting
	Increased risk to public health if there is extensive damage to the water supply or if it becomes contaminated
Fuel supplies	Increased risk of fire or explosion from ruptured fuel lines
	Risk of asphyxiation from natural gas leaks in confined areas

The Community Emergency Response Team (CERT) concept was originally developed and implemented by the City of Los Angeles Fire Department after the 1987 Whittier Narrows earthquake. They realized that citizens would likely be on their own at least during the early stages of a catastrophic disaster, and thus there was a need for a Disaster Preparedness program. So far, thousands of people and hundreds of teams have been trained.

Disaster Mitigation

When examining how to mitigate the effects of a disaster, safety precautions and preparation must be considered first, that is, personal safety, home preparation, and community preparation. Individual safety and home preparation need to be dealt with on a personal level. Focusing on both natural disasters, such as earthquakes and floods, and man-made disasters, each family or community should develop a Preparedness Plan. In addition, each healthcare facility must have its own Preparedness Plan, developed enough to implement under the chaotic circumstances of a disaster.

The purpose of this chapter is to focus on natural and man-made disasters, such as a terrorism event, and how the medical community, specifically nurses, could develop their own Preparedness Plan to cope with a mass casualty disaster.

Community Response Plan

Apart from personal safety and home preparation before a disaster, a planned community response is a critical element. A CERT that is trained and prepared to intervene will do more to mitigate disaster outcomes than any other planned approach. A CERT organizational structure would look like this:

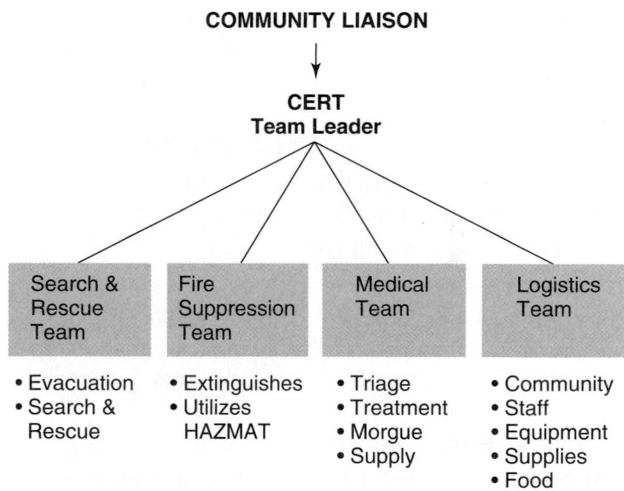

Strategic Plan for Responding to Biological or Chemical Terrorism

The CDC has formulated a Strategic Planning Workgroup to combat the deliberate dissemination of biological or chemical agents. The plan encompasses detection and surveillance, laboratory analysis, emergency response, and communication systems. Success of the plan hinges on the relationship between medical and public health professionals working together for emergency management.

Five Focus Areas in the CDC's Strategic Plan

- *Preparedness and Prevention:* Emergency coordinated preparedness teams are to be developed in all cities and states in order to respond effectively. The CDC will assist in developing tools and strategies to prevent and mitigate illness and injury.
- *Detection and Surveillance:* Early detection is critical for prompt responding. The CDC will develop disease surveillance systems, as well as mechanisms for detecting, evaluating, and reporting suspicious events. This will be done in partnership with front-line medical–hospital emergency professionals. Reporting of unexplained injuries and illnesses will be part of routine surveillance systems.
- *Diagnosis and Characterization of Biological–Chemical Agents:* The CDC and its partners will create a multilevel laboratory response network to analyze biological agents. Diagnostic technology will be disseminated to state laboratories for diagnostic confirmation and reference support for terrorism response teams.
- *Response:* The CDC will develop a comprehensive public health response to a terrorist event that will encompass investigation, medical treatment, prophylaxis for infected persons, and disease prevention and decontamination measures.
- *Communication Systems:* The ability of the United States to be prepared and intervene effectively when a terrorist event has been identified is dependent on well-trained healthcare and public health professionals having access to emergency information via state-of-the-art communication systems. Effective communication with the public is also essential. Through this sophisticated communication network, the CDC will disperse information regarding disease outbreaks, dissemination of diagnostic results, and emergency health information.

In 2004, the Homeland Security Council, in partnership with the Department of Homeland Security and federal, state, and local agencies, developed a series of planning scenarios for various types of disasters. They included a general description, timeline dynamics, secondary events, key implications, interventions, and recovery. These scenarios were designed to provide the foundation structure for the development of national preparedness standards from which capabilities can be measured. Please check the Homeland Security Web site for more information about disaster planning for your facility.

Home Emergency/Disaster Kit*

- Prescription medications (to last a minimum of 1 month)
- First aid kit and handbook; gloves for work and protection
- Bottled water (1 gallon/person/day; minimum 15 days)
- Nonperishable foods that do not have to be prepared; comfort snack foods high in protein and calories; can opener
- Extra pet food
- Battery or hand-cranked radio, extra batteries
- Emergency lighting (flashlights, oil lamps)
- Cellular phone or CB radio
- Emergency cash in small bills
- Emergency phone numbers
- Tools and supplies: whistle (to alert rescuers to your location); wrench (to turn off water and gas); duct tape (for broken windows, etc.); buckets and heavy plastic bags for waste
- Blankets, sleeping bags, warm clothing, rain gear
- Comfort items (games, books, teddy bears, etc.)
- Special items for adults (contact lens equipment, glasses) and children (formula, diapers, powdered milk)
- Place items in waterproof containers that are easily accessible
- Replace perishable items (water, food, medications, batteries) yearly

*The Department of Homeland Security (DHS) has developed the READY.gov Web site. You can find an emergency planning and preparation guide on this site.

The Joint Commission Standards

The Joint Commission has focused on security management and has developed a plan that describes how the organization will establish and maintain a security program to protect those involved. The plan provides for designation of personnel who will report and investigate security incidents, provide identification for participants, and control access and egress to sensitive areas. As of 2005, this plan has been modified to include communication and coordination between healthcare organizations. Now, to meet The Joint Commission standards, hospital emergency departments are expected to include four specific phases of disaster management: mitigation, preparedness, response, and recovery. They are also expected to participate in at least one annual drill.

The Joint Commission, together with Homeland Security, has insisted that hospitals strengthen their disaster plans. Hospitals that are renovating or expanding must include new features like decontamination showers, personal protective equipment, hurricane-resistant glass windows, and better power generators. Hospitals must also develop a plan to recover from a disaster and return to predisaster status.

Hospitals Must Be Disaster Ready

A major step in creating a disaster plan is to evaluate the individual hospital's vulnerability in different situations. For example, a hospital on the San Andreas fault in northern California would be vulnerable in different ways than a hospital on the Florida coast. These aspects should be taken into account when a disaster plan is formulated. The plan should also be open, up-to-date, and frequently examined. One consultant on

TABLE 15-1 Disaster Preparation

	Focus of Concern-Safety	Preparation and Coping
Power	Electricity—Millions may lose power for days Gas—Natural gas, the main source of heat for many, will be lost when gas lines rupture Gas may leak into homes, especially from fallen water heaters Oil—Damaged oil refineries or oil lines could catch on fire—no oil available	Have flashlights and batteries or oil lamps on hand Turn off gas if you smell it Carefully anchor a gas-powered water heater Have wood available to burn for heat if you are in a cold climate
Structures	Homes—could become uninhabitable, especially after an earthquake Inspect any damage before living in structure Schools—Many do not yet meet current standards for seismic retrofitting	Bolt down home to foundation or refit to meet seismic requirements Have buildings inspected and subsequently reinforced Attach large pieces of furniture to the wall Plan safe areas in the home (basement) for tornadoes, high winds, or hurricanes Protect window glass with wood shutters, etc. Keep an ax close in case you have to break out of structure
Communication	Land lines—Most may survive, but if there is an earthquake or flood, they will be interrupted Power grid—If down, no calls will go through Wireless—Mobile phone towers could topple, leaving dead zones	Have at least one phone that does not require electricity Keep extra charged battery for cell phone Have wind-up radio or extra battery-powered radio to receive information after disaster
Water	If water comes into the home by pipeline, these could be interrupted or destroyed for weeks or months Wells could be destroyed by a disaster	Keep 1 gallon pure water/person/day for a minimum of 15 days Have a portable water purifier on hand to make potable water from pools, ponds, creeks, etc.

disaster planning says if the plan cannot be reduced to a one-page flowchart, it is probably too complicated.

DISASTER MANAGEMENT

Everyday communication systems are likely to be overwhelmed in a disaster. Preparing for this eventuality by establishing backup and redundant communication systems is essential.

First responders will be local. They will work in conjunction with the state and federal organizations, and therefore, there must be an integrated system of in-hospital and out-of-hospital team members with state and federal agencies.

Local systems, both in and out of the hospital, will comprise the critical human infrastructure for responding to weapons of mass destruction (WMD) incidents. Communication coordination will be an essential component in this infrastructure system. One measure is to include a 24-hr wireless radio dedicated communication system to communicate with other healthcare facilities if telephone lines and the Internet do not function.

Communication among the triage team (out-of-hospital) establishing victim care priorities, the hospital or treatment staff (in-hospital), and state and federal agencies' forensic investigation needs must also be established as a cooperative effort. Training through drills and scenarios would provide practice so that these vital communication functions would be implemented instantly if there were to be a WMD incident.

Following from the local communication structure, where there should be one single community-identified person or small group in command acting as liaison agent, the state and federal response teams will be integrated into the communication system. An example of a local system used nationally might be the Incident Command System (ICS), commonly used among EMS personnel. It is a logical management command and control structure that should be part of hospital planning. Specific roles and positions carry specific duties and responsibilities. Each position has a prioritized list of tasks that are checked off as they are completed. When an emergency occurs, the "incident commanders" take command. They can, in turn, appoint liaison or safety officers or any other position to communicate back to any local or regional ICS, according to the needs created by the emergency. This system organizes emergency responses in five categories: command, planning, operations, logistics, and administration.

A new program introduced by the CDC expands on the ICS. This program, National Incident Management System (IMS) or NIMS, includes guidelines that all community organizations, including healthcare facilities, are required to follow if they receive grant funds for disaster preparation. All employees who will be involved in disaster response must show evidence of having learned about the NIMS guidelines.

Hospital Evacuation Plans

Evacuation plans must be in place with a designated authority who will order the implementation. There are several types of evacuation:

- *Shelter in Place:* Staying where everyone is may be the safest plan, especially if there is a known contaminant released in the area or it is too dangerous to leave due to a storm, hurricane, etc.
- *Moving Either Up or Down Levels:* Moving all people (clients, staff and visitors) to another, safer level. Examples are moving up to avoid flood waters or down to the basement to take shelter from an airborne attack.
- *Total Evacuation:* Removing all people from a building and relocating them to a safe area.

Once the evacuation plan is in place, the staff must be drilled on a regular basis so that the plan may be carried out in safety.

The hospital should also have a plan to accommodate special populations if they must evacuate the hospital. For example, if they must evacuate babies, they should have on hand special aprons that hold several babies in pockets.

Internal (or In-Hospital) Communication

Hospitals will have to expand their sphere of influence to include community-level teams. They must have an ongoing, open channel of communication with emergency response

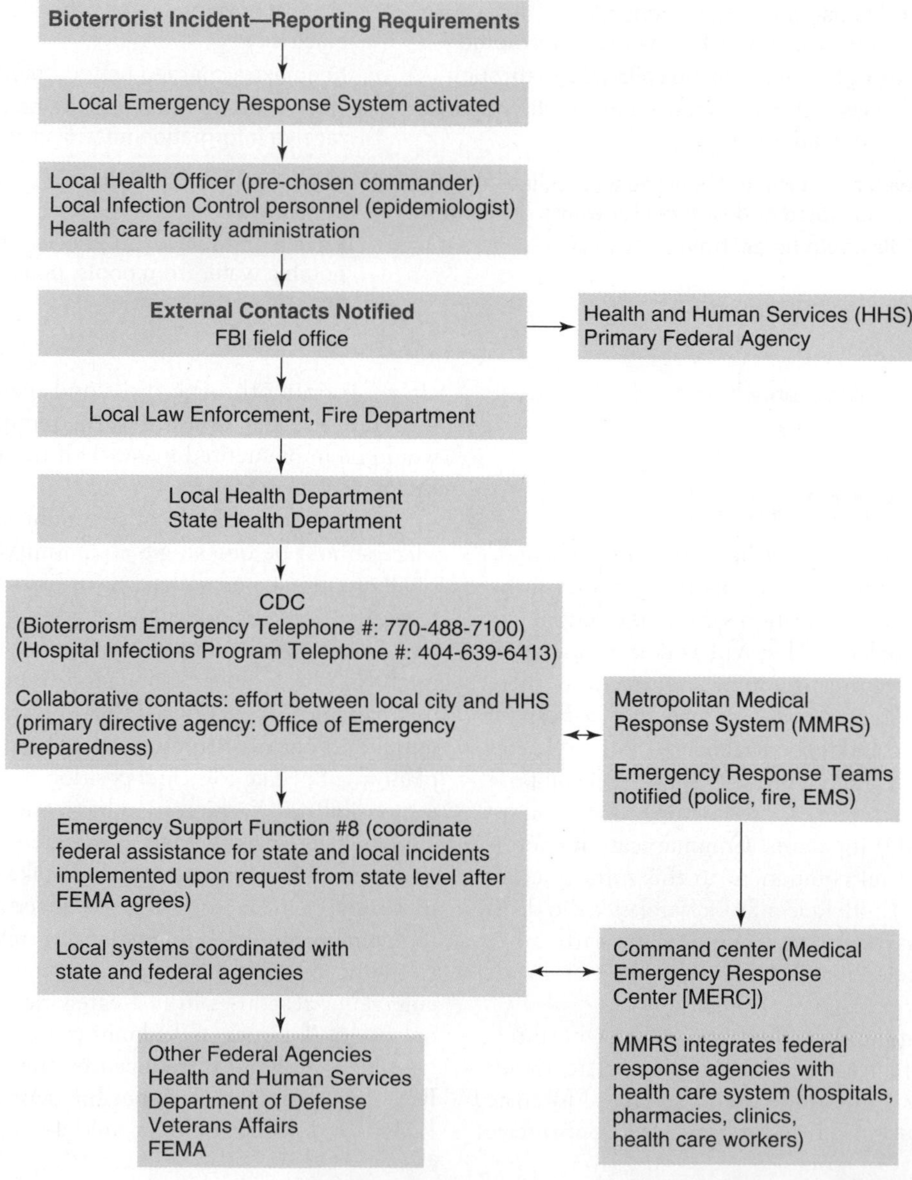

teams who will have been notified first of a mass casualty incident. A community-wide network, all using the same channel of communication, is necessary.

Family and friends, calling to learn about their loved ones after the arrival of casualties, will rapidly overload the system and isolate the hospital. To cope with this eventuality, a single communication site for obtaining victim and locator information should be established. The Red Cross or comparable organization could serve as this third-party, off-site source of information.

A clear and open information system, using both telecommunications and a position-to-position cascade in the event of the primary system being overloaded, is necessary. This cascade should be designated by position (e.g., emergency room supervisor), not person, due to turnover, multiple shifts, and personnel reassignment during a disaster. One hospital instituted a text message alert system by pager that could be sent to many personnel at one time. In addition to a communication system being established, adequate equipment, such as cell phones, walkie-talkies, even runners, must be available because current phone land lines may be totally overwhelmed.

TRIAGE SYSTEMS

Triage is from a French word (*trier*) meaning to sort. It is a medical process of prioritizing treatment urgency. One example of a triage system is START, an acronym for "simple triage and rapid treatment." This is a standardized system that provides a framework for triage decisions, especially useful for triaging large numbers of victims at an emergency incident. START was developed in the 1980s in California as a way of preparing for a disaster.

Emergency department personnel use the triage system to quickly assess large numbers of people with multiple problems. Rapid identification in the hospital is important to determine which clients require immediate treatment and which can safely wait.

The three-level triage system has been used for years to differentiate the levels of emergency cases waiting to be seen. Now, the five-level system appears to be preferred because it decreases the ambiguity of the middle level of emergency care (where the majority of casualties would fall).

There are several methods of categorizing casualties according to the three-level system. One option is as follows:

1. **Emergent** triage refers to a life-threatening or potentially life-threatening condition that requires immediate treatment. These conditions could include multisystem failure, cardiopulmonary arrest, bleeding, airway loss, multiple trauma, severe shock, cervical spine injury, and so on.
2. **Immediate** or Urgent triage is not life-threatening or acute, but refers to clients who need treatment as soon as possible (within 2 hr). These clients have stable vital signs and there is no immediate crisis. This category would include fever, minor burns, lacerations, significant pain, and fractures.
3. The third category is **Nonemergent** or Nonurgent, including clients who have a condition that would not be affected by a delay in treatment. These are clients with chronic or minor injuries, strains, rash, back pain, and so on.

A second way of implementing the three-level strategy of triage is as follows:

1. **Immediate (I)**—the victim has a life-threatening injury (airway, bleeding, or shock) that demands immediate attention (the same as Emergent).
2. **Delayed (D)**—an injury that does not jeopardize the victim's life if definitive treatment is delayed.
3. **Dead (DEAD)**—no respiration after two attempts to open airway. (CPR is not performed in a disaster environment because it demands extensive resources, including personnel time.)

The above strategy will probably be the one used (if a three-level system is adopted) if there is a mass casualty disaster, because **the goal of triage is to do the greatest good for the greatest number**. Triage must occur as quickly as possible after victims are located.

Field Triage

An example of a five-level system of triage is the Emergency Severity Index (ESI), developed by two physicians in the late 1990s who found that a five-level triage system was more reliable than the three-level. The assessment begins with whether the client has a life-threatening condition or if the problem is potentially fatal. Included in this assessment is vital signs and, for the lower acuity casualty, the number of resources required. A level from 1 (most acute) to 5 (least acute) is assigned. Some U.S. hospitals have switched from a three- to a five-level system and have developed their own criteria. A five-level system improves client flow and allows nonacute clients to be screened, but not take space in an ED bed. Because of this, hospitals feel that this system is more effective and reliable than the former three-level system for handling disaster casualties.

Emergency Severity Index

Level	1	Most Acute	Life-threatening—potentially fatal
	2		Includes vital sign assessment
Level	3	Lower Acuity	Resources required from this level to 5
	4		
Level	5	Least Acute	Not life-threatening—minimal resources

During a disaster, instead of a finite number of victims coming to emergency departments that are able to utilize all of the hospital's resources, victims arrive in huge numbers and overwhelm the emergency department. In this case, there are actually so many injured, triage must occur in the field, thus the term *field triage*.

Field triage would be used in case of a major disaster—either natural (earthquake, tornado, hurricane), or one caused by man, including events such as a chemical spill, plane crash, explosion, fire, or a terrorist event. The numbers of injured would exceed the resources of any emergency medical personnel at the scene. Thus decisions will be triage driven, not treatment driven. These victims would be classified according to a color-coding tag system.

Colored Tags		Classification
Red	=	Emergent
Yellow	=	Immediate
Green	=	Urgent
Blue	=	Psychological Support or First-Aid level
Black	=	Dead or Imminently Terminal

Catastrophic Triage

When events are cascading out of control or disaster has wiped out primary treatment resources, the choice of triage system will be limited. Basically, there are two options. One option is to follow first and second steps and the other is severely limited to those who have the potential to survive—they will be Red Tagged. Thus triage categories change during a disaster. The primary assessment is one of acuity, but the victim must have the ability to survive. Making these decisions will be terribly difficult, but this system seems to be the only realistic method of categorizing thousands of victims from a deadly disaster.

First Step The most direct and expedient method of field triage would be to evaluate victims according to these categories:

I	=	Immediate
D	=	Delayed
Dead	=	Dead

Everyone must be tagged.

Second Step Treat victims immediately.

Check airway and breathing rate	▶	Initiate airway management
Check circulation	▶	Initiate bleeding control
Check mental status	▶	Treat for shock

Document Results

Necessary for effective deployment of resources

Information on location of victims

Quick record of number of casualties by degree of severity

Triage Victim Flow

From triage, victims are taken to a designated medical treatment area (Immediate Care, Delayed Care, or Morgue), and from there, transported out of the disaster area (see flowchart below). There are various methods of implementing triage that include minimal to massive numbers of victims. Whichever triage method or strategy is chosen, the community or identified team must be aware of the specific categories.

TRIAGE VICTIM FLOW CHART*

Incident Location	Triage	Medical Treatment	Transportation
		Delayed Care Area	Air Transportation
Search and Rescue	Triage Team	Immediate Care Area	Transportation Manager
		Morgue	Ground Transportation

*CERT Training: Participant Handbook.

Decontamination

Every facility should have a protocol and site for decontamination, both outside and inside. Rooms with negative pressure are especially important for toxic areas and soiled infectious areas. For example, if there is a pandemic flu, that client should be isolated and the air in that room exhausted to the outside to prevent it from contaminating the rest of the facility.

Triage and Decontamination

While triage is an essential component of disaster management, decontamination prioritization is also critical. This is a process to determine the need for and order of victim decontamination. Both processes may be implemented simultaneously. The same triage rule of thumb applies; namely, **providing the greatest benefit for the greatest number**.

If there are mass casualty victims inside a "hot zone," the Incident Commander may assign personnel to manage both medical triage and decontamination. The first step may be to group victims into ambulatory and nonambulatory categories. Prioritization of these victims may be done using the medical triage system, START.

The highest priority for Ambulatory decontamination (classified as *Immediate*) casualties includes:

- Victims closest to the point of release
- Those who report exposure to aerosol
- Victims with evidence of liquid deposits on skin or clothing
- Those who are clinically symptomatic (i.e., shortness of breath) but were not as close to point of release
- Victims evidencing conventional injuries, such as open wounds

Nonambulatory casualties includes:

- Victims who are unconscious or unresponsive and will remain in place while further prioritization for decontamination occurs
- Those triaged as *Delayed* (casualties who may have serious injuries, but can wait without compromising the outcome)

Triage Categories for Use During a Disaster

Field Triage

Red	=	Emergent (hyperacute—1st priority)
Yellow	=	Immediate (serious—2nd priority)
Green	=	Urgent (injured—3rd priority)
Blue	=	First aid
Black	=	Dead or dying

Catastrophic Triage (First Option)

I	=	Immediate (life-threatening)
D	=	Delayed (may delay treatment without death)
Dead	=	Dead

Catastrophic Triage (Second Option)

Red Tag = Potential to survive

No other victims tagged.

START Categories

Color Tag		Decontamination Priority
Red Tag	= Immediate	1. Serious signs/symptoms Known agent contamination
Yellow Tag	= Delayed	2. Moderate-to-minimal signs/symptoms Known agent or aerosol contamination Close to point of release
Green Tag	= Minor	3. Minimal signs/symptoms No known exposure to agent
Black Tag	= Deceased/ Expectant	4. Very serious signs/symptoms Grossly contaminated Unresponsive

Highest priority for overall decontamination includes casualties:

- Who are medically triaged as *Immediate*
- In need of lifesaving medical procedures that can be performed on the spot
- Who have been exposed to nerve agents—decontamination as soon as possible may be lifesaving

Post-Triage Organization

After evaluation and prioritizing victims into treatment groups and providing immediate lifesaving measures, clients will be transported to three locations: Immediate Treatment, Delayed Treatment, and the Morgue.

Treatment area personnel will then:

1. Perform additional *triage* as needed.
2. Complete *physical assessment* (head-to-toe) to determine extent of injuries.
3. Render *first aid* if needed.

After this post-triage assessment, personnel will provide immediate treatment for burns, open wounds, fractures, sprains, hypothermia, frostbite, and so on. After triage and post-triage assessment, it is essential to document the number of victims in each category (immediate, delayed), as well as the dead victims. See Unit 3 for skills in Post-Triage.

The number of victims may exceed local capacity for treatment. Survivors will assist others, but it cannot be assumed they will know how to give lifesaving aid or post-disaster survival techniques. Therefore, outside resources will be requested. For example, the U.S. government has an action plan in place.

This federal response plan includes a stockpile of specialized medical supplies assembled in eight guarded secret warehouses nationwide. More than 100 air cargo containers (each one fills a Boeing 747) are ready to be sent to any city in the United States within 12 hr. State and local officials will be able to track the cargo sent by ground transport to a final, local destination.

When the CDC, in consult with local officials, agrees that an attack has occurred and the local system is insufficient to cope, a container of supplies will be dispersed, as well as physicians and health personnel, if needed.

WEAPONS OF MASS DESTRUCTION

Biological Agents

Biological terrorism is the use of specific agents to cause harm or kill people, and includes the use of organisms such as bacteria, viruses, and toxins. The use of biological agents as weapons poses a difficult problem for public health officials because these agents present with an insidious onset and mimic natural epidemics of influenza. Symptoms may take days to develop before victims seek medical care.

These agents are classified as a threat to national security because they possess unique characteristics:

- Agents that are easily disseminated or transmitted person to person and could be dispersed over a wide geographical area
- Agents that cause high mortality with the potential for major public health impact
- Agents that require specific actions in order that public health preparedness is secured

Biological weapons have a history that goes back as far as the sixth century. Recent history reveals the fact that many nations have biowarfare capability with agents such as anthrax, plague, and smallpox. In spite of the fact that the Geneva convention prohibited use of biological and chemical warfare, and in 1972 many nations agreed to stop research, the United States remains vulnerable to a biowarfare attack.

A biological agent cannot be detected directly. The way it will be identified is when victims arrive at clinics and hospitals and, either through the awareness and perception of professionals who correlate the unusual influx of victims with similar symptoms, or through a retrospective of "putting the pieces together," the biological cause will be identified.

To accomplish the goal of identifying a biological attack, several steps need to be taken.

TABLE 15-2 Bioterrorism Agents

Disease	Signs & Symptoms	Incubation Period	Person-to-Person Transmission
Anthrax (Inhalational) Organism—*Bacillus anthracis*	Nonspecific flulike, with fever, malaise, fatigue, cough Delayed symptoms—severe respiratory distress	1–7 days (usually 48 hr) Can be 6 weeks	No
Botulism (Inhalational) Organism—*Clostridium botulinum* toxin	Increasing muscle weakness, drooping eyelids, blurred vision, difficulty speaking and swallowing; progresses down body to paralysis	12–36 hr after exposure	No
Pneumonic Plague Organism—*Yersinia pertis*	Sudden onset of high fever, chills, chest pain, headache, and cough with bloody sputum. Possibly vomiting and diarrhea. Advanced: skin lesions, respiratory failure.	2–3 days (1–6 days after exposure)	Yes, through droplet, aerosol
Smallpox Organism—*Variola virus*	Sudden onset of high fever, headache, and backache. Then, painful rash of small, red spots starts on face and spreads over entire skin surface. Progresses from macules to papules.	7–17 days after exposure (average is 12 days)	Yes, airborne, droplet or direct contact with skin lesions (until scabs fall off—3–4 weeks)
Typhoid Tularemia Organism—*Francisella tularensis*	Sudden onset of high fever, weakness, weight loss, chest pain, and cough	3–5 days after exposure	No
Viral Hemorrhagic Fevers (Filoviruses, such as Ebola and Marburg, and arenaviruses, such as Lassa and Junin)	Sudden onset of fever, muscle aches, and profound weakness, followed by circulatory compromise	2–21 days after exposure	Yes, risk higher during late stages of disease

1. Set up bioterrorism education programs and training for healthcare professionals who must be able to recognize signs and symptoms of a biological attack.
2. Prepare and distribute educational materials that will inform and remind healthcare professionals of the signs and symptoms of various biological weapons.
3. Establish communication systems to ensure that accurate information is delivered.
4. Recognize the signs and symptoms of major high-priority agents. For example:
   - *Variola major* (smallpox)
   - *Bacillus anthracis* (anthrax)
   - *Francisella tularensis* (tularemia)
   - *Yersinia pestis* (plague)
   - *Clostridium botulinum* toxin (botulism)

Chemical Agents

Chemical terrorism is the deployment of chemical weapons with the intention of causing havoc, harm, and death to the recipients. The release of these weapons will quickly cause death, especially if released in an enclosed space. The U.S. Army Medical Research Institute of Chemical Defense has classified these agents as potential weapons. These chemical weapons can be pulmonary agents (phosgene, chlorine), cyanide agents (hydrogen cyanide), vesicant agents (mustard, oxime), nerve agents (tabun, sarin, VX), or incapacitating agents (agent 15, BZ). These weapons will inflict painful external and internal injuries, psychological devastation, and death. An act of chemical terrorism is likely to be overt because the effects of these agents on people are immediate and obvious; the agents are absorbed through the skin, mucous membranes, or pulmonary system.

Perhaps the most dangerous of these agents are nerve gases (sarin, tabun, VX), which are extremely toxic and easy to disseminate in the air. These nerve agents are designed to kill people by binding up a compound known as acetylcholinesterase, which is the body's "off" switch. When acetylcholinesterase is significantly decreased or absent in the body, the glands and voluntary muscles continue to be stimulated, eventually wear out, and the body can no longer sustain healthy function.

Decontamination of some chemical agents is time- and labor-intensive and requires tremendous resources. However, if chemical agents are widely dispersed, every one of thousands of persons affected cannot be individually decontaminated. Also, decontamination may not be required for certain chemical incidents. The triage team may remove victims to an uncontaminated area and/or send victims home to shower.

TABLE 15-2 Bioterrorism Agents (*Continued*)

Treatment	Death Rate if Untreated	Death Rate if Treated	Isolation Precautions/ Standard Precautions
Antibiotics, including ciprofloxacin 500 mg PO q12 hr. Doxycycline 100 mg PO q12 hr; also, combined IV and PO.	High	Improved chances for survival. Once symptoms appear, treatment is less effective.	Standard Precautions
Antitoxin—requires skin testing. Supportive care and ventilate until victim can breathe on his own.	High	Low, if breathing can be supported for duration of illness (weeks to months, in some cases)	Standard Precautions
Antibiotics, including ciprofloxacin 400 mg IV q12 hr. Doxycycline 200 mg PO, then 100 mg PO q12 hr.	Almost always fatal	Treatment is highly effective if taken within 24 hr of first symptoms	Bubonic form: Standard Precautions. Pneumonic form: Standard Precautions plus Droplet Precautions until 48–72 hr after antibiotic treatment
Vaccination is effective if given within 3–4 days of exposure; passive immunization with VIG if 3 days post-exposure.	3–30%.	If vaccinated, less than 1%.	Strict Isolation Precautions: Airborne (includes N95 mask) and Contact, in addition to Standard Precautions
Antibiotics, including doxycycline and ciprofloxacin	33%	1–3% if treated within 24 hr of exposure.	Standard Precautions
Little is known. Antiviral agents, such as ribavirin, may be useful.	15–90%	Unknown. Including negative-pressure room with anteroom.	Strict Isolation Precautions

Radiation

The threat of terrorists using nuclear or radioactive materials in the United States is considered to be real. While we cannot predict which form this terrorist event might take, we can prepare to cope with the situation should it arise.

Radiation presents unique characteristics, in that exposure may occur without individuals coming in direct contact with the source of radiation. With other bioterrorism agents, the victim must be in contact with the material, either through inhalation, ingestion, or through the skin.

Radioactive substances emit radiation in the form of rays (waves) or extremely small particles. *Waveforms* are x-ray and gamma rays; *particle forms* are alpha, beta, and neutron. Ionizing radiation is radiation that has enough energy to cause atoms to lose electrons and become ions. Charged particles are emitted from ionizing radiation. These particles (alpha and beta) are the most likely to be dispersed after a terrorist attack. They may adhere to airborne dust particles or attach to clothing, and could be inhaled, causing internal contamination. Beta rays are found in "fallout" and alpha particles are emitted from plutonium. Gamma rays, also an example of ionizing radiation, are emitted in a nuclear blast and have high penetration potential, causing severe damage to the individual, but do not require decontamination. In the event of a nuclear attack, both rays and particle forms are likely to be dispersed.

A cell that has been exposed to any type of radiation is damaged and may die. If a terrorist event causes radiation to be released, it could result in either external or internal hazards that could be major or insignificant.

Internal–External Exposure Exposure to radiation from a source outside the body is external exposure; exposure from inside the body is internal. Internal exposure occurs when radioactive material is assimilated into body tissues. This occurs from inhalation, ingestion, or insertion, such as a radioactive implant of iodine-131. A critical point of discrimination is whether the victim was exposed to or contaminated by radiation. If exposed, the victim is *not* a hazard to others. The radiation is absorbed by or passes through the body, but does not result in radioactive contamination.

Radioactive contamination as radioactive particulate material is a major cause for concern. The source of contamination, resulting from spillage, leakage, deliberate dispersal, or attached to dust particles in the air, can be passed on to healthcare workers. If this were to occur, it could become an internal exposure hazard as it is incorporated into the body, as well as an external exposure.

Measuring Radiation The term *RAD* (radiation absorbed dose) is a unit of measure for radiation exposure; 1 RAD results in absorption of 100 ergs of energy/gram of tissue exposed. The international system now measures the unit of exposure by Gray (Gy); thus the amount of absorbed radiation is more commonly measured by the Gray, rather than RAD (1 Gy equals 100 RADs).

Radiation dose is a specific calculated measurement of the amount of energy deposited in the body. The unit of dose is called REM, which takes into account the type of radiation. It is not necessary for the reader to understand the technical specifics of exposure and dose. It is important to know how to measure external radiation levels and to understand the dangers of exposure.

A survey instrument measures radiation levels. The readout is in units of R (which can be either RAD or REM), which is exposure or dose. An instrument reading of 50R/hr tells the healthcare worker that if he stays in the exposed area for 1 hr, he will receive a 50-RAD exposure. Some instruments measure dose over time, called radiation dosimeters; these instruments should be worn by personnel working in a contaminated area. A radiation detection device (film badge) should be worn by personnel who come in contact with the exposed area or victims. Both survey instruments and dosimeters have limitations. In the case of survey instruments, they need to be recalculated at regular intervals and, because they use batteries, should be checked and replaced periodically. Dosimeters also must be zeroed and checked at regular intervals.

Health Effects of Radiation A victim contaminated by radiation is at risk—how much risk is dependent on how much radiation is absorbed. Victims who absorb less than 0.75 Gy will not experience symptoms of exposure. Those who absorb 8 Gy could die. Between 0.75 and 8 Gy, the victim could develop acute radiation syndrome (ARS). See box on page 487.

Low exposures do not cause major damage, such as bone marrow damage or birth defects. High exposure may kill cells and significantly increases the incidence of cancer. Regardless of the type of exposure, triage must focus on life-threatening injury before radiological injury.

Background Radiation We are all exposed to a certain amount of radiation from our daily environment. This is known as background radiation and is derived from natural sources such as radiation from outer space; industrial, academic, or military uses of radiation; and radiation used in medicine. All these sources combine to give us a background radiation dose of 0.360 REM per person per year.

A possible terrorism event involving radiation dispersal could be:

- An attack on a nuclear facility or detonated nuclear weapon
- A radiation dispersal device: "dirty bomb" (embedding radioactive material in a conventional explosive)
- Radioactive material dispersal

American Nurses Association Response to Disaster Planning

- RN should notify employer in writing of any disaster or emergency preparedness education
- RN should request written approval for participation on an emergency response team
- RN should provide employer with ongoing documentation of all continuing education related to disaster preparedness
- RNs who are preapproved members of emergency preparedness team should give written notice to employer of deployment to emergency team

ETHICAL CONSIDERATIONS

When we consider the profession of nursing, a central theme must be the ethical considerations of the practice of nursing. Under the chaotic and challenging conditions of a terrorist event, ethics may seem unimportant; while they may not be addressed overtly during a disaster, ethical considerations form the bedrock of nursing interventions.

In the midst of a crisis, when resources are limited or unavailable, and the emergency medical and nursing staff do not have the capability of handling the disaster, decision making, nursing judgments, indeed, even functioning ability will rest on one's code of ethics. To review the Nurses Code of Ethics, see chapter 1, page 2.

DIVERSITY CONSIDERATIONS

If a mass casualty terrorist event were to occur in the United States, many citizens could potentially be harmed. Because approximately 30% of our population is nonwhite, it is important for nurses to be aware of the impact of culture, beliefs, and values on responses to a disaster. Cultural competence in disaster nursing should be addressed because nurses may be called upon to perform in areas where they are not familiar with the diverse client population. They may not speak the language of the ethnic groups and may not be familiar with the cultural components. They can, however, convey concern, empathy, and the willingness to communicate with the victims who are suffering the effects of a disaster. Nurses who travel to a disaster area should learn from and model local helpers so that their actions are culturally sensitive. Simply being aware of diversity within populations will assist the emergency team to recognize different responses to a mass casualty incident and to relate in a sensitive, appropriate manner.

During the initial assessment after a disaster, the nurse should be aware of the following cultural components:

- Language—(non–English-speaking) communication
- Cultural background and beliefs
- Values, patterns relating to health practices
- Religious practices—limitations
- Nutritional parameters
- Assessment variances for people of color

SUMMARY

In November 2001, 800 public health and military professionals participated at a joint conference. They identified the chief challenge in formulating a strategic plan for preparedness response as "lack of training among front-line responders—physicians and nurses—and inadequate planning at the local, state, and federal levels." Combining these deficit areas—lack of planning, identified skills, and training—helps us to design a framework for nurses to acquire the knowledge necessary for strategic planning and preparedness. Nurses are a vital part, along with physicians and other healthcare professionals, of preparedness programs throughout the country. Nurses must identify their own skill level and the skills necessary to participate as members of the medical response team.

The term "*skill*" may be applied to performance. A complex series of actions to accomplish a task may be called skilled performance. A skill can be learned, but it takes experience in performing step-by-step actions before a well-defined response pattern is accomplished. In addition, the change from hesitant responses in the middle of performing a skill to a competent, automatic response takes place only with practice. Thus the skills necessary to participate in a medical response system when there has been a disaster caused by a WMD must be identified, practiced, and mastered.

This chapter identifies certain skills, drawn from performance-based learning objectives, that nurses must acquire to become high-level task performers on a disaster response team.

Note to Readers

The skills in this chapter have been formulated according to the latest information and protocols available at the time of publication. Because events change, please check periodically with the appropriate government sources (i.e., CDC, DHS, NIOSHA, AHA, APIC, The Joint Commission, FEMA, etc.) for the latest information and updates on procedures and protocols.

TABLE 15-3 Terrorism Response Drill: What Did They Learn?

Problems	Solutions
Communication	
Implemented Hospital Emergency Incident Command System (HEICS) but failed to identify a "point person"; communication between the ED and command center was inadequate.	Appoint individual to be "point" who will maintain communication between command center and ED. Secure two-way radios for hospital staff.
Patient Management	
Tracking victims from arrival in ED to admission or discharge difficult. Comparing identification number for incoming patients from the field to hospital also inadequate.	Implement a patient tracking form and use ID bands to track unidentified patients.
Pediatric Patients	
Difficult to track young children with no ID and no parents available.	Use ID bands and instant photos to identify children and match with parents. Request extra social workers.
Clinical Protocols	
Staff did not suspect which infectious disease was used in bioterrorism attack and did not have a treatment protocol identified.	Create an up-to-date clinical protocol of all potential bioterrorism agents and their treatment and distribute to all staff in the ED and hospital.
Supplies	
Lack of food and water for the emergency staff. Also deficient supplies of garbage cans, linens, IV equipment, and disaster packets.	Have necessary supplies on hand and develop standardized procedures for obtaining extra supplies during disaster.
Facilities Management	
Lack of adequate security to secure the ED; not enough space in the morgue.	Plan to call in extra security immediately after disaster is recognized; assign extra space for dead victims. Request government to suspend the EMTALA law to reroute "worried well" patients not in immediate need of treatment.

Source: Walker-Cillo, G. (2006, April). Bioterrorism: We put our plan to the test. *New Jersey Hospital Association RN Magazine* 69(4), 36–41.

NURSING DIAGNOSES

The following nursing diagnoses appropriate to use on client care plans when the components relate to a client who requires treatment related to a disaster.

NURSING DIAGNOSIS	RELATED FACTORS
Ineffective Community Coping	Disaster-overwhelmed community resources Lack of access to healthcare facilities Infrastructure (services) not functioning at 100% Deficits in social support
Deficient Knowledge	Lack of information about bioterrorism agent, triage, decontamination methods, treatment
Ineffective Protection	First responders' and healthcare personnel protection not appropriate for identified bioterrorism agent
Ineffective Role Performance	First responders and healthcare personnel unclear or unable to function in designated roles
Ineffective Therapeutic Regimen Management	First responders and healthcare personnel unclear about or unable to function in designated roles Communication network inadequate for crisis

CLEANSE HANDS The single most important nursing action to decrease the incidence of hospital-based infections is hand hygiene. *Remember to wash your hands or use antibacterial gel before and after each and every client contact.*

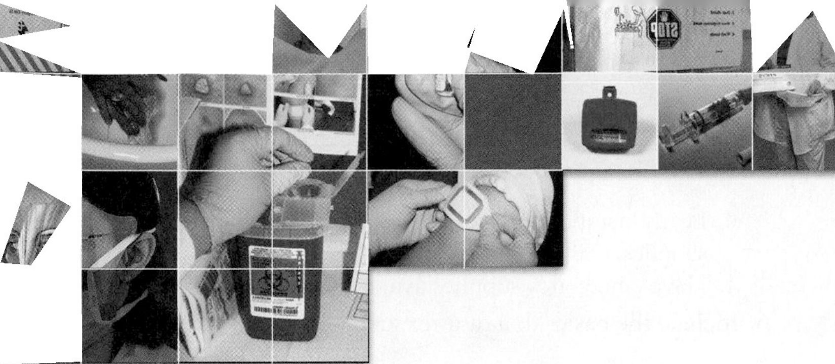

Chapter 15

UNIT 1

Natural Disasters

Nursing Process Data

ASSESSMENT Data Base

- Identify need for information on creating a safety plan for disasters.
- Determine components of a safety plan, including a disaster supply kit.
- Assess need for teaching earthquake safety.
- Identify epidemiologic features of diarrhea-related diseases.
- Assess knowledge of preventive techniques for diarrhea-related diseases.

PLANNING Objectives

- To assist client to create a safety plan for disasters
- To include components of a disaster supply kit
- To identify major challenges (medical/health and infrastructure) after a natural disaster
- To teach earthquake safety to appropriate clients
- To prevent diarrhea-related diseases

IMPLEMENTATION Procedures

EVALUATION Expected Outcomes

- Clients are taught how to create a safety plan for disasters.
- Clients learn how to prepare for an emergency.
- Clients know what to include in a disaster kit.
- Earthquake safety principles are taught to nurses and clients.
- Diarrhea-related diseases are identified early with subsequent interventions.

Pearson Nursing Student Resources

Find additional review materials at
nursing.pearsonhighered.com

Prepare for success with NCLEX®-style practice questions and Skill Checklists

Creating a Safety Plan for Disasters

Procedure

1. Hold a meeting with family members to make a plan if a disaster occurs.
2. Pick two places to meet, one outside the house and the other outside the neighborhood.
3. Choose someone in another state whom all members of the family can check in with during a disaster.
4. Formulate an evacuation plan so everyone will know how to leave the area.
5. Prepare your home for an emergency.
   a. Teach family how to turn off all utilities (especially gas).
   b. Post emergency numbers near the phone.
   c. Put smoke detectors in every room and have fire extinguishers accessible.
   d. Fix potential hazards in the home (anchoring water heater, heavy bookcases, etc.).
   e. Learn first aid and take a CPR course and have supplies available.
   f. Have emergency supplies available and a disaster kit.
6. Include the basics in a disaster supply kit.

Critical/Survival Issues

Lack of safe shelters

No safe food or water

No access to needed medicines (insulin, heart drugs)

No access to medical care for injuries or diseases

Chaos in the streets

Lack of normal resources

Disaster Supply KIT

- Water—1 gallon/person/day for a minimum of 1 to 2 weeks
- Food—selection of ready-to-eat foods, high in protein, for 1 to 2 weeks
- First aid kit with bandages, gloves, soap, H_2O_2, OTC medications for pain, stomach ills, etc.
- Prescription drugs (with copies of prescriptions) that are essential for health (insulin, heart meds [1 month supply], etc.)
- Supplies—radio (battery-operated) with extra batteries, flashlights or oil-burning lamps, wood for heat in a fireplace, personal maintenance items (contact lens supplies, feminine products, denture needs, extra glasses, etc.)
- Clothing and bedding supplies—warm clothing for winter, blankets, sleeping bags, rain protection gear, etc.
- Family documents—personal identification, all records that are essential (passport, wills, trusts, insurance records)
- Credit card and cash

Check and replenish supplies and kits once a year, practice evacuation procedures, and check your disaster plan.

Teaching Clients Earthquake Safety

Procedure

1. Make a plan for you and your family if an earthquake should occur. Create a disaster-preparedness plan. (See above.)
2. Create a disaster kit, both for the home and car. (See above.)
3. Identify potential hazards in the home and have them fixed. ▶ ***Rationale:*** A toppled water heater could cause a fire, and loose, large furniture could be a hazard.
4. Teach how to protect self during severe shaking.
   a. Indoors: drop to floor, take cover and hold on; find a space beside a couch or table. ▶ ***Rationale:*** Earthquake specialists advise taking cover beside the item, not under it (such as a car) because when items fall they create a "triangle safe space" beside the large object.
   b. Avoid exterior walls, windows, hanging objects, and cabinets filled with items.
   c. Outdoors: move to a clear area; avoid buildings, power lines, trees.
   d. Driving: Pull over and stop; set brake. Wait beside the car (not under it) until shaking stops.
5. After the quake, check for injuries and damage (fire, gas leaks, damaged electrical wiring, downed utility lines, chemical spills, damaged structures).
6. Follow disaster plan after earthquake: listen to communication for safety advisories; pay attention to safety precautions; check food and water supplies.

Preventing Diarrhea-Related Diseases After a Natural Disaster

Procedure

1. Recognize early clinical features.
   a. Early symptoms: abrupt, painless watery stool, vomiting; diarrhea may be mild or fulminating.
   b. Delayed symptoms: water and electrolyte depletion leading to thirst, oliguria, and, if untreated, circulatory collapse.
2. Identify cholera as the diagnosis.
   a. Know incubation is 1 to 3 days.
   b. Mode of dissemination—ingestion of contaminated water is most common.
3. Teach preventive techniques.
   a. Purify all drinking water; boil, chlorinate, or use water purification tablets.
   b. Wash all vegetables, fruit, and fish in clean water and cook thoroughly.
   c. Properly dispose of human excrement.

Major Challenges Following a Natural Disaster

Medical/Health

Contaminated food and water (sewage)
Sanitation—decomposing bodies
Interruption of existing/traditional medical/health care
Ease of disease transmission
Infections such as malaria and cholera and secondary infections (pneumonia)
Insect infestation
Skin infections from open wounds and dirty water
Diseases from animal carcasses and spilled chemicals in homes and companies
Contamination from gas/oil in water
Possible epidemics—malaria, cholera, typhoid; and hepatitis A
Mental health concerns—posttraumatic stress disorder

Infrastructure

Destroyed infrastructure contributing to the above issues
Structural damage to homes, hospitals, and other structures
Downed power lines/no electricity
No public transportation
No communication on land lines/cell towers down

TABLE 15-4 Monitoring Survivors of Natural Disasters for Signs of Illness*

Potential Illness	Causative Conditions	Occurrence of Symptoms	Manifested Symptoms	Mode of Transmission
West Nile Virus	Standing water (3 to 4 weeks for mosquito production)	3 to 14 days after mosquito bite	Meningitis, encephalitis, fever, headache, rash, fatigue, muscle aches	Not spread person to person
Leptospirosis	Exposure to infected animals (dogs, rodents, etc.) or water contaminated with urine of infected animals	2 days to 4 weeks	Symptom range: none to high fever, severe headache, jaundice, muscle aches	Not spread person to person
Vibrio vulnificus	Bacteria living in brackish water	Short time after exposure to rapid progression	Pain, redness, swelling, infected wounds, shock	Not spread person to person; susceptible are those with weakened immune systems
Norovirus	Cramped spaces of shelters	Acute onset after exposure	Vomiting, diarrhea, fever, headache, cramps (lasts 3 to 4 days)	Acutely contagious, spread person to person.
Tuberculosis	Cramped spaces of evacuation centers	4 to 12 weeks after exposure	Cough lasting more than 3 weeks, chest pain, fatigue, weight loss, fever, night sweats, chills	Spread through droplet of infected person

***NOTE:** These are the most commonly detected conditions/illnesses following a disaster where thousands of survivors are gathered.

DOCUMENTATION for Natural Disasters

- Safety plan presented to clients
- A basic disaster supply kit is discussed and presented to clients
- Principles of earthquake safety taught to clients
- Clinical features and preventive techniques of diarrhea-related diseases

CRITICAL THINKING Application

Expected Outcomes

- Clients are taught how to create a safety plan for disasters.
- Clients learn how to prepare for an emergency.
- Clients know what to include in a disaster kit.
- Earthquake safety principles are taught to nurses and clients.
- Diarrhea-related diseases are identified early with subsequent interventions.

Unexpected Outcomes	Alternative Actions
Clients and staff do not acknowledge need for a safety plan.	Hold meetings and bring in consultants to present rationale and need for a safety plan for both man-made and natural disasters.
Clients and staff do not have a disaster supply kit.	Discuss need for a supply kit and the components so that clients and staff will follow through and implement the plan.
Staff and clients are not aware of the major challenges after a natural disaster.	Hold meetings to discuss the major challenges so that all are prepared.
People do not understand the need to learn about earthquake safety.	Hold discussion groups about the components of earthquake safety for both clients and hospital staff.
Diarrhea-related diseases occur after a natural disaster (similar to Katrina).	Include the signs and symptoms of these diseases in the preparedness plan so staff will be able to recognize them. Institute preventive measures to combat these diseases immediately after a disaster. Hold meetings to discuss preventive techniques and have the necessary items available (e.g., water purification tablets).

Chapter 15

UNIT 2

Bioterrorism Agents, Antidotes, and Vaccinations

Nursing Process Data

ASSESSMENT Data Base

- Identify epidemiologic features.
  - Rapidly increasing incidence of specific signs and symptoms.
  - Unusual number of clients seeking care, especially with flulike symptoms, fever, respiratory complaints.
  - An endemic disease that rapidly emerges.
  - Clusters of clients from one area.
  - Large numbers of fatalities.
- Identify mode of dissemination and incubation period.
- Assess the appropriate therapy/antidotes necessary to treat victims of a bioterrorist attack.
- Determine clients who could be in a high-risk group for smallpox vaccination.
- Assess need for smallpox vaccination.
- Observe post-vaccination reactions and compare with adverse reactions.
- Assess client's understanding of post-vaccination evaluation.
- Assess need for collecting a clinical specimen to identify a specific bioterrorism agent.
- Identify acute radiation syndrome.
- Assess radiation dose exposure of client.

PLANNING Objectives

- To recognize a possible terrorist attack
- To provide clinical knowledge to recognize features of a biological–chemical–nuclear attack
- To enhance ability to detect a biological attack by distinguishing signs and symptoms of various agents
- To participate in an effective medical response to a terrorist attack
- To provide focused educational content for healthcare professionals as knowledge base
- To possess the skills to initiate an effective response to a terrorist event
- To identify the steps of reconstituting smallpox vaccine
- To be able to recognize post-vaccination reactions (expected and adverse) and instruct clients in these reactions
- To identify need for *vaccinia* immune globulin (VIG)
- To know how to collect and transport a clinical specimen
- To be able to respond to a nuclear disaster

IMPLEMENTATION Procedures

EVALUATION Expected Outcomes

- Epidemiologic features of disease are identified.
- Preparedness plans for hospitals are in place and staff are aware of the components.
- If smallpox vaccinations are imposed, staff are knowledgeable about the procedure.
- Smallpox vaccinations are given with no untoward effects.
- Radiation dose remains at safe levels.
- Healthcare workers learn how to respond safely to a nuclear event.
- Victims of a man-made disaster (chemical, biologic, or nuclear) are treated according to protocols.

Pearson Nursing Student Resources

Find additional review materials at **nursing.pearsonhighered.com**

Prepare for success with NCLEX®-style practice questions and Skill Checklists

Identifying Agents of Biological Terrorism

ANTHRAX

Definition: An acute infectious disease caused by *Bacillus anthracis*, a spore-forming gram-positive bacillus. Human anthrax occurs in three forms: inhalation (the form most dangerous), cutaneous, or gastrointestinal.

Procedure

1. Recognize clinical features. The first line of defense for an outbreak of anthrax is rapid identification.
   a. Inhalation or pulmonary form.
      1. Early signs and symptoms: developing within days, nonspecific flulike illness with malaise, dry cough, mild fever, and headache.
      2. Delayed signs and symptoms: severe respiratory distress, hemodynamic collapse—victim may die, even with antibiotic treatment.
   b. Cutaneous form.
      1. Early signs and symptoms: local skin involvement with intense itching; painless, papular lesions (commonly seen on head, forearms, or hands).
      2. Delayed signs and symptoms: papular lesion turned vesicular, developing into black eschar with edema.
   c. Gastrointestinal form (from contaminated meat).
      1. Early signs and symptoms: abdominal pain, nausea and vomiting, severe diarrhea.
      2. Delayed signs and symptoms: gastrointestinal bleeding and fever; usually fatal after progression to toxemia and sepsis.
2. Know mode of dissemination and incubation period.
   a. Inhalation of spores: aerosol—no person-to-person transmission. Incubation: 2–60 days (usually 48 hr).
   b. Cutaneous: direct contact with skin lesions.
   c. Gastrointestinal ingestion of contaminated food: no person-to-person transmission; incubation: 1–7 days.
3. Manage decontamination.
   a. Remove contaminated clothing.
   b. Instruct clients to shower thoroughly with soap and water.
   c. Instruct personnel to use Standard Precautions.*
   d. Decontaminate environment with 0.5% diluted bleach (1 part to 9 parts water), or EPA-approved germicidal agent.
4. Institute isolation precautions.
   a. Inhalation—Standard Precautions,* wash victim thoroughly (use 0.5% diluted bleach for visible contamination); store clothing in sealed plastic bag with biohazard label.
   b. Cutaneous—contact precautions (gown and gloves).
   c. Gastrointestinal—Standard Precautions.*
5. Assign client placement.
   a. Private room placement *not* necessary.
   b. Airborne transmission does *not* occur.
   c. Skin lesions may be transmitted by direct skin contact only.

*Standard Precautions: See Chapter 14, pg. 410.

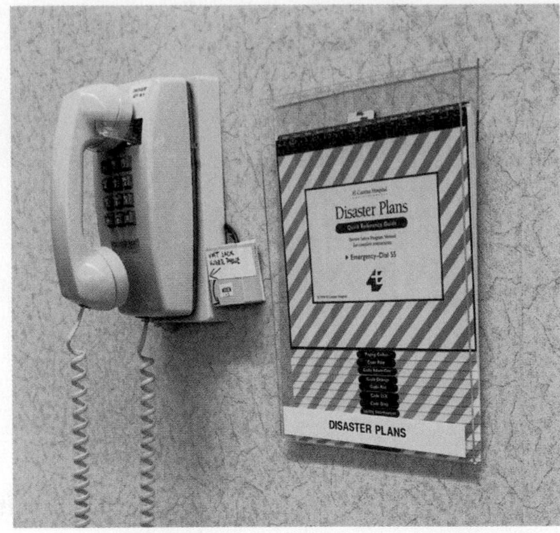

▲ Be familiar with disaster and preparedness plan in the hospital. Perform mock disaster scenarios to maintain skill level and knowledge of procedures if disaster occurs.

Understand the Danger of Biologically Toxic Agents

1. Biological incidents will be the most difficult of all attacks for the community to recognize and effectively coordinate a response.
2. Most viruses are useful as bioterror agents—they cause unique signs and symptoms that require intervention and isolation of the victims to prevent spread.
3. Specific incapacitating viral or bacterial agents slowly produce signs and symptoms.
   a. Signs and symptoms are nonspecific and difficult to recognize; onset of incident may remain unknown for days before symptoms appear.
   b. It may be necessary to identify "clusters" of illness—many victims in one location become sick within a short period of time.
4. If agents are detected early, most can be treated with antibiotics or antivirals.
5. The most common form of agents that could be used in a bioterror attack are bacteria.

6. Implement therapy for anthrax infection.
   a. Ciprofloxacin 400 mg IV q8–12 hr; 500 mg PO q12 hr; doxycycline 200 mg IV (1 dose); 100 mg IV q8–12 hr; or 100 mg PO q12 hr, or amoxicillin may also be ordered.
   b. Continue treatment for 60 days.
   c. Mass casualty—oral therapy with standard doses.

Plague

Definition: Acute, severe bacterial infection, caused by gram-negative bacillus. Seen in bubonic or pneumonic form; caused by bacillus *Yersinia pestis*. A bioterrorism outbreak could be airborne, causing pneumonic plague.

Procedure

1. Recognize clinical features.
   a. Bubonic form.
      1. Swollen, tender lymph nodes (femoral or inguinal commonly most involved).
      2. High temp 103.1–105.8°F (39.5 to 41°C), chills.
      3. Pulse rapid, hypotension.
      4. Extreme exhaustion.
   b. Pneumonic form.
      1. High fever, chills, tachycardia, headache.
      2. Cough with foamy hemoptysis.
      3. Tachypnea and dyspnea.
2. Know mode of dissemination and incubation period.
   a. Transmitted from rodents to humans by infected fleas; incubation 2–8 days.
   b. Human-to-human transmission occurs by inhaling droplets through cough; incubation 1–6 days.
   c. Bioterrorism-related through dispersion of aerosol; incubation: 1–3 days.
3. Manage decontamination—procedure should be done in a room designed for this purpose or at a special site outside the hospital.
   a. Instruct clients to remove clothing and store in closed plastic biohazard bags.
   b. Instruct clients to shower thoroughly with soap and water—include all crevices.
   c. Home decontamination: employ Standard Precautions (gloves, gown, face shield, when necessary).
   d. Use 0.5% diluted bleach or EPA-approved germicidal agent.
4. Institute isolation precautions.
   a. Bubonic form—routine aseptic (Standard) Precautions.
   b. Pneumonic form—add droplet precautions to Standard Precautions (eye protection and surgical mask when within 3 feet of client) until 72 hr of antimicrobial therapy.
5. Assign client placement.
   a. Bubonic form—private isolation room or cohort with clients with similar symptoms.

A Holistic Approach to Coping With Plague

Athens, 200 B.C.: Hippocrates uses precious oils to protect and treat his patients. It is known that essential oils, volatile molecules, float in the air and enter the olfactory system where the limbic system is stimulated to release chemical messages that activate a physical response. Oils have the ability to oxygenate, transport nutrients, and heal. One particular oil blend, "Thieves," was created from research looking back to the fifteenth century when four thieves used clove, rosemary, lemon, cinnamon, and eucalyptus to protect themselves while robbing plague victims in England. The thieves did not die from plague, while hundreds of thousands did. These oils may be used today to protect oneself from certain diseases.

Source: Young, D., & Gary, N. D. (2002). *An introduction to young living essential oils* (10th ed.). Payson, UT: Young Living.

   b. Maintain at least 3 feet between clients when cohorting is not possible.
   c. Do not place client with immunosuppressed client.
6. Implement therapy.
   a. Doxycycline 100 mg 2× daily.
   b. Ciprofloxacin 500 mg 2× daily.

Botulism

Definition: A muscle-paralyzing disease caused by an anaerobic gram-positive bacillus that produces a potent neurotoxin. Food-borne botulism is the most common form; inhalational botulism is most likely to occur through a bioterrorist release of aerosol.

Procedure

1. Recognize clinical features.
   a. Food-borne botulism.
      1. Gastrointestinal symptoms: nausea, vomiting, diarrhea.
      2. Leads to symptoms of inhalational botulism.
   b. Inhalational botulism.
      1. No fever—client is responsive.
      2. Symmetric cranial nerve paralysis: drooping eyelids, blurred vision, diplopia, difficulty swallowing, dry mouth.
      3. Symptoms progress to paralysis of arms, respiratory muscles, and legs.
      4. Symptoms may be confused with Guillain-Barrè syndrome or myasthenia gravis.
2. Know mode of dissemination and incubation period.
   a. Food-borne botulism: generally transmitted through toxin-contaminated food; incubation is 12–36 hr after ingestion.
   b. Inhalational botulism: transmitted through aerosolization of the toxin. Incubation is 24–72 hr postexposure.

3. Manage decontamination.
   a. Client does not require decontamination.
   b. Contaminated clothing washed with commercial soap.
4. Institute isolation precautions.
   a. No evidence of person-to-person transmission.
   b. Standard Precautions for clients.
5. Assign client placement: client room selection and care according to facility policy. Client-to-client transmission does not occur.
6. Implement therapy.
   a. Early recognition of botulism important for administration of antitoxin that may stop or reduce paralysis.
   b. Administer trivalent botulinum antitoxin (per CDC orders); requires skin testing due to 95% hypersensitivity reactions.
   c. Monitor client for respiratory failure and provide supportive care.

Typhoidal Tularemia

Definition: A disease caused by *Francisella tularensis* bacterium. It is extremely infectious and can be transmitted via aerosol or contaminated water or food.

Procedure

1. Recognize clinical features.
   a. Early symptoms: headache, cough, fever, and chills, malaise.
   b. Delayed symptoms: pharyngeal ulcers, pleuritic chest pain, pneumonia, pericarditis—may progress to respiratory failure.
2. Know mode of dissemination and incubation period.
   a. Bioterrorism mode is aerosol.
   b. This disease may not be recognized unless a bioterrorism attack is suspected.
   c. Incubation period: 2–12 days (average 3–5 days) after exposure.
3. Manage decontamination: general decontamination measures for clothing of infected person—shower with soap or use 0.5% diluted bleach. Because there is no person-to-person transmission, no other measures are necessary.
4. Institute isolation precautions.
   a. This disease is not transmitted person to person, so isolation measures are not required.
   b. Standard Precautions recommended.
5. Assign client placement: cohort clients and do not place with immunosuppressed clients.
6. Implement therapy: ciprofloxacin 250 mg PO q12 hr × 14 days, streptomycin 15 mg/kg BID IM × 10–14 days, or gentamicin 1.5 mg/kg q8 hr IV × 10–14 days.

Viral Hemorrhagic Fever (VHF)

Definition: An infection caused by agents such as Ebola, Marburg, Lassa, Argentine, yellow, and dengue fevers. These viruses could be life-threatening (moderately high lethality) and could be delivered by aerosol in a biological attack.

Procedure

1. Recognize clinical features.
   a. Each illness has unique clinical manifestations; however, some features are similar.
   b. Characterized by abrupt onset of fever, myalgia, headache, prostration.
   c. Other signs and symptoms are nausea and vomiting, diarrhea, pain in abdomen and chest, cough, and pharyngitis.
   d. A maculopapular rash, prominent on the trunk, develops in most clients 5 days after onset of illness.
   e. Bleeding manifestations may occur as the disease progresses. Even though it is rare for this life-threatening condition to occur, bleeding (intracranial hemorrhage) could result, hence the term hemorrhagic fever.
2. Know mode of dissemination and incubation period.
   a. Viruses are zoonotic (animal-borne), but can be spread person-to-person.
   b. All viruses (except dengue fever) could be spread by aerosol in a biological attack.
   c. Incubation period: usually 5–10 days, with a range of 2–21 days.
3. Manage decontamination: the virus is transmitted person-to-person; decontamination with overt attack: victim undresses, showers with soap or 0.5% diluted bleach.

EVIDENCE-BASED PRACTICE

Lessons Learned From a Full-Scale Bioterrorism Exercise

In May 2000, three hospitals in metropolitan Denver and officials from local, state, and federal agencies participated in a simulated bioterrorism attack exercise involving the simulated release of *Yersinia pestis* aerosol that infected 2,000 people. During the attack, decision making became inefficient and many problems were identified. The single most important lesson learned from this experience was that three aspects must receive equal effort: controlling the spread of disease, triage, and treatment of ill persons.

In April 2005, there was a federal terrorism response exercise developed by the U.S. Department of Homeland Security. The drill involved 84 acute-care hospitals in New Jersey and Connecticut, nearly 10,000 simulated deaths, and more than 22,000 volunteers. (See results, pg. 467.)

Source: Hoffman, R., & Norton. J. (2000, Dec.). Colorado Dept. of Public Health and Environment. *Emerging Infectious Diseases*, 6(6), 652–653. Walker-Cillo, G. (2006, April). Bioterrorism: We put our plan to the test. *RN Magazine* 69(4), 36–41.

4. Institute isolation procedures.
   a. Communicable person-to-person; risk is highest after infection has progressed. Isolation precautions (including airborne and contact), including respirators, face shields, gowns, gloves, shoe and head covers.
   b. Negative-pressure ventilated rooms with an anteroom.
5. Assign client placement.
   a. Clients should be under strict isolation precautions, including a negative-pressure room with anteroom.
   b. Only clients with the same form of hemorrhagic infection should be cohorted.
6. Implement therapy.
   a. Primarily supportive.
   b. Ribavirin, 30 mg/kg IV × 1 dose; 15 mg/kg IV q6 hr × 4 days.

Q Fever

Definition: A rickettsial organism (*Coxiella burnetii*) naturally found in sheep, cattle, and goats. Bioterrorism mode of dissemination will be aerosol or food supply sabotage.

Procedure

1. Recognize clinical features.
   a. Early signs and symptoms: headache, fever, chills, malaise, diaphoresis, anorexia; insidious onset with nonspecific flulike symptoms.
   b. Delayed signs and symptoms: double vision, sore throat, cough, chest pain, nuchal rigidity, encephalitis, hallucinations, weight loss.
   c. Differential diagnosis: atypical pneumonias.
2. Know mode of dissemination and incubation period.
   a. Aerosol or food supply.
   b. Incubation period: 10–40 days (average 10–14 days).
3. Manage decontamination.
   a. Have victim undress and shower thoroughly with soap. May use 0.5% diluted bleach.
   b. Clean environment with 0.5% diluted bleach.
4. Institute isolation precautions: none required. Rarely transmitted person to person. Use Standard Precautions.
5. Assign client placement: transmissibility rare, so clients can be cohorted.
6. Implement therapy.
   a. Tetracycline 500 mg PO q6 hr × 5–7 days; doxycycline 100 mg PO q12 hr × 5–7 days.
   b. Continue treatment for 2 days post-febrile condition.

Ricin Toxin

Definition: Produced from the castor bean plant and secreted in castor seeds; *Ricinus communis* is a cytotoxin that blocks protein synthesis, killing the cell.

Procedure

1. Recognize clinical features.
   a. Signs and symptoms depend on route of exposure. Diagnosis is difficult. ELISA test of blood will identify ricin.
      1. Ingestion: nausea, vomiting, diarrhea, and severe abdominal cramps occur before vascular collapse (GI bleeding), leading to death on third day.
      2. Aerosol—inhalation: cough, fever, hypothermia, and hypotension (usually nonspecific symptoms); cardiovascular collapse leads to death in 36–48 hr.
   b. This biotoxin has been used by assassins; causes death within minutes when placed on the skin. In 2003, ricin was found in a terrorist cell in England—potential use unknown.
2. Know mode of dissemination and incubation period.
   a. Ricin will be delivered via the castor bean through a chemical process (ingested) or through inhalation method.
   b. Incubation period is within hours to days (ingestion: 3 days; inhalation 3–4 days).
3. Manage decontamination.
   a. Ingested biotoxin does not require decontamination.
   b. Aerosol exposure—victim should shower with soap or use 0.5% diluted bleach.
4. Institute isolation precautions. This toxin is not transmitted to others, but Standard Precautions should be implemented.
5. Assign client placement. There is no communicability person to person or transport through the skin, so placement is planned to protect client's immune system.
6. Implement therapy. There is no approved antitoxin treatment or prophylaxis (vaccination) at this time.
   a. Therapy is supportive; give oxygen and hydration.
   b. If there is ingestion, GI decontamination would be implemented.

Smallpox

Definition: An acute viral disease caused by the *variola virus*. It was eradicated worldwide in 1977, and in the early 1980s, routine vaccinations were discontinued. Because there is a large nonimmune population, authorities fear it could be a bioterrorism weapon, transmitted via the airborne route as aerosol or by infected human vectors.

Procedure

1. Recognize clinical features.
   a. Initially, symptoms resemble an acute viral illness like influenza with high fever, myalgia, headache, and backache.
   b. Rash appears (when smallpox becomes most contagious), progressing from macules to papules (in 1 week) to vesicles, and scabs over in 1–2 weeks.
   c. Distinguishing rash from varicella (chicken pox): smallpox has a synchronous onset on face and extremities, rather than arising in "bunches," starting on the trunk.

Dangers of Smallpox Vaccination: The Debate Continues

Smallpox vaccination results in 2–4 deaths per million—as many as 1,000 deaths could occur if everyone in the United States were to be vaccinated. In 2003, there were 300 million doses of vaccine available, enough to vaccinate everyone in the United States. Live virus is dangerous, especially to those who have a compromised immune system, those with cardiovascular conditions, and those with skin diseases, such as eczema and psoriasis. Those who were already vaccinated 30 years ago have been tested and some have been found to have what appears to be a significant level of immunity, but is it enough? Others who received vaccinations in the 1970s and earlier are believed to have no useful immunity. There is still a debate: Should the vaccinations be voluntary? Should only first responders and emergency personnel receive vaccinations? Should only those who were never vaccinated receive vaccinations?

2. Know mode of dissemination and incubation period.
   a. Smallpox is transmitted by large and small respiratory droplets; thus both respiratory and oral secretions spread the disease, as well as lesion drainage and contaminated objects such as bed linens.
   b. Clients are considered more infectious if they are coughing or have a hemorrhagic form of the disease.
   c. Vaccination effective if given within 3–4 days.
   d. Incubation: 7–17 days; average is 12 days.
3. Manage decontamination.
   a. Decontamination of clients is not indicated with smallpox.
   b. Careful management using contact precautions of potentially contaminated equipment and environmental surfaces—clean, disinfect, and sterilize when possible.
   c. Dedicated or disposable equipment for each client should be used.
4. Institute strict isolation precautions *immediately*.
   a. Airborne and contact precautions in addition to Standard Precautions; includes gloves, gown, eye shields, shoe covers, and correctly fitted masks (very important).
   b. Airborne precautions: Microorganisms transmitted by airborne droplet nuclei (particles 5 μm or smaller).
      1. Respiratory protection when entering client's room (particulate respirators, N95); must meet National Institute for Occupational Safety and Health (NIOSH) standards for particulate respirators.
      2. Isolate in room under negative pressure with high-efficiency particle air filtration.
   c. Contact precautions: Clients known to be infected or colonized with organisms that can be transmitted by direct contact or indirect contact with contaminated surfaces.
      1. Wash hands using antimicrobial agent when entering and leaving room.
      2. Don gloves when entering room.
      3. Wear gown for all client contact or contact with client's environment.
      4. Wear gown when entering room and remove before leaving isolation area.
5. Assign client placement.
   a. Rooms must meet ventilation and engineering requirements for airborne precautions.
      1. Monitored negative air pressure with 6–12 air exchanges/hr.
      2. Appropriate discharge of air to outdoors or high-efficiency filtration of air.
   b. Door to room must remain closed; private room is preferred. Clients with same diagnosis may be cohorted.
   c. Limit transport of clients; use appropriate mask if unavoidable.
6. Implement therapy.
   a. Post-exposure immunization (*vaccinia* virus) is available.
      1. Vaccination alone if given within 3–4 days of exposure.
      2. Passive immunization (VIG) if greater than 3 days post-exposure.
      3. VIG given at 0.6 mL/kg IM. See administration skill, pg. 480. Check with CDC for up-to-date recommendations.
   b. Prophylactic care with precautions.

Prioritizing High-Risk Groups for Smallpox Vaccination

Procedure

1. Identify healthcare workers. ▶ ***Rationale:*** All persons potentially exposed to the virus must be evaluated for possible vaccination.
   a. Personnel involved in evaluation, care, or transportation of confirmed, probable, or suspected smallpox clients.
   b. Laboratory personnel involved in collection or processing of clinical specimens.
   c. Other persons with increased likelihood of contact with infectious materials from a smallpox client (laundry or medical waste handlers).

   d. Other persons or staff who have a reasonable probability of contact with smallpox clients or infectious materials (e.g., selected law enforcement, emergency response, or military personnel).
   e. Because of potential for greater spread of smallpox in a hospital setting due to aerosolization of the virus from a severely ill client, all individuals in the hospital may be vaccinated.
2. Identify clients exposed to the smallpox virus. ▸ ***Rationale:*** The sooner clients are identified, the earlier they can receive smallpox vaccination, which must be given within 4 days to be effective.
   a. Persons who were exposed to initial release of the virus.
   b. Persons who had face-to-face, household, or close-proximity contact.
3. Determine contraindications for vaccination of noncontacts. ▸ ***Rationale:*** Persons with certain medical conditions are known to have a higher risk of developing severe complications after vaccination with *Vaccinia* vaccine.
   a. Persons with diseases or conditions that cause immunodeficiency, such as HIV, AIDS, leukemia, lymphoma, persons with cardiac conditions, therapy with alkylating agents, antimetabolites, radiation, or large doses of corticosteroids.
   b. Persons with serious, life-threatening allergies to the antibiotics polymyxin B, streptomycin, tetracycline, or neomycin. ▸ ***Rationale:*** Dryvax contains trace amounts of these antibiotics.
   c. Persons who have ever been diagnosed with eczema, even if the condition is mild or not presently active.
   d. Women who are pregnant.
   e. Persons with other acute or chronic skin conditions such as atopic dermatitis, burns, impetigo, or varicella zoster (shingles). These persons should not be vaccinated until the condition resolves.

Clinical Alert

A household member who has eczema or a history of eczema who has been exposed to a recently vaccinated household member is at higher risk for developing a post-vaccine complication from the vaccination site of the vaccinated person.

Reconstituting *Vaccinia* Vaccine for Smallpox

Equipment

Vial of vaccine (Dryvax)
Prefilled syringe of diluent
Clean or latex-free gloves
Biohazard bag and label

Procedure

1. Remove vaccine vial from refrigerated storage and allow vial to come to room temperature. ▸ ***Rationale:*** Vaccine must be at room temperature to be reconstituted.
2. Wash hands and don gloves. ▸ ***Rationale:*** Personnel must be protected from touching vaccine.
3. Lift tab of aluminum seal of vaccine vial. DO NOT BREAK OFF OR TEAR DOWN TAB.
4. Place vaccine vial upright on a hard, flat surface.
5. Remove cap from prefilled syringe of diluent. ▸ ***Rationale:*** Diluent is required for reconstitution before administration.
6. Inject 0.25 mL of diluent into vaccine vial. ▸ ***Rationale:*** This amount of diluent reconstitutes vaccine.
7. Withdraw needle and syringe and discard in appropriate biohazard sharps container. ▸ ***Rationale:*** This needle and syringe are now contaminated with the vaccine.
8. Allow vaccine vial to stand undisturbed for 3–5 minutes. Then, if necessary, swirl vial gently. ▸ ***Rationale:*** Complete reconstitution of vaccine must take place.
9. In the space provided on vaccine vial label, record date and time diluent was added. The vaccine is now ready for use. ▸ ***Rationale:*** Use reconstituted vaccine for time period recommended by manufacturer if stored at 35.6–46.4°F (2–8°C) when not in actual use.
10. Dispose of diluent syringe, needle used for diluent reconstitution of vaccine, and any gauze or cotton that came in contact with vaccine as follows: in a biohazard bag labeled to burn, boil, or autoclave before final disposal. ▸ ***Rationale:*** Staff could be inadvertently inoculated by touching these items.

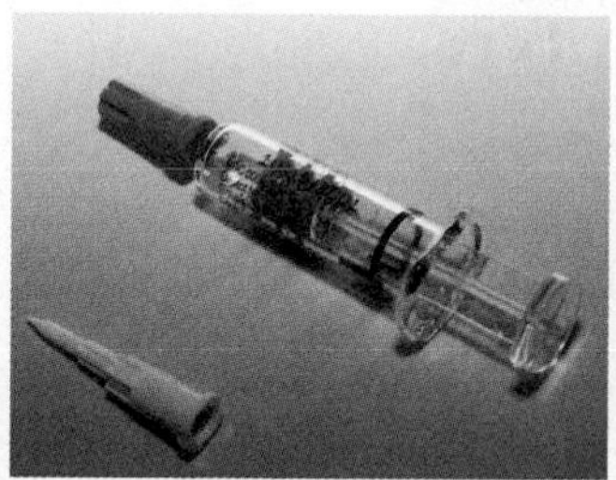

▲ Prefilled syringe of diluent. This will be injected into vaccine vial to reconstitute.

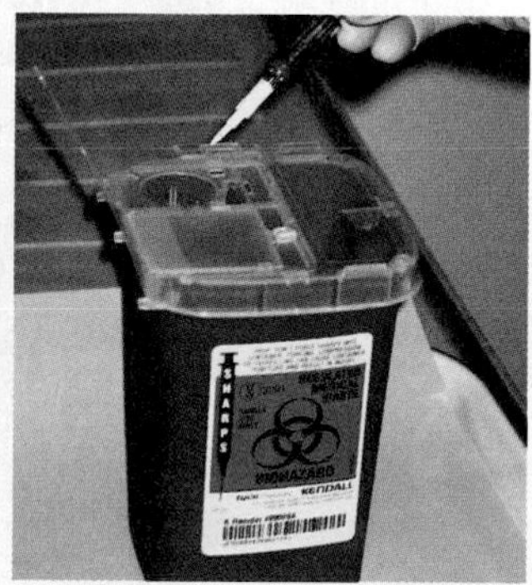

▲ After injecting diluent into vaccine vial, discard syringe into biohazard container.

Administering Reconstituted Smallpox Vaccine

Equipment

Clean or latex-free gloves
Vaccine vial
Sterile container
Swab if necessary
Sterile bifurcated (two-pronged) needle
Sterile gauze
4 × 4 gauze bandage
Tape

Preparation

1. Identify client(s) to be vaccinated according to public health protocol.
2. Issue information client must receive before smallpox vaccination.
   a. Preapproved vaccine information entitled "What You Need to Know about Smallpox Vaccinations."
   b. An 11-minute CDC video describing the process and results of a vaccination.
   c. The understanding that vaccination is voluntary.
   d. Personal information packet and signed permission form.
3. Obtain reconstituted *Vaccinia* vaccine vial from pharmacy. (Public Health Centers are issued vials that hold 100 doses that are administered at scheduled times.)
4. Inspect vaccine for particulate matter or discoloration; if present, do not use.
5. Gather equipment.
6. Perform hand hygiene.

NOTE: Vaccinators must attend classes, read appropriate material, and watch a CDC video before administering vaccination.

Procedure

1. Don clean or latex-free gloves.
2. Remove rubber stopper from vaccine vial and place in sterile container. ▸ ***Rationale:*** Stopper should remain sterile as it will be used to recap the vial containing vaccine.
3. Choose site of vaccination—one that is easily accessible for vaccination and evaluation of vaccine "take" on post-vaccination day 7. The outer aspect of the upper right arm over the insertion of the deltoid muscle is the standard (and CDC recommended) vaccination site. ▸ ***Rationale:*** This prevents confusion with vaccination site from a previous vaccination.
4. Ask client if he/she has applied lotion or anything on upper arm. If so, wash with soap and water.
5. Clean vaccination site only if grossly contaminated. Let dry thoroughly. Under no circumstances apply alcohol to the skin (per CDC 2002). ▸ ***Rationale:*** Alcohol will inactivate vaccine deposited on skin.
6. Dip point of a sterile bifurcated needle into vial of reconstituted vaccine and withdraw needle perpendicular to the floor.

NOTE: Needles are designed to hold designated dose of vaccine (2.5 μL) between needle prongs to allow delivery to skin surface.

7. Hold skin of upper arm taut and place wrist firmly on the arm.
8. Hold needle at a 90° angle (perpendicular) to skin and apply up-and-down (perpendicular) strokes rapidly within a 5-mm diameter area.
   a. First-time smallpox vaccination recipients: Deliver 3 strokes with a bifurcated needle. Observe for blood appearing within 15–30 seconds. If blood does not appear, deliver 3 additional punctures with the same needle *without* reinserting needle into the vaccine vial. ▸ ***Rationale:*** New guidelines from the Advisory Committee on Immunization Practices (APIC) were

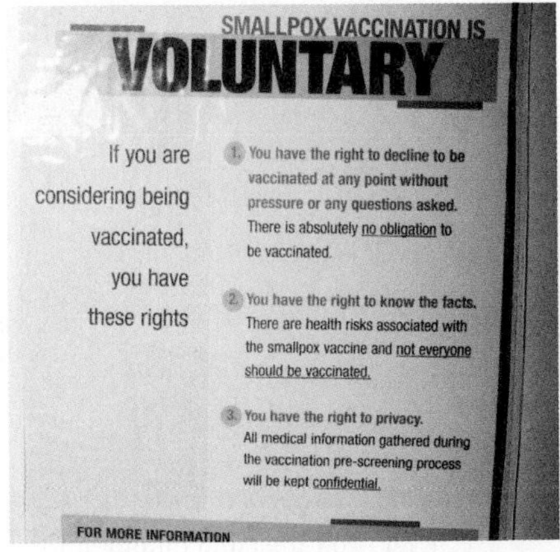

1 It is important that client understand that smallpox vaccination is voluntary.

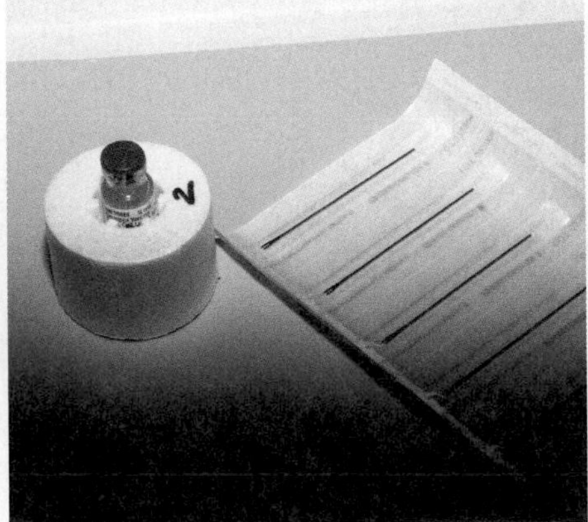

2 Obtain reconstituted vaccine vial (which was stored at 2° to 8°C) from pharmacy.

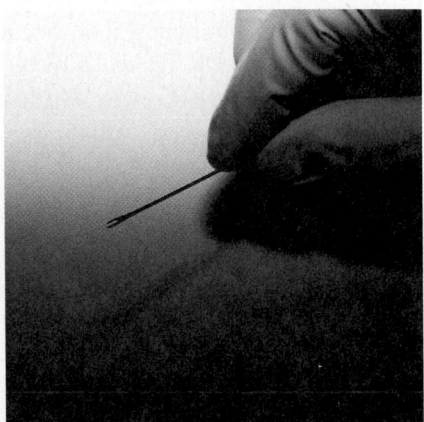

3 Sterile bifurcated (two-pronged) needle is provided individually wrapped.

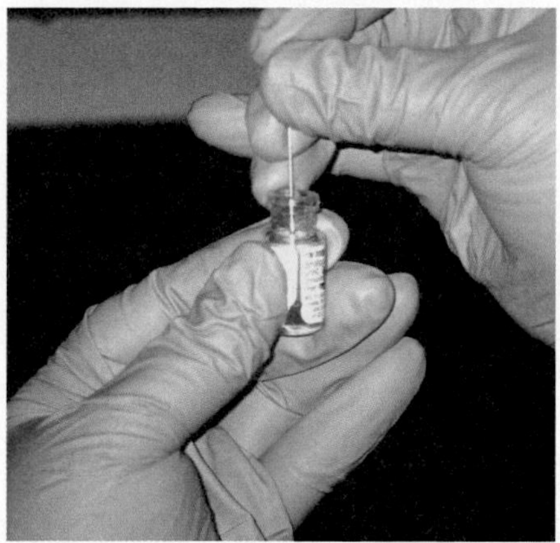

4 Dip point of bifurcated needle into vial of reconstituted vaccine.

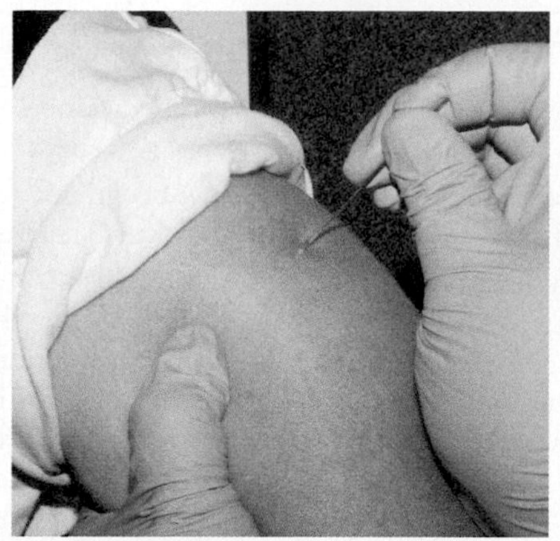

5 Hold needle at 90° angle and apply rapid strokes within a 5-mm diameter.

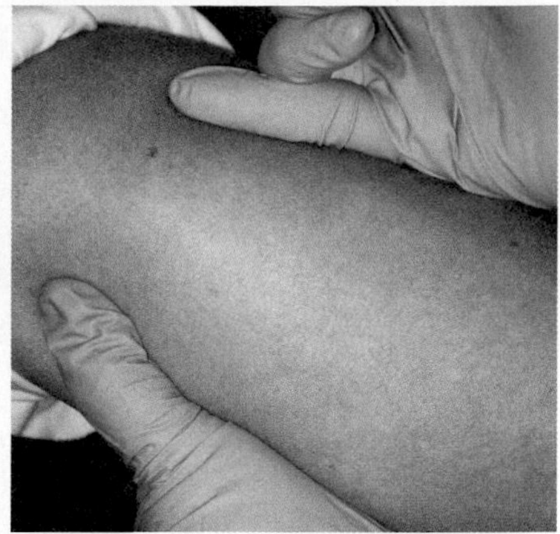

6 Wait for a trace of blood at site to indicate successful vaccine delivery.

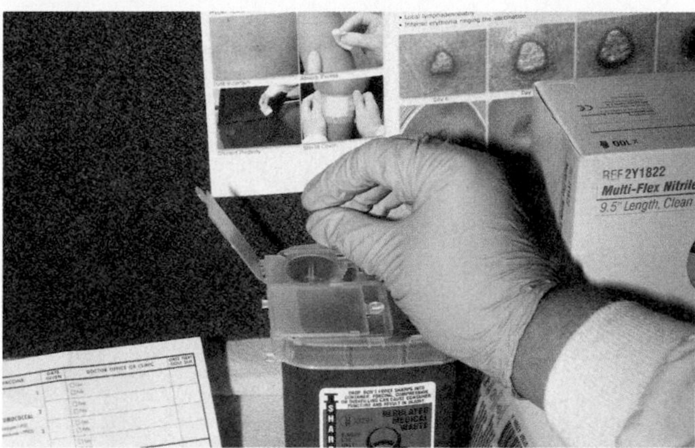

7 Dispose of bifurcated needle in puncture-resistant medical waste sharps container.

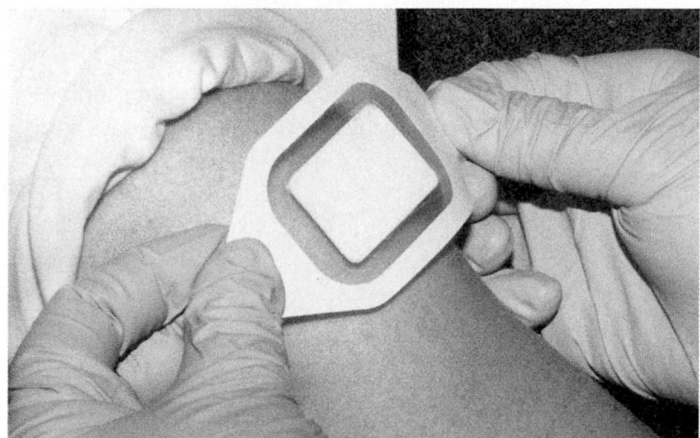

8 Cover vaccination site with semipermeable dressing.

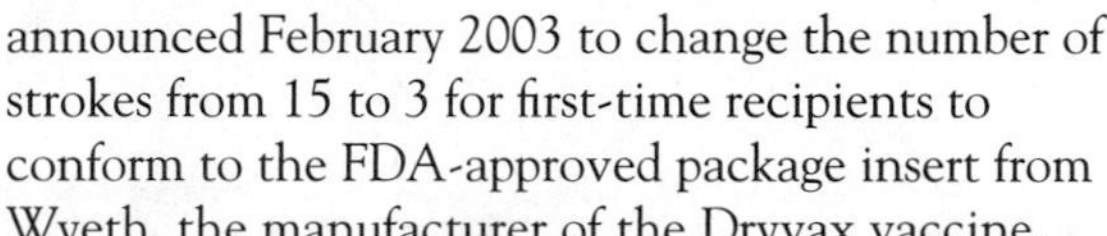

announced February 2003 to change the number of strokes from 15 to 3 for first-time recipients to conform to the FDA-approved package insert from Wyeth, the manufacturer of the Dryvax vaccine.

   b. Revaccination recipients: Deliver 15 up-and-down strokes with a bifurcated needle.

9. Examine for a trace of blood at vaccination site, which usually takes 15 to 30 seconds to appear. ▸ ***Rationale:*** This indicates successful vaccine delivery.
10. Cover vaccination site with gauze bandage and tape or semipermeable dressing. ▸ ***Rationale:*** This prevents contact transmission of virus to unvaccinated persons (people with contraindications to vaccination) or inadvertent inoculation of another body site.
    a. Keep vaccination covered until scab separates.
    b. Change dressing if exudate builds up. The CDC recommends changing dressing daily, or every 3 days.

NOTE: The CDC recommends using a semipermeable dressing (Tegaderm) when at a work site, in public, or for showering. When site is totally blocked from air, skin at site might soften and wear away.

Clinical Alert

Do not redip needle into vaccine vial if needle has touched skin. This contaminates the vial.

Clinical Alert

When administering smallpox vaccination, strokes should be made rapidly and be sufficiently vigorous to elicit a trace of blood at vaccination site. If trace of blood does not appear, strokes have not been sufficiently vigorous and procedure should be repeated.

11. Dispose of bifurcated needle in a puncture-resistant medical waste sharps container. ▸ ***Rationale:*** Bifurcated needle is for single usage only.
12. Instruct client to keep site dry and not to rub or scratch vaccination site.

NOTE: Vaccinia virus may be recovered from vaccination site, beginning at the time of development of a papule (2–5 days postvaccination) until scab separates from skin (14–21 days postvaccination) and underlying skin has healed.

13. Recap vial with sterile rubber stopper and store capped vial at 35.6–46.4°F (2–8°C.) Note number of doses left in vial. ▸ ***Rationale:*** This temperature will allow vaccine to be saved for subsequent use.
14. Remove gloves, discard in appropriate hazardous waste receptacle, and perform hand hygiene.

Understanding Post-Vaccination Reactions

Procedure

1. Identify persons who should be revaccinated. ▶ ***Rationale:*** If the vaccination did not take, the individual will remain vulnerable to the smallpox virus.
   a. They will have delayed type of skin sensitivity consisting of *erythema only* within 24–48 hr.
   b. This represents a response to inert protein in a previously sensitized person and can occur in a highly immunized person or in individuals with little or no immunity; it is indistinguishable from the immediate or immune reaction.
2. Confirm successful vaccination and enter results in client's record. ▶ ***Rationale:*** So that the client will not have to be revaccinated.
   a. Presence of a pustular lesion in previously unvaccinated persons.
   b. Pustular lesion or an area of definite induration or congestion surrounding a central lesion 7 days after revaccination in a previously vaccinated person.
   c. Vaccinees who do not exhibit a "major" reaction at vaccination site on day 7 should be revaccinated.
3. Recognize adverse reactions. ▶ ***Rationale:*** Identifying an adverse reaction is important so that VIG may be administered.
   a. The overall risk of serious complications after vaccination with *vaccinia* vaccine appears to be low.
   b. Complications occur more frequently in persons receiving their first dose of vaccine, and among young children.
   c. The *most frequent* complications of vaccination are inadvertent inoculation, generalized vaccinia, eczema vaccination, progressive vaccinia, and post-vaccination encephalitis.
   d. Unexpected cardiovascular complications resulted in reevaluation of the vaccination program in 2003.
4. Document results on vaccination record in client's chart.

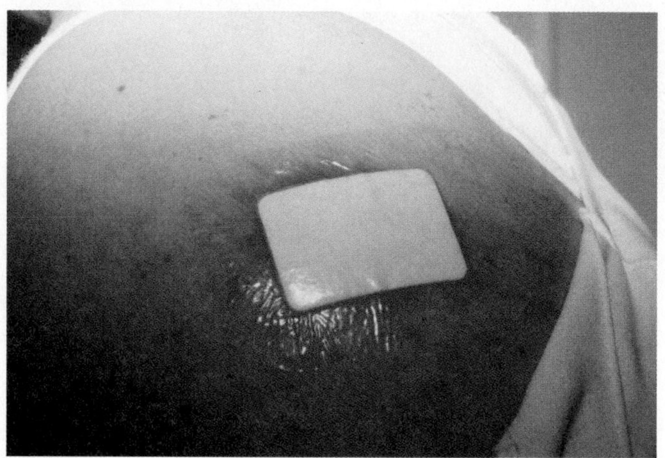

1 Example of semi-permeable dressing covering site at eighth day post-vaccination.

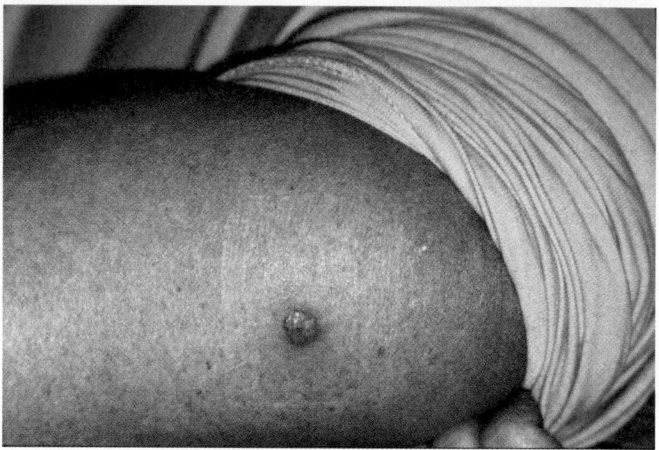

2 Example of pustular lesion 8 days following revaccination in a previously vaccinated person.

Instructing Client in Post-Vaccination Evaluation

Procedure

1. Tell client that successful vaccination is normally associated with tenderness, redness, swelling, and a lesion at the vaccination site.
2. Instruct client that vaccination may also be associated with fever for a few days, malaise, and enlarged, tender lymph nodes in the axilla of the vaccinated arm.

NOTE: These symptoms are more common in older children and clients receiving their first dose of vaccine (15%–20%) than in persons being revaccinated (0%–10%).

3. Check for inoculation site becoming reddened and pruritic 3–4 days after vaccination and every 3 days following; place results in the record. ▶ ***Rationale:*** This is a primary reaction after vaccination.
   a. A vesicle surrounded by a red areola enlarges, becomes umbilicated, and then pustular by the 7th to 11th day after vaccination.
   b. The pustule begins to dry, redness subsides, and lesion becomes crusted between 2nd and 3rd week.

4. Inform client that by the end of the 3rd week, scab falls off, leaving a permanent scar that at first is pink in color, but eventually becomes flesh-colored.
5. Instruct person who has been previously vaccinated (a partially immune person) that an attenuated primary vaccine site reaction will occur with the following characteristics.
   a. Absence of fever or constitutional symptoms.
   b. Papule by 3rd day that becomes vesicular by 5th to 7th day and dries shortly thereafter.
   c. A relatively small vesicle and areola.
   d. Scar, if present, is usually insignificant and disappears within 1–2 years.

Clinical Alert

Instruct client to wash hands thoroughly after touching vaccination site to prevent inadvertent inoculation at another site.

EVIDENCE-BASED PRACTICE

Complications From Inadvertent Inoculation

Inadvertent smallpox inoculation at other sites accounts for about 50% of all complications after primary and revaccination. This complication of vaccinia vaccination occurs at a rate of about 1 in 2,000 primary vaccinations and usually results from autoinoculation when virus is transferred by hand from the site of vaccination to other areas. The most common sites involved are the face, eyelid, nose, mouth, genitalia, and rectum. Most lesions will heal without specific therapy.

Source: Vaccination guidelines for state and local health agencies (2002). Centers for Disease Control, U.S. Department of Health and Human Services.

Identifying Indications for *Vaccinia* Immune Globulin (VIG) Administration

Procedure

1. Identify post-vaccination complications for which VIG may be indicated. ▸ ***Rationale:*** VIG is indicated for some complications, but not others.
   a. Eczema vaccinatum.
   b. Progressive *vaccinia* (*vaccinia* necrosum).
   c. Severe generalized *vaccinia* if client has a toxic condition or serious underlying illness.
   d. Inadvertent inoculation of eye or eyelid without vaccinial keratitis.
2. Check physician's orders for VIG treatment of complications due to *vaccinia* vaccination.
3. Administer VIG intramuscularly (IM) as early as possible after onset of symptoms.
4. Give VIG in divided doses over a 24–36-hr period. Doses may be repeated at 2–3-day intervals until no new lesions appear. ▸ ***Rationale:*** Because the therapeutic dose of VIG may be large (e.g., 0.6 mL/kg body weight), it is given in divided doses.
5. Instruct staff that VIG is not indicated for treatment of post-vaccination encephalitis and is contraindicated for vaccinial keratitis.

Possible Adverse Reactions to Smallpox Vaccination

- *Inadvertent Inoculation at Another Site*: Virus is transferred by hand from vaccination site to another body area. Most lesions heal without therapy.
- *Generalized Vaccinia*: Bloodborne dissemination of *Vaccinia* virus resulting in vesicular rash of varying extent (occurs 1 in 5,000 vaccinations). Usually self-limiting.
- *Eczema Vaccinatum*: Skin lesions that cover area affected by eczema or a chronic skin condition. Illness (fever, lymphadenopathy) is usually mild, but can be fatal (occurs 1 in 26,000 primary vaccinations).
- *Progressive Vaccinia*: Severe and potentially fatal; occurs in persons with immune deficiencies. Characterized by failure of lesion to heal with progressive necrosis. VIG is used to treat this condition.
- *Post-Vaccination Encephalitis*: All symptoms of encephalitis occur between 8 and 15 days post-vaccination. Incidence is 1 in 300,000 vaccinations, and there is no cure.
- *Cardiac complications*: Heart inflammation (myocarditis, pericarditis), angina, and a few heart attacks have occurred. Incidence is 1 in 20,000 individuals vaccinated for the first time. Experts are evaluating the connection.

Collecting and Transporting Specimens

Equipment

Disposable gown
1 N95 mask
Eye shield
Shoe covers
2 pair gloves
2 zip-closure plastic bags
2 biohazard bags
Label for specimen and chain of custody form

Procedure

1. Acquire and follow specific recommendations for diagnostic sampling of the specific agent.
   a. Perform all sampling according to Standard Precautions. ▸ ***Rationale:*** For protection of healthcare workers.
   b. Check that laboratory has capacity and equipment to handle specific sample. There are four laboratory levels.

NOTE: Proposed laboratory levels (A through D): local clinical labs for minimal identification of an agent; county or state labs; state and other large labs with advanced capacity for testing; and level D, CDC, or select Department of Defense labs with Bio Safety Level (BSL) testing capacity.

2. Wear protective gear when entering environment where potential for exposure exists. ▸ ***Rationale:*** It is important to safeguard health and safety of persons collecting specimen.
   a. Disposable gown.
   b. Properly fitted N95 mask.

NOTE: Mask will not protect males with beards.

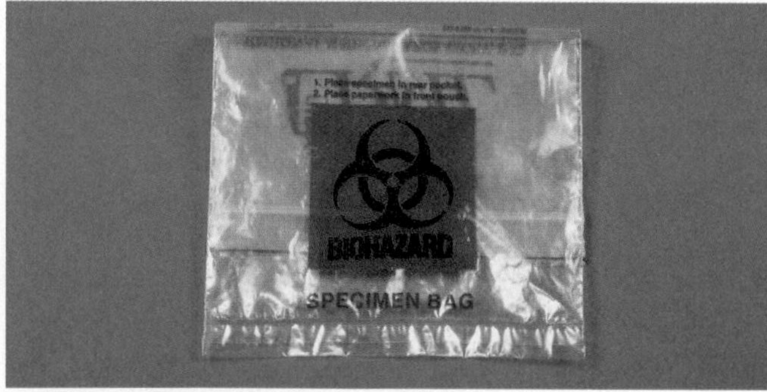

▲ Biohazard specimen bag.

   c. Gloves.
   d. Eye shield.
   e. Shoe covers if indicated.
3. Choose gown with sleeve cuffs that can be covered by stretching gloves up and over cuff. ▸ ***Rationale:*** No skin should be exposed.
4. Collect specimen and place in appropriate container (zip-closure plastic bag, sealed).
5. Remove original gloves handling specimen, and place in biohazard container. ▸ ***Rationale:*** These gloves may have been contaminated.
6. Don new pair of gloves.
7. Place specimen bag in second zip-closure bag and seal, or if specimen is large, in trash bag.
8. Remove protective gear and place in biohazard bag. ▸ ***Rationale:*** Protective equipment may be contaminated.
9. Label specimen on outside of bag with appropriate label: date, person collecting specimen, location, and contact person.
10. Wash hands or complete hand hygiene.
11. Document specimen collection in duplicate, fill out worksheet, "Possible Biological Agent Exposure Contact." ▸ ***Rationale:*** This will warn staff who transport specimen to protect themselves.
12. Give to person designated for this location.
13. Collect an acute phase serum sample, as well as a later convalescent serum sample. ▸ ***Rationale:*** The two samples will be compared as follow-up study.
14. Transport specimens by coordinating with local, state health departments, and the FBI.
    a. Include a chain of custody form with specimen information from moment of collection, completed each time specimen is transferred to another party.
    b. Plan ahead for care of specimens by having appropriate packaging materials and transport media available.

Clinical Alert

Be careful not to contaminate outside of either of the two disposal bags during handling.

Identifying Chemical Agent Exposure

Procedure

NOTE: Chemical agents may be solid, liquid, or gas; there are numerous ways of disseminating the agent.

1. **Pulmonary agents:** such as chlorine, chloropicrin, or phosgene, when inhaled produce pulmonary edema with little damage to other pulmonary tissues (with resulting hypoxemia) and hypovolemia.
   a. Immediate symptoms are irritation of eyes, nose, and upper airways—often not distinctive enough to be recognized as chemical agent exposure.
   b. Two to 24 hr later, victim develops chest tightness, shortness of breath with exertion (later, at rest).

c. Cough produces clear, frothy sputum, fluid that leaked into lungs.
d. If symptoms begin soon after exposure, death may occur within hours.

2. **Cyanide agents:** may be gases or solids, such as hydrogen cyanide or cyanogens chloride; with high concentrations, death occurs in 6–8 minutes.
   a. Initial symptoms are burning irritation of eyes, nose, and airways, and smell of bitter almonds.
   b. Victim's skin may be acyanotic, cherry-red (oxygenated venous blood), or normal.
   c. Large amount of gas inhaled: hyperventilation, convulsions, cessation of breathing (3–5 minutes), and no heartbeat (6–10 minutes).
3. **Vesicant agents:** cause vesicles or blisters. Common agents are sulfur mustard and lewisite. More lethal than pulmonary agents and cyanide.
   a. Mustard—initial symptoms not observable. Effects begin hours after exposure: erythema, burning and itching with blisters; burning of eyes; airway pain, sore throat, nonproductive cough.

Clinical Alert

Suspect a chemical agent exposure if healthcare facility is presented with several nontrauma clients with similar symptoms.

   b. Lewisite—oily liquid that results in topical damage. Vapor causes immediate pain, burning, and irritation of eyes, skin, and upper airways.

NOTE: This is distinguishing feature of lewisite versus mustard when initial symptoms are not observable.

   Cellular damage occurs that can result in hypovolemic shock.

4. **Nerve agents:** liquids or vapors that are the most toxic of all chemical agents. Common agents are Sarin, tabun, Soman, GF, and VX.
   a. Nerve agents block the enzyme acetylcholinesterase, so activity in organs, glands, muscles, smooth muscles, and central nervous system cannot turn off; body systems wear out.
   b. Effects of nerve agent depends on route (vapor or droplet) of exposure and amount; it is felt within seconds.
      1. Felt first on face: eyes, nose, mouth, and lower airways—watery eyes, runny nose, increased salivation, and constriction of airways, shortness of breath.
      2. Large concentration of vapor: loss of consciousness, convulsions, no breathing.

Clinical Alert

The most common sign of nerve vapor exposure is constricted pupils (miosis) with reddened, watery eyes.

Triaging for Chemical Agent Exposure

Procedure

1. **Pulmonary agents.**
   a. Victim complaining of dyspnea within 6 hr of exposure requires immediate intervention—bedrest (no exertion) and oxygen.
   b. Continued care.
      1. Continue airway support with oxygen.
      2. Monitor for hypovolemia and correct acidosis.
      3. If symptoms are not present within 12 hr, and x-ray, physical exam, and ABGs normal, client may be discharged.
2. **Cyanide agents.**
   a. Antidotes should be administered within minutes of inhalation if client has seizures or respiratory symptoms.
   b. Mild symptoms: give supportive care and monitor.
3. **Vesicant agents.**
   a. Almost all victims will have delayed treatment for skin, eyes, and airway injuries.
   b. Clients with severe airway injury (dyspnea) require intensive pulmonary care.
4. **Nerve agents.**
   a. Victims exposed to liquid nerve agent who show signs of nerve exposure must be decontaminated immediately. ▶ ***Rationale:*** Rapid decontamination will decrease reaction, but not prevent it.
   b. Administer antidotes immediately according to symptoms—multiorgan involvement, respiratory difficulty, convulsions.
   c. Victims suspected of exposure, but who present with no symptoms, may have delayed treatment.

Triage in the Hot Zone After a Chemical Agent Terrorist Attack

- First responders will probably not be able to identify the exact agent.
- Early intervention is critical for nerve agents and cyanide.
- Pulmonary agent exposure will be treated later.
- Intervention in the hot zone generally has to do with airway, breathing, and circulation (ABCs); add antidotes for nerve agents.

Managing Care After Chemical Agent Exposure

Procedure

1. **Pulmonary agents:** Client with pulmonary edema must be on immediate bedrest with no exertion and receive oxygen.
2. **Cyanide agents:** Administer antidotes.
   a. Client inhales amyl nitrite, or is given sodium nitrite IV (10 mL; 300 mg); frees bound cyanide from hemoglobin to allow O_2 transport.
   b. Sulfur thiosulfate IV (50 mL; 12.5 gm); sulfur converts cyanide to form a nontoxic substance.
   c. Give antidotes sequentially and slowly, titrated to monitor effects; ventilate with oxygen and correct acidosis.
3. **Vesicant agents.**
   a. Mustard: Immediate decontamination (within 1 minute) will minimize damage; longer will be too late. Irrigate affected skin areas and eyes frequently and apply antibiotics to skin 3 to 4 times/day.
   b. Lewisite: Similar to mustard. Immediate decontamination is important. An antidote for systemic lewisite is British anti-Lewisite (BAL), a drug given IV for heavy metal poisoning.
4. **Nerve agents.**
   a. Personal protection equipment is necessary when decontaminating victims. Decontamination must take place first, before management begins.
   b. Antidotes:
      1. *Atropine* 2–6 mg (average dose 2–4 mg) IM; 2 mg more may be administered in 5–10 minutes if no improvement. A high initial dose is necessary to block excess neurotransmitter, especially if victim is unconscious.
      2. *Protopam*, an oxime, 600 mg given slowly IV to counteract nerve agent by removing agent from the enzyme.
      3. *Valium* might be used for prolonged convulsions.
   c. The military has a device (Mark I Auto-Injection Kit) that holds two spring-powered injectors containing two antidotes, atropine and Protopam, that can be used effectively and quickly to administer antidotes.

Chempacks, which include chemical weapon antidotes, are being shipped to all states from federal stockpiles. Each pack will treat 1,000 clients and will be available to medical facilities within 12 hr of an emergency.

Source: Office of Terrorism Preparedness and Emergency Response, CDC, 2006.

Identifying Acute Radiation Syndrome

Procedure

1. Assess for an acute illness characterized by manifestations of cellular deficiencies. ▸ ***Rationale:*** Early recognition of the body's reaction to ionizing radiation is important.
   a. Prodromal period: loss of appetite, nausea, vomiting, fatigue, and diarrhea.
   b. Latent period: symptoms disappear for a period of time.
   c. Overt illness follows the latent period—infection, electrolyte imbalance, diarrhea, bleeding.
   d. The final phase is a period of recovery or death.
2. Determine the radiation dose, if possible.
3. Attempt to identify dose exposure of client. ▸ ***Rationale:*** Treatment is according to dose exposure.
   a. Dose less than 2 Gy (200 RADS) is usually not severe; nausea and vomiting seldom experienced at 0.75–1 Gy (75–100 RADS) of penetrating gamma rays.
      1. Hospitalization unnecessary at less than 2 Gy, thus outpatient care indicated.
      2. Closely monitor and administer frequent CBC with differential blood tests.
   b. Dose greater than 2 Gy (200 RADS).
      1. Signs and symptoms become increasingly severe with increased dose.
      2. See box on page 487 for description of four syndromes.

▲ Wear film badge when likely to be exposed to radioactive material.

Clinical Alert

The higher the radiation dose, the greater the severity of early effects and possibility of late effects.

c. Give supportive care—treat gastric distress with H_2 receptor antagonists (Tagamet, Pepcid, etc.).
d. Prevent and treat infections—monitor viral prophylaxis.
e. Consult with hematologist and radiation experts.
f. Observe for erythema, hair loss, skin injury, mucositis, weight loss, and fever.

4. Identify if radiation dose includes radioactive iodine. ▸ ***Rationale:*** Uptake of this isotope could destroy thyroid tissue.
5. Administer potassium iodide before exposure, if possible, or as soon as available (within 4 hr). ▸ ***Rationale:*** Blocks uptake of specific damaging isotope which protects thyroid tissue.

Dealing With a Nuclear Disaster

Procedure

1. Move away from blast area as soon as possible. ▸ ***Rationale:*** Downwind contamination and dispersed radioactive material will contaminate.
2. Travel in a direction that keeps wind to left or right. ▸ ***Rationale:*** If wind is blowing from blast toward you, this will give you the least exposure.
3. Cover your face with cloth or mask. ▸ ***Rationale:*** This will help you avoid inhaling radioactive dust.
4. Remove your outer clothing and shower as soon as you are in a safe area. ▸ ***Rationale:*** Fallout dust is dangerous because it emits radiation energy that can go through clothing.
5. Find a shelter with enough mass (thickness) to shield you from penetrating radioactive dust. ▸ ***Rationale:*** The denser the shelter mass or walls, the more effective at blocking (thickness required to stop 99% of radiation is 5 inches of steel, 16 inches of brick or concrete blocks filled with sand or mortar, 2 feet of packed earth, or 3 feet of water).

Acute Radiation Syndromes

- *Hematopoietic syndrome*: Characterized by deficiencies of red blood cells, lymphocytes, and platelets, with immunodeficiency; increased infectious complications, including bleeding, anemia, and impaired wound healing.
- *Gastrointestinal syndrome*: Characterized by loss of cells lining intestinal crypts and loss of mucosal barrier with alterations in intestinal motility; fluid and electrolyte loss with vomiting and diarrhea; loss of normal intestinal bacteria, sepsis, and damage to the intestinal microcirculation, along with the hematopoietic syndrome.
- *Cerebrovascular–central nervous system syndrome*: Primarily associated with effects on the vasculature and resultant fluid shifts. Signs and symptoms include vomiting and diarrhea within minutes of exposure; confusion, disorientation, cerebral edema, hypotension, and hyperpyrexia. Fatal in short time.
- *Skin syndrome*: Can occur with other syndromes; characterized by loss of epidermis (and possibly dermis) with "radiation burns."

Source: Oak Ridge Institute for Science and Education. (2002). Guidance for Radiation Accident Management, "Managing Radiation Emergencies." www.orau.gov/reacts/syndrome.htm.

DOCUMENTATION for Bioterrorism Agents, Antidotes, and Vaccinations

Agents of Bioterrorism Identified

- Clinical features of agent (anthrax, plague, botulism, typhoid, VHF, Q fever, smallpox, ricin)
- **Incubation period**
- **Decontamination, if necessary**
- **Client placement and isolation precautions implemented**
- Therapy–treatment implemented

Clients to Whom *Vaccinia* Smallpox Vaccine Administered

- Post-vaccination reactions noted
- Adverse reactions of smallpox vaccination assessed
- Client to whom *vaccinia* immune globulin (VIG) administered
- Specimens collected and destination of transport (Lab)

Chemical Agents Identified (Pulmonary, Cyanide, Vesicant, Nerve)

- Triaging, if necessary, for chemical exposure
- Treatment administered to chemically exposed client

Acute Radiation Syndrome Identified

CRITICAL THINKING Application

Expected Outcomes

- Epidemiologic features of disease are identified.
- Preparedness plans for hospitals are in place and staff are aware of the components.
- If smallpox vaccinations are imposed, staff are knowledgeable about the procedure.
- Smallpox vaccinations are given with no untoward effects.
- Radiation dose remains at safe levels.
- Healthcare workers learn how to respond safely to a nuclear event.
- Victims of a man-made disaster (chemical, biologic, or nuclear) are treated according to protocols.

Unexpected Outcomes	Alternative Actions
Epidemiologic features of disease cannot be identified.	• Examine clusters or unusual numbers of clients with similar signs and symptoms by communicating with other hospitals in the community. • Gather specimens and send them to the appropriate laboratory. • Institute Standard Precautions plus airborne and contact precautions until specific agent is identified.
An effective community response to a terrorist attack is unlikely (hospital does not have a Preparedness Plan in place).	• Form a hospital committee to prepare a Preparedness Plan. • Collect educational materials to fill in areas of content the response team requires to function effectively in the event of a disaster. • Set up practice sessions with post-evaluation to increase response effectiveness. • Establish a communication network so it is already in place in the event of a terrorist attack; assign roles and a command center spokesman.
The U.S. government orders your hospital staff to vaccinate a targeted population for smallpox.	• Collect the necessary material to identify high-risk clients and have the knowledge base to perform the skill of administering smallpox vaccinations. • Practice administering smallpox vaccinations without using the actual vaccine until staff is proficient in the skill.
Client receives smallpox vaccination and inadvertently inoculates another site (face, eyelid, nose, etc.).	• Request orders to administer VIG IM for complications, if client is appropriate. • Assess that no new lesions appear after VIG doses given over 24–36 hr.

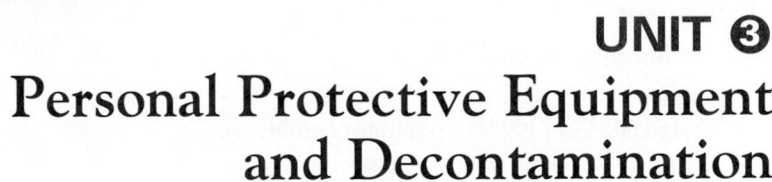

Chapter 15

UNIT 3

Personal Protective Equipment and Decontamination

Nursing Process Data

ASSESSMENT Data Base

- Identify clients who present risk to healthcare professionals.
- Assess need for special equipment (biohazard bags, specimen bags, etc.).
- Determine type of protection equipment required according to an identified biohazard (biological, chemical, or radiological).
- Assess need for decontaminating victims before triage.
- Assess strategy for decontamination at site of incident.
- Assess need for mass casualty decontamination.

PLANNING Objectives

- To select and utilize appropriate personal protection equipment
- To demonstrate Standard Precaution techniques
- To demonstrate behaviors that help to ensure personal safety
- To understand containment principles to avoid spreading contamination
- To prevent further spread of biological–chemical–radiological agents with appropriate decontamination procedures
- To understand principles of decontaminating via triage
- To prevent spread of bioterrorism agents by following guidelines of mass casualty decontamination

IMPLEMENTATION Procedures

EVALUATION Expected Outcomes

- Infection control protocols are followed.
- Staff is familiar with protective equipment and the protocols to use it.
- Staff knows decontamination procedures and implements them safely.
- Decontamination procedures for mass casualty disasters are implemented.
- Radiation exposure is controlled.

Implementing Hospital Infection Control Protocol

Equipment

Handwashing material
Gloves
Masks (HEPA or N95 for respiratory problems, pneumonia, plague, smallpox, etc.)
Eye shields or face shields
Gowns
Disinfecting material

Procedure

1. Utilize Standard Precautions for all clients admitted to or arriving at the hospital. For specific protocols and skills, see Chapter 14, Infection Control. ▶ ***Rationale:*** Agents of bioterrorism are generally not transmitted person to person.
2. Follow routine client placement for normal number of admissions.
   a. Isolate suspicious cases.
   b. Group similar cases.
3. Utilize alternative placement for large numbers of clients.
   a. Co-group clients with similar syndromes in a designated area.
   b. Establish designated unit, floor, or area in advance.
   c. Place clients based on patterns of airflow and ventilation with respirator problems, smallpox, or plague. ▶ ***Rationale:*** Transmission is through droplets (touching).
   d. Place clients after consultation with engineering staff. ▶ ***Rationale:*** Adequate plumbing and waste disposal must be available.
4. Control entry to client designated areas. ▶ ***Rationale:*** Minimizes possibility of transmission to other clients and staff.
5. Transport bioterrorism clients as little as possible—limit to essential movement. ▶ ***Rationale:*** This practice will reduce opportunity for microorganism transmission within facility.
6. Clean, disinfect, and sterilize equipment according to principles of Standard Precautions.

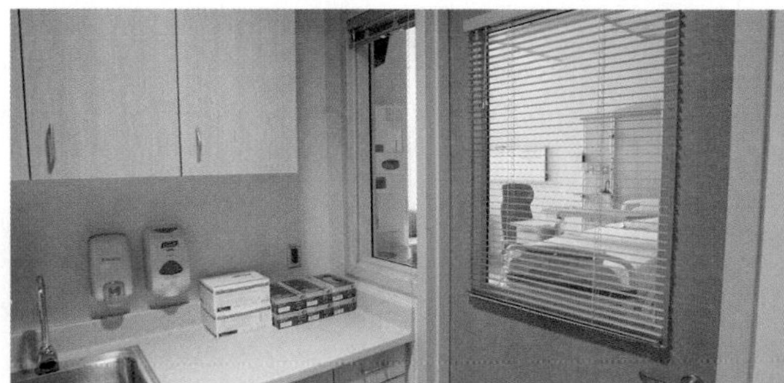

▲ Clients who are placed in isolation require a room with a directional airflow, negative-pressure ventilation system with minimum of 6 to 12 air exchanges per hour. An anteroom entry is preferred to maintain isolation protocol.

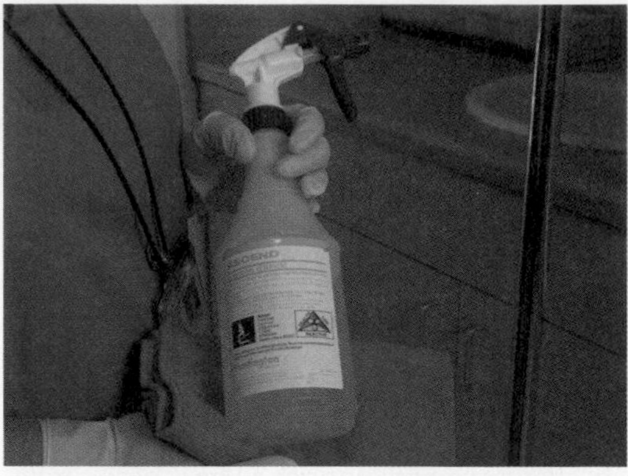

▲ Clean all reusable large equipment thoroughly with antimicrobial or antiseptic agent as required by hospital policy.

   a. Use procedures facility has in place for routine cleaning and disinfection.
   b. Have available approved germicidal cleaning solutions.
   c. Contaminated waste should be sorted and disposed of in accordance with biohazard waste regulations. See Handling Biohazard Waste in Chapter 14, page 415.
   d. For clients with bioterrorism-related infections, use Standard Precautions for cleaning unless infecting organism indicates special cleaning.

Glove Protection From Toxic Chemicals

- OSHA's new PPE standard requires companies to perform a hazard assessment to determine the need for protective clothing.
- Wide variations in chemical resistance of gloves and protective clothing make equipment selection difficult.
- Many factors affect the performance of gloves during actual use. Toxic chemicals such as pesticides, aromatic amines, and isocyanates can permeate gloves and protective clothing. In addition, flexing, stretching, pressure, and abrasion are physical factors that can cause premature breakthrough.
- A new generation of products produce a color change when permeation occurs, thus providing a method for field validation of the efficacy of protective clothing.
- PERMEA-TEC™ sensors are an example—they are attached to hands before gloving. The detector is placed on thumb, middle finger, and palm, as these areas represent the highest area of contact and abrasion.
- Sensors should be checked hourly to determine when breakthrough occurs, indicating gloves must be changed.

Source: Colormetric Laboratories Inc. (© 1999—modified April 8, 2002). www.clilabs@clilabs.com.

Standard Precautions

Hand hygiene	Use antimicrobial soap or waterless antiseptic agent to clean hands.	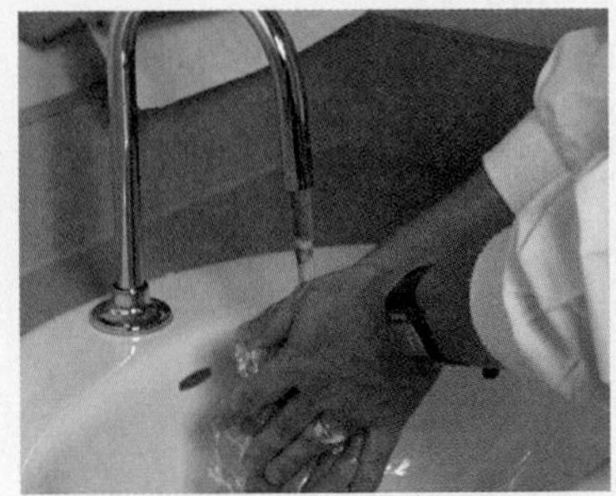
Donning gloves	Wear clean nonsterile gloves to protect healthcare personnel from touching blood, body fluids, secretions, excretions, and contaminated items.	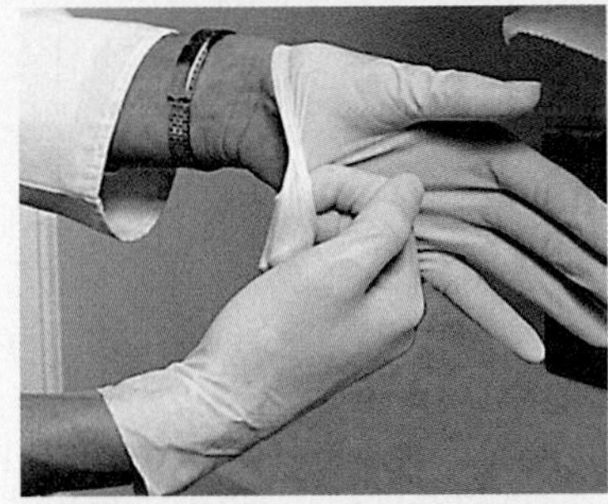
Donning a gown	A clean, nonsterile gown will protect skin and prevent soiling of clothes.	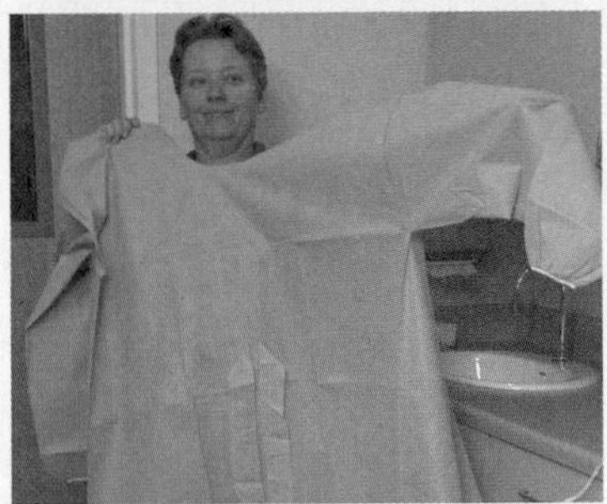
Wearing a mask	Wear a mask to protect mucous membranes of nose and mouth for workers and victims.	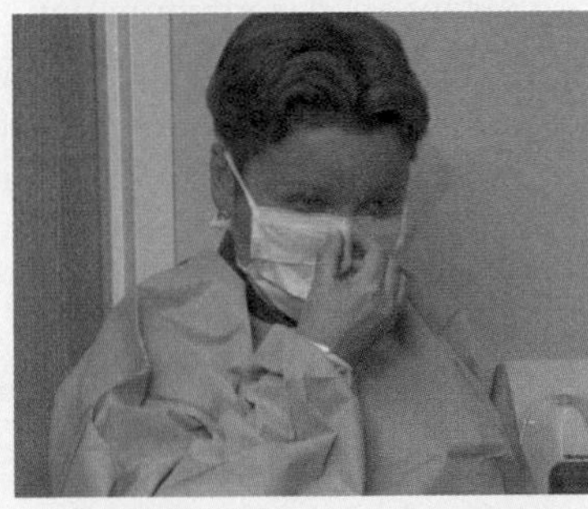
Wearing special masks: HEPA or particulate filter respiratory mask	When bioterrorism agent is suspected and is transmitted via aerosol or airborne, special masks are indicated. Individually fit each mask.	
Wearing eye or face shield	Shield will protect mucous membranes of eyes from splash or spray of victim's body fluids.	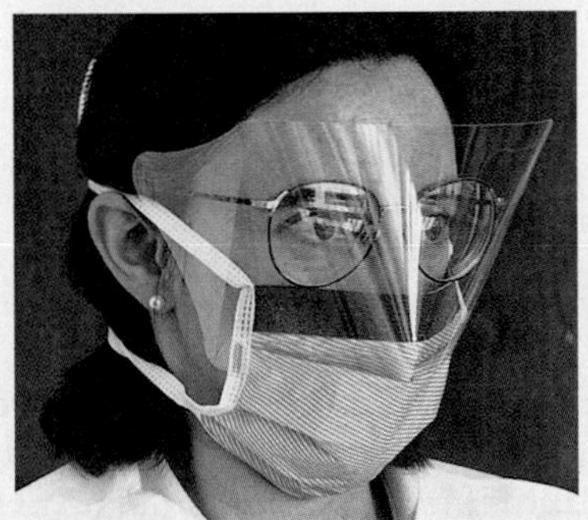

NOTE: See more complete explanation of Standard Precautions in Chapter 14, Infection Control.

Decontaminating via Triage

Equipment

Personal protection equipment including clothing
Water source
Soap
0.5% sodium hypochlorite (HTH chlorine or diluted bleach) cleaning solution
Towels
Waste container for contaminated clothes
Masking tape, 2 in wide
Body bags
Film badge or chemical agent detector

Procedure

1. Decontaminate at scene of incident (hot zone). ▶ ***Rationale:*** Prevents hospital system from absorbing contaminated victims and protects healthcare providers and uncontaminated casualties.
2. Familiarize emergency personnel with stages of decontamination. ▶ ***Rationale:*** Effective decontamination is essential for victim and staff protection.
   a. Gross decontamination.
      1. Decontaminate those who require assistance.
      2. Remove and dispose of exposed victim's clothing. ▶ ***Rationale:*** This will remove 70%–80% of contaminant.
      3. Perform a thorough head-to-toe tepid water rinse. ▶ ***Rationale:*** Cold water can cause hypothermia and hot water can result in vasodilation, speeding distribution of the contaminants.
   b. Secondary decontamination.
      1. Perform a full-body rinse with clean tepid water. ▶ ***Rationale:*** Water is an effective decontaminant because of rapidity of application.
      2. Wash rapidly from head to toe with cleaning solution (HTH chlorine is effective) and rinse with water. ▶ ***Rationale:*** HTH chlorine can decontaminate both chemical and biological contaminants.

NOTE: Undiluted household bleach is 5.0% sodium hypochlorite.

   c. Definitive decontamination.
      1. Perform thorough head-to-toe wash and rinse.
      2. Dry victim and don clean clothes.

Salvageable Victims

First Priority: Decontaminate exposed victims with no symptoms.
Second Priority: Decontaminate exposed victims with minor injuries who require minimal resources.
Third Priority: Decontaminate exposed victims needing maximum medical care.
Last to decontaminate are deceased victims.

3. Initial decontamination may be accomplished by the fire department with hoses spraying water at reduced pressure. ▶ ***Rationale:*** This will remove a high percentage of contaminant at an early stage.
4. Decontaminate salvageable clients first. ▶ ***Rationale:*** The goal is to decontaminate victims who have been exposed, yet are salvageable. Clients who are dead or unsalvageable have lowest priority for decontamination.
5. Reduce extent of contamination in facility by decontaminating clients before receiving in healthcare facility. ▶ ***Rationale:*** Necessary to ensure safety of clients and staff.
   a. Establish decontamination site outside facility using a decontamination tent before needing it. ▶ ***Rationale:*** To protect clients and staff inside facility.
   b. Set up procedures for decontamination, depending on infectious agent.
6. Implement procedure for decontaminating client.
   a. Don appropriate personal protective gear before assisting clients to decontaminate.
   b. Remove contaminated clothing and place in appropriate double biohazard bags.
   c. Instruct or assist client to shower with soap and water. ▶ ***Rationale:*** Bathing clients in bleach may be potentially harmful. For specific infections, diluted bleach 0.5% is indicated.
   d. Use clean water, normal saline, or ophthalmic solution for rinsing eyes.

Guidelines for Setting Up Site for Decontamination

- Establish upwind from contamination area.
- Set up site on a downhill slope, if possible, or on flat ground (so that runoff can be captured).
- Have water source available and, if possible, decontamination solution.
- Have decontamination equipment available, if possible.
- Supply personal protection equipment for healthcare personnel.
- Notify healthcare facilities nearby to be available, if possible.
- Maintain security and privacy for site.
- Institute post-decontamination monitoring and checks.

Source: Maniscalco, P., & Christen, H. (2002). *Understanding terrorism and managing the consequences.* Upper Saddle River, NJ: Pearson Education.

Choosing Protective Equipment for Biological Exposure

Equipment

Listed below in procedure

Procedure

1. Plan for protection from biological hazards.
   a. First responders to a biological hazard may be exposed to bacteria, viruses, or toxins via inhalation (through respiratory tract) or ingestion (contact with mucous membranes of eyes, nasal tissues, or open cuts).
   b. Biological weapons are particles and will not penetrate proper protective equipment.
   c. Respirators—type selected according to hazard identified and its airborne concentration.
      1. High level of protection: Self-contained breathing apparatus (SCBA) with full facepiece. Provides highest level of protection against airborne hazards when used correctly. ► ***Rationale:*** Reduces exposure to hazard by a factor of 10,000.
      2. Minimal level of protection: Half-mask or full facepiece air-purifying respirator with particulate filters like N95 (used for TB) or P100 (used for hantavirus).
   d. Protective clothing includes gloves and shoe covers—necessary for full protection. ► ***Rationale:*** Prevents skin exposure and/or contamination of other clothing.
      1. Level A Protective Suit used when a suspected biological incident occurs and type, dissemination method, and concentration are unknown.
      2. Level B Protective Suit used when biological aerosol is no longer present.
      3. Full facepiece respirator (P100 or HEPA filters) used if agent was *not* aerosoled or dissemination was by letter or package that could be bagged.
   e. If possible, have biological detection equipment in place—SMART tickets are a handheld point detection system developed by the Navy Medical Institute. Instrument captures antigen and changes color according to eight different biological agents detected.
2. Identify *anthrax* precautions.
   a. Implement and maintain Standard Precautions (gowns, gloves, and mask). Use Contact Precautions for cutaneous anthrax.
   b. Isolation or decontamination is not implemented. ► ***Rationale:*** Anthrax is not transmitted by person-to-person contact.
   c. If client has been exposed and clothing may be contaminated, decontamination is advised.
3. Identify *plague* precautions.
   a. In a bioterrorism attack, bacterium (*Yersinia pestis*) may be spread by inhalation of droplets, aerosols, or disseminated via infected fleas or other biting insects. ► ***Rationale:*** Droplet precautions are used until client has been treated for 2–3 days (gown, gloves, and mask).
   b. Strict isolation until client has been treated for 2–3 days. ► ***Rationale:*** So that airborne contaminants do not spread throughout the hospital or community.
   c. Decontamination precautions: soap/shower; 0.5% diluted bleach for visible contamination.
   d. Disinfect environment: 0.5% diluted bleach or EPA-approved detergent.
4. Identify *botulism* precautions.
   a. A bioterror attack could disseminate an aerosol of the bacterium or purified neurotoxins. Therefore, use Standard Precautions. ► ***Rationale:*** If toxin is used, there is no danger of person-to-person transmission.
   b. Decontamination procedures: toxin may be removed from skin by soap and water.
   c. Place contaminated clothes in sealed plastic bag for biohazard disposal.
   d. Other precautions:
      1. Environment: diluted bleach 0.5%, 15–20 seconds, or EPA-approved germicidal detergent.
      2. Boil water for 15 minutes.
      3. Cook food at 176°F for 30 minutes.
5. Identify *smallpox* (*variola*) virus.
   a. Spread through airborne or direct contact with skin lesions or secretions. Use Standard Precautions with airborne (respiratory isolation; N95 or P100 mask) and contact precautions (gown and gloves). ► ***Rationale:*** Virus is spread through droplet or contact; therefore, isolation decontamination precautions are used.
   b. Isolate and quarantine victim immediately and place in negative pressure room with HEPA filtration or direct exhaust to the outside.
   c. All direct contacts are quarantined for at least 17 days. ► ***Rationale:*** Incubation period is 7–17 days.
   d. Cleanse with soap/shower; use 0.5% diluted bleach for gross or visible contamination.
   e. Place mask on victim, if not in isolation. ► ***Rationale:*** Virus is spread through airborne method so mask will protect others.

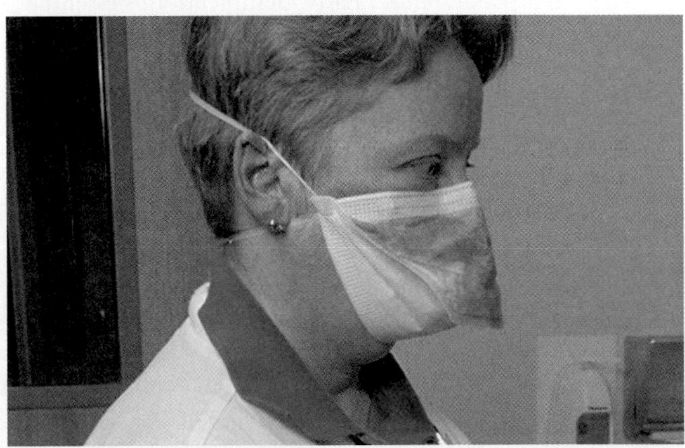

▲ For minimal protection, use particulate filter N95 or HEPA filter respirator when you may be exposed to an unknown biological hazard.

f. Healthcare workers maintain standard/airborne/contact precautions for minimum 17 days (until all scabs separate). ▸ ***Rationale:*** When scabs separate, client is no longer contagious.

g. All bedding and clothing must be autoclaved or laundered in hot water and bleach.

6. Identify *brucellosis* precautions.
   a. Bioterrorism mode of dissemination could be aerosol or food supply sabotage. Standard Precautions indicated. If lesions are draining, use contact precautions.

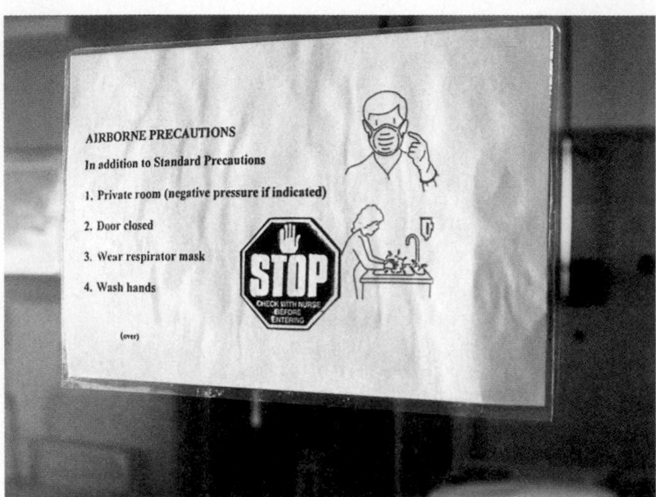

▲ Institute airborne precautions when certain bioterrorism agents such as plague and smallpox are suspected.

   b. Decontamination—victim should undress and use soap/shower.
   c. Environment: 0.5% bleach.
7. Identify *typhoidal tularemia* precautions.
   a. Bioterrorism mode of dissemination would probably be aerosol with nontransmission. Use Standard Precautions.
   b. Isolation/decontamination precautions. Victim should undress, use soap, and shower. For visible contamination, use 0.5% bleach.
   c. Environment: 0.5% bleach.
8. *Viral encephalitides* precautions.
   a. Bioterrorism mode of dissemination is aerosol. Use Standard Precautions.
   b. Isolation/decontamination precautions. Victim should undress, use shower with soap and large quantity of water.
   c. Mosquito control × 72 hr.
   d. Environment: 0.5% bleach.

The U.S. Government is now launching an early warning system that detects bioterrorism agents released into the air. Adapting 3,000 existing monitors that now are used for air pollution, this system could detect biological agents, such as smallpox or anthrax. Results of early warnings could be confirmed at a network of laboratories within 24 hr using DNA analysis.

Choosing Protective Equipment for Chemical Exposure

Equipment

Listed below in procedure.

Procedure

1. Identify victims who were exposed to chemical substance. ▸ ***Rationale:*** Early identification is essential to save lives, especially from nerve agents or cyanide.
2. Cover all skin surfaces with protective clothing impervious to chemicals. ▸ ***Rationale:*** Necessary for protection until exact chemical agent is identified.
   a. Use Mission-Oriented Protective Posture (MOPP) suit, if available (chemical protection suit).
   b. Use fire department chemical suits as alternative.
3. Don masks with filtered respirator. (HEPA filter respirator—P100 with full facepiece—and fit-tested N95 meet CDC performance criteria for chemical exposure.) ▸ ***Rationale:*** Chemicals can be inhaled.
4. Wear boots or boot covers. ▸ ***Rationale:*** Feet should be covered to prevent tracking contaminant.
5. Initiate decontamination procedures with trained personnel.

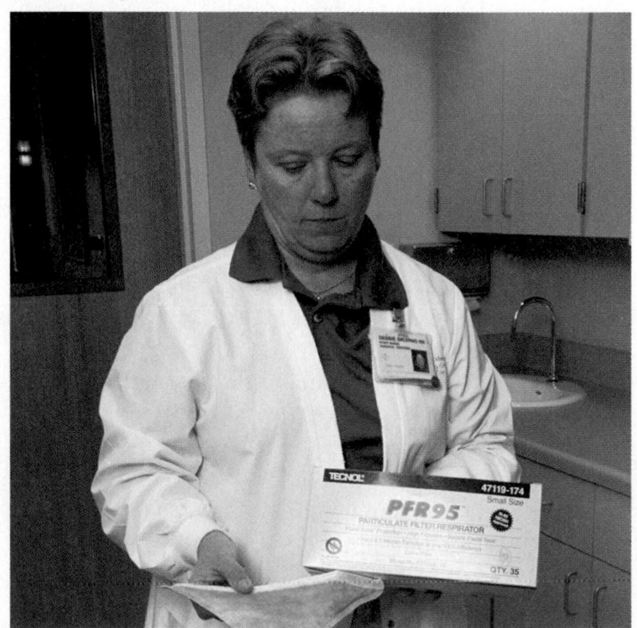

▲ For chemical or certain biological exposure, masks with HEPA filtered respirator or N95 should be used.

   a. Decontaminate at site, if possible.
   b. Otherwise, decontaminate outside of facility.
6. Use chemical detection devices, if available. ▶ ***Rationale:*** Devices would validate presence or absence of agent.
   a. M8 Paper: Sheet of chemically treated paper—if colored spots appear within 20 seconds, chemical agent is present.
   b. M9 Tape: Affix adhesive-backed paper to equipment or protective clothing—color changes when exposed to chemical agent.
   c. M2S6A1 Chemical Agent Detector Kit: Can detect nerve, blister, or blood agent vapors; a glass ampule contains substance that, when placed on test spot, changes color.
   d. Chemical Agent Monitors (CAMs): Contain a microprocessor chip that identifies presence of certain nerve and blister agents.

Choosing Protective Equipment for Radiological Attack

Equipment

Listed below in procedure.

Procedure

1. Identify victims contaminated by radiation. ▶ ***Rationale:*** If victim is contaminated, clothes, skin, etc., can transmit contamination to others.
   a. If victim was exposed to ionizing radiation (most common are alpha, beta particles, and gamma rays), contamination occurred.
   b. The higher the dose of radiation, the greater the severity of contamination.
2. Don protective clothing: basic gear will stop alpha and some beta particles, not gamma rays. ▶ ***Rationale:*** Necessary to protect responders from exposure and to prevent cross-contamination, exposing other clients.
   a. Scrub suit.
   b. Gown and cap.
   c. Mask.
   d. Eye shield.
   e. Double gloves—one pair under cuff of gown and taped to close all entry; second pair can be removed and/or replaced.
   f. Masking tape, 2 ins. wide.
   g. Shoe cover with all seams taped.
   h. Radiation detection device: able to detect energy emitted from a radiation source. Several detectors available: Geiger counters, dosimeters, etc.
   i. Film badge.
3. Transport victim to facility.
   a. If victim is not decontaminated at site, set up portable decontamination unit before entering facility.
   b. Double-bag all victim's clothing in sealed biohazard plastic bags marked "Radioactive."
4. Institute decontamination procedures.
   a. Open wounds or nonintact skin: irrigate with sterile water or normal saline (NS); cover with dry, sterile dressing.
   b. Eyes: irrigate with sterile water of NS according to skill, "Irrigating the Eyes," Chapter 18.
   c. Intact skin: wash skin with soap and warm water. Bleach, 0.5%, may also be used.
   d. Radiation burns: treat as other burns are treated.
5. Recheck radiation levels at each stage of treatment until reduced to background levels.
6. Dispose of used protective gear appropriately. ▶ ***Rationale:*** This gear is radiologically contaminated waste, and to prevent cross-contamination, it must be treated as such.

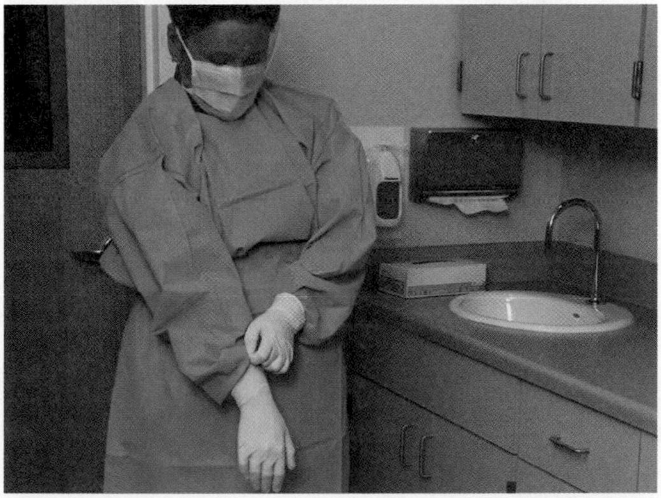

▲ When exposed to radiological material, double gloves that cover all skin exposure should be worn.

New Trends: Tiny Radiation Detector Saves Lives

Because the greatest threat to our national security is the use of a nuclear device, this matchbook-size detector that you can keep on your key chain could save your life. This device, called a NukAlert, measures levels of radiation (like a Geiger counter) and lets you know the areas that are safe or dangerous by emitting a chirp sound. The more chirps, the greater the danger. This device is reasonably priced—you may contact KI4U in Texas for more information.

Decontaminating Victims After a Biological Terrorist Event

Equipment

Protective clothing for healthcare worker
Biohazard bags
Soap and water; diluted sodium hypochlorite (bleach)

Procedure

1. Don protective clothing and adhere strictly to Standard Precautions for emergency personnel. ▶ ***Rationale:*** This will prevent secondary contamination of personnel.
2. Identify dermal exposure, if possible. ▶ ***Rationale:*** Biological agents are difficult to detect.
3. Remove victim's clothing as soon as possible and place in biohazard bags. ▶ ***Rationale:*** If victim was exposed, clothing is contaminated.
4. Cleanse exposed areas using soap and tepid water (large amounts) or diluted sodium hypochlorite (0.5%).
5. Send victims home, if possible, to continue decontamination procedure by washing thoroughly with soap and water.
   a. Instruct victims to monitor for signs and symptoms of agent.
   b. Inform victim of result of lab analysis as soon as possible.

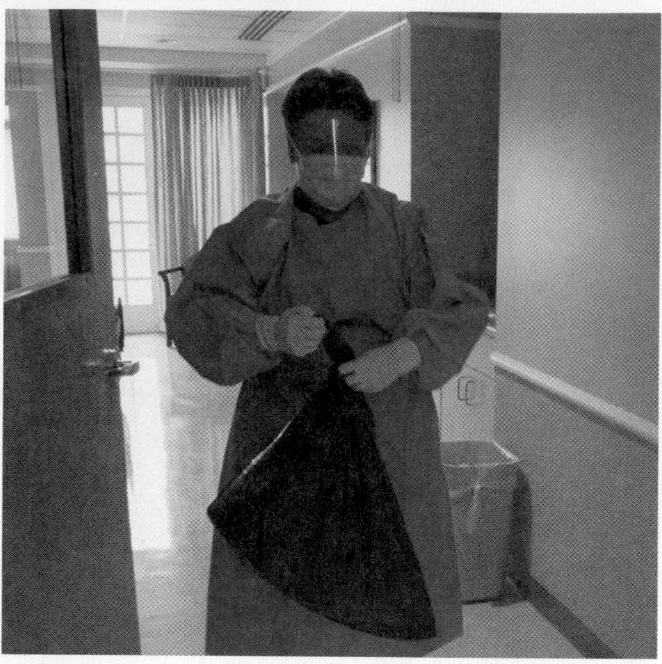

▲ Dispose of all contaminated clothing in appropriate biohazard bags.

Decontaminating Victims After a Chemical Terrorist Event

Equipment

Protective equipment for healthcare workers
Biohazard bags
Soap and water; diluted sodium hypochlorite (bleach)
Saline or isotonic bicarbonate
Chemical agent monitor or M8 paper

Procedure

1. Know general principles to guide actions after a chemical agent incident.*
   a. Expect a 5:1 ratio of unaffected:affected casualties.
   b. Decontaminate immediately (ASAP).
   c. Disrobing is decontamination, head to toe; the more removal, the better.
   d. Large-volume water flush is best decontamination method.
   e. After exposure, first-responders must decontaminate immediately to avoid serious effects.
2. Practice triage guidelines for Mass Casualty Decontamination.* ▶ ***Rationale:*** Chemical exposure can be deadly, so early decontamination is critical. Decontaminate according to:
   a. Casualties closest to point of release.
   b. Casualties reporting exposure to vapor or aerosol.
   c. Casualties with liquid deposits on clothing or skin.

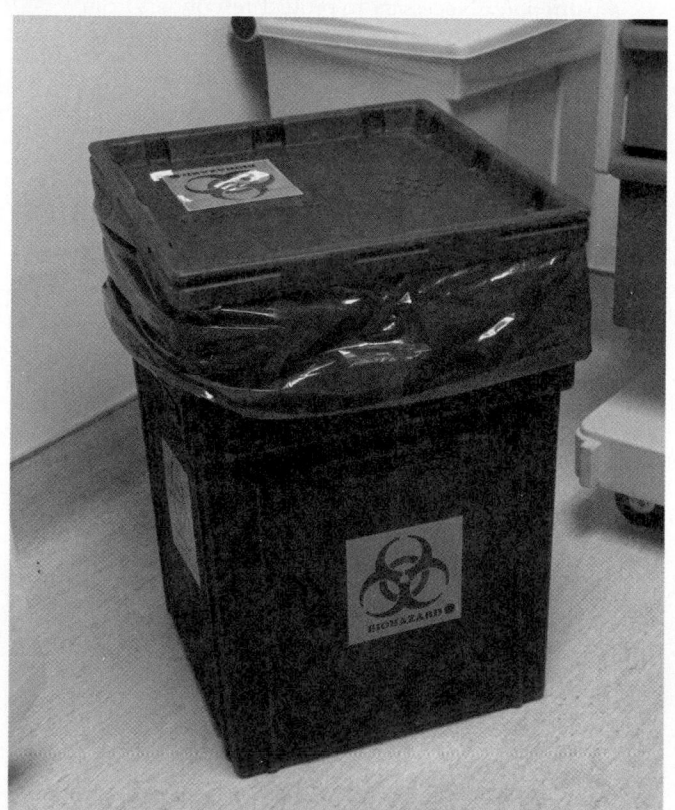

▲ Place contaminated clothing in bins or biohazard bag labeled "RADIOACTIVE" if that is source of contamination.

d. Casualties with serious medical conditions.
e. Casualties with conventional injuries.

3. Decontaminate victims as early as possible. ▶ ***Rationale:*** Requirements differ according to type of chemical agent used: sarin dissipates quickly in the air; VX remains lethal for hours.
   a. Nerve agents may be absorbed on all body surfaces—must be removed quickly to be effective.
   b. Vesicant (blister) agents are not always identified due to latent effects.
4. Treat eyes and mucous membranes with special protocol.
   a. Flush with copious amounts of water. ▶ ***Rationale:*** Eyes and mucous membranes are too sensitive to use other skin decontaminant solutions.
   b. If available, isotonic bicarbonate (1.26%) or saline (0.9%) may be used as a flushing agent.
5. Monitor victim for remains of agent or contaminant using chemical agent monitor (CAM) or M8 paper for chemical agents. ▶ ***Rationale:*** To validate removal of contaminant.

NOTE: Skin decontamination kits (M258A1) designed for chemical decontamination are available. They hold wipes that contain a solution that neutralizes most nerve and blister agents.

**Source:* Guidelines for Mass Decontamination During a Terrorist Chemical Agent Incident. U.S. Army Soldier and Biological Chemical Command, January 2000. Available at http://orise.oran.gov/reacts/resources/guide/management.htm

Decontaminating Victims After Radiation Exposure

Equipment

Personal protection equipment including self-contained breathing equipment and flash suits, if indicated
Surgical attire or disposable garments, shoe covers, eye shield, gloves, and masks with respirators
Water source and container to catch runoff
Bins for contaminated clothing
Biohazard bags
Vacuum cleaner with HEPA filter
Radiation dose meter

Procedure

1. Determine cause of incident to identify radiation exposure or contamination. ▶ ***Rationale:*** Exposure does not necessarily indicate need for decontamination.
   a. First responders may be told by those requesting assistance that there has been a radiation-exposure event.
   b. First responders may recognize radiation exposure from observation at incident site.
2. Understand difference between exposure and contamination.
   a. Exposed victim: presents no hazard, requires no special handling, and presents no radiological threat to personnel. ▶ ***Rationale:*** This is no different from client who has had diagnostic x-rays.
   b. Externally contaminated victim: may mean individual has come in contact with unconfined radioactive material. ▶ ***Rationale:*** Any person or object contaminated by radioactivity must be considered contaminated. Steps should be taken to minimize contamination.
   c. Internal contamination: occurs by inhalation or ingestion (airborne radioactive particles) or through an open wound. *Usually* this form of contamination is not a hazard to others.
3. Use appropriate personnel protection equipment (PPE). ▶ ***Rationale:*** This will protect personnel who may come in contact with contaminated victim.
   a. If radiation incident is suspected, self-contained breathing apparatus (SCBA) and flash suits are indicated. ▶ ***Rationale:*** This will reduce potential exposure of healthcare providers. Inhalation of radioactive particles is cross-contamination hazard.
   b. If SCBA suits not available:
      1. Use surgical attire or disposable garments (such as those made of Tyvek).
      2. Use eye protection and double gloves.
      3. Use masks with respirators. ▶ ***Rationale:*** These will protect healthcare workers from inhaling radioactive particles leading to internal contamination.
   c. It is important to recognize that external radiation (such as penetration by gamma rays) is *not* dangerous to emergency personnel the only exception to this rule is a rare neutron radiation exposure. ▶ ***Rationale:*** Gamma ray radiation is absorbed by or passes through the body, but does not leave radioactive contamination.
   d. If monitoring for radiation is not available, consider all clients contaminated.
   e. Personnel should minimize time in radiation zone. ▶ ***Rationale:*** Radiation exposure depends on time, distance, and shielding.

4. Triage client's medical condition first, regardless of radiation exposure. ▸ ***Rationale:*** First priority is delivery of emergency medical services, including transport.
   a. Administer emergency medical treatment to radiation-exposed clients.
   b. Decontaminate clients who have been contaminated on the scene before transport.
5. Complete decontamination of victims. ▸ ***Rationale:*** Until decontamination is complete, victims are an exposure risk to selves, staff, and others.
   a. Remove client's clothing and have client do a total body wash, scrubbing skin with soap and soft brush. ▸ ***Rationale:*** Removal of victim's clothing will reduce 80% of the contamination.
   b. Place contaminated clothing in bins or biohazard bag labeled "Radioactive."
   c. Capture runoff of water; contain and label "Radioactive."
   d. Wash area down between washing victims. ▸ ***Rationale:*** This will prevent transfer of contaminated material.
   e. Capture material with vacuum cleaner with HEPA filter, if appropriate. ▸ ***Rationale:*** This prevents release of radioactive material into the air.
   f. Monitor client with radiation meter to measure radiation.
6. Implement isolation techniques for contaminated victims. ▸ ***Rationale:*** To confine contamination and protect personnel.
7. Determine source of radiation, type of radioactive material, length of time of exposure, if possible. ▸ ***Rationale:*** This is valuable data for long-term interventions, but does not alter immediate handling and transport of victim.

Controlling Radiation Contamination

Equipment

Soap and water
Disposable client equipment
Biohazard bags
Wide tape
White tape
Heavy, wide paper
Plastic-lined containers
Radiation meter

Procedure

1. Decontaminate all victims; remove all clothing and complete a full body wash. ▸ ***Rationale:*** This will reduce most of the contamination.
2. Institute isolation techniques. ▸ ***Rationale:*** This will confine contamination and protect others.
3. Decontaminate equipment touched by client.
   a. Gurney used to transfer client.
   b. Equipment used in client care (BP cuff, stethoscope, etc.)
   c. Ambulance.
4. Decontaminate care providers who touched or moved client. ▸ ***Rationale:*** Protective clothing may be contaminated.
5. Examine surrounding area (walls, floor that client may have touched).
6. Control entry and exit of victims. ▸ ***Rationale:*** Radioactive particles adhere to dust, may become airborne, and can contaminate other clients and personnel.
   a. Mark entry area with white tape to differentiate areas.
   b. Restrict access to controlled area.
   c. Monitor everyone leaving controlled area—have persons cleared by radiation safety officer.
7. Cover floor areas with rolls of heavy, wide paper and tape securely to floor. ▸ ***Rationale:*** To prevent tracking of contaminants.
8. Control waste by using large plastic-lined containers for contaminated articles.
9. Monitor radiation by using meter.

DOCUMENTATION for Personal Protective Equipment and Decontamination

- Specific infection control protocols implemented (i.e., Standard or Airborne Precautions)
- Personal protection gear and equipment used
- Decontamination site established
- Decontamination procedure used for biological or chemical event
- Radiation exposure decontamination procedure

CRITICAL THINKING Application

Expected Outcomes

- Infection control protocols are followed. Staff is familiar with protective equipment and the protocols to use it.
- Staff knows decontamination procedures and implements them safely.
- Decontamination procedures for mass casualty disasters are implemented.
- Radiation exposure is controlled.

Unexpected Outcomes	Alternative Actions
Mass casualty disaster occurs with hundreds of victims affected in one area.	• Don protective gear before approaching WMD site. • Identify weapon or agent used to create disaster, if possible. • Institute field triage (triage first done at site before victims sent to community healthcare facilities). • Decontaminate victims at site before transporting to treatment facility.
Type of personal protection equipment is unknown for agent exposure.	• It is critical that response team be fully protected; thus choose highest level of equipment; that is, assume you need: 1. airborne protection with respirators—self-contained breathing apparatus (SCBA) with full face piece. 2. full Level A protective suit. 3. shoe covers and double gloves. 4. biological detection device, if available.
Clients are admitted with potential radiation exposure.	• Determine if radiation is exposure or contamination; if the latter, use protective gear and radiation dose meter. • Decontaminate clients by removing all clothing and giving a full body wash—institute isolation techniques. • Decontaminate all equipment, surfaces, and personnel that came in contact with client. • Administer treatment according to dose exposure: supportive care, frequent blood tests (CBC and differential), and prevent infection.

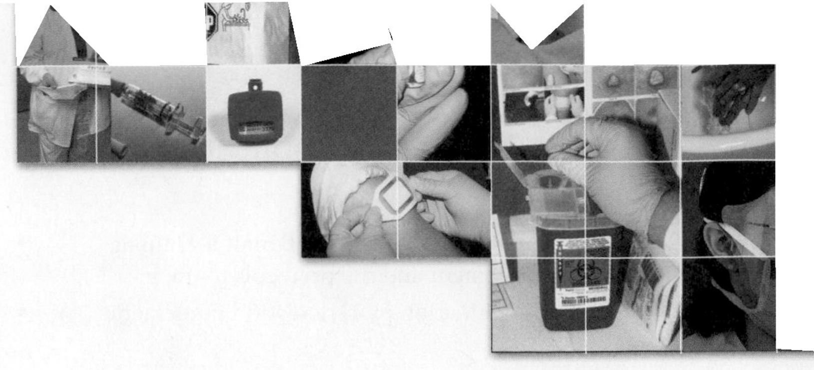

Chapter 15

UNIT 4 Triage, Treatment, and a Communication Matrix

Nursing Process Data

ASSESSMENT Data Base

- Assess the need to establish triage treatment areas.
- **Validate that public health parameters are established.**
- **Observe that the steps of triage are followed.**
- **Assess that victim is not in immediate danger or, conversely, requires immediate intervention.**
- **Assess vital signs of victims.**
- **Assess the treatment steps necessary to treat life-threatening conditions.**
- Observe for signs of respiratory distress.
- Assess need for establishing an airway.
- Observe for amount and source of bleeding and need for intervention.
- Recognize shock state and need for intervention.
- **Assess victims post-triage and observe for any signs or symptoms that indicate major injury.**
- **Identify victims having a severe psychological reaction to bioterrorism event.**
- **Assess possibility of post-traumatic stress syndrome developing.**
- **Assess that lines of communication are established and activated.**
- **Assess that Federal Response Plan is activated.**
- Assess that external, internal, and collaborative communication networks are in place.

PLANNING Objectives

- To establish a triage site taking into account public health parameters
- To establish triage treatment areas appropriate to number and injuries of victims
- To follow steps of triage
- To observe for any signs/symptoms that indicate major injury
- To treat life-threatening conditions
- To care for clients with major psychological reactions to bioterrorism event
- To prevent post-terrorism trauma
- To develop a communication network including external, internal, and collaborative communication

IMPLEMENTATION Procedures

EVALUATION Expected Outcomes

- Triage treatment areas are established within public health parameters.
- Staff follows appropriate steps of triage protocol.
- Life-threatening conditions are identified and treated.
- Post-triage assessment is completed.
- Post-traumatic stress disorder (PTSD) is identified and clients are referred appropriately.

Establishing Triage Treatment Areas

Procedure

1. Assign roles to personnel in treatment areas.
2. Select a site as soon as possible—advance planning is essential.
   a. Select safe area, free of hazards and debris.
   b. Position site upwind of hazard zone.
   c. Determine whether site is accessible to transportation vehicles (ambulances, trucks, helicopters).
   d. Be sure site is able to expand.
3. Protect treatment area and delineate area using tarps, etc. If possible, do not contaminate a crime scene.
4. Set up signs to identify subdivisions of area.
   a. I = Immediate care.
   b. D = Delayed care.
   c. Dead = Dead for morgue.
5. Establish I and D areas close together. ▶ ***Rationale:*** Facilitates verbal communication between workers who can also share medical supplies and transfer victims quickly when status changes.
6. Position victims in head-to-toe configuration, with 2–3 feet between victims. ▶ ***Rationale:*** This system will effectively use space and personnel.
7. Establish morgue site secure and away (and not visible) from medical treatment areas.

Clinical Alert

Survey entire scene, including area above you, for threats to your safety before beginning triage or team work.

Establishing Public Health Parameters

Equipment

Soap and water; antibacterial gel
Gloves
Mask and goggles
Biohazard waste disposal containers
Plastic bags
Water purification equipment
Search and rescue equipment

Procedure

1. Assign personnel to monitor public health concerns where disaster victims are sheltered. ▶ ***Rationale:*** To avoid or minimize spread of disease.
2. Have available search and rescue safety equipment.
   a. Helmet or hardhat.
   b. Goggles.
   c. Sturdy work gloves and shoes.
   d. Clothing appropriate for weather conditions.
   e. Dust mask or appropriate filtered mask (see Protection section).
   f. Rescue whistle.
3. Maintain proper hygiene by washing hands and using gloves.
   a. Wash hands with soap and water if dirty or antibacterial gel between victims.
   b. Wear gloves at all times.
   c. Change gloves between victims if possible. If not, clean them between victims in a bleach and water solution (1 part bleach to 9 parts water).
4. Wear a mask and goggles.
5. Avoid direct contact with body fluids.
6. Maintain sanitation.
   a. Mark and have available specific biohazard waste disposal containers where bacterial sources (gloves, dressings, etc.) are discarded.
   b. Place waste products in plastic bags and bury them in designated area.
   c. Bury human waste.
7. Purify water for drinking, cooking, medical use, if potable water is not available.
   a. Boil water at rolling boil for 10 minutes.
   b. Use water purification tablets.
   c. Use unscented liquid bleach (16 drops per gallon of water or 1 teaspoon per 5 gallons; mix and let stand for 30 minutes).

Developing a Communication Network

Procedure

1. Understand lines of communication. ▶ ***Rationale:*** When lines of communication are compromised, effective triage and intervention cannot take place.
   a. Mass casualty incident occurs.
   b. Local public health official notifies FBI—lead agency for crisis plan.
   c. FBI notifies DHS, HHS, CDC, and FEMA.
   d. State health agency requests CDC to deploy response teams if needed.

2. Understand the network of communication that will be activated in response to a suspected or actual bioterrorism event.
   a. Emergency response team:
      Local and state public health officials.
      Infection control personnel in notified facilities.
      FBI field offices (Department of Homeland Security).
      CDC.
      Local emergency medical services (EMS).
      Local police and fire departments.
   b. In turn, the Federal Response Plan will be activated.
3. Activate Federal Response Plan. ▸ ***Rationale:*** When the local area cannot cope with the disaster, federal assistance is available.
   a. Department of Health and Human Services (HHS) is primary agency.
   b. Office of Emergency Preparedness is action agency.
   c. Emergency Support Function N8 coordinates federal assistance to supplement state and local resources (directed by HHS).
   d. Implemented when state requests assistance and FEMA agrees.

EVIDENCE-BASED PRACTICE

Who Can You Count On?

Research has repeatedly shown that disasters result in increased pro-social behavior, where cooperation and consensus are present during the emergency response phase, and self-interested activity is set aside.

Source: Tierney, K., Lindell, M., & Perry, R. (2001). *Facing the unexpected: Disaster preparedness and response in the United States.* Washington, DC: Joseph Henry Press.

Establishing Viable Communication

Procedure

1. Set up **external communication** system designated spokesperson.
   a. A viable system will minimize disruption.
   b. All communication goes through designated spokesperson—no staff will communicate with the public, press, or outside persons.
2. Report to appointed community-wide regional spokesperson or small group designated as being in command throughout the incident. Spokesperson will be in charge of coordination of all media relations. ▸ ***Rationale:*** One person or small group in charge will minimize confusion.
3. Set up a single community site for family and friends to obtain victim-locator information. ▸ ***Rationale:*** More than one site will lead to mass confusion.
   a. Provide clear, consistent, and verifiable information to clients and general public.
   b. Plan in advance methods and channels of communication to be used to inform the public.
4. Establish **internal communication**.
   a. Determine position (not person) that will be in charge (i.e., emergency department supervisor, called "incident commander"). ▸ ***Rationale:*** Position, rather than person, will negate confusion when there is staff turnover, multiple shifts, or reassignment of staff.
   b. Communicate only through established lines of communication with designated commander or liaisons.
5. Establish a **collaborative communication system**.
   a. Establish ongoing, open channels of communication with emergency response teams. ▸ ***Rationale:*** Response teams may have first awareness of the disaster and will need to communicate with the hospital.
   b. Appoint person (reporting to spokesperson) to collaborate with response team and link to community representative.
   c. Develop a community-wide communications network. ▸ ***Rationale:*** If different organizations cannot communicate with each other, precious time will be lost.

NOTE: Local areas are beginning to establish their own interconnected networks to facilitate communication. For example, all of New York City's hospitals are connected via the Internet, so if victims begin to funnel into several facilities, their symptoms can be quickly correlated to establish a diagnosis.

   d. Test the communications network so overload does not occur in the event of a mass casualty incident.
6. Develop clear communication systems that have access to telecommunications as well as a person-to-person communication system. ▸ ***Rationale:*** This position-to-position or person-to-person system is necessary if telecommunications are overwhelmed or unavailable.
   a. Use pagers, walkie-talkies, and the Internet via e-mail as substitutes for communication network during a disaster.
   b. Develop horizontal and vertical relationships between organizations, governmental and private, that will have to work together in a mass casualty event.

Clinical Alert

The goal of disaster medical interventions is to do the greatest good for the greatest number of victims.

Carrying Out Steps of Triage

Procedure

1. Evaluate the disaster area: stop, look, listen, check safety, and designated treatment areas.
2. Don protective gear (based on type of disaster) for your safety.
3. Quickly assess conditions for triage before beginning.
4. Conduct voice triage—tell victims to move, if they are able, to designated areas of triage.
   a. Immediate triage for life-threatening conditions.
   b. Delayed triage for those who can wait to be treated.
5. Treat immediate victims (airway, bleeding, and shock).
6. Tag all victims, even those who are dead.
7. Document results.

Treating Life-Threatening Conditions

Equipment

Protective gear
Dressings/bandages
Tourniquets
Stethoscope
Tongue blades
Automated external defibrillator (AED), if available

Procedure

1. Implement Simple Triage and Rapid Treatment (START). ▸ ***Rationale:*** This is the first step for treating multiple casualties in a disaster.
2. **Check breathing immediately**.
   a. Open airway. ▸ ***Rationale:*** If airway is obstructed, victim cannot get oxygen.
   b. Move fast—time is critical. ▸ ***Rationale:*** Heart function will be affected within minutes, and brain damage is possible after 4 minutes.
   c. Check if tongue is obstructing airway. ▸ ***Rationale:*** This is the most common airway obstruction (especially when victim is positioned on back).
3. Use head-tilt/chin-lift method if victim is not breathing and airway is not obstructed.
   a. Touch victim and shout, "CAN YOU HEAR ME?" ▸ ***Rationale:*** To ensure victim has not fainted.
   b. If victim does not respond, place one hand on forehead, two fingers of other hand under chin, and tilt jaw upward and head back slightly. ▸ ***Rationale:*** This position opens airway.
   c. Look for chest to rise, listen for air exchange, and feel for abdominal movement. ▸ ***Rationale:*** Reliable indicator of open airway is feeling or hearing air movement.
   d. If no response (victim does not start breathing), repeat procedure. (If AED is available, may apply to victim.)
   e. If victim does not respond after second attempt, move on to next victim. ▸ ***Rationale:*** Goal of disaster intervention is to do the greatest good for the greatest number of victims.
   f. If the victim begins breathing, maintain airway (hopefully with a volunteer holding airway open) or place soft object under victim's shoulders to elevate them, keeping airway open.
4. **Control bleeding.** ▸ ***Rationale:*** If bleeding is not controlled within a short period of time, victim will go into shock. Loss of 1 liter of blood—out of a total of 5 in the human body—will present risk of death.
5. Identify type of bleeding.
   a. Arterial bleeding (spurting blood)
   b. Venous bleeding (flowing blood)
   c. Capillary bleeding (oozing blood)
6. Choose appropriate method to control bleeding.
   a. Direct local pressure—place direct pressure over wound (using clean or sterile pad) and press firmly. ▸ ***Rationale:*** 95% of bleeding can be controlled by direct pressure with elevation.
   b. Maintain compression by wrapping wound firmly with pressure bandage.
   c. Elevate wound above level of heart.
   d. Use pressure point to slow blood flow to wound, brachial point for arm, femoral point for leg. ▸ ***Rationale:*** Using pressure on a pulse point on a major artery will slow blood flow.
7. Use tourniquet if bleeding cannot be controlled by other methods (consider this a last resort). ▸ ***Rationale:*** Tourniquets can pose serious risks to affected limbs.
   a. Incorrect material or application can cause more damage and bleeding; if too tight, nerves, blood vessels, or muscles may be damaged.
   b. If tourniquet is left in place too long, limb may be lost.
   c. If tourniquet is applied, leave in plain sight and affix label to victim's forehead, stating time tourniquet was applied.
   d. Notify physician to remove tourniquet.
8. **Recognize and treat shock.** ▸ ***Rationale:*** If the victim remains in shock, it will lead to death of cells, tissue, and organs.
   a. Body will initially compensate for blood loss, so signs of shock may not be observable.
   b. Continually evaluate victim's condition.

Steps of Trauma Assessment Applied to Triage

1. Perform a rapid systematic assessment. ▶ *Rationale:* Trauma is a multisystem condition so all systems must be assessed.
2. Complete a primary trauma assessment. ▶ *Rationale:* To identify victim's primary and critical problem.
   a. Airway
   b. Breathing capability
   c. Shock—circulation and bleeding
   d. Neurologic—level of consciousness, mental status
   e. Exposure to contaminate
   f. Disability
   g. Evacuation necessity
3. Complete a secondary assessment (post-triage) that includes a focus assessment.

Clinical Alert

Experts agree that 49% of disaster victims could be saved by providing simple medical care for life-threatening conditions: airway obstruction, bleeding, and shock.

9. Observe for signs/symptoms of shock:
   a. Rapid, shallow breathing
   b. Cold, pale skin (capillary refill)
   c. Failure to respond to simple commands
10. Administer treatment for shock:
    a. Position victim supine with feet elevated 6–10 in.
    b. Maintain open airway.
    c. Maintain body temperature (cover ground and victim).
    d. Avoid rough or excessive handling, and do not allow victim to eat or drink.

Assessing Victims Post-Triage

Procedure

1. Perform head-to-toe assessment, always in the same order. ▶ *Rationale:* Performing assessment in same way every time will enable you to complete it more quickly and accurately.
   a. Head
   b. Neck
   c. Shoulders
   d. Chest
   e. Arms
   f. Abdomen
   g. Pelvis
   h. Legs
   i. Back
2. Complete assessment before beginning any treatment. ▶ *Rationale:* In order to prioritize treatment interventions, a complete assessment must be done.
3. Observe for any sign/symptom that indicates major injury.
   a. Assess how person received injury (mechanism of injury)
   b. Airway obstruction
   c. Signs of shock
   d. Labored or difficult breathing
   e. Excessive bleeding
   f. Swelling/bruising
   g. Severe pain
4. Provide immediate treatment. During treatment, reclassify victim, if necessary.

Cultural Awareness

During a disaster, it remains a priority for staff to address ethnic, religious, and cultural customs of diet, death, and burial.

5. Assess that victim is not in immediate danger. If available staff, continue to assess for signs of head, neck, and spinal injury.
   a. Change in level of consciousness (unconscious, confused)
   b. Unable to move body part
   c. Severe pain in head, neck, back
   d. Tingling or numbness in extremities

Phases of Death Due to Trauma

Phase 1	Death within minutes due to overwhelming and irreversible damage to vital organs.
Phase 2	Death within several hours due to excessive bleeding.
Phase 3	Death within several days or weeks due to infection or multiple system failure (not from injury per se).

Experts agree that more than 40% of disaster victims in Phases 2 and 3 of death could be saved by providing basic medical care.

Source: American College of Surgeons.

   e. Difficulty breathing or seeing
   f. Heavy bleeding/blood in eyes or nose
   g. Seizures
   h. Nausea, vomiting
   i. Possible closed compression injury (e.g., victim found under collapsed structure)
6. Immobilize head, neck, or spine by keeping spine in straight line, putting cervical collar on neck, or placing victim on board—if equipment is available.
7. Document who person is and relevant medical information.
   a. Available identifying data
   b. Description, clothing
   c. Injuries
   d. Treatment
   e. Transfer location

Caring for Those Who Died

Procedure

1. Tag victims pronounced DOA (dead on arrival).
   a. Add special tag "not to remove personal effects."
   b. Incorporate special instructions for people performing autopsies, preparing bodies for burial or transportation.
2. Place bodies in cordoned-off area for field triage. ▸ ***Rationale:*** Decontamination may have to be completed before transport.
3. Notify those performing post-mortem care of victim's diagnosis. ▸ ***Rationale:*** For protection of staff handling post-mortem care.
   a. Autopsies performed carefully using all personal protective equipment and Standard Precautions, including use of masks and eye protection.
   b. Incorporate any special instructions about biological–chemical–radiological agent present.
4. Complete a record for all bodies including identification, name of person declaring death, diagnosis, if known, name of agency removing body, etc.

Caring for Clients With Psychological Reactions

Procedure

1. Expect major psychological reactions of fear, panic, anger, horror, paranoia, unrealistic concerns about infection, fear of contagion, social isolation, demoralization, etc., after a bioterrorism event.
2. Plan prior to such an event for professional and educated volunteers to be on site.
3. Minimize fear and panic in staff.
   a. Provide educational materials that include risks to healthcare workers, accurate information of bioterrorism facts, plans for protecting workers, and how to use personal protection equipment.
   b. Encourage team participation in disaster drills. ▸ ***Rationale:*** Experience in handling a disaster will build confidence and allay anxiety.
4. Cope with psychological reactions of fear and anxiety.
   a. Minimize panic by clearly explaining care given with explanations.
   b. Offer rapid evaluation and treatment and avoid isolation, if possible. ▸ ***Rationale:*** Waiting for evaluation and treatment (as well as isolation) will cause anxiety.
5. Treat major anxiety reactions in unexposed persons with factual information, reassurance, and medication, if indicated. ▸ ***Rationale:*** Anxiety is communicable; prompt intervention will allay group anxiety. ("Worried well" persons could overwhelm hospitals if they leave disaster area and go to closest healthcare facility.)
6. Prevent post-terrorism trauma. ▸ ***Rationale:*** Early intervention may reduce stress disorder.
   a. Gather victims into a group with a skilled therapist soon after event (within 24 hr) to prevent a major post-trauma reaction.
      1. Early opportunity for catharsis will help prevent suppression of traumatic event emotions.
      2. Group victims according to age and experience.
   b. Follow initial group meeting with subsequent meeting within 1 week to discuss feelings about event. ▸ ***Rationale:*** Research has found that group meetings after traumatic event have eliminated 80% of post-traumatic stress disorder.

EVIDENCE-BASED PRACTICE

Studies on mass casualty incidents have reported enormous stress and pressure faced by health workers. Effective response to the crises requires considerable support services for themselves.

Source: Caro, D. (1999). Towards integrated crisis support of regional emergency networks. *Health Care Management Review, 24*(4), 7–19.

Clinical Alert

If a disaster occurs, be alert to signs of disaster trauma in yourself and/or coworkers and take steps to alleviate stress before it becomes incapacitating.

Identifying Post-Traumatic Stress Disorder (PTSD)

Procedure

1. Recognize possibility of existing condition.
   a. Traumatic event occurs and is reexperienced as flashbacks, dreams, or memory state.
   b. Abreaction occurs: vivid recall of painful experience with original emotions.
   c. Individual cannot adjust to event.
2. Assess signs and symptoms of anxiety and depression.
   ▸ ***Rationale:*** Early recognition will assist in therapeutic intervention.
   a. Emotional instability, withdrawal, and isolation.
   b. Nightmares, difficulty sleeping.
   c. Feelings of detachment or guilt.
3. Assess aggressive or acting-out behavior; may be explosive or impulsive behavior.
4. Assist client to go through recovery process.
   ▸ ***Rationale:*** Client may have to be assisted through recovery steps to reach adjustment.
   a. Recovery—reassure client that he is safe after experience of the traumatic event.
   b. Avoidance—client will avoid thinking about traumatic event; support client.
   c. Reconsideration—client deals with event by confronting it, talking about it, and working through feelings.
   d. Adjustment—client rehabilitates and adjusts to environment after event; client functions well and is able to view future positively.

Post-Traumatic Stress Syndrome (PTSD) After a Natural Disaster

After the Katrina disaster, one third of the people hardest hit could develop PTSD. Disaster-related mental problems such as anxiety, substance abuse, and depression could also occur.

The major contributors to the risk of psychological trauma and later PTSD are:

- Severity of person's exposure to the tragedy
- Threat to life
- Severity of property damage or loss
- Degree of injuries to self or family members
- Degree of panic during disaster
- Separation from family members
- Amount of financial loss
- Predisaster history of mental illness or those already under stress
- Lack of resources (social, family, or financial) after disaster
- Statistics reveal that females over males, ethnic minorities, and adults age 40 to 60 are more challenged by a disaster

Nurses doing psychological triage after a disaster need to evaluate the individuals based on risk assessment. They need to identify potential danger to self or others and intervene accordingly.

EVIDENCE-BASED PRACTICE

Post-Traumatic Stress Syndrome (PTSD) After a Natural Disaster

In 1992, after Hurricane Andrew, one study found that 36% of South Florida subjects exposed to the disaster met the criteria for new onset of PTSD 6 months after the storm, and 30% suffered major depression.

Source: David, D., Mellman, T. A., Mendoza, L. M., Kulick-Bell, R., Ironson, G., & Schneiderman, N. (1996). Psychiatric morbidity following Hurricane Andrew. *J Trauma Stress* 9(3), 607–612.

DOCUMENTATION for Triage, Treatment, and Communication Matrix

- Triage treatment areas established—note site and subdivisions
- Triage format for assessing victims
- Public health parameters followed
- Protection equipment used for site selection and maintenance
  Sanitation procedures
  Purified water procedure
  Search and rescue procedures
- Protection gear and equipment used for triaging victims
- Procedures implemented for individual life-threatening conditions
- Post-triage assessment of victim
- Assessment of psychological reactions
- Interventions for identifying post-traumatic stress disorder
- Communication network established:
  Internal communication lines
  External communication lines
  Collaborative communication lines

CRITICAL THINKING Application

Expected Outcomes

- Triage treatment areas are established within public health parameters.
- Staff follows appropriate steps of triage protocol.
- Life-threatening conditions are identified and treated.
- Post-triage assessment is completed.
- Post-traumatic stress disorder (PTSD) is identified and clients are referred appropriately.

Unexpected Outcomes	Alternative Actions
Triage site does not conform to public health requirements.	• Assign additional personnel to monitor for public health concerns (in addition to triage and treatment). • Collect waste in disposable containers for human waste or place in plastic bags and bury. • Boil water or use water-purifying tablets if potable water is not available. • Use diluted bleach (0.5%) to decontaminate surfaces.
Multiple casualties exhibit life-threatening conditions.	• Implement triage principles—simple triage and rapid treatment (START)—check breathing, control bleeding, and treat shock. • Assess and treat victims post-triage and post-initial interventions, then refer to community facility.
Large group of victims are experiencing major psychological reactions of fear, panic, and horror.	• Assign personnel and/or volunteers to separate and group victims according to age and degree of reaction. • Assign skilled therapist to work with group at least 15–30 minutes, allowing them to talk about their fears and feelings. • Refer victims to post-trauma group to prevent post-traumatic stress disorder.

GERONTOLOGIC Considerations

Under the circumstances of a bioterrorism event, all victims will be triaged and treated according to the system established. The elderly will be included in general triage decisions according to their injuries, not age.

For natural disasters, elderly victims will be treated according to the triage system used. The first responders will, however, have to take into account certain principles when dealing with elderly casualties.

- Number of elderly residents in nursing homes expected to double by 2030 to 3.2 million
- Elderly are more vulnerable to disaster conditions—aging immune system, mobility, and physical limitations
- Special concerns for elderly in disaster situations due to:
  Mobility impairment
  Chronic health issues
  Slowed response time
  Need for multiple meds
  Sensory changes
  Memory changes
  Communication barriers

MANAGEMENT Guidelines

Delegation

- Pre-emergency/disaster planning and coordination will have (should have) occurred before the terrorist event.
- Personnel roles and lines of authority will have been previously delineated so healthcare workers will refer to the Preparedness Plan posted in each facility and report to the designated superior or Incident Command Center.
- Each member of the responder team should have an identified role, have practiced actions necessary to perform in this role, studied the educational materials, and demonstrated knowledge necessary to perform in this designated role.
- Role responsibilities must be decided before a disaster occurs. For example, in one disaster scenario, the nursing supervisor is responsible for setting up the command center, the administrator will be in contact with outside resource organizations, and the director of nursing will do the administrator's functions.

- Because emergency response teams must work together as a team, be flexible and adapt to the requirements of a changing situation, team response must have practice sessions.
- Duties of command center designated person:

  Find adequate nursing personnel and assign roles and responsibilities

  Assign responsible person to switchboard

  Limit all routine nonemergency admissions

  Refer all public information calls and media to designated place

Communication Matrix

Once a disaster has been declared, the information flow is delineated in the Preparedness Plan.

- Reporting of the incident takes place (see Reporting Requirements on page 460).
- The community liaison notifies Community Emergency Response Team (CERT) team leader (out-of-hospital staff), who notifies medical–nursing group (in-hospital staff).
- Federal agencies notified.
- A community-wide network is established—all using the same channels of communication.
- Position-to-position (not person) cascade of communication (community liaison ► command center person ► team leader) is established.
- A single off-site communication center for family and friends of victims must be established to avoid overloading system.

CRITICAL THINKING Strategies

Scenario 1

Your hospital has not developed a total Preparedness Plan, including specific recommendations and strategies.

1. What are the implications of this situation under disaster conditions? Include a list of several consequences.
2. What strategies would you suggest to increase hospital administration awareness?
3. Describe the steps you would suggest to alter this situation so that a viable Preparedness Plan is in place.

Scenario 2

A Russian organized crime syndicate has stolen radioactive isotopes from an unprotected nuclear research facility and sold the material to an al-Qaeda group. This terrorist group smuggled the material into the United States via Canada. At a professional football game, this group detonates the weapon, creating a small explosion that rapidly spreads radiological material. The firefighters and police who rushed to the site had no radiation detectors, so they were exposed to radiological fallout. HAZMAT teams were sent to the area, detected radiation, and set up decontamination equipment.

You are part of the Preparedness Plan team for the local hospital in charge of the command center. Upon being notified of the disaster:

1. What additional information does your team need to make decisions about coping with this disaster?
2. What are the priority actions you would take?
3. What further assessment of contamination is necessary?
4. Describe the special protective equipment your team would require.

Scenario 3

You are tasked with developing a disaster kit for people to carry in their cars in case of a disaster that occurs when they are away from home.

1. What items would you suggest be included in a car disaster kit?
2. Add a rationale for including each item.

NCLEX® Review Questions

Unless otherwise specified, choose only one (1) answer.

1. During an earthquake, the best rationale for finding a space *beside* a large piece of furniture or a car (rather than *under* it) is
   1. To protect your head if the car or furniture caves in.
   2. That research has shown this will be a triangle of safe space.
   3. A large piece of furniture may not completely cover you.
   4. That it is easier and quicker to get beside the item rather than under it.
2. The best definition of a disaster is an event that
   1. Is unexpected and occurs with little warning.
   2. Is of great magnitude which disrupts and overwhelms current resources.
   3. Places the public and environment in danger.
   4. Carries an immediate threat to public health.

3. If a weapon of mass destruction strike occurs in the United States, the most difficult type or agent to identify would be
   1. A nuclear attack.
   2. Smallpox.
   3. Sarin gas.
   4. A biological agent.
4. The most Grays (units of exposure to radiation) that a person can absorb before experiencing symptoms of radiation poisoning are
   1. Over 8 Gy.
   2. Between 0.75 and 8 Gy.
   3. Less than 0.75 Gy.
   4. Over 10 Gy.
5. Which of the following biological agents might be used by terrorists to cause a mass casualty incident? ***Select all that apply.***
   1. Anthrax.
   2. Botulism.
   3. Radiation.
   4. Smallpox.
   5. Typhoid.
   6. Sarin gas.
6. In triage, the rationale for choosing a 5-level system over the more common 3-level is that
   1. The 5-level system decreases ambiguity of the middle level of emergency cases.
   2. More rapid identification of the client condition can be made.
   3. There is more variety in categorizing client conditions.
   4. This method is more appropriate for categorizing large numbers of victims.
7. You are assigned to establish a site for decontaminating victims. Place the steps of setting up the site in order.
   1. Set up the site on a downhill slope.
   2. Establish the site upwind from the contamination area.
   3. Supply personnel protection equipment for all health personnel.
   4. Find a source for water.
8. An indication that *vaccinia* immune globulin (VIG) should be administered is
   1. Encephalitis.
   2. Cardiac complications.
   3. The client is pregnant.
   4. Eczema vaccinatum.
9. Which of the following weapons of mass destruction would fall into the category of chemical agent?
   1. Q fever.
   2. Cyanide.
   3. Ricin.
   4. Smallpox.
10. When administering a smallpox vaccination, the nurse will evaluate the success of the procedure by observing
    1. A lump where the vaccine was administered.
    2. No blood at the site.
    3. A trace of blood at the site.
    4. A needle mark where the needle entered the skin.

16

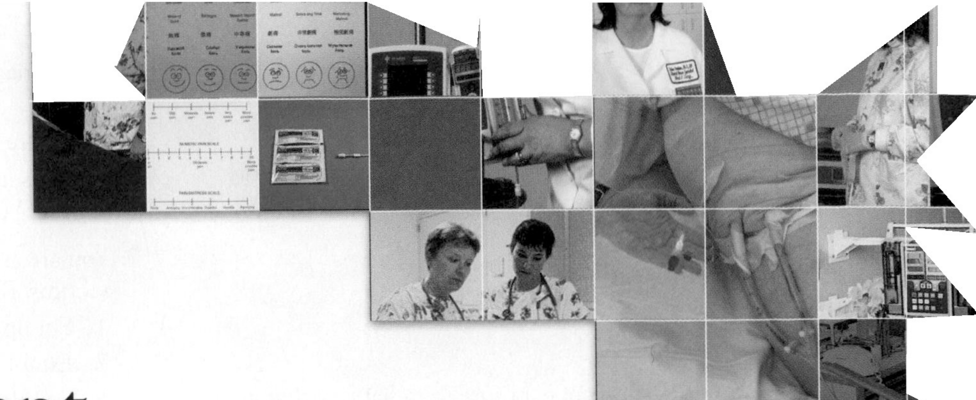

Pain Management

LEARNING OBJECTIVES

1. Discuss what is meant by the experience of pain.
2. Explain how natural endorphins work for pain control.
3. Describe the body's physiologic response to pain.
4. Identify the most important information elicited from the client regarding pain.
5. Discuss what it means for the nurse to be the client's advocate in relation to pain control.
6. Discuss the main components of The Joint Commission's Standards for Pain Management.
7. Compare assessing pain by quality and intensity.
8. Outline the main points of one nonpharmacological method of relieving pain.
9. Select a comfort measure for a client in acute pain and for a client in chronic pain.
10. Describe two different pain scales.
11. Describe the behavioral responses to mild versus severe pain.
12. Discuss two advantages of epidural narcotic analgesia.
13. Describe the potential side effects of narcotic medications via IV or epidural route.
14. List three criteria for client selection for patient-controlled analgesia (PCA).
15. Explain the steps involved in loading, priming, and changing a PCA syringe.
16. Describe the steps of teaching PCA to a client.
17. Discuss two components of pain management.

CHAPTER OUTLINE

TERMINOLOGY

Acupressure Chinese method of treatment that involves compression of certain areas of the body by following a system of meridians or energy flow.

Adaptive reaction a response by which the person attempts to improve or alter his or her condition in relation to the environment.

Alleviate to make more bearable; reduce (pain, grief, or suffering).

Angina a sense of suffocation with symptoms of severe, steady pain and feeling of pressure in region of the heart.

Arrhythmia irregular rhythm.

Arthritis inflammation of a joint, usually accompanied by pain and, frequently, deformity.

ATC around-the-clock medication for persistent pain.

Autogenic training a method of deep muscle relaxation that enables one to reduce the stress response, regain homeostasis, and prepare to handle additional stress.

Autonomic nervous system the part of the nervous system that regulates the functioning of internal organs and glands; it controls such functions as digestion, respiration, and cardiovascular activity.

Behavior the manner in which one acts.

Biofeedback a training technique that uses monitoring instruments to assist people to control stress-related disorders through self-regulation of internal functions.

Booster dose an additional dose given to a client on a PRN basis. Ordered by physician, administered by RN.

Brady prefix indicating slow.

Bradycardia slowed heart action, below 60 beats/min.

Capnography (side-stream) a module attached to PCA to detect client hypoventilation and/or a change in respiratory status.

Cardiovascular pertaining to the heart and blood vessels.

Cerebral cortex the extensive outer layer of gray tissue of the cerebral hemispheres (brain), responsible for higher nervous functions.

Coping mechanisms means by which an individual adjusts or adapts to a threat or a challenge; actions that assist in maintaining homeostasis.

Diaphoresis profuse sweating.

Dynamics of homeostasis danger or its symbols, whether internal or external, resulting in the activation of the sympathetic nervous system and the adrenal medulla. The organism prepares for fight or flight.

Emotional affected by strong feelings, as of joy and sorrow.

Endorphins a naturally occurring body chemical similar to morphine but many times stronger.

Fight or flight one's immediate response to stress that is, although archaic and often inappropriate, part of our central nervous system biologic heritage.

Four (4)-hour limit (mL) the maximum amount of drug that can be administered to client during a 4-hour period.

Gastrointestinal pertaining to the stomach and the intestine.

General adaptation syndrome a general theory of stress response formulated by Dr. Hans Selye; describes the action of stress response in three stages: the alarm reaction, the stage of resistance, and the stage of exhaustion.

Health the state of physical, psychologic, and sociologic well-being.

Hypertension a condition in which the client has a higher blood pressure than judged to be normal.

Illness a state characterized by the malfunction of the biopsychosocial organism.

Insomnia inability to sleep.

Ischemic local and temporary anemia due to obstruction of the circulation to a part.

ISMP Institute for Safe Medication Practices is a nonprofit organization that focuses on preventing medication errors by providing medication safety information to healthcare practitioners.

Loading dose (optional) initial dose given to client as ordered by physician.

Lockout interval period during which the PCA cannot be activated and no analgesic can be delivered by client. (A booster dose can be given during lockout interval if ordered.)

Meditation the act of reflecting on or pondering; contemplation.

Musculoskeletal pertaining to the muscles and the skeleton.

Nausea inclination to vomit, usually preceding emesis.

Opioid (narcotic) addiction pattern of compulsive drug use characterized by continued craving for the narcotic—creates both a psychological and physiological dependence.

Pain a sensation in which a person experiences discomfort, distress, or suffering. There are three main types of pain: acute, chronic, and malignant.

Parasympathetic nervous system a division of the autonomic nervous system that regulates acetylcholine and conserves energy expenditure; it slows down the system.

PCA—Patient-controlled analgesia a method of delivering pain medication via IV pump. Within physician-ordered parameters, the client can control the medication amount necessary to manage his or her pain level.

Physiologic concerning body function.

Psychogenic of mental origin.

Referred pain pain felt in a part removed from its point of origin.

Regression a turning back or return to a former state.

Relaxation a lessening of tension or activity in a part.

Resistance opposition to or the ability to oppose.

Stamina constitutional energy; strength; endurance.

Stress a nonspecific response of the body to any internal or external event or change that impinges on a person's system and creates a demand.

Stressor a specific demand that gives rise to a coping response.

Sympathetic nervous system a division of the autonomic nervous system that controls energy expenditure and mobilizes for action when confronted with a threat.

Tachy prefix meaning fast.

Tachycardia abnormal rapidity of heart action; above 100 beats/min.

TENS—Transcutaneous electrical nerve stimulation a noninvasive method to relieve pain that involves stimulation to the skin via a mild electric current.

The Joint Commission sets standards of care and accredits healthcare facilities (formerly JCAHO).

Traction determining the concentration of a solution.

Tolerance a larger and larger dose of an opioid is required to have the same effect.

Touch a tactile sense.

Visceral pertaining to internal organs.

Wellness a state of physical, psychologic, and sociologic well-being of a whole person.

COPING WITH PAIN

Pain is now considered the fifth vital sign and, according to The Joint Commission's Standards for Pain Management, is essential to regularly assess and manage in order to maintain the client's homeostasis and quality of life.

The experience of pain is direct and personal. In this culture we tend to view pain as a negative condition and often go to any lengths to avoid the sensation. The positive aspect of pain is that it is an early warning system; its presence triggers an awareness that something is wrong in the body. Without the sensation of pain we could not survive, because pain provides the cues that allow us to modify our reactions and direct our behavior. One perspective of pain is that it is a message to our conscious self to check out any pain sensation before it gets worse, for that is the nature of pain. Without intervention the condition may well get worse.

Margo McCaffery, a nurse–researcher who writes about caring for the client in pain, defines pain as "whatever the patient experiencing pain says it is, existing whenever he says it does." The nurse is totally dependent on the client to describe the sensation of pain, identify the location, and tell about what kind of pain is being experienced.

The most important information in pain assessment, then, is the client's report. The pain experience is totally subjective. The onset of acute pain stimulates the sympathetic nervous system "fight or flight" response that results in certain signs or symptoms. While observation of these symptoms provides objective data, it cannot be considered conclusive evidence to the identification of pain—that must come from the client.

The sensation of physical pain arouses some specific responses in the client. The sympathetic nervous system response is usually stimulated by superficial pain, and the parasympathetic nervous system response is usually stimulated by deeper pain and results in the slowing down of all the systems to conserve energy.

Theories of Pain

The neurophysiologic basis of pain can be explained by several theories, none of which is mutually exclusive nor totally comprehensive.

Specificity Theory This theory suggests that certain pain receptors are stimulated by a specific type of sensory stimuli that sends impulses to the brain. This theory dealt with the physiologic basis for pain but did not take into account the psychologic components of pain, nor the degree of pain tolerance.

Pattern Theory This theory attempts to include factors that were not adequately explained by the specificity theory. This theory suggests that pain originates in the dorsal horn of the

Types of Pain

Acute pain	Pain that occurs only in a defined period of time (6 months or less) and is caused by specific stimuli that damage the tissue. Usually of recent onset and varies in intensity.
Chronic pain	Prolonged, persistent nonmalignant pain that occurs over a 6-month period or longer. Pain varies in intensity and may serve no useful function.
Malignant pain	Recurrent, acute episodes of pain, which may also include chronic pain. This pain may vary in intensity and have rapid or slow onset. It may last longer than 6 months and be intractable.
Intractable pain	Severe and constant, usually resistant to relief measures.

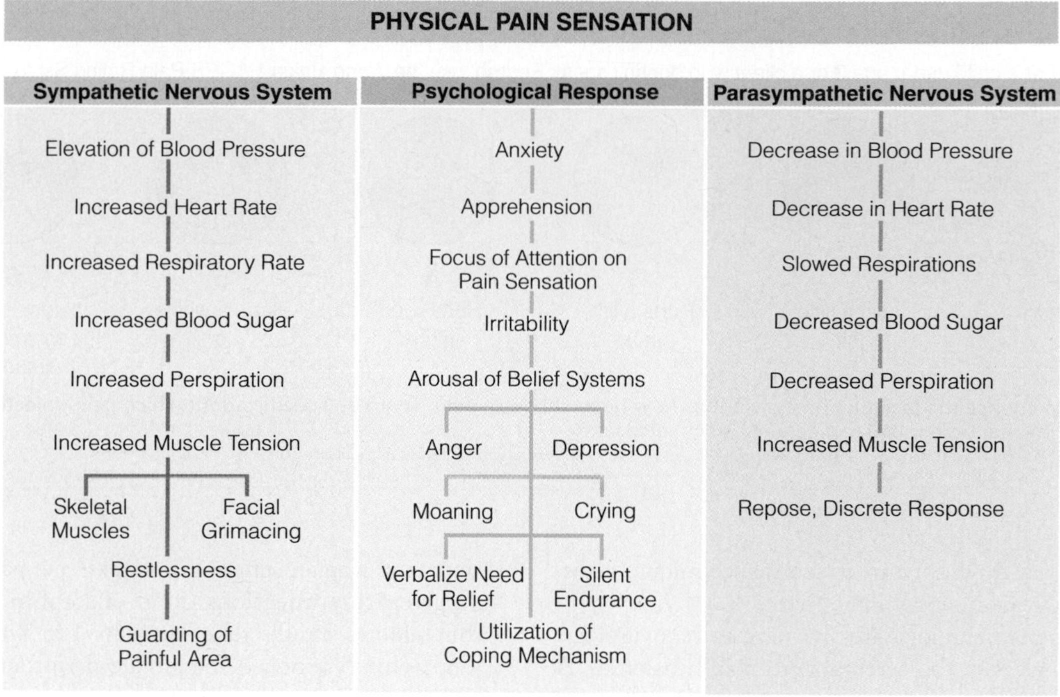

spinal cord. A certain pattern of nerve impulses is produced and results in intense receptor stimulation that is coded in the central nervous system (CNS) and signifies pain. Like the specificity theory, the pattern theory does not explain the psychologic factors of pain.

Gate Control Theory One of the most popular and credible concepts is the gate control theory. The first premise of the gate control theory is that the actual existence and intensity of the pain experience depends on the particular transmission of neurologic impulses. Second, gate mechanisms along the nervous system control the transmission of pain. Finally, if the gate is open, the impulses that result in the sensation of pain are able to reach the conscious level. If the gate is closed, the impulses do not reach the level of consciousness and the sensation of pain is not experienced.

Three primary types of neurologic involvement affect whether the gate is open or closed. The first type involves activity in the large and small nerve fibers that affect the sensation of pain. Pain impulses travel along small-diameter fibers. The large-diameter nerve fibers close the gate to the impulses that travel along the small fibers. The technique of using cutaneous stimulation on the skin, which has many large-diameter fibers, may help to close the gate to the transmission of painful impulses, thereby relieving the sensation of pain. Interventions that apply this theory to practice include massage, hot and cold applications, touch, acupressure, and transcutaneous electric nerve stimulation. These interventions are described in detail later in this chapter.

The second form of neurologic involvement is the impulses from the brainstem that affect the sensation of pain. The reticular formation monitors in the brainstem regulate sensory input. If the person receives adequate or excessive amounts of sensory stimulation, the brainstem transmits impulses that close the gate and inhibit pain impulses from being transmitted. If, on the other hand, the client experiences a lack of sensory input, the brainstem does not inhibit the pain impulses, the gate is open, and the pain impulses are transmitted. Interventions that apply to this part of the gate control theory are those

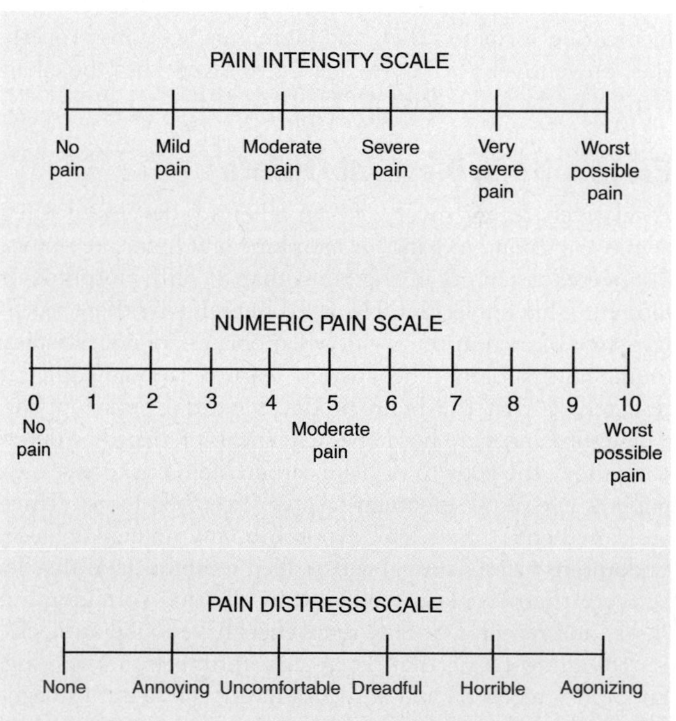

▲ Acute Pain Management: Operative or medical procedures and trauma.

Source: U.S. Department of Health and Human Services, Public Health Service.

Wong-Baker FACES Rating Scale

For a child under age 3 or a client who doesn't speak English, use the Wong-Baker FACES Pain Rating Scale

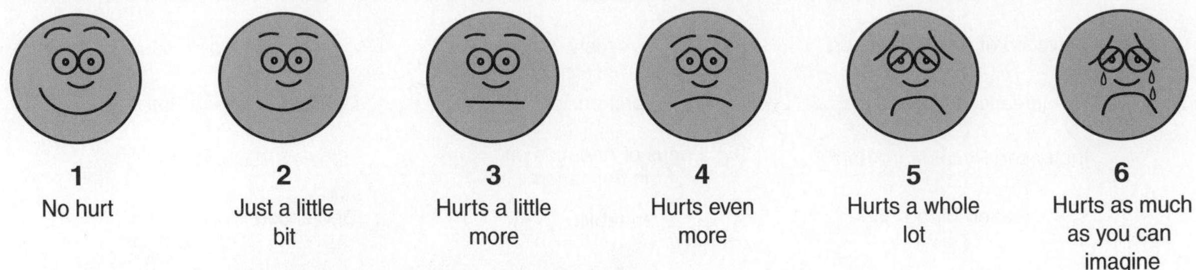

▲ Ask the client to choose the face that best describes how he or she feels pain. Try to be specific about which pain (injection or incision), where it hurts, and what time (now, earlier, after lunch, etc.).
Source: Wong-Baker FACES Pain Rating Scale (from Wong, D. L., et al. (1999). *Nursing care of infants and children* (6th ed). St. Louis: Mosby.

related in some way to sensory input, such as techniques of distraction, guided imagery, and visualization.

The third type of neurologic involvement is the neurologic activities or impulses in the cerebral cortex and thalamus. A person's thoughts, emotions, and memories may activate certain impulses in the cortex that trigger pain impulses, which are transmitted to the conscious level. Past experiences relating to pain affect how the client responds to current pain. For this reason, it is important to explore the client's previous experiences and teach the client what to expect from the present situation. Interventions that apply to this part of the gate control theory include using and teaching various relaxation techniques, teaching the client about what expectations to have about pain as related to a specific illness, allowing the client to feel he or she has some control over the taking of medication for pain relief, and giving medications properly (i.e., preventively, before the pain is so severe that the client fears he or she will receive no relief).

Endorphins, Natural Opiates

A relatively recent theory of pain relief was developed when Avron Goldstein, looking for morphine and heroin receptors, discovered receptors in the brain that fit only morphine or morphine-like molecules. He asked himself why these receptors were located in the brain, when opiates are not naturally found in this area. The answer, learned through diligent research, is that the brain produces natural brain opiates. These substances are hormones, chemicals produced by different parts of the body to regulate certain biologic processes. At present, five of these natural opiates have been found. Three are called endorphins, one dynorphin, and one enkephalin. Endorphins fit into special cells, called receptors, and thereby activate their regulating powers. In addition to endorphin "keys" and receptor "locks," researchers have found antilocks, called antagonists, that keep endorphins from working. Endorphin receptors and antilocks have been found throughout the body—in the stomach, intestines, pancreas, spinal cord, and bloodstream, as well as the brain.

A beta-endorphin is 50 times stronger than morphine, and a dynorphin is 190 times stronger than morphine. In one test, 14 men and women suffering from extreme pain from cancer were given tiny injections of an endorphin. All felt relief within minutes and the relief lasted for 1 to 3 days.

Endorphins are now being produced synthetically, but they are very expensive and at this time are used only for research. Researchers must discover how the body makes and releases endorphins before a method is developed to encourage the body to produce more of its own endorphins to control pain.

Pain Pathways

The pathway to pain is a complicated, fascinating expression of how our amazing bodies work. First there is the source of pain, a direct causative factor. Stimulation of a pain receptor may be mechanical, chemical, thermal, electric, or ischemic. The sensation travels along the sensory pathways and ascends the spinal cord to the thalamus. The autonomic nervous system is activated, and sensations travel to the sensory area of the cerebral cortex. Pain reception occurs in the thalamus, where awareness and integration take place, and pain interpretation occurs in the cerebral cortex. Once awareness of pain takes place and it has been interpreted by the cerebral cortex, the person becomes aware and the response patterns are activated.

The Pain Experience

The pain experience is a mixture of physical sensations, physiologic changes, and psychosocial (including psychological, sociocultural, and environmental) factors. The client's interpretation of the physical sensation is influenced by the client's culture, previous experiences with and without pain, beliefs about self, interpretation of the future, present environment, and the persons in that environment. The intensity of pain is influenced by what the sensation means to the client, the client's level of anxiety, degree of fatigue, and the number of stressors in the client's environment.

There are several methods of assessing the degree or level of pain a client may be experiencing. Note the examples of pain scales you may use to assess your client's pain. After explaining the scale you are using, ask your client what level of pain he or she is experiencing at the moment. You may use a numeric scale of 1 to 10, an intensity scale with 3 or more categories to

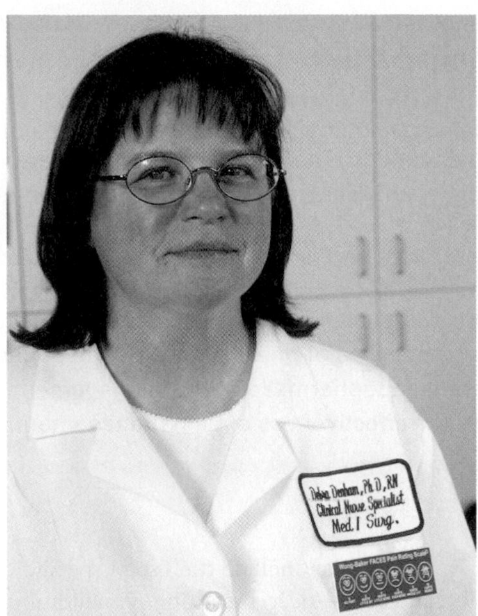

▲ Nurse's badge with Wong-Baker FACES Pain Rating Scale reminds both nurse and client to pay attention to pain level.

rate client pain, a pain distress scale, or the Wong-Baker FACES scale. Note the photo in which the nurse is wearing a FACES scale badge. The FACES pain scale is very important for pediatric clients, since children may have difficulty verbalizing the degree of pain they are experiencing. The different faces help them relate to pain by how sad the face appears, thus identifying for the nurse the level of pain they are feeling. Whichever scale is chosen, maintain its use throughout the course of pain control.

The Joint Commission Standards for Pain Management

In 2000, The Joint Commission described the appropriate standards for pain management for all healthcare facilities. The standards below were adapted from the comprehensive accreditation manual for hospitals.

- *Recognize that clients have the right to appropriate assessment and management of pain.* Pain assessment is to be considered a priority; in fact, it is now considered by many facilities and several states to be the fifth vital sign. This will enable the client's pain level to be assessed as frequently as vital signs.
- The facility must provide appropriate pain assessment tools (see pain scales and faces), and *pain levels should be recorded so that regular reassessment and follow-up can be done.*
- *Policies will be in place so that clients will be treated for pain, and adequate doses of opioids to relieve pain without unacceptable side effects will be given. Clients will be involved in their own pain management.*
- *If a facility, such as a long-term home care facility, cannot treat the client adequately for pain, the client should be referred to an appropriate facility.*
- *Facilities should collect data to monitor the effectiveness of pain management.*
- *Facility staff should receive education so they are competent in pain assessment and management.*
- *Clients and their families should be informed about pain management and client's needs for symptom control, and these should be included in discharge planning.*

Again, in 2001, The Joint Commission released revised standards for the assessment and management of pain. They stated that all healthcare facilities are expected to comply with these standards and that accreditation will be granted only on this basis. Margo McCaffery, an expert on pain management, believes that these revised standards may do more to

COMMUNITY HOSPITAL

PAIN ASSESSMENT

CONFIDENTIAL INFORMATION

SECTION I — TO BE COMPLETED BY PATIENT / RESPONSIBLE ADULT (PRE-PROCEDURE)

Describe current pain on pain scale. Circle number.

0	2	4	6	8	10
No Hurt	Hurts Little Bit	Hurts Little More	Hurts Even More	Hurts Whole Lot	Hurts Worst

0	1	2	3	4	5	6	7	8	9	10
No Pain		Mild Pain		Moderate Pain		Severe Pain		Very Severe		Worst Possible

Wong-Baker FACES Pain Rating Scale from Wong DL, Hockenberry-Eaton M, Wilson S, Winkelstein ML, Schwartz, P.: Wongs Essentials of Pediatric Nursing, ed. 6, St. Louis, 2001; Mosby, p. 1301. Copyright Mosby. Reprinted with permission.

Where? Mark drawing with an X

PLEASE RATE YOUR PAIN BY CIRCLING THE ONE NUMBER THAT BEST DESCRIBES YOUR PAIN RIGHT **NOW**.	PLEASE RATE YOUR PAIN BY CIRCLING THE ONE NUMBER THAT BEST DESCRIBES YOUR PAIN AT ITS **LEAST** IN THE LAST 24 HOURS.
0 1 2 3 4 5 6 7 8 9 10 (No Pain … Worst Pain Imaginable)	0 1 2 3 4 5 6 7 8 9 10 (No Pain … Worst Pain Imaginable)
PLEASE RATE YOUR PAIN BY CIRCLING THE ONE NUMBER THAT BEST DESCRIBES YOUR PAIN AT ITS **WORST** IN THE LAST 24 HOURS.	PLEASE RATE YOUR PAIN BY CIRCLING THE ONE NUMBER THAT BEST DESCRIBES YOUR PAIN AT ITS **AVERAGE** IN THE LAST 24 HOURS.
0 1 2 3 4 5 6 7 8 9 10 (No Pain … Worst Pain Imaginable)	0 1 2 3 4 5 6 7 8 9 10 (No Pain … Worst Pain Imaginable)

DURATION: ☐ Constant ☐ Intermittent

TYPE OF PAIN: ☐ Burning ☐ Dull ☐ Sharp ☐ Cramping ☐ Pressure ☐ Heavy ☐ Other ______

WHAT HELPS THE PAIN: ☐ Rest ☐ Heat ☐ Cold ☐ Alternative Therapy (Massage) ☐ Medication Specify ______

WHAT MAKES THE PAIN WORSE: ☐ Deep breath ☐ Coughing ☐ Activity Specify ______

HOW MUCH RELIEF ARE YOU OBTAINING FROM YOUR CURRENT METHODS OF PAIN MANAGEMENT (Please Circle)
0% 10% 20% 30% 40% 50% 60% 70% 80% 90% 100%

HAVE YOU EXPERIENCED DECREASED FUNCTION OR DECREASED QUALITY OF LIFE DUE TO PAIN ☐ Yes ☐ No

PATIENT OR RESPONSIBLE ADULT SIGNATURE	DATE

SECTION II — TO BE COMPLETED BY REGISTERED NURSE

PRE-OP PAIN MANAGEMENT INSTRUCTIONS GIVEN (BOOKLET) ☐ Yes ☐ No

EXPECTED COMFORT GOAL POST PROCEDURE — **AT REST**
0 1 2 3 4 5 6 7 8 9 10

EXPECTED COMFORT GOAL POST PROCEDURE — **WITH ACTIVITY**
0 1 2 3 4 5 6 7 8 9 10

DOES PATIENT HAVE NEEDS RELATED TO COMFORT ☐ Yes ☐ No ☐ Acute Pain ☐ Chronic Pain

PAIN SCALE PATIENT PREFERS ☐ Numeric Pain Distress Scale ☐ Faces Scale ☐ Translation Scale

NURSE'S SIGNATURE	DATE	TIME

▲ Pain assessment form.

How to Measure Pain

Location	Ask the client to locate pain on or within the body—exactly where is the pain felt?
Intensity	Determine strength, power, or force of the pain the client is experiencing. Use numeric or verbal scales or the faces pictures.
Quality	Determine the features or characteristics that distinguish this pain, such as searing, dull, throbbing, sharp, burning, etc.
Pattern	Ask client how pain changes and timing of the pain, such as is it continuous, steady, intermittent, transient?

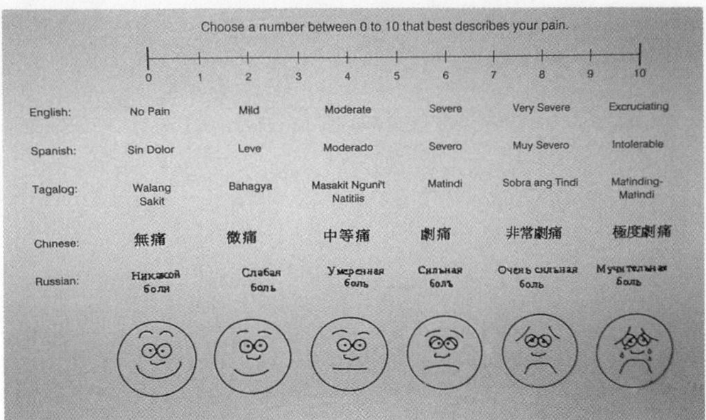

▲ A multilanguage pain chart facilitates an accurate description of pain.

improve pain management than any other development in managing pain.

NONINVASIVE PAIN RELIEF

When a method to relieve pain is noninvasive, it is safer and results in fewer potential side effects for the client. Such measures are becoming the pain control choice of the future.

Current practice for controlling pain is to use both drugs and nondrug options because both, separately or combined, meet the objectives of relieving pain and making the client more comfortable.

Nondrug options may include the use of specific cognitive–behavioral techniques—deep breathing, visualization, imagery; physical agents—electric stimulators, massage–vibration, and biofeedback systems; and various adjunct therapies—cold therapy, heat therapy, or counterirritants.

The nonpharmacological approach (Table 16-1) is appropriate for clients who are receptive to alternative methods; who have a high level of anxiety around the issue of pain; who would benefit from reducing dependence on drug therapy; who anticipate long-term or have chronic pain; or who receive inadequate pain relief from pharmacological interventions.

Recommendations for Pain Management

The University of Iowa has developed guidelines for acute pain management, including a set of major recommendations. The main topics covered are:

- Complete a baseline pain assessment, including pain level.
- Educate client and family about pain management.
- Monitor the acute pain the client is experiencing, including intensity, duration, and effect of pain.
- Follow guidelines of pharmacological management.
- Implement nonpharmacological management.
- Assess the effectiveness of pain management.

Characteristics of Pain

Location

- Area of the body
- Diffuse or localized
- Radiates and area involved

Quality

- Stabbing, knife-like
- Throbbing
- Cramping
- Vise-like, suffocating
- Searing, burning
- Superficial, deep

Intensity

- Rate on scale: 0–10 (0 = no pain, 10 = most pain ever experienced)

Factors Associated With Pain

- Nausea
- Vomiting
- Bradycardia, tachycardia
- Hypotension, hypertension
- Profuse perspiration
- Apprehension or anxiety

Precipitating Factors

- Motion affecting incision area (e.g., coughing, turning, deep breathing)
- Fear and emotional distress
- Inflammation or infection
- Trauma
- Disease state

Aggravating Factors

- Position changes
- Environmental stressors
- Fatigue
- Inadequate pain relief measures

Alleviating Factors

- Position change
- Medications
- Biofeedback
- Visualization
- Relaxation techniques
- TENS
- Massage

The Nurse's Role

Pain reduction methods include a wide range of techniques and medications. Rarely is pain relief successfully achieved with only one method. Even massive doses of narcotics do not always control pain effectively—especially when it has been allowed to escalate.

One of the most important influences on pain relief is the relationship that exists between nurse and client. With most methods (the exception is PCA), the nurse has the power to relieve pain or to withhold pain relief. This knowledge creates anticipatory anxiety for the client. The client may request less medication when the nurse is supportive, caring, and assists with pain management.

The single most critical factor in achieving pain relief is for the nurse to be the client's advocate. The comfort of the client is the nurse's primary concern.

Nursing interventions that provide effective pain relief, in addition to pain medication, are those that encourage behaviors that assist the client not to focus on pain. For example, when the client is talking about something of great interest or pleasure, he or she is not thinking about pain. Teaching the client techniques, such as deep, slow breathing and relaxation, lessens pain, whereas muscle tension and anxiety increase it. If the nurse teaches pain relief techniques before surgery, the client can more easily implement them when the pain is intense. The nurse may also encourage the client to use techniques that he or she has already found effective, no matter how "unscientific" they may be. Whatever method or technique the nurse uses to assist the client with relieving pain, the single most critical intervention is a caring and supportive attitude.

To provide pain management effectively to clients from other cultures, the nurse must understand a client's culture and how it affects the client's response to pain. To accomplish this, the nurse must take into account a client's religious beliefs and the external influence these may have on the client's pain experience.

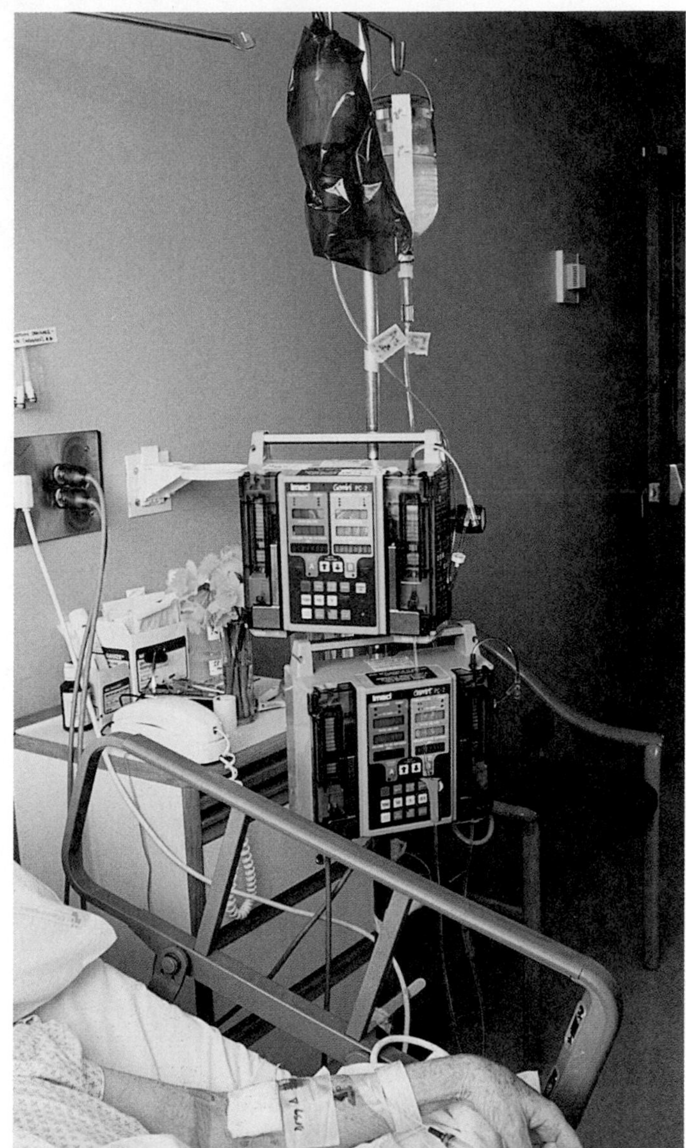

▲ Continuous IV narcotic drip for pain control.

TECHNIQUES FOR PAIN CONTROL

IV Patient-Controlled Analgesia (PCA)

One of the most successful methods of pain relief, introduced in the 1970s, was patient-controlled analgesia (PCA). The primary purpose of PCA is to allow the client to self-administer an analgesic dose of medication predetermined by the physician. PCA enables the client to assess and control his or her own pain level. This method of pain control has been found to be very efficacious because the client feels in more control of his or her life situation, there is no significant difference in the amount of analgesic medication used (if anything, it is usually less), there is better pain control than IM injections, and this method of pain control is less time-consuming for the nurse.

Epidural Pain Control

An effective technique for controlling pain is the use of an epidural catheter inserted into the epidural space. The advantage of epidural pain control is that the narcotic moves directly from the epidural space into the spinal fluid and binds with opiate receptors in the spinal cord, blocking reception of pain. Administered by this method, the required drug dose is considerably lower because it is not metabolized in the liver.

Direct IV Pain Control

In addition to the new methods of pain control, a client may receive a continuous infusion via direct IV. The dosage may be titrated to achieve pain relief with the lowest dose (10 mg or

> **Pain—the Fifth Vital Sign**
>
> Many states have passed into law the requirement that pain be considered the fifth vital sign. It must be assessed and documented at the time other vital signs are taken. The Veterans Administration, as well as other states and facilities, has incorporated pain on their vital signs graphic record.

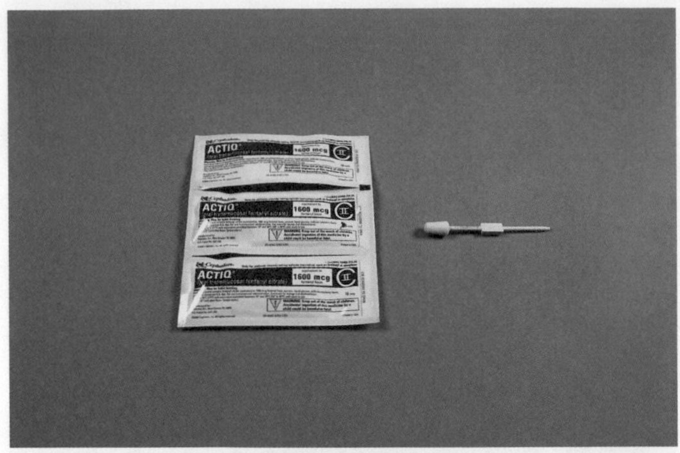

▲ A method for managing breakthrough pain is oral transmucosal, delivering medication via a lozenge on a stick.

1/6 g of morphine sulfate). The dose is individualized according to the client's needs, tolerance, and response. When pain relief is not achieved, increments of at least 25% of the previous dose should be implemented. When morphine is administered IV, a dark bag should be placed over the narcotic bag because the medication is light-sensitive.

Breakthrough Pain Control

There are two major types of pain—continuous and breakthrough. Many clients with cancer experience long periods of persistent pain and may also experience severe flare-ups that occur even when the client is on around-the-clock (ATC) medication. Studies suggest that nearly 70% of cancer clients experience breakthrough pain. These episodes typically last about 30 minutes, but tend to totally decimate the client.

Generally, breakthrough pain occurs as two types:

- Incident pain—caused by movement or activity (for example, sitting up, walking, or coughing).
- Spontaneous pain—does not seem to be linked to any specific source, but occurs with no warning or relation to activity or movement.

Breakthrough pain can be managed by different protocols, some of which are listed below.

- Increasing the dose of ATC so that breakthrough pain is eliminated—this method is not always advisable because sedation and other side effects of the drug may occur.
- Changing the ATC so that relatively constant analgesia occurs (use long-acting oral opioids or fentanyl patches).
- Prescribing a supplemental dose of a short-acting morphine-like drug so that it is taken 30 minutes before incident pain when this type of pain is predictable.
- When spontaneous pain occurs, instruct the client to take the dose as soon as possible after onset. At this point in pain control, this is the best plan, even though there may be a "pain gap." New drugs, currently being researched in clinical trials, may solve this problem.
- A new delivery method, oral transmucosal, delivers fentanyl citrate via a sucker. An example of this drug is Actiq, 1,600 mcg/sucker. This has the advantage of being quickly absorbed through the mucous membrane of the mouth and working rapidly to control breakthrough pain. This medication should be taken only by clients already taking prescription opioid (narcotic) drugs on a regular schedule.

Analgesic Patches

Two types of patches are now available to assist in pain management. One, the size of a credit card, uses a slight electric current to deliver medication through the skin of the arm or chest. In a survey of postsurgical clients, 77% rated this method good to excellent (*Journal of American Medical Association*, March 17, 2000). The second type of patch is transdermal, may be placed at the point of chronic pain (for example, a ruptured disc in the back), and delivers fentanyl (Duragesic).

The Institute for Safe Medication Practices (ISMP) suggests that serious adverse reactions can occur when new transdermal patches (for example, opioids for pain relief) are applied without the removal of existing patches. To avoid a potential overdose, the site and time should be clearly charted on the medication record when the patches are applied and removed.

CULTURAL AWARENESS

Healthcare personnel working in a variety of settings maintain that pain is a culturally influenced phenomenon. How pain is experienced and expressed varies by cultural group. For example, some cultures (such as the Italians and Jewish people) encourage open expression of feelings like pain, while others (the stoic English, Irish, and Chinese) believe that pain is something to be ignored or endured in silence. This was demonstrated by Zborowski's study done as early as the 1950s. While these general conclusions may lead to stereotyping, it is important to consider the impact of the individual's culture in the assessment of pain level.

Source: Spector, R. (2001). *Cultural diversity in health and illness* (5th ed.). Upper Saddle River, NJ: Prentice Hall Health

NURSING DIAGNOSES

The following nursing diagnoses may be appropriate to include on client care plans when the components are related to alleviating pain in a client.

NURSING DIAGNOSIS	RELATED FACTORS
Anxiety	Anticipation of discomfort, fear, helplessness, inability to relax
Compromised Family Coping	Family members have difficulty dealing with client's pain, functions as proxy for pain relief (see Table 16-3 for proxy explanation)
Ineffective Coping	Poor adjustment to pain/illness, fear
Fear	Long-term disability, terminal disease, hospitalization, invasive procedures, lack of knowledge, surgery and its outcome
Acute or Chronic Pain	Trauma, immobility, surgery, chronic illness

CLEANSE HANDS The single most important nursing action to decrease the incidence of hospital-based infections is hand hygiene. *Remember to wash your hands or use antibacterial gel before and after each and every client contact.*

IDENTIFY CLIENT Before every procedure, check two forms of client identification, not including room number. These actions prevent errors and conform to The Joint Commission standards.

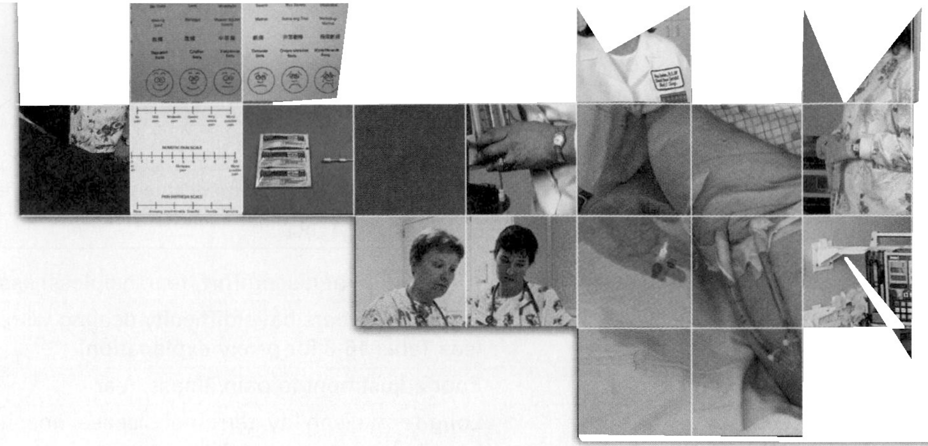

Chapter 16

UNIT 1

Pain Assessment

Nursing Process Data

ASSESSMENT Data Base

- See skill Assessing Pain, page 521

PLANNING Objectives

- To determine presence of pain in terms of type, location, quality, intensity, and level of discomfort
- To identify associated symptoms
- To identify a database that will assist in formulating a plan for pain management
- To increase client's satisfaction with pain management

IMPLEMENTATION Procedures

EVALUATION Expected Outcomes

- Pain level of client is identified and a plan for decreasing pain is formulated.
- Client is able to experience decreased pain level after interventions.
- Client's anxiety level is decreased in relation to pain.

Pearson Nursing Student Resources

Find additional review materials at **nursing.pearsonhighered.com**

Prepare for success with NCLEX®-style practice questions and Skill Checklists

Assessing Pain

Procedure

1. Assess type of pain, and ask client to describe pain using his or her own words.
   a. Acute pain: short duration of a few seconds/minutes to 6 months.
   b. Chronic pain: prolonged, persistent pain, 6 months to years.
   c. Intractable pain: severe and constant, resistant to relief measures.
   d. Malignant pain: recurrent, acute episodes, which may include chronic pain and may last longer than 6 months.
2. Assess location.
   a. Ask client to point to area of the body or verbalize location of pain.
   b. Ask if pain is superficial or deep.
   c. Ask if pain is diffuse or localized.
   d. Ask if pain radiates and where it goes.
3. Assess quality.
   a. Stabbing, knife-like.
   b. Throbbing.
   c. Cramping.
   d. Vise-like, suffocating.
   e. Searing or burning.
4. Assess intensity.
   a. Ask client to indicate intensity of pain using a pain scale; for example, a scale of 0–10. Use the same pain scale comparing intensity before and after interventions.
   b. Ask client what measures have reduced the level of pain on the scale.
5. Assess onset of pain and aggravating factors.
   a. What triggers the pain?
   b. How does movement affect pain?
   c. Does coughing affect pain?
   d. What is impact of emotion on pain?
   e. How does position or fatigue affect pain level?

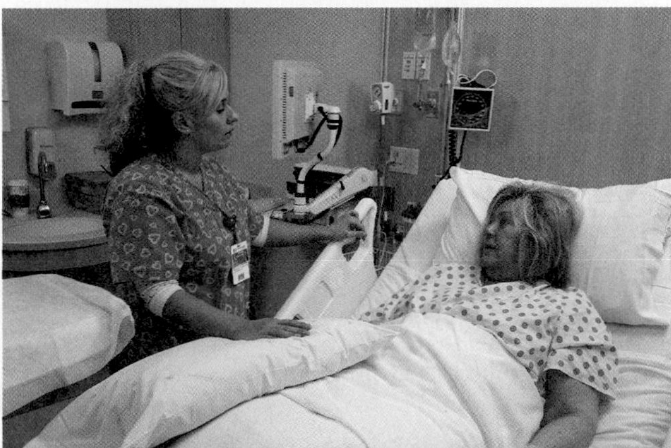

▲ Assist client to describe pain in detail so that your assessment is complete.

6. Assess associated factors.
   a. Nausea and vomiting.
   b. Hypotension/hypertension.
   c. Profuse perspiration.
   d. Apprehension or anxiety.
   e. Respiratory and heart rate.
7. Assess alleviating factors.
   a. Position.
   b. Elevation of extremity.
   c. Techniques used at home for pain relief.
   d. What pain medications does client use?
8. Assess client's behavioral responses to pain.
   a. No pain—relaxed, calm, and alert. (0)
   b. Mild pain—stressed, tense, occasional grimace or frown. (1–3)
   c. Moderate pain—stoicism, squirming, grimacing, more reassurance to comfort. (4–6)
   d. Severe pain—moaning, restless, muscle twitching, difficult to comfort. (7–9)
   e. Worst pain—crying, constant moaning, withdrawn, unable to comfort. (10)
9. What is the client's level of sedation and is it safe to administer the next pain medication?
   a. Is the client awake and responsive? (1)
   b. Is the client frequently drowsy? (2)
   c. Is the client continually falling asleep, even in mid-sentence? (3)
   d. Is the client difficult to arouse? (4)
   e. Is the client somnolent—unable to arouse? (5)
10. By checking the level of sedation above, determine the level of response by number.
   a. Level 1 and 2—generally safe to administer the next pain medication.
   b. At level 3, it may be dangerous to administer the next pain medication.
   c. At levels 4 and 5, it would be dangerous to administer the next pain medication. Notify physician.

Clinical Alert

Assess the sedation level of the client before administering a pain medication, even if it is within the time limit allowed by physician's orders (e.g., every 2 hr) or risk CNS depression. See Assessment Scale (9. and 10.) above.

11. When to reassess for follow-up pain medication administration.
   a. Post-op client—every 2 hr or until pain is controlled.
   b. Client experiencing pain—every 4 hr.
12. After pain medication is given, the appropriate follow-up time for reassessment is as follows:
   a. Injection—5–30 minutes.
   b. Oral medication—60–90 minutes.
   c. Sustained-release analgesic or transdermal patch—4 hr.

Assessing Pain in a Cognitively Impaired or Nonverbal Client

Procedure

1. Assess client's level of understanding (i.e., Alzheimer's client may still be able to answer questions about pain he or she is experiencing).
2. Assess nonverbal cues if a verbal response is not elicited.
   a. Facial expressions.
   b. General behavior.
   c. Unusual movements, twisting or turning, restlessness, pacing, immobility.
   d. Vocal sounds—moaning, crying, gasping, groaning.
   e. Muscle contractions especially around the eyes.
3. Evaluate changes after pain relief intervention to determine whether further assessment is indicated.

Assessing Pain in Young Children

Procedure

1. Assess unidimensional indicators.
   a. Increase in heart rate.
   b. Elevation is blood pressure.
   c. Sweating.
   d. Changes in skin color.
2. Assess multidimensional indicators.
   a. High-pitched cry.
   b. Baby or child is inconsolable.
   c. Awake continuously—not able to sleep.
   d. Fussy.
   e. Grunting sounds.
3. Assess behavioral responses.
   a. Facial movement.
   b. Bulging of area between eyebrows.
   c. Tightly closed eyes.
   d. Rigid mouth and tongue.

DOCUMENTATION for Assessing Pain Level

- Describe client's pain, including all of the assessment parameters.
- Describe pain level, including behavioral and verbal manifestations used to determine level for the cognitively impaired or nonverbal client.
- Describe behavioral cues used to assess pain level in a young child.

CRITICAL THINKING Application

Expected Outcomes

- Pain level is assessed adequately.
- Pain level in a cognitively impaired or nonverbal client is adequately assessed.
- Pain in a young child is assessed correctly.

Unexpected Outcomes	Alternative Actions
Pain level is incorrectly or inadequately assessed.	• Begin again to assess pain level after all of the steps of assessment. • Pay close attention to client's report of pain level.
Client reports new level of pain or pain not relieved by previously effective strategies.	• Do not attribute this report to preexisting cause, but let this report trigger a diagnostic evaluation.
Pain level in a cognitively impaired or nonverbal client is not assessed correctly as facial expressions and behavior indicates.	• Reassess according to the steps of assessment. • Request a consult from a pain expert. Try an alternative method of pain control.
Pain level in a child is not assessed adequately.	• Reassess pain level, paying close attention to behavioral expressions. • Request a consult with the physician to change pain medication.

Chapter 16

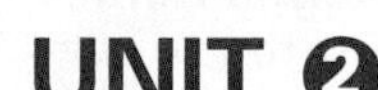

Nonpharmacological Pain Relief

Nursing Process Data

ASSESSMENT Data Base

- Assess type of pain.
  - Acute pain: short duration of a few seconds to 6 months
  - Chronic pain: longer duration of 6 months to years
  - Malignant pain: severe and constant and resistant to relief measures
- Choose a pain-intensity scale and identify the level or degree of pain the client is experiencing.
- Assess nonverbal indications of pain.
- Assess client's behavioral responses to pain.
  - Depression, withdrawal, or crying
  - Stoicism or expressive
- Assess location, quality, intensity, onset, duration, pattern, aggravating factors, associated factors, and relief or alleviating factors. (See *Physical Pain Sensation* chart, page 513.)

PLANNING Objectives

- To relieve pain or prevent pain from escalating by relaxing muscles; muscle tension increases the pain
- To decrease client's anxiety that present and future pain relief will not be achieved
- To bring pain relief to a level acceptable to the client
- To educate clients to communicate their pain level
- To improve client satisfaction with pain management

IMPLEMENTATION Procedures

EVALUATION Expected Outcomes

- Pain is controlled through nonpharmacological methods such as massage, relaxation techniques, or TENS.
- Client is satisfied with level of pain control.
- Client receives adequate pain medication; pain level does not interfere with client's activity.
- Client's anxiety level is lowered in relation to pain.

Pearson Nursing Student Resources

Find additional review materials at **nursing.pearsonhighered.com**

Prepare for success with NCLEX®-style practice questions and Skill Checklists

EVIDENCE-BASED PRACTICE

Herbal Remedies Used for Pain Control

This review of the literature summarizes existing studies of herbal remedies used to relieve pain for the period of 1966–2005. The most common natural products were echinacea, ginseng, ginkgo biloba, and garlic. Pain relief was the most frequently cited reason for seeking alternative medicine. The results indicated few well-controlled studies and also documented limited efficacy of herbal therapies.

Source: Wirth, J. H., Hudgins, J. C., & Paice, J. (2005). Use of herbal therapies to relieve pain: A review of efficacy and adverse effects. *Pain Management Nursing*, Vol. 6, No. 4, Dec 05, pp. 145–167.

Nonpharmaceutical Treatment for Chronic Pain

Norman Shealy, MD, PhD, is director of the Shealy Pain Institute and has treated more than 30,000 clients for chronic, disabling pain. Many clients' pain was the result of back surgery failures; others suffered from migraines, arthritis, compression fractures, nerve or cord injury, and cancer. The focus of treatment in this clinic was alternative—acupuncture, TENS, biofeedback, autogenic training, and ancillary techniques such as massage, exercise, and nutrition. Dr. Shealy has a success rate of 85%, and 70% for clients with long-term chronic pain.

Alleviating Pain Through Touch (Massage)

Equipment

Body lotion
Massage oil
Towel or drape

Procedure

1. Establish a quiet, private environment.
2. Determine whether client achieves more relief from pain with massage over painful area, near painful area, or from foot rub, back rub, or hand rub.
3. Warm your hands by rubbing them together or rinsing in warm water.
4. Warm lotion to be used by holding closed bottle under warm running water.
5. Massage area of client's choice with slow and steady motion.
6. Use deep pressure or light stroking motion, whichever is more comfortable for the client. ▶ ***Rationale:*** Relaxed muscles result in a decreased pain level.

Using Relaxation Techniques

Equipment

A printed relaxation technique (the nurse can read slowly until client learns technique)
CD and disc or cassette recorder and tape

Procedure

1. Help client assume a comfortable position.
   a. If lying, place support under knees, lower legs, and under head. Be sure body is in good alignment.
   b. If sitting, sit comfortably positioned with both feet on the floor, hands on knees, back straight, and head balanced comfortably straight.
2. Instruct client to inhale deeply, hold breath for a moment, then exhale deeply. Repeat several times.
3. Give the following instructions to client, using a slow, soothing voice.
   a. Continue to breathe in and out slowly. Concentrate on my voice and follow my words.
   b. Find a point of tension in your body.
   c. As you identify the tension, tense the area up even more.
   d. Then relax the area, letting all the tension drain out.
4. Continue with these instructions until the client has had time to relax all points of tension.
5. To end the process, instruct the client to open eyes slowly and say, "I feel relaxed and awake."

NOTE: For more relaxation skills, see "Teaching Controlled Breathing," "Teaching Body Relaxation," and "Using Meditation," Chapter 17, pages 565–566.

TABLE 16-1 Nonpharmacological Approaches to Pain

Physical Methods	Advantages
TENS—stimulating skin with mild electric current—provides pain relief by blocking pain impulses to the brain	Noninvasive method Higher level of activity Studies show more effective for postoperative pain Gives staff confidence they can assist client with pain Choice for chronic pain
Acupuncture—ancient Chinese form of treating diseases and pain through insertion and manipulation of needles at specific points on the body	Insertion of thin needles is not painful to the client Pain relieving capacity extends beyond actual procedure Method may provide relief when no other method works
Biofeedback—electric monitoring device that feeds back effect of behavior so client can control internal processes (e.g., heartbeat)	Noninvasive method Completely controlled by client Promotes stress reduction as well as pain relief After mastery, instruments are not needed to achieve result
Vibration or massage—hands-on manipulation of muscles or electrical form of massage (vibration)	Noninvasive method—electrically alleviates pain by numbness or paresthesia or through touch Increases circulation and endorphins to area Relaxes muscles and reduces tension on nerves and promotes relaxation Useful only for light to moderate pain
Cold therapy—cold wraps, gel packs, cold therapy, ice massage; do not use on irradiated tissue or when clients have peripheral vascular disease	Relieves pain faster than heat therapy Numbs nerves and decreases inflammation and spasms Effective for nerve, abdominal, and lower back pain Alters pain threshold Decreases tissue injury response
Heat therapy—hot wraps, dry heat, moist heat; do not use on irradiated tissue or tumors	Noninvasive method Decreases pain by reducing inflammation Promotes relaxation of muscles Increases vasodilation and blood flow to area Facilitates clearance of tissue toxins and fluids
Counterirritants—mentholated ointments or lotions (Ben-Gay or Icy Hot)	May contain salicylates (reduces inflammation) but dangerous if client has potential bleeding problems May be irritating to the skin—potential skin breakdown
Acupressure application—based on the ancient Chinese method of acupuncture, this method involves using specific points located on meridians at various places on the body	Noninvasive method Redirection of energy flow through pressure on meridian points Reduces pain and increases endorphins
Chiropractic adjustment	Manipulation of muscles and realignment of spinal column Nerve function is restored Structural integrity and balance are restored
Cognitive–Behavioral Methods	**Advantages**
Relaxation—body relaxation of muscles used with imagery, therapist instruction	Relaxes tense muscles and reduces stress Effective in reducing pain Easy to learn and implement techniques for self-mastery Reduces fear and anxiety connected to pain
Imagery—visualization technique of forming sensory images, or seeing in the "mind's eye" an image that distracts from the sensation of pain	Effective in reducing pain Client can control use and timing of technique Reduces high-level anxiety connected to pain
Deep breathing—techniques using breath to control pain	Effective in reinforcing body relaxation and visualization Reduces pain through breath control; increases oxygen utilization
Hypnosis—creating a state of altered consciousness so that client is susceptible to instruction	Effective with a client who is suggestive and who experiences tension and anxiety accompanying pain

NOTE: Other alternative techniques are presented in Chapter 17.

DOCUMENTATION for Nonpharmacological Pain Relief

- Describe the client's pain, including onset, pattern, location, quality, intensity, precipitating factors, associated factors, and aggravating factors
- Describe alleviating factors, including what the client does to relieve pain as well as nursing assistance
- Describe behavioral changes due to pain relief or the absence of objective changes in response to nursing interventions
- If there is a poor response to therapy, state what other measures will be attempted, and chart results
- Continue to document attempts to relieve pain until relief occurs and the client is satisfied

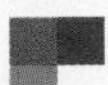

CRITICAL THINKING Application

Expected Outcomes

- Pain is controlled through nonpharmacological methods such as massage, relaxation techniques, or TENS.
- Client is satisfied with level of pain control.
- Client receives adequate pain medication; pain level does not interfere with ambulation, getting out of bed, etc.
- Client's anxiety level is lowered in relation to pain.

Unexpected Outcomes	Alternative Actions
Client achieves no relief from massage.	• Try combining method with use of medications (i.e., while waiting for the medication to take effect). • Client has to trust the technique before it can be effective. Have client talk to another person who has found technique helpful.
Client cannot focus on relaxation technique.	• Start with very simple breathing techniques and progress slowly to relaxation and visualization (see Chapter 17 for specifics).

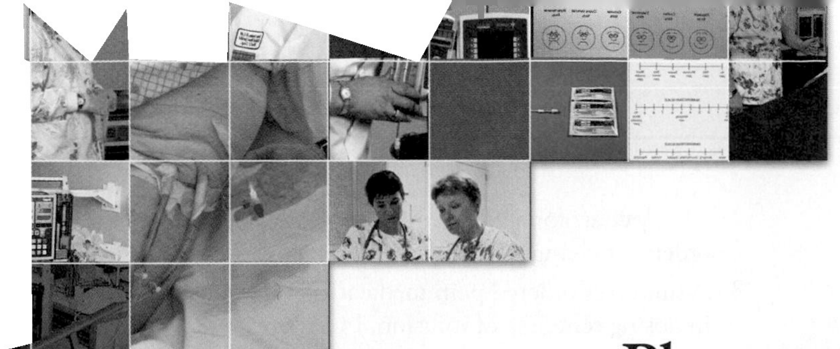

Chapter 16

UNIT 3

Pharmacological Pain Management

Nursing Process Data

ASSESSMENT Data Base

- Assess client's type, description, rating (use a pain-intensity scale), and level of pain.
- Assess vital signs for baseline comparison.
- Assess allergy to ordered pain medication.
- Assess patency of IV lines or epidural catheter.
- Assess sedation level of client on epidural analgesia.
- Assess insertion site for drainage, inflammation, etc.
- Assess potential use of PCA as method of pain control.
- Assess PCA risks.
- Assess reliability of candidate—ability to self-administer PCA.
- Assess client throughout PCA therapy (every 2 hr during first 24 hr, then every 4 hr).

PLANNING Objectives

- To implement strategies to decrease pain
- To prevent pain from retarding recovery
- To prevent pain from causing nausea and vomiting, a decrease in fluid intake which results in fluid and electrolyte imbalance
- To prevent pain from causing undue fatigue
- To prevent pain from inhibiting moving, ambulating, turning, and coughing; pain increases the possibilities of secondary problems from inactivity (e.g., pneumonia, emboli)
- To provide a consistent level of pain control without unacceptable side effects
- To enable the client to feel in control of his or her pain management
- To decrease the client's anxiety around the pain control issue
- To allow the client, according to needs for pain control, to self-administer pain medication via PCA

IMPLEMENTATION Procedures

Managing Pain With Patient-Controlled Anesthesia (PCA)

EVALUATION Expected Outcomes

- Client feels competent to self-administer pain medication via PCA.
- PCA infuser works efficiently to administer medication.
- IV site or epidural site remains free of complications.
- Pain is controlled to client's satisfaction.
- Client's anxiety level remains low or manageable around issue of pain control.
- Family and friends (proxy) are educated not to interfere with pain relief protocols.

Administering Pain Medications

Equipment

Pain-Assessment Scale

Ordered pain medication

Procedure

1. Assess pain according to the parameters of pain assessment and select a pain tool based on client's preference.
   a. Verbal description scale.
   b. Numeric rating scale.
   c. FACES pain scale.
2. Check chart for any allergy to pain drug and physician's orders for changes in pain medication.
3. Administer ordered pain medication or request change in dosing schedule of infusion, PCA, etc.
4. Ensure analgesic is individualized to client, taking into account type of pain, intensity, and potential for toxicity (age, renal impairment, peptic ulcer, etc.).
5. Record results and set schedule for follow-up reassessment.

See chart on Narcotic Analgesics, page 529.

TABLE 16-2 Pain Management

Effective Pain Management	Barriers to Effective Pain Control
Listens to and believes clients when they describe the level of pain they are experiencing. This is the single most important pain assessment tool.	Insensitive response or not believing the client's subjective experience of pain.
Intervenes or administers the pain medication when it is needed.	Nurse wants reassurance the pain really necessitates medication—does not just respond to the client's request.
Does not allow the pain to escalate but anticipates when pain medication is needed.	Believes drug tolerance will make the medication less effective, so the less medication given, the better.
Works with the client to control the pain and requests different medications or dosages from the physician when needed.	Believes the physician knows best about the amount of pain medication for the client.
Is not concerned about addiction when administering pain medication. (The incidence of opioid addiction in hospitalized clients is less than 1%.)	Concerned about drug dependence or addiction—believes it is more important than effective pain management.
Understands the various actions of drugs and their role in pain control.	Inadequate knowledge about pain medications, so dosage, duration of action, or synergistic drug interactions are miscalculated.

Improving Client Satisfaction With Pain Control*

Procedure

1. Identify client receiving pain medication using two forms of client ID.
2. Inform client you will be asking questions to determine his/her level of satisfaction with pain medication protocol.
3. Ask, on a scale of 1 to 5 with 1 being very satisfied, "Can you tell me how satisfied are you with our pain control program?"
4. Ask, on the same scale, 1 to 5, "How do you rate nurse intervention for your pain control?"
5. Determine how often in hours during a 24-hr period they experience pain.
6. Ask, "During which shift of the three 8-hr shifts do you experience the most pain?"
7. Ask, "How long does it take you to receive pain relief when you have requested it?"

**These are only guideline questions. Your hospital may wish to develop its own short questionnaire to increase client satisfaction with pain control and meet The Joint Commission Pain Standards.*

EVIDENCE-BASED PRACTICE

Preoperative Preparation for Pain Management

Researchers studied 38 post-op clients who underwent knee replacement surgery. A control group viewed a 10-minute video that described how to manage their pain; the intervention group watched a 15-minute video that described how to manage their pain as well as how to specifically describe it. Subjects in the intervention group reported greater pain relief and less pain interference.

Source: McDonald, D. D., Thomas, G. J., Livingston, K. E., & Severson, J. S. (2005). Assisting older adults to communicate their postoperative pain. *Clinical Nursing Research, 14*(2), 109–126.

Medications Used for Pain and Postoperative Care

Narcotic Analgesics Used for Pain Relief

A. Pharmacological action—reduces pain and restlessness.

B. General side effects.
   1. Drowsiness
   2. Urinary retention
   3. Sedation
   4. Respiratory depression
   5. Nausea and vomiting
   6. Constipation
   7. Pruritus

C. Given at 3- to 4-hr intervals for first 24–48 hr for consistent action and pain relief.

D. Types of analgesics.
   1. Opioids (narcotics)
      a. Morphine sulfate—potent analgesic.
         (1) Specific side effects: miosis (pinpoint pupils) and bradycardia
         (2) Usual dosage: 10 mg IM/PO every 4–6 hr PRN
      b. Hydromorphone (Dilaudid)—potent analgesic.
         (1) Specific side effects: hypotension, constipation, euphoria
         (2) Usual dosage: 1.5–2 mg PO, IM, or IV every 4–6 hr
      c. Oxymorphone (Numorphan)—potent analgesic.
         (1) Specific side effects: urinary retention, ileus, euphoria
         (2) Usual dosage: 1–1.5 mg subcutaneously or IM every 4–6 hr; 0.5 mg IV every 4–6 hr.
      d. Hydrocodone (Vicodin)—potent analgesic.
         (1) Specific side effects: dizziness, drowsiness, sedation, nausea, and vomiting
         (2) Usual dosage: 10 mg orally every 3–4 hr
      e. Codeine sulfate—mild analgesic.
         (1) Specific side effect: constipation
         (2) Usual dosage: 30–60 mg every 3–4 hr IM. (May be combined with Tylenol 300 mg.)
      f. Oxycodone HCl; also Percocet (with acetaminophen) and Percodan (with aspirin).
         (1) Potent opioid analgesic that is very addictive, especially with high dosage and long-term use
         (2) Usual dosage is 20–30 mg PO every 3–5 hr
         (3) This drug is very popular "on the street" and is dangerous because of its addictive quality.
   2. Synthetic opiate-like drugs.
      a. Demerol (meperidine)—potent analgesic (rarely used as of 2000)
         (1) Specific side effects miosis or mydriasis (dilatation of pupils), hypotension, and tachycardia
         (2) Usual dosage: 25–100 mg every 3–4 hr IM.
         (3) Used less frequently today.
      b. Talwin (pentazocine)—potent analgesic.
         (1) Specific side effects: gastrointestinal disturbances, vertigo, headache, and euphoria
         (2) Usual dosage: 50 mg oral tablets every 3–4 hr; 30 mg IM every 3–4 hr PRN

Pain Management Options

Medications Approved for Pain Relief

DepoDur (morphine) an MS extended-release liposome injection to treat pain after major surgery. Lasts up to 48 hr; 5–15 mg given by lumbar epidural injection.

Hydromorphone (Palladone) opioid drug available as extended-release tablets. Used for clients already taking opioid medications; 12–32 mg.

Current Standards of Pain Care

Continuous IV infusion of pain medication PCA—combination of continuous infusion with client-controlled bolus dosing for breakthrough pain

Epidural analgesia (continuous infusion or PCA analgesia)

Adjunctive medications, i.e., anti-inflammatory, antiemetics to enhance effects of opioids

Transition to long-acting oral meds before discontinuing IV analgesics

Transdermal pain patches for chronic moderate-to-severe pain

Administering Epidural Narcotic Analgesia

NOTE: Many hospitals require specific certification before the RN can administer narcotics via an indwelling epidural catheter. A student nurse should not administer solutions via epidural catheter. Verify the regulations and role parameters for each healthcare worker. All nurses should, however, be aware of the safety precautions.

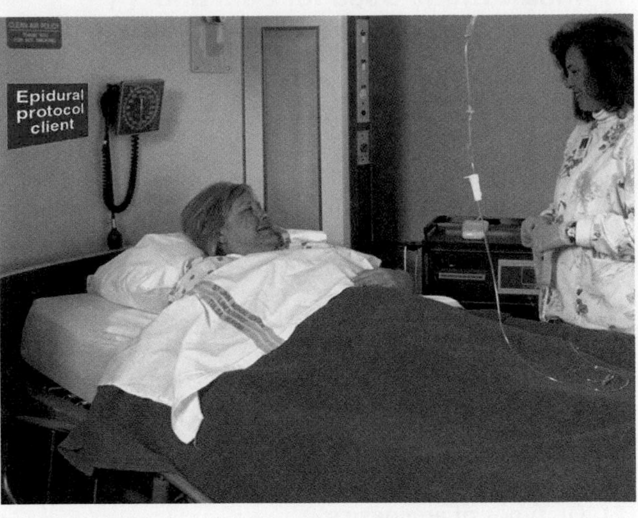

▲ When a client is receiving epidural analgesia, there should be a sign over the bed stating "Epidural Protocol Client."

Equipment

Labels for safety precautions:
- At head of bed: "Epidural Protocol Client"
- At end of catheter: "Epidural Catheter"

3-mL syringe and ampule of naloxone hydrochloride (Narcan: 0.4 mg) as ordered at bedside

Ambu bag at bedside

Respiratory record, apnea monitor, or pulse oximeter

Sterile gloves

Tape

For Bolus Injection

Prescribed medication solutions prepared by pharmacy in prefilled syringe or bag

Antimicrobial swabs (alcohol should NEVER be used)

Sterile 2 × 2 gauze

For Continuous Infusion

Infusion pump

IV Epidural infusion tubing

Prediluted preservative-free narcotic container/syringe or bag

Preparation

1. Check physician's orders for epidural narcotic indicating minimum and maximum dosage.
   a. Preservative-free narcotic, preordered from pharmacy; preservative-free saline and amount ordered.
   b. Interval between doses.
   c. Infusion rate and concentration, if appropriate.
2. Check that safety sign is over bed: "Epidural Protocol Client." ▸ ***Rationale:*** Identifies client to all staff as having epidural tubing.

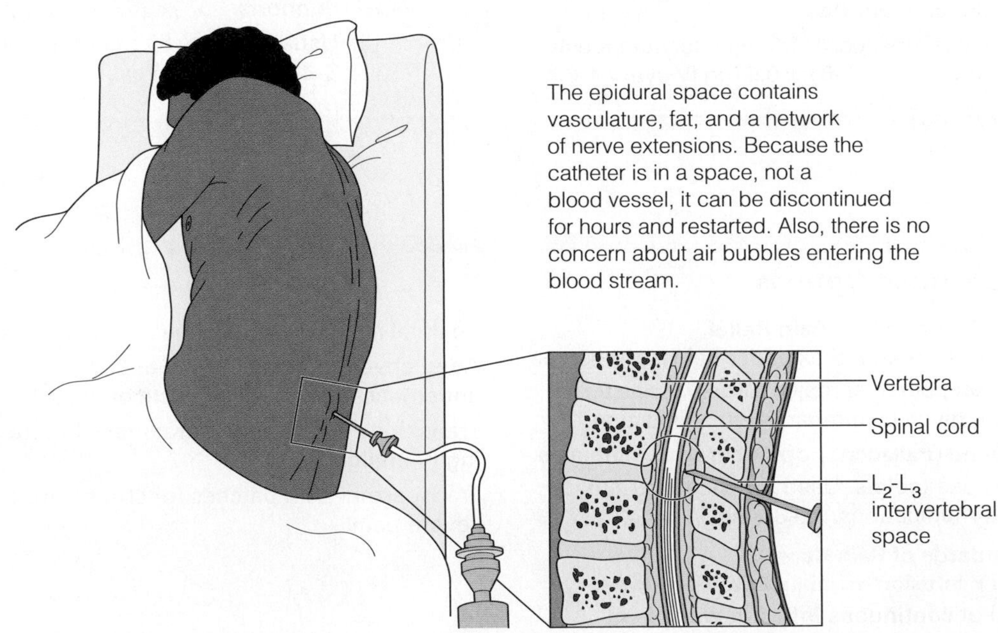

The epidural space contains vasculature, fat, and a network of nerve extensions. Because the catheter is in a space, not a blood vessel, it can be discontinued for hours and restarted. Also, there is no concern about air bubbles entering the blood stream.
Vertebra
Spinal cord
L_2-L_3 intervertebral space

▲ Placement of indwelling catheter in the epidural space.

3. Check that catheter is labeled "Epidural catheter." ▸ ***Rationale:*** Identifies catheter and avoids confusing epidural catheter with IV tubing.
4. Check that a Narcan ampule and 3-mL syringe are at bedside. ▸ ***Rationale:*** Respiratory depression can be treated with IV Narcan, a narcotic antagonist.
5. Check that there is IV access for administration of Narcan. ▸ ***Rationale:*** It may be necessary to quickly administer a narcotic antagonist if respiratory depression occurs.

NOTE: *IV should be accessed with needleless syringe.*

6. Check that Ambu bag is available on unit. ▸ ***Rationale:*** Necessary for complication of respiratory depression.
7. Check if an apnea monitor or pulse oximeter is ordered. ▸ ***Rationale:*** It is important that clients be monitored closely (at least for the first 12 hr) because of dangerous side effects, especially respiratory depression.
8. Assemble equipment.
9. Perform hand hygiene, and maintain strict aseptic technique. ▸ ***Rationale:*** Maintaining sterility of insertion site, administered solutions, and infusion lines decreases potential for complications.
10. Check two forms of client identification.
11. Position client on side in knee-chest position or leaning over bedside table.

Procedure

For Bolus Injection

1. Put on sterile gloves and maintain sterile technique.
2. Check again that preprepared narcotic is preservative-free, nonbacteriostatic opioid, as ordered. ▸ ***Rationale:*** Preservatives are toxic to neural tissues.

Clinical Alert

If client is elderly, the dose should be adjusted downward (25% to 50%) initially, then titrated according to client response.

Clinical Alert

Place IV line as far as possible from an epidural catheter and label epidural catheter to avoid mistaking it for IV catheter—this could be a *fatal* mistake. Some catheters are specifically labeled. For example, the DuPen permanent epidural catheter has a yellow band near the Luer-Lok tip that has a sign "Epidural catheter—not an IV access."

3. Verify narcotic with a second nurse before administering. ▸ ***Rationale:*** It is important to take every precaution to prevent inadvertent administration of a drug that could cause spinal cord damage.
4. Check epidural pump function and report any problems.
5. Continue assessment of client's pain level and volume of medication delivered every 8 hr (per policy).
6. Monitor insertion site.
7. Disinfect catheter injection port (Luer-Lok port or the injection cap) with nonalcohol antimicrobial wipe. ▸ ***Rationale:*** Alcohol must *never* be used because it is extremely toxic to the spinal cord.
8. Dry injection cap or port with sterile 2 × 2 gauze.
9. Insert cannula into injection cap or port, and attempt to aspirate for 30 seconds. ▸ ***Rationale:*** See Clinical Alert above.

Narcotic Administration

Narcotics Commonly Administered Via Epidural Continuous Infusion

- Preservative-free Morphine sulfate (Duramorph: 0.2–1.0 mg/hr)
- Hydromorphone hydrochloride (Dilaudid: 0.05–0.3 mg/hr)
- Fentanyl (50–150 μg/hr)

EVIDENCE-BASED PRACTICE

Pain Relief for the Elderly

Researchers analyzed the records of 709 elderly clients who were hospitalized for hip fracture. While around-the-clock PRN medication was recommended, only one-third of 87% of the nurses believed this method should be used. Also, in spite of this study finding that 75% of the nurses were aware that meperidine use should be avoided in the elderly (because it may cause seizures) and other drugs are more appropriate, 57% of the clients received at least one dose.

Source: Titler, M. G., Herr, K., Schilling, M. L., Marsh, J. L., Xie, X. J., Ardery, G., Everett, L. Q. (2003). Acute pain treatment for older adults hospitalized with hip fracture: Current nursing practices and perceived barriers. *Applied Nursing Research*, *16*(4), 211–227.

Clinical Alert

If more than 1 mL of fluid or blood is returned during aspiration of the catheter, the procedure *must be terminated* (because the catheter may have migrated) and physician notified.

What's a Smart Pump?

Infusion pumps have revolutionized the way nurses administer IV therapy. Now they have become "smarter." The pump's "brain" includes software that contains a drug library and alerts you if a medication is outside the recommended parameters, such as dose, dosing unit, rate, or concentration. Smart pumps also log data about all these alerts. As required by The Joint Commission, smart pumps include safety features that will prevent unintentional overdoses of a medication or fluid. The smart pumps available include Alaris System with Guardrails Safety Software (Cardinal Health), Colleague CX with Guardian feature (Baxter), Outlook 100-400 Safety Infusion Systems with Dose Guard (B. Braun Medical), PlumA+ and Life Care infusion system with Hospira MedNet Software (Hospira).

Smart Pump Protocol

- Turn on the smart pump and designate the specific client care area you're going to use it in. (The pump will automatically configure itself to give you the infusion parameters for that area, e.g., Pediatrics.)
- Program the pump by choosing the intended drug and concentration from the pump's list.
- Enter the ordered dose and infusion rate. (The pump checks this information against the drug library.)
- If what you've programmed is outside the allowed parameters, the pump will alert you. The pump will sound a "soft" alarm, which you can override to allow the infusion to begin, or a "hard" alarm. This will require you to reprogram the pump to be within the facility's specified limits.
- The pump logs and tracks all alerts to provide the hospital with data to shape current practice guidelines.

Integrating a Smart Pump With Bar Coding

When a hospital integrates a smart pump with a bar-code medication administration system (BCMA), it will address all five "rights" of medication administration.

The FDA mandated that, by 2006, drug manufacturers must label most prescription drugs and certain OTCs with a machine-readable bar code.

General Steps of Using a Bar Code

- Check the client's electronic medication record (which tells you which IV meds were ordered and time of administration).
- Enter client's room with scanning device and scan bar codes on the medication, the client's ID, and your own ID badge.
- The bar-code label on the drug is then programmed into the pump. Software ensures medication in bar-coded drug vial is consistent with hospital guidelines. When all scanned information is received, the pump will allow you to begin the infusion.
- The pump will automatically communicate with a computer in the pharmacy so that an up-to-date status of your client is available.

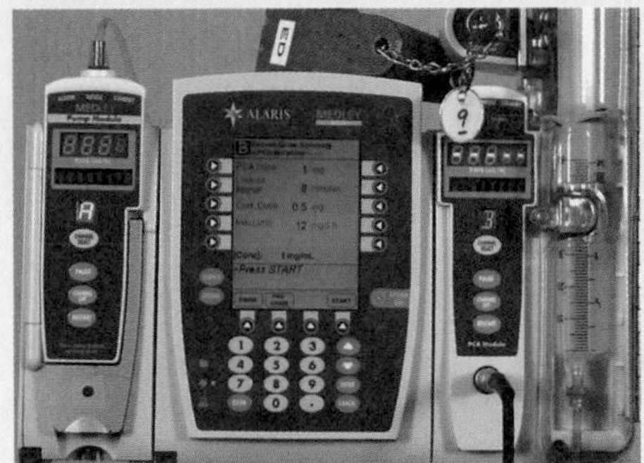

▲ Alaris Smart Pump with attached modules.

10. Inject medication slowly.
11. Remove cannula from injection cap or port.
12. Dispose of syringe in appropriate container.
13. Check that a sterile, occlusive dressing is over insertion site. Dressing is changed every 72 hr (certified RN or MD to change dressing) or when wet.
14. Tape all injection ports on epidural line if there is no continuous infusion. ▸ ***Rationale:*** This will prevent injecting a solution meant for the IV line into the epidural line.
15. Closely monitor respirations every 1 hr for 24 hr or use apnea monitor or pulse oximeter. ▸ ***Rationale:*** Due to risk of respiratory depression, close monitoring after administration of an epidural narcotic is essential.
16. Monitor vital signs: BP and pulse every 30 minutes for 1 hr after initial epidural dose, then every 8 hr.

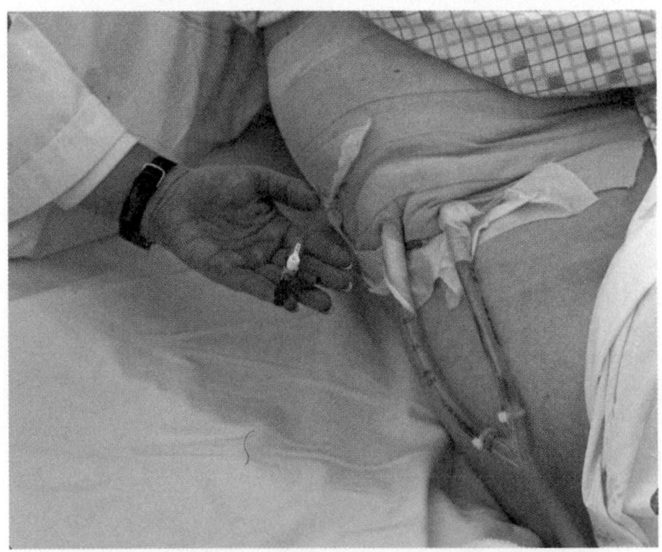

▲ Intrapleural catheter may be used for pain medication instillation.

17. Monitor for possible side effects of narcotic administration: respiratory depression, urinary retention, nausea and vomiting, and pruritus.
18. Document dose and client status.

For Continuous Infusion

1. Check physician's orders for epidural narcotic.
2. Check that safety signs are near bed and label is on catheter.
3. Complete hand hygiene and don gloves.
4. Attach container of narcotic to infusion pump tubing.
5. Prime tubing (see Chapter 28 for step-by-step instruction).
6. Attach proximal end of tubing to pump and distal end to epidural catheter.
7. Tape all connections securely.
8. Set infusion pump to ordered calibration.
9. Observe for side effects of narcotic or client response and pain level.
10. Dispose of gloves and complete hand hygiene.
11. Chart pump reading every hour for 12–24 hr or as dictated by institutional policy.
12. Record narcotic on appropriate sign-out sheet.

Clinical Alert

Low-molecular-weight heparin (LMWH) should NOT be used concurrently with epidural or spinal analgesia.

Managing Pain With Patient-Controlled Analgesia (PCA)

Qualifying the Client for PCA

Procedure

1. Determine whether physician wishes to use PCA for pain control.

NOTE: The greatest use of PCA is in the management of pain after surgery. There are 73 million surgical procedures performed annually in U.S. hospitals, with 86% of postoperative clients reporting pain in the moderate-to-severe level.

2. Determine whether client is a candidate for PCA.
   a. Check criteria for client selection.
   b. After explaining PCA, determine whether client wishes to use this method of pain control.
3. Determine which type—electronic or mechanical—PCA unit is appropriate.
   a. A mechanical device is fed by gravity rather than electricity; it is simple, inexpensive, disposable, and does not interfere with the client's mobility.
   b. A pump or electronic device has a computer for dosage monitoring, is more flexible, and can be reset as necessary.
4. Assess any allergy to prescribed pain medication.
5. Perform basic physical assessment before initiating PCA.
   a. Establish baseline vital sign chart.
   b. Specifically assess client's respiratory system for ongoing evaluation during PCA therapy.

Clinical Alert

Determine whether client is allergic to pain medication prescribed—usually morphine, hydromorphone, Dilaudid, or fentanyl.

Criteria for Client Selection for PCA

- Clients requiring parenteral analgesic treatment.
- Clients requiring postoperative pain relief.
- Trauma clients who have clear sensorium.
- Clients suffering from chronic pain (terminal cancer).
- Clients who are mentally alert and able to understand and comply with procedure instructions.
- Clients without a handicap that impairs ability to use PCA.
- Clients with no prior addiction to drugs or alcohol.
- Eighteen years of age is the usual minimum age for PCA use, but it has been used in children as young as 7 years of age.

Preparing for PCA IV Administration

Equipment

NOTE: This skill applies to the ALARIS Medley System. Specific steps of administering PCA vary with different manufacturers' equipment (ALARIS is used only as an example for teaching).

- Specific physician's orders for PCA
- Gloves
- PCA central unit, infuser pump, and PCA module
- PCA administration tubing
- IV start kit, tubing, catheter, and ordered fluid
- Extension set with Luer-Lok adapter
- Analgesic medication cartridge and injector (vial injector)
- PCA administration record
- PCA booklet for client

Procedure

1. Check that physician's orders, including medication orders for PCA, are complete.

NOTE: Morphine is available in 30-mL vial injectors (concentration of 1 mg/mL or 5 mg/mL; hydromorphone concentration 0.2 mg/mL; fentanyl concentration 50 mcg/mL).

2. Check PCA medication recommendations for dose and lockouts.
   a. Morphine: 1 mg, lockout is 8 minutes.
   b. Hydromorphone: 0.2 mg, lockout is 8 minutes.
   c. Fentanyl: 10 mcg, lockout is 6 minutes.
3. Check two forms of client ID.
4. Assemble IV administration set (refer to Chapter 28, Preparing the Infusion System).
   a. Perform hand hygiene and don gloves.
   b. Start IV line. ▸ ***Rationale:*** This establishes venous access for PCA.
5. Assemble PCA module following manufacturer's instructions.

Administering IV PCA to a Client

Equipment

Follow machine steps to know how to set various parameters, i.e., loading dose, lockout intervals, etc.

Procedure

1. Administer loading dose if ordered. ▸ ***Rationale:*** This initiates pain relief to client.
2. Set lockout interval on pump.
3. Set volume to be delivered using dose-volume control.
4. Press and release loading-dose switch.
5. Now set parameters for dosage control following physician's orders.
6. Calculate volume of medication needed to deliver ordered dose (example: 30 mg morphine per 30-mL vial).
7. Set dose volume which is the amount of fluid and medication.
8. Set rate as ordered if client is receiving continuous infusion (basal rate). **NOTE:** Basal rate is no longer being used in many hospitals.
9. Set lockout interval—minimum time between doses. ▸ ***Rationale:*** Prevents drug overdose.
10. Set 4-hr limit by pushing control switch. ▸ ***Rationale:*** Limits volume to be given in any 4-hr period.
11. Check dose given to client every 1–2 hr by pressing total dose switch. ▸ ***Rationale:*** To prevent excessive sedation and CNS depression.
12. Monitor client's pain level and sedation level. ▸ ***Rationale:*** To check if pain level is being controlled and sedation level is within acceptable limits.

Loading PCA—Alaris Model

Procedure

1. Open syringe barrel clamp (clear piece) until it clears syringe chamber.
2. Raise drive head (gray) to fully extended position.
3. Insert syringe barrel flange between barrel flange grippers.
4. Twist gripper control clockwise, lower drive head, and lock (anchor) plunger in place with plunger grippers.

NOTE: Be sure you complete these steps according to manufacturer's directions.

5. Explain ongoing procedure to client. (You have already completed client teaching regarding pain management with use of PCA infuser.)
6. Leave PCA booklet with client for referral during pain control time.

Clinical Alert

To administer blood or any other medication incompatible with pain medication, you must establish a second IV site.

PCA Infuser Pump

PCA infuser pumps are made for home or hospital use. These special pumps allow the client to control three parameters of medication delivery:

- Stopping and starting a continuous infusion.
- Titrating the hourly dose within a preset range of milligrams per hour.
- Administering a bolus dose within preset parameters.

Priming PCA

Procedure

1. Attach administration set to syringe.
2. Prime the administration set.
   a. Priming manually, express air from the administration tubing set.
   b. Priming using PCA module, view screen and press OPTIONS, then press PRIME SET WITH SYRINGE.
3. Close slide when tubing set is primed. ▸ ***Rationale:*** Closing slide clamp maintains prime and prevents air entry.
4. Press SYSTEM ON KEY.
5. Select YES or NO to new client.
6. Select appropriate PROFILE.
7. Press CHANNEL SELECT KEY.
8. Set key to program position.
9. Press CONFIRM TIME setting.
10. Choose correct syringe type and size; choose correct medication and concentration. ▸ ***Rationale:*** Medication and dose must match physician's orders.
11. Press OPTIONS KEY to prime.
12. Press PRIME SET WITH SYRINGE. (See 2b above.)
13. Press and hold PRIME KEY to prime tubing.

NOTE: Do not prime while attached to client.

14. Press EXIT when priming is complete.
15. Choose desired infusion mode and follow on-screen prompts.
16. Close and lock door.
17. Attach administration set tubing to client.
18. Review settings and press START.

Clinical Alert

There is a high rate of errors associated with PCA according to MEDMARX error reporting system of U.S. Pharmacopeia (USP). When pumps are involved, client harm increases threefold. Most common errors are:

1. Improper dose and quantity (39%).
2. Unauthorized/wrong drug (18%).
3. Omitting a dose (18%).

The Joint Commission has issued a *Sentinel Event Warning* about client harm and death with PCA pumps. There were more than 6,000 errors reported with 460 resulting in death or some level of harm to the client.

Changing Syringe on PCA

Procedure

1. Press PAUSE.
2. Close tubing clamp.
3. Use key and unlock door.
4. Remove old syringe.
5. Press SILENCE.
6. Attach new syringe to tubing.
7. Load new syringe.
8. SET KEY to "program" position and close door.
9. Press CHANNEL SELECT.
10. Choose correct syringe type and size.
11. Press CONFIRM.
12. Press RESTORE if same drug and dose is issued.
13. Verify drug and concentration.
14. Verify current settings.
15. Lock door and open tubing clamp. ▸ ***Rationale:*** Door must be locked for PCA to begin.
16. Review settings and press START.

Changing Program/Mode

Procedure

1. Press CHANNEL SELECT key.
2. Press PROGRAM.
3. SET KEY to "program" position or enter authorization code.
4. Press CHANNEL SELECT key.
5. Choose desired infusion mode and follow on-screen prompts.

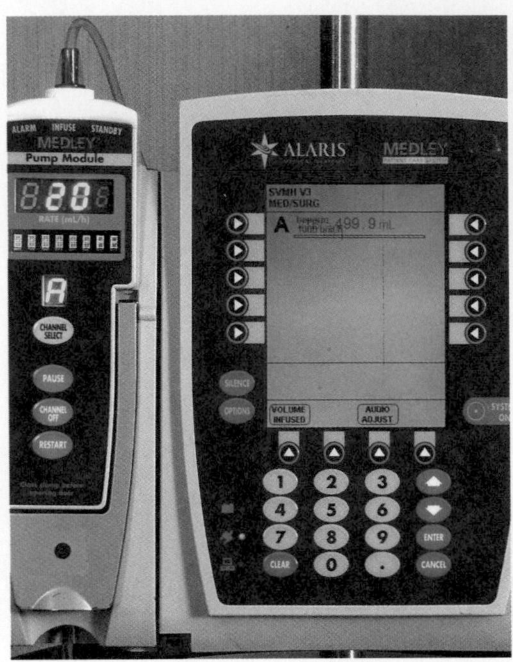

▲1 Alaris Central Processing Unit (smart pump).

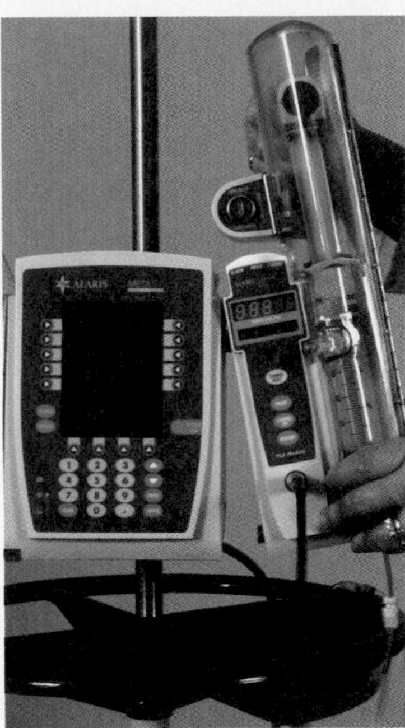

▲2 Attach PCA module to central unit.

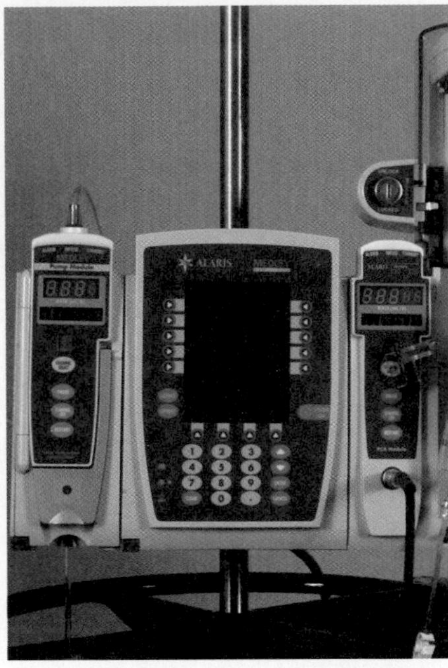

▲3 Load syringe (50 mL) into module.

Checking PCA at Shift Evaluation

Procedure

1. Press CHANNEL SELECT key.
2. Verify syringe type and size.
3. Verify drug, concentration settings, and medication use.
   ▶ ***Rationale:*** Narcotics must be accounted for when used in PCA.
4. Inspect the IV site to ensure the medication is being delivered into the vein, not surrounding tissue.
5. Press START key.

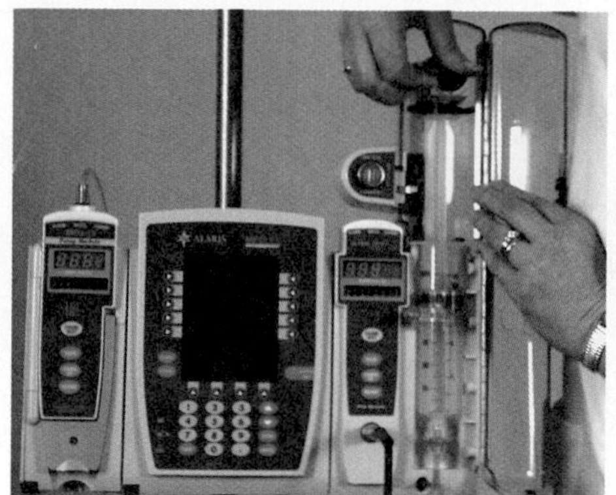

4 Anchor syringe/plunger in three steps; be sure plunger is anchored according to manufacturer's directions.

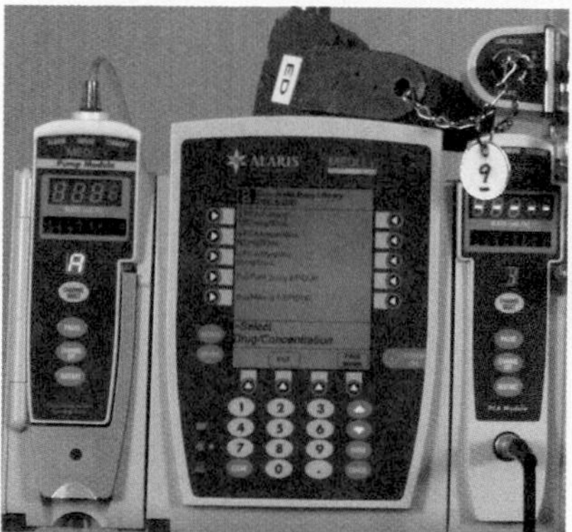

5 Set key to "program" position and check drug library on screen.

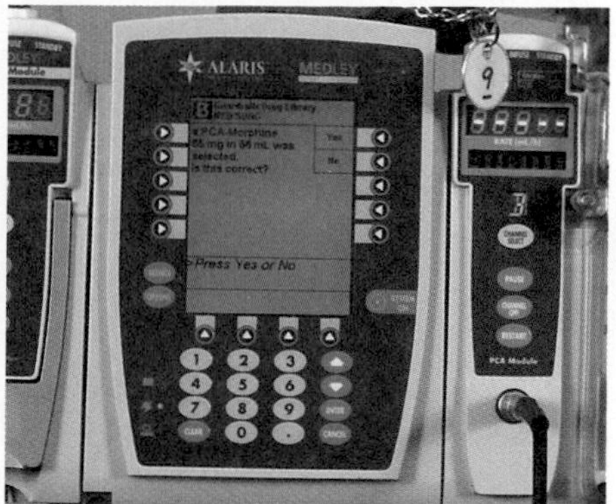

6 Recheck drug selected and confirm by pressing "yes."

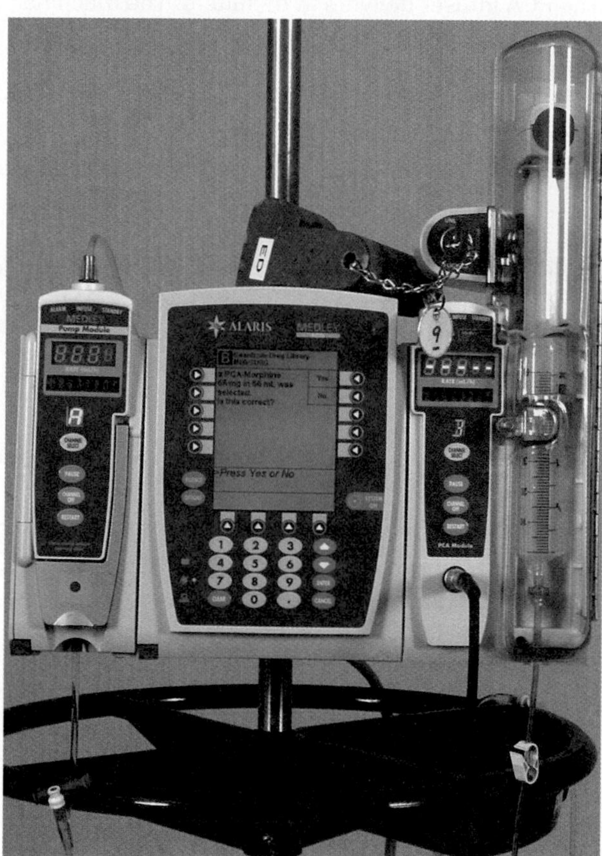

7 Close and lock door.

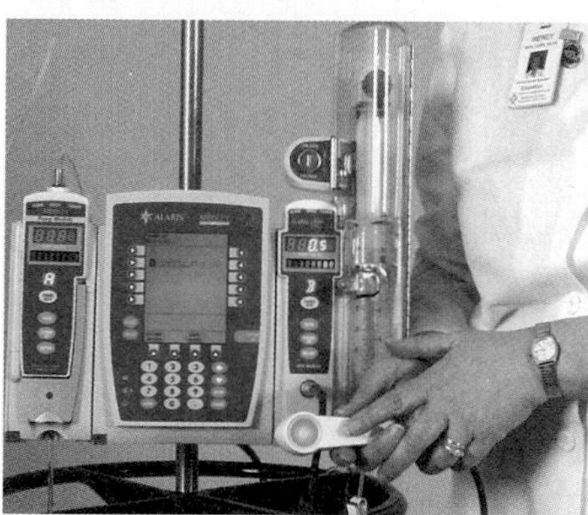

8 Pass client control button to client.

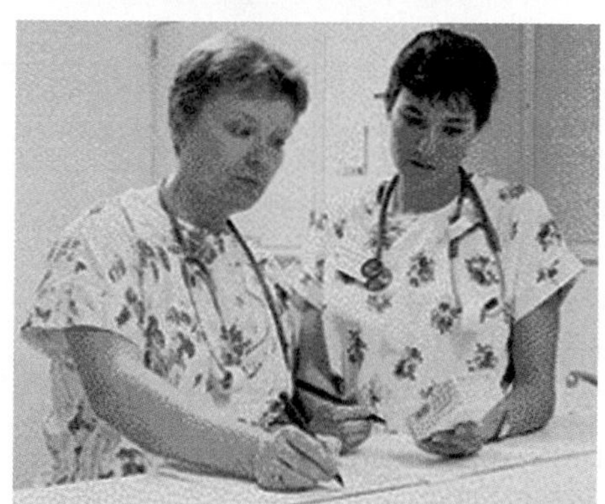

9 Check narcotic dose with a second nurse.

EVIDENCE-BASED PRACTICE

In 2007, a hospital with 9,000 PCA clients a year looked at the source of its 56 PCA-related errors:

- Misprogramming—71% (common errors were misplaced decimal)
- Wrong entering—(basal rate where bolus dose should be entered)
- Wrong selection of lockout settings
- Selecting the wrong concentration
- Confusing words (milliliter for milligram)

Source: Institute for Safe Medication Practices. (June 14, 2007). *Safety Issues with Patient-Controlled Analgesia.* Available at: www.ismp.org

Giving Bolus Dose

Procedure

1. Press CHANNEL SELECT key.
2. Press BOLUS DOSE.
3. SET KEY to "program" position or enter authorization code.
4. Enter bolus dose amount.
5. Lock door.
6. Press CONFIRM.
7. Review settings and press START.

Stopping Bolus, Loading, or PCA Dose

Procedure

1. Press CHANNEL SELECT key.
2. Press STOP bolus/loading or PCA.
3. Press YES or NO.

Dose Calculation

- The PCA infuser delivers in milliliters. The machine calculates the number of milliliters needed for the correct milligram dose. Examples: 10 mg (1 mL) every 10 minutes; 40 mg (4 mL) every 10 minutes.
- The maximum rate of administration is 20 mL/hr.

Ten Profiles of PCA Use

Pediatrics and Peds ICU
Medical–Surgical
Post-operative
Chronic pain, High-dose PCA
Progressive Care
ICU–NICU

TABLE 16-3 PCA Risks and Strategies

PCA Risks	Risk Reduction Strategies
Wrong or improper drug or dose	Standardizing the drugs for PCA use Standardizing PCA order sheets Use prefilled syringes and bags with standardized concentrations Integrating bar coding on medications for PCA use Limiting the concentration of drugs New protocols for infusion of meds
Side effects of medication—toxicity, respiratory distress, over-sedation	Continual respiratory monitoring Adding pulse oximetry (S_pO_2) and capnography ($EtCO_2$) to the same module monitoring adverse responses Monitoring level of consciousness
Improper client selection	Use standard protocol for client selection
Programming errors of meds	Safety software for dosing and safety limits Have nurses annually demonstrate entering correct PCA settings from standard orders
PCA by proxy	Proxy (intervening in established pain relief protocols) is usually family and friends intervention, so better education of family and client is indicated

Ongoing Assessment of the PCA Client

Procedure

1. Check pulse oximetry readings—when Spo2 is less than 90% with decreased respiratory rate (less than 10), client status requires intervention.
2. Monitor respiratory status often with a prescribed time interval. ▸ ***Rationale:*** It is a key indicator of adverse response to opioid infusion.
3. Keep naloxone (Narcan) and positive pressure ventilation on hand. ▸ ***Rationale:*** These items will be needed to reverse respiratory depression due to over-sedation.
4. Check heart rate, respiratory rate, oxygen level, end-tidal C02 if PCA has capnography module. ▸ ***Rationale:*** These criteria are important to assess and monitor status of the client.

NOTE: Intermittent monitoring may not pick up ventilatory depression that occurs between monitoring times.

Due to PCA sentinel event warnings, recent studies suggest using side-stream capnography (together with pulse oximetry) to provide continuous recordings of heart rate, oxygen saturation, respiratory rate, and end-tidal C02 from which they can monitor for respiratory depression. A change in respiratory status is a leading indicator of adverse client response to opioid infusion, and capnography can detect hypoventilation. The newer PCA pumps have integrated capnography and pulse oximetry.

Teaching PCA to a Client

Preparation

1. Determine whether client is a candidate for PCA (see skill in this chapter *Qualifying the Client for PCA*).
2. Allow client to directly handle equipment and practice using a "dummy" PCA button. ▸ ***Rationale:*** This reduces fear of technology and teaches basic steps of PCA.

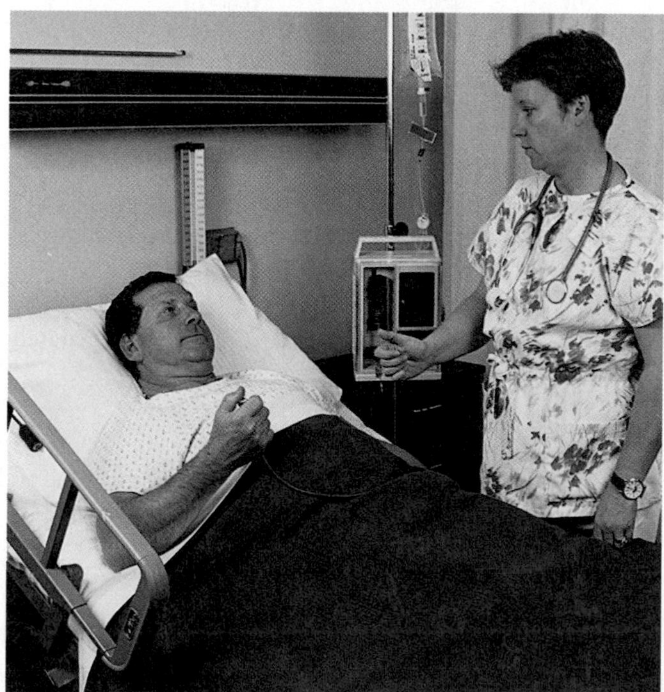

▲ Teach PCA procedure to client.

Procedure

1. Demonstrate how PCA device works.
   a. Set the pump's controls to deliver pain medication.
   b. Instruct client that if amount of medication is not sufficient to control pain, he or she may press a button to deliver an additional bolus.
   c. Tell client that after each bolus, client must wait a minimum amount of time (usually 5–10 minutes) before delivering another dose. ▸ ***Rationale:*** This protects client from receiving too much medication.
   d. Dose may be adjusted to maintain pain control. ▸ ***Rationale:*** When clients control their own medication dose, studies indicate usage is not excessive.
   e. Have client explain and demonstrate PCA use before initiating therapy.
2. Clarify with client how he or she administers medication dose when pain is felt. ▸ ***Rationale:*** Self-control of pain medication has been found to be very successful with clients and less time-consuming for the nurse. There is no significant difference in amount of medication used.
3. Program PCA infuser for continuous infusion plus a bolus dose.
   a. Establish amount of narcotic needed to control client's pain (i.e., give 1–5 mg morphine every 10 minutes until pain is relieved).
   b. Set pump's hourly infusion rate to equal total milligrams per hour needed to control pain.

4. Reassure client that PCA will control, but not totally abolish, pain. ▸ ***Rationale:*** Continuous infusion supplemented by small boluses provides steady relief (more so than IM injections) but does not eliminate pain.
5. Teach client how to evaluate pain level on a five-point scale. If client's pain is not sufficiently relieved, medication dose is increased. ▸ ***Rationale:*** When clients know they can control their pain level, they feel less helpless and more empowered.

   1 = Pain relieved

   2 = Occasional discomfort

   3 = Decreased pain intensity, e.g., able to walk, cough

   4 = Minimal pain relief

   5 = No pain relief
6. Evaluate client's response to medication schedule. ▸ ***Rationale:*** It is important to check for adverse effects of sedation to avoid complications or necessity of revising dose parameters.
7. Reassess client's ability to control pain level and effectiveness of medication dosage to control pain.
8. Teach client importance of not letting family member (or anyone other than client) activate PCA pump. ▸ ***Rationale:*** PCA by proxy (family members) has caused critical events of overdosing.
9. Teach client potential adverse effects (sedation, respiratory depression) if anyone other than client activates pump.
10. Instruct client to notify staff if machine malfunctions (alarm sounds or message display indicates a problem), pain is not controlled or changes in severity, or if he or she has any questions.

DOCUMENTATION for Pharmacological Pain Management

- Pain assessment: onset, pattern, description, location, intensity
- Amount and type of pain medication administered
- Sedation level of client
- Interventions, level of pain relief
- Side effects—pruritus, nausea, and vomiting
- Vital signs

For Epidural Analgesia

- Pain relief from medication
- Side effects—pruritus, nausea, and vomiting
- Condition of insertion site
- Vital signs

For PCA

- Assess and chart on client using PCA infuser every 4 hr (after initial 24 hr), unless otherwise ordered.
- Describe respirations every 2 hr and compare to baseline assessment sheet.
- Record sedation and pain legend every 4 hr. Include degree of pain relief obtained from PCA.

  1 = Wide awake

  2 = Drowsy

  3 = Dozing intermittently

  4 = Mostly sleeping

  5 = Only awakens when disturbed
- Initiate new PCA administration record for each narcotic vial injector used.

For PCA Record

- Chart appropriate entries throughout your shift. To determine amount of medication administered, press TOTAL DOSES and multiply by number of milliliters prescribed.
- Chart LOADING DOSE and time administered separately on medication record.
- Chart wasted narcotic—cosigned per hospital policy.
- Verify and document that calculated volume remaining and actual volume remaining in syringe are the same. Report any discrepancy and follow hospital procedure for incorrect narcotic count.

CRITICAL THINKING Application

Expected Outcomes

- Client feels competent to self-administer pain medication via PCA.
- PCA infuser works efficiently to administer medication.
- IV site used to administer PCA remains free of complications.
- Pain is assessed at the appropriate level and controlled to client's satisfaction.
- Medication administration for pain is monitored at an appropriate level.
- Client's anxiety level remains low or manageable around issue of pain control.
- Family and friends are educated not to interfere with pain relief protocols.

Unexpected Outcomes	Alternative Actions
For Administering Pain Medication	
Client says that pain medication is not helping the pain.	• Reassess tolerance level of client (check if client has previously been on high doses of a narcotic, thus developing a high tolerance level). • Check that pain dose is adequate for pain management. • Request consultation with physician to increase or change pain medication (remember, the nurse is the client's advocate).
Client appears overly sedated.	• Hold the next pain medication until client can be evaluated—notify the physician. • Check other drugs client is taking—there may be a synergistic effect.
For Epidural Analgesia	
Client develops constipation from regularly administered narcotic preparations.	• Obtain order for and administer stool softener and peristaltic stimulant. • Encourage intake of high-fiber diet, if not contraindicated. • Encourage adequate fluid intake.
Client develops respiratory depression and appears to be sedated.	• Check sedation level (drug may have been absorbed by systemic vasculature and epidural veins and ended up in high concentrations in the brain). • Reduce rate of epidural and notify physician. • Check on other drugs the client is taking—there may be a synergistic effect. • Nursing assessment: respirations, ability to cough and deep breathe, auscultate chest, arterial blood gases. • Check that Narcan is at the bedside—may be ordered if respirations are too slow (this drug reverses analgesia so monitor for high pain level returning).
Client develops nausea and vomits.	• Assess cause of problem—consider pain, ileus, as well as reaction to drug. • Administer antiemetics as ordered, and protect client from aspiration. • Keep client NPO until cause of problem is discovered.
Client complains of numbness in legs and motor weakness but has no pain.	• Turn epidural infusion off until normal sensations return, then restart infusion at 2 to 4 mL/hr lower than original rate. • Monitor for pain relief. • Chart nursing actions and client response.
Catheter insertion site is red and warm to touch, and drainage is noted.	• Check temperature and vital signs and notify physician.
For PCA	
Alarm Alert—PCA no longer infusing.	• Check if hourly maximum limit reached. • Check if maximum amount of drug was delivered based on PCA programmed setting. • Use SILENCE key to end alarm tone. **NOTE:** Alarm tone will re-sound if additional dose is requested if drug has reached maximum limit.

Unexpected Outcomes	Alternative Actions
Near end of infusion, ALERT message appears on screen.	• PCA module will remain silent until syringe is empty, then alarm will sound. • PCA module remains functional and will continue to infuse.
Client exhibits bradypnea, hypotension, nausea, vomiting, or dizziness.	• Monitor sedation level—remember the goal of PCA is to control pain without sedation. • Report to physician that medication parameters are resulting in oversedation.
Client experiences breakthrough pain.	• Readjust the medication or dosage level or bolus level (according to orders) so that breakthrough pain does not occur.
Client is insecure and anxious about using PCA mode of pain control.	• Determine which steps client feels insecure about completing, and reteach procedure while demonstrating steps.
Medication, either type or dose, is not sufficiently controlling client's level of pain.	• Reevaluate medication and dose parameters with physician.
Client is receiving too much pain medication.	• Install bar codes on all PCA meds. • Double-check module set-up and maintenance of pump. • Re-educate client and family about proper use of PCA.

NOTE: Refer to Table 16-3 PCA Risks and Strategies on page 538.

GERONTOLOGIC Considerations

The Incidence of Pain in the Elderly Has Not Been Well Studied and This Population Presents Several Pain Management Problems

- Elderly people often suffer acute and chronic painful diseases or have multiple diseases, thus they often have more than one source of pain.
- Elderly are at increased risk for drug as well as disease interactions.
- Studies show the incidence of pain is twofold higher in those over 60. Acutely painful conditions affect the elderly disproportionately (herpes zoster, arthritis, polymyalgia rheumatica, peripheral vascular disease).
- Elderly may have impaired senses (vision, hearing) and an impaired ability to express themselves.

Pain Assessment Is More Complex and Difficult With the Elderly

- The elderly may report pain differently (not as clearly) than younger clients due to physiologic, psychologic, and cultural changes associated with aging.
- Clinicians often hold the mistaken belief that the elderly have increased pain thresholds; they may be more stoic about experiencing, and thus reporting, pain.
- Cognitive impairment (which may occur in as many as 50% of the institutionalized elderly) may interfere greatly with the assessment of pain. Even though behavior may be assessed (restlessness, groaning, agitation), it is nonspecific and subject to interpretation.
- See Gerontologic Considerations for Medications in Chapter 18 for specific guidelines for drug use with the elderly.

Traditional Approaches to Pain Control May Not Work With the Elderly

- Universal use of pain protocols may not be possible with visual, hearing, and motor impairments.
- Clients may report pain initially, but recall (due to cognitive impairment) may not be possible.
- Pain assessment may require frequent monitoring. Monitoring may have major implications for quality of care and quality of life, so facilities with limited staff may result in poor pain control in the elderly.
- The elderly are at risk for over- and undertreatment. Adverse drug reactions are more prevalent with the elderly.
- Attitudes among healthcare professionals may also impede appropriate care (partially due to belief that acute and chronic pain are a normal component of aging).

MANAGEMENT Guidelines

Each state legislates a Nurse Practice Act for RNs and LVN/LPNs. Healthcare facilities are responsible for establishing and implementing policies and procedures that conform to their state's regulations. Verify the regulations and role parameters for each healthcare worker in your facility.

Delegation

- Noninvasive pain management techniques can be delegated to any staff member who feels comfortable performing and/or has experience in using touch (massage) or relaxation techniques. If TENS is used for pain control, the nurse must understand the basic principles of how this method works.
- The nurse, RN or LVN/LPN, is the primary individual who is responsible for pain management. He or she does this through the nurse–client relationship by becoming the client's advocate. Therefore, a professional nurse must manage the client's pain in order to identify the intensity, codify the degree, and evaluate the response to pain medication and intervene as necessary with the physician to change the medication protocol.
- Administration of epidural narcotic analgesia *must* be done by an RN and, in many hospitals, the nurse must have special certification. This skill may *not* be delegated to a nonprofessional staff member.
- Initial administration of PCA must be done by an RN or experienced LVN/PN. It may not be delegated to a UAP, nor may the UAP administer a booster dose.
- PCA may be managed and taught to the client by an RN or LVN/LPN *if* two parameters exist: (1) The Nurse Practice Act and agency protocol in the state allows it, and (2) the nurse has the information and experience to qualify the client and teach the procedure (under physician's orders). Nonprofessional staff may *not* perform this skill.

Communication Matrix

- It is critically important that the RN inform all staff where epidural narcotic analgesia is being used.
- Safety precautions (written labels) *must* be placed in the appropriate places, such as "Epidural Protocol Client" at the head of the bed, and the catheter labeled "Epidural Catheter" to avoid injuring the client.
- It is also imperative that the RN communicate to other nurses through the client's written records, labeling the IV line, and verbally through report that the client is receiving epidural anesthesia, and that the IV line be placed as far as possible from the epidural catheter. If an epidural catheter is mistaken for an IV line, it could be a *fatal* mistake.
- Because the nurse is the client's advocate in pain control, he or she must receive adequate feedback from all staff who interact with the client so that a viable pain management program can be implemented. It is the nurse's responsibility to inform the auxiliary staff caring for the client to report how the client is managing pain.

CRITICAL THINKING Strategies

Scenario 1

The client assigned to you has a diagnosis of advanced Alzheimer's disease and cancer with bone metastases. He is a 65-year-old man recently hospitalized. You know he is in pain, but he is unable to relate the degree of pain clearly to the staff or his family.

1. What is the most appropriate method of assessing pain in this client?
2. When considering this client, what is unique about the pain assessment in this situation?
3. What are some possible plans/goals to deal with this client's pain?
4. What are some of the risks in implementing the plan?

Scenario 2

The client has a PCA in place but constantly complains that the pain medication is not working. When asked if he uses the bolus dose, he says that he is constantly "locked out."

1. What further assessment, if any, is necessary with this client?
2. Describe the goals and strategies you would devise to handle this situation.
3. What are the best actions you can carry out to meet these goals?

Scenario 3

A female client has been admitted to the nursing unit with the diagnosis of acute abdominal pain. You are assigned to admit her to room 113. The chart only contains the following demographic data: lives locally, is 28 years old, recently married. Her husband is at the bedside and is very concerned with his wife's pain. As you walk in the room to complete the admission process, she is writhing in pain and crying loudly.

1. To prepare for the admission interview, what will you do first? Why?
2. State how you will ask the client to describe her pain.
3. What questions might be appropriate to ask regarding the abdominal pain?
4. What assessment data is priority for this client?
5. How is this information utilized in the development of a client plan of care?

NCLEX® Review Questions

Unless otherwise specified, choose only one (1) answer.

1. Which of the following theories of pain is the most recent and accepted as the most likely explanation of pain?
   1. Pattern theory.
   2. Specificity theory.
   3. Endorphin theory.
   4. Gate control theory.
2. Which of the following characteristics are most important when you are measuring the degree of pain? ***Select all that apply.***
   1. Location.
   2. Intensity.
   3. Quality.
   4. Pain pathway.
   5. Pattern.
   6. Amount of pain relief needed.
3. What is the best explanation of why pain is now considered the fifth vital sign?
   1. Pain is as important to assess as blood pressure and other vital signs.
   2. Considered as a vital sign, pain will be measured and documented when other vital signs are taken.
   3. As a vital sign, the presence of pain will result in an intervention.
   4. As a vital sign, assessing pain allows the effectiveness of pain management to be measured.
4. The primary purpose of using a nonpharmacological method of pain relief over a pharmacological one is that it:
   1. Is noninvasive.
   2. Works better.
   3. Works faster.
   4. Is preferred by clients and physicians.
5. When a client is receiving epidural narcotic analgesia, the priority safety issue is:
   1. Respiratory depression.
   2. Checking that the apnea monitor is working.
   3. Assessing for migration of the catheter.
   4. Mistaking the epidural catheter for an IV catheter.
6. Which of the following is the most important rationale for qualifying a client for patient-controlled analgesia (PCA)?
   1. To determine whether this pain method will relieve the client's pain.
   2. To evaluate whether the client is mentally alert and able to comply with the instructions.
   3. To assess the level of pain the client is experiencing.
   4. To assess whether the client's pain is chronic.
7. You are assigned to care for a client receiving PCA. When you assess the client, you find that he is experiencing bradypnea, hypotension, and nausea. What is the priority intervention?
   1. Assess the medication level.
   2. Determine whether the medication is relieving the client's pain.
   3. Monitor client's sedation level and request that the physician evaluate dose parameters.
   4. Terminate the PCA.
8. When monitoring a client with PCA, which of the following are common dangers when IV pumps are involved? ***Select all that apply.***
   1. Improper dose and quantity.
   2. Unauthorized/wrong drug.
   3. Poor pain relief results.
   4. Omitting a dose.
   5. Drug administration by proxy.
9. You have a client who is to receive epidural narcotic analgesia. As a team leader, you may safely assign this client to which of the following staff members?
   1. An LVN/PN or an RN.
   2. A nonprofessional.
   3. Any staff member.
   4. Only an RN.
10. A client with recurrent acute pain is instructed on pain management. Successful compliance to the plan is reflected by which of the following statements?
    1. "I take the pain medication faithfully every 4 hours."
    2. "The best time to take my medication is after I shower and dress."
    3. "The medication works best when I take it soon after the pain begins."
    4. "I take the pain medication whenever the pain is a 7 on the scale of 10."

17

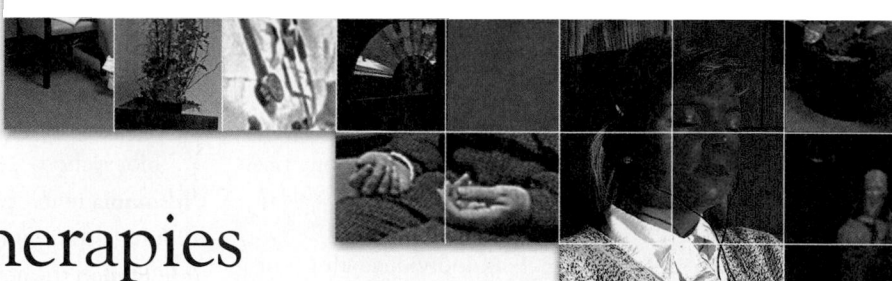

Alternative Therapies and Stress Management

LEARNING OBJECTIVES

1. Define the term *stress* according to Hans Selye.
2. Discuss the psychologic effect of stress on the body.
3. Describe the body's physiologic response to stress, and include at least two body systems.
4. List at least three different categories of stressors.
5. Identify at least five danger signals of stress.
6. Discuss a specific alternative method used to control stress.
7. Discuss complementary and alternative medicine (CAM) and how it can be applied to nursing.
8. Choose two alternative therapies, discuss the major components, and relate how you use them with clients.
9. Practice breathing techniques and discuss how you would teach this to a client.
10. Discuss why herbs could be dangerous.
11. List two herbs that could be dangerous when taken with a specific medication.

CHAPTER OUTLINE

TERMINOLOGY

Adaptive reaction a response by which the person attempts to improve or alter his or her condition in relation to the environment.

Alleviate to make more bearable; reduce (pain, grief, or suffering).

Anxiety a state of uneasiness and distress; diffuse apprehension.

Apathy indifference; insensibility; without emotion; sluggish.

Apprehension a fearful or uneasy anticipation of the future; dread.

Ataraxia the absence of all anxiety.

Autonomic nervous system the part of the nervous system that regulates the functioning of internal organs and glands; it controls such functions as digestion, respiration, and cardiovascular activity.

Cerebral cortex the extensive outer layer of gray tissue of the cerebral hemispheres (brain), responsible for higher nervous functions.

Complementary/alternative medicine (CAM) a set of practices that encompass many treatments and ideologies outside of mainstream medicine.

Coping mechanisms means by which an individual adjusts or adapts to a threat or a challenge; actions that assist in maintaining homeostasis.

Defense mechanisms conscious or unconscious processes used to protect oneself from threats or to alleviate anxiety.

Dynamics of homeostasis danger or its symbols, whether internal or external, resulting in the activation of the sympathetic nervous system and the adrenal medulla. The organism prepares for fight or flight.

Emotional strong feelings, as of joy and sorrow.

Fight or flight one's immediate response to stress that is, although archaic and often inappropriate, part of our central nervous system's biologic heritage.

General adaptation syndrome a general theory of stress response formulated by Dr. Hans Selye; describes the action of stress response in three stages: the alarm reaction, the stage of resistance, and the stage of exhaustion.

Hallucination false perception having no relation to reality and not accounted for by external stimuli.

Health the state of physical, psychologic, and sociologic well-being.

Herbal preparations the use of plants to make medicines used for healing various conditions.

Holistic a way of looking at individuals and organisms as a whole rather than a sum of the parts.

Homeostasis the maintenance of a constant state in the internal environment through self-regulatory techniques that preserve an organism's ability to adapt to stress.

Hypertension a condition in which the client has a higher blood pressure than judged to be normal.

Illness a state characterized by the malfunction of the biopsychosocial organism.

Insomnia inability to sleep.

Lifestyle the manner in which one is accustomed to living.

Meditation the act of reflecting on or pondering; contemplation.

Musculoskeletal pertaining to the muscles and the skeleton.

Pain a sensation in which a person experiences discomfort, distress, or suffering.

Parasympathetic nervous system a division of the autonomic nervous system that regulates acetylcholine and conserves energy expenditure; it slows down the system.

Perspective subjective evaluation of relative significance; a view.

Psychogenic of mental origin.

Relaxation a lessening of tension or activity in a part.

Stamina constitutional energy; strength; endurance.

Stress a nonspecific response of the body to any internal or external event or change that impinges on a person's system and creates a demand.

Stressor a specific demand that gives rise to a coping response.

Sympathetic nervous system a division of the autonomic nervous system that controls energy expenditure and mobilizes for action when confronted with a threat.

Tachycardia abnormally rapid heart action; above 100 beats per minute.

Tranquilizer a drug that acts to reduce tension and anxiety without interfering with normal mental activity.

Wellness a state of physical, psychological, and sociologic well-being of a whole person. Synonym for health.

STRESS

Stress is a universal phenomenon; all human beings in all cultures experience it as a part of their everyday existence. Although stress is a natural component of life, it can sap energy and contribute to the presence of disease. The concept of stress has been with us since the beginning of time, but it was not until William Osler and Walter Cannon began their investigations in the early 1900s that stress was actually linked to illness. By 1950, Hans Selye, a Canadian endocrinologist and biologist, scientifically demonstrated that stress plays a major role in certain diseases, such as gastric ulcers and high blood pressure. Since Selye's early research, authorities from medicine as well as all areas of science have studied and written thousands of articles on this subject. With the undeniable fact that stress affects an individual's total life, nurses should have a basic understanding of this phenomenon, its effect on humans, how humans cope and adapt to stress, and how the nurse can deal with his or her own stress and help clients deal with theirs. To examine stress and its influence on human beings in this culture, we have to examine the total scope of life experience. The stress of life is life itself according to Dr. Barbara Brown, a nurse–author.

Western medicine is entering an era of transformation. The whole context of the medical profession is changing. Clients and professionals alike are examining alternatives to traditional patterns of treatment and are devising new modes of healthcare delivery. These changes are occurring at a time when the healthcare system in this country, and indeed the world, desperately needs a new structure to deal with health and illness.

Perhaps the greatest impetus for these changes has developed in response to new knowledge about the role of stress in our lives. Selye, the acknowledged expert on stress, believed that efforts to manage and find cures for diseases is ineffective as an approach to wellness. He and other prominent scientists think that a viable answer is to examine our ability to cope and adapt to stress. Arnold Fox, MD, stated that stress is either the main cause or a strong contributing factor in all diseases of humankind. In fact, most scientists now attribute 70%–80% of all diseases to stress and lifestyle.

The view that disease is caused by invading microorganisms, or that ill people are merely victims, or even that all disease can be cured by modern science, is misleading and limiting. New definitions of existing problems necessitate finding new solutions. The current emphasis on stress is relevant to our times, and nurses need to recognize and understand stress and its influence on individuals, on the profession, and, most particularly, on clients.

Stress is a difficult term to define precisely, for it does not have a single specific source or one definite response. Selye stated that stress may be viewed as the common denominator of all the body's adaptive reactions. Stress may be grief as well as joy, pleasure as well as unhappiness, cold as well as heat, fear as well as elation. In fact, stress covers the total range of mental, emotional, and physical demands on the body and causes the body to respond with predictable biochemical and general adaptation changes. If the body is in a state of balance and the whole organism functions in harmony, the body is healthy. Stress can be defined as a state of arousal or agitation that throws the body out of balance. Although a certain amount of stress is necessary for survival, when it becomes prolonged and intense, our adaptive responses weary, and the negative aspects begin to take their toll on our bodies and our minds. When this occurs, it can be said that disease has overtaken the body and an unhealthy state exists.

The Effect of Stress

Physiologically, stress may be viewed as the experience an individual has when the demands placed on the body exceed the ability to cope, and the body is thrown out of balance. Chemically, stress initiates certain bodily processes, such as the "fight-or-flight" mechanism, which result in a threat to homeostasis. Early in the 1900s, Walter Cannon, a Harvard physiologist, coined the term *homeostasis*. As a result of his work, certain adjustment mechanisms of the body, such as blood sugar level, temperature, and hydration, were identified. According to Cannon, the stress response resulted in these mechanisms being activated, which in turn threw the body out of balance.

Rather than a specific response, Hans Selye focused on a general adaptation process as a response to stress. This process is the body's attempt to adapt and maintain homeostasis. Selye further defined stress as the rate of wear and tear on the body and stated that the only freedom from stress is death.

Selye's *general adaptation syndrome* occurs in three stages. The first stage, the *alarm stage*, occurs when the generalized response throughout the body responds to stressors, such as trauma, infection, pain, cold, heat, and fear. The purpose of the alarm reaction is to mobilize the body's defenses to meet the stressor. Biochemically, during the alarm stage, the adrenal cortex produces the anti-inflammatory hormones, the adrenocorticotropin hormones (cortisone and cortisol), and the proinflammatory hormones (aldosterone and desoxycorticosterone). This is called the shock phase because it is when the autonomic nervous system comes into full play.

The second stage, *resistance*, occurs when the body's defenses are mobilized to produce hormones to cope with the alarm stage. The body chemistry either repels or adapts to the stressor. During this phase the organism may be successful in adapting to the stressor, and, if so, the biochemical changes resulting from the alarm phase return to the prealarm stage. Any life change causes alarm and resistance, and the stress accrued through life reduces the body's adaptive abilities.

The *final stage* occurs when the stress is prolonged and the body can no longer cope effectively. The result is exhaustion, and the body may become ill with disease. The organism's adaptive abilities are depleted, and the organism loses its ability to deal with the stress. The organism goes into shock, and if the stress is not alleviated, the result may be death of the organism. The general adaptation syndrome varies widely in intensity. Reaction to positive stimuli, such as getting married or a job promotion, also activates a stress response. The response may, however, result in less damage than a negative stressor, even though it does temporarily throw the body out of balance. Furthermore, a person does not respond with the same intensity to all negative stressors. For example, one doesn't respond with the same degree of intensity to jumping in a cold pool as to turning a corner and seeing a man with a gun.

The *local adaptive syndrome* is the manifestation of stress in a limited part of the body. The body responds locally to the stressor, such as a burn or cut to a finger. The local response may also trigger a general response if the ability of the body to respond to the specific area is greatly affected by the condition of the whole organism. An upper respiratory infection causes a much different response within a healthy child than in a child with cystic fibrosis. The better the organism as a whole adapts to stress, the more effective the local adaptive response.

Individual Responses to Stress

Responses to stress, then, can be categorized into several different patterns: the *physiologic response*, in which there is loss or gain in weight over time, hormone levels increase, blood pressure increases, or possibly a somatoform (psychosomatic) symptom appears; the *psychologic response*, which may also result in a psychosomatic illness or psychiatric manifestations, such as depression, mania, withdrawal from reality, or anxiety; and, the *behavioral response*, in which one hits out, becomes aggressive (fights), or withdraws; one may also become immobilized, or turn inward (physical or emotional flight). The *interpersonal mode* can reflect stress when communication effectiveness decreases, relationships deteriorate, trust in others diminishes, and the ability to form and maintain close, intimate, loving ties with another person decreases. Finally, the affective response may be present when one's emotions are affected so that anxiety is high and

TABLE 17-1 Selye's Stress Adaptation Syndrome

Stage	General Function	Interpersonal	Behavioral	Affective	Cognitive	Physiological
1 Alarm reaction	Mobilization of body defenses	Interpersonal communication effectiveness decreases	Task oriented Increased restlessness Apathy Regression Crying	Feelings of anger, suspiciousness, helplessness Anxiety level increases	Alert Thinking becomes narrow and concrete Symptoms of thought blocking, forgetfulness, and decreased productivity	Muscle tension Increase in epinephrine and cortisone Stimulation of adrenal cortex and lymph glands Increase in blood pressure, pulse, blood glucose
2 Stage of resistance	Adaptation to stresses Resistance increases	Interpersonal communication self-oriented Uses interpersonal relationships to meet own needs	Automatic behaviors Self-oriented behaviors Fight or flight behavior apparent	Increased use of defense mechanisms Emotional responses may be automatic or exaggerated	Thought processes more habitual than problem-solving oriented	Hormonal levels return to prealarm stage if adaptation occurs Physiological responses return to normal or are channeled into psychosomatic symptoms
3 Stage of exhaustion	Depletion or exhaustion of organs and resources Loss of ability to resist stress	Disintegration of personal interactions Communication skills ineffective and disorganized Self-oriented	Restless, withdrawn, agitated; may become violent or self-destructive Diminished productivity	Depressed, flat or inappropriate affect Exaggerated or inappropriate use of defense mechanisms Decreased ability to cope	Thought disorganization, hallucinations, preoccupation Reduced intellectual processes	Exhaustion, with increased demands on organism Adrenal cortex hormone depletion Death, if stress is continuous and excessive

emotions are unstable, labile, unpredictable, and inappropriate to the situation. All of the above-mentioned modes of response relate to the negative elements of response patterns. Of course, these modes can be used in a positive way so that stress becomes nondetrimental. There is no way to eliminate stress completely, but individuals can learn to minimize the harmful effects and use their response modes in a positive way.

Stressors may be chemical, physical, developmental, and emotional. Graduating from nursing school, being promoted, failing to be promoted, having arguments, and playing a tough game of racquetball are all stressful events and require adaptation and change at some level. By understanding stress, we can more easily identify stress factors and their effects on clients who need or seek health care. Whether a client is having a baby, undergoing open-heart surgery, or seeking counseling for emotional problems, each of these individuals is experiencing stress in his or her own particular manner. How the individual adapts or fails to adapt depends on several factors: personality and emotional makeup and past experiences in dealing with stress (response repertoire).

People are able to create many different forms of disease as well as emotional and spiritual scars. And the more we use up our reserves of adaptation energy, the more likely we are to age and hasten our death. In fact, Selye warned that there is no evidence that the basic reserves of energy for adaptation can be restored. These may be genetically programmed. The more reserves we use handling everyday stress, the less we have for major crises or for growing older. The latest research indicates that there is a direct relationship between the amount of stress encountered in everyday life and aging.

Stress and Disease

Stress and an individual's method of handling it have been associated with the risk of developing heart disease, cancer, and other illnesses. Although stress is an inevitable part of life, excessive amounts of it can contribute to poor health. When one goes through a very stressful period, it is important to work through that stress, rather than ignore it.

The mechanisms by which stress leads to disease may differ for heart disease and cancer. Perceived stress leads to a release of adrenaline, cortisol, and other hormones within the body. These substances, in turn, increase the heart rate, blood pressure, cholesterol level, and platelet stickiness. When stress becomes chronic, these physiologic changes can accelerate atherosclerosis, the process that causes coronary heart disease.

Individuals with Type A behavior are known to be at increased risk of heart disease. Type A behavior is defined as having a constant sense of time urgency and a feeling of free-floating anger at the world in general. These behavior patterns can be seen as a maladaptive way of dealing with chronic

TABLE 17-2 Signals of Stress

Physiologic	
Fatigue, lethargy	Pain—backache, teeth grinding
Muscle tension—neck, back, legs, and so forth	Excessive sweating
Frequent headaches—tension, migraine	Heart problems—palpitations, racing, variable heartbeat, chest pain
Shaking, trembling, spasms	Breathing complications—hyperventilation
Cold extremities, poor circulation	High blood pressure
Digestion disturbances—acid, nausea, gas, cramps, colitis	Skin eruptions—rash, hives, itching, eczema, acne
Eating disorders—compulsive eating, loss of appetite	Sexual difficulties—impotence, low libido (desire), nonorgasmic, elimination disorders—diarrhea, constipation, vaginitis
Sleep problems—insomnia, nightmares, excessive sleep, early awakenings	Amenorrhea (absence of menstrual period)
Psychologic	
Anxiety	Confusion
Panic disorder	Helplessness
Depression	Apathy
Pessimism	Alienation
Melancholy	Isolation
Impatience	Numbness
Anger	Self-consciousness
Irritability	Purposelessness
Boredom	
Behavioral Indicators	
Restlessness	Indecisiveness
Loss of memory, poor concentration	Tardiness
Nervous mannerisms—tics, grimaces, finger tapping, hair twisting	Inflexibility
Speech difficulties—stuttering, stammering	Nonproductivity
Hyperactivity	Poor problem solving
Disorganization	Alcohol and drug abuse
Passivity	Phobic responses
Aggressiveness	Overeating

stress. The famous study of the causative factors in heart disease, the Framingham study, examined many aspects of heart disease. Results revealed that males who were classified as Type A developed chest pains three times as often as their more peaceful Type B counterparts. Another fascinating conclusion was that those who remained calm and serene (Type B personalities) rarely developed high cholesterol levels regardless of their diet.

Chronic stress causes changes in the immune system that can interfere with its ability to recognize and destroy cancerous cells. Several researchers have shown that cancer clients have a characteristic personality pattern years before the cancers are diagnosed. Part of this personality pattern involves difficulty dealing with stress and turning conflict inward instead of confronting it directly.

It is important to remember that the stress syndrome can be both positive and negative. Any change or alteration in the balance of life can create stress. The Holmes and Rahe stress scale is an excellent example of the varying conditions in life that result in stress. (See Holmes and Rahe's Social Readjustment Rating Scale in *Instructor's Manual for Clinical Nursing Skills*, 8th ed.) We are all unique individuals, and we respond differently to various stressors. Thus it does not matter whether the stress is positive or negative, light or severe. What matters is how we develop adaptive mechanisms to cope with these stressors. The ability to cope or solve a problem can be translated as the ability to withstand stress and create life experiences that do not work against us. The implications of stress theory—that by being able to withstand stress, by coping with it, diluting it when it occurs,

Danger Signals of Stress

- Depression, lack of interest in life
- Uncontrolled hyperactive behavior
- Lack of concentration, inability to focus
- Feelings of unreality
- Loss of control, emotional instability
- Pervasive high anxiety level
- Physical manifestations
  Irregular heartbeats
  Tremors, tics
  Gastrointestinal disturbance
  Skin disturbance
  Changes in respiratory patterns
- Insomnia
- Disease
- Increased dependence on alcohol, drugs
- Feelings of dread

or eliminating it, we can actually affect our life—are tremendously exciting. It means that we are not doomed to inevitable illness later in life, nor are we preprogrammed for premature aging. In fact, every individual controls his or her own health. To quote the *Journal of the American Medical Association*, "Nature did not intend us to grow old and ill; we were designed to die young in old age but free of disease." In other words, even when we are old we should feel "young" (healthy) and be free of disease.

Alternative Methods to Reduce Stress

- Biofeedback
- Massage
- Progressive muscle relaxation
- Meditation
- Audio tapes on stress reduction, music
- Yoga, t'ai chi
- Physical exercise
- Friends or groups to discuss feelings

Along with coping with one's own stress, it is the responsibility of the nurse to be aware that clients suffer from stress phenomena and that part of the nurse's role is to assist clients to adapt and cope with stress.

Guidelines for Implementing Stress Objectives in Nursing

The nurse must have an understanding of the role of stress.

- Understand and accept the theory of stress—what it is and what effect it has on the body.
- Be aware of how stress manifests: tiredness, apathy, frequent illness, lack of interest or liveliness, unwillingness to seek out new challenges, inability to cope with change, and many other symptoms.

Stress and a Satisfying Life

Understanding stress teaches you critical principles for creating a healthy and satisfying life. Consider the following principles, and reflect on how you can use stress in your life to positive advantage.

- **Stress does not come from the outside; you generate it totally within yourself.** In Hans Selye's definition, stress is the nonspecific reaction to any demand. An upcoming exam may be a stressor; your reaction may or may not be stress. A specific response to the exam (assuming you want to get a good grade in the course) is to study extra hard. But nonspecific reactions, which do not serve specifically to resolve the imbalance of having an upcoming exam and wanting to do well, may also include a certain amount of fear, even panic. You might eat more, smoke cigarettes, pace the floor, or have difficulty sleeping. You yourself, not the exam, have generated these reactions—they are the symptoms of stress.
- **You cannot see stress directly; you can only experience its symptoms.** No one can see love, but we all know its symptoms: the fluttering heart, butterflies in the stomach, inability to concentrate on other things, tendency to think about a loved one all the time. You must discover your personal characteristic symptoms of stress. You might overeat or get headaches or skin rashes. You might become short-tempered. Learn to recognize your symptoms as not actual problems but bodily warning lights signaling an imbalance. Merely seeking immediate relief from the symptoms through drugs, sex, or other distractions is like painting over the warning light to keep it from bothering you. You must look deeper within your system to discover and correct the imbalance.
- **Your attitude plays a significant role in illness and wellness.** While working at the University of Chicago with professionals who experienced constant pressure, researcher Susanne Kobasa demonstrated that the primary difference between those who became ill and those who stayed well was attitude. Those who stayed well tended to be committed to their jobs, viewed problems as challenges not obstacles, and felt a sense of control—they believed their actions and presence actually made a difference. Your attitude, beliefs, and conceptualization of what is happening to you determine your internal reaction to those events and, therefore, determine your stress level.

The challenge is to shift your attitudes so that you look for the positive side of events—not a phoney positive attitude that turns one into a "Pollyanna" who fails to recognize painful situations or major problems, but a "can do" attitude.

- **Stress is essential to everything you enjoy.** We all love the feeling of victory, and this feeling of achievement is proportional to the challenge. Think about what makes you feel happiest, most excited and enthusiastic. Having your team win a football game in the final two minutes is more exciting and memorable than when the team wins by a large margin over a poor team. When you have learned a subject well, how much better it feels to handle successfully a challenging set of final exam problems rather than a bunch of boring multiple-choice questions that test only a small part of what you've learned in the course.

Coping with stress requires exploring the inner you, utilizing and reinforcing your creativity, skill, and strength. Stressful events and periods in our lives can help us grow to be better able to make the most of our lives. Learning to truly celebrate your successes will increase your joy, personal satisfaction, and enthusiasm.

- **A healthy life is a balance of stress and relaxation.** In nature, stress and tension alternate with relaxation. Your heart contracts and relaxes to keep your blood flowing. Your breath enters and leaves. Your busy, complex world provides plenty of stress; most of us must work diligently to find relaxation techniques and time to balance this stress. Few aspects of our culture really encourage us to acknowledge the importance of relaxation. Can you imagine one of your professors, as the assignment is being collected, asking if you made sure to do your 20-minute meditation last night?
- **You must take responsibility for your own life, including its stress.** Only you can really make your life better. No one else can feel or deal with your symptoms of stress. Take responsibility for dealing effectively with stressors. Focus on wellness, not illness. Practice self-awareness, self-education, and self-responsibility. Create a stress management program, motivate yourself to follow it, and update it regularly until it becomes an automatic part of your life.

Emmett E. Miller, MD

Source Emmett E. Miller, MD, is a leading practitioner of psychophysiological medicine, which relates mental processes to physical health and optimal performance. Dr. Miller has developed a unique series of self-improvement audio tapes and experiential videotapes relating to stress management, self-improvement, and health and wellness. He is a frequent guest speaker at health conferences and workshops. Dr. Miller maintains a private practice in hypnotherapy, preventive medicine, and psychotherapy in Los Altos, California.

- Recognize the factors that increase stress, both positive and negative (illness, hospitalization, pain, marriage, family pressures, etc.).
- Assist in making a plan and implementing it, designing specific actions to reduce stress, such as relaxation methods, meditation, exercise.
- Work out a plan with the individual about how to control, alter, or change stressors in his or her life.

The nurse may carry out specific behaviors in the hospital setting to reduce stress.

- Identify the stressors affecting the client now.
- Counsel the client and family on the theory of stress; together, examine how the client's particular stressors affect his or her lifestyle.
- Reinforce the client's adaptive process by meeting his or her needs, listening to concerns, administering care, and providing emotional support.
- Assist the client to alter adaptive behaviors to cope more effectively with stress.
- Remember that laughter decreases stress, so maintain a light rather than a depressed or morbid attitude.

A NEW PARADIGM FOR HEALTH

The way the Western world views health is undergoing a change. Even the terms we use to describe health are changing; new terms, like *holistic health* and *alternative, unconventional,* or *complementary medicine* are being heard more frequently in both medical and nonmedical circles. In the past, good health meant the absence of disease. The new definition of health goes beyond physical health to encompass the health of the whole person, including mental, emotional, and spiritual health. The World Health Organization (WHO) formulated a new definition of health in 1970 that has significantly influenced the medical model of health care. WHO described health as "a state of complete physical, mental, and social well-being, not merely the absence of disease or infirmity." What made this definition innovative is that it took into account the mind as well as the body. In fact, this new interpretation of health almost enters the spiritual dimension. Though critics have pointed out that by this definition no one is truly healthy, it is the beginning of a view of health as an open system in a holistic framework. A holistic redefinition of health emphasizes high-level wellness or going beyond the absence of disease toward one's maximum health potential. This section focuses on the connection among mind, body, spirit, and environment and discusses how one can use this connection to reach the possible highest level of health and wellness.

A Holistic Approach to Health

From the 1990s into the new century, we are witnessing a significant growth in many dimensions of health. As shown in a recent Gallup survey completed for *American Health Magazine*, many people in society now include a very broad range of issues in the concept of personal health. Certainly their top health concern is still oriented toward personal health—"staying free of disease." The third-highest priority, however—"living in an environment with clean air and water"—expresses a much more global health perspective. Many of their top concerns show not only physical status but also mental and emotional status as important components of personal health. Today's significant health goals may even include having a positive outlook on life and sharing love with friends and family. Wellness can be thought of as a state of being; holistic health is the means of achieving it.

The term *holistic* implies wholeness; a harmonious individual that integrates mind, body, and spirit into a functioning unit. A holistic stress model implies modifying all parts of one's life so that stress is both encountered and alleviated from an integrated perspective.

In the modern era, holistic medicine postulates a constant interchange between mind and body, psyche and soul. Carl Jung was one of the first physicians and therapists to discuss the prevention of illness in terms of using one's inner resources. He discussed the inner self and themes of self-renewal in relation to growth, spirituality, and health. As our body of research knowledge grows, more and more physicians are employing spiritual growth techniques as a health tool. For example, Dr. Carl Simonton has been using meditation and imagery as adjunct therapy for clients with cancer and has shown that clients recover faster and have less pain when guided imagery is used. He has also demonstrated that cancer clients showed a heightened immune response. Dr. Joan Borysenko at the Harvard Mind–Body Clinic is also using meditation as a medical tool; Dr. Norman Shealy, founder of the American Holistic Medical Association and the Shealy Institute for Comprehensive Pain and Healthcare, has used alternative methods of health care for many years. The current literature, much of it authored by prominent healthcare providers, exemplifies today's trend toward the holistic, or alternative, model.

The holistic paradigm suggests that the body, psyche, and environment are one and interact as an open system. This idea can assist us to view our client's health as well as our personal health from a new dimension. In the holistic view, health care includes three types of actions: disease and injury prevention, treatment, and health promotion.

There are more than 200 alternative modalities—from bee sting therapy for multiple sclerosis to essential healing oils. Some probably do not work, except for a placebo effect, but others definitely are being shown by research to work. An example is stress reduction for heart disease and angina.

Alternative treatments may include treatments that require involvement on the client's part, such as changes in eating patterns and other lifestyle behaviors; or physical treatments, such as acupuncture or vitamin therapy. The client is counseled to take the initiative and assume responsibility for his or her own health, and the role of the nurse and physician is to guide clients to various healthcare options. Truly holistic treatment involves an integrated assessment of all aspects of health.

COMPLEMENTARY AND ALTERNATIVE MEDICINE (CAM)

The terms "complementary" and "alternative" medicine are often used interchangeably, even though they may have slightly different meanings. Complementary medicine refers more directly to treatment methods, such as acupuncture, nutrition, and physiotherapy, that complement mainstream medicine and are often used in conjunction with it. Alternative medicine, on the other hand, refers to treatment modalities that exist outside of the established medical system (for example, herbalism, massage, and naturopathic medicine).

Alternative, or complementary, medicine is not nearly as unknown, untried, or unaccepted as traditional physicians believed. For the first time, in 1993, physicians learned, through the *New England Journal of Medicine*, that Americans made 425 million visits to alternative providers, compared with 388 million visits to all other mainstream primary care physicians. Many physicians, on learning the results of this survey, were stunned because they had no idea Americans were seeking alternative therapies in such numbers. Now it is estimated that Americans spent an estimated $33.9 billion out-of-pocket on CAM products and services in 2007, which totals 11.2% of all out-of-pocket healthcare spending. The most commonly used therapies include prayer, natural products such as herbs and oils, deep breathing exercises, meditation, and chiropractic care. Research notes that 38% of those using alternative care chose to do so because they felt conventional treatment would not help them with their health problems. Researchers also say that women and those with higher education are more apt to use complementary medicine.

The National Institutes of Health (NIH), a conservative, scientifically based organization, gave nearly $130 million in 2010 to the National Center for Complementary and Alternative Medicine. This office was founded because of congressional pressure to investigate new approaches to the degenerative diseases killing Americans. It is one of 27 NIH centers.

Several national insurance companies now reimburse their clients for selected alternative treatments. Among the companies are Blue Cross–Blue Shield, Alliance for Alternatives in Health Care, Inc., Oxford Health Plan, and Aetna US Life. Alternative treatments reimbursed include acupuncture, massage therapy, and body therapies such as Rolfing, chiropractic, stress reduction, and homeopathic therapy.

Legal Implications of Alternative Therapy

Several bills were passed in the U.S. House of Representatives and the Senate that will allow authorized healthcare providers to give alternative treatments, provided the client is fully informed about the type of treatment, the risks and benefits, and conventional therapy that is available. Written consent is necessary only if the therapy is invasive (acupuncture) or can cause the client harm.

If the client does request information about alternative approaches to illness, the nurse should discuss this request with the client's physician and unit manager or supervisor. The nurse may even contact the client advocate or ombudsman and ask them to talk with the client and honor the request. In many states, there are staff personnel and physicians who are open to alternative therapy and even encourage the client's right to take responsibility for their own health. In such a situation, the personnel may work as a team in conjunction with the client to explore all of the available treatment options, including alternative therapy.

Over the past few years, many hospitals have opened alternative clinics so that clients who wish to combine mainstream medicine with alternative treatment methods can do so. A national poll completed in 2007 showed that 40% of hospitals offered at least one CAM therapy. Another interesting statistic, showing a trend toward including alternative treatment methods in traditional therapies, is that CAM courses have become a requirement in almost 90% of medical schools in the United States. This is for the academic year 2007–2008, compared with 30% for the 2001–2002 year. Integrated programs in hospitals are being customized to meet the needs of both the hospital's clients and the community; thus this appears to be the direction of health care in the country today.

Alternative Treatment Methods

A new direction in alternative medicine is called *integrative medicine*, a blending of the best of conventional methods with high-tech and alternative therapies. This method combines drugs, surgery, high-tech treatments, and mind–body practices, as well as alternative treatments. It remains client-centered.

Following is a short sampling of the more than 200 alternative treatment methods that may be used alone or in tandem with conventional medical treatments. Alternative methods may be classified as lifestyle (holistic medicine; nutrition), botanical (homeopathy, herbal, aromatherapy), energy/manipulative (chiropractic, acupressure and acupuncture, reflexology, massage), and mind–body (meditation, guided imagery, biofeedback, color healing, and hypnotherapy).

Acupuncture An ancient Chinese method of relieving pain and treating disease, acupuncture is based on the belief that energy, or *qi*, flows along 12 lines or meridians in the body, creating a balance between two principles of nature called yin and yang. Each meridian is connected to a particular organ or system. It is believed that lack of energy flow or blocked energy along the meridians leads to illness or disease. Acupuncture treatment involves inserting sharp needles under the skin along the meridian lines, thereby unblocking energy, stimulating flow, and restoring balance and health of internal organs. Since the 1960s in the United States, Chinese doctors, as well as some U.S. physicians, have performed major surgery with acupuncture as the only anesthetic.

Applied Kinesiology Applied kinesiology is a form of evaluation based on the theory that the condition of a person's muscles reflects certain internal disorders or problems. Body imbalances or disorders are identified when certain muscle groups are tested and appear weak. Certain foods, medications, or herbs are held in a person's hand or placed next to their skin. If the substance is not appropriate for the body, the muscles respond to testing by appearing weak. When the substance is removed, the muscles regain their strength. Based on identifying weak muscles, various treatments, such as vitamins, herbs, diet therapy, acupressure, or chiropractic, are suggested.

Aromatherapy Essential oils are the aromatic liquids extracted from herbs, plants, and flowers. These oils have been used to treat various conditions and have been an important part of medical lore for thousands of years. For example, there are 188 references to essential oils in the Bible. Modern aromatherapy became known in the 1930s, but it was not until the 1990s that aromatherapy emerged as a major mode of alternative treatment.

Essential oils can be included in the genre of vibrational therapy because specific oils have their own vibrational level or life force and, as such, work differently in the body. Dr. Robert Becker, in his book *The Body Electric*, discusses the fact that the human body has an average electrical frequency and the health of a person depends on their particular body frequency. Research at the State University in Cheny, Washington, determined that the average body frequency is 62–68 hertz (Hz). When the frequency drops, the immune system is compromised and various illnesses may ensue. Based on this research, scientists found that pollutants lower the body frequency. For example, canned or processed foods have a frequency of zero, fresh produce 15 Hz, and essential oils start at 52 Hz and go as high as 320 Hz (which is organic, pure rose oil). Essential oils have the ability to penetrate the human body through either the skin or olfactory receptors. Supporters of this form of alternative therapy believe that essential oils are a most effective healing agent and they are noninvasive. Examples of commonly used oils are lemon and thyme oil, used to kill strep, staph, and TB; lavender, used as a relaxing or sleep-enhancing oil; and peppermint, used to aid digestion. This mode of treatment would be used to supplement, not replace, other treatment methods.

Ayurveda A form of medicine that originated in India, ayurveda, meaning the science of life, has been practiced in India for over 5,000 years and has just recently become known in the West. This system is based on the concept of three metabolic body types: slim, athletic, and heavy. Each body type utilizes food and herbs in a different way; thus treatment includes dietary changes, herbs, and exercise, as well as specific practices, such as yoga, meditation, massage with herbal remedies, and medicated inhalations. This form of medicine has recently gained popularity in the West after several Indian physicians opened clinics based on this system of treatment. Notable among them is Dr. Deepak Chopra, an endocrinologist, who has written many popular books on the subject.

Biofeedback This technique employs an instrument to monitor physiologic processes of the body and to "feed back" measurements to the individual being monitored. A scale, thermometer, and pulse monitor are common feedback devices, as are more technically sophisticated machines having electronic sensors and digital readouts. Recent research has confirmed that many people can influence or control their autonomic processes (heart rate, blood pressure, temperature, digestive functions, etc.). As the client becomes more adept at controlling body responses, the need to use monitoring devices decreases—and the mental skills can be used independently.

Chiropractic Originating in ancient Greece and literally meaning "done by the hands," chiropractic suggests that one cause of disease and dysfunction in the body is a misalignment of the spinal column that interferes with proper nerve function.

These conditions cause or contribute to some diseases and lower the body's resistance to others. Spinal adjustments and manipulation restore structural integrity, thus enabling the body to heal itself. Studies have shown that chiropractic can relieve pain and structural disorders in the joints and muscles. The focus of treatment is general and includes correction of such disorders as headaches; allergies; pain in the back, hip, or spinal column; or gastrointestinal problems.

Energy Medicine This contemporary aspect of health views the human body as comprised of electronic vibrations. Interventions involving the energy field will interface with environmental, spiritual, and vibrational aspects of healing. Special high and low frequencies of sound and light are already being used for healing. For example, sound therapy is used to speed healing through a cast; full-spectrum light frequencies are being used to affect moods such as seasonal affective disorder (SAD). Other examples of energy/vibrational/frequency healing are Reiki healing, in which the healer has progressed through two or three weekend education levels; Therapeutic Touch, the founders of which are Dolores Krieger and Janet Mentgen, also entails learning the techniques via a seminar or educational program; and energy healing, which may be the transmission of the healer's energy into the client's body, or the empowerment of the client to heal herself/himself. Documented studies have shown that certain individuals have this ability to transmit healing energy to others. In fact, a special photographic process called Kirlian photography has shown the energy moving from healer to client.

Herbal Medicine There is a growing interest in herbal products, as more and more clients become interested in healing themselves.

For more information on herbs and plants, see Table 17-3.

Homeopathy Based on the work of the German physician Dr. Samuel Hahnemann in the early 1800s, homeopathy is a system of treatment that rests on the theory that extremely minute doses of certain substances, usually herbal or chemical, cause a response in a person that mimics a particular disease. These substances, or homeopathic remedies, are administered to a person with a disease exhibiting a similar symptom pattern, stimulating the body's natural healing response. This is called "treatment by similars, or like cures like." The practice of homeopathy is becoming more popular; there is even a software package designed to assist physicians in the homeopathic diagnosis and treatment of disease.

Massage Of all the alternative treatments, massage may be the oldest form of medicine known to man. Historical records indicate that the Chinese, in 3000 B.C., wrote about massage, and both the Greeks and Romans considered massage a therapy. Massage was introduced to the United States in 1877 by Dr. S. Mitchell, and schools of massage proliferated in both the United States and Britain.

With the introduction of electrical treatments, the application of massage began to diminish as a part of recommended physiotherapy. However, today, the application of touch to the skin to relieve tension in muscles, ligaments, tendons, and joints is an accepted nonpharmacological approach to decrease pain.

Naturopathy Founded almost 100 years ago, this form of medicine includes natural therapeutics such as nutrition, herbs, homeopathy, massage, exercise, and even acupuncture. Drugs are not in this repertoire. Naturopathy school of thought believes that diseases are the body's attempt to heal itself through release of impurities. Treatments are designed to increase the client's "vital force" by eliminating toxins, thus allowing the body to heal.

Nutrition The holistic approach dictates that an individual pay close attention to nutritional status as a critical component of wellness. Research strongly points to diet as a major contributor to health or disease. This is especially so when a person has a diet of high saturated fat, refined sugars, additives, preservatives, or junk food. It is also current thinking that a high-carbohydrate diet contributes to obesity. Nutrition can also play a major role in prevention of disease; more and more emphasis is currently being placed on the role of antioxidants (vitamins C, E, beta-carotene, pycnogenol, etc.) in preventing such diseases as cancer and heart disease.

There is much controversy today over whether the average American consumes a diet that provides enough of the essential nutrients to prevent disease and aging. The pro argument group says that if you follow the USDA Revised Food Pyramid, you do not need to supplement your diet. (See Chapter 19.) The opposing argument says that the quality of food today (unless you are eating a majority of organic/natural foods) is so deficient in nutrients that you cannot sustain a healthy diet.

To follow preventive guidelines for better health, most alternative physicians and healthcare workers advocate supplementing diet with a broad-based multiple vitamin/mineral capsule daily, preferably with natural, food-based (not synthetic) nutrients. This prescription would include basic vitamins, all the minerals (including trace minerals), antioxidants, essential fatty acids (Omega 3 and 6), the carotinoids, coenzyme Q10, nutrients for the eyes such as lycopene and lutein, and bioflavonoids.

Prayer and Spirituality in Health People have used both prayer and spiritual practices for thousands of years. These two areas are currently included in the arena of alternative medicine because it is built on a foundation of mind–body–spirit.

In a major survey of complementary medicine, when prayer was included in the definition, 62% had used this practice for dealing with a health problem. In fact, research shows that it is the therapy most commonly used among all alternative therapies. In one study at Harvard Medical School, analyzed data on the use of prayer showed that among 3,055 participants, 57% used prayer for health concerns or specific medical conditions and 75% prayed for wellness. (See Evidenced-Based Practice, page 557.)

Reflexology Also called "zone therapy," reflexology is a method of treatment that proposes that diseases and organ dysfunction can be both diagnosed and treated by pressing on certain areas of the hands or feet. Each area of the body is represented by a corresponding area on the feet or hands; pressing on specific points is said to stimulate blood, nutrient, and energy flow to the diseased area of the body.

Relaxation and Visualization Stress experts have carefully studied the effects of deep relaxation on the mind and

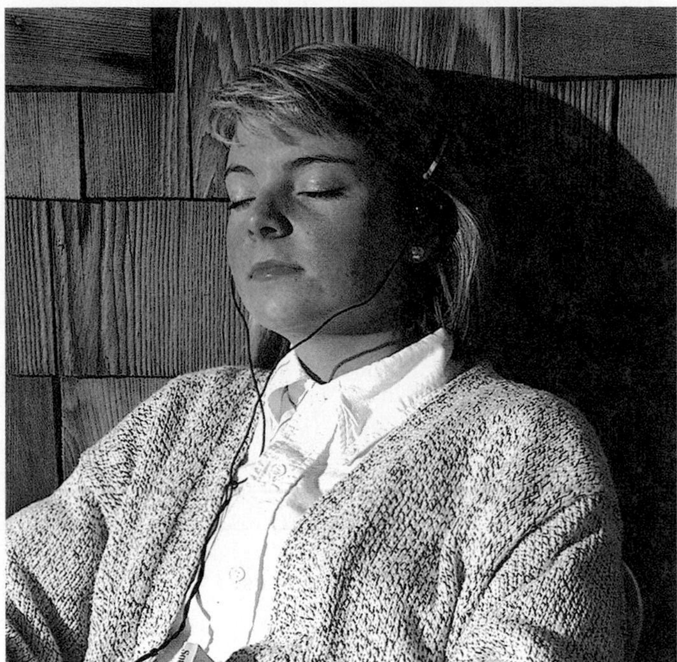

▲ Sound and visualization are alternative treatment methods.

body. They found that individuals who regularly practice relaxation exercises experience less stress than people who don't. The relaxation response is actually the physiologic opposite of the stress response. People adept at invoking the relaxation response use their minds to control their autonomic nervous system—oxygen consumption, respiratory rate, heart rate, blood pressure, and muscle tension. Their alpha brain waves, the waves associated with feelings of well-being, increase. Effective body relaxation techniques have existed for centuries. Several have gained significant popularity in recent years. In the United States, about 12% of adults use deep breathing exercises and 8% use meditation as complementary to their health care. The following short descriptions should familiarize you with the leading techniques.

1. *Deep Breathing:* Emphasized by virtually all relaxation exercises, deep breathing is a key to reducing stress. When you are tense, your breathing becomes rapid, irregular, and shallow. Healthy *deep* breathing increases the amount of oxygen in your blood, cleanses your system of carbon dioxide and other waste chemicals, relaxes your muscles, increases the endorphin release, and encourages your heart rate to return to normal. Learning to take deep, slow, full breaths and exhale completely effects mastery of this key relaxation technique. B. K. S. Iyengar, a world-class yoga teacher, suggests a breathing technique for stress reduction. Try it and instruct your clients in this technique.
   - Inhale as you normally do.
   - Exhale as you normally do.
   - Pause as long as comfortable.
   - Repeat the first three steps.

   Simple? Yes. Effective? Yes. This technique allows lungs to empty more completely, continuing the normal exhalation process. Why is this simple exercise effective? Because the completed exhalation enables the mind to quiet—a rest from the jumble of one thought upon another. Iyengar says that if you learn this "secret," you can control stress. It also provides the foundation for meditation.
2. *Autogenic Training:* In this form of relaxation, warmth and heaviness are visualized: two physical sensations associated with the relaxed state. The warmth represents increased blood flow throughout the body, and heaviness is perceived as relaxation of the skeletal muscles. During progressive relaxation, specific muscles or groups of muscles are tensed and released throughout the body. This technique is especially effective for clients who are fearful and stressed.
3. *Meditation:* Originating thousands of years ago, meditation is based on Eastern cultures and religions. The effects of meditation are similar to those associated with deep relaxation. Meditation is the process of bringing the mind to stillness. It sounds easy, but if you have tried meditation, you know from experience how difficult and frustrating this process can be. There are many methods of meditation, from the traditional transcendental meditation (TM) and Zen meditation to the repetition of a word such as "one," advocated by Dr. Herbert Benson of Harvard University. TM is a structured form of meditation popularized in the United States in the 1960s by Maharishi Mahesh Yogi. In TM, a mantra is selected (a word or sound) that is repeated mentally while the person is seated quietly in a tranquil place.

   Perhaps the easiest meditation technique is to sit in a comfortable position with the spine straight (the lotus position is perfect if the legs can stand it), eyes closed, and to relax. While meditating, one concentrates on relaxing the muscles and organs throughout the body, then focuses on breathing. One is to inhale fully, then exhale, watching the breath come out "in one's mind's eye." If a thought comes in, it should be made to slip away and one should continue inhaling and exhaling. No thoughts should be allowed to rush in to break the concentration.
4. *Visualization:* Visualization is a proven technique for healing, stress management, and positive goal attainment. When a mental picture is created, the body responds as if it were a real experience. Visualization can assist a client to feel more confident in circumstances filled with uncertainties. It can also assist with reducing pain. Teach the client to first relax (through one of the techniques mentioned in this chapter), then deep breathe, and finally to see the pain in the mind's eye becoming less and less severe.

T'ai Chi Ch'uan This slow, graceful Chinese technique for relaxation is actually a system to both stimulate and balance subtle life energies. Thirty minutes a day devoted to the gentle, flowing movements of t'ai chi is relaxing, centering, and invigorating—a great way to relax and an interesting alternative to energetic Western exercise.

Yoga Yoga is an ancient Indian discipline that begins with postures, or asanas, that stretch and strengthen muscles.

It progresses to meditative relaxation or breathing techniques. Yoga is not sport or exercise as such; nor does it have to be a religion. The system is devised completely for health and well-being. The best way to begin yoga is to find an experienced teacher who can correct postures and guide the individual through the breathing and relaxation exercises.

All cultures from ancient times onward have used herbs to cure illness. Indeed, many drugs commonly used today are derived from herbs. Nearly one-fourth of all medications have at least one ingredient that is plant-based. The WHO estimates that 80% of the world population includes herbal medicines as part of their health practices.

Other countries are far ahead of the United States in integrating herbal products into mainstream medicine. WHO's *Guidelines for the Assessment of Herbal Medicine* state that historical use is a valid way to document safety and efficacy in the absence of scientific evidence to the contrary. European herbs are among the world's best-studied medicines. Some are even prescribed by physicians in Europe because they are so effective in treating diseases. In the United States, more and more holistic physicians are incorporating herbs into their medical practice, both because they are effective and because they have far fewer side effects than drugs.

Following is a listing of the most common herbs used today.

TABLE 17-3 The Most Common Herbs and Plants and What They Can Do for You

Aloe
A plant that has been used for centuries. It is a proven healer for skin problems and burns and has been used for gastrointestinal distress and as a daily tonic.
Bilberry
A European berry used by British Royal Air Force pilots flying night missions during World War II for improving night vision. This berry also relieves eye strain and helps to prevent eye disorders.
Black Cohosh
A remarkable herb for females because it helps to maintain normal hormone balance, especially during menopause. This herb is powerful and will increase the effect of synthetic hormones.
Cayenne
Anyone who has eaten a chili pepper has experienced the power of cayenne pepper. Capsaicin, the main ingredient, is used topically as a pain reliever and is useful for arthritis. This herb also reduces inflammation and increases circulation.
Chamomile
Produced from the chamomile flowers, this herb renews the skin or, used in a tea, is helpful for digestive upset or insomnia.
Echinacea
A favorite herb because of its immune-boosting properties. It is very effective for colds, flu, and coughs. It is not good to use on a long-term basis.
Elderberry
An ancient remedy for colds and one of the best herbal medicines for the flu. It is available in capsule, tincture, or extract form.
Feverfew
Many holistic physicians recommend this herb as a preventive measure for migraine headaches. Studies have shown that feverfew decreases the severity and intensity of headaches.
Garlic
A common plant Italians love to use in cooking, but it is also a remedy for many disorders. Garlic keeps immunity high, lowers cholesterol, and can be used for ear infections.
Ginger
A medicinal as well as a cooking herb that is useful for nausea, stomach upset, and intestinal gas. Also, taken after meals, it helps digestion and reduces allergies.
Ginkgo
Traced back in time to the age of dinosaurs, this amazing tree is the oldest known species in existence. The many uses include improving circulation, helping memory and attention deficit disorder, relieving tinnitus, and accelerating stroke recovery.
Ginseng
American, Chinese, and Siberian are all forms of this famous root. The Chinese form (Panax) is a warming herb that can increase energy and sex drive. American and Siberian forms are cooling herbs that fight fatigue and decrease stress. This herb also helps to normalize blood pressure and cholesterol.
Goldenseal
Extracted from a root, this bitter herb is excellent for colds, sore throats, ear infections, and as a cream useful for skin infections.

TABLE 17-3 The Most Common Herbs and Plants and What They Can Do for You (*Continued*)

Green Tea
The leaves of this plant have become very popular because they contain some of the most powerful antioxidants known which help the body to eliminate free radicals. Used as a tea, tincture, tablet or capsule, this herb can be taken as a cancer preventive or detoxification agent.
Hawthorn
A tonic made from berries, hawthorn can be used for a variety of heart disorders—lowering blood pressure, congestive heart failure, angina, and cardiomyopathy. Clients should seek medical consultation when using it with other heart medications.
Milk Thistle
Liver disease is one of the country's major health problems. This seed, known for its restoration of liver function, is one of the best-studied herbs for liver disease. Silymarin is the main ingredient in milk thistle. It is one of the most liver-protecting substances known to protect intact liver cells.
Pau D'Arco
Extracted from the bark of a tree in the Amazon Rain Forest, this potion in tea or capsule form has amazing uses—for infections, cancer, killing parasites or candida overgrowth.
Saw Palmetto
Made from berries grown on a small palm tree, this extract is a popular substance for men with an enlarged prostate. It relieves symptoms of benign prostatic hyperplasia and has been confirmed as the most researched and helpful substance for the prostate.
St. John's Wort
This herb, from which both the flowers and whole plant are used, enhances the production of key neurotransmitters. It works for mild to moderate depression and to decrease stress. With considerably fewer side effects than antidepressant drugs, it should not be used with pharmaceutical medications.
Turmeric
Known and used for centuries as a basic ingredient in Indian cooking, turmeric (from curcuma) is best used as an anti-inflammatory herb. It is also useful for arthritis, as a digestive aid, and for its antitumor qualities.
Valerian
A root that is used to relax nerves, promote peaceful feelings, and assist in sleeping. It is also used for spasms and pain.

HERB–DRUG INTERACTIONS

Millions of Americans are using herbal preparations instead of prescription and over-the-counter drugs. Other millions are combining herbs and medications. A survey by *Prevention* magazine in 2000 estimated that more than 50 million persons were using herbal remedies, and there are even more using them now.

Since use of herbs among nonprofessionals has greatly increased in the past few years, healthcare professionals must be aware of the potential danger, especially when combined with medications. In addition there is no regulation, standardization, quality control, or even efficacy with herbal preparations. When nurses are completing admission assessments, questions should include asking about herbal preparations the client is now taking. The following table of herb–drug interactions will cover some of the most popular herbs and their interactions with specific drugs.

EVIDENCE-BASED PRACTICE

Herbal Remedies and Interaction With Drugs

A review of herbal remedies and their interactions with drugs found that warfarin was the drug most likely to be involved in adverse effects. St. John's wort was the herbal remedy most likely to cause an adverse interaction with other drugs.

Source: Fugh–Berman, E. (2003). *Natural medicine comprehensive database.*

TABLE 17-4 Herb–Drug Interactions Chart

Herb	Action	Side Effects	Drug Interaction	Drugs Affected
Black Cohosh	An herb for females, especially during menopause for hot flashes—maintains healthy levels of luteinizing hormone Decreases menstrual discomfort Sedative, diuretic Lowers blood pressure	Overdose may cause nausea, vomiting, headache, dizziness, tremors, and depressed heart rate	Increase effects of drugs—especially synthetic hormones **Clients with congestive heart failure and pregnant women should not use this herb**	Hormone replacement therapy (HRT) Contraceptives Heart/cardiac medications

(*Continued*)

TABLE 17-4 Herb–Drug Interactions Chart (*Continued*)

Herb	Action	Side Effects	Drug Interaction	Drugs Affected
Echinacea	Immunostimulant Treatment for colds (URIs) and influenza Bladder infections Blood purifier Helps preserve white cells during radiation treatment	Possible, but not common: nausea, vomiting, diarrhea, heartburn, skin rash, allergic reactions	Stimulates immune system—may alter effect of certain drugs; do not use with clients using immunosuppressants, or those who have AIDS, TB, or are pregnant	Anabolic steroids Amiodarone Methotrexate Ketoconazole
Ephedra (Ma Huang)	Promotes weight loss and acts as a stimulant (asthma) Considered toxic by FDA	Stimulant, insomnia, headaches, nervousness, seizures, death	Heart attack, seizure or death Additive effect; increased thermogenesis (related to stimulants/coffee) Elevation of BP (related to MAO inhibitors) Reduces drug action—may cause arrhythmias Increased steroid drug clearance may reduce effectiveness	Decongestants (Actifed, Dristan, Sinutab, Sudafed) Stimulants—caffeine MAO inhibitors Beta-blockers Cardiac glycosides Steroids (anti-inflammatories)
Feverfew	Eases pain and nausea of migraine headaches Prevents blood vessel spasms Interferes with action of platelets (which clump together to form clots) Lowers blood pressure	Gastrointestinal symptoms, nervousness, insomnia, and tiredness	Severe bleeding **Pregnant women, children under age 2, and people taking drugs as listed should not take this herb**	Anticoagulants—Warfarin Aspirin NSAIDs (ibuprofen)
Garlic	Contains allicin, natural antibiotic—effective against bacteria and viruses Lowers total cholesterol and increases HDL Reduces blood pressure Reduces blood clot formation (when arteries are narrowed)	Intestinal problems—upset stomach, heartburn, garlic odor	Excessive thinning of blood (bleeding) when used with blood thinners. Those who have blood disorders should use this herb conservatively	Anticoagulants—Warfarin Coumadin Aspirin Antihypertensives Saquinavir
Ginger	Relieves nausea associated with seasickness, motion sickness, or anesthesia Digestive aid; increased secretion of bile Reduces side effects of chemotherapy Reduces congestion and fevers Supports cardiovascular system	Heartburn	Excessive thinning of blood (bleeding) when used with blood thinners Interferes with platelet action Increases gut absorption (may increase drug bioavailability)	Anticoagulants—Warfarin Take cautiously with all cardiac or diabetic medications; Antihypertensives
Ginkgo Biloba	Improves circulation by thinning blood Enhances flow of oxygen and blood to brain Improves memory and mental function (dementia) May delay progression of Alzheimer's (jury still out) Asthma	Headache Indigestion, nausea, vomiting Nervousness Allergic skin reactions	Anticoagulant effect and may cause spontaneous or excessive bleeding **Those with blood clotting disorders should not take this drug**	Anticoagulants Coumadin Warfarin Aspirin NSAIDs Cox-2—inhibitors Anticonvulsants Vitamin K antagonists Diuretics Thiazides

TABLE 17-4 Herb–Drug Interactions Chart (*Continued*)

Herb	Action	Side Effects	Drug Interaction	Drugs Affected
Siberian Ginseng	Tonic, boosts energy and stamina Reduces stress, fatigue Improves sexual performance,regulates hormones Strengthens immune system Raise "good" cholesterol, HDL Protects against heart attacks Preventative for aging Improves blood sugar and diabetic symptoms (could reduce amount of insulin needed)	Insomnia, hypertension Diarrhea Low blood glucose Allergy symptoms Increased alcohol clearance Affects insulin level	Increases anticoagulant effect and bleeding Headache, manic behavior may occur when other drugs are taken Monitoring effect of drug may be difficult—may increase digoxin levels Stimulates alcohol metabolism **Those who have blood clotting problems, high blood pressure, asthma, emphysema, and children and pregnant women should not take this herb**	Anticoagulants Warfarin Coumadin Aspirin NSAIDs Nardil (MAO inhibitor) Digoxin (Lanoxin) Alcohol Insulin Antidepressants (phenelzine sulfate)
Kava Kava	Sedative effect to treat anxiety	GI problems, liver problems (even liver failure has been reported) Allergic skin reaction	Sedation, and even coma when taken with certain drugs	Alprazolam Sleeping meds Antipsychotics Alcohol Xanax (antidepressant) Drugs treating Parkinson's disease
Licorice Root	Helps steroid drug withdrawal Helps to heal gastric ulcers Diuretic effect	Raises blood pressure Headache Lethargy Cardiac dysfunction	Potentiates drug levels and offsets effects of NSAIDs Antibiotics reduce herb activity Diuretic effect could result in decreased potassium leading to electrolyte imbalance Increased sensitivity to digoxin or other cardiac glycosides **Women who are pregnant or nursing, and people with glaucoma, hypertension, stroke, or heart disease should not take this herb**	Corticosteroids Thiazides Oral contraceptives Antibiotics
Saw Palmetto	Supports health of prostate gland, benign prostatic hypertrophy (BPH) Improves urine flow Maintains healthy testosterone metabolism Anti-inflammatory	Relatively few: mild nausea, gastro intestinal disturbance, hypertension, headache	The safety profile of this herb is very good—no known drug interactions	
Silymarin (Milk Thistle)	Increases liver detox capacity in general Supports liver function Protects liver from drug damage	Nausea, GI disturbance	Reduces drug toxicity to liver and protects liver from drug damage Reduces toxic side effects of chemotherapy Potentially dangerous for transplant clients—reduces levels of immunosuppressives	Aspirin Alcohol Chemotherapy

(*Continued*)

TABLE 17-4 Herb–Drug Interactions Chart (*Continued*)

Herb	Action	Side Effects	Drug Interaction	Drugs Affected
St. John's Wort	Relieves mild to moderate depression by countering monamine oxidase (avoid same foods as if taking MAO inhibitor drug) Immune-stimulating properties—useful with AIDS because it is antiviral Helps bruises and hemorrhoids	Dry mouth, dizziness, fatigue, digestive problems (fewer side effects than prescription antidepressants) Sensitivity to light	Decreases immunosuppressant therapy Additive serotonin-like effects—serotonin syndrome (serious condition: fever, dizziness, sweating, etc.) Could affect action of epilepsy drugs **Clients with hypertension and those on immunosuppressive therapy should not use this herb**	Tetracyclines Cyclosporin Digoxin Oral contraceptives Zoloft and antidepressants Other SSRIs Anticonvulsants Warfarin
Valerian	Quiets and calms neurological system Promotes sleep Used for headache, anxiety, and nervousness	Restlessness, headache, giddiness, nausea, and blurred vision	Effect may be altered by alcohol or barbiturates—use cautiously Not for children under 2 years Effect may be enhanced with sleeping tablets Additive effect—may be used to wean off drugs (diazepam)	Alcohol Barbiturates Sleeping tablets Benzodiazepines

Source: Adapted from Herb/Drug Interaction Chart in Smith, S. F. (2009). *Sandra Smith's review for NCLEX-RN* (12th ed). Sudbury, MA: Jones and Bartlett Publishers.

Top five herbs your clients take but do not tell their physician:

Black Cohosh
Echinacea
Ginkgo Biloba
Saw Palmetto
St. John's Wort

Source: Crock, R. (2003, September). Herbal medicine consultant.

CULTURAL AWARENESS

Allowing for a religious or spiritual component in the care plan will enhance the client's ability to cope. Benson (1997) found that when religious beliefs were added to relaxation response procedures, worries and fears improved greatly.

Source: Fontaine, K. (2000). *Healing practices*. Upper Saddle River, NJ: Prentice Hall.

NURSING DIAGNOSES

The following nursing diagnoses may be appropriate to include in a client care plan when the components are related to decreasing stress and promoting adaptation.

NURSING DIAGNOSIS	RELATED FACTORS
Anxiety	Increased stress; for instance, illness, trauma, loss
Defensive Coping	Denial of problem, rationalization of failure, such as increased demands on individual
Ineffective Coping	High stress on person; for example, individual inability to adapt, length and duration of stressor
Disturbed Energy Field	Decreased immune response, increased stress level, poor integration of mind–body energy.
Ineffective Health Maintenance	High stress level, from illness, abuse, or psychologic factors
Deficient Knowledge	Lack of exposure to alternative methods, lack of interest in change (Relaxation Techniques)
Acute or Chronic Pain	Trauma, immobility, illness, or disease
Trauma, Risk for	Reexperiencing a traumatic event, exhibiting altered lifestyle, psychic numbness
Disturbed Sleep Pattern	Stressful thoughts, anxiety
Social Isolation	Maladaptive coping to stressor, such as long-term or high level of stress

CLEANSE HANDS The single most important nursing action to decrease the incidence of hospital-based infections is hand hygiene. *Remember to wash your hands or use antibacterial gel before and after each and every client contact.*

IDENTIFY CLIENT Before every procedure, introduce yourself and check two forms of client identification, not including room number. These actions prevent errors and conform to TJC standards.

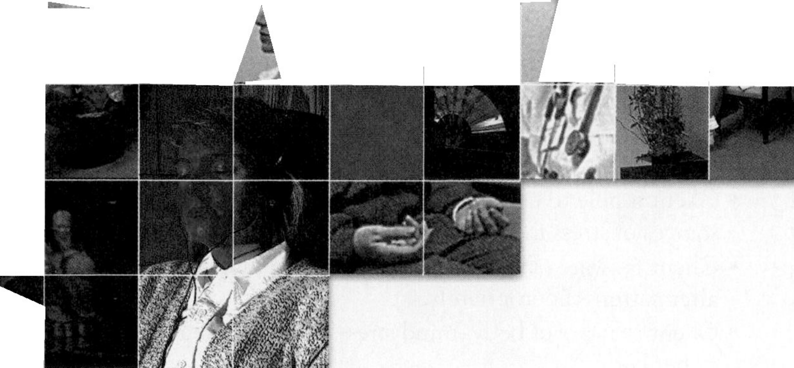

Chapter 17

UNIT 1

Stress and Adaptation

Nursing Process Data

ASSESSMENT Data Base

- Identify the client who demonstrates stressed behavior.
- Evaluate, with the client, the past and present stressors that the client has experienced.
- Evaluate the stressors' effect on the client's body and signs of distress in the body.
- Examples of physiological stress effects:
  Cardiovascular system: increased pulse and blood pressure, evidence of angina, arrhythmias, migraine headaches, disturbance of heat and cold mechanisms
  Gastrointestinal system: ulcers, ulcerative colitis, constipation or diarrhea, imbalance in sugar absorption
  Musculoskeletal system: backache, tension headaches, arthritis, proneness to accidents
  Autoimmune system: infections, flu, allergies, rheumatoid arthritis, cancer
- Assess client's level of energy and the degree to which it is depleted.
- Evaluate client's awareness of thoughts, attitudes, values, and beliefs that influence stress response and adaptation.
- Assess present level of distress in the client's body.
- Assess possible causes of stress that are affecting client:
  Environmental stressors: input overload, such as sights, sounds, smells; actions and demands of others in the environment; or monotony
  Physical stressors: hunger, heat or cold, dangerous environment, injury, or pain
  Emotional stressors: loss of something of value, frustrations of needs and drives, threats to self-concept
  Psychosocial stressors: Conflicting cultural values (e.g., the American values of competition and assertiveness vs the need to be dependent)
  Future shock: physiologic and psychological stress resulting from an overload of the organism's adaptive systems and decision-making processes brought about by too rapidly changing values and technology
  Cultural shock: stress developing in response to the transition from a familiar environment to unfamiliar one; involves unfamiliarity with communication, technology, customs, attitudes, and beliefs (e.g., immigrating, being confined in a hospital or prison); crowding, and urban life
  Job choice and the work environment (About 80% of the workers in our country are estimated to be unhappy in their jobs.)
- Assess the factors that influence how the client responds to stress:
  Characteristics of the stressful event: magnitude, intensity, duration
  Client's biologic and psychologic inclinations
  Appropriateness of support system
- Life changes according to a stress scale (Holmes & Rahe, 1967).
- Assess current coping strategies.

PLANNING Objectives

- To identify presence of stress in client
- To identify how stress affects the body
- To identify the current sources that result in stressed behavior
- To determine the client's response to stress
- To evaluate stress interventions that have a positive effect on stressed client

IMPLEMENTATION Procedures

EVALUATION Expected Outcomes

- Client is able to evaluate the general stressors and identify sources of stress in his or her life.
- Client is aware of response patterns to stress and is able to alter patterns appropriately.
- Client is aware of body–mind stress and its influence on his or her body.
- Client is able to reduce environmental stressors.
- Client is able to identify and alleviate stress caused by mental concerns.

Determining the Effect of Stress

Hans Selye's Definition of Stress

- Stress is a specific syndrome that consists of all nonspecifically induced changes within the biologic system.
- The body is the common denominator of all adaptive responses.
- Stress is manifested by measurable changes in the body.
- Stress causes a multiplicity of changes in the body.

Procedure

1. Identify client's stress tolerance level.
   a. Recognize the body's alarm signals (see major signals in assessment).
   b. Assess signal correctly as signifying high level of stress.
2. Discuss the concept of stress to elicit understanding of the effect on client.
   ▶ ***Rationale:*** Stress may be physical, chemical, or emotional and may cause bodily or mental tension that may be a factor in disease causation.
3. Encourage client to feel free to discuss life patterns that relate to stress.
4. Discuss the effect of stress. ▶ ***Rationale:*** Directing the conversation to the emotional, mental, and social sources of stress assists the client in examining its total effect and promotes self-awareness.
5. Assist the client in formulating a plan to reduce or eliminate at least some sources of stress. ▶ ***Rationale:*** Promotes client self-empowerment.

Determining Response Patterns

Procedure

1. Evaluate adaptation factors that influence stress management.
   a. *Age:* adaptation is greatest in youth and young middle life and least at the extremes of life.
   b. *Environment:* does environment support managing stress?
   c. *Time:* the client can more easily adapt to stress over a period of time than suddenly.
   d. *Flexibility:* degree of flexibility of the individual influences survival.
   e. *Expenditure of energy:* the individual usually uses the adaptation mechanism that is most economic in terms of energy.
   f. *Presence of illness:* disease decreases the person's capacity to adapt to stress.
2. Assess the effects of stress on the client.
   a. Feelings resulting from stress:
      1. Anxiety.
      2. Anger.
      3. Helplessness and hopelessness.
      4. Guilt, shame and disgust.
      5. Fear and frustration.
      6. Depression.
   b. Behaviors resulting from stress:
      1. Apathy, regression, withdrawal.
      2. Crying, demanding.
      3. Physical illness.
      4. Hostility, manipulation.
      5. Senseless violence, lashing out.

EVIDENCE-BASED PRACTICE

The Opposite of a Stress Response

In many studies, Herbert Benson, MD, author of *The Relaxation Response*, found that the opposite of a stress response (physiological response) can be achieved by completing only two steps: repeating a prayer, word, sound, phrase, or movement, and disregarding all other thoughts (as in meditation, yoga, etc.).

Source: Benson, H. (1984). *The relaxation response*. New York: Times Books.

Managing Stress

Procedure

1. Discuss the client's body response to stress.
   a. The body's response to stress is a self-preservation mechanism that automatically and immediately becomes activated in times of danger.
   b. Assist client to understand response patterns.
2. Teach client to be aware of stress sensations in his or her body—recognize physical symptoms.
3. Suggest that client frequently monitor thought patterns to identify those thoughts that cause automatic tensing responses (tight muscles, increase in heartbeat, butterflies in stomach).
4. Assist client to decide whether these thoughts are essential to survival or if they can be changed, eliminated, or replaced.
5. Assist client in planning to set aside periods each day for self-stress evaluation.
6. Provide problem-solving assistance so the client can examine new, more appropriate response patterns.
7. Refer client to resources (therapy classes, books, relaxation tapes) that will assist in developing new responses.

EVIDENCE-BASED PRACTICE

Managing Stress

The results of 153 studies on stress management were analyzed to determine whether there was consensus in definitions and therapy protocols. Most studies endorsed either a cognitive–behavioral approach to stress-coping skills (77%) (examples are problem-focused skills, self-monitoring of stress intensity, record keeping, time management, assertiveness training) or a less structured approach, breathing, relaxation, imagery, meditation, yoga, and massage therapy (85%).

Source: Ong, L., Linden, W., & Young, S. (2004). Stress management, what is it? *Journal of Psychosomatic Research*, 56(1), 133–137.

Manipulating the Environment to Reduce Stress

Procedure

1. Modify client's external environment so that adaptation responses are within his or her capacity.
2. Support the efforts of the client to adapt or to respond.
3. Provide client with the materials required to maintain constancy of his or her environment.
4. Understand the body's mechanisms for accommodating stress.
5. Prevent additional stress.
6. Reduce external stimuli and input through senses.
7. Reduce or increase physical activity depending on the cause of and response to stress.

Teaching Coping Strategies

Procedure

1. Analyze client's stress status.
   a. Estimate total amount of stress client is experiencing—too high a level of stress indicates need for intervention.
   b. Recognize where in body or mind the stress is manifesting.
2. Discuss various options for reducing stress—which alternatives fit with client.
3. Suggest client use diversion methods of coping.
   a. *Physical diversion:* jogging, swimming, cooking, cleaning.
   b. *Mental diversion:* reading, painting, going to a movie, or simply thinking about a pleasant memory.

4. Plan with client how to use rest as a way to cope with stress.
   a. Vacation, leave of absence from job, frequent naps.
   b. Eliminate or decrease major stressors so result is rest from stress input.
   c. Plan with client how to manage time so that input can be reduced and goals limited.
5. Teach client how to use concentration, body relaxation, breathing, or meditation techniques to relieve mind stress.
6. Remind client that laughter is a great tranquilizer and healer as well as a stress reducer, and assist client to plan how to use this method.

Suggestions for Coping With Stress

- Rank tasks to be completed, and identify activities that need to be accomplished.
- Forget unimportant details; do not try to remember too many things. Concentrate on the essential issues and details.
- Eliminate past unpleasant events from the mind and focus on the present.
- Do not cling to unpleasant experiences and emotions that impair emotional ability to respond to here and now.
- Discard habit of anticipating negative outcomes, which is often worse than the actual event.
- Do not yearn for things relating to the past or the future; focus attention on present desires.

Managing Stress Using a Holistic Model

Procedure

1. Manage stress through exercise.
   a. Poor physical condition becomes a stressor—this state contributes to lethargy, a constant fatigue level, and low resistance for illness and lessens adaptive responses.
   b. Good physical condition results in stamina, reserves necessary to withstand stress, and protection against unpredictable stress periods.
   c. Exercise prepares the body physically for stress caused by environmental conditions.
   d. Consistent exercise prepares body to handle stress emotionally.
2. Manage stress through diet.
   a. Certain foods and drug substances (caffeine, alcohol, sugar, junk foods, preservatives, tobacco) are potent stressors to our bodies.
   b. Consuming high-stress foods results in negative body changes, such as hypertension, high cholesterol, labile blood sugar levels, and a rapid, bounding pulse rate.
   c. Consuming a low-stress diet results in more energy and stamina to cope with stress. Teach client that a low-stress diet includes reducing saturated fat and limiting protein intake to 10%–15% of consumed calories. Remainder of intake should be raw or barely cooked vegetables, fruits, whole grains, nuts, low-fat dairy products, and plenty of liquids. Eliminate sodas, caffeine products, and most alcohol. Exclude refined sugars and carbohydrates and convenience or processed foods.
   d. Encourage the use of vitamin supplements: vitamin C, B-complex, mineral supplements. Assist client to examine diet and experiment with different vitamin–mineral supplements.
3. Manage stress by altering lifestyle patterns.
   a. Counsel clients to eliminate unnecessary stressors in their life—change parts of life that are particularly stressful.
   b. Assist client to develop personal methods for coping with stress: walking in the woods, painting, listening to music, reading, or practicing yoga.
   c. Encourage client to assess lifestyle periodically and alter habits as necessary to reduce stress.
4. Manage stress through use of prayer and/or meditation.

EVIDENCE-BASED PRACTICE

Prayer as Alternative Medicine

According to a survey by the National Institutes of Health (NIH) of more than 31,000 adults, prayer is the most commonly used alternative medicine. Fifty-five percent of Americans use prayer for health reasons: 52% prayed for their own health, 31% asked others to pray for them, and 23% prayed for health in a prayer group.

Source: Harper, J. (May, 2004). *Washington Times*, National Institutes of Health, Washington, D.C.

Teaching Controlled Breathing

Procedure

1. Instruct client to sit so that his or her back is well supported, with spine straight but not rigid.
2. Have client place feet flat on floor and place hands on legs.
3. If client is lying down, have him or her place hands at side.
4. Suggest client find a comfortable position, close eyes, and take a deep, slow breath through nostrils.
5. Continue giving the client the following instructions.
   a. Extend your abdominal muscles.
   b. Hold your breath for the count of four. Then very slowly release the air through slightly parted lips, making a "whoosh" sound.
   c. When you think that all the air is out, hold your stomach in to push out even more air.

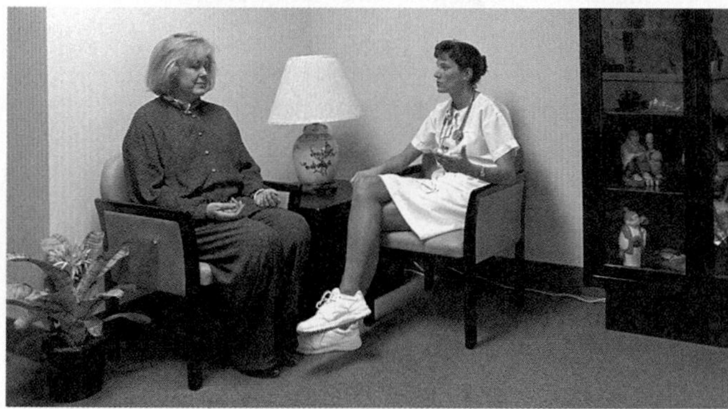

▲ Find a quiet room to teach relaxation process.

   d. Repeat this breathing pattern several times so that your body relaxes.
   e. Breathe in through your nostrils to the count of four— 1-2-3-4. Hold it—1-2-3-4—and expel the breath all the way out slowly, slowly releasing the air through your mouth.
   f. As the air goes out, feel all of the tension drain out with it.
   g. Now double the count and breathe in slowly, filling your lungs all the way to the top to the count of eight. 1-2-3-4-5-6-7-8. Hold it—1-2-3-4—and now slowly release the breath—5-6-7-8.
   h. Again breathe in slowly to the count of 10 and count for the client—1-2-3-4-5-6-7-8-9-10. Hold it to the count of eight—1-2-3-4-5-6-7-8—and slowly release the air through your mouth to the count of 10—1-2-3-4-5-6-7-8-9-10. Pause.
   i. Continue with your regular breathing pattern, letting the air breathe for you.
6. Stop the process by having the client open his or her eyes.

If you are motivated to learn CAM techniques, there are numerous classes available. In fact, to implement certain CAM therapies such as Reiki, therapeutic touch, acupressure, or acupuncture, you will need specialized classes/training.

Teaching Body Relaxation

Procedure

1. Place client in a comfortable position.
   a. Have client sit so that back is well supported and spine is straight. Have client put both feet on the floor and hold hands comfortably in lap.
   b. If sitting is uncomfortable, have client lie on a bed and support areas of the body so that he or she is comfortable.
2. Instruct client to concentrate on each key muscle of the body, tensing and relaxing each muscle until it is totally relaxed.
3. Ask client to tense and release the muscles in the left toes, left foot, left calf, left thigh, and left leg.
4. Now have the client continue the process on the right leg, trunk, upper torso, arms, shoulders, neck, and face. Then have the client check to see that every muscle is relaxed.
5. Ask the client to check for tight areas, any tension, any uncomfortable areas or sensations and then to let it all go. Ask the client if he or she is willing to let all of the tension go.
6. Ask client to practice being totally relaxed.

Using Meditation as an Alternative Therapy

Procedure

1. Meditation is the process of relaxing the body and focusing and quieting the mind. The essence of this method depends on the ability to concentrate on an object, a word, or nothing at all.
2. The process of meditation begins with slow, quiet breathing and deep muscle relaxation. (See Alleviating Stress Using Controlled Breathing and Body Relaxation.)
3. Instruct the client in meditation techniques—suggest books or tapes that focus on meditation.
4. Encourage the client to begin meditation—suggest positive outcomes.
   a. During meditation, there is a decrease in oxygen consumption, blood pressure, pulse rate, respiration, brain wave activity, and blood lactate level (high in anxious people).
   b. Research indicates that meditation has a measurable effect on stress-related conditions.

DOCUMENTATION for Stress and Adaptation

- Identification of stressed behavior observed in client
- Separation of physical from emotional and environmental stressors
- How client is responding to stress
- Pertinent verbalizations of client related to stress
- Nursing interventions related to stress reduction

CRITICAL THINKING Application

Expected Outcomes

- Client is able to evaluate the general stressors and identify sources of stress in his or her life.
- Client is aware of response patterns to stress and is able to alter patterns appropriately.
- Client is aware of body–mind stress and its influence on his or her body.
- Client is able to reduce environmental stressors.
- Client is able to identify and alleviate stress caused by mental concerns.

Unexpected Outcomes	Alternative Actions
Client moves into the stage of exhaustion, and stress becomes dangerous to health.	• Immediately take measures to remove stressors through medication, complete rest, and so forth. • Implement specific stress-reducing measures, such as relaxation processes, visualization, and biofeedback.
Client refuses to acknowledge that stress is affecting his or her life.	• Attempt to elicit feelings of client before giving information about the role of stress and effect on one's body. • Refer client to resources, articles, and knowledgeable persons who can discuss the effect of stress and the importance of eliminating stressors.

GERONTOLOGIC Considerations

The Influence of Stress on Aging is Significant and Affects Response and Coping Ability

- Nearly 23% of older people living in the community have some degree of disability.
- Elderly have less resistance to stressors: mental, emotional, environmental, and physical.
- Homeostatic imbalance is more common in the elderly and causes additional stress on the body.
- Adaptation to stress lessens with age (depends in part on genetic makeup and personal learning to deal with life crises).
- Many elderly suffer from depression.
- Nursing care should focus on adaptive responses to stress—assist client to develop mechanisms to deal with the stress of illness and hospitalization.

Risk Factors That Influence Stress Levels and Psychosocial Adaptation

- Lowered economic resources
- Unanticipated events such as death of a spouse
- Poor coping mechanisms
- Unrealistic appraisal of conditions
- Physical illness

Symptoms to Evaluate That Indicate High Stress Levels

- Insomnia
- High anxiety level
- Abuse of drugs, alcohol, or tobacco
- Hypertension, tachycardia, irregular heartbeat
- Depression, chronic fatigue
- Chronic pain
- Physical complaints
- Lack of any pleasure in life

MANAGEMENT Guidelines

Each state legislates a Nurse Practice Act for RNs and LVN/LPNs. Healthcare facilities are responsible for establishing and implementing policies and procedures that conform to their state's regulations. Verify the regulations and role parameters for each healthcare worker in your facility.

Delegation

- Stress assessment should be completed by an RN or LVN with experience evaluating stress in clients and one who understands Selye's model of stress.
- An LVN/LPN assigned to a client who needs coping strategies for stress should check the care plan with an RN or team leader.
- Teaching a client body relaxation, controlled breathing, or meditation should be done by an experienced nurse—RN or LVN/LPN.

Communication Matrix

- Integrating stress reduction and coping strategies into a client's care plan should be shared by the total staff interacting with the client to maintain a consistent approach.
- The staff approach should have outcome behaviors designated so that the strategies can be evaluated as to effectiveness and efficacy for the client.

CRITICAL THINKING Strategies

Scenario 1

Robert Warren is 40 years old and works as an administrative assistant for a senator in Washington, D.C. Before his admission to the hospital, he had no history of heart trouble and had no other major health problems. He is overweight by 30 pounds, complains of difficulty sleeping for several years, and has admitted to several brief depressive episodes that he has handled by either working longer hours or becoming intoxicated with alcohol. He does admit to overuse of alcohol on a daily basis.

Robert complains of burnout related to his work. Although he admires and supports his boss, he also competes with him and secretly believes he would make a better senator. Another area of concern is his marriage, which he says is dull except for an explosive argument every few weeks. Robert has been having affairs with other women regularly for the past few years. He and his wife have no children. Robert's admission diagnosis is acute myocardial infarction.

1. What are the consequences of Robert's adhering to this lifestyle behavior?
2. Which assessment parameters for stress are important for this client? Be specific about the areas of stress in the assessment.
3. In what ways can you assist this client to improve his coping with stress? (Robert's nutrition and exercise plans are deferred because he is currently in a cardiac rehabilitation program which daily monitors his diet and exercise.)
4. How might you test the result of stress reduction behaviors?

Scenario 2

The nurse is admitting a 60-year-old client to the unit. He is scheduled to undergo a series of tests to determine why he is fatigued, dizzy, and has constant digestive complaints. He had one seizure and was started on Dilantin until a diagnosis is made. As the admitting RN, you are completing an assessment.

1. Excluding the physical assessment parameters and signs and symptoms, what additional assessments will you make?
2. Based on the information you receive from the client, what teaching does this client require?

NCLEX® Review Questions

Unless otherwise specified, choose only one (1) answer.

1. Which of the following terms indicate signals of stress the nurse should be aware of?

   Select all that apply.

   1. Fatigue, lethargy.
   2. Eating disorder.
   3. Anxiety.
   4. Anger.
   5. Restlessness.

2. Which of the following is the best definition of holistic when referring to a holistic approach to health?
   1. The term implies wholeness.
   2. Holistic refers to the whole body, including mind and psyche.
   3. The term parallels wellness and means if the person is holistic, they are healthy.
   4. The term suggests that the body, mind, and spirit are one and interacts as an open system with the environment.

3. The World Health Organization (WHO) estimates that 80% of the world's population uses which of the following alternative practices as a part of their health care?
   1. Herbal medicine.
   2. Chiropractic.
   3. Energy medicine.
   4. Homeopathy.

4. Which of the following adaptation factors influence stress management?

   Select all that apply.

   1. Age.
   2. Environment.
   3. Degree of flexibility of the individual.
   4. Religion.
   5. Presence of illness.
   6. Expenditure of energy needed.

5. Which of the following is a therapeutic suggestion for coping with stress?
   1. Pay attention to unimportant details.
   2. Rank tasks to be completed in order of importance.
   3. Consider unpleasant past events and figure out what went wrong.
   4. Anticipate negative outcomes before they occur.

6. What is the best rationale for including nutrition/diet as an alternative treatment method.
   1. Diet is a major contributor to health or disease.
   2. Nutrition influences how long we live.
   3. Diet can cure disease.
   4. The quality of food influences well-being.

7. A client requests information about alternative treatments. Choose the most appropriate response.
   1. "I think that you should ask your doctor about this."
   2. "Perhaps it would be better to stick to mainstream medicine."
   3. "Let's get your doctor and my supervisor together to discuss your question."
   4. "I'll bring you information about alternative treatments."

8. Which of the following statements does not fit into Hans Selye's definition of stress?
   1. Stress is a specific syndrome.
   2. Stress is manifested by specific changes in the body.
   3. Stress can only be controlled by changes in thought patterns.
   4. Stress causes a multiplicity of changes in the body.

9. Which one of the following statements about stress is inaccurate?
   1. Chronic stress causes changes in the immune system.
   2. Stressors may be chemical, physical, developmental, or emotional.
   3. The stress syndrome can be both positive and negative.
   4. The danger signals of stress are easy to observe.

10. A client tells the nurse that he is constantly under stress. The nurse could teach the client a stress reduction technique such as:
    1. Counting to 10 before getting angry.
    2. Sitting relaxed and quiet, clearing the mind, and breathing deeply.
    3. Jumping up and down on a trampoline.
    4. Saying a mantra or one word over and over again.

18

Medication Administration

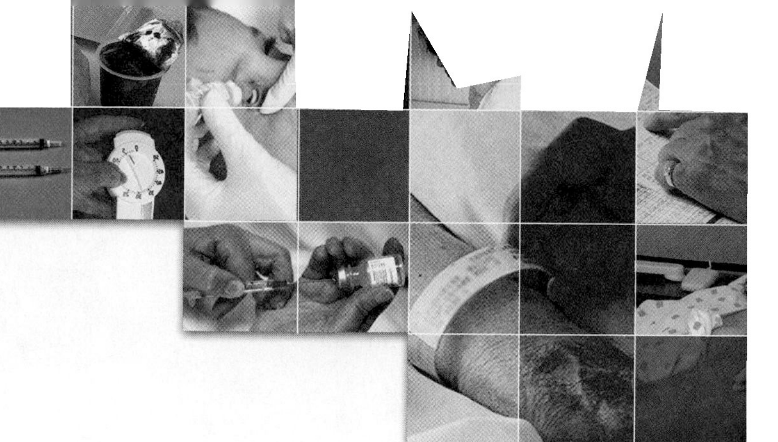

LEARNING OBJECTIVES

1. Explain the concepts of drug absorption, distribution, biotransformation, and excretion.
2. List the seven parts of a medication order.
3. State the "five rights" for administering medications.
4. Describe the medication cart and its purpose.
5. Identify three nursing actions to prevent medication errors.
6. Outline steps for applying a transdermal medication.
7. List factors to assess before applying medications to the skin or mucous membranes.
8. Describe steps for instilling eyedrops.
9. Outline the process of eye and ear irrigations.
10. Contrast the procedure for instilling ear medication in adults and children.
11. Outline steps used when preparing parenteral medications.
12. Demonstrate correct calculation and preparation of a complex medication order.
13. Compare insulin types, their onset, peak, and duration of action.
14. List four important factors to assess when administering parenteral medications.
15. State four techniques to alleviate pain with parenteral injections.
16. Describe the Z-track method of intramuscular injection.
17. List steps for inserting a rectal or vaginal suppository.

CHAPTER OUTLINE

TERMINOLOGY

Absorption the passage of a substance from administration site into the bloodstream.

Actuation propellant-driven medication dose.

Addictive causing enslavement to some habit.

Adverse reaction undesirable, usually unpredictable medication effect; may be immediate or take months to develop.

Allergy an antigen–antibody reaction or hypersensitivity to a substance.

Anaphylaxis a shock state due to an antigen/antibody reaction to a foreign substance (e.g., medication).

Anesthesia partial or complete loss of sensation with or without loss of consciousness as a result of injury, disease, or administration of a drug.

Aseptic sterile; condition free from germs and infection.

Aspirate to remove by suction.

Biotransformation metabolic conversion of a drug into inactive metabolites that are readily excreted from the body.

Bronchodilation dilation of the airways.

Cerumen protective secretion produced by the outer ear canal.

Circulation movement of blood in a circular course, exiting through the aorta and coming back into the heart via the venae cavae.

Compatible able to mix with another substance without destructive changes.

Congestion the presence of an excessive amount of blood or fluid in an organ or in tissue.

Contaminate to soil, stain, or pollute; to render impure.

Contraindication any circumstance indicating the inappropriateness of a form of treatment otherwise advisable.

Dosage the amount of medicine to be administered to a client at one time.

Drug any substance that, when taken into the living organism, may modify one or more of its functions.

Dyspnea a subjective feeling of difficulty in breathing.

Ecchymosis irregularly formed hemorrhagic area of the skin; a bruise.

Enteral administration administration through the gastrointestinal tract via a tube, catheter, or stoma to deliver nutrients/medications distal to the oral cavity.

Generic common or general name for a drug as opposed to a brand name.

Instillation slowly pouring or dropping a liquid into a cavity or onto a surface.

Intradermal within the dermal layer of the skin; injection here used for testing allergies, immune responses.

Intramuscular within a muscle; injected medication is rapidly absorbed due to rich vascular supply.

Intravenous administration into a vein for immediate drug action.

MAR medication administration record.

Medicine a drug or remedy.

Metabolism the biological process of changing a substance so that it (a) is less active, and (b) can be excreted.

Narcotic a controlled substance that depresses the central nervous system, thus relieving pain and producing sedation.

Nebulizer a device for breaking a drug into small particles to produce a mist or fog for inhalation.

Ophthalmic topical route for administering eye medications.

Otic topical route for administering ear medications.

Parenteral absorption route for administering medications other than the GI tract requiring injection.

Peristalsis a progressive, wavelike movement that occurs involuntarily in the intestines of the body.

Side effect predictable, unavoidable secondary effects produced by the medication at the usual dose (e.g., constipation, nausea, drowsiness).

Subcutaneous third layer of skin, which contains fat, with few blood and lymph vessels; route for injected medication. Results in slower absorption.

Sublingual under the tongue.

Systemic pertinent to the whole body rather than one specific area.

Therapeutic having medicinal or healing properties.

Tonicity state of normal tension (e.g., muscular) or normal osmolality (body fluid).

PHARMACOLOGIC AGENTS

The term "medication" refers to approved therapeutic (pharmacologic) agents applied to or introduced into the body to produce specific local or systemic physiologic effects. Medications are chemical compounds that are produced in a pharmaceutical laboratory and prescribed by a physician to be administered to a client to prevent, treat, or cure illness. These agents should be differentiated from over-the-counter (OTC) products such as vitamins, minerals, nutritional supplements, and botanical agents (herbs, phytomedicines), which also affect the body. While such OTC products are available to the public and commonly used for self-treatment, they are not officially regulated or monitored in the United States. It is important to assess the client's use of pharmaceutical agents as well as over-the-counter products or supplements, since there is potential for dangerous interactive effects.

Pharmacologic agents have a generic (patented official) name (e.g., acetaminophen), and a trade or brand name (created by the particular manufacturer) which is capitalized (e.g., Tylenol). Generic formulations are usually less expensive than brand-name products.

BIOLOGIC EFFECTS OF DRUGS

The ultimate effect of a drug is influenced by four biologic processes: absorption, distribution, metabolism (biotransformation), and excretion. These processes determine the onset, duration, and intensity of a drug's action.

Absorption This process refers to the movement of the drug from the administration site into the bloodstream. The route of administration determines whether or not a drug is confined to one area of the body to exert a *local effect*, or is absorbed by the vascular system and distributed to body tissues for a *systemic effect*. The oral route (PO, per os) is most frequently used for drug administration. Drugs may be given PO to exert a local effect (e.g., cough medicine, antacid), but more commonly the drug dissolves and is absorbed by the GI tract to exert a systemic effect. Liquid forms are absorbed more quickly. Most drugs are absorbed in the small intestine via the large vascular mucosal surface. The alkaline environment of the intestines enhances this absorption process. GI absorption is influenced by the pH, the presence or absence of food, concomitant ingestion of other drugs, solubility of the drug, and blood flow to the absorption site. In general, bioavailability of oral drugs is decreased because after absorption, the drug is circulated to the liver (first pass) and metabolized before reaching the circulation.

Medications applied "topically" to the skin (dermal) or eye (ophthalmic) or into the ear canal (otic) are often administered for local action. The skin is also used for transdermal (percutaneous) absorption of drugs by diffusion via patches, which release a medication continuously into capillaries of the epidermis for a systemic effect.

Mucous membranes provide a variety of convenient sites for drug administration to achieve a local or systemic effect by absorption. Sites include sublingual and buccal areas, the nose or respiratory tract (by inhalation), the eye, vagina, and rectum.

The parenteral route (by injection) provides the most direct, reliable, rapid drug absorption. Methods of parenteral administration include intradermal (ID), subcutaneous (Sub Q), intramuscular (IM), and intravenous (IV). Site selection depends on the drug, its action, and client factors. For example, a client with a severe allergic reaction receives epinephrine IV (directly into the bloodstream) because this route bypasses the process of absorption and provides immediate distribution and drug action in an emergency situation.

Distribution Distribution refers to the process by which a drug is transported by the blood to the site of action. Some of the drug binds to plasma protein and may compete with other drugs for this storage site. The rest is transported in "free" form through the circulation. It is the "free" form that is pharmacologically active. The "free" drug crosses cell membranes and as it is metabolized and excreted, the protein-bound drug is freed for action. Lipid-soluble drugs are distributed to and stored in fat and then released slowly into the bloodstream when drug administration is discontinued. The distribution process requires adequate cardiac output and tissue perfusion, while the rate of diffusion is influenced by the drug's protein-binding capacity, its solubility, the amount of drug in the plasma, and the presence of physiologic barriers such as the blood–brain and placental barriers.

Metabolism Metabolism or biotransformation refers to the enzymatic process by which a "free" drug is converted to an inactive and harmless form that can be excreted. Most drugs are metabolized in the liver, where some drugs are converted into metabolites that are more pharmacologically effective than their "parent" form. Some drugs given orally are significantly inactivated by "first passing" through the liver before entering the general circulation to be transported to the site of action. Oral doses of these drugs must be higher than parenteral doses, and some drugs totally inactivated by "first pass" must be given parenterally. Other sites of drug metabolism include the lungs, kidney, plasma, and intestinal mucosa.

Excretion This is the final process by which the drug is eliminated from the body. The kidneys are the most important route of excretion because they eliminate both the pure drug as well as metabolites of the parent drug. During excretion, substances are filtered through the glomeruli, secreted by the tubules, and then either reabsorbed by the tubules or directly excreted and eliminated through urine. Other routes of excretion include the lungs (by exhalation), GI tract, saliva, sweat, and breast milk.

Medication biodynamic processes and the individual client's response to drug therapy are influenced by many factors, including a client's body weight, body mass index, age, sex, acid–base and fluid and electrolyte balance, biorhythms, and general health and nutritional status. In addition, ethnic origin and genetic and immunologic factors affect biodynamics, as do psychological, emotional, and environmental influences. The term "drug polymorphism" is applied to these variations in clients' response to medications.

Seven Parts of Medication Orders

- Client's name
- Date medication was ordered
- Name of medication
- Medication dosage
- Route of administration and any special instruction for administration
- Time and frequency medication is to be given
- Signature of individual ordering the drug

Common communication breakdowns leading to medication errors include:

- Unapproved or unclear abbreviations (see box, p. 628)
- Illegible writing
- Misplaced or unnoticed decimals (e.g., .2 rather than 0.2)
- "Verbal orders"
- Incomplete orders

Source: Institute for Safe Medication Practices. www.ismp.org.

ADMINISTERING MEDICATIONS SAFELY

A medication must have physician's order or prescription before it can be legally administered to a client. If a written order is illegible or is questionable for any reason, the physician must be notified for clarification. In many agencies it is the pharmacist's responsibility to contact the prescriber to clarify unclear or questionable orders. Since verbal (using words) orders may be written or spoken, it is important to specify the mode of communication. If a medication order is spoken aloud (VO) or over the phone (TO), there is greater risk of error. Verbal (spoken) orders should not be taken if the prescriber is present and the chart is available, nor are they appropriate for complex therapeutic protocols (e.g., chemotherapy).

If the order is communicated by telephone, always repeat the order to avoid misinterpretation. Have the prescriber spell out the name of the medication and dosage, and have another person listen to the order as well. Get the prescriber's phone number, then record the order onto the client's chart directly (rather than transcribing from scrap paper). This order must be signed by the prescriber within 24 hr. Some agencies restrict telephone orders to emergencies only. To avoid error, it is better to have the prescriber e-mail or fax the medication order.

Medication orders may be *routine* (administered as ordered until discontinued by the prescriber), *one-time-only*, "*stat*" (immediately), or PRN (administered when the client needs the medication within the specified time interval, e.g., q4h). The continued validity of any medication order should be evaluated since prescribers sometimes forget to discontinue medications no longer appropriate for the client's condition.

While the physician prescribes the medication and the pharmacist dispenses it, the nurse is responsible for validating, preparing, and administering medications safely and in accordance with agency policies and procedures. The nurse should understand why the particular medication is prescribed for the particular client and clarify concerns about its use. The nurse who prepares the medication must also give it to the client, then document the medication, time, dosage, and route on the client's record. In addition, the nurse assesses and documents the client's response to the drug administered. If the client is allergic to a medication, an anaphylactic reaction may occur. This is a life-threatening medical emergency requiring immediate administration of epinephrine.

Safe administration requires adherence to the "Six Rights" (originally five) each time a medication is given in order to decrease the risk of a medication error.

Safety Precautions

When administering medications, follow established safety rules, known as "The Six Rights." These rules are to be carried out each time you give a medication to a client.

The Six Rights

- **Right medication.** Compare medication container label to the medication sheet (MAR) **three** times (when obtaining the medication, when preparing the medication, and after preparation). Note medication expiration date. Know action, dosage, and method of administration. Know side effects of the medication and any *allergies* the client might have.
- **Right client.** Check the room and bed number and client's Ident-A-Band: validate correct client with two identifiers other than room number (e.g., stated name and date of birth).

- **Right time.** Medication given 30–45 minutes before or after time ordered is acceptable (according to agency policy).
- **Right method or route of administration.** If a change in route is indicated, request new orders from physician.
- **Right dose.** Validate calculations of divided doses with another nurse. Have another nurse double-check your preparation of insulin, potassium chloride, morphine, hydromorphone HCl, heparin, and warfarin sodium (The Joint Commission high-alert drugs). Know the usual dose and question any dose outside safe range.
- **Documentation.** After administration may be considered to be the sixth right; the nurse should document the name of the drug, the dose and route, time administered, and the client's response to the medication administered.

In the event of a medication error, the physician must be notified immediately so that potential adverse client outcomes can be prevented or minimized. Follow your agency's unusual occurrence or variance reporting procedure to facilitate audits that help identify and rectify sources of medication errors.

Some agents within drug classes are more effective than others for different populations. Asians metabolize psychotropic agents more slowly than other ethnic groups, so lower doses may be indicated.

The nurse should obtain a list of each client's current medications as well as any alternative therapies used so that possible untoward interactions can be prevented.

CULTURAL AWARENESS

Cultural and genetic factors affect how a client reacts to medications. Physiologic rhythms, use of alcohol, and stress may either inhibit or accelerate drug biodynamics.

Cultural acceptance factors include values and beliefs, educational level, previous experiences, family influence, and physician/client relationship.

The concomitant use of "natural" remedies can also alter the client's response to drug therapy.

One genetic factor noted to differ among ethnic groups is variation in metabolic pathways that may accelerate or slow drug metabolism. It is also thought that the pathophysiology of various disease states may differ among populations based on genetic determination. For example, black clients respond differently to different antihypertensives than whites do. Blacks respond better to diuretics than they do to beta-blockers and angiotensin-converting enzyme (ACE) inhibitors for hypertension.

NURSING DIAGNOSES

The following nursing diagnoses are appropriate to use on client care plans when the components relate to a client who requires treatment with medications.

NURSING DIAGNOSIS	RELATED FACTORS
Ineffective Health Maintenance	Lack of education or readiness to learn, cognitive impairment, lack of equipment, inadequate support systems, inadequate financial resources, religious beliefs, cultural beliefs/values
Enhanced Self Health Management, Readiness for	Client seeks supervision and practices self-administration of MDI/DPI Client expresses interest in use of insulin pump/delivery system and seeks counseling for diabetes management with Certified Diabetes Educator Client seeks supervision and practices self-injection of anticoagulant before discharge
Risk for Injury	Altered clotting factors due to anticoagulant therapy Altered regulatory function due to side effects of medications (e.g., drowsiness) Altered biochemical function due to interactive effects of prescribed or nonprescribed medications/herbal supplements/vitamins Allergic/anaphylactic reaction to administered medication Medication error on part of nursing staff
Deficient Knowledge	Inadequate understanding of condition, medication regimen or self-care skills Inadequate understanding of rationale for follow-up laboratory monitoring related to prescribed medications
Ineffective Therapeutic Regimen Management	Impaired ability to perform tasks, side effects of therapy, nontherapeutic environment, denial of condition, lack of information or finances, poor self-esteem, nonsupportive family

CLEANSE HANDS The single most important nursing action to decrease the incidence of hospital-based infections is hand hygiene. *Remember to wash your hands or use antibacterial gel before and after each and every client contact.*

IDENTIFY CLIENT Before every procedure, introduce yourself and check two forms of client identification, not including room number. These actions prevent errors and conform to The Joint Commission standards.

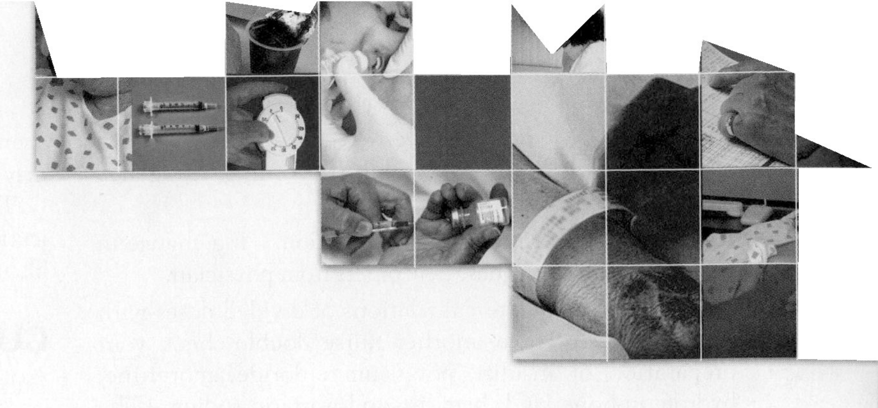

Chapter 18

UNIT 1

Medication Preparation

Nursing Process Data

ASSESSMENT Data Base

- Validate medication to be given with physician's order and client's MAR.
- Know desired therapeutic action of the drug, side effects, and adverse reactions.
- Assess for potential drug interaction with client's other medications or contraindication to administration (allergy, lab data, vital signs, unsafe dose).
- Identify route for drug administration.
- Recognize need to calculate drug dosage and seek verification of calculation by another nurse.
- Validate drug and dosage of certain critical drugs with another nurse or pharmacist.

PLANNING Objectives

- To understand the drug's action and rationale for administration to the client (desired therapeutic effect)
- To prepare the appropriate medication to be given by the correct route
- To have another nurse double-check dosage calculations and preparation of high-alert medications
- To anticipate potential side effects or adverse client reactions and be prepared to take corrective actions

IMPLEMENTATION Procedures

EVALUATION Expected Outcomes

- Rationale for medication administration is clear.
- Client's MAR matches physician's orders.
- Dosage calculations are accurate.
- Medication sign-out sheet matches remaining stock.
- Medication is administered according to the "Six Rights."

Pearson Nursing Student Resources

Find additional review materials at **nursing.pearsonhighered.com**

Prepare for success with NCLEX®-style practice questions and Skill Checklists

Preparing for Medication Administration

Equipment

Reference resource (e.g., *Physicians' Desk Reference*, pharmacology textbook, drug handbook)
Calculator (if indicated)
Medication administration record sheet (MAR)
Client's chart

Procedure

1. Check physician's orders and client's MAR for medications client is to receive (drug, dosage, route of administration, time intervals).
2. Identify any unfamiliar drugs.
3. Research unfamiliar drugs using appropriate reference.
   a. Generic and trade name.
   b. Drug classification and major uses.
   c. Pharmacologic actions.
   d. Safe dosage, route, and time of administration.
   e. Side effects; adverse reactions.
   f. Nursing implications.
   g. Complete client teaching as needed.

Clinical Alert

Individual drugs are designed to be administered by specific route—be sure to check drug labels for appropriate route of administration.

4. Review client's record for allergies, lab data, any factor (e.g., NPO status, planned procedures) that contraindicates administration of ordered medications.

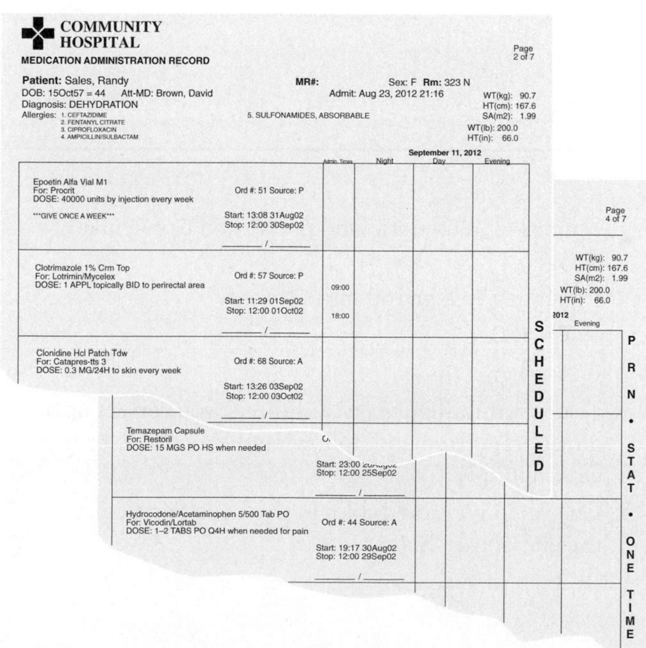

COMMUNITY HOSPITAL
MEDICATION ADMINISTRATION RECORD
Page 2 of 7

Patient: Sales, Randy   MR#:   Sex: F Rm: 323 N
DOB: 15Oct57 = 44   Att-MD: Brown, David   Admit: Aug 23, 2012 21:16
Diagnosis: DEHYDRATION
Allergies: 1. CEFTAZIDIME 2. FENTANYL CITRATE 3. CIPROFLOXACIN 4. AMPICILLIN/SULBACTAM 5. SULFONAMIDES, ABSORBABLE
WT(kg): 90.7 HT(cm): 167.6 SA(m2): 1.99 WT(lb): 200.0 HT(in): 66.0

September 11, 2012

		Admin. Times	Night	Day	Evening
Epoetin Alfa Vial M1 For: Procrit DOSE: 40000 units by injection every week ***GIVE ONCE A WEEK***	Ord #: 51 Source: P Start: 13:08 31Aug02 Stop: 12:00 30Sep02 ____ / ____				
Clotrimazole 1% Crm Top For: Lotrimin/Mycelex DOSE: 1 APPL topically BID to perirectal area	Ord #: 57 Source: P Start: 11:29 01Sep02 Stop: 12:00 01Oct02 ____ / ____	09:00 18:00			
Clonidine Hcl Patch Tdw For: Catapres-tts 3 DOSE: 0.3 MG/24H to skin every week	Ord #: 68 Source: A Start: 13:26 03Sep02 Stop: 12:00 03Oct02 ____ / ____				

SCHEDULED

Page 4 of 7
WT(kg): 90.7 HT(cm): 167.6 SA(m2): 1.99 WT(lb): 200.0 HT(in): 66.0
2012 Evening

Temazepam Capsule For: Restoril DOSE: 15 MGS PO HS when needed	Start: 23:00 Stop: 12:00 25Sep02 ____ / ____
Hydrocodone/Acetaminophen 5/500 Tab PO For: Vicodin/Lortab DOSE: 1–2 TABS PO Q4H when needed for pain	Ord #: 44 Source: A Start: 19:17 30Aug02 Stop: 12:00 29Sep02 ____ / ____

PRN • STAT • ONE TIME

▲ Example of a medication administration record.

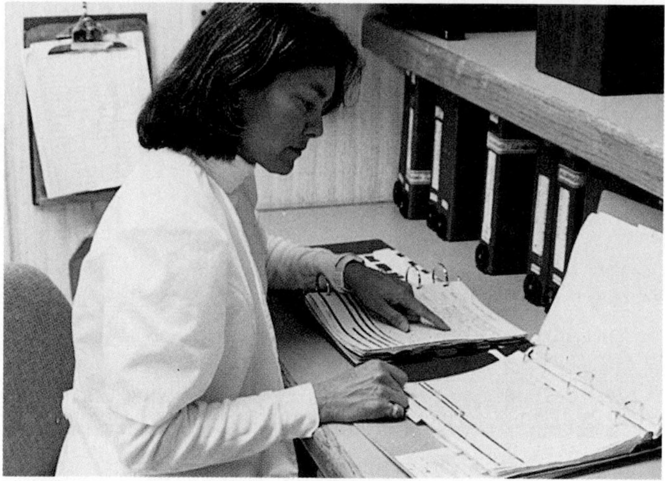

▲ Check physician's order against medication administration record (MAR).

5. Check client's daily MAR with previous day's MAR every 24 hr for each drug's dosage, route, and time to be given. ▶ ***Rationale:*** Pharmacy produces each daily MAR sheet. Any new medications, discontinued medication, or altered dosage must be identified and verified with the physician's orders.
6. Validate carefully that MAR is consistent with physician's most recent order for each medication. ▶ ***Rationale:*** Some medication dosages are adjusted on a daily basis. Errors in transmission of intentions may occur between physician, pharmacy, and client's MAR.
7. Perform hand hygiene.
8. Take medication to client's room.
9. Open medication cart; take out client's medication drawer.
10. Starting at the top of the MAR, check each medication in order against the medication packages in the client's drawer.

Alternately, obtain client's medication from the automated dispensing system.

11. Retrieve medication to be given and compare drug label with MAR. ▶ ***Rationale:*** This is a safety check to ensure the right medication is selected.
12. Inspect label for expiration date, and ensure that medication is indicated for ordered route of administration. ▶ ***Rationale:*** Different preparations of the same medication are used for different routes of administration.

Clinical Alert

If client assessment is indicated before administering drug to client (e.g., BP), make note on wrapper as a reminder to do so.

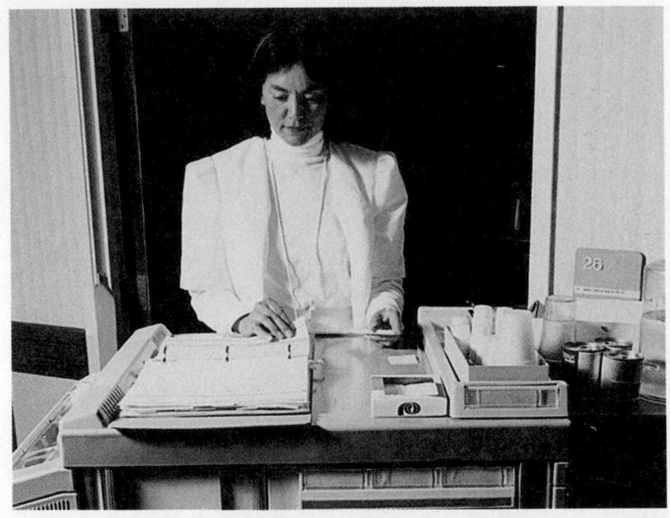

▲ Take medication cart to client's room.

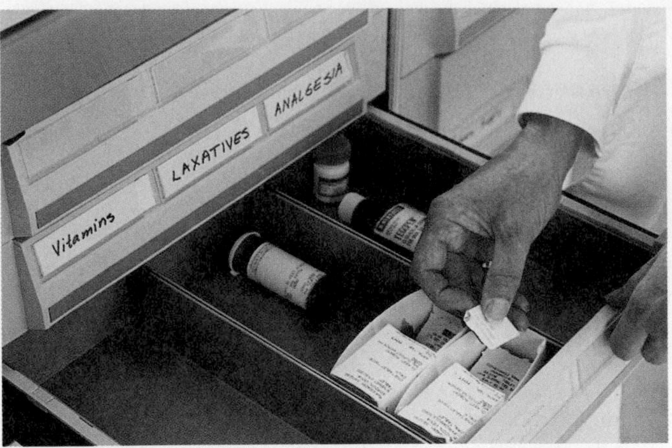

▲ Locate medications in client's drawer. Retrieve medication to be given and inspect label.

Clinical Alert

Check medication label three times before administering the medication:

- When retrieving the medication from storage area.
- When preparing the medication.
- When returning the medication to storage area.

13. Determine if any calculation is necessary to prepare the correct dosage.
14. Calculate client's dosage based on strength of medication, if indicated. Have another nurse double check your calculation. (See page 626 for formulas.)
15. Prepare medication as indicated for nonparenteral or parenteral route, checking drug label before, during, and after preparation.

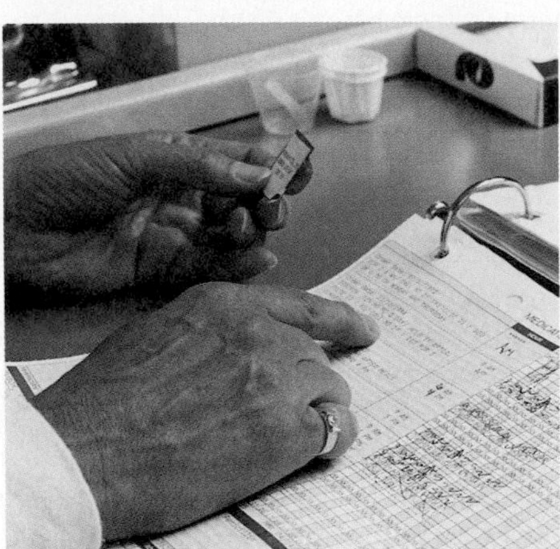

▲ Check individually wrapped medication against client's MAR.

Converting Dosage Systems

Procedure

1. To make conversions from the metric to apothecaries' or household systems, it is necessary to memorize or refer to equivalency tables.
2. To convert milligrams to grains, use the following formula:

$$\frac{\text{1 grain}}{\text{milligrams per grain}} = \frac{\text{Dose desired}}{\text{Dose on hand}}$$

$$\frac{1}{60} = \frac{X}{180}$$

$$60X = 180$$

$$X = 3 \text{ grains}$$

3. You may also use ratio and proportion to calculate dosage:

$$1 \text{ gr}:60 \text{ mg} :: X \text{ gr}:180 \text{ mg}$$

$$60X = 180$$

$$X = 3 \text{ gr}$$

4. To convert milligrams to milliliters, you can set up a direct proportion and, following the algebraic principle, cross multiply.
5. Check Conversion Tables in the Drug Supplement at the end of the chapter.

Calculating Dosages

Equipment

Orders for dosage of medication needed

Dosage of medication on hand

Procedure

1. To calculate oral dosages, use the following formula. (D and H must be in same unit of measure.)

$$\frac{D}{H} = X$$

where D = dose desired; H = dose on hand; and X = dose to be administered.

Example: Give 500 mg of ampicillin sodium when the dose on hand is in capsules containing 250 mg.

$$\frac{500 \text{ mg}}{250 \text{ mg}} = 2 \text{ capsules}$$

2. To calculate dose when in liquid form, use the following formula:

$$\frac{D}{H} \times Q = X$$

where D = dose desired; H = dose on hand; Q = quantity; and X = amount to be administered

Example: Give 375 mg of ampicillin when it is supplied as 250 mg/5 mL.

$$\frac{375 \text{ mg}}{250 \text{ mg}} \times 5$$

$$1.5 \times 5 = 7.5 \text{ mL}$$

3. To calculate parenteral dosages, use the following formula:

$$\frac{D}{H} \times Q = X$$

Example: Give client 40 mg gentamicin C complex sulfate. On hand is a multidose vial with a strength of 80 mg/2 mL.

$$\frac{40}{80} \times 2 = 1 \text{ mL}$$

4. To calculate dosages for infants and children using BSA:

$$\frac{\text{BSA*}}{1.7} \times \text{adult does} = \text{pediatric dose}$$

*BSA = body surface area.

See *Pediatric Nursing*, 3rd ed., by Jane Ball and Ruth Bindler, 2003, Prentice Hall, for complete description of method to determine body surface area.

5. To calculate dosages for infants and children using Clark's weight rule:

$$\text{Child's dose} = \frac{\text{Child's wt. in lbs.}}{150} \times \text{Adult dose}$$

6. Check your calculations before drawing up the medications.

NOTE: Calculation of Solutions is in the Drug Supplement section at the end of the chapter.

Using the Narcotic Control System

Equipment

Medication record sheet

Narcotic sign-out sheet

Medication

Procedure

For Client Administration

1. Check client's medication sheet for narcotic order.
2. Check dose and time last narcotic was administered.
3. Unlock and open narcotic drawer and find appropriate narcotic container.
4. Count the number of pills, ampules, or prefilled cartridges in container.
5. Check the narcotic sign-out sheet, and check that the number of narcotics in drawer matches the number on specific narcotic sign-out sheet. ▸ ***Rationale:*** Laws on controlled substances require careful monitoring of narcotics.
6. Correct any discrepancy before proceeding with narcotic administration.
7. Sign out for the narcotic on the narcotic sheet after taking narcotic out of drawer.
8. Lock drawer after dispensing medication.
9. Administer medication according to specific oral or parenteral procedure.
10. Document narcotic on client's medication record according to agency procedure. Include client's sedation level and pain rating (e.g., 8/10) before and after narcotic administration according to agency policy.

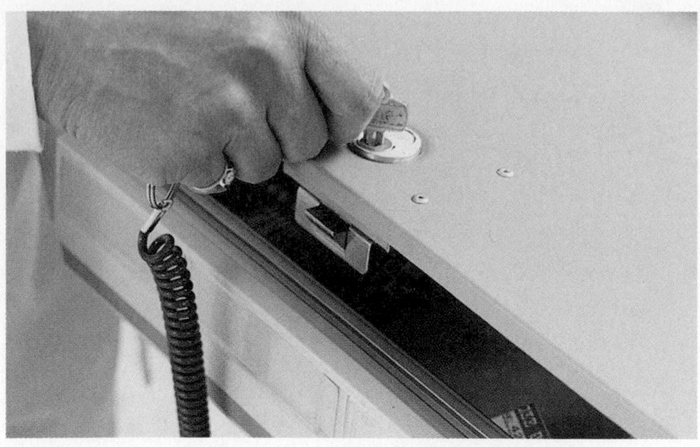

▲ Lock narcotic drawer after removing medication. Keep key with you at all times.

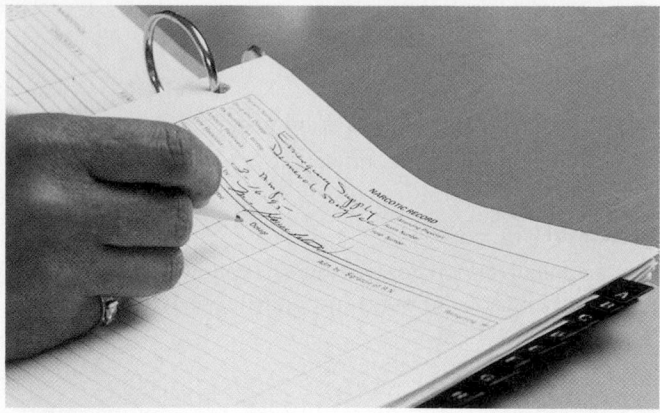

▲ Sign on specific narcotic sign-out sheet after taking narcotic out of drawer.

For Unit Narcotic Stock

11. Check narcotic counts every 8 hr. One off-going and one on-coming *licensed* nurse must check the narcotics together. The number on each narcotic sign-out sheet must match the number of that particular narcotic remaining in the drawer.
12. Explore any discrepancy in stock and recorded dispensed narcotic numbers. ▶ ***Rationale:*** Counts must balance. It is the nurse's responsibility to account for all controlled substances dispensed.
13. Licensed nurses cosign the narcotic record if the count is accurate.

Clinical Alert

If the narcotic depresses breathing, note client's level of sedation and respiratory rate before administering, and document assessment.

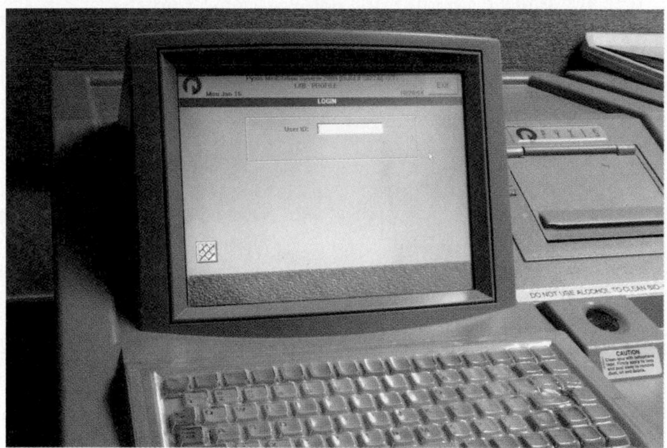

▲ User ID and password or scanned fingerprint control access to medications.

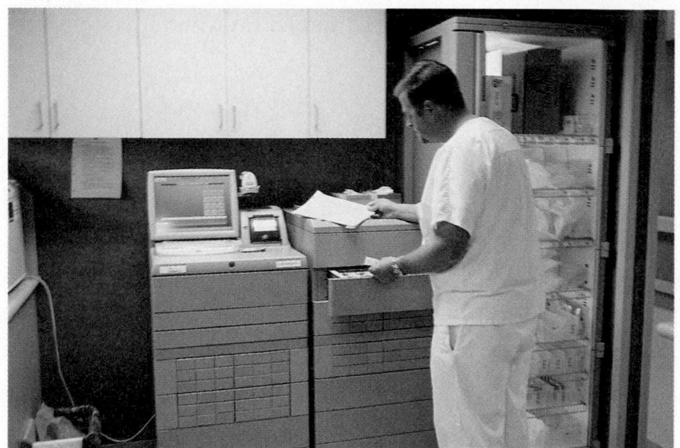

▲ Validate that client's MAR matches selected medications and dose on screen.

Using an Automated Dispensing System

Equipment

Automated dispensing system (e.g., PYXIS)
Client's medication record

Preparation

See Medication Preparation (Unit 1), all procedures.

Procedure

1. Touch the screen to activate the system.
2. Enter your ID code number and user password or scanned fingerprint. ▶ ***Rationale:*** This process controls access to medications.
3. From the main menu, select command on medication management station (e.g., *remove*, *waste*, *return*).

4. Select client's room number, medication, and name and additional identifiers (e.g., *birth date*, *hospital number*).
5. Touch/select medication desired from client's displayed list of ordered medications.
6. Validate that client's medication record matches selected medication and dose on monitor screen.

Clinical Alert

The usual checks and balances between nurses and pharmacists may be bypassed with automated dispensing systems, increasing the risk for medication errors.

Dispensing Medications—Safe Practices

No technology system eliminates the risk for error.

Never become complacent about what technology can do to support safe practice.

No computer has your ability to think critically, to understand whether an ordered drug is appropriate for your client.

Technology (e.g., bar codes) increases the amount of time spent administering medications, but does reduce time spent in documentation.

7. Type in quantity (#) of doses desired if indicated by a range of possible doses ordered.
8. Enter a witness ID/scan (by another nurse) to validate wasted medication (if partial dose is needed).
9. Remove the medication from the automated delivery system.

Medication Safety Measures

- Accurately and completely reconcile the client's medications across the continuum of care.
- Keep all medications in locked carts or cabinets.
- Limit access to and use special safeguards with "high alert" drugs (those causing significant client harm if used in error; e.g. hypoglycemic, anticoagulant, anesthetic agents, narcotics, paralytic agents, chemotherapy drugs, certain cardiac drugs). This list is periodically updated by the Institute for Safe Medication Practices (ISMP).
- Keep narcotics in double-locked cabinets or PYXIS. Count all narcotics with oncoming staff at the end of each shift.
- Separate topical medications from parenteral or oral medications.
- Clearly label all prepared medication containers (syringes, medicine cups, solutions).
- Check with another nurse (1) mathematical calculations for dosages and (2) dispensed/prepared "high alert" drugs and those for high-risk clients (e.g., insulin, anticoagulants, concentrated electrolytes, digoxin, and hemodynamic agents if not premixed).
- Do not leave any medication at client's bedside unless there is a specific physician's order to do so.
- Report any errors in drug administration to charge nurse and client's physician immediately. Monitor the client closely for adverse effects. Document the drug given, and complete an anonymous written variance report.
- Provide complete instruction to clients regarding medications to be used at home.

Hazardous Waste Disposal

Health care produces biohazardous waste, chemical waste, pharmaceutical waste, and other toxins, with each source having environmental consequences. Scientists have found concentrations of antibiotics, hormones, antineoplastic agents, and other chemical products in our water supplies due to improper disposal of pharmaceuticals into the sink, toilet, or trash. Best practice waste management is consistent with regulations mandated by the Environmental Protection Agency:

- Discard pharmaceutical waste into a Medical Waste receptacle (black box):
  1. Any unused oral medication not in package
  2. Unused IV medication that has been partially infused (unused IV fluid with electrolytes and TPN are excluded)
  3. Unused medication in syringes or vials (empty vials, empty IV bags and tubing are discarded in the trash)

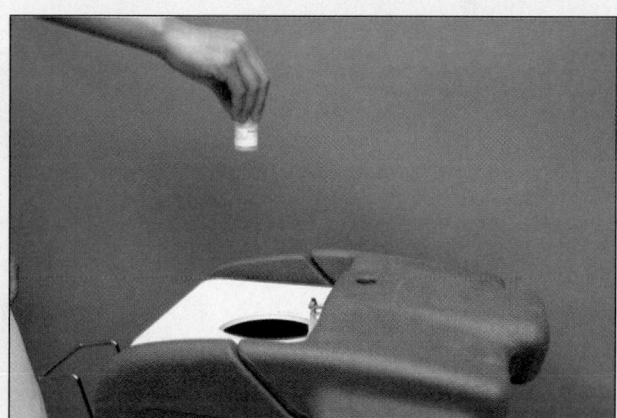

▲ Discard pharmaceutical waste into Medical Waste receptacle (black box).

- Chemotherapy Waste Container (yellow) is used to discard any trace chemotherapy (containers, tubing, contaminated PPE).

10. Close drawer/storage door, and exit the system.
11. Prepare medication and administer according to route.

NOTE: Certain medications (e.g., cough syrup and other client-specific multiple-dose medications) may be dispensed by pharmacy and placed in the client's medication drawer rather than being accessed through the automated system.

Clinical Alert

All Joint Commission–accredited agencies must have protocols developed for documenting and reconciling medications across the continuum (admission, transfer, discharge). A list of the client's home medications is compared with the admitting medication orders. Upon transfer, medications being taken are compared with orders in the new unit. Upon discharge, medications taken in the hospital are compared with the discharge medication orders. Verification, clarification, and reconciliation of discrepancies help prevent adverse drug events throughout the client's hospitalization.

Administering Medication Protocol

Equipment

Prepared medication
Gloves (if indicated)
Stethoscope and sphygmomanometer, if indicated

Preparation

See Preparation (Unit 1), all procedures.

Procedure

1. Check client's name and room number against the medication record and lock the medication cart before entering client's room, if cart is used. ▸ ***Rationale:*** Locking cart is a safety measure.
2. Check client's Ident-A-Band and ask client to state name and birth date.
3. Provide privacy.
4. Explain procedure and purpose of medication to client.
5. Assist client to appropriate position for medication administration.
6. Check client's vital signs if indicated before administering medication. ▸ ***Rationale:*** Medication's effects may cause hemodynamic instability if client's vital signs are at the high or low extreme of normal.

Clinical Alert

Use at least two client identifiers other than room number when administering medications or providing treatments (e.g., stated name and birth date or hospital number).

7. Perform hand hygiene and don gloves if indicated. ▸ ***Rationale:*** Parenteral and enteral medication administration may require the use of gloves, as well as preparation and administration of oral antineoplastic agents.

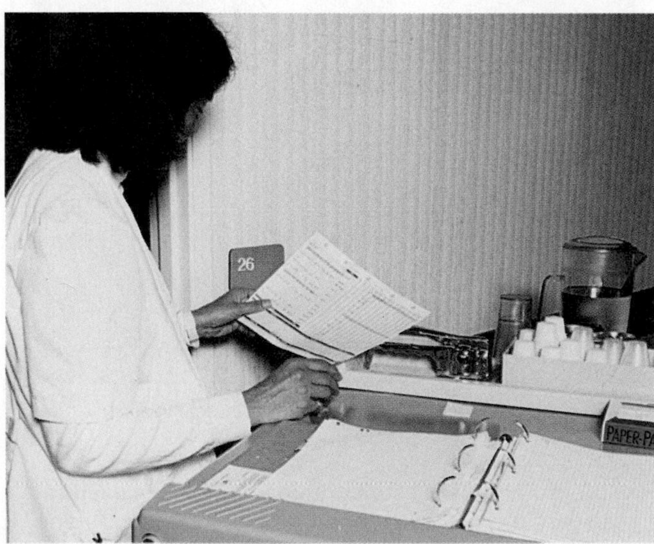

▲ Check client's name and room number against medication record.

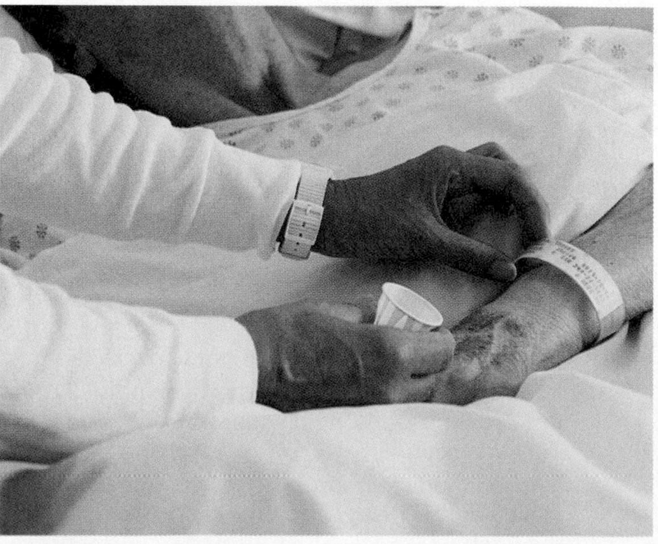

▲ Check client's Ident-A-Band and ask client to state name and birth date.

8. Administer medication according to route procedure and adhering to the "six rights" of medication administration.
9. Dispose of equipment appropriately; then remove gloves, if used, and wash your hands.
10. Record administered medications in client's record; the time, medication given, dosage, and route (including site of injection); and any relevant assessment findings.

EVIDENCE-BASED PRACTICE

Medication Errors—A Growing Problem

- Medication errors originate across the spectrum of care: prescribing, 39%; transcribing, 17%; dispensing, 11%; and administering, 38%. Nurses must identify errors before administering medications: both the mistakes of others, and their own.

Source: Cohen, H. (2008, April). Let's work together to improve medication safety. *Nursing*, 38(4), 6.

Medication Administration Errors

- In a study involving 400 staff nurses, 30% of full-time staff reported making at least one error in a 28-day period, and another 33% reported a near error. The majority of errors or near errors involved medication administration. Of these events, 25% involved giving the wrong dose, with nurses citing interruptions and distractions during preparation.

Source: Professional Update (2005). *RN*, 68(3), 20.

EVIDENCE-BASED PRACTICE

Wristband Placement

It is best to place all wristbands on the same arm, but best practice requires the nurse to check both arms, and also the ankles since placement here may be required.

Source: Cizek KE, Estrade N, Allen J, Elsholz T. A crystal clear call to standardize color-coded wristbands. *Nursing 2010*; 40 (5) 57-59.

Bar Code Medication Administration

Medication administration errors account for 34% of preventable adverse drug events. Bar code medication administration (BCMA) technology can improve client safety by reducing these errors. The central feature of this point-of-care system is barcode labeling of medications and client wristbands. In order to facilitate implementation, vendors and hospitals usually customize these systems to interface with existing electronic medical records.

Failure to adhere to the steps of the BCMA process may expose the nurse to fraud charges. Hazardous shortcuts ("workarounds") may lead to patient harm and legal pitfalls.

Steps to take before medication administration:

- Compare the medication order in the client's medical record against each medication on the eMAR.
- Obtain medication from the automated dispensing cabinet.
- Perform a "five rights" check against the eMAR while removing the medication. *Note:* The sixth right is *documentation* and does not apply here.

Steps to perform at the client's bedside:

- Check client's Ident-A-Band and ask client to state name and birth date.
- Perform a second "five rights" check of selected medications against the eMAR.
- Scan barcode on client's Ident-A-Band, then scan bar code on *unopened* medication packaging and bar code on client's Ident-A-Band.
- Obtain confirmation of bar code matching by the software system and attend to any alarms or cues.
- Prepare scanned medication.
- Administer the medication promptly.
- Document medications administered.

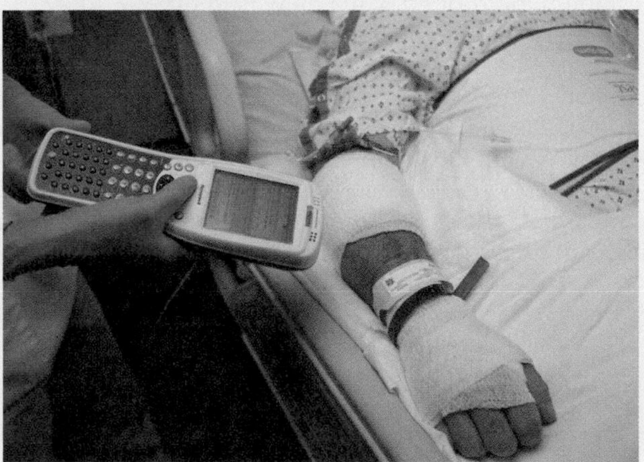

▲ Scan the bar code on the client's ID band.

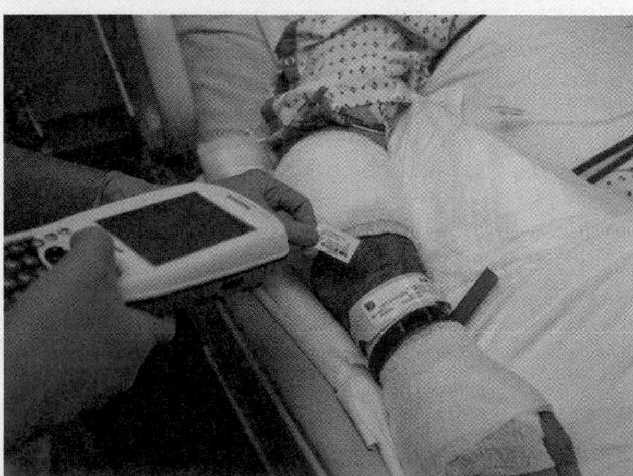

▲ Scan the bar code on the unopened medication packaging to confirm matching.

EVIDENCE-BASED PRACTICE

Interuptions Linked to Medication Errors

This study of 98 nurses administering 4,271 medications to 720 adult clients showed that nurses who are interrupted while preparing and administering medications may have increased risk of making medical errors. Interruptions require switching from one task to another, completing the interrupting task and then returning to the interrupted task. For each interruption there is an increase in procedural (e.g., technique) and clinical error (e.g., dosage). Frequency of interruption was associated with increased severity of error. While some interruptions are excusable when directed toward provision of safe patient care, there is a need to better understand the reasons for high interruption rates.

Source: Barclay, Laurie (2010). Interuptions linked to medication errors by nurses. *Archives of Internal Medicine, April 26, 2010.*

Clinical Alert

Report any actual or potential error (e.g., look-alike/sound-alike drug names, confusion over abbreviations) to the Institute for Safe Medication Practices at 1-800-FAIL-SAF(E) or complete the form at www.ismp.org/orderforms/reporterrortoISMP.asp. All communications are kept confidential. This agency publicizes warnings and notices in response to submitted information to help alert other professionals to potentially dangerous medication pitfalls.

Source: Nurse Advise-ERR, July 2009.

Legal Considerations

Transcription Error and Reconciliation Failure (*Robert Ferguson v. Baptist Health System, Inc, 2005*)

Robert Ferguson brought medical malpractice action against Baptist after experiencing drug toxicity due to a medication (Dilantin) transcription error on the part of the pharmacist and failure on the part of the nurse to conduct reconciliation between the MAR entry and the doctor's order. The physician's order was for Dilantin, 300 milligrams "po QHS." The MAR was generated by pharmacy for Dilantin, 300 milligrams, "t.i.d." The agency policy dictated that any time a new medication order was entered, the nurse initially undertaking to administer the medication was responsible for comparing the MAR to the actual order to "reconcile" the two. In this case, the pharmacy error was not detected by the reconciliation process. Subsequent erroneous doses were administered, but none of the nurses administering the Dilantin detected the error "due to the fact that there were no additional checks, balances, or other safeguards in place to prevent the repetition of the error." No one ever checked the original physician's order "despite the unusually large amount of Dilantin being administered." None of the nurses suspected that Ferguson's symptoms represented Dilantin toxicity. Ferguson was awarded compensatory damages and punitive damages.

McMunn v. Mount Carmel Health et al, 1998

Plaintiff was awarded $433,415.00 for wrongful death of William Muncey, age 39, resulting from improper administration of morphine and failure to monitor and guard the client from adverse effects of the drugs he received, those known to cause respiratory depression. The client presented to Mount Carmel ED at 1635 with severe pain due to kidney stones. He received 5 mg of morphine IV at 1653, at 1700, and again at 1740. His respiratory rate was 24 and SpO_2 was 92%.

He then received additional 5 mg of intravenous morphine at 1805 and 1820, whereupon his SpO_2 dropped to 86%. The client was placed on oxygen therapy and by 1935 his SpO_2 had increased to 94%.

At 2015 he was admitted as an inpatient. His vital signs were taken at that time, but not again for the evening shift. The nurse had not been advised that the client's O_2 saturation had dropped while he was in the ED. At 2215, the nurse administered 15 mg of morphine sulfate and 50 mg Phenergan by injection. At 2300 it was documented that the client was sleeping, but no vital signs were taken.

At 0105, the nurse was notified that Mr. Muncey was unresponsive and had no pulse or respirations. A "Code Blue" was called, Narcan was given, but the client died. At autopsy, spinal fluid and blood levels of morphine were supportive of death from a respiratory depressant effect of morphine, with levels unusually high explained by the *combination* of depressant drugs he had received.

Three areas of nursing care were found to fall below the accepted standard: coordination and communication of assessment and care, monitoring of a client receiving narcotics, and documentation of assessments for a client receiving narcotics.

CRITICAL THINKING Application

Expected Outcomes

- Rationale for medication administration is clear.
- Client's MAR matches physician's orders.
- Dosage calculations are accurate.
- Medication sign-out sheet matches remaining stock.
- Medication is administered according to the "Six Rights." *Note:* Six rights is correct here because it includes documentation.

Unexpected Outcomes	Alternative Actions
Medication or dosage on MAR does not fit client's clinical picture.	• Compare new MAR with previous MAR. • Compare new MAR with recent physician's orders. • Discuss concerns with agency pharmacist. • Contact physician for clarification.
Nurse is unsure of dosage calculation.	• Utilize helpful calculation formulas. • Use a calculator. • Request that another nurse check calculation or conversion. • Seek agency pharmacist's assistance.
Medication sign-out sheet does not correspond to remaining stock.	• Check with other nurses who may have dispensed stock medication. • Check MARs for unclaimed stock that may have been administered. • Complete discrepancy report if sign-out sheets and stock cannot be reconciled.
Client receives the wrong medication.	• Document the medication administered on client's MAR. • Monitor client closely for potential undesired effects and document findings. • Notify client's physician and document. • Complete anonymous variance report according to agency policy. • Always check two client identifiers before administering medication.

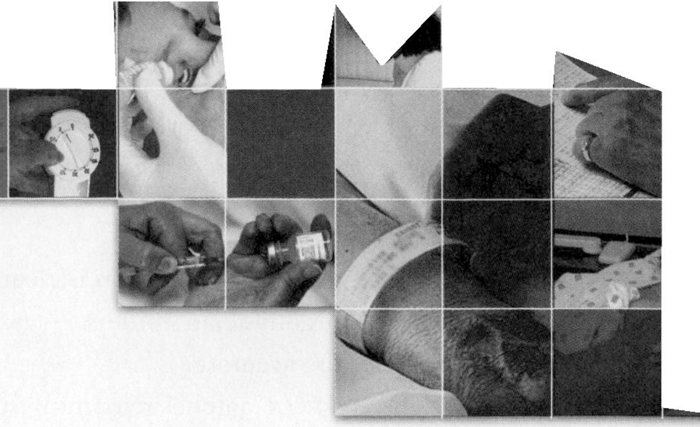

Chapter 18

UNIT 2

Oral Medication Administration

Nursing Process Data

ASSESSMENT Data Base

- Check that medication is to be given by oral route.
- Determine that client is not NPO.
- Determine that client is able to take medication orally.
  - Client is alert.
  - Swallow/gag reflex is present.
  - No risk of aspiration exists.
  - Client is not nauseated/vomiting.
- Determine that medication can be safely altered if necessary for administration.

PLANNING Objectives

- To provide an easy, inexpensive, and convenient route for administering medications
- To ensure that client is able to take oral medication
- To safely administer an altered oral medication
- To facilitate administration of oral medication to the client with swallowing difficulty (dysphagia)
- To administer oral medication to an adult or child

IMPLEMENTATION Procedures

EVALUATION Expected Outcomes

- Client takes medication orally without difficulty.
- Client experiences intended therapeutic drug effect.

Pearson Nursing Student Resources

Find additional review materials at **nursing.pearsonhighered.com**

Prepare for success with NCLEX®-style practice questions and Skill Checklists

Preparing Oral Medications

Equipment

Oral medication: tablet, capsule, or liquid from bottle or unit dose.

Client's preference of water, juice, milk, or other vehicle (e.g., jelly, yogurt, pudding) to assist swallowing (if not contraindicated for drug absorption)

Mortar and pestle to crush or pill cutter to divide medication if necessary

Measuring spoon, *calibrated* dropper, syringe or medicine cup

Gloves, for oral antineoplastic agents

Preparation

1. Follow all steps for Medication Preparation (Unit 1).
2. Perform hand hygiene.

Procedure

For Liquid Medications

1. Remove bottle lid and place topside down to avoid contamination.
2. Hold bottle with label facing palm to avoid dripping medication onto label.
3. Set medication cup on firm surface and pour liquid medication; read fluid dispensed at eye level, *read at lowest point of meniscus.* ▸ ***Rationale:*** This reading ensures accurate dose of medication.
4. Wipe bottle lip before replacing cap. Check medication label again. ▸ ***Rationale:*** This safety check ensures correct drug and dosage.
5. Return multidose bottle to storage area. Sign out for any narcotic dispensed on narcotic sheet with date, client's name, room number, physician's name, dosage, your signature, and any wasted narcotic (co-signed by another nurse/witness).
6. Remember to check the label three times:
   a. When taking the medication container from storage place.

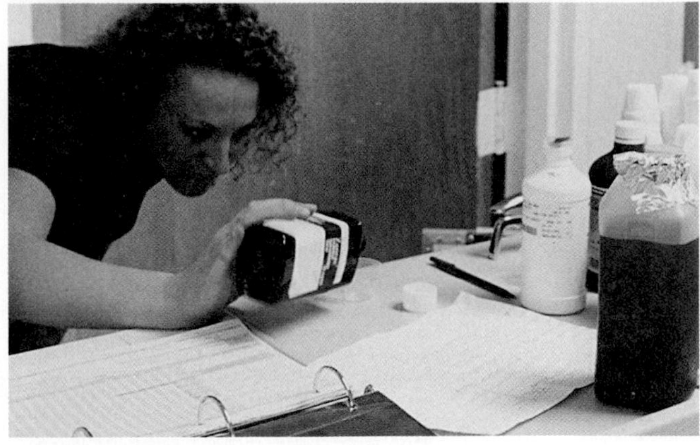

▲ Pour liquid at eye level to read dose correctly.

   b. When placing medication into medicine cup.
   c. When returning medication container to storage place.

For Crushing or Altering Medications

1. Leave pill in unit dose packaging and place on firm surface. ▸ ***Rationale:*** Labeled packaging maintains identity and prevents loss of medication. If client does not take medication, it can be returned to drawer.

   Or:
2. Place pill between two soufflé cups and pound with pestle or other tool to crush, pulverizing thoroughly ▸ ***Rationale:*** The cups confine the medication. *Note: This is the preferred method for crushing medication to be given enterally.*
3. Remove any uncrushed pill coating if medication is to be given per feeding tube. ▸ ***Rationale:*** To prevent tube clogging.
4. Check orders for partial dose medication. Place tablet in pill cutter or break tablet if scored.
5. If giving orally, mix pulverized medication (or powder from opened capsule) carefully in small amount of soft food (pudding, jelly, applesauce). ▸ ***Rationale:*** For many clients with swallowing difficulty, soft food is easier to swallow than liquid.

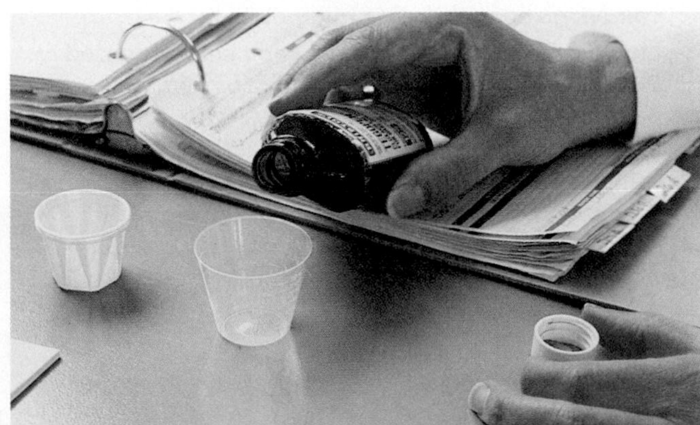

▲ Palm the label while pouring liquid medication.

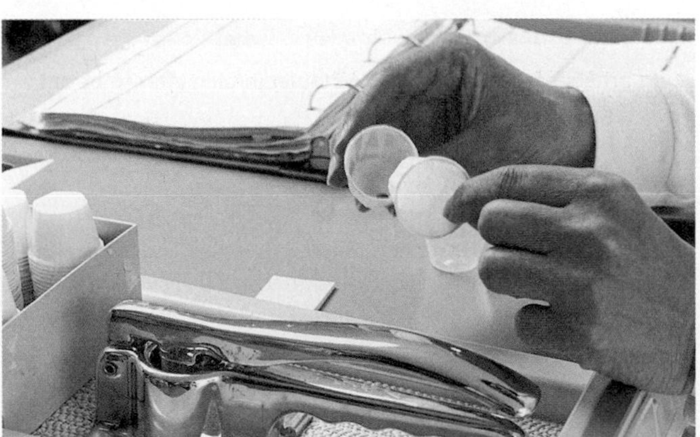

▲ Place med cups with tablet between to pulverize with crusher.

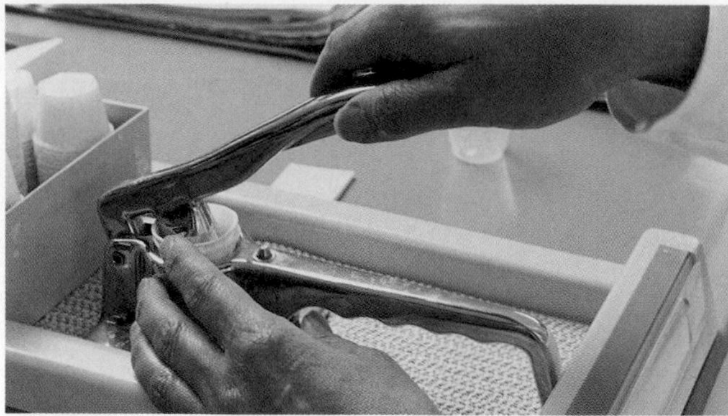

▲ Place pill in crusher to crush tablet, or pulverize/crush pill in unit dose container.

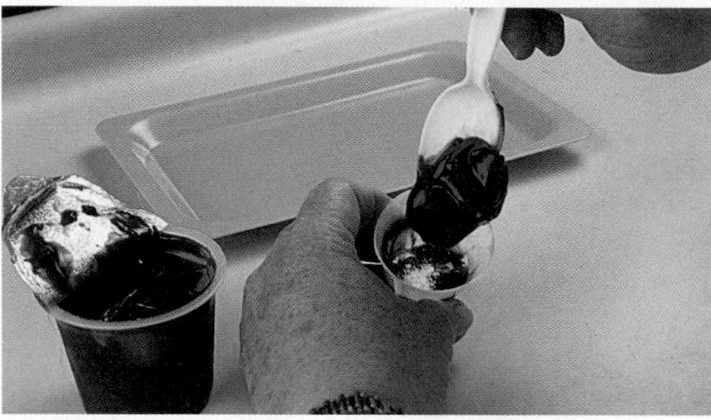

▲ Mix pulverized medication (for powder from opened capsule) carefully in *small* amount of soft food (pudding, jelly, applesauce).

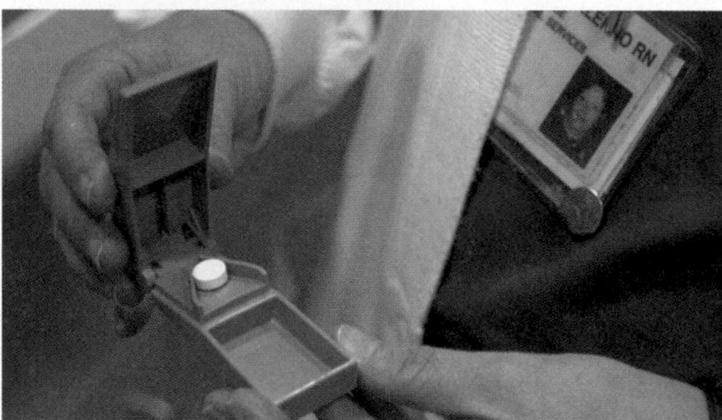

▲ If partial dose is ordered, place tablet in pill cutter to be cut in half.

6. Open capsule and sprinkle "beads" over soft food to administer. Warn client not to chew the "beads." ▶ ***Rationale:*** Beads are formulated for a sustained timed release therapeutic effect.
7. Ensure client has received all of medication.
8. Offer liquid or food to cleanse palate.

General Precautions for Altering Oral Medications

Unsafe Actions

- *Do not* crush enteric coated or gel-coated tablets. ▶ Rationale: Coatings allow intestinal absorption of the drug, protect the medication from stomach acid, or protect the stomach from the medication.
- *Do not* crush long-acting tablets. ▶ Rationale: Sustained action over hours is the advantage of extended-release versions of drugs. Crushing could yield a toxic dose and eliminate the sustained action needed through the day.
- *Do not* try to open sealed capsules.
- *Do not* crush contents of capsules (e.g., spansule) with beads or pellets. ▶ Rationale: These are intended for sustained-release action.
- *Do not* give sublingual formulations orally. ▶ Rationale: Ingredients may be inactivated by stomach acid.
- *Do not* crush sublingual formulations.
- *Do not* give oral medications sublingually. ▶ Rationale: This could yield a toxic dose since the medication would be absorbed directly into the bloodstream and skip intended first pass through the liver for early metabolism before entering the bloodstream.
- Do not alter (crush, split) tablets or open capsules of antineoplastic agents. ▶ Rationale: To avoid sending drug particles into the air where they could be inhaled.

Safe Actions

- Scored tablets may be split. Unscored tablets may be cut unless they are:
  - extended release
  - a combination product
  - a critical dose product
  - film-coated
  - crumbled with cutting

Note: Dispose of unused medication in the Medication Waste receptacle.

- Chewable medications *can be* crushed safely.
- If a capsule opens easily, powder from the capsules *can be* mixed with food or liquid.
- Liquid-filled capsule contents *can be* (a) squeezed out through a hole punched with a large gauge needle, or (b) aspirated, then mixed with food or liquid. *Liquid-filled capsule contents should not be administered sublingually.*
- Beads from readily opened capsules *can be* sprinkled over soft food to administer, *but should not be chewed.*
- A sublingual formulation still *can be* given sublingually if the client is NPO.

Administering Oral Medications to Adults

Equipment

See Equipment for Preparing Oral Medications.

Preparation

1. Follow steps for Administering Medication Protocol, Unit 1.
2. Follow procedure for Preparing Oral Medications.
3. Perform hand hygiene.

Procedure

1. Take medication tray/cart to client's room; check room and bed number against medication record.
2. Check client's Ident-A-Band and ask client to state name and birth date so you are sure you have correct client.
3. Assist client to sitting position.
4. Explain type of medication you are giving and purpose.
5. Determine if specific assessment is indicated before administering medication (e.g., vital signs) and assess client.
6. Remove medication from packet and place into medication cup.
7. Hand medication cup to client if assessment findings do not contraindicate administration.
8. Offer water or other liquid. ▶ ***Rationale:*** Aids swallowing, dilution, and absorption of medication.
9. Make sure client swallows medication.
10. Discard used medicine cup.
11. Record medication on client's record, including assessment findings, if indicated.
12. Continue to assess client for desired drug action and possible side effects or adverse reactions.

Administering Medications per Enteral (NG/NI) Feeding Tube

Equipment

See Equipment for Preparing Oral Medications.
Sterile water for diluting and flushing
50-mL irrigating piston (oral) syringe
Clean gloves

Preparation

1. Follow steps for Administering Medication Protocol in Unit 1.
2. Stop any continuous tube feeding for 15 minutes and flush tube with 15 mL of sterile water.

▲ Administer each medication separately, flushing before with 15 mL sterile water. Allow to flow through tube by gravity, then flush tube again with 15 mL sterile water.

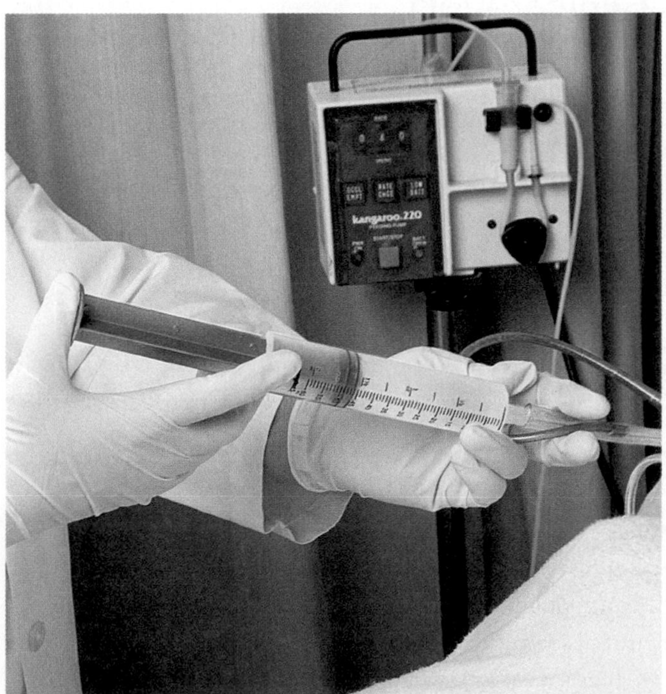

▲ Flush tube with 15 mL sterile water after each medication and record total amount on I&O sheet.

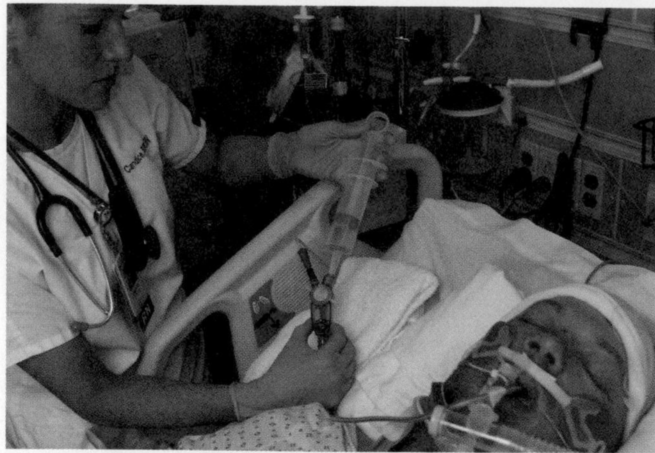

▲ For closed system, use medication/irrigation port. Administer each medication separately, flushing before and after with 15 mL sterile water or saline.

3. Follow procedure for Preparing Oral Medications.
4. Obtain liquid dosage form of medication if available.
5. Dilute each medication (crushed tablet, powder from capsule, or liquid medication) separately in 30 mL of warm sterile water (*considering client's fluid balance status*).

NOTE: Do not mix medications together. Do not add medication directly to an external feeding formula. ▸ ***Rationale:*** Reduces the risk of physical and chemical incompatibilities, tube obstruction, and altered drug responses.

6. Perform hand hygiene.

Clinical Alert

Consult with pharmacist before deciding to alter the form of *any* medication. Have pharmacist substitute liquid form of medication if available, or substitute a short-acting formulation that can be safely crushed for administration. Contact the physician for a substitute medication if formulation alternatives are unavailable.

Clinical Alert

Never use a parenteral (Luer-Lok) syringe for enteral tube administration. It may then be mistakenly administered IV. Oral syringes are incompatible with IV ports to prevent this hazard.

Procedure

1. Don gloves.
2. Disconnect NG tube from feeding delivery system or select port for decompression.
3. Insert 50-mL oral syringe into NI tube or NG tube decompression port, and aspirate to check residual volume. Return residual and flush tube with 15 mL of sterile water. ▸ ***Rationale:*** To validate enteral capacity for receiving medication.

NOTE: Do NOT administer medication through blue pigtail of Salem sump tube (See Chapter 19.)

4. Administer each medication separately, allowing to flow through tube by gravity.
5. Flush tube with 15 mL of sterile water after each medication, monitoring amount of flush to record on I&O sheet. ▸ ***Rationale:*** Flushing reduces risk of drug incompatibilities and tube clogging.
6. Restart tube feeding at appropriate time. ▸ ***Rationale:*** to avoid altering bioavailability of medication and to avoid compromising client's nutritional therapy.
7. Rinse and replace syringe to storage area at client's bedside.
8. Remove gloves and perform hand hygiene.

(**NOTE:** See also Chapter 19.)

DOCUMENTATION for Oral Medications

Client's Medication Record

- Name of medication
- Vital signs if indicated
- Dosage
- Route
- Time administered
- Initials of nurse administering medication
  - *Intake and Output record: Amount of sterile water used for medication dilution and administration.*
- Signature of nurse identifying initials

Nurses' Notes

- Client's assessment parameters
- Record PRN, STAT, and one-time-only medications
- Name of medication, dosage, route, time administered
- Client's response
- Signature of nurse

Legal Considerations

Nimodipine capsules were dispensed to the clinical area where they were used for patients who could not swallow. In one case, a nurse softened the gelatin capsule in hot water, withdrew the medication into a parenteral syringe, and the dose was inadvertently administered as IV instead of via a feeding tube. Subsequently, the patient died. A boxed warning has now been added to the nimodipine labeling to caution about this type of administration error.

Source: ISMP Medication Safety Alert, *Nurse Adviser*, April 2010.

CRITICAL THINKING Application

Expected Outcomes

- Client takes medication orally without difficulty.
- Client experiences intended therapeutic drug effect.

Unexpected Outcomes	Alternative Actions

Client has an allergic or anaphylactic response to medication.	• Immediately stop or hold medication.
	• Notify physician at once; prepare to administer epinephrine to dilate bronchi and support blood pressure.
	• If reaction is severe:
	  • Keep client flat in bed with head elevated.
	  • Take vital signs every 10–15 minutes; stay with client.
	  • Assess for hypotension or respiratory distress.
	  • Establish airway, if necessary.
	  • Have emergency equipment available.
	  • Provide psychologic support to client to alleviate fears.
	  • Record type and progression of reactions.

Client has difficulty swallowing medication.	• Offer water before administering oral medication. • Crush medications if appropriate and administer mixed with food such as applesauce, pudding, or jelly. • Consult pharmacist to dispense same medication in liquid form. • If difficulty continues, consult physician for altered route of medication delivery (rectal, parenteral). • Request swallow study.
Client is nauseated and oral medications have not been taken.	• Hold medication. Notify physician for antiemetic medication order and alternate route for administering necessary medications. • Administer antiemetic if ordered, then administer medication when client's nausea is relieved.

Chapter 18

UNIT 3

Topical Medication Administration

Nursing Process Data

ASSESSMENT Data Base

- Assess for proper route of medication administration.
- Observe skin for open lesions, rash, or redness.
- Determine drug manufacturer's recommended site for transdermal application.
- Assess that area for transdermal application is dry, hairless, intact.
- Assess for allergies as reported by client or noted in client's chart.
- Assess condition of ear or eye and surrounding area.
- Determine purpose for eye or ear irrigation.
- Assess client's ability to cooperate with eye/ear medication administration or irrigation.

PLANNING Objectives

- To provide local anesthetic, anti-inflammatory, or anti-infective effect to a specified part of the body
- To provide slow continuous transdermal absorption of medication
- To decrease intraocular pressure
- To prevent unwanted systemic effect of topically applied eye medication
- To provide pupil dilation to facilitate eye examination or therapeutic procedure
- To remove debris or neutralize chemical action and minimize eye injury
- To soften and remove cerumen (ear wax)

IMPLEMENTATION Procedures

EVALUATION Expected Outcomes

- Topical medication has intended effect.
- Client self-administers eye medication according to instructions.
- Ear canal irrigation removes cerumen.

Pearson Nursing Student Resources

Find additional review materials at **nursing.pearsonhighered.com**

Prepare for success with NCLEX®-style practice questions and Skill Checklists

Applying Topical Medications

Equipment

Medication container (tube or jar)
Soap and water to cleanse skin
Clean gloves
Tongue blade
Gauze or transparent dressing (as indicated)
Tape
Pen (to label dressing, if indicated)

Preparation

See Medication Preparation (Unit 1).

Procedure

1. Take medication container and dressing supplies to client's room.
2. Check room and bed number against client's record and check client's Ident-A-Band, asking client to state name and birth date.
3. Provide privacy.
4. Explain procedure and purpose to client.
5. Perform hand hygiene and don clean gloves.
6. Cleanse skin site with soap and water and dry thoroughly.
7. Squeeze medication from tube or use a tongue blade to take cream/ointment from medication container.
8. Spread small quantity of medication smoothly and evenly with gloved hand over client's skin following direction of hair follicles. ▸ ***Rationale:*** Gloves facilitate smooth application.
9. Apply dressing if indicated. ▸ ***Rationale:*** Dressing may ensure that medication is not rubbed off.
10. Label dressing with date, time, and your initials.
11. Remove gloves and perform hand hygiene.
12. Check that client is comfortable.
13. Return medication container to storage area.

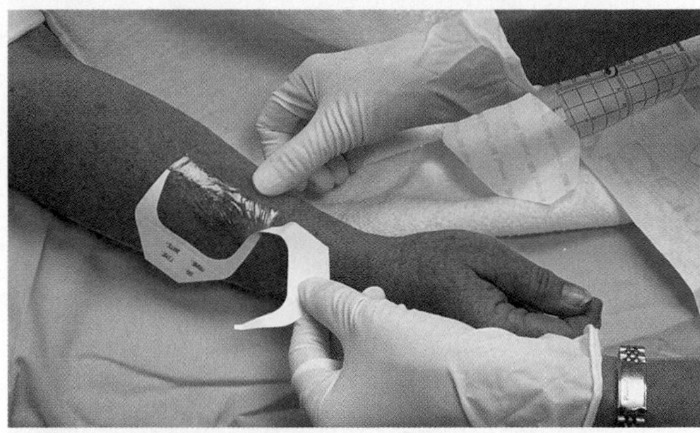

▲ Apply dressing; then label with date, time, and initials.

Clinical Alert

Systemic absorption of topical medication from open lesions can result in toxic reactions.

Applying Creams to Lesions

Equipment

Medication container (tube or jar)
Sterile normal saline for cleansing
Sterile gauze for cleansing site
Sterile tongue blade
Mask (see agency policy)
Sterile gloves
Sterile gauze or transparent dressing (or commercially prepared burn dressing)
Kerlix gauze wrap or stretch net to secure dressing
Pen for labeling dressing

Preparation

See Applying Topical Medications.

Procedure

1. Take medication to client's room; check room and bed number against medication record.
2. Check client's Ident-A-Band and ask client to state name and birth date.
3. Provide privacy.
4. Perform hand hygiene, don mask and clean gloves.
5. Remove previous dressing if present.
6. Note characteristics of site and cleanse area as ordered with sterile gauze pads and saline. Remove gloves.
7. Open medication container.
8. Don sterile gloves.
9. If no dressing is ordered, use gloved hand to apply medication directly to lesion; apply medication sparingly to 1/16-inch thickness. ▸ ***Rationale:*** To provide an occlusive effect.
10. If dressing is ordered, apply thin layer of medication to sterile gauze, then apply dressing to lesion area.
11. Secure dressing with Kerlix wrap or net if large area is involved.
12. Label dressing with date, time, and your initials.

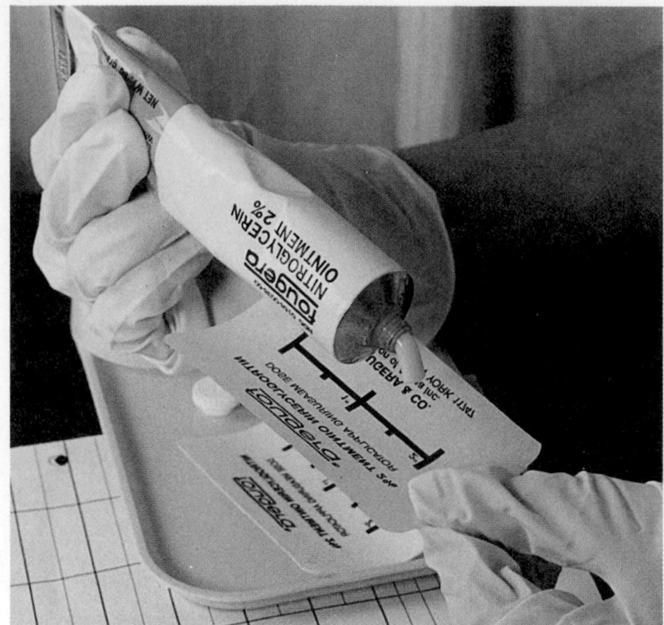

▲ Use premeasured paper to measure medication dosage.

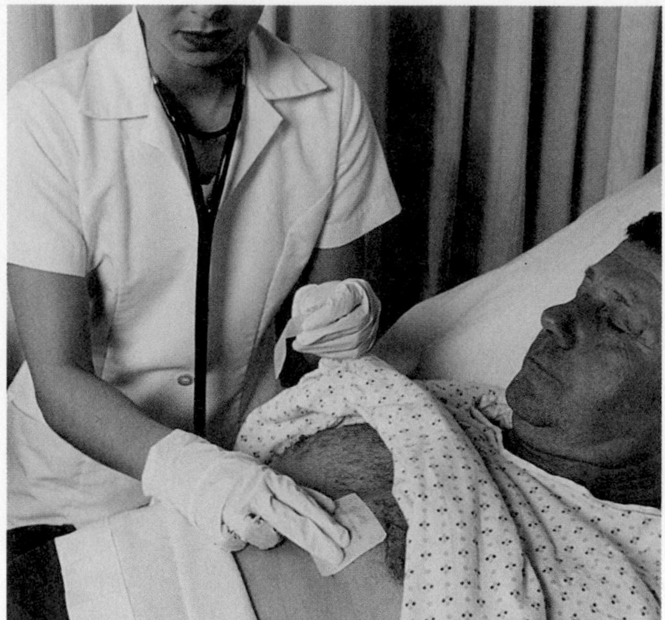

▲ Wear gloves to prevent drug absorption through fingertips.

13. Check to ensure that client is comfortable after procedure.
14. Remove gloves and perform hand hygiene.
15. Return medication container to appropriate storage area.

Applying Transdermal Medications

Equipment

Medication patch or tube
Gloves
Premeasured medication administration paper
Soap and water
Clear plastic wrap (optional)
Tape and pen for labeling dressing

Preparation

See Medication Preparation (Unit 1).

1. Obtain transdermal patch or premeasured paper that accompanies medication tube.
2. Carefully read the manufacturer's directions for application. ▶ ***Rationale:*** Directions as well as application areas of the body differ.

Procedure

1. Take medication to client's room, and check room and bed number against medication record.
2. Check Ident-A-Band, and ask client to state name.
3. Provide privacy.
4. Perform hand hygiene.

Clinical Alert

- Never cut a transdermal patch. Doing so releases the entire dose of medication to the client at once. Overdose and accidental death may occur.
- Manufacturers' directions for application of transdermal agents differ significantly. Body temperature and blood flow to different regions influence the suggested application site. Always adhere to the manufacturer's specific guidelines and precautions when administering these systems.

5. Don gloves. ▶ ***Rationale:*** Gloves prevent you from absorbing transdermal medication.
6. Alternate areas with each dose of medication to prevent skin irritation. Remove previous medicated paper/patch, fold patch in half with sticky side in, and discard in biohazard box.
7. Cleanse area before applying new dose at another site.
8. Place prescribed medication directly on paper (usually ½–1 in. strip).
9. Apply medicated paper to clean, dry, hairless, intact skin.
10. Use paper to spread medication paste over a 2-in. area. Secure paper with tape or cover medicated area with plastic wrap and tape.

Clinical Alert

The use of heating pads or hot tubs can increase the absorption rate of transdermal medications.

The nonadhesive backing of some drug patches contains metal that may not be visible. These may become heated during MRI and can cause second-degree burns. Warnings may be missing from patch labels. Patches should be removed before MRI.

Self-improvement patches purporting to deliver herbs or other substances (marketed on TV or the Internet) are not FDA regulated. Counterfeit patches also endanger clients. Refer clients to www.fda.gov/counterfeit.

11. For patch, remove protective covering and immediately apply patch to clean, dry, hairless, intact skin.
12. Press patch with palm for 30 seconds to attain a good seal.
13. Remove gloves and perform hand hygiene.

Clinical Alert

Dispose of used transdermal patch by folding sticky sides together and discarding in Medical Waste receptacle to protect others from exposure to medication. Do not flush used patches down the toilet because trace amounts of the drug may appear in treated water.

14. Label patch or paper with date, time, and your initials.
15. Return medication tube to appropriate storage area.

Instilling Ophthalmic Drops

Equipment

Eye medication in Ocumeter container
Gloves
Tissues

Preparation

1. See Medication Preparation (Unit 1).
2. Gather necessary equipment.
3. Compare the label on the medication container to the medication record. ▸ ***Rationale:*** This is a safety check to ensure that medication is for ophthalmic instillation.

Procedure

1. Take medication to client's room; check room and bed number against medication record.
2. Check Ident-A-Band, and ask client to state name and birth date.
3. Perform hand hygiene and don gloves.
4. Explain procedure and purpose of medication to client.
5. Tilt client's head slightly backward and ask client to look up. ▸ ***Rationale:*** The cornea is protected as client looks up.
6. Uncap Ocumeter, placing cap on its side.
7. Give tissue to client for wiping off excess medication.

Clinical Alert

Apply pressure to inner canthus for 2 minutes to prevent rapid drug absorption if eyedrops have potential systemic effects (e.g., bradycardia due to timolol maleate [Timoptic] drops for glaucoma).

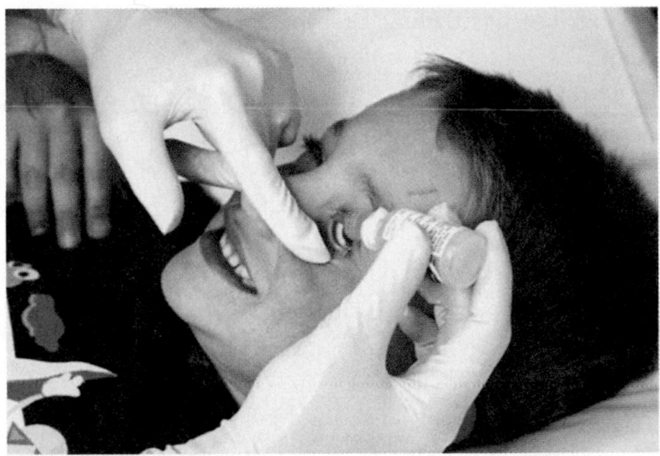

▲ Use nondominant hand to pull lower lid down. Drop eye medication in the center of lower conjunctival trough.

Clinical Alert

Occult blood developer bottles are the same size and shape as eyedrop bottles. Never leave occult blood developer in the client's room where it could be confused with the client's ophthalmic drops.

8. Place Ocumeter ½–¾ in. above eyeball with dominant hand. ▸ ***Rationale:*** This position reduces risk of dropper touching eyeball and causing injury.
9. Place nondominant hand on cheekbone and hand holding dropper on top.
10. Expose lower conjunctival trough by pulling lower lid down on cheek.
11. Drop prescribed number of drops into center of conjunctival trough. ▸ ***Rationale:*** Placing medication directly on cornea could cause injury to cornea.

12. Apply pressure to inner canthus, if indicated.
13. Ask client to close eyelids and move eyes. ▸ ***Rationale:*** This distributes solution over conjunctival surface.
14. Very gently massage closed lid for client who cannot cooperate (e.g., comatose client).
15. Remove excess medication with tissue.
16. Remove gloves and perform hand hygiene.
17. Replace medication in appropriate place.

Clinical Alert
Promoting Safe Practice

Abbreviations for eye medication administration should not be used as they may be mistaken for ear administration (OS as AS, OD as AD, and OU as AU). Always check that the medication label states ***ophthalmic*** for use in the eye (ISMP 2006: www.ISMP.org).

Administering Ophthalmic Ointment

Equipment

Eye ointment in tube
Tissues
Gloves

Preparation

See Instilling Ophthalmic Drops.

Procedure

1. Take medication to client's room, check room and bed number against medication record.
2. Check Ident-A-Band and ask client to state name and birth date.
3. Explain procedure and purpose to client.
4. Perform hand hygiene and don gloves.
5. Take protective guard off medication tube and lay on its side.
6. Expose conjunctival trough by pulling lower lid down on cheek or grasping lower lid below client's eyelashes to form a trough.
7. Instruct client to look upward. ▸ ***Rationale:*** To keep cornea out of way of medication administration area.
8. Place medication tube tip ½–¾ in. above exposed conjunctival trough.
9. Squeeze ribbon of ointment along middle third of lower lid trough.
10. Ask client to close eyelids and move eyes or gently massage closed lid to distribute medication.
11. Remove excess medication from client's eye area with tissue.
12. Caution client that ointment will cause vision to be temporarily blurred.
13. Recap and replace medication.
14. Remove gloves and perform hand hygiene.

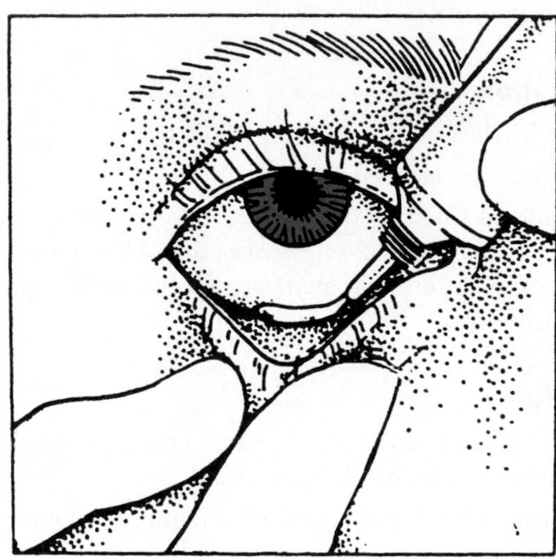

▲ Squeeze ointment along middle third of lower conjunctival trough and ask client to close eyes.

Irrigating the Eye

Equipment

500 mL bag of sterile normal (isotonic) saline *or* bottle of sterile pH-balanced commercial eye irrigating solution (e.g., Dacriose)
IV administration tubing
IV fluid pole for elevation
Nasal cannula (as for oxygen delivery)
Tape
Sterile gauze pads
Absorbent pad or towel
Clean gloves

Preparation

1. Check physician's order for irrigation.

2. Perform hand hygiene.
3. Gather equipment.
4. Warm irrigating solution to body temperature by placing container in dry heating pad.

Procedure

1. Take equipment to client's room, and check room and bed number against medication record.
2. Check client's Ident-A-Band and ask client to state name and birth date.
3. Provide privacy.
4. Explain procedure and purpose to client.
5. Place client in semi-Fowler's position, turned to side of client's affected eye.
6. Have client hold curved basin on cheek under affected eye.
7. Don gloves.
8. Using your thumb and forefinger, open client's eye to expose lower conjunctival trough by pulling the lower lid down toward cheek.
9. Place eye irrigation bottle spout tip ¾ in. above client's inner canthus, pointing downward toward the outer canthus.
10. Squeeze bottle, allowing irrigating solution to flow into client's conjunctival trough to remove debris.
11. Continue irrigating for 10 minutes or until eye is cleansed completely.
12. Note results of debris returned with irrigation.
13. Wipe client's eyelid with gauze, wiping from inner to outer canthus.
14. Dispose of equipment in appropriate area.
15. Remove gloves and perform hand hygiene.
16. Assist client to comfortable position.
17. Document irrigation and results.

For Bilateral Irrigation

1. Spike saline bag with IV tubing and hang bag on pole.
2. Affix end of IV tubing to nasal cannula, then fit cannula around client's head (or around ears as for oxygen administration) securing prongs at bridge of client's nose with tape.
3. Start flow of saline solution from IV bag and allow to flush client's eyes to neutralize a chemical exposure.
4. Increase flow rate, then continue wide open irrigation until 500 mL has been used over a 10-minute period.
5. Follow steps 12–17 above.

Administering Otic Medications

Equipment

Ear wick, if ordered
Prescribed ear medication
Dropper for instilling medication
Gloves (optional)

Preparation

1. See Medication Preparation (Unit 1).
2. Gather necessary equipment.
3. Remove the medication from the medication cart.
4. Compare the label on the medication bottle to the medication record. ▶ ***Rationale:*** Safety check.
5. Before preparing medication for administration, warm medication bottle to body temperature. ▶ ***Rationale:*** Instillation of cold medication can cause vertigo.

Procedure

1. Take medication to client's room, and check room number against medication card or sheet.
2. Check Ident-A-Band, and ask client to state name and birth date.
3. Explain procedure and purpose to client.
4. Perform hand hygiene.
5. Don gloves.
6. Position client on side, with ear to be treated in the uppermost position. ▶ ***Rationale:*** This position allows medication to enter external ear canal by gravity.
7. Fill medication dropper with prescribed amount of medication.
8. Prepare client for instillation of ear medication as follows:
   a. *Infant.* Draw the pinna gently downward and backward. ▶ ***Rationale:*** This separates the drum membrane from the floor of the cartilaginous canal.

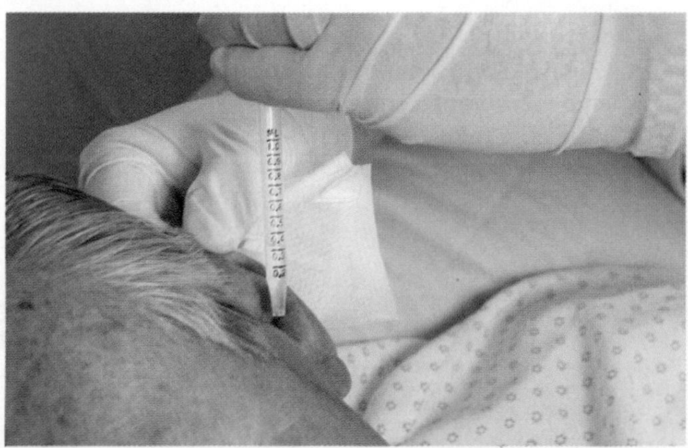

▲ Lift pinna upward and backward to instill eardrops in an adult.

b. *Adult.* Lift pinna upward and backward. ▸ ***Rationale:*** This position straightens the ear canal.

9. Insert ear wick if ordered. ▸ ***Rationale:*** Medication is absorbed into the ear wick. Ear wick enhances medication delivery directly to the entire ear canal.
10. Instill medication drops, holding dropper slightly above ear. ▸ ***Rationale:*** This position protects dropper from contamination.
11. Instruct client to remain on side for 5–10 minutes after instillation. ▸ ***Rationale:*** Prevents medication from escaping and facilitates distribution.
12. Dispose of gloves and perform hand hygiene.

NOTE: The ear wick normally extrudes spontaneously in 12–36 hr (after edema subsides).

Irrigating the Ear Canal

Equipment

Asepto or irrigating syringe
Prescribed irrigating solution or tap water
2 basins: round basin, curved basin
Absorbent pad or towel
Cotton ball

Preparation

(Client may have instilled wax-softening eardrops several hours before irrigation.)

1. See Medication Preparation (Unit 1).
2. Perform hand hygiene.
3. Gather equipment.
4. Warm irrigating solution to body temperature. ▸ ***Rationale:*** Cold solution can precipitate nausea and vertigo.

Procedure

1. Take equipment to client's room, and check room and bed number against medication record.
2. Check client's Ident-A-Band and ask client to state name and birth date.
3. Provide privacy.
4. Explain procedure and purpose to client.
5. Don clean gloves.

Clinical Alert

Ear canal irrigation should be performed only when the tympanic membrane can be visualized because of the risk that debris may cover an unseen perforation.

6. Place client in Fowler's position and place absorbent towel over client's chest and shoulders.
7. Pour irrigating solution into round basin.
8. Place curved basin under ear to catch irrigating solution.
9. Fill syringe with irrigating solution.
10. Open and straighten client's ear canal by pulling the pinna up and backward for adult or down for an infant or child. ▸ ***Rationale:*** This action allows the solution to flow into ear canal.
11. Hold irrigating syringe at entrance to ear canal without occluding meatus. ▸ ***Rationale:*** Entering ear canal can cause impaction.
12. Push plunger, directing flow of solution toward the top of the canal. ▸ ***Rationale:*** This action allows the flow to reach the entire length of canal.
13. Note return flow throughout procedure.
14. After solution has ceased to flow, dry outside of ear.
15. Return client to comfortable position and place cotton ball in ear canal to absorb excess fluid. ▸ ***Rationale:*** This reduces risk of external otitis.
16. Return used equipment to appropriate area.
17. Remove gloves and perform hand hygiene.
18. Document irrigation and results.

Clinical Alert

Ensure that client's tympanic membrane is intact before irrigating the ear. Water should not be used to irrigate the ear to remove an organic foreign body (e.g., insect or bean) since water may cause the object to swell.

DOCUMENTATION for Topical Medications

Client's Medication Record

- Time administered
- Name of medication
- Dosage
- Route and site of application
- Initials of nurse administering medication
- Signature by nurse which identifies initials

Nurses' Notes

- Record PRN, STAT, and one-time-only medications
- Time administered, name of medication, dosage, route, site
- Client's response to application
- Condition of area treated
- Signature of nurse

CRITICAL THINKING Application

Expected Outcomes

- Topical medication has intended effect.
- Client self-administers eye medication according to instructions.
- Ear canal irrigation removes cerumen.

Unexpected Outcomes	Alternative Actions
Client develops adverse reaction to topical medication (e.g., itching, inflammation).	• Rotate sites of medication system application. • Consult physician or pharmacist for alternative route of medication administration (e.g., oral).
Obese client fails to obtain pain relief from topical analgesic patch.	• Consult pain management team. • Consider weight-based dosage. • Change route of analgesic administration since adipose tissue has decreased perfusion and topical medication uptake is unpredictable.
Client is reluctant to use eye medication ointment because it causes "blurred vision."	• Suggest client apply eye ointment at bedtime. • Assist client to create safe means for urination at night (e.g., night lighting, safety rails, bedside commode, urinal).
Client complains of nausea and vertigo after ear irrigation.	• Warm irrigating solution to body temperature. • Consult physician to order wax-softening eardrops to instill before irrigation to facilitate removal of cerumen and shorten process.

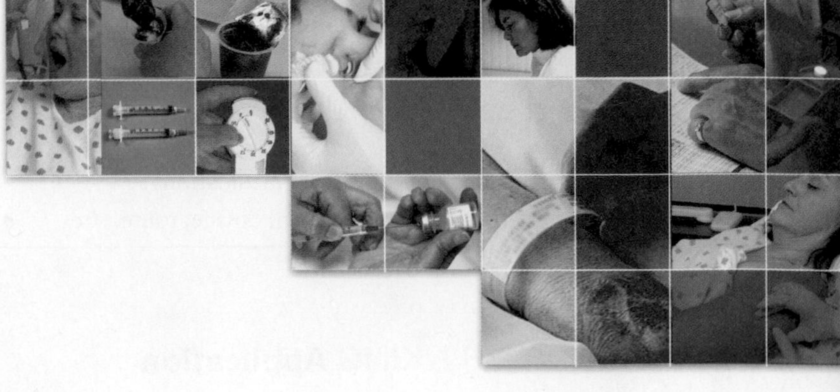

Chapter 18

UNIT 4

Mucous Membrane Medication Administration

Nursing Process Data

ASSESSMENT Data Base

- Assess that drug can be administered sublingually.
- Assess client's ability to understand and follow directions.
- Assess vital signs, SpO_2, relevant to medication action.
- Assess for dyspnea, labored breathing, wheezing.
- Determine possible undesired systemic effects of inhaled agents (tremor, nausea, tachycardia).
- Review physician's orders for medication and diluent to be administered, and frequency of treatments.
- Observe amount and character of expectorated sputum.
- Determine need for other respiratory techniques.
- Assess client's breath sounds before and after each treatment.
- Assess client's bowel elimination pattern.

PLANNING Objectives

- To provide appropriate surface for rapid absorption of medication for systemic effect
- To confine drug action to a local area
- To facilitate ease and consistency of self-administration of medication
- To decrease client's work of breathing
- To provide alternate route of medication administration when client is NPO/nauseated
- To promote bowel elimination
- To combat infection
- To deliver aerosolized medications
- To temporarily decrease the work of breathing
- To promote better ventilation
- To loosen secretions

IMPLEMENTATION Procedures

EVALUATION Expected Outcomes

- Chest pain is relieved due to rapid systemic response to sublingual medication administration.
- Desired local effect of medication is achieved without undesired side effects.
- Suppository has desired effects/results.

Administering Sublingual Medications

Equipment

Sublingual medication (e.g., nitroglycerin tablets in a dark bottle). *Tablets lose potency when exposed to light; opened bottle should be replaced in 3 months.*

or

Nitrolingual aerosol spray in canister

Preparation

1. See Medication Preparation (Unit 1).
2. Assess vital signs if administering sublingual nitroglycerin. (*Systolic BP should not be lower than 90 mmHg.*)
3. Place client in a sitting position.

Procedure

1. Follow steps for preparing and administering oral medications, *except*:
   a. Explain that client must not swallow drug or eat, smoke, or drink until medication is completely absorbed.
   b. Ask client to place tablet under the tongue or to hold tongue up so tablet can be placed under tongue. ▶ ***Rationale:*** Absorption is rapid and complete due to the vast network of capillaries in this area.
   c. Alternate: hold Nitrolingual canister vertically with spray opening as close to mouth as possible. Deliver 1 or 2 metered sprays onto or under tongue, then have client close mouth immediately. Tell client not to inhale medication.

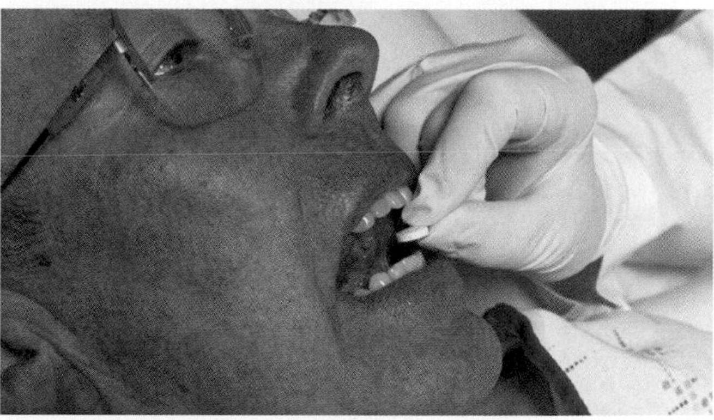

▲ Sublingual medication is placed under client's tongue for rapid absorption.

2. Evaluate client for drug action and possible side effects (e.g., headache).

Clinical Alert

Assess client's chest discomfort: quality, location, radiation, intensity, duration and precipitating factors. When administering rapid-acting (sublingual) nitroglycerin, monitor client's response and vital signs. If chest discomfort is not relieved in 5 minutes, notify physician. Obtain order for opiate analgesic (morphine sulfate), EKG, ST-segment monitoring, and cardiac biomarkers. No more than 3 doses of nitroglycerin should be administered in a 15-minute period because of potential hypotensive effect (BP ≤90 mmHg) or bradycardia (HR ≤50) as this would preclude adequate dosage of morphine sulfate for pain control.

EVIDENCE-BASED PRACTICE

ACC/AHA Guidelines—Nitroglycerin

It is recommended by the American College of Cardiology and the American Heart Association that clients who have been previously prescribed nitroglycerin be advised to take ONE dose sublingually promptly for chest discomfort/pain. If symptoms *do not* improve, or worsen in 5 minutes after ONE nitroglycerin dose, the client should call 9-1-1 immediately to access EMS. For clients with chronic stable angina, if symptoms are significantly improved after ONE nitroglycerin dose, repeat nitroglycerin dose every 5 minutes for a total of 3 doses and call 9-1-1 if symptoms have not totally resolved.

Source: Antman, E.M., Anbe, D. T., Armstrong, P. W., Bates, E. R., Green, L. A., Hand, M., ... Ornato, J. P. (2004). ACC/AHA guidelines for the management of patients with ST-elevation myocardial infarction: A report of the American College of Cardiology/American Heart Association Task Force on Practice Guidelines. *Journal of American College of Cardiology, 44*(3): E1–E211 (http:// www.acc.org/clinical/guidelines).

Instilling Nose Drops

Equipment

Medication bottle

Dropper

Tissues

Preparation

1. See Medication Preparation (Unit 1).
2. Perform hand hygiene.

Procedure

1. Take equipment to client's room; check room and bed number against medication record.
2. Check client Ident-A-Band and have client state name and birth date.
3. Place client in sitting position with head tilted back or in supine position with head tilted back over pillow.
4. Fill dropper with prescribed amount of medication.

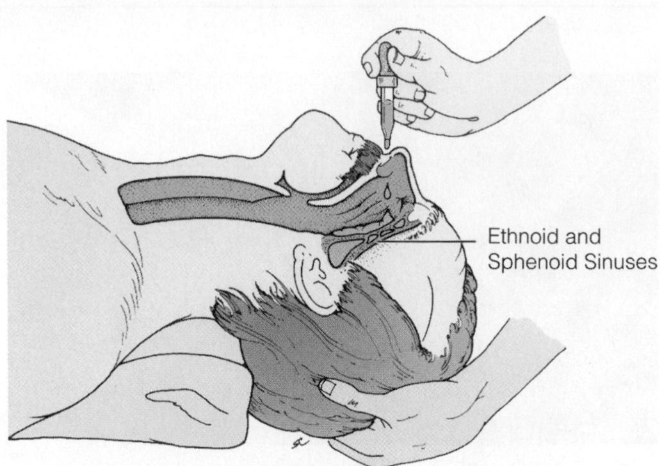

▲ Instruct client to tilt head backwards and place dropper inside nares when instilling nose drops.

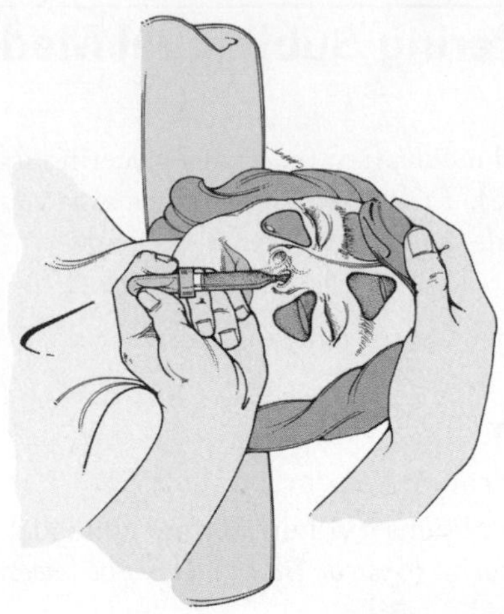

▲ Tilt client's head back for nose drops to reach maxillary and frontal sinuses.

5. Place dropper just inside the naris and instill correct medication dosage. Repeat procedure in other naris.
6. Wipe away any excess medication with tissue.
7. Instruct client not to sneeze or blow nose and to keep head tilted back for 5 minutes to prevent medication from escaping.
8. Check to see that client is comfortable before leaving room.
9. Perform hand hygiene.
10. Return medication to appropriate storage area.

Administering Metered-Dose Inhaled (MDI) Medications

Equipment

Prescribed medication canister
Metered-dose inhaler (MDI) dispenser (actuator or holder)
Spacer or holding chamber (if ordered)
Tissues

Clinical Alert

Check inhaler medication label for number of actuations (propellant-driven medication doses, e.g., 200). Have client maintain a record of actuations and discard after the number indicated. Final puffs may be nothing but propellant, which would not dilate airways in an emergency situation.

EVIDENCE-BASED PRACTICE

MDI Canister Actuations—Client Monitoring

A study evaluated how clients determined that their MDI canisters were empty. Of the clients studied, 74% did not know how many actuations were in their canisters and used their MDIs until they could no longer "hear" the medication when actuating. Additionally, while 78% knew to shake the canister before actuating, only half did so. The conclusion was that clients are likely to use the medication for up to twice the intended duration, using canisters with no active ingredients more than 50% of the time. The authors concluded that dose counters appear to be the only practical solution.

Source: Rubin B., & Durotoye, L. (2004). How do patients determine that their metered-dose inhaler is empty? *Chest*, *126*, 1134–1137.

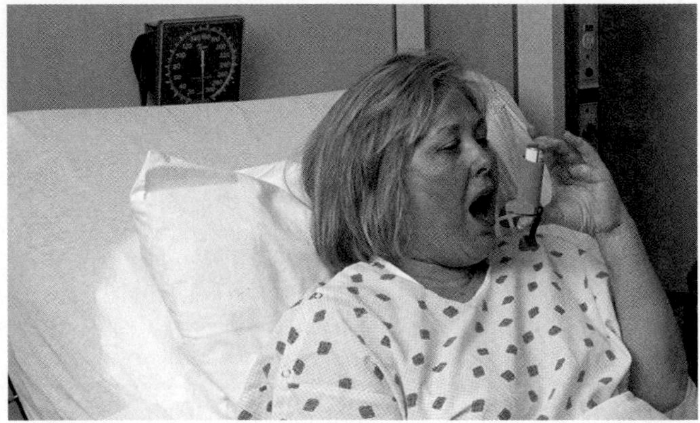

▲ Depress inhalation device while inhaling slowly (3–5 seconds) and deeply through mouth.

Preparation

1. See Medication Preparation (Unit 1).
2. Perform hand hygiene.
3. Gather equipment.
4. Compare label of drug canister to client's medication record.

Procedure

1. Take medication canister and MDI dispenser to client's room.

Client Teaching

- Canister must be shaken before each puff so that propellant and medication are adequately combined. Priming sprays are performed only with a new canister (canister volume allows for this).
- Prime new MDI by spraying into the air four times. Prime inhaler that has not been used for 4 weeks by spraying once into the air.
- Tell client to keep track of number of puffs (actuations) used in order to plan for refill of prescription.

2. Check client's Ident-A-Band and have client state name and birth date.
3. Provide privacy.
4. Explain procedure and purpose to client.
5. Assist client to standing or sitting position.
6. Insert canister (stem down) into longer part of metered-dose dispenser. (For new canister, test spray [prime] MDI into air one or two times. ▶ ***Rationale:*** This is done *only* with new canister to ensure patency of unit.)
7. Shake MDI with canister to mix medication and propellant. (*Shake canister before each MDI puff*). ▶ ***Rationale:*** Without shaking propellant, little or no medication will be delivered.

NOTE: Canisters typically contain propellants and other inert ingredients in addition to the actual drug; a client may believe a canister contains medication when none is actually present.

8. Instruct client to remove mouthpiece and hold inhaler 2 in. away from mouth (following manufacturer's instructions). Mist is to be *inhaled* into airways. **Alternately,** place mouthpiece in mouth, holding canister upright.
9. Instruct client to exhale through pursed lips. ▶ ***Rationale:*** Exhaling through pursed lips increases exhaled volume, allowing room for a greater *inspiratory* volume.
10. Instruct client to depress inhalation device, releasing a puff of medication while inhaling slowly and deeply (3–5 seconds). ▶ ***Rationale:*** With slow deep inhalation, medication goes to lower respiratory tract.
11. Tell client to hold breath for 10 seconds, then remove unit and slowly exhale through pursed lips. ▶ ***Rationale:*** Holding the breath allows time for the medication to be absorbed.
12. Assess client's breathing and reaction to medication. ▶ ***Rationale:*** With certain drugs, heart rate may increase.
13. Provide tissues. ▶ ***Rationale:*** Inhaled medication may stimulate coughing.
14. Instruct client to wait 1 or 2 minutes between inhalations and to *shake canister* before each puff. ▶ ***Rationale:*** Waiting between doses helps prevent paroxysmal bronchospasm.
15. Have client replace mouthpiece cap.
16. Caution client not to increase dose without physician's order. ▶ ***Rationale:*** Potential side effects of an increased dose could be serious.
17. Have client rinse mouth after using MDI that contains steroids.
18. Teach client to remove canister and to clean mouthpiece *daily*, washing with soap and water and allowing to air dry. ▶ ***Rationale:*** These devices are sites for microbial growth.
19. Instruct client to rinse mouth after use and to not swallow the water.
20. Review medication side effects with client. ▶ ***Rationale:*** Client continues home therapy and should be aware of self-monitoring needs.
21. Perform hand hygiene.
22. Document procedure and results.

Inhaled Medications

- Inhaled medications provide relief for bronchospasm, wheezing, asthma, or allergic reactions.
- Medications include bronchodilators, steroids, and antimediators.
- Common systemic side effects include tremors, nausea, tachycardia, palpitations, nervousness, and dysrhythmias.

Using MDI With Spacer

Equipment

See Administering Metered-Dose Inhaled (MDI) Medications.

Preparation

1. See Administering Metered-Dose Inhaled (MDI) Medications.
2. Perform hand hygiene.

Procedure

1. Assemble medication canister in MDI.
2. Insert MDI mouthpiece into spacer. ▸ ***Rationale:*** Research indicates an MDI inhaler fitted into a spacer improves airway delivery of medication because large drops do not fall into the mouth.
3. Remove mouthpiece cover from spacer.
4. Hold upright and shake MDI with spacer to mix medication and propellant.
5. Instruct client to exhale slowly through pursed lips.
6. Instruct client to close lips around spacer mouthpiece. ▸ ***Rationale:*** Spacer eliminates need for simultaneous hand action and mouth inspiration coordination.
7. Activate MDI canister, pressing down with fingers, pushing it farther into plastic adapter. ▸ ***Rationale:*** This releases metered dose of medication into spacer.
8. After activation, instruct client to inhale slowly and deeply through mouth and hold breath for 10 seconds.
9. Instruct client to exhale and relax.
10. Provide water mouth rinse after inhaled corticosteroids. ▸ ***Rationale:*** To prevent oral candidiasis.
11. Remove drug canister and clean mouthpiece and spacer daily, washing with soap and water.

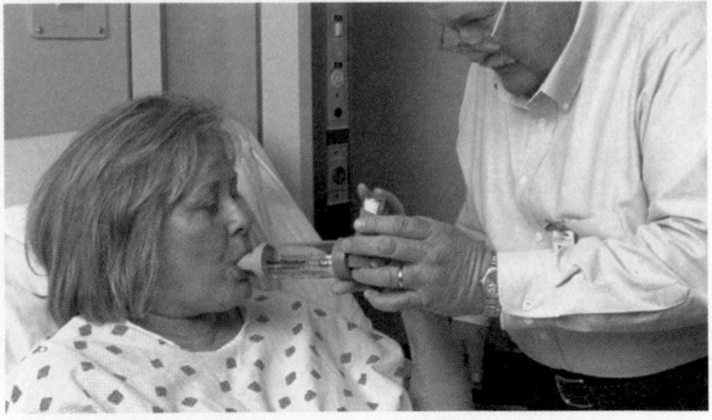

▲ Hold canister upright when using MDI with spacer.

EVIDENCE-BASED PRACTICE

Why Use a Spacer With MDI?

Only 10%–15% of inhaled (MDI) medications reach the small airways, but use of a spacer can increase this by about 12%.

Source: Togger, D., & Brenner, P. (2001). Metered dose inhalers. *American Journal of Nursing, 101*(10), 29.

Clinical Alert

If several types of medications are used, follow this sequence: Quick-acting bronchodilator (e.g., albuterol sulfate); slower-acting bronchodilator (e.g., ipratropium bromide [Atro-vent]); antimediators (e.g., steroids).

Administering Dry Powder Inhaled (DPI) Medication

Equipment

Dry powder capsule intended for oral inhalation
Medication package insert (instructions)
Handheld inhalation device intended for medication to be given

Preparation

1. See Administering Metered-Dose Inhaled (MDI) Medications.
2. Review medication package insert instructions.
3. Perform hand hygiene.

Procedure

1. Take dry powder capsule package and inhalation device to client's room.
2. Check client's Ident-A-Band and have client state name and birth date.
3. Provide privacy.
4. Explain procedure and purpose to client.
5. Assist client to a sitting position.
6. Remove capsule from package, peeling back foil cover to expose only one capsule. ▸ ***Rationale:*** Capsules should be used immediately; unused capsules exposed to air may lose effectiveness.
7. Open the outer cap of inhaler device (pull cap upward).
8. Open the mouthpiece.
9. Insert the capsule into center of chamber of the inhalation device.

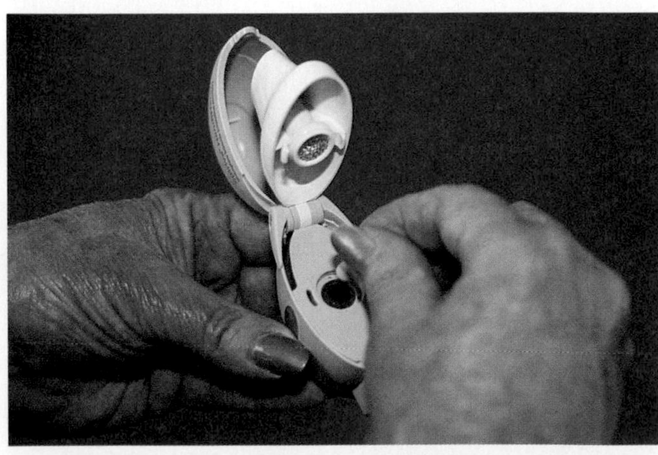

▲ Insert capsule into center of chamber of the inhalation device.

10. Hold the device upright, and, leaving the outer cap open, close mouthpiece/lid firmly until a click is heard and leave the outer cap open.
11. Press the side mounted piercing button in completely, then release. ▶ ***Rationale:*** The piercing button punctures the capsule, allowing medication to be released upon inhalation.
12. Have the client breathe out completely.
13. Have the client keep his/her head in upright position and place lips tightly round the mouthpiece.
14. Have client breathe slowly and deeply with sufficient energy to hear the medication capsule vibrate. ▶ ***Rationale:*** As long as the capsule rattles, the client's inhalation is fast enough.

NOTE: Some DPIs require a fast initial inhalation to activate the medication distribution.

15. Have the client hold the deep breath as long as comfortable, then return to normal breathing.
16. Have client repeat Steps 12 through 15 if indicated in medication package insert. ▶ ***Rationale:*** Repeating the steps may be necessary to get the full dose of medication.
17. Open mouthpiece and discard remaining capsule.
18. Close mouthpiece and outer cap and store at client's bedside.
19. Clean unit only as necessary, using warm water and allowing device to air dry *thoroughly* before next use. ▶ ***Rationale:*** No cleaning agents should be used and the device should not be wet when used.

Administering Medication by Nonpressurized (Nebulized) Aerosol (NPA)

Equipment

Nebulizer medication chamber
T-piece, mouthpiece or mask
Corrugated tubing
Air flow tubing
Prescribed medication (e.g., bronchodilator)
Prescribed diluent (normal saline)
Wall source (or other source) for compressed air, or oxygen with flowmeter

Preparation

1. See Medication Preparation (Unit 1).
2. Perform hand hygiene.
3. Dilute medication as ordered and place in nebulizer chamber.
4. Attach one end of tubing to compressed air source.
5. Attach other end of tubing to nozzle at side or bottom of nebulizer.
6. Keep nebulizer chamber vertical, and connect top of chamber to mask or T-piece sidearm.
7. Hold mouthpiece in its protective cover, and attach to one end of T-piece.
8. Attach corrugated tubing to other end of T-piece.

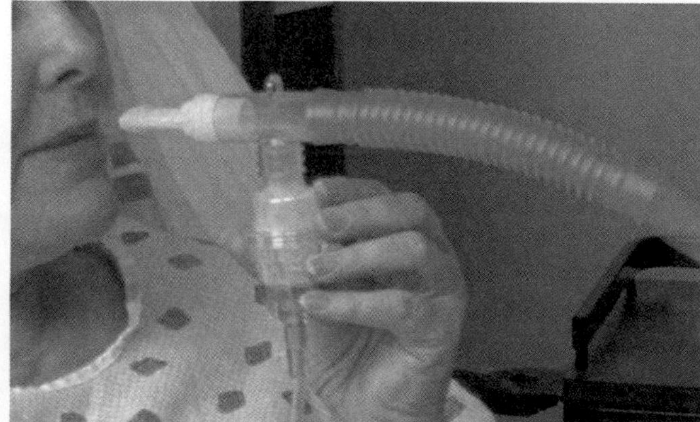

▲ Nonpressurized aerosol (NPA) treatment in progress.

Procedure

1. Turn on air or oxygen (8 L/min) source, and observe for mist flow.
   a. If the client is receiving 3 L/min or less of oxygen therapy, deliver aerosolized medications with compressed air (yellow wall outlet).
   b. If the client is receiving 4 L/min or more of oxygen therapy, deliver the aerosol medication with the oxygen flowmeter (green wall outlet) set at 8 L/min.
2. Have client place mouthpiece in mouth and close lips.

Clinical Alert

The plastic containers with respiratory medications for nebulizers are similar to the plastic containers for single-dose eyedrops. Both products have the drug name molded into the plastic, but it is difficult to see.

3. Instruct client to breathe normally in and out of mouthpiece or mask.
4. Have client take a deep breath and hold for several seconds, then exhale slowly every 3–5 breaths. (Treatment is complete when all medication is used and no mist is seen.)
5. Turn power (air or O_2 flow) off, and unplug compressor (if used), or reset prescribed O_2 flow rate.
6. Clean mouthpiece, and place equipment in plastic bag at bedside. (Dispose of and replace components according to agency policy.)

Administering Rectal Suppositories

Equipment

Suppository as ordered from refrigerator
Clean gloves
Water-soluble lubricant
Paper towel

Preparation

1. See Medication Preparation (Unit 1).
2. Compare the medication record with the most recent physician's order.
3. Perform hand hygiene.
4. Gather necessary equipment.
5. Retrieve medication from refrigerator if indicated.
6. Compare the medication label with client's MAR.
7. Place suppository, lubricant, and paper towel on a tray if not using medication cart.

Procedure

1. Take equipment to client's room.
2. Check room number against client's MAR.
3. Check client's Ident-A-Band and have client state name and birth date.
4. Explain procedure and purpose to client.
5. Provide privacy.
6. Place client in dorsal-recumbent or side-lying position.
7. Squeeze dollop of lubricant onto paper towel.
8. Remove foil wrapper from the suppository.
9. Moisten suppository tip with warm water or lubricant to facilitate insertion.

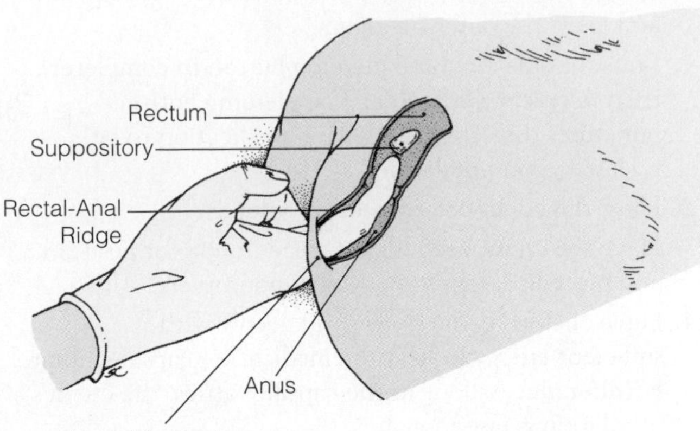

▲ Insert rectal suppository beyond the anal–rectal ridge to ensure it is retained.

10. Don clean gloves and inspect anal area for hemorrhoids.
11. Instruct client to bear down to identify anal opening and insert the suppository about 1½ in. into the rectal canal beyond the anal sphincter. ▶ ***Rationale:*** Prevents suppository from slipping out.
12. Instruct client to lie quietly for 15 minutes while medicine is absorbed and that suppository may take up to 1 hour to be effective.
13. Dispose of equipment and gloves and perform hand hygiene.
14. Return after 15 minutes to ensure client is comfortable.
15. Chart medication and results obtained.

Administering Vaginal Suppositories

Equipment

Prescribed vaginal suppository
Client's applicator (should be kept in client's room)
Clean gloves

Preparation

1. See Medication Preparation (Unit 1).
2. Compare the medication record with the most recent physician's order.
3. Perform hand hygiene.
4. Gather necessary equipment.
5. Remove the medication from medication cart.
6. Compare the medication label to the client's MAR.

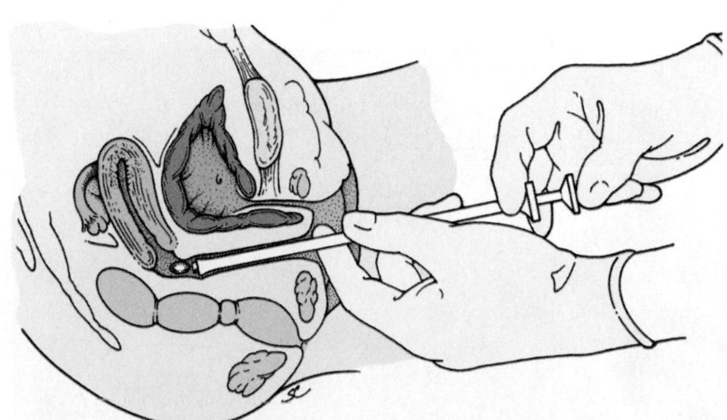

▲ Insert vaginal suppository at least 2 inches into vaginal canal using applicator as shown.

Procedure

1. Take equipment to client's room, and check room number against client's MAR.
2. Check client's Ident-A-Band and ask client to state name and birth date.
3. Provide privacy.
4. Explain procedure and purpose to client.
5. Don gloves.
6. Place client in dorsal recumbent or side-lying position.
7. Remove foil wrapper from suppository. Insert into applicator.
8. Don clean gloves.
9. Insert applicator with suppository into the vaginal canal at least 2 in. ▶ ***Rationale:*** Prevents suppository from slipping out.
10. Instruct client to lie quietly for 15 minutes until the suppository is absorbed.
11. Discard equipment, wash applicator, and return to appropriate place in client's room.
12. Remove gloves and perform hand hygiene.
13. Chart medication and assessment findings (e.g., discharge, odor).

DOCUMENTATION for Mucous Membrane Medications

Client's Medication Record

- Time
- Medication administered
- Route of administration
- Initials of nurse administering medication
- Signature of nurse identifying initials

Nurses' Notes

- Time
- Name of medication, dosage, route pre- and post-administration assessment findings (chest discomfort, vital signs, SpO_2, breath sounds)
- Physician notification, if done
- Results of suppository action

CRITICAL THINKING Application

Expected Outcomes

- Angina is relieved with ONE dose of sublingual nitroglycerin.
- Chest pain is relieved due to rapid systemic response to sublingual medication administration.
- Desired local effect of medication is achieved without undesired side effects.
- Suppository has desired effects/results.

Unexpected Outcomes	Alternative Actions
Client's chest discomfort is not relieved with ONE dose of sublingual nitroglycerin.	• Provide anticipatory instructions. • Check bottle for expiration date—potency is lost 3 months after opening bottle. • Recognize associated symptoms of acute MI such as dyspnea, nausea, cold sweat, lightheadedness. (www.nhlbi.nih.gov/actintime). • Don't take a "wait and see" approach or deny symptoms indicative of acute MI.
Client's discomfort is not relieved with sublingual nitroglycerin.	• Check bottle for expiration date—potency is lost 3 months after opening bottle. • Administer second tablet in 5 minutes—if discomfort continues, administer opiate analgesic, call Rapid Response Team, notify physician, and obtain stat ECG. • Administer no more than three tablets/sprays in a 15-minute period. • Monitor for blood pressure effect—hold medication if systolic BP is less than 90 mmHg. • Consult with physician for blood test for possible myocardial injury and need for continuous cardiac monitoring.

Client states that breathing has not improved after using inhaler.	• Place client in Fowler's position. Validate that MDI/spacer/NPA device is functioning properly (e.g., canister shaken before use). • Check number of actuations left in MDI canister. • Validate that client's lips have tight fit around MDI mouthpiece so mist is inhaled. • Instruct client to hold breath 10 seconds after MDI use and to wait 2 minutes between puffs.
Client using MDI reports painful white patches in mouth.	• Instruct client to use spacer with MDI steroid medication. • Instruct client to rinse mouth with water and expectorate after administering MDI steroid. • Notify physician of findings.
Client fails to have BM post-laxative suppository administration.	• Reassess abdomen and check client for rectal fecal impaction. • Consult with physician to order oil-retention enema or cleansing enema. • Teach client ways to prevent constipation.
Client is unable to retain vaginal suppository.	• Administer vaginal suppository at bedtime to prevent medication leakage.

Chapter 18

UNIT 5

Parenteral Medication Administration

Nursing Process Data

ASSESSMENT Data Base

- Check that appropriate method for administration of drug was ordered.
- Assess condition of administration site for presence of lesions, rash, inflammation, lipid dystrophy, ecchymosis.
- Assess client's understanding of medication action.
- Check client's written history and ask for oral history for past allergic reactions. (Do not rely solely on client's chart.)
- Review client's chart noting previous injection sites.

PLANNING Objectives

- To ensure proper route of drug administration
- To protect self from harm when administering parenteral injections
- To administer medication parenterally according to the "Six Rights"
- To reduce discomfort with medication injection
- To alternate injection sites for consistent absorption of medication
- To observe and report side effects/adverse reactions of drug administration

IMPLEMENTATION Procedures

EVALUATION Expected Outcomes

- Injection is administered without complications.
- Injection is as painless as possible.
- Medication therapeutic effect is achieved.

Pearson Nursing Student Resources

Find additional review materials at **nursing.pearsonhighered.com**

Prepare for success with NCLEX®-style practice questions and Skill Checklists

Preparing Injections

Equipment

Medication in vial or ampule
Vial of compatible diluent (if necessary)
Syringe of closest capacity to hold medication.
Filter needle for withdrawing medication from ampule or rubber-topped vial
Appropriate-size needle for injection
Antimicrobial wipe
Dry gauze sponge
Label for prepared injection

Preparation

See Medication Preparation (Unit 1).

Procedure

1. Perform hand hygiene.
2. Obtain equipment.
3. Assemble the syringe and filter needle, maintaining sterility.
4. Fill syringe with medication
5. Attach appropriate-size needle for injection, considering route, desired site, client's size, and viscosity of medication. ▶ ***Rationale:*** The larger the gauge number, the *smaller* the needle lumen. Larger gauges produce less tissue trauma and are used for aqueous solutions. Smaller gauges are required for viscous solutions such as hormones.
6. Unless administering immediately, apply identifying label to prepared syringe. ▶ ***Rationale:*** Lack of labeling has been cited as a major risk for medication administration errors.

Clinical Alert

Federal needlestick safety legislation **requires** healthcare facilities to implement devices that protect against accidental needlesticks.

EVIDENCE-BASED PRACTICE

Needlestick Injuries

Six percent of needlestick injuries involve safety devices with shielding, retracting, or blunting safety features. Most injuries occur after use and before disposal. In some cases, the protective features are not activated. Puncture-proof sharps disposal containers continue to play an important role in preventing injury.

Source: Jagger, J., & Perry, J. (2002). Realistic expectations for safety devices. *Nursing 2002*, *32*(3), 72.

Clinical Alert

Change needle after withdrawing medication from ampule or vial.

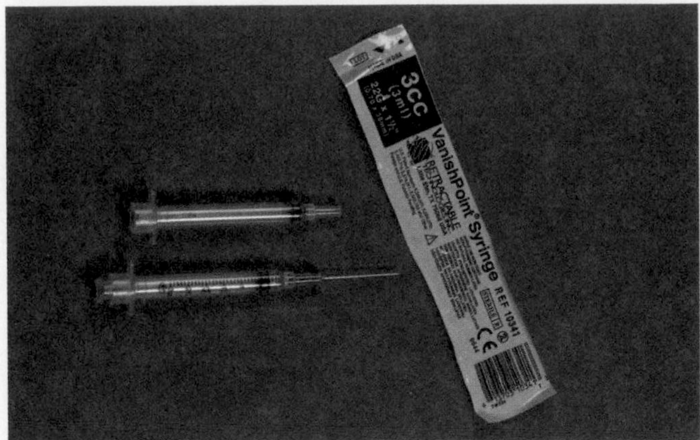

▲ Health care facilities must use safety needles to conform to needlestick safety legislation.

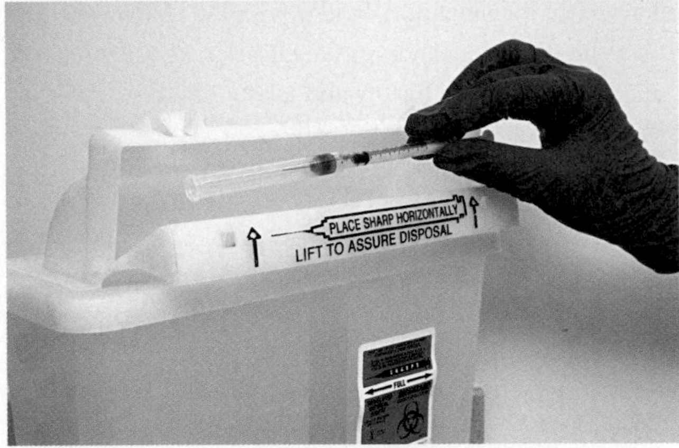

▲ Discard syringe in biohazard container following injection.

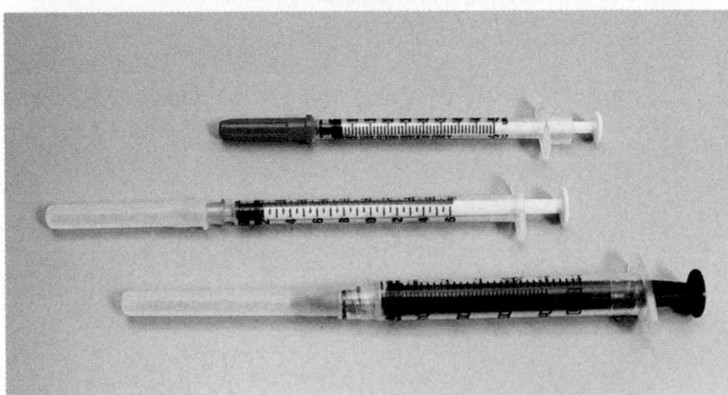

▲ Three types of syringes: tuberculin, insulin, and 3-mL.

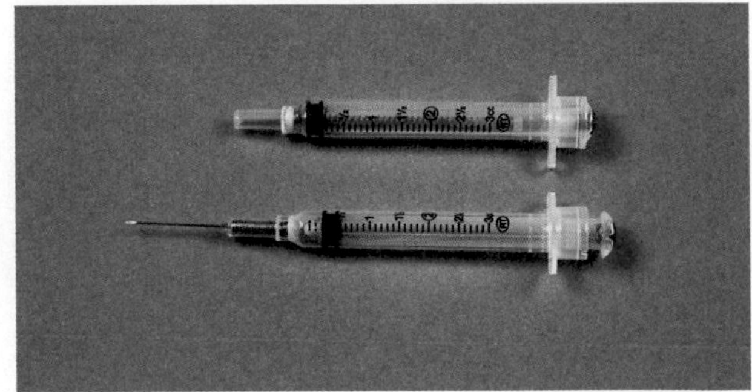

▲ Safety syringe with retractable needle (bottom image) and needle retracted into barrel (top image).

Sites for Injections

Site is the single most consistent factor associated with complications and injury. One must consider client's age, size, medication type, and medication volume.

Intradermal Injections

- Injection sites: inner aspect of forearm or scapular area of back; upper chest; medial thigh.
- Purpose: to test for antigens (tubercle bacillus, allergens).
- Amount injected: ranges from 0.01 to 0.1 mL.
- Absorption rate: slow.

Subcutaneous Injections

- Injection sites: fatty tissue of abdomen, lateral and posterior aspects of upper arm or thigh, scapular area of back, upper ventrodorsal gluteal areas.
- Purpose: for medications that are absorbed slowly.
- Amount injected: variable—no more than 2 mL. If repeated doses are necessary, alter site accordingly.

Intramuscular Injections

- Purpose: to promote rapid absorption of the drug; to provide an alternate route when drug is irritating to subcutaneous tissues.
- Amount injected: variable—may be large amount of fluid. If more than 5 mL for adult or 3 mL for child and 1 mL for infant, divide dose into two syringes.
- Absorption rate: depends on circulatory state of client.
- Injection sites:

Ventrogluteal Injection Site (preferred site for IM injection for all clients over age 7 months)

1. Place client in side-lying or supine position.
2. Use right hand for left anterior hip, or left hand for right anterior hip.
3. Identify greater trochanter and place palm at site.
4. Keep palm on greater trochanter and point index finger toward client's anterior superior iliac spine and fan out other three fingers.
5. Form "V" area with index finger separated from other three fingers.
6. Inject medication at 90° angle within "V" area.

Vastus Lateralis Injection Site

1. Place client in supine position with thigh exposed.
2. Identify greater trochanter and lateral femoral condyle.
3. Using middle third and anterior *lateral* aspect of thigh, select site.
4. Inject medication directly into muscle at 90° angle.

Deltoid Injection Site (solution must be nonirritating)

1. Expose client's upper arm.
2. Deltoid site is two fingerbreadths below acromion process.
3. Place left hand on acromion process and right index finger two fingerbreadths below.
4. Inject limited medication volume (0.5–1 mL) in deltoid IM site at 90° angle.

Clinical Alert

Do Not Use These Sites

- The dorsogluteal site is no longer recommended for IM injection. There is a high risk for injury to the sciatic nerve and major blood vessels due to difficulty palpating appropriate bony landmarks in this area. Variation of thickness of subcutaneous tissue at this site makes inadvertent injection into subcutaneous tissue, altered drug absorption, and tissue injury possible.
- Do not use the rectus femoris (anterior thigh) muscle for injection.

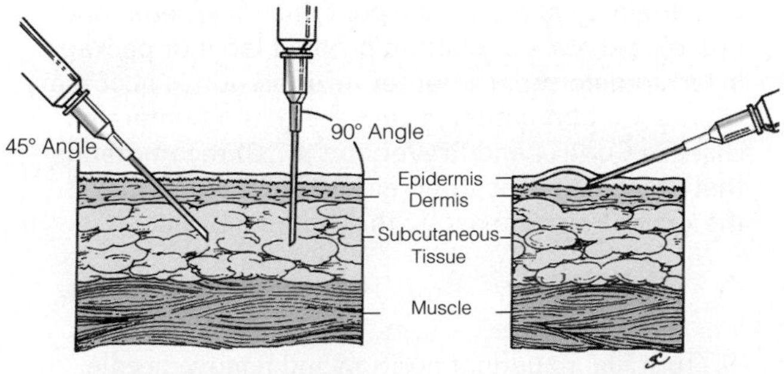

45° Angle
90° Angle
Epidermis
Dermis
Subcutaneous Tissue
Muscle

▲ Insert needle at 45° or 90° angle into tissue for subcutaneous injection.

▲ Insert needle at 15° angle just under the epidermis for intradermal injection.

Selecting the Appropriate-Size Needle for Injection

- *Intradermal injections*: 1 mL tuberculin syringe with short bevel, 25–27 gauge, 3/8–1/2 in. needle.
- *Subcutaneous injections*: 0.5–3 mL syringe with 25–29 gauge, 3/8–5/8 in. needle.
- *Intramuscular injections*: 1–5 mL syringe with needle gauge and length appropriate for muscle site and fat thickness; deltoid muscle requires 23–25 gauge, 5/8–1 in. needle; needle sizes for the vastus lateralis and ventrogluteal muscle vary from 18 to 23 gauge, needle lengths, 1–1½ in.

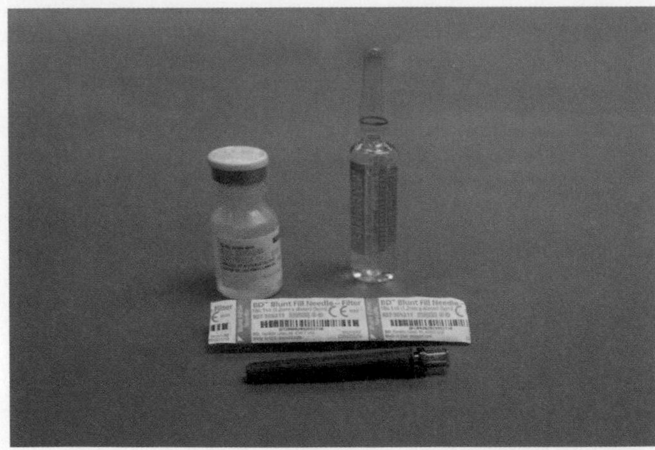

▲ A special filter needle should be used to prevent aspirating particulate matter when withdrawing solution from an ampule or vial.

For Withdrawing Medication From a Vial

1. Remove the vial cap.
2. Open antimicrobial wipe, and cleanse the rubber top of the vial. ▸ ***Rationale:*** Manufacturer does not guarantee sterility of rubber top.
3. Tighten filter needle to syringe. Remove needle guard.

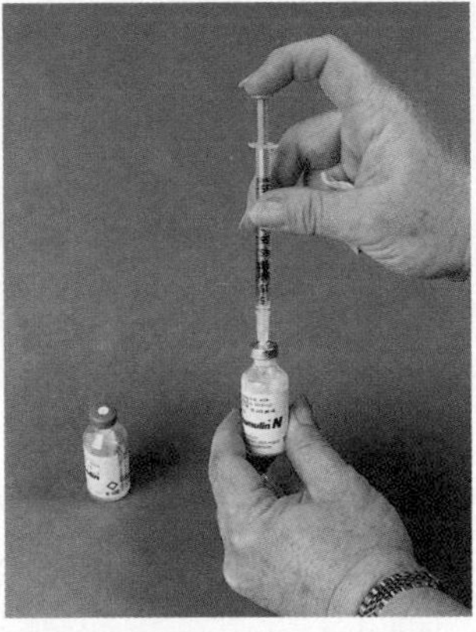

▲ Inject prescribed amount of air into vial.

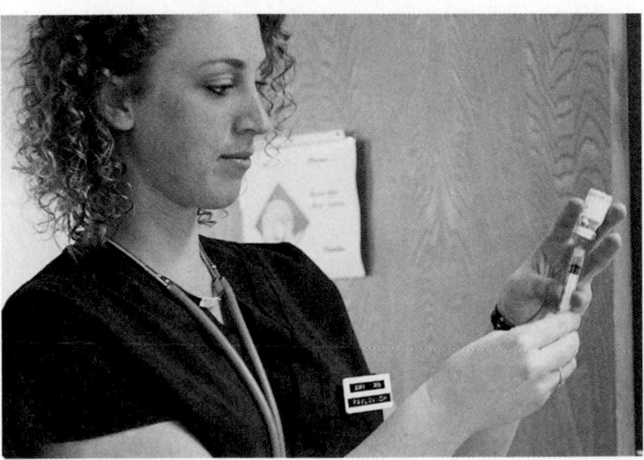

▲ Invert vial to extract desired amount of medication.

4. Pull back on plunger to fill syringe with an amount of air equal to amount of solution to be withdrawn. ▸ ***Rationale:*** The displacement of solution with air is necessary to prevent the formation of a vacuum in the sealed vial.
5. Insert filter needle into upright vial. Inject air into vacant area of vial, keeping needle bevel above surface of medication. ▸ ***Rationale:*** Air creates positive pressure within vial, allowing accurate withdrawal of medication.
6. Invert vial, and pull plunger to extract desired amount of medication. Touch only syringe barrel and plunger tip. ▸ ***Rationale:*** This prevents contamination of the plunger, inside of barrel, and medication.
7. Expel any air bubbles from syringe at this time by tapping the side of syringe sharply with your finger or pen below the air bubble. ▸ ***Rationale:*** Air bubbles form in syringe due to dead air space in needle hub. Removing air bubbles while needle remains within the inverted vial avoids accidental contamination of needle and facilitates easy removal of air and accurate withdrawal of solution.
8. Recheck amount of medication in syringe.

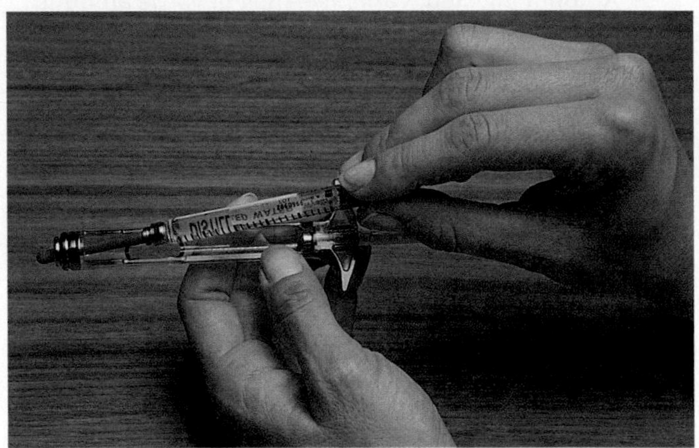

▲ Slide prefilled, sterile cartridge into syringe barrel; then turn and lock.

Clinical Alert

If multiple-use vials are opened, they must be marked with the date and time the container is entered and nurse's initials. Consult the product label or package insert to determine whether refrigeration is necessary. Unless contamination is suspected, the Centers for Disease Control and Prevention (CDC) recommends that the vial be discarded either when empty or on the expiration date set by the manufacturer.

9. Turn vial to upright position and remove needle. ▸ ***Rationale:*** Removing needle from inverted vial may cause leaking of medication from needle insertion site.

10. Replace filter needle with needle for injection.
11. Recheck medication label and dosage against medication record and any dosage calculation. ▸ ***Rationale:*** This is a second safety check.
12. Replace or dispose of medication vial, checking label once again. ▸ ***Rationale:*** This is a third safety check.

For Combining Medications in One Syringe Using Two Vials

1. Prepare both vials by removing caps and cleansing tops with separate antimicrobial wipes.
2. Draw air into syringe equal to amount of solution to be removed from *second* vial. Inject air into *second* vial. Do not withdraw medication at this time. ▸ ***Rationale:*** Air creates positive pressure within the vial, allowing withdrawal of solution.

Clinical Alert

Check appropriate text or consult agency pharmacist to ensure compatibility of medications before combining in a syringe for injection.

Reconstituting Powdered Medication

- Insert filter needle into upright powdered medication vial.
- Remove the amount of air equal to desired quantity of diluent; this provides space for the diluent.
- Inject diluent into upright powdered medication vial.
- Remove needle and cover with guard.
- Rotate powdered medication vial with diluent between palms. Do not shake vial because shaking creates air bubbles and may cause difficulty withdrawing medication dose.
- Withdraw medication from vial.
- Replace filter needle with needle for injection.

3. Draw air into syringe equal to amount of solution to be removed from *first* vial and inject it into *first* vial.
4. Invert first vial and withdraw ordered amount of medication without removing syringe.
5. Expel all air bubbles from syringe.
6. Recheck amount of solution and remove syringe from vial.
7. Insert needle into *second* vial, invert, and carefully withdraw exact amount of solution ordered. ▸ ***Rationale:*** Withdrawing excess solution from second vial results in an inaccurate dosage of medication. If this occurs, syringe must be discarded and procedure begun again.
8. Replace filter needle with needle for injection.

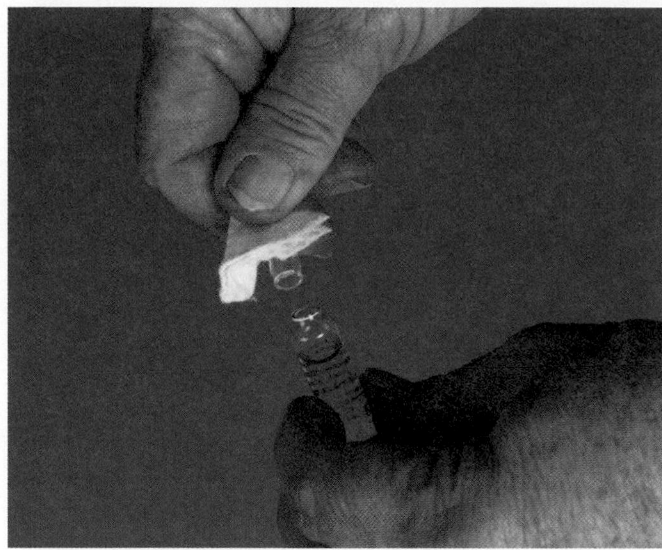

▲ Using alcohol swab or dry gauze square, grasp and snap off stem of ampule, breaking away from you.

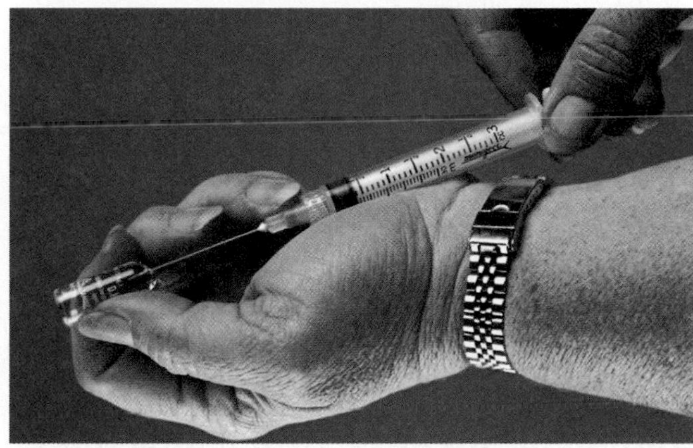

▲ Tilt or invert ampule to withdraw appropriate amount of medication, using filter needle.

For Withdrawing Medication From an Ampule

1. Move solution from neck to body of ampule by tapping stem sharply or holding neck of ampule between thumb and forefinger and flicking wrist.
2. Using a pad, grasp neck (stem) of ampule between thumb and forefinger of one hand and grasp body of ampule with other hand. Break stem away from you. (If ampule is not scored, partially file neck of ampule.) ▸ ***Rationale:*** Gauze pad protects hands, and breaking away from you prevents injury from glass fragments. Alternatively, slip a nipple from a baby bottle over the stem to prevent injury.
3. Set the ampule upright. It is not necessary to add air before withdrawing the medication.
4. Use a special filter needle to withdraw solution. ▸ ***Rationale:*** Filter needle prevents aspiration of glass when withdrawing solution from ampule, especially if the ampule is inverted.

5. Remove needle guard and insert needle into ampule without touching sides of ampule and withdraw medication. Alternatively, invert ampule and withdraw appropriate amount of medication. ▸ ***Rationale:*** Surface tension prevents solution from leaking out of inverted ampule.
6. Withdraw needle with ampule in upright position.
7. Tap syringe barrel below bubbles to dislodge air bubbles to hub of syringe.
8. Eject air with syringe in an upright position. If amount of solution is overdrawn, invert syringe and remove excess solution into the Medical Waste (black box) receptacle. ▸ ***Rationale:*** Appropriate waste disposal is mandated by the EPA.
9. Cover needle with guard, using scoop method.

For Combining Medications Using Alternative Method

1. Draw up ordered dose from each vial or ampule into two separate syringes. First syringe must be able to hold entire volume of combined medications.
2. Remove needle from first syringe.
3. Pull back plunger of first syringe to allow space for volume of second medication to be added.
4. Insert needle of second syringe into hub of first syringe.
5. Slowly inject medication of second syringe through first syringe hub, then withdraw needle.
6. Attach new needle to first syringe.
7. Discard needles and second syringe.

For Preparing Prefilled Medication Cartridge

1. Hold barrel of cartridge syringe (e.g., Tubex) in one hand and pull back on plunger with other hand.
2. Insert prefilled medication cartridge, needle first, into cartridge barrel.
3. Twist cartridge syringe flange clockwise until it is secure.
4. Screw plunger rod onto screw at bottom of medication cartridge until it fits firmly and tightly into rubber stopper.
5. Remove needle guard and any air bubbles.
6. Determine if dosage in cartridge is greater than required amount. If so, invert Tubex and gently expel excess medication into Medical Waste receptacle, being careful to maintain sterility of needle. ▸ ***Rationale:*** If permanent needle is contaminated, the cartridge becomes contaminated and must be discarded.
7. Replace needle guard, using scoop method.

Administering Intradermal Injections

Equipment

Medication (e.g., 0.1 mL Purified Protein Derivative Antigen for tuberculin testing)

Unit dose (1 mL) tuberculin syringe with 1/4–3/8 in. 27-gauge needle

Antimicrobial wipes

Gauze sponge

Clean gloves (if indicated)

Pen to mark injection site

▲ Insert needle with bevel up for intradermal injection.

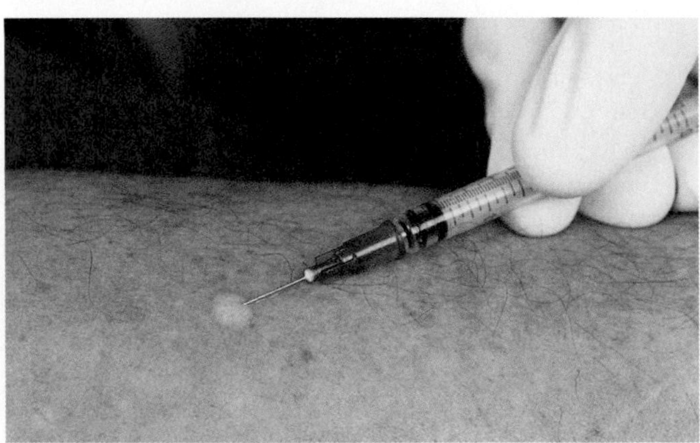

▲ Inject solution to form wheal on skin.

Preparation

Follow steps for Preparing Injections.

Procedure

1. Take prepared injection to client's room, checking room and bed number against client's medication record.
2. Check client's Ident-A-Band and ask client to state name and birth date.
3. Explain procedure and purpose to client.
4. Perform hand hygiene and don gloves if exposure is anticipated.
5. Select lesion-free injection site on undersurface, upper third of forearm for skin testing.
6. Cleanse area with antimicrobial wipe and allow to dry.
7. Remove needle guard.
8. Grasp the client's dorsal forearm to gently pull the skin taut on ventral forearm.
9. Holding syringe almost parallel to skin, insert needle at a 10°–15° angle with bevel facing up, about 1/8 in. Needle point should be visible under skin. DO NOT ASPIRATE.
10. Inject medication slowly, observing for a wheal (blister) formation and blanching at the site. ▶ ***Rationale:*** This indicates that the medication was injected within the dermis. If no wheal develops, injection was given too deeply.
11. Withdraw needle at same angle as inserted. Pat area gently with dry gauze sponge, but DO NOT MASSAGE. ▶ ***Rationale:*** Massaging could disperse medication.
12. Activate needle safety feature and discard syringe unit in puncture-proof container.
13. Mark injection site with pen for future assessment.
14. Return client to comfortable position.
15. Dispose of gloves and perform hand hygiene.
16. Record site and antigen in client's record.

Clinical Alert

For tuberculin testing, instruct client to return and have the site checked by the healthcare provider in 48–72 hr.

Administering Subcutaneous Injections

Equipment

Nonirritating medication
3-mL syringe with 5/8-inch needle (usual 25–27 gauge)
Antimicrobial wipe
Dry gauze sponge
Clean gloves if indicated

Preparation

See steps for Preparing Injections.

Procedure

1. Take prepared injection to client's room, checking room and bed number against client's medication record.
2. Check client's Ident-A-Band and ask client to state name and birth date.
3. Explain procedure and purpose to client.
4. Perform hand hygiene and don gloves.
5. Select fatty site for injection (e.g., abdomen, avoiding 2-in. radius around umbilicus), alternating sites for each injection. ▶ ***Rationale:*** This prevents repeated trauma to tissue.
6. Cleanse area with antimicrobial wipe and allow to dry.
7. Remove needle guard.
8. Use thumb and forefinger and gently grasp loose area ("pinch an inch") of fatty tissue on appropriate site (e.g., posterior-lateral aspect, middle third of arm). ▶ ***Rationale:*** This ensures insertion of medication within subcutaneous tissue, not muscle.

Gloving Protocol for Injections

The CDC has no regulations concerning the wearing of gloves during injections. OSHA recommends that gloves are not necessary when administering IM or subcutaneous injections, as long as bleeding that could result in hand contact with blood (or other potentially infectious material) is not anticipated.

The practice of whether or not to wear gloves for subcutaneous or IM injections is based on judgment. Hospital policy may dictate gloving protocol for injections.

If wearing gloves for mass inoculations, nurses must change gloves between clients and perform hand hygiene. Therefore, nurses may choose *not* to wear gloves in these situations (OSHA & CDC).

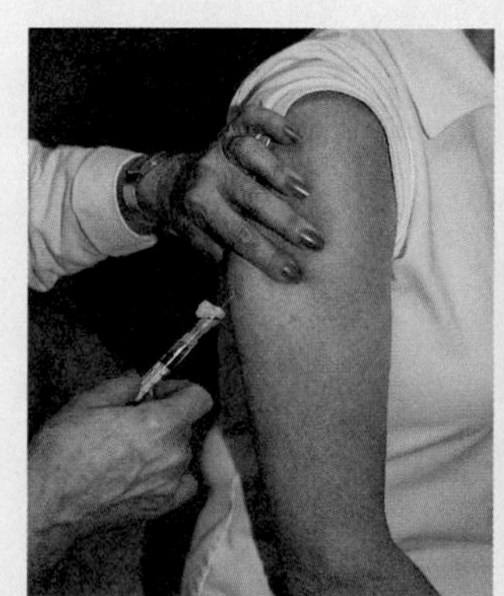

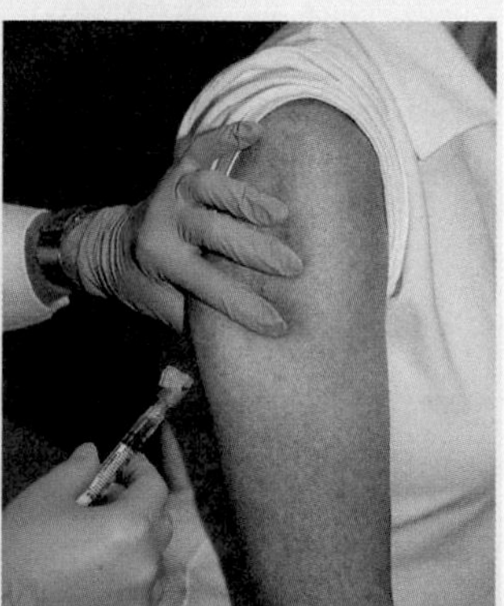

NOTE: This action is not necessary when there is substantial fatty tissue.

9. Hold syringe like a dart between the thumb and forefinger.
10. Insert needle at a 45° or 90° angle. A 90° angle is used more commonly due to short needles on prepackaged syringes. ▸ ***Rationale:*** Angle varies with the amount of subcutaneous tissue, selected site, and needle length.
11. Continue to hold tissue and aspirate 5 to 10 seconds by pulling back on plunger with thumb of dominant hand. If no blood appears, administer injection. If blood appears, withdraw needle, activate safety feature and discard, then prepare a new injection. ▸ ***Rationale:*** Blood indicates needle has entered a blood vessel. Injecting the drug IV may be dangerous.
12. Inject medication slowly, 10 seconds per mL.
13. Wait 10 seconds, then withdraw needle and activate needle safety feature.
14. Release tissue and massage area with dry gauze sponge (if indicated). ▸ ***Rationale:*** Massaging area aids absorption.

Clinical Alert

Irritating medications such as Vistaril must not be administered subcutaneously, as or tissue necrosis may result. Such medications should be administered intramuscularly in the ventrogluteal site using the Z-track method.

15. Discard needle/syringe unit in puncture-proof container.
16. Return client to position of comfort.
17. Discard gloves and perform hand hygiene.
18. Record medication and site used.

Preparing Insulin Injections

Equipment

Insulin(s) vials

Unopened vials of insulin should be stored in refrigerator

Opened vial of insulin may be refrigerated or kept at room temperature; recommend discard after 28 days

Insulin should not be exposed to light, or to temperatures over 80° F

Do not use insulin that has clumping, frosting, or precipitation

Insulin syringe: available in 3/10 mL, ½ mL, and 1 mL sizes (*Note:* syringes are no longer called U40, U100, etc.)

Needles: 29–31 gauge short needles

Antimicrobial swab

Dry gauze sponge

Clean gloves if indicated

Preparation

1. Follow steps for Preparing Injections.
2. Obtain client's blood glucose level *before preparation* to determine appropriate administration of insulin. See Chapter 20 (Specimen Collection) for finger stick blood.

For Newly Diagnosed Diabetic Client

a. Explain to client that the dose of short-acting insulin must be adjusted according to blood glucose test results.
b. Explain that there is a variation in levels—the lowest blood glucose level is before meals and highest 1–2 hr after meals.
c. Goal of treatment is to eliminate wide swings in glucose levels.

Procedure

For One Insulin Solution

1. Perform hand hygiene.
2. Turn intermediate or long-acting (cloudy) insulin vial top-to-bottom 10 times. ▸ ***Rationale:*** This brings cloudy insulin solution into suspension. Clear insulins do not require this.

▲ Select site on lateral aspect of mid-upper arm for subcutaneous injection.

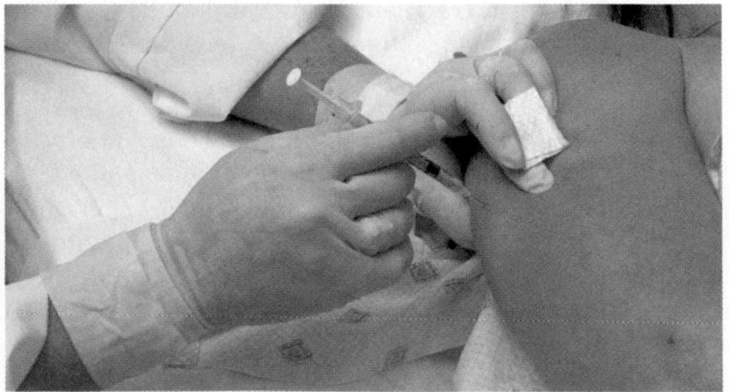

▲ Insert needle at 45° or 90° angle, using short needle for subcutaneous injection.

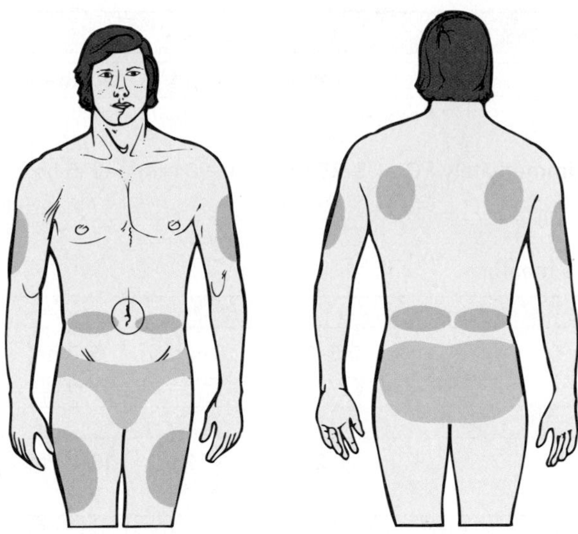

▲ Sites for subcutaneous injections given routinely. (Avoid umbilicus area.) Abdomen site preferred for insulin injection as absorption is more predictable.

3. Wipe top of insulin bottle with antimicrobial swab.
4. Remove needle guard and place on tray.

Clinical Alert

Hypoglycemia (blood sugar <60) is the most common adverse effect of insulins. Client should wear Med-Alert bracelet/ID to alert others. The client should be instructed to carry at least 15 g of fast-acting sugar (e.g., glucose tablet, 1 T sugar, jelly, honey) to be taken in the event of a hypoglycemic reaction.

Clinical Alert

Do not shake insulin vial, as this destroys insulin potency. Rolling the vial fails to bring insulin into suspension. Turn the vial top to bottom 8 to 10 times instead.

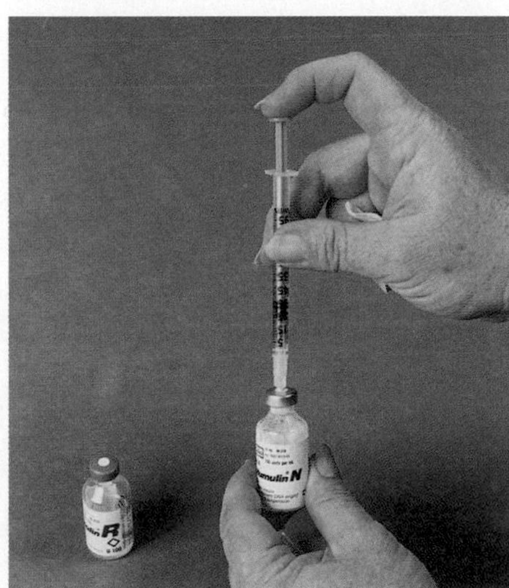

▲ Types of insulin syringes used based on unit dosages required.

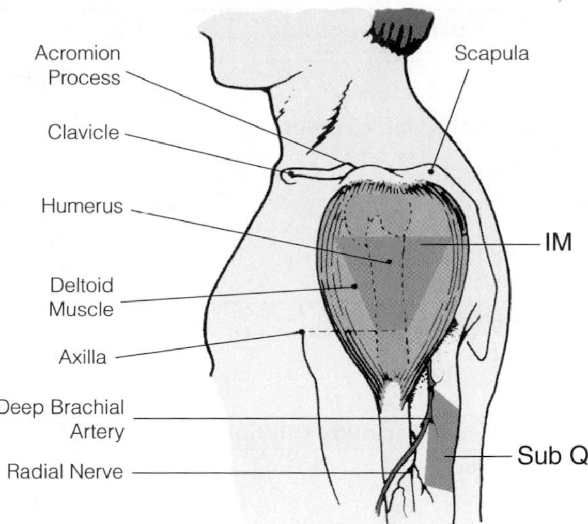

▲ Use upper shaded triangle for IM injection in upper arm; use lower shaded area for subcutaneous injection.

5. Pull plunger of syringe down to desired amount of medication (e.g., 12 units). With vial upright, inject amount of air into air space, not into insulin solution. ▸ ***Rationale:*** Injecting air directly into insulin solution causes bubbles.
6. Withdraw ordered amount of insulin into syringe.
7. Validate medication record, insulin bottle, and prepared syringe with an RN for accuracy. ▸ ***Rationale:*** Double-checking insulin helps safeguard against errors.
8. Remove needle from vial and expel air from syringe.
9. Replace needle guard.
10. Take medication to client's room.
11. Follow steps for administration of medications by subcutaneous injection.

For Two Insulin Solutions

1. Check medication orders.
2. Perform hand hygiene.
3. Follow steps for combining medications in one syringe using two vials.
4. Turn cloudy insulin **Bottle (A)** top to bottom 8–10 times. ▸ ***Rationale:*** This brings cloudy solution into *suspension.*
5. Wipe top of both insulin bottles with alcohol swab.
6. Take needle guard off and place on tray.

Clinical Alert

The IV route is superior for administering RAPID OR SHORT-ACTING insulin to an obese client. Adipose tissue slows onset of insulin action.

Clinical Alert

Long-acting insulin, LANTUS (glargine) and Levemir (detemir), are clear solutions. These are *not* to be mixed with any other type of insulin or solution. They are administered subcutaneously and are not intended for IV use.

TABLE 18-1 Insulin Types and Therapeutic Action (in Minutes/Hours*)

Types	Inject**	Onset	Peak	Duration
Very Rapid Acting (clear solution)				
Humalog® (lispro) NovoLog® (aspart)	Within 15 min AC or immediately PC Within 5–10 min AC	5–15 min	30–90 min	3–5 hr
Apidra® (glulisine)	15 min AC or within 20 min after *starting* a meal			
Short Acting (clear solution)				
Novolin R Humulin R	Per order Within 30–60 min AC	0.5–1 hr	2–4 hr	5–7 hr
Intermediate Acting (cloudy solution)				
Humulin N (NPH) Novolin N (NPH)	Per order Per order	1–2 hr	6-10 hr	16–24 hr
Mixtures (cloudy solution)				
Novolin 70/30 (70% NPH, 30% Regular) Humulin 70/30 (70% NPH, 30% Regular) Humulin 50/50 (50% NPH, 50% Regular)	Per order Within 30–60 min AC	30 min 15 min	R- 2–4hrs N-6–10 hr 1 hr	24 hr
Humalog 75/25 *(75% lispro protamine suspension, 25% lispro)* Humalog 50/50 *(50% lispro protamine suspension, 50% lispro)* NovoLog 70/30 *(70% aspart protamine suspension, 30% aspart)*	Within 15 min AC Within 15 min AC Within 15 min AC			
Long Acting				
Lantus (glargine) (*clear solution*) Levemir (detemir) (*clear solution*)	Daily	4–6 hr	No peak	24 hr

*The time of insulin action may vary significantly in different clients and in the same client at different times.

**AC = before meals; PC = after meals.

Insulin is biologically engineered through the process of recombinant-DNA technology. Insulin is produced by different companies who use different names for short-, intermediate-, or long-acting forms of insulin or their mixtures.

NPH = neutral protamine Hagedorn

7. Pull plunger of syringe down to prescribed units of cloudy insulin.
8. Insert needle and inject air equal to cloudy dose into upright **Bottle A** (*cloudy*) insulin.
9. Withdraw needle.
10. Pull plunger of syringe down to prescribed units of clear insulin.
11. Insert needle and inject air equal to clear dose into upright **Bottle B** (clear) insulin.
12. Invert vial and withdraw medication. ▶ ***Rationale:*** Withdrawing *clear* insulin first prevents inadvertent injection of intermediate-acting insulin into rapid- or short-acting insulin bottle, which would slow its rapid action.
13. Double-check your preparations with another nurse.
14. Withdraw needle from bottle and expel all air bubbles.
15. Invert **Bottle A** and insert needle. Take care not to inject any rapid or short-acting (*clear*) insulin into intermediate-acting (*cloudy*) insulin bottle. This can be avoided by holding steady pressure on plunger when inserting needle into bottle.
16. Pull back on plunger to obtain exact prescribed amount of intermediate or long-acting insulin. The total insulin dose now includes both the clear insulin, previously drawn up into syringe, and the intermediate cloudy insulin you have just drawn up.

Clinical Alert

Do not massage site after injection of certain drugs such as insulin or heparin because this hastens absorption and drug action and may cause tissue irritation.

17. Withdraw needle from bottle and replace needle guard.
18. Follow protocol for administration of medications by subcutaneous injections.

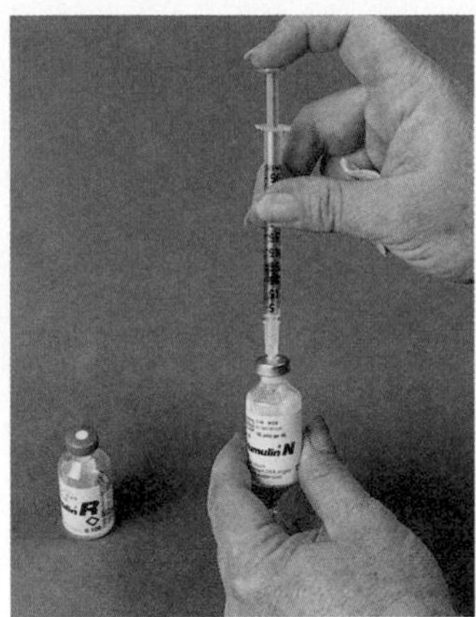

▲ Step 1: Inject prescribed amount of air into intermediate-acting (cloudy) insulin vial—withdraw needle without needle touching solution.

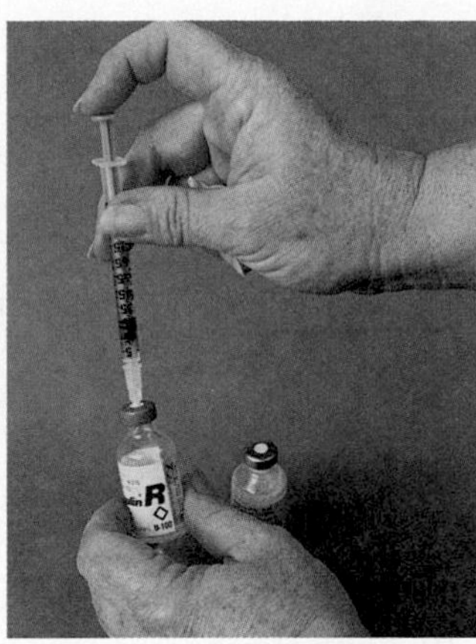

▲ Step 2: Inject prescribed amount of air into rapid- or short-acting (clear) insulin vial. Do not withdraw needle.

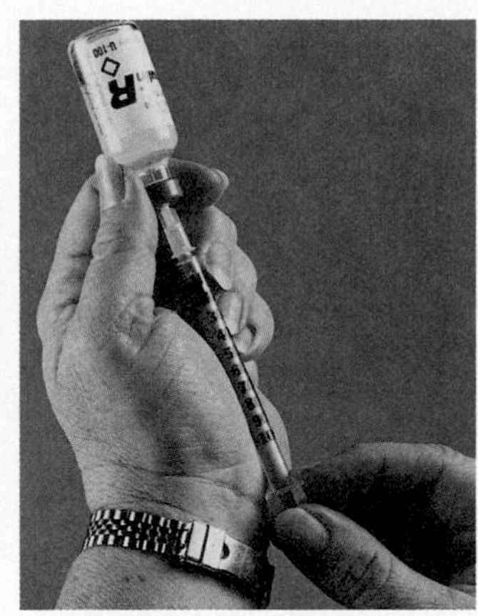

▲ Step 3: Invert vial of rapid or short-acting insulin; withdraw prescribed amount of medication and withdraw needle from vial.

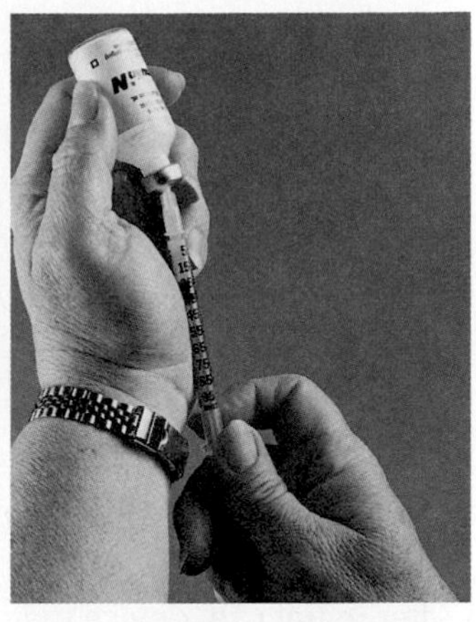

▲ Step 4: Invert intermediate-acting insulin vial and withdraw exact amount without injecting insulin into bottle.

Premixing Types of Insulin

- Mixtures of rapid-acting (Humalog) and intermediate- or long-acting insulin should be administered within 10 minutes before a meal.
- Mixtures of NPH and regular (short-acting) insulin should be administered 20 to 30 minutes before a meal.
- Mixtures may be stored in refrigerator for up to 30 days and should be gently resuspended before injection.

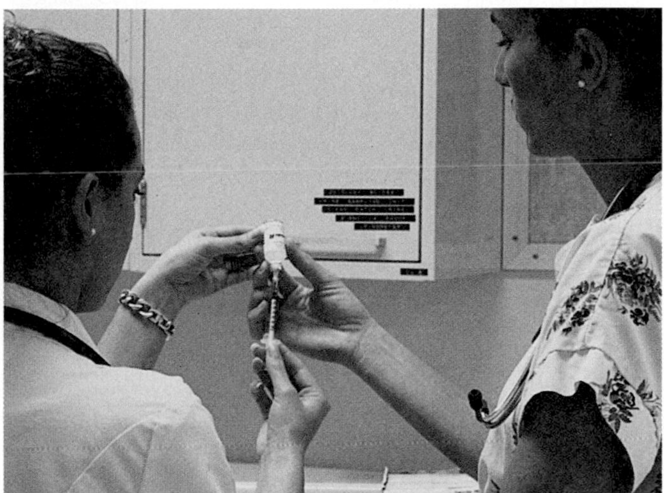

▲ Double-check insulin dose with a second nurse to help prevent errors in preparation.

Clinical Alert

Insulin type and brand should remain consistent for an individual client.

EVIDENCE-BASED PRACTICE

The Importance of Double-Checking Drug Dose

- Double checks have revealed that up to 4.2% of *prescriptions* are filled erroneously.
- Double checks help the nurse identify mistakes that are difficult for someone alone to recognize.
- Double checks work best when each nurse calculates desired dosages *independently* rather than having another nurse "*verify*" what has been prepared.

Source: Cohen, M. (2002). Double checking for errors. *Nursing 2002, 32*(3), 18.

Using an Insulin Pen

Equipment

Insulin delivery device labeled with client's name: Prefilled pen or cartridge with correct insulin type with instructions for use

Device-compatible needle

Antimicrobial swab

Clinical Alert

Insulin injection "dial a dose" pens contain a prefilled multidose cartridge available with various types of insulin.

- The pen is intended for single-client use.
- Do not aspirate contents out of the pen cartridge with a needle as pen calibration will no longer be accurate.
- A sterile disposable needle is attached for each injection.
- An "air shot" primes the needle before the appropriate dose (units) of insulin is dialed for injection.

After initial use, device may be kept for 28 days. Most devices are not to be stored in the refrigerator nor to be exposed to excessive heat.

Preparation

1. Perform hand hygiene.
2. Identify client.
3. Complete the first "Five Rights" validation again before administering insulin. Note: The sixth right is documentation and is not indicated here. ▸ ***Rationale:*** The client may be receiving more than one type of insulin.

Procedure

1. Remove pen cap and insert insulin cartridge (if indicated).
2. Turn pen up and down at least 10 times if indicated. ▸ ***Rationale:*** To create suspension of cloudy insulin.
3. Wipe pen's rubber stopper with antimicrobial swab before placing pen needle.
4. Remove needle cap and screw needle onto the pen immediately before injecting.
5. Pull cover off needle.
6. Hold pen with needle up and tap cartridge to move air bubbles to top of cartridge.
7. Dial pen dose selector to 2 units.
8. Keeping needle pointing upward, press push button until dose selector returns to "0". ▸ ***Rationale:*** This will allow an "air shot" to clear cartridge of air and prime needle before injection. A drop of insulin should show at the needle tip. *Do not recap after priming needle*.
9. Check that dose selector is set at "0", then dial required number of insulin units to be injected; listen for a click for each unit dialed.
10. Swab client's injection site.
11. Insert needle perpendicular (90° angle) to the skin, maintaining constant pressure. The needle is in the subcutaneous tissue when the shield completely retracts (1/2 in.) and touches the insulin reservoir.
12. Using your thumb, press pen "push button" completely and keep depressed, counting to 10 after plunger has returned to "0" position before removing needle from skin.

NOTE: There may be a drop of residual fluid left on skin after injection due to fall back into shield with priming.

13. Do not massage the area.
14. Remove retracted pen needle from device and dispose in sharps container. ▸ ***Rationale:*** A new needle must be used for each injection.
15. Replace pen/device cap and store according to directions.

Clinical Alert

An FDA alert reminds healthcare providers that single-patient insulin pens and insulin cartridges must not be used for multiple patients, even if needles are changed, due to risk of transmitting bloodborne pathogens.

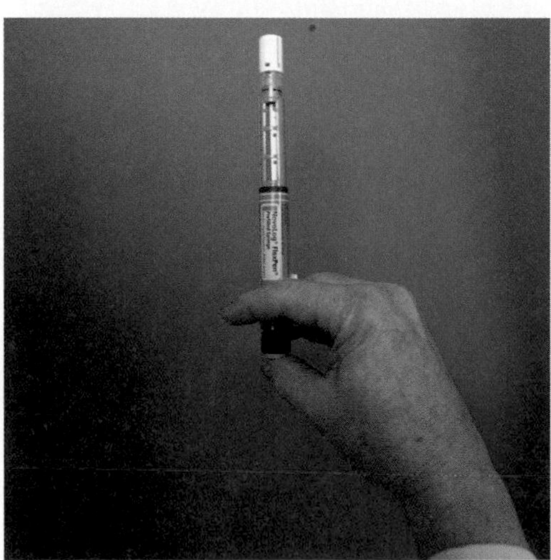

▲ Air shot clears cartridge and needle of air and primes needle for injection.

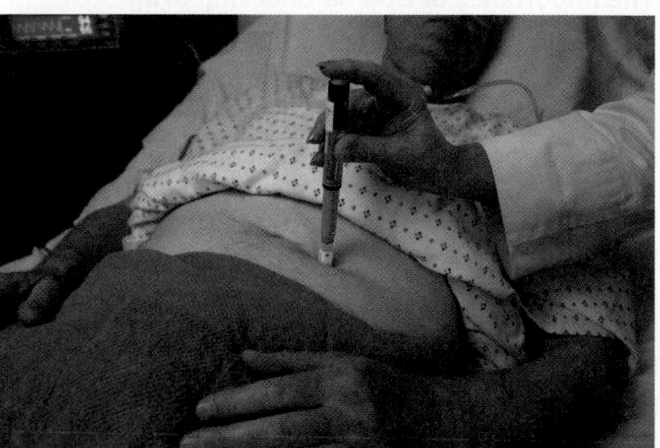

▲ Press pen firmly on client's abdomen to engage needle; inject dialed units and hold 10 seconds before releasing. Remove needle, dispose in sharps receptacle. Recap and return pen to storage area for future use.

The Client With an Insulin Pump

- Continuous Subcutaneous Insulin Infusion (CSII) is a form of intensive insulin therapy utilized as an alternative to multiple daily injections in an attempt to achieve optimal glycemic control and decrease risk of long-term complications of diabetes. Insulin pumps are manufactured by a number of companies that provide 24-hr emergency and clinical specialists to assist clients with start-up of their pump. All models consist of a battery-powered pump with insulin reservoir, an infusion catheter, and microcomputer that allows programming to deliver basal and bolus doses according to the physician orders. Only rapid-acting or short-acting insulin is used.
- CSII more closely mimics release of insulin by the pancreas with continuous-delivery basal and bolus insulin infusion.
- Basal rate/rates: amount of insulin delivered (units per hour) to keep blood glucose levels in target range between meals and overnight.
- Bolus: additional amount of insulin delivered immediately before meals or for episodes of hyperglycemia, the greatest risk associated with insulin pump therapy.
- The client should be referred to a certified diabetes educator before the start of pump use. Insulin boluses will be based on blood glucose readings and carbohydrate grams intake.

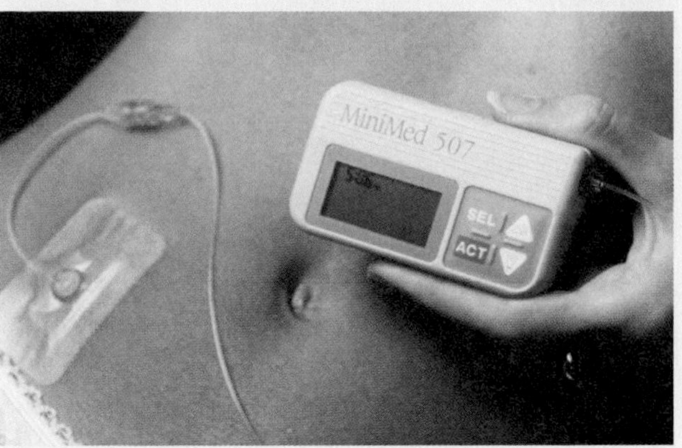

▲ MiniMed 507 Insulin Pump attached to infusion set. Abdominal site is preferred because insulin absorption is faster and most predictable.

- The client performs frequent fingerstick blood glucose checks: before adjusting any insulin dose, fasting, before meals, 2 hr after eating, at bedtime, and at 3 AM weekly.
- Lifestyle advantages: flexibility; insulin needs can be tailored to changes in schedule (meal time, exercise, or sleep).

Clinical Alert

Insulin pump management and education should be done by a certified diabetes educator who is also a certified insulin pump trainer.

Clinical Alert

If insulin must be discontinued (e.g., for MRI, CT scan), the pump should be disconnected. Blood glucose level should be checked before disconnecting and upon reconnecting. Ketoacidosis can occur within 2 hr if insulin delivery is interrupted.

Administering Subcutaneous Anticoagulants (Heparin, LMWH, Arixtra)

Equipment

Heparin in vial (*carefully note units per mL*)

1-mL tuberculin syringe or unit-dose syringe with small (25–29) gauge needle

or

Low-molecular-weight heparin (LMWH) or Arixtra in prefilled syringe

Antimicrobial swab

Dry gauze sponge

Gloves (if indicated)

Preparation

1. See Preparing Injections.
2. Double-check heparin calculated dose with another nurse.
3. Perform hand hygiene.

NOTE: To avoid loss of drug, do not clear prefilled syringe needle of air before injecting LMWH or Arixtra

Clinical Alert

Heparin is available in a variety of strengths (e.g., 1,000, 2,500, 5,000, 10,000, 25,000 units per mL vials). *Carefully* check vial units per mL before drawing into syringe and have another nurse double-check your calculations and prepared injection.

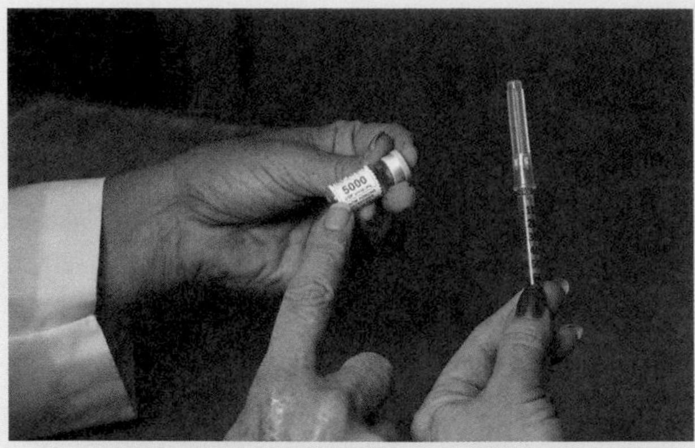

Clinical Alert

Subcutaneous injection of low-molecular-weight heparin (LMWH) *or* Arixtra involves low doses that help prevent clot formation but do not alter blood coagulation studies and do not require coagulation monitoring as does unfractionated heparin.

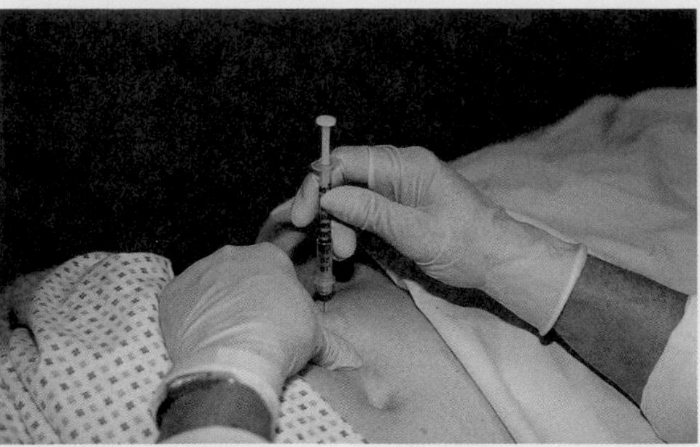

Clinical Alert

To prevent tissue damage and bruising, do not aspirate or massage anticoagulant injections.

Procedure

1. Check client's record for site of previous injection. ▸ ***Rationale:*** Injections should be rotated to prevent local post-injection complications.
2. Take prepared injection to client's room, and check room and bed number against client's MAR.
3. Check client's Ident-A-Band, and ask client to state name and birth date.
4. Provide privacy.
5. Explain procedure and purpose to client.
6. Don gloves (if indicated).
7. Assist client to supine position.
8. Select site on client's lower abdomen (at least two fingerbreadths from umbilicus) or select area of fatty tissue above iliac crest. ▸ ***Rationale:*** Anticoagulants should not be administered IM or in the extremities.

▲ Activate needle safety feature; then, dispose of syringe in sharps container.

9. Avoid ecchymotic area or lesions.
10. Cleanse site gently with antimicrobial swab, and allow to dry.
11. Gently pinch an inch of subcutaneous tissue (fat roll) between thumb and forefinger of nondominant hand and hold fat pad throughout injection.
12. Hold syringe between thumb and forefinger of dominant hand and insert full length of needle into skinfold at a 90° angle.
13. Inject medication slowly *without* aspirating first. ▸ ***Rationale:*** Aspiration can rupture small vessels and increase risk of bleeding into tissue.

    Note: Press prefilled syringe plunger rod firmly as far as it will go.
14. Wait 10 seconds before gently withdrawing needle at same angle in which it entered skin. ▸ ***Rationale:*** This allows medication to absorb into tissue and minimizes bruising.

NOTE: Release of Arixtra plunger will cause needle to retract into the security sleeve as it automatically withdraws from the skin.

15. Press and hold dry gauze sponge over injection site. ▸ ***Rationale:*** This prevents back-tracking of medication.
16. Do not massage area. ▸ ***Rationale:*** This may cause bruising.
17. Activate needle safety feature and discard syringe in puncture-proof container.
18. Return client to position of comfort.
19. Remove gloves and perform hand hygiene.
20. Document injection.

Administering Intramuscular (IM) Injections

Equipment

Medication vial or ampule
3-mL syringe with 1–1½ in. needle (21–23 gauge)
Antimicrobial swab
Dry gauze sponge
Gloves (if indicated)

Preparation

See Preparing Injections.

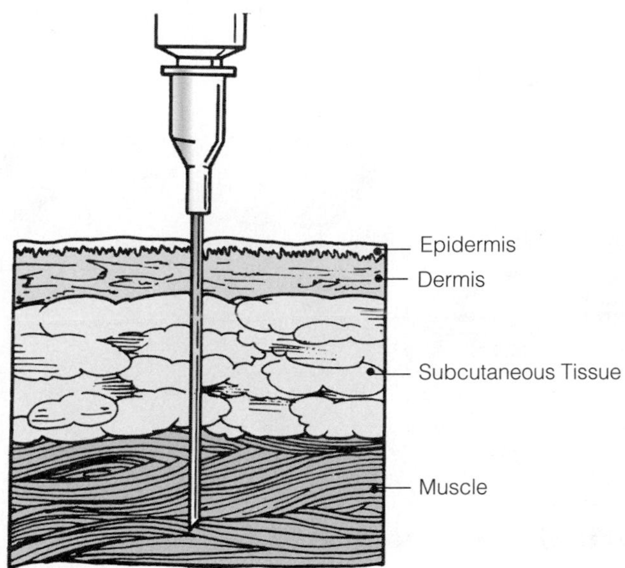

▲ Insert needle at 90° angle for IM injections into muscle.

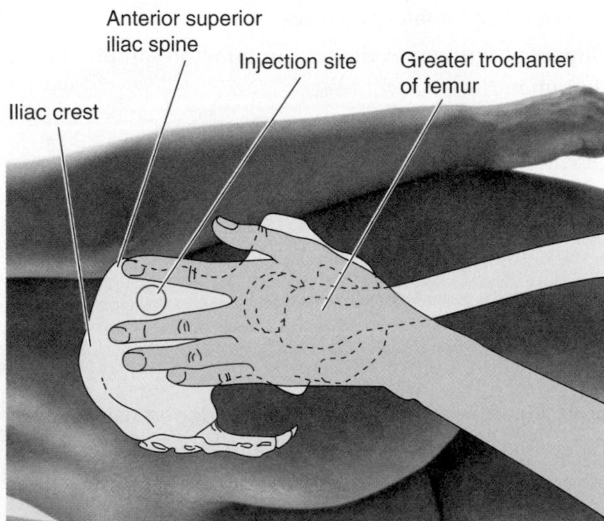

▲ Overlay of hand shows area of injection into ventrogluteal site for IM injections (client's right side).

Procedure

1. Check client's record for site of previous IM injections. ▸ ***Rationale:*** IM injections should be rotated to prevent local post-injection complications.
2. Take prepared injection to client's room. Check room and bed number against client's MAR.
3. Check client's Ident-A-Band, and have client state name and birth date.
4. Explain procedure to client.
5. Provide privacy for client.
6. Perform hand hygiene and don gloves, if indicated.
7. Select injection site, identifying bony landmarks. Consider client's size and amount and viscosity of medication being injected. Alternate sites each time injections are given.
8. Cleanse area with antimicrobial swab and allow to dry.
9. Spread skin taut between thumb and forefinger (grasping muscle is acceptable in pediatric and geriatric clients with less fatty tissue) to ensure needle placement in muscle belly.

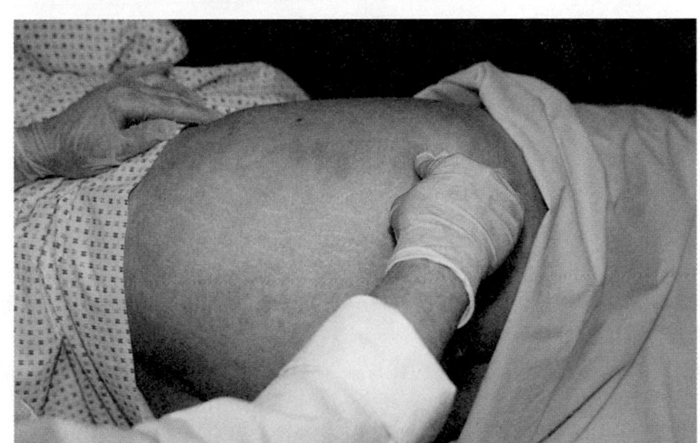

▲ Locate greater trochanter and anterior superior iliac spine.

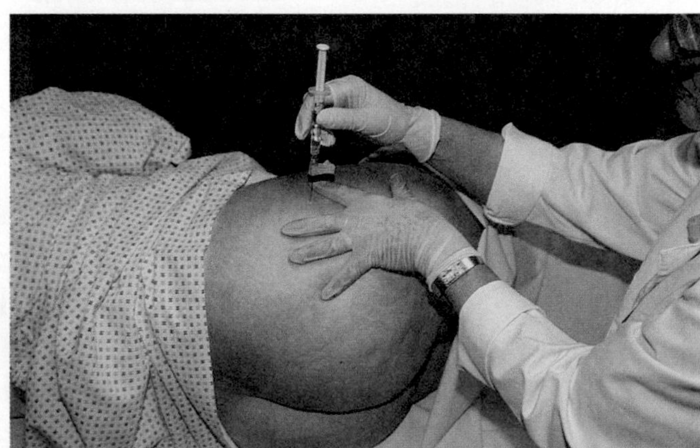

▲ Place palm at trochanter and index finger at anterior superior iliac spine; fan remaining fingers posteriorly.

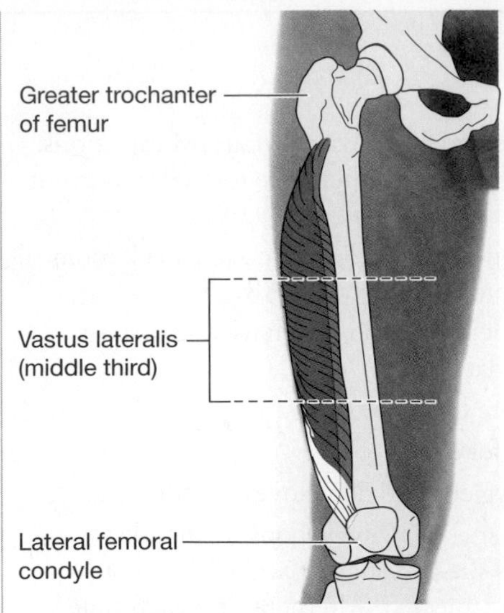

▲ Shaded area indicates site location for vastus lateralis injection.

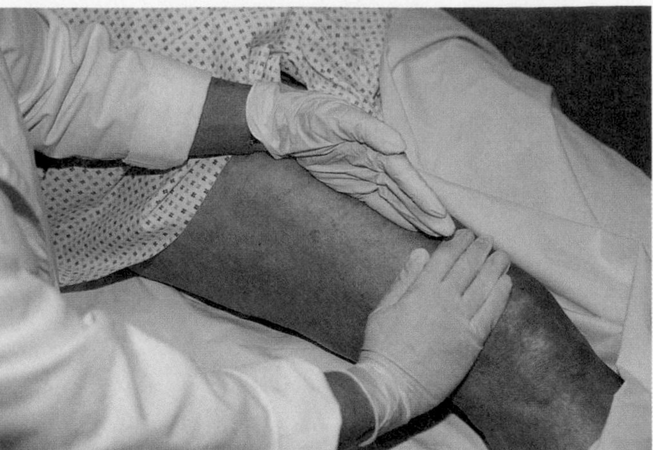

▲ Site is middle third an anterior-lateral aspect of thigh. Avoid the rectus femoris muscle (anterior thigh).

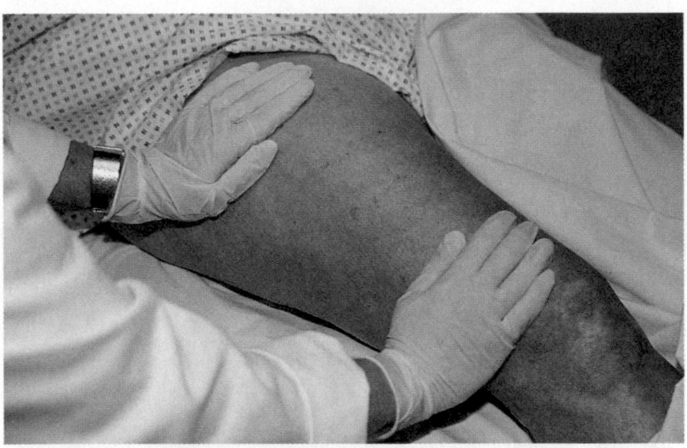

▲ Select site one hand breadth below greater trochanter and one hand breadth above knee for vastus lateralis injection.

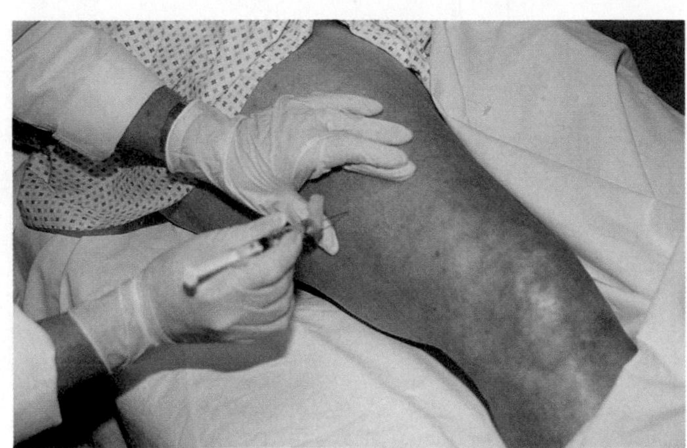

▲ Inject medication at 90° angle directly into muscle.

10. Insert needle perpendicular (90° angle) to the muscle, using a quick, darting motion. ▸ ***Rationale:*** This angle facilitates medication reaching muscle.
11. Pull back on plunger for 5 to 10 seconds; if blood returns, discard and prepare a new injection. ▸ ***Rationale:*** The appearance of blood indicates needle has entered a blood vessel. Medication must not be injected directly into bloodstream.
12. Inject medication slowly (10 seconds per mL). ▸ ***Rationale:*** This allows time for medication to disperse through tissue.
13. Hold needle in place for 10 seconds, then withdraw needle and massage area with dry gauze sponge.
14. Activate needle safety feature.
15. Dispose of syringe/needle unit in puncture-proof container.
16. Return client to comfortable position.
17. Discard gloves and perform hand hygiene.
18. Chart medication and site of injection.

Techniques for Minimizing Pain During IM Injections

- Encourage client to relax.
- Use a new needle for injection.
- Place client on side with upper knee flexed for ventrogluteal injection.
- Have client place hand on hip to relax deltoid muscle.
- Avoid injecting into sensitive or hardened tissue.
- Apply pressure to site for 10 seconds before injecting.
- Ensure that needle length reaches muscle for IM injection.
- Prevent antiseptic from clinging to needle during insertion by waiting until skin prep is dry.

- Reduce puncture pain by "darting" needle quickly into muscle.
- Use as small a gauge needle as possible.

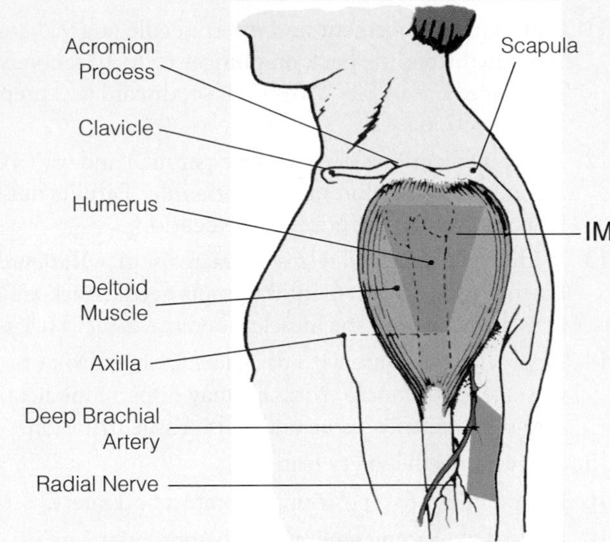

▲ Locate deltoid site in the area between two fingerbreadths below the acromion process and anterior axillary fold.

- Inject medication slowly (10 seconds per mL).
- Hold needle in place for 10 seconds after injecting medication.
- Maintain grasp on syringe; do not move needle once inserted.
- Withdraw needle quickly after injection.
- Use Z-track technique.
- EMLA cream may be applied 30 to 40 minutes before injection.

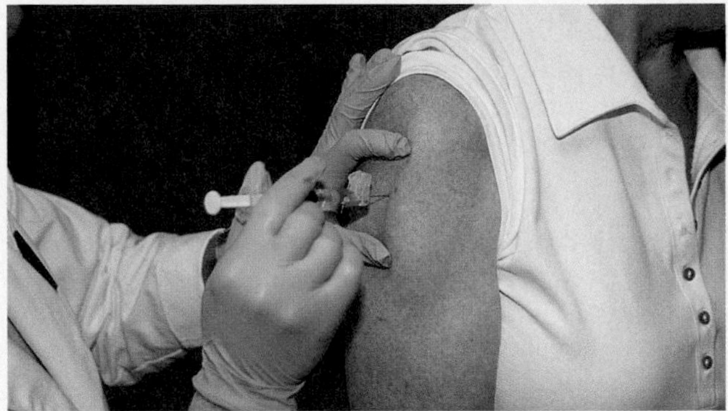

▲ Inject medication into deltoid area site.

EVIDENCE-BASED PRACTICE

Choose the Right Needle Size

A 5/8-in. needle won't reach deltoid muscle in 17% of men and 50% of women. A 1-in. needle is better for men (130–260 lb) and women (132–198 lb).

Source: Zuckerman, J. N. (2000, November 18). The importance of injecting vaccines into muscle. Different patients need different needle sizes. *BMJ, 321*(7271), 1237–1238.

Using Z-Track Method

Equipment

Syringe
Filter needle for preparation
2-in. needle for injection
Medication
Antimicrobial swab
Dry gauze sponge
Gloves (if indicated)

Preparation

See Preparing Injections.

Procedure

1. Use filter needle to draw up prescribed medication into syringe.

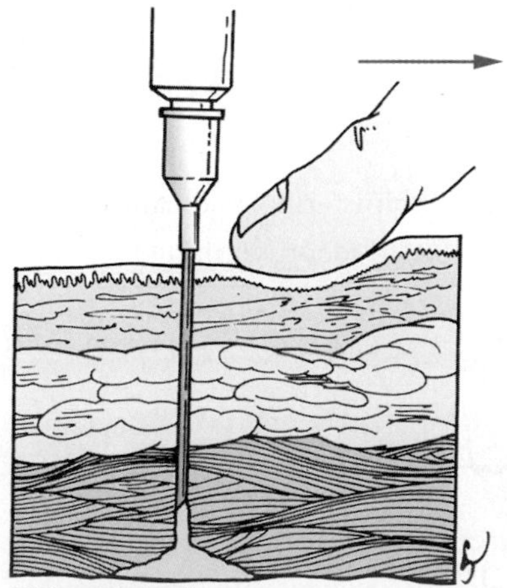

▲ Z-track injection. Maintaining displacement, insert needle at 90° angle. Aspirate by pulling back on plunger, checking to see if needle is in blood vessel. If blood is aspirated, discard and prepare new injection.

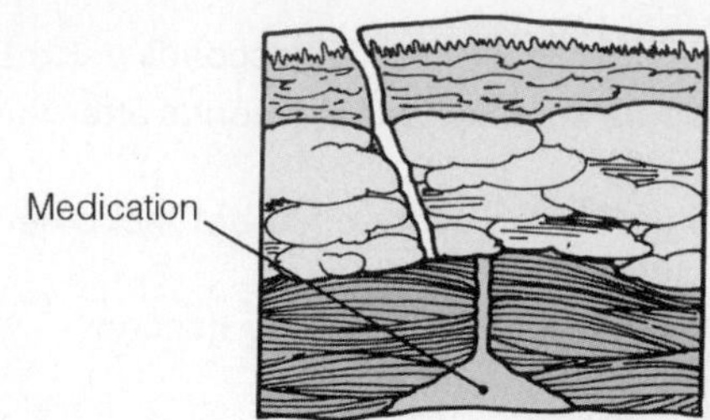

▲ Z-track injection, after displacement released. Method is used to prevent backflow of medications into subcutaneous tissue.

2. Attach new 2-in. sterile needle to syringe. ▸ ***Rationale:*** A new needle prevents introducing medication that could be irritating to tissue. A long needle allows medication to go deep into the muscle.

Clinical Alert

The Z-track method prevents "tracking" and is recommended for administering medications into the ventrogluteal or vastus lateralis sites.

3. Take medication to client's room; check room number against MAR.
4. Check Ident-A-Band, and ask client to state name.
5. Provide privacy.
6. Explain procedure and purpose to client.
7. Perform hand hygiene and don gloves (if indicated).
8. Position client for ventrogluteal or vastus lateralis injection.
9. Cleanse site with antimicrobial swab.
10. Pull skin 1–1½ in. laterally away from injection site. ▸ ***Rationale:*** This tissue displacement creates a track that keeps medication from seeping into subcutaneous tissue.
11. Maintain displacement and insert needle at a 90° angle. Aspirate by pulling back on plunger (5 to 10 seconds) to see if needle is in blood vessel. If so, discard and prepare new injection.
12. Inject medication slowly (10 sec per mL) and wait 10 seconds, keeping skin taut. ▸ ***Rationale:*** Permits muscle relaxation and absorption of medication.
13. Withdraw needle and release retracted skin. ▸ ***Rationale:*** Lateral tissue displacement interrupts needle track and seals medication in the muscle when the tissue is released.
14. Apply light pressure with dry gauze sponge. Do not massage. ▸ ***Rationale:*** Massage may disperse medication into subcutaneous tissue and cause tissue irritation.
15. Activate needle safety feature.
16. Return client to a position of comfort and safety.
17. Discard gloves and equipment in appropriate area.
18. Perform hand hygiene.
19. Document administration of medication in the medication record.

Clinical Alert

If client is obese, use a 2–3-in. needle so that medication is absorbed into muscle (not fat) tissue and blood level of drug is achieved.

DOCUMENTATION for Parenteral Medications

Client's Medication Record

- Time administered
- Name of medication
- Dosage
- Route
- Injection site
- Initials of nurse administering medication
- Signature by nurse (to identify initials)

Nurses' Notes

- Record PRN, STAT, intradermal, and one-time-only medications
- Name of medication, dosage, route, site, time administered
- Client's pre- and post-injection assessment findings (sedation and pain rating, any relevant laboratory data)
- Signature of nurse

CRITICAL THINKING Application

Expected Outcomes

- Injection is administered without complications.
- Injection is as painless as possible.
- Medication therapeutic effect is achieved.

Unexpected Outcomes	Alternative Actions
Ecchymosis occurs after heparin injection.	• Rotate injection site. Do not inject medication into ecchymotic area. • Do not aspirate before injection or massage site after needle withdrawal. • Do not pinch tightly when forming fat pad in preparation for injection site. • Apply ice to area before injecting heparin.
Client experiences pain with IM injection.	• Use Z-track method for ventrogluteal or vastus lateralis sites to prevent medication from leaking into subcutaneous tissue. • Use new needle for injection. • Inject medication slowly (10 sec/mL) to allow medication to diffuse. • Hold needle in place for 10 seconds after injection. • Use a dry gauze sponge to apply pressure to site after withdrawing needle.
Medication is administered using wrong parenteral route.	• Notify physician; medications may need to be administered to reverse the action of the medication. • Monitor client's response closely and report adverse findings immediately. • Medication administered IM or IV rather than subcutaneous route leads to faster absorption rates; therefore ongoing assessment must be done to determine effects. (IV administration has immediate action.) • Complete unusual occurrence report according to agency policy.
Client has allergic or anaphylactic response to medication.	• Call rapid response team immediately. • Maintain a patent airway and follow ABCs of emergency care. • Notify client's physician. • Document incident; place allergy alert bracelet on client. • Complete unusual occurrence report according to agency policy.
Obese client fails to obtain pain relief from subcutaneous injection.	• Consult pain management team. • Consider weight-based dosage. • Obtain order to change to IV route for analgesic administration since adipose tissue has decreased perfusion and subcutaneous medication uptake is unpredictable.

GERONTOLOGIC Considerations

Older clients take more medications than any other age group, largely because of chronic illness. Risk of adverse drug events rises with comorbidity. *Major problems with prescriptive drugs in the elderly include the following:*

- Drug–drug interactions—seniors may use multiple physicians and pharmacies, each unaware of what others have prescribed, creating risk of taking two or more medications to treat the same condition.
- Medication errors—the more medications a person takes, the greater risk of medication error (people over age 75 take an average of 17 prescriptions annually).
- Poor adherence—not taking right dose at right time or discontinuing drug without consultation; common due to lack of understanding about reason to take drug and general knowledge base of drug action. Elders may have difficulty reading labels and directions and opening medicine containers.
- Unpredictable drug action—age-related physiologic changes and comorbid conditions affect drug utilization (absorption, distribution, metabolism, and elimination).
- Drug side effects not recognized—elderly not aware or do not understand potential dangerous side effects of drugs.
- Inadequate monitoring—elderly are often alone or not monitored consistently, so drug problems are not identified.
- Cost of drugs—multiple medications are costly for many elderly, so they may reduce the frequency of dosing or stop taking a drug.

The Elderly Are at Risk for Drug Toxicity

- Drug absorption is altered; oral route is slower, but complete; topical route absorption may increase due to thin skin.
- Drug distribution is altered; increased percentage of body fat in the elderly results in longer storage of fat-soluble medications. The elderly have proportionately less body water, so blood levels of a water-soluble drug may be higher than usual.
- Decreased blood flow through the liver slows medication metabolism.
- Altered renal excretion, slows drug excretion.
- Reduced protein level (increased ratio of fat to muscle) decreases medication binding and increases free circulating drug levels.
- Increased CNS sensitivity to drugs that interfere with neurotransmitters that regulate brain function.

Drugs the Elderly Should Avoid:

- Sedatives/hypnotics
- Tranquilizers (antianxiety medications)
- Anticholinergics (belladonna alkaloids, antispasmodics)

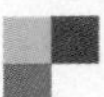

MANAGEMENT Guidelines

Each state legislates a Nurse Practice Act for RNs and LVN/LPNs. Healthcare facilities are responsible for establishing and implementing policies and procedures that conform to their state's regulations. Verify the regulations and role parameters for each healthcare worker in your facility.

Delegation

- Registered and licensed vocational nurses are responsible for administering oral and parenteral medications to clients. In some nonacute facilities, such as residential homes, geriatric technicians may administer medications following standard procedures.
- Individuals administering medications must be knowledgeable about the RATIONALE for their use. This insight cues the need for specific pre- and post-administration individual client assessment (responses such as vital signs, lab values, adverse reactions) as an integral part of this deceptively simple skill.
- Unlicensed assistive personnel are not trained (or expected) to obtain and interpret essential client data necessary for decision making when administering medications. However, if they are assigned to administer daily care, they should be informed what to observe for and report to the RN or LVN/LPN.

Communication Matrix

- *Immediately report to physician:*

  All errors in medication administration (and complete agency variance report)

  Ineffective client responses to medication including adverse responses (vital signs, rash, paradoxical reaction, etc.)

  Reports of abnormal relevant lab data (e.g., toxic drug levels)
- *Report to relief staff:*

  All of the above PLUS:

  Any new or discontinued medication orders PRN, STAT, and one-time-only medications given

  Effectiveness of medication therapy

Drug Supplement

Calculations of Solutions

Types of Solutions

1. Volume to volume (vol/vol): a given volume of solute is added to a given volume of solvent.
2. Weight to weight (wt/wt): a stated weight of solute is dissolved in a stated weight of solvent.
3. Weight to volume (wt/vol): a given weight of solute is dissolved in a given volume of solvent, which results in the proper amount of solution.

Preparing Solutions

Solutions of Varying Strengths

Determine the strength of the solution, the strength of the drug on hand, and the quantity of solution required.

Use this formula for preparing solutions:

$$\frac{D}{H} \times Q = X$$

where D = desired strength; H = strength on hand; Q = quantity of solution desired; and X = amount of solute.

Example: You have a 100% solution of hydrogen peroxide on hand. You need a liter of 50% solution.

$$\frac{50}{100} \times 1{,}000 \text{ mL} = 500 \text{ mL (solute)}$$

If the strength desired and strength on hand are not in like terms, you need to change one of the terms.

Example: You have 1 L of 50% solution on hand. You need a liter of 1:10 solution. 1:10 solution is the same as 10%.

$$\frac{10\%}{50\%} \times 1{,}000 \text{ mL} = 200 \text{ mL (solute)}$$

Add 200 mL of the drug to 800 mL of the solvent to make a liter of 10% solution.

Volume-to-Volume Solutions

Use the formula:

$$\frac{D}{H} \times Q = X$$

Example: Prepare a liter of 5% solution from a stock solution of 50%.

$$\frac{5\%}{50\%} \times 1{,}000 \text{ mL} = 100 \text{ mL}$$

Add 100 mL to 900 mL of diluent to make 1 L of 5% solution.

Solutions From Tablets

Use the formula:

$$\frac{D}{H} \times Q = X$$

where X = amount per number of tablets used.

Example: Prepare 1 L of a 1:1000 solution, using 10-gr tablets.

$$\frac{1/1000}{10 \text{ gr}} \times 1{,}000 \text{ mL} = X$$

First convert 10 gr to grams so the numerator and denominator are in the same unit of measure. 1 g = 15 gr; therefore 10 gr = 2/3g. Now substitute the new numbers in the formula and solve for X.

$$\frac{1/1000}{2/3} \times \frac{1000}{1} \text{mL} = X$$

$$\frac{3}{2000} \times \frac{1000}{1} = X$$

$$X = 2/3 \text{ or } 1\tfrac{1}{2} \text{ tablets}$$

Place $1\frac{1}{2}$ tablets into the liter of solution and dissolve.

Abbreviations and Symbols

aa	of each
a.c.	before meals
ad lib.	freely, as desired
BID	twice each day
$\bar{c}$	With
C	Carbon
Ca	Calcium
Cl	Chlorine
dr *or* ʒ	Dram
et	And
GI	Gastrointestinal
gt *or* gtt	drop(s)
H_2O	Water
H_2O_2	hydrogen peroxide
IM	Intramuscular
K	Potassium
lb *or* #	Pound
m	Meter
mcg	Microgram
mEq	Milliequivalent
mg	Milligram
mL	Milliliter
mmol	Millimole
Na	Sodium
NA	not applicable
NG	Nasogastric
NPO	nothing by mouth
oob	out of bed
oz	Ounce
p.c.	after meals
per	by, through
PO	by mouth
prn, or PRN	whenever necessary
q.h.	every hour
q.i.d.	four times each day
q.s.	as much as required, quantity sufficient
q2h	every 2 hours
q3h	every 3 hours
q4h	every 4 hours
Rx	treatment, "take thou"
$\bar{s}$	Without
STAT	Immediately
TID	three times each day
tsp	Teaspoon
WBC	white blood count
°	Degree
–	minus, negative, alkaline reaction
+	plus, positive, acid reaction
%	Percent
v	Roman numeral 5
vii	Roman numeral 7
ix	Roman numeral 9
xiii	Roman numeral 13

Abbreviation Alert

Abbreviations to Avoid: Entries marked* are prohibited by The Joint Commission

@ (at) misinterpreted as a 2. Write out "at."

AU (each ear) misinterpreted as OU (each eye). Do not use AU. Also avoid AD (right ear) and AS (left ear).

cc (cubic centimeter) misinterpreted as units. Write "mL" for milliliters.

D/C misinterpreted as discharge or discontinue. Write out "discharge" or "discontinue."

Dram symbol (ʒ) misinterpreted as a 3. Write out "dram."

Per os (orally) misinterpreted as OS (left eye). Use "PO."

IN (intranasal) misinterpreted as IM (intramuscular) or IV (intravenous), or as inhaled. Write out "intranasal" and "inhaled."

*IU (international unit) misinterpreted as IV. Write "international unit."

Large doses without properly placed commas (e.g., 100000). Place commas appropriately.

*MS, MSO_4, or $MgSO_4$ confused for one another. Write "morphine sulfate," "magnesium sulfate."

*Q.D. (each day) misinterpreted as qid (four times a day). Write "daily."

*Q.O.D., (every other day) misinterpreted as four times a day. Write "every other day."

qhs (at bedtime) misinterpreted as qh (every hour). Write "at bedtime."

SC or SQ, sub q (subcutaneous) misinterpreted as SL for sublingual. "sub q 2 hours before surgery" has been misinterpreted as "every 2 hours before surgery." Write "subcutaneously."

$\overline{ss}$ (one-half) misinterpreted as 55. Write "one-half."

SSRI (sliding scale regular insulin) misinterpreted as selective-serotonin reuptake inhibitor Write out.

*Trailing zero after a decimal point (e.g., 5.0). Use a zero before a decimal point, never after.

*U (unit) misinterpreted as cc, or 0. Write "unit."

µg (microgram) mistaken for milligram. Write "mcg."

X4d (for 4 days) misinterpreted as times three doses. Write out "for four days."

Conversion Tables

Household Equivalents (Volume)

Metric	Apothecary	Household
0.06 mL	1 minim	1 drop
5(4) mL	1 fluid dram	1 teaspoonful
15 mL	4 fluid drams	1 tablespoonful
30 mL	1 fluid ounce	2 tablespoonfuls
240 mL	8 fluid ounces	1 glassful

Apothecary Equivalents (Volume)

Metric		Apothecary
1 mL	=	15 minims
0.06 mL	=	1 minim
4 mL	=	1 fluid dram
30 mL	=	1 fluid ounce
500 mL	=	1 pint
1,000 mL (1 L)	=	1 quart

Apothecary Equivalents (Weight)

Metric		Apothecary		
1.0 g	*or*	1,000 mg	=	gr xv
0.6 g	*or*	600 mg	=	gr x
0.5 g	*or*	500 mg	=	gr viiss
0.3 g	*or*	300 mg	=	gr v
0.2 g	*or*	200 mg	=	gr iii
0.1 g	*or*	100 mg	=	gr ½
0.06 g	*or*	60 mg	=	gr 1
0.05 g	*or*	50 mg	=	gr ¾
0.03 g	*or*	30 mg	=	gr ½
0.015 g	*or*	15 mg	=	gr ¼
0.010 g	*or*	10 mg	=	gr ⅙
0.008 g	*or*	8 mg	=	gr ⅛
4 g			=	1 dr
30 g			=	1 oz
1 kg			=	2.2 lb

CRITICAL THINKING Strategies

Scenario 1

Your client has recently suffered a "brain attack" (stroke), which has caused him to have difficulty swallowing (dysphagia) and places him at risk for aspiration. When the previous shift nurse attempted to have him take his oral medications with water, he coughed and choked violently, so the nurse discontinued efforts to complete his medication administration. One of this client's most important medications is Inderal LA 80 mg, a timed-release capsule that is given once a day. This long-acting capsule cannot be opened and its contents emptied for convenient administration without interfering with the timed-release property of its formulation.

1. What types of consult would provide assistance in decision making about this client's swallowing problem and medication administration?

2. What actions would facilitate this client's swallowing and decrease the risk of aspiration?
3. What alternative method is there for administering the Inderal LA?
4. How will the nurse communicate adjustments in administration to the other staff members?

Scenario 2

This is Nancy Drew's third hospitalization for diabetic ketoacidosis this year. She has been an insulin-dependent diabetic for 5 years (since age 9). For several years, Nancy has controlled the condition using two daily insulin injections, a combination of regular and NPH (intermediate-acting) before breakfast and dinner.

This year Nancy made the cheerleading A squad—quite an achievement and an honor—requiring practice before and after school, enrollment in gymnastics class, and participation at evening and weekend games, some of which were out of town. In addition, Nancy must attend cheerleading camp this summer and is preparing for all-state competition trials.

Nancy's condition is stabilized during hospitalization, and shortly before discharge she confides in you that she hates needles, that "the shots really hurt," and, in fact, she prepares the syringes and sometimes just throws them away. In addition, she has experienced low blood sugar on occasion while cheerleading and knows that something happens with her insulin "overreacting" at these times; it makes her uncoordinated and "confused," but she just can't take time out to ingest sugar. She is afraid of losing her position on the A squad—she worked so hard to get there.

1. Based on this data, identify Nancy's psychosocial needs and developmental tasks at age 14.
2. What are the implications of insulin absorption and action as influenced by exercise and site of administration?
3. Describe actions that can decrease pain associated with medications.
4. Suggest an alternative way for Nancy to maintain her insulin coverage without discomfort and erratic absorption rates.

Scenario 3

Your elderly client takes many medications at the same time, all for a variety of chronic disorders. She sees several physicians for these various conditions and uses several pharmacies to have prescriptions filled.

When you visit her, she asks you how she can remember to take all her medications, states that she doesn't take all the pills she should each day, and says that she feels fine anyway, without taking her medications.

1. Why do the elderly take so may medications (polypharmacy)?
2. Identify drugs that frequently cause adverse effects in the elderly.
3. Why are the elderly more susceptible to adverse drug events?
4. Identify some ways to protect elderly clients from adverse drug events due to polypharmacy.
5. How can the client's medication regimen be simplified to help prevent adverse drug events?

NCLEX® Review Questions

Unless otherwise specified, choose only one (1) answer.

1. The most common cause of injury due to medications errors is
   1. The wrong client.
   2. The wrong medication.
   3. The wrong dosage.
   4. The wrong route.
2. Before administering a medication that appears to be inappropriate for the client, the nurse should
   1. Consult the pharmacist.
   2. Consult the ordering physician.
   3. Consult the drug manufacturer.
   4. Recheck the medication against the MAR.
3. In general, agents that lower the blood pressure should be held if the client's systolic blood pressure is less than
   1. 110 mmHg.
   2. 100 mmHg.
   3. 95 mmHg.
   4. 90 mmHg.
4. Which of the following alterations of oral medications are acceptable?
   Select all that apply.
   1. Capsules should never be opened.
   2. Beads from capsules may be chewed.
   3. Liquid from capsules can be mixed with food.
   4. Sublingual tablets may be given to the client who is NPO.
   5. Gel-coated tablets can be dissolved to ease swallowing.
5. The inner canthus is pressed to slow absorption of eye drops which
   1. Can cause systemic effects.
   2. Cause a burning sensation.
   3. Dilate the pupil.
   4. Treat eye infections.
6. When administering ear drops to an adult, the nurse positions the pinna
   1. Upward and backward.
   2. Downward and backward.

3. Upward and forward.
4. Downward and forward.

7. Bony landmarks for administering a ventrogluteal injection include
Select all that apply.
   1. Acromion process.
   2. Anterior superior spine of iliac crest.
   3. Posterior superior spine of iliac crest.
   4. Greater trochanter.
   5. Gluteal fold.
   6. Upper outer quadrant of buttocks.

8. Clients should keep track of the number of MDI actuations performed because
   1. The canister's remaining contents may have expired.
   2. The canister's remaining contents may be active ingredient only.
   3. The canister's remaining contents may be propellant only.
   4. Clients become drug tolerant before the canister is empty.

9. When preparing an insulin injection using two solutions, the following order should be used
   1. Add equivalent amount of air to the clear insulin.
   2. Add equivalent amount of air to the cloudy insulin.
   3. Withdraw the cloudy solution.
   4. Withdraw the clear solution.

10. The greatest risk associated with use of an insulin pump is
   1. Site infection.
   2. Lipodystrophy.
   3. Insulin shock.
   4. Ketoacidosis.

19

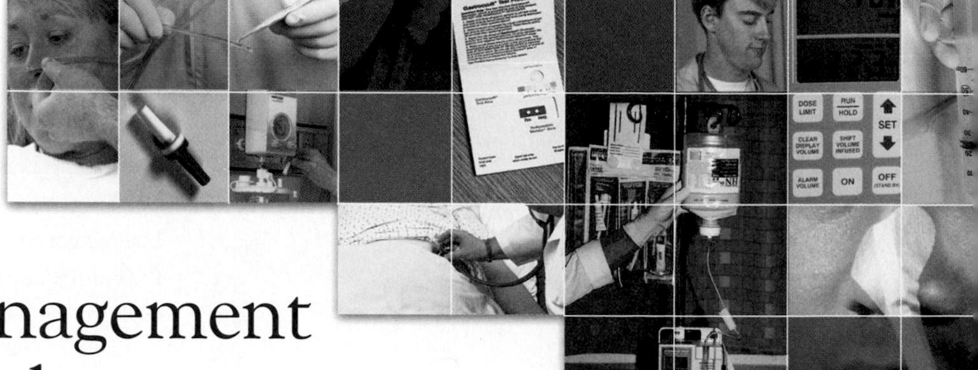

Nutritional Management and Enteral Intubation

LEARNING OBJECTIVES

1. List the essential nutrients necessary to sustain life.
2. Describe the functions of the gastrointestinal system and accessory organs.
3. Identify the categories important for a total nutritional assessment.
4. Discuss feeding techniques and precautions used for dysphagic clients.
5. Identify clients who are candidates for modified diets.
6. List foods that are restricted or supplemented for clients who are receiving modified diets.
7. Outline steps for inserting a nasogastric tube.
8. Describe ways to determine placement of a nasogastric/intestinal tube.
9. Outline the steps of administering a tube feeding.
10. List possible complications of GI tract decompression.
11. Describe emergency management to decontaminate the GI tract of toxins/poisons.
12. Compare and contrast aspects of gastric versus intestinal tube feedings.
13. Discuss problems that may occur with tube feedings.

CHAPTER OUTLINE

TERMINOLOGY

Alimentary of or pertaining to nutrition.

Anabolism reaction in which small molecules are put together to form larger ones—repairing or building up cells.

Anorexia loss of appetite for food.

Aspirate to remove fluids or gases by suction.

Aspiration accidental inspiration of fluid or a foreign body into the airway.

Calorie the amount of heat necessary to raise the temperature of 1 kilogram of water 1°C. This is the "small" calorie. The dietary, or large, Calorie represents 1,000 of these calories, or 1 kilocalorie.

Carbohydrates a group of chemical substances, including sugars, glycogen, starches, dextrins, and celluloses, that contain only carbon, oxygen, and hydrogen.

Cardio prefix pertaining to the heart.

Carina point at which the trachea divides into the right and left bronchi.

Cardiovascular term that pertains to the heart and blood vessels as cardiovascular system.

Catabolism reaction in which large molecules are broken down into smaller ones—process of breaking down cells.

Diabetic one who has inadequate production and/or use of insulin.

Diet liquid and solid food substances regularly consumed.

Digestion the process by which food is broken down mechanically and chemically in the gastrointestinal tract.

Diverticulosis diverticula of the colon without inflammation or symptoms.

Dumping syndrome symptoms that develop due to rapid entry of undigested food into the jejunum.

Dysphagia difficulty swallowing.

Emaciation a condition characterized by extreme leanness or thinness.

Emesis the act of vomiting.

Enteral nutrition provision of nutrients via the gastrointestinal tract (includes oral feedings).

Enterostomy opening into the stomach or jejunum through which a feeding tube can be inserted.

Fat substance made up of carbon, hydrogen, and oxygen, occurring naturally in most foods but especially in meat and dairy products.

Food supplement a preparation added to the regular diet that aids nourishment.

Gavage introduction of nourishment into the GI tract by mechanical means.

Gastrointestinal term that pertains to the stomach and intestines.

Hematemesis vomitus containing blood.

Hydrogenation a chemical process by which hydrogens are added to monounsaturated or polyunsaturated fats, making the fats more saturated, termed *trans fats*.

Hyperalimentation the process of nourishing the body through parenteral means.

Hyperglycemia condition characterized by an increase in blood sugar.

Hypertonic solution having a higher osmotic pressure or tonicity than a solution to which it is compared.

Hypoglycemia condition characterized by a deficiency of sugar or glucose in the blood.

Ileus obstruction of the intestine caused by paralysis of the intestinal muscles.

Ingest the process of taking material into the gastrointestinal tract.

Jejunostomy surgical creation of a permanent opening into the jejunum.

Kwashiorkor a type of protein-energy malnutrition primarily associated with hypermetabolic acute illness such as burns, trauma, sepsis.

Lavage to wash.

Lumen the inner open space of a tube.

Malnutrition a condition characterized by a lack of necessary food substances or improper absorption and distribution of food substances in the body.

Marasmus a type of protein-energy malnutrition due to long-term calorie and protein deprivation resulting in cachexia or severe muscle/fat depletion (COPD, HF, cancer, AIDS).

Minerals inorganic elements or compounds.

Nasogastric tube a tube that is passed through the nose and into the stomach.

Nasointestinal tube small-bore flexible tube passed through the nose and advanced to the proximal intestine to be used for short-term feeding.

Nausea a feeling of sickness accompanied with the urge to vomit.

Nutrient nourishing; food item that supplies the body with necessary elements.

Obstruction blocking of a structure that prevents it from functioning normally; obstacle.

Parenteral nutrition process of providing nutrition via a route other than the alimentary canal, such as intravenous.

PEG percutaneous endoscopic gastrostomy.

Polyunsaturated term usually referring to a fat, indicating that the carbon chain has more than one double bond. These fats tend to have higher densities (HDL) than saturated fats.

Projectile vomiting the expulsion of vomitus with great force.

Proteins substances that contain amino acids essential for growth and repair of tissues.

Renal term that pertains to the kidney.

Saturated fatty acid fatty acid carrying the maximum possible number of hydrogen atoms.

Sepsis Systemic inflammatory response to an infection or cellular injury process.

Trans fat a partially hydrogenated mono- or polyunsaturated fat.

Trauma an injury or wound.

Unsaturated fatty acid fatty acid that lacks hydrogen atoms and has at least one double bond between carbons (includes polyunsaturated and monounsaturated fatty acids).

Uremia toxic condition associated with end-stage renal disease and the retention of nitrogenous substances in the blood.

Vitamin organic substance essential for life.

NUTRITIONAL MANAGEMENT

Food is undeniably necessary for maintenance of life, and is, as a symbol, equally important to man's psychological health. Food has powerful social meaning as it promotes hospitality, companionship, and kinship, and perpetuates ethnic heritage and traditional customs. While these emotional and social aspects are influential in food choices, they are not necessarily based on an awareness of the importance of nutrition in health.

Nutrition is the science of foods, the nutrients and other substances they contain and how they act in our body. These include carbohydrates, fats, proteins, fat-soluble and water-soluble vitamins, minerals, and water, all of which are necessary for life. The body requires a proper balance of nutrients, vitamins, and minerals for energy, growth and development, tissue repair and regulation, and maintenance of body processes. Malnutrition occurs when this balance is disrupted.

TABLE 19-1 Body Mass Index (BMI) Table

	Normal						Overweight					Obese					
BMI	**19**	**20**	**21**	**22**	**23**	**24**	**25**	**26**	**27**	**28**	**29**	**30**	**31**	**32**	**33**	**34**	**35**
Height	Weight (in pounds)																
4′10″(58″)	91	96	100	105	110	115	119	124	129	134	138	143	148	153	158	162	167
4′11″(59″)	94	99	104	109	114	119	124	128	133	138	143	148	153	158	163	168	173
5′ (60″)	97	102	107	112	118	123	128	133	138	143	148	153	158	163	168	174	179
5′1″(61″)	100	106	111	116	122	127	132	137	143	148	153	158	164	169	174	180	185
5′2″(62″)	104	109	115	120	126	131	136	142	147	153	158	164	169	175	180	186	191
5′3″(63″)	107	113	118	124	130	135	141	146	152	158	163	169	175	180	186	191	197
5′4″(64″)	110	116	122	128	134	140	145	151	157	163	169	174	180	186	192	197	204
5′5″(65″)	114	120	126	132	138	144	150	156	162	168	174	180	186	192	198	204	210
5′6″(66″)	118	124	130	136	142	148	155	161	167	173	179	186	192	198	204	210	216
5′7″(67″)	121	127	134	140	146	153	159	166	172	178	185	191	198	204	211	217	223
5′8″(68″)	125	131	138	144	151	158	164	171	177	184	190	197	203	210	216	223	230
5′9″(69″)	128	135	142	149	155	162	169	176	182	189	196	203	209	216	223	230	236
5′10″(70″)	132	139	146	153	160	167	174	181	188	195	202	209	216	222	229	236	243
5′11″(71″)	136	143	150	157	165	172	179	186	193	200	208	215	222	229	236	243	250
6′ (72″)	140	147	154	162	169	177	184	191	199	206	213	221	228	235	242	250	258
6′1″(73″)	144	151	159	166	174	182	189	197	204	212	219	227	235	242	250	257	265
6′2″(74″)	148	155	163	171	179	186	194	202	210	218	225	233	241	249	256	264	272
6′3″(75″)	152	160	168	176	184	192	200	208	216	224	232	240	248	256	264	272	279

Source: Adapted from Evidence Report of Clinical Guidelines on the Identification, Evaluation, and Treatment of Overweight and Obesity in Adults, 1998. NIH/National Heart, Lung, and Blood Institute (NHLBI). Centers for Disease Control and Prevention, United States Department of Health and Human Services.

The body can make some but not all nutrients, and some are made in insufficient amounts. Therefore, it is essential that a person obtain and consume the essential nutrients from exogenous sources. A deficiency of one nutrient causes abnormalities that will usually disappear if the deficiency is corrected. Deficiencies may be the result of decreased dietary intake, a disease condition, or even drug interactions.

RDAs and DRIs

Standards have been established that recommend the amounts of energy, nutrients, other dietary components, and physical activity that best support health. These recommendations are called Dietary Reference Intakes (DRIs), which consist of several component values such as Recommended Dietary Allowances (RDAs). Established Energy Recommendations for dietary energy intake (kilocalories per day) have also been established. These recommendations are based on the requirements of an average healthy person of a particular age, gender, weight, height, and physical activity level so that energy intake does not exceed energy needs in order to help prevent obesity (excess amount of body fat). Obesity is associated with increased morbidity and mortality. It is recommended that body mass index (weight in kilograms, divided by height in meters squared, or weight in pounds multiplied by 704, divided by height in inches squared) should be kept within the range of 18.5 to 24.9.

Energy-producing nutrients, called macronutrients, include carbohydrates, fats, and proteins. The percentage of each macronutrient range recommended to provide adequate energy and nutrients, and to reduce risk of chronic diseases, follows:

45%–65% from carbohydrate	(4 kilocalories per gram)
20%–35% from fat	(9 kilocalories per gram)
10%–35% from protein	(4 kilocalories per gram)

The recommended intakes for nutrients are generous and probably should not be exceeded. Food labels now incorporate a column providing macronutrient and micronutrient (vitamins A and C, calcium, and iron) "% Daily Value." This assists in calculating the particular food's stated serving size energy-yielding nutrient contribution to the total diet (based on a 2,000-kilocalorie daily recommendation).

MACRONUTRIENTS

Carbohydrates

Carbohydrates are the chief source of energy and contain carbon, hydrogen, and oxygen. Carbohydrates include simple sugars, starches, and cellulose. Simple sugars (refined carbohydrates) such as white sugar, white rice, and white flour are easily digested. They cause fluctuations in blood sugar and create a feeling of hunger that can lead to overeating. Starches, which are more complex, require more sophisticated enzyme processes and are more slowly reduced to glucose, the end product of carbohydrate metabolism. Examples include whole grains and some fruits and legumes.

Glucose (converted sugars and starches) appears in the body as blood sugar and is "burned" as fuel by the tissues. Glucose is the only energy source for red blood cells and is the preferred energy source for the central nervous system, placenta, and fetus. A minimum of 100 grams of carbohydrate is essential for daily brain function and to prevent ketosis. Some glucose is processed by the liver, converted to glycogen, and stored by the liver for later use.

The acceptable macronutrient range for carbohydrate is 45%–65% of total calories. Ingesting too many carbohydrate (sugars) supplies calories, but few if any nutrients. The greater the number of high-carbohydrate foods consumed, the more difficult it is to take in essential nutrients without weight gain. It is recommended that individuals select fiber-rich fruits and vegetables and whole grains often, and prepare food with little added sugar. Too few carbohydrates may lead to loss of energy, depression, ketosis, and a breakdown of body protein.

Fats

Fats or lipids are the second important group of nutrients. When oxidized, fats are the most concentrated sources of energy and, as such, furnish the calories necessary for survival. Fats also act as carriers for the fat-soluble vitamins, A, D, E, and K. The optimal percentage of fat in the diet is 20%–35% of our daily caloric intake. Consuming too much fat can lead to weight problems. High-fat diets may increase the risk of developing atherosclerotic cardiovascular disease and cancer.

Fatty acids are the basic components of fat and comprise two main groups: saturated fatty acids and unsaturated fatty acids. Saturated fatty acids usually come from animal sources.

Essential Body Nutrients

- Carbohydrates
  - Monosaccharides
    - Glucose, fructose, galactose
  - Disaccharides
    - Sucrose, lactose, maltose
  - Polysaccharides
    - Starch, dextrin, glycogen, cellulose, hemicellulose
- Fats
  - Linoleic acid, linolenic acid, arachidonic acid
- Proteins
  - Amino acids
    - Phenylalanine, lysine, isoleucine, leucine, methionine, valine, tryptophan, threonine, and histidine (required by infants, not adults)
- Vitamins
  - Fat-soluble
    - Vitamins A, D, E, and K
  - Water soluble
    - B and C vitamins
- Minerals
  - Calcium, chloride, iron, magnesium, phosphorus, potassium, sodium, sulfur
- Water
  - Trace elements

It is recommended to limit total fat and trans fat intake and *substitute* saturated (hydrogenated) fats with polyunsaturated and monounsaturated fats. Saturated fats typically are solid at room temperature and should not exceed 10% of calories; cholesterol and trans fat consumption should be limited to less than 300 mg daily. Unsaturated fatty acids primarily come from vegetables, nuts, or seed sources. The unsaturated group provides two essential fatty acids: linoleic and linolenic acid. These acids are called "essential" because they are necessary for health and growth and the body cannot manufacture them. They must therefore be obtained from the diet.

Proteins

Proteins, the third essential group of nutrients, are complex organic compounds that contain amino acids. Proteins are critical to all aspects of growth and development, necessary for building muscles, blood, skin, internal organs, hormones, and enzymes, and are also a source of energy when there is insufficient carbohydrate or fat in the diet. Protein is either used for tissue repair and maintenance or converted by the liver and stored as fat.

When digested and broken down, proteins form 20 amino acids. Amino acids are then absorbed from the intestine into the bloodstream and carried to the liver for synthesis into tissues and organs of the body. If just one amino acid is missing, protein synthesis is impaired. All but nine of the amino acids are produced by the body. These nine must be obtained from the diet. Eight essential amino acids are required by all, while infants require one more, histidine. If all are present in a particular food, the food is a "complete protein." Foods that lack one or more of these essential amino acids are called "incomplete proteins." Most meat and dairy products are complete proteins, and most vegetables and fruits are incomplete. When several incomplete proteins form the major portion of a person's diet, they should be combined carefully so that the result is a balance yielding complete protein. For example, the combination of beans and rice is balanced to give a complete protein food.

It is difficult to determine the exact amount of protein needed to supply all of the essential amino acids because there are many variables. Height and weight, level of activity, and nutritional and health status all influence the amount of protein necessary for any individual. The National Research Council recommends that 0.42 gram (g) of protein be consumed per day per pound of body weight or 56 g/day for men and 45 g/day for women. The optimal healthy diet should be 10% to 12% protein.

Protein deficiency can affect the entire body—organs, tissues, skin, and muscles—as well as certain body processes. If a child is deficient in protein, he or she may suffer from kwashiorkor, a disease resulting in physical and mental impairment and, if severe enough, death. If an adult is deficient in protein, ability to recover from illness or surgery may be affected.

Protein is very plentiful in the body. It is an integral part of all cells and essential for growth and development. Just like fats and carbohydrates, adequate protein must be consumed in balance with other nutrients for human survival.

Water

Although not specifically a nutrient, water is essential for survival. Water is involved in every body process, from digestion and absorption to excretion. It is a major portion of circulation and is the transporter of nutrients throughout the body.

Body water performs three major functions: it gives form to the body, constituting 50%–75% of the body mass; it provides the necessary environment for cell metabolism; and it maintains a stable body temperature.

Almost all foods contain water that is absorbed by the body. The average adult body contains about 53 liters of water and loses 2.8 liters a day. If a person suffers severe water depletion, dehydration can result and can eventually lead to death. A person can survive several weeks without food, but only days without water. In order to prevent dehydration (water loss exceeding water intake), a general requirement is to drink 2–3 liters of water daily, or 1 mL/kcal expenditure. Measures of intake and output assist the healthcare team in identifying and correcting body water imbalances.

MICRONUTRIENTS

Vitamins

Vitamins are organic food substances and are essential in small amounts for growth, maintenance, and the functioning of body processes. Vitamins are found only in living things—plants and animals—and usually cannot be synthesized by the human body.

Vitamins can be grouped according to the substance in which they are soluble. The fat-soluble group includes vitamins A, D, E, and K. Excessive amounts of vitamins A and E can be quite toxic. The water-soluble vitamins include eight B complex vitamins, vitamin C, and the bioflavonoids. These are usually measured in milligrams.

Vitamins have no calorie value, but they are as necessary to the body as any other basic nutrient. Currently, there are about 20 substances identified as vitamins, but recent research is concerned with identifying even more of these substances since they are so essential to survival.

Minerals

Minerals are inorganic substances, widely prevalent in nature, and essential for metabolic processes. Minerals are grouped according to the amount found in the body. *Major minerals* include calcium, magnesium, sodium, potassium, phosphorus, sulfur, and chlorine, all of which are measured in milligrams. A second group—*trace minerals*—include iron, copper, iodine, manganese, cobalt, zinc, fluorine, selenium, and molybdenum. These minerals are measured in micrograms. Minerals form 60%–90% of all inorganic material in the body and are found in bones, teeth, soft tissue, muscle, blood, and nerve cells.

Minerals act as catalysts for many metabolic processes, and all minerals work synergistically with other minerals; their actions are interrelated. A deficiency of one mineral, therefore, affects the action of others in the body. It is essential that adequate minerals be ingested because a mineral deficiency can result in serious illness. A balanced diet that includes a variety of foods provides most fat-soluble and water-soluble vitamins and minerals.

Refined foods such as rice, pasta, cereals, and products that include these may suffer loss of nutrients during processing. To compensate for these losses, many foods are *enriched* with iron, thiamin, riboflavin, and niacin. Since the 1940s, all grain products are enriched, with folate being added in 1996 to help prevent birth defects. Food labels indicate such enrichment. Additionally, some foods are *fortified* by the addition of nutrients that are not present or are present in insignificant amounts in a food, such as orange juice fortified with calcium and vitamin D.

While some nutritionists and biochemists recommend taking a daily basic vitamin–mineral supplement to ensure adequate levels, the intake of supplements in excess of the Tolerable Upper Level Intake can have toxic systemic effects. Tolerable Upper Intake levels represent the maximum amount of a nutrient that is safe for most people on a daily basis.

As new knowledge surfaces about the importance of nutrients for basic health, the recommended intake reflects this increased awareness.

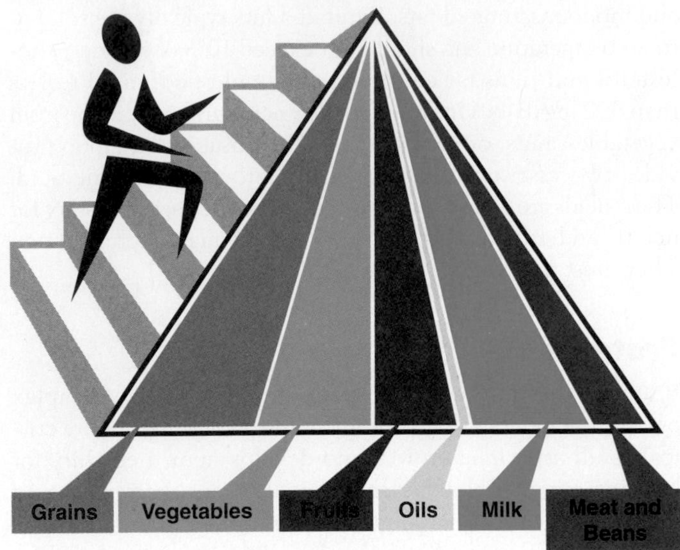

▲ Pyramid symbolizes a personal approach to healthy eating and exercise. *Source:* MyPyramid.gov; USDA, 2005.

NUTRITIONAL ASSESSMENT

Healthy individuals can satisfy essential nutrient recommendations by following a personalized approach to healthy eating and exercise. The *Dietary Guidelines for Americans 2005* MyPyramid, published by the U.S. Department of Agriculture, includes daily intake recommendations for the five food groups (grains, vegetables, fruits, milk, and meat and beans) and liquid oils, symbolized by color bands of different widths. A figure climbs steps up the pyramid as a reminder of the importance of regular physical activity. Color bands emphasize a variety of food groups. The wider base represents foods with little or no solid fats or added sugars. These should be selected more often than the foods at the narrow tip of the pyramid, which contain added sugars and solid fats. More active individuals can add more of these pyramid tip foods to their diet.

These recommendations consider an individual's size, age, and activity level, then estimate daily calorie needs, serving sizes, and activity requirements to prevent weight gain and sustain weight loss, as well as to reduce risk for major chronic diseases. Endorsement of a diet rich in fruits and vegetables provides greater than the median requirement of vitamins and minerals so that supplemental therapy of micronutrients is not necessary. The MyPyramid Food Guidance System provides options to help individuals make healthy food choices and to incorporate physical activity into daily living. Web-based interactive and print materials for consumers are available at www.mypyramid.gov.

No single parameter is sufficient to determine a client's nutritional status. Initial screening of the hospitalized client is performed by the professional nurse on admission.

In general, the nurse asks the client about a recent change in body weight of 10 pounds or more in the last 6 months, nausea, vomiting, diarrhea lasting more than 5 days, any declining food intake, difficulty chewing or swallowing, and time/duration of recent hospitalizations. If results of this initial screening (within 24 hr of hospital admission) classify the client at "nutrition risk," dietitian consult is indicated. Unfortunately, many clients are unable to provide the essential subjective information.

Objective measures of nutritional status include weight in relation to height (body mass index), monitoring dietary intakes with calorie counts, examination for signs of micronutrient deficiencies, and laboratory tests such as serum albumin, transferrin, and prealbumin; tests of cellular immunity; and total lymphocyte count. Other measures include evaluation of body composition by visual inspection or anthropometric measurements (triceps skin fold, midarm muscle circumference). See Nutritional Assessment Parameters, Table 19-2.

EVIDENCE-BASED PRACTICE

The Mini Nutritional Assessment (MNA) is an assessment tool that helps identify older adults who are at risk of malnutrition. A PDF is available, and a video demonstration is posted by the source listed below.

DiMaria-Ghalili, Rose Ann, & Peggi A. Guenter, (February 2008). *The American Journal of Nursing*, 108(2): 50–59.

TABLE 19-2 Nutritional Assessment Parameters

Clinical Assessment	Normal	Abnormal
Dietary Data		
Appetite	Remains unchanged	Increased or decreased recently Particular cravings
Nutritional intake	Adequate foods and fluids to supply body nutrients Nonallergic response to major food groups	Elimination of certain food categories that results in limited nutrients Emphasis on some food groups (sugar) to the exclusion of others (vegetables) Allergic response to certain foods
Caloric intake	Average 28 kcal/kg/day	Constant use of fad diets to lose weight Use of drugs or chemicals that interfere with appetite or nutrient assimilation
Meal patterns	3–6 home-prepared meals/day Adequate time and calm atmosphere for meals	Fast-food or packaged foods Missed meals, constant snacking, or overeating Eating “on the run” or hurried
General Appearance		
	Alert, responsive, healthy-appearing eyes and skin	Listless, dull, nonresponsive Skin and eyes appear unhealthy
Physical factors	Adequate chewing and swallowing capability Mouth and gums healthy so food can be ingested Physical exercise adequate for calorie intake	Teeth or gums in poor condition or ill-fitting dentures Swallowing impairs ingestion Inadequate physical exercise to burn calories
Presence of disease	No disease process that interferes with nutrient assimilation No congenital condition or postsurgery condition that interferes with nutrient assimilation	Disease present that interferes with ingestion, digestion, assimilation, or excretion Congenital condition, rehabilitation phase, or postsurgery that interferes with food assimilation
Elimination schedule	Regular, adequate elimination of foods Absence of constant flatus, discharge, or mucus	Irregular or painful elimination Presence of constant flatus Presence of discharge, blood, or mucus
Anthropometric Measurements		
Height	For bedridden clients, measure arm span—fully extend arms 90° angle to body and measure from tip of one middle finger to the tip of other middle finger for estimated height	Loss of 2–3 inches in height may indicate osteoporosis
Weight—compared to ideal and usual body weight.	Ideal body weight 100 lb (female); 106 lb (male) for 5 feet height + 5 lb for each 1 inch over 5 feet (female) and 6 lb for each 1 inch over 5 feet (male). Small frame minus 10% Large frame plus 10%	Changed—markedly increased or decreased recently: important indicator of changed nutritional status Loss of more than 10% weight for prior 6 months should be clinically evaluated
Body Mass Index Ratio of weight in kilograms and height in meters.	18.5–24.9	Less than 18.5—underweight 25–29—overweight 30–39—obese
Triceps skinfold measurement (mm)	Standard values—male to female 12.5–16.5	If values change over months, may indicate a chronic condition
Circumference of upper arm (cm)	29.3–28.5	
Midarm muscle circumference (cm)	25.3–23.2	Hydration status may influence results

Continued

TABLE 19-2 Nutritional Assessment Parameters (*Continued*)

Clinical Assessment	Normal	Abnormal
Biochemical Assessments*		
Serum albumin	3.5–5.0 g/dL	Examples of possible disease conditions: Decrease signifies lowered nutritional status—protein deficient
Serum transferrin binds iron to plasma and transports to bone marrow	200–430 mg/dL	Reduced levels may indicate chronic diseases and protein deficiency Elevated levels—anemias, liver damage, lead toxicity
Hemoglobin	Male—13.5–17 g/dL Female—12–15 g/dL	Decreased related to iron deficiency (anemias and leukemia)
Prealbumin (PA) serum	20–50 mg/dL	Decreased—protein wasting diseases, malnutrition (<10.7 indicates severe nutritional deficiency) Elevated—Hodgkin's disease
Blood urea nitrogen/creatinine	10:1–20:1	Nitrogen imbalance, inadequate renal functioning; ratio increased in heart failure, decreased renal perfusion.
24-hr urinary nitrogen	Positive balance	Inadequate protein intake
Sociocultural Data		
Cultural–religious factors	Ability to afford adequate foods in all food categories Cultural beliefs that do not eliminate whole food groups Religious beliefs that do not eliminate whole food groups	Economic position that precludes purchase of adequate food Religious or cultural beliefs that interfere with receiving balanced diet (macrobiotic diets) Inadequate knowledge, experience, or intelligence to prepare healthy meals
Ethnicity	Traditional foods that do not eliminate whole food groups	Beliefs and ethnic preference that eliminate major nutrients from the diet
Lifestyle	Well-balanced meals that include all nutrients Food does not lose all nutrient value in preparation	Fast-paced stressful lifestyle that incorporates fast food or convenience foods deficient in nutrients or imbalanced (high-fat)

*Laboratory test parameters differ among laboratories. Check the reference range for the specific lab where the client's blood or urine was tested.

ASSIMILATION OF NUTRIENTS

Nutrients must be broken down by the body. This process is called digestion. It starts in the mouth and continues in the stomach and small intestine.

The total daily energy requirement of an individual is the number of calories needed to replace the energy loss from the metabolic rate, plus loss from a person's physical, emotional, and mental output. The number of calories ingested should be directly related to maintaining an adequate energy level and supporting the body's metabolic processes.

Gastrointestinal System

The gastrointestinal system is comprised of the mouth, esophagus, and intestines, plus accessory organs. The main functions of the gastrointestinal system are the secretion of hormones, enzymes, and hydrochloric acid to digest ingested materials; the movement of the ingested contents through the system; their absorption into the blood; and the storage or elimination of the end products of digestion.

Mechanical digestion begins with chewing of food. When food reaches the stomach, both mechanical and chemical digestive processes occur.

The average meal remains in the stomach for 3 hr, where digestion continues. The stomach's secretion of hydrochloric acid and pepsin break down proteins, while the *acid pH* environment helps protect against ingested pathogens. Vomiting or suction removal of *acid* gastric contents (primarily HCl, Na, and K) can lead to fluid and electrolyte imbalance with metabolic *alkalosis* (high bicarbonate and elevated pH on arterial blood gases [ABGs]). H_2 receptor antagonists (e.g., cimetidine) make gastric secretions less acid, so their administration reduces the risk of metabolic alkalosis and electrolyte disturbance in clients who require gastric secretion suction (decompression).

The stomach's mechanical processes occur with intervals of peristalsis and relaxation of the pyloric sphincter as gastric content (chyme) moves into the small intestine (duodenum). Digestive processes continue within the small intestine (duodenum, jejunum, ileum) as enzymes break down protein to amino acids, fats to glycerol and fatty acids, and carbohydrates to monosaccharides. Here, most nutrients and water are absorbed into the circulation. While 7–10 liters of electrolyte-rich secretions mix with the chyme, only 600–800 mL enters the large intestine. Small intestine secretions have an *alkaline pH*, making this environment more vulnerable to bacterial invasion. *Alkaline* intestinal fluid loss (e.g., due to diarrhea, intestinal decompression) can lead to fluid and electrolyte imbalance with metabolic *acidosis* (low bicarbonate and low pH on ABGs).

The ileocecal valve separates the small intestine from the large intestine. In the large intestine, fluids and electrolytes continue to be absorbed to solidify the stool, and mucus is secreted to lubricate waste as it moves toward the rectum for storage and final elimination of stool, which contains approximately 200 mL water.

The Accessory Organs

The accessory organs of the gastrointestinal tract also play an important role in the utilization of nutrients.

The liver has a major role in the metabolism of carbohydrates, fats, and proteins. In carbohydrate metabolism, the liver converts glucose to glycogen and stores it. The liver then can reconvert glycogen to glucose when the body requires higher blood sugar. The process of releasing carbohydrates (end products) into the bloodstream is called glycogenolysis.

The liver metabolizes fats through the process of oxidation of fatty acids and the formation of acetoacetic acid. Also, the liver forms lipoproteins, cholesterol, and phospholipids and converts carbohydrates and protein to fats.

The liver metabolizes proteins by deamination of amino acids. In this process, the urea and plasma proteins are formed.

The gallbladder functions as a reservoir for bile, which is produced by the liver. When food enters the duodenum, it releases cholecystokinin, which causes the gallbladder to contract and release bile, while the sphincter of Oddi relaxes so that bile enters the duodenum. Here, the bile acids emulsify and digest lipids, which are then absorbed by the intestine.

The pancreas secretes enzymes into the small intestine for the digestion of carbohydrates, fats, and proteins. The enzyme trypsin acts on proteins to produce peptones, peptides, and amino acids. Pancreatic amylase acts on carbohydrates to produce disaccharides, and pancreatic lipase acts on fats to produce glycerol and fatty acids.

In summary, the gastrointestinal tract's primary function is to provide the body with a continuous supply of nutrients by the processes of ingestion, digestion, and absorption.

GASTROINTESTINAL DYSFUNCTIONS

Dysphagia

The voluntary and involuntary actions of swallowing require coordination of several muscles and brain areas. Dysphagia (difficulty swallowing) commonly affects the elder population, especially those in nursing home facilities. Difficulty may be due to dysfunction of neurologic pathways or from dysfunction of muscles of the swallowing tract such as occurs with stroke, dementia, and Parkinson's disease. Dysphagia resulting from stroke is usually temporary, whereas it progresses as part of a general decline in those with dementia or Parkinson's disease. Others who experience dysphagia are those with esophageal obstructive disorders or reflux, and chronic neurologic disorders such as cerebral palsy, multiple sclerosis, polio, amyotrophic lateral sclerosis, and myasthenia gravis.

The most serious complication of dysphagia is aspiration of oropharyngeal secretions, liquid, or food into the lungs, creating an environment conducive to bacterial growth (aspiration pneumonia). This occurs in more than 50% of those with dysphagia. A protective cough normally prevents aspiration, but 50% of clients who aspirate do so silently, *without* coughing, so aspiration goes undetected until pneumonia develops. A complex disorder, dysphagia requires an individualized diagnosis and management by collaborative experts: speech–language pathologist, dietitian, radiologist, and occupational therapist.

GI Hemorrhage

The gastric blood from GI hemorrhage is an irritant that usually triggers vomiting, which may aggravate the bleeding. Clients with impaired liver function are an example of those most likely to experience a gastric bleed, but these clients are also unable to process the protein load created by digestion and absorption of blood. The digestion of blood can cause a precipitous rise in serum ammonia, which can lead to altered neurologic function (somnolence, loss of coordination, coma). Lavage (washing) per gastric intubation removes blood to prevent this "metabolic encephalopathy," and also allows estimation of the client's acute blood loss.

Intestinal Obstruction

When gastrointestinal processes are disrupted, intestinal "obstruction" develops. Cessation of peristalsis (ileus) due to neurogenic impairment (traumatic stress), abdominal pathology, electrolyte imbalance (hypokalemia), or bowel manipulation (as in surgery) may alter GI movement and absorption, allowing secretions and gas to accumulate. The small intestine is the first site to regain motility after surgery (24 hr), then the stomach (2–4 days), and finally the colon (3–7 days). The presence or absence of bowel sounds, however, does not relate to feeding tolerance. Early postoperative nasointestinal or direct small bowel feeding is thought not only to be safe, but also important for maintaining bowel integrity and preventing sepsis. Temporary decompression to remove fluids and gas *may* be necessary in some instances because progressive accumulation of gases and fluid distends the bowel, compresses bowel wall capillaries, and can lead to septic shock, as well as hypovolemic shock. Decompression *may* also alleviate pain, nausea, and vomiting, and reduce the possibility of aspiration.

Decompression Decompression requires the insertion of a nasogastric tube, which is connected to continuous or intermittent negative pressure suction while the client is kept NPO and given IV fluids. Since gastrointestinal secretions are isotonic with extracellular fluid, a guideline for fluid replacement is to administer a volume of normal saline (or one-half normal saline with KCl) equivalent to the previous day's drained secretions. A unique feature of the GI tract is that its nutrition is derived directly (rather than from the bloodstream), so early ambulation, termination of decompression, and resumption of PO intake are recommended. The passage of flatus, bowel movement, and tolerance of oral intake are indicators that GI function has returned and is able to accommodate PO intake.

NORMAL AND THERAPEUTIC NUTRITION

Normal nutrition is based on recommended daily dietary allowances designed for the maintenance of health. While these standards have been established for nutrition requirements of an average healthy person, therapeutic modification of nutritional needs may be based on a client's disease condition associated with an excess or deficiency of a particular nutrient. Therapeutic diets may include alterations of minerals, vitamins, proteins, carbohydrates, fats, and fluids, as well as alterations of their consistency to facilitate the client's intake. Whether a normal or therapeutic diet has been ordered based on the client's physiologic status, the client's cultural, socioeconomic, and psychologic influences must also be taken into account. The nutritional requirements must be considered within the context of the total needs of the individual client.

Eating and mealtime are considered by many to be a "social" event. Hospitalized clients, however, may be isolated from others, so that eating is not a pleasure. Painful or uncomfortable procedures should be planned so that they are not immediately before or after meals. The client should be in a position as near to normal as possible: sitting in a chair or with the head of the bed elevated 90°. The environment should be bright and free of offensive odors. Client allergies should be noted; personal preferences and cultural or religious restrictions should be honored. Food trays should be checked for compliance with the physician's order. If the client is NPO, a sign may be posted on the unit door so that the client does not receive a tray.

When you are preparing to assist the client to eat, lower the side rail and place the tray table over the client's lap low enough so that he or she can see what is on it. If the tray is not neatly arranged, rearrange it. Food appearance and presentation influence appetite. Assist the client with whatever is needed, such as cutting meat. If the client is unable to drink from a glass, provide a straw or special cup.

Be sensitive to the client's response to food, and continually attempt to orient feeding to meet the client's needs. If the client has impaired vision but is able to self-feed, tell the client what is on the tray and the position of each item. Often, it is clearer to describe position of foods by a clock; for example, chicken at 12, green beans at 3 o'clock.

When therapeutic diets are ordered, it is critical to be sensitive to the client's acceptance of any restrictions or supplements and to help the client understand their purpose. The nurse is most closely involved with the client and can best determine the client's actual intake. The nurse should ensure that the client is not receiving inappropriate foods from other sources and that the client is actually eating the foods prescribed.

Nutrition Problems in the Hospital

Nutrition may be overlooked as a vital component of a hospitalized client's care. For clients who seem to be stable on admission and give no history of nutrition-related problems, the usual hospital diet is adequate; however, all clients must be reassessed periodically to detect and prevent nutritional problems. Fear, anxiety or depression, poorly fitting dentures, and even medications and therapies may limit a client's ability to eat or may interfere with his or her appetite. Some clients may have the desire to eat and have a good appetite, but shortly after eating certain food, experience cramps, pain, or diarrhea or feel nauseated or vomit. This may lead to decreased food intake. Clients may become more malnourished the longer they remain in a hospital for a variety of reasons that limit food intake.

Well-nourished clients can tolerate a short period of caloric balance deficit such as that occurring with a brief illness or surgery, because the body's fat stores provide calories during such periods. Nutrient guidelines for healthy persons, however, are not meant to meet the needs of clients whose nutritional status is altered by illness that affects oral intake and nutrient digestion, absorption, or utilization. Protein-energy malnutrition is widely seen in hospitalized clients due to acute illness and protein-deficient diets (kwashiorkor) or long-term calorie and protein deprivation with cachexia or severe muscle/fat depletion (marasmus). Protein-energy malnutrition is commonly seen in the obese or diabetic client as well, and while the client may not appear to be malnourished visually, nutrition parameters reveal a malnourished state.

Studies indicate that malnutrition (protein-energy deficiency) is present in as many as 50% of hospitalized clients and that clients become more malnourished the longer the hospital stay. Clients with negative nitrogen balance (reduced serum albumin, reduced prealbumin) have already lost structural and functional proteins and have poor surgical outcome, increased infection rates, and prolonged hospital stays. As malnutrition progresses, all major organ systems, fluids and electrolytes, and immune system dysfunction develops.

Enteral Feeding for Nutritional Support

Enteral nutrition may be prescribed for clients who are unable or unwilling to eat or those who need a supplement to ingested food, as well as for clients in catabolic states with intensive caloric requirement (e.g., burn, trauma clients).

Enteral feeding is preferred over parenteral (intravenous) nutrition because it is safer, less expensive, and associated with fewer complications. It helps to maintain GI function and speeds regeneration of the small intestine, which receives its nutrition from food directly rather than from the bloodstream. Enteral nutrition preserves production of humoral antibodies, reduces gut bacterial overgrowth, and, by helping to maintain the gut's protective mucosal barrier, promotes gut motility, and reduces risk of sepsis. Since the small intestine is less prone to ileus than the stomach and large intestine, postoperative feeding into the small intestine is feasible even though the client is NPO.

Enteral formulas come in powder form to reconstitute or as ready-to-use liquids. They contain all or just one of the following: protein, carbohydrates, fat, electrolytes, and vitamins and minerals, depending on the client's needs. Isotonic formulas provide 1 cal/mL and are most commonly used. Modified formulas are available for clients with specific nutritional requirements: lactose-free or lactose-containing, fiber-containing, elemental (predigested), or modular formulations that provide additional macronutrient components (lipid, carbohydrate, or protein). Specialized formulas are also available for trauma clients or those with pulmonary disease, renal failure, diabetes, liver failure, or immune deficiency.

Many types of nasogastric/nasointestinal tubes are available for enteral feeding. Large-bore nasogastric tubes are inserted for short-term (1 week) intermittent feedings which are delivered by gravity through a syringe or by an infusion pump 4–6 times daily. If nutritional support is indicated for an extended period (4 weeks), a long, soft, flexible, small-bore tube made of silastic or polyurethane is placed naso or orointestinally (advanced beyond the pylorus). Small-bore tubes are more comfortable for the client. Since feeding is by continuous infusion using a pump, the client's position must be kept with head of bed elevated 30° or greater to decrease risk of aspiration. Feeding into the small intestine is associated with greater risk of infection due to the intestine's alkaline (less protected) environment.

For clients with a history of gastric reflux or tube feeding–related aspiration pneumonia, a small-bore jejunostomy tube may be placed surgically or by laparoscopy. Special "dual-purpose tubes" (e.g., Moss tube) can be placed at the time of surgery to provide gastric decompression and simultaneous (early postoperative) feeding into a functional small intestine while the client is NPO.

For *extended nutritional support* (feeding over 4 weeks), tube enterostomies are created surgically through the abdominal wall, directly into the stomach (gastrostomy, percutaneous endoscopic gastrostomy [PEG], or small intestine jejunostomy). Directly placed tubes are secured by stabilizing bars (bumpers), a large mushroom tip, or a balloon inflated with water (similar to a urinary retention catheter).

CULTURAL AWARENESS

Cultural Accommodations for Special Diets

When a special diet is prescribed, it should be consistent with the client's cultural preferences and religious practices. For example, Jewish people do not combine certain foods. So, to comply with kosher laws, do not combine meat and dairy products at the same meal.

Food Is One of the Most Interesting Aspects About Any Culture

- American acculturation tends to replace traditional habits, tastes, and preferences with a detrimental switch to highly processed foods.
- This may account for increased rates of illness and death from heart disease and cancer in some populations.
- While not all cultural food habits are healthy, they are usually higher in fiber and vitamins than the typical American diet and should be encouraged.

General Recommendations

- Food preferences should be maintained.
- Focus education on food practices and preparation, possible health hazards, and importance of role modeling for children.

NURSING DIAGNOSES

The following nursing diagnoses are appropriate to use on client care plans when the components are related to nutritional problems or nutritional health maintenance.

NURSING DIAGNOSIS	RELATED FACTORS
Aspiration, Risk for	CVA, neuromuscular disease, NG intubation, artificial airway, decreased level of consciousness, oral/cervical surgery
Dentition, Impaired	Poor oral hygiene, oral surgery, injury, ill-fitting dentures
Knowledge, Deficient	Lack of appropriate dietary information, misinterpretation of information, cognitive limitation, inadequate motivation
Noncompliance	Chronic illness, disease-related symptoms, side effects of therapy, financial status, cultural practices
Imbalanced Nutrition: Less Than Body Requirements	Impaired swallowing, faulty metabolism, altered level of consciousness, inadequate absorption, eating disorders
Imbalanced Nutrition: More Than Body Requirements	Lack of basic nutritional knowledge, excessive intake in relation to metabolic requirements, decreased activity patterns, decreased metabolic needs, eating disorders
Impaired swallowing	Esophageal obstructive disorder, chronic neurologic disorder (multiple sclerosis, ALS, myasthenia gravis), muscle dysfunction (stroke, dementia, Parkinson's dsisease)

CLEANSE HANDS The single most important nursing action to decrease the incidence of hospital-based infections is hand hygiene. *Remember to wash your hands or use antibacterial gel before and after each and every client contact.*

IDENTIFY CLIENT Before every procedure, check two forms of client identification, not including room number. These actions prevent errors and conform to the Joint Commission standards.

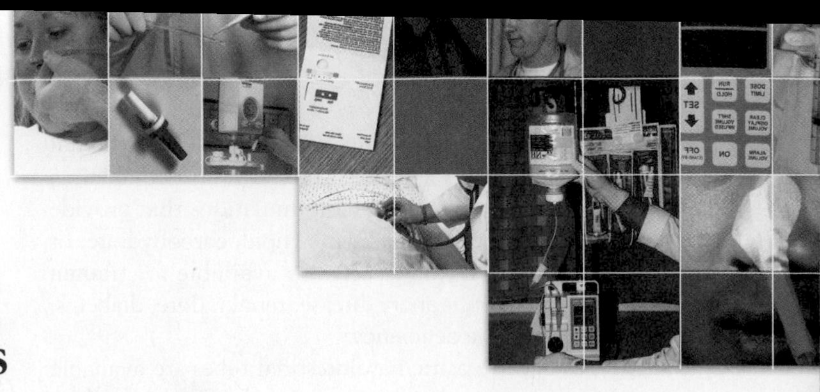

Chapter 19

UNIT 1

Modified Therapeutic Diets

Nursing Process Data

ASSESSMENT Data Base

- Refer to general assessment parameters (physical and laboratory findings) in chapter introduction.
- Assess client's dietary preferences.
- Assess client's health status that necessitates diet modification.
- Identify disease state, which may necessitate dietary modification (e.g., cardiac, pulmonary, renal disease).
- Determine whether registered dietitian has consulted to assist with diet design.

PLANNING Objectives

- To meet nutritional needs of clients with altered health status
- To provide a therapeutic diet that is acceptable to client's taste and cultural orientation
- To provide specialized dietary information to promote client's adherence

IMPLEMENTATION Procedures

EVALUATION Expected Outcomes

- Therapeutic diet assists in management of client's altered health status.
- Client accepts therapeutic diet prescribed to help manage altered health status.
- Client demonstrates understanding (verbalized knowledge) of dietary information provided.

Restricting Dietary Protein

1. A **restricted protein diet** is used for clients with renal insufficiency, hepatic coma, and cirrhosis (according to individual requirements).
   a. Control end products of protein metabolism (nitrogenous waste) by limiting protein intake.
   b. Protein allowance is decreased to 0.5–0.6 gm/kg/day (pre-dialysis).
   c. Limits high-protein foods, such as eggs, meat, milk, and milk products.
2. A **PKU diet** is an amino acid metabolism abnormality diet used for phenylketonuria (PKU), galactosemia, and lactose intolerance.
   a. Reduce foods that contain compounds that cannot be metabolized correctly.
   b. Avoid milk and milk products.
   c. Provide substitutes to meet daily allowances.

Restricting Dietary Fat

1. A **restricted fat diet** is used to reduce risk for and to manage cardiovascular diseases, diabetes mellitus, and high serum cholesterol levels. It focuses on restriction of saturated (hydrogenated) fats, trans fats (found in fast and fried foods), and cholesterol to treat dyslipidemia and reduce risk for atherosclerosis. These fats are solid or semi-solid at room temperature.
   a. Lipid levels goals = total cholesterol <200mg/dL, LDL-C<100 mg/dL, HDL-C> 45 males and 55 females mg/dL, and triglycerides < 150 mg/dL.
   b. Restrict total fat to less than 30% of calories, achieve normal body weight by reducing calorie intake; restrict saturated fat to 7% of calories and reduce cholesterol to 200 mg per day.
   c. Higher percentage may be allowed if saturated and trans fats are substituted with monosaturated fats found primarily in plant products (olive oil, canola oil, avocados, pecans, almonds); use low-fat or nonfat products; increase intake of fruits and vegetables, whole grains, legumes, and seeds.
   d. Limit high-cholesterol foods found in animal products, such as egg yolk, red meat, shellfish, organ meats, bacon, and pork.
2. A **modified-fat diet** is used according to individual tolerance in malabsorption syndromes (cystic fibrosis, gallbladder disease, obstructive jaundice, pancreatitis, and liver disease).
   a. Attempt to lower fat content in diet when there is inadequate absorption of fat or when excessive fat aggravates a condition.
   b. Avoid such foods as gravies, fatty meat and fish, cream, fried foods, rich pastries, whole-milk products, cream soups, salad and cooking oils, nuts, and chocolate. Allow eggs (3–5 per week), lean meat, and small amount of butter or butter substitute.

Restricting Mineral Nutrients (Sodium, Potassium)

1. A **restricted sodium diet** is used to manage hypertension, liver disease, heart failure (edema), and renal insufficiency.
   a. Correct or control the retention of sodium and water in the body by limiting sodium intake. May include restriction of salt in the diet or in combination with medications.
   b. Sodium restriction may allow lower dosage of diuretic use.
   c. Restrict salt in cooking or at the table. May prohibit any product containing sodium, such as soda bicarbonate (typical diet provides 4–6 g of sodium/day).
   d. Explain sodium restrictions in diet.
      Mild: 2–3 g of sodium (no added salt provides 2–3 g of sodium/day)
      Moderate: 1,000–1,500 mg of sodium
      Strict: 500 mg of sodium
      Be aware of sodium content of some medications (e.g., antacids).
2. Potassium may be restricted for the renal client.

Foods High in Sodium and Potassium

Foods High in Sodium
- Table salt and all prepared salts, such as celery salt
- Smoked meats and salted meats
- Most frozen vegetables or canned vegetables with added salt
- Butter, margarines, and cheese
- Quick-cooking cereals
- Shellfish and frozen or salted fish
- Seasonings and sauces
- Canned soups
- Chocolates and cocoa
- Beets, celery, and selected greens (spinach)
- Anything with salt added, such as snack chips, popcorn

Foods High in Potassium
- Fruit juices, such as orange, grapefruit, banana, raw apple
- Instant, dry coffee powder
- Egg, legumes, whole grains
- Fish, fresh halibut, codfish
- Pork, beef, lamb, veal, chicken
- Milk, skim and whole
- Dried dates, prunes
- Bouillon and meat broths
- Salt substitute

Providing Consistent Carbohydrate Diets

1. Nutrition is one of the cornerstones of treatment for diabetes.
   a. Foods included on the diet are balanced and provide protein, fat, and carbohydrates in relation to an individual's needs.
   b. Foods limited are refined or simple sugars.
   c. Counting grams of carbohydrates and using the glycemic index (describes how much blood glucose level rises with a specific food when compared with an equivalent amount of glucose) are nutritional tools for managing diabetes.
   d. Equal (consistent) amount of carbohydrate is provided at each meal to ease management of blood sugars.
2. Reactive hypoglycemia occurs when the pancreas over-secretes insulin post-prandially and most of the glucose moves from blood into cells, resulting in abnormally low blood glucose levels.
   a. Foods prescribed are a combination of foods high in protein and a variety of complex carbohydrates, consumed in five or six small meals per day.
   b. Foods restricted are simple carbohydrates; for example: juices, white sugar, white rice, and white flour.

Providing Nutrient-Enhanced Diets

1. An **increased potassium diet** is used to compensate for potassium loss due to certain diuretics or steroids, burns, vomiting, fever, and COPD and may have an antihypertensive effect.
   a. Replace potassium loss from the body with specific foods high in potassium or a potassium supplement. Severe loss is managed with intravenous replacement therapy.
   b. Avoid no specific foods unless there is a sodium restriction (some foods high in potassium are also high in sodium).
   c. Reduced sodium intake reduces potassium loss.

Refeeding Syndrome

The *refeeding syndrome* first noted in individuals refed after famine and war is a potentially life-threatening complication of aggressive specialized *nutrition repletion*/support. This complication can occur regardless of the route of feeding, whether parenteral, enteral, or even oral. Semistarved marasmic or fasting clients, those with morbid obesity, anorexia nervosa, or chronic alcoholism whose bodies have adapted to using free fatty acids and ketone bodies for energy can develop hypophosphatemia, hypokalemia and hypomagnesemia, altered glucose metabolism, and fluid shifts associated with hematologic, neuromuscular, cardiac, and respiratory dysfunction when large amounts of carbohydrate feedings are reintroduced. Sudden expansion of extracellular (intravascular) fluid can result in cardiac decompensation, and administration of dextrose can result in hyperglycemia with osmotic diuresis and dehydration.

When nutritional support therapies are initiated in malnourished clients, caloric goals should be achieved gradually (3–4 days) while the client's cardiopulmonary response, serum electrolytes, and glucose are closely monitored.

Source: Gottschlich, M., ed. (2001). Chapter 9: Complications of Enteral Nutrition Therapy. *The Science and Practice of Nutrition Support*. American Society for Parenteral and Enteral Nutrition. Dubuque, Iowa: Kendall/Hunt Co.

2. A **high-iron diet** is used to manage anemias (blood loss, nutritional), and malabsorption syndrome.
   a. Replace a deficit of iron caused by inadequate intake or chronic blood loss.
   b. Include foods high in iron content, such as meats (especially organ meats), egg yolks, seafood (especially shellfish), and plant-based sources such as whole-wheat products, leafy vegetables, nuts, dried fruit, and legumes.
   c. Vitamin C enhances absorption of plant-based iron.
3. A **high-calcium diet** is used to prevent osteoporosis and prevent and treat hypertension.
   a. Increases normal adult intake of 1 g/day to 1.5 g/day for postmenopausal female.
   b. Recommends use of *fortified* low-fat and nonfat dairy products, fruit juices, and oatmeals.
   c. Clients who are lactose intolerant should use leafy green vegetables and nonliquid dairy products (cheese, yogurt) or lactose-free dairy products, fish products, and almonds.

Providing Progressive Diets

For Dietary Fiber

1. There are two types of fiber: Insoluble fiber found in cell walls of plants does not dissolve in water, so it speeds elimination of waste products, and soluble fiber (oat bran) dissolves in water and decreases intestinal speed, decreases blood cholesterol levels, and slows absorption of glucose, so blood sugar levels are reduced in diabetes.
2. A *low-fiber diet* is used during phases of intestinal diseases and may be used preoperatively and postoperatively during transition to a regular diet.
   a. Long-term fiber restriction is discouraged.
   b. Inform client that low-fiber foods are ground meat, fish, broiled chicken without skin, limited fat, refined strained cereals, white bread, and possibly limited milk products.
3. A *high-fiber diet* is prescribed to treat constipation and diverticulosis.
   a. Includes foods high in fiber such as beans, fruits, vegetables, nuts, whole grain breads and cereals, and especially unrefined bran.
   b. Fluid intake should be increased as fiber is increased in the diet.

For Postoperative Diet Progression

1. A special postoperative surgical diet may be necessary to promote wound healing, to avoid hypovolemia due to decreased plasma proteins and circulating red blood cells, and to prevent edema.
   a. For tissue repair and extensive stress states, energy needs should be determined by a specialist for tissue repair needs and extensive stress states.
   b. Fluid intake is 2–3 liters per day for uncomplicated surgery and 3–4 liters for sepsis. Clients with extensive wound drainage may require more fluid intake.

Nutrient Requirements for Healing*

- Total calories per day:
  1. 2,800 for tissue repair
  2. 6,000 for extensive repair
- Protein:
  1. 40–50 g/day average person
  2. 50–75 g/day early in postoperative period
  3. 100–200 g/day if needed for new tissue synthesis
- Carbohydrates:
  1. 55%–60% of calories—sufficient in quantity to meet calorie needs and allow protein to be used for tissue repair
- Fat:
  1. 25%–30%—not excessive as it leads to poor tissue healing and susceptibility to infection
- Vitamins:
  1. Vitamin C—up to 1 g/day for tissue repair
  2. Vitamin B—increased above normal for stress management
  3. Vitamin A—adjuncts autoimmune system
  4. Vitamin E—increases O_2 to tissues
- Minerals:
  1. Zinc—tissue repair
  2. Selenium—cell repair
  3. Calcium/magnesium—relaxes nerves and maintains electric function

*This is an example of nutrients necessary for healing. Each diet should be individualized and a dietary consult is required.

2. Diet progression may consist of nothing by mouth (NPO) the day of surgery and advance to a regular diet as soon as tolerated. A progressive diet may include the following diets:
   a. **Clear liquid diet** 1,000–1,500 mL/day of liquid foods such as water, tea, broth, gelatin, and pulp-free juices or clear carbonated beverages.
   b. **Full liquid diet** lacks many nutrients, so is used temporarily. Includes any food that is liquid at room temperature—clear liquids, milk and milk products, custard, puddings, creamed soups, sherbet, ice cream, and any fruit juice.
   c. A **surgical soft diet** is full liquid plus pureed vegetables, eggs (not fried), milk, cheese, fish, fowl, tender beef, veal, potatoes, and cooked fruit. Include foods that are easy to chew and digest and limited in fiber; do not include gas-formers.
   d. **General diet:** Take into consideration client's tolerance and preferences.

Providing Altered Food Consistency Diets

For Bland Diet

1. A bland diet is used to promote the healing of the gastric mucosa by eliminating food sources that are chemically and mechanically irritating. Bland diets may be used to manage duodenal ulcers, gastric ulcers, and postoperative gastric surgery.
   a. Instruct client that bland diets are presented in stages with the gradual addition of certain foods.
   b. Provide frequent, small feedings during active stress periods.
2. Establish regular meals and food patterns when condition permits.
3. Foods allowed include:

   milk, butter, eggs (not fried), custard, vanilla ice cream, cottage cheese
   cooked refined or strained cereal, enriched white bread
   gelatin; homemade creamed, pureed soups
   baked or broiled potatoes
4. Examples of foods that are eliminated include:

   spicy and highly seasoned foods
   raw foods
   very hot and very cold foods
   gas-forming foods (varies with individuals)
   coffee, alcoholic beverages, carbonated drinks
   high-fat-content foods (some butter and margarine allowed)

For Mechanical Soft Diet

1. A mechanical soft diet is used when clients
   a. Are edentulous.
   b. Have poorly fitted dentures.
   c. Have difficulty chewing.
   d. Do not chew food thoroughly.
2. Any food that can be easily digested can be included in this diet. It allows clients variations in tastes that are not allowed on a soft diet (chili beans).

For Pureed Diet

1. A pureed diet provides food that has been mashed, minced, or ground.
   a. Used for clients with dysphagia.
   b. Used for clients with limited chewing ability.
2. When assisting clients with this type of diet, talk with them about the meal, describing the different foods. When the texture is all the same, distinguishing between foods is difficult.
3. Do not mix all pureed food together or feed out of one bowl or dish. Try to keep foods separate and feed alternately, with dessert last.

For Blenderized Liquid Diet

1. Contains food and liquid that are blenderized to liquid form.
2. Used for persons who cannot chew, swallow, or tolerate solid food; or may be used for gastrostomy feeding.

DOCUMENTATION for Modified Therapeutic Diets

- Type of diet provided
- Client's daily weight
- Intake and output
- Client's understanding of dietary restriction
- Any client or family teaching provided
- Nutritional consult requested
- Client's tolerance of diet progression
- Community agency referral offered

CRITICAL THINKING Application

Expected Outcomes

- Therapeutic diet assists in management of client's altered health status.
- Client accepts therapeutic diet prescribed to help manage altered health status.
- Client demonstrates understanding (verbalized knowledge) of dietary information provided.

Unexpected Outcomes	Alternative Actions
Client does not adhere to diet.	• Elicit client's feelings to determine reason for nonadherence. • Check method of diet preparation and administration to see if it is attractive and appealing. • Ensure that environment is conducive to eating. • Notify dietitian to discuss diet with client.
Client with sodium-restricted diet states that food has no taste.	• Recommend use of lemon, herbs, and spices to add flavor to foods. • Encourage client to avoid processed foods, frozen entrees, salty snacks. • Inform client that salt craving decreases over time with change in diet. • Consult physician for recommendation of potassium-containing salt substitute.
Client states that fat is fat and all fats are to be avoided in preference to carbohydrates.	• Suggest client remove all visible fat from and limit intake of red meats. • Encourage to substitute poultry (skin removed) and fish for red meat. • Limit intake of butter, salad dressings, trans fat (partially hydrogenated) products. • Use low-fat or nonfat products. • Increase intake of fruits, vegetables, and legumes.
Postmenopausal client has lactose intolerance but is concerned about need for increased calcium to prevent osteoporosis.	• Consult with registered dietitian. • Encourage intake of nonliquid dairy products (yogurt, cheese) or lactose-free dairy products. • Suggest intake of leafy vegetables, canned fishes. • Calcium carbonate supplements are best absorbed. • Recommend calcium carbonate supplement in low dose (500 mg or less), several times/day for better absorption and efficacy.

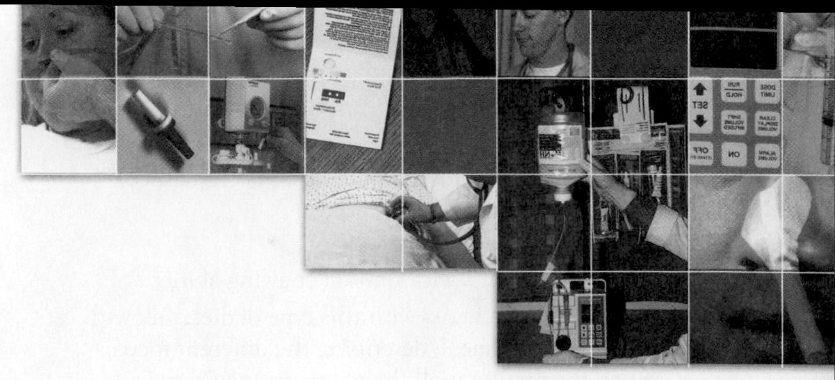

Chapter 19

UNIT 2

Nutrition Maintenance

Nursing Process Data

ASSESSMENT Data Base

- Check physician's or consultant's diet order.
- Determine client's sociocultural orientation.
- Obtain client's diet history and determine eating habits and food preferences.
- Determine if client is candidate for dietitian or speech pathologist consultation.
- Assess client's risk for aspiration.
- Check for specific instructions for positioning and feeding technique for the dysphagic client.

PLANNING Objectives

- To provide a diet that meets nutritional requirements and is acceptable to client
- To assist the visually impaired client to self-feed
- To assist the dysphagic client to eat

IMPLEMENTATION Procedures

EVALUATION Expected Outcomes

- Diet meets nutritional requirements and is acceptable to client's taste and cultural orientation.
- Visually impaired client is able to self-feed.
- Dysphagic client is able to eat using adaptations to prevent aspiration.

Serving a Food Tray

Equipment

Diet slip completed
Diet tray
Over-bed table
Utensils
Protective covering (e.g., towel)

Preparation

1. Check client's chart for physician's diet order.
2. Obtain dietary consult, if necessary, to meet client's needs.
3. Elicit food preferences of the client.
4. Check all diet trays before serving to ensure the diet provided is the one ordered.
5. Ensure that hot food is hot and cold food is cold.
6. Keep food trays attractive. Avoid spilling liquids on tray.
7. Assist client to empty bladder (if needed) and perform hand hygiene.
8. Remove unpleasant objects from area.

Procedure

1. Identify client by checking Ident-A-Band and having client state name and birth date.
2. Perform hand hygiene and assist client to do so.
3. Assist client to sit in a chair, or elevate the head of the bed to 90°.
4. Place protective covering over client's chest.
5. Place food tray on over-bed table and adjust the table so client can see the food.
6. Assist client as needed (cut meat, open containers).
7. Leave call light in client's reach and check on client periodically.
8. Reposition tray table at bedside when meal is completed.
9. Assist client with hand and oral hygiene if desired.
10. Position client for comfort.
11. Note percentage and type of food eaten.
12. Remove food tray from room.
13. Document percentage and type of food eaten and, if indicated, amount of liquid intake on I&O record.
14. Perform hand hygiene.

Clinical Alert

Clients sensitive to latex have potential for serious allergic reactions to some plant proteins. Cross-reactivity to latex has been shown with foods such as avocado, banana, papaya, chestnuts, kiwi, potatoes, and tomatoes. Clients with allergy to these foods may have latex allergy and vice versa.

Assisting the Visually Impaired Client to Eat

Procedure

1. Check client chart for ordered diet.
2. Identify client and check allergy band.
3. Perform hand hygiene.
4. Raise head of bed to HIGH position, or assist client to sit in chair if possible.
5. Assist client to perform hand hygiene.
6. Place protective covering over client's chest.
7. Place food tray on client's over-bed table and adjust to client and caregiver's comfort.
8. Stand or sit facing client.
9. Assist client by using the following technique:
   a. Use the clock face to describe food arrangement on the plate.
   b. Tell the client the time on the clock at which each food item is placed; for example, "The corn is at 4 o'clock, chicken is at 8 o'clock."
   c. Encourage the client to feed self, but remain with client if possible.
10. Encourage the client to hold glass, bread, finger foods.
11. Allow client time to chew and swallow.
12. Provide fluids throughout meal.
13. Alternate foods; rather than one complete item at a time.
14. Allow client to rest at intervals during the meal.
15. Talk with client during meal. ▸ ***Rationale:*** Talking makes mealtime more pleasant and promotes relaxation.
16. Reposition tray table at bedside when meal is completed.
17. Assist client with hand and oral hygiene if desired.
18. Raise side rail if it has been lowered.
19. Position bed for comfort. Lower bed if it is raised.
20. Note percentage of food eaten.
21. Remove food tray from room.
22. Perform hand hygiene.
23. Document amount eaten. If necessary, record fluid intake on I&O record.
24. Place call bell within client's reach.

Assisting the Dysphagic Client to Eat

Equipment

Provision for oral care and hand hygiene
Towel
Penlight to inspect oral cavity
Oral suction catheter connected to suction source

Preparation

1. Note specific instructions for feeding technique (diet and positioning) prescribed by speech or swallowing specialist; for example, cornstarch, Thickit, or rice cereal to thicken food, as prescribed. ▸ ***Rationale:*** Clients with swallowing problems find it easier to swallow thickened liquids.
2. Check if client is receiving both oral and enteral feeding; stop the enteral solution about 1 hr before oral feeding.
3. Check that client has not recently received sedating medication.
4. Eliminate environmental distractors such as television, radio.
5. Provide a 30-minute rest period before mealtime.
6. Ensure that temperature of food is appropriate.

Procedure

1. Complete hand hygiene.
2. Check client's Ident-A-Band and allergy bracelet and have client state name and birth date.
3. Provide client privacy.
4. Maintain bed in LOW position.
5. Assist client to sit upright (90°) in a chair, or in bed with hips flexed, shoulders and face slightly forward, and chin parallel to the floor or slightly tucked. ▸ ***Rationale:*** Gravity assists proper bolus movement to the stomach.

NOTE: Prescribed position is different for specific forms of dysphagia. Some types of dysphagia necessitate client positioning to one side, or with head rotated toward the stronger or weaker side, or even side-lying. Instructions should be placed in client's record, care plan, and posted at client's head of bed.

6. Assist client to perform hand hygiene before eating.
7. Place towel over client's chest.
8. Place tray on over-bed table and towel under plate. ▸ ***Rationale:*** This stabilizes plate while feeding.
9. Suction oral secretions before feeding, if necessary.
10. Sit at client's side, or sit facing client.
11. Encourage self-feeding.
12. Instruct client to take (or offer) small portions of food at first (0.5 to 1 tsp at a time), bites manageable in size but large enough to require chewing.
13. Instruct client to eat food first, without accompanying liquid, reserving *all* liquid intake until after finishing food. ▸ ***Rationale:*** Using liquids to wash down boluses of food pushes the food down too rapidly, although some authorities recommend alternating solids with liquids.
14. Instruct client to perform an exaggerated sucking motion at the beginning of each swallow with chin tucked slightly. ▸ ***Rationale:*** Decreases risk of aspiration.

NOTE: Clients with advanced dementia may not remember how to chew or swallow. Demonstrating chewing and gently stroking the area under the client's chin with a downward motion during swallowing may be helpful cues.

15. Allow client to concentrate on swallowing *without* distractions such as conversation or television. ▸ ***Rationale:*** For the dysphagic client, swallowing takes concentration; talking increases risk for aspiration.
16. Avoid rushed or forced feeding and make sure client is swallowing every mouthful.
17. Visually inspect oral cavity and under dentures for retained food. ▸ ***Rationale:*** Buildup may occur on weak side of mouth or pharynx.
18. Observe client closely for evidence of aspiration (e.g., cough, drooling, voice change such as hoarseness or a gurgling noise after swallowing), and suction oropharynx if indicated.
19. Help with feeding only if client shows signs of weakness, fatigue.
20. Provide positive reinforcement for accomplishment.
21. Assist with oral care and hand hygiene after meal. ▸ ***Rationale:*** To reduce oral colonization with pathogens and risk of aspiration pneumonia.
22. Remove food tray and raise side rails as indicated.
23. Place call bell in reach.
24. Record percentage of food eaten and amount of liquid intake (if indicated).
25. Maintain client's sitting position for 30 minutes after eating.
26. Carefully observe client with impaired communication for 30 minutes after the first few servings.

Clinical Alert

The use of a straw increases risk of aspiration because the dysphagic client has less control over the amount of fluid intake. Similarly, the dysphagic client should not be fed with a syringe.

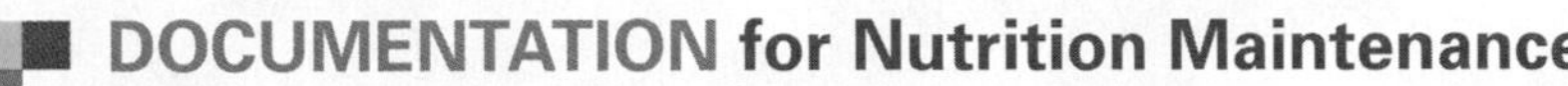

DOCUMENTATION for Nutrition Maintenance

- Appetite
- Food intake (percentage eaten)
- Tolerance to diet
- Weight
- Liquid intake
- Feeding techniques for the dysphagic client

CRITICAL THINKING Application

Expected Outcomes

- Diet meets nutritional requirements and is acceptable to client's taste and cultural orientation.
- Visually impaired client is able to self-feed.
- Dysphagic client is able to eat using adaptations to prevent aspiration.

Unexpected Outcomes	Alternative Actions
Client is nauseated and vomits.	• Withhold food if client is nauseated or vomiting. • Provide antiemetic or client's preferred comfort measures (cold cloth to throat, soda drink). • Identify potential sources for nausea: specific foods or odors, experience of pain, side effects of medication (e.g., morphine sulfate), or positional changes.
Visually impaired client only eats food on one half of food tray.	• Client may have *homonymous hemianopia* due to stroke and is unable to see the half of the tray on client's paralyzed side. • Move food tray so that ignored side is within client's restricted range of vision (move tray leftward if client has had a left CVA and right side of tray has been ignored). • Encourage client to turn head so that client's visual field includes the half of tray with food that has not been seen or eaten.
Client has signs of aspirating food (coughing, drooling, hoarseness, noisy breathing).	• Request speech pathologist consult for swallow evaluation. • Ensure that assistive personnel are following individualized feeding instructions/precautions (e.g., client positioning, use of thickening agents, and avoiding use of straws). • Remind client not to talk while eating and to concentrate on swallowing.

Chapter 19

UNIT ❸

Nasogastric Tube Therapies

Nursing Process Data

ASSESSMENT Data Base

- Validate order for NG tube type and purpose.
- Assess overall status necessitating NG decompression (gastric surgery, intestinal obstruction).
- Assess status of GI function (presence of nausea, vomiting, abdominal distention, presence/absence of passage of flatus or bowel movement).
- Assess patency of nares.
- Assess risk for aspiration.
- Assess client's I&O balance and relevant lab data (electrolytes, hemoglobin and hematocrit, coagulation studies).
- Assess type of IV fluid replacement therapy client is receiving.

PLANNING Objectives

- To remove fluid and gas from the gastrointestinal tract
- To maintain decompression tube patency
- To perform gastric lavage to remove blood, fluid, or particles, or to prevent digestion and absorption of poison

IMPLEMENTATION Procedures

EVALUATION Expected Outcomes

- NG tube is placed without complication.
- NG tube functions effectively (gastric contents are decompressed).
- Toxic substances are removed by lavage/not absorbed.

Pearson Nursing Student Resources

Find additional review materials at **nursing.pearsonhighered.com**

Prepare for success with NCLEX®-style practice questions and Skill Checklists

Inserting a Large-Bore Nasogastric (NG) Tube

Equipment

Tapered plug for tube (if indicated for single-lumen tube)
Single-lumen Levin tube or double-lumen Salem sump tube with anti-reflux valve (30–36 in.)
Water-soluble lubricant
Tape (2.5 cm or 1 in.) or commercial tube holder
pH chemstrip or Gastroccult test card and developer
Towel
Emesis basin
Tissues
Safety pin and rubber band
Tongue blade
Glass of water with straw
50-mL catheter-tip syringe
Clean gloves
Indelible pen or piece of tape for marking tube
Spindle adapter
Suction tubing and suction source

Preparation

1. Check physician's order and client care plan for inserting an NG tube.
2. Check client's Ident-A-Band and have client state name and birth date.
3. Discuss procedure with client. ▶ ***Rationale:*** Demonstration and display of items to be used helps to allay client's fear and to gain cooperation.
4. Provide privacy.
5. Gather equipment.

Procedure

1. Perform hand hygiene. Don clean gloves.
2. Position client at 45° angle or higher with head of bed elevated.
3. Examine nostrils, and select the most patent nostril by having client breathe through each one. ▶ ***Rationale:*** The nostril with greater airflow should be chosen for insertion.
4. Place a towel over client's chest, an emesis basin and tissues within reach; establish a cueing signal for client to use to stop you momentarily. ▶ ***Rationale:*** Client may experience discomfort or gag during tube insertion.

Clinical Alert

Nurses never insert or withdraw an NG tube for clients recovering from gastric surgery. The suture line could be interrupted, and hemorrhage could occur. The physician should be notified of dislodgement.

Never insert an NG tube in a client after nasal, craniofacial, or hypophysectomy surgery.

Gastric (Salem) Sump Tube

This gastric tube is a double-lumen radiopaque plastic tube. One lumen is used for decompression. The blue lumen with a blue pigtail provides an air vent to allow atmospheric pressure to enter the stomach to prevent tube adherence to gastric mucosa when the tube is attached to suction. It is NOT used for irrigation, obtaining a specimen, etc. However, if the vent lumen is blocked and requires flushing, after the flush, the pigtail should be cleared with an injection of 20 mL air. The pigtail should be kept above the level of the client's stomach to prevent stomach contents from siphoning into the air vent lumen, making it dysfunctional.

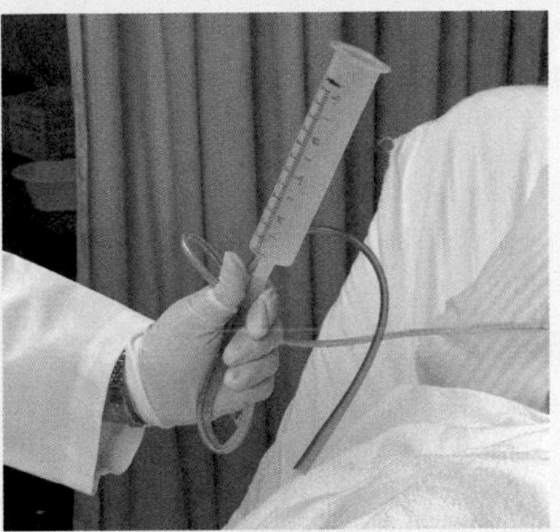

Salem Sump Tube With Gientri Port

This nasogastric system has selector knobs to allow a change in modes for suctioning (decompression), feeding, irrigating, and medication administration all through one closed port. The anti-reflux valve/air vent lumen allows atmospheric air to enter the stomach similar to the way the double lumen tube with blue pigtail functions.

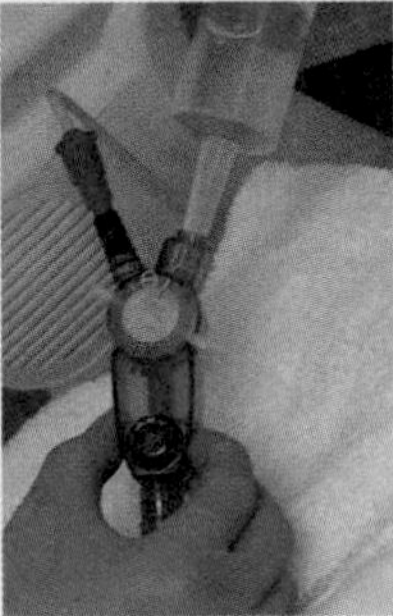

▲ Salem Sump with Gentri port.

5. Measure from tip of client's nose to earlobe to xiphoid (NEX) process of sternum to determine appropriate length for tube insertion.
6. Mark determined distance on tube with tape or pen if tube does not have markings.
7. Coil end of tube over fingers. ▸ ***Rationale:*** This softens tube and facilitates insertion.
8. Lubricate first 4 in. of tube with water-soluble lubricant. ▸ ***Rationale:*** Oil-based lubricant could cause respiratory complications.
9. With client's head slightly extended, carefully insert tube through nostril to back of throat. Aim the tube toward the ear on that side and downward toward the nasopharynx. ▸ ***Rationale:*** Advancing tube this way conforms to anatomic passageways.
10. Instruct client to flex head forward. ▸ ***Rationale:*** This position helps prevent tube entering clients airway.
11. Suggest client sip water while advancing tube until predetermined mark is reached. ▸ ***Rationale:*** Swallowing opens upper esophageal sphincter and allows tube to enter esophagus.
12. Listen at tube end for air exchange at 25-cm (carina) level; if no sound is heard, advance tube. ▸ ***Rationale:*** If sound is heard, tube may be advancing into airway and should be removed.
13. Continue advancing tube, having client dry swallow or giving client sips of water, until mark is reached.
14. Determine tube placement by aspirating gastric contents with 50-mL syringe to check color and pH. See page 668, Determining Gastric pH; if it is 5 or less, color is green or clear with tan *mucus shreds*, tube is in stomach. (Small bowel aspirate indicates a pH range of 6–7 and color is golden yellow to brownish green, consistency is thick. Pulmonary tree aspirate indicates pH of 6 or greater and color is white or pale yellow and watery consistency.) ▸ ***Rationale:*** The outcome of pH testing is useful only if the fluid aspirated tests acidic (<5).

Clinical Alert

Coughing and choking are normal responses for some clients; however, choking and coughing plus *cyanosis* or inability to speak indicate that the tube may be in the airway.

EVIDENCE-BASED PRACTICE

Determining Proper NG Tube Placement

A number of methods have been proposed to determine whether a tube has been inadvertently placed into the pulmonary tree, including air insufflation, observation of respiratory symptoms, pH testing of aspirated fluid, visual inspection of aspirated fluid, detection of carbon dioxide in the tube, and x-ray tube location verification. The best method of confirming the location of a blindly inserted gastrointestinal tube is by chest/abdominal x-ray.

Rauen, C. A., Chulay, M., Bridges, E., Vollman, K. M., & Arbour, R. (2008). Seven evidence-based practice habits: putting some sacred cows out to pasture. *Critical Care Nurse*, 28(2), 98–123.

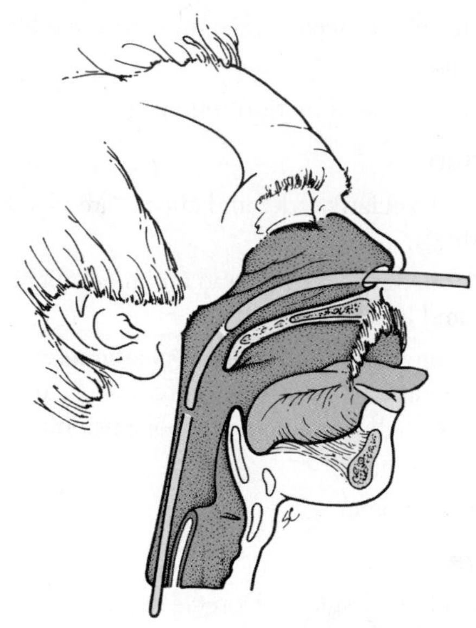

▲ NG tube inserted through naris to stomach.

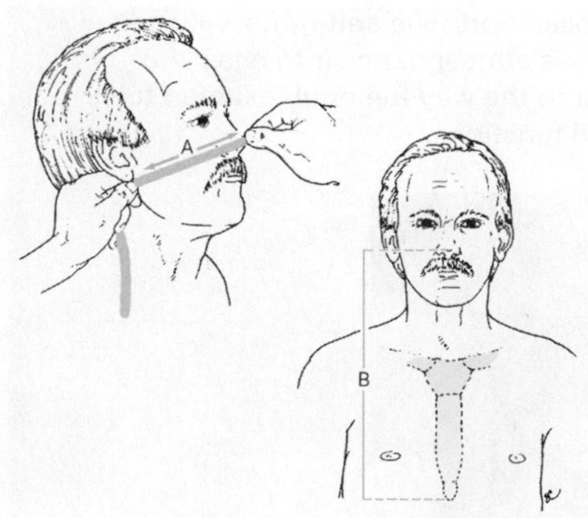

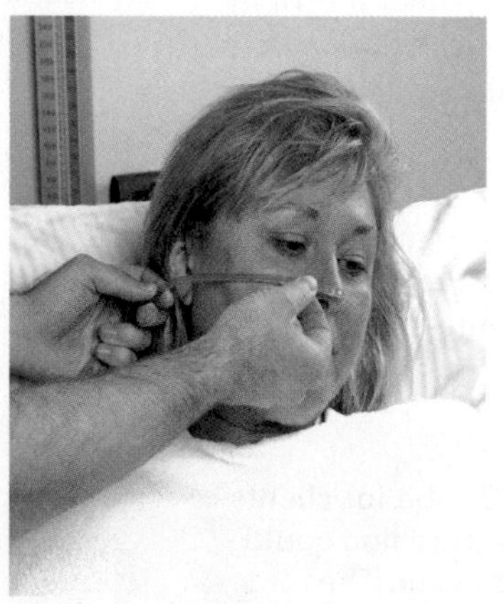

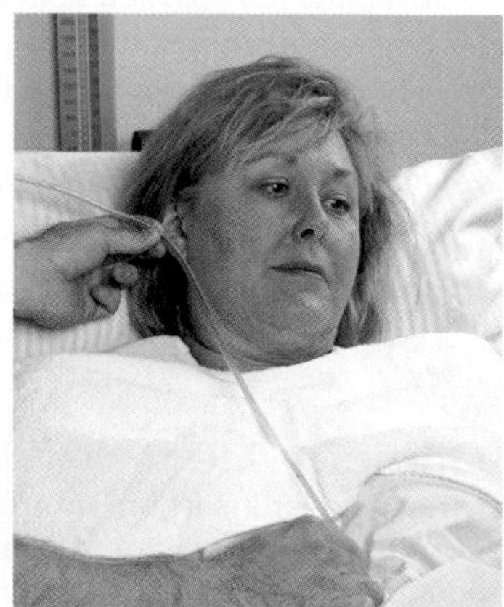

▲ NG tube-measuring (A) Nose to earlobe, (B) Earlobe to xyphoid.

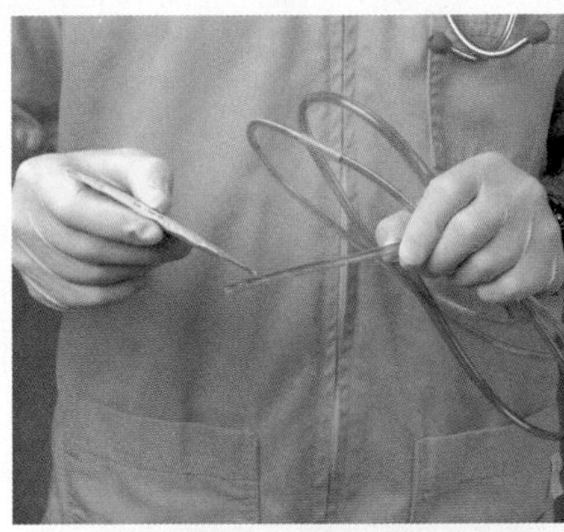

3 Lubricate first 4 inches of NG tube with water-soluble lubricant.

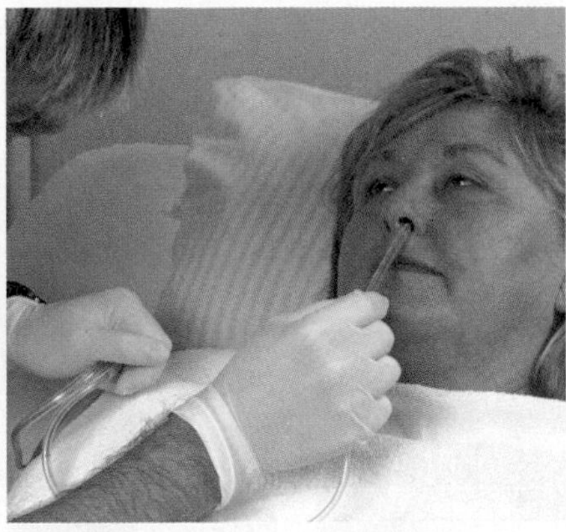

4 Insert NG tube through client's more patent nostril.

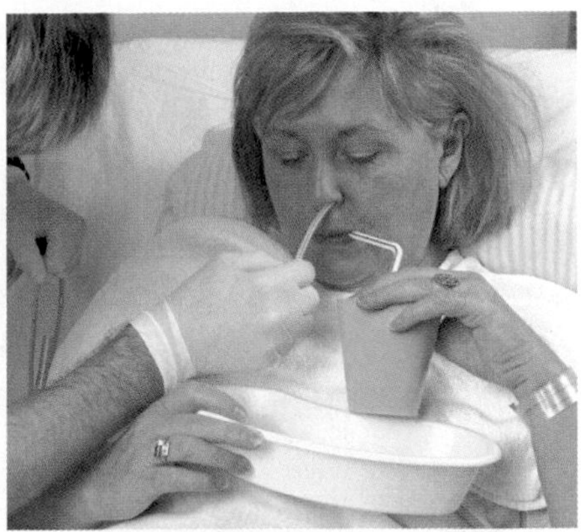

5 Instruct client to flex head forward and take sips of water as tube is advanced.

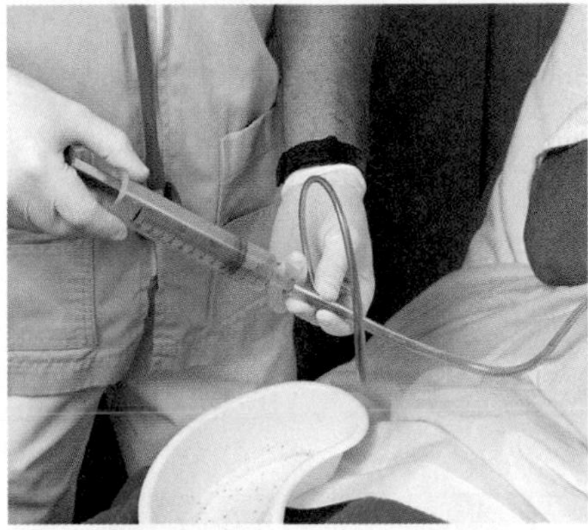

6 Aspirate gastric contents to check color and pH.

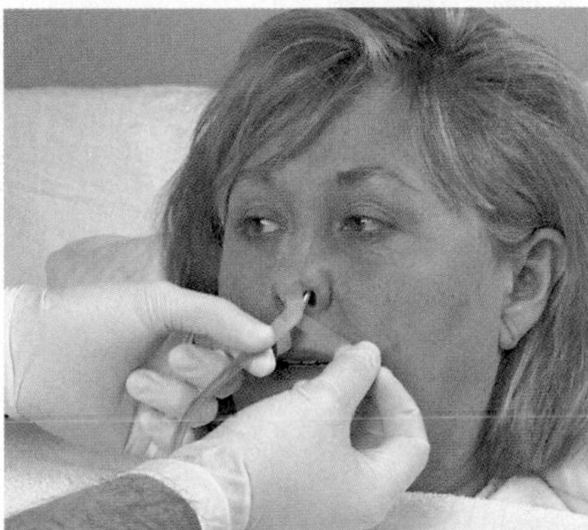

7 Tape tube securely to client's nose to prevent tube migration.

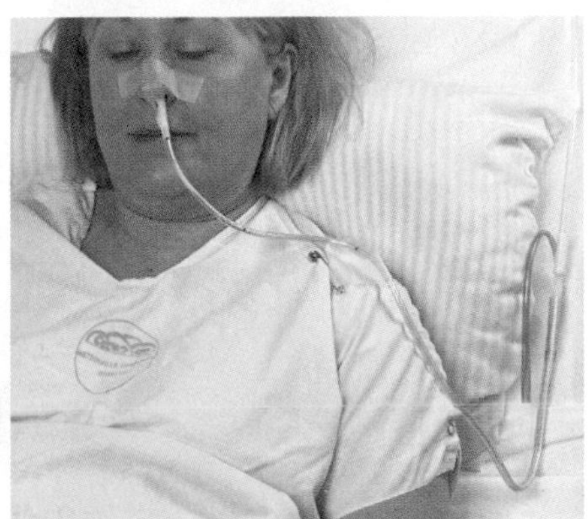

8 Secure tube by pinning to client's gown so blue pigtail is stabilized.

For Testing Blood in Gastric Specimen

a. Note *color* of secretions. ▶ ***Rationale:*** Coffee ground appearance may represent digested blood, while bright red color may indicate active bleeding or ingestion of red food.

b. Place one drop of aspirate onto Gastroccult test area. (See photo in Method of Determining Gastric pH in Unit 4.)

c. Apply two drops of Gastroccult developer directly over the sample in the Gastroccult test area.

d. Read occult blood results within 60 seconds; any blue color indicates presence of blood.

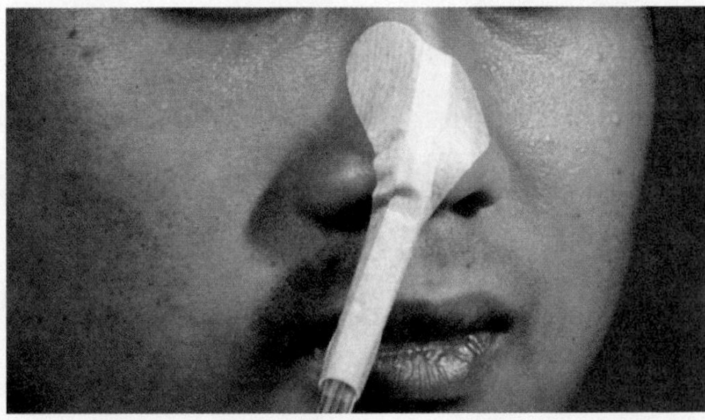

9 StatLock-NG Securement Device prevents tissue trauma.

NOTE: To determine if reagents in developer are functioning properly, add one drop of developer between positive and negative areas. The positive Performance Monitor area should turn blue within 10 seconds and the negative area should not turn blue.

15. Tape tube securely to nose or use an attachment device. (StatLock-NG Securement Device is flexible, yet resistant to tearing and adheres strongly to skin.) ▶ ***Rationale:*** When tube is taped securely, tissue trauma caused by pull on sides of nostril will be minimized.
    a. Cut tape about 3 in. long.
    b. Split half of tape lengthwise.
    c. Place unsplit end of tape over bridge of nose, with bifurcated ends hanging free.
    d. Wrap each end of tape around the tube where it exits from the nose.
16. Plug end of tube or connect it to suction tubing using tapered adapter.
17. Mark tube at client's nostril. ▶ ***Rationale:*** To note possible tube migration.

For Decompressing the GI Tract

a. Connect suction tubing to suction source.

b. Set suction on *intermittent low* (40 mmHg) for decompression. ▶ ***Rationale:*** Intermittent suction allows gastric tube suction force to be intermittently released, thereby reducing risk of mucosal erosion.

Or

c. Connect clear lumen of Salem sump tube to *continuous low* suction (30–40 mmHg) or to *intermittent high* suction (120 mmHg). ▸ ***Rationale:*** Continuous suction can be used because air vent lumen prevents excessive negative pressure from developing in stomach.

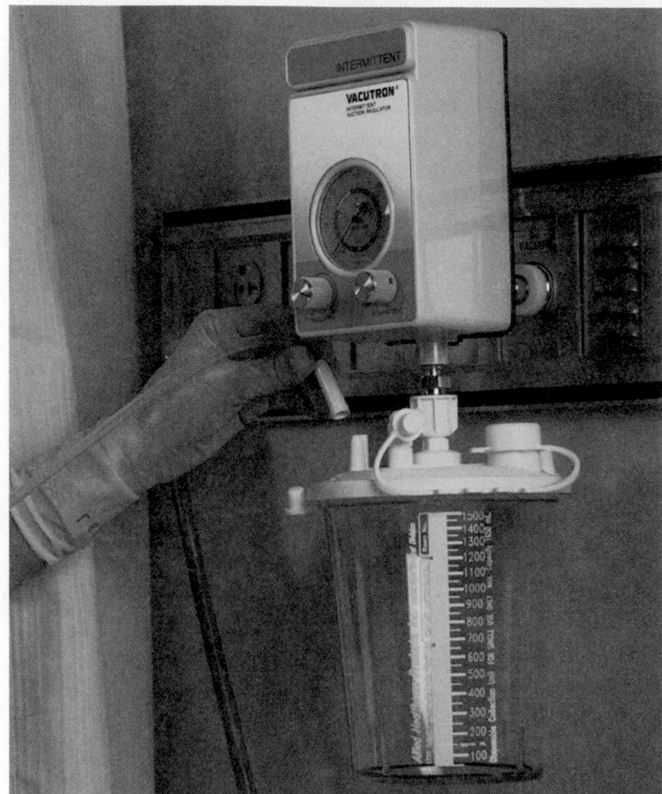

▲ Connect suction tubing to suction source.

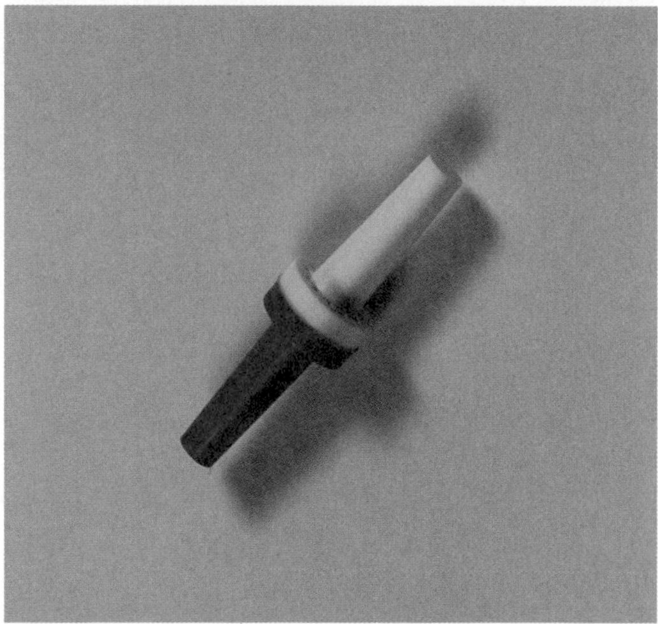

▲ Insert blue side of anti-reflux valve into Salem sump tube blue pigtail.

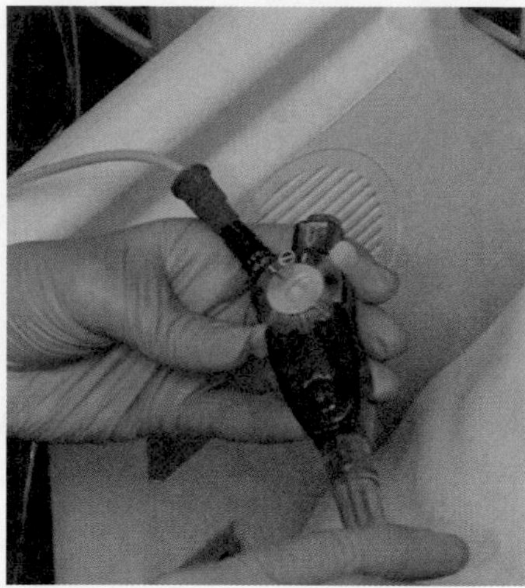

▲ Closed all-in-one enteric system port allows feeding, suctioning, irrigating, and medication administration. The built-in antireflux valve prevents gastric wall invagination during suction, replacing blue "pigtail" function.

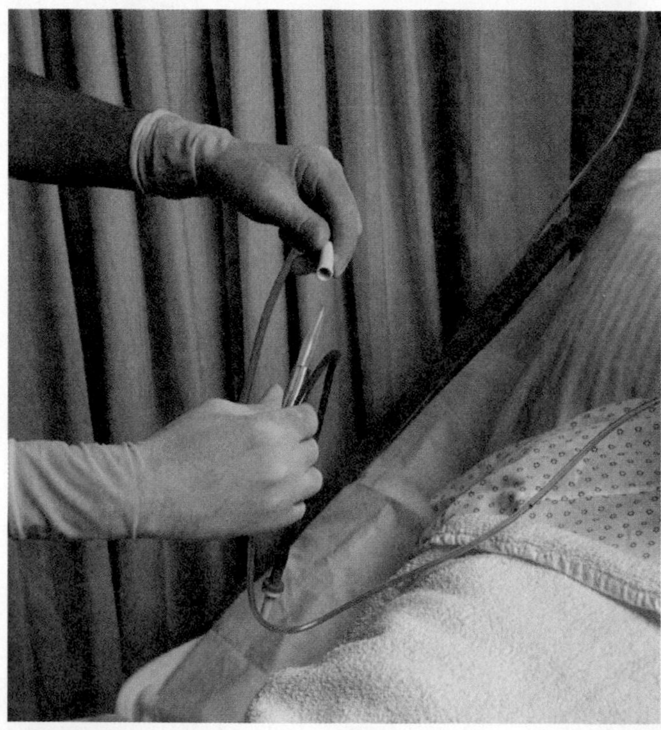

▲ Tapered adapter is inserted to connect NG tube to suction tubing.

Oral/Nasal Hygiene for NG/NI Tube Clients

- Clients who are unable to ingest food or take fluids by mouth should receive regular oral and nasal hygiene to keep mucous membranes moist and to help prevent infection of the parotid glands.
- Oral hygiene also reduces the risk of aspiration pneumonia, as it decreases the number of pathogens in oropharyngeal secretions.
- Chewing gum or sucking on sugar-free candy also helps stimulate salivation, but excessive use can stimulate gastric secretions and cause electrolyte imbalance.

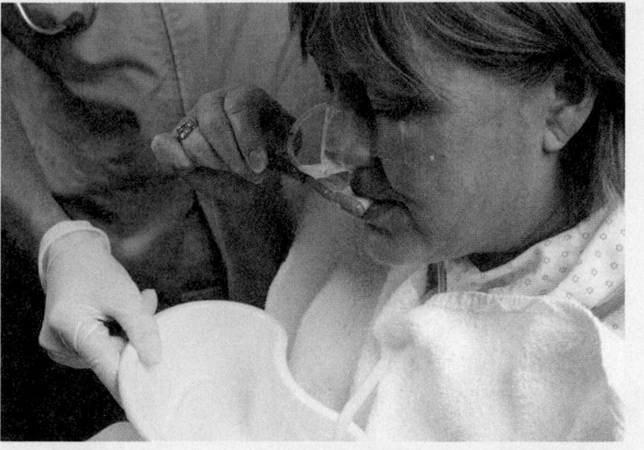

▲ Provide regular nasal and oral hygiene to keep mucous membranes moist and help prevent parotiditis and bacterial colonization of the upper respiratory tract.

18. Secure tube with tape/rubber band pinned to client's gown, leaving slack for head movement.
19. Implement procedure below when double-lumen (Salem sump) tube is used.
    a. Stabilize blue pigtail above level of stomach. ▸ ***Rationale:*** Helps to prevent siphoning into sump (pigtail) tubing.
    b. Insert anti-reflux valve (blue tip) into blue pigtail of Salem tube. ▸ ***Rationale:*** Anti-reflux valve allows air to enter tube, yet prevents leakage of gastric secretions.
20. Provide oral and nasal hygiene.
21. Remove gloves and perform hand hygiene.
22. Position client for comfort.

Flushing/Maintaining Nasogastric (NG) Tube

Equipment

Disposable irrigation set with 50-mL syringe with catheter tip
Emesis basin
Towel
Normal saline irrigation solution
I&O record sheet
Clean gloves

Preparation

1. Check orders and client care plan.
2. Perform hand hygiene.
3. Check client's Ident-A-Band and have client state name and birth date.
4. Provide privacy.
5. Explain procedure to client.
6. Place client in semi-Fowler's position.

Procedure

1. Don clean gloves.
2. Disconnect NG tube from suction source if used.
3. Place towel under NG tube to protect sheets and place emesis basin nearby.

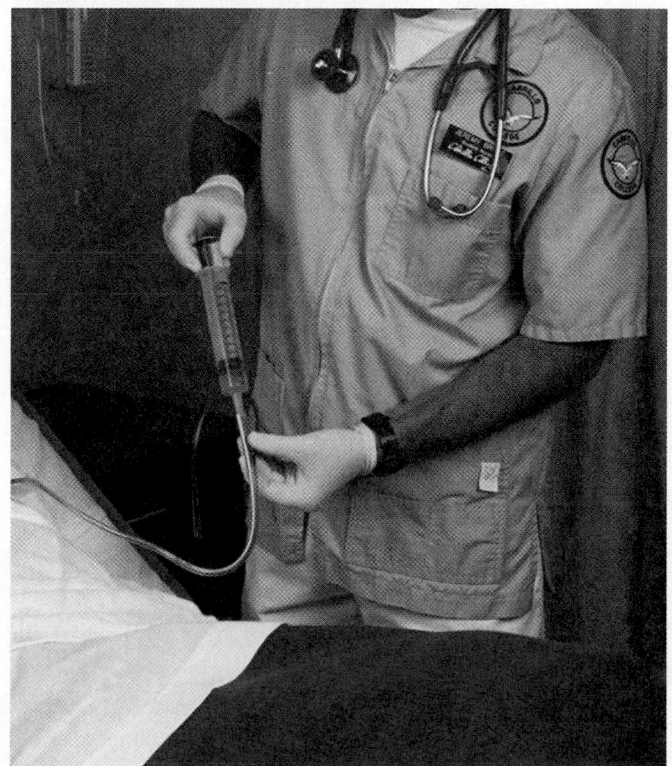

⚠ Aspirate secretions to check tube placement before instilling saline solution.

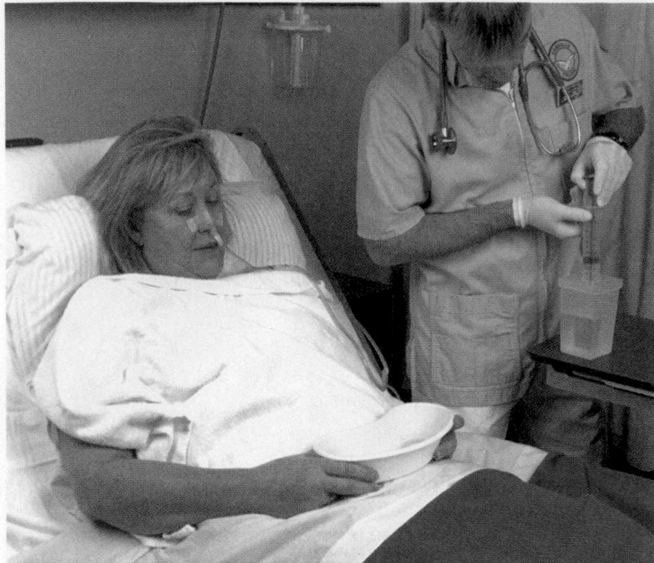

2 For irrigating NG tube, draw up 20–30 mL normal saline into irrigating syringe.

4. Check for NG tube placement by following Step 14 in previous skill. ▶ ***Rationale:*** Solution could be instilled in lungs if NG tube is not in the stomach.
5. Draw up 20–30 mL normal saline into irrigating syringe.

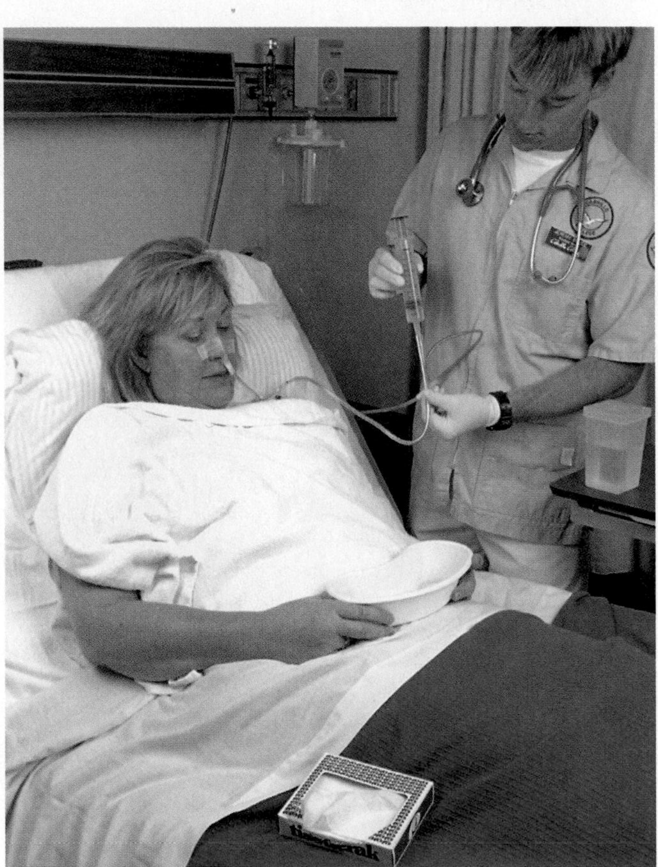

3 Gently instill normal saline into NG tube by syringe, or allow to flow by gravity.

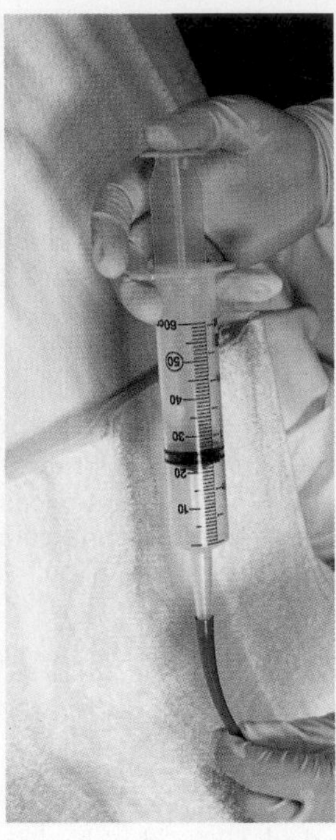

4 Follow Salem tube irrigation with injection of air into blue pigtail to clear; then reinsert blue end of antireflux valve.

Clinical Alert

- If water rather than normal saline is used to flush enteral decompression tubes, the production of gastric secretions will increase and increasing amounts of electrolytes will be washed out. Similarly, if the client is NPO but ingests ice chips ad lib, electrolyte imbalance due to washout can occur, causing metabolic alkalosis.
- Limit the use of ice chips by substituting chips made from an electrolyte solution, and provide oral hygiene to keep the client's mucous membranes moist for comfort.
- If the client is receiving adequate parenteral hydration (IV fluids), excessive thirst should not be experienced.

6. Gently instill normal saline into NG tube or remove syringe plunger, pour NS into syringe barrel, and allow solution to flow in by gravity.
7. Repeat procedure if necessary.
8. Reconnect NG tube to suction or plug tube.
9. Record instilled amount on I&O record.
10. Remove gloves and perform hand hygiene.
11. Reposition client for comfort.

Clinical Alert

If secretions siphon into blue vent lumen, clear it by instilling 20 mL of normal saline followed by 20 mL of air. Air vent must be cleared of secretions to restore proper functioning.

Performing Gastric Lavage

Equipment

Large-bore (37–40 Fr) soft Ewald or orogastric tube (client must have cuffed endotracheal tube in place if comatose)

Large irrigating syringe with adapter

Container for aspirate

Lavage fluid, normal saline, or lukewarm water

Activated charcoal for drug/toxin adsorption

Container for specimen

Water-soluble lubricant

Standby suction available

Towel

Pen and tape

Gloves

Preparation

1. Check physician's orders for gastric lavage and solution to be used.
2. Determine if client is alert or comatose.
3. Gather equipment.
4. Perform hand hygiene and don gloves.

Procedure

1. Per agency protocol (physician may insert) measure for tube insertion using the following guidelines:
   a. Measure distance from bridge of nose to earlobe to xiphoid process (NEX).
   b. Mark with pen or tape.
2. Place client in head-down, left side-lying position. ▸ ***Rationale:*** This reduces risk of aspiration if client vomits.
3. Lubricate tube with water-soluble lubricant.
4. Insert tube nasogastrically or orogastrically (about 50 cm or 20 in.).
5. Aspirate gastric contents with syringe before instilling solution. **Save specimen for analysis.**

> **Clinical Alert**
>
> Gastric lavage used to remove unabsorbed poison or drug ingestion is generally ineffective if more than 60 minutes have passed, and the procedure may delay administration of activated charcoal or antidotes; therefore, it is not recommended to manage overdose. It is not used for corrosive agents or petroleum distillates due to risk of aspiration, and induced vomiting is no longer considered safe.

6. Repeatedly instill 50–100 mL normal saline or water and aspirate contents ▸ ***Rationale:*** Some authorities recommend water to lavage the stomach of blood since it breaks up clots more easily than saline solution, is less expensive, and is readily available.
7. Carefully monitor volume instilled and character and volume of aspirated contents. ▸ ***Rationale:*** This will assist in determining net volume if there is blood loss.
8. Continue repeating process until gastric return is clear, or as ordered.
9. Stomach will be left empty for decontamination. Activated charcoal may be instilled (as ordered) or a saline cathartic may be given. ▸ ***Rationale:*** Activated charcoal adsorbs drugs in the stomach or intestine.
10. Pinch tube for removal, wrap in towel, and dispose of equipment.
11. Remove and dispose of gloves and perform hand hygiene.
12. Record vital signs frequently and monitor client's response closely.

EVIDENCE-BASED PRACTICE

Erythromycin, 250 mg IV bolus given 20 minutes before upper GI endoscopy (EGD), speeds gastric emptying and is first-line choice for clearing gastric contents in clients with GI bleed.

Source: DiMaio, D. J., & Stevens, P. D. (2007). Nonvariceal upper gastrointestinal bleeding. *Gastrointestinal Endoscopy Clinics of North America, 17*(2), 253–272.

Administering Poison Control Agents

Equipment

Large (37–40 Fr) Soft Ewald tube (physician may insert); comatose client must have endotracheal tube in place.

Lukewarm tap water or saline for lavage

Container for aspirated contents

Large irrigating syringe with catheter tip

60–100 g of activated charcoal in aqueous slurry consistency to administer orally or through gastric tube

Or

Balanced polyethylene glycol–electrolyte solution (e.g., GoLYTELY) for mechanical bowel cleansing.

Preparation

See Preparation for Inserting a Nasogastric Tube

Procedure

1. Place comatose *intubated* client in a head-down, left side-lying position or place cooperative alert client on commode.
2. Insert large bore (37–40 Fr) flexible tube nasogastrically or orogastrically.
3. Aspirate gastric contents and save specimen for analysis.
4. Lavage repeatedly with 50–100 mL of fluid until return is clear.

Activated Charcoal for Ingested Poisons

Activated charcoal adsorbs significant amounts of certain poisons in the stomach and intestines. The earlier charcoal is given, the more effective it is. The amount given is 60–100 g orally or per gastric tube. Repeated doses (20–30 g) may be given every 3–4 hr.

Clinical Alert

For a known toxin, one should call a regional poison control center by dialing 800-222-1222.

5. Administer activated charcoal slurry and repeat if ordered or, for cooperative client, administer balanced electrolyte solution per NG tube at a rate of 1–2 L/hr until rectal run-out is clear.

Removing an NG or Nasointestinal (NI) Tube

Equipment

Towel, paper towel
Stethoscope
Container of sterile normal saline solution
50-mL syringe with catheter tip
Tissues
Gloves
Tube plug

Preparation

1. Check physician's orders for NG tube removal.
2. Assess client to determine presence of bowel sounds (auscultate to right of umbilicus as alternative to all four sites). Signs more indicative of GI function include passage of flatus, bowel movement, absence of nausea or vomiting, and presence of hunger.
3. Prepare client for tube removal by explaining that it may cause some nasal discomfort, coughing, sneezing, or gagging.
4. Perform hand hygiene and don gloves.

Procedure

1. Provide tissues and place towel over client's chest.
2. Disconnect NG tube from suction tubing if indicated.
3. Flush NG tube with 20 mL normal saline (sterile water or saline for NI tube). ▸ ***Rationale:*** To clear tube so that GI contents do not inadvertently drain into esophagus on tube removal.

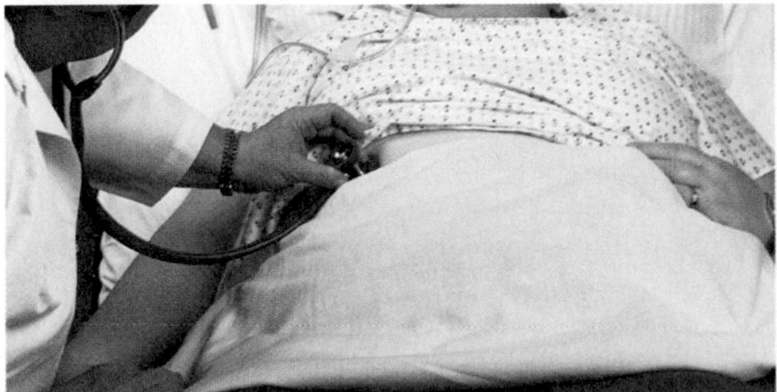

1 To determine return of GI function, assess client for presence of bowel sounds passage of flatus or bowel movement, absence of nausea, presence of hunger.

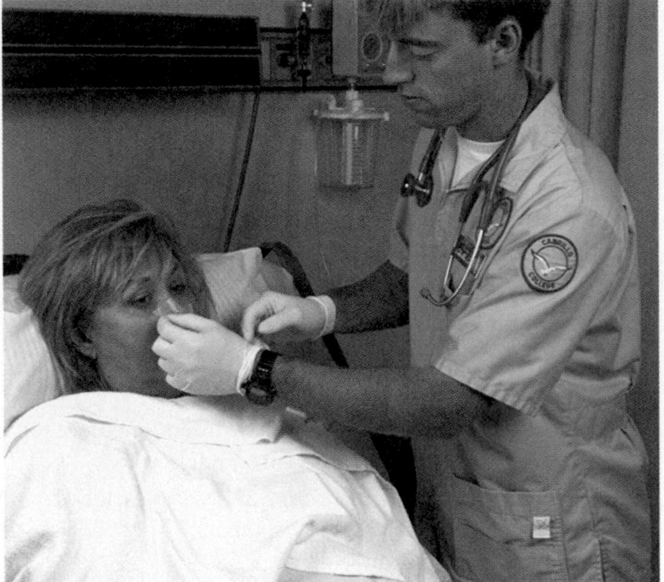

2 Clamp tube, unpin tube from gown, and loosen tape on nose securing NG tube.

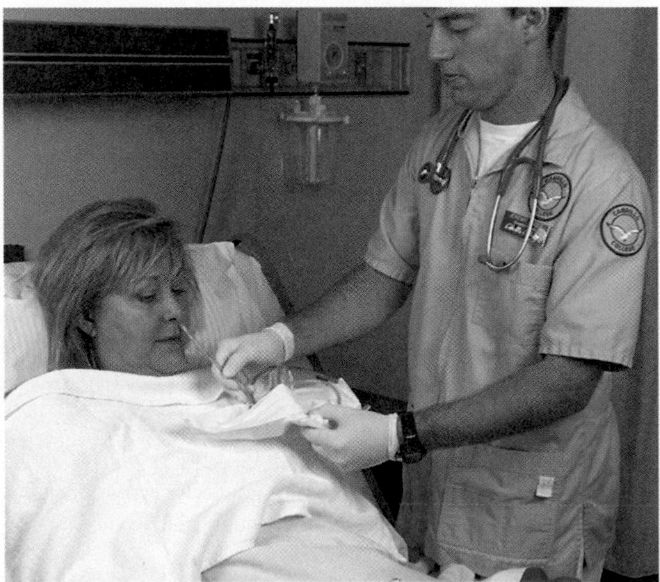

3 Have client hold breath and remove NG tube with continuous steady pull.

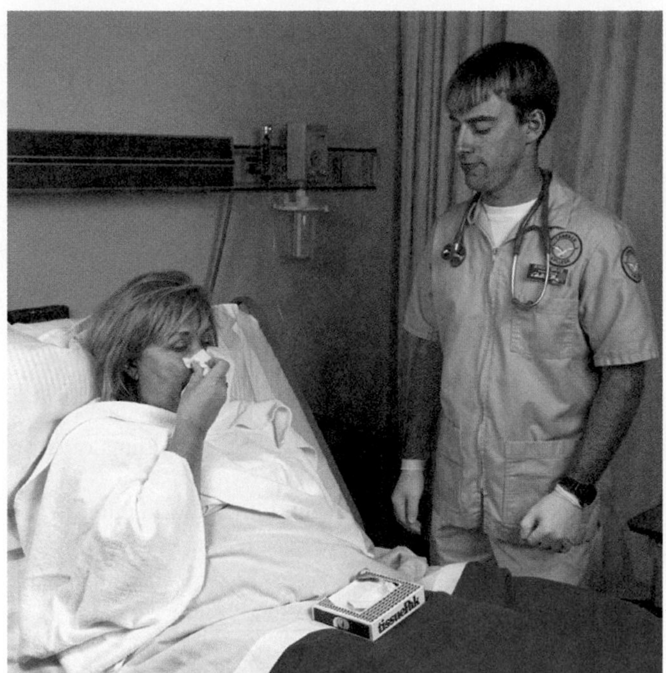

4 Offer oral and nasal hygiene after removing tube.

4. Follow saline flush with a bolus of air. ▶ ***Rationale:*** To free tube from stomach/intestinal lining.
5. Unpin tube from client's gown and loosen tape that secures tube to client's nose.
6. Plug tube or clamp it by folding it over in your gloved hand.
7. Pinch tube close to client's naris, have client take a deep breath and hold it while you withdraw the tube. ▶ ***Rationale:*** Holding breath closes glottis and helps prevent aspiration.
8. Wrap tube in paper towel to remove from client's view.
9. Offer oral and nasal hygiene.
10. Empty and record amount and character of drainage.
11. Discard disposable equipment and return reusable equipment to appropriate area.
12. Remove and dispose of gloves and perform hand hygiene.

EVIDENCE-BASED PRACTICE

Postoperative GI Motility

Nurses in this practice project discontinued bowel sound assessment to determine the return of gastrointestinal motility after abdominal surgery, since bowel sounds reflect the normal activity of the small intestine alone but do not represent return of functional GI motility. Primary indicators of the return of GI motility include return of flatus, bowel movement, client's tolerance of oral intake without nausea or vomiting, return of appetite, and absence of abdominal distension, bloated feeling, and cramps. Recent work on early feeding and reducing the routine use of nasogastric tubes has also contributed to a growing body of evidence on recovery of postoperative GI motility.

Source: Madsen, D., Sebolt, T., Cullen, L., Folkedahl, B., Mueller, T., Richardson, T., & Titler, M. (2005). Listening to bowel sounds: An evidence-based practice project. *The American Journal of Nursing*, *105*(12), 40–49.

DOCUMENTATION for Nasogastric Tube Therapies

- Type of tube inserted
- Technique used to assess NG tube placement
- Character and amount of drainage
- Type of suction and pressure setting used
- Frequency and solution used for flush or irrigation
- Gastrointestinal assessment findings (e.g., passage of flatus, bowel movement)
- Net return for lavaged client (amount of irrigant instilled subtracted from amount of aspirated return)
- Frequent vital signs (if indicated)
- Nasal and oral hygiene measures
- Client's tolerance of decompression
- Results of gastric specimen testing (blood, pH)
- Decontaminating agents instilled

CRITICAL THINKING Application

Expected Outcomes

- NG tube is placed without complication.
- NG tube functions effectively (gastric contents are decompressed).
- Toxic substances are removed by lavage/not absorbed.

Unexpected Outcomes	Alternative Actions
NG tube is difficult to advance.	• Select more patent nostril: Have client compress each nostril and breathe in to determine which is more patent. • Rotate tube or withdraw slightly, then try to advance, but do not force. • Relubricate tube and try again. • Curl tube around fist and hold under warm running water to soften for easier insertion. • Have client hold ice chips in mouth for a few minutes to numb nasal passage and suppress gag reflex.
Client coughs, is unable to speak and becomes cyanotic during tube insertion.	• Remove tube immediately as these indicate that tube is being advanced into client's airway.
Salem sump pigtail leaks gastric contents.	• Flush pigtail with normal saline, then with air to clear. • Keep blue pigtail at level above client's stomach. • Maintain anti-reflux valve plug insertion (blue side into blue pigtail lumen).
Client has ingested a large number of tablets which cannot be removed by lavage.	• Whole bowel irrigation is more effective for ingestion of enteric coated or sustained-release tablets. • Repeated dose of activated charcoal may be indicated to speed drug elimination. • Prepare for possible arrangement for hemodialysis.

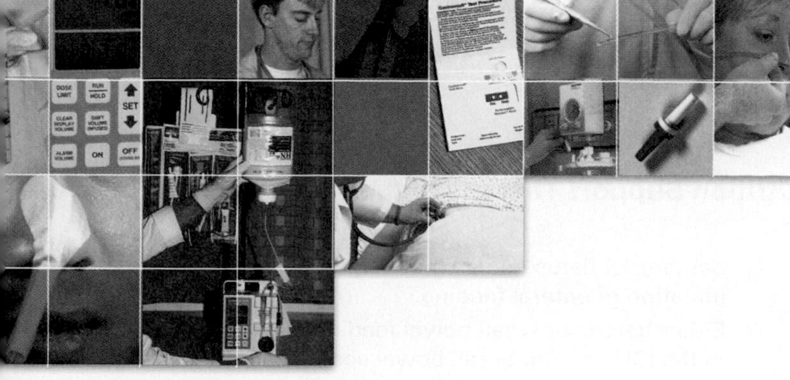

Chapter 19

UNIT 4

Enteral Feeding

Nursing Process Data

ASSESSMENT Data Base

- Assess client's nutritional status.
- Check physician's order for enteral feeding.
- Determine rationale for prescribed enteral feeding.
- Ensure appropriate placement of NG/NI tube using a variety of means.
- Assess client's gastrointestinal status (passage of flatus, bowel movement).

PLANNING Objectives

- To provide nutrients to the client who is temporarily unable to ingest food
- To correct nutritional deficiency in selected clients
- To provide nutrients to the client who requires continuous enteral feeding
- To maintain gastrostomy tube site

INTERVENTIONS Procedures

EVALUATION Expected Outcomes

- Client's nutritional needs are met with nasogastric feeding.
- Client's nutritional needs are met with continuous enteral feeding.
- Gastrostomy tube site is free of signs of irritation/inflammation.

Guidelines for Provision and Assessment of Nutrition Support Therapy in the Adult Critically Ill Client

1. Traditional nutrition assessment tools (albumin, prealbumin, and anthropometry) are not validated in critical care. Before initiation of feedings, assessment should include evaluation of weight loss and previous nutrient intake prior to admission, level of disease severity, co-morbid conditions, and function of the GI tract.
2. Nutrition support therapy in the form of enteral nutrition should be initiated in the critically ill client who is unable to maintain volitional intake.
3. Enteral nutrition is the preferred route of feeding over parenteral nutrition for the critically ill client who requires nutrition support therapy.
4. Enteral feeding should be started early within the first 24–48 hr following admission. The feedings should be advanced toward goal over the next 48–72 hr.
5. In the setting of hemodynamic compromise (clients requiring significant hemodynamic support including high dose catecholamine agents, alone or in combination with large volume fluid or blood product resuscitation to maintain cellular perfusion), enteral nutrition should be withheld until the client is fully resuscitated and/or stable.
6. In the ICU client population, neither the presence nor absence of bowel sounds nor evidence of passage of flatus and stool is required for the initiation of enteral feeding.
7. Either gastric or small bowel feeding is acceptable in the ICU setting. Small bowel access should be used in clients at high risk for aspiration, or those with repeated high gastric residual volumes.
8. Inappropriate cessation of enteral nutrition should be avoided. Holding enteral nutrition for gastric residual volumes <500mL in the absence of other signs of intolerance should be avoided. NPO periods for diagnostic tests or procedures should be minimized to prevent inadequate delivery of nutrients and prolonged periods of ileus.
9. If early enteral nutrition is not feasible or available the first 7 days following admission to the ICU, no nutrition support therapy should be provided. In the patient who was previously healthy prior to critical illness with no evidence of protein-calorie malnutrition, use of parenteral nutrition should be reserved and initiated only after the first 7 days of hospitalization.
10. If there is evidence of protein-calorie malnutrition on admission and enteral nutrition is not feasible, it is appropriate to initiate parenteral nutrition as soon as possible.

Journal of Parenteral and Enteral Nutrition, 33(3), May–June 2009, 277–316.

Administering an Intermittent Feeding via Large-Bore Nasogastric Tube

Equipment

Pen to mark date and time on equipment
Prescribed nutritional formula/product (check expiration date)
Calibrated container for measuring formula
Irrigating syringe (50 mL) with catheter tip (date and discard in 24 hr)
pH indicator strip
Warm water for flushing, towel
Antimicrobial swab
Gloves
Clean dressing for gastrostomy site, if needed

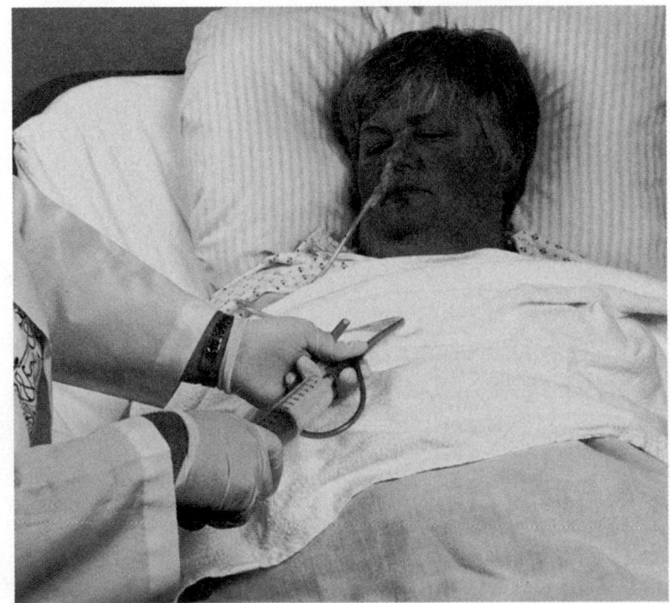

▲ Aspirate gastric contents to determine residual volume; then return contents to stomach to prevent electrolyte imbalance.

Preparation

1. Check physician's order for type, amount, and frequency of feeding.
2. Wipe unopened formula container top with swab.
3. Pour prescribed amount of formula into container (if refrigerated, warm formula by placing container in hot water; do not use microwave to warm formula).

4. Cover, date, and refrigerate opened formula (discard in 24 hr).
5. Perform hand hygiene.
6. Maintain artificial airway cuff inflation during feeding (if indicated).

Procedure

1. Check client's Ident-A-Band and have client state name and birth date.
2. Provide privacy and explain procedure and purpose to client.
3. Assess that client does not have abdominal distention, nausea or pain, and has bowel elimination or flatus.
4. Check mark on tube at exit site. ▸ ***Rationale:*** To check for possible migration of tube.
5. Don gloves.
6. Elevate client's head of bed 30°–45° angle or high Fowler's.
7. Place towel under work area.
8. Remove white tip of antireflux valve from NG tube if indicated.

Clinical Alert

Always flush the NG tube with warm water after checking residual volume to prevent tube clogging.

9. Insert syringe into NG tube to validate gastric placement. ▸ ***Rationale:*** Tube could have migrated between feedings.
   a. Check color, character, and test pH of aspirate (once every 8 hr after first 24 hr of tube placement).
   b. Aspirate gastric contents to determine residual volume. ▸ ***Rationale:*** Further client assessment is indicated if residual volume is greater than 500 mL and client shows other signs of intolerance.

Residual Volume Considerations

Gastric residual volumes do not correlate well to incidence of pneumonia, measures of gastric emptying, or to incidence of regurgitation and aspiration. There is potential for inadequate nutrition support when feedings are delayed or withheld based on residual volumes under 500 mL. Assessment of tolerance should include absence of abdominal distention, nausea, pain, and presence of bowel elimination/flatus.

Source: McClave, S. A., Martindale, R. G, Vanek, V. W., McCarthy, M., Roberts, P., Taylor, B., ... Cresci, G. (2009). Guidelines for the provision and assessment of nutrition support therapy in the adult critically ill patient: Society of Critical Care Medicine (SCCM) and American Society for Parenteral and Enteral Nutrition (A.S.P.E.N.). *Journal of Parenteral and Enteral Nutrition*, *33*(3), 277–316.

   c. Return aspirated contents to stomach. ▸ ***Rationale:*** This helps prevent electrolyte imbalance.
10. Pinch tubing. ▸ ***Rationale:*** This procedure prevents air from entering stomach.
11. Remove plunger from barrel of syringe, and attach barrel to NG tube.
12. Flush tube before feeding with 30 mL of warm water.
13. Fill syringe barrel with formula.
14. Hold container no more than 18 in. above client's stomach. ▸ ***Rationale:*** Holding container too high increases flow rate; rapid infusion can cause diarrhea/aspiration.

EVIDENCE-BASED PRACTICE

Aseptic Technique for Enteral Feeding

Enteral feeding should always adhere to principles of medical asepsis; however, *surgical* asepsis may be more appropriate for critically ill or immune suppressed clients.

Source: Padula, C., Kenny, A., Planchon, C., & Lamoureux, C. (2004). Enteral feedings: What the evidence says. *The American Journal of Nursing*, *104*(7), 62–69.

15. Allow formula to infuse slowly (between 20 and 35 minutes) through the tubing. Clamp tubing or continue to fill syringe before syringe empties; do not allow syringe to "run dry." ▸ ***Rationale:*** If syringe runs dry before the addition of more formula, air enters stomach.
16. Follow tube feeding with 30 mL warm water flush. ▸ ***Rationale:*** Water cleans tube and prevents obstruction with formula.
17. Reinsert antireflux valve.
18. Maintain head of bed elevation at least 1 to 2 hr.
19. Wash, rinse, and dry equipment after each feeding. Mark date and *change syringe daily*.
20. Return equipment to client's bedside.
21. Give prescribed amount of water between feedings, if tube feeding is sole source of nutrition.
22. Provide regular oral hygiene.
23. Remove gloves and perform hand hygiene.

For Intermittent Feedings via Gastrostomy Tube

1. Check length of exposed tubing.
2. Aspirate to check residual volume. ▸ ***Rationale:*** Increased residuals may indicate delayed gastric emptying or that gastrostomy tube's internal stabilizer has migrated and is obstructing pyloric outlet.
3. Hold syringe no higher than 18 in. above client's stomach and administer 30 mL of warm water to flush and test patency of tubing. Clamp tubing by folding before syringe empties. ▸ ***Rationale:*** To prevent administering air into client's stomach.

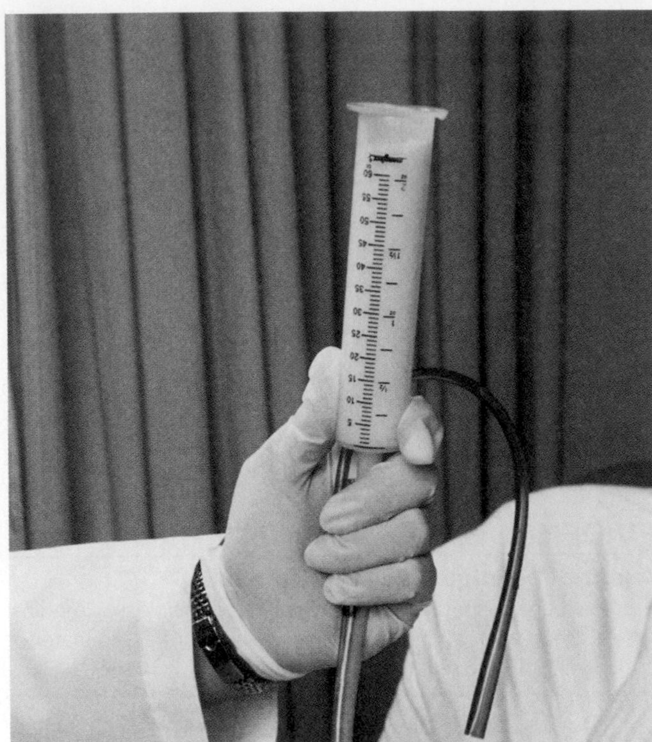

▲ Allow feeding to flow by gravity and clamp tubing before syringe empties, or continuously fill syringe before it completely empties.

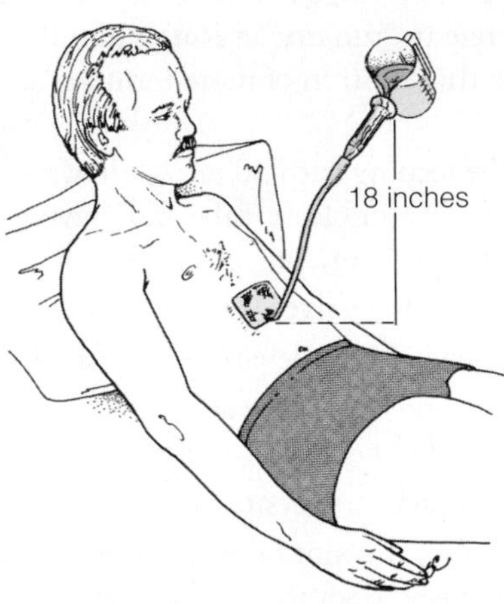

▲ Allow feeding to flow by gravity through gastrostomy tube.

4. Remove plunger, insert empty syringe barrel into gastrostomy tube, and administer feeding no higher than 18 in. above client's stomach, allowing formula to flow slowly by gravity.
5. Proceed as in previous skill with flushing, then reinsert tube plug.

NOTE: Gastrostomy site may be left open to air.

Clinical Alert

If gastrostomy tube residual is unobtainable, the tube may be displaced between client's stomach and abdominal wall, in which case administration of feeding could result in peritonitis.

6. Remove dressing (if present) around gastrostomy site.
7. Wash, rinse, and dry skin. Assess skin condition.
8. Apply clean dressing. (See Dressing the Gastrostomy Tube Site.)
9. Maintain head of bed elevation for 1–2 hr.

Clinical Alert

The use of blue food coloring as a marker for aspiration and use of glucose oxidase strips to test tracheal secretions for glucose are invalid measures to test for aspiration of enteral formulations.

EVIDENCE-BASED PRACTICE

- **Safety Issues for Gastric Feeding**
  Studies show that clients receiving gastric feedings require intact gag and cough reflexes and adequate gastric emptying. Small bowel access for continuous enteral nutrition should be obtained for clients with tracheal aspiration, reflux esophagitis, gastroparesis, gastric outlet obstruction, or previous gastric surgery. Prokinetic drugs (metoclopramide and erythromycin) or narcotic antagonists (naloxone, alvimopan) should be initiated to promote motility where clinically feasible.

Source: McClave, S. A., Martindale, R. G, Vanek, V. W., McCarthy, M., Roberts, P., Taylor, B., ... Cresci, G. (2009). Guidelines for the provision and assessment of nutrition support therapy in the adult critically ill patient: Society of Critical Care Medicine (SCCM) and American Society for Parenteral and Enteral Nutrition (A.S.P.E.N.). *Journal of Parenteral and Enteral Nutrition, 33*(3), 277–316.

- **PEG Tube Feedings Influence on Health Status**
  In a study of 150 patients (mean age of 78.9), 70% of those receiving PEG tube feedings had no significant improvement in functional, nutritional, or overall health status.

Source: Callahan, C. M., Haag, K. M., Weinberger, M., Tierney, W. M., Buchanan, N. N., Stump, T. E., & Nisi, R. (2000). Outcomes of percutaneous endoscopic gastrostomy among older adults in a community setting. *Journal of American Geriatric Society, 48*(9), 1048–1054.

- **Enteral Feedings—Gastric pH**
  Studies show that normal gastric pH (1.5–2.5) destroys ingested organisms. More alkaline secretions (pH >3.5) promote bacterial proliferation and may increase risk of nosocomial infection.

Source: Padula, C., Kenny, A., Planchon, C., & Lamoureux, C. (2004). Enteral feedings: What the evidence says. *The American Journal of Nursing, 104*(7), 62–69.

TABLE 19-3 Comparison of Enteral Tube Feeding Methods

	Advantages	Disadvantages
Nasogastric	• Easily placed. • Intermittent feeding is possible, so client is less confined. • Large-volume feeding may be delivered less often. • Tube placement does not require x-ray confirmation. • Acid environment may reduce infection. • Less risk of dumping syndrome. • Uses normal gastric emptying, preventing intestinal overload. • Less expensive; no feeding pump required.	• Limited to 1 wk use. • Gastric retention, reflux, and aspiration are possible. • Requires x-ray confirmation of placement before feeding unless aspirate is definitely acidic (<5 pH). • Large tube is uncomfortable and visible to others. • Naris ulceration may occur. • Allows regurgitation by interfering with normal upper and lower esophageal sphincter function. • Gastric ulceration or fistulae may occur.
Gastrostomy or PEG	• Long-term use is possible. • Allows intermittent feeding. • Normal gastric emptying occurs. • Tube is not visible to others. • Medication administration is easier. • Less risk of infection. • Client can ambulate. • Esophageal irritation is avoided.	• Requires surgical placement with sedation or local anesthetic. • Requires local skin care. • May ulcerate gastric mucosa.
Nasointestinal	• Smaller tube is more comfortable. • Less risk of reflux and aspiration.	• Requires x-ray confirmation before feeding or flushing. • Tube is more difficult to place. • Client is still at risk for aspirating nasopharyngeal and gastric contents. • Elevated position must be maintained. • Constant infusion used; intermittent feeding not recommended because of osmotic response of small intestine. • Cramping, vomiting, distention, and diarrhea more common. • Requires pump; more expensive. • Tube can displace back into stomach (with constant infusion, this increases risk of aspiration). • Medication administration is difficult (liquid form preferred). • Greater risk of infection due to alkaline environment. • Limited to 4-wk use.
Jejunostomy	• Tube position is guaranteed. • Tube is not visible. • Possibly less risk of reflux and aspiration.	• Requires general anesthesia for placement. • Continuous infusion is required. • Local skin care is required. • Cramping, vomiting, distention, and diarrhea are more common. • Other disadvantages associated with nasointestinal feeding.

Determining Gastric pH

Gastric pH is used to help determine NG tube placement, to assess gastric contents, and to evaluate and treat certain disease conditions. It is useful to determine placement only if aspirated secretions are acidic.

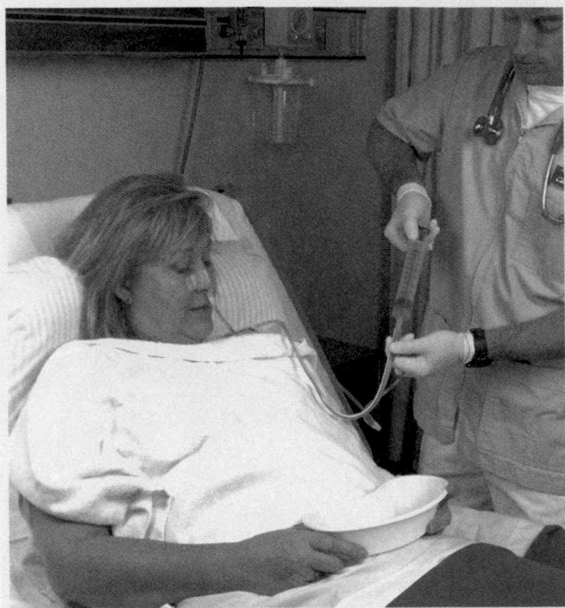

1 Aspirate 5–10 mL of gastric secretions to test pH.

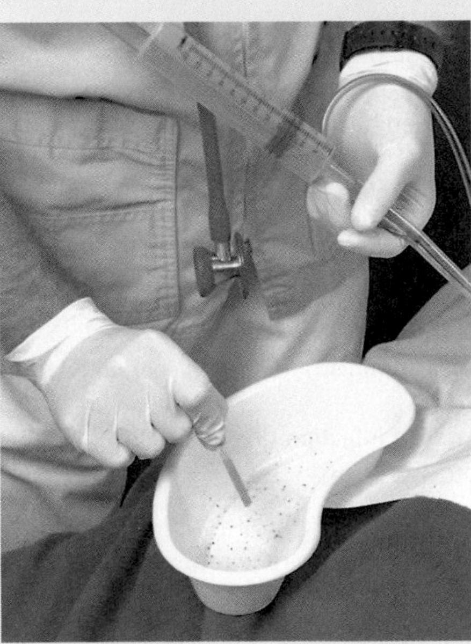

2 Dip test paper into gastric secretion to test pH. *Note:* Normal gastric pH is 1.5 to 2.5.

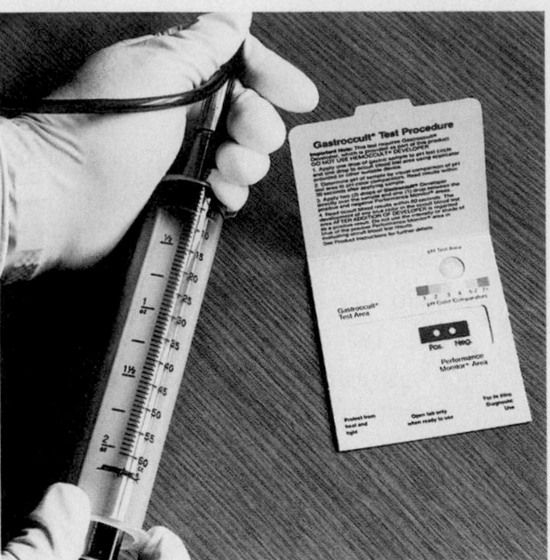

3 Place small drop of secretion on card to check pH.

Equipment

50 mL syringe with catheter tip
Emesis basin
Applicator
pH test paper (e.g., Gastroccult card)

Procedure

- Complete initial steps as for any procedure: gather equipment, explain procedure to client, perform hand hygiene, and don gloves.

  Note: When testing for pH, wait at least 1 hr after administering medication or an NG feeding.
- Attach a 50-mL syringe with catheter tip to the NG tube and flush with 20 mL of air.
- Aspirate 5–10 mL of gastric secretions.
- Note color of secretions—gastric secretions are greenish to tan or off-white; respiratory secretions are clear to light yellow with mucus; duodenal samples are usually deep yellow. *Color of secretions does not guarantee correct placement.*
- Place 5 mL of gastric aspirate into a small cup or emesis basin and dip test pH paper into the cup, place a sample on the pH test paper, or using applicator, apply one drop of gastric sample to pH test area on Gastroccult card.
- Read chemstrip pH within 30 seconds by comparing the color of the paper with the pH color guide.
- Gastric contents are usually pH 5 or less. If the NG tube is in the pulmonary tree, it will be 6 or more. If the NG tube has passed into the small intestine, the pH is more than 6 and could be 7.0–8.0.
- If clients are receiving medications that raise gastric pH, or have gastric bleeding or esophageal reflux, pH measurement may be unreliable.
- Document result of gastric specimen (pH).

Dressing the Gastrostomy Tube Site

Equipment

Normal saline; dated and initialed container left at client's bedside.

4 × 4 gauze squares or swabs

Protective skin barrier (if indicated)

Prepared split gauze dressing (occlusive dressing encourages fungal growth)

Gloves

Tape

Pen to label dressing

Preparation

1. Gather equipment.
2. Perform hand hygiene.

Procedure

1. Check client's room number and Ident-A-Band and have client state name and birth date.
2. Provide privacy and explain procedure and purpose to client.
3. Don gloves.

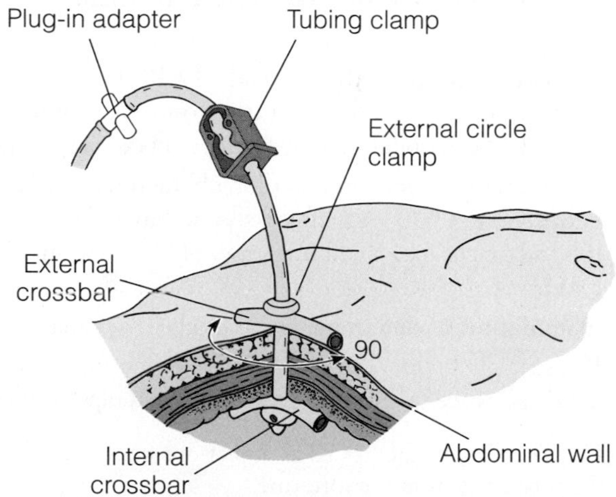

▲ Change tube dressing when wet, or daily, placing dressing over external crossbar.

4. Remove old dressing and discard.
5. Inspect exit site for signs of irritation or leakage.
6. Open packet of gauze squares and saturate with normal saline.
7. Cleanse around exit site, then rotate external bumper 90°. ▶ ***Rationale:*** To prevent skin irritation, ulceration beneath bumper.
8. Dry site.
9. Apply thin layer of protective skin barrier paste to site (if irritated). ▶ ***Rationale:*** To protect the skin from leakage.
10. Place split dressing over (*not under*) external bar. ▶ ***Rationale:*** Dressing placed under the external bar can cause erosion of gastric tissue or abscess of the abdominal wall due to pressure on the internal bar within the stomach.
11. Secure dressing with tape (if necessary) and if external tube is long, secure it to dressing with tape. ▶ ***Rationale:*** To prevent tube drag and erosion or ulceration of the internal mucosa from tension on the inner retaining piece.
12. Mark dressing with initials, date, and time.
13. Remove gloves and perform hand hygiene.
14. After 1 week, cleanse site with soap and water and leave open to air, according to physician's orders.

Low-Profile Gastrostomy Tube

Clients requiring *sustained* enteral feeding may prefer a low-profile gastrostomy tube. These tubes are inserted several (3+) months after the gastrostomy tract (stoma) has healed. They fit close to the skin, so are less apt to be pulled out or get in the way of daily activities. In addition, some incorporate a one-way anti-reflux valve that opens for feedings and also prevents backflow of gastric contents.

Since products differ, refer to the manufacturer's instructions for the specific tube your client has had inserted.

Inserting a Small-Bore Feeding Tube

Equipment

Small-bore (8–12 Fr) radiopaque enteral feeding tube (43–60 in.) with stylet

Administration set with pump or controller

60 mL catheter tip syringe

Sterile water or saline

Clean gloves

Water-soluble lubricant (if needed)

Tape or other device to secure tube

Glass with water and straw, if appropriate

Towel and tissues

Safety pin or clip

Emesis basin

pH chemstrip

Pen for marking tube

Prepared prokinetic agent (metaclopramide by IV injection or Erythromycin by IV infusion) if ordered

Antimicrobical swab

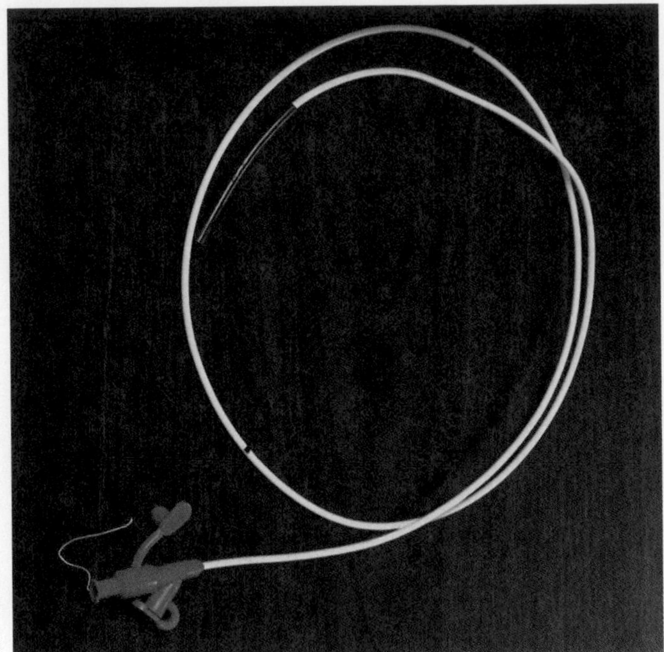

▲ Check that guidewire (stylet) does not protrude through holes in feeding tube. Reposition guidewire if necessary.

Clinical Alert

This skill may be performed using surgical asepsis for critically ill or immune-suppressed clients.

Preparation

1. Validate physician's orders.
2. Gather equipment.
3. Check client's room number and Ident-A-Band. Have client state name and birth date.
4. Provide privacy.
5. Administer prokinetic agent injection or infusion (if ordered for duodenal advancement) 10 minutes before tube insertion.

Procedure

1. Perform hand hygiene.
2. Explain procedure to client.
3. Elevate head of bed at least 45°. Place towel over chest; provide tissues and emesis basin.
4. Determine length of tube for insertion into stomach. Use distal end of feeding tube, and measure from tip of nose to earlobe to xiphoid process (NEX) for gastric placement.

NOTE: For small bowel placement, all but 10 cm of tube is inserted.

5. Note NEX marking on tube and place tape or mark with pen.
6. Seat stylet connector firmly into tube connector.
7. Check that guidewire does not protrude through holes in feeding tube. Reposition guidewire if necessary. ▶ ***Rationale:*** This prevents trauma to mucosa during placement.

NOTE: Use of stylet is optional and may not be necessary in a conscious cooperative client.

8. Don clean gloves.
9. Lubricate tip of feeding tube with water-soluble lubricant, or for tube with surface lubricant, moisten tip in water to activate lubricant.
10. Assess nares to determine patency. ▶ ***Rationale:*** Select the more patent nare for tube insertion.
11. Instruct client to momentarily hyperextend neck.
12. Insert feeding tube through patent nostril, gently advancing tube—advance parallel to nasal septum.
13. Ask client to flex head forward and swallow when tube reaches pharynx. ▶ ***Rationale:*** Hyperextension at this stage may open airway, and tube could advance into the trachea.
14. Pull back on tube if client begins to cough or shows signs of respiratory distress or cyanosis. ▶ ***Rationale:*** Tube may have entered trachea. Wait several seconds, then advance tube asking client to swallow sips of water with tube advancement.
15. Listen at tube end for air exchange at carina level. ▶ ***Rationale:*** If air exchange is heard, tube may be in respiratory tract. If no sound is heard, advance tube.
16. Advance tube to premeasured (NEX) position.
17. Tape tube securely in place.
18. Flush tube side port with 30–50 mL of AIR then attempt to slowly aspirate gastric contents; reposition client to *left side* and repeat aspiration if necessary to obtain a specimen.
19. Test aspirated specimen for color, character, and pH. ▶ ***Rationale:*** Gastric specimen should have pH <5. As tube advances into small intestine, pH becomes higher (>5).
20. Obtain x-ray to determine feeding tube placement.
21. If gastric placement is confirmed, use a rotating motion to gently advance tube to all but 10 cm and retape securely.

NOTE: This may be facilitated by injections of 30 mL of air to free the tube away from the intestine.

22. For stylet removal, activate internal lubricant before removing stylet. Cap access port and flush tube through the stylet connector with 10 mL sterile water. ▶ ***Rationale:*** Reinsertion of stylet into the enteral tube.

Clinical Alert

Do not initiate feeding or any flush until desired placement is confirmed and guidewire is removed. *Most tubes migrate into small intestine in 24 hr; advancement may be facilitated manually.*

Clinical Alert

Presence of an endotracheal tube may tend to guide feeding tube into the trachea. The use of glucose oxidase reagent strips to monitor pulmonary secretions for aspiration lacks adequate specificity.

should not be attempted because this can perforate tube and client's esophagus.

23. Once desired position is validated, swab feeding tube port, and attach administration set.
24. Swab port, then *gently* flush feeding tube (side port) with 20 mL of sterile water (using 60-mL catheter tip syringe) every 4 hr, and before and after each medication administered. ▸ ***Rationale:*** To maintain patency of the tube. Smaller syringe and vigorous flushing could cause pressure exceeding bursting pressure of the tube.
25. Check tape that secures tube to nose daily. Keep nares clean. Provide slack, securing tube by pinning or clipping to client's gown.
26. Replace small-bore tube every 4 weeks or as ordered, alternating nostrils. ▸ ***Rationale:*** Small-bore tubes can become contaminated or obstructed.
27. Provide frequent and regular oral hygiene. ▸ ***Rationale:*** Prevents parotiditis and respiratory complications.
28. Remove gloves, perform hand hygiene, and make client comfortable.

Safety Concerns: Continuous Enteral Feedings

Limit formula hang to 8 hr for an open system and 48 hr for a closed system if sterile technique is used.

Change administration sets and syringes used for flushing daily.

Do not add new formula to any formula remaining from previous administration. Flush bag with tap water before refilling.

Disinfect ports with antiseptic swab before and after handling.

Clinical Alert

The pH method for determining tube placement may not be useful during *continuous* NG/NI feeding because the infused formula raises gastric pH and lowers intestinal pH. The continuous-feeding aspirate will look like formula; it may be curdled or bile stained. A sudden increase in residual volume may indicate that a nasointestinal tube has become displaced upward into the stomach.

Clinical Alert

Potential Feeding Contamination

Open systems or opening a "closed system" (formula exposed to the environment) can invite contamination by numerous exogenous sources, hands being the main source. Do not touch any part of the system that contacts formula.

Source: Padula, C., Kenny, A., Planchon, C., & Lamoureux, C. (2004). Enteral feedings: What the evidence says. *The American Journal of Nursing, 104*(7), 62–69.

EVIDENCE-BASED PRACTICE

Client Positioning for Tube Migration

Positioning clients right side-lying has *not* been demonstrated to increase spontaneous tube migration into the small bowel. Prokinetic agents given before, but not after, tube insertion may facilitate tube passage into the small bowel.

Source: Journal of Parenteral and Enteral Nutrition (2002, Jan-Feb.). Section VIII, Access for administration of nutrition support.

EVIDENCE-BASED PRACTICE

Feeding Tube Positioning

Studies have shown that x-ray confirmation of *feeding tube* tip position should be obtained after placement of a small bore feeding tube and before any flushing or feeding is initiated.

Rauen, C. A., Chulay, M., Bridges, E., Vollman, K. M., & Arbour, R. (2008). Seven evidence based practice habits: Putting some sacred cows out to pasture. *Critical Care Nurse, 28*(2), 98–123.

Providing Continuous Feeding via Small-Bore Nasointestinal/Jejunostomy Tube

Equipment

Prescribed formula in closed container ready to infuse system (preferred). Note expiration date.

Antimicrobial swabs

Formula reservoir or bag if necessary for open system (date and replace daily)

Container of ready to use sterile formula (cover, label for client, refrigerate unused portion, and discard in 48 hr) or closed-system formula

Administration tubing compatible with pump (replace daily)

Infusion pump (not to exceed 40 psi)

Label or pen

60-mL sterile syringe

Sterile water or saline

Gloves

Mask (if caregiver has URI)

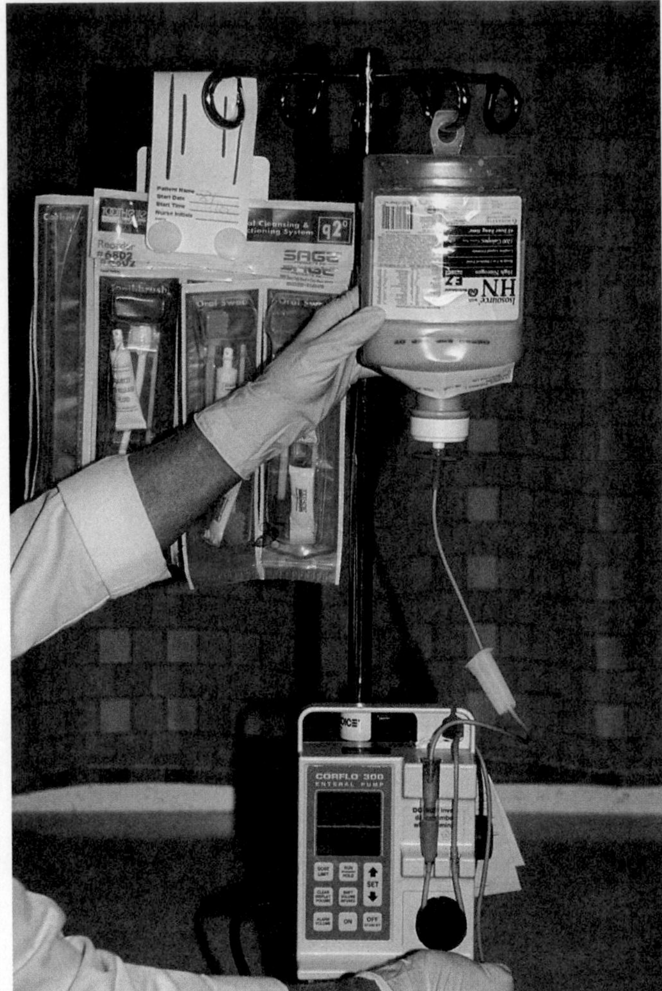

▲ Closed system formula can hang for 48 hours if sterile technique is used.

Clinical Alert

Obese clients cannot efficiently mobilize fat stores, but use protein as a primary source of energy, have marked loss of muscle and lean body mass, and become nutrient-depleted when critically ill. Nutrient support, however, can cause *refeeding syndrome* in these as in other protein-deficient clients. This adverse response is characterized by volume overload, heart failure, pulmonary edema, glucose intolerance, excess carbon dioxide production (by-product of glucose metabolism), increased respiratory work, and respiratory failure.

Preparation

1. Check physician's order for feeding formula type and rate of administration.
2. Check x-ray report. ▸ ***Rationale:*** Validates desired tube placement.
3. Check length of exposed tubing. ▸ ***Rationale:*** An increase in length may indicate tube tip has dislocated upward, from duodenum to stomach, or from stomach into the esophagus.
4. Perform hand hygiene.
5. Gather equipment.
6. Don clean gloves and mask if indicated.

Procedure

1. If using reservoir or bag for continuous intestinal feeding, rinse bag with sterile water, and fill with enough formula to limit hang time to 8 hr. *Note: Bring unused formula to room temperature before use*. ▸ ***Rationale:*** To reduce risk of infection. Advancement of tube to intestine places it in less protected (alkaline) environment.
2. Disinfect ports with antiseptic swab before and after handling.
3. Connect administration tubing to formula reservoir (container or bag) and prime tubing per manufacturer's instructions.
4. Thread tubing through pump per manufacturer's instructions.
5. Note mark on client's feeding tube to determine if migration has occurred.
6. Connect primed formula tubing to client's small-bore feeding tube. Initiate feeding with isotonic (300 mOsml) or slightly hypotonic formula. ▸ ***Rationale:*** To prevent dumping syndrome (cramping and diarrhea).

NOTE: Alternate method is to connect formula tubing to client's surgically established jejunostomy feeding tube.

7. Start feeding at slow constant infusion rate (25–50 mL/hr). ▸ ***Rationale:*** Slow increase in feeding volume is better tolerated. (Maximum rate is 100–150 mL/hr.)

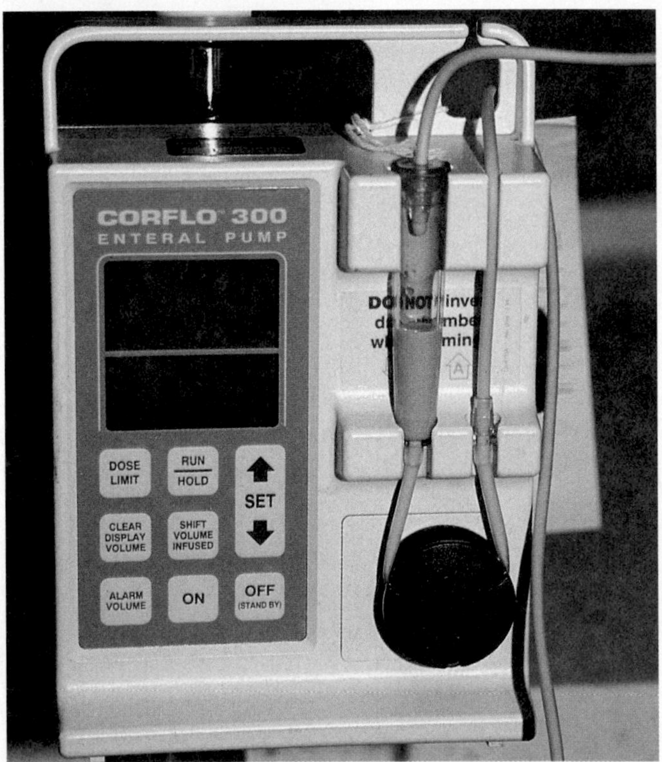

▲ Thread tubing through pump per manufacturer's instructions. Pump must not exceed 40 psi.

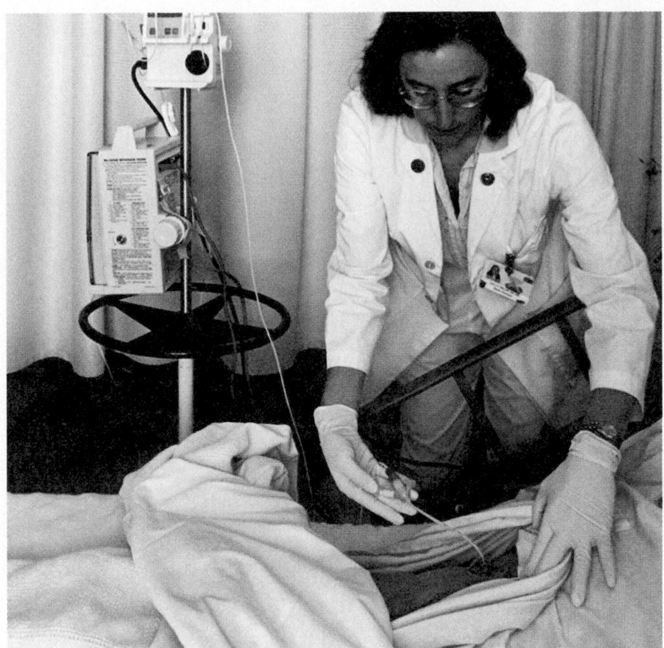

▲ Connect continuous feeding system to client's surgically placed jejunostomy tube.

8. If client tolerates feeding, increase rate in 8–24 hr (increase by 25–50 mL/hr to prescribed rate).

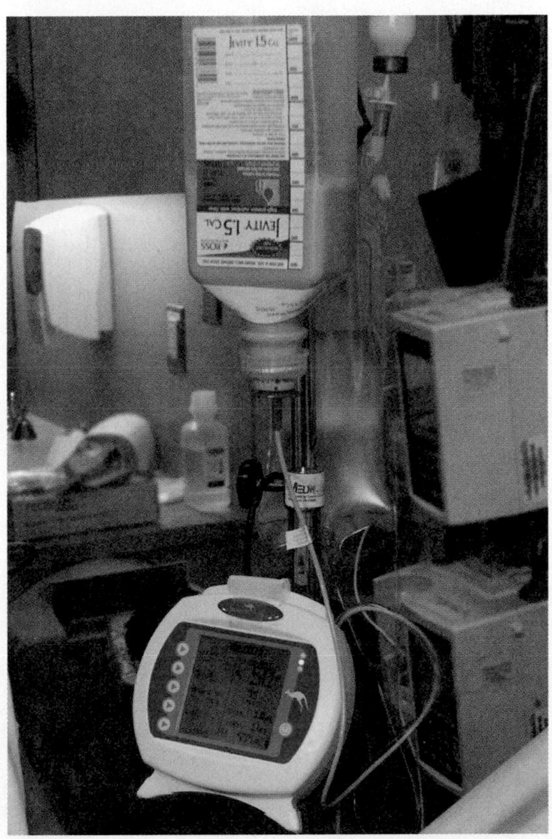

▲ The Kangaroo enteral feeding pump provides a preset water flush volume at programmed time intervals reducing need of manual flush and risk of misconnecting various devices.

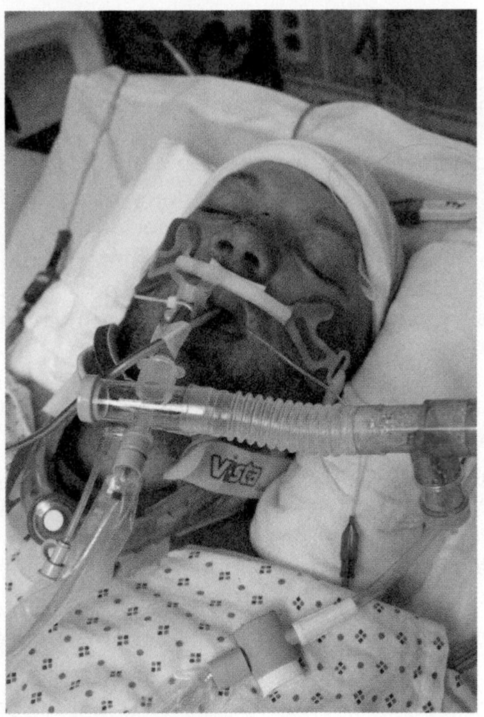

▲ Maintain head of bed elevation at 30–45° to reduce risk of aspiration in clients receiving continuous enteral feeding.

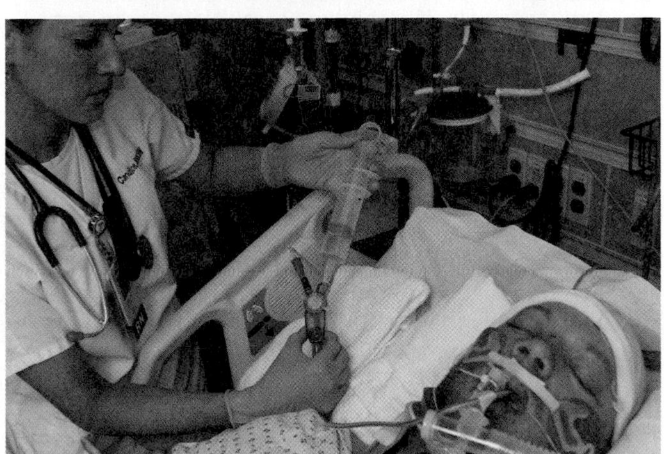

▲ Use 60 mL syringe to flush tube with 15 mL sterile water or saline every 4 hours and before and after each medication administered. Do not use tap water.

9. Keep client's head of bed elevated at 30–45°, or maintain obese client in reverse Trendelenburg position. ▸ ***Rationale:*** To lower intra-abdominal pressure and reduce risk of aspiration.
10. Prep side port with antimicrobial swab and, using 60 mL syringe, flush small-bore continuous feeding tube with 20–30 mL sterile water or saline every 4 hr; flush before and after each medication administered with 15 mL sterile water or saline. ▸ ***Rationale:*** To prevent tube clogging.
11. Check residual volume regularly. ▸ ***Rationale:*** Small-bore feeding tube residuals are usually less than 10 mL. Residuals as much as 50 mL may indicate upward displacement from the bowel into the stomach.

Safety Alert for Enteral Feeding

- Prefilled enteral feeding containers should be accompanied with enteral administration sets and should be labeled "Non-IV Compatible."
- Use only enteral feeding sets/pumps so that IV pumps are not used for enteral delivery.
- Enteral pumps should feature an automatic flush mode so that there is no need to manually flush lines and to reduce risk of misconnecting adapters or Luer devices.
- Use oral syringes rather than Luer syringes to draw up and deliver medications into the enteral feeding system.
- Identify and confirm a solution's label (3-in-1 parenteral nutrition solution may look similar to an enteral nutrition formulation bag).
- Label bags with bold statements "WARNING! For Enteral Use Only – Not for IV Use."

Clinical Alert

Enteral nutrition via naso/orointestinal infusion should be withheld if the client is hypotensive (MAP < 60 mmHg), especially if receiving catecholamine agents to maintain hemodynamic stability. Signs of intolerance may indicate gut ischemia.

Clinical Alert

Many devices, both enteral and parenteral are the color purple. While *enteral* connectors have gone to purple in an attempt to have the nurse note that this is not an IV device color, two manufacturers' PIC catheters use purple and thus the risk for enteral misconnection may be increased. *American Society for Parenteral and Enteral Nutrition (A.S.P.E.N.) 2006.*

Minimizing Risk of Misconnections

- Only those knowledgeable about the device should make a connection/reconnection.
- Enteral equipment should not mate with female Luer connectors—avoid GI tubes with female Luer connectors.
- Ensure that all connections are made under proper lighting conditions.
- IV and feeding devices should not be modified/adapted (this may compromise the safety features incorporated into their design).
- Trace line back to their origins when making connections.
- Recheck connections and trace all tubes when the client arrives at a new setting or as part of a hand-off process.
- Route IV lines toward the client's head; route enteric lines toward the client's feet.
- "Package" all parts needed for enteral feeding; reduce availability of additional adapters and connectors to reduce risk of improperly connecting dissimilar tubes or catheters.
- Label feeding tubes and connectors.

Guenter, P., Hicks, R. W., & Simmons, D. (2009). Enteral feeding misconnections: An update. *Nutrition in Clinical Practice*, *24*(3), 325–334.

Clinical Alert

- If client is receiving continuous feeding, maintain HOB elevation at 30°– 45° at all times. Turn off feeding 1 hr before client must be repositioned at less than 30° elevation for any procedure or transport.
- Transition from nutrition support to oral feeding requires careful monitoring. Enteral tubes or parenteral access should not be removed until the client has tolerated oral nutrition for 2–3 days.

DOCUMENTATION for Enteral Tube Feedings

- Date and time of procedure
- Placement of small-bore enteral tube and x-ray validation of proper placement
- External length of exposed tubing
- Methods of validating tube placement
- Quantity and character of aspirated residuals (color, pH, other tests)
- Amount and type of formula administered
- Head of bed elevation during and after feeding
- Frequency of tube irrigation and irrigant used
- Abdominal assessment findings (distention, nausea, vomiting, flatus, bowel movement)
- Bowel elimination pattern and characteristics
- Daily weight
- Intake and output
- Tube exit site assessment
- Application of dressing to exit site
- Oral hygiene provided

CRITICAL THINKING Application

Expected Outcomes

- Client's nutritional needs are met with intermittent nasogastric feeding.
- Client's nutritional needs are met with continuous enteral feeding.
- Gastrostomy tube site is free of signs of irritation/inflammation.

Unexpected Outcomes	Alternative Actions
NG tube feedings are delayed/skipped due to large residual volumes.	• Assess for adequate GI function (no abdominal pain or distention; no nausea or vomiting, presence of flatus, bowel movement). If residual is <500 mL, continue feeding but closely monitor client's response. • Change to continuous rather than intermittent feeding. • Continue measures to prevent aspiration. • Consider post-pyloric feeding.
Client develops diarrhea with enteral feeding.	• Use closed system if possible to prevent contamination. • Don clean gloves when setting up or opening system; use sterile technique if client is immunocompromised or critically ill. • Flush bag before refilling with formula. • Use prepackaged, ready-to-use sterile feeding formulas. If using open system, cover, label, and refrigerate unused formula and discard in 24 hr. • Disinfect ports before and after any handling. • Consult dietitian about osmolarity of formula (hyperosmolar or high-fiber formula may cause diarrhea).
Small-bore feeding tube fails to advance into duodenum.	• Determine if gastric feeding is acceptable (client does not have gastroparesis, reflux esophagitis, high risk for aspiration, absence of gag or cough reflex). • Administer prokinetic agent before rather than after tube insertion. • Suggest tube be advanced under fluoroscopy.
Small-bore feeding tube becomes clogged; occlusion alarm sounds.	• Do not let formula bag run dry. • Use warm sterile water in 50-mL syringe with a gentle push/pull technique for flushing tube. Do not use vigorous pressure. • Do not flush with cola or acidic pH juices such as cranberry juice, as this can precipitate protein and cause tube clogging. • Papain, combinations of activated pancreatic enzymes, and sodium bicarbonate mixed with water may declog the tube. • Flush tube with sterile water every 4–6 hr and before and after any medication administered. • Crush medications fully—ensure proper dilution and administer each medication separately. • Consider use of papain and sodium bicarbonate with water for flush. • Use declogging system suggested by tube manufacturer—do not reinsert guidewire to unclog tube. • Replace long-term tube every 4 weeks using alternate nostril.
Gastrostomy tube site becomes irritated.	• Apply plain antacid (e.g., Mylanta) to area if condition is mild. • Use skin prep barrier followed by antifungal powder followed by skin prep barrier. • Request tube with external bar or disc be replaced with plain tube that is sutured into place (bars and discs may embed into skin).

GERONTOLOGIC Considerations

Dietary Needs of the Elderly

Energy (caloric) requirement: 2,000–2,400 kcal/day (may adjust to energy expenditure and physical activity).

Protein: 10% of energy requirement, increases to 20% of energy requirement during periods of stress (surgery, infection, burn).

Fiber: 20–35 g/day of fiber (five servings of fruit per day).

Fluids: 1,500–2,000 mL of water/day or 30 mL/kg body weight.

Vitamins: same as for younger adult except for vitamins D, B_6, and B_{12}. *Significant deficiencies in serum levels of vitamins and minerals are rare in healthy older adults.*

Vitamin D requirement is 10 mg/day for adults 51–70 and 15 mg/day for those over age 70.

Vitamin B_6 intake should be 1.7 mg/day for men and 1.5 mg/day for women over age 51 (25% of elderly are deficient in vitamin B_6).

Vitamin B_{12} intake should be 2.4 mg for all adults over age 51 (about 15% of elderly are deficient in vitamin B_{12}).

Minerals: increased need—10 mg/day of iron.

The elderly are at high risk for malnutrition due to age-related physiologic changes, healthcare status, and lifestyle factors.

Physiologic Changes Associated With Aging

- Between ages 25 and 70, percentage of body fat doubles and lean body mass decreases by about one-third.
- Metabolic rate decreases 20% in men and 13% in elderly women; energy requirements decrease, there is reduced hunger and increased satiety due to increased levels of cholecystokinin, so food intake decreases.
- Esophageal and intestinal motility decrease.
- Saliva production decreases.
- Gastric secretions decline by 30% in adults over age 65, increasing risk for malabsorption of vitamin B_{12}, calcium, iron, folate, and possibly zinc.
- Lactose intolerance (more prevalent in elderly than younger adults) increases risk for calcium and vitamin D deficiency.
- Gastric emptying is slowed.
- Protein reserves may be inadequate for periods of stress, sepsis, or injury, leading to protein–calorie malnutrition.
- Loss of sense of smell (in more than 50% of those age 65–80 and 75% of those older than age 80).
- Decline in thirst drive (risk for dehydration).

Health Status Factors

- Poor dentition (up to 37% of elderly are edentulous). Loss of dentition is not due to the normal aging process but to improper oral hygiene and or inadequate nutrition beginning at an earlier age.
- Ill-fitting dentures causing pain limiting variety and quantity of intake.
- Swallowing or self-care deficit disorders (e.g., neuromuscular disorders, Parkinson's, Alzheimer's).
- Psychological changes (depression, cognitive impairment).
- Effect of medications (altered metabolism, anorexia, nausea, diarrhea, cognitive disturbance).
- Inappropriate diet prescription (low-salt, low-cholesterol, or low-calorie diet).
- Medical conditions (e.g., COPD, heart failure, cancer resulting).

Lifestyle Factors

- Alcoholism
- Inadequate income
- Decreased physical activity, lack of transport, isolation
- Cultural values
- Lack of monitoring/caregiving

  Assessment parameters for nutritional status of the elderly client in addition to the above risk factors include:
- Anthropometric values:

  Ideal body weight = men should weigh 106 lb for 5 feet plus 6 lb for each additional inch in height. Women should weigh 100 lb for 5 feet plus 5 pounds for each additional inch in height. Significant weight loss is more than 10% of body weight over the last 6 months or more than 7.5% over the last 3 months or more than 5% over the last month.

  Body mass index risk for malnutrition:

  Mild = BMI is 17.0–18.4

  Moderate = 16.0–16.9

  Severe = less than 16.0
- Biochemical indicators of *malnutrition* include:

  Serum albumin below 3.5 mg/L (increased risk for infection, pressure ulcers, prolonged hospitalization)

  Low serum cholesterol
- Serum creatinine (reflects muscle mass)

  Moderate deficit if 60%–79% of predicted

  Severe deficit if less than 60% of predicted

MANAGEMENT Guidelines

Each state legislates a Nurse Practice Act for RNs and LVN/LPNs. Healthcare facilities are responsible for establishing and implementing policies and procedures that conform to their state's regulations. Verify the regulations and role parameters for each healthcare worker in your facility.

Delegation

- The professional nurse is responsible for the client's basic nutritional assessment (an evaluation tool) if a dietician is not available. An unlicensed (CNA or UAP) is not trained to assess this information. A periodic nutritional assessment should be completed for any client who is hospitalized for a long period of time.
- The UAP (unless specifically trained by a swallowing specialist) should not be allowed to feed or assist in feeding the dysphagic client. The licensed professional should monitor and evaluate the UAP's adherence to client-specific feeding instructions.
- Generally, serving a food tray or feeding a client is assigned to the unlicensed staff. These staff should be reminded to report any unusual complaints or poor intake of food based on the client's care plan.
- Insertion of NG tubes is performed by a physician, an RN, or an LVN/LPN. A CNA or UAP may measure and record drainage from an NG tube and provide oral hygiene.
- Enteral feedings should be given by professional nurses, but some facilities do allow trained nonprofessionals to administer the feedings.
- If medication is administered through a (double lumen) tube, refer to agency protocol to determine who may administer the medication. According to some facilities, it is only an RN or LVN/LPN who may administer medication.

Communication Matrix

- Changes in GI therapy or nutritional support orders as well as significant changes in client data regarding tolerance of nutritional therapies (including laboratory data client's elimination pattern) should be communicated to all staff.
- NPO or positioning requirements should be posted at the client's head of bed (HOB) and communicated to all attending staff (orally and by written plan of care).
- Specific instructions and special techniques for feeding the dysphagic client should be posted at the client's HOB.
- The UAP should report to the nurse when a feeding pump alarm sounds, or when additional formula is needed.
- The UAP should report to the nurse if a client's NG tube is leaking or if the client becomes nauseated or vomits.
- Clients who are taking enteral feedings should be working with a Nutrition Support Team (NST) in accordance with the American Society for Parenteral and Enteral Nutrition. The nursing staff should work with and communicate through this team, because they are trained to follow this aspect of the care plan.
- The nurse assigned to the client is the essential link between the client and the team; thus both verbal and written reports are important for continuity of care and assessment of the nutritional status of the client.
- It is also important for the nurse to teach the client and his or her family about the need for and aspects of nutritional support through enteral feedings.
- After initial nutrition screening by the admitting nurse or speech pathologist, the Nutrition Support Team for individualized assessment of clients should be contacted. Referral concerns include:

  Nutrition risk on initial screening

  Extended ICU stay

  Any nutrition support (tube feeding, TPN)

  Latex allergy

  75 years and older and having surgery

  Liquid diet or NPO for more than 72 hr

  Pregnant or lactating but not admitted for delivery

CRITICAL THINKING Strategies

Scenario 1

Mrs. Ramsey, age 62, has been admitted to the hospital with complaints of painful abdominal distention and signs of dehydration after 2 days of vomiting. She is diagnosed with small bowel obstruction due to adhesions (scar tissue) from a remote abdominal hysterectomy.

1. What are the pathophysiologic effects of intestinal obstruction?
2. What potential fluid and electrolyte problems occur with small bowel obstruction?
3. How does the loss of gastric secretions differ from the loss of intestinal secretions?
4. What are the body's normal compensatory mechanisms for acid–base imbalances due to loss of gastrointestinal fluids?
5. What interventions help to correct these imbalances?

Scenario 2

An elderly client (age 64) is admitted to the hospital for a hip replacement. When you are taking a history, you note that she appears to be malnourished.

1. What additional dietary information would be important to include in the database for this client?
2. Evaluate the assessment parameters in terms of the nutritional needs of the elderly and examine how this client fits into the model.

3. Identify the primary parameters to be included in the discharge plan for this client.

Scenario 3

Mr. Bradley has been diagnosed with cancer of the liver and is admitted to the hospital with brain metastases. He complains of no appetite, refuses most meals, and is becoming significantly malnourished with drastic weight loss. Impairment of his hepatic and neurologic status has caused intermittent periods of nonresponsiveness and inability to eat.

Mr. Bradley's family is asking about alternative nutrition options and the physician is requesting that they make decisions about the treatment options.

1. If nutritional support is indicated, what are the processes normally followed?
2. Who has the primary decision-making power about medical treatments such as nutritional support?
3. Do healthcare providers have an obligation to provide extraordinary care?
4. Once initiated, can healthcare providers discontinue artificial feeding?
5. In what ways can healthcare providers provide symbolically significant care?

NCLEX® Review Questions

Unless otherwise specified, choose only one (1) answer.

1. Trans fats are polyunsaturates and monounsaturates that
   1. Have been hydrogenated.
   2. Are unsaturated.
   3. Primarily come from vegetables, nuts, and seeds.
   4. Come from animal sources.
2. Which of the following clients would mostly likely be placed on a potassium restricted diet?
   1. Heart failure client
   2. Renal failure client
   3. COPD client
   4. Burn client
3. Which of the following are helpful for the dysphagic client?
   Select all that apply.
   1. Swallowing liquid foods.
   2. Eating food accompanied by liquids.
   3. Swallowing thickened liquids.
   4. Eating food without accompanying liquid.
   5. Using a straw for liquids.
   6. Being fed with a syringe.
4. The purpose of the Salem NG decompression tube's blue lumen is to
   1. Prevent esophageal reflux of gastric contents.
   2. Allow siphoning of gastric contents if they stagnate.
   3. Provide a port for continuous feeding.
   4. Prevent tube adherence to the gastric mucosa.
5. Which of the following is the least reliable indicator of the return of bowel function?
   1. Appetite
   2. Bowel sounds
   3. Presence of flatus
   4. Bowel movement
6. The best way to determine NG tube placement with continuous feeding is to
   1. Auscultate for injected air sound over the epigastrium.
   2. Aspirate secretions and check for an acid pH.
   3. Note the character of aspirated secretions.
   4. Use capnography to detect presence of carbon dioxide.
7. An intermittent NG tube feeding should be withheld if the residual volume is
   1. 50 mL.
   2. 100 mL.
   3. 150 mL.
   4. >200 mL.
8. The best way to prevent clogging of a small bore feeding tube is to
   1. Flush frequently with cola.
   2. Flush frequently with cranberry juice.
   3. Flush frequently with warm water.
   4. Replace the tube weekly.
9. The most effective way to promote small bore feeding tube advancement into the small intestine is to
   1. Place the client right side-lying.
   2. Place the client left side-lying.
   3. Administer prokinetic medication before tube insertion.
   4. Reinsert guidewire to advance the tube.
10. The most appropriate method for extended nutritional support is
    1. Nasogastric tube feeding.
    2. Nasointestinal tube feeding.
    3. Gastrostomy tube feeding.
    4. Parenteral nutrition.

20

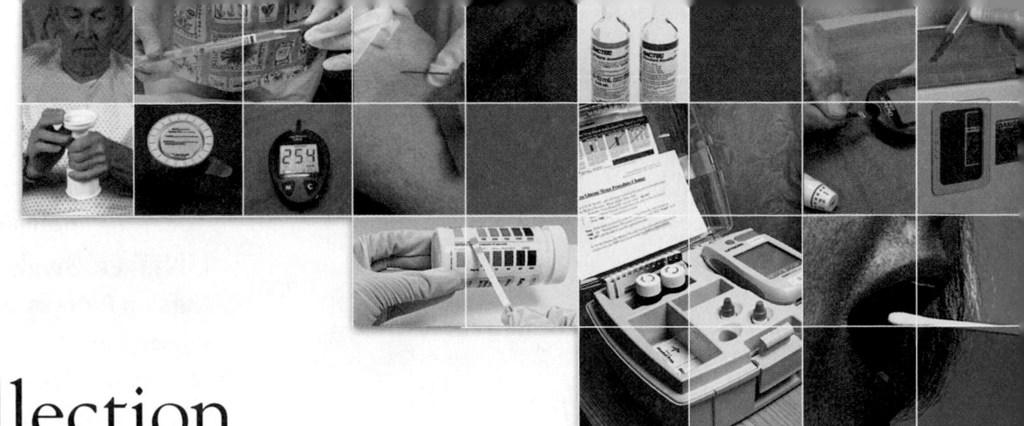

Specimen Collection

LEARNING OBJECTIVES

1. Discuss the nursing responsibilities for reporting abnormal laboratory values.
2. Describe the major client instructions that ensure an uncontaminated midstream urine specimen.
3. State the purpose for testing urine for ketone bodies.
4. State two objectives for obtaining a stool specimen.
5. List four precautions that must be carried out when obtaining a stool specimen for parasite identification.
6. Demonstrate the procedure for testing for occult blood.
7. State necessary documentation when collecting a stool specimen.
8. Explain the objectives for collecting a sputum specimen.
9. Outline the steps of collecting a sputum specimen from a suction trap.
10. Compare and contrast obtaining an aerobic and anaerobic culture.
11. State purpose for obtaining a blood specimen for glucose testing.
12. Write two nursing diagnoses that are relevant for specimen collection.
13. Demonstrate the removal of blood using a Vacutainer.
14. List specimen collections requiring specific consent forms.
15. State two critical-thinking solutions for the problem of blood not flowing into the syringe when withdrawing blood.
16. State the nursing action when a hematoma occurs at the puncture site.
17. Describe procedure for testing presence of HIV antibodies.

CHAPTER OUTLINE

TERMINOLOGY

Aerobe a microorganism that lives and grows in the presence of free oxygen.

Albuminuria the presence of albumin in the urine.

Anaerobe an organism that lives and grows in the absence of molecular oxygen.

Antimicrobial an agent that prevents the multiplication of microorganisms.

Antimicrobic preventing the development or pathogenic action of microbes.

Asepsis prevention of contact with microorganisms.

Aspiration the removal of fluids or gases from a cavity by the application of suction.

Autolet a small instrument with lancet used to obtain a capillary blood specimen; usually used to measure blood glucose level.

Bacteria unicellular plant-like microorganisms lacking chlorophyll.

Cannula a tube for insertion into a duct or cavity.

Culture to grow microorganisms or living tissue cells in a special medium.

Dermis synonym for corium; the skin layer beneath the epidermis; contains vascular connective tissue.

Excoriation a breakdown of the epidermis.

Expectorant an agent that facilitates the removal of the secretions of the bronchopulmonary mucous membrane.

Exudate material obtained from a wound as the result of the inflammatory process.

Genitourinary pertaining to the genital and urinary systems.

Glucose a monosaccharide, the end product of carbohydrate metabolism; also known as dextrose; found in the normal blood.

Glycosuria the presence of sugar in the urine.

Granulocytes a granular leukocyte.

Hematuria blood in the urine.

HIV antibodies produced by the immune system and present in the blood when individual is exposed to HIV.

Hypovolemia diminished circulating fluid volume.

Inflammatory process localized response when injury or destruction of tissue has occurred; destroys, wards off, or dilutes the causative agent or the injured tissue.

Intracellular inside the cell.

Micturition the process of emptying the urinary bladder; voiding.

Occult blood blood in minute quantities, can be recognized only by microscopic examination or by chemical means.

Parasite an organism that lives within, on, or at the expense of another organism, known as the host.

Patency the state of being freely open.

Pathogen disease-producing organism.

Pinworm oxyurid parasite of the intestine, usually *Enterobius vermicularis*. Commonly found in children. Piperazine is drug of choice.

Polyuria the excessive production and elimination of urine.

Purulent containing pus, or caused by pus.

Pus an inflammation product containing leukocytes and exudate.

Septic pertinent to pathologic organisms or their toxins.

Septicemia presence of pathologic bacteria in the blood.

Skin turgor the tension or fullness of the cells and resistance against deformation.

Specific gravity weight of a substance compared with an equal volume of water. Water is 1.000.

Specimen a sample taken to show or to determine the character of the whole, as a specimen of urine.

Sputum substance expelled by coughing or clearing the throat.

Stool waste matter discharged from the bowels.

Transtracheal passage of a tube or needle through the wall of the trachea.

Urinary tract infection (UTI) an infection of the urinary tract, including all or part of the organs and ducts participating in the secretion and elimination of urine.

Vacutainer a plastic adapter that fits onto a double-ended needle for obtaining a venous blood sample.

Venipuncture puncture of a vein with a needle or catheter.

Venous pertaining to the veins; unoxygenated blood.

Viscosity resistance offered by a fluid; property of a substance that is dependent on the friction of its component molecules as they slide by each other.

LABORATORY TESTS

Laboratory tests are an adjunct for diagnosing healthcare problems and assessing the health status of clients. Test findings can reveal occult problems, determine the stage of disease, estimate the activity of the disease process, and measure the effect of therapy. Multiple laboratory tests are usually ordered not only to assist in diagnosing problems, but also to rule out certain disease states.

Laboratory tests can be analyzed individually or as a part of a screening panel. For example, a routine urinalysis screens for the chemical makeup of the urine, as well as color, clarity, and presence of abnormal cells. Blood chemistry components can be tested individually, as well as in combination through a multiparameter test. These tests provide data on 8, 12, or 16 different elements of blood, depending on the laboratory equipment. It is more cost-effective when all the tests are run simultaneously with one blood specimen. For example, a "panel 12" analyzes the following tests: total protein, albumin, calcium, inorganic phosphorous, cholesterol, glucose, blood urea nitrogen (BUN), uric acid, creatinine, total bilirubin, alkaline phosphatase, and serum glutamic oxaloacetic transaminase (SGOT).

Every laboratory establishes its own normal values for each test. The normal values are generally printed on each laboratory slip to facilitate comparisons with the client's findings. Healthy clients do not always fall within the calculated laboratory norms. The physician, considering other variables, must judge the value and diagnostic implications of these tests.

Point-of-Care Testing (POCT)

An important component of client care has always been bedside nursing. Now, and in the future, this will include procedures to obtain laboratory results at the bedside. Immediate lab results will save crucial time and allow for quick decision making. For example, if the nurse knows, through POCT, that a critically ill client's glucose level is elevated, an immediate intervention of IV insulin and monitoring may immediately improve the client's status.

The most common POCT performed at the bedside are glucose levels, coagulation, blood gas, electrolytes, pregnancy tests, and urine dipstick tests. Most POCT in facilities are coordinated by a laboratory according to regulatory protocols. For example, the Clinical Laboratory Improvement Amendment regulates at the federal level who may perform the test and which ones may be included in POCT.

The Joint Commission and the College of American Pathologists set additional standards. More tests will, in the future, be incorporated into these protocols because their immediate results at the bedside will greatly improve client outcomes.

Nursing Responsibility

Nursing responsibilities associated with the collection of specimens range from client education to reporting abnormal laboratory findings to the appropriate health team member. When specimens are ordered, it is essential that the client understand the full importance of how and why the specimen is to be obtained. If sterile or clean technique is required, client teaching can provide an understanding of the process. If the client is involved with obtaining the specimen, precise instructions should be given.

To prevent unnecessary lost time and cost to the client, the nurse must be well informed of the correct procedure for obtaining, handling, and processing each specimen. If the nurse is unfamiliar with the procedure, he or she should refer to the nursing procedure or laboratory manual for the healthcare facility. Specific directions are written for most tests performed by the laboratory. If there is any question about the procedure, the laboratory should be called for directions before obtaining the specimen.

The physician should be notified immediately of any abnormal laboratory findings that could be potentially life-threatening. Verbal communication is the most appropriate and efficient method. When the nurse leaves written messages on the chart, several hours may elapse before the physician sees the findings.

The nurse should also document when abnormal results are reported to the physician. Documentation should include date, time, tests, and the orders taken. If results were left with another person such as office personnel, the name of the person receiving results should be documented.

All clients admitted to a healthcare facility have at least one laboratory specimen collected during their hospitalization. The most frequent laboratory tests ordered are those involving the urine and blood.

It is the nurse's responsibility to be aware of any and all legal implications of specimen collection. Reporting certain tests, such as HIV testing, requires a specific consent; likewise, certain test results are required to be reported to ensure public safety. It is important to remember that all client information, including laboratory results, is confidential.

Urine Tests

Nursing responsibilities include collecting, temporarily storing, and performing tests on the urine specimen. Timed urine specimens are usually left in the nursing unit until completion of the test. When urine specimens are retained in the nursing unit, the nurse must take special care in the storing and handling of the specimen to ensure reliable results. Generally, urine specimens collected over a period of hours must be refrigerated or have preservatives added to the specimen to ensure accurate results. Preservatives, such as hydrochloric acid or thymol, prevent deterioration of the specimen.

Most urine specimens are collected as clean-catch, or midstream, specimens and sent directly to the laboratory. Single urine specimens are obtained through random sampling. It is best to obtain the first voided specimen in the morning for routine urine tests. This specimen is more concentrated, and the pH is more acidic. The midstream method of urine collection necessitates that proper instructions be given to the client in cleansing the genitalia and obtaining the specimen.

When timed specimens are ordered, the nursing role encompasses not only the handling of the urine specimen, but also precise instructions to the client for collecting the specimen. The collection of urine needs to start and finish at the designated time. Timed tests vary from 2 hr to 24 hr. Assessment for amylase and bilirubin can be done on a 2-hr collection. Creatinine clearance and estriol determination require a 24-hr specimen. A 24-hr urine specimen that is started at 9 AM must be finished at 9 AM the next day in order to obtain accurate results. Instructions to the client include voiding at 9 AM, discarding that urine specimen, and collecting the rest of the urine at 9 AM the next morning.

Clinitest, Acetest, and the test for specific gravity are usually performed by the nurse and are not done by the laboratory. Nurses should follow the specific procedures for each test to obtain accurate results.

Blood Tests

Even though blood studies are carried out on venous, capillary, or arterial blood, the usual sample is obtained from venous blood. Capillary blood specimens are usually used to obtain specimens from infants and neonates. In adult clients, blood glucose and hemoglobin levels can be determined from capillary blood. Arterial samples are obtained for blood gas determination and cultures.

Venipunctures must be carried out keeping in mind that hemoconcentration and hemolysis can occur if the procedure is done improperly. Hemoconcentration results from prolonged use of a tourniquet. Hemolysis may occur from using a small-bore needle for the venipuncture of rapidly infusing blood into the specimen tubes. Using a larger bore needle for performing the venipuncture and taking the cap off the specimen tubes is recommended to prevent hemolysis.

If a needle and syringe are used for drawing blood, the top may be removed from the blood tube. After removing the top, slowly inject the blood into the test tube to prevent hemolysis.

Blood specimens are placed in specific blood tubes according to the type of test ordered and sent to the laboratory for analysis. Each healthcare facility has a list of blood tests that are analyzed from blood in a specific color-top test tube. The colored top on the test tube indicates whether or not the tube contains a preservative. When whole blood is required for the test, an anticoagulant, such as heparin or trisodium citrate, is placed in the test tube to keep the blood from clotting. When serum is needed for the laboratory test, no preservative is added to the blood as the clot is used for the test. If the test tube contains a preservative, the tube should be gently rotated back and forth with palms of hands to prevent the blood from clotting.

Some blood tests require that the client fast for several hours before obtaining the specimens. Other blood tests have no special requirements for collection. Blood studies requiring a fasting specimen for accuracy include fasting blood sugar, lipid panels, glucose tolerance tests, and insulin levels.

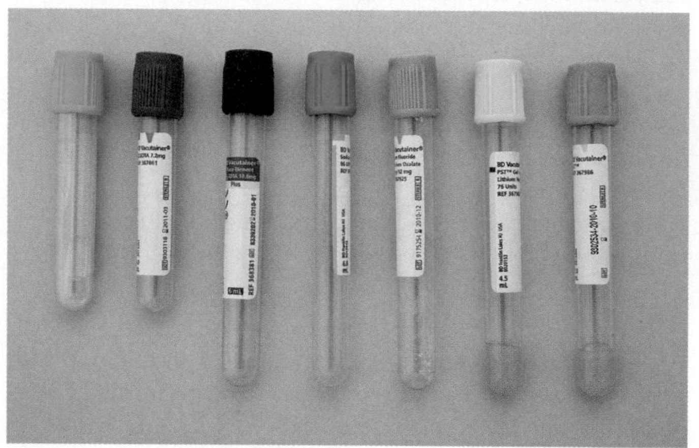

▲ These are examples of color-identified blood specimen tubes. Each color indicates the specific test ordered and contains the appropriate additive/preservative.

TABLE 20-1 Collection Blood Sample Types

Purpose	Common Tests	Tube Color	Draw Volume	Additives
Whole blood studies	Blood culture	Yellow*	12 mL	Acid citrate Dextrose/nutrient Broth or preservative
Prothrombin times (PT)	Coagulation studies on plasma	Blue (or black)	3 to 5 mL	Sodium citrate (Sodium oxalate)
Chemistry, therapeutic drug monitoring, blood type	Serum studies	Red	2 to 20 mL	None
Chemistry (including lipids)	Plasma	Green	2 to 15 mL	Lithium heparin
Hematology CBC – CSR	Whole blood studies	Purple/ Lavender	2 to 10 mL	K_2 or K_3 EDTA anticoagulant
Glucose on serum or plasma	Plasma	Gray	3 to 10 mL	Anticoagulant Sodium flouride Sodium oxalate

*Requires sterile technique.

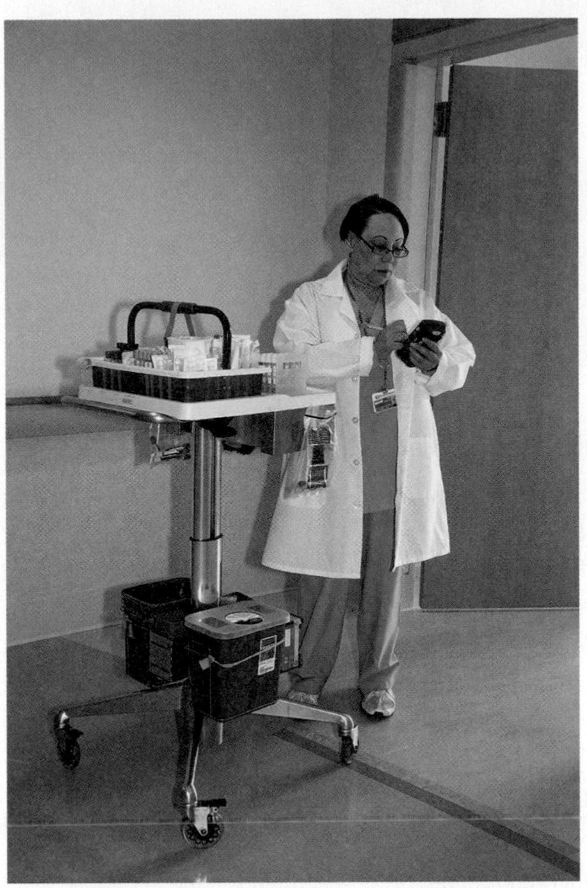

▲ Blood specimens are usually drawn by a special technician according to the physician's orders.

Clinical Alert

Order of tube draw is important because there may be a small amount of residual or tube coating, called "carryover," which could invalidate the results.

Tube Order: Yellow (Sterile), Blue, Red, Green, Purple, Gray.

Cultures

Specimens from the throat, eyes, nose, vagina, wounds, sputum, stool, urine, and blood are often ordered to be cultured for pathogens. Special tubes or containers with culture media are used for organism growth. The culture is prepared in the laboratory according to the type of test ordered. It is essential that the proper technique be used to place the specimen in the appropriate container to ensure accurate results. Specimens obtained for culture and sensitivity require immediate processing and must be sent directly to the laboratory after they are obtained. If a time lapse occurs, the specimen may need to be discarded and a new one obtained. If the specimen is allowed to dry before the examination, the organism cannot be transferred to the slide and thus to the culture medium.

NURSING DIAGNOSES

The following nursing diagnoses may be appropriate to include in a client care plan when the components are related to collecting specimens.

NURSING DIAGNOSIS	RELATED FACTORS
Anxiety	Dread of unknown outcome, results of specimen tests
Ineffective Coping	Fear, external stress, situational crisis
Infection, Risk for	Invasive procedure, contamination from poor technique of specimen collection
Deficient Knowledge	Inaccurate collection of specimen (e.g., instruction not clear, unable to hear or see well enough to complete collection)
Noncompliance	Inadequate understanding of the purpose or value of diagnostic test (e.g., language and cultural barriers)
Acute Pain	Invasive procedure, altered body function, recent surgery

CLEANSE HANDS The single most important nursing action to decrease the incidence of hospital-based infections is hand hygiene. *Remember to wash your hands or use antibacterial gel before and after each and every client contact.*

IDENTIFY CLIENT Before every procedure, check two forms of client identification, not including room number. These actions prevent errors and conform to the Joint Commission standards.

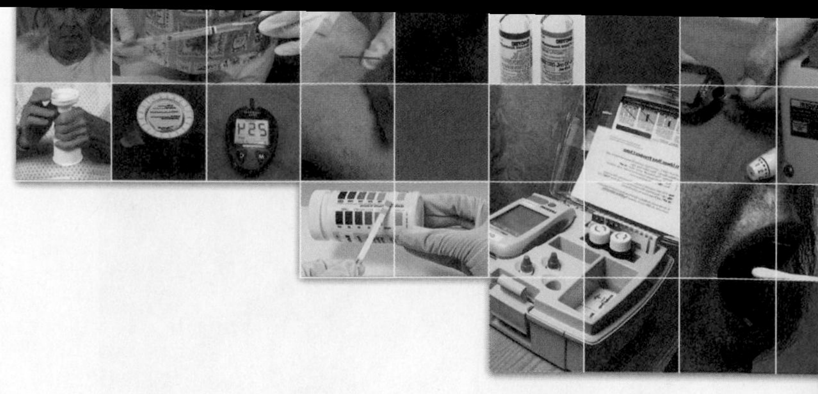

Chapter 20

UNIT ❶

Urine Specimens

Nursing Process Data

ASSESSMENT Data Base

- Assess client's ability to understand instructions and to obtain specimens properly.
- Identify if signs and symptoms of urinary tract infections are present: frequency, urgency, dysuria, hematuria, flank pain, fever, and cloudy urine with sediment.
- Determine the purpose for which the specimen is being obtained.
- Determine how the collection is to be obtained.
- Assess parents' understanding of the purpose for collecting infant's urine.
- Assess client's ability to test own urine for ketone bodies.

PLANNING Objectives

- To instruct the client in the method for obtaining a specimen
- To obtain an uncontaminated urine specimen for culture and sensitivity
- To obtain urine specimen for routine hospital admission or as a preoperative urine sample
- To maintain the collection of urine for 24 hr
- To successfully teach client to test urine for ketone bodies

IMPLEMENTATION Procedures

EVALUATION Expected Outcomes

- Client understands rationale and procedure for collecting urine specimen.
- Uncontaminated urine specimen is collected.
- Collection of 24-hr urine specimen is successful.
- Client learns how to test for ketone bodies.
- A clean, uncontaminated urine specimen is collected from a child.

Collecting Midstream Urine

Equipment

Soap and water or hand cleanser
Cleaning swab or bactericidal soap
Sterile specimen container
Label for container
Clean gloves

Procedure

1. Gather equipment.
2. Perform hand hygiene.
3. Identify client by checking two forms of client ID.
4. Explain procedure to client.
5. Don clean gloves and provide perineal care as needed.
6. Instruct client to collect specimen in bathroom or place on bedpan.
7. Instruct client to clean the urinary meatus and obtain urine specimen. (See procedure below: *For a Female*, a-e.)

> **Clinical Alert**
> Do not use alcohol-containing wipes for cleansing before collecting urine for suspected drug abuse.

For a Male

a. Don clean gloves and open container.
b. Cleanse end of penis with cleansing swab using circular motion and moving from middle toward outside. ▸ ***Rationale:*** Always swab from clean to dirty area to decrease bacteria levels.

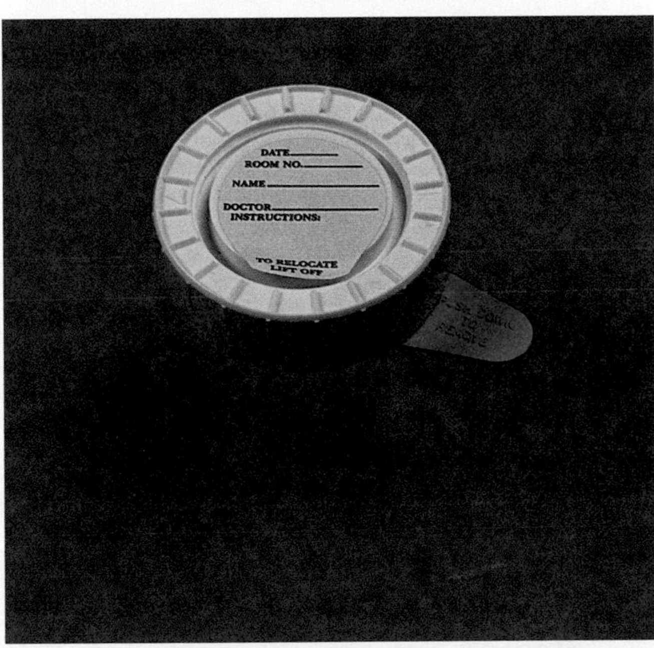

▲ Sterile urine specimen container.

c. Ask client to initiate urine stream.
d. After single stream achieved, pass specimen bottle into stream and obtain urine sample. At least 30 mL must be obtained for adequate specimen. ▸ ***Rationale:*** The microorganisms which accumulate at the urinary meatus have been flushed out with the original stream of urine and are not collected in the specimen.

For a Female

a. Don clean gloves and open container.
b. Spread labia minora with nondominant hand.
c. Cleanse area with disinfectant swab, beginning above the urethral orifice and moving posteriorly.
d. Ask client to initiate urine stream. Hold labia open throughout the voiding process.
e. After single stream achieved, pass specimen bottle into the stream and obtain sample of at least 30 mL (half full).

8. To prevent contamination of specimen with skin flora, instruct the client to remove the bottle before the flow of urine stops and before releasing the labia or penis.
9. Instruct client to completely empty bladder.
10. Wipe off outside of container after replacing cap.
11. Remove gloves and perform hand hygiene.
12. Label the specimen (as appropriate) with client's name, room number, medical record number, date, time, and physician's name.
13. Take specimen to laboratory within 15 minutes. If this is not possible, refrigerate specimen. ▸ ***Rationale:*** Delays in testing may decrease glucose ketone, bilirubin, and urobilinogen values. Falsely elevated bacteria counts can also occur if specimen is not refrigerated.

> **Clinical Alert**
> A contaminated specimen is the single most common reason for inaccurate reporting on urinary cultures and sensitivities. To prevent contamination, place cap of container with sterile side up while collecting specimen and do not touch inside of container.

Collecting 24-Hour Urine Specimen

Equipment

Urine specimen container
Preservative, if required
Requisition slip
Label for specimen
Sign that urine collection is in progress
Container with ice, if needed

NOTE: 24-hour urine specimens must be collected for the entire time ordered. To obtain accurate finding, the laboratory needs the entire urine specimen. The start and stop dates and times should be reported at change of shift.

> **Clinical Alert**
> Note any dietary restriction or medication precautions in preparation for 24-hr urine collection.

Procedure

1. Explain procedure to client and check two forms of client ID. Stress the importance of saving all urine for 24 hr.
2. Place sign in client's bathroom stating that 24-hr urine specimen is in progress, with start and stop date and time.
3. Collect urine specimen and discard it. ▶ ***Rationale:*** The first specimen is considered "old urine" or urine in the bladder before test began. Test begins with an empty bladder.
4. Record date and time of first specimen on label, and place bottle in appropriate area. Depending on hospital protocol, specimens may be refrigerated, placed on ice, or left in the client's bathroom.
5. Add preservative, if required.
6. Post sign in appropriate place, if other than client's bathroom.
7. Place all urine voided in specimen container. Instruct client *not* to urinate directly into the large collection container.
8. Request client to void exactly 24 hr after first specimen was obtained. Place voided urine in container.
9. After the last voided specimen is placed in the container, cover and send entire specimen to the lab with the proper requisition.
10. Remove sign, and remind client that the test is completed.
11. If a specimen is accidentally discarded, obtain a new container, note the new date and time, and restart the procedure. Notify lab of lost urine.

NOTE: For creatinine clearance test: Instruct client to avoid caffeine-containing drinks including coffee, tea, and most soft drinks. Drink plenty of water before and during 24-hr collection.

Collecting a Specimen From an Infant

Equipment

Cleansing solution
Towel
Pediatric urine collector
Diapers
Appropriate specimen containers
Clean gloves (2 pair)
Clean specimen container
Label for specimen

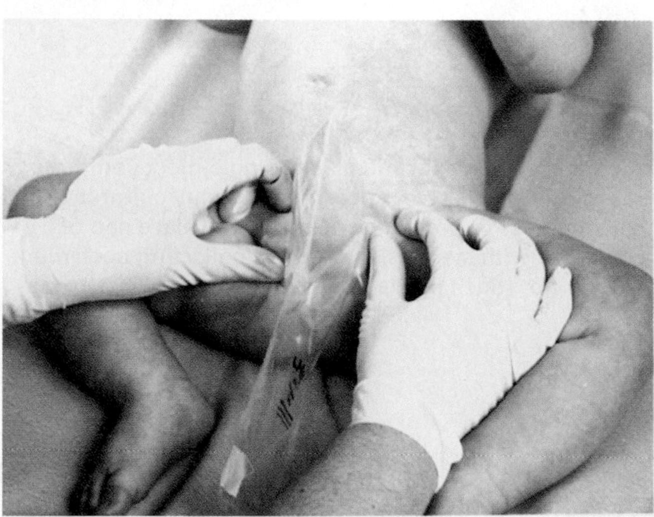

▲ Remove adhesive backing from urine collection bag and place securely over penis.

Procedure

1. Gather equipment.
2. Perform hand hygiene. Don clean gloves.
3. Identify correct child by checking two forms of infant ID.
4. Cleanse and dry child's perineum.
5. Remove paper backing from the adhesive on the urine collector.
6. Apply urine collector to child's perineum, avoiding extension over anus to prevent contamination.
   a. *Male:* Place child's penis through the opening of the collector.
   b. *Female:* Place the opening of the collection bag over the child's urinary meatus.
7. Remove gloves.

8. Place a diaper on the child to help hold the collector in place.
9. Perform hand hygiene.
10. Check the collector every 15 minutes until a specimen is obtained.
11. Don clean gloves.
12. Remove the collector and place in a urine specimen container.
13. Place clean diaper on child.
14. Send the urine specimen to the lab by either placing the urine collection bag in a urine container or pouring urine from collection bag into the urine container.
15. Remove gloves and perform hand hygiene.
16. Label the container with the child's name, date and time of collection, and the initials of the nurse doing the collection.

Teaching Clients to Test for Urine Ketone Bodies

Equipment

Urinal or container
Test tube
Urine testing kit (test tube, dropper)
Color charts
Paper towel
Watch for timing

Procedure

1. Type 1 diabetics, when blood glucose is over 200, will need to check urine for ketone bodies.
2. Instruct client to void in urinal or container to collect urine specimen. ▸ ***Rationale:*** Specimen should be fresh because urine collected overnight will not accurately reveal concentration of ketone bodies.
3. Empty small amount of urine into test tube or dip Keto-Diastix strip into urine. Wait 15 seconds.

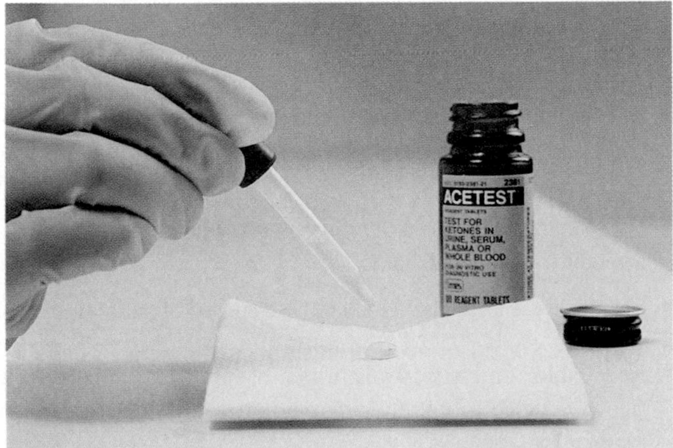

▲ Place one drop of urine on Acetest tablet to check for ketone bodies.

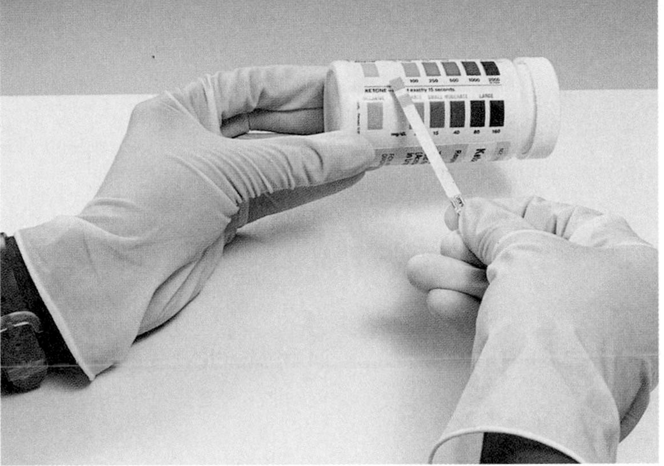
▲ Keto-Diastix strips are checked against the chart for ketone bodies.

4. *Alternative method:* Place ketone (Acetest) tablet on a piece of paper towel. ▸ ***Rationale:*** White towel reflects color and absorbs more efficiently.
   a. Wait 30 seconds.
   b. Compare color of tablet and chart.
5. Compare strip against color chart and note findings. ▸ ***Rationale:*** Instruct the client to notify client's physician if ketone bodies are moderately present.

Clinical Alert

Ketones in urine may be negative or present in small, moderate, or large amounts. If there are more than moderate ketones and the client does not feel good or has nausea and vomiting, client should immediately contact physician.

DOCUMENTATION for Urine Specimens

- Method used to obtain specimen
- Color, consistency, and odor of urine
- Amount of urine obtained (record this amount on the intake and output record also)
- Time specimen sent to laboratory
- Refrigeration, if required
- Exact time for 24-hr specimen
- Results of client teaching to test for ketone bodies

CRITICAL THINKING Application

Expected Outcomes

- Client understands rationale and procedure for collecting urine specimen.
- Uncontaminated urine specimen is collected.
- Collection of 24-hr urine specimen is successful.
- Client learns how to test for ketone bodies.
- A clean, uncontaminated urine specimen is collected from a child.

Unexpected Outcomes	Alternative Actions
Client is unable to assist with obtaining a sterile specimen.	• Place female client in bed and, after cleaning perineum thoroughly, place on sterile or clean bedpan. Cleanse perineal area with swab and obtain specimen according to procedure. • Assist client into bathroom. Assist client to cleanse perineum, instruct to start urine stream, and place the sterile specimen container under the stream to collect specimen. • For male clients, cleanse the penis, and place a sterile or clean urinal under the client. Instruct to start stream of urine and then place sterile container under stream. • Notify physician. Consider catheterization.
Urine specimen contaminated with feces or toilet paper.	• Instruct client on need for accuracy and compliance to urine collection.
Client cannot void on command at completion of test.	• Instruct client to void as close to time as possible. • Chart exact time when last specimen collected on both urine bottle and lab slip. Notify lab of findings.
Urine specimen discarded before 24-hr sample collected.	• If time period is close to 24 hr, call laboratory to determine whether test can be completed on sample collected. • If 24-hr sample must be started again, instruct client of necessity to save all urine. • Place signs indicating 24-hr test collection in progress on bathroom door and client's bedside stand. • Mark in bold or underlined print in Kardex indicating 24-hr urine collection in progress.
Infant's urine specimen is lost because collector does not adhere.	• Obtain a new collection bag and repeat the procedure. • Tape bag in place with nonallergenic paper tape if necessary.
Infant specimen is lost because collection bag is the wrong size.	• Obtain appropriate size bag and repeat the procedure.
Infant specimen cannot be obtained with a collection bag.	• Notify the physician that you are unable to obtain urine specimen. • If possible, keep diapers off and observe when infant urinates; attempt to obtain specimen.
Strips or tablets are discolored or moist.	• Sensitivity is lost. They need to be disposed of and new strips or tablets used. • Keep tablets and strips away from moisture by keeping them in tightly covered container (original bottle for tablets and baby food jar for tape). • Always check tablet before using to ensure accurate results.
Ketones are present in urine specimen.	• Check expiration date on strip; an expired product will not yield accurate results. • Check that client understands what actions to take if moderate or above ketones are present in the urine. • Be sure client is aware that a low-carbohydrate or a high-fat diet may cause false-positive results; certain drugs may also cause a false positive.

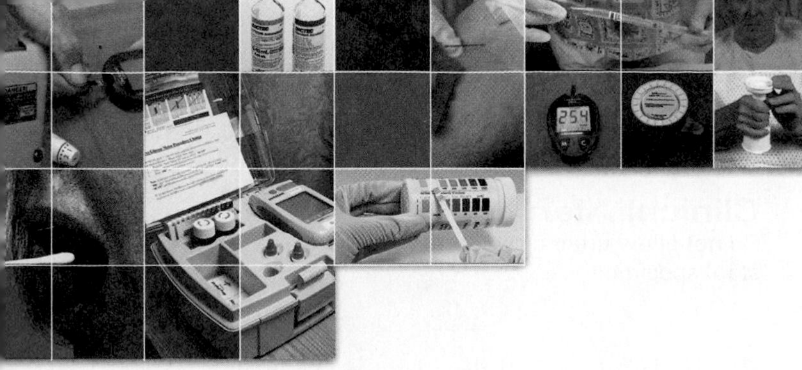

Chapter 20

UNIT 2

Stool Specimens

Nursing Process Data

ASSESSMENT Data Base

- Determine the purpose for the test.
- Check whether the specimen must be sent to the laboratory immediately.
- Determine the eliminatory status of the client (i.e., liquid vs. formed stools).
- Assess gastrointestinal tract dysfunction.

PLANNING Objectives

- To obtain stool specimens for diagnosing dysfunction in bowel elimination
- To assess for perforation or bleeding from a gastric ulcer
- To detect presence of ova and parasites
- To determine presence of pinworms

IMPLEMENTATION Procedures

EVALUATION Expected Outcomes

- Client understands purpose of test.
- Client is able to follow procedure of collection when appropriate.
- Dietary restrictions (if appropriate to test) were adhered to by client before test.
- Specimen collected is adequate for test.

Pearson Nursing Student Resources

Find additional review materials at **nursing.pearsonhighered.com**

Prepare for success with NCLEX®-style practice questions and Skill Checklists

Collecting Adult Stool Specimen

Equipment

Waxed cardboard or plastic container with cover
Tongue blade
Label for container
Clean bedpan or bedside commode
Clean gloves
Two signs for over client's bed and in bathroom stating, "Save All Stool."

Procedure

1. Check two forms of client ID, and explain the procedure to the client.
2. Determine if dietary restrictions are required before specimen collection.
3. Before collecting stool specimen, ask the client to void. Tell client not to void on the specimen. ▶ ***Rationale:*** This prevents contamination of specimen with urine, which could result in inaccurate test results.
4. Don gloves.
5. Clean out all urine from the bedpan or bedside commode.
6. Raise the head of the bed so that client can assume a squatting position on the bedpan, or help client sit on the bedside commode.

> **Clinical Alert**
> Do not allow urine or water to come in contact with the stool specimen.

7. Provide privacy until client has passed a stool.
8. Remove the bedpan or bedside commode. If necessary, help the client clean perineum.
9. Use tongue blade to obtain and place a small portion (2 teaspoons) of the formed stool in a waxed cardboard or plastic container. (For some tests you may need to collect the entire specimen.) Do not contaminate inside of container.
10. Wrap tongue blade in paper towel, discard remaining stool, and clean bedpan or bedside commode.
11. Remove gloves, and perform hand hygiene.
12. Label container with client's name.
13. Fill out laboratory request for appropriate test.
14. Take specimen to laboratory immediately. ▶ ***Rationale:*** Specimen may need to be refrigerated or examined immediately after collection.

Collecting Stool for Ova and Parasites

Equipment

Waxed cardboard or plastic container with cover
Tongue blade
Label for container
Clean bedpan or bedside commode
Clean gloves

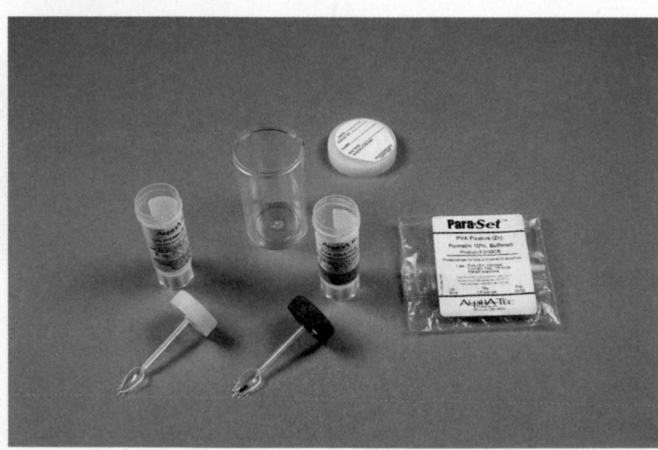

▲ Equipment necessary for collection ova and/or parasite specimen.

Procedure

1. Follow the steps for *Collecting Adult Stool Specimen*. Don clean gloves to collect stool specimen.
2. Collect exudate, mucus, and blood with all specimens.
   a. Place stool into container (with a preservative fluid).
   b. Mash the specimen in the container until mixed well with preservative. ▶ ***Rationale:*** Parasites thrive in this type of medium.
3. Replace and tighten cup. Shake the contents until mixed well.
4. Keep specimens at body temperature to be examined within 30 minutes. ▶ ***Rationale:*** Organisms must be seen in their active stages, as loose, fluid stools are likely to contain trophozoites or intestinal amoebas and flagellates.
5. There is usually no need to maintain well-formed or semiformed stool specimens at body temperature or to examine them quickly even though they may contain ova or cystic form of parasites.

6. Collect complete stools after purgative medications are administered.
7. When the presence of tapeworms is suspected, all stools must be examined in their entirety in order to find the head of the parasite.
8. Do not give barium, oil, and laxatives containing heavy metals that interfere with the extraction process for 7 days before stool examination. ▶ ***Rationale:*** Ova or cysts are not revealed.
9. Use only normal saline solution or tap water if an enema must be administered to collect specimens. Do not use soap suds or other substances.
10. Do not contaminate the specimen with urine as it kills amoeba.
11. Collect three random, normally passed stool specimens to ensure accurate test results.
12. Provide air freshener, if needed.

Collecting Infant Stool Specimen

Equipment

Diaper
Plastic diaper liner
Waxed cardboard or plastic container with cover
Cotton swabs
Label for container
Clean gloves

Procedure

1. Perform hand hygiene and identify infant using two forms of ID.
2. Place a clean, disposable diaper on the child or infant.
3. Check diaper frequently so that you obtain a specimen that is not contaminated with urine.
4. If child is passing liquid stools, place a plastic liner inside the diaper.
5. Don clean gloves before taking diaper off child and collecting specimen.
6. Use cotton swabs to procure the specimen.
7. Place specimen in stool container.
8. Remove gloves, perform hand hygiene, label, and send to lab immediately with client's name and medical record number.

Testing for Occult Blood

Equipment

Clean bedpan or bedside commode
Tongue blade
Guaiac test (Hemoccult) or gamma Fe-Cult packet
Guaiac solution
Glacial acetic acid
Hydrogen peroxide
Clean gloves

Procedure

1. Explain need for stool specimen to client and check two forms of client ID.
2. Provide privacy.
3. Position client on bedpan or commode.
4. Don clean gloves.
5. Take stool specimen to bathroom or utility room.
6. Prepare slide for testing according to packet instructions:

For Gamma Fe-Cult Plus

a. Smear thin layer of stool on panel number 1.
b. Obtain second specimen from a different part of stool specimen and smear thin layer on panel number 2.
c. Turn packet over, and remove perforated flap (marked Not to Be Opened by Patient).
d. Add 2 drops of Fe-Cult developing solution to test area over smear of stool.

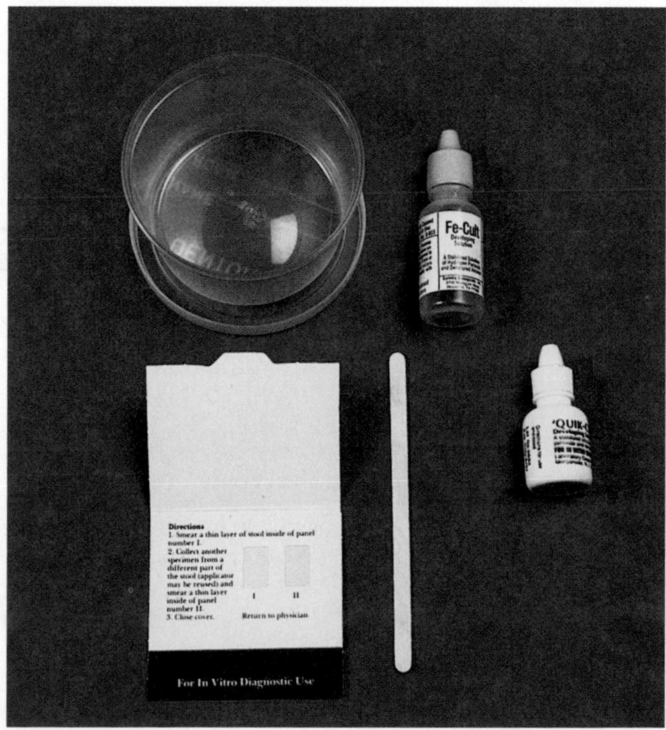

▲ Supplies needed for testing stool for occult blood.

e. Read and record test results within 30 seconds. ▸ ***Rationale:*** Color reaction fades within 2–3 minutes. Any trace of blue indicates a positive result. No trace of blue indicates a negative result.

For Hemoccult

a. Follow steps a and b for Fe-Cult Plus test.
b. Wait 3–5 minutes before processing test.
c. Turn packet over, and lift flap.
d. Apply two drops of Hemoccult developer over each smear.
e. Read and record test results within 60 seconds.
f. Apply 1 drop of Hemoccult developer between the + and − quality monitor test strip (orange section at bottom of packet).
g. Interpret results within 10 seconds. If the positive side turns blue, the test slide is accurate.

7. Discard filter paper or packet.
8. Remove gloves and perform hand hygiene.
9. Check facility policy for testing. Some laboratories conduct studies.
10. Document stool smear results and confirm quality monitor test.

For Gastroccult

NOTE: See procedure in chapter 19, Nutrition Management and Enteral Intubation, p.655.

Clinical Alert

Overt bleeding from hemorrhoids or menstrual bleeding renders the Hemoccult test inaccurate.

Clinical Alert

A hemoccult processing test cannot be used for gastric contents. A Gastroccult test must be used.

Collecting Stool for Bacterial Culture

Equipment

Waxed cardboard container with cover
Tongue blade
Label for container
Clean bedpan or bedside commode
Clean gloves

Procedure

1. Follow steps for *Collecting Adult Stool Specimen*. Don clean gloves before collecting stool specimen.
2. Collect exudate, mucus, and blood with all specimens.
3. Place a small amount of feces in a waxed cardboard container (if entire specimen is not needed).
4. Remove gloves, perform hand hygiene, and send entire specimen to the laboratory immediately after collection. If there is any delay, the specimen must be iced.
5. Report and calculate on the basis of daily output any stool specimens that are to undergo chemical analysis.

Teaching Parents to Test for Pinworms

Equipment

Specimen container with paddle
Clean gloves

Procedure

1. Explain procedure to child and parent.

NOTE: This test is rarely done or seen in hospital settings, so if pinworms are suspected, the parents can be taught how to obtain specimen at home.

2. Parents may choose to wear clean gloves.
3. Instruct parents to make collection upon arising in the morning before bathing, cleansing, or passing a bowel movement.

NOTE: For very active children, specimens may be collected a few hours after going to bed, while the child is sleepy and more cooperative. ▸***Rationale:*** Pinworms, when present, migrate out of the anus to lay eggs during sleep.

4. Remove cap in which is inserted a plastic paddle with one side coated with a nontoxic, adhesive material. This side is marked "sticky side." Do not touch this side with fingers.
5. Separate buttocks and press the sticky side against several areas around anus using moderate pressure.
6. Replace the paddle in tube. Be sure there is no stool on paddle.

7. Label container with your full name, medical record number, and date.
8. Keep specimen at room temperature until all specimens are collected (on consecutive days). Return all tubes to the doctor.

Clinical Alert
After treatment (drug of choice is mebendazole) and to prevent reinfection, use meticulous cleaning practices and teach parents of child to do the same.

DOCUMENTATION for Stool Specimens

- Date and time specimens collected
- Date and time specimens sent to laboratory
- Number of specimens sent to laboratory
- Description of stool: color, amount, odor, and any purulent patches or blood noted
- Dietary restrictions imposed
- Condition of perianal skin, if client is having diarrhea
- If serial stool specimens are needed, record each specimen on the Kardex card as well as the chart

CRITICAL THINKING Application

Expected Outcomes

- Client understands purpose of test.
- Client is able to follow procedure of collection when appropriate.
- Dietary restrictions (if appropriate to test) were adhered to by client before test.
- Specimen collected is adequate for test.

Unexpected Outcomes	Alternative Actions
Client is embarrassed by having to give stool specimen.	• Place a bedpan or other collection device under the toilet seat in bathroom to obtain specimen. • If client is confined to bed, pull sheets over client's legs and draw curtains around the bed until procedure is completed. • If odor occurs from passage of stool, spray room with air freshener.
Client is unable to pass adequate stool for specimen collection.	• Notify physician to obtain order to give a normal saline or tap water enema.
Client passes liquid stools.	• Determine if part or entire specimen is required for test. • Obtain a plastic container with a cover and several large cotton swabs. Dip cotton swabs into the liquid stool. Place swabs in plastic container. After procedure, pay close attention to skin care. A protective ointment may be necessary to protect skin from liquid stools.

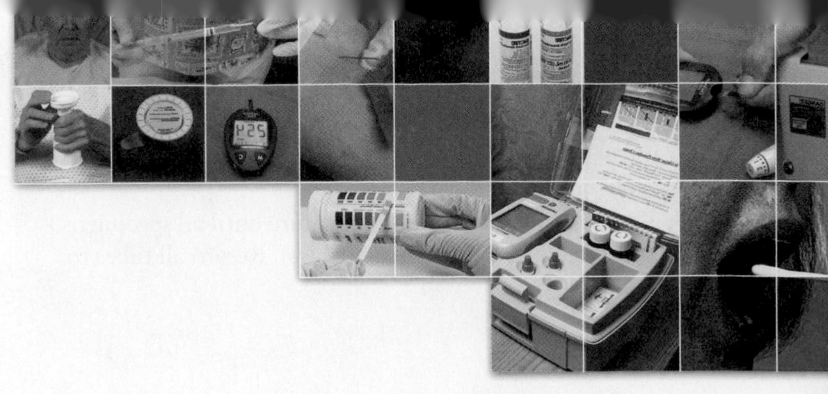

Chapter 20

UNIT 3

Blood Specimens

Nursing Process Data

ASSESSMENT Data Base

- Check order for blood withdrawal in client's chart.
- Note specific requirements for the test (e.g., fasting or administration of medications before the test).
- Check to see if the test is routine or urgent.
- Assess veins for venipuncture site.

PLANNING Objectives

- To obtain an uncontaminated blood specimen
- To obtain a blood sample without complications, such as hematoma formation or excessive oozing at the site
- To obtain specimens of blood that can be used to diagnose the client's illness
- To obtain and transfer specimens without destroying red blood cells
- To ensure accurate test results by making sure the client follows all requirements for the test (e.g., fasting)
- To ensure accurate test results by selecting the right tube for the right test
- To ensure that uncontaminated blood specimen for culture is obtained
- To obtain an accurate blood glucose level

IMPLEMENTATION Procedures

EVALUATION Expected Outcomes

- Blood sample is collected without complications. Uncontaminated blood specimen is collected.
- Blood is collected according to designated test tube colored top.
- Client follows all requirements for test (for example, fasting before collection).
- Client understands and learns steps of procedure when necessary (glucose levels).
- Accurate blood glucose level is obtained.

Pearson Nursing Student Resources

Find additional review materials at **nursing.pearsonhighered.com**

Prepare for success with NCLEX®-style practice questions and Skill Checklists

Withdrawing Venous Blood (Phlebotomy)

Equipment

5-mL or 10-mL safety syringe
20-gauge 1-in. needle(s)
Antimicrobial wipe (with blood alcohol specimen, use nonalcohol solution)
Appropriate plastic laboratory tubes
Dry, sterile sponges
Tourniquet
Absorbent pad or towel
Clean gloves
Laboratory slip

Preparation

1. Check physician's orders for tests to be obtained.
2. Perform hand hygiene.
3. Gather equipment.
4. Open sterile packages.

Procedure

1. Identify client by two identification methods; introduce yourself and explain the procedure.
2. Don clean gloves (see box on OSHA protocols).
3. Place extremity straight and in dependent position, if possible.
4. Place absorbent pad or towel under arm. ▸ ***Rationale:*** This prevents soiling the linen with blood.
5. Place equipment close to work area.
6. Place a tourniquet 4–6 in. above the client's elbow. Tighten the tourniquet and tell the client to open and close fist. ▸ ***Rationale:*** Muscle contraction increases blood flow to arm.
7. Cleanse antecubital fossa (inner aspect of elbow) with antimicrobial wipe starting at vein site and moving in a circular motion about 2 in. away from vein. ▸ ***Rationale:*** A larger vessel is more appropriate than a smaller vessel for blood draw.
8. Let site dry. ▸ ***Rationale:*** This reduces bacteria on skin surface when dry.
9. Hold skin taut with nondominant hand. Perform a venipuncture with bevel of needle pointed up at a 30° angle.
10. Lower needle toward skin after needle has entered vein. ▸ ***Rationale:*** This decreases risk of accidentally penetrating the other side of vein.
11. Thread needle along path of vein. Watch for backflow of blood in syringe.
12. Pull syringe plunger back gently, and check for placement of the needle in the vein. If placement is correct, release tourniquet, wait a few seconds to allow fresh blood to flow into the vein, and then pull back gently on the plunger.
13. Fill syringe to desired amount.
14. Remove needle from vein, cover venipuncture site with a sterile sponge, and press the sponge firmly on the site for 2–3 minutes. (Client may be able to hold sponge in place.)
15. Choose one of two methods to transfer specimen.
    a. Do not remove top from laboratory tube. Place needle straight through top. ▸ ***Rationale:*** Needle can be inserted through rubber stopper of test tube if 20-gauge needle is used.
    b. Gently eject blood down the side of the tube. Do not allow blood to foam or splash. ▸ ***Rationale:*** Red blood cells can be destroyed if the blood sample is not handled carefully.
    c. Rotate blood gently to mix blood with tube contents.

▲ Clamp vein down by placing forefinger below puncture site and insert needle at 15–30° angle.

Clinical Alert

If client has a fistula or has an IV inserted, place the tourniquet *on the other arm.*

OSHA Glove Protocol When in Contact With Blood Pathogens

- Routine gloving for phlebotomies is not necessary.
- Gloves are required when:
  1. The employee has cuts, scratches, or other breaks in the skin.
  2. Hand contamination with blood may occur.
  3. The employee is receiving training in phlebotomy.

Source: Standard OSHA Protocol. http://www.osha.gov

16. *Alternate method.*
    a. Remove top of test tube(s).
    b. Remove needle from syringe and gently inject blood down side of tube. ▸ ***Rationale:*** Inject blood slowly to prevent hemolysis of red blood cells.
    c. Gently rotate tube back and forth to mix additive.
17. Label tube promptly. Write client's name, date, and time. You may also need to write initials of the person who drew the specimen if this information is required by hospital policy.
18. Check client's venipuncture site for oozing. Continue to press sponge firmly over site if clots have not begun to form at site.
19. Dispose of shielded needle and syringe in biohazard receptacle.
20. Remove gloves, perform hand hygiene.
21. Take blood specimens to a designated station or laboratory according to hospital procedure.

Using Vacutainer System

Equipment

Vacutainer assembly with shielded or blunting needle
Antimicrobial wipe (with blood alcohol specimen, use nonalcohol solution)
Plastic vacuum blood collection tubes, placed in order of collection
Dry, sterile sponges
Double-ended needle that screws into the adapter
Clean gloves
Tourniquet
Tape
Laboratory slip

Preparation

1. Check physician's orders for tests to be obtained.
2. Perform hand hygiene.
3. Obtain plastic adapter, double-ended needle that screws into the adapter, and appropriate vacuum specimen tubes.
4. Screw the double-ended needle into the plastic adapter, with the shorter needle facing the plastic adapter.
5. Explain procedure to client.
6. Don clean gloves.

▲ When blood begins to fill tube, tell client to relax fist and release tourniquet.

Procedure

1. Follow steps 1–12 in Withdrawing Venous Blood.
2. Once the needle is positioned inside vein and blood return is visualized, insert blood collection tube into plastic holder while holding the plastic adapter steady. Press the vacuum tube firmly into the short needle so that it pierces the top of the tube. Blood should begin to spurt quickly into the tube until the tube is filled or vacuum is used.
3. Instruct client to relax fist and release tourniquet. ▸ ***Rationale:*** Hemolysis occurs with prolonged tourniquet use.

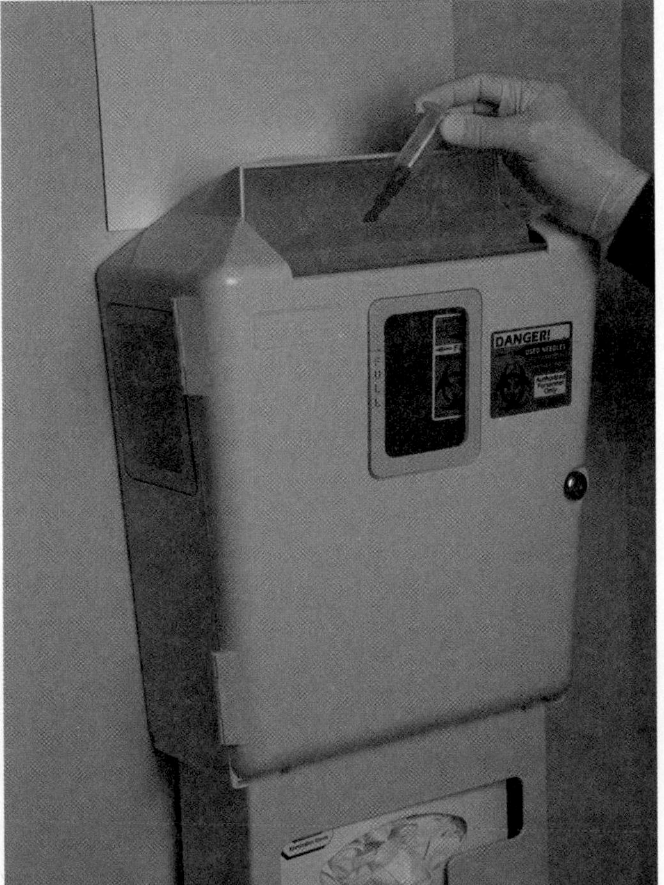

▲ Place vacutainer with safety needle attached into biohazard container.

4. Release the tube, and set it aside. Attach another tube to Vacutainer, or prepare to remove needle.
5. Place sponge over needle site, and remove needle while applying gentle pressure to site.
6. Hold sponge on site for 2–3 minutes. Do not have client bend elbow. ▸ ***Rationale:*** Bending the elbow can facilitate formation of a hematoma.
7. Place Vacutainer with needle in biohazard container.
8. Check if tube contains additive, gently invert to mix and label specimen tubes.
9. Remove gloves, and perform hand hygiene.
10. Complete laboratory slip, and take specimen to designated station or laboratory.

TABLE 20-2 Routine Blood Chemistry Tests

Test	Purpose	Normal Values
Erythrocytes		
Red blood cell count (RBC or erythrocytes)	Determines actual number of formed blood elements in relation to volume Identifies abnormalities; monitors RBC count	Males: 4.5–6.2 million/mm^3 Females: 4.0–5.5 million/mm^3 Children: 3.2–5.2 million/mm^3
Hematocrit (HCT)	Measures percentage of red blood cells per fluid volume of whole blood	Males: 40–54/100 mL Females: 37–47/100 mL Children: 29–54/100 mL
Hemoglobin (Hgb)	Measures amount of hemoglobin/100 mL blood to determine oxygen-carrying capacity; assists in diagnosing anemia	Males: above 13–18 g/100 mL Females: above 12–16 g/100 mL
Platelet count	Determines number of platelets	Adults: 150,000–450,000/mm^3
Prothrombin time (PT)	Evaluates thrombin generation or how long it takes for a fibrin clot to form Detects deficiencies in extrinsic clotting mechanism; monitors anticoagulant therapy	10–13 seconds Prolonged values seen in liver disease, vitamin K deficiency, specific drugs, etc.
Activated partial thromboplastin time (APTT)	Evaluates adequacy of plasma-clotting factors—intrinsic clotting mechanism	20–38 seconds Prolonged values indicate coagulation factor deficiency, cirrhosis, vitamin K deficiency
Thrombin time	Screening test to detect abnormalities in thrombin fibrinogen reaction (Conversion to fibrin in stage 3 of clotting sequence)	10–15 seconds
Leukocytes		
White blood cell count (WBC or leukocytes)	Establishes quantity and maturity of white blood cell elements	Adults: 4,500–11,000/mm^3 Children: 5000– 13,000/mm^3 Neutrophils: 3000–7500/mm^3 Band neutrophils: 150–700/mm^3 Basophils: 25–150/mm^3 Eosinophils: 50–450/mm^3 Lymphocytes: 1,500–4,500/mm^3 Monocytes: 100–800/mm^3
Erythrocyte sedimentation rate (ESR)	Measures rate of red blood cells settling from plasma—reflects inflammatory conditions	*Wintrobe Method* Males: 0–9 mm/hr Females: 0–15 mm/hr Children: 0–13 mm/hr *Westergren Method* Males: 0–15 mm/hr Females: (under 50 years) 0–20 mm /hr; (over 50 years) 0–30 mm/hr; Children: 0–20 mm/hr

Source: Smith, S. F. (2010). *Sandra Smith's Review for NCLEX-RN (12th ed)*. Los Altos, CA: National Nursing Review.

Understanding Blood Chemistry Tests

1. Read results of laboratory blood tests that were completed.
2. Evaluate client's test results and compare with normal values. (See Table 20-2, Routine Blood Chemistry Tests.)
3. Report abnormal values to team leader or physician.
4. Check Chem 7 (SMA 7) values—tests fluid balance, renal function and acid–base status. ▸ ***Rationale:*** When combined with the CBC, these tests give a view of how the entire body is functioning.
5. Standard values of Chem 7 (may vary from lab to lab; check own facility values).
   a. Potassium: 3.5–5.3 mEq/L.
   b. Sodium: 135–145 mEq/L.
   c. Chloride: 98–106 mEq/L.
   d. CO_2: 23–30 mmol/L.
   e. Glucose (fasting): 65–110 mg/dL.
   f. BUN: 7–18 mg/dL.
   g. Creatinine: 0.6–1.3 mg/dL.

Withdrawing Arterial Blood

Equipment

A commercial ABG kit containing all of the equipment *OR* 3-mL syringe with 22-gauge 1-in. needle with safety guard
Syringe cap/stopper
1:1000 solution heparin, 1 mL ampule
Antimicrobial swabs (2)
2 × 2 gauze pad
Nonallergenic tape
Plastic bag filled with crushed ice
Clean gloves
Goggles and mask
Laboratory requisition
Label for syringe
Adhesive bandage

▲ An arterial blood sample requires puncture of the brachial, radial, or femoral artery or a sample from an arterial line.

Preparation

1. Check physician's orders for test to be performed. (Usual test is arterial blood gases.)
2. Call laboratory to apprise them of specimen being sent for ABGs according to hospital policy.
3. Assemble equipment.
4. Perform hand hygiene.
5. Wipe top of heparin bottle with antimicrobial swab.
6. Uncap needle and insert into heparin bottle.
7. Withdraw 0.5 to 1 mL of heparin solution into syringe.
8. Prepare syringe by pulling plunger back entire length of syringe; rotate syringe to allow heparin to coat syringe sides.
9. Express excess heparin into sink.

Procedure

1. Take equipment into room and place on over-bed table and check two forms of client ID.
2. Explain procedure and purpose of test.
3. Ask if client is taking aspirin or anticoagulant therapy. ▸ ***Rationale:*** These drugs will affect test results and should be documented.
4. Don clean gloves, goggles, and mask.
5. Palpate selected radial site (the site most frequently used) with fingertips. ▸ ***Rationale:*** To determine best site for puncture.

NOTE: Allen's test should precede an arterial puncture if there is a question of poor collateral circulation.

6. Hyperextend wrist slightly. ▸ ***Rationale:*** This position will stabilize radial artery.
7. Cleanse puncture site with antimicrobial swab using a circular motion beginning over the artery site. Place swab on inside of packet and in close proximity to site.
8. Keep fingertip of nondominant hand over puncture site. ▸ ***Rationale:*** To maintain puncture site location.
9. Pick up syringe and hold needle bevel in uppermost position and insert needle into artery at a 30 to 45° angle.

10. Do not advance needle once blood is observed flowing into syringe.
11. Hold needle steady and allow blood to automatically fill syringe. Collect 1–5 mL of blood. Pulsations from artery will assist in filling syringe. Do not draw back on syringe. ▶ ***Rationale:*** Drawing back on syringe can cause air bubbles to fill syringe and inaccurate ABGs results will occur.
12. Place 2 × 2 in. gauze next to needle site and withdraw needle when syringe is filled.
13. Immediately apply pressure over site with gauze. Maintain pressure for 5–10 minutes. ▶ ***Rationale:*** Prolonged pressure over arterial puncture site will prevent bleeding.
14. Monitor puncture site for signs of oozing. When bleeding has stopped, place 2 × 2 gauze over site and apply adhesive bandage as you would for a pressure dressing.
15. Expel any air bubbles from syringe. Activate needle guard. Syringe contents should be airtight.
16. Label syringe.
17. Place syringe in plastic bag filled with ice. Close plastic bag.
18. Remove gloves and perform hand hygiene.
19. Complete laboratory requisition slip. Indicate client's temperature and oxygen percentage as necessary.
20. Take specimen to laboratory immediately.

Clinical Alert

If client is receiving anticoagulant therapy, apply pressure for 10 to 15 minutes after arterial puncture.

Allen's Test

Allen's test is performed to determine adequacy of collateral perfusion before arterial blood stick.

- Ask client to rest hands facing upward.
- Observe color changes in palm.
- Ask client to make a tight fist (to force blood from hand).
- Compress the radial and ulnar arteries by applying direct pressure using index and middle fingers (obstructs blood flow to hand).
- Ask client to clench and unclench fist several times.
- Ask client to relax hand in a slightly flexed position. Hand should appear blanched due to absence of blood flow.
- Release pressure on ulnar artery and note if fingers and palm flush within 5 minutes. This is a positive test for patency.
- If fingers and palm remain pale, do not use this site for arterial puncture; test other extremity.

Understanding Arterial Blood Gases (ABGs)

Procedure

1. ABG values are most often ordered for clients who have the following diagnoses: chronic obstructive pulmonary disease, pulmonary edema, myocardial infarction, pneumonia, or acute respiratory distress syndrome.
2. Check client's values against normal arterial values.
   a. Oxygen saturation—93%–98%.
   b. PaO_2—95 mmHg
   c. Arterial pH— 7.35–7.45 (7.4).
   d. pCO_2—35–45 mmHg (40).
   e. HCO_3 content—22–26 mEq/L.
   f. Base excess— −3 to +3 (0).
3. Check acid–base imbalances (acid–base balance is the ratio of acids and bases in the body necessary to maintain a chemical balance conducive to life). See Table 20-3.
   a. Acid–base ratio is 20 base to 1 acid.
   b. Values are measured by an arterial blood sample and recorded as blood pH. Normal range is 7.35 to 7.45.

TABLE 20-3 Acid–Base Imbalances

Respiratory Acidosis	Metabolic Acidosis
a. pH—7.32. b. pCO_2—52 mmHg. c. pO_2—90 mmHg. d. HCO_3—24 mEq/L.	a. pH—7.30. b. CO_3—16 mEq/L. c. pCO_2—38 mmHg. d. pO_2—95 mmHg. e. Cl—120 mEq/L. f. K—5.5 mEq/L.
Respiratory Alkalosis	**Metabolic Alkalosis**
a. pH—7.51. b. pCO_2—32 mmHg. c. pO_2—95 mmHg. d. HCO_3—24 mEq/L.	a. pH—7.50. b. HCO_3—26 mEq/L. c. pCO_2—38 mmHg. d. pO_2—95 mmHg. e. K—3.0 mEq/L. f. Cl—88 mEq/L.

Collecting a Blood Specimen for Culture

Equipment

Two sets of paired culture media bottles (aerobic and anaerobic)
Blood withdrawal equipment (e.g., tourniquet, two needles, and syringe with attached needle)
Povidone–iodine (Betadine) swab
Two antimicrobial swabs
Additional needles
Clean gloves
Laboratory request form and biohazard transport bag
Small adhesive bandages

Preparation

1. Check physician's orders.
2. Perform hand hygiene.
3. Gather equipment. Check expiration dates on culture bottles.
4. Don clean gloves.
5. Explain procedure to client and check two forms of client ID.

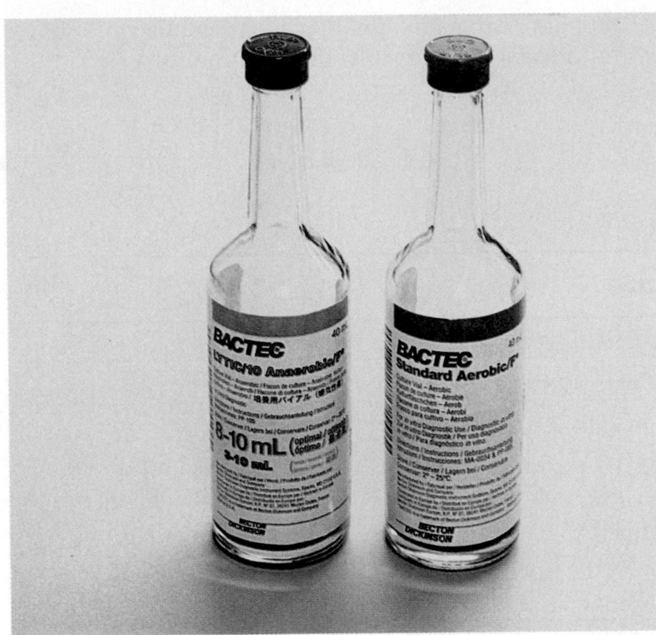

▲ Inject blood into both aerobic and anaerobic culture bottles.

Procedure

1. Cleanse skin with antimicrobial wipe. Allow skin to dry.
2. Prepare skin with povidone–iodine. Cleanse starting at vein site and moving in circular motion outward 2 in.
3. Allow skin to dry.
4. Remove povidone–iodine with antimicrobial wipe.
5. Perform venipuncture.
6. Withdraw 10–20 mL of blood from vein without IV. Do not draw specimen through catheter. ▸ ***Rationale:*** Fluid from IV alters results.
7. Remove needle used for venipuncture and replace with new sterile needle. ▸ ***Rationale:*** Contamination may result if needle used to puncture skin is reused.
8. Swab top of paired blood culture bottles with povidone–iodine swab and then antimicrobial swab, and inject 5–10 mL blood into each bottle according to hospital policy. Gently rotate bottle to mix well. Change needle each time so new sterile needle is used for each bottle.
9. Draw a second sample of blood after 15 minutes or according to hospital policy. Use percutaneous stick if required by hospital policy. (Prepare skin with povidone–iodine solution again.)
10. Place in second set of paired blood culture bottles, using single sterile needle technique.
11. Remove gloves and perform hand hygiene.
12. Place bandage over puncture site.
13. Label bottles with your name, date, and time of collection and transport to lab immediately. Include site where blood specimens were obtained.
14. Discard syringes, needles, and gloves in appropriate container.

Clinical Alert

Check with physician—blood culture may be ordered prior to client beginning antibiotic therapy.

Calibrating a Blood Glucose Meter (One Touch Ultra)

Equipment

Blood glucose meter
Chemstrips including calibration strip
Dry cotton ball
Clean gloves

Procedure

1. Obtain container of Chemstrips and remove calibration strip. Check expiration date on strips.
2. Compare lot numbers on calibration strip to lot number on side of Chemstrip bottle. These must match.

3. Place calibration strip in meter by opening door and inserting top of strip into slot on right side of meter.
4. Insert strip until you hear a "click."
5. Close door.
6. Push ON/OFF button. Numbers 888 should appear on screen.
7. Open door of monitor.
8. Push black button on the left side of door, and slide Chemstrip under strip guide with test pads facing up.
9. Close door quickly. Numbers 000 should be displayed on screen indicator. If not, open and close door again.
10. Open door and remove strip. Leave door open.
11. Don clean gloves and prepare to obtain blood specimen.

Obtaining Blood Specimen for Glucose Testing (Capillary Puncture)

Equipment

Automatic lancet (i.e., Autolet or Glucolet)
Penlet
Soap and water
Cotton ball, sterile sponges
Clean gloves

Preparation

1. Gather equipment and take to bedside.
2. Perform hand hygiene.
3. Don gloves.
4. Identify client using two forms of client ID.

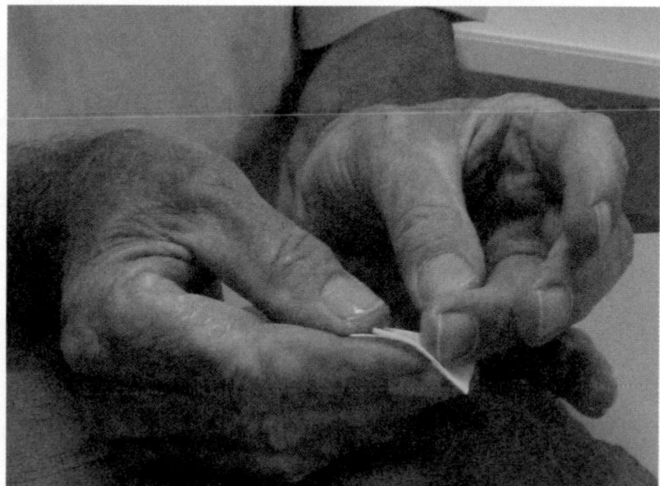

1 Use soap and water or swab to cleanse finger before puncture.

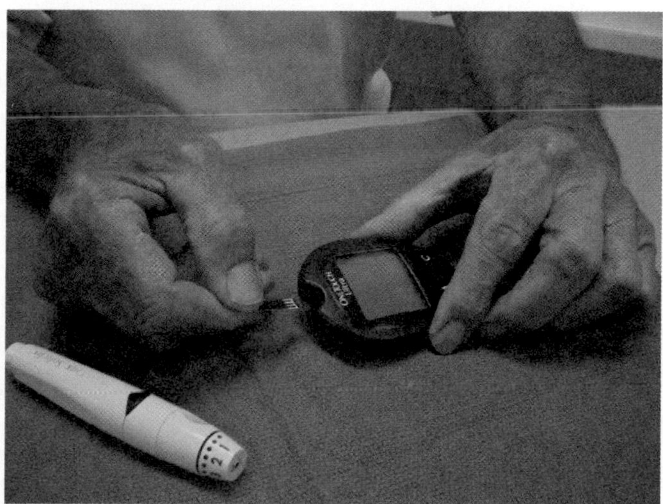

2 Insert test strip into monitor (you have 30 seconds to obtain a reading).

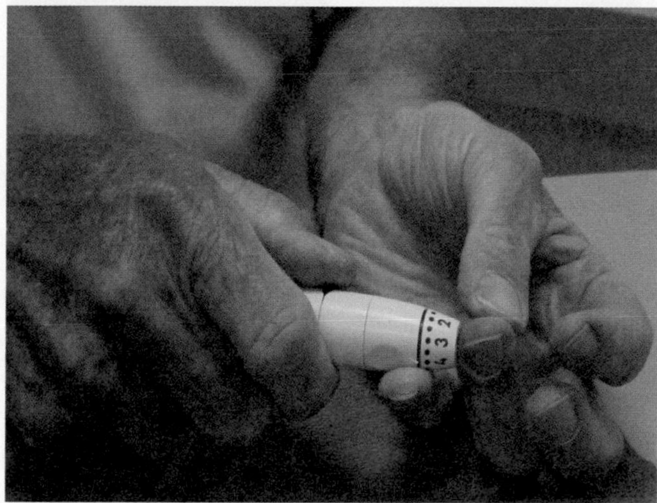

3 Adjust penlet depth, place on side of finger, and release.

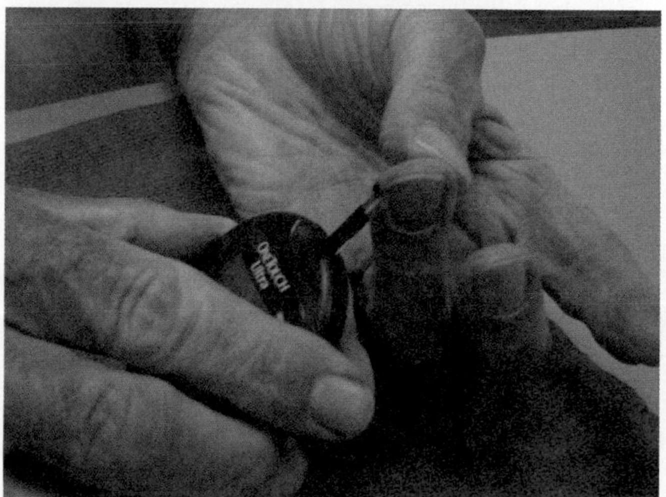

4 After gently massaging finger, place large drop of blood on test strip.

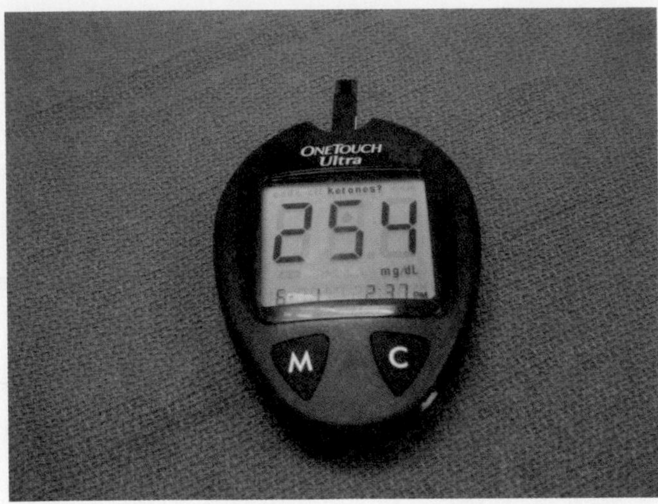

5 Wait 30 seconds and note reading on monitor.

Procedure

1. Wash client's fingertip (especially side of finger where lancet will puncture, or heel for infant) with soap and water and dry. ▶ ***Rationale:*** Use soap and water if repeated sticks are to be done, as alcohol toughens skin.
2. Insert test strip into monitor. (You have 30 seconds to obtain reading.)
3. Gently manipulate finger or heel to determine whether good blood supply is available.
4. Adjust Penlet to depth.
5. Place Penlet on side of finger and release. The lancet punctures the skin immediately.
6. Gently massage the base of the finger, stroking toward the puncture site. Do not squeeze or apply pressure to site. ▶ ***Rationale:*** Massaging increases blood flow to the fingertip.
7. Wait a few seconds to allow blood to collect at puncture site.
8. Place a large drop of blood onto test strip. (You have 30 seconds to obtain a reading.)
9. Wait 30 seconds and note reading on monitor.
10. Rotate finger tips when doing capillary punctures.
11. Wipe puncture site with cotton ball to seal.
12. Remove gloves and perform hand hygiene.
13. Document results.

NOTE: Many hospitals have changed to blood glucose meters that can "download" results, such as the Sure Step Flexx BG meter.

Monitoring Glucose: Sure Step Flexx

Equipment

Sure Step Flexx blood glucose monitor
Blood glucose test strips
High and low control solutions
Single use blood-letting device
Antimicrobial skin preparation pad
Lint free cloth, such as 2 × 2 gauze
Prepackaged disinfectant towelette, moistened with 1:10 dilution of 5.25% sodium hypochlorite, i.e., "Gluco-Chlor" towelette
Clean gloves

Procedure

For Quality Control

1. Turn on the meter.
2. Check the battery status to ensure adequate power.
3. Press "continue."
4. Select Quality Control (QC) Test from main menu by touching appropriate area on the screen.
5. Select Control Test by touching "HIGH" or "LOW" area on the screen to indicate which control test is to be done.
6. Enter operator ID assigned by specific facility.
7. Select Control Solution Lot Number from list displayed, or enter it manually. Verify lot number on control solutions.
8. Select Test Strip Lot number (and code) from this list displayed, or enter in manually. Verify lot number (and code) on test strips.

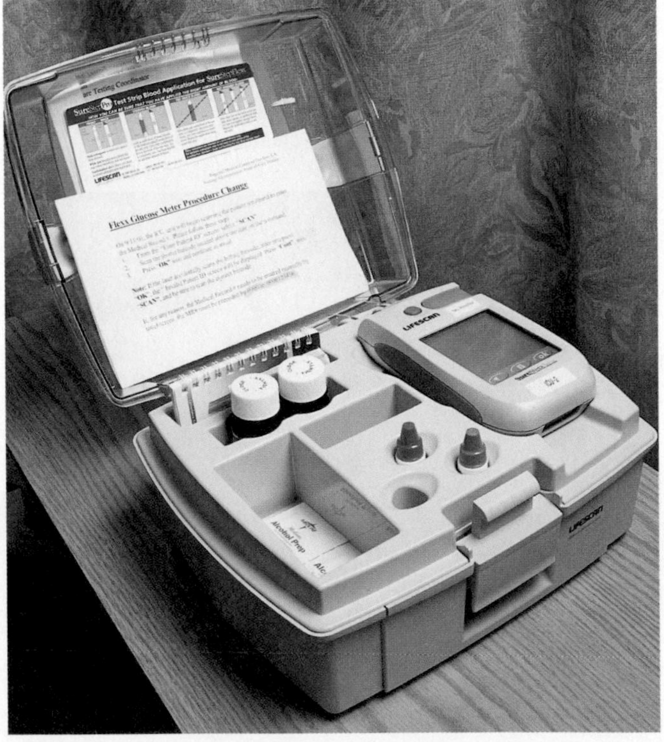

▲ Sure Stepp Flexx blood glucose monitoring equipment.

Clinical Alert
Quality control for the Flexx (with documentation) is required on a regular basis to verify test results when client data are entered.

9. Shake Control Solution vial gently. Check confirmation dot on back of test strip to ensure it is completely blue.
10. Apply one drop of Control Solution to pink test square on test strip.
11. Insert test strip into test holder within 2 minutes of applying Control Solutions. The white side of test strip tip should be facing up. Firmly push strip into meter.
12. Check result, which appears in approximately 30 seconds. Control Solution test results should fall within expected ranges printed on test strip bottle. If Control Solution test results fall outside expected control range, press "ENTER NOTE" and follow recommendations.
13. Remove test strip and dispose of it according to facility policy and procedure.
14. Quality Control test must be completed for both "HIGH" and "LOW" controls.

For Monitoring Blood Glucose

1. Perform hand hygiene and don gloves.
2. Press power button to turn on meter.
3. Check battery status as status screen appears.
4. Press "CONTINUE." Select "PATIENT TEST" from Main Menu.
5. Enter operator ID and press "OK."
6. Check to ensure Code Number displayed on meter matches code number on test strip bottle.
7. Enter client's ID (medical record number), and press "OK."
8. Select Test Strip Lot Number (and code) from list displayed, or enter in manually. Verify lot number (and code) displayed on screen.
9. Follow steps in Obtaining Blood Specimen for Glucose Testing.
10. Apply drop of blood to test strip by carefully touching pink test square on test strip. Check "Confirmation Dot" on back of test strip to verify that it has turned completely blue.

Clinical Alert
The test strip must be *completely* inserted to receive accurate results.

11. Use 2 × 2 gauze pad and apply direct pressure to puncture site to control bleeding.
12. Insert test strip completely into test strip holder within 2 minutes of applying blood. ▶ ***Rationale:*** Strip must be completely inserted to receive accurate results.

NOTE: Meters are institution specific—may require users to be certified once a year to use meters.

13. Check results which appear in approximately 30 seconds.
14. Evaluate client results that fall above or below the Critical Lab Values limit.
    a. Press "ENTER NOTE" and choose one to three comments, if indicated, that correspond to client's current situation.
    b. Follow appropriate nursing actions as determined by facility policy and procedure.
15. Press "OK" and remove test strip from meter.
16. Remove gloves and dispose of gloves and test strip according to facility policy.

Principles of Measuring Blood Glucose
- Bedside glucose testing is used only to monitor progress of treatment and not to establish a diagnosis of diabetes.
- Specimens used for glucose testing must be whole blood (capillary, arterial, or venous).
- Appropriate nursing actions need to be taken whenever client results exceed critical lab values (check facility policies).
- For a critical value, the FIRST action is to repeat the test.
- Test strip bottle should be dated when opened and recapped firmly between uses to protect strips.

DOCUMENTATION for Blood Specimens

- Date and time of blood withdrawal
- Date and name(s) of test(s) for which blood was drawn
- Any unusual conditions in either the client or specimen
- Site where blood cultures were obtained for capillary specimen
- Results of blood glucose reading
- Insulin administered: type, amount, location of injection
- Notification of physician of critical lab values, orders, or interventions

CRITICAL THINKING Application

Expected Outcomes	
• Blood sample is collected without complications. • Uncontaminated blood specimen is collected. • Blood is collected according to designated test tube colored top.	• Client follows all requirements for test (for example, fasting before collection). • Client understands and learns steps of procedure when necessary (glucose levels). • Accurate blood glucose level is obtained.

Unexpected Outcomes	Alternative Actions
Veins roll away from needle when performing a venipuncture.	• Stabilize vein by applying traction to skin below needle insertion site. • Common occurrence in elderly. Use a 5°–15° angle when inserting needle into vein as elderly clients' veins are superficial.
Blood does not flow into the syringe.	• Check the position of the needle in the vein. • Pull needle back slightly away from the wall of the vein. Rotate needle gently. Do not pull excessively on the plunger, especially if the vein is small, since this movement may cause the vein to collapse.
Blood does not flow into the vacuum tube.	• Check the position of the needle in the vein. If vacuum in the tube is lost or if the vein is not large enough, discard the tube and get another. • If there is pressure on the vein for vacuum pull, select a larger vein or use a syringe and needle instead of the Vacutainer method.
Unable to get blood sample with Autolet.	• Check that fingertip or heel is not toughened with overuse of alcohol sponges. Should use soap and water to clean area. • Choose an alternative site and repeat the stick. • Stroke gently from base of finger toward the tip. Do not apply firm massage as it can interfere with blood flow.
Meter shows not enough blood.	• Remove test strip, and insert new strip. • Obtain new blood drop. • Ensure blood drop is sufficient to form a round, shiny drop that covers entire strip. • Complete procedure.

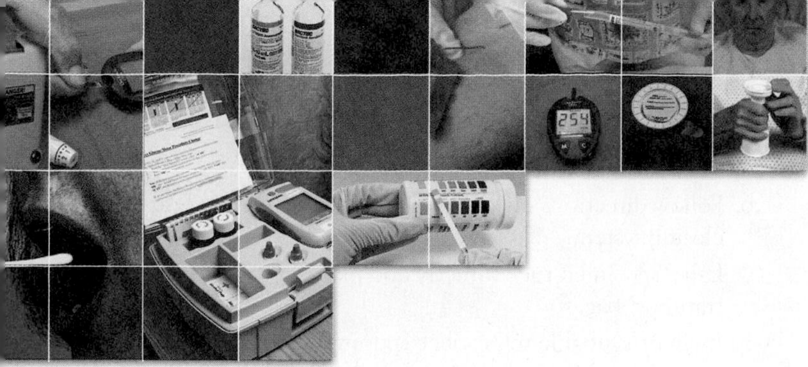

Chapter 20

UNIT 4

Sputum Collection

Nursing Process Data

ASSESSMENT Data Base

- Check diagnosis for indication of need for specimen.
- Observe client's ability to cough up specimen. You may need to assist the client while obtaining a specimen, or suction equipment may be necessary.
- Determine the degree of pain the client can tolerate.
- Check client's understanding of procedure so sputum and not saliva is obtained.

PLANNING Objectives

- To obtain adequate sputum specimen for laboratory examination
- To identify predominant organisms, if respiratory disease is present
- To maintain client's respiratory status during and after procedure

IMPLEMENTATION Procedures

EVALUATION Expected Outcomes

- Client understands and participates in specimen collection.
- Adequate amount of specimen is collected for the test ordered.
- Specimen collected is uncontaminated.

Obtaining Sputum Specimen

Equipment

Sputum specimen container and label
Biohazard bag for delivery of specimen to laboratory
Tissues
Laboratory requisition slip
Clean gloves
Gown, mask (HEPA or N95 if client has TB), goggles, if needed

Preparation

1. Identify client with two forms of ID.
2. Gather equipment.
3. Perform hand hygiene.
4. Provide privacy.
5. Place client in sitting position.

Procedure

1. Explain procedure and rationale to client.
2. Have client rinse mouth before coughing to remove any oral contaminants.
3. Don clean gloves. Don mask, gown, goggles if client requires assistance with procedure.
4. Instruct client to breathe in and out deeply 2 to 4 times, then give a series of low, deep coughs to raise sputum from the lungs. ▸ ***Rationale:*** Deep coughs produce sputum rather than saliva.
5. Obtain 1–2 teaspoons of sputum in container; close and seal lid.
6. Follow directions on specimen container to complete closing system.
7. Label specimen tube directly and place in biohazard transport bag.
8. If client is unable to produce sputum specimen, assist client by placing palms of your hands or a rolled pillow around incision area if client is inhibited by pain. ▸ ***Rationale:*** Wrapping a sheet around chest or abdomen also provides support for body walls during coughing.
9. Remove gloves, gown, mask, and goggles and perform hand hygiene.
10. Evaluate client's status after procedure.
11. Deliver sputum to the laboratory within 30 minutes after collection. Obtain specimen during treatment if client is receiving IPPB or PVD.

Clinical Alert

A first specimen obtained in the early morning before eating or drinking provides the best sputum sample. Chest physiotherapy may be helpful in mobilizing secretions just before sputum collection.

Clinical Alert

Know what test the sputum is being collected for:

- Routine culture—sterile container
- Acid-fast bacilli (AFB)—sterile container
- Cytology—container contains a preservative warning: preservative is poisonous

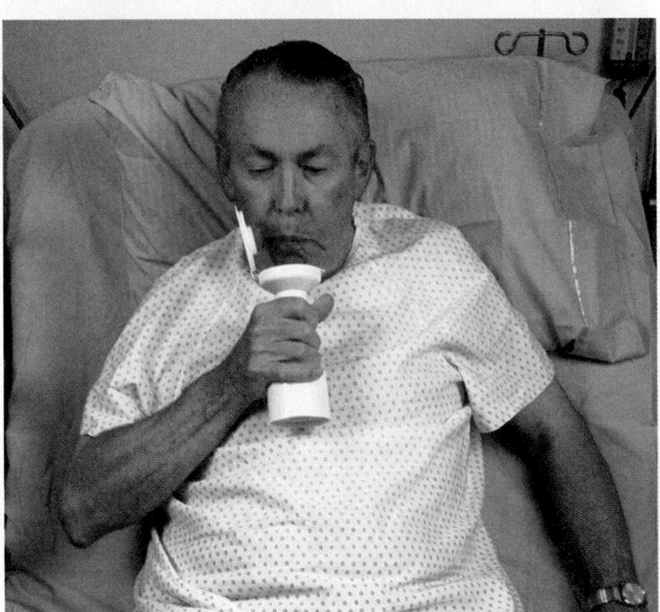

▲ Instruct client to lift hinged lid of sputum collection system, and expectorate directly into sterile container.

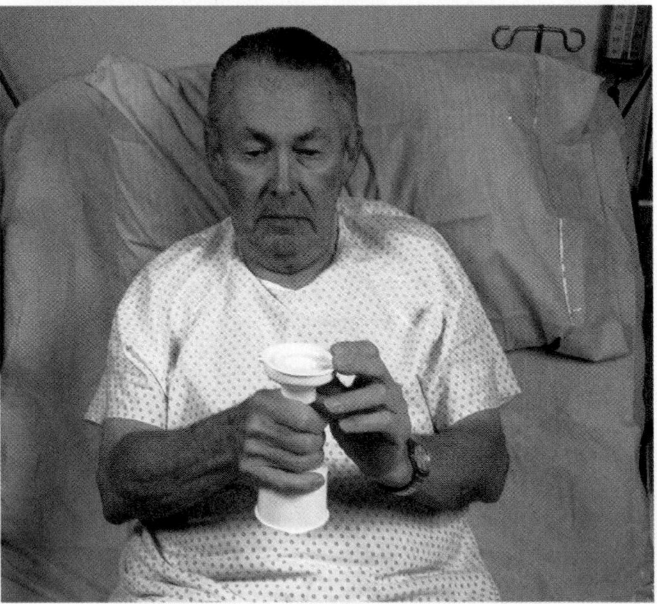

▲ Instruct client to obtain 1–2 teaspoons of sputum, close and seal lid of container.

Using Suction Trap

Equipment

Suction machine
Sterile catheter and glove
Sterile saline
Sterile sputum trap
Culture tube
Biohazard disposal bag
Clean gloves
Gown, mask, goggles

Preparation

1. Check physician's orders and client care plan for type of equipment needed.
2. Perform hand hygiene.
3. Gather equipment.
4. Explain procedure to client and check client's identity with two forms of ID.
5. Provide privacy.
6. Don clean gloves, goggles, gown, and mask as appropriate.

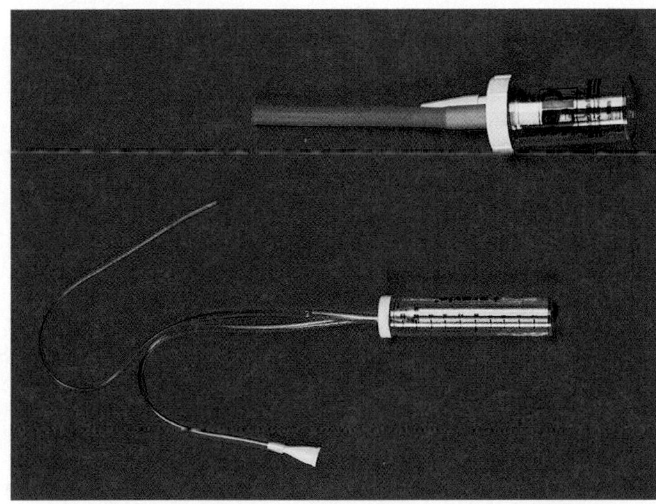

▲ Two common types of suction traps used in client care.

Procedure

1. Set up suction equipment.
2. Attach sputum trap between suction catheter and tubing. Maintain trap in upright position throughout procedure.
3. Complete suctioning as for naso-oropharyngeal suctioning using sterile technique.
4. Place your thumb on top of sputum trap to monitor; remove your thumb and provide intermittent suction, lifting thumb at intervals until 3–5 mL specimen is collected.
5. Suction no more than 10 seconds at a time.
   ▸ ***Rationale:*** This prevents removal of too much oxygen.
6. Turn off wall suction.
7. Label specimen container: client's name, date, time, and physician.
8. Cap suction trap and place it in biohazard bag. Follow agency protocol for double-bagging specimens before transporting to laboratory.
9. Remove gloves and other equipment (mask, gown, and goggles if used) and dispose of in appropriate receptacle.
10. Send specimen that was collected in trap to laboratory. (In many hospitals suction tube is also sent to the lab with specimen.)
11. Place client in a comfortable position.
12. Perform hand hygiene.

Collecting Specimen by Transtracheal Aspiration (Done by Physician)

Equipment

No. 14 needle with polyethylene tubing or small intracatheter (IV catheter)
Sterile saline and 3–5 mL syringe
Skin-cleansing solution dictated by hospital policy
Xylocaine injection
Clean gloves

Procedure

1. Explain procedure and check identity with two forms of ID.
2. Collect equipment.
3. Provide privacy for client.
4. Perform hand hygiene and don gloves.
5. Position client by hyperextending client's neck and placing a pillow under shoulders.
6. Cleanse cricothyroid area of neck with antimicrobial solution.
7. Physician will anesthetize area with Xylocaine.
8. Physician will insert 14-gauge needle into cricothyroid area, thread polyethylene tubing through needle, withdraw needle, and leave tubing in place.
9. Attach syringe (3–5 mL) with 1–2 mL sterile saline into polyethylene tubing.

10. Inject saline into polyethylene tubing to initiate coughing response.
11. To obtain specimen, immediately pull back on barrel of syringe.
12. Withdraw catheter and apply pressure over puncture site.
13. Place sputum secretions in sterile container, label container, and send it to laboratory.
14. Remove gloves and perform hand hygiene.
15. Position client for comfort.

DOCUMENTATION for Sputum Collection

- Date and time of collection
- Amount, color, and consistency of sputum
- Mechanical sputum trap used for collection
- Client's tolerance of procedure

CRITICAL THINKING Application

Expected Outcomes

- Client understands and participates in specimen collection.
- Adequate amount of specimen is collected for the test ordered.
- Specimen collected is uncontaminated.

Unexpected Outcomes	Alternative Actions
Pain inhibits client from coughing.	• If diagnosis permits, support painful area with rolled pillows or tight sheets so that external pressure equals internal pressure, thus minimizing pain and discomfort. • Before beginning procedure, ask client to take several deep breaths. These breaths may trigger the cough reflex and aerate the lungs. • Give client pain medication as ordered 15–30 minutes before obtaining the specimen.
Client develops coughing spasms during procedure.	• Press your third finger lightly over the client's trachea in the cricoid hollow. This pressure releases the nerve that innervates the coughing reflex. • Report to physician to obtain an order for nebulization.
Unable to obtain sputum specimen.	• Notify physician for orders: bronchodilator drugs, nebulization treatment. • Perform chest physiotherapy to mobilize secretions for expectoration before obtaining sputum specimen. • Attempt procedure early in the morning when mucus has collected during the night and is more easily expectorated. • Obtain order for aerosol therapy.

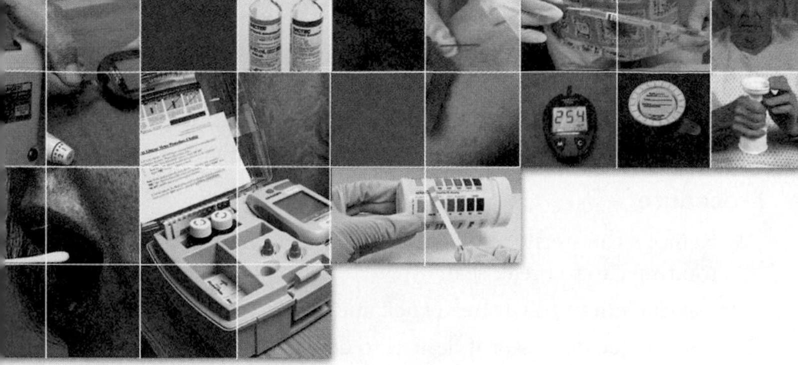

Chapter 20

UNIT 5

Swab Specimens

Nursing Process Data

ASSESSMENT Data Base

- Identify appropriate container for specimen swabs or material.
- Determine time frame for expediting specimen to lab.
- Assess exact area for specimen.
- Assess client's ability to cooperate with procedure.
- Assess wound and drainage.

PLANNING Objectives

- To obtain an uncontaminated specimen for study
- To place specimen swab or material in container using appropriate techniques
- To send specimen to laboratory within specified time frame

IMPLEMENTATION Procedures

EVALUATION Expected Outcomes

- Uncontaminated specimen is collected.
- The proper container (aerobic or anaerobic) is used for specimen collection.
- Specimen is sent to the lab within specified time.

Obtaining a Throat Specimen

Equipment

Tongue depressor
Culture tube with applicator stick
Light source
Clean gloves
Laboratory request form and biohazard transport bag, if indicated

Preparation

1. Check physician's orders.
2. Gather equipment.
3. Explain procedure to client and check two forms of client ID.
4. Position client in Fowler's position.
5. Place treatment light or face client toward natural light source to provide good lighting.
6. Perform hand hygiene and don clean gloves.

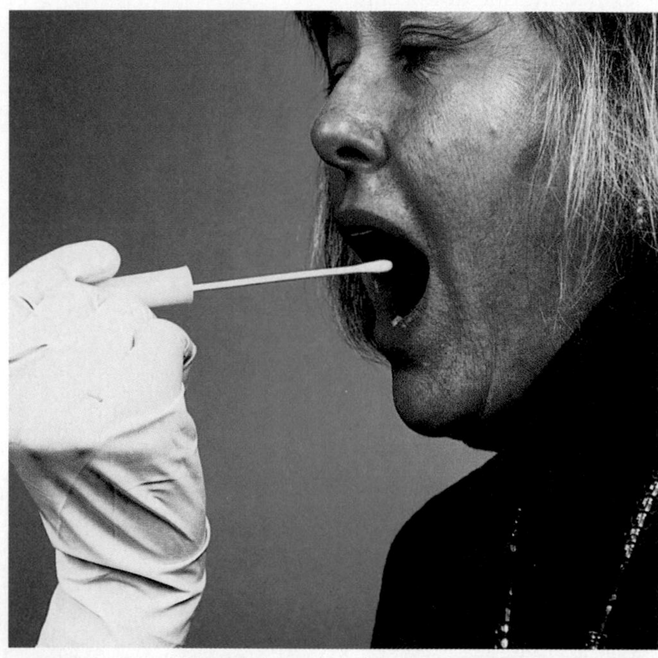

▲ After swabbing throat, remove applicator stick, being careful not to touch any part of the mouth.

Procedure

1. Remove the sterile applicator from the culture tube by rotating cap to break seal.
2. Ask the client to tilt head back and open mouth.
3. Use tongue depressor if desired to depress tongue. ▸ ***Rationale:*** Prevents tongue from contaminating the swab.
4. Swab the back of the throat along the tonsillar area from left to right. ▸ ***Rationale:*** Swab only one side of the throat. A second specimen of the other side may be taken; check hospital protocol.
5. Remove the applicator stick, and place in the specimen tube.
6. Push the stick into the tube until the swab is saturated with culture medium and cap reaches black dot. ▸ ***Rationale:*** This places the applicator tip into the culture medium to preserve bacteria until laboratory can complete test.
7. Position client for comfort.
8. Remove gloves and perform hand hygiene.
9. Label specimen tube, and send to laboratory immediately. ▸ ***Rationale:*** To ensure accurate identification of microorganisms.

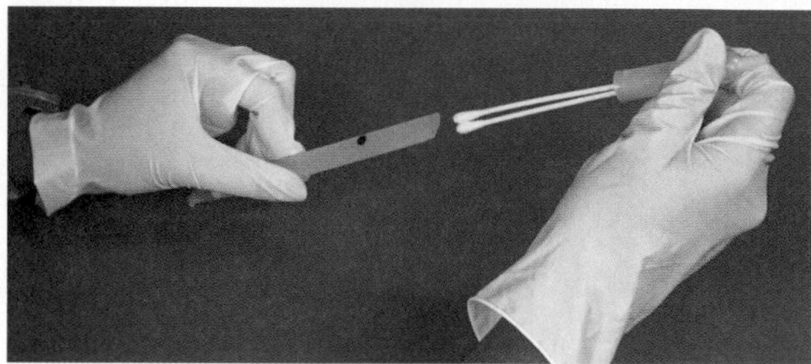

▲ Push applicator stick into specimen tube, being careful not to contaminate stick.

Obtaining a Gum Swab for HIV Antibodies

Equipment

One of four testing kits:
- OraQuick Advance Rapid HIV-Antibody Test
- Reveal B_2 Rapid HIV-Antibody Test
- Uni-Gold Recombigen HIV Test
- Multispot HIV-1/HIV-2 Rapid Test

Clean gloves

Procedure

1. Perform hand hygiene and don gloves.
2. Check two forms of client ID.
3. Swab outer gum with device included in kit. ▸ ***Rationale:*** Device contains absorbent pad to absorb saliva.
4. Insert swab into vial containing special solution.

5. Check window display on device, and if antibodies are present, two red-purple lines will appear. ▶ ***Rationale:*** When a person is exposed to HIV, the immune system will produce antibodies.
6. Following preliminary positive results, instruct client to confirm results with a blood test (the Western blot analysis is the gold standard for HIV testing).
7. Refer client to appropriate consultation if results are positive.

Obtaining Wound Specimen for Aerobic Culture

Equipment

Culture transport swab with transport medium (sterile)
Laboratory slip
Clean gloves, 2 pair
Sterile gloves
Dressing material
Disposal bag
Biohazard bag

Preparation

1. Check physician's orders and client care plan.
2. Perform hand hygiene.
3. Gather equipment.
4. Explain procedure to client and check two forms of client ID.
5. Open all sterile dressing material, and arrange for easy access during dressing change.

Procedure

1. Don clean gloves.
2. Remove and discard soiled dressing from wound into disposal bag.
3. Remove gloves, discard into disposal bag, and don clean gloves.
4. Rinse wound thoroughly with sterile normal saline. ▶ ***Rationale:*** Decreases risk of culturing normal flora, exudate, or eschar.
5. Remove swab, and wipe swab in wound avoiding wound edges. Obtain culture from active drainage area. ▶ ***Rationale:*** Touching skin edges or other surfaces will contaminate swab.
6. Return swab to container.
7. Crush transport medium vial, and push swab tip into contact with transport medium. ▶ ***Rationale:*** Specimen should be covered by medium.
8. Close container.
9. Place specimen in sealed biohazard bag. Label with specific anatomic site from which culture was taken.
10. Write any recent antibiotic or antifungal therapy on laboratory requisitions. ▶ ***Rationale:*** These drugs may lead to false-negative results from the culture.
11. Remove clean gloves and perform hand hygiene.
12. Don sterile gloves and replace dressing.
13. Remove gloves, discard, and perform hand hygiene.
14. Transport specimen to laboratory within 30 minutes. Do not refrigerate. ▶ ***Rationale:*** This ensures organisms are still viable.

NOTE: Determine whether wound should be cleaned with normal saline or whether area around wound should be cleaned with alcohol swab (do not use alcohol if client has a perineal wound, because it is irritating) before obtaining specimen.

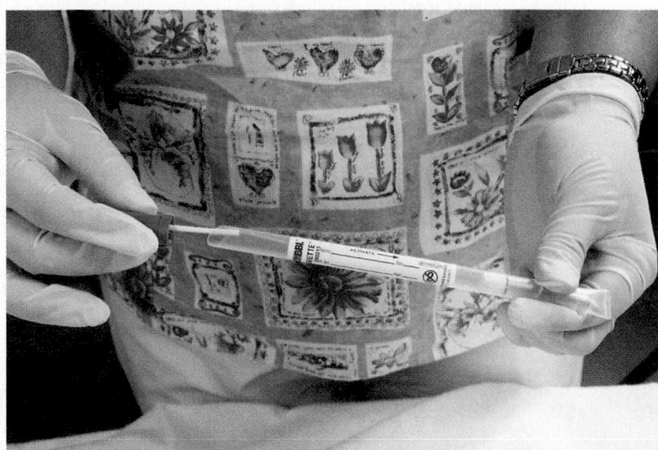

▲ Push tip of swab into liquid culture medium.

Clinical Alert

Large wounds should have separate cultures taken from different areas of the wound.

Obtaining Wound Specimen for Anaerobic Culture

Equipment

Anaerobic transport medium kit with swab
Laboratory slip
Clean gloves
Sterile gloves
Dressing material
Disposal bag
Plastic bag

Preparation

1. Check physician's orders and client care plan.
2. Perform hand hygiene.
3. Gather equipment.
4. Explain procedure to client and check two forms of client ID.
5. Open all sterile dressing material, and arrange for easy access during dressing change.

Procedure

1. Don clean gloves.
2. Remove dressing from wound, and discard in disposal bag.
3. Remove gloves and don clean gloves.
4. Rinse wound thoroughly with sterile normal saline. ▸ ***Rationale:*** Increases chance of culturing microorganisms rather than normal flora or other exudate.
5. Remove specimen swab, insert deeply into wound, rotate it gently, and remove. Be sure you do not tip the anaerobic transport medium tube because it contains carbon dioxide. ▸ ***Rationale:*** Tipping "spills" the gas out, making it useless to transport anaerobic organisms.
6. Return swab to container. *Do not* touch sides of container with applicator.
7. Fill out or affix label to specimen and place specimen in sealed biohazard bag.
8. Write any recent antibiotic or antifungal therapy on laboratory requisition. ▸ ***Rationale:*** These drugs can lead to false-negative results.
9. Transport specimen to laboratory *immediately*. Do not refrigerate specimen.
10. *Alternative method:*
    a. Draw up 1 to 5 mL of exudate in sterile 10 mL syringe with all air expelled or have a physician aspirate the wound.
    b. Inject drainage into anaerobic culture tube.
    c. Transport specimens to laboratory *immediately*. ▸ ***Rationale:*** Anaerobic organisms may appear on gram stain even though they are not grown in the culture.
11. Remove clean gloves, perform hand hygiene, don sterile gloves.
12. Replace sterile dressing following protocol.
13. Remove sterile gloves.
14. Perform hand hygiene.

Clinical Alert

Obtain wound specimen for both aerobic and anaerobic organisms during scheduled dressing change before any medication or antimicrobial agents have been applied.

Using an Anaerobic Specimen Collector

Anaerobic specimens must be transported in tubes filled with carbon dioxide, because most anaerobes die when exposed to oxygen. A special carbon dioxide–filled, rubber-stopped container with a small inner tube and a swab attached to a plastic plunger is used.

Before specimen collection, the inner tube is held in place with the plunger rubber stopper. After collecting the specimen, quickly replace the swab into the inner tube, and push on the plunger. This will force the inner tube down, away from the plunger, and into the carbon dioxide environment of the outer tube. The rubber stopper will maintain the overall tube seal.

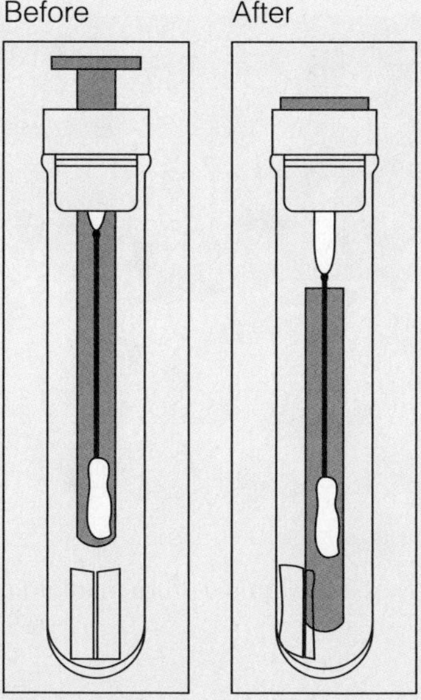

▲ Anaerobic specimen collector tube.

Collecting an Ear Specimen

Equipment

Normal saline solution
2 × 2 gauze pads
Gloves
Sterile swabs
Labeled sterile culture tube with medium
Laboratory request form
Biohazard transport bag

Procedure

1. Perform hand hygiene and don gloves.
2. Check two forms of client ID.
3. Cleanse ear with normal saline and gauze pad.
4. Insert sterile swab into ear canal and rotate gently along ear walls without pressing on eardrum.
5. Withdraw swab and place into sterile culture tube.
6. Remove gloves and complete hand hygiene.
7. Complete laboratory request form and send biohazard bag to the laboratory.

NOTE: If a middle ear specimen is ordered, the physician will puncture the eardrum with a needle and aspirate fluid into a syringe, which will be sent in a container to the laboratory.

DOCUMENTATION for Obtaining Specimen for Culture

- Assessment of wound and drainage
- Date and time specimen collected
- Type of culture obtained (aerobic or anaerobic)
- Site where culture obtained
- For wound specimens, document an assessment of wound and drainage
- Time specimen sent to lab

CRITICAL THINKING Application

Expected Outcomes

- Uncontaminated specimen is collected.
- The proper container (aerobic or anaerobic) is used for specimen collection.
- Specimen is sent to the lab within specified time.

Unexpected Outcomes	Alternative Actions
Inner surface of collection container contaminated while inserting swab into the culture medium container.	• Obtain new specimen and send to laboratory.
Swab becomes contaminated.	• Touch only sterile items with replaced swab. • Obtain new specimen.
Anaerobic specimen not sent to laboratory immediately.	• Obtain new specimen and send to laboratory.
Anaerobic specimen not sent in appropriate container with hydrogen gas.	• Obtain appropriate container and send new specimen to laboratory.
Wound culture produces false-negative results.	• Check if antibiotics or antifungal medications had been administered. If so, notify laboratory and provide specific drugs administered.
Testing kit for HIV antibodies shows positive.	• Counsel client to repeat test. • Refer client to appropriate entity for treatment and support.

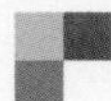

GERONTOLOGIC Considerations

- Elderly clients may not clearly hear and understand the directions given regarding specimen collection. Ask specific questions to ensure compliance.
- Determine client's ability to follow directions for obtaining specimens such as urine and stool. Hearing and vision may be impaired, thereby interfering with their ability to follow through on specimen collection.
- Assess client's ability to accurately use blood glucose–monitoring equipment. Finger dexterity may be altered due to stroke, arthritis, or other chronic conditions, thus preventing them from being able to use the equipment or obtain the blood specimen.
- Residual urine may increase as a result of changes in the bladder tone, leading to urinary stasis and potential bacterial proliferation. This leads to bladder infections, necessitating accurate identification of bacteria. This is accomplished through analysis of urine obtained from specimens free of contamination. Ensure client understands the procedure for obtaining an uncontaminated urine specimen. The nurse may need to obtain the specimen if the client is unable to do so without contaminating it.
- Avoid obtaining blood specimens from client's arm if neurological or vascular alterations are present.
- Clients receiving anticoagulant/antiplatelet therapy require a longer pressure time over the venipuncture site to prevent bleeding.
- Elderly clients have large rolling veins that make it appear easier to perform a venipuncture. In fact, the veins tend to collapse and rupture quite easily. Elderly clients may not require a tourniquet for venipuncture.
- Minimize the amount of tape used over IV site to prevent skin breakdown.

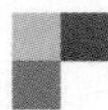

MANAGEMENT Guidelines

Each state legislates a Nurse Practice Act for RNs and LVN/LPNs. Healthcare facilities are responsible for establishing and implementing policies and procedures that conform to their state's regulations. Verify the regulations and role parameters for each healthcare worker in your facility.

Delegation

- CNAs can be assigned to obtain specimens that are nonsterile and noninvasive. Examples of these specimens include urine and stool collections.
- Unlicensed Assistive Personnel (UAP) and CNAs have been instructed in some areas to take blood measurements using the Accu-Chek and Glucometer machines. You will need to check with the facility policy and procedure manual for directions. Most states consider this an invasive technique and do not allow this level of healthcare worker to perform the task.
- LVN/LPNs can obtain most specimen collections except withdrawing blood. This task requires that they have additional education and be IV certified in order to obtain the blood specimens.

Communication Matrix

- It is very important that all staff members be aware of clients needing specimen collection. Many of the specimens, particularly blood specimens, require fasting. Shift and team reports should identify those clients with special needs relative to obtaining all specimens.
- When 24-hr specimens are being collected, ensure that signs are posted in the client's room to remind all healthcare workers to save the specimens. This is usually for a 24-hr urine specimen collection.
- Remind LVN/LPN to notify the RN of blood glucose findings, even if they are administering the insulin. It is the RN's responsibility to know these facts and to document because there are legal aspects to these interventions.
- Remind all healthcare workers to notify the nurse manager when any specimen has been collected. Follow the procedure for the facility for sending the specimen to the laboratory. Some facilities have personnel who pick up specimens from the nursing unit; others require the unit staff to take the specimen to the laboratory.
- Inform the healthcare workers about specimens that must be taken to the laboratory immediately after collection.

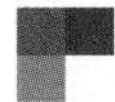

CRITICAL THINKING Strategies

Scenario 1

You have been assigned to collect specific specimens on several clients. Ms. Saunders is scheduled to have a 24-hr urine specimen collected.

1. When will you start collecting the specimen? List parameters necessary for accurate collection.
2. If the 24-hr urine specimen becomes contaminated with stool, what nursing action is indicated?

Scenario 2

Mrs. Block has orders for a stool specimen to be collected for presence of amoeba. When you collect the specimen from her, urine is mixed with the stool.

1. What is the nursing action?

Scenario 3

Mr. Jarvis has recently been diagnosed with diabetes, and you are assigned to collect a blood specimen for glucose testing.

1. Describe the activities you would perform to complete this assignment.
2. If the results exceed critical lab values, what is the implication of this result?
3. What actions will you take?

NCLEX® Review Questions

Unless otherwise specified, choose only one (1) answer.

1. The nurse is teaching a client how to obtain a sputum sample. Which one of these statements is a critical factor in the instruction?
   1. Rinse the mouth before obtaining the sample.
   2. Obtain the sample in the morning after breakfast.
   3. Have client hold breath before coughing up sputum.
   4. Take an expectorant to help facilitate the cough.
2. When collecting a blood specimen for culture, the nurse should
   1. Draw the blood from the IV line.
   2. Wipe the sample site with alcohol.
   3. Wear gloves during the procedure.
   4. Use the venipuncture needle to inject blood into culture bottle.
3. A 4-year-old child with vomiting and diarrhea is admitted to the hospital. Which one of these statements regarding collecting stool specimens for ova and parasites is correct?
   1. Specimen or culture must be from first stool of the day.
   2. Clean-catch technique is used to collect stool sample.
   3. Specimen can be refrigerated up to 24 hr.
   4. Samples can be affected by laxatives containing heavy metals.
4. A client asks the nurse about the purpose of a guaiac test. The best response by the nurse is that it
   1. Detects the presence of bacteria.
   2. Tests for fat in the stool.
   3. Tests for hidden or occult blood.
   4. Determines whether pinworms are present.
5. During a 24-hr urine collection, the client discards a recent void. The nurse should
   1. Stop the collection.
   2. Extend the collection by 2 hr.
   3. Call laboratory to report the loss.
   4. Reinforce to the client to save urine.
6. A female client has collected a clean-catch urine sample. The sample is 50 mL, cloudy, odorless, and light yellow. Which one of the specimen's characteristics would be considered abnormal?
   1. Color.
   2. Clarity.
   3. Amount.
   4. Odor.
7. The nurse is withdrawing a venous blood sample from the antecubital fossa using a Vacutainer system. Which one of these statements would indicate the nurse is using correct technique in obtaining the sample?
   1. Place tourniquet 1–2 in. above client's elbow.
   2. Instruct client to keep fist clenched until needle is withdrawn.
   3. After needle removal, have client bend elbow and hold gauze on site.
   4. Cleanse site with antimicrobial wipe and allow to dry.
8. When drawing an arterial blood sample, the nurse should
   1. Flex the wrist to stabilize the vessel.
   2. Draw back on the syringe when blood is observed.
   3. Apply pressure for 1–2 minutes after needle is withdrawn.
   4. Perform Allen's test before arterial puncture.
9. The nurse is teaching a male client how to monitor his blood glucose using a One Touch meter. When observing his technique, which one of these actions would be cause for further instruction?
   1. Places the lancet on the lateral side of his finger.
   2. Washes his hands with soap and water.
   3. Adds additional blood to strip after test begins.
   4. After stick, strokes gently from base of finger to tip.
10. A client has a large, draining wound and the nurse is to obtain a specimen for an aerobic culture. When performing this procedure, the nurse should
    1. Note antibiotic or antifungal therapy on lab requisition.
    2. Wipe several areas of the wound with one swab.
    3. Place specimen in a paper cup to transport.
    4. Refrigerate specimen if unable to take immediately to lab.

21

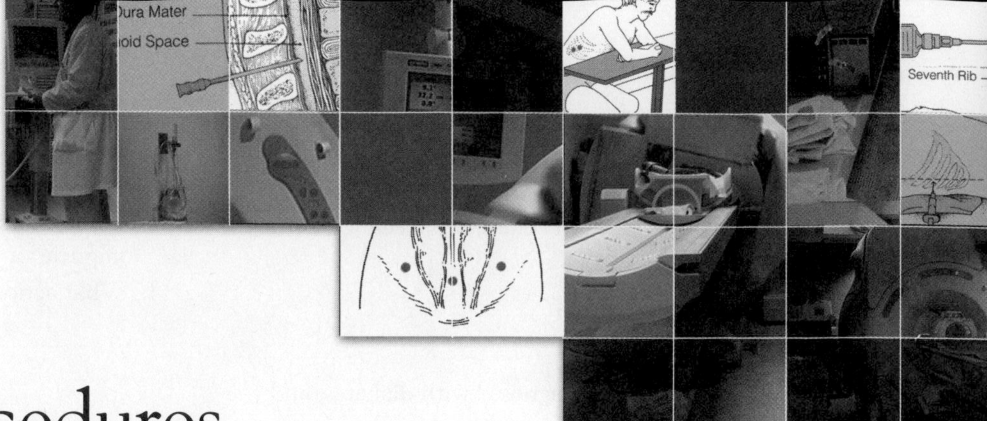

Diagnostic Procedures

LEARNING OBJECTIVES

1. Describe the major components of client teaching for diagnostic studies.
2. Define interventional radiology (IR) and the nurse's role in IR.
3. List at least three preparatory functions for clients undergoing diagnostic studies.
4. Explain the importance of determining allergic responses to shellfish before clients undergo contrast media studies.
5. List the signs and symptoms that occur when the client experiences an allergic reaction.
6. Explain the reason for giving blocking agents before administering radioisotopes to clients.
7. Outline the nursing care responsibilities when a client returns from myelography.
8. Discuss the nursing care responsibilities when a client returns from arteriography.
9. Describe the care necessary after cardiac catheterization to prevent postprocedure complications.
10. Explain the steps you would take if a client is given medication before a GI series.
11. Describe client positions for at least four diagnostic procedures commonly performed at the bedside.
12. Compare and contrast postprocedure nursing observations for clients undergoing liver biopsy, paracentesis, and thoracentesis.
13. Explain the nurse's role during procedures that use fiberoptic scopes.
14. Describe how ultrasonography is used for diagnostic studies.
15. Describe the data that should be included in the charting for clients undergoing diagnostic procedures.
16. Describe the preparation clients must complete before an MRI.

CHAPTER OUTLINE

TERMINOLOGY

Abscess a localized collection of pus in any part of the body.

Allergy an altered reaction of body tissues to a specific substance; essentially an antibody–antigen reaction and may be due to the release of histamine.

Amniocentesis puncturing the amniotic sac, usually by using a needle and syringe, to remove amniotic fluid for assessment of fetal maturity.

Antiemetic an agent that prevents or arrests vomiting.

Arteriography study using radiopaque dye injected into an artery to assess arteries.

Barium a radiopaque compound used in roentgenography of the gastrointestinal tract.

Bone densitometry Test used to determine bone mineral content and density; used to diagnose osteoporosis.

Bronchoscopy a visualization of the larynx, trachea, and bronchi through a flexible scope.

Catheterization use or passage of a catheter, a tube for evacuating or injecting fluids.

Centesis perforation or puncture through the skin to obtain fluid.

Cholangiography x-ray examination of the bile ducts.

Cholecystogram x-ray picture of the gallbladder.

Computed tomography (CT scan) a scanning technique that provides a series of detailed visualizations.

Contrast medium a radiopaque substance used during x-ray examination to provide a contrast in density between the tissue being filmed and the medium.

Contusion an injury in which the skin is not broken.

Craniotomy incision involving the skull.

Crepitus a crackling breath sound caused by air pockets in the subcutaneous tissue.

Diagnosis method or art of identifying the disease or condition a person has or is believed to have.

Diaphoresis profuse sweating.

Dissipate to scatter, disperse, dispel, disintegrate.

Dyspnea shortness of breath.

Endoscopy visualization of body organs and cavities using an endoscope (tubular instrument with light source and viewing lens).

Enema introduction of a solution through a tube into the rectum or colon.

Fiberoptic scope flexible scope that uses fiberoptic materials for visualization. These materials transmit light along its course by reflecting it from the side or wall of the fiber. Devices using fiberoptic materials are used in endoscopic examinations.

Fluoroscopy type of examination using a screen to view shadows with the aid of x-rays.

Interventional radiology procedures formerly completed in perioperative settings that are now performed in radiology departments.

Lithotomy incision into the bladder for removing a stone.

Lumbar pertaining to the loins and lower vertebrae in the back.

Magnetic resonance imaging (MRI) a noninvasive test that uses a magnetic field with radio frequency waves to produce cross-sectional images of the body.

Mammography x-ray examination of breast used to detect breast cancer.

Myelography x-ray inspection of the spinal cord by the use of radiopaque medium.

Neoplasm a new and abnormal formation of tissue, as a tumor or growth.

NPO nothing by mouth.

Oliguria diminished amount of urine formation.

Paracentesis puncture of the abdominal cavity for the removal of fluid.

Peripheral outer part or surface of a body.

PET Scan imaging technique used to scan entire body or its various regions.

Pyelo pertaining to the pelvis of the kidney.

Pyelography x-ray study of the renal pelvis and ureter.

Scintillation the emissions from radiographic substances; a subjective sensation of seeing sparks.

Septicemia blood poisoning; septic products in blood and tissue.

Tachycardia fast pulse above 100 beats/min.

Thoracentesis surgical puncture of the chest wall for the removal of fluid.

Tumor uncontrolled new growth or tissue forming an abnormal mass that performs no physiologic function.

Urticaria a vascular reaction of the skin characterized by the eruption of pale, elevated wheals that are associated with severe itching.

Ventro denoting the abdomen or ventral (anterior) surface of the body.

Vertigo sensation of moving or having objects move when they are actually still.

CLIENT PREPARATION

Diagnostic tests play a major role in the diagnosis and care of clients. Diagnostic testing is as important as a thorough history and physical examination. The results from diagnostic tests can confirm or eliminate client diagnosis. In addition to assisting with the identification of disease states, diagnostic tests assist with monitoring diseases as interventions and treatments are established. With cost containment a major issue in health care today, it is imperative that tests be scheduled appropriately, the client be prepared for the tests, and specimens, if any, be collected and disseminated efficiently. Many tests are completed on an outpatient basis; therefore, very explicit information must be provided to the client. Many procedures begin the preparation 1 or 2 days in advance of the actual test. Clients must thoroughly understand this and be able to comply with the instructions in order to obtain an accurate result.

Nurses play a major role in client preparation for diagnostic tests. Client education is one of the most important means to promote an accurate test result. The educational process begins with a discussion of the test itself, the preparation necessary for an accurate result, and the posttest interventions if any.

Many types of diagnostic tests are being utilized in the healthcare industry today. This chapter contains only a few of the most common tests. There is a brief overview of pretest preparation and any posttest interventions commonly done after the test. As client education is a major role of the nurse, it is highlighted throughout the chapter.

The responsibility of the nurse begins with the initial scheduling of the test and continues after the results of the test are explained to the client. The physician explains the results of the test, but the nurse answers questions, interprets terminology, and listens to the client express his or her feelings or apprehensions.

The preparation of clients for diagnostic tests must be done on an individual basis. Some clients are well informed about the test they are scheduled to take. They know about diet and fluid restrictions, what to expect during the procedure, whether or not there is any discomfort with the test, and how long the procedure takes. Others need a great deal of explanation. Also, some clients prefer not to be given any explanation about the test. Nurses need to respect the client's preferences and provide only information requested, unless it in some way is a danger to the client.

Undergoing diagnostic tests can be frightening for clients; they are often unaware of what the procedure involves and worry about the outcome. Communication involves an active, verbal interchange of ideas, as well as an astute observation of the client's nonverbal cues, and can be hindered by this fear. One effective way to allow clients time to think about questions is to provide a printed form explaining the diagnostic test. The form may cover such information as how long a test takes, equipment used for the test, and any sensations experienced during the test. Leaving the form at the bedside can stimulate interest and prompt the shy, reserved client to ask questions when you return later.

Most diagnostic procedures are done on an outpatient basis. This makes it imperative that the nurse provide the necessary information about the procedure. Instructions are sent home with the client that include preprocedural preparation. When the client arrives for the diagnostic test, time should be allotted to answer questions, reassure the client, and determine if the preprocedure preparation was followed.

Another important aspect of teaching involves the way in which the nurse approaches the client. The nurse should avoid giving the impression that she/he is in a hurry and that she/he has no time to answer any questions. On the other hand, be aware of the client's ability to pay attention to what you have to say. If the client seems distracted, he or she may be worried about finances, about who is watching the children, or whether or not their job will be waiting after discharge from the hospital. This preoccupation may prevent assimilation of knowledge and the client may be unprepared for the events that follow.

Remember, the client probably does not know medical jargon; therefore, explain procedures in terms the client can understand. If the client looks puzzled and does not ask any questions, evaluate how you presented the information.

Feedback is the only way in which you can evaluate the learner's knowledge. Feedback can be in the form of direct questioning about certain aspects of the test. Feedback can also be determined through direct observation of facial expressions, posturing, and activities.

X-Ray Studies

Many x-rays use the normal contrasts of the body, such as air, water in soft tissues, fat, and bone. These four densities observe varying degrees of radiation. Air has less density, causing dark images on the film, whereas bone has high density, producing light images. Plain radiology is performed without contrast material. These include x-rays of chest, skull, abdomen, and bones. Some tests do require a contrast medium. Several types of contrast media are used routinely, including barium sulfate, helium, carbon dioxide, iodized oils, and organic iodides.

One of the major problems with the use of some contrast media is the adverse reaction or sensitivity that can occur. This is more common when iodine preparations are used. The degree of reaction varies from mild (such as nausea) to severe (such as cardiovascular collapse). The usual symptoms include urticaria, hives, dyspnea, nausea, vomiting, and decreased blood pressure.

Clients allergic to food, especially shellfish, or drugs are often allergic to some dyes used in diagnostic studies, particularly those that are iodine-based. After injections of iodine dye, many tests are abnormal for varying lengths of time. Urine sodium, specific gravity, protein, and osmolality are abnormal for 16 hr. Urine catecholamines are also abnormal for 16 hr.

Barium sulfate is a radiopaque substance that blocks the passage of x-rays and provides excellent contrast to body structures. It can cause some uncomfortable feelings and problems with the gastrointestinal tract, but with proper postprocedure care, this condition can be greatly reduced. It is not used as frequently now as it was previously, due to the newer diagnostic equipment now available.

Fluoroscopy, x-rays that pass through the body to a fluorescent viewing screen, a sequence of x-ray films each representing a section of tissue at different levels, have been very important in diagnosing and confirming clients' conditions. Two very common uses of fluoroscopy are upper GI barium swallow studies and angiography procedures to guide catheters to predetermined positions, such as in cardiac catheterization.

Computed tomography (CT) of various organs, particularly abdominal and renal organs, are noninvasive x-ray procedures used to diagnose pathologic conditions such as tumors, cysts, abscesses, inflammation, perforation, obstruction, and calculi. The CT scan image results from passing x-rays through the abdominal organs using several angles. CT scans are used as a guide to aspirate fluid from organs to obtain cultures and biopsies. There are newer scanners that can visualize the blood flow and degree of vascularity of the organ through arterial injection of dye to specific organs in the abdomen. This is termed dynamic CT scanning. A second scan, the helical CT scan, obtains images as the client passes through the scanner. A large advantage to this type of scanning is the speed with which the client passes through the scanner. A CT scan of the abdomen or chest is completed in less than 30 seconds. The procedure can be completed with the client holding only one breath.

Ultrasound Studies

Ultrasonography can be done alone or with other procedures. Sound waves produced by ultrasound differentiate normal from diseased tissue. The sound waves are transmitted through fluid, but not bone, air, or contrast material. It is usually performed in physicians' offices or outpatient settings. Ultrasound is painless, requiring only that the client lie quietly during the 15–30-minute procedure. There is no risk to the procedure; therefore, it can be repeated frequently without side effects. This procedure needs to precede barium studies because barium impedes transmission of sound waves. It requires that a gel be placed over the site of the organ to be tested. This provides an air-free barrier between the probe (which holds the transducer) and the skin. The probe, or transducer, is passed over the specific body area, and ultrasonic waves are transmitted through the tissue. The transducer converts the echoes to electric impulses and transforms them into visual images. There is no preprocedural or postprocedural care for the client because it is a noninvasive procedure, except for an ultrasound of pelvic organs. The client needs to drink four glasses of water to promote a full bladder. The full bladder enhances transmission of sound waves and thus improves visualization of organs.

Echocardiography is a procedure similar to ultrasound. It is a painless, noninvasive technique that uses transducers and oscilloscopes similar to those in ultrasound procedures. The echocardiogram records heart motion, not heart outline. There is no preparation or postprocedure alteration in activity for this procedure.

Doppler ultrasonography is used to evaluate blood flow through carotid arteries or peripheral blood vessels. Deep vein thrombosis and peripheral vascular disease are diagnosed using this diagnostic test. A handheld transducer transmits high-frequency sound waves to an artery or vein. The sound waves strike the moving RBCs and are reflected back to the transducer, which amplifies the sound and produces a graphic recording.

Nuclear Scanning

Radioisotopes distribute uniformly through normal tissue, but unevenly in pathologically involved or diseased tissue. The radionuclide atom emits radioactive particles (photons in the gamma radiation range), which have short half-lives. The most commonly used are gallium, thallium, and iodine. A scanning procedure involves less radiation exposure than a chest x-ray.

Radioisotopes tend to concentrate in specific organ tissues and thus are more effective when administered for scanning a particular organ. For example, technetium-99m is specifically used for thyroid scanning, while thallium-201 (^{201}Tl) is used to evaluate blood flow through vessels that are too small to visualize with a cardiac catheterization procedure. This is often termed a *myocardial perfusion scan*. Technetium-99m is also used for cardiac scanning. The newer thallium imagery is three-dimensional; the camera moves around the client in a 180°–360° arc. The three-dimensional view is more precise in identifying abnormalities. Scanning allows visualization of organs that are unobservable by x-ray alone. Tumors present as areas of reduced radioisotopic activity. Radioisotope studies are contraindicated with pregnancy, breast-feeding mothers, or persons who are allergic to the radioisotopes.

The radioactive isotopes are administered intravenously or orally to the client. A specified time elapses before the scanning is done. This allows time for the radioactive material to reach the specific tissue under study. Then, a scanning device is used to record the concentration of radiation that emerges from the radioisotope. Equal or gray distribution is normal, but lighter or brighter areas, termed "hot spots," indicate hyperfunction, and darker areas, "cold spots," indicate hypofunction.

Some clients are given blocking agents before the administration of the radioisotope. This prevents the radioactive material from entering organs other than those being studied. A common blocking agent is Lugol's solution, which is given to a client who is having a study done on an organ other than the thyroid gland.

Microscopic Studies

Microscopic studies are necessary for diagnosis and treatment of many diseases and infectious processes. Specimens are collected from tissues, blood, organ biopsies, and secretions, in addition to other sources such as blood and urine.

Biopsies involve the physician's taking a piece of tissue from the designated area to be used for microscopic evaluation. Biopsies can be done on endometrial tissue, the lung and liver, and bone marrow aspiration, to name a few areas. Information obtained from the biopsy can indicate pathologic conditions, diseases, and treatment for infections.

Endoscopic Studies

An endoscopy refers to inspection of an internal body organ and cavities by introducing an instrument called an endoscope. Biopsies of suspicious tissue, removal of abnormal growths, injection of blood vessels, dilation and stent procedures, and surgical procedures can all be accomplished through the endoscope.

Endoscopes are either rigid or flexible and have a light source and viewing lens that allows the physician to observe the specified area. Scopes can be inserted through body orifices or through small incisions. Rigid scopes are used mostly for operative laparoscopic procedures. Flexible fiberoptic scopes are used in pulmonary and GI endoscopy. Because the scope is flexible, light can be transmitted around corners and thus provide a view of body structures not visible by older rigid scopes.

Fluid Analysis Studies

Normal body fluids can provide information concerning the client's health status. Body fluids frequently studied include CSF analysis and condition of the fetus and its environment. Abnormal accumulation of fluids within the body can be analyzed by aspirating the fluid and sending it to the laboratory for studies. The most common areas where fluid needs to be removed include the abdomen and pleural space. Most often, the fluid is removed for therapeutic purposes, although it may be removed for diagnostic purposes. Once fluid is removed, it is measured and samples are sent to the laboratory for analysis.

Magnetic Resonance Imaging (MRI)

The MRI procedure has revolutionized diagnostic medicine. It is a method of looking inside the body. It replaces the use of x-rays. The procedure identifies the distribution of hydrogen molecules in the body using a three-dimensional process. The images are translated by computer and differentiate normal from abnormal tissue structure and blood flow. It uses a strong magnetic field in conjunction with radio frequency waves to transmit signals from body cells to the computer. The computer produces cross-sectional images of the body. The procedure is noninvasive and does not involve harmful exposure to radiation. The MRI detects and describes soft tissue abnormalities and yields information about the chemical nature of the cells. Gray and white brain matter can be differentiated and brain tumors and vascular abnormalities identified. The MRI is the most sensitive technique for defining the structures of internal organs and for detecting edema, infarction, hemorrhage, tumors, and infection.

Even though the full usefulness of the MRI has not been totally determined, the MRI is the diagnostic procedure of choice for detecting most brain abnormalities and shows great promise in identifying abnormal blood flow through coronary arteries, assessing kidney flow, heart defects, and a myriad of other abnormalities and defects. This procedure has replaced the need for arthrography and myelography. It has been used as a diagnostic tool in the diagnosis of multiple sclerosis; however, it has limited ability to detect plaque as the client ages. The MRI scan may require the use of a contrast agent administered IV to assist in visualization of certain structures in the body.

Interventional Radiology

With the technological advances and changes in health care, many procedures performed exclusively in the perioperative settings are now being performed in the radiology department. The usual procedures completed in the radiology department are those that have minimal incisions, are low risk, entail low pain, and have a short recovery time.

Interventional radiologists do the following: biopsies, cryotherapy, embolization, stenting, thrombolysis, vascular access procedures, and vertebroplasty.

The radiology team consists of the physician, technologist, and nurse. Selected radiology departments employ physician's assistants and nurse practitioners.

Role of the RN in Radiology The nurse working in the radiology department is a critical care RN who manages clients during interventional radiology procedures. This nurse must have experience in ICU or ER and be certified in both ACLS and administration of moderate sedation. Responsibilities include completing preprocedure assessments and preparation, intraprocedure monitoring and procedural sedation, postprocedure recovery from sedation, and monitored anesthesia care. The RN works in all modalities of radiology, including CT scan, ultrasound, PET, vascular radiology, MRI, and interventional radiology procedures including abdominal, bone, neurovascular, and thoracic.

Assisting the Physician During Tests

Nurses are frequently called on to assist the physician with procedures at the bedside. The procedures presented in this chapter are the most common ones performed in the hospital unit. It is important that the nurse be aware of the correct client positioning in order to facilitate the procedure, decrease complications, and decrease the time it takes to complete the procedure.

Some diagnostic tests frequently used in the past are used less frequently today. One such procedure is the lumbar puncture. Removal of fluid from the spinal tract may cause the brain, because of edema, to herniate down through the tentorium. Because of this complication, a lumbar puncture is not done on a client with head trauma or potential increased intracranial pressure. The CT scan is now frequently used to determine intracranial bleeding. If a lumbar puncture is ordered, the client may have the procedure done in the x-ray department.

CULTURAL AWARENESS

A cross-culture assessment questionnaire should be offered to clients who may have difficulty in understanding or following directions in preparation for diagnostic procedures. In some cultures, it is difficult for clients to admit they do not understand what is being said to them. Westerners are bold and direct when asking questions so they expect the same from clients of different cultures.

With the "push" to get clients in and out of procedure rooms, communication and understanding can be compromised. However, while preparing for the procedure, talking with the client can provide the comforting measures necessary to allow them to participate appropriately during the procedure. Ask clients which family member should be included in the discussion and client teaching regarding the diagnostic procedure. Pay close attention to what family members say.

They can provide valuable information regarding the client's understanding or fear of the procedure. In some cultures words such as cancer, surgery, or death are not used. In many Middle Eastern cultures you do not speak of death; it is viewed as a breach in the nurse–client relationship. Modesty is an issue with some cultures. This varies greatly among cultures and individuals within those cultures. Be sensitive to this issue and allow the client to undress in private if at all possible.

Source: Heinekine, J., & McCoy, N. (2000, January). Establishing a bond with clients of different cultures. *Home Healthcare Nurse, 18*(1), 45.

NURSING DIAGNOSES

The following nursing diagnoses may be appropriate to include in a client care plan when the components are related to clients undergoing diagnostic procedures.

NURSING DIAGNOSIS	RELATED FACTORS
Anxiety	Apprehension regarding test or procedure outcome
Fear	Results of diagnostic test, change in health status, threat to self-concept
Risk for Deficient Fluid Volume	Reaction to contrast media, NPO status, side effects of medication
Deficient Knowledge	Misunderstanding of instructions or information, inadequate data or explanation of procedure (maintaining position after spinal tap, liver biopsy)
Noncompliance	Inability to follow directions as a result of poor health status, cultural influences, or patient's value system

CLEANSE HANDS The single most important nursing action to decrease the incidence of hospital-based infections is hand hygiene. *Remember to wash your hands or use antibacterial gel before and after each and every client contact.*

IDENTIFY CLIENT Before every procedure, introduce yourself and check two forms of client identification, not including room number. These actions prevent errors and conform to the Joint Commission standards.

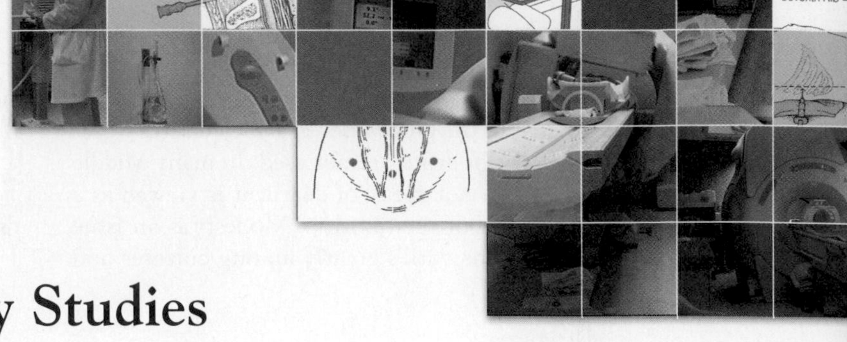

Chapter 21

UNIT ❶

Contrast Media and X-Ray Studies

Nursing Process Data

ASSESSMENT Data Base

- Assess client's knowledge of procedure to be done.
- Identify any history of drug or food allergies.
- Evaluate client's ability to follow directions before and during the test.
- Assess vital signs and document for baseline data.

PLANNING Objectives

- To determine if the client is physically prepared for the test
- To determine if the client is psychologically prepared for the test
- To determine if the client is at risk for an allergic reaction
- To determine if the client is able to cooperate with the preparation and completion of the test

IMPLEMENTATION Procedures

EVALUATION Expected Outcomes

- Client acknowledges understanding of the scheduled procedure.
- Client is calm and emotionally prepared for procedure.
- Client is well prepared for x-ray study after client teaching.
- Client completes x-ray study without complications.
- Client did not experience allergic reaction to contrast media.
- Client describes posttest care upon discharge.

Preparing for X-Ray Studies

Equipment

Signed consent form
Pajama bottoms and hospital gown
Allergy Ident-A-Band, if needed
Wheelchair

> **Clinical Alert**
> Ensure that female client is not pregnant nor is there a chance of being pregnant before performing any diagnostic tests using x-rays.

Procedure

For All X-Ray Studies

1. Identify the specific diagnostic test to be performed (Table 21-1).
2. Determine if any tests must precede others in order to schedule test appropriately.
3. Obtain client's history to determine allergies to food or drugs, and note these on the chart. Notify physician of findings.
4. Identify specific preparations that need to be carried out before the studies.
5. Monitor food and fluid restrictions that need to be altered for the studies.
6. Obtain special consent forms for all invasive diagnostic studies after the physician has explained the study to the client. The consent form must be signed before any medication is administered.
7. Provide client teaching regarding the purpose of the study, including any special preparation required and restrictions imposed by the study.

> **Clinical Alert**
> Clients taking metformin hydrochloride (Glucophage, Glucophage XR, or Riomet) are at risk for acute renal failure and lactic acidosis with iodinated contrast media. Instruct the client to STOP the metformin for 48 hr before and after the studies.

8. Provide psychological support and reassurance to the client.
9. Obtain orders regarding medications or nutrition for clients with special problems, such as diabetes or seizure disorders.
10. Carry out safety precautions immediately before the study:
    a. Check two forms of client identification.
    b. Have client void if necessary.
    c. Remove client's hairpins, jewelry, and dentures if necessary.
    d. Chart premedication given.
    e. Monitor safe transfer from the bed to gurney or wheelchair.
    f. Accompany client to x-ray department if needed. (Usually, nurses accompany critically ill clients.)

> **Clinical Alert**
> Clients scheduled for a diagnostic test using contrast media must have BUN and creatinine tests completed before the scheduled study. Nephrotoxicity is a side effect of the contrast media, particularly iodinated dyes.

For Oral Cholecystography

1. Explain purpose for procedure to client—x-ray provides visualization of gallbladder.
2. Identify allergies to shellfish or iodine. Notify physician if allergy is noted.

TABLE 21-1 Contrast Media and X-Ray Studies

Diagnostic Test	Rationale	Contrast Media
Oral cholecystography	To visualize shape and position of the gallbladder and to identify the presence of stones	Yes
Intravenous pyelography	To visualize structures of the urinary tract	Yes
Myelography	To visualize the subarachnoid space to identify abnormalities	Yes
Arteriography	To visualize abnormalities or obstructions in specific blood vessels	Yes
Computed tomography	To visualize a cross-section of the brain, chest, and abdomen to precisely localize lesions	Yes/No
Cardiac catheterization	To measure oxygen concentration, provide blood samples, determine cardiac output, and visualize coronary arteries	Yes
Bone densitometry	To determine bone mineral density and strength of bone	No
Magnetic resonance imaging	To visualize inner structures of body	Yes/No
Mammography	To determine presence of breast pathology	No

Informed Consent

- Informed consent indicates clients have received a full explanation of the procedure, including risks, complications, benefits, and alternatives.
- Obtaining informed consent is the responsibility of the physician. It is the nurse's responsibility to check that the consent is signed before the procedure.
- The nurse can be asked to witness the signature. Before witnessing the signature, the nurse must have been present during the client/physician discussion.

Clinical Alert

Symptoms of contrast media reactions:

- Urticaria, hives
- Nausea, vomiting
- Respiratory distress
- Decreased blood pressure

Clients allergic to food or drugs may also be allergic to contrast media used for diagnostic studies.

3. Obtain consent form.
4. Instruct client to eat low-fat meal evening before test.
5. Administer iodine radiopaque medication 2 hr after dinner. Drug: iopanoic acid (Telepaque). ▸ ***Rationale:*** It takes 12–14 hr for the dye to be concentrated in the gall bladder.
   a. Number of tablets administered is based on client's weight.
   b. Tablets are given 5 minutes apart with 8 oz. of water for each tablet. Usually six tablets are given.
   c. Inform client that diarrhea is a common side effect.
6. Keep client NPO after administration of contrast medium. ▸ ***Rationale:*** This prevents contraction of gallbladder and expulsion of radiopaque dye.
7. Take client to x-ray department.
8. Explain details of procedure to client.
   a. X-ray client in standing and lying positions for good visualization of gallbladder and common bile duct. Test takes about 1 hr.
   b. Feed client a fatty meal to test ability of the gallbladder to contract.
   c. If visualization does not occur, additional medications may be given and the test repeated the following day, or an IV cholangiogram may be done.

Clinical Alert

Do not schedule cholecystogram after barium study because the barium precludes visualization of gallbladder.

Clinical Alert

Ultrasound has replaced the oral cholecystogram test in most cases. It may still be used, however, if ultrasound results are inconclusive.

9. Explain postprocedure care to client.
   a. Mild dysuria can occur. ▸ ***Rationale:*** Dye is excreted through the kidneys.
   b. Observe for allergy symptoms from dye.

For Intravenous Pyelography (IVP)

1. Follow steps as appropriate in Preparing for X-Ray Studies.
   a. Give client clear liquid diet the evening before the IVP and maintain NPO status after 12 midnight. Some facilities allow clear liquid diet in morning.
   b. Give laxative or cathartic as ordered, usually the night before test. A cleansing enema may be ordered the morning of the test (check facility policy). ▸ ***Rationale:*** To eliminate feces and gas to provide better contrast.
   c. Identify allergies to shellfish or iodine. ▸ ***Rationale:*** Other contrast material will be used in place of iodine contrast media.
   d. Obtain consent.
   e. Take baseline vital signs.
   f. Take client to x-ray department when notified.
2. Explain details of procedure to client.
   a. Client is positioned in supine position.
   b. Flat plate of abdomen taken. ▸ ***Rationale:*** Ensure no residual stool, which could interfere with visualization of renal system.
   c. Test dose of contrast medium may be injected intradermally for clients with a history of allergies. The contrast material is administered if there is no reaction within 15 minutes of test dose.
   d. IV is inserted and contrast medium injected as a large single dose.
   e. X-rays are taken over period of 30 minutes to 1 hr to determine extent to which dye is filtered through the kidneys.
3. Warn client that contrast medium can cause feelings of nausea, shortness of breath, and a hot, flushed effect.
4. Instruct client to void at end of test. An x-ray is taken to visualize residual dye in kidneys.
5. Return client to room and resume ordered activity level.
6. Encourage fluids, and resume usual diet. Fluids should include at least 24 ounces of water. ▸ ***Rationale:*** Increasing fluid intake prevents osmotic diuresis from contrast medium.
7. Monitor client for at least 24 hr for signs and symptoms of reactions to contrast medium such as oliguria, nausea, and vomiting.

For Myelography

1. Follow steps as appropriate in Preparing for X-Ray Studies.
   a. Explain procedure to client—test identifies abnormalities of spine and subarachnoid space.
   b. Client may have cleansing enema ordered.
   c. Identify allergies to shellfish, iodine, or other contrast media.
   d. Keep client NPO for 4–8 hr before test.
   e. Obtain baseline levels of motor and sensory function and vital signs.
   f. Assess for signs of increased ICP. ▸ ***Rationale:*** This test is contraindicated for clients with ICP. Brain herniation can occur.
   g. Obtain consent form.
   h. Medicate with sedative if ordered. ▸ ***Rationale:*** This provides client comfort.
   i. Take client on gurney to x-ray department.
2. Explain details of procedure to client.
   a. Client is placed either in prone position with pillow under abdomen or side-lying with knees drawn up to abdomen and chin on chest on fluoroscopic table, and secured to table with several straps. ▸ ***Rationale:*** This position allows physician to visualize ruptured disc or neoplasms.
   b. A lumbar puncture needle is inserted between the vertebrae into the subarachnoid space.
   c. A small amount of cerebrospinal fluid is sent to lab for study.
   d. Contrast medium is injected, and client is tilted on table to allow flow of dye to designated areas of spine to visualize it by x-rays.
   e. Oil-based contrast medium, Pantopaque, is removed through aspiration. Explain to client that sudden sharp pain in legs may occur.
   f. Water-based contrast medium, metrizamide, is absorbed and excreted through kidneys. It is not removed by aspiration. Most facilities now use Omnipaque. ▸ ***Rationale:*** It has far fewer side effects.
   g. Procedure lasts about 1 hr.
   h. Client is returned on gurney to room.
3. After the test:
   a. Keep client in prone position or supine position for 8 hr for water-based or 12 hr for oil-based contrast. May turn side to side. ▸ ***Rationale:*** This position prevents a headache and CSF leaks.
   b. Keep head of bed elevated 30°–50° for 8 hr. If procedure has included water-soluble dye medium, client may be on bedrest for up to 24 hr. ▸ ***Rationale:*** This position reduces rate of upward displacement of dye.
4. Observe for seizure activity if metrizamide used for procedure. It can precipitate seizures. Do not give medications that can decrease seizure threshold.
5. Monitor vital signs and motor and sensory function.
   a. Cervical myelogram: Check upper and lower extremities and bladder function.
   b. Lumbar myelogram: Check lower extremities and bladder function.
6. Medicate for pain as ordered, usually with a mild sedative.
7. Increase fluids to at least 2,500 mL each day for 2 days. ▸ ***Rationale:*** Fluids rehydrate and replace cerebrospinal fluid and may prevent headache after procedure. Offer diet.
8. Monitor output, and observe for distention.
9. Observe puncture site for 24 hr for bleeding, hematoma, or edema.
10. Observe for complication of chemical or bacterial meningitis: fever, stiff neck, photophobia or delayed reaction to dye.
11. Use comfort measures and relaxation techniques when needed.

Clinical Alert

A myelogram is performed less frequently today because of the wide use of the MRI and CT scanning. The MRI is more accurate for viewing spinal cord and surrounding structures.

For Arteriography

1. Follow steps as appropriate in Preparing for X-Ray Studies.
2. Explain purpose of procedure to client—examination of arteries to determine abnormalities in blood flow.
3. Identify allergies to shellfish, iodine, or any contrast media. Ask client if taking anticoagulants.
4. Obtain baseline CBC, PT/PTT, and APTT, BUN, and creatinine. Anticoagulants must be discontinued before procedure.
5. Obtain consent form.
6. Keep client NPO for 2–8 hr or as ordered.
7. Shave and scrub puncture site when ordered.
8. Have client void before procedure. Remove dentures and metallic objects.
9. Obtain vital signs and check peripheral pulses. ▸ ***Rationale:*** To provide comparison data after procedure.
10. Administer preprocedure medications 1 hr before test, if ordered, and transport client to x-ray department.
11. Explain details of procedure to client.
    a. Client is positioned supine on x-ray table.
    b. IV for fluid administration may be started. ▸ ***Rationale:*** For use in emergency situations.
    c. Puncture site will be scrubbed and a local anesthetic administered. Catheter is inserted into brachial or femoral artery.
    d. Contrast medium will be injected to visualize abnormalities or obstruction to specific vessels. Inform client that a warm flush may be felt when dye injected.

e. Client may be instructed to hold breath for x-rays. Procedure takes about 1–2 hr if an automatic film changer is used.
f. Catheter is removed and pressure dressing applied over site.

12. Monitor vital signs, pulses, and puncture site, as with surgical clients. ▸ ***Rationale:*** To identify potential complications.
13. Observe for signs of shock and presence of pain, which indicate hemorrhage or thrombosis.
14. Observe for symptoms of delayed allergic reaction to dye, such as nausea, vomiting, tachycardia, sweating, rash, or hives. ▸ ***Rationale:*** Delayed reactions can occur up to several hours after the procedure.
15. Notify physician immediately if unusual symptoms are present. ▸ ***Rationale:*** Immediate medical intervention is necessary to prevent anaphylaxis.
16. Do not flex the involved extremity.
17. Maintain bedrest with head elevated slightly for at least 6–8 hr depending on site of puncture. Check hospital policy for time.
18. Offer fluids and diet as ordered and tolerated. Fluids should be 1 to 2 liters. ▸ ***Rationale:*** To facilitate elimination of contrast media.
19. Provide comfort measures as needed.

For Computed Tomography (CT Scan)

1. Explain purpose of procedure to client—CT scans give outlines of bone tissue and fluid structures due to tumors and hematomas. Tomography can be performed on abdomen, brain, chest, or bones and joints.
2. Identify allergies to shellfish or iodine if contrast medium is used.
3. Obtain consent if contrast medium is used or facility requires.
4. Place client on NPO for 4 hr if contrast medium is used. ▸ ***Rationale:*** Dye can cause nausea; NPO prevents emesis and potential aspiration.
5. Administer preprocedure medication if ordered. A mild sedative may be ordered for client to alleviate anxiety.
6. Remove all metal objects, such as hair clips, necklace, and jewelry. ▸ ***Rationale:*** Metal objects block bony structures on the film.
7. Take client on gurney to x-ray department.
8. Explain equipment and procedure to client.
9. Explain client will have IV injection of contrast material if enhanced study is to be done. Explain that a warm, flushed feeling or nausea can occur.
10. Explain that client will be placed in an encircling body scanner.
11. Instruct client to lie very still during the procedure and to not touch area to be scanned. Scan takes 15 minutes. ▸ ***Rationale:*** Movement causes artifact on the image.
12. Return client to room.

Xenon Computed Tomography

This test is used to evaluate cerebral blood flow. This technique precisely measures blood flow to various areas of the brain. It can define the degree and extent of ischemia in acute neurologic conditions such as stroke. This technology detects changes hours to days before changes can be seen on the MRI or CT. The client inhales a xenon/oxygen gas mixture for approximately 4–5 minutes, during which time CT data are obtained. The xenon gas travels to regions of the brain where it is distributed to tissue in proportion to blood flow and lipid content (xenon is fat soluble). A computer actually calculates blood flow to many different areas of the brain, and within minutes the computer provides precise measurements of cerebral blood flow. This scan is used to determine brain death.

13. Provide diet and encourage fluids to 3,000 mL or as ordered. ▸ ***Rationale:*** Increasing fluids assists in eliminating the contrast medium more quickly.
14. Observe for signs of delayed allergic reaction if contrast study is done.

For Cardiac Catheterization

1. Explain purpose and risk factors of procedure to client—to visualize heart structures and coronary blood flow and measure oxygen saturation, cardiac output and heart pressures. Angioplasty or stent placement is done through cardiac catheterization. Used most often to determine the cause of chest pain in adult clients. Procedure takes about 1 hr.
2. Obtain consent form.
3. Identify allergies to drugs, iodine, shellfish, or any other contrast media.
4. Check if client is on anticoagulants. Contact physician for instructions related to drug administration.
5. Complete prep and shave of groin or brachial area (or both). Mark peripheral pulses for post catheterization assessment.
6. Establish baseline data for vital signs, peripheral pulses, coagulation studies (PTT, PT), ACT, BUN, creatinine, renal function tests, and ECG pattern.
7. Place client on NPO 6–8 hr before test.
8. Keep client NPO for medications 6–8 hr before test, unless physician orders otherwise. Oral anticoagulants are discontinued or dosage reduced. ▸ ***Rationale:*** To prevent bleeding.
9. Before procedure, obtain vital signs, take weight, and have the client void. ▸ ***Rationale:*** Weight is used to calculate amount of dye required for the test.
10. Administer preprocedure medication, usually Valium and atropine, 30 minutes to 1 hr before procedure.

11. Remove dentures.
12. Take client on gurney to cardiac catheterization lab.
13. Explain equipment and details of procedure to client.
    a. Client is strapped onto a table. ECG leads and blood pressure equipment are applied.
    b. IV is started using D5W at TKO rate. ▸ ***Rationale:*** For use in emergency.
    c. ECG monitoring is initiated to monitor heart rate and rhythm.
    d. Groin or brachial area is scrubbed and injected with Xylocaine.
    e. Catheter is placed in femoral or brachial artery and advanced to cardiac chambers.
    f. When contrast medium is injected for coronary artery visualization, explain to client that a warm, flushed feeling, shortness of breath, or nausea can occur.
    g. Instruct client to report any chest pain immediately.
    h. Client is asked to hold breath about 10 seconds during contrast medium injection.
    i. Reinforce that client will not fall off table as he or she may be turned on side for cineangiography. Total procedure takes 30 minutes to 3 hr.
    j. After catheterization, pressure is applied to puncture site for 10–15 minutes.
14. Transport client on gurney to room.
15. Provide post–cardiac catheterization care.
    a. Monitor vital signs, puncture site, heart and lung sounds, and peripheral pulses as with a surgical client.
    b. Elevate extremity used for catheterization site. Keep extremity extended. ▸ ***Rationale:*** Position promotes blood supply back to heart and prevents thrombus formation.
    c. Apply pressure dressing to puncture site if bleeding continues.
    d. Encourage fluids and diet when vital signs are stable and no evidence of nausea or drowsiness is present.

Procedures Done During Cardiac Catheterization

Transluminal Coronary Angioplasty: Specially designed catheter is introduced into the coronary arteries and placed across the stenotic area of the artery. The artery is then dilated by controlled inflation of the balloon for a few seconds. Coronary stents can be placed at the site of the stenosis after angioplasty. The stent is used to keep the coronary artery patent.

Laser Arterectomy: Permanent procedure to open coronary arteries that have plaque deposits using laser therapy.

Angioplasty: Catheter is placed in a stenotic area and a balloon is inflated and forcefully dilates the stenotic area. The client is monitored during the procedure using ECG tracings. If myocardial ischemia is present during the procedure, the balloon is removed.

    e. Monitor for signs and symptoms of allergic response.
    f. Monitor for signs of clot induced stroke or myocardial infarction.
    g. Administer analgesics for pain.
16. Position client for comfort. Place on back for several hours after the procedure, then turn from side to side.

For Bone Densitometry

1. Discuss procedure with client before scheduled test and ask pertinent questions for the record.
    a. Determine whether barium studies have been done within last 10 days. ▸ ***Rationale:*** Barium may falsely increase bone density of lumbar spine.
    b. Instruct client that no specific pretest fasting, blood work, or sedation needs to be done. A consent form may be required.
    c. Instruct client to go to outpatient x-ray or hospital facility according to instructions (there are no preparations for study, so it is usually not important to come early for test).
    d. Instruct client not to wear jewelry, belt buckles, or zippers to x-ray department and to remove coins and keys from pocket; clothing need not be removed for test.
    e. Determine whether client has had previous bone density tests or fractures. Document findings for physician.
2. Explain that there is no pain or discomfort associated with test. It is used to detect early osteoporosis. The bones usually examined include lumbar spine, neck of femur, and heel. Test takes approximately 30–60 minutes.
3. Explain that false-positive results can include previous fractures and previous bone scans.
4. Explain procedure to client.
    a. Client will be placed on an imaging table with legs supported on padded box. ▸ ***Rationale:*** Position flattens pelvis and lumbar spine. Radiation source is below, with detector above the table that measures the bone's radiation absorption.
    b. Images of lumbar and hip bones are projected on a computer monitor.
    c. Each machine scans the bones of the finger, heel, and forearm differently, so specific instructions will be given according to machine descriptions.
    d. After computer screen calculates bone mineral density, it is compared with existing data from healthy 25–35-year-old women and a T score is determined. The T score indicates the strength of the bone. The positive T score indicates a bone that is stronger than normal. A negative T score indicates the bone is weaker than normal. Z scores are also obtained. These scores compare clients matched for age, sex, race, height, and weight.
5. Instruct client that no specific postprocedural care is required. There are no side effects or complications associated with the test.

For Magnetic Resonance Imaging (MRI)

1. Evaluate client for following conditions.
   ▸ ***Rationale:*** These conditions exempt clients from having MRI because the magnet can move and displace metal, such as clips and staples, or cause a malfunction.
   a. Clients with pacemakers, insulin pumps, nerve stimulating devices, or implanted devices (i.e., Port-a-Cath, PAS Port).
   b. Clients with hip prostheses, cardiac surgery, or metal implants.
   c. Clients with vascular clips and staples from recent surgery.
   d. Pregnant clients should not be scanned even though there is no definitive evidence of harm to fetus.
   e. Clients with cardiac or respiratory complications may be excluded.
2. Check for allergies if contrast medium is to be used. Two common contrast mediums are gadodiamide and gadolinium Magnevist.
3. Instruct client to remove all metal or magnetically sensitive objects: jewelry, glasses, wallets, watches, hair clips, credit cards. ▸ ***Rationale:*** The magnetic field can damage watches.
4. Describe MRI machine and procedure to client—it provides a clear picture of the inner structures of the extremities, brain, and spinal cord, and it clearly reproduces soft tissue, ligaments, and nerves; often used for determining response to radiotherapy and chemotherapy.

NOTE: Newer implanted devices may be compatible with the use of MRI. Each client needs to be assessed for type of device.

Vessel Closure Devices

There are several arterial closure devices on the market; however, the Perclose ProGlide Suture-Mediated Closure System is the most commonly used. These devices provide a monofilament suture knot that is easily advanced to the opening in the artery and delivers a pretied knot to close the access site in the femoral artery after a catheterization procedure. If needed, the physician can easily reopen the access site in the vessel for repeat or additional procedures.

This secure stitch provides rapid hemostasis (the cessation of bleeding) and allows a shorter recovery time. This is more cost effective for the facility.

However, in spite of using this device, not all clients should be considered for early discharge. Suture-mediated closure is not risk-free. There are complications associated with the procedure.

NOTE: Newer implanted devices may be compatible with use of MRI. Each client needs to be assessed for type of device.

Clinical Alert

Clients who are extremely claustrophobic may require conscious (moderate) sedation or may be moved to a nonenclosed MRI. If sedated, client must be monitored for at least 1 hr before discharge. The open MRI is also used for obese clients, confused clients, or a child. Clients must remain still. This MRT uses a lower-field magnet; therefore, lesser quality images are usually produced.

   a. Client is placed in a padded plastic cradle or on a pillow. The table then slides into the scanner so that the whole body is encased in the machine.
   b. Client needs to lie flat, still, and relax inside the tube magnet. ▸ ***Rationale:*** Movement can produce artifact on image.
   c. The client is instructed to hold his/her breath for up to 30 seconds.
   d. Explain that during the procedure the client will hear rapidly repeating, loud thumping noises coming from the walls of the scanner. ***Rationale:*** Noises are caused by changing magnetic fields.
   e. During the time the client is in the machine he/she can talk to and hear staff. Prism glasses may be worn so client can see outside scanner.
   f. Inform client he or she will have ear plugs in place but will be able to communicate with MRI staff through microphone. ▸ ***Rationale:*** This allays feelings of claustrophobia.
   g. Instruct client in relaxation techniques.
   h. Procedure lasts 20–90 minutes.
5. Instruct client to void before procedure. ▸ ***Rationale:*** This prevents the need for client to void while undergoing procedure.
6. Administer premedication as ordered, usually Valium.

Claustrophobia has been thought to be the reason that clients are uncomfortable and not able to lay still while in the MRI. Through new research, it has shown that the amount of distress is caused by the mattress pads currently available on the MRI, PET, CT nuclear medicine, and x-ray tables. Traditional pads wear out quickly and fail to provide sufficient support and comfort for the client. The Tempur® material has been incorporated into the Patient Comfort Systems Pads, knee wedges, and positioners. The pads mold into the client's body shape and contour; pressure is redistributed away from the weight-bearing contact points, thus reducing pressure on the body. The redistribution improves blood flow, which reduces the client's overall pain and discomfort.

Source: Kusza, J. Seeing Solace: Leading MRI facilities benefit from comfort pads. Patient Comfort Systems. www.patientcomfortsystems.com.

Infection Control in the MRI Suite

Challenges in Preventing MRSA and Other Infections in the MRI Suite

Infection occurs as a result of hospitals prohibiting cleaning crews from entering to clean the pads and the suite due to its high magnetic field. Most facilities just change the sheet on the table and the pillow case. This will not prevent contamination of the pads. An average MRI scans 3,000–5,000 clients each year. Many of these clients are infected with MRSA, and 30%–50% of all clients carry less virulent staphylococcus on their skin. Direct contact with personnel also leads to the spread of infection. Most clients undergoing an MRI have IVs inserted, which can lead to blood getting onto the sheets.

To prevent the spread of infection, hand hygiene must be completed frequently and the pads cleaned with antiseptic solutions after each client. To check efficacy of the cleansing process, the pads can be visualized under ultraviolet wavelengths, which detect biological material such as blood, bacteria, and bodily fluids.

Rothschild, P. (2007). Sick sense. Advances for imaging and oncology administrators. MRI Infection Control Paper. http://www.mrinet.net/cpcommerce/product

7. Place client in a comfortable position on table.
8. Instruct client on feelings of warmth or shortness of breath if contrast medium is used during procedure.
9. Transport client to room after procedure.
10. Observe for symptoms of delayed reaction to contrast material if used during procedure.

For Mammography

1. Instruct client to not wear deodorant, ointments, or talcum powder. ▶ ***Rationale:*** It can interfere with the reading of the mammogram, and false-positive results can occur.
2. Instruct client not to wear jewelry around neck.
3. Review client's history regarding breast implants or previous breast surgery, lumps, or unusual findings on monthly examinations. ▶ ***Rationale:*** Included on health record so radiologist has an accurate assessment of mammogram findings. The mammogram is contraindicated for pregnant clients.

Clinical Alert

Mammography only suggests a possible diagnosis of breast cancer. The diagnosis must be confirmed with histological examination of breast tissue obtained through a biopsy.

Digital Mammography

Digital mammography is a newer method of breast imaging in which images are captured electronically and viewed on a computer monitor. The radiologist is able to manipulate the contrast and brightness of the images, which increases the chance of identifying cancers. Portions of the breast image can be magnified with computer manipulation rather than with repeated films.

Standardization of Mammography Reports

Class I: Negative

Class II: Benign

Class III: Benign; short-term follow-up suggested

Class IV: Suspicious for cancer; further evaluation suggested

Class V: Cancer highly suspected

Recommendation of the American College of Radiology (ACR).

4. Explain procedure to client—may cause some momentary discomfort when x-ray cone compresses breast tissue; discomfort does not last after release of cone. ▶ ***Rationale:*** Compression of breast provides better visualization of breast tissue.
5. Explain that there is minimal radiation exposure from this procedure.
6. Instruct client to take off clothing above waist, including bra, and put x-ray gown on so it ties in front.
   a. One breast is placed on x-ray plate and the cone is brought down on breast to compress it.
   b. The breast will be placed in different positions to view the entire breast tissue.

Nuclear Medicine Breast Imaging (Scintimammography)

Scintimammography is a nuclear medicine breast imaging test that is considered supplemental to a breast exam and mammography. The test is often referred to as the Miraluma Tc-99m test. It assists the physician to determine the presence of cancer in the breast. It is used in some clients to investigate breast abnormalities, especially if the client has dense breast tissue, which makes it difficult to interpret. It is also used if the client has a palpable mass or when multiple tumors are suspected. A radioactive tracer is injected intravenously; the dye accumulates differently in noncancer and cancer tissues.

c. The second breast is done in same manner.
d. The test takes 15–30 minutes.

7. Instruct client to wait when mammography is finished until films are processed. ▸ ***Rationale:*** Sometimes additional films will need to be taken; this prevents client from having to return to the department.
8. Instruct client in self breast examination, if necessary, and answer questions before client leaves.
   a. Test results are usually mailed to client.
   b. If the mammography is being done for diagnostic purposes, the mammogram may be read and results are immediately available for client.

EVIDENCE-BASED PRACTICE

Diagnostic Performance of Digital Versus Film Mammography for Breast Cancer Screening

A study of 49,528 asymptomatic women had screening mammography at 33 sites in the United States and Canada. They underwent both digital and film mammography. Of these clients, 86.3% had all relevant information available for the study.

The mammograms were interpreted by two radiologists. A breast biopsy was completed 15 months after the start of the study or a follow-up mammogram was obtained at least 10 months after the initiation of the study.

The accuracy of digital mammography was significantly higher than film mammography among women under the age of 50, women with heterogeneously dense or extremely dense breasts on mammography, and premenopausal or perimenopausal women.

Source: Pisano, E. D., Gatsonis, C., Hendrick, E., Yaffe, M., Baum, J. K., Acharyya, S., ... Rebner, M. (2005). Diagnostic performance of digital versus film mammography for breast-cancer screening. *The New England Journal of Medicine, 17*(353), 1773–1783.

DOCUMENTATION for X-Ray Studies

- Client's history
- Preparation completed (e.g., NPO, clear liquid dinner)
- Client teaching completed
- Medication administered
- Allergies noted
- Unusual anxiety or fears of client
- How client transported to test
- Time sent and returned from test
- Postprocedure care
- Appearance of dressing or puncture sites

CRITICAL THINKING Application

Expected Outcomes

- Client acknowledges understanding of the scheduled procedure.
- Client is calm and emotionally prepared for procedure.
- Client is well prepared for x-ray study after client teaching.
- Client completes x-ray study without complications.
- Client did not experience allergic reaction to contrast media.
- Client describes posttest care upon discharge.

Unexpected Outcomes	Alternative Actions
Client has allergic reaction.	• Follow protocol or standing orders for allergic reactions. • Start O_2 at 6 L/min unless otherwise contraindicated. Use nasal cannula. • Place in semi- or high-Fowler's position if not contraindicated. • Administer medications as outlined in protocol or according to physician's orders. • Provide reassurance and encouragement. • Have client take slow, deep breaths. • If nausea or vomiting occur, obtain an order for an antiemetic from the physician.
Client is given meal when on NPO status.	• Call x-ray and change time of test. If possible, arrange for test to be done later in the day to avoid additional hospitalization, or return visit. • Instruct client on what NPO means.

(Continued)

Unexpected Outcomes	Alternative Actions
Client very apprehensive and refuses test at last minute.	• Identify reasons for anxiety and attempt to allay fears. • Notify physician and ask if he or she wants to cancel or postpone test to later time. Do not attempt to "talk client into it." • Discuss use of sedation during test.
Bleeding or hemorrhage occurs from arteriogram puncture site.	• Notify physician. • Apply direct pressure until pressure dressing can be applied. • Monitor amount of blood loss and possible signs and symptoms of shock. • Elevate and keep extremity in extension position. • Monitor vital signs.
Client develops irregular pulse after cardiac catheterization.	• Notify physician immediately • Start IV if not in place. • Prepare for possible code and IV administration of medication. • Monitor vital signs frequently.
Bleeding occurs at catheter insertion site after cardiac catheterization.	• Apply pressure dressing. • Elevate extremity. • Monitor peripheral pulse and vital signs. • If bleeding does not subside, notify physician. • Monitor ECG findings.

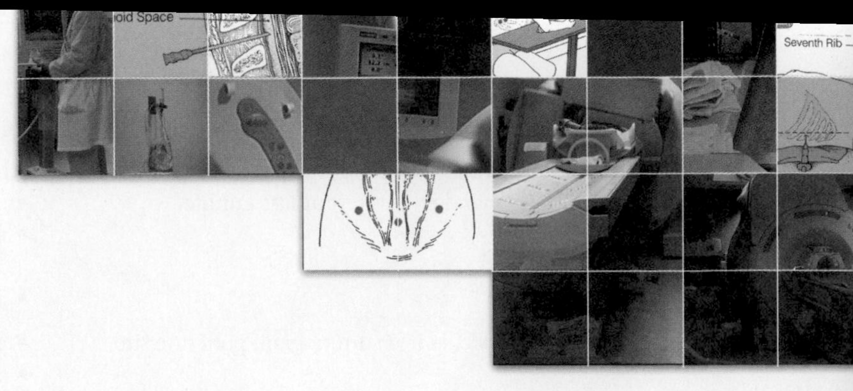

Chapter 21

UNIT ❷

Nuclear Scanning

Nursing Process Data

ASSESSMENT Data Base

- Assess client's understanding of nuclear imaging and the specific diagnostic test he or she is to receive.
- Assess client's ability to tolerate procedure (e.g., swallowing iodine solution, fasting).
- Determine client's psychologic needs in relation to the nuclear scan.
- Identify any allergies the client may have to radioactive materials.
- Assess need to remain with client during procedure.
- Assess vital signs and document for baseline data.

PLANNING Objectives

- To diagnose tumors, metastatic disease, abnormal conditions, and cardiac and other organ abnormalities via noninvasive method
- To prepare the client physically for the nuclear diagnostic test
- To prepare the client psychologically to prevent undue stress
- To complete client teaching to ensure the client understands the procedure

IMPLEMENTATION Procedures

EVALUATION Expected Outcomes

- Client is physically and psychologically prepared for the scan.
- Client demonstrates understanding of the purpose of the test and potential side effects from the radionuclide material.
- Client completes procedure without complications.

Preparing for Nuclear Scans

Equipment

Signed consent form
IV equipment (for most scans)
Hospital gown and pajama bottoms

Preparation

1. Identify the specific diagnostic test that is to be performed (Table 21-2).
2. Determine if any tests must precede others in order to schedule test appropriately.

NOTE: Technetium-99m, gallium, thallium, and iodine are used commonly for scanning. Technetium-99m is used extensively because it has a 6-hr half-life and emits low levels of gamma rays.

3. Identify specific preparations that need to be carried out before the studies. Check for recent exposure to radionuclides. ▸ ***Rationale:*** May interfere with current study.
4. Monitor fluid alterations that need to precede the studies.
5. Obtain special consent forms if required by facility after the physician has explained the study to the client.
6. Provide client teaching regarding the study, including any special preparation required for the study.
7. Provide psychologic support and reassurance to the client.
8. Explain that radiation exposure is minimal and limited.
9. Record client's height and weight.
10. Carry out safety precautions immediately before the study:
    a. Check two forms of client identification.
    b. Check for allergies.
    c. Chart premedication if given.
    d. Monitor safe transfer from the bed to gurney or wheelchair.
    e. Accompany client to nuclear medicine department if needed. (Usually, nurses accompany critically ill clients.)

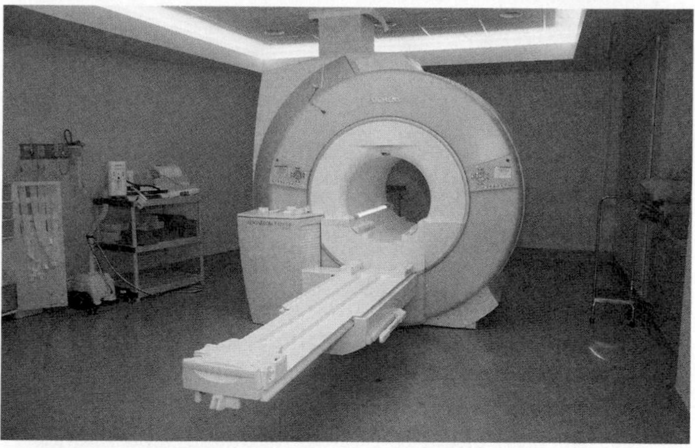

▲ Magnetom Large Bore MRI, 1.5 magnet strength.

For Bone Scan

1. Follow steps as appropriate in *Preparing for Nuclear Scans.*
    a. Explain purpose of procedure to client—usually done to detect metastatic cancer, early bone disease, osteomyelitis, detect fractures or abnormal healing of fractures. If client is of child-bearing age, determine whether she is pregnant. If so, test cannot be done.
    b. No fasting or sedation is required.
    c. Have client ready for injection of radionuclide material, probably technetium-99m, 1–3 hr before scan.
    d. Force fluids between injection of isotope and scan.
    e. Have client void before going to x-ray.
    f. Take client to nuclear medicine department.
2. Explain procedure.
    a. Client is positioned supine under scintillation camera (camera records radiation emitted by skeleton).
    b. Instruct client to remain very still for 20 minutes to ensure observation of bone abnormalities.
    c. Client will be repositioned to prone and lateral positions during scan.
    d. Return client to room.

TABLE 21-2 Nuclear Studies

Diagnostic Test	Rationale
Bone scan	To diagnose metastatic bone disease, osteomyelitis, or fractures
Lung scan	To diagnose pulmonary embolism or pneumothorax or to assess pulmonary status before lung surgery
PET scan	To scan whole body or its various areas; used in diagnosis; especially useful in diagnosing epilepsy
Cardiology scan	To diagnose coronary artery disease, cardiomyopathy, valvular heart disease, or to assess cardiac status and analyze ventricular function
Thyroid scan	To diagnose thyroid nodules, abnormal function, or thyroid cancer

3. Instruct client to resume activities and diet. ▸ ***Rationale:*** There is no problem with radiation exposure because only tracer doses of radioisotopes are used.
4. Force fluids for 2–3 hr after scan. ▸ ***Rationale:*** To promote renal filtering of excess tracer. Trace elements are excreted in 6–24 hr.

For Lung Scan

1. Follow steps as appropriate in Preparing for Nuclear Scans.
   a. Explain purpose of procedure—used to detect pulmonary embolism, tumors, COPD.
   b. Obtain consent if required.
   c. Obtain chest x-ray 24–48 hr before scan.
   d. Transport client to nuclear medicine department.
   e. Ensure all jewelry is removed.
2. Explain details of procedure.
   a. Explain equipment to client:
      Closed-breathing system is used when ventilation scan is done.
      Scintillation camera.
   b. Client is injected intravenously with a tracer amount of radioactive material—usually, radionuclide-tagged MAA (macroaggregated albumin with technetium) is used.
   c. Client is positioned in several ways to obtain clear images.
   d. Client is instructed to breathe through a closed system until all radioactive gas is cleared from the system.
   e. Instruct in use of mouthpiece or nose clips if used.
   f. Client is instructed to lie quietly for 30 minutes as radiography is completed—gamma ray detector is passed over client, records radionuclide uptake on film.
3. Transport client on gurney to room.
4. Instruct client to resume prestudy activities.

For PET Scan

1. Follow steps as appropriate in Preparing for Nuclear Scans.
2. Explain that purpose of test is to scan the whole body or its various regions for early detection of recurrent tumor or cancer that has spread. PET scans can determine what heart tissue is still alive after a suspected heart attack. It aids in determining focal area for seizure activity and is used to help diagnose epilepsy. It is also useful in determining brain region for surgical removal of affected area when medication resistance is present.
3. Assess client and take complete history to determine if client is pregnant. Determine if client is claustrophobic or anxious. ▸ ***Rationale:*** Test cannot be performed if client is pregnant. Client must be able to lie still during the entire process, including a minimum of 45 minutes with his or her head inside scanner.

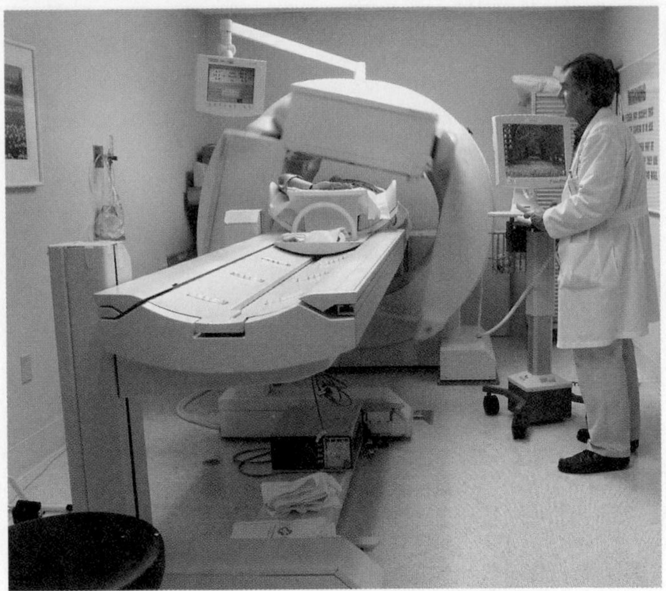

▲ Nuclear scanner used for cardiac thallium scans.

4. Premedicate with nonaspirin analgesia if client has arthritis or lower back pain that could prevent client from lying still for prescribed time. ▸ ***Rationale:*** Sedatives are avoided if at all possible because they alter metabolism. If necessary, chloral hydrate could be used; it has fewest adverse effects.
5. Instruct client to stay NPO for 6–8 hr.
6. Instruct client to void 1–2 hr before the test.
7. Instruct client to avoid caffeine, alcohol, and nicotine for 24 hr before test.
8. Explain procedure:
   a. Reassure client that there is no discomfort except lying on a hard surface for up to 3 hr.
   b. Ensure client has not taken aspirin or other anticoagulants for several days before scan.
   c. Explain that an arterial line will be inserted to obtain blood samples.
   d. Explain that a peripheral intravenous catheter will be inserted to inject radioisotope. One hour after injection, client will be placed in scanner.
   e. Instruct client to lie quietly for 45 minutes. Lights will be dim. ▸ ***Rationale:*** This is time for radioisotope uptake to occur, as isotopes are circulating to the brain.
   f. Monitor vital signs as indicated.
   g. Explain that actual scan time is about 15–75 minutes. He or she must remain quiet with head in scanner during this entire time. ▸ ***Rationale:*** Any motion, moving, or talking can detract from the quality of image.

h. Explain that arterial blood samples may be drawn from arterial line during scan.
i. Place blindfold on client to keep client from being distracted during certain brain studies. The head is also placed in a holder to restrain movement.
j. Place Velcro straps on clients with heart or abdominal studies. ***Rationale:*** To prevent movement.

9. Provide postprocedural instructions.
   a. After scan, IV and arterial lines will be discontinued.
   b. Client can resume normal activities and meals.
   c. Monitor for signs of seizure activity or adverse effects if seizure did occur during scan.
   d. If sedative was given, do not allow client to drive or engage in any hazardous activities until sedative has worn off. Instruct client to have someone drive him/her home.

For Nuclear Cardiography

1. Follow steps as appropriate in Preparing for Nuclear Scans.
2. Instruct client that radioactive tracer substances are used to detect and evaluate cardiovascular abnormalities. Alterations of left ventricular muscle function and coronary blood flow are evaluated.
3. Instruct client in specific activities related to the test (i.e., exercise on a treadmill, holding certain medications, fasting). See Step 2 for specific cardiology test.
4. Explain that short fasting time may be necessary.
5. After isotope injection, scan will be performed 15 minutes to 4 hr later.
6. Instruct client in nuclear medicine department.
   a. Gamma ray detector is placed over heart.
   b. Detector is placed in several positions during scan.
   c. Scan records images of heart.
7. Evaluate client's status after the scan.
   a. Encourage fluids to excrete isotopes.
   b. Apply pressure over venipuncture site if necessary.

For Thyroid Scan

1. Follow steps as appropriate in Preparing for Nuclear Scans.

PET provides information about the body's metabolism, unlike CT scans or MRIs, which only show body structure. Metabolic change occurs before structural changes. Some studies have shown that up to 60% of invasive tests or surgeries can be eliminated using the PET scan.

Source: Valk, P. (2000). Randomized controlled trials are not appropriate for imaging technology evaluation. *Journal of Nuclear Medicine, 41*(7), 1125–1126.

Common Tests in Nuclear Cardiology

Technetium pyrophosphate scan. This binds with calcium and creates an area of increased radionuclide uptake. The client receives an injection into the antecubital vein. He or she then waits 2 hr while the renal system clears the drug. A special camera scans the heart to identify areas of increased uptake of the radioisotope. The radioisotope accumulates in damaged areas of the heart and shows any evidence of a recent MI. Scan is also called a myocardial infusion scan.

Thallium scan. A medication (^{201}Tl) is injected into the antecubital vein and scanning is done within 4–10 minutes. Necrotic or ischemic tissue does not reflect the radioisotope as tissue with normal blood supply and healthy cells does. To detect myocardial scarring and perfusion, an acute or chronic MI, or the evaluation of prior cardiac surgery are the primary purposes for this test.

Thallium scan with exercise. When this test involves exercise, it takes 1 hr and 15 minutes; 3 hr later, a 30-minute resting scan is performed. Imaging with exercise may demonstrate perfusion problems not apparent when the client is at rest.

Gated cardiac blood pool scan. The client receives an intravenous injection of a red blood cell tagging agent, and ECG leads are positioned on him or her. The computer is then synchronized with the ECG reading. This test evaluates left ventricular function.

2. Purpose of scan is to diagnose thyroid nodules, abnormal thyroid function, or thyroid cancer.
3. Explain procedure to client.
   a. Instruct client not to consume any iodine compounds (vitamin or mineral supplements that may contain iodine or iodized table salt) or eat any foods that contain iodine—especially seafood, which has a high iodine content, for at least 3 days. ▸ ***Rationale:*** Consuming iodine products interferes with the test.
   b. Instruct client not to take thyroid or antithyroid drugs or x-ray contrast medium before the test, usually 3 days before test. ▸ ***Rationale:*** These materials interfere with the thyroid scan.
   c. Instruct client to remain NPO for 2 hr after oral iodine administration.
   d. Tell client that after the initial oral radioactive technetium he or she must return to the lab 24 hr later. Some labs do scanning after 2 hr of ingestion of technetium.
   e. Instruct client that no isolation is needed after scan.

Teaching for Nuclear Scans

Procedure

1. Inform client that test is to be performed in the nuclear medicine department.
   a. The department name alone may be frightening to the client.
   b. Taking the client to the department ahead of time may help to decrease anxiety.
   c. Instruct client to remove jewelry or metal objects in the area of the study.
2. Explain to the client that he or she will be receiving an injection of a radioisotope through a vein. The exceptions to this procedure are a lung scan in which the isotope is administered through an oxygen mask and a gastric-emptying scan in which the isotope is given orally with food.
   a. Inform client that this isotope emits a harmless amount of radiation.
   b. Inform client that the camera used for scanning does not emit radiation. The camera detects a small and harmless amount of radiation from the isotope as it is lodged in the part of the body being imaged.
   c. The radioactive substance usually leaves the body in 6–24 hr.
3. Explain to the client that he or she will be lying on a table (he or she will not be confined in an enclosed space) while the camera is positioned above or below the table. He/she may be asked to change positions during the test.
4. Assure the client that someone will be with him or her throughout the test, contrasting this procedure with x-rays for which the technician must leave the room or with the MRI for which the client enters a tube-like structure.
5. Tell the client that if he or she is in pain, he or she may receive an analgesic during the procedure, as he or she must remain still while the camera is scanning the body.
6. The scanning usually takes 30–60 minutes.

DOCUMENTATION for Nuclear Scanning

- Client teaching completed
- Client's emotional state
- Any radioisotopes given on the unit
- Preprocedural preparation completed (i.e., enema or laxative)
- History regarding earlier tests or studies
- NPO status
- Means by which client transported to nuclear medicine department
- Time client sent to and returned from scan

CRITICAL THINKING Application

Expected Outcomes

- Client is psychologically and physically prepared for the scan.
- Client demonstrates understanding of the purpose of the test and potential side effects from the radionuclide material.
- Client completes procedure without complications.

Unexpected Outcomes	Alternative Actions
Client appears not to understand purpose of diagnostic test.	• Observe for nonverbal cues or misunderstandings in order to clarify purpose of the test. • Provide alternative teaching aids. • Show client the equipment if necessary. • Ask client to repeat explanation to you.
Client is unable to cooperate during the procedure.	• If not contraindicated by condition, ask physician for sedation order. • Nursing staff members may be asked to help client remain quiet. If so, wear lead apron shield.
Client is uncomfortable during procedure.	• Reposition client for comfort if possible. (It may not be possible depending on area of body to be scanned.) • Provide support by propping client in position needed for scanning. • Assist client to focus on other things (e.g., the ball game, weather, or something pleasant).

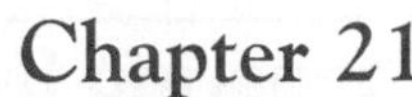

Chapter 21

UNIT 3

Barium Studies

Nursing Process Data

ASSESSMENT Data Base

- Assess results of laxative and enema administration to ensure a clean colon for the study. Notify physician if client is unable to "hold" enema solution.
- Evaluate client's ability to cooperate with test.
- Evaluate client's knowledge of test.

PLANNING Objectives

- To determine the client's ability to understand the preparatory process
- To clean out colon in order to ensure visualization of colon
- To prepare the client psychologically for the test

IMPLEMENTATION Procedures

EVALUATION Expected Outcomes

- Client is able to cooperate with test.
- Client's bowel is clean and free of stool, promoting an accurate barium study.
- Client is prepared and knowledgeable about what to expect during procedure.
- Client's study is completed without complications.
- Client successfully expels barium following test.

Preparing for Barium Studies

Equipment

Signed consent if agency requires
Enema tube and bag
Ordered solution for enema
Laxative
Wheelchair

Procedure

1. Identify the specific diagnostic test that will be performed (Table 21-3).
2. Explain purpose of procedure to client.
3. Obtain consent for specific test to be performed.
4. Instruct client to refrain from smoking for 8–12 hr.
5. Instruct client to withhold medications for 8 hr before test unless otherwise indicated. Narcotics and anticholinergics are withheld for 24 hr. ▶ ***Rationale:*** To avoid intestinal immobility.
6. Instruct client to prepare for test.
   a. Stay on low-residue diet 2 to 3 days before test and a clear liquid diet from lunch the day before test. No dairy products.
   b. Take one glass of water or clear fluid every hour for 8–10 hr.
   c. Administer one full bottle (10 oz) of magnesium citrate or X-prep at 2 PM day before test.
   d. Administer three 5-mg Dulcolax tablets at 7 PM, evening before test.
   e. Keep NPO after Dulcolax tablets.
   f. Administer a suppository or a cleansing enema (or both if necessary) in early morning on day of test. Ensure bowel is clear; liquid return should be clear. If not, notify x-ray department.
7. Carry out safety precautions immediately before the procedure:
   a. Check two forms of client identification.
   b. Monitor safe transfer from bed to gurney or wheelchair.

For Barium Enema

1. Transport client to radiology department, usually via wheelchair.
2. Explain details of procedure to client.
   a. A balloon rectal tube is inserted and balloon is tightly inflated against anal sphincter. ▶ ***Rationale:*** To keep barium in rectum during study.
   b. Client is turned side to side while dripping barium into rectum using gravity flow for infusion.
   c. Barium flow is monitored by fluoroscopy continuously and colon is examined as barium goes through colon.
   d. Barium is drained out and an x-ray is taken to determine whether barium has been expelled.
   e. Entire procedure takes 15 minutes to 1 hr.
3. Transport client to room.
4. Force fluids with electrolytes unless contraindicated.
5. Administer laxative or enema as ordered. ▶ ***Rationale:*** To facilitate bowel evacuation.
6. Ensure client has bowel movement within 2–3 days.

For Barium Swallow Study

1. Explain purpose of procedure to client.
2. Instruct client to stay on low residue diet 1–3 days before procedure, if ordered and to stay NPO for 8 hr before test.

Clinical Alert

If client has suspected bowel obstruction, no cathartics are given.

Clinical Alert

Barium studies should follow IVPs, ultrasound examinations, and arteriograms because barium interferes with visualization of other structures. Barium enema should precede barium swallow.

Small Bowel Enema

Barium is injected into a tube positioned in the small bowel. This procedure provides better visualization of the entire small bowel because the barium solution is not diluted by juices from the GI tract. This test is used when bowel obstruction is suspected.

TABLE 21-3 Barium Studies

Diagnostic Test	Rationale
Lower GI Studies	
Barium Enema	To visualize the lower GI tract for contour, patency, position and mucosal pattern of colon
Upper GI Studies	To visualize the upper GI tract; pharynx, esophagus, and stomach
Barium Swallow	To visualize the esophagus
Small Bowel Follow-Through	To visualize the duodenum, jejunum, and ileum

Clinical Alert

Gastrografin, a water-soluble contrast material, should be used if there is a risk of leakage of contrast material through a perforation of the GI tract. Usual dose is 16–20 ounces.

3. Administer laxative or enema the evening before procedure, particularly if this test follows barium enema study.
4. Instruct client not to smoke. ▸ ***Rationale:*** Smoking causes an increase in flow of digestive juices.
5. Transport to radiology department.
6. Explain details of procedure to client.
   a. Client is instructed to drink a cup of flavored barium, usually in milkshake-like form, under fluoroscopic exam.
   b. Client is instructed to turn to several positions while x-rays are obtained.
   c. X-rays are taken every 30 minutes as barium advances. Procedure can take up to 4–6 hr.

Clinical Alert

Obtain specific orders for enemas when client has severe abdominal pain, ulcerative colitis, or history of megacolon. Do not follow general preprocedural orders.

NOTE: Upper GI series, or barium enema, provides better visualization of the bowel. Large tumors and perforations of the bowel can be identified with the CT scan.

For Small Bowel Follow-Through

   a. Barium swallow may be extended to examine duodenum and small bowel.
   b. Films can be taken as long as 24 hr later.

7. Transport client to room.
8. Force fluids unless contraindicated.
9. Administer cathartic.
10. Ensure bowel movement within 2–3 days. Enema may need to be administered.

DOCUMENTATION for Barium Studies

- Laxative administered
- Type, amount of fluid, number of enemas administered
- Enema result, consistency of stool, color of returning enema solution
- Unusual symptoms such as pain, bleeding, or nausea associated with enemas
- Color of stool after test

CRITICAL THINKING Application

Expected Outcomes

- Client is able to cooperate with test.
- Client's bowel is clean and free of stool, promoting an accurate barium study.
- Client is prepared and knowledgeable about what to expect during procedure.
- Client's study is completed without complications.
- Client successfully expels barium after test.

Unexpected Outcomes	Alternative Actions
Barium is unable to be expelled even after administration of laxatives and enemas.	• Obtain order for and administer oil-retention enema. • Administer tap water enema following oil-retention enema. • Continue to administer laxatives until barium is expelled.
Laxatives or enemas (or both) are ordered for clients with ulcerative colitis or severe abdominal pain.	• Do not administer either the laxative or enema without checking with the physician. • If physician confirms order, carefully administer small amount of enema fluid, and observe and document effects on client. • Chart the type of pain, if any, characteristics of stool, and any symptoms noted while enema is administered. • If client complains of excruciating pain, stop procedure and notify the physician.
Client's medications are administered in error.	• Notify x-ray department, and ask for specific orders regarding what action needs to be taken regarding the test. • Inform physician, complete a medication error form, and send to nursing office. An unusual occurrence may need to be completed as well. • If this is a frequent problem on the unit or in the hospital, an in-service education program should be given that includes a discussion of when medications should be given and when held.

Chapter 21

UNIT 4

Endoscopic Studies

Nursing Process Data

ASSESSMENT Data Base

- Assess vital signs before and during studies, if indicated. Some studies require general anesthesia or conscious (moderate) sedation, and scope is used that could result in perforation and bleeding.
- Assess client's knowledge of procedure to be done.
- Evaluate baseline laboratory tests, particularly those for potential bleeding problems, if biopsy is to be done.
- Evaluate if client is at risk for complications, especially infection (antibiotics may need to be ordered).
- Assess biopsy site for indications of bleeding.
- Evaluate for signs of infection after procedure.

PLANNING Objectives

- To provide information regarding procedure to decrease client's anxiety
- To determine if previous studies were completed using barium
- To evaluate potential for complications following procedure
- To position client on table correctly to facilitate optimal visual outcome and aid in diagnosing condition

IMPLEMENTATION Procedures

EVALUATION Expected Outcomes

- Client is prepared psychologically and physically for endoscopic procedure.
- Client experiences no sequelae after moderate sedation.
- Client does not experience pain or discomfort with procedure.
- Client diagnosis is confirmed with endoscopic study.

Pearson Nursing Student Resources

Find additional review materials at **nursing.pearsonhighered.com**

Prepare for success with NCLEX®-style practice questions and Skill Checklists

TABLE 21-4 Endoscopic Procedures

Diagnostic Test	Rationale
Arthroscopy	To evaluate meniscus cartilage or ligament injury; to differentiate arthritic inflammation from injury
Bronchoscopy	To visualize larynx, trachea, bronchi, and alveoli; to diagnose bleeding sites and obtain sputum specimens
Colonoscopy	To visualize rectum and colon; to obtain tissue biopsy and remove polyps
Cystoscopy	To visualize urethra, bladder, ureters, prostate; to place stents
Gastrointestinal tract endoscopy (EGD)	To visualize esophagus, stomach, and duodenum; to obtain specimen for cell studies
Laparoscopy	To visualize abdominal cavity; to perform surgical interventions
Sigmoidoscopy	To visualize anus, rectum, sigmoid colon; to remove polyps, obliterate hemorrhoids

Preparing for Endoscopic Studies

Procedure

1. Identify client using two forms of identification and explain test to client.
2. Obtain signed consent form.
3. Complete preparation according to endoscopic test being performed.
4. Place on NPO status for 8–12 hr for gastroscopy and as directed for other procedures.
5. Remove dentures for bronchoscopy, gastroscopy procedures.
6. Provide bowel prep for laparoscopy, sigmoidoscopy, or colonoscopy to cleanse all fecal material from colon. ▸ ***Rationale:*** Allows adequate visualization of mucosa.
7. Obtain lab results for CBC, bleeding and clotting factors, Hgb, Hct, electrolytes if potential bleeding could occur or possible biopsy will be done with endoscopy.
8. Withhold medications that interfere with coagulation, such as ASA, NSAIDS, iron medications, and alcohol 1 week before test.
9. Complete physical assessment to determine risk factors for possible complications and allergies.
10. Notify special procedure room staff and physician of potential problems with client's condition that could interfere with procedure.

Clinical Alert

Conscious sedation is a preferred method for anxiety and pain relief during therapeutic and diagnostic procedures, particularly in the radiology department.

Versed is the most common drug used for sedation, and fentanyl is commonly administered for pain control.

Both are short-acting drugs with duration of 30–60 minutes.

See also Moderate Sedation, chapter 26, p. 983.

For Arthroscopy

1. Follow steps in Preparing for Endoscopic Studies as it applies to this procedure.
2. Explain that arthroscopy allows direct visualization of specific anatomic site (i.e., knee joint). Small trocars are placed into joint and surgical procedure is completed with direct vision of a camera attached to arthroscope.
3. Explain that client usually receives local anesthesia and procedure takes 30 minutes to 2 hr.
4. Instruct client to remain NPO from midnight if general anesthesia is to be given.
5. Instruct client in use of crutches, if necessary.
6. Shave hair 6 in. above and below involved joint, if ordered.
7. Explain procedure to client.
   a. Anesthesia is given, either local or general.
   b. Leg is scrubbed, elevated, and wrapped in elastic bandage from toes to lower thigh. ▸ ***Rationale:*** Reduce blood flow from lower extremity.
   c. Physician places tourniquet or instills saline solution in client's knee before insertion of scope. ▸ ***Rationale:*** To reduce bleeding.
   d. Knee is placed at 45° angle.
   e. Small incision is made in skin around knee and scope is inserted into joint space.
   f. Procedure is completed, joint is irrigated, and medication to decrease inflammation is injected into knee.
   g. Sutures or butterfly tapes are placed on skin with pressure dressing applied over site.
8. Assess client's neurovascular status immediately after procedure.
9. Assess vital signs and observe site for potential complications (i.e., bleeding, edema, or excessive drainage).
10. Provide discharge teaching.
    a. Elevate knee at all times when sitting, minimize use of joint for several days.
    b. Apply ice packs according to physician's orders.

c. Instruct client to observe for potential complications: fever, redness around site, excess drainage, or alteration in color of drainage, pain, increased edema.
d. Ambulation with crutches is usually allowed on same day as surgery.
e. Remind client to make postop physician appointment according to orders.

For Bronchoscopy

1. Follow steps for Preparing for Endoscopic Studies as it applies to this procedure.
2. Explain purpose of procedure to client.
3. Explain that test provides endoscopic visualization of larynx, trachea, and bronchi through insertion of flexible fiberoptic bronchoscope. Biopsies may be taken and cultures obtained during procedure. Procedure is done under local anesthetic.
4. Place client on NPO for 6–8 hr before procedure. ▸ ***Rationale:*** This decreases risk of aspiration while gag reflex is blocked during the procedure.
5. Instruct client to practice good oral hygiene.
6. Remove dentures. ▸ ***Rationale:*** This prevents damage or lodging of dentures in the throat during procedure.
7. Remove contact lenses and jewelry.
8. Obtain baseline data: vital signs and respiratory assessment. ▸ ***Rationale:*** This provides comparison data after procedure.
9. Premedicate client with sedative and atropine if ordered. ▸ ***Rationale:*** These medications inhibit vagal stimulation, suppress gag reflex, and decrease the client's anxiety.
10. Assist client to relax and decrease anxiety. Instruct client to breathe through nose.
11. Client is placed in sitting or supine position in operating room or special procedure room.
12. Explain procedure to client.
    a. Physician sprays nasopharynx and oropharynx with topical anesthetic. ▸ ***Rationale:*** This prevents laryngospasm, depresses gag reflex, and prevents discomfort when scope is inserted.
    b. Client is instructed to avoid swallowing anesthetic agent. Instruct client to expectorate into emesis basin.
    c. Bronchoscope is inserted into mouth and advanced to trachea and bronchi.
    d. Tissue specimens or secretions are collected and sent to laboratory for study.
    e. Bronchoscope is removed. Procedure takes about 1 hr.
13. Cleanse client's nose of lubricant after removal of scope.
14. Provide postprocedure care.
    a. Monitor vital signs and respiratory status as with a surgical client. ▸ ***Rationale:*** To identify possible complications, such as bleeding or hypoxia.
    b. Assess for respiratory difficulties (dyspnea, wheezing, apprehension, and decreased breath sounds). Call physician if this occurs.
    c. Elevate head of bed, place in side-lying position if not alert.
    d. Monitor for bloody sputum. ▸ ***Rationale:*** Bleeding can occur as a result of the bronchoscopy. Notify physician immediately if this occurs.
    e. Instruct client not to eat or drink until gag reflex returns, usually 1–2 hr. ▸ ***Rationale:*** Aspiration can occur when gag reflex is absent.
    f. Explain hoarseness and/or sore throat can occur after procedure.

For Colonoscopy

1. Follow steps in Preparing for Endoscopic Studies as it applies to this procedure.
2. Explain that procedure visualizes rectum, colon, and small bowel to detect pathologic conditions. It is used for cancer screening. Ensure barium studies were completed 10–14 days before fast. ▸ ***Rationale:*** Barium can decrease visualization of colon.
3. Place client on liquid diet and Dulcolax tabs 2 days before procedure, if ordered. May use just 1-day prep with Colyte. Keep on NPO for 8 hr.
4. Instruct client to drink electrolyte laxative solution (Go-lytely or Nu-lytely) the day before procedure. Take according to directions, usually 8 ounces every 15 minutes until 1 gallon taken. Entire gallon should be taken in 4 hr. Solution should be chilled (more palatable) and swallowed quickly. ▸ ***Rationale:*** This osmotic solution works quickly and produces a clear colon in about 4 hr if directions are followed accurately. Watery diarrhea usually begins 30–60 minutes after first glass taken.

NOTE: If client has diabetes, an implantable cardioverter defibrillator, pacemaker, or prosthetic heart valve, instruct him/her to call physician before buying bowel prep.

5. Explain side effects of nausea and fluid and electrolyte imbalance to client, especially elderly clients.
6. Instruct client to not take any routine or PRN medications when drinking electrolyte solution. ▸ ***Rationale:*** The medications will not be digested.
7. Obtain baseline vital signs.
8. Start peripheral IV and medicate client with a narcotic analgesic (usually Versed) as ordered.
9. Take client to special procedure room. Procedure takes 15–60 minutes.
10. Explain procedure to client.
    a. Position client on left side with legs drawn up.
    b. Flexible fiberoptic or video colonoscope is inserted through rectum and advanced through the sigmoid, descending, transverse, and ascending colon.
    c. Client may experience discomfort when air is instilled into colon to open colon and advance scope.
    d. Monitor vital signs and oxygen saturation during procedure, if needed.
    e. Valium may be administered if client is anxious.

f. Biopsy forceps or brush is inserted through scope to obtain specimens for study.
g. Tissue or secretions obtained are placed in specimen container.
h. Scope is removed and rectal area cleaned and dried.

11. Instruct client in discharge teaching: to report any rectal bleeding, abdominal pain, distention, or purulent rectal drainage. ▸ ***Rationale:*** These symptoms indicate possible bowel perforation or hemorrhage.
    a. Instruct client to resume normal diet and force fluids after test.
    b. Instruct client that he or she may experience flatulence from air instillation.
12. Monitor vital signs as with any client. ▸ ***Rationale:*** Vital sign changes indicate complications, especially increased temperature and pulse and decreased blood pressure.

EGD and ERCP

The esophagogastroduodenoscopy (EGD) can be used therapeutically for cautery and injection of sclerosing agents on bleeding varices.

Endoscopic retrograde cholangiopancreatography (ERCP) provides visualization of the bile and pancreatic ducts. Stones can be removed and stents placed in the bile ducts to drain bile.

For Cystoscopy

1. Follow steps in Preparing for Endoscopic Studies as it applies to procedure. Review assessment to determine if cystitis or prostatitis is present. ▸ ***Rationale:*** Sepsis could occur; therefore, antibiotics may be ordered.
2. Explain that cystoscopy is used to evaluate conditions associated with urinary tract: urethra, bladder, lower ureters. It is used for both diagnostic and therapeutic procedures. Test takes 30–60 minutes.
3. Instruct in bowel prep, if ordered.
4. Keep client NPO for 8 hr if general anesthesia is given. Otherwise, a full liquid breakfast can be given. Several glasses of water may also be ordered.
5. Administer preprocedural medications 1 hr before test. Ensure consent form was signed before giving medication.
6. Place client in lithotomy position. Provide covering to preserve modesty and prevent chilling.
7. Prepare external genitalia with antimicrobial swabs.
8. Explain procedure to client.
    a. Local anesthetic may be instilled into urethra before scope is inserted if under local anesthesia.
    b. Cystoscope is inserted through the urethra to inspect bladder and urethral wall and facilitate a biopsy.
    c. Bladder is filled with sterile irrigating solution to assist in distending the bladder and irrigating bladder of clots. ▸ ***Rationale:*** Irrigation allows for better visualization of bladder.
    d. Biopsy forceps may be passed through cystoscope to obtain tissue.
    e. Bladder is emptied, and scope removed.
9. Provide posttest instructions. Instruct client to:
    a. Observe closely for signs of septicemia (i.e., chills, fever, flushed feeling).
    b. Force fluids unless contraindicated.
    c. Monitor urine for persistent bright red color. ▸ ***Rationale:*** Bleeding can occur; if present, notify physician.
    d. Assess for severe pain (colicky pain is normal with urethral catheterization), continual burning, and frequency.
10. Monitor vital signs.
11. Palpate client for bladder distention and ensure client voids before discharge. ▸ ***Rationale:*** Urinary retention can be caused by edema from instrumentation.
12. Monitor urine output for 48 hr. If client's output is less than 200 mL in 8 hr, increase fluid intake. ▸ ***Rationale:*** Anuria can indicate urinary retention due to blood clots or urethral stricture.

For Gastrointestinal Tract Endoscopy

1. Follow steps in Preparing for Endoscopic Studies as it applies to this procedure.
2. Explain that this procedure is used to visualize upper GI tract by inserting flexible fiber-optic–lighted scope.
3. Keep NPO for 6–12 hr.
4. Remove dentures.
5. Explain procedure to client.
    a. Client taken to special procedure room.
    b. Client is awake during procedure, usually takes 20–30 minutes.
    c. Cardiac monitoring and pulse oximetry are done.
    d. Throat is anesthetized by swabbing with local anesthetic, usually Xylocaine. ▸ ***Rationale:*** To decrease gag reflex.
    e. Client is sedated with intravenous medication (usually Valium or Versed). Atropine may be administered to decrease secretions.
    f. Client is placed in left lateral recumbent position.
    g. Endoscope passed through esophagus to the duodenum. Can evaluate all structures as scope goes through the GI tract (termed EGD).
    h. Air is introduced through scope to distend upper GI tract. ▸ ***Rationale:*** To maximize visualization.
    i. Specimens may be taken and sent to lab.
6. Provide postprocedure care.
    a. Monitor vital signs as for surgical client.
    b. Check for signs and symptoms of bleeding or perforation. ▸ ***Rationale:*** Sharp, intense pain in stomach or chest and cool, pale skin indicate perforation.

c. Check gag reflex. ▸ ***Rationale:*** May take 2–3 hr before gag reflex returns.
d. Keep side rails up until effects of medications have subsided.
e. Provide ice chips or throat lozenges for sore throat.

For Laparoscopy

1. Follow steps in Preparing for Endoscopic Studies as it applies to this procedure. Ensure consent form is signed.
2. Explain that scope is inserted through abdominal wall and into peritoneum to visualize abdominal and pelvic organs—used to assist in diagnosing pathologic conditions of pelvic and abdominal area.
3. Instruct client to discontinue anticoagulant therapy 5–7 days before test.
4. Complete bowel prep as ordered.
5. Instruct in NPO status after midnight. Client receives general anesthesia.
6. Shave and prep abdomen as ordered.
7. Start a peripheral IV as ordered. Medications may be given during procedure.
8. Have client void just before surgery. ▸ ***Rationale:*** To prevent accidental penetration of distended bladder during procedure.
9. Insert Foley catheter and NG tube before or after anesthesia administration, according to facility policy. ▸ ***Rationale:*** To prevent complications associated with penetration of distended stomach or bladder with needle placement.
10. Explain procedure to client.
    a. Client is placed in supine position on operating room table.
    b. Skin preparation is completed using antimicrobial swabs.
    c. Blunt-tipped needle is inserted through small incision in periumbilical area and into peritoneal cavity.
    d. Peritoneal cavity is filled with CO_2. ▸ ***Rationale:*** Separates abdominal wall from intra-abdominal viscera to allow better visualization of pelvic and abdominal structures.
    e. Laparoscope with light camera is inserted through trocar and procedure completed.
    f. Scope is removed and CO_2 is allowed to escape. It takes 24 hr to be totally eliminated.
    g. Incision is closed with butterfly tape, spray tape, or sutures and covered with transparent dressing.
11. Provide general postop care.
12. Instruct client in discharge teaching.
    a. Observe site for signs of infection, bleeding, increased pulse rate or fever. Notify physician immediately if these signs occur.
    b. Instruct client that he or she will have shoulder or subcostal discomfort for 24 hr. Medicate for pain as needed.
    c. Instruct client not to do physical exercise for 4–7 days.

For Sigmoidoscopy

1. Follow steps in Preparing for Endoscopic Studies. Ensure consent form is signed.
2. Explain that test allows for visualization of rectum and sigmoid colon. Used for screening for colon polyps.
3. Ensure barium studies have not been given up to 3 days before test.
4. Administer tap water or disposable (e.g., Fleet's) enema as ordered the morning of the procedure. Clients with ulcerative colitis will not have an enema ordered. Oral cathartic may also be given.
5. Provide light dinner the night before test and then place client on NPO. Avoid heavy meat, vegetables, and fruit for 24 hr before test.
6. Have client void before procedure.
7. Explain procedure to client.
    a. Client is placed on special table in special procedure room or in physician's examining room.
    b. Position in a knee–chest position if using examination table and rigid scope. Place on left side with right leg bent and placed over left leg if using flexible scope.
    c. Drape client to provide for modesty and warmth.
    d. Physician examines the rectum digitally first.
    e. Lubricated flexible sigmoidoscope is advanced through anus into the rectum to visualize any abnormality of rectum, sigmoid colon, and large bowel.
    f. Client may feel pressure and need to have a bowel movement. Assure client this is usual feeling.
    g. Air may be introduced to increase visualization of bowel wall.
    h. Suction equipment passed through the scope may be used to remove secretions for better visualization of colon.
    i. Biopsy may be obtained by passing a snare through scope.
    j. Scope is removed, and client's rectal area is cleaned and dried.
    k. Gloves are applied if nurse is assisting with cleaning. Remove gloves and wash hands.
    l. Have client remain flat for 10–15 minutes before leaving room. Procedure takes 15–30 minutes.
8. Instruct client in discharge teaching.
    a. Resume preexamination activities.
    b. Monitor stools for bleeding. Bloody stools are normal first 1–2 days after test.
    c. Instruct client to avoid enema or barium studies for at least 1 week.
    d. Observe for signs of increased abdominal distention, increased tenderness, or rectal bleeding. ▸ ***Rationale:*** These are symptoms of bowel perforation.

DOCUMENTATION for Endoscopic Studies

- Test preparation completed
- Client teaching completed and client's ability to understand procedure evaluated
- Client's tolerance of procedure
- Preprocedure and postprocedure vital signs, if required
- Record type of specimen taken and sent to lab
- Specific postprocedure care given and client's response to treatment
- Specific signs and symptoms indicating potential complications

CRITICAL THINKING Application

Expected Outcomes

- Client is prepared psychologically and physically for endoscopic procedure.
- Client experiences no sequelae after moderate sedation.
- Client does not experience pain or discomfort with procedure.
- Client diagnosis is confirmed with endoscopic study.

Unexpected Outcomes	Alternative Actions
Lower gastrointestinal tract not clear and sigmoidoscopy not completed.	• Repeat laxative and enemas per physician orders. • Observe results of enema; if solution not clear, notify physician.
Vertigo occurs while maintaining knee–chest position during sigmoidoscopy.	• Have client lie in supine position for few minutes. • Have client assume standing position slowly. • Have client assume Sims' position.
Upper gastrointestinal bleeding begins when scope inserted.	• Insert nasogastric tube, and apply suction. • Monitor vital signs for evidence of shock. • Place in semi-Fowler's position.
Potential colon perforation after endoscopic procedure.	• Assess for abdominal distention, tenderness, and pain. • Notify physician immediately. • Ensure client has a patent IV line, if not, insert peripheral line.
Potential infection after cystoscopy.	• Instruct client to force fluids to maintain constant flow of urine and prevent accumulation of bacteria in bladder. • Instruct client on signs and symptoms of sepsis: fever, flushing, chills, increased pulse rate, and feeling faint. Instruct client to notify physician immediately if any of these occur. • If client has been given prophylactic antibiotics, instruct in taking them as ordered. Do not stop taking the medication; take entire prescription.
Client goes from minimal sedation to anesthesia when administering Versed for conscious sedation.	• Call the Rescue Team. • Have Code Cart available. • Maintain respirations with Ambu bag or rescue breathing. • Infuse additional IV fluids. • Administer flumazenil as an antidote if ordered.

Chapter 21

UNIT 5

Fluid Analysis and Microscopic Studies

Nursing Process Data

ASSESSMENT Data Base

- Assess vital signs before, during, and after the procedure.
- Assess client's ability to maintain position necessary for procedure.
- Assess client's knowledge of the procedure to be performed.
- Review pertinent laboratory tests before procedure.
- Evaluate signs and symptoms that indicate a potential problem could exist if test performed.

PLANNING Objectives

- To provide reassurance for clients undergoing diagnostic tests
- To position the client in a manner that facilitates the introduction of a needle through the skin surface to obtain a fluid or tissue sample
- To obtain tissue or fluid to determine presence of infection or diseases
- To obtain body fluids for specific disease analysis
- To aspirate fluid to relieve pressure on body organs

IMPLEMENTATION Procedures

EVALUATION Expected Outcomes

- Client is prepared psychologically and physically for procedure.
- Diagnostic tests performed with minimal discomfort and no untoward effects.
- Specimens from studies sent to laboratory according to hospital policy, in appropriate container and in a timely manner.

Pearson Nursing Student Resources

Find additional review materials at **nursing.pearsonhighered.com**

Prepare for success with NCLEX®-style practice questions and Skill Checklists

TABLE 21-5 Diagnostic Procedures

Diagnostic Test	Rationale
Lumbar puncture	To obtain a cerebrospinal fluid specimen to determine presence of microorganisms, RBCs, or WBCs
Liver biopsy	To obtain a specimen to determine presence of tumor or disease
Thoracentesis	To remove fluid from the thoracic cavity; to obtain a specimen for cell study
Paracentesis	To remove fluid from the abdominal cavity; to obtain a specimen for cell study
Bone marrow aspiration	To study cells obtained from the specimen
Vaginal examination and Papanicolaou smear	To determine cell changes through a smear; to obtain a specimen for venereal disease identification
Amniocentesis	To remove amniotic fluid for studies of fetal maturity and genetic abnormalities

Assisting With Lumbar Puncture

Equipment

Diagnostic tray or equipment specific for procedure
Bath blanket
Sterile collection bottles or test tubes if indicated and not on tray
Sterile gloves
Xylocaine injection or EMLA cream if not on tray
Examining light
Clean gloves
Dressing or band aid

Procedure

1. Identify client using two forms of identification and explain that a lumbar puncture (LP) is used for diagnosis of tumors, hemorrhage, infection, and autoimmune diseases involving CNS.
2. Explain procedure—a hollow core needle is placed in the subarachnoid space at L3–4 or L4–5 to facilitate measuring CSF pressure and obtaining fluid for testing.
3. Obtain history of client's complaints, including known allergies and current medications.

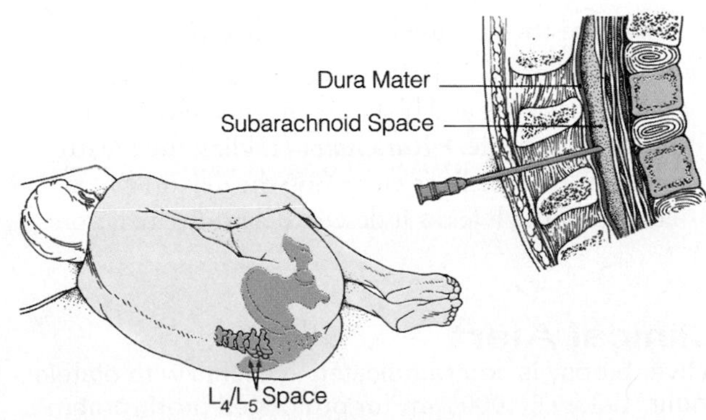

▲ Place client in Sims' position to facilitate needle insertion for lumbar puncture.

Clinical Alert

This procedure is contraindicated in clients with increased intracranial pressure. A reduction in pressure may cause a herniation of the brainstem. It is also contraindicated if infection is present at puncture site or client is uncooperative.

4. Obtain consent.
5. Instruct client to empty bowel and bladder.
6. Perform hand hygiene.
7. Obtain tray and any additional equipment needed, such as sterile gloves, bath blanket.
8. Position client in lateral recumbent position with back at the edge of the examining table. Cover with bath blanket, exposing only client's back.
9. Open sterile tray if requested by physician. Pour antiseptic solution into sterile medicine cup if needed.
10. Instruct client to pull knees up to abdomen and flex chin on chest. Assist client to maintain position, by nurse standing in front of the client, reaching across to support client behind neck and knees. ▶ ***Rationale:*** This position widens the space between the spinous processes of the lower lumbar vertebrae for ease of needle insertion.
11. Place pillows between knees. ▶ ***Rationale:*** This prevents upper legs from sliding off lower legs.
12. Assist client in relaxation exercises or instruct in deep, slow breathing through the mouth.
13. Use Xylocaine or EMLA cream around site before needle insertion by physician.
14. Explain that he or she must remain still without movement during test.
15. Assist physician with the Queckenstedt's test when requested. After opening pressure is obtained, apply compression to neck veins with your fingers.
16. Don clean gloves and assist physician as directed.

Clinical Alert

Queckenstedt's test is used to identify blockage of CSF flow in the spinal subarachnoid space. Generally when neck pressure is applied, there is a rapid rise in pressure level on the manometer with a return to normal within seconds when pressure is released.

17. Label cerebrospinal fluid samples with number on each specimen container.
18. After removal of needle, apply Band-Aid to puncture site.
19. Remove gloves and perform hand hygiene.
20. Fill out lab slips for appropriate test (i.e., cell count, serology).
21. Instruct client to lie flat for 4–24 hr, depending on hospital policy. Head is to remain flat and even with position of body. ▸ ***Rationale:*** To reduce CSF leakage.
22. Encourage fluids if not contraindicated by client's condition. ▸ ***Rationale:*** To reduce chance of headache.
23. Observe for spinal fluid leak from puncture site.
24. Check for headaches or alterations in neurologic status.
25. Document cerebrospinal fluid (CSF) characteristics, including color and clarity. Record opening pressure.

Assisting With Liver Biopsy

Equipment

Same as for Assisting With Lumbar Puncture

Procedure is often done through ultrasound to guide the needle to pathologic site.

Tray with equipment, sterile gloves, 2 × 2 dressing, and tape

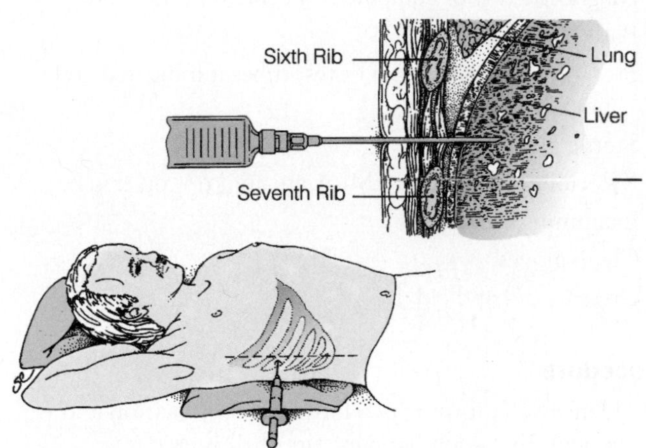

▲ Instruct client to raise arm over head to facilitate needle insertion for liver biopsy.

Preparation

1. Obtain lab values before scheduled test: prothrombin time, bleeding time, and platelet count if ordered. ▸ ***Rationale:*** Liver is vascular and if these lab results are abnormal, bleeding may occur after procedure.
2. Determine if a blood typing and crossmatching is needed.
3. Determine if client is to be NPO. Need to be NPO for 6 hr.
4. Identify client using two forms of identification and explain that tissue will be removed after special needle is inserted into liver. Tissue will be studied to determine presence of disease.
5. Obtain consent.
6. Assess whether client has any allergies to topical anesthetic agents.

Procedure

1. Perform hand hygiene.
2. Take vital signs. ▸ ***Rationale:*** This provides baseline data to compare with postprocedure data.
3. Administer sedative as ordered.
4. Obtain tray and any additional equipment needed, such as sterile gloves, sandbag, bath blanket.
5. Place client in supine position at the right edge of the bed. Raise right arm and extend it over the left shoulder behind the head. If possible, turn head to left side. ▸ ***Rationale:*** This position provides maximal exposure of right intercostal space.

NOTE: Left lateral position can be used for biopsy.

6. Open sterile tray if requested by physician.
7. Local anesthesia is used around puncture site.
8. Instruct client to inhale and exhale deeply several times and then exhale and hold breath while physician inserts the biopsy needle. ▸ ***Rationale:*** Holding the breath prevents the needle from tearing the diaphragm or lacerating the liver as it descends during exhalation.

Clinical Alert

A liver biopsy is contraindicated in clients with platelet counts below 50,000/mm^3 or prolonged prothrombin time. Bleeding can occur after the procedure.

9. Instruct the client to breathe normally after the physician removes the needle.
10. Don clean gloves and place Band-Aid or small dressing over puncture site.
11. Position client on right side for 2–4 hr. A folded blanket may be placed under client's right side to provide hemostasis. ▶ ***Rationale:*** This position compresses the liver against the chest wall, thereby decreasing risk of hemorrhage.
12. Remove gloves and perform hand hygiene.
13. Instruct client to remain on bed rest for 24 hr.
14. Assess for signs of hemorrhage at least every hour for 12 hr.
15. Monitor vital signs as you would for a surgical client (e.g., every 15 minutes for 1 hr).
16. Assess rate, rhythm, and depth of respirations.
17. Assess breath sounds and check for signs of dyspnea and restlessness. ▶ ***Rationale:*** Lung may be punctured during biopsy.
18. Send specimen to lab.

Assisting With Thoracentesis

Equipment

Same as for Assisting With Lumbar Puncture

Vacutainer

Interventional radiologist may perform biopsies using CT or ultrasound (paracentesis and thoracentesis) for better visualization of organs.

Sterile gloves

Sterile pressure dressing and tape

Preparation

1. Identify client using two forms of identification and explain purpose of procedure to client.
2. Explain that needle is inserted into pleural space for removal of fluid for either diagnostic tests or to relieve pleural pressure.
3. Obtain consent.
4. Ensure chest x-ray film has been taken. ▶ ***Rationale:*** This film is used to compare with the film taken after the procedure.
5. Assess if client has any allergies to topical anesthetic agents.
6. Explain that movement or coughing must not be done during procedure to prevent lung or pleural damage.
7. Ensure client has IV for emergency medication administration.

Procedure

1. Perform hand hygiene.
2. Take vital signs, and complete a respiratory assessment. ▶ ***Rationale:*** This information provides postprocedure comparisons and early identification of potential complications.
3. Administer sedative as ordered.
4. Position client on edge of bed with arms crossed and resting on the overbed table. ▶ ***Rationale:*** This position provides good access to the intercostal spaces and facilitates fluid removal.

NOTE: Client can be placed in side-lying position on unaffected side if unable to sit up.

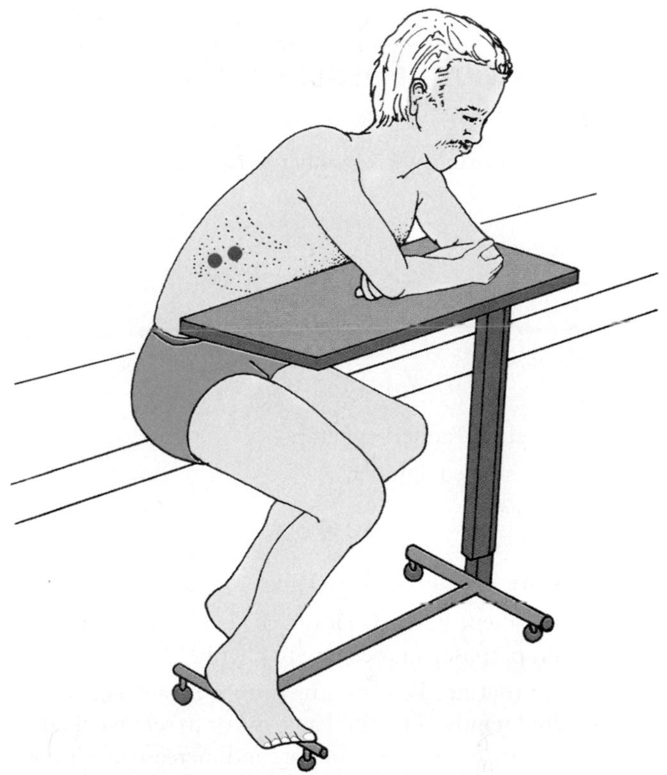

▲ Place client in a leaning forward position to expose intercostal space for thoracentesis.

5. Provide adequate warmth and covering for client using bath blanket.
6. Place unwrapped sterile tray on bedside stand.
7. Open sterile gloves as indicated. Maintain sterile technique throughout procedure.
8. Assist physician as needed with skin prep.
9. Don clean gloves. Instruct client not to cough, take a deep breath, or move during placement of needle by the physician.
10. After insertion of needle into pleural space, observe client for pallor, dyspnea, tachycardia, chest pain, or vertigo. Report these findings immediately to the physician. ▶ ***Rationale:*** These symptoms occur with a pneumothorax.

11. Connect tubing to vacutainer, allowing fluid to be drawn from cavity.

NOTE: Blunt-tip, soft catheter-over-needle is used more often than a needle to prevent pneumothorax.

12. Apply pressure dressing (as determined by policy) after fluid and needle are removed. Remove gloves and perform hand hygiene.
13. Observe client every 5 minutes for half hour for pulmonary edema (blood-tinged sputum), crepitus, cardiac distress (changes in respirations, pulse, or color), or a shift in the mediastinum.
14. Place client on unaffected side with head elevated 30° for at least 1 hr.
15. Monitor vital signs and breath sounds as with postoperative clients for 2 hr.
16. Observe dressing, change as needed. ▸ ***Rationale:*** Drainage is a common occurrence after a tap.
17. Obtain chest x-ray after procedure to check for pneumothorax.
18. Record color, amount, consistency, and samples of fluid obtained.
19. Complete lab slips, and send specimen to lab.

Assisting With Paracentesis

Equipment

Same as for Assisting With Lumbar Puncture

- Sterile tray
- Vacutainer
- Chair
- Drape
- Sterile gloves
- Bucket
- Dressing-elastic adhesive patch
- Blood pressure equipment
- Clean gloves

Preparation

1. Identify client using two forms of identification and explain purpose of procedure to client.
2. Explain that needle is inserted into peritoneal cavity and fluid removed for fluid analysis or to remove fluid from cavity to promote comfort and increase respiratory status.
3. Obtain consent.
4. Assess whether client has any allergies to topical anesthetic agents.
5. Assess whether client has coagulation abnormalities or bleeding tendencies. (Procedure is contraindicated in these clients.)
6. Perform hand hygiene.
7. Assess client's abdominal girth and bowel sounds. ▸ ***Rationale:*** This information provides postprocedure comparisons and early identification of potential complications.
8. Have client empty bladder. ▸ ***Rationale:*** This prevents accidental puncture of the bladder during the procedure.
9. Weigh client. ▸ ***Rationale:*** This information can be used to assess fluid loss after the procedure.

Procedure

1. Place client in Fowler's position on chair or on edge of bed with legs spread apart.
2. Drape client, and provide adequate warmth and covering with a bath blanket.
3. Obtain vital signs, and observe client for pallor and vertigo during procedure. ▸ ***Rationale:*** These symptoms are indicative of shock.
4. Position and open tray on over-bed table.
5. Open sterile gloves if needed.
6. Assist physician in preparing skin with antiseptic solution and topical anesthesia or as needed.
7. Don clean gloves.
8. Physician inserts trocar needle, or cannula through small incision. Plastic tubing is attached to cannula

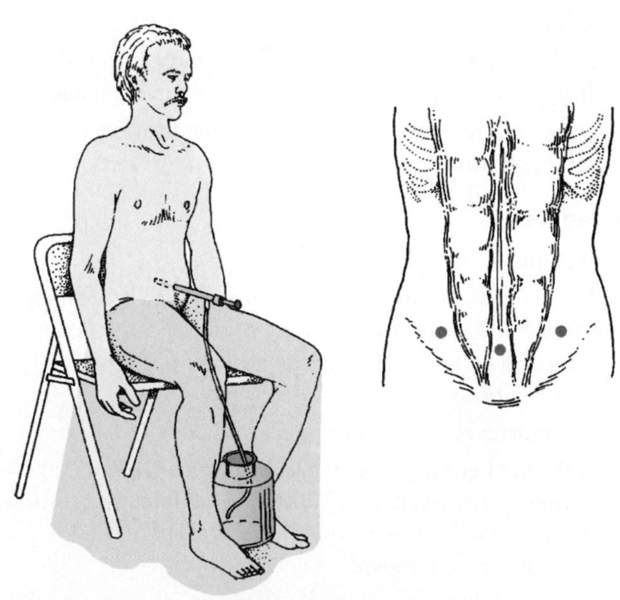

▲ Position client in chair to facilitate trocar insertion and drainage for paracentesis.

and other end of tubing is placed in the collection receptacle. Vacutainer may be used to provide gentle suction of fluid from cavity.

9. Observe total amount of fluid aspirated. Usually no more than 2000 mL (2 L) is removed at one time. ▸ ***Rationale:*** Removing larger amounts of fluid can lead to hypotension and hyponatremia.
10. Apply pressure dressing after removal of needle. ▸ ***Rationale:*** This prevents bleeding from puncture site.
11. Remove gloves, and place in appropriate receptacle.
12. Perform hand hygiene.
13. Return client to bed and place in semi- to high-Fowler's position. ▸ ***Rationale:*** These positions usually are most comfortable for client and promote lung expansion.
14. Observe for leakage at puncture site or scrotal edema in male client.
15. Monitor vital signs and observe closely for signs of hypotension. Monitor urine output and color and dressing every 15 minutes for at least 2 hr; every hour for 4 hr; every 4 hr for 24 hr.
16. Assess bowel sounds, and measure abdominal girth. ▸ ***Rationale:*** To monitor for signs of perforated bowel or peritonitis.
17. Weigh client when vital signs are stable. ▸ ***Rationale:*** This prevents hypotension.
18. Reinforce or change dressings as needed.
19. Monitor serum protein and electrolytes, particularly sodium. ▸ ***Rationale:*** Fluid contains high levels of protein that is removed with this procedure.
20. Record color, amount, consistency, and samples obtained from paracentesis, and send to laboratory.

Assisting With Bone Marrow Aspiration

Equipment

Same as for Assisting With Lumbar Puncture
Two slides
Green or lavender top tube
Preservative spray
Sterile gloves

Procedure

1. Identify client using two forms of identification and explain purpose of procedure.
2. Explain procedure.
3. Client will experience discomfort or pressure when needle is inserted.
4. Obtain consent
5. Obtain tray and provide any additional equipment needed, such as specimen container.
6. Assess coagulation studies and report unusual findings to physician.
7. Premedicate client with prescribed drugs.
8. Position client in supine position if sternum or anterior iliac crest is the biopsy site or prone if posterior iliac crest is the biopsy site. Place a sandbag under iliac crest area if physician requires.
9. Open tray on over-bed table.
10. Assist physician as needed.
11. Physician injects local anesthetic at site.

NOTE: A large-bore needle containing a stylus is inserted into bone, about 3 mm deep. Stylus is removed and 10-mL syringe is attached to needle. About 0.5 to 2 mL of bone marrow is removed as specimen, spread on slides, and sprayed with preservative. Remainder is placed in green or lavender top tube.

12. Perform hand hygiene and don sterile gloves.
13. Apply direct pressure for 5–15 minutes after removal of needle. ▸ ***Rationale:*** To prevent bleeding.
14. Cover puncture site with sterile pressure dressing. Ice pack may be applied to help control bleeding.
15. Remove gloves and perform hand hygiene.
16. Monitor vital signs, and observe puncture site for drainage, edema, or pain, as with surgical client. ▸ ***Rationale:*** To monitor for signs of infection. Call physician for temperature above 101°F.
17. Position the client for comfort.
18. Properly label specimens and send to laboratory.
19. Evaluate client for signs of hemorrhage, shock, or infection.

Assisting With Vaginal Examination and Papanicolaou (PAP) Smear

Equipment

Two slides
Cytology container
Fixative agent
Vaginal speculum, several sizes
Gloves
Water-soluble lubricant jelly
Examining light

Preparation

1. Identify client using two forms of identification and explain purpose of procedure.

2. Explain that test is performed to detect neoplastic cells in cervical and vaginal secretions. Procedure takes 10 minutes.
3. Instruct client not to douche, insert vaginal medications, or take tub bath for 24 hr before exam.
4. Instruct client that test should be done 2 weeks after start of last menses.
5. Instruct client to refrain from sexual intercourse for 24–48 hr before exam, according to physician's orders.
6. Foods or fluids are not restricted.

Procedure

1. Instruct client to empty bladder.
2. Assist client to examination room.
3. Instruct client to remove clothing including underwear and don gown.
4. Position client on examining table in lithotomy position using stirrups.
5. Provide adequate coverings to preserve modesty and prevent chilling.
6. Open speculum package, gloves, and lubricant. Place on tray. Place cytology slides and container on tray.
7. Label two slides with client's name and area from where specimen is obtained.
8. Position light for good exposure.
9. Stay with client if she is a child or physician is a male.
10. Assist physician as needed. A lubricated speculum is inserted into vagina.
11. Instruct client that material is collected from cervical canal by rotating either a cotton swab moistened with saline or a wooden spatula.
12. Wipe swab across a clean glass slide to disperse cells.
13. Affix to slide either by immersing the slide in equal parts of 95% alcohol and ether or by using a commercial hair spray. ▸ ***Rationale:*** Secretions must be fixed before drying to prevent abnormal interpretation of smears.
14. Place slides in cytology container and send to the lab. Complete all cytology forms. Client's medical history and reason for examination are written on request form.
15. Assist client in perineal care.
16. Provide perineal pad if bleeding occurs.
17. Assist client to dress if necessary.

Assisting With Amniocentesis

Procedure

1. Identify client using two forms of identification and explain purpose of procedure to client.

NOTE: Test is to withdraw fluid for analysis to check fetal maturity status, sex of fetus, genetic or chromosomal abnormalities, hereditary metabolic disorders, anatomical abnormalities, or fetal distress.

2. Obtain consent, both client and her partner.
3. Explain that foods and fluids are not restricted. Have client void before test. ▸ ***Rationale:*** This prevents injury to the bladder. Before 20 weeks of gestation, bladder may be kept full to support the uterus.
4. Transport client to treatment room.
5. Instruct client to lie quietly in supine position for 30 minutes.
6. Obtain fetal heart tones and mother's blood pressure.
7. Open amniocentesis tray and gloves. Place Xylocaine nearby if not included on tray. ▸ ***Rationale:*** Procedure is performed under sterile conditions to prevent infection.
8. Explain details of procedure to client.
   a. Physician prepares abdomen with antiseptic solution or alcohol.
   b. Xylocaine injection provides local anesthesia for needle insertion area.
   c. Placenta and fetus are located manually or by ultrasound.
   d. A 22-gauge spinal needle with a stylet is inserted through the midabdominal wall and 5 to 15 mL of amniotic fluid is withdrawn.
   e. Amniotic fluid is placed in light-resistant specimen container and labeled with client's name. Appropriate lab slips are completed. ▸ ***Rationale:*** To prevent breakdown of bilirubin.
   f. Procedure takes about 10 minutes.
9. Perform hand hygiene and don sterile gloves and place small dressing or Band-Aid over needle site.
10. Remove gloves and perform hand hygiene.
11. Monitor fetal heart tones and observe for signs of labor.
12. Observe puncture site for bleeding or other drainage.
13. Instruct client to notify physician of any unusual occurrences, signs of labor, or signs of infection.
14. Give RhoGAM if woman is Rh-negative. ▸ ***Rationale:*** There is a risk of immunization against fetal blood (hemolytic disease).
15. Explain that test results will be available in 2 weeks.

DOCUMENTATION for Fluid Analysis and Microscopic Studies

- Preparation completed for test
- Client teaching completed and client's ability to understand procedure evaluated
- Consent form signed
- Client's tolerance of procedure
- Fluid or specimens sent to laboratory for analysis
- Preprocedure and postprocedure vital signs if required
- Color and amount of fluid withdrawn from paracentesis, thoracentesis, or lumbar puncture
- Fetal heart tones before and after amniocentesis
- Type of dressing applied
- Specific position assumed after procedure as indicated
- Abnormal findings after procedure indicating potential complications

CRITICAL THINKING Application

Expected Outcomes

- Client is prepared psychologically and physically for procedure.
- Diagnostic tests performed with minimal discomfort and no untoward effects.
- Specimens from studies sent to laboratory according to hospital policy, in appropriate container and in a timely manner.

Unexpected Outcomes	Alternative Actions
Client has spinal fluid leak after lumbar puncture.	• Keep client in supine position. • Notify physician. • Keep sterile dressing over puncture site. Do not allow dressing to become wet. • If leak persists, physician may place client in Trendelenburg's position to prevent headache. This position is contraindicated in clients with increased intracranial pressure or after a craniotomy.
Client complains of shortness of breath or expectorates blood-tinged sputum after a thoracentesis.	• Place client in Fowler's position. • Assess vital signs. • Administer oxygen. • Monitor breath sounds. • Notify physician and check on order for chest x-ray. • Have chest tube insertion tray available. • Allay client's fears and provide emotional support.
Urine output is blood-tinged after paracentesis or amniocentesis.	• Notify physician at once; bladder may have been punctured during procedure. • Monitor vital signs for shock. • Maintain client on bed rest. • Observe for urine output.

GERONTOLOGIC Considerations

Elderly Clients Requiring Diagnostic Tests Are at Risk for the Following Problems:

- Dehydration can result from fluid restriction, use of contrast agents for the tests, and bowel preparation using enemas. Osmolar imbalances and hypovolemia can result from the dehydration.
- Extracellular fluid volume excess can occur if large volumes of fluid are required for the test. Renal studies, which usually require the use of large volumes of fluid, should not be considered if the client is at risk for circulatory overload. Elderly clients may have a compromised cardiorespiratory status. A secondary choice of tests may need to be considered, such as a CT scan.
- Renal dysfunction resulting from multiple tests using contrast agents should be avoided. Acute renal failure can result from multiple tests with contrast agents in elderly clients who already have a compromised renal system. Spacing tests over time helps prevent this problem.

Nursing Responsibilities for Elderly Clients Requiring Diagnostic Tests Should Include the Following:

- Carefully monitor fluid and electrolyte balance.
- Adequately hydrate client before and after tests unless contraindicated.

- Monitor laboratory tests, such as electrolytes and osmolarity.
- Monitor intake and output frequently.
- Monitor vital signs.
- Weigh clients who are at risk for fluid volume disturbances.
- Complete physical assessment, including mental status, each shift, and report unusual findings to physician.

MANAGEMENT Guidelines

Each state legislates a Nurse Practice Act for RNs and LVN/LPNs. Healthcare facilities are responsible for establishing and implementing policies and procedures that conform to their state's regulations. Verify the regulations and role parameters for each healthcare worker in your facility.

Delegation

- LVNs/LPNs and RNs may both be assigned to care for clients undergoing diagnostic tests. Nurses are frequently working in x-ray and diagnostic procedure laboratories today and assisting physicians with invasive procedures. Technicians are also educated to work in areas such as cardiac catheterization labs. These technicians are not nursing personnel. In most cases, radiologic technologists assist with the various procedures within the x-ray and diagnostic procedure labs.
- When invasive procedures such as liver biopsy and paracentesis are performed on the nursing unit, either an LVN/LPN or RN is assigned to assist the physician.
- Preprocedure and postprocedure interventions are assigned to the LVN/LPN or RN for direct responsibility. A CNA may assist the nurse by taking vital signs.
- Only RNs can transport clients who have received conscious sedation for a procedure.

Communication Matrix

- All staff members must be aware of clients undergoing diagnostic tests. This information is disseminated through shift and team reports. It is also written on the Kardex card or is on the client's information sheet on the computer. If premedication is required, this information is found on the Medication Administration Record as well. If the client is NPO for the test, a sign must be placed in the client's room indicating this status.
- Specific directions must be given to the staff member assigned to the client to inform them of their client care responsibilities both pre- and postprocedure.
- The RN must assess the knowledge base of the staff member assigned to assist the physician with any procedure being performed on the unit. This is to ensure safety for the client.
- The RN collaborates with the physician to identify any specific equipment or needs he or she may have for the procedure being performed on the unit.

CRITICAL THINKING Strategies

Scenario 1

Mr. Michael Spicer, a 72-year-old retired fireman, is scheduled for the following diagnostic procedures as an outpatient. He has started his testing with a barium enema. You have been asked to call him and instruct him about the procedures.

Diagnostic Tests to be Completed

- IV pyelography
- Bone scan
- Sigmoidoscopy

1. What is the priority question you should ask? Provide rationale for your answer.
2. When beginning the discussion about the IVP, what is your priority question? Provide rationale for your answer.
3. Identify the most important postprocedure client education regarding the IVP. Provide rationale for your answer.
4. The client asks you if he will be radioactive and a risk to his family after the bone scan. What is your best response?
5. Briefly explain the preprocedure prep for the sigmoidoscopy.

Scenario 2

A young 30-year-old client has been referred to the surgeon for further evaluation of a lump in the upper, outer quadrant of her left breast. You work with the physician and are obtaining the history from the client. She tells you she noticed the lump about 1 month ago. When you examine the breast you feel a quarter size lump without dimpling of the nipple.

1. The client asks you how will they know if it is benign or malignant? Your best response is:
2. She is very anxious and asks you questions about the various procedures that they do now to determine whether surgery is necessary. Explain the various diagnostic tests that are completed and prioritize the tests according to usual protocol for completion of the tests.
3. Describe the preprocedural instructions for the procedures listed in #2.

NCLEX® Review Questions

Unless otherwise specified, choose only one (1) answer.

1. Nurses' major responsibility with interventional radiology is related to
   1. Assisting the radiologists in preparing the client for the procedure.
   2. Managing procedural sedation, monitoring, and postprocedure recovery.
   3. Monitoring vital signs during the procedure.
   4. Providing client education about the procedure.
2. Dynamic CT scanning is best defined as
   1. Visualizes blood flow and degree of vascularity of organs via dye injection to specific organs.
   2. Using sound waves produced by ultrasound to differentiate normal from diseased tissue.
   3. Observation of internal body organs and cavities by introducing the endoscope and then obtaining scans of the organs or cavities.
   4. A scan that uses a strong magnetic field in conjunction with radiofrequency waves to transmit signals from body cells to the computer.
3. Which one of the following preparations would not be included in the procedure for x-ray studies?
   1. Determine, if several studies are ordered, which one needs to be completed first.
   2. Ensure informed consent form is signed.
   3. Inform the client there is no restriction to food or fluid necessary before the tests.
   4. Determine need for withholding medications before the x-ray.
4. What are the client instructions when undergoing an intravenous pyelography (IVP)?
   Select all that apply.
   1. "You should not eat anything after 6 PM but you can take fluids until early morning."
   2. "Do you have any allergies to shellfish or iodine?"
   3. "Dye injection material can cause nausea, shortness of breath, and a hot, flushed feeling."
   4. "Drink at least 24 ounces of water immediately after the IVP."
5. Which of the following baseline lab values need to be obtained before an arteriography?
   1. Hemoglobin and hematocrit.
   2. WBC, RBC, SGOT, SGPT.
   3. BUN, creatinine, PT/PTT, APTT.
   4. MVP, platelets, blood smear.
6. You are obtaining a history before scheduling the client for a bone scan. The most important question to ask is
   1. "Have you had a barium study done in the last 10 days?"
   2. "You have had a bone scan before; do you have any questions?"
   3. "Do you suffer from claustrophobia?"
   4. "Do you have someone who can take you home after the test?"
7. Printed instructions frequently provided a client scheduled for a mammogram include
   1. Remain NPO for at least 6 hr before the test.
   2. Refrain from wearing deodorant.
   3. Remove jewelry from neck and wrists.
   4. Wear easy to remove clothing as it must all be removed.
8. As you observe the catheter insertion site after a cardiac catheterization, which of the following interventions would be considered a priority to implement?
   1. Apply a pressure dressing over the site.
   2. Call lab to order a CBC, HGB, and HCT.
   3. Elevate the extremity.
   4. Monitor peripheral pulses.
9. A major reason why PET scans are used in place of the CT scan or MRI is
   1. It is not necessary to have an IV or dye injection for the PET scan.
   2. Metabolic changes, which are visualized on the PET scan, occur before structural changes.
   3. It takes only a few minutes for a PET scan, whereas it can take up to 75 minutes for an MRI.
   4. Foods or fluids do not need to be restricted with the PET scan.
10. A client is very fearful and asks you about the arthroscopy he is scheduled to have in the afternoon. Which of the following responses would be most appropriate?
    1. "You will receive general anesthesia, not local anesthesia, so you will not experience any pain."
    2. "The procedure will take about 2 to 3 hours."
    3. "The incision will probably be under the knee cap and you will have sutures to hold the tissue in place."
    4. "You will most likely be able to ambulate with crutches the same day."

22

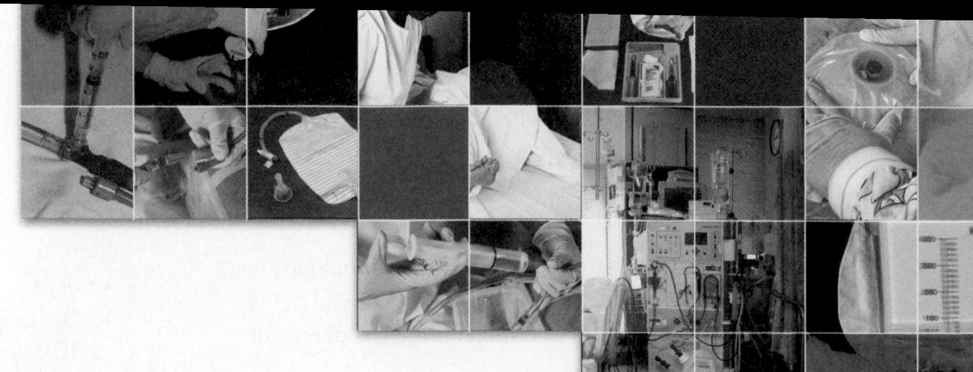

Urinary Elimination

LEARNING OBJECTIVES

1. Describe the process of urine production.
2. List four alterations that result in urinary elimination problems.
3. State two nursing diagnoses that relate to urine elimination.
4. Complete an intake and output bedside record.
5. Compare and contrast the steps for inserting a straight catheter in a male and female client.
6. Describe the major parameters needed to preserve a sterile environment when inserting a catheter.
7. Demonstrate the clamping protocol used for clients with suprapubic catheters.
8. Explain how a catheter is attached to a leg bag.
9. Identify the most important advantages of a suprapubic catheter.
10. List the major steps of irrigating by opening a closed urinary system.
11. Outline the steps necessary to obtain a urine specimen from a closed urinary drainage system.
12. Outline the steps for applying a urinary diversion pouch.
13. Describe rationale for renal replacement therapy.
14. List safety precautions for maintaining a fistula or graft for vascular access for hemodialysis.

CHAPTER OUTLINE

TERMINOLOGY

Albuminuria the presence of albumin in the urine.

Anemia a condition in which the number of circulating red blood cells, or hemoglobin, is reduced.

Antibiotic a substance that inhibits or kills bacteria.

Antidiuretic Pituitary hormone that causes water reabsorption by the distal tubule of the nephron.

Anuria suppression of urine production (less than 100 mL/day).

Arteriovenous extracorporeal circuit created with arterial to venous blood flow. The client's blood pressure forces blood through a hemofilter and back to a venous return access.

A-V fistula anastomosis of a vein with an artery as an access site for hemodialysis.

Azotemia increased levels of BUN and creatinine in the blood.

Bactericidal able to kill bacteria.

Calyx cuplike portion of the kidney pelvis.

Catheterization insertion of a tube for the injection of or removal of fluids from a vessel or body cavity.

Coude Catheter an elbowed catheter used for draining urine from bladder.

Dehydration the process of losing excessive water.

Dialyzer artificial kidney.

Distention stretching or inflating a structure such as the bladder.

Diuresis the excessive production of urine.

Dysuria painful urination.

Edema a condition of excess fluid in the interstitial space.

Electrolyte a substance that develops an electrical charge when dissolved in water.

End-stage renal disease the loss of 90% of kidney nephrons resulting in accumulation of nitrogenous wastes in the blood and uremia necessitating dialysis.

Excoriation a breakdown of the epidermis.

Foley catheter a self-retaining indwelling tube that is used to provide continuous drainage, usually from the bladder.

Genitourinary pertaining to the genital and urinary systems.

Hemodialysis process of removing excess fluid and accumulated wastes and electrolytes from the blood.

Hydrostatic pressure pumping force created by the mean arterial blood pressure, or a pump.

Incontinence inability to retain urine.

Indwelling urethral catheter a retention, or Foley, catheter.

Infection condition in which the body or a part is invaded by pathogens.

Irrigation the flushing of a tube or area with solution.

Micturition the process of emptying the urinary bladder; voiding.

Nocturia urination during the night.

Oliguria diminished production of urine (400 mL/day).

Patency the state of being freely open.

Peri prefix meaning around or about.

Peristalsis a progressive wavelike movement that occurs involuntarily in hollow tubes in the body.

Polyuria the excessive production of urine (output >2 liters/day).

Pyuria the presence of pus in the urine.

Renal pertaining to the kidney.

Sediment a substance settling at the bottom of a liquid.

Sepsis presence of pathogens or their toxins in the blood.

Septicemia presence of pathogens in the blood.

Shock a state of inadequate tissue perfusion.

Specific gravity weight of a substance compared with an equal volume of water. Water is 1.000.

Stoma surgically created opening.

Ultrafiltrate fluid collection from the blood which is isotonic and devoid of red blood cells or protein.

Urethra a canal for the discharge of urine from the bladder to the outside.

Urinary diversion an alternate route for urine elimination.

Urinary tract infection (UTI) an infection of the urinary tract, including all or part of the organs and ducts.

Venovenous extracorporeal circuit created using a dual-lumen hemodialysis catheter inserted into a central vein. Blood flow through the dialysis circuit is pump-controlled.

URINARY SYSTEM

The structures of the urinary system are the kidneys, ureters, bladder, and urethra. Each kidney produces urine, which is carried to the bladder by a ureter that is about 25 cm (10 in.) long and 0.6 cm in diameter. Peristaltic waves, pressure, and gravity propel urine through the ureters so that it can be discharged into the bladder.

The bladder serves as a reservoir for urine until voiding takes place. When voiding, or urination, occurs, urine passes through two sphincters and is transported from the bladder to the external environment through the urethra. The kidneys are essential to life, but the urine collection system is not.

The anatomic position of the bladder and the structure of the urethra differ in males and females. The bladder is posterior to the symphysis pubis. In a female the bladder is anterior to the vagina and the neck of the uterus. In a male the bladder is anterior to the rectum. The urethra of the female is about 4 cm (1.5 in.) long, and the male urethra is 20 cm (8 in.) long.

The urethra, bladder, ureters, and kidney pelves are lined with a continuous layer of mucous membrane. Because there is continuity of the lining, bacteria introduced into the normally sterile system can spread throughout the urinary tract. When the bladder is empty, its lining falls into folds that provide pockets where bacteria can multiply. Since the membrane is highly vascular, bacteria can easily enter the bloodstream and septicemia can result.

Urine Production

Nephrons, the functional units of the kidneys, produce urine. Each nephron consists of a renal corpuscle (Bowman's capsule) and a renal tubule, which is surrounded by a capillary bed. Each kidney has approximately a million nephrons.

Urine formed in the renal tubules enters collecting ducts, which empty urine into the kidney calyx. As urine collects in the renal pelvis, it flows to the bladder. If movement of urine from the pelvis is interrupted, infection, hydronephrosis, or formation of calculi may occur.

Blood is circulated to kidneys by way of the renal artery. This artery branches into arterioles, which supply a capillary tuft (glomerulus) filter. Under the influence of blood pressure, plasma is forced through the glomerulus and enters renal tubules. Filtered blood then passes from the glomerulus through an efferent arteriole and finally a capillary system that surrounds the renal tubules (peritubular capillaries). Kidneys filter approximately 140 liters of blood each day, but only 1500 mL of urine is produced. As blood pressure falls, urine production decreases.

The plasma that is filtered into the renal tubule contains water, glucose, electrolytes, and nitrogenous wastes. This "filtrate" is then modified as it moves through the tubular system. Substances such as medications are secreted from the peritubular capillaries and into the filtrate for elimination. Most of the plasma fluid is reabsorbed into the bloodstream

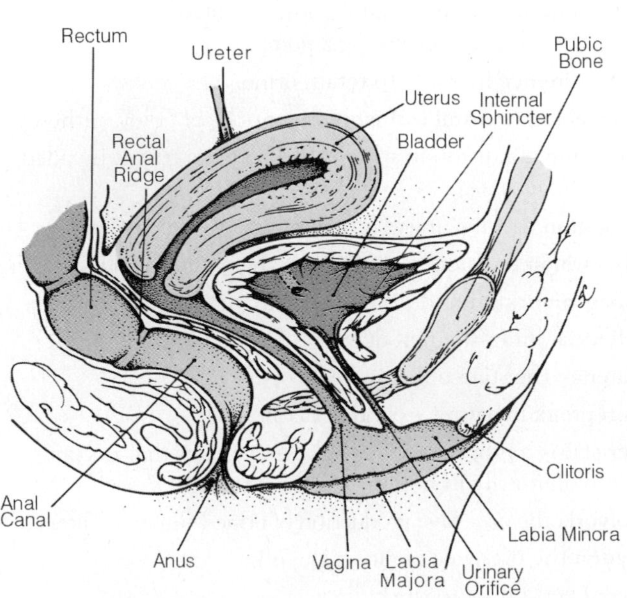

▲ Female genitourinary system.

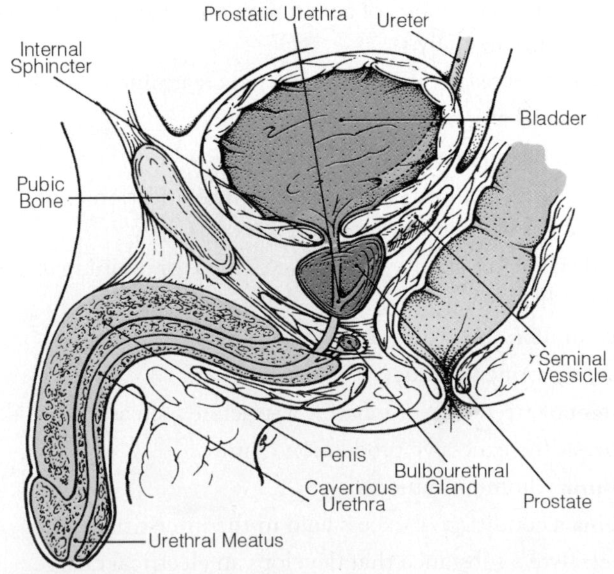

▲ Male genitourinary system.

TABLE 22-1 Tubular Alterations of Filtrate

Proximal tubule and descending limb	Obligatory water reabsorption, which accounts for about 80% of the absorption of water, occurs in the proximal tube and descending limb. Glucose, amino acids, vitamins, and sodium are actively reabsorbed. Chloride, sulfate, phosphate ions, and urea are passively reabsorbed. Bicarbonate is actively reabsorbed in relation to systemic pH. Water is reabsorbed with these substances, leaving the filtrate osmotic pressure unchanged.
Loop of Henle	Sodium is actively transported from the filtrate in the ascending limb into the medullary interstitial fluid, thus raising its osmotic pressure. This rising pressure causes more water to be reabsorbed from the descending limb and the collecting duct and results in the concentration of the urine.
Distal tubule and collecting ducts	Facultative or optional reabsorption of water, which accounts for about 10%–15% of the absorption of water, occurs in the distal tubule and collecting ducts. Sodium is actively reabsorbed in exchange for secreted potassium or hydrogen. As water continues to be reabsorbed, the filtrate becomes more concentrated and its volume is greatly reduced.

by way of peritubular capillaries, and excess fluid is removed along with acid waste products (urea, creatinine, hydrogen ion) in the form of urine. Through this process, kidneys maintain fluid and electrolyte and acid–base balance. In addition to urine production, kidneys play an important role in maintenance of blood pressure by secreting renin, activation of vitamin D to facilitate calcium absorption, and stimulation of red blood cell production by erythropoietin. It is easy to appreciate that loss of kidney function has a profound and widespread effect on homeostasis since it influences elimination of waste products, bone metabolism, blood pressure, tissue oxygenation (RBC production), acid–base balance, and fluid and electrolyte balance.

Micturition

Micturition (urination or voiding) is a voluntary response to pressure changes within the bladder. When urine begins to collect, the muscular walls of the bladder are relaxed, with little change in pressure. After about 300 mL of urine accumulates, pressure increases. This rising pressure stimulates receptors in the bladder wall, which send impulses to the spinal cord. After 400–500 mL of urine is collected, the bladder walls contract and the internal sphincter relaxes, causing a sense of needing to void. Under voluntary control, urine enters the urethra, the external sphincter relaxes, and voiding occurs.

Micturition can occur sooner if the tone of the bladder is increased because of such factors as emotional stress or infection. Micturition can be delayed by voluntary contraction of the external sphincter or pelvic floor muscles. Once the volume of urine reaches about 700 mL, however, most individuals lose their ability to delay micturition.

If an individual is unable to void, as much as 1000 mL of urine can accumulate in the bladder. When a large volume of urine is retained, the bladder's lining and blood vessels can be damaged by the increased stretching and pressure. When this happens, an individual experiences pain, restlessness, chilling, flushing, headache, diaphoresis, and a rise in blood pressure.

ALTERATIONS IN URINARY ELIMINATION

Alterations in urinary elimination can result from changes in the intake and output of fluids, obstructions to the flow of urine, changes in the secretion of antidiuretic hormone (ADH), and changes in blood volume or blood pressure.

Alterations Related to Fluids

The average person takes in approximately 2600 mL of fluid each day: 1200 mL from drinking, 1100 mL from the water content of food, and 300 mL from metabolism. An increase or decrease in fluid intake results in a parallel increase or decrease in urine output.

Healthy individuals rarely experience decreases in urine output because they take in more fluids whenever they are thirsty. Individuals who are ill, however, may experience decreases in urine output because they are unable to respond to thirst, their intake is limited due to testing that requires NPO preparations, or their IV fluid intake is insufficient to balance fluid losses.

Fluid is lost from the body not only through urine, but also through respiration, perspiration, and feces. On a daily basis, most individuals lose approximately 2400 mL of fluid: 1500 mL through urine output, 200 mL through respiration, 600 mL through perspiration, and 100 mL through the elimination of feces. Individuals who are ill may also lose fluids through vomiting, bleeding, wound drainage, and suctioning/decompression.

Alterations Related to Obstructions

A decrease in the output of urine may also be caused by an obstruction (tumor, clot, tissue hypertrophy) to the flow of urine from the bladder. If the obstruction is great enough, the bladder does not empty completely. Instead, it retains fluid and, over time, becomes distended. Individuals who have urinary outlet obstructions experience the need to void more frequently. When they do void, however, they eliminate only very small amounts of urine.

Alterations Related to Aldosterone and Antidiuretic Hormone

Changes in the secretion of ADH and aldosterone also alter urine output since these hormones control the amount of water that is reabsorbed in the distal renal tubules and collecting ducts. Common factors that increase the secretion of ADH and aldosterone and reduce urine output include the physiologic stress response to accidental or surgical trauma, pain, hemorrhage, decreased cardiac output, anesthesia, and drugs, such as morphine and barbiturates. Factors that reduce the secretion of ADH and thus increase urine output include alcohol, caffeine, cold, and disease states and medications such as diuretics.

Alterations Related to Changes in Blood Volume

Because the production of urine is influenced by the volume of blood perfused to the kidneys, decreases in perfusion lead to reduction in the output of urine. Hemorrhage, dehydration, and shock reduce the flow of blood to the kidneys and cause decreased glomerular filtrate. If the volume of filtrate is reduced substantially, oliguria, or even anuria and accumulation of nitrogenous wastes (azotemia), may occur.

Other factors that may increase or decrease urine production include pathophysiologic states of the kidneys or other body systems, drugs, treatment modalities, diet, and metabolic rate.

Alterations in Disease States

Urinary outlet diversion is required when the bladder is obstructed or has been removed due to disease or trauma. Diversion can be created anywhere along the urinary pathway, and is named for the structure involved in the diversion. The most common urinary diversion is the ileal conduit, named because it uses the ileum of the bowel to form the conduit. A segment of the ileum close to the ileocecal valve is resected with its mesentery intact to create the conduit. The proximal end of this segment is closed and the distal segment is brought out through the lower quadrant of the abdominal wall to form the stoma. The ureters are anastomosed to the ileal segment at the proximal end or side of the conduit. This type of diversion is an incontinent urinary diversion. Clients with incontinent diversions must wear a pouch for urine collection.

TABLE 22-2 Urine Exam: What to Look For

Urine color: pale yellow to amber
Clarity and odor: clear with minimal odor
Urine pH: 4.5–8
Urine specific gravity: 1.005–1.020
Protein, glucose, and ketone bodies
Urine sediment: abnormal; red and white blood cells, casts, crystals, and bacteria

Ileal reservoirs are continent diversions that do not require the use of a collection device. The ileal reservoir is created with valves that allow it to function as a "bladder," which is regularly emptied by client self-catheterization through the abdominal stoma.

The "neo bladder" is created by connecting the ureters to a segment of ileum that is connected to the urethra. The client has no stoma; therefore, no collection device is required. The "bladder" is emptied by timed voiding or urethral self-catheterization.

Alterations Related to Chronic Renal Failure

A number of disease states and socioeconomic factors place clients at risk for chronic renal failure. Nephron loss is irreversible as it progresses through five stages of deterioration marked by a declining glomerular filtration rate, glomerular leakage of protein into urine, and the retention of nitrogenous wastes in the blood (rise in the serum creatinine).

The presence of microalbuminuria (Stage 1) is the initial indicator to manage risk factors (e.g., diabetes and blood pressure control). With stage progression, proteinuria worsens and the glomerular filtration rate is reduced from a normal 120 to below 15 mL per minute (Stage 4). Unfortunately, the chronic decline in renal function is often asymptomatic until the client has reached this fourth stage when the kidneys are unable to maintain their homeostatic role and are unable to excrete wastes or excess water. It is at this stage that the client is usually referred to a nephrologist to prepare for lifelong renal replacement therapy (hemodialysis, peritoneal dialysis, or transplantation).

In the final fifth stage, the client has become uremic, having lost 90% of nephrons. The retention of nitrogenous wastes and loss of renal homeostatic processes alters all body system functions and is responsible for a constellation of signs and symptoms. *End-stage renal disease* is a term used for clients treated with dialysis or transplantation (renal replacement therapy), but does not actually define a stage of severity of renal disease.

NURSING INTERVENTIONS

The primary purpose for performing nursing interventions associated with urinary elimination is to maintain the integrity of the urinary system, which eliminates excess fluid and wastes and thereby promotes homeostasis.

Aseptic technique is essential whenever performing procedures that could introduce bacteria into the urinary tract. Handwashing, using sterile gloves, and maintaining a closed urinary collection system decrease the incidence of ascending bladder contamination and subsequent urinary tract infection. Maintaining aseptic technique throughout dialysis procedures is necessary to prevent infection in grafts, fistulae, and catheters.

Indwelling Catheters

Millions of Americans have bladder dysfunction every year. Twenty-five percent of these individuals are older adults in acute-care hospitals; 7% of clients are in long-term care facilities. Due to the dysfunction, they require urinary drainage systems (UDS) to drain and collect urine. The median time of UDS usage in home care is 3 to 4 years.

Preventing antibiotic resistance by avoiding catheter-associated urinary tract infections (CAUTIs):

- Unnecessary use and misuse of antibiotics leads to antibiotic resistance.
- CAUTIs comprise the largest institutional reservoir of antibiotic-resistance pathogens.
- Hospital-acquired urinary tract infections (UTIs) account for more than 40% of all hospital-acquired infections.
- More than 70% of HAIs are resistant to at least one of the drugs most commonly used to treat them.
- Clients infected with drug-resistant organisms are prone to longer hospitalization and require treatment with second or third choice drugs that may be less effective, more toxic, and/or are more expensive.
- Use of anti-infective Foley catheters with silver alloy coating and hydrogel decreases the incidence of CAUTIs.
- Use of the silver alloy coating and anti-infective catheters reduces the use of antibiotics by 40% to 50%.

Indwelling catheters are invasive devices with significant complications. Infection and encrustation are common. Long-term use of catheters provides access for bacteria from a contaminated environment. As a result, catheter-associated urinary tract infections (CAUTIs) occur. Eighty percent of infections are the result of *Escherichia coli*.

ADAPTATIONS FOR HOME CARE

Home care clients who require assistance with emptying their bladders are usually placed on intermittent clean catheterization protocols rather than having an indwelling catheter. This procedure assists in preventing penoscrotal abscess formation, overwhelming infection, and altered body image. Fluid intake needs to be monitored and restricted to 1500 mL per day to avoid bladder distention. If spontaneous voiding returns, frequency of catheterizations can be extended to every 12 hr and discontinued when the residual urine is consistently less than 100 mL in 24 hr.

When an indwelling catheter is used, it is important to be aware that it may lead to urinary tract infection. The nurse must teach the client and family to observe for signs and symptoms of urinary tract infections and sepsis. They should note odor, color, and consistency of the urine; burning pain; and flank pain. Catheter changes are the responsibility of the nurse and are usually performed once a month. Encouraging fluids becomes a major role assumed by family members and monitored by the nurse. Urinary antiseptics are adjunctive measures when catheterizations are required.

Home care dialysis is common in many areas of the country. The principles and procedures are similar to those in a hospital or free-standing dialysis unit. The major change is the advent of portable dialysis methods such as continuous ambulatory peritoneal dialysis (CAPD) and continuous cycling peritoneal dialysis (CCPD). These procedures allow individuals to participate in a normal lifestyle. However, use of these methods requires monitoring by the nurse and specific teaching of the essential components to prevent complications and promote health. Peritoneal dialysis (PD) reflects more normal kidney function than hemodialysis. Fluid and electrolytes are removed gradually and, therefore, clients have fewer complications with blood pressure alterations and disequilibrium syndrome. There are fewer dietary and fluid restrictions, allowing clients to lead a more normal life. PD provides the client with a more flexible schedule, allowing him or her to work, travel, and participate in activities. One major restriction, besides ensuring the ordered number of exchanges each day, is the monthly appointment at the dialysis center for lab work and consultation with the physician or nurse.

The catheter is placed in a dependent position in the peritoneal cavity to minimize the chance of catheter obstruction or erosion into other abdominal organs. The other end of the catheter is placed outside of the abdomen to decrease infections. There are several devices that are placed around the catheter that prevent fluid leak from the peritoneal cavity. These devices impede the migration of bacteria.

There are three types of PD: continuous ambulatory peritoneal dialysis (CAPD), continuous cycling peritoneal dialysis (CCPD), and intermittent peritoneal dialysis (IPD). The two most common types for home care clients are CAPD and CCPD.

CAPD does not require a machine and can be done almost anywhere that is clean and well lighted. The client performs 4–5 exchanges daily that take approximately 30–45 minutes for each exchange. Each exchange allows a prescribed amount of a dextrose solution, termed *dialysate*, 1500–2000 mL for adults, to flow into the abdomen. The dialysate remains in the abdomen, called dwell time, for approximately 4 hr, and then it is drained out of the abdomen for about 10 minutes. The last exchange of the day is before bedtime. The dialysate remains in the abdomen overnight.

CCPD requires a portable machine that connects to the catheter and automatically fills and drains the dialysate from the abdomen at night while the client sleeps. This procedure usually takes 10–12 hr every night.

IPD is similar to CAPD except that it is done for about 10 hr each day for 3–4 days each week. The exchanges take place hourly, with approximately 2 liters of fluid for each exchange. This type of dialysis is usually done in an outpatient setting.

CULTURAL AWARENESS

- African-Americans have a more rapid decline in glomerular filtration rate than do Caucasians.
- Hypertensive African-Americans have decreased renal excretion of sodium, making sodium restriction an important factor in treatment.
- Hypertension, diabetes, and end-stage renal disease (ESRD) are 3–4 times more common in African-Americans and American Indians than in Caucasians.

NURSING DIAGNOSES

The following nursing diagnoses may be appropriate to use on client care plans when the components are related to promoting urine elimination.

NURSING DIAGNOSIS	RELATED FACTORS
Disturbed Body Image	Alteration in body appearance, urinary diversion stoma, use of appliance, catheter presence, fear of rejection, psychosocial factors
Ineffective Coping	Poor adjustment to illness or treatment, chronic disease state Inadequate knowledge base, denial of health status, cultural or spiritual beliefs
Deficient Fluid Volume	Increased urine output, decreased fluid intake
Excess Fluid Volume	Decreased urine output, renal system dysfunction, decreased cardiac output
Infection, Risk for	Vascular access site, altered immunity, urine retention, presence of catheter, malnutrition
Noncompliance	Inadequate knowledge base, inability to manage equipment for irrigation, denial of health status, cultural or spiritual beliefs
Impaired Urinary Elimination	Inability to retain urine related to stress, surgery, anatomical or functional problems, infection, motor or sensory impairment
Stress Urinary Incontinence	Inability to retain urine related to stress, surgery, anatomical or functional problems, infection, motor or sensory impairment
Urinary Retention	Inability to void, bladder distention or atony, surgical repair

CLEANSE HANDS The single most important nursing action to decrease the incidence of hospital-based infections is hand hygiene. *Remember to wash your hands or use antibacterial gel before and after each and every client contact.*

IDENTIFY CLIENT Before every procedure, introduce yourself and check two forms of client identification, not including room number. These actions prevent errors and conform to The Joint Commission standards.

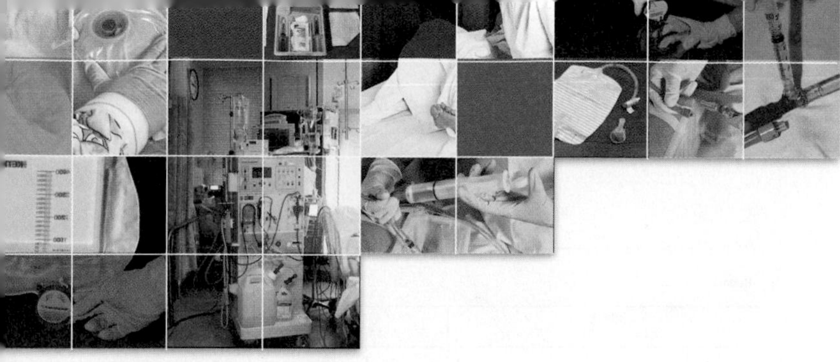

Chapter 22

UNIT 1

Intake and Output

Nursing Process Data

ASSESSMENT Data Base

- Assess whether strict measurement of intake and output is ordered.
- Assess client's ability to assist in keeping intake and output record.
- Assess all potential sources of intake (e.g., IVs, oral fluids, tube feeding) and output (e.g., urine, emesis, diarrhea, drainage from tubes).
- Observe color, clarity, and odor of urine.
- Assess for signs of dehydration or fluid excess.
- Evaluate weight changes (most accurate assessment of fluid balance).

PLANNING Objectives

- To accurately measure all sources of fluid intake
- To accurately measure all sources of fluid output
- To identify alterations in fluid balance
- To record data on appropriate records

IMPLEMENTATION Procedures

EVALUATION Expected Outcomes

- All sources of fluid intake and output are recorded.
- Client's intake and output balance.

Pearson Nursing Student Resources

Find additional review materials at **nursing.pearsonhighered.com**

Prepare for success with NCLEX®-style practice questions and Skill Checklists

Measuring Intake and Output

Equipment

I&O bedside form
Client's own graduated container
Bedpan, urinal, or underseat basin for toilet ("hat")
Hourly inline urine measurement device for client requiring frequent monitoring
Clean gloves

Preparation

1. Perform hand hygiene
2. Explain purpose of keeping I&O record to client.
3. Instruct client to keep record of all fluids taken orally. Keep an I&O record at the bedside for the client to document intake.
4. Instruct client to void into bedpan, urinal, or underseat basin for toilet.
5. Instruct client not to place toilet tissue in bedpan or defecate in bedpan.

Procedure

Fluid Intake

1. Measure all fluid intake (including oral, IV, fluid medications, and tube feedings) according to hospital values (e.g., cup = 150 mL, glass = 240 mL).
2. Record time and amount of fluids in the appropriate space on bedside form.
3. Check bedside I&O record for approximate amounts of fluid containers.
4. Total 8-hr fluid intake on bedside I&O record.
5. Complete 24-hr intake record by adding together all three 8-hr totals.

Fluid Output

1. Don clean gloves to measure output from all sources.
2. Empty urinal, bedpan, or drainage bag into client's graduated container. ▸ ***Rationale:*** Measurement is only approximate from drainage bag or "hat." (Include other sources of output such as drainage, diarrheal stools, draining wounds, or emesis on output record.)
3. To drain urine collection bag:
   a. Use client's individual (labeled) graduated receptacle.
   b. Slide port opener clockwise to allow urine to drain.
   c. Turn port opener counterclockwise to close.

If using drainage tube with plastic clips:

a. Raise drainage tube to drain urine into collection bag.
b. Hold bag over receptacle, squeeze green plastic pieces together gently. The clips will come out off edge of holder.

BEDSIDE INTAKE AND OUTPUT RECORD

Name ______________ Date ________

Room # ______

	Intake			Output		
	Oral	IV		Urine	Emesis	Drainage
7 am – 3 pm			7 am – 3 pm			
Total			Total			
3 pm – 11 pm			3 pm – 11 pm			
Total			Total			
11 pm – 7 am			11 pm – 7 am			
Total			Total			
24hr Total			24hr Total			

Measurements

Glass 240cc
Cup 150cc
Bowl 150cc
Juice Glass 100cc
Coffee Pot 240cc

Ice Cream 100cc
Jello 100cc
Ice Chips 5cc/Cube

▲ Bedside intake and output record.

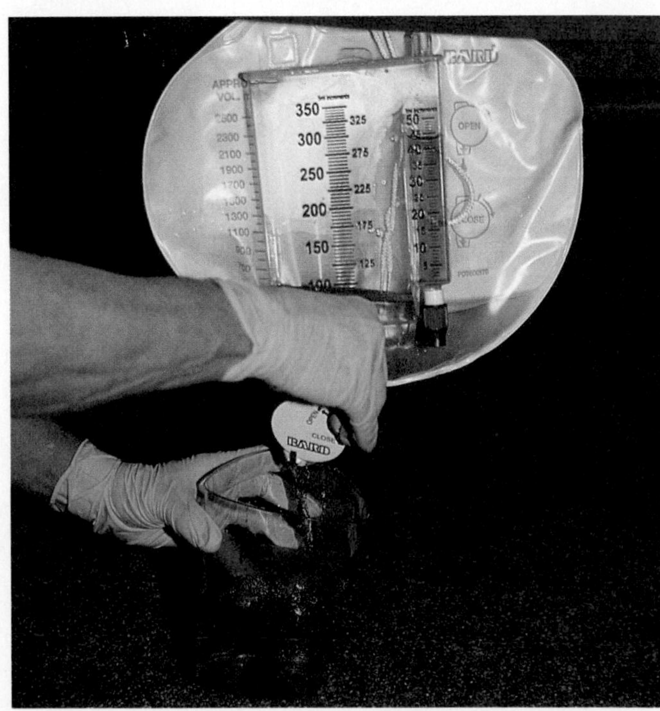

▲ Empty urinal, bedpan, or Foley drainage bag into clients individual (labeled) graduate and note amount of urine.

c. Slide green tube out of holder and point into receptacle.
d. Open metal clamp by pushing down on bottom metal pieces and wait until all urine has drained from bag.
e. Close clamp by pressing metal pieces together. Listen for click sound. ▶ ***Rationale:*** Clamp is now closed.
f. Clip drainage tube back into holder.

4. Remove gloves and perform hand hygiene.
5. Record time and amount of output on bedside I&O record.
6. Complete 24-hr output record by adding together all intermediate output totals during that 24-hr period, and place total on graphic sheet.
7. Notify physician of any significant imbalance; more intensive monitoring may be indicated.

Clinical Alert

Hourly urine output less than 30 mL/hr for 2 consecutive hours or 24-hr urine output less than 500 mL can indicate dehydration or internal bleeding and can result in acute renal failure.

Methods to Stimulate Voiding

- Have client drink a cup of hot fluid such as coffee or tea.
- Run water in sink.
- Massage the lower abdomen.
- Place a hot washcloth on the abdomen.
- Pour warm water over the perineum with client positioned on toilet or bedpan.
- Obtain order for sitz bath.
- Put oil of wintergreen on a cotton ball in the bedpan or urinal.

Clinical Alert

Use client's own graduated receptacle when measuring output. Change gloves and perform hand hygiene between each client. The CDC calls for decontamination of hands after removing gloves. Gloves should also be *changed* and hands decontaminated when moving from a contaminated body site to a clean one on the same client.

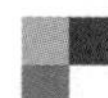

DOCUMENTATION for Intake and Output

- Time and amount of all oral fluid intake
- 8-hr totals of all IV and enteral fluids
- 24-hr total of all fluid intake
- Time and amount of all urinary output
- Time and amount of all drainage (e.g., NG)
- 8-hr totals of all fluid output
- 24-hr total of all fluid output

CRITICAL THINKING Application

Expected Outcomes

- All sources of fluid intake and output are recorded.
- Client's intake and output balance.

Unexpected Outcomes	Alternative Actions
Client voids in toilet.	• Document "voided in toilet" on I&O record. • Review instructions for accurate I&O monitoring with client. • Post sign above toilet: "All urine must be measured and recorded." • Place "hat" receptacle in toilet.
Family members obtain fluids for client without notifying staff.	• Post sign indicating need to record all fluid intake. • Remind family of importance of I&O monitoring; provide cups with measured increments and paper for them to record fluids given (unless fluids are restricted).

Fluid intake and output do not balance (intake greater than output).	• Initiate daily weight measurement (weigh before breakfast, after voiding, same scale, same clothing). • Compare losses or gains with client's daily weight measurement. • Fluid intake and output generally are relatively equal (assuming numbers are accurate). Output should be about 500 mL less per 24 hr due to insensible fluid loss. • Determine whether treatment goal is to rehydrate or diurese the client. • Use graduated container to accurately measure output in "hat." • Search for sources of unmeasured output (fever, wound drainage, diarrhea).
Fluid output is greater than intake.	• Analyze whether treatment goal (rehydration, diuresis) has been achieved. • Reposition client cautiously, monitoring for possible orthostatic hypotension. • Identify when "dry weight" has been achieved (intake balances output after therapy received). • Search for sources of unrecorded intake (family offerings, flush solutions, ice chips, full-liquid foods).

Chapter 22

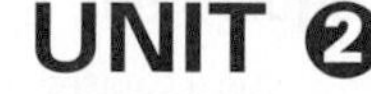

UNIT 2

External Urine Collection System

Nursing Process Data

ASSESSMENT Data Base

- Assess that client is able to empty bladder completely and spontaneously.
- Assess the genital area for signs of irritation and edema during the use of condom catheter for urine collection.
- Assess activity level of client to determine when a leg bag or a continuous drainage system is necessary.

PLANNING Objectives

- To provide a means for managing incontinence
- To provide a means of collecting urine in a system that allows client ambulation
- To prevent skin breakdown due to incontinence of urine
- To prevent urinary tract infections in clients who are at risk and require a method of urine collection

IMPLEMENTATION Procedures

EVALUATION Expected Outcomes

- Client remains dry with condom catheter for urine collection.
- Skin irritation does not occur with condom catheter use.

Pearson Nursing Student Resources

Find additional review materials at **nursing.pearsonhighered.com**

Prepare for success with NCLEX®-style practice questions and Skill Checklists

Applying a Condom Catheter for Urine Collection

Equipment

Soap, water, towel, washcloth
Commercial condom catheter; select appropriate size
Leg bag or bedside drainage system
Skin barrier prep
Clean gloves
Drape
Scissors

Preparation

1. Check physician's orders and client care plan.
2. Gather equipment.
3. Identify client and explain procedure.
4. Perform hand hygiene and provide privacy.
5. Raise bed and lower side rail on working side of bed. Place client flat supine.
6. Don clean gloves.
7. Drape for privacy.
8. Wash genital area with soap and water, and dry area thoroughly. (If client is uncircumcised, gently attempt to retract foreskin, cleanse shaft beneath it, then replace foreskin to normal position.)
9. Clip hair from base of penis if necessary. ▸ ***Rationale:*** To avoid catching in adhesive strip.

Procedure

1. When commercial condom catheter is used, apply protective coating to skin on penile shaft and allow to dry completely (60 seconds).
2. If adhesive strip is required, peel off paper from one side of the adhesive strip according to product instructions. Spirally wrap the adhesive strip around the penile shaft starting behind the glans, then peel outer paper from adhesive strip.

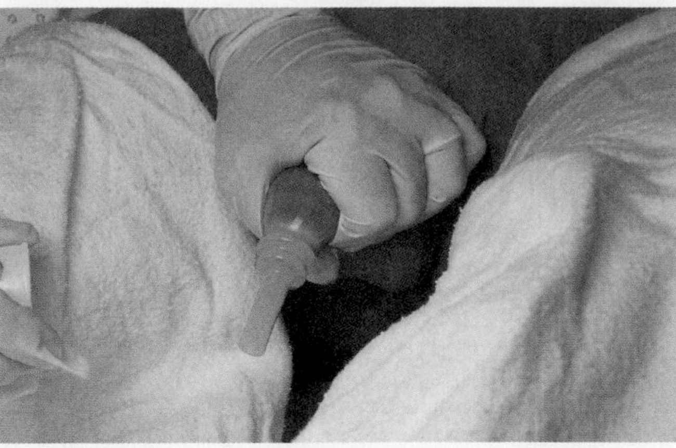

▲ After unrolling condom onto penis, apply pressure to ensure smooth fit.

3. Take the condom catheter and place the prerolled sheath so funnel is against the glans, but *not* rubbing it.
4. Unroll the condom up the penis until it is completely over the adhesive strip.
5. Gently squeeze condom against strip to seal it after sheath is completely rolled over the penis. Do not wrinkle as wrinkles cause urine to leak through catheter.
6. Clip rolled portion of condom if necessary to prevent constriction at base of penis.
7. Connect condom to a drainage system. The drainage system can be a leg bag or a bedside drainage system depending on activity level and condition of client.
8. Lower bed, and raise side rail and/or assist client out of bed if he is to be ambulated.
9. Remove gloves and perform hand hygiene.
10. Assess penis 30 minutes after condom applied to check for edema, discoloration, and urine flow. ▸ ***Rationale:*** This detects complication with application.

Attaching Urine Collection Condom Catheter to Leg Bag

Equipment

Leg bag with Velcro straps (or stockinette to secure bag)
Antimicrobial swabs
Clean gloves

Preparation

1. Obtain order for leg bag from physician.
2. Gather equipment.
3. Identify client and explain procedure.
4. Provide privacy.
5. Raise bed, and lower side rail on working side of bed.
6. Perform hand hygiene and don clean gloves.

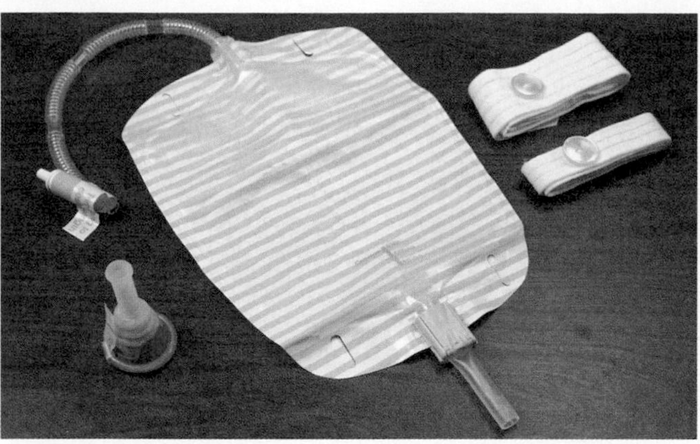

▲ Leg bag with Velcro straps to secure to leg.

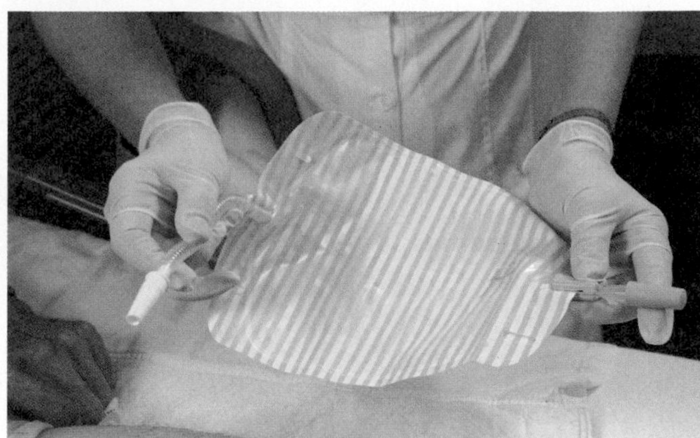

▲ Connect longer tube from leg bag to condom catheter.

Procedure

1. Remove protective cap from connecting tube on top of leg bag.
2. Disconnect drainage tubing from indwelling or condom catheter.
3. Cap bedside drainage tubing end with protective cap from leg bag. ▶ ***Rationale:*** To maintain sterility of connecting parts.
4. Wipe leg bag and catheter connectors with swab, if not already sterile.
5. Connect tip of leg bag into catheter.
6. Secure leg bag to thigh by placing Velcro strap through bag and around leg. Alternately, secure with stockinette.
7. When removing leg bag, disconnect catheter from leg bag and wipe each connection end with antimicrobial wipes.
8. Take leg bag cap off drainage tubing and replace it onto leg bag.
9. Connect catheter to bedside drainage tubing.
10. Lower bed and raise upper side rails.
11. Rinse leg bag in warm soap and water, and place in bathroom to dry.
12. Remove gloves and perform hand hygiene.

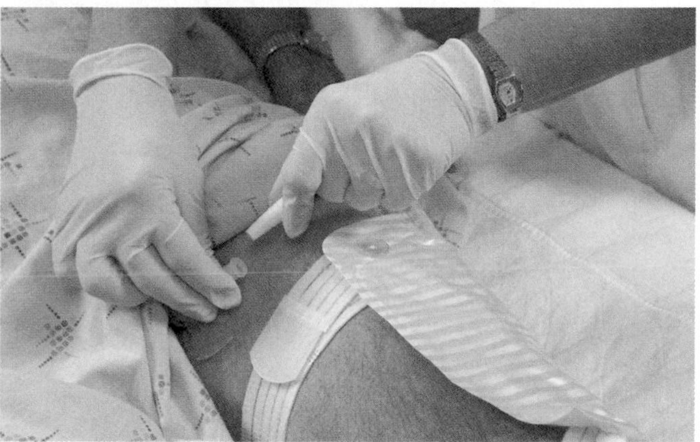

▲ Maintain sterility when placing the tip of leg bag into condom catheter.

Clinical Alert

Use of an external urine collection system is recommended for incontinent men without urine retention. These devices are comfortable, and there is less chance of a urinary tract infection than with indwelling catheters.

DOCUMENTATION for External Urine Collection System

- Type and size of condom catheter applied
- Condition of genital area
- Protective coating (prep) applied to skin
- Type of drainage collection device attached
- Amount, color, and odor of urine obtained
- Client's tolerance of procedure and ability to perform self-care

CRITICAL THINKING Application

Expected Outcomes

- Client remains dry with condom catheter for urine collection.
- Skin irritation does not occur with condom catheter use.

Unexpected Outcomes	Alternative Actions
Condom catheter leaks.	• Use smaller size condom to provide *wrinkle-free* fit. • Replace adhesive strips for better condom adherence. • Make sure penis is thoroughly dry before applying condom system. • Ensure that drainage collection system is dependent of condom tubing to promote gravity flow. • Consider using a retracted penis pouch.
Penis becomes reddened with condom catheter use.	• Remove condom. • Notify wound care specialist/physician for topical medication order. • Apply adult brief and change frequently until problem resolves. • Make sure penis is clean and dry and protective coating is applied before condom application. • Clip rolled portion of condom to prevent constriction at base of penis.

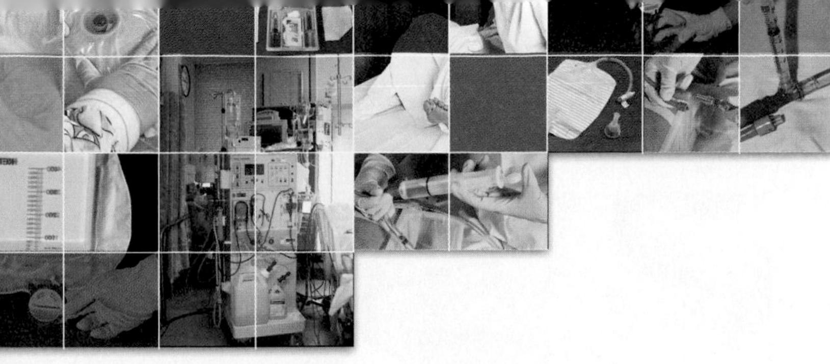

Chapter 22

UNIT 3

Catheterization

Nursing Process Data

ASSESSMENT Data Base

- Assess the client's bladder for distention.
- Assess purpose of catheterization or urine output monitoring.
- Check physician's orders for method of catheterization to be done.
- Assess urinary meatus for exudate or inflammation.
- Assess character and amount of urine.
- Note client's I&O balance.

PLANNING Objectives

- To prevent or relieve discomfort due to bladder distention
- To promote urinary elimination
- To obtain a sterile urine specimen
- To instill medication or provide continuous urinary bladder drainage
- To provide bladder irrigation
- To measure the amount of residual urine (post void)
- To monitor the output of a critically ill client

IMPLEMENTATION Procedures

EVALUATION Expected Outcomes

- Catheterization is avoided with use of bladder scanner.
- Sterile technique is maintained throughout catheterization procedure.
- Catheter enters bladder as evidenced by urine outflow.
- Client remains free of urine leakage around retention catheter.
- Urinary tract infection does not occur secondary to catheterization.

Pearson Nursing Student Resources

Find additional review materials at **nursing.pearsonhighered.com**

Prepare for success with NCLEX®-style practice questions and Skill Checklists

Using a Bladder Scanner

Equipment

Ultrasound BladderScan device
Ultrasound conducting gel
Tissues

Preparation

1. Check physician's order to evaluate client's bladder.
2. Identify client and explain procedure and purpose.
3. If female, ask client if she has had a hysterectomy or is pregnant. If a hysterectomy is not documented, and settings are adjusted appropriately, results may be inaccurate. ▸ ***Rationale:*** Scanner is not indicated for pregnant clients.
4. Provide privacy.
5. Determine time and amount of last void or assist client to empty bladder if residual volume is to be evaluated.
6. Determine that client does not have an indwelling catheter. ▸ ***Rationale:*** Scanner reflects off the catheter bulb, giving an echo reading.
7. Perform hand hygiene.
8. Place client flat and supine, and palpate client's bladder to locate appropriate site.

Procedure

1. Turn the device on and press "SCAN."
2. Apply conducting gel to scanner head.
3. Select MALE or FEMALE mode on scan unit. Select *MALE MODE* if female client has had a hysterectomy.
4. Fanfold linens to expose client's suprapubic area.

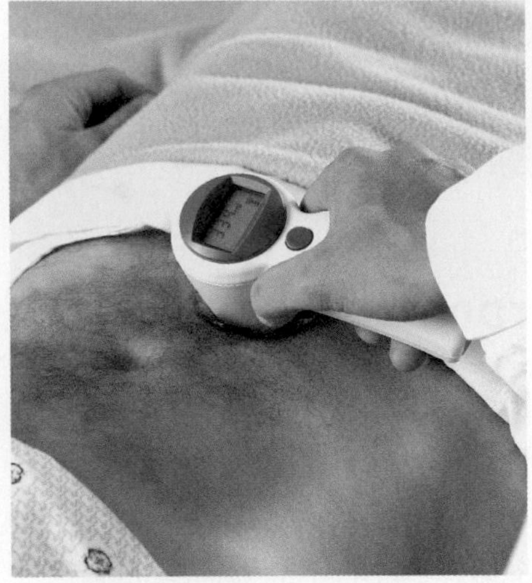

▲ Handheld portable untrasound bladder scanner.

5. Place head of scanner 3 cm above client's symphysis pubis, directed toward the bladder, and align the icon.
6. Press scan head button and hold scanner still until a beep is heard.
7. Scan until bladder image is lined up on cross-hairs.
8. Take several scans at different angles and press DONE when finished.
9. Press PRINT for a printout of client's bladder volume in milliliters.
10. Wipe gel from client's skin.
11. Reposition client for comfort.
12. Wipe ultrasound probe with antiseptic solution.
13. Perform hand hygiene.

Draping a Female Client

Equipment

Bath blanket

Procedure

1. Bring bath blanket to bedside.
2. Identify client, and explain procedure.
3. Provide privacy.
4. Perform hand hygiene.
5. Place bed in HIGH position, and lower side rail nearest you.
6. Place bath blanket over client's top linen so that one corner of the blanket is pointed toward the client's head to form a diamond shape over the client.
7. Instruct client to hold onto bath blanket. Fanfold linen to foot of bed and place on chair.

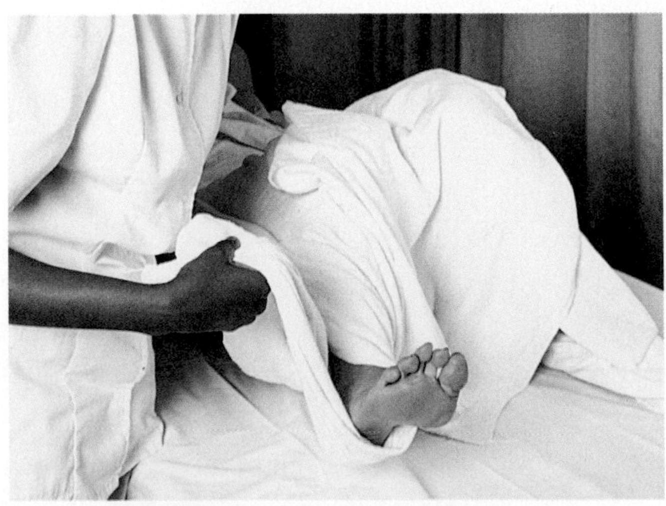

▲ Use bath blanket to drape client before catheterization.

8. Request that client flex knees and keep them apart with feet firmly on bed.
9. Wrap lateral corners of bath blanket around feet in a spiral fashion until they are completely covered.
10. The corner of the blanket between knees and extending over perineum can later be folded back over the abdomen. ▸ ***Rationale:*** Draping provides for warmth and prevents unnecessary exposure of genital area until procedure is performed.

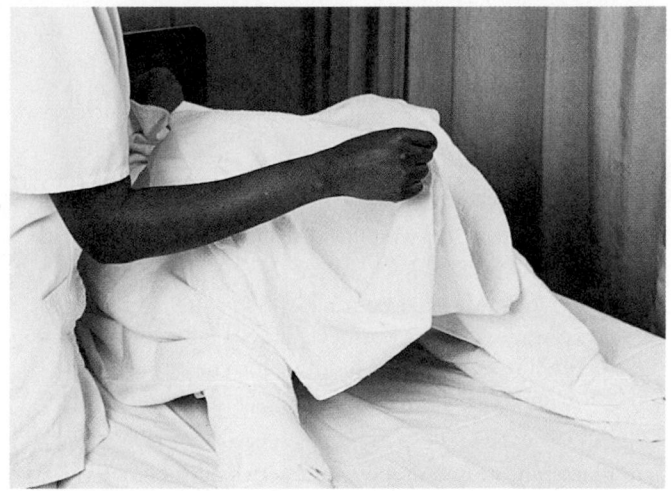

▲ Corner of blanket is folded back over abdomen to expose perineum.

Inserting a Straight Catheter (Female)

Equipment

Disposable catheterization tray with straight catheter (14 Fr), and specimen cup. Determine type of catheter to use. See Table 22-3, page 776.

Biohazard specimen transport bag

Bath blanket or turn sheet

Additional light source, if needed

If necessary for cleansing, towel, washcloth, basin with warm water and soap

Clean gloves

NOTE: If bladder scanner is not available, this skill may be indicated after client voids to determine residual volume.

Preparation

1. Bring equipment to client's room.

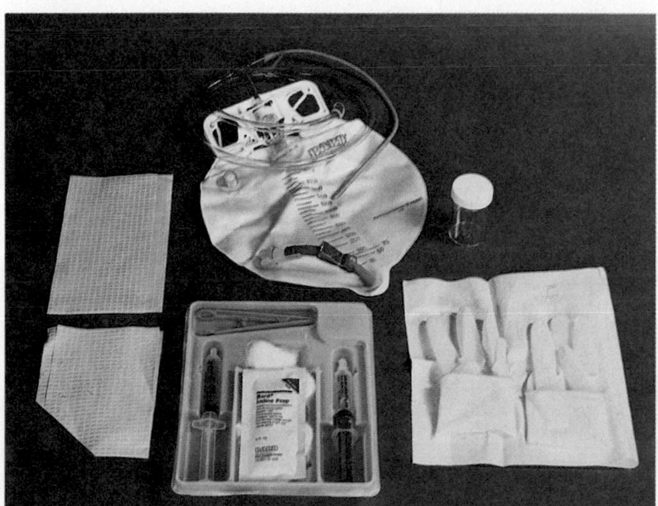

▲ Disposable kit includes equipment necessary for performing a catheterization. (Retention catheter/Foley is shown above).

2. Check lighting source.
3. Identify client, and explain procedure and need for client to keep knees positioned during procedure.
4. Provide privacy.
5. Perform hand hygiene.
6. Place bed in HIGH position, and lower side rail on working side.
7. Fold linens to foot of bed and cover client's lower body with bath blanket drape.
8. Provide perineal care, if necessary, with soap and water using clean gloves. Dry perineum thoroughly.
9. Discard towels and water and replace basin.
10. Dispose of gloves and perform hand hygiene.
11. Drape the client (see Draping a Female Client).
12. Have client bring knees up and out. May need assistance to keep knees in this position. ▸ ***Rationale:*** This position provides for good visualization of urinary meatus.
13. Fold up bath blanket drape corner to expose perineum.
14. Adjust light source to ensure that meatus is adequately visualized.

EVIDENCE-BASED PRACTICE

Regaining Voiding Ability

In hip surgery patients, those receiving intermittent catheterization regained satisfactory voiding quicker than those with an indwelling catheter.

Source: Cravens, D., & Zweig, S. (2000). Urinary catheter management. *American Family Physician, 61*(2), 369–375.

Procedure

1. Open sterile catheter set package by tearing the package on the lined edge of plastic wrap. Place plastic wrap at foot of bed for waste disposal.
2. Place catheter set on bed between client's legs.
3. Fold back drape to expose perineum.
4. Open white outer wrap away from sterile package with last turn toward client.
5. Remove sterile absorbent pad, and position plastic side down under client's buttocks. Have client lift buttocks if able. Position pad by holding corners of pad only. ▶ ***Rationale:*** Pad creates a sterile field.
6. Put on sterile gloves.
7. Place fenestrated drape over client's perineum, exposing meatus (optional).
8. Place tray on sterile field, which may be enlarged by utilizing sterile wrapping, with care not to contaminate sterile field.
9. Open package, and pour antiseptic solution over cotton balls or open package of antiseptic-soaked swabs with stick ends up, according to hospital policy.
10. Uncap syringe filled with lubricant, or tear open lubricant package, pick up catheter tip, and lubricate the tip of the catheter generously. ▶ ***Rationale:*** Removing catheter from sterile container (tray) increases risk of contamination.
11. If specimen is required, uncap sterile specimen container.
12. Move catheter tray close to client on sterile field.
13. Prep client's meatus according to hospital policy.
    a. Separate the client's labia minora with your nondominant hand (maintain separation throughout prep).
    b. With your dominant hand, *use forceps* to pick up an absorbent ball that has been saturated with antiseptic solution. (If Betadine swabs are used, pick up one swab.)
    c. Cleanse client's meatus using the procedure in the above note, or with one downward stroke of forceps or swab. ▶ ***Rationale:*** Using a downward stroke cleans from least contaminated to most contaminated area.
    d. Discard absorbent ball or swab in the plastic cover at foot of bed. ▶ ***Rationale:*** Using a new cotton ball or swab with each downward stroke prevents transfer of microorganisms.
    e. Repeat Step c at least three to four times.
    f. Continue to hold client's labia apart until you insert catheter. ▶ ***Rationale:*** This prevents contamination of urinary meatus.
14. Using sterile gloved hand, pick up lubricated catheter, keeping drainage end in collection container, and insert 2 in. or until urine begins to flow.
15. Move nondominant hand from holding labia open to hold catheter in place.

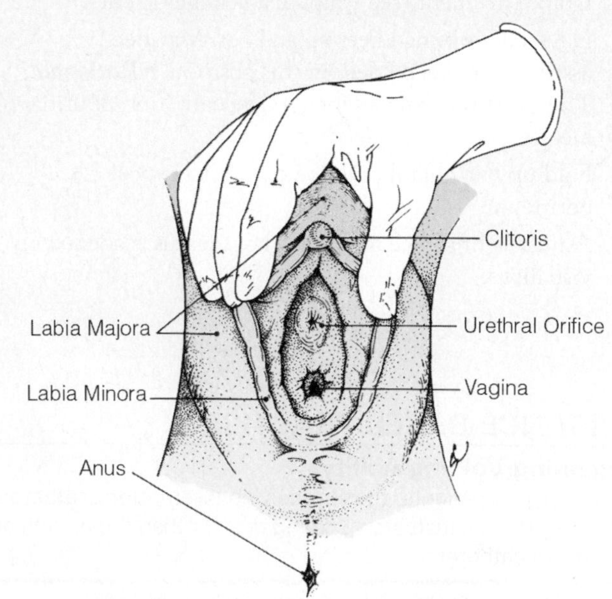

▲ Anatomical view of female perineal area showing urethral orifice.

Estimating Bladder Fullness

- The bladder is not normally palpable until it contains more than 150 mL of urine.
- Normally, suprapubic percussion produces a hollow sound. A dull or flat sound indicates bladder distention.
- A bulge may be noted in the suprapubic area when the bladder contains 500 mL.
- Pain is often felt after bladder capacity has been reached, commonly after 400–500 mL.
- Subjective symptoms are not reliable indicators of bladder fullness.

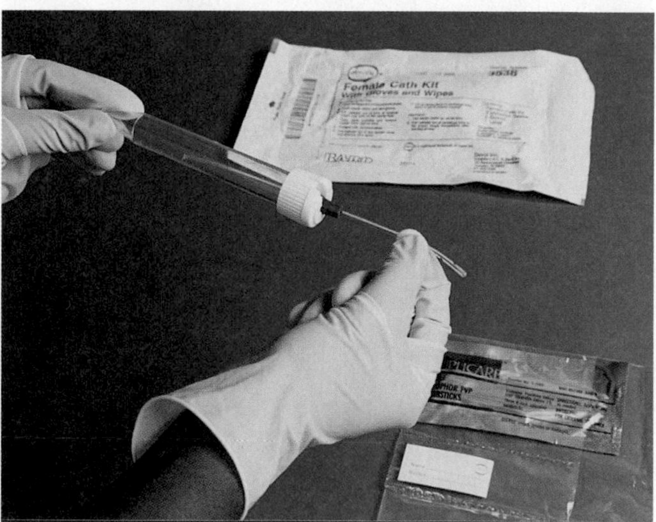

▲ Female mini-catheter used to obtain sterile urine specimen.

16. Instruct client to take a deep breath. While client is exhaling, insert catheter. ▸ ***Rationale:*** Sphincter will relax, decreasing discomfort and resistance to insertion of catheter.
17. Place sterile specimen container under drainage end of catheter if specimen is needed, and fill container with approximately 30 mL of urine.
18. Replace catheter drainage end into collection container, and allow urine to flow until it ceases.
19. Pinch catheter closed when urine ceases to flow, and remove gently and slowly.
20. Remove drapes and dry the perineum.
21. Position client for comfort, put the bed in LOW position with the upper side rails raised.
22. Measure and record urine output on I&O bedside record.
23. Discard gloves and equipment appropriately.
24. Perform hand hygiene.
25. Label specimen, place in transport bag, and send to lab.
26. Document procedure.

EVIDENCE-BASED PRACTICE

Expert opinions indicate there is no advantage in using antiseptic preparation for cleansing the urethra before catheter insertion. Urethral trauma and discomfort will be minimized by cleansing with sterile, single-use lubricant or anesthetic gel.

Source: Dunn, S., Pretty, L., Reid, H., & Evans, D. (2000). *Management of Short Term Indwelling Urethral Catheters to Prevent Urinary Tract Infection: A Systematic Review.* Adelaide, Australia: The Joanna Briggs Institute For Evidence Based Nursing.

Inserting a Straight Catheter (Male)

Equipment

Same as for Inserting a Straight Catheter (Female)

15–20 mL, 2% lidocaine gel for lubricant, if ordered

Preparation

1. Follow Steps 1 through 6 in Inserting a Straight Catheter (Female).
2. Place client in a supine position with knees slightly apart. ▸ ***Rationale:*** This position relaxes abdominal and perineal muscles.
3. Drape client by placing a bath blanket or draw sheet over chest area and fanfold top linen down to cover lower extremities, exposing only genital area.
4. Don clean gloves, and wash genital area if necessary.
5. Remove gloves and perform hand hygiene.

Procedure

1. Open sterile package by tearing the package on the lined edge of plastic wrap. Place plastic wrap at foot of bed for waste disposal.
2. Place sterile kit at client's side near thigh.
3. Open outer wrap away from sterile package.
4. Don sterile gloves.
5. Place first drape over thighs and under penis.
6. Place fenestrated drape over penis.
7. Open antiseptic package and pour solution over cotton balls or open package of antiseptic-soaked swabs with stick ends up, according to hospital policy.
8. Open lubricant packet or syringe—eject onto prep tray, unless using procedure in Step 13b of procedure Inserting a Straight Catheter (Female) on page 774.
9. If specimen is required, uncap the specimen container.
10. Hold penis upright with your nondominant hand.

Clinical Alert

A Coudé or 12-Fr catheter may be easier to insert if the client has an obstruction.

11. With your dominant hand, use forceps to pick up cotton ball saturated with antiseptic solution or pick up Betadine swab.
12. Cleanse meatus with circular expanding stroke using cotton ball or swab. Discard cotton ball or swab into plastic bag at foot of bed.
13. Repeat circular cleansing motion prep around tip of penis. Cleanse three times using a new cotton ball or swab each time.
14. Continue to hold penis with your nondominant hand.
15. Discard forceps into plastic bag.
16. Lubricate catheter about 3–4 in. using generous amount of lubricant.
17. *Alternate Method:* Insert tip of lubricant syringe at urethral opening and instill lubricant (or 2% lidocaine gel if ordered) directly into urethra. (If cath tray does not have syringe, place sterile syringe on tray before gloving.) ▸ ***Rationale:*** Lidocaine gel facilitates catheter placement by expanding, anesthetizing, and lubricating the urethra.
18. Pick up catheter with sterile gloved hand about 8–10 cm (3–4 in.) from tip of catheter.
19. Lift penis to a 90° angle (perpendicular to body) and exert slight traction by pulling upward. ▸ ***Rationale:*** This

movement straightens the urethra for easier insertion of catheter.

20. Instruct client to take a deep breath and while client is exhaling, insert catheter. ▸ ***Rationale:*** Sphincter will relax, decreasing discomfort and resistance to insertion of catheter.
21. Insert catheter about 24.5 cm (10–12 in.) or until urine is obtained.
22. If catheter meets resistance, decrease angle of penis to 45° or less, and ask client to take a deep breath. ▸ ***Rationale:*** Taking a deep breath helps relax external sphincter. If persistent resistance is felt and catheter cannot be inserted without difficulty, remove catheter and notify physician.
23. Fill sterile specimen container from drainage end of catheter if specimen is needed.
24. Pinch tubing, and transfer end of catheter into collection container.
25. Allow urine to drain into collection container until flow stops.
26. Remove catheter, and place lid on specimen bottle.

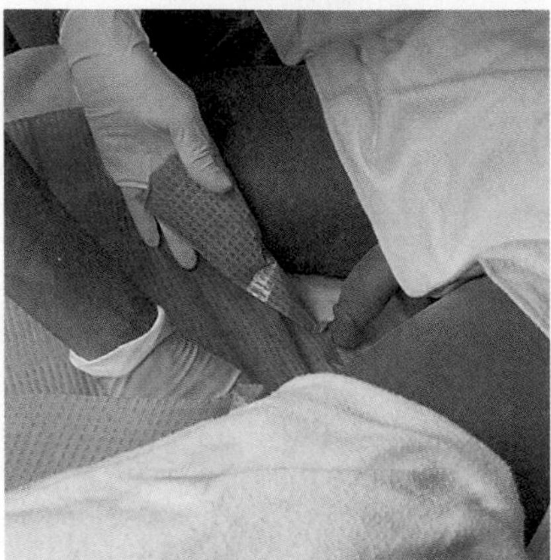

1 Place absorbent pad, with plastic side down, under penis to establish sterile field.

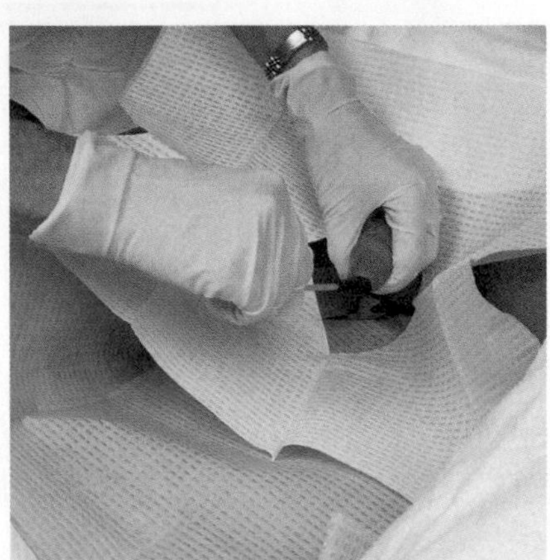

2 Prep head of penis, starting at meatus and cleansing outward in a circular motion.

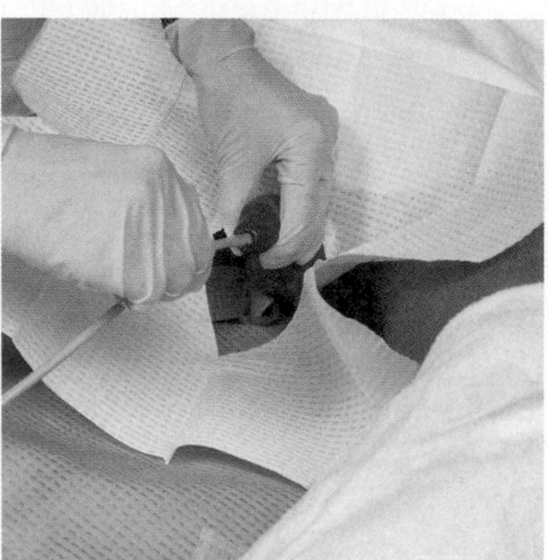

3 Insert amply lubricated catheter 10–12 inches.

TABLE 22-3 Types of Catheters

Latex	Rubber, ideal for forming the core of an indwelling catheter, due to its flexibility. Comfortable for client. Can cause urethral trauma. Latex swells as it absorbs body fluids.
100% Silicone	Larger drainage lumen due to having a coating. Biocompatible with urethra mucosa and is resistant to encrustation. Major advantage is hypoallergenic. Less flexible than latex. Up to 50% water loss from balloon can occur due to gas diffusion. Can stay in place up to 12 weeks. Used for clients with latex hypersensitivity. Discomfort in removal can occur as a result of incomplete cuff deflation of the balloon.
Latex Catheter Coated With Hydro Gel	Gel is a polymer that absorbs water and forms a smooth surface on catheter. It is resistant to encrustation and settlement of bacteria, which diminishes risk of infection. Can stay in place up to12 weeks. Used for clients with latex hypersensitivity.
Silicone–Elastomer	Coated latex catheter that is biocompatible and reduces urethra mucosal irritation. Flexibility provides comfort and can remain up to 12 weeks. Useful for clients with latex hypersensitivity.
PTFE Coated Catheter	Teflon is fixed onto a latex core to form a catheter; used short term. Client is more comfortable, decreased incidence of urethritis and encrustation. Can stay in place 28 days. Loss of balloon water occurs. Clients with latex hypersensitivity can use this catheter.
Silver Alloy	Lower incidence of bacteriuria than with silver oxide catheter. Clinically effective in reducing Catheter Associated Urinary Tract Infection (CAUTI) if used short term (14 days). Silver is an antiseptic and inhibits growth of gram-positive and gram-negative bacteria. Silver-coated catheters may reduce catheter-related infections and have a low risk for generating antibiotic resistance.
Antiseptic-Impregnated or Antimicrobial-Coated	Significantly prevents or delays onset of CAUTI. Both the outer wall and inner drainage lumen are impregnated with an antibacterial agent that exudes from the catheter over time.

27. Dry penis and remove drapes.
28. Make client comfortable. Place bed in LOW position with upper side rails raised.
29. Discard equipment in appropriate container.
30. Remove gloves and perform hand hygiene.
31. Send specimen to lab and document procedure.

EVIDENCE-BASED PRACTICE

Care Variances With Male Catheterization

At University of Colorado Hospital, there had been two cases involving care variances with male patient catheterization. While the nursing staff searched for evidence on why this occurred (since the nurses' competency had been verified), they consulted urology experts to document their best practices for male catheterization procedures.

This evidence-based project revealed that some nursing literature at the time of the study contained outdated facts about male catheterization, including out-of-date information on the distance to insert the catheter (6 to 8 in. when it should be 10 to 12 in.) and the "fact" that return of urine means the catheter is properly placed (incorrect, since there will be a residual urine return even when a catheter is not fully and properly placed). This evidence-based practice study was reported in *MedSurg Nursing.*

Source: Internet: CE Course 359, *Nurse Week*. (2005, Feb. 28).

EVIDENCE-BASED PRACTICE

Using Silver-Coated Catheters

In a base-case analysis, use of silver-coated catheters led to a 47% relative decrease in incidence of symptomatic UTI from 30 to 16 cases per 1,000 clients, and a relative decrease in the incidence of bacteremia from 4.5 to 2.5 cases per 1,000 clients, compared with standard catheters. Use of the silver alloy catheters reduces the cost savings of $4.09/client compared with standard catheters. Silver-coated catheters provide clinical benefits over standard catheters in all cases.

Source: Saint, S., et al. (2000). The potential clinical and economic benefits of silver alloy urinary catheters in preventing urinary tract infections. *Archives of Internal Medicine, Sept. 25, 2000, 160*(17), http://archinte.ama-assn.org/cgi/content/full.

Inserting a Retention Catheter (Female)

Equipment

Disposable retention catheter kit with appropriate size catheter (size 14–16 Fr for adult female, size 16–18 Fr for adult male with 10 mL balloons) and preconnected closed-system 2000-mL drainage bag with MONO-FLO antireflux device

Closed drainage set with or without urimeter or urometer, if indicated

Label for urine specimen if indicated

Biohazard bag for specimen if indicated

Additional lighting if needed

Bath blanket or turn sheet

Towels, washcloth

Clean gloves

Basin with warm water

Soap

Tape or commercial catheter securement (Bard Catheter leg strap, Dale Anchor Strap, Statlock Foley)

Catheter tip shapes are either Coudé or Tiemann, and size of lumen is based on French scale (each unit equals 0.33 mm of internal lumen).

Preparation

Same as for Inserting a Straight Catheter (Female).

Procedure

1. Open sterile package by tearing the package on the lined edge of plastic wrap. Place plastic wrap at foot of bed for waste disposal.
2. Place catheter kit on bed between client's legs.
3. Open closed drainage set bag and place on bed near client (if indicated).
4. Fold back corner of bath blanket to expose perineum.
5. Open white outer wrap away from package with last turn toward client.
6. Remove sterile absorbent pad, and position under client's buttocks plastic side down. Have client lift buttocks if able. Position pad by holding corners of pad only. ▸ ***Rationale:*** Holding onto the edges keeps the center sterile.
7. Don sterile gloves.
8. Position fenestrated drape over the client to expose the genitalia (optional).

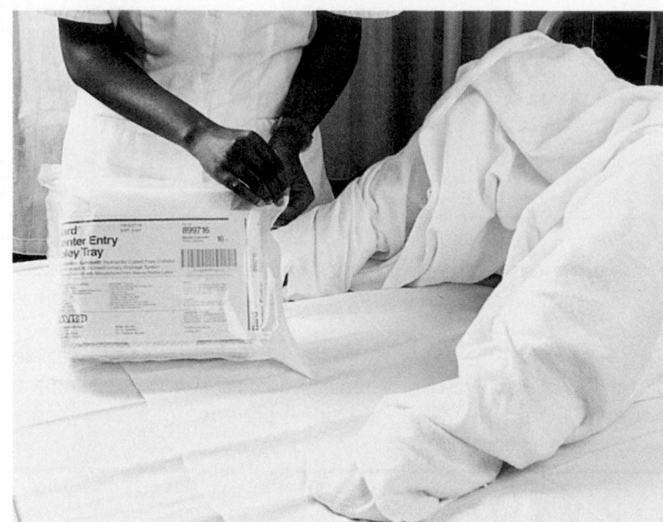

1 Open sterile package by tearing it along lined edge of plastic wrap.

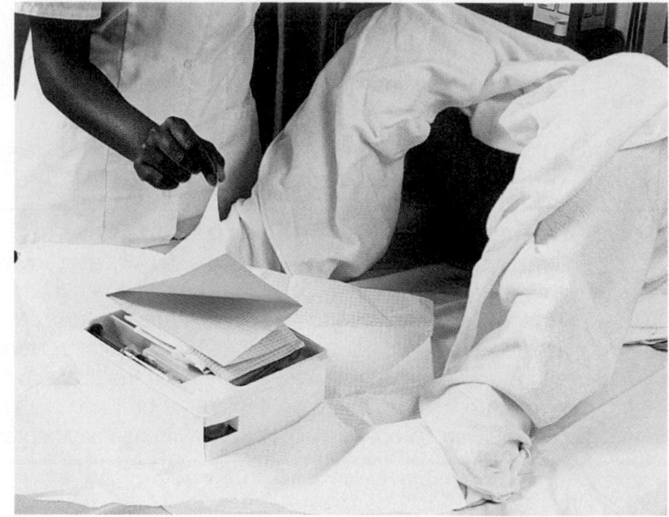

2 Remove sterile absorbent pad and place it under client's buttocks.

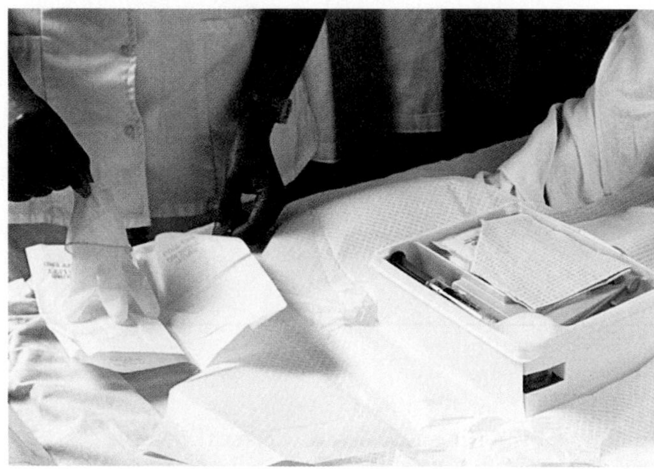

3 Put on sterile gloves, being careful not to contaminate sterile field.

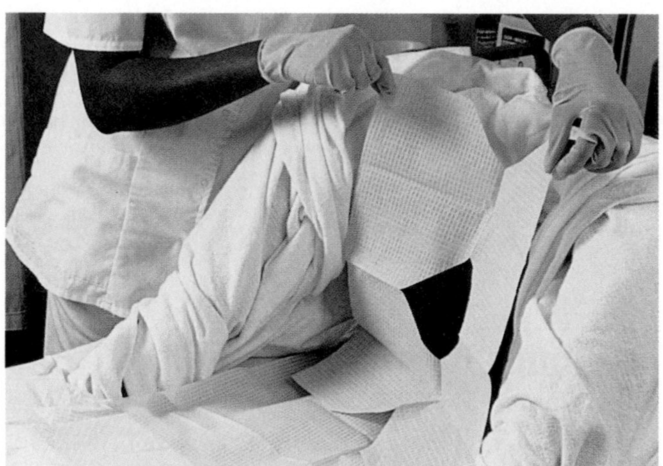

4 Position sterile fenestrated drape over client to expose genitalia (optional).

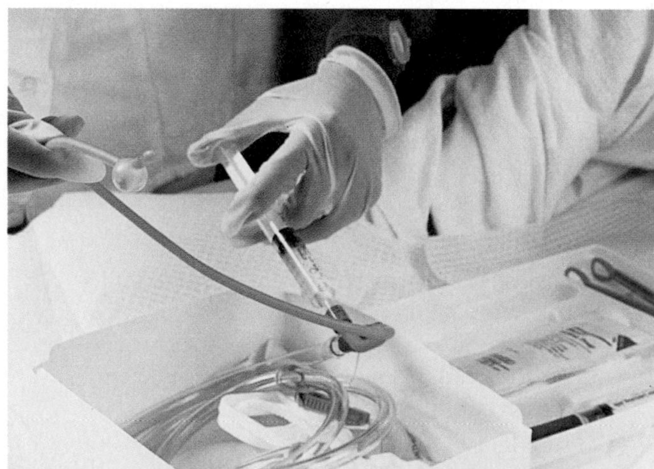

5 Test catheter balloon by inserting prefilled syringe and injecting sterile water through catheter side port, unless silicone catheter, and according to hospital policy.

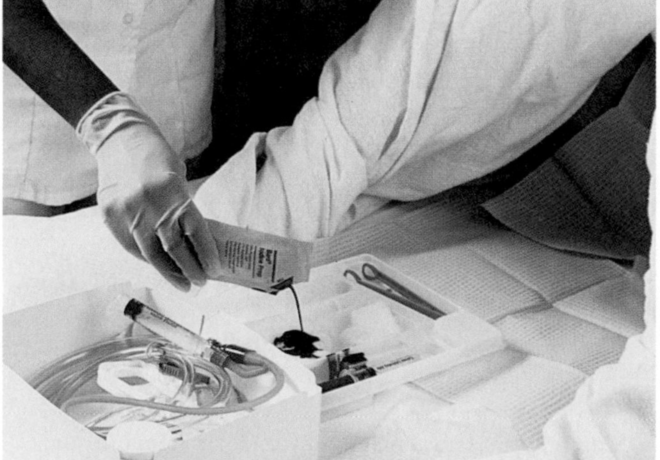

6 Pour antiseptic solution completely over cotton balls. Use type of solution according to facility policy.

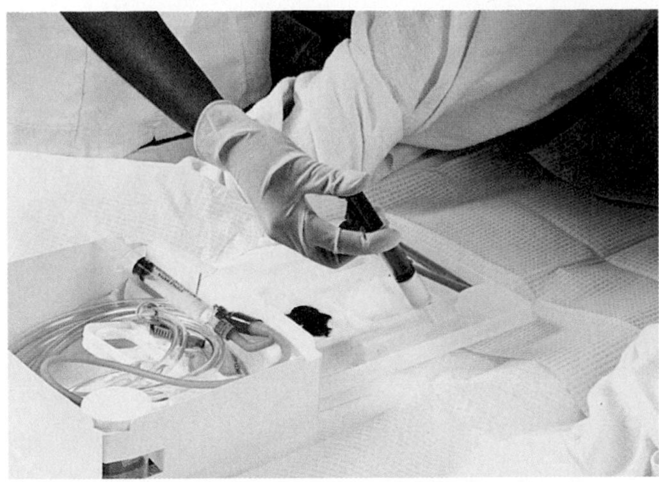

7 Uncap lubricant syringe and squeeze lubricant onto tray.

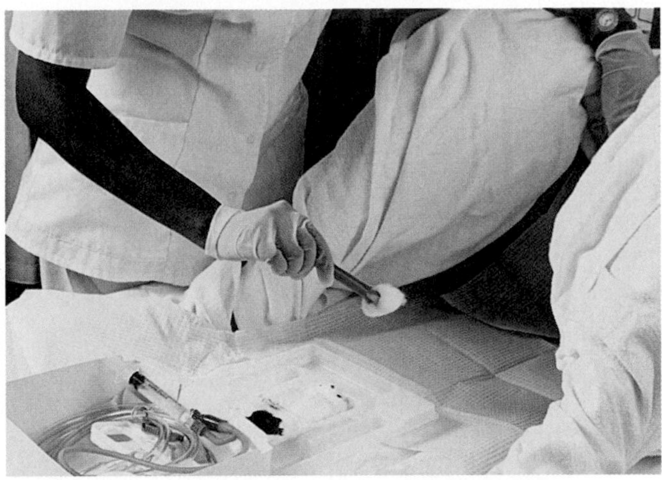

4 Cleanse meatus by using downward strokes with cotton balls or use single-use lubricant or anesthetic gel.

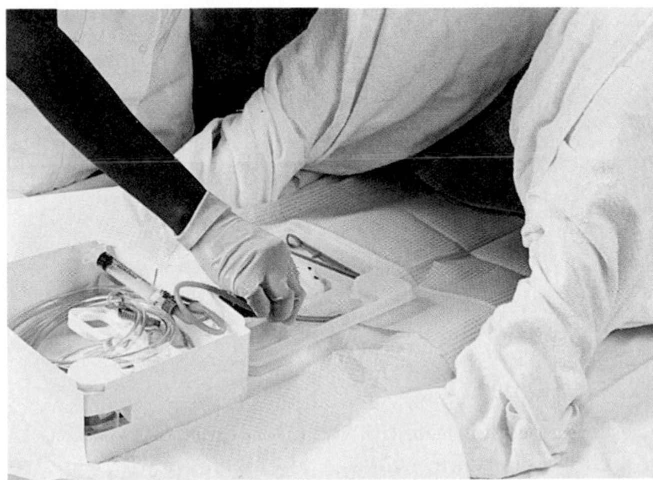

9 Lubricate tip of catheter to facilitate insertion without trauma

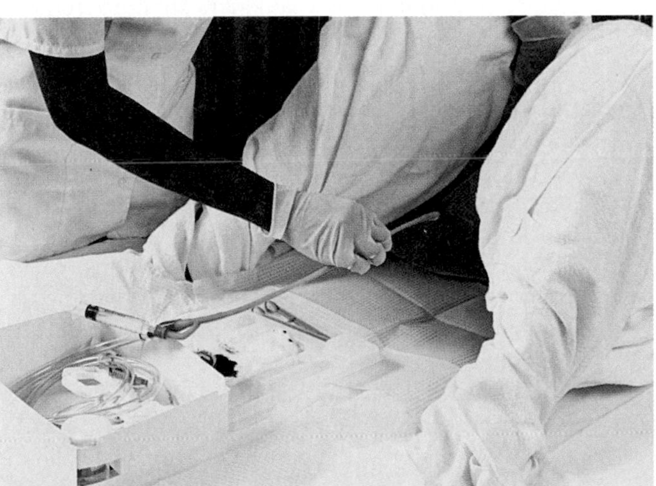

10 Hold labia apart while inserting catheter to prevent contamination.

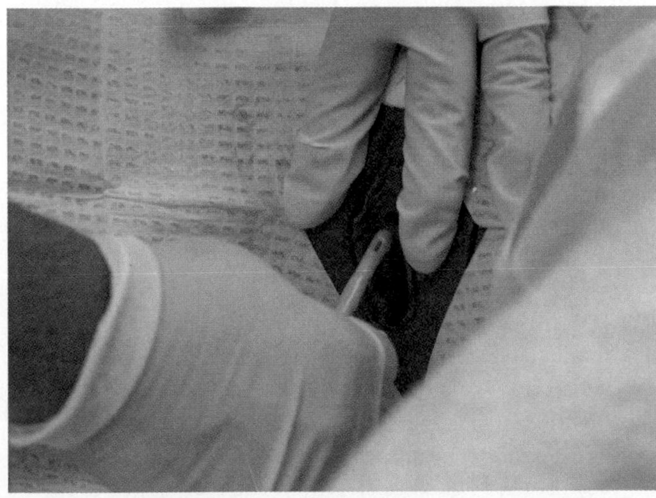

11 Insert catheter gently into meatus until urine begins to flow; then advance another 1-2 inches (2.5-5 cm).

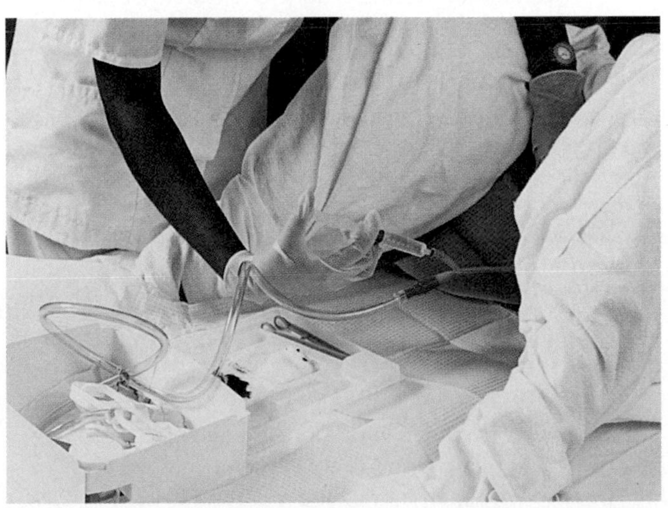

12 Inject water from prefilled syringe into catheter balloon after inserting catheter.

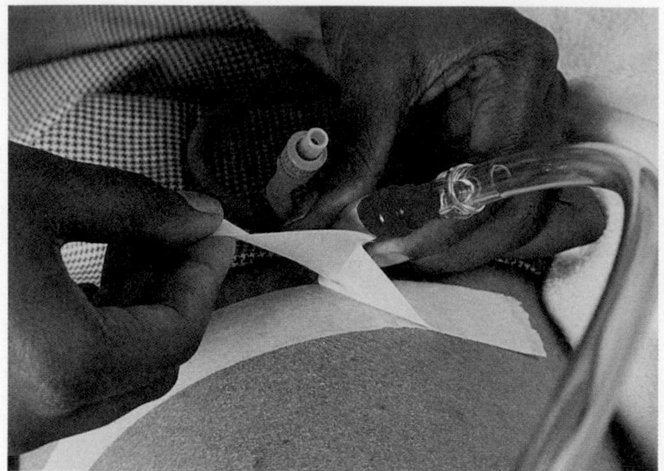

13 Tape catheter to side of client's thigh using nonallergenic tape.

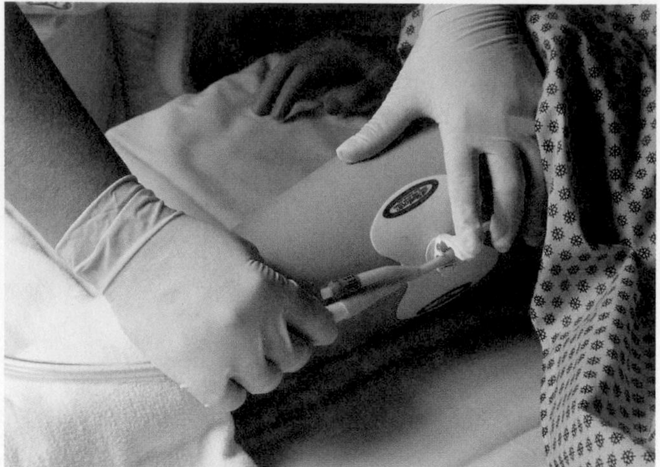

14 Securement device (StatLock Foley) stabilizes catheter to minimize urethral trauma.

9. Separate prep tray from container, placing prep tray with cotton balls, antiseptic solution packet or according to hospital policy and lubricant onto sterile field toward client.
10. To test catheter balloon (check hospital policy, and brand of catheter to determine need for inflating balloon before insertion):

    NOTE: Certain manufacturers of the balloon catheters (i.e., Bard) are now alerting facilities to instruct their staff NOT to pre-inflate to test the balloon before insertion, because it is pretested during the manufacturing process.

    a. Remove rubber protector and insert tip of prefilled sterile water syringe into catheter side arm to inflate balloon.
    b. Inject 10 mL of sterile water to inflate balloon to test balloon integrity. ▸ ***Rationale:*** The catheter can fall out if not secured with appropriately inflated balloon.
    c. If balloon malfunctions with testing, obtain a new sterile retention catheter before continuing with procedure.
    d. After testing balloon, pull back on plunger to remove fluid and deflate balloon, leaving syringe in place. ▸ ***Rationale:*** Testing is done to ensure that balloon inflates without leaking.

Clinical Alert

A silicone coated Foley catheter is not pre-inflated for testing before insertion because a ridge is present in the balloon when it is deflated, and ridges can lead to irritation of the urethra. Silicone catheters are used for clients with latex allergies. They are also used if a urethral stricture is present, and during radical prostatectomy surgery, as there is less meatus.

11. Open package and pour antiseptic solution over cotton balls.
12. Uncap syringe filled with lubricant and eject onto prep tray to lubricate catheter tip at time of catheter insertion, or open lubricant packet and insert catheter tip into lubricant, keeping catheter in tray.
13. Remove cap from specimen cup if indicated.
14. Prep client's meatus:
    a. Separate client's labia minora with your nondominant hand.
    b. With your dominant hand, *use forceps* to pick up an absorbent cotton ball that has been saturated with antiseptic solution, according to hospital policy. See 13c, page 774.
    c. Cleanse client's meatus with one downward stroke of forceps or swab. Discard absorbent cotton ball or swab in plastic bag at foot of bed.
    d. Repeat Step c at least three times.
    e. Continue to hold the client's labia apart until you insert the catheter.
15. Discard forceps in plastic bag at foot of bed.
16. With uncontaminated hand, take catheter from container, lubricate tip, and insert gently into meatus 2 in. or until urine starts to flow.
17. Guide the catheter gently 1–1.5 in. just beyond the point at which urine begins to flow. ▸ ***Rationale:*** Inserting catheter further into bladder ensures it is beyond neck of the bladder.
18. Inject entire contents of prefilled (10–30 mL sterile water) syringe into the side arm of the catheter used for balloon inflation. ▸ ***Rationale:*** Underinflation can cause balloon distortion and catheter tip deflection.

Clinical Alert

Chronic irritation and inflammation of bladder mucosa due to long-term (more than 8 months) presence of an indwelling catheter (urethral or suprapubic) is associated with an increased risk for bladder cancer.

19. If client complains of pain on balloon inflation, immediately aspirate the sterile water. ▸ ***Rationale:*** The catheter may be in the urethra rather than the bladder.
20. Gently retract the catheter until you feel resistance. ▸ ***Rationale:*** This indicates the balloon is resting against the bladder neck and in the correct position.
21. Obtain urine specimen before attaching catheter to drainage tubing, if indicated.

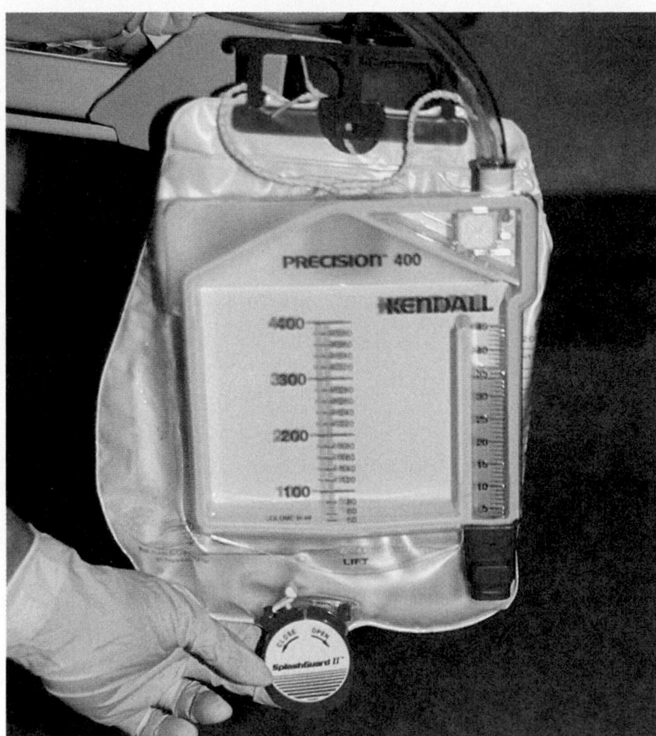

15 Attach urine collection bag to nonmovable part of bed. Do not allow tubing to hang below collection bag.

22. Remove protective cap from drainage tubing and attach securely to catheter, if indicated.
23. Apply catheter holder or tape catheter to client's upper thigh. Place one piece of tape on thigh. Take second piece of tape and encircle catheter, leaving two "tails" on tape. Secure "tails" from tape on catheter to tape on leg. ▶ ***Rationale:*** To stabilize catheter and minimize urethral trauma and avoid tension on bladder neck.
24. Attach drainage bag to bed frame (not side rails); coil tubing to allow free gravity flow of urine.
25. Remove drapes.
26. Reposition client for comfort; put bed in LOW position with upper side rails up.
27. Remove equipment, including gloves, and discard disposable trash in appropriate container.
28. Perform hand hygiene.
29. Record urine output on I&O.

TABLE 22-4 Indications for an Indwelling Catheter

- Short term for acute urinary retention.
- Sudden and complete inability to void.
- Need for immediate and rapid bladder decompression.
- Temporary relief of bladder outlet obstruction secondary to:
  - Enlarged prostate gland
  - Urethral stricture
  - Obstructing pelvic organ prolapse
  - Urologic or prolonged surgical procedure
- Chronic urethral obstruction or urinary retention and surgical interventions and/or the use of intermittent catheterization has failed or is not feasible.
- Irreversible medical conditions are present (e.g., metastatic terminal disease, coma, end states of other conditions).
- Presence of stage III or IV pressure ulcers that are not healing because of continual urine leakage.
- Instance where a caregiver is not present (usually in home care setting) to provide incontinence care.

Source: Newman, D. (2007). The indwelling urinary catheter: principles for best practice. *Journal of Wound, Ostomy and Continence: Nursing, 34*(6), 655–661.

30. Label specimen and place cup in biohazard transport bag.
31. Send urine specimen to lab and document procedure.

NOTE: The optimal drainage system is a closed system with a one-way valve between the bag and tubing. ▶ ***Rationale:*** This system reduces UTIs for clients with a short-term indwelling urinary catheter.

Clinical Alert

Immediate assessment and documentation of the amount of urine obtained after inserting the retention catheter is important to document. If the client has urinary retention, it may alter clinical decisions.

Clinical Alert

Do not obtain a urine specimen from the catheter drainage bag. Pathogens in drainage bag do not necessarily represent those present in lower urinary tract.

Inserting a Retention Catheter (Male)

Equipment

Same as for Inserting a Retention Catheter (Female)

Preparation

1. Follow Steps 1 through 6 in Inserting a Straight Catheter (Female).
2. Place client in a supine position with knees slightly apart. ▶ ***Rationale:*** This position relaxes abdominal and perineal muscles.
3. Drape client by placing a bath blanket or turn sheet over chest area and fanfold top linen down to cover lower extremities, exposing only perineal area.

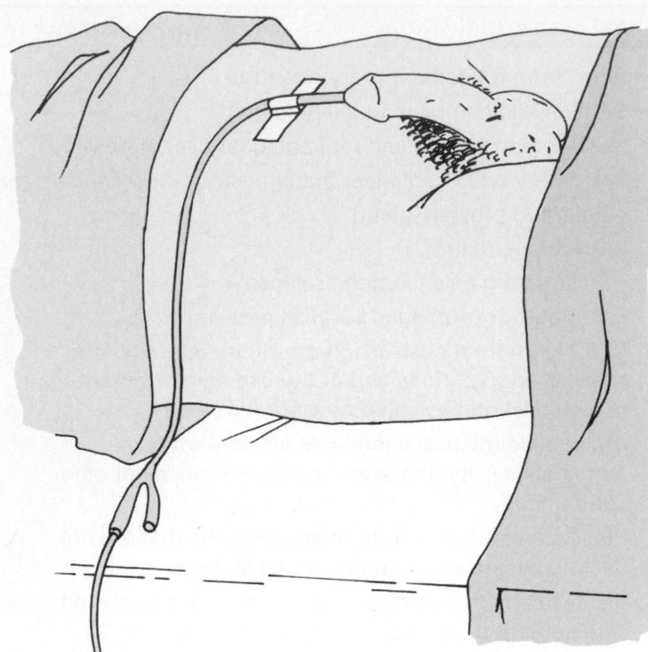

▲ Tape catheter to abdomen to prevent pressure in penoscrotal angle if client on bedrest.

4. Don clean gloves and wash client's perineal area if necessary.
5. Remove gloves and prepare for catheterization.

Procedure

1. Open sterile package by tearing package on lined edge of plastic wrap. Place plastic wrap at foot of bed for waste disposal.
2. Place sterile kit on bed at client's side near thigh.
3. Open closed drainage set and place on bed near work area.
4. Open outer white wrap away from sterile package.
5. Place sterile drape over thighs and under penis.
6. Don sterile gloves and set fenestrated drape aside on sterile field.
7. Separate prep tray from container, placing prep tray with cotton balls, antiseptic solution packet, and lubricant onto sterile field toward client.
8. Test catheter balloon according to hospital policy:
   a. Remove rubber protector and insert tip of prefilled sterile water syringe into catheter side arm to inflate balloon.
   b. Inject 10 mL of sterile water to inflate balloon to test balloon integrity. ▶ ***Rationale:*** The catheter can fall out if not secured with appropriately inflated balloon.
   c. If balloon malfunctions with testing, obtain a new sterile retention catheter before continuing with procedure.
   d. After testing balloon, pull back on plunger to remove fluid and deflate balloon, leaving syringe in place. ▶ ***Rationale:*** Testing is done to ensure that balloon inflates without leaking.
9. Open package and pour antiseptic solution over cotton balls according to hospital policy.
10. Remove cap from specimen cup if indicated.
11. Uncap syringe filled with lubricant and eject onto rolling prep tray, or open lubricant package.
12. Lubricate catheter generously about 3–4 in., keeping catheter in tray, or, if using alternate method, insert lubricant directly into the urethra using a prefilled syringe.
13. Position fenestrated drape over the penis.
14. Hold penis upright with your nondominant hand. Hold sides of penis to prevent closing of urethra.
15. With your dominant hand, use forceps to pick up cotton ball saturated with antiseptic solution or pick up swab.
16. Cleanse meatus first with expanding circular stroke using the cotton balls held by forceps or Betadine swab. Check hospital policy for Betadine use.
17. Discard swab into plastic wrap at foot of bed.
18. Repeat circular prep around head of penis. Cleanse three times using a new cotton ball or Betadine swab each time. ▶ ***Rationale:*** Using a circular motion around head of penis prevents bacteria from entering urinary meatus.
19. Continue to hold penis with your nondominant hand.
20. Discard forceps into plastic bag.
21. Pick up catheter with sterile hand about 8–10 cm (3–4 in.) from tip of catheter.
22. Lift penis to a 90° angle (perpendicular to body) and exert slight traction by pulling upward. ▶ ***Rationale:*** This movement straightens the urethra for easier insertion of catheter.
23. Insert catheter about 10–12 in.
24. If resistance is met, lower angle of penis to 45° and ask client to take a deep breath. ▶ ***Rationale:*** Taking a deep breath helps relax external sphincter.
25. Guide catheter gently 1–2 in. beyond point at which urine begins to flow. ▶ ***Rationale:*** Inserting catheter further into bladder ensures it is beyond neck of bladder.

Foley Catheter Cautions

Some studies have shown that the standard Foley catheter with a solitary drainage hole at its tip (1.5 cm above the base of the balloon) allows residual urine to accumulate. This may lead to inaccurate measurement of urine output, and may increase risk for urinary tract infection.

Source: Fallis, W. (2005, April.) Indwelling Foley catheters: Is the current design a source of erroneous measurement of urine output? *Critical Care Nurse, 25*(2), 44–46, 48–51.

26. Inject entire contents of prefilled sterile water syringe into side arm of catheter for balloon inflation.
27. Gently retract catheter until you feel resistance of the balloon at neck of bladder.
28. Obtain urine specimen if indicated.
29. Remove protective cap from drainage tubing and attach securely to catheter if indicated.
30. Tape catheter to abdomen with 1-in. tape if client is not ambulatory, or use securement device made with Velcro strap. ▸ ***Rationale:*** This prevents pressure on the penoscrotal angle and ventral urethral meatus. Tape catheter to upper thigh if client is ambulatory.
31. Attach drainage bag to bed frame (not side rails).
32. Reposition client for comfort; put bed in LOW position with upper side rails raised.
33. Remove all equipment, including gloves, and discard disposable trash in the appropriate container.
34. Measure and record urine output in I&O bedside record.
35. Perform hand hygiene.
36. Label specimen cup, place in biohazard transport bag, and send to lab.
37. Document procedure, including amount of urine obtained.

Types of Securement Devices

Categories of securement devices for short- and long-term indwelling catheters:

- Improvised devices using adhesive tape, safety pins, and sutures.
- Manufactured devices with an adhesive backing and a mechanism for attaching catheter.
- Nonadhesive devices that incorporate Velcro and straps to secure the catheter to the upper thigh.

Note: Securement products developed specifically to hold indwelling catheters include the nonadhesive products that secure to the upper thigh or abdomen with a soft closure strap. These products are latex-free with hypoallergenic backing with the Velcro locking system that holds the catheter securely in place. Reusable leg anchors are available from several companies (Bard Medical Division, Posey Company, Dale Medical, Venetec, McJohnson).

Clinical Alert

Maintaining a sterile continuously closed and sealed urinary drainage system is critical to prevent CAUTI.

Optimal management of an indwelling catheter includes securing catheter to thigh or abdomen to prevent catheter or balloons from exerting excessive force on bladder neck or urethra.

Providing Catheter Care

Equipment

Soap and water
Washcloth
Towel
Clean gloves
1-in. tape or commercial catheter holder

Preparation

1. Check client care plan.
2. Gather equipment.
3. Identify client.
4. Provide privacy.
5. Perform hand hygiene.
6. Explain procedure to client.
7. Raise bed, and lower side rail on working side.

Procedure

1. Place client in supine position, and expose perineal area to easily visualize the meatus.
2. Remove catheter securing tape.
3. Don clean gloves.

For Female

a. Cleanse urinary meatus using circular motion moving outward with washcloth, soap, and water.
b. Dry area with towel.
c. Re-secure retention catheter with tape or commercial holder.

For Circumcised Male

a. With mitten washcloth, soap, and water, cleanse around urinary meatus.

Clinical Alert

Almost all clients will be bacteriuric after 1 month of catheterization. Indwelling urinary catheters promote UTIs by creating a portal of entry for microorganisms, and nosocomial UTIs increase mortality rate threefold. The client should be assisted to urinate by using noninvasive techniques before resorting to catheterization.

b. Dry area with towel.
c. Using separate washcloth, clean area between scrotum and rectal area, then dry.
d. Place soiled linen in hamper.

For Uncircumcised Male

a. Retract foreskin back away from catheter.
b. With mitten washcloth, soap, and water, cleanse around urinary meatus.
c. Dry penis with towel.
d. After drying, pull foreskin back around the catheter.
e. Place soiled linen in hamper.

4. Remove gloves and discard. Re-tape catheter.
5. Position client for comfort.
6. Lower bed and raise upper side rail.
7. Perform hand hygiene.

Complications Associated With Long-Term Indwelling Catheter Placement

- Urinary tract infections
- Catheter leaks
- Bladder spasms
- Urethral erosion
- Urethritis
- Epididymitis
- Prostatitis
- Scrotal abscess
- Prostatic abscess
- Urinary stones
- Urethral sphincter damage
- Bladder cancer

EVIDENCE-BASED PRACTICE

Cranberry for Urinary Tract Infection Prophylaxis

There is a growing accumulation of evidence-based information in support of use of cranberry in UTI prevention. Its beneficial effect is not by acidifying urine, but by inhibiting adherence of *E. coli* and other gram-negative uropathogens to urinary tract epithelial cells. A recent randomized controlled trial demonstrated that one tablet of concentrated cranberry extract (300–400 mg) twice daily or 8 oz of pure unsweetened cranberry juice three times daily is safe and effective for up to 12 months. Cranberry may increase urinary oxalate levels and so may increase risk of kidney stone formation in patients with a history of oxalate calculi.

Cranberry also seems to inhibit the aggregation of dental plaque bacteria.

Source: Lynch, D. (2004). Cranberry for prevention of urinary tract infections. *American Family Physician, 70*(11), 2175.

Removing a Retention Catheter

Equipment

10-mL syringe without needle
Paper towel
Clean gloves
Client's calibrated graduate

Preparation

1. Check physician's orders for removing catheter.
2. Perform hand hygiene.
3. Gather equipment.
4. Explain procedure to client.
5. Provide privacy.
6. Don clean gloves.

Procedure

1. Remove tape attaching catheter to client.
2. Insert syringe into balloon port of catheter. Do not cut port with scissors. ▸ ***Rationale:*** Balloon may not totally deflate if inflation port is cut.

Clinical Alert

Do not aspirate balloon vigorously. Doing so may collapse inflation lumen and prevent balloon deflation.

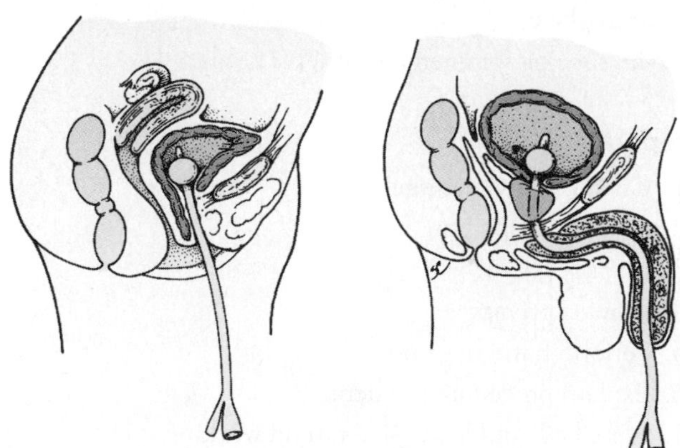

▲ Balloon must be deflated before removing to prevent damage to urethra.

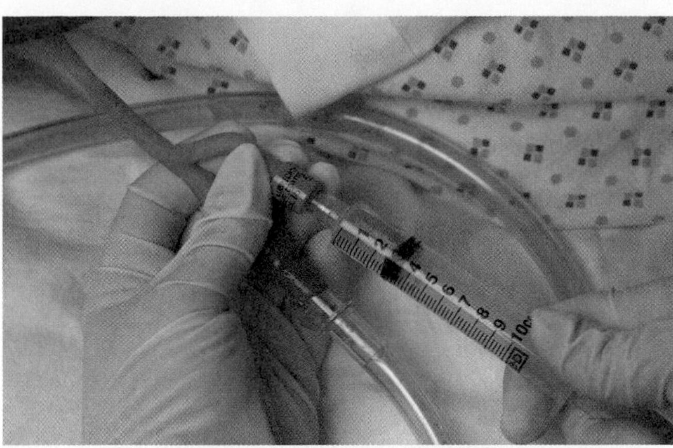

▲ Insert syringe hub into balloon port and withdraw fluid from retention catheter balloon.

3. Withdraw fluid from balloon (usually 10 mL of water in balloon).
4. Pull gently on catheter to ensure balloon is deflated before attempting to remove. ▶ ***Rationale:*** Damage to urethra can occur if balloon is not totally deflated.
5. Hold paper towel under catheter with your nondominant hand.
6. If resistance is not met, slowly withdraw catheter, allowing it to fall into paper towel.
7. Disconnect urine drainage bag from bed frame.
8. Empty drainage bag into graduate and measure.
9. Record output on I&O bedside record.
10. Dispose of catheter in appropriate receptacle.
11. Position client for comfort.
12. Remove gloves and perform hand hygiene.
13. Instruct client to drink oral fluids as tolerated and observe for symptoms of urinary tract infection (burning, frequency, urgency).
14. Offer bedpan or urinal after removing catheter, until voiding occurs. Keep accurate I&O record of time and amount of postcatheterization voidings.
15. Report to physician if client has not urinated in 8 hr or is uncomfortable.

EVIDENCE-BASED PRACTICE

Reminder Reduces Urinary Catheterization Use

This study demonstrated that catheter use could be decreased if physicians received automatic computerized (or written) reminders that their clients had catheters and how long they had been in place. Because urinary catheters are a major source of nosocomial infection, their use should be as brief as possible.

Source: Saint, S., Kaufman, S. R., Thompson, M., Rogers, M. A., & Chenoweth, C. E. (2005). A reminder reduces urinary catheterization in hospitalized patients. *Journal on Quality and Patient Safety, 31*(8), 455–462 .

DOCUMENTATION for Catheterization

- Time and purpose
- Type and size of catheter
- Amount, color, and odor of urine obtained
- Client's tolerance of procedure
- Specimen sent to lab (if ordered)
- Catheter care provided
- Catheter removed
- Voiding: time and amount after catheter removal
- Intake and output
- Residual volume amount and time since last void

CRITICAL THINKING Application

Expected Outcomes

- Catheterization is avoided with use of bladder scanner.
- Sterile technique is maintained throughout catheterization procedure.
- Catheter enters bladder as evidenced by urine outflow.
- Client remains free of urine leakage around retention catheter.
- Urinary tract infection does not occur secondary to catheterization.

Unexpected Outcomes	Alternative Actions
Bladder scan does not give reading.	• Make certain adequate conducting gel has been used. • Have obese client bend knees so that feet are flat on the bed. • Have thin client partially sit up to compress abdomen. • Apply more pressure with scan head, depressing 1–2 in. into client's abdomen.

Catheter is contaminated during procedure.	• Obtain new kit (or sterile catheter) and repeat procedure. • Keep catheter tip in lubricant packet until ready to catheterize. • If catheter has tear-away sleeve, leave catheter within it while catheterizing client.

Catheter is inserted into female client's vagina.	• Leave the catheter in place and follow these actions:
	  • Have someone obtain a new sterile catheter and gloves.
	  • Reposition fingers to better visualize urethral meatus.
	  • Obtain an assistant to provide direct lighting.
	  • Insert new catheter pointing upward (toward client's umbilicus), as downward angle insertion tends to follow vaginal inlet.
	  • Place obese client in side-lying position and flex upper leg for catheterization.

Catheter cannot be inserted into male client.	• Obtain new catheter kit and follow these actions:
	  • Obtain order for intraurethral lidocaine gel.
	  • Hold penis vertical to client's body, insert lidocaine gel.
	  • Insert catheter while applying slight traction by gently pulling upward on the shaft of the penis.
	  • If resistance encountered, rotate catheter, increase traction, and lower angle of penis.
	  • Ask client to cough.
	  • Try using a Condé or 12-Fr catheter.

Urine leaks around retention catheter.	• Obtain order for catheter irrigation to ensure patency of catheter. • Inflate catheter balloon with full amount of sterile water in syringe (10 mL) to fill balloon and catheter inflation lumen as well. • Do not increase catheter size, as this increases bladder irritation, spasm, and leakage. • Obtain urine culture and sensitivity, as leakage may be sign of urinary tract infection. • Obtain order for anticholinergic medication to relieve bladder spasms.
Client develops urinary tract infection while catheterized.	• Remind physician that client has a catheter; reevaluate need for continued use. • Keep urine collection system below level of client's bladder—avoid any chance of bacteria entering system caused by retrograde flow from collections bag to bladder. • Encourage fluid intake of 2–3 L/day unless contraindicated. • Maintain client and system positioning so that continuous urine drainage is unobstructed. • Make certain that catheter is secured properly (thigh of female, abdomen of male). • Maintain/coil drainage tubing to allow straight drainage into urine collection bag. • Provide daily perineal care with soap and water only. • Don clean gloves to empty urine collection bag; avoid contamination of drain port. • Suggest external collection system (condom catheter) for male client.

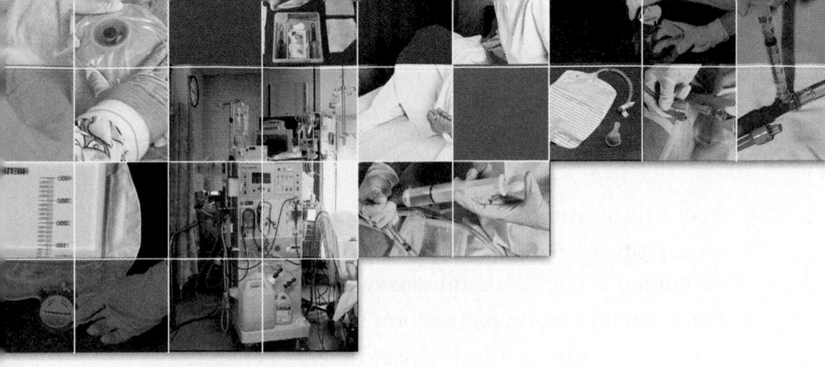

Chapter 22

UNIT 4

Bladder Irrigation

Nursing Process Data

ASSESSMENT Data Base

- Determine rationale for irrigation.
- Note rate of urine flow from bladder, color of urine, presence of clots or debris.
- Assess for distended bladder.
- Assess for bladder discomfort.
- Note client's I&O balance.

PLANNING Objectives

- To remove blood clots from client's bladder
- To ensure patency of drainage system
- To relieve bladder spasm discomfort

IMPLEMENTATION Procedures

EVALUATION Expected Outcomes

- Continuous bladder irrigation is maintained to prevent clot formation and catheter obstruction.
- Client does not experience discomfort.

Irrigating by Opening a Closed System

Equipment

Sterile irrigation set with catheter tip syringe (new set for each irrigation)
Clean gloves
Sterile normal saline irrigant (or solution as ordered)
Catch basin
Antiseptic swab
Absorbent pad
Sterile protective cap for tubing
Pain or antispasmodic medication
Tape for securing catheter

Preparation

1. Check physician's order for system irrigation.
2. Gather equipment.
3. Identify client.
4. Explain procedure and rationale to client.
5. Perform hand hygiene.
6. Premedicate client as indicated. ▸ ***Rationale:*** Manual irrigation causes painful bladder spasms.
7. Provide privacy and place client in a comfortable position. The dorsal-recumbent position is most convenient if client can tolerate this position. Raise bed and lower side rail if needed.

Procedure

1. Fanfold linen to expose catheter.
2. Palpate client's bladder to check for distention.
3. Open sterile irrigant container on overbed table. Maintain sterility of inside of the container.
4. Don clean gloves.
5. Place an absorbent pad under connection of tubing and catheter. ▸ ***Rationale:*** This will form a working field for irrigating catheter.
6. Pour irrigant into sterile solution container.
7. Uncap tip of irrigation syringe and place into solution container. Do not contaminate syringe tip.
8. Place catch basin on pad to form working field.
9. Disconnect catheter from drainage tube. Place sterile protective cap over the end of the drainage tube. ▸ ***Rationale:*** This will prevent contaminating tip of tubing.
10. Coil tubing on bed.
11. Place catheter end into sterile irrigation set catch basin. ▸ ***Rationale:*** If end of catheter touches covers, underpad, exposed skin surfaces, or drainage tube, it will be contaminated.
12. Insert irrigating syringe into catheter and attempt to aspirate any obstructing debris. ▸ ***Rationale:*** If irrigation is performed without removing debris, debris can be forced into bladder and result in infection.
13. Withdraw irrigating solution into syringe.
14. Instill 30–50 mL of irrigant into catheter with a gentle pressure.
    a. Aspirate instilled solution.
    b. Continue to irrigate client's bladder with 30–50 mL of irrigant until fluid returns are clear.
15. Remove the protective cap from drainage tube.
16. Wipe end of catheter with an antiseptic sponge and reconnect the catheter to the drainage tube.
17. Ensure straight line from tubing to drainage bag. Curl excess tubing loosely on bed and secure tubing to linen. ▸ ***Rationale:*** If tubing hangs below drainage bag, urine will stagnate, increasing risk of urinary tract infection.
18. Tape catheter to inner thigh for a female and to abdomen for a male.
19. Lower bed and raise side rails.
20. Discard equipment and remove gloves.

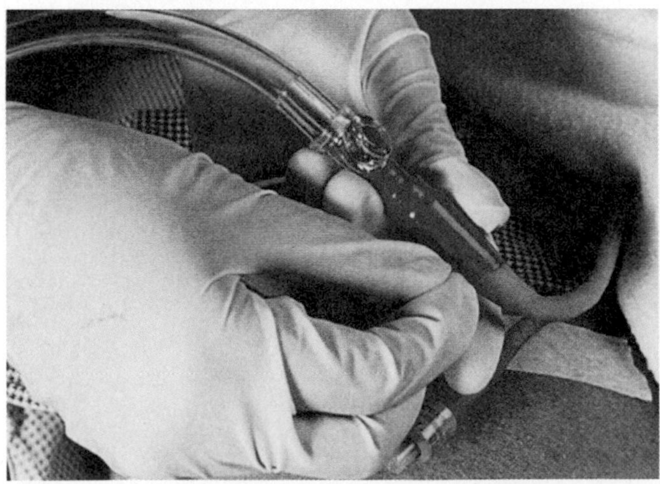

⚠1 Carefully remove sealing tape to access catheter.

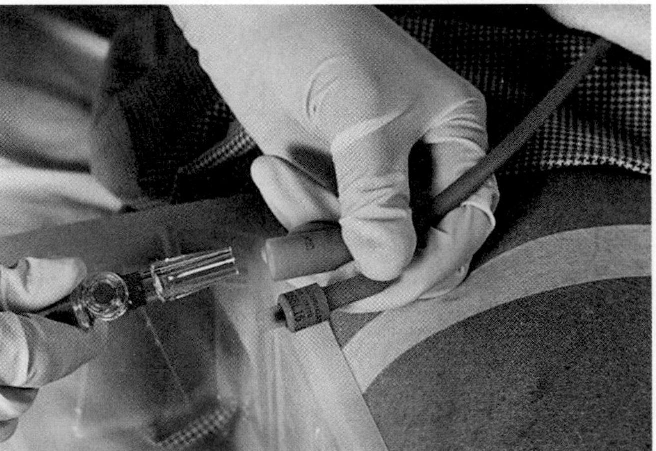

⚠2 Disconnect catheter from drainage tubing; cover tubing end with sterile cap.

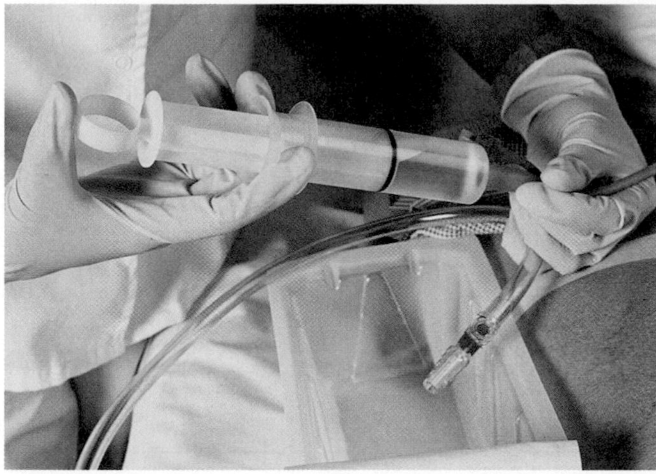

3 Instill 30–50 mL of irrigant into catheter to irrigate an open system.

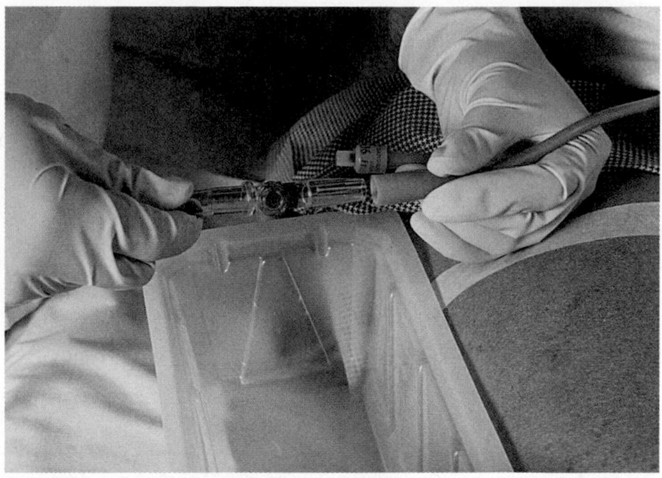

4 Reconnect catheter to drainage tubing using aseptic technique.

21. Make sure client is clean and comfortable.
22. Perform hand hygiene.
23. Measure amount of return. Subtract amount of irrigating solution used to irrigate.
24. Record net amount on client's I&O record.

Clinical Alert

Opening a closed urinary drainage system is indicated as a last resort to reestablish catheter patency. Manual irrigation should be done carefully for a client with transurethral resection of a bladder tumor due to risk of bladder rupture.

Irrigating a Closed System

Equipment

Irrigation set
30-mL syringe with needleless cannula
Antiseptic swabs
Ordered irrigating solution (sterile saline)
Clamp for drainage tubing
Clean gloves
Prepared pain medication, if ordered

Preparation

1. Check physician's order and client care plan.
2. Identify client. Explain procedure and rationale.
3. Premedicate client if ordered.
4. Gather equipment.
5. Perform hand hygiene.
6. Provide privacy, and place client in dorsal-recumbent position, if tolerated.
7. Raise bed, and lower side rail on working side of bed.
8. Don clean gloves.
9. Empty client's urinary drainage bag and record amount.

NOTE: This method is less effective because most clots are larger than the cannula utilized for aspiration.

Procedure

1. Open sterile container. Maintain sterility on inside of the container.
2. Place absorbent pad under end of catheter to form a working field.
3. Pour irrigant into solution container.
4. Clamp tubing just distal to injection port.
5. Swab tubing injection port with antiseptic swab.
6. Insert the needleless cannula into tubing injection port.

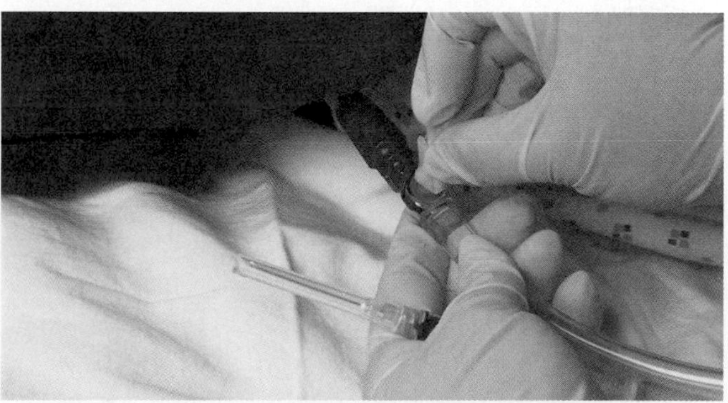

▲ Prep injection port on catheter drainage tubing before inserting needleless cannula.

7. Attempt to aspirate obstructing clot or debris.
   ▸ ***Rationale:*** Irrigation without first attempting removal of debris can force it into bladder, resulting in infection.
8. Withdraw irrigating solution into syringe.
9. Swab injection port again.
10. Inject solution slowly into port.
11. Remove syringe from injection port.
12. Unclamp drainage tube and lower catheter to allow solution to drain. ▸ ***Rationale:*** This facilitates drainage.
13. Repeat irrigation steps until return is free of clots and debris.
14. Lower bed and raise side rail.
15. Dispose of equipment and remove gloves.
16. Perform hand hygiene.
17. Measure amount of return. Subtract amount of irrigating solution to determine urine output.
18. Record net urine output on client's I&O record.

Maintaining Continuous Bladder Irrigation

Equipment

Irrigating solution (2000 mL of sterile normal saline, or less than drainage bag volume) as prescribed
IV tubing with roller clamp
IV pole
Antiseptic swabs
Clean gloves

Procedure

1. Check physician's orders and client care plan.
2. Note if client has triple-lumen indwelling catheter and drainage bag.
3. Identify client.
4. Explain procedure to client and provide privacy.
5. Perform hand hygiene and don clean gloves.
6. Remove protective covering from spike on tubing, and insert spike into insertion port of solution container. Use aseptic technique.
7. Hang irrigating solution container on IV pole and prime tubing. Height of pole is usually 24–36 in. above bladder.
   a. Remove protective cover from end of tubing using aseptic technique.
   b. Open roller clamp, and allow irrigating solution to run through tubing until all air is expelled.
      ▸ ***Rationale:*** This prevents air from entering bladder and causing discomfort.
   c. Close roller clamp.
8. Connect tubing to catheter irrigating (indwell) lumen using aseptic technique.
9. Check for patency of catheter; ensure there is an absence of clots or foreign bodies that may obstruct catheter.
10. Remove gloves.
11. Adjust drip rate of irrigating solution by adjusting the clamp on the tubing to increase or decrease based on urine outflow color.
    a. Infuse continuously to keep urine drainage pink to clear.
    b. When drainage is dark red or contains tissue or blood clots, irrigate manually, then increase drip rate.
       ▸ ***Rationale:*** Increased drip rate will clear the drainage and flush out debris and clots.

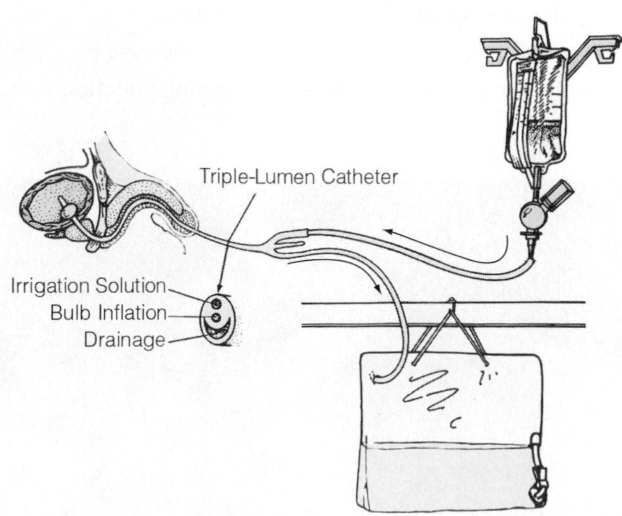

▲ Maintain continuous bladder irrigation by using a triple-lumen catheter for procedure.

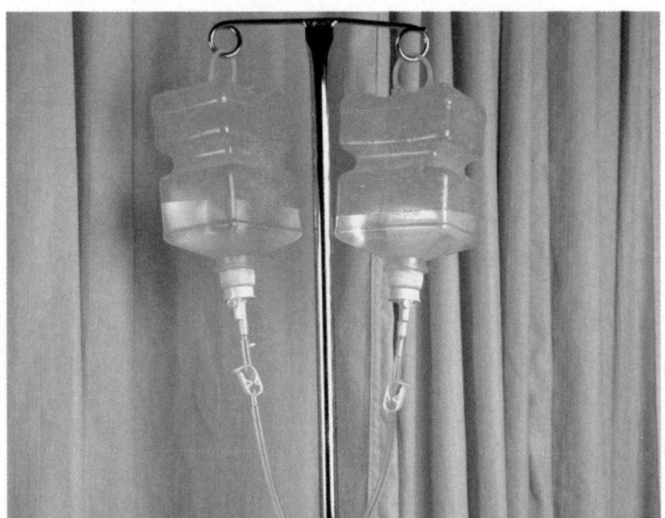

▲ Hang irrigating solution on IV pole at height of 24–36 inches above bladder.

c. Change irrigation solution bottle using aseptic technique.

12. Check for bladder distention or abdominal pain; note urine color.
13. Monitor urine output at least every hour to observe patency of system.
14. Empty drainage bag as needed. Subtract amount of irrigant infused from total output to obtain urine output and record.
15. Maintain catheter traction if taped to thigh.
    ▸ ***Rationale:*** This promotes venous hemostasis.
16. Remove gloves and perform hand hygiene.

NOTE: Procedure is done to flush clots and debris from bladder or obstruction of catheter after prostatic surgery and to prevent catheter obstruction and promote patency. Immediately report bright red urine outflow, as this indicates an arterial bleed.

DOCUMENTATION for Bladder Irrigation

- Type and amount of solution administered for irrigation
- Rate of administration of irrigating solution
- Description of urinary output, including color and presence of clots or debris
- Any statements of discomfort or cramping
- Medication given for pain
- Amount of actual urine output (total urine output minus amount of irrigant instilled)

CRITICAL THINKING Application

Expected Outcomes

- Continuous bladder irrigation is maintained to prevent clot formation and catheter obstruction.
- Client does not experience discomfort.

Unexpected Outcomes	Alternative Actions
Irrigation flow is not infusing at prescribed rate.	• Raise or lower IV standard with attached irrigation bag to assist in regulating flow using gravity. • Move flow adjuster clamp to new site on tubing. • Suspect obstruction.
Irrigation outflow is less than expected.	• Suspect obstruction: a. Check tubing for kinks. b. Have client change position. c. Maintaining sterile technique, disconnect catheter outflow port, and gently aspirate solution from catheter to remove clots. d. Instill 30–50 mL of irrigating solution to free clots. e. Reconnect drainage system and observe for 30 minutes; bladder spasms may block outflow of urine. f. Notify physician if problem is not resolved or client develops nausea, hypertension, bradycardia (client may develop TURP syndrome due to absorption of hypotonic irrigating solution). • Increase irrigation inflow rate; monitor vital signs. • Do not allow client to cough.
Client's urine outflow is dark pink with blood clots.	• Keep client's catheter-taped leg straight to maintain traction on catheter inflation bulb. • Suspect obstruction. • Increase irrigation rate. • Notify physician if problem continues.
Client experiences painful bladder spasms during irrigation.	• Notify physician to obtain order for urinary antispasmodic medication. • Assist client to change position.

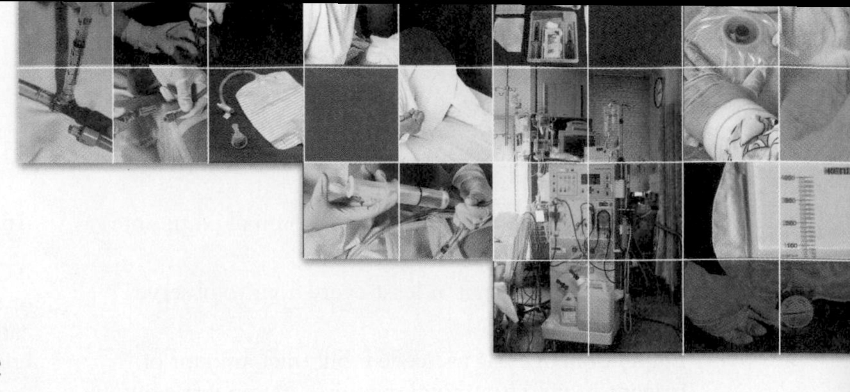

Chapter 22

UNIT 5

Suprapubic Catheter Care

Nursing Process Data

ASSESSMENT Data Base

- Observe for urine flow through catheter.
- Observe for excessive bleeding through catheter or at insertion site.
- Check that suture site is clean, dry, and intact.
- Check that straight drainage is maintained.
- Assess that fluid intake is at least 2000 mL daily.
- Assess client for pain, bladder distention, or spasms.
- Assess client's ability to assist with clamping procedure.
- Assess client's ability to tolerate catheter being clamped.

PLANNING Objectives

- To prevent urinary tract infection when a suprapubic catheter is inserted
- To maintain a patent suprapubic catheter
- To monitor the catheter clamping procedure
- To prevent infection at catheter insertion site
- To provide discharge teaching if catheter is to remain in place when client is discharged

IMPLEMENTATION Procedures

EVALUATION Expected Outcomes

- Suprapubic catheter remains intact.
- Client remains free of urinary tract infection.

Pearson Nursing Student Resources

Find additional review materials at **nursing.pearsonhighered.com**

Prepare for success with NCLEX®-style practice questions and Skill Checklists

Providing Suprapubic Catheter Care

Equipment

Closed drainage system, including Foley catheter tubing and bag
Catheter clamp and plug
Dry sterile dressing and tape if ordered
Cleansing solution
Clean gloves
Sterile gloves

Preparation

1. Check physician's orders and client care plan.
2. Identify client and explain purpose of catheter.
3. Describe procedure for continuous or intermittent urinary drainage.
4. Perform hand hygiene.
5. Provide privacy.

Procedure

1. Observe catheter for patency. ▸ ***Rationale:*** The most common problem with suprapubic catheters is occlusion with sediment or clots.
   a. First 24 hr: check the catheter every hour to detect possible obstruction. Urine output should be in excess of 30 mL/hour.
   b. Second day: check the catheter every 8 hr.
   c. Third day: check the catheter when the catheter is unclamped.
2. Maintain a closed drainage system. Do not open system to irrigate or obtain urine sample.
3. Observe for signs of urinary tract infection (color, odor, presence of sediment).
4. Keep the dressing dry around site of insertion. Apply a new dressing, maintaining sterile technique, every morning and as necessary.
   a. Place bed in high position.
   b. Perform hand hygiene and don clean gloves.
   c. Remove old dressing, discard gloves, and dispose in appropriate container.
   d. Perform hand hygiene and open sterile supplies.
   e. Open cleansing solution and pour over sterile gauze.
   f. Don sterile gloves.
   g. Assess skin surrounding suprapubic catheter.
   h. Cleanse area with cleansing solution. Allow to dry.
   i. Apply sterile dressing and secure with tape.
   j. Remove gloves and supplies and discard in appropriate container.
   k. Perform hand hygiene.
   l. Replace bed in low position.
5. Perform clamping protocol according to physician orders for intermittent urinary drainage.
   a. Explain the clamping procedure and ask client to help monitor the clamping.
   b. Instruct client to report if he or she feels fullness in the bladder during clamping.
   c. Don clean gloves.
   d. Clamp the catheter.
6. Empty the drainage bag or remove drainage tubing from catheter, maintaining aseptic technique.
   a. Place drainage tubing in sterile package to maintain sterility.
   b. Place catheter plug in catheter end.
   c. Remove gloves and perform hand hygiene.
   d. Record urine output on I&O record.
   e. Leave the catheter clamped or plugged for 3–4 hr depending on client's level of comfort and physician's orders.
7. At 3- to 4-hr intervals, or when client feels bladder fullness, ask client to void normally. Don clean gloves to measure the urine and record output on I&O bedside record.
8. Immediately after client voids, unclamp catheter and leave unclamped for 5 minutes, collecting the residual urine.
   a. Don clean gloves to measure the residual urine after unclamping of the catheter.
   b. Reclamp catheter.
   c. If ordered, send a urine specimen to laboratory after the first clamping. ▸ ***Rationale:*** This checks for the presence of microorganisms.
9. Repeat clamping protocol every 3–4 hr according to physician orders. The catheter may be open to drainage from bedtime until 6 AM.
10. When the client is voiding normally, clamp the catheter throughout the night in preparation for its removal.
11. When the client's residual urine output is less than 100 mL or retains less than 20% of residual urine on two successive checks, notify the physician for removal of the catheter.
12. Cleanse insertion area with antimicrobial swab.

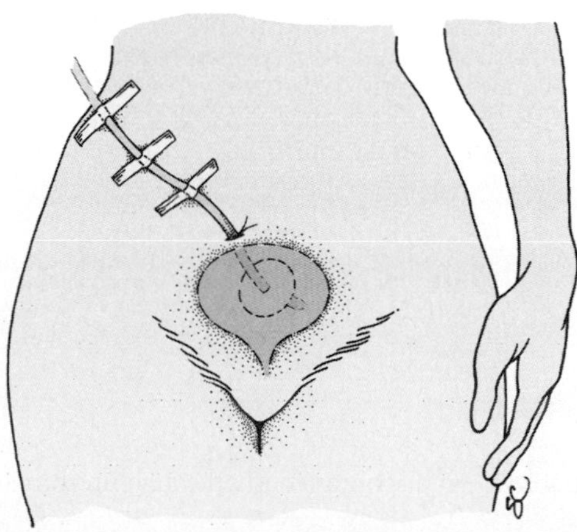

▲ Tape catheter and connect to a closed system.

13. Deflate balloon and remove catheter, if order written for nurse to remove.
14. Apply a 2 × 2 sterile dressing over the insertion site.
15. Dispose of the catheter in biohazard bag.
16. If the client is discharged from the hospital with the catheter, provide the following teaching for home care:
    a. Instruct the client to drink one glass of fluid every hour while awake.
    b. Instruct client to follow clamping procedure when awake or as instructed by physician.
    c. Instruct the client to leave the catheter open to the drainage system at night. (Drainage system may be urinary tubing and bag or leg bag.)
    d. Tell client to notify physician if dysuria occurs when voiding or if urine becomes cloudy, odorous, or has sediment.

For Removing the Suprapubic Catheter

a. Don clean gloves.
b. Prep the catheter and the insertion site with Betadine or antiseptic prep.
c. Deflate balloon: Insert syringe into inflation tube of catheter and withdraw fluid from balloon, which will deflate.
d. Gently withdraw catheter.
e. Place 2 × 2 sterile dressing over the insertion site.

For Reinserting at Established Suprapubic Catheter Site

NOTE: In selected hospitals, nurses are now allowed to reinsert suprapubic catheters per physician's orders.

a. Obtain same size suprapubic catheter as used previously. (Check size at distal end of catheter.)
b. Insert new catheter 1.5–2 in. or add length if large amount of adipose tissue. There may or may not be urinary return with insertion of catheter.
c. Inflate balloon with appropriate volume of sterile water.

DOCUMENTATION for Suprapubic Catheter Care

- Time catheter clamped
- Length of time clamped
- Client's ability to void spontaneously
- Client's feelings of fullness
- Time specimen sent to laboratory
- Color, amount, and odor of urine obtained
- Color, amount, and odor of residual urine

CRITICAL THINKING Application

Expected Outcomes

- Suprapubic catheter remains intact.
- Client remains free of urinary tract infection.
- Client is able to void naturally.

Unexpected Outcomes	Alternative Actions
Suprapubic catheter becomes dislodged.	• Place sterile dressing over catheter insertion site; do not attempt to replace catheter. • Notify physician. • Obtain new catheter to prepare for insertion by physician.
Client develops urinary tract infection.	• Note signs and symptoms of UTI: cloudy malodorous urine with sediment, bladder discomfort/spasms, elevated temperature. • Notify physician to obtain order for urinalysis and antimicrobial therapy. • Increase fluid intake to at least 2–3 L/day (unless contraindicated). • Maintain continuous urine drainage per suprapubic catheter.
Client is unable to void spontaneously through urethra.	• Maintain suprapubic urine drainage. • Notify physician.

Chapter 22

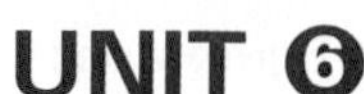

Specimens From Closed Systems

Nursing Process Data

ASSESSMENT Data Base

- Assess the type of specimen needed.

  Note: From a closed system, all will be sterile specimens—voided urine is a clean specimen.
- Identify amount of urine needed for specimen.
- Check to see if the closed urinary system has a port for obtaining a specimen.

PLANNING Objectives

- To prevent urinary infection by obtaining a urine specimen without interrupting a closed urinary drainage system
- To determine the specific microorganism causing a urinary tract infection
- To obtain a urine specimen for diagnostic purposes.

IMPLEMENTATION Procedures

EVALUATION Expected Outcomes

- Urine specimen is obtained from the closed urinary drainage system.
- Urine specimen remain sterile.

Pearson Nursing Student Resources

Find additional review materials at **nursing.pearsonhighered.com**

Prepare for success with NCLEX®-style practice questions and Skill Checklists

Collecting Specimen From a Closed System

Equipment

Catheter tubing clamp or rubber band
Kova specimen trap syringe *or* syringe with blunt cannula
Sterile specimen container with label if necessary
Label
Biohazard bag
Antimicrobial swab
Clean gloves

Procedure

1. Gather equipment.
2. Identify client using two forms of identification.
3. Explain the procedure and rationale to the client.
4. Clamp (or crimp and bind) retention catheter drainage tubing a few inches distal to sample access port (approximately 15 minutes to allow urine to collect in tube). ▸ ***Rationale:*** This ensures urine specimen is adequate.
5. Perform hand hygiene and don gloves.
6. Wipe the sample access port of the drainage tubing with the antimicrobial swab.
7. Insert cannula of specimen trap syringe into port. Alternately, insert blunt cannula of syringe, or engage uncapped Luer-Lok syringe with port. ▸ ***Rationale:*** Different manufacturers recommend different equipment use with their products.
8. Aspirate urine sample (at least 2 mL) by gently pulling back on syringe plunger, then remove syringe.

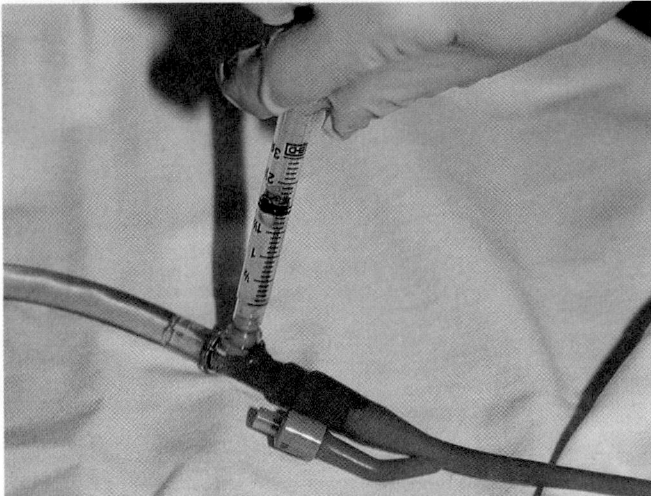

Ⓐ1 Luer-Lok syringe: Obtain specimen using Luer-Lok syringe and transfer urine to sterile specimen cup.

9. For Kova specimen syringe, cap syringe, completely retract plunger, snap it off from end of syringe barrel, and discard.
10. Apply identifying label to specimen syringe.
11. For syringe with blunt cannula or Luer-Lok syringe, transfer urine sample into specimen container and apply client label.
12. Remove drainage tubing clamp.
13. Remove gloves and perform hand hygiene.
14. Send specimen syringe or container in biohazard bag to laboratory as soon as possible, or place in unit refrigerator.

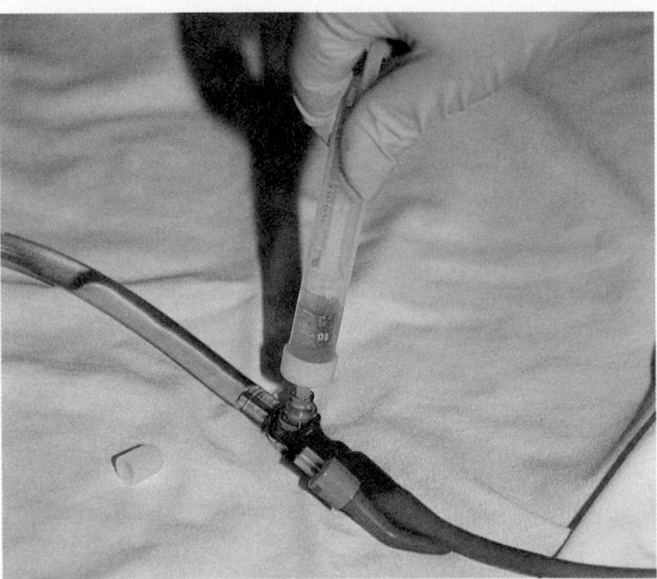

Ⓐ2 Specimen trap syringe: Insert specimen collection syringe cannula into aspiration port and gently pull back on plunger to aspirate urine.

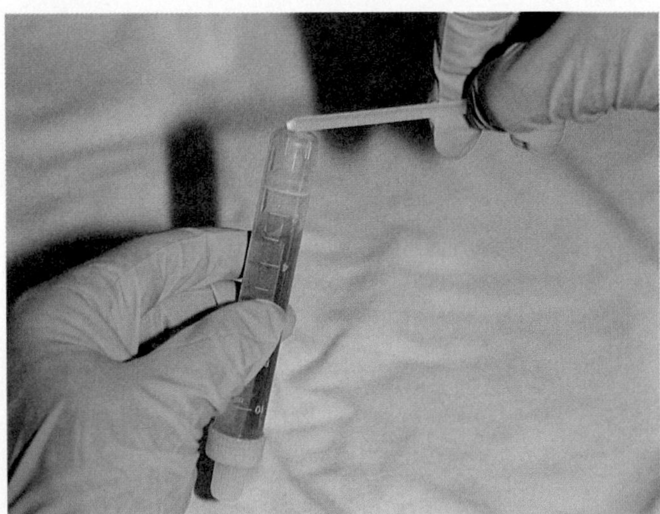

Ⓐ3 Kova specimen syringe: Snap off plunger of Kova specimen collection syringe, place in biohazard bag, and send as self-contained unit to lab for urine analysis.

DOCUMENTATION for Specimens From Closed Systems

- Type and amount of specimen obtained
- Type of specimen container/syringe used to obtain specimen
- Color, consistency, and odor of urine
- Time of urine collection
- Time specimen sent to laboratory

CRITICAL THINKING Application

Expected Outcomes

- Urine sample is obtained from closed urinary drainage system.

Unexpected Outcomes

Insufficient amount of urine is obtained when collection is attempted.

Alternative Actions

- Check that client has had sufficient fluid intake.
- Check for kinking of catheter.
- Clamp catheter tubing for 45 minutes before specimen collection.
- Reposition client.

Chapter 22

UNIT 7

Urinary Diversion

Nursing Process Data

ASSESSMENT Data Base

- Assess location of stoma on client's abdomen. (Depends on type of diversion.)
- Determine type of urinary diversion.
- Observe stoma color (same color as mucous membrane lining the mouth).
- Assess skin for condition.
- Assess presence of ureteral stents for new ileal conduit.
- Assess most appropriate pouching system for client. (System depends on client's age, manual dexterity, size of stoma, stoma location, presence of skin folds, and bony prominences.)
- Assess client's ability to manage self-care.
- Assess urine output (amount and character).

PLANNING Objectives

- To provide a pouching system that prevents skin irritation
- To instruct the client in self-care
- To monitor stoma for viability
- To obtain a sterile urine specimen

IMPLEMENTATION Procedures

EVALUATION Expected Outcomes

- Pouching system does not leak.
- Client demonstrates self-care skills.
- Urine specimen is readily obtained from urinary diversion system.
- Peristomal skin remains intact and healthy.

Applying a Urinary Diversion Pouch

Equipment

One- or two-piece urinary pouch with skin barrier, flange, and spigot at bottom of pouch to empty urine
Items to clean stoma (e.g., soft cloth or gauze sponges) and warm water
Plastic bag for disposal of used equipment
Gauze for drying skin and for wicking stoma
Underpad to protect bedding
Scissors if indicated
Protective barriers such as skin prep, skin gel, or protective barrier film if necessary
Stoma measuring guide
Clean gloves

Preparation

1. Check physician's order and client care plan. Pouch should be changed every 3–7 days.
2. Gather equipment.
3. Perform hand hygiene.
4. Identify client and explain procedure.
5. Provide privacy.
6. Place client in a position that promotes visualization and self-care.
7. Place protective pad under client.
8. Place bath blanket over client's chest and position top covers over lower abdomen without impeding client's visualization of procedure.

Procedure

1. Don clean gloves.
2. Empty, then remove entire ostomy appliance by pushing the skin gently away from the appliance and peeling the appliance downward. Discard in plastic bag.
3. Wash stoma and peristomal skin with warm water and soap if needed, rinse well, and pat skin dry.▸ ***Rationale:*** Chemical or perfumed wipes can irritate skin or may interfere with pouch seal.

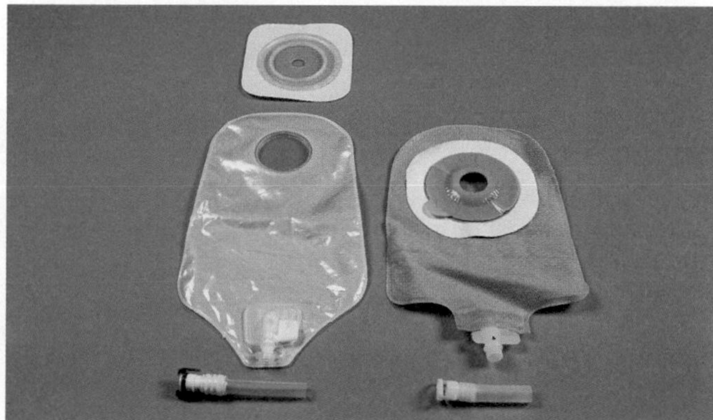

▲ One-piece and two-piece urinary diversion pouches.

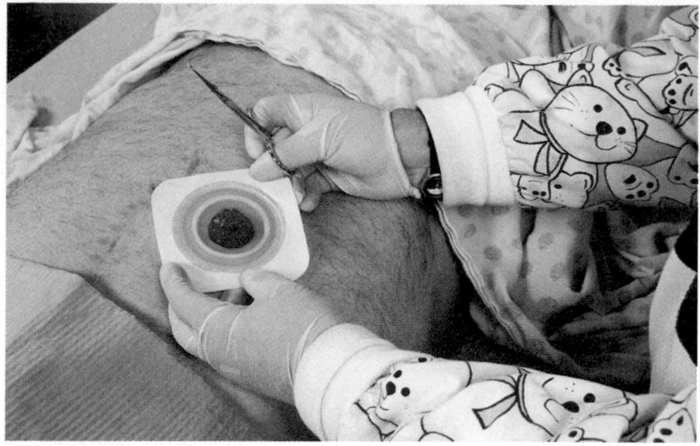

▲ Cut wafer opening slightly larger than stoma.

NOTE: Stoma may bleed slightly when wiped.

4. Check stoma for healing; it should be bright but not dark red and moist, and raised 0.5–1 in. above skin surface (or may be flush). Check for mucocutaneous separation, ulceration, encrustation, and signs of infection, and sensitivities or allergies.
5. Check skin surrounding stoma to ensure urine hasn't been draining under wafer, causing skin irritation.
6. Prepare new urinary pouch. Place gauze over stoma to prevent urine from oozing onto skin. A wick can be placed in stoma, if needed. Measure stoma site with measuring guide, unless pouch has precut opening. ▸ ***Rationale:*** To keep urine from contact with skin during pouch change.
7. Trace size of stoma on wafer and cut 1/16 1/8 in. larger than size. ▸ ***Rationale:*** This small opening prevents leakage of effluent onto skin; however, the size is large enough to prevent pressure on the stoma from the wafer rubbing on skin.
8. Apply protective barrier (only if indicated) to skin surrounding stoma or to wafer. Do not use lotion. ▸ ***Rationale:*** Protective barriers contain alcohol and

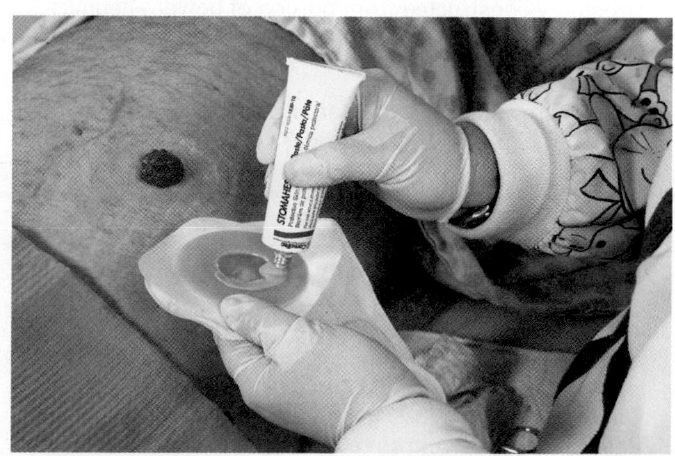

▲ Apply protective paste to wafer, only if indicated.

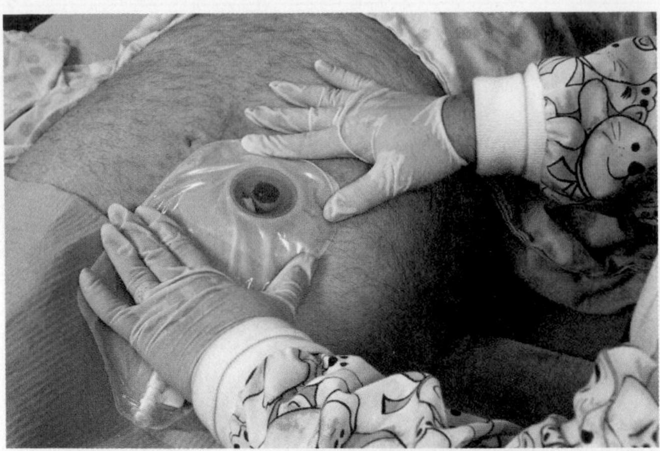

▲ Apply pouch and press firmly to facilitate seal.

cause burning and may interfere with seal. In addition, barrier must be removed with adhesive remover.

9. Let site dry thoroughly.
10. Remove paper from adhesive on wafer of one- or two-piece appliance.

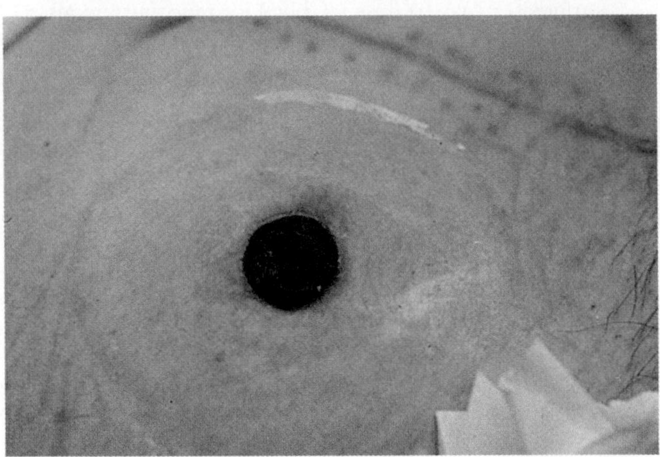

▲ Cleanse stoma and periostomal skin; dry thoroughly.

11. Remove wick and center wafer over stoma; apply to dry skin, starting at bottom, and working up around stoma. Press wafer on skin for 3 minutes. ▶ ***Rationale:*** To promote adherence to skin. If two-piece pouch, attach pouch to wafer flange.
12. Remove air from clean pouch and close spout. Attach pouch to gravity drainage bag only while client is in bed. Empty pouch when one-third full.
13. Discard equipment in appropriate receptacle.
14. Remove gloves and perform hand hygiene.

Clinical Alert

Thin plastic tubes (stents) may be placed in each ureter during surgery. These exit stoma and remain in place for up to 10 days. They serve to maintain patency until swelling has subsided at ureteroileal anastomosis site (6–10 days). Their presence and length of exposure should be documented. The surgeon should be notified when they wash out into collection pouch.

Client Teaching for Emptying Pouch

Instruct client to:

- Empty pouch when one-third full.
- Use bathroom if possible.
- Place distal end of pouch between thighs or stand over toilet.
- Open drainage port to allow urine to drain.
- Dry drainage port with toilet paper.
- Close drainage port.
- Perform hand hygiene.

Types of Urinary Diversion	Nursing Considerations
I. Ileal or Colonic Conduit	
• Urostomy constructed from portion of bowel—ileum is resected and an internal conduit formed and attached to abdominal wall.	• Care of urinary pouch. • Monitor peristomal skin for breakdown.
• Ureters are connected to internal conduit. • An external pouch collects urine.	• Monitor stoma.
II. Continent Urostomy	
A. (Kock's Reservoir)	
• Reservoir is constructed from ileum and ascending colon. Two nipple valves are created by pulling ileum back onto itself. • Ureters are implanted near internal nipple valve (valve prevents reflux). • Outlet valve is attached to abdominal wall and stoma. • Reservoir is catheterized to drain urine.	• Instruct in clean intermittent self-catheterization every 2–4 hr.

Types of Urinary Diversion	Nursing Considerations
B. Indiana Pouch	
• Internal pouch is created from the ascending colon and terminal ileum. • Pouch is larger than Kock's reservoir. • Reservoir is catheterized to drain urine.	• Instruct in clean intermittent self-catheterization every 2–4 hr. • Monitor for electrolyte imbalance; reservoir may absorb urea and electrolytes.
III. Neo Bladder	
• Created from cecum or ileum with ureters attached. • Has no stoma. • Requires no external appliance. • Urine exits via urethra. • Preserves normal body image.	• Client may eliminate with timed voiding. • May require self–urethral catheterization.

Obtaining Urine Specimen From an Ileal Conduit

Equipment

Sterile catheter kit
Prep solution
Sterile saline or water
Underpad
New urinary pouch
Supplies necessary to apply new pouch
Bath blanket, towels
Clean gloves
Soap and water
Pitcher of water and glass
Biohazard bag

Preparation

1. Check physician's orders and client care plan.
2. Gather equipment.
3. Perform hand hygiene.
4. Explain procedure to client.
5. Provide privacy.
6. Place bath blanket over client's chest and position top covers over lower abdomen.
7. Place towels around stoma. ▶ ***Rationale:*** Urine will leak around catheter.
8. Don gloves.

Procedure

1. Open sterile packages.
2. Remove pouch or snap pouch off wafer flange.

NOTE: Do not use pouch contents to obtain urine specimen. Remove gloves.

3. Put on sterile gloves.
4. Place sterile drape over stoma.
5. Remove lid from specimen container and place end of catheter into container.
6. Apply lubricant to catheter.
7. Use forceps to pick up cotton ball and prep stoma with solution and rinse with sterile saline or water.
8. Insert tip of catheter into stoma approximately 1.5 in.
9. When urine specimen is obtained (usually not more than 5–25 mL), remove catheter. If no urine is obtained, have client drink water.
10. Return lid to specimen container and apply label.
11. If wafer removed, wash and dry peristomal area.
12. Replace pouch or apply new pouch.
13. Remove gloves and perform hand hygiene.
14. Place specimen container in biohazard bag and send specimen to lab immediately or refrigerate.

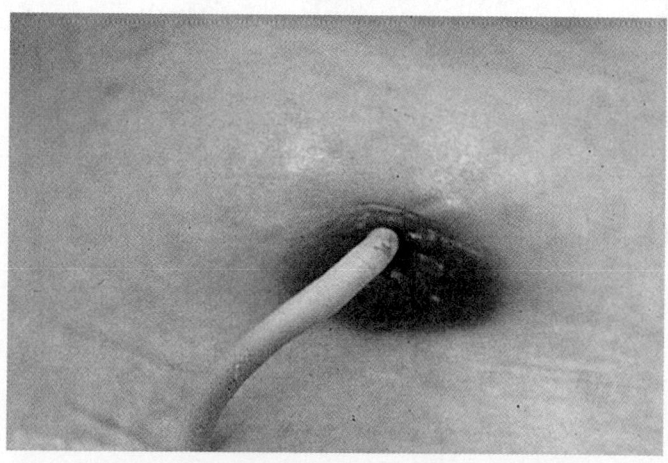

▲ Catheter is used to obtain specimen from ileal conduit.

Catheterizing Continent Urinary Reservoir

Equipment

Sterile catheter (if client hospitalized)
Water-soluble lubricant
Clean gloves
Bedpan (if client unable to use toilet)
Warm water and soap
Washcloth, towel

Preparation

1. Check physician's orders and client care plan.
2. Gather equipment.
3. Identify client and explain procedure.
4. Perform hand hygiene and don gloves.
5. Provide privacy.
6. Position client on chair facing toilet or place bedpan next to client if on bedrest.

Procedure

1. Open lubricant packet.
2. Lubricate tip of catheter, maintaining sterility.
3. Insert catheter 1.5–2 in. into stoma. Place distal end of catheter over toilet or bedpan.
4. Instruct client to take deep breath and gently insert catheter through nipple valve until urine returns. ▸ ***Rationale:*** When the abdominal muscles are relaxed, it is easier to advance catheter through nipple valve.
5. Hold catheter in place until urine stops draining.
6. Remove catheter.
7. Wash and dry peristomal area with soap and water.
8. Assist client back to bed, or position for comfort.
9. Remove gloves and perform hand hygiene.

Clinical Alert

Irrigation: During the immediate postoperative period after formation of a continent reservoir, irrigation of the reservoir must be done. A mucous plug can block the catheter, leading to over-distention of the reservoir and perforation or disruption of the surgical reconstruction. Teach the client with a continent reservoir (Kock's or Indiana) to irrigate the reservoir with warm water daily using catheter and bulb or piston syringe to remove collected mucus. ▸ ***Rationale:*** Mucus produced by the bowel segment will accumulate in the reservoir.

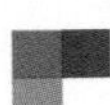

DOCUMENTATION for Urinary Diversion

- Color and amount of urine obtained from catheterizing continent reservoir
- Catheter size used for catheterization
- Status of ureteral stents, if present
- Peristomal skin and stoma condition
- Client's acceptance of stoma, participation in self-care
- Type and method of drainage pouch applied
- Specimen sent to lab

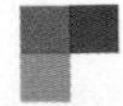

CRITICAL THINKING Application

Expected Outcomes

- Pouching system does not leak.
- Client demonstrates self-care skills.
- Urine specimen is readily obtained from urinary diversion system.
- Peristomal skin remains intact and healthy.

Unexpected Outcomes

Pouching system leaks.

Alternative Actions

- Check area for crease or dip in skin, which allows urine to pool and leak out.
- Fill in dip area with skin barrier to prevent pooling.
- Apply belt to improve fit.
- Apply another type of pouch (e.g., convex).
- Change more frequently if leak is due to dissolving of skin barrier—or use different barrier.
- Advise client to avoid using soaps or wipes to clean area because they interfere with pouch adhesion.

Client is unable to manage own urinary diversion.	• Simplify pouch procedure if possible. • Provide detailed instruction in more simplified manner. • Include caregiver in teaching to assist and support client. • Refer client to home health agency for follow-up care.
Client is offended by odor in urine collection system.	• Recommend urine-acidifying agent (e.g., vitamin C, 500 mg BID to TID); avoid alkaline ash citrus juices. • Wash reusable equipment with mild soap and water and rinse in vinegar weekly or use commercial deodorant. • Inform client that certain foods and drugs (asparagus, vitamin B complex) give odor to urine. Empty pouch frequently if these are ingested. • Inform client that cloudy urine and strong odor may indicate urinary tract infection. Advise physician and collect sterile urine specimen.
No urine is obtained from conduit.	• Rotate catheter, or position client on side to allow urine to flow into catheter. As little as 1 mL is needed for urine culture and sensitivity testing. • Have client drink water.
Erythematous vesicular rash appears on peristomal skin.	• Suspect possible allergic reaction; obtain patch test for allergy. • Avoid use of chemical wipes and perfumed soaps. • Suspect yeast infection; report to physician.

Chapter 22

UNIT 8

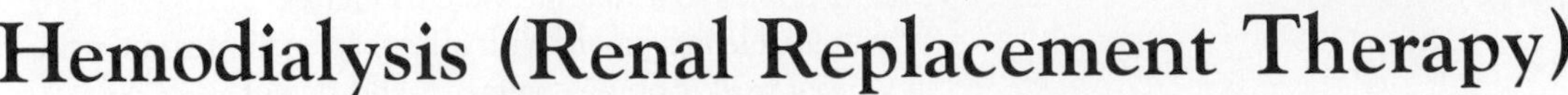

Hemodialysis (Renal Replacement Therapy)

Nursing Process Data

ASSESSMENT Data Base

- Review dialysis orders.
- Assess patency of vascular access.

  Femoral vein catheter: dual-lumen vascular device used for immediate vascular access in life-threatening situations.

  Central venous dual-lumen catheter (DLC): vascular device placed in internal jugular vein used for temporary access for acute hemodialysis clients.

  Permanent dual-lumen catheter (PDLC): vascular device inserted through internal jugular vein and advanced to superior vene cava (SVC).

  Arteriovenous fistula: surgically created internal anastomosis between an artery and vein; used for clients undergoing chronic hemodialysis.

  Arteriovenous graft: surgically implanted synthetic material (Gortex) or biologic material (human umbilical vein) used for anastomosis between an artery and vein for clients undergoing chronic hemodialysis.
- Review chart and laboratory reports for factors that may alter management of dialysis (especially potassium, sodium, calcium, and phosphorus levels; albumin; hemoglobin; hematocrit levels; BUN; and creatinine).
- Assess vital signs.

  Assess causes of hypotension: fluid loss, hypoalbuminemia, large interdialytic weight gain.

  Check serum electrolytes, BUN, and creatinine before and after dialysis according to physician orders.

  Weigh client before and after dialysis to determine fluid loss.

PLANNING Objectives

- To remove end products of protein metabolism: urea, creatinine, and uric acid
- To remove excess fluid, thereby reestablishing fluid balance
- To maintain or restore normal level of electrolytes in the body
- To maintain a patent access site for hemodialysis
- To maintain patent catheters centrally placed
- To instruct the client in self-care

IMPLEMENTATION Procedures

EVALUATION Expected Outcomes

- Dialysis proceeds without complication (excess fluids and wastes removed from blood).
- Vascular access site remains patent.
- Client demonstrates self-care after teaching.

Pearson Nursing Student Resources

Find additional review materials at
nursing.pearsonhighered.com

Prepare for success with NCLEX®-style practice questions and Skill Checklists

Providing Hemodialysis

Equipment

Dialyzer (types are hollow fiber or cellulose acetate)
1000-mL bag of 0.9% normal saline IV solution
Machine blood lines
Fistula needles, 15/16 gauge, 1–1.5 in. in length
Sterile gauze pads, alcohol swabs, and povidone–iodine or ChloraPrep swabs
Two 3-mL syringes
Two 20-mL syringes
Drape
Client mask
Hemostats, cannula clamps
Tape
Sterile gloves and clean gloves
Gown
Protective goggles and face mask or visor shield
12-mL syringe
Heparin solution 1000 U/mL
Hemastix

Preparation

1. Obtain dialysate bath composition as ordered.
2. Set up 1000-mL IV of normal saline using IV tubing in blood line set.
3. Load heparin pump (e.g., 8 mL heparin) per manufacturer's instructions. ▶ ***Rationale:*** Heparin is added to system just before blood enters dialyzer to prevent clotting. The clotting mechanism is activated when blood moves outside body and is in contact with foreign substances.
4. Check location of nearest emergency power outlet. ▶ ***Rationale:*** To maintain electric current if routine power fails.
5. Test dialysis machine for presence of bleach with Hemastix. ▶ ***Rationale:*** This detects presence of caustic agents that could result in client complications.
6. Prime dialyzer and arterial and venous blood lines with saline.
7. Hang additional IV solution of saline. ▶ ***Rationale:*** Saline infusions must be available immediately for rapid reversal of hypotension or discontinuation of dialysis.
8. Connect pressure monitor lines to both arterial and venous drip chambers. ▶ ***Rationale:*** This monitors the amount of hydrostatic pressure exerted on blood in the ultrafiltration process used to extract fluid throughout dialysis treatment.
9. Set the alarm pressures—high and low.
10. Connect air leak detector to venous drip chamber.
11. Test all machine alarms—venous and arterial pressure, air detector, and blood leak detector.

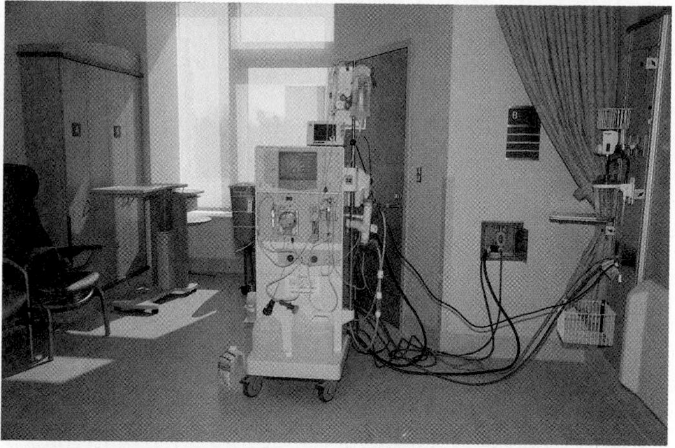

▲ Hemodialysis unit used to treat renal failure clients.

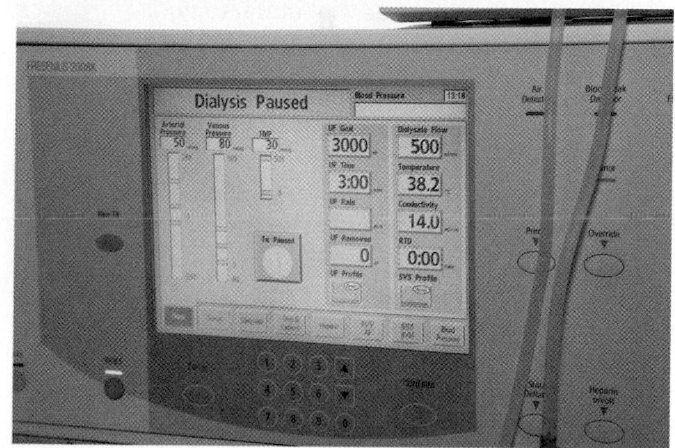

▲ Dialysis panel indicates settings and values.

12. Connect arterial and venous lines for recirculation with adapter, and turn blood pump to 200 mL/min.
13. Document alarm checks in dialysis log.

Procedure

For AV Fistula or Graft

1. Place blood line at the same level as the bed.
2. Don mask and gown. Put on goggles and perform hand hygiene.
3. Don clean gloves and remove dressing, if used. Remove and discard gloves and perform hand hygiene.

Clinical Alert

When a hemodialysis client is hospitalized:

1. Place an identifying bracelet on access arm.
2. Post safety precautions at head of bed (e.g., "Do not use access arm for blood pressure or venipuncture," and "Fluid restriction specified").
3. Notify dialysis specialty nurse of client's admission to hospital.

The Hemodialysis Process

Hemodialysis works by removing blood from the client's arterial access site (graft, fistula, or catheter). It travels through a blood pump and an arterial pressure monitor to a dialyzer (filter). In the dialyzer, the blood is separated from the dialysate by a synthetic semipermeable membrane. The dialysate (bath) runs against the blood flowing on the opposite side of the semipermeable membrane, leading to osmosis, diffusion, and ultrafiltration. Fluid, electrolytes, and toxins are removed from the blood. The blood then flows from the dialyzer through a tubing system to the client's venous access site. Fluid is removed through the use of hydrostatic pressure applied to the blood and a negative hydrostatic pressure applied to the dialysate bath. The difference between these two pressures is termed *transmembrane pressure,* and this results in the process of ultrafiltration.

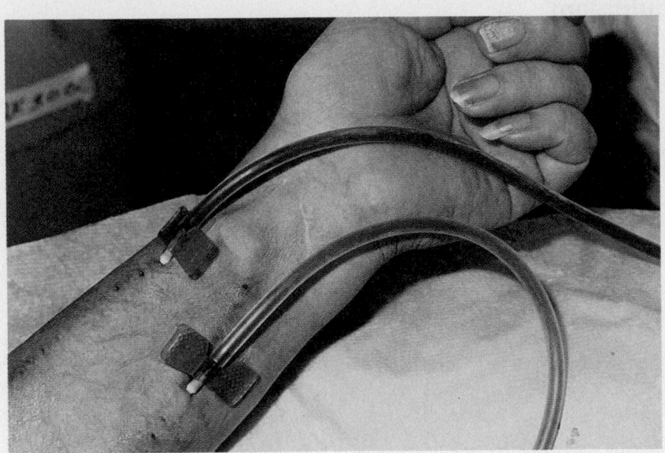

▲ Arterial and venous needles placed in graft for hemodialysis.

4. Don sterile gloves.
5. Clean access site using ChloraPrep or alcohol swab, then povidone–iodine swab. Using a circular motion, cleanse from needle insertion site outward. Allow to dry. ▸ ***Rationale:*** Cleansing occurs from cleanest to dirtiest area, preventing contamination of the site.
6. Insert needles into fistula or graft. Tape securely to extremity.
7. Obtain blood for predialysis blood samples as ordered by the physician. (Usually electrolytes, hematocrit, clotting time, etc.)
8. After blood is drawn for lab work, heparin bolus should be given to client according to physician's order—start heparin pump at ordered rate.
9. Prime the extracorporeal circuit with blood.
   a. Connect arterial tubing of the blood line to client's arterial site.
   b. Connect venous tubing.
   c. Unclamp venous blood line.
   d. Unclamp arterial blood line.
   e. Clamp saline infusion line.
10. Note time of dialysis initiation.
11. Tape all connections securely; secure blood tubing to client's extremity.

Blood Flow for Dialysis

An adequate vascular access should permit blood flow to the dialyzer of 200–400 mL/min. Optimal blood access and blood flow to the dialyzer influences dialysis efficiency.

Safety Precautions for Fistula or Graft

- Feel for vibration (thrill) over access site regularly.
- Do not measure blood pressure on extremity.
- Do not perform venipuncture in extremity.
- Counsel client not to wear constrictive clothing on extremity.
- Counsel client to avoid lying on extremity.
- Avoid carrying heavy loads with access extremity.
- Immediately report swelling, discoloration, drainage, or coldness, numbness, or weakness of hand.

12. Set alarm pressures—high and low.
13. Establish blood flow rate (usually 200–400 mL/min) and the dialysate rate of 500 mL/hr. ▸ ***Rationale:*** These flow rates allow the imbalances in fluids and electrolytes to be corrected rapidly (3–4 hr per run and 2–3 times/week).
14. Ensure that access connections are visible.
15. Check client's blood pressure and pulse once dialysis has been initiated, then every 30 minutes unless otherwise indicated.
16. Assess client at least every 30 minutes for vital signs and potential complications.
17. Administer any ordered medication through the venous line. ▸ ***Rationale:*** Medication infuses into client, not machine.
18. Turn heparin infusion off last 30–60 minutes or as ordered.

Assessing Arteriovenous Fistula

- Perform hand hygiene.
- Position client's arm so fistula is easily accessed.
- Palpate the area to feel for thrill (vibration). This indicates arterial to venous blood flow and fistula patency.
- Auscultate with a stethoscope to detect a bruit (swishing noise). This indicates a patent fistula.
- Palpate pulses distal to fistula to check circulation.
- Observe capillary refill in extremity digits.
- Assess for numbness, tingling, coldness, pallor, or alteration in sensation in digits of fistula extremity.
- Assess for signs and symptoms of infection: redness, edema, soreness, warmth, or increased temperature.

Note: Vascular access promotes more efficient removal and replacement of blood during dialysis and fewer complications occur. Vascular access should be prepared weeks or months before using it for dialysis. This will stabilize the graft site and ensure adequate blood flow when used for dialysis.

Providing Ongoing Care of Hemodialysis Client

Procedure

1. Limit fluid intake to prescribed amount (e.g., 1500 mL/day).
2. Maintain individualized diet as prescribed: high-quality protein 1.1 g/kg ideal body wt/day; sodium 70 mEq/day; potassium, average 70 mEq/day.
3. Check blood pressure for hypertension/hypotension; check temperature for possible infection.
4. Auscultate heart and lung sounds for signs of fluid overload (pulmonary edema and pericarditis).
5. Provide access site care.
6. Observe mental status—indicative of fluid and electrolyte imbalance.
7. Administer Epogen, if ordered, to improve hemoglobin level (given at time of dialysis).
8. Encourage regular rest periods.
9. Weigh daily to assess fluid accumulation.
10. Use antibacterial soap and lotion to bathe. ▶ ***Rationale:*** This decreases risk of staphylococcal infections.
11. Determine that client understands when and how to take medications (e.g., Tums with meals).
12. Provide continued emotional support.
    a. Allow for expression of feelings about change in body image and role performance.
    b. Encourage expression of fears.
    c. Encourage caregiver support.
    d. Give support for required change in lifestyle.
13. Instruct client to prevent obstruction to blood flow on fistula arm.

NOTE: Dialysis adequacy is improved with increased prescription, conversion of catheters to grafts or fistulas, and by not shortening treatments.

Terminating Hemodialysis

Equipment

Clean gloves
Gown
Goggles
Mask
Nonsterile pads
Tubing clamps

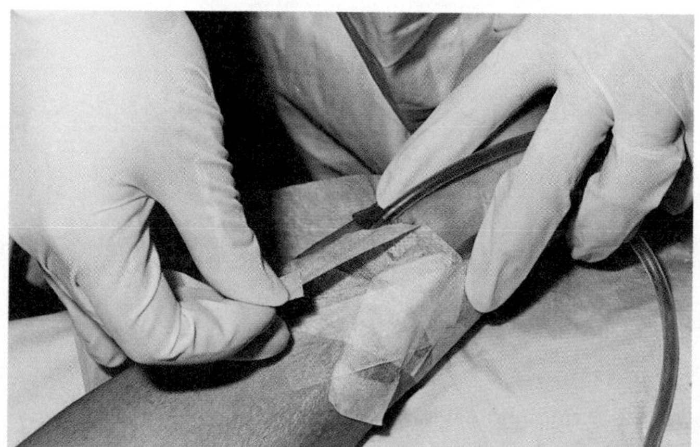

▲ Carefully remove tape from needle sites when terminating dialysis.

Procedure

1. Don gloves, gown, goggles, and protective mask.
2. Remove tape and dressing to visualize needle insertion site.
3. Place pads under connectors.
4. Open IV of normal saline to return blood on the arterial side of tubing.

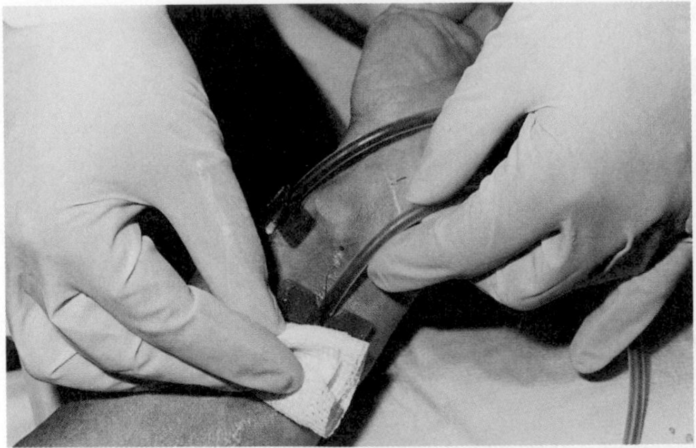

▲ Remove arterial and venous needles, using needle safety shields.

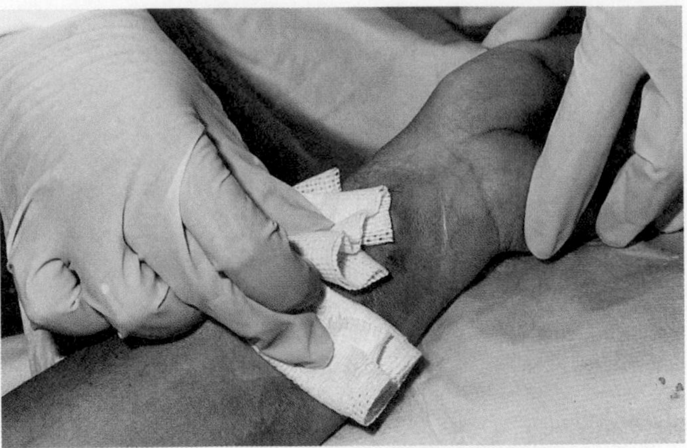

▲ Apply pressure over needle site for 5 to 10 minutes.

5. Start blood pump at 200 mL/min.
6. Return venous blood.
7. Clamp lines.
8. Remove needles according to unit protocol and apply pressure to sites.
9. Apply sterile dressing to needle sites maintaining aseptic technique. ▸ ***Rationale:*** Sepsis is the primary cause of client death for acute renal failure clients.
10. Remove protective gear, discard, and perform hand hygiene.
11. Measure and record postdialysis vital signs and weight.

EVIDENCE-BASED PRACTICE

Survival Rate in Hemodialysis Clients

This study revealed that elderly ESRD clients receiving hemodialysis during morning hours have a higher survival rate than those undergoing dialysis in the afternoon. Previously identified risk factors for this study did not account for these differences.

Source: Bliwise, D., Kutner, N. G., Zhang, R., & Parker, K. P. (2001). Survival by time of day of hemodialysis in an elderly cohort. *Journal of the American Medical Association*, *286*(21), 2690–2694.

Maintaining Central Venous Dual-Lumen Dialysis Catheter (DLC)

Equipment

Heparin 1000 U/mL
Sterile normal saline for injection
Betadine spray
Sterile 4 × 4 gauze pads
Sterile transparent occlusive dressings if indicated
Tape
Luer-Lok catheter caps
Nonsterile drape
Two 3-mL syringes
Two 20-mL syringes
Clean gloves
Two masks
Sterile gloves

Preparation

1. Perform hand hygiene.
2. Fill two 20-mL syringes with 20 mL each of normal saline, and two 3-mL syringes with 3 mL of 1000 μ/mL of heparin.
3. Mask client and self, and don clean gloves.
4. Place drape under catheter lumens.
5. Remove gauze wrap from lumens, if present, and discard in appropriate receptacle.
6. Remove gloves and perform hand hygiene.

Clinical Alert

Femoral dialysis DLCs are only temporary and are rarely seen outside of the ICU setting. The client is not allowed to flex leg or ambulate.

Procedure

1. Open sterile supplies.
2. Holding corner of 4 × 4, place under catheter lumens.
3. Spray lumens with Betadine and allow to dry.
4. Don sterile gloves.
5. Remove old lumen caps.
6. Use 4 × 4 gauze to pick up new caps and place on lumens.

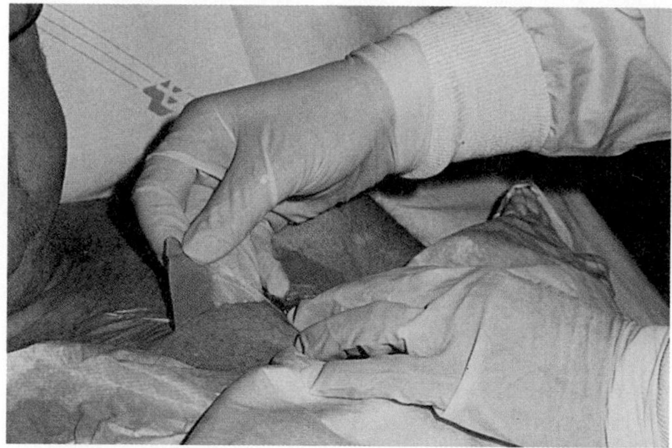

▲ Maintain sterility while carefully removing dressing from dual-lumen catheter.

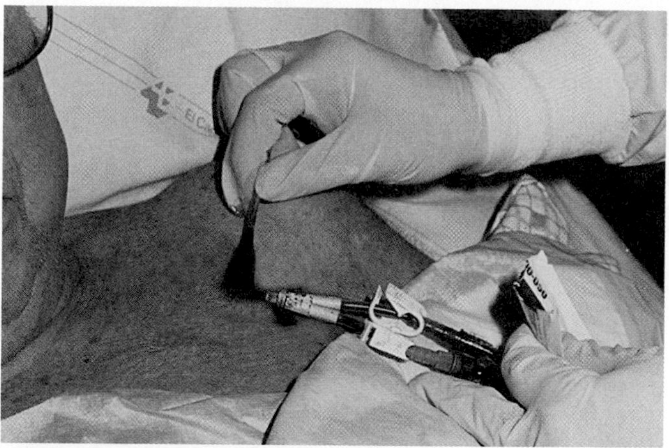

▲ Cleanse catheter insertion site with antimicrobial swabs.

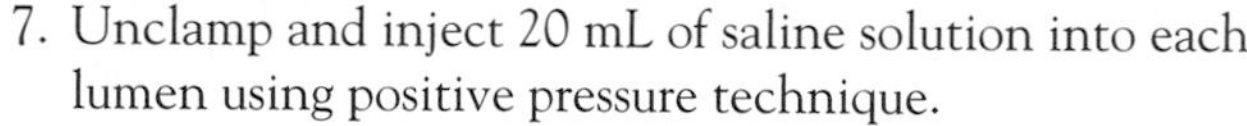

7. Unclamp and inject 20 mL of saline solution into each lumen using positive pressure technique.
8. Inject 3 mL of heparin into each catheter using positive pressure technique.
9. Reclamp lumens.
10. Remove old dressing and discard in biohazard receptacle.
11. Cleanse area surrounding catheter with antimicrobial swabs.
12. Place sterile transparent dressing over catheter insertion site.

NOTE: Provide catheter site care after each dialysis treatment. Dressing is not required after permanent catheter site epithelializes around catheter (about 2 weeks).

13. If desired, wrap lumens in gauze and tape. ▸ ***Rationale:*** To prevent skin irritation from lumen clamps.
14. Dispose of equipment in biohazard receptacle.
15. Remove gloves and mask and discard.
16. Perform hand hygiene.
17. Monitor daily for signs of infection, bleeding, or displacement of catheters.

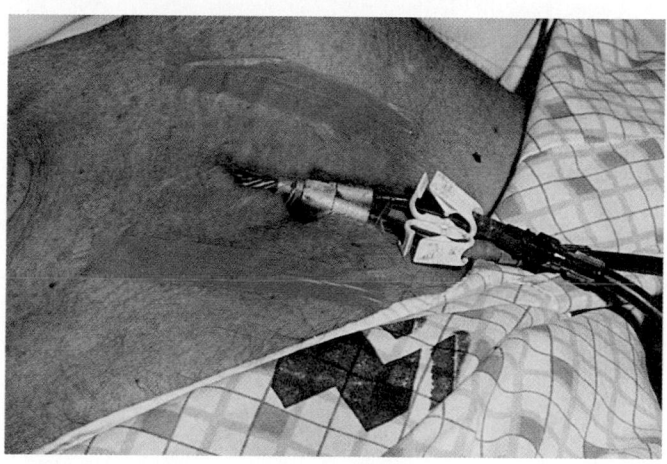

▲ Monitor frequently for signs of infection, bleeding, or catheter displacement.

Clinical Alert

Central venous dual-lumen dialysis catheter (DLC) maintenance (heparin "pack" and site dressing) is performed *only* by the nephrology nurse after a dialysis treatment. These catheters are not maintained the way CVADs are. Instead, they are "packed" with *undiluted* heparin after dialysis, then "unpacked" (3 mL of blood withdrawn from catheter) before the next dialysis treatment.

DOCUMENTATION for Hemodialysis

- Predialysis assessment, subjective and objective data
- Status of fistula, graft, or catheter access site and distal circulation
- Time dialysis initiated and terminated
- Dialyzer type and dialysate used
- Volume of blood processed
- Any complications during procedure and actions taken
- Client symptoms at 30-minute intervals
- Vital signs every 30 minutes
- Postdialysis assessment

CRITICAL THINKING Application

Expected Outcomes

- Dialysis proceeds without complication (excess fluids and wastes removed from blood).
- Vascular access site remains patent.
- Client demonstrates self-care after teaching.

Unexpected Outcomes	Alternative Actions
Hypotension occurs during dialysis.	• Administer normal saline, concentrated saline bolus, or albumin into extracorporeal circuit. • Place client in shock position if tolerated. • Consider using smaller volume dialyzer, less ultrafiltration, or intermittent normal saline doses to maintain BP in future dialysis sessions. • Consider possible dialyzer reaction or myocardial infarction; notify physician for further assessment/diagnostic testing.
Alarms sound during dialysis.	• Before dialysis, become familiar with alarm sounds, functions, and troubleshooting options.
Bleeding occurs during dialysis.	• If blood leak alarm sounds, observe dialysate. If no blood is apparent, check dialysate with Hemastix since air bubbles can cause false alarms. • If bleeding or blood leak is present, discontinue dialysis without returning client's blood.
Client develops restlessness, confusion, seizures, headache, nausea, vomiting, or hypertension near end of dialysis session.	• Suspect dialysis disequilibrium syndrome (usually only occurs in new clients). • Consult physician and implement orders to slow blood flow rate or discontinue dialysis. • Administer medications as ordered (hypertonic saline or mannitol) to relieve symptoms. • For future sessions, consider earlier dialysis before BUN rises excessively or shorten the dialysis treatment and increase number of runs/week.
Client states hand feels weak; neither thrill nor bruit can be assessed in fistula or graft.	• Notify physician of potential clotting of fistula/graft (declotting should be attempted ASAP). • Prepare to possibly send client to radiology for vascular procedure. • Review safety precautions to prevent constriction of blood flow in access extremity.
Client gains 7 pounds between dialysis sessions; blood pressure is elevated.	• Assess client's understanding of fluid restriction (1500 mL/day); advise of hidden fluid in certain foods (ice cream, watermelon, etc.). • Encourage client to control blood sugar (if diabetic) to help relieve thirst; decrease salt intake, but avoid salt substitute (KCl). • Encourage client to weigh daily.
Client's predialysis phosphorus level is excessively elevated.	• Review foods high in phosphorus (colas, red meat, dairy products, eggs). • Encourage client to continue calcium and vitamin D supplement as prescribed. • Remind client to take phosphorus binder medication with meals; if not taking, inquire if constipation is reason and recommend stool softener.
Client develops hypothermia and experiences chills while on dialysis.	• Place warm blanket on client. • Place warmer on blood return line to client. Ensure client's room is set at a comfortable temperature.

Chapter 22

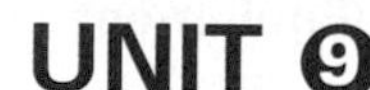

Adaptation to Home Care

Nursing Process Data

ASSESSMENT Data Base

- Assess the client's bladder for distention.
- Assess the client's physical ability to cooperate with positioning.
- Assess urinary meatus and catheter for exudate, edema, inflammation, and general cleanliness.
- Assess need for perineal care before catheterization procedure.
- Assess dialysate solution for clarity.
- Assess dialysis returns for cloudiness.
- Assess family's ability to use gloving technique and maintain asepsis when needed.
- Assess need for suprapubic catheter care.
- Assess need for catheterization procedure.
- Assess for proper function of dialysis machine.

PLANNING Objectives

- To prevent or relieve discomfort due to bladder distention
- To promote urinary elimination
- To identify family's knowledge related to signs and symptoms of dialysis-related infections.
- To prevent urinary tract infections through aseptic catheter care
- To prevent infection at peritoneal catheter site
- To use aseptic technique when instituting CAPD
- To identify client's and family's knowledge base regarding CAPD or CCPD

IMPLEMENTATION Procedures

EVALUATION Expected Outcomes

- Catheterization performed using aseptic technique.
- Bladder emptied when client is unable to void.
- Urinary tract infection prevented through aseptic catheter care.
- Aseptic peritoneal dialysis procedure used.
- Catheter site remains free of infection.
- Suprapubic catheter care is completed and client is free of urinary tract infections.

Pearson Nursing Student Resources

Find additional review materials at **nursing.pearsonhighered.com**

Prepare for success with NCLEX®-style practice questions and Skill Checklists

Using Clean Technique for Intermittent Self-Catheterization

Equipment

Straight catheters in clean container, plastic bag, or wrapped in aluminum foil
Washcloth, soap, water
Water-soluble lubricant (K-Y; Surgilube)
Plastic bags
Basin or container
Mirror

Procedure

For Female Client

1. Attempt to urinate. If unable to do so, continue to follow these steps.
2. Perform hand hygiene and gather equipment. (Keep equipment in one large container.)
3. Assume sitting position on the bed or commode. (Place plastic under towel if bed is used.)
4. Separate labia with one hand while cleaning with soap and water front to back with other hand.
5. Position mirror to visualize urinary meatus.
6. Remove catheter from container (plastic bag or aluminum foil).
7. Lubricate end of catheter with water-soluble lubricant and place other end in container to catch urine.
8. While holding labia apart with one hand, insert catheter about 3 in. or until urine flows.
9. Press down with abdominal muscles to promote bladder's emptying.
10. Pinch off catheter after all urine has drained and withdraw gently, holding tip of catheter upright.
11. Wash and dry perineal area.
12. Wash catheter in warm, soapy water.
13. Rinse with clear water and dry outside with paper towel.
14. Place in plastic bag for storage.
15. Use catheters for 2–4 weeks and then discard.
16. Perform hand hygiene.

For Male Client

1. Attempt to urinate. If unable to do so, continue to follow these steps.
2. Perform hand hygiene and gather equipment. (Keep equipment in one large container.)
3. Assume sitting position on the bed or commode. (Place plastic under towel if bed is used.)
4. Retract the foreskin, if present, and wash tip of penis with soap and water.
5. Remove catheter from container (plastic bag or aluminum foil).
6. Lubricate the first 7–10 in. of catheter with water-soluble lubricant. Place other end in container to catch urine.
7. Hold penis at right angle to body, keeping foreskin retracted. Insert catheter 7–10 in. into penis or until urine begins to flow. Then insert catheter 1 in. further.
8. Press down with abdominal muscles to promote bladder's emptying.
9. Pinch off catheter after all urine has drained and gently withdraw, holding tip of catheter upright.
10. Wash and dry area. Replace foreskin, if present.
11. Wash catheter in warm, soapy water.
12. Rinse with clear water and dry outside with paper towel.
13. Place in plastic bag for storage.
14. Use catheters for 2–4 weeks and then discard.
15. Perform hand hygiene.

Providing Suprapubic Catheter Care

Equipment

Catheter plug and clamp
Closed drainage system
Sterile dressings if necessary
Clean gloves
Receptacle to drain urine from drainage bag
Normal saline solution or mild soap and water
White vinegar
Applicator sticks
4 × 4 gauze pads
Paper tape

Procedure

1. Instruct client to gather equipment for specific skill to be done.
2. Perform hand hygiene and don gloves.
3. Clean around catheter site with normal saline solution or mild soap and water. Use applicator sticks to remove material from around catheter opening.

4. Ensure catheter is not pulling on exit site. Tape catheter to skin so a gentle curve is present to prevent tugging on catheter.
5. Empty catheter bag. Some clients use leg bags. Empty into container and then dispose of contents in toilet or, if removing bag, empty directly into toilet.
6. Clean drainage bags with warm water and soap every day or two. Place one teaspoon of vinegar in rinse water to reduce odor.
7. Replace catheter bag on catheter.
8. Remove gloves and perform hand hygiene.
9. Instruct client in bladder testing:
   a. Wash hands and catheter connections with soap and water.
   b. Clamp the suprapubic tube so it does not drain. Use catheter plug or clamp.
   c. Have client attempt to void when client feels urge to urinate. Measure amount of urine.
   d. Unclamp the suprapubic tube immediately after voiding; empty urine into container and measure residual urine amount.
   e. Instruct client to keep a log of each voiding and residual amount.
   f. Call physician with findings when residual amount is less than 20% voided amount. Usually, this amount is about 60 mL. Usually, the suprapubic tube is removed when client is able to urinate without complications.
10. Instruct client to monitor carefully for signs of urinary tract infection and notify physician immediately. Check for bladder pain, bleeding, temperature over 100°F, chills, cloudy urine, drainage or edema around the suprapubic tube.

Administering Continuous Ambulatory Peritoneal Dialysis (CAPD)

Equipment

Sterile dialysate solution, 1–2 bags, warmed
Heating pad
Transfer set, either Y tubing or straight, and cap
Hook on wall of room used for dialysis
Clamp
Paper towels
Low stool or table
Intake and output record
Two pairs of sterile gloves
Mask
Antibacterial soap
Cleansing solution for catheter
Medication, if ordered

Preparation

1. Perform hand hygiene thoroughly; dry using paper towel.
2. Obtain container of sterile dialysate.
3. Check that strength and amount of solution are accurate as ordered.
4. Take equipment to clean area for assembly.

Procedure

For Draining Fluid

1. Perform hand hygiene and don gloves. ▸ ***Rationale:*** Infection control precaution for caregiver when there is potential contact with blood or body fluids.
2. Don mask.
3. Uncap catheter maintaining aseptic technique.
4. Attach sterile bag and transfer set to catheter for draining dialysate.
5. Place bag on low stool or table below level of client's abdomen. ▸ ***Rationale:*** This position allows fluid to drain by gravity from client's peritoneal cavity.
6. Unclamp tubing.
7. Allow fluid to drain into bag from abdomen until flow ceases, approximately, 10–20 minutes.
8. Reclamp tubing.
9. Examine drainage for discoloration or cloudiness. ▸ ***Rationale:*** Change in color may indicate presence of infection, or if white gelatin-like material is present, it indicates shredding of the peritoneal lining's old skin; an increase in this fibrin indicates potential peritonitis.
10. Disconnect tubing from drainage bag while maintaining aseptic technique. Unscrew catheter from tubing and attach Mini Cap, according to clinic's instruction. ▸ ***Rationale:*** The glucose in the dialysate solution predisposes the client to infections.
11. Weigh drainage bag on scale. Effluent should weigh at least 4.5 pounds. This is equal to 2 liters of fluid. ▸ ***Rationale:*** To ensure all fluid is drained from abdomen.
12. Dispose of effluent into toilet.
13. Double bag tubing and drainage bag. Place biohazardous label on bag. Discard by placing in biohazardous container. Tubing is usually disposed of after each exchange.
14. Remove and discard gloves and mask.
15. Perform hand hygiene.
16. Check blood pressure and pulse. ▸ ***Rationale:*** Rapid fluid shift may cause hypotension.

NOTE: Mini Cap disinfects dialysis tubing between exchanges.

Transfer Sets

Transfer sets are tubing that connects bag of dialysate solution to catheter. There are two types used for CAPD.

Straight Tubing

Straight tubing stays connected to the catheter. For each exchange, the "free" end is connected to the solution. With this type of transfer set, the empty bag from solution is rolled up and worn under clothing. That bag is then unrolled, placed on the floor, and used to drain dialysate from the abdomen. After draining is completed, tubing is disconnected from the straight transfer set and a new solution bag and tubing are connected to the catheter.

Y-Set Tubing

This type of tubing is disconnected between exchanges. The base of the Y is connected to the catheter. One branch of the Y is connected to a new bag of solution and the other to an empty bag. The base of the Y is closed, and a small amount of solution is drained from the full bag into the empty bag. This is done to rid the transfer set of any bacteria that might be in the tubing. The branch that leads to the empty bag is then closed, and the solution flows into the abdomen. Once the solution bag is empty, the Y-set is disconnected from the catheter. This removes the need to wear the bag around the waist while solution is in abdomen. The catheter is then reconnected to the Y-set and solution is drained into an empty bag to discard. A new bag of solution is hung and the process continues. The Y-set is filled with disinfectant when not in use. The disinfectant is flushed out with the used dialysate. The Y-set can be reused for several months.

Principles of Peritoneal Dialysis

- Works on principle of diffusion and osmosis.
  - Diffusion—particles move through semipermeable membrane from area of high to low solute concentration.
  - Osmosis—fluids move through a semipermeable membrane from an area of low solute concentration to an area of high solute concentration from the blood, creating a high osmotic gradient.
- Peritoneal dialysis—used for chronic states of renal failure. Acute renal failure clients do not benefit due to the fact that it is not efficient or rapid enough to adequately remove the waste products such as urea when it accumulates in catabolic acute renal failure clients.

For Infusing Dialysate

1. Warm dialysate. The bag can be encased in a heating pad for 1 hr. DO NOT PLACE IN MICROWAVE. ▶ ***Rationale:*** Microwave heating will produce uneven heating and can cause burning in the client.
2. Perform hand hygiene for 3 minutes with antibacterial soap. ▶ ***Rationale:*** To prevent contamination.
3. Gather equipment and don gloves.
4. Open plastic wrap on dialysate solution and inspect solution bag for expiration date and color and consistency of dialysate and assess bag for possible leaks.
5. Add medications as ordered. Maintain sterile technique in this step. ▶ ***Rationale:*** Some clients add routine drugs to dialysate, such as insulin.
6. Connect tubing to dialysate bag by removing protective cover from port and spiking into dialysate bag. Maintain sterility throughout this step. Each manufacturer has a slightly different mechanism for connecting the tubing and bag. Follow manufacturer's directions. See Transfer Sets box.
7. Hang new dialysate bag on hook, which is positioned above client at shoulder height.
8. Open clamp and adjust height to ensure inflow of solution by gravity over a 10- to 20-minute period.
9. Clamp tubing.
10. Discard empty dialysate bag or place in a holding pouch at client's waist, according to type of transfer set being used.
11. Allow fluid to remain in peritoneal cavity approximately 4 hr.
12. Remove gloves.
13. Perform hand hygiene.
14. Repeat procedure four times daily, the last time at bedtime, allowing fluid to remain in peritoneal cavity overnight.
15. Ensure that client and caregiver are knowledgeable in strict aseptic technique.
16. Instruct client to notify physician if there is evidence of infection.
17. Document findings and bring to physician at each visit.

Changing Dressing for CAPD Client

Equipment

Dressing according to facility policy
Antimicrobial swabs or sterile 4 × 4 dressings and Betadine solution
Tape
Sterile gloves (two pair)
Forceps (optional)
Povidone iodine ointment
4 × 4 gauze pads and pre-cut drain dressings
Warm soapy water, if needed

Procedure

1. Perform hand hygiene.
2. Don sterile gloves.
3. Remove old dressing with sterile gloves.
4. Remove any dried blood or drainage with warm, soapy water.
5. Saturate 4 × 4 dressings with Betadine solution or use swabs and clean skin around catheter, moving in concentric circles from the catheter site outward. Remove crusted material, if present.
6. Inspect site for infection (erythema, edema, warmth, exudate).
7. Apply povidone iodine ointment to catheter site using sterile dressings.
8. Change gloves.
9. Place two precut drain dressings over catheter site, and tape dressing. ▸ ***Rationale:*** Secure dressings to prevent infection at site.
10. Remove gloves and perform hand hygiene.

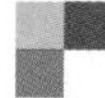

DOCUMENTATION for Home Care

Use Appropriate Home Care Documentation Forms.

- Client's assessment appropriate for skill; suprapubic catheter care and catheterization
- Peritoneal catheter site assessment
- Peritoneal dialysis site fluid assessment
- Complications associated with skill
- Client's response to interventions
- Ability of client and family to participate in skill

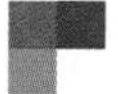

CRITICAL THINKING Application

Expected Outcomes

- Client's peritoneal dialysis is efficient and promotes urinary waste removal.
- Client remains infection free from catheterizations and catheter changes.
- Peritoneal catheter site remains infection-free.

Unexpected Outcomes	Alternative Actions
Client's peritoneal catheter becomes occluded.	• Check tubing. • Raise bag to higher level above abdomen to increase the inflow. • Turn client to side-lying position to facilitate drainage.
Instruct client and family on specific positions and interventions to increase dialysis outflow.	• Notify physician to check position of catheter, or fibrin can be occluding catheter.
Vital signs are increased above normal.	• If BP is elevated, check for retention of dialysate solution in abdomen. • Temperature and pulse increase may be result of peritonitis. • Instruct client and family on how to promote sterile technique when assisting with dialysis.
Client experiences respiratory distress.	• Increased respirations and/or distress are a result of increased pressure in peritoneal cavity. • Evaluate dialysate output.

Client experiences constipation.	• Caused by inflow-outflow complications. • Administer stool softener or laxative.
Client experiences CAUTIs.	• Determine whether client can urinate without catheter. • Promote toileting every 2 hr. • Use external condoms for men instead of indwelling catheters. • Use intermittent catheterization using sterile technique.

GERONTOLOGIC Considerations

Some changes in the urinary system that occur naturally with aging may be difficult to differentiate from pathologic processes.

Changes seen with aging include:

- Reduced activation of vitamin D results in decreased absorption of calcium from the gut.
- Reduction in glomerular filtration rate by 1 mL/min each year after age 40. The diabetic client loses 5 mL/min per year.
- Medications eliminated by the kidneys may require dosage modification; the elderly client should be monitored closely for signs of drug toxicity.
- Lower specific gravity of urine occurs due to decreased ability to concentrate urine; may cause nocturia.
- Any acute fluid loss may cause renal insufficiency.
- The bladder has reduced holding capacity, weaker smooth muscle contractility, and decreased sphincter tone, but lack of bladder control is *not* a normal part of aging.
- Urgency as well as urge incontinence and nocturia are common among all elderly clients due to decreased bladder capacity.
- In the elderly, postvoiding residual volume increases, but remains within the normal range, usually no more than 50 mL.
- Prostatic enlargement in men causes obstruction with resultant urinary retention, frequency, urgency, and UTIs.
- Reduced estrogen levels in women lead to atrophy of tissues that line and surround the urethra, bladder outlet, and vagina, contributing to urinary incontinence.
- Many elderly have coexistent urge and stress incontinence.
- Women may experience weakening of pelvic muscles, causing urethral shortening and urinary retention.

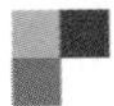

MANAGEMENT Guidelines

Each state legislates a Nurse Practice Act for RNs and LVN/LPNs. Healthcare facilities are responsible for establishing and implementing policies and procedures that conform to their state's regulations. Verify the regulations and role parameters for each healthcare worker in your facility.

Delegation

- CNAs may document intake and output findings on bedside records. Some facilities allow CNAs to chart these findings on flow sheets. Check the facility policies and procedures regarding this.
- UAPs may apply condom catheters and provide catheter care.
- Unlicensed Assistive Personnel (UAPs) may perform the same tasks as the CNA. In addition, many states are allowing "clean" catheterization on clients requiring long-term procedures. It is advisable to check the policy and procedure manual to determine the tasks UAPs may perform.
- Technicians may be trained to perform certain tasks in hemodialysis units. They may initiate the dialysis treatment and monitor clients while they are on dialysis but may not give medications or make nursing judgments.
- LVN/LPNs are assigned to care for clients requiring catheterization and instillation of medication into the bladder and irrigating a closed urinary system with a physician's order.
- LVN/LPNs may be assigned to clients with urinary diversion. They may change pouches and empty continent ileostomies.
- LVN/LPNs can work in a hemodialysis unit with additional training, much like the RN, but can make limited nursing judgments.

Communication Matrix

- It is very important that all staff be informed about which clients require intake and output recordings. I&O records should be at the bedside to remind everyone to record the findings.
- Hemodialysis grafts/fistulas and distal circulation of the involved extremity must be assessed frequently after the initial placement and regularly thereafter.
- Healthcare team members should report any complaints of pain or discomfort from the client, as well as unusual odor,

color, or abnormal findings from urinary catheter drainage systems.

- Urinary diversion pouches should be emptied when one-third full. If the facility policy does not allow ancillary personnel to complete this task, the nurse will instruct them to observe the amount of urine in the pouch and report when it needs to be emptied.
- Hemodialysis technicians must be instructed on client's parameters while on dialysis. They should be instructed to immediately report deviations from the norm to the RN. The RN is ultimately responsible for the care of all clients, regardless of who is assigned to monitor the dialysis treatment.

CRITICAL THINKING Strategies

Scenario 1

Your 55-year-old neighbor confides in you that every time she coughs or sneezes she loses urine. She asks if this is normal since so many of her friends have the same problem.

1. Describe various types and causes of urinary incontinence.
2. What lifestyle changes help to correct stress incontinence?
3. What noninvasive measures help to correct stress incontinence?

Scenario 2

Mrs. Christofferson, a 64-year-old female client, is a first-day postoperative client. She had a bowel resection yesterday. The physician ordered her Foley catheter discontinued at 8 AM this morning. His additional order is to check for residual urine after her first voiding.

1. The client has not voided since the Foley catheter was removed 2 hr earlier. What is your priority nursing intervention?
2. The client voids 600 mL of urine 6 hr after the Foley catheter was removed. What further actions should the nurse take at this time?
3. Checking for residual urine, you obtain 120 mL of urine. What is your next intervention? What alternative action might you take if you suspect the client may exceed the normal amount of residual urine?

NCLEX® Review Questions

Unless otherwise specified, choose only one (1) answer.

1. The amount of urine production is directly related to
   1. Renal perfusion.
   2. Fluid intake.
   3. Bladder capacity.
   4. Metabolic rate.
2. A scanner is useful to reflect the client's bladder volume but is not reliable for assessing.
   Select all that apply.
   1. Obese clients.
   2. Catheterized clients.
   3. Clients with hysterectomy.
   4. Pregnant clients.
   5. Male clients.
   6. Children.
3. For male catheterization, the catheter is inserted
   1. 2-4 in.
   2. 4-6 in.
   3. 6-8 in.
   4. 8-10 in.
4. For female catheterization, the catheter is inserted
   1. 1 in.
   2. 2 in.
   3. 3 in.
   4. 4 in.
5. Urine leakage in the client with a urinary retention catheter indicates
   1. The need for a larger size catheter.
   2. An additional 10 mL of water should be added to the retention balloon.
   3. A possible urinary tract infection.
   4. The client is now able to urinate normally.
6. Common causes of urinary tract infection associated with retention catheters are
   Select all that apply.
   1. Long-term use.
   2. Break in aseptic technique.
   3. Inadequate catheter stabilization.
   4. Insufficient balloon inflation.
   5. Drainage tubing dependent of collection bag.
   6. Urine specimen sampling.

7. The purpose of continuous bladder irrigation (CBI) after prostate surgery is to prevent
   1. Catheter obstruction.
   2. Bladder infection.
   3. Bladder spasms.
   4. Postoperative bleeding.
8. When applying a urinary diversion pouch, a protective barrier product should be used
   1. Only if absolutely necessary.
   2. For the client with sensitive skin.
   3. To ensure pouch adherence.
   4. Only with a two-piece pouch.
9. A client with end-stage renal disease
   1. Has no functioning nephrons.
   2. Receives renal replacement therapy.
   3. Produces no urine.
   4. Is uremic.
10. The nurse avoids taking blood pressure or performing venipuncture in the arm with a graft/fistula used for hemodialysis because
    1. Phlebitis and blood clot may occur.
    2. There is increased risk for infection.
    3. Undue pressure can cause graft/fistula rupture.
    4. There is insufficient blood flow in the extremity.

23

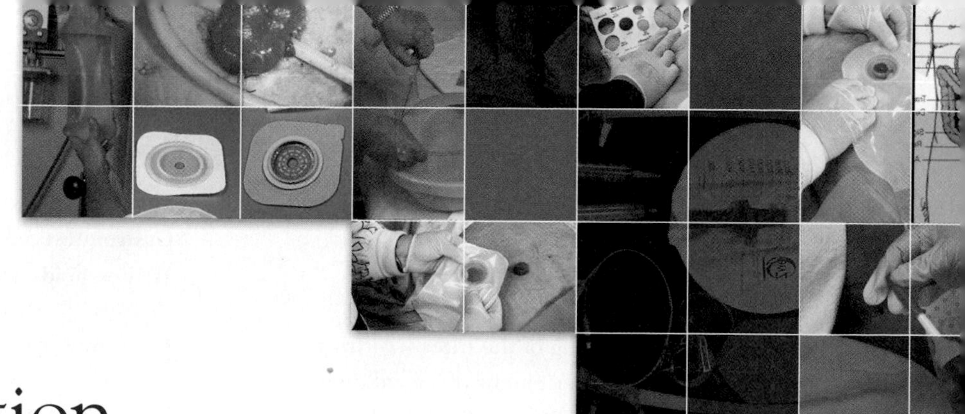

Bowel Elimination

LEARNING OBJECTIVES

1. Explain both the mechanical and chemical aspects of digestion.
2. Compare and contrast hypermotility with hypomotility.
3. Discuss what is meant by obstruction of the bowel.
4. Describe the anatomic locations for an ileostomy, cecostomy, or colostomy.
5. List the components of a good bowel training program.
6. Outline the essential steps in administering a tap water or saline enema to an adult client.
7. Describe the precautions necessary when performing digital stimulation to remove a fecal impaction.
8. Compare and contrast stoma care of an ileostomy and a colostomy.
9. Outline the steps for developing a regular bowel routine.
10. Describe at least three interventions used when skin is denuded from leakage.
11. Describe at least three precautions necessary when applying a fecal ostomy pouch.
12. Discuss the corking and intubation procedure for a client with a continent ileostomy.
13. Describe the precautions necessary when using a rectal tube.
14. Discriminate between clients who should have a rectal tube or bowel management system (BMS) in place.
15. Compare and contrast nursing interventions for clients with alterations in bowel elimination in home care and hospital.

CHAPTER OUTLINE

TERMINOLOGY

Anal fissure a small linear ulcerated area in the anal area.

Bacteria unicellular plantlike microorganisms lacking chlorophyll.

Bowel the intestine.

Bowel movement the emptying of the intestinal tract.

Bowel management system placement of a fecal diversion to manage flow of loose stool, prevent contamination of wounds, and prevent skin breakdown.

Carminative an agent that removes gases from the gastrointestinal tract.

Cathartic a drug to induce emptying of the intestinal tract; a laxative.

Chyme the viscous, semifluid contents of the stomach present during digestion of a meal. Chyme then passes through the pylorus into the duodenum, where further digestion occurs.

Colitis inflammation of the colon.

Colon the large intestine, which extends from the cecum to the anus.

Colostomy an artificially created opening from the colon to the abdominal surface for the elimination of waste.

Constipation difficulty or straining in defecation and infrequent bowel movements over an extended period of time.

Defecation elimination of waste products of digestion from the body by evacuation of bowel.

Diarrhea the passage of unformed liquid stools.

Digestion the process by which food is broken down, mechanically and chemically, in the gastrointestinal tract.

Diverticulitis inflammation of diverticula in the intestinal tract causing stagnation of feces in the small, distended sacs (diverticula).

Diverticulum an outpouching of the mucous membrane of the intestine.

Emulsification the breaking down of large fat globules in the intestine to smaller, uniformly distributed particles.

Enema the introduction of fluid through a tube into the lower intestinal tract.

Fecal incontinence an involuntary or inappropriate passing of liquid or solid stool.

Feces intestinal waste products consisting of bacteria and secretions of the liver, in addition to a small amount of food residue.

Fistula an abnormal tubelike passage from a normal cavity or tube to a free surface or another cavity.

Flaccid relaxed, flabby; having defective or absent muscle tone.

Flatulence excessive gas in the stomach and intestines.

Gastrointestinal having to do with the stomach and intestines.

Hemorrhoids abnormally distended rectal veins due to a constant increase in venous pressure.

Hypermotility unusually quick motility in the gastrointestinal tract.

Hyperreflexia increased action of reflexes.

Hypertonic having a higher osmotic pressure than normal body fluid.

Hypomotility unusually slow motility of the gastrointestinal tract.

Ileostomy an artificially created opening from the ileum to the abdominal surface for the elimination of wastes.

Impaction condition of being tightly wedged into a place, as of feces in the bowel.

Integumentary relative to a covering, as the skin.

Laxative a mild-acting drug to induce emptying of the intestinal tract.

Mucosa mucous membrane.

Necrosis death of areas of tissue or bone caused by enzymatic action or lack of circulation.

Obstipation the act or condition of obstructing; extreme constipation due to obstruction.

Occlude to block off, obstruct.

Occult blood blood in such minute quantities that it can only be detected by a microscope or chemical means.

Ostomy a surgically formed artificial opening that serves as an exit site for the bowel or intestine.

Parasite an organism that lives within, on, or at the expense of another organism, known as the host.

Perforation the act or process of making a hole, such as that caused by an ulcer.

Peristalsis a progressive wave-like movement that occurs involuntarily as in the gastrointestinal tract.

Reflux a return of or backward flow.

Sphincter circular band of muscle fiber constricting a natural orifice.

Stoma an artificially created opening between two passages or between a passage and the body surface.

Stool waste matter discharged from the bowels.

Suppositories semisolid substances for introduction into the rectum, vagina, or urethra where they dissolve; serves as a vehicle for medicines to be absorbed.

Villi short filamentous processes found on certain membranous surfaces.

ANATOMY AND PHYSIOLOGY

The gastrointestinal system converts food into products that can be used as nutrients on the cellular level and disposes of wastes incurred in the process. The primary structures in this system include the mouth, esophagus, stomach, small intestine, and large intestine.

The mouth, esophagus, and stomach are the structures of the upper gastrointestinal tract, where the process of digestion begins. The small intestine, where digestion is completed and most absorption takes place, is a 12-foot tube composed of the duodenum, jejunum, and ileum. The large intestine is made up of the cecum, colon, and rectum. The cecum contains the ileocecal valve and the appendix. The colon is divided into the ascending, transverse, descending, and sigmoid colon. The rectum extends from the sigmoid colon to the anus. The terminal end of the rectum is called the anal canal and is guarded by the internal and external sphincter muscles. The chief functions of the colon are to reabsorb water and sodium and to store wastes.

Digestion is accomplished mechanically and chemically. Food is mechanically churned through the intestinal tract by sharp contractions, or peristaltic waves, of the circular and longitudinal muscles of the intestinal wall. Muscular sphincters and valves are located at strategic points throughout the intestinal tract. These structures help propel the food bolus or feces at appropriately timed intervals in a process called rhythmic segmentation. The sphincters and valves, when functioning properly, prevent reflux of contents. Peristaltic waves, coupled with rhythmic segmentation, allow maximal contact between food and the bowel wall so that chemical reactions can accomplish digestion and absorption can take place.

The chemical aspects of digestion in the small intestine begin in the duodenum with the introduction of pancreatic juices and bile. Pancreatic juices are rich in enzymes, which work to break down proteins and fats and to complete the transformation of starch to sugar. Bile, secreted from the liver, aids in the emulsification and absorption of fats. These substances work in an alkaline medium that combines with the acidity of chyme to provide a neutral pH in the duodenum, thereby protecting the duodenal mucosa.

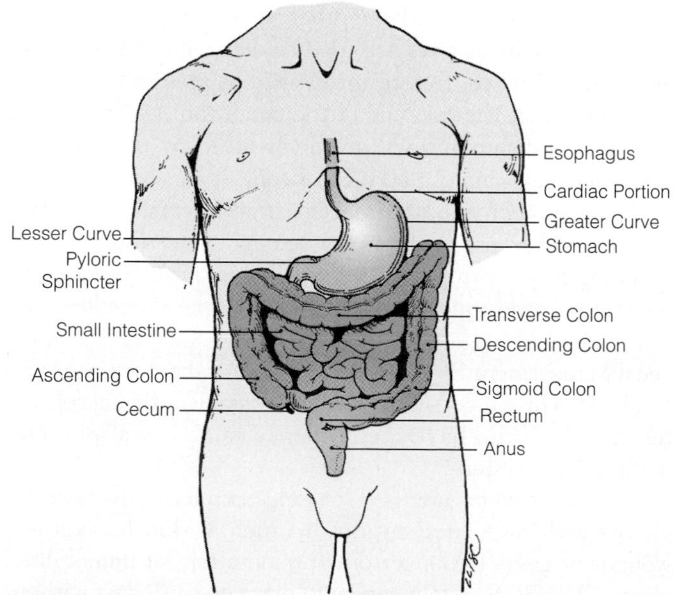

▲ Anatomy of the gastrointestinal tract.

In the 20 feet of jejunum and ileum, approximately 3000 mL of digestive enzymes are secreted. These enzymes, which are secreted by the mucus glands of the intestines, complete the digestive processing of food before absorption. Again, the alkaline nature of these secretions works to protect the mucous membrane of the intestinal tract.

The peristaltic activity of the gastrointestinal tract, as well as its secretory functions, is governed, to a large degree, by parasympathetic and sympathetic nerve fibers. Stimulation of the parasympathetic system increases the activity of the intestinal tract, while stimulation of the sympathetic nervous system inhibits activity in the tract. The internal anal sphincter, however, is activated by sympathetic stimulation, whereas the external anal sphincter is under voluntary control.

Absorption, another primary function of the small bowel, is the passage of prepared materials from the gastrointestinal lumen to the blood and cells. Most absorption in the small intestine results from the churning action of the bowel. Chyme is continually exposed to the circular folds of the mucosal surface, which is lined with thread-like projections called villi. Villi serve as the sites of absorption of fluid and nutrients. The duration of contact between chyme and the mucosal surface of the bowel is very important in absorption. Hypermotility in the small intestine can result in decreased contact with the mucosal wall and deficient absorption; hypomotility can result in increased absorption of fluids, as well as problems with elimination.

The circulatory system delivers nutrients to tissue cells and transports the waste products of metabolism. Arterial circulation to the small bowel and colon is via the superior and inferior mesenteric arteries. Blood that contains absorbed nutrients is carried from the gastrointestinal tract by the superior and inferior mesenteric veins, which become a part of the portal system delivering blood to the liver. Each villus on the intestinal wall contains a network of small capillaries, which absorb sugar and amino acids, and a central lymph channel, which absorbs fatty acids and glycerol. When circulation is compromised, absorption is decreased and cells are lost.

By the time chyme reaches the ileocecal valve—the junction between the small and large intestines—most nutrients have been absorbed. Whereas 3 L of fluid passes through the small bowel, only 500 mL actually passes through the ileocecal valve. The semiliquid material received by the large intestine consists of living and dead bacteria, undigested food and residue, and cell debris. As residue is slowly passed along the colon by peristaltic-like mass movements, fluid is absorbed. These movements occur relatively infrequently (perhaps two or three times per day) and are stimulated by the entrance of food into the stomach by the gastrocolic reflex.

Absorption of fluid in the colon takes place primarily in the ascending and transverse colon. Fecal masses are stored in the sigmoid colon and move into the rectum with mass peristaltic movement. When the rectum fills and becomes sufficiently distended, centers in the sacral area of the spinal cord facilitate a defecation reflex, which contracts the rectum and relaxes the internal and external anal sphincters. The resulting urge, facilitated by the autonomic nervous system, leads to contraction of the abdominal, perineal, and diaphragmatic muscles. Willful defecation is a coordinated, learned habit. Voluntary inhibition of the act returns the stool to the sigmoid colon.

DEFECATION

Defecation is defined as elimination of waste products of digestion from the body by evacuation of the bowel. Excreted waste products are termed feces or stool. The pattern of defecation varies with each individual. It can occur from several times each day to two to three times each week. The type and amount of stool evacuated is also individualized. It is determined by such factors as diet and normal changes in the intestinal flora. Additional factors that influence bowel patterns include age, fluid intake, exercise, psychologic factors, alterations in lifestyle, and medications.

For healthy bowel elimination, the client needs to have sufficient bulk (cellulose and fiber) to produce adequate fecal volume. Food intake at specified times and food that does not produce flatulence are also important for healthy elimination. Daily fluid intake of 2000 to 3000 mL is essential to promote adequate urine output, as well as maintain a soft stool for easy elimination. Daily exercise stimulates peristaltic activity, facilitating bowel movements.

Normal feces are composed of about 75% water and 25% solid material. The stool is soft, but formed, and the color ranges from light to dark brown. The color of the stool is due to the presence of stercobilin and urobilin, derived from bilirubin. In the absence of bile pigment the stool takes on a characteristically clay-colored or white appearance. The action of bacteria in the colon plays a role in the color of the stool. Ingestion of certain foods, drugs, and vitamins can alter the color and consistency of the stool. The nurse must complete an accurate bowel history to determine normal or abnormal findings. Conclusions should not be made on observation alone. Iron supplements, vitamins with iron, beets, red peppers, licorice, grape juice, and spinach affect the color of the stool, which could lead to an incorrect conclusion of blood in the stool. Feces that are red or black in color can be a direct result of ingestion of these foods. Medications can also affect the color and consistency of the stool. General anesthetics block parasympathetic stimulation to the colon, leading to potential constipation. In addition to consistency and distinct color of the feces, there is an odor associated with the feces. The odor is a result of the action of microorganisms on the chyme.

Abnormal characteristics of the feces include the presence of exudate, parasites, fat, and large amounts of mucus. Large amounts of mucus are generally associated with an inflammatory process of the bowel. The stool appears slimy in this condition. Diseases, such as ulcerative colitis or Crohn's disease, produce a stool with large amounts of pus when inflammation is present. Stools with abnormally high fat content are foul-smelling and float to the top of the water. Children with cystic fibrosis commonly produce this type of stool.

Constipation

Because many factors influence the development of constipation, the management of it is also individualized according to each client's need. There is acute and chronic constipation, each a result of certain problems and each requiring their own form of management.

Acute constipation is usually managed with suppositories, enemas, or osmotic laxatives to clear the rectum. A bowel program is usually indicated after the initial treatment. Usually, there is a modification of the diet and fluid intake in addition to education about bowel habits.

Chronic constipation requires the use of bulk-forming agents if the client has a low dietary fiber and no specific underlying cause for the constipation. Osmotic agents may be effective for immediate results, but the goal of the bowel management program is to establish regular bowel habits, using only small doses of laxatives.

Bowel (Fecal) Incontinence

Normal bowel function is based on the client having functioning muscles and nerves, a healthy bowel structure and tissues, normal bowel organisms, proper diet, adequate fluids, and physical activity.

Bowel incontinence can occur when any of these factors are not functioning properly. It can also be caused by disease, injury, stress, poor elimination habits, and side effects of medications. Structure and functional changes as a result of aging can result in bowel incontinence. Structural changes include rectal prolapse, surgical interventions of the bowel, colectomy, and prostate or rectal surgery. Functional causes are often related to an individual's lifestyle or behaviors. These causes may be related to medication effects or nerve damage. Common causes include severe diarrhea, leakage due to chronic constipation, stress, chronic laxative use, and general functional damage from a stroke or other debilitating condition.

Several medical tests are used to determine the cause of fecal incontinence. Before interventions are discussed, it is imperative that the etiology of the condition be determined. Examples of common tests include proctoscopy, ultrasonography, electromyography, and colonoscopy.

An older approach, the placement of a rectal tube, is not encouraged because of the major trauma to the anus and surrounding tissue with prolonged use. Three of the newer treatments for bowel incontinence are the Secca Procedure, the Zassi Bowel Management System (BMS), and the FlexiSeal Fecal Management System (FMS). A surgical procedure is also available. This procedure inserts an inflatable artificial sphincter in clients who have incontinence caused by a sphincter dysfunction or injury.

The new systems are used for long-term fecal diversion for clients with associated conditions such as skin breakdown, wounds or grafts in danger of contamination, or immobilized clients. The BMS system can be in place up to 29 days without removing and changing the catheter.

ALTERATIONS IN ELIMINATION

By-products of digestion must be continually eliminated to maintain normal body function. Alterations in normal elimination can result from changes in motility, obstruction of the lumen of the bowel, circulatory deficiencies, disease process, and surgically induced alterations to the structures of the intestinal tract.

Changes in Motility

Normal motility of the bowel provides peristaltic activity that pushes and churns food and chyme through the upper tract and feces through the lower tract at timed intervals.

Hypermotility may be caused by direct stimulation or irritation of the autonomic nervous system, as well as by inflammatory processes in the gastrointestinal tract. Stimulation of parasympathetic nerves promotes peristalsis and increases bowel muscle tone. Increased peristalsis speeds the propulsion of chyme through the upper tract, resulting in deficient absorption of nutrients. When increased peristalsis speeds the propulsion of feces through the lower tract, diarrhea occurs.

Stimulation of the autonomic nervous system may be psychic in origin. Anxiety, for example, may be mediated through either parasympathetic nerves, with resultant diarrhea, or through sympathetic nerves, with resultant constipation. The action on the parasympathetic nervous system of certain drugs may also cause hypermotility of the intestine. Antihypertensive drugs, such as reserpine, and cholinergic drugs can cause diarrhea by their stimulation of parasympathetic nerves.

Hypermotility caused by the stimulating effect of an irritant on intestinal peristalsis may arise from infectious agents, chemical agents, or inflammatory disease processes. The most common intestinal irritants are the products of certain bacteria that release toxins in the digestive tract. Chemical agents that irritate the intestinal mucosa include cytotoxic drugs, castor oil, and quinidine. Ulcerative and inflammatory disease processes include diverticulitis, tuberculous lesions, ulcerative colitis, and Crohn's disease.

Hypomotility may be caused by direct stimulation or blockage of the autonomic nervous system, intestinal muscle weakness, and chemical agents that inhibit peristalsis and induce flaccidity in the intestinal tract. Decreased peristalsis causes chyme to move sluggishly through the upper tract so that fluids are overabsorbed. Decreased peristalsis also slows the propulsion of feces through the lower tract and causes constipation, fecal impaction, and obstruction.

Stimulation or blockage of the autonomic nervous system may be congenital in origin, as is the case in Hirschsprung's disease, where the absence of parasympathetic nerve ganglia results in failure of peristalsis of the affected portion of the bowel. The effects of trauma or toxins on autonomic innervation of the intestine, which occur with paralytic (adynamic) ileus, inhibit motility to the point of obstruction.

Intestinal muscle weakness that results from disease processes, old age, or a lack of essential vitamins (notably the B group) or electrolytes (particularly potassium) may all contribute to hypomotility. Certain drugs, such as codeine and morphine, can also cause hypomotility by relaxing the smooth muscles of the digestive tract and by increasing spasms of the intestinal sphincters.

Obstruction of the Lumen of the Bowel

Obstruction of the lumen of the bowel may be partial or complete. The severity of the obstruction depends on the region of the bowel that is affected, the degree to which the lumen is occluded, and the degree to which the circulation in the bowel wall is disturbed.

A small-bowel obstruction that occurs as a consequence of persistent vomiting (reverse peristalsis) can cause severe disturbances in the electrolyte balance of the body. Large-bowel obstructions, even if complete, are not as dramatic, provided that the blood supply to the colon is not disturbed.

The causes of intestinal obstruction are varied. In rare instances, obstruction may result when a foreign body, such as a large fruit stone or a mass of parasitic worms, becomes lodged in the bowel. Intestinal obstruction is more frequently caused by strictures, adhesions, hernias, volvulus, intussusception, polyps, neoplasms, and fecal impaction.

The physiology of an obstruction in the lumen of the bowel is generally the same, regardless of cause. As the lumen of the bowel is blocked, the body attempts to overcome the obstruction by increasing peristalsis. During this process, liquid feces move past the site of obstruction and cause diarrhea and increased obstruction, which leads to constipation. Within several hours peristalsis is reduced, and the bowel becomes flaccid. As intraluminal pressure builds up, fluid is retained and absorption decreases. The increased intraluminal pressure then leads to the compression of the bowel wall and its capillaries, which causes necrosis of the bowel wall.

Circulatory Deficiencies

An adequate circulatory flow is essential for maintaining the structure of the bowel and for carrying on cellular nutrition. Any interruption of the arterial blood supply inhibits the bowel function. An occlusion of the circulatory flow, also called an intestinal infarction, results in gangrene of the bowel unless surgical intervention is carried out. A partial occlusion of the mesenteric arteries due to atherosclerosis can cause intestinal angina, a condition that occurs when the blood supply is increasingly interrupted.

Surgically Induced Alterations in Bowel Elimination

When alterations in bowel elimination become life-threatening and medical management fails, surgical intervention becomes necessary. Diversionary surgical procedures of the bowel include cecostomy, ileostomy, and colostomy.

An ostomy may be temporary or permanent, depending on the etiology. The most common indication for a permanent ostomy is low cancer of the rectum or advanced metastatic cancer involving the colon. A temporary ostomy is usually created with the intent of reconnecting it in the future. The anatomy of the GI system is left intact. Many of these ostomies

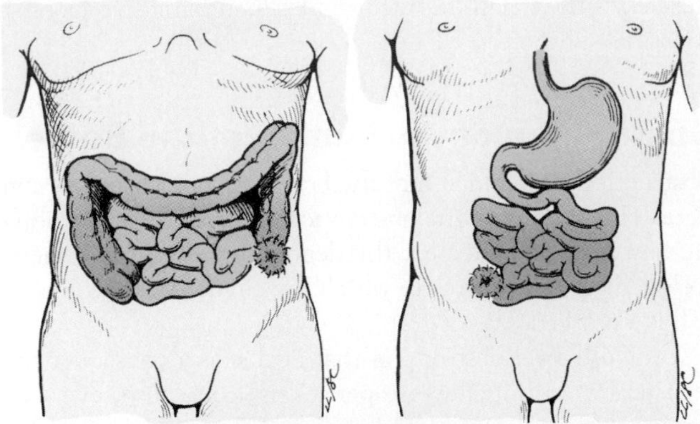

▲ A sigmoid colostomy. An ileostomy.

are done as an emergency. The temporary ostomy may be performed because a bowel prep could not be done due to obstruction and/or perforation, or to protect a distal surgery of the colon. Reversal, or re-anastomosis, can be done at a later time when infection is unlikely and healing can take place. Ileostomy and colostomy are the most frequent type of fecal diversion. Today, both of these ostomies can be reversed as long as the anatomy of the GI system is left intact. Children with certain congenital intestinal disorders may require an ostomy. These are usually temporary and reversed once the child reaches a certain weight.

A cecostomy is a surgically created opening from the cecum through the abdominal wall. This procedure is a quick and temporary method to decompress the right side of the colon. This is usually done with the insertion of a catheter into the colon. This catheter requires frequent irrigation to ensure patency. If stool leaks around the site, a pouch should be applied to collect the output.

An ileostomy is a surgically created opening from the terminal ileum through the abdominal wall. The entire large intestine is bypassed or removed. Permanent ileostomies are usually performed on clients with Crohn's disease of the entire large intestine and those clients with a weakened rectal sphincter, which would leak stool if a pull-through procedure was performed. The stoma is smaller than the colostomy stoma as it is formed by the small intestine. The tip of the small intestine is brought to the skin's surface and folded back on itself. The stoma size is about the size of a quarter or fifty-cent piece. The effluent is a paste-like consistency, although it can be more liquid if fluid intake is abnormally high.

In recent years, new surgical procedures have eliminated many permanent ileostomies. Clients with polyposis or ulcerative colitis may choose to have a continent ileostomy or Kock Continent Ileostomy or Kock pouch, an internal reservoir of the ileum constructed at the rectum. The Kock reservoir consists of an internal pouch with two limbs of the ileum, one forming an internal valve. Continence occurs as a result of the stool collecting in the internal pouch. The pouch must be intubated four to six times a day to evacuate the stool. The rectal reservoir is created by joining the ileum to the anus after the colon is removed. The client will have four to ten stools a day and must have good sphincter control. Any of the surgeries that remove or bypass the large intestine produce a soft-to-watery effluent that contains water and many digestive enzymes that have not yet been absorbed by intestinal villi. The daily output varies from 500 to 2000 mL. Another type of continent internal reservoir is the Barnett Reservoir (BCIR). The pouch is made from the ileum, the last segment of the small intestine. A self-sealing valve mechanism and "living collar" is constructed from the intestine, which prevents leaking from the pouch.

The pouch stores liquid waste and is drained several times each day using a small catheter. The catheter is inserted through the opening on the abdomen into the pouch. The pouch holds about 1000 mL after a few months following surgical intervention.

A colostomy is a surgically created opening from the colon through the abdominal wall and can be created using any segment of the large intestine. With a colostomy, the diseased portion of the colon is bypassed or removed and a portion of healthy colon is brought to the outside of the abdomen to form a stoma. The type of stoma is named after the segment of bowel used to form the stoma; most colostomies are sigmoid colostomies. The farther to the right side of the colon the stoma is placed will determine the type of output from the stoma.

The most common surgery performed for cancer of the colon is a low anterior resection. In this procedure a wide excision of the tumor and surrounding lymph nodes is made and the remaining colon is reconnected. The client may have a diverting ostomy proximal to the resected area to protect the surgical site from leakage.

Abdominal–perineal resections with permanent sigmoid colostomy are usually done only when the tumor is located too low in the rectum for the client to maintain continence. Output from colostomies on the left side of the intestine will eventually become formed and firm, since most of the water has been absorbed by the time the feces reaches these portions of the colon.

A descending colostomy is usually temporary. It is seen frequently in children with congenital disorders. Adults may have a descending colostomy after trauma or severe diverticulitis when perforation is present.

A transverse colostomy can be located anywhere along the transverse colon. It is also usually temporary and is done for either a bowel obstruction or perforation.

Potential Postoperative Complications

- Hemorrhage
- Shock
- Thrombophlebitis
- Pulmonary embolism
- Sepsis
- Paralytic ileus
- Intestinal obstruction
- Impaired intestinal absorptive capability
- Leaky anastomosis
- Stoma necrosis

TABLE 23-1 Comparison Chart for Ostomies

Colostomy	Ileostomy
Etiologic Factors	
Cancer of colon	Ulcerative colitis
Traumatic or congenital disruption of intestinal tract	Crohn's disease (regional ileitis)
Diverticulitis	Birth defects Trauma Protect distal surgery Distal obstruction
Surgical Procedure	
Portion of colon brought through abdominal wall	Portion of ileum brought through abdominal wall
Bowel Control	
Sigmoid—Sometimes	None
Ascending—No	
Stool Consistency	
Sigmoid—Formed	Liquid to semisoft
Ascending—Semiformed	
Irrigation for Bowel Control	
Sigmoid or descending colon, but rarely used	No
Use of Appliance	
Yes, use nondrainable, but only if evacuation pattern is not achieved	Yes
Nursing Care Priorities	
Maintain skin integrity a. Keep skin clean and dry b. Provide skin barrier c. Ensure proper fit of appliance	Same as colostomy
Fluid Requirement	
Sigmoid—Normal intake	8–10 glasses per day
Transverse—8–10 glasses per day	
Diet Control	
Avoid gas-forming foods	Same as colostomy
Eat in moderation odor-forming foods	
Chew food well	
Medications	
Sigmoid—none	Same as colostomy
Transverse—Avoid enteric coated meds	B_{12}
May need Na replacement	
Vitamins, especially K minerals	
Psychosocial	
Promote self-image	Same as colostomy
Refer to Ostomy Club	

Colostomies can also be named for the way they are constructed. A loop colostomy is a very quick surgical procedure to exteriorize the bowel. A loop of intestine is brought out to the surface of the abdomen and some type of plastic bridge is placed under the loop to prevent it from falling back inside the abdomen. This bridge is left in place for 7–14 days until the abdominal wall has sealed. In any of the surgeries in which the rectum is left the client can expect to pass any old stool remaining from before surgery, plus mucus produced by the lining of the intestine on an ongoing basis. A double-barrel colostomy is one that has two stomas. One is the proximal or functional stoma. The second is the distal stoma that connects the remaining stoma and rectum. This stoma is often referred to as a mucus fistula. It may put out mucus or old stool from before surgery, especially if the client is totally obstructed distal to the stoma.

An end colostomy has only one stoma, which originates from the proximal portion of the bowel. The distal end of the colon is either resected or is closed off with sutures and remains in the abdomen. This can also be called a Hartman's procedure. All of these ostomies can be reversed once the distal site is healed and an adequate bowel prep can be done.

Another type of colostomy is the Pelvic Pouch or Ileo-Anal Pull-through, better known as the J Pouch, S Pouch, or W Pouch, depending on the stoma location in the intestine. There is no external stoma. An internal pouch is constructed from the rectum, allowing waste products to accumulate before being expelled in the normal manner, although bowel movements will be more watery and more frequent than usual. If the rectum is too diseased and the anal sphincter muscle was removed, the client is not a candidate for this pouch procedure. The J Pouch is also not recommended for those with Crohn's disease as the disease can return and infect the pouch, requiring removal of the pouch.

Colostomy irrigations are not commonly used today to establish regularity of bowel elimination. Clients usually reestablish bowel habits similar to those before the surgery. There may still be some clients who do perform daily irrigations; however, there are situations when irrigations must not be done. Irrigations are always contraindicated in clients with unstable fluid and electrolyte balance and in those clients in whom vagal stimulation is dangerous. Irrigations are also contraindicated when clients are receiving radiation therapy or are experiencing chemotherapy-induced diarrhea.

ADAPTATION FOR HOME CARE

The actual care of clients requiring interventions for altered bowel elimination is basically the same for hospitalized clients as home care clients. Equipment may be slightly different, but it is similar enough to make it easy to teach clients and family members to perform the skills.

A major responsibility of the nurse is to provide client and family education in the care and management of the ostomy, bowel elimination interventions, and how to administer an enema. At the time of discharge from the hospital, most clients and family members need support in the management of an ostomy. The home care nurse will need to not only demonstrate and evaluate the performance and outcome of the ostomy care, but will need to provide emotional support as well.

CULTURAL AWARENESS

When providing nursing care for clients requiring an intervention for bowel elimination, remember that many cultures are very modest and do not like to talk about elimination issues. Respectful approaches and providing privacy during the procedure are critical for all clients, but especially for some cultures, in order for them to feel comfortable with the task that needs to be completed. This is especially true for Chinese-Americans, who may request to use the toilet and not a bedpan. Arab-Americans prefer to wash rather than use toilet paper after every urination and bowel movement. They may insist on using a bidet to wash up. Muslims may require additional bathing rituals.

NURSING DIAGNOSES

The following nursing diagnoses may be appropriate to use on client care plans when the components are related to alterations in bowel elimination.

NURSING DIAGNOSIS	RELATED FACTORS
Disturbed Body Image	Presence of stoma, fear of rejection, psychosocial factors
Constipation, Risk for	Inadequate intake of fluid or bulk, decreased exercise, disease states, medication, personal habits
Diarrhea	Nutritional intake, medication, disease state
Deficient Fluid Volume	Effluent from ileostomy is watery to semisoft; excessive use of enemas or laxatives
Grieving	Loss of body contiguity, operative procedure (colostomy, ileostomy)
Ineffective Health Maintenance	Cognitive impairment, depression, immobility, cultural beliefs, lack of social support
Deficient Knowledge	Inability to manage ostomy, constipation
Noncompliance	Inability to manage equipment, impaired manual dexterity, poor vision
Impaired Skin Integrity	Skin irritation or breakdown, poor pouching techniques, incontinence or diarrhea, poor-fitting equipment, economic situation

CLEANSE HANDS The single most important nursing action to decrease the incidence of hospital-based infections is hand hygiene. *Remember to wash your hands or use antibacterial gel before and after each and every client contact.*

IDENTIFY CLIENT Before every procedure, introduce yourself and check two forms of client identification not including room number. These actions prevent errors and conform to The Joint Commission standards.

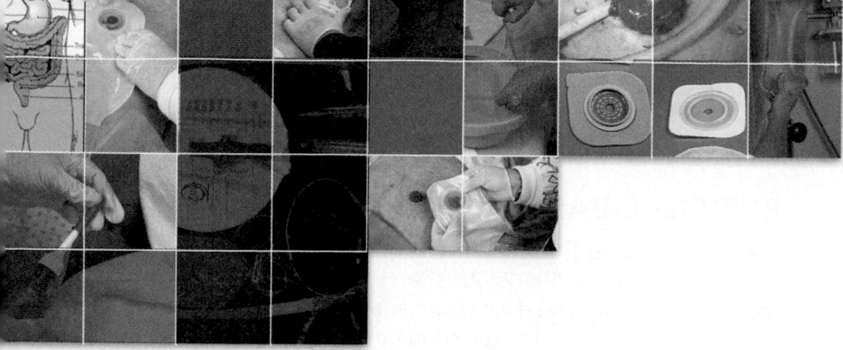

Chapter 23

UNIT 1

Bowel Management

Nursing Process Data

ASSESSMENT Data Base

- Assess for symptoms indicating presence of impaction: nausea; headache; abdominal pain; malaise, abdominal distention, or bloating.
- Evaluate client's diet.
  Amount of high-bulk foods.
  Amount of fluid intake daily.
- Evaluate client's physical status.
  Extent of physical exercise performed daily.
  Ability to ambulate (i.e., spinal cord injury, CVA).
  Ability to perform bed exercises, abdominal exercises.
  Extent of disease process.
  Medications routinely taken.
- Assess effectiveness of drugs, such as stool softeners, bulk formers, suppositories.
- Assess time of day client usually evacuates bowels, any changes in normal routine.
- Identify client's ability to adapt and psychologic readiness for the above program.
- Identify position most effective for bowel evacuation.
- Assess consistency and amount of stool for abnormal findings (diarrhea, fecal impaction, thin pencil-like stool, or blood in stool).
- Assess when client had last bowel movement.
- Assess perianal area for tears, ulcerations, or excoriation.
- Assess for fecal contamination of wounds or grafts.
- Assess for postoperative constipation.
- Assess the need for colostomy irrigation for home care client.

PLANNING Objectives

- To promote regular bowel evacuation
- To prevent constipation
- To promote removal of flatulence
- To remove a fecal impaction
- To promote colostomy evacuation at same time each day
- To establish a bowel program to which the client can easily adapt
- To develop a bowel program that the client can perform him or herself
- To prevent skin breakdown and/or wound contamination from fecal incontinence
- To manage stool elimination for clients with mobility issues
- To relieve pain and discomfort

IMPLEMENTATION Procedures

EVALUATION Expected Outcomes

- Client establishes regular bowel evacuation program.
- Constipation is prevented.
- Fecal impaction is removed.
- Client is able to evacuate bowel at a convenient and consistent time.
- Client is free of pain, flatus, and discomfort.
- Digital stimulation is performed without cardiac complications.
- Rectal tube insertion relieves flatus.
- Colostomy irrigation promotes routine daily bowel evacuation.
- BMS is effective to prevent skin excoriation for clients with diarrhea.

Pearson Nursing Student Resources

Find additional review materials at **nursing.pearsonhighered.com**

Prepare for success with NCLEX®-style practice questions and Skill Checklists

Providing Assistive Digital Evacuation

Equipment

Clean gloves, 2 or 3 pair
Water-soluble lubricant
Absorbent pad
Washcloth and towel
Bath blanket
Bedpan
Basin of warm water

Preparation

1. Check physician's order for impaction removal if the client is at risk for possible complications from vagal stimulation (i.e., cardiac or spinal cord injured client). ▸ ***Rationale:*** Vagal stimulation can result from manual removal of feces. It should be used only as a last resort and with specific physician's order. It causes a decreased pulse rate by decreasing conductivity at the sinoatrial (S-A) node and decreasing the rate of impulse firing at the node.
2. Gather equipment.
3. Introduce yourself, identify the client using two forms ofidentification, and explain procedure.
4. Provide privacy.
5. Perform hand hygiene.

Procedure

1. Obtain baseline pulse and blood pressure.
2. Place client on left side with knees flexed. ▸ ***Rationale:*** Positioning on left side allows easier access to sigmoid colon.
3. Place absorbent pad on bed. Cover client with bath blanket.
4. Place bedpan next to client's buttocks.
5. Don gloves, and lubricate fingers of dominant hand. You may want to double-glove dominant hand to prevent contamination if glove tears.
6. Ask client to take a slow, deep breath and exhale slowly through the mouth as your index finger is gently inserted into rectum moving toward the umbilicus. ▸ ***Rationale:*** Encouraging breathing assists in relaxing the sphincter.

Clinical Alert

Removal of fecal impaction is usually performed in small steps to reduce the risk of injury to the rectal tissue. A series of suppositories may be given between manual removal attempts to assist in clearing the bowel.

Clinical Alert

Stimulation of rectum could result in excessive vagal nerve (in rectal wall) stimulation with subsequent cardiac arrhythmias.

EVIDENCE-BASED PRACTICE

Assisted Bowel Evacuation

In a report by Powell in 2000, she stated that 8% of clients required assisted digital evacuation. In a published document in the Royal College of Nursing (London 2000), a list of indications for assisted evacuation was outlined. These indications included fecal impaction, inability to defecate, neurogenic bowel dysfunction, and clients with spinal cord injury. Very little is written about manual evacuation of stool. It is considered a nursing function, although there is a risk to the procedure, particularly vagal nerve stimulation, leading to bradycardia.

Even though manual fecal removal is a well-established procedure for clients with spinal cord injury, it is suggested by this author that further research into long-term bowel management in general and manual evacuation should be studied.

Source: Powell, M., & Rigby D. (2000). Management of bowel dysfunction: Evacuation difficulties. *Nursing Standard, 14,* 47–51.

7. Gently massage around stool and remove the hardened stool by working the forefinger into and around the mass to break it up. ▸ ***Rationale:*** Smaller pieces allows for easier expulsion of stool.
8. Allow client to rest between digital removal if any untoward effects, such as palpitations or faintness, are exhibited.
9. Obtain vital signs if client complains of any discomfort.
10. Provide hygienic care, as needed.
11. When stool is removed, change gloves; wash and dry buttocks thoroughly.
12. Dispose of stool in toilet or send stool specimen to laboratory.

Clinical Alert

Due to risk factors, manual evacuation should be considered an acute intervention, not a regular intervention. Risk factors include autonomic dysreflexia, rectal trauma or perforation, rectal bleeding, and history of abuse.

Even though manual evacuation of stool is considered within the scope of practice for a registered nurse, nurses receive little or no training to perform the procedure. At a minimum, the practitioner should:

- be knowledgeable regarding the anatomy and physiology of the lower rectum.
- demonstrate awareness of common perineal and anal conditions.
- be able to discuss constipation management options.
- utilize critical synthesis of evidence-based practice and relevant literature.
- demonstrate professional accountability.

13. Clean bedpan and replace in appropriate area.
14. Remove gloves and perform hand hygiene.
15. Position client for comfort.
16. Perform hand hygiene.
17. Follow physician's orders for administering a cleansing enema or inserting a suppository. ▸ ***Rationale:*** These procedures will assist in the removal of any remaining feces.
18. Instruct client in management of simple constipation, if appropriate. Include diet, exercise, and laxatives and/or stool softeners.

NOTE: An oil retention enema may be used before removing the impaction. ▸ ***Rationale:*** Helps soften and lubricate stool.

Providing Digital Stimulation

Equipment

Bath blanket (optional)
Clean gloves, 1 or 2 pair
Lubricant
Bedpan or commode
Absorbent pad
Washcloth and towel
Medication if ordered
Toilet tissue

Procedure

1. Check physician's orders and client care plan. Determine client's usual bowel habits and time of evacuation.
2. Perform hand hygiene.
3. Gather equipment.
4. Identify the correct client and explain procedure.
5. Provide privacy and place absorbent pad on bed as necessary.
6. Place client in position in the bed for bowel evacuation (bedpan in place). Place client in either left or right lateral position (if on right side, sigmoid is uppermost) and assist with feces removal.
7. Place bath blanket over client if appropriate.
8. Don gloves, and lubricate fingers of nondominant hand. You may want to double-glove to prevent contamination if gloves tear. ▸ ***Rationale:*** Lubrication reduces resistance by fingers moving through anal sphincter.
9. Insert finger into rectum 1.5–2 in.
10. Move your finger from side to side in a circular motion to slightly stretch the rectal wall. Move toward the spine and not the bladder to prevent injury to the bladder. ▸ ***Rationale:*** Stimulates lower bowel and helps relax sphincter.

> **Clinical Alert**
> A daily routine should be set up for at least 2–3 weeks to establish a pattern.

11. Instruct client to take slow, deep breaths during procedure.
12. Continue stretching the rectal wall for 1–3 minutes until the internal sphincter muscle relaxes.
13. Work with client to discover an associated stimulus to help establish a good bowel routine. ▸ ***Rationale:*** Abdominal massage, coughing, deep inhalations, and tightening of abdominal muscles, in conjunction with digital stimulation, assist in bowel evacuation.
14. Repeat digital stimulation for 1–3 minutes at 5-minute intervals up to 20 minutes if a bowel movement does not occur.
15. Use two fingers if necessary to break up hard stool for evacuation to occur.
16. Place stool in bedpan as it is removed.
17. Assess vital signs if prolonged digital removal is required. ▸ ***Rationale:*** Vagal nerve stimulation can occur.
18. Assess for bleeding.
19. After bowel evacuation occurs, assist the client with cleaning and drying perineum.
20. Remove equipment from room.
21. Wash equipment and return to storage area.
22. Discard gloves and perform hand hygiene.
23. Position the client for comfort.

Developing a Regular Bowel Routine

Equipment

Clean gloves, 1 or 2 pair
Lubricant
Bedpan or commode
Absorbent pad
Specific enema if ordered
Washcloth and towel

Preparation

1. Check physician's orders and client care plan.
2. Identify the correct client and explain procedure.
3. Identify time of day client usually evacuates bowels.
4. Evaluate diet, exercise, and former use of medications for bowel evacuation.
5. Administer the following drugs as ordered:
   a. Stool softener (Colace, Dialose, DCS, Coloxyl) daily.
   b. Bulk former (Metamucil or FiberCon)—daily to TID.
   c. Mild laxative (Senokot, Doxidan, Dulcolax) 8 hr before program.
   d. Suppository (glycerin or Dulcolax) just before digital stimulation.
6. Perform hand hygiene.

Procedure

1. Don gloves. You may want to double-glove to prevent contamination if glove tears.
2. Perform digital stimulation one half hour after dinner or breakfast or according to client's time schedule for evacuation (see previous intervention).
   ▸ ***Rationale:*** Food stimulates bowel activity.
3. Place client on toilet or commode. (Use bedpan if client is on bedrest.) ▸ ***Rationale:*** Assuming normal posture for bowel movement facilitates evacuation.
4. Encourage client to contract abdominal muscles or bend forward while bearing down. ▸ ***Rationale:*** Increases abdominal pressure and helps evacuate the bowel.
5. Remove gloves.
6. Perform hand hygiene.
7. Provide privacy and sufficient time for evacuation.
8. Don gloves.
9. Wash and dry perineal area if client is unable to do so.
10. Remove gloves.
11. Place client in wheelchair or bed and position for comfort.
12. Perform hand hygiene.
13. Wean client away from suppositories and laxatives when spontaneous bowel movements occur with digital stimulation.

Bowel Training

Good bowel training programs include:

- Initiation of defecation on demand with digital stimulation and abdominal massage.
- Evacuation at same time each day; best time 20–40 minutes after a meal.
- Proper diet, increased fiber and fluids.
- Daily physical exercise regimen.
- Client and family education.

Recommendations for Preventing Constipation in the Older Adult Population

- Assess constipation by obtaining the client's history, including information regarding the amount of fluid intake, food ingested, and dietary fiber.
- Review medications associated with an increased risk of developing constipation; screen for polypharmacy.
- Identify bowel patterns using a bowel diary.
- Increase fluids to 1500–2000 mL/day; minimize caffeine and alcohol intake.
- Promote regular consistent toileting.
- Tailor physical activity to client's physical abilities.

Source: Registered Nurses Association of Ontario. (2005, March). Prevention of Constipation in the Older Adult Population (revised). Toronto, Canada: Author. Available at: www.guidelines.gov.

EVIDENCE-BASED PRACTICE

Management of Constipation in Older Adults

Studies conducted in Britain and the United States indicate that between 10% and 18% of otherwise healthy adults have frequent straining on defecation. Constipation appears to be more common in women than men, and about 20% of the elderly identify the problem. Constipation is not a physiological consequence of the aging process; however, decreased GI motility is a contributing factor to the prevalence in older adults. Constipation may occur secondary to other conditions, such as colorectal cancer or strictures. It is also associated with contributing factors such as inadequate fluid intake, absence of dietary fiber, caloric intake, and lack of exercise. In a recent study of clients who considered themselves constipated, 40% were using over-the-counter medications known to cause constipation. In addition to these factors, clients in the hospital may have a lack of privacy and inconvenience or lack of toilet facilities, which can lead to constipation.

A variety of products have been studied to determine whether any of them prevent constipation. Some studies support the effectiveness of supplementing the diet with bran, but its effectiveness has not been supported by randomized controlled trials.

Other studies suggest that fiber may be effective in improving bowel movement frequency in the ambulatory client, while stimulant and osmotic laxatives may be more effective than bulk-forming agents for the immobilized client. A current study supports establishing a bowel training program to establish regularity. Additional studies support incorporating regular exercise to reduce the risk of constipation.

Source: (a) (1999). Management of constipation in older adults, *Best Practice*, 3(1). (b) Hsieh, C. (2005). Treatment of constipation in older adults. *American Family Physician*, 72(11), 2277–2284.

Administering a Suppository

Equipment

Clean gloves
Lubricant
Bedpan or commode
Absorbent pad (optional)
Suppository as ordered
Washcloth and towel
Paper towel

Procedure

1. Check physician's orders and MAR.
2. Perform hand hygiene.
3. Gather equipment.
4. Identify the correct client and explain procedure.
5. Provide privacy. Place client in Sims' position with upper leg flexed.
6. Place bed protector on bed if necessary. Fold back top bed covers.
7. Remove suppository foil; lubricate tip of suppository. ▸ ***Rationale:*** This prevents tissue damage and promotes easy insertion of suppository.
8. Don gloves; lubricate fingers of nondominant hand.
9. Place small amount of lubricant on paper towel.
10. Lift upper buttock to expose the rectal area.
11. Instruct client to breathe through mouth. ▸ ***Rationale:*** This relaxes anal sphincter.
12. Gently insert suppository (usually glycerin) with pointed end first, and place high in rectum beyond external and internal sphincters, approximately 3–4 in. (approximately 10 cm). ▸ ***Rationale:*** This prevents expulsion of suppository.
13. Push the suppository against the side of the rectal wall. Ensure it is not placed into fecal mass. ▸ ***Rationale:*** It is ineffective if placed in feces because it cannot be absorbed.
14. Withdraw finger and press client's buttocks together for a few minutes. ▸ ***Rationale:*** To prevent expulsion of suppository.
15. Instruct client to stay in Sims' position for at least 5 minutes. ▸ ***Rationale:*** This position helps retain the suppository.
16. Remove gloves by turning inside-out and discarding in appropriate receptacle.
17. Perform hand hygiene.
18. Place client on toilet or commode. If bowel movement does not occur in 30 minutes, perform digital stimulation. A suppository is usually effective within 30 minutes.
19. Repeat with stronger suppository if ordered (Dulcolax) after 30 minutes if there are no results. Follow steps for inserting the suppository including donning gloves.
20. Allow client to retain Dulcolax suppository for 30 minutes. If no results, do digital stimulation again.
21. After bowel evacuation, cleanse and dry perineal area.
22. Remove gloves and perform hand hygiene.
23. Position client in wheelchair or bed.

Clinical Alert

If client has a spinal cord injury, observe for signs of autonomic hyperreflexia (goose pimples, pounding headache, hypertension, perspiration above level of spinal cord injury).

If signs and symptoms of autonomic hyperreflexia occur, discontinue digital stimulation, apply Nupercainal and Xylocaine ointment around anus and rectum as ordered. This anesthetizes the area and decreases the stimulation that caused the response. Wait 10 minutes for symptoms to decrease, and then gently remove the feces.

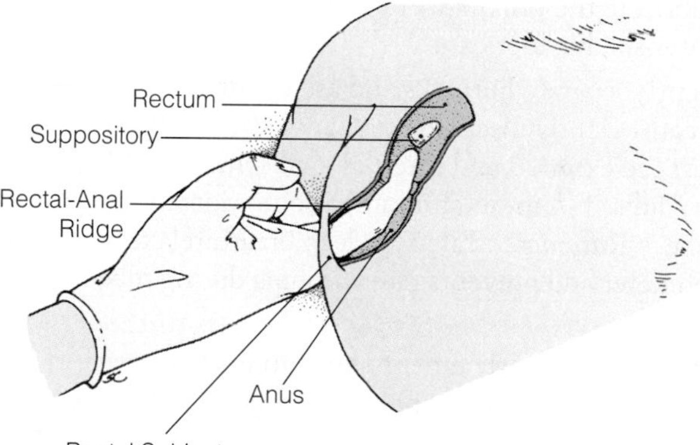

▲ Insert rectal suppositories beyond the rectal-anal ridge for retention.

EVIDENCE-BASED PRACTICE

Trial to Investigate Properties of Six Skin Protectants

In the treatment of incontinence dermatitis, a skin protectant primarily prevents skin breakdown due to moisture and biological irritants found in urine and feces. Six currently available skin hydration properties were studied in a controlled three-phase study in the United Kingdom. Eighteen volunteers addressed each product's efficacy against a known irritant, skin hydration potential, maintenance of skin barrier, and barrier efficacy against maceration. Each of the six products tested had different performance properties. Products containing petrolatum demonstrated protection against irritants and maceration and provided some skin hydration. Overall, only the water-in-oil petrolatum-based product performed efficiently in oil-tested parameters. This study suggested further testing and use of barrier products to provide additional evidence for appropriate product selection.

Source: Hoggarth, A. (2005). A controlled, three-part trial to investigate the barrier function and skin hydration properties of six skin protectants. *Ostomy/Wound Management, 51*(12), 30–42.

Inserting a Rectal Tube

Equipment

Rectal tube: size 22–24 straight (French) for adults and size 12–18 French for children
Small plastic bag or stool specimen container
Hypoallergenic paper tape
Water-soluble lubricant
Bed protector
Clean gloves, 2 pair
Washcloth and towel

Procedure

1. Check physician's orders and client care plan.
2. Perform hand hygiene.
3. Gather equipment.
4. Identify the correct client with two forms of identification and explain the procedure.
5. Provide privacy. Place client on left side in a recumbent position and drape. ▸ ***Rationale:*** This position facilitates insertion of tube following the normal curve of rectum and sigmoid colon.
6. Place bed protector under client.
7. Tape the plastic bag around the distal end of the rectal tube or insert the tube into the stool specimen container.
8. Vent the upper side of the plastic bag to prevent inflation.
9. Don gloves.
10. Lubricate the proximal end of the rectal tube with water-soluble lubricant.
11. Gently separate buttocks and ask client to take a deep breath. Gently insert the tube into the client's rectum, past the external and internal anal sphincters (2–4 in. in adults, 1–3 in. in children). Do not force the rectal tube. ▸ ***Rationale:*** Taking a deep breath relaxes the anal sphincter and prevents tissue trauma during tube insertion.
12. With adults, gently tape the tube in place, using hypoallergenic paper tape. With children, hold the tube in place manually.
13. Remove gloves and place in appropriate receptacle. Perform hand hygiene.

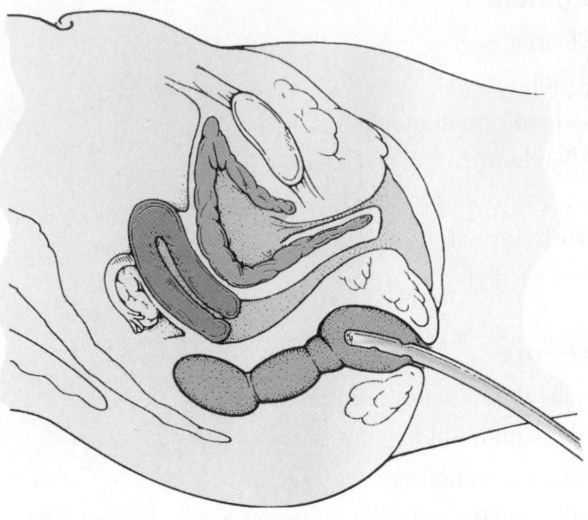

▲ Insert rectal tube past the external and internal anal sphincters.

14. Take client's pulse. ▸ ***Rationale:*** Alterations in pulse rate can indicate a vagal stimulation and the rectal tube may need to be removed. This can occur particularly in a client with a cardiac condition.
15. Leave the tube in place no longer than 20 minutes. ▸ ***Rationale:*** Prolonged stimulation of the anal sphincter may result in a loss of the neuromuscular response. The prolonged presence of a catheter may cause pressure necrosis of the mucosal surface.
16. Don gloves.
17. Remove the tube and provide perianal care.
18. Help the client assume a comfortable position.
19. Clean the tubing, and replace in bathroom if to be reused. Remove and discard the plastic bag.
20. Instruct client that chewing gum, sucking on candy, drinking liquids through a straw, carbonated beverages, and smoking tend to promote the swallowing of air and increase abdominal distention.
21. Remove gloves and perform hand hygiene.

Clinical Alert

Rectal tubes should not be used to manage diarrhea, only for removal of flatus.

Instructing Client in Colostomy Irrigation

Equipment

Solution container with 1000 mL warm water
Irrigating tubing with cone
Three pair of clean gloves
Irrigating sleeve cut long enough to reach water level in toilet
Items to clean skin and stoma (e.g., washcloths or gauze sponges)
Plastic bag for disposal of used pouch
Clean pouch and closure device
Skin barriers
Water-soluble lubricant
Hook near toilet

Procedure

1. Instruct client in benefits of relaxing and taking periodic deep breaths.
2. Perform hand hygiene and don clean gloves.
3. Remove and dispose of used pouch in plastic bag.
4. Clean stoma and skin with warm water and soft cloth. Assess skin for signs of irrigation or breakdown.
5. Apply irrigation sleeve to peristomal skin, and place belt around waist.
6. Fill container with 1000 mL lukewarm water (500 mL for first irrigation). ▸ ***Rationale:*** Lukewarm water temperature is 105°–110°F. This temperature prevents injury from hot solutions and cramping from cold solutions.
7. Suspend container on bathroom hook at level of client's shoulders (no higher than 18 inches above stoma).
8. Open roller clamp and allow solution to run through tubing; close clamp. ▸ ***Rationale:*** This removes air from tubing and prevents discomfort for client.
9. Assist client to sit on toilet or on chair in front of toilet.
10. Place sleeve between client's thighs and direct end into toilet.
11. Lubricate cone tip with water-soluble lubricant.
12. Position cone in sleeve by placing through top opening. If cone cannot be inserted easily do not force it.
13. Hold cone snugly against stoma. ▸ ***Rationale:*** This prevents back flow of solution.
14. Open roller clamp on tubing and allow water to run through cone while inserting cone into stoma.
15. Instill solution (750–1000 mL) over 5–10 minutes. ▸ ***Rationale:*** The container height and rate of water flow affect results obtained. If client complains of feeling light-headed or has vertigo, take pulse and stop instillation. ▸ ***Rationale:*** These are symptoms of a vagal response.

Clinical Alert

Colostomy irrigations are done only if normal bowel evacuation cannot be achieved.

Instructing Home Care Client in Colostomy Irrigation

Procedure

1. Instruct client and family on ostomy care.
2. Provide telephone number and address of supply vendors.
3. Refer client to community support groups for psychological support as needed.
4. Review infection control measures when carrying for ostomy pouches or dressings. Dispose of used equipment in appropriate receptacle.
5. Review potential skin and/or infection signs and symptoms and when to report findings to healthcare provider.

Implementing the Zassi Bowel Management System

Equipment

One hydrocolloid dressing, cut in half
Two pieces of tape, 2-cm width
One irrigation set
One 20-mL syringe
Bowel Management System Catheter; 4 cm or 6 cm
Retention cuff
Large-capacity collection bag
Gloves, 2 pair
Water-soluble lubricant
Container with 100 mL of water
500 mL of lukewarm irrigant (water or saline)

Preparation

1. Identify the client using two forms of identification.
2. Review client history to determine whether a contraindication to catheter placement has occurred.
   a. Severe strictures of distal rectum or anal canal.
   b. Presence of impacted or formed stool. ▸ ***Rationale:*** Client must have loose stool flow before insertion of BMS.
   c. Recent history of rectal anastomosis (less than 6 weeks)
   d. History of recent anal or sphincter reconstruction.
   e. Compromised rectal wall integrity.
3. Explain procedure to client. RNs or MDs may insert catheter.
4. Determine need for analgesia. If analgesia is necessary, notify MD or check orders to determine appropriate medication.

Procedure

1. Perform hand hygiene and don clean gloves.
2. Position client in left lateral, knee-chest position. ▸ ***Rationale:*** Provides maximal sphincter relaxation.
3. Perform digital rectal exam.
   a. Assess rectum and anal canal for pathology, size, stool, fecal impaction.
   b. Rectum must be cleared of stool.

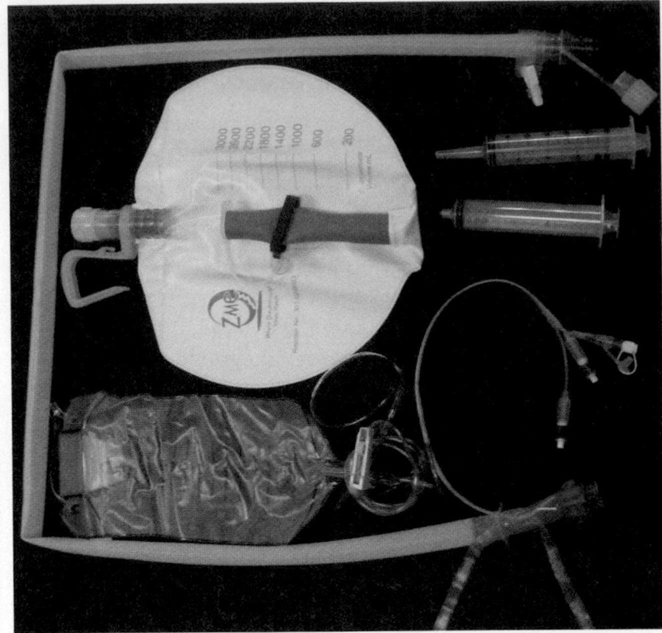

▲ Equipment needed for inserting and managing Bowel Management System.

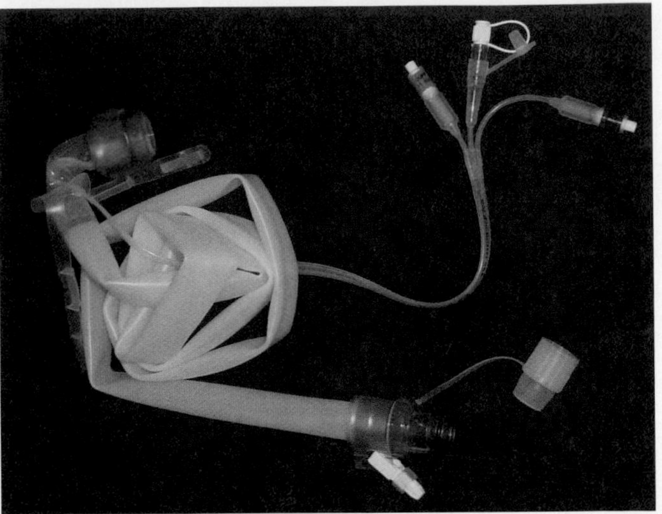

▲ Bowel Movement System Catheter.

c. Determine length of anal canal. If 2.5 cm or less, a 4-cm BMS is used. If greater than 2.5 cm, a 6-cm BMS is used. Follow directions on package.

4. Apply lubricant to perianal and anal canal.
   ▸ ***Rationale:*** Aids in pre-dilation of anal canal.
5. Remove gloves and discard. Don new clean gloves.
6. Open package containing catheter and bag.
7. Check catheter for appropriate functioning of system:
   a. Draw up 20 mL of air in syringe.
   b. Inflate intraluminal balloon (red connector) with 20 mL of air. Disconnect syringe. Status of connector pilot balloon indicates inflated state of intraluminal balloon.
   c. Fill syringe with 35–40 mL of water. Fill retention cuff (blue connector) with 35–40 mL of water. Disconnect syringe. Verify that pilot balloon indicates inflated state of retention cuff.
   d. Inspect cuff and balloon for leaks and check pilot balloons to indicate the inflated state of the intraluminal balloon or retention cuff.
   e. After verifying proper function, insert syringe and slowly and completely aspirate ALL fluid from cuff and balloon. Disconnect syringe. Connector pilot balloons indicate deflated state of intraluminal balloon and retention cuff.
   f. Inject water through the irrigation lumen (clear connector) to confirm lumen patency. Close white tethered cap and continue with preparations for insertion.
   g. Ensure the system does not come into contact with sharp edges such as lubricating packet. This could damage the system.
8. Connect end of catheter drain tube to collection bag by inserting catheter connector into bag connector and twisting clockwise to lock in place after closing off collection bag drain tube with red clamp.
9. Draw up 25 mL of air into syringe, attach syringe to intraluminal balloon, and inflate balloon via red connector. Disconnect syringe.

NOTE: An additional 5 mL of air is infused for added rigidity to perform the introducer function. Normal inflation is 20 mL of air.

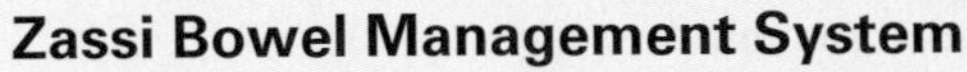

Zassi Bowel Management System

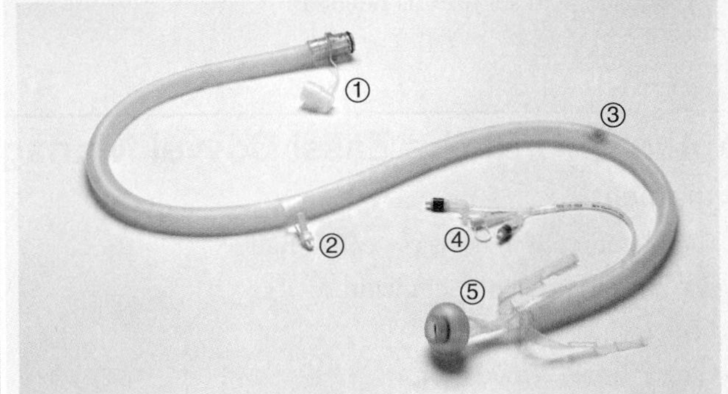

1. Drain tube connector and cup used to prevent leakage when bag disconnected.
2. Adjustable sheet clamp used to maintain the position of the drain tube.
3. Flush/Sampling port provides access for specimen collection and catheter cleaning.
4. Connectors are color coded and accept Luer-tip syringes. Pilot balloons on the intraluminal balloon and retention cuff indicate inflation status of catheter.
5. Transsphincteric catheter zone allows normal sphincter function during use and after removal.

Source: Courtesy of Zassi BMS/Zassi Medical.

10. Apply water-soluble lubricant generously over inflated intraluminal balloon, and fully collapse retention cuff around anus and anal canal.
11. Grasp the lubricated catheter directly behind the retention cuff with triple lumen connector tubing oriented anteriorly. At the time of maximum sphincter relaxation, insert the balloon end of the catheter into the distal rectum.
12. Maintain anterior orientation of the triple lumen connector tubing throughout insertion.
13. Fill the syringe with 35–40 mL of lukewarm water and insert into retention cuff via blue connector. Disconnect syringe. Connect catheter to collection bag.
14. After catheter placement insert syringe into red connector and aspirate 25 mL of air from intraluminal balloon. Disconnect syringe.
15. Confirm pilot balloon is fully collapsed.
16. Confirm catheter fit is tension-free with gentle tug and recoil to "seal" retention cuff (fit of 1 cm or greater gap between anchor strap faceplate and anus).
17. Secure catheter with anchor straps to "seat" retention cuff on rectal floor.
    a. Apply hydrocolloid dressing to each buttock.
    b. Check that catheter is not twisted, anchor straps are lateral, and triple lumen connector is anterior.
    c. Tape anchor straps to hydrocolloid dressing.
    d. Ensure straps do not apply tension on catheter.
18. Hang collection bag and position catheter to facilitate gravity drainage. ▸ ***Rationale:*** This allows for unobstructed flow of fecal matter from catheter to collection bag.
19. Secure catheter drain tube to sheet using sheet clip.
20. Maintain system by verifying system patency with open flow configuration (intraluminal balloon deflated) and irrigate with 50 mL of water.
21. Ensure client is in comfortable position.
22. Remove gloves and discard.
23. Perform hand hygiene.

For Maintaining Bowel Management System

1. Maintain system throughout catheter insertion. Catheters can remain in place up to 29 days.
2. Follow strict Stool Modification Plan and irrigation protocol.
3. Monitor deflated state of intraluminal balloon (via pilot balloon) at least three times per day.
4. Rinse catheter two times per day with 60 mL of water at room temperature, using the flush/sampling port.
5. Check BMS every 2 hr to ensure it is not occluded as a result of client lying on tube or tube being twisted.
6. Inspect BMS drainage tube near anus every 8–12 hr to verify that no column of irrigant and/or feces is in catheter. If irrigant or feces is present, milk into collection bag. Change bag every 8–12 hr.
7. Assess perianal region every 12 hr to observe for mucus or feces leakage in region. Cleanse area and place absorbent pad over area.

Clinical Alert

The BMS is contraindicated for use in clients with impacted stool. The BMS catheter must be removed and then the impaction removed before continuing use of the BMS.

8. Check retention cuff volume weekly or according to physician orders by aspirating all fluid from retention cuff and disconnect syringe; observe that cuff is deflated by checking pilot balloon; refill retention cuff with 35–40 mL of room temperature water.
9. Provide the following interventions to maintain a stool modification plan. ▸ ***Rationale:*** To maintain a functioning BMS system.
    a. Add fiber either in a tube feeding or through use of bulk laxatives.
        1. Citrucel (methyl cellulose), psyllium, prune juice, 6 oz every 8 hr.
        2. Add water to the diet when administering fiber.
    b. Add stool softeners such as docusate (Colace) 100–200 mg every 12 hr.
    c. Administer osmotic laxatives such as Lactulose 30 mL every 12 hr or MiraLax, 17 grams daily for 14 days.

NOTE: Increasing the frequency and/or dose of stool-modifying agents may improve results.

For Irrigating Bowel Management System

Equipment

60-mL Luer-tip syringe
Irrigation bag with connector
Lukewarm irrigant 300 to 1000 mL per order

Procedure

1. Perform hand hygiene and don clean gloves.
2. Empty collection bag unless it can accommodate additional 2 L of irrigant.
3. Fill irrigation bag with 300–1000 mL lukewarm tap water or saline and hang from IV pole 50–100 cm above client's anus.
4. Position client in Sims' or left side position with knees up and bed tilted to a slight head down position.
5. Connect irrigation bag administration set to clear connector. Ensure the irrigation bag is connected to correct catheter connector.
6. Draw up 20 mL of air into syringe, and inflate intraluminal balloon via red connector. Inflate with 20 mL air only.
7. Infuse 500 mL of water in approximately 10 minutes. If flow rate is less than optimal, attempt to squeeze gravity bag to clear occlusion.
8. After irrigant infusion, allow solution to dwell for 5 to 10 minutes.
9. Connect syringe to red connector. Aspirate the 20 mL of air from the intraluminal balloon. Disconnect syringe and confirm pilot balloon is fully collapsed. ▸ ***Rationale:*** This allows drainage of fluid and feces out of rectum and colon.
10. Position client with head slightly raised and feet in downward position to facilitate gravity drainage, if necessary.

Clinical Alert

If the client experiences cramping or leakage, the irrigation solution may be too hot or too cold, or the infusion rate is too fast. Check the solution temperature and monitor the rate of infusion carefully. You may need to stop the infusion until the cramping is alleviated. If leakage occurs, infuse additional water into retention cuff (blue connector) to prevent leakage.

11. Disconnect administration set from clear connector upon completion of irrigation procedure.
12. Attach syringe to blue connector and completely aspirate all water from retention cuff and then refill to 35 to 45 mL of water if additional water was added to prevent leakage.
13. Milk all remaining feces and irrigant in catheter, from anchor straps to collection bag. Empty contents of bag.
14. Remove and dispose of gloves and perform hand hygiene.

For Emptying Collection Bag

1. Perform hand hygiene and don clean gloves.
2. Remove drain tube plug.
3. Remove drain tube clamp from holster by sliding upward.
4. Open drain tube clamp and empty bag into secondary container.
5. Reclamp drain tube and return clamp to holster after emptying completed.
6. Replace drain tube plug.
7. Dispose of contents according to facility policy, maintaining standard precautions.
8. Dispose of gloves and perform hand hygiene.

For Removing Catheter

1. Perform hand hygiene and don clean gloves.
2. Insert 20-mL syringe into intraluminal balloon via red connector and inflate with 20 mL of air. Disconnect syringe.
3. Insert 60-mL syringe into blue connector of catheter retention cuff and deflate by slowly aspirating all water from the retention cuff. Disconnect syringe.
4. Verify state of retention cuff by confirming blue connector pilot balloon is collapsed.
5. Grasp catheter at external retention faceplate, ask client to bear down, and apply steady traction to slide catheter out the anal orifice.
6. If catheter does not come out easily, add water-soluble lubricant to anal canal and attempt to slide catheter again.
7. Discard catheter in biohazard container, maintaining standard precautions.
8. Remove and discard gloves and perform hand hygiene.

DOCUMENTATION for Bowel Management

- Type and number of suppositories used
- Digital stimulation used
- Approximate time used for digital stimulation
- Amount, consistency, characteristics of stool
- Protocol for bowel evacuation for client
- Untoward complications of bowel training program
- Nursing interventions needed to correct complications
- Time rectal tube inserted, size of tube
- Amount, color, and consistency of feces collected
- Time rectal tube removed
- Presence, absence, or change in abdominal distention
- Client's reaction to procedure
- Any unexpected outcomes and measures taken to treat these outcomes
- Take pulse rate before and during procedure
- Colostomy irrigation, amount, color, and concentration of return solution
- BMS insertion and maintenance
- Interventions related to stool modification plan
- Irrigation solution; type and amount

CRITICAL THINKING Application

Expected Outcomes

- Client establishes regular bowel evacuation program.
- Constipation is prevented.
- Fecal impaction is removed.
- Client is able to evacuate bowel at a convenient and consistent time.
- Client is free of pain, flatus, and discomfort.
- Digital stimulation is performed without cardiac complications.
- Rectal tube insertion relieves flatus.
- Colostomy irrigation is effective in promoting consistency in daily evacuation time.
- BMS is effective to prevent skin excoriation for clients with diarrhea.

Unexpected Outcomes	Alternative Actions
When digital stimulation is performed, client exhibits reflex spasm that prevents stool expulsion.	• Apply local anesthetic around rectum and anus, if ordered. • Wait for spasm to relax, and then proceed with stimulation.
Client develops diarrhea.	• Identify possible cause of diarrhea. • Observe dietary intake for possible cause. Provide for bulk. • Hold the laxatives and stool softeners temporarily. • Instruct client to eat yogurt and drink milk if not contraindicated by condition. • Inform physician of diarrhea and obtain orders for Kaopectate. Administer 2 teaspoons after each loose stool for 24 hours. • Check with physician if medications should be readjusted for bowel training as needed.
Client exhibits signs and symptoms of vagal response during removal of fecal impaction.	• Immediately discontinue procedure. • Place client in shock position. • Monitor vital signs every 5–15 minutes until condition is stable. • Notify physician of findings and request medication order for antispasmodic such as atropine. • Be prepared for "Code" situation, even though it is not likely to occur.
Effective bowel evacuation program is not established.	• Ask dietitian for altered diet (including more fruits and vegetables). • Check if contraindication exists for increasing fluids to 3000 mL daily. • Obtain order from the physician to administer a different stool softener and bulk former or increase dosage. • Have client increase physical activity, especially exercise of the abdominal muscles if not contraindicated by condition. • Ensure that client begins bowel training program one half hour after a meal.
No relief of abdominal distention.	• Reposition client at an angle that raises the lower part of the body (e.g., in a prone position with the foot of the bed raised). • Instruct client to circle, raise, and lower his or her legs. • Reinsert the tube after 2–3 hr. • Remove the tube and check for feces that may be clogging the outlet. Clean tube, and reinsert.
Fecal impaction lower in rectum prevents insertion of rectal tube.	• Perform digital examination with gloved finger and water-soluble lubricant. • Break up impaction if present. • Position client on left side in Fowler's position. • Reinsert the rectal tube.
Client is impacted with stool even after stool modification program is instituted.	• Irrigate aggressively to loosen stool. • Irrigate every 8–12 hr if necessary to maintain loose stool. • Administer enema and/or laxatives.
Stool becomes liquid when using the BMS.	• Obtain physician's order for antidiarrheal agent.
Irrigant will not infuse or infuses slowly through BMS.	• Use large-bore syringe to clear occlusion. • Place 100–200 mL of irrigant into catheter through flush/sampling port, milk across anal canal, and douche to clear occlusion.
BMS catheter is expelled.	• Ensure that no external traction is applied to catheter (i.e., catheter is caught in bed linen). • Clean catheter and reinsert but increase retention cuff pressure.

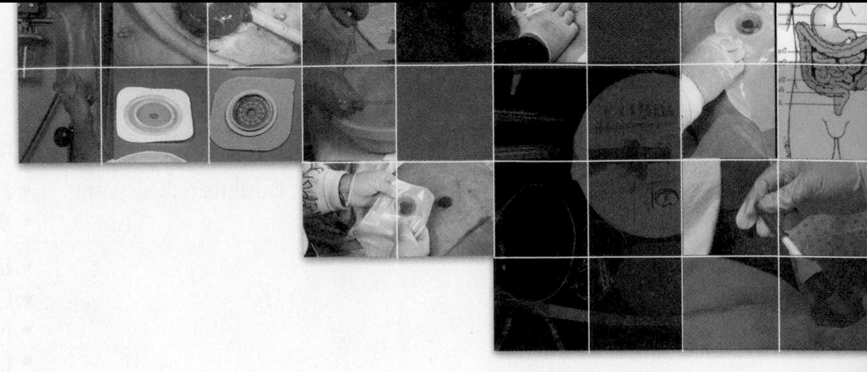

Chapter 23

UNIT 2

Enema Administration

Nursing Process Data

ASSESSMENT Data Base

- Review client's present and past eliminatory status.
- Assess the need for an enema.
- Evaluate amount of solution a client can tolerate.
- Assess if fecal impaction is present.
- Assess the degree of abdominal distention.
- Assess degree of sphincter control.
- Assess current medical regimen.
- Assess dietary history.
- Assess vital signs before and after procedure, as necessary.

PLANNING Objectives

- To relieve constipation
- To relieve fecal impactions
- To cleanse the bowel before surgery or diagnostic examination
- To evacuate the bowel in clients with neurologic dysfunction
- To provide nutrients
- To introduce an exchange resin
- To relieve abdominal distention
- To stimulate peristalsis

IMPLEMENTATION Procedures

EVALUATION Expected Outcomes

- Client experiences increased comfort and relief from abdominal distention.
- Enema administered without difficulty.
- Returns are clear if preparing client for diagnostic examination or surgery.
- Relief obtained from fecal impaction or constipation.
- Return of solution plus formed, soft feces is complete.

Pearson Nursing Student Resources

Find additional review materials at
nursing.pearsonhighered.com

Prepare for success with NCLEX®-style practice questions and Skill Checklists

Administering a Large-Volume Enema

Equipment

Fluid container with attached rectal tube (size 22–30, straight, or French, for adults)
Normal saline, tap water, soap (750–1000 mL of solution)
Water-soluble lubricant
Bath blanket, if desired
IV pole
Clean bedpan, commode, or toilet
Bed protector pad
Skin care items (e.g., soap, water, towels)
Two pair of clean gloves
Toilet tissue

Preparation

1. Check physician's orders and client care plan.
2. Gather equipment.
3. Identify correct client and explain the procedure. Explain the benefits of relaxing and taking periodic deep breaths and that he/she will need to hold solution for specified time.
4. Provide privacy.
5. Perform hand hygiene.

Procedure

1. Fill water container with 750–1000 mL of lukewarm solution, 105°–110°F. ▸ ***Rationale:*** Solutions that are too hot or too cold or solutions that are instilled too quickly can cause cramping, damage to rectal tissues, and extreme shock.
2. Allow solution to run through tubing until air is removed. Clamp tube. ▸ ***Rationale:*** If air is instilled during procedure, client experiences discomfort as a result of distension of the colon.
3. Hang container on IV pole next to bed. Solution should hang 18 to 24 in. above buttocks.
4. Raise bed to HIGH position, and lower side rails on side where you will be working.
5. Don gloves.
6. Place bed protector under client.
7. Place bedpan within easy reach, or place commode near bed.
8. Place client on left side in Sims' position. ▸ ***Rationale:*** To facilitate flow of solution using contour of bowel.
9. Provide privacy, and drape client with bath blanket.
10. Lubricate tip of tubing 2–4 in. with generous amount of water-soluble lubricant.
11. Gently spread buttocks, instruct client to take a slow breath, and insert tubing 3–4 in.
12. Raise the solution container to a maximum height of 18 in. above rectum when giving a high enema and 12–18 in. when giving a low enema. ▸ ***Rationale:*** To assist in fluid movement, turn client to supine position midway through procedure, then to right side.
13. Open regulating clamp and allow solution to flow slowly. ▸ ***Rationale:*** If the flow is slow, client experiences fewer cramps. The client will also be able to tolerate and retain a greater volume of solution. If cramping occurs, lower container to slow influx of

▲ Fill bag to 750 or 1000 mL with tepid solution.

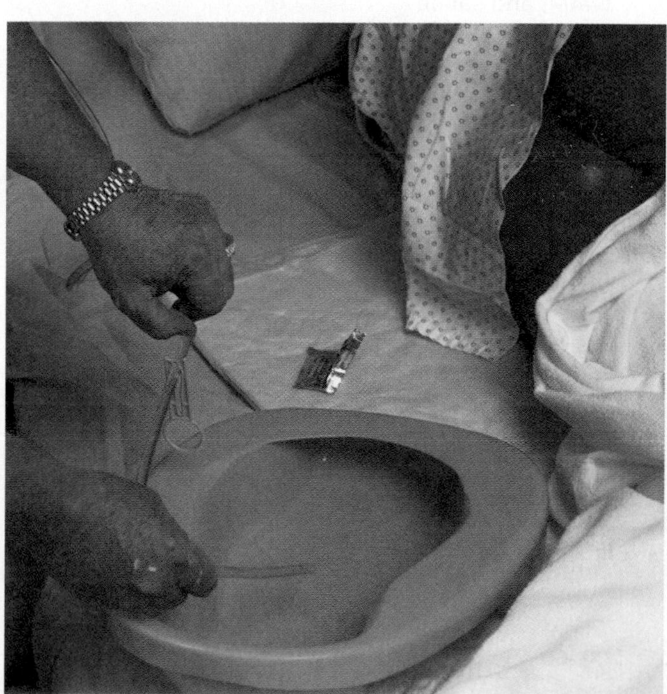

▲ Allow solution to run through tubing to expel air.

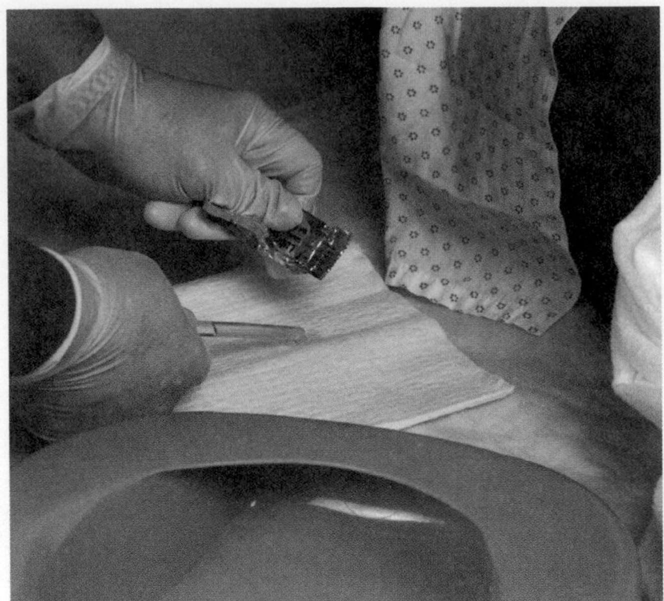

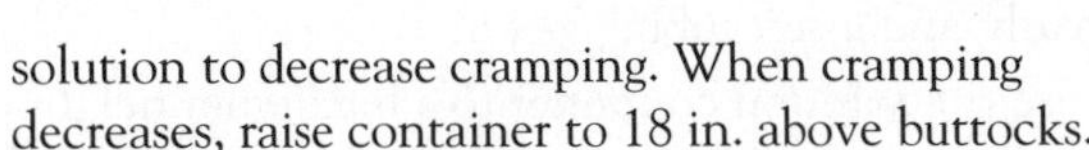

▲ Lubricate tip of tubing to prevent rectal injury.

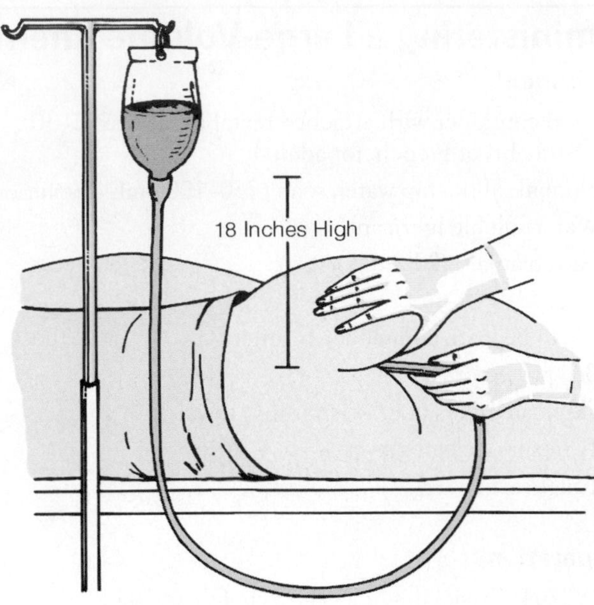

▲ Place enema solution container no more than 18 inches above rectum for safety.

solution to decrease cramping. When cramping decreases, raise container to 18 in. above buttocks.

14. Hold tubing in place in client's rectum at all times. Keep a bedpan nearby.

15. Lower solution container or momentarily clamp tubing if client experiences cramping, is unable to retain solution, or exhibits anxiety. Resume infusion of solution after a few minutes.

Types of Enemas

Cleansing

- Stimulates peristalsis through irritation of colon and rectum and by distention. Agents: Soap suds, tap water, and saline.
- *Soap suds*: Mild soap solutions stimulate and irritate intestinal mucosa. Strong soap solutions can cause severe irritation of the mucous membrane of the colon. Dilute 3–5 mL of mild soap in 1000 mL of water.
- *Tap water:* Give with caution to infants or to adults with altered cardiac and renal reserve. Tap water is a hypotonic solution.
- *Saline:* For normal saline enemas, use a smaller volume of solution. Hypertonic solutions draw fluid into the colon from the body tissues. These solutions are mildly irritating to the mucous membrane of the colon.

Retention

- Solution or nutrient is retained for specified time. Agents: mineral oil, olive oil, cottonseed oil, liquid petrolatum. Nutrient agent: dextrose solution.
- *Emollient (Oil):* Lubricates the rectum and colon, protecting the intestinal mucous membrane. Feces absorb oil and become softer and easier to expel. Client retains enema for prescribed time, usually 30–60 minutes.
- *Nutritive:* Provides nourishment in temporary or emergency situations. Enema is retained.

Distention Reduction

- Provides relief from flatus causing distention. It improves ability to expel flatus. Types: carminative and return flow.
- *Carminative:* Two common types include: 1-2-3 enema (30 g of magnesium sulfate, 60 g of glycerin, and 90 mL warm water) and milk and molasses (180–240 mL of equal amounts).
- *Return flow:* Harris flush most common. Mild colonic irrigation using 100–200 mL of enema solution. After instillation, enema container is lowered and solution siphoned back into container.

Medicated

- Enemas containing drugs used for reducing bacteria or removing potassium. Agents: Kayexalate and neomycin.
- *Kayexalate:* A resin is introduced into the large intestine, removing the excess potassium by exchanging it for sodium ions.
- *Neomycin:* Antibiotic solution used to reduce bacteria before bowel surgery.

16. After you have instilled the solution, gently remove the tubing. Instruct client to hold solution for 10–15 minutes or as long as tolerated. ▸ ***Rationale:*** The longer the solution is retained, the more effective the results.
17. Clean and dispose of equipment.
18. Place client on bedpan, elevate the head of the bed so that client can assume a squatting position on bedpan, or assist to commode.
19. Remove gloves and perform hand hygiene.
20. Provide privacy until client has expelled total volume of instilled solution.
21. Don clean gloves before removing bedpan, or assist client to bed.
22. Remove bedpan when client is ready, and immediately empty, clean, and replace to proper storage area.

TABLE 23-2 Fluid Volume for Enema Administration

Infant	50–150 mL
Toddler	250–350 mL
Child	300–500 mL
Adolescent	500–750 mL
Adult	750–1000 mL

23. Assist client with perineal care, and help client to assume a comfortable position.
24. Lower bed and raise side rails.
25. If client is on strict I&O, measure returns. ▸ ***Rationale:*** To make sure total volume of the solution is expelled.
26. Remove gloves and perform hand hygiene.

Administering an Enema to a Child

Equipment

Water container with attached rectal tube (size 14–18 straight [French] for children, and size 10–12 French or infant enema syringe with bulb for infants)
Normal saline, tap water, soap solution
Water-soluble lubricant
Clean potty chair for children
Bed protector
Skin care items (e.g., soap, water, towels)
Clean gloves

Preparation

1. Check physician's orders and identify client using two forms of identification.
2. Gather equipment.
3. Provide privacy for child.
4. Perform hand hygiene.
5. Identify correct client, and explain procedure to child or family. Inform an older child he/she will feel like he has to go the bathroom while the solution is flowing in. Take time to calm a frightened child and to answer the child's questions.
6. If child is toilet trained, place potty chair next to crib or bed.

Procedure

1. Fill water container with 100°F solution, using appropriate volume according to age.
2. Open clamp and allow solution to run through the tubing so that air is removed.
3. Clamp tube and hang solution container on IV pole.
4. Place bed protector under child.
5. Place child on left side or in knee–chest position. ▸ ***Rationale:*** To facilitate flow of solution using contour of bowel.
6. Don clean gloves.
7. Lubricate tip of tubing or infant enema syringe with bulb.
8. Gently separate buttocks and insert catheter or syringe into child's rectum (1–1.5 in. for infants, 2–3 in. for children) at an angle pointing toward the navel.
9. If there is resistance when inserting the tip or solution, carefully withdraw the tip and try a different angle.
10. Elevate solution container no more than 12–18 in. above the child's hips, according to hospital policy. ▸ ***Rationale:*** Height increases pressure of solution entering colon—too much pressure may damage colon.
11. Open clamp and allow solution to flow slowly for 10–15 minutes. If the solution starts to ooze out of rectum, briefly squeeze child's buttocks firmly together around the tube.
12. After you have instilled the solution, close clamp and gently remove the tubing or syringe.
13. Hold child's buttocks together or tape them with hypoallergenic paper tape.
14. Retain solution 10–15 minutes for cleansing enemas.
15. Place the child on a potty chair or bedpan to expel solution.
16. Remove gloves and place in trash receptacle. Perform hand hygiene.
17. If there are no contraindications, you may gently massage child's abdomen to help child expel returns.
18. If the child wants to be left alone while expelling returns, provide privacy. Child should expel the total volume of the instilled solution.
19. Don gloves.
20. Remove the potty chair or bedpan.

21. Clean the child's perineal area, and help child assume a comfortable position.
22. Estimate returns of solution. ▸ ***Rationale:*** To determine that the child expelled the total volume of the solution.
23. Clean all equipment, and replace in appropriate area.
24. Remove gloves and perform hand hygiene.

Administering a Small-Volume Enema

Equipment

Commercially prepared enema
Water-soluble lubricant
Bedpan, commode, toilet
Two pair of clean gloves
Bed protector
Skin care items (e.g., soap, water, towels)

Preparation

1. Check physician's orders and identify client using two forms of identification.
2. Gather equipment.
3. Perform hand hygiene.
4. Identify correct client and explain the procedure. Explain the benefits of relaxing and taking periodic deep breaths.
5. Place bed protector under client.
6. Place client on left side in a Sims' position.
7. Provide privacy.
8. Read directions on enema container.
9. Don clean gloves.

Procedure

1. Fold linen down to expose buttocks.
2. Lubricate with water-soluble lubricant if necessary. (Usually rectal tube is self-lubricated.)
3. Expose the anal opening to assist you in inserting the tube without traumatizing the tissue.
4. After inserting rectal tube, gently squeeze the container, and empty entire 120 mL of hypertonic solution.
5. Keep pressure on container while removing from rectum. ▸ ***Rationale:*** To prevent solution from being drawn back into container.
6. Instruct client to hold solution 5–7 minutes.
7. When ready to expel solution elevate the head of the bed so that the client can assume a squatting position on the bedpan. If able, client may expel solution in toilet.
8. Remove and dispose of gloves.
9. Provide privacy until the client has expelled the total volume of the instilled solution.
10. Don gloves and remove bedpan if client using bedpan.
11. Assist client with perineal care, and help client to assume a comfortable position.
12. Measure returns if on strict I&O.
13. Dispose of equipment, and remove gloves.
14. Perform hand hygiene.

▲ Remove cap from container and ensure that it is lubricated.

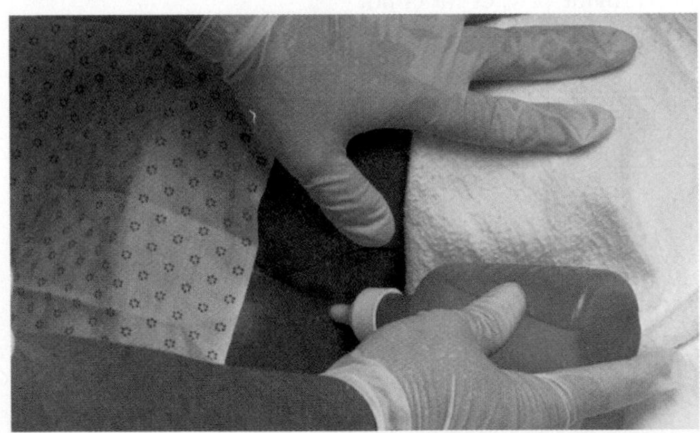

▲ Insert tip of container gently into rectum and expel all fluid.

Administering a Retention Enema

Equipment

Commercially prepared disposable oil retention enema
Oil: Adult 150–200 mL, child 75–100 mL, 91°F
Water-soluble lubricant
Bedpan or commode
Bed protector
Skin care items (e.g., soap, water, towels)
Clean gloves

Preparation

1. Identify and prepare client as for any enema.
2. Provide privacy.
3. Gather equipment—disposable oil retention enema is administered like a small enema. Read directions on enema container.

Procedure

1. Explain steps of procedure to client.
2. Raise bed to HIGH position.
3. Perform hand hygiene and don gloves.
4. Place bed protector on bed.
5. Expose anal opening, and gently insert rectal tube tip of container 3–4 in. Commercially prepared enemas are prelubricated.
6. Squeeze contents slowly, and empty entire amount into rectum.
7. Keep container compressed and remove rectal tube gently. ▸ ***Rationale:*** To prevent solution from being drawn back into container.
8. Lower bed.
9. Discard equipment and gloves, following Standard Precautions. Perform hand hygiene.
10. Explain to client that oil should be retained for 30–60 minutes before it is expelled. ▸ ***Rationale:*** Purpose of enema is to soften stool.
11. A cleansing enema may need to be given to remove oil and stimulate defecation.
12. Don gloves and provide hygienic care if needed. Discard washcloth and towel in laundry.
13. Remove gloves, discard in appropriate container, and perform hand hygiene.

Administering a Return Flow Enema

Equipment

Fluid container with attached rectal tube
Normal saline or tap water at 105°–110°F
Water-soluble lubricant
Clean bedpan
Bed protector
Skin care items (e.g., soap, water, towels)
Clean gloves

Preparation

1. Check physician's orders and identify client using two forms of identification.
2. Gather equipment.
3. Provide privacy.
4. Perform hand hygiene.
5. Fill fluid container with 100–200 mL of ordered solution; check that temperature is between 105°–110°. ▸ ***Rationale:*** Cool solutions increase cramping.
6. Allow solution to run through tubing so that air is removed. ▸ ***Rationale:*** If air is instilled during procedure, client experiences discomfort.
7. Hang container on IV pole.

Procedure

1. Explain procedure to client. Explain the benefits of relaxing and taking periodic deep breaths during procedure.
2. Raise bed to HIGH position, and lower side rails.
3. Don gloves.
4. Place bed protector under client.
5. Place client on left side in Sims' position with right leg flexed as much as possible. ▸ ***Rationale:*** This position facilitates instillation of fluid.
6. Lubricate tip of tubing with water-soluble lubricant.
7. Gently spread buttocks, and insert tubing 3–4 in. into client's rectum, past external and internal sphincters. Avoid traumatizing hemorrhoids during insertion. ▸ ***Rationale:*** Vagal nerve stimulation from enemas may cause cardiac arrhythmias.
8. Raise water container to a maximum height of 12–8 in. above rectum.
9. Open clamp and allow 200 mL of solution to flow slowly into rectum and sigmoid colon. If cramping occurs, clamp tube for a few minutes and then continue infusion.
10. Lower solution container 12–18 in. below level of rectum and allow all fluid to flow back into container.

11. Raise container 12–18 in. above rectum and allow solution to flow back into rectum.
12. Repeat inflow–outflow process 5–6 times, changing solution when it becomes thick with feces.
    ▸ ***Rationale:*** This assists in stimulating intestinal peristalsis with expulsion of flatus.
13. Provide privacy until client has expelled total volume of instilled solution after last inflow–outflow series.
14. Assist client with perineal care, and help client assume a comfortable position.
15. If client is on strict I&O, measure returns to make sure total volume of solution is expelled.
16. Clean all equipment, and replace in bathroom or appropriate location.
17. Remove gloves and perform hand hygiene.
18. Lower bed and raise side rails.

DOCUMENTATION for Enema Administration

- Purpose of enema
- Time enema given
- Volume and type of solution used
- Results obtained: amount, consistency, and color
- Any unexpected outcomes and measures taken to remedy problems
- Client's reactions to procedure
- Relief of flatus and distension

CRITICAL THINKING Application

Expected Outcomes

- Client experiences increased comfort and relief from abdominal distention.
- Enema administered without difficulty.
- Returns are clear if preparing client for diagnostic examination or surgery.
- Relief obtained from fecal impaction or constipation.
- Return of solution plus formed, soft feces is complete.

Unexpected Outcomes	Alternative Actions
Client expels solution prematurely.	• Calm and ease client's distress by reassuring him or her as you clean the equipment. • Place bedpan under client. Place client in semi-Fowler's position with knees flexed. • Hold the rectal tube in client's rectum between thighs. Slow the water flow, and continue with the enema.
Client complains of severe and sudden abdominal pain, nausea, and distention.	• Remove tubing and notify physician immediately of possible perforation. (This is an uncommon complication.) • Assess vital signs. If you suspect cardiac dysrhythmias, remove bedpan and notify physician immediately. • Be prepared to administer emergency drugs, such as atropine. • If an IV is not in place, start an IV of 5% dextrose in water (D_5W) using a large-bore needle for emergency use.
The flow of water is impeded or an obstruction is felt.	• Open clamp on tubing. Allow a small amount of solution to flow. (The warm solution may help relax the internal sphincter.) • Withdraw tube slightly and reinsert. • Gently perform a digital examination for the possibility of fecal impaction. Break up impaction if present. Ask physician for order to give a retention enema, followed by a cleansing enema 2–3 hr later.

Client cannot return enema solution.	• Gently massage client's abdomen if not contraindicated. • Replace rectal tube. Lower the enema bag below the level of the bed. • If client is not uncomfortable, do nothing. If client complains of discomfort or pain, notify physician.
Enema returns are not clear before surgery or diagnostic testing.	• Repeat enema. If, after three enemas, returns are still not clear, notify physician of findings. • May need to give an enema with a stronger solution. • Physician may need to order magnesium citrate or electrolyte solution (i.e., GoLYTELY).
Fecal impaction is not relieved.	• Check orders for oil retention enema. • Check catheter size needed. • Obtain order for and use digital stimulation and manual extraction of feces if not contraindicated by diagnosis of cardiac or neurologic involvement.

Chapter 23

UNIT ❸

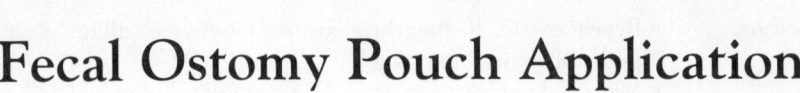

Fecal Ostomy Pouch Application

Nursing Process Data

ASSESSMENT Data Base

- Assess type and location of stoma (section of bowel used to create stoma).
- Observe stoma color, which should be beefy red and moist.
- Inspect client's abdomen for creasing, firmness, softness, contour, scars, folds, and incisions.
- Inspect client's peristomal skin for signs of erythema, excoriation, ulceration, and fistula formation.
- Assess how far stoma protrudes above skin surface; it should be 0.5–1 in.
- Assess size of stoma.
- Assess output of effluent including amount, consistency, odor.
- Assess client's learning abilities, age, manual dexterity, and visual acuity.

PLANNING Objectives

- To assist client to feel more confident that colostomy will not evacuate once appliance is intact
- To collect effluent for accurate assessment of output in the hospital
- To collect effluent for the comfort of the client
- To contain stool and odors to facilitate the client's return to a productive lifestyle, including the resumption of satisfying and meaningful relationships.
- To protect peristomal skin from erythema, excoriation, and infection
- To protect the client's clothing

IMPLEMENTATION Procedures

EVALUATION Expected Outcomes

- Pouch remains intact without leakage for 3–5 days.
- Pouching system provides maximal skin protection.
- Pouching system remains odor-proof for 3–5 days.
- Client gradually assumes an active role in applying the pouch.
- Client's skin remains free of erythema or excoriation and infection.

Pearson Nursing Student Resources

Find additional review materials at
nursing.pearsonhighered.com

Prepare for success with NCLEX®-style practice questions and Skill Checklists

Applying a Fecal Ostomy Pouch

Equipment

One- or two-piece transparent ostomy pouch with adhesive wafer
Warm water and mild soap
Soft cloths
Bath blanket
Plastic bag for pouch disposal
Tail closure or night adaptor for pouch
Clean gloves
Graduate or bedpan
Measuring guide
Tissues
Ostomy scissors and dark marking pen

Preparation

1. Check client care plan and identify client using two forms of identification.
2. Determine exact supplies client uses.
3. Gather equipment.
4. Explain procedure to client.
5. Provide privacy.
6. Raise bed to high position.
7. Perform hand hygiene and don gloves.

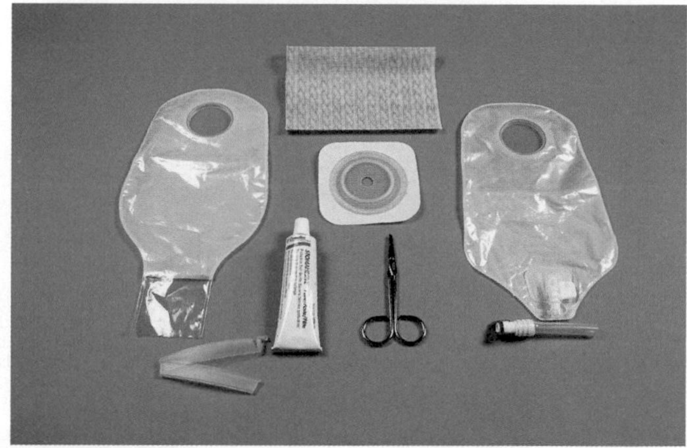
▲ Supplies needed to change two-piece pouches.

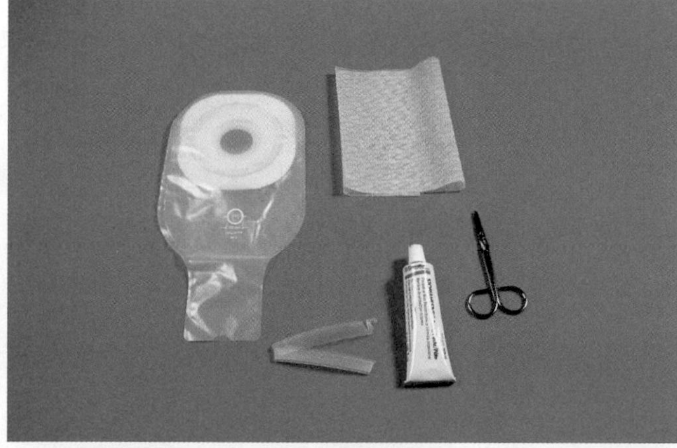
▲ Supplies needed to change one-piece pouches.

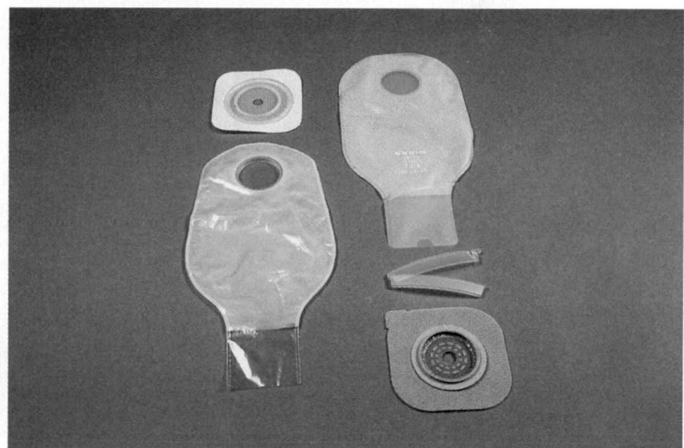
▲ Two-piece fecal pouches.

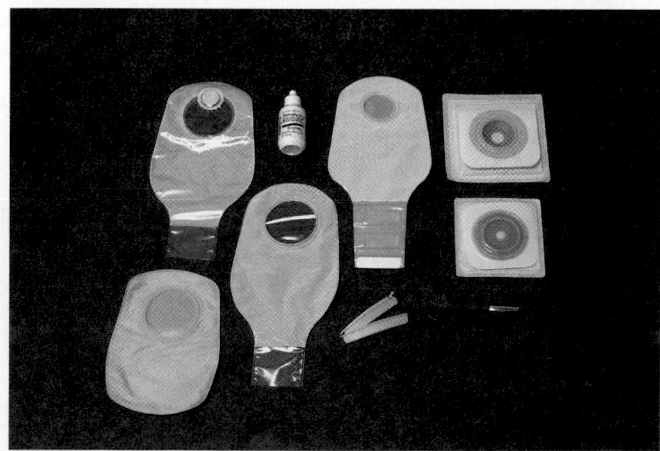
▲ Fabric pouches, convexity faceplates, pouch with filter.

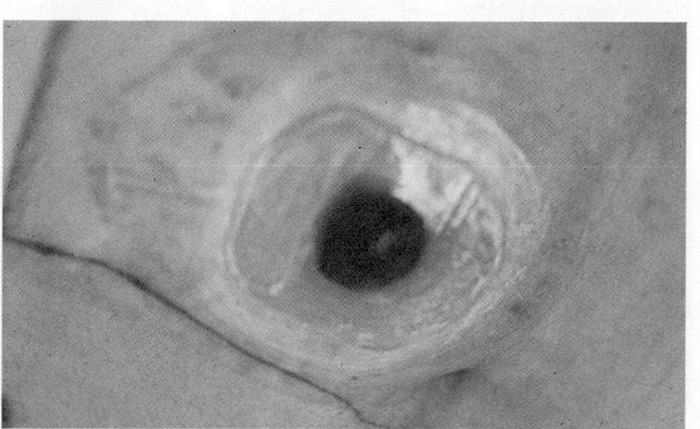
▲ Viable stoma.

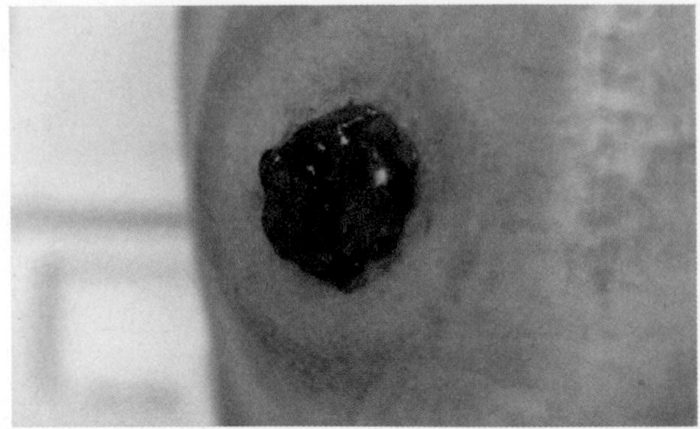

▲ Nonviable parastomal hernia.

Procedure

1. Place bath blanket over client. Place absorbent pad or towels under client. ▶ ***Rationale:*** To protect bed from spillage.
2. Observe placement of stoma. ▶ ***Rationale:*** To determine normal amount of output and consistency. (Immediately after surgery, all stomas will have very liquid stool and high flatus output.)
3. Empty old pouch into graduate, bedpan, or toilet.
4. Remove old pouch by pushing against skin as you pull backing from skin and discard in plastic bag. Save tail closure on bottom of pouch.

Changing One-Piece Fecal Ostomy Pouch

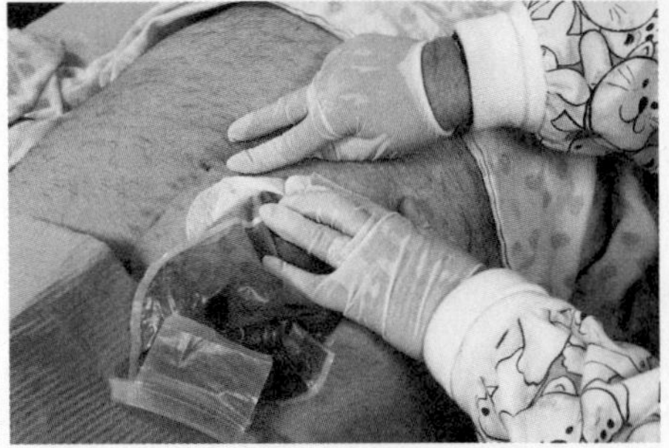

1 Starting at upper corner, remove old pouch.

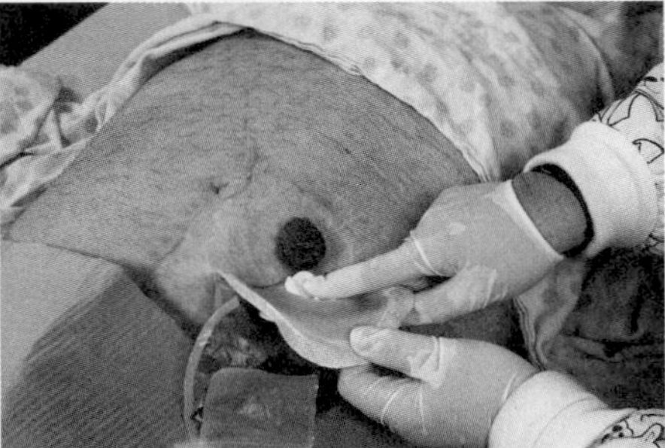

2 As you remove old pouch, push against skin while pulling down on pouch.

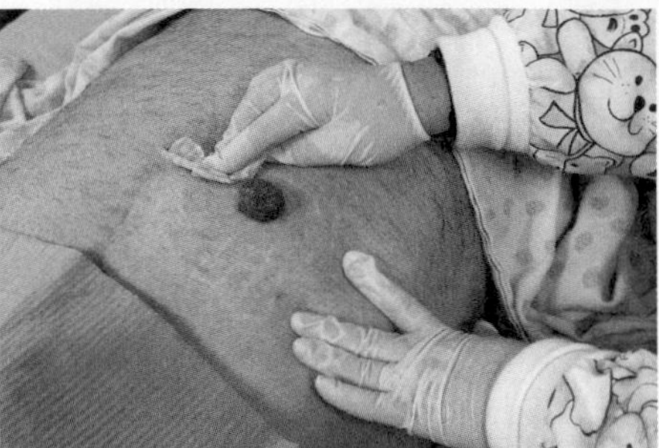

3 Clean skin with warm water,; dry well.

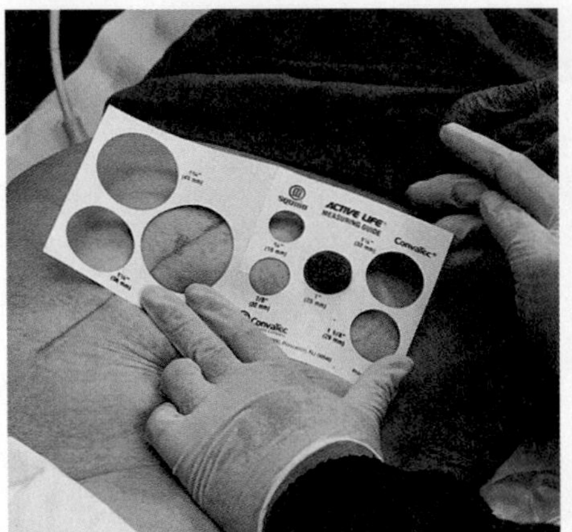

4 Measure stoma size.

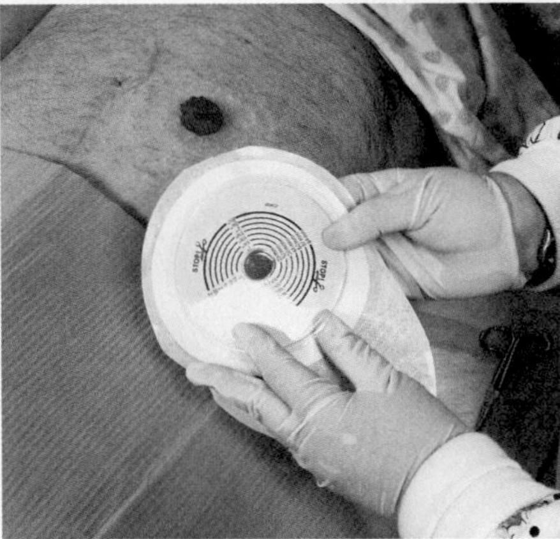

5 Remove plastic covering from one-piece pouch.

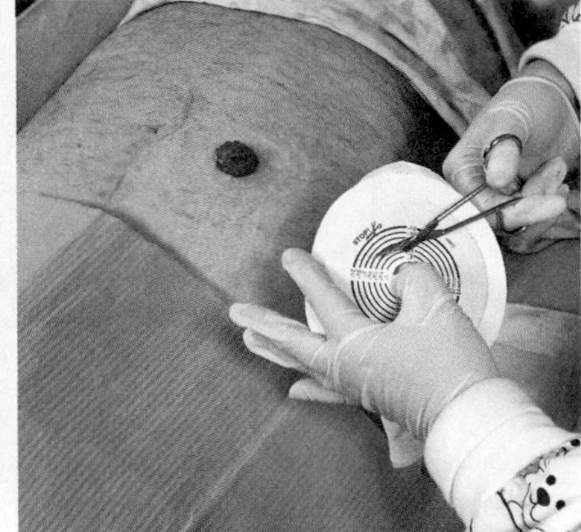

6 Cut pouch opening to exact size of stoma.

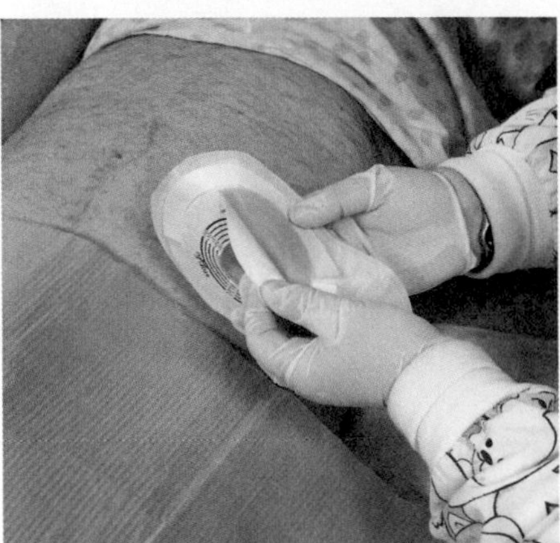

7 Remove paper from inner wafer. Save pattern for future pouch changes.

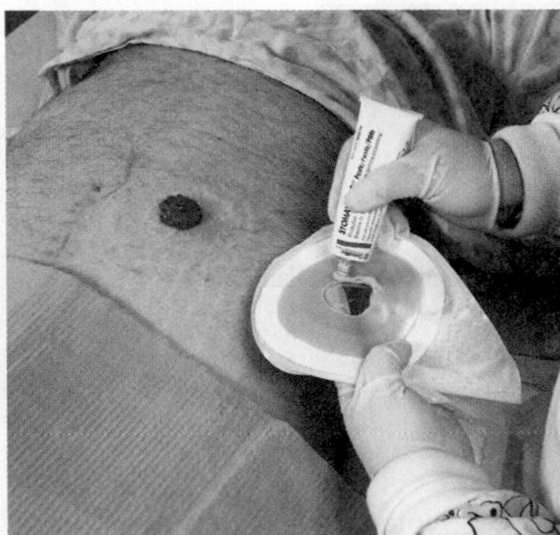

8 Apply ring of paste to opening on pouch.

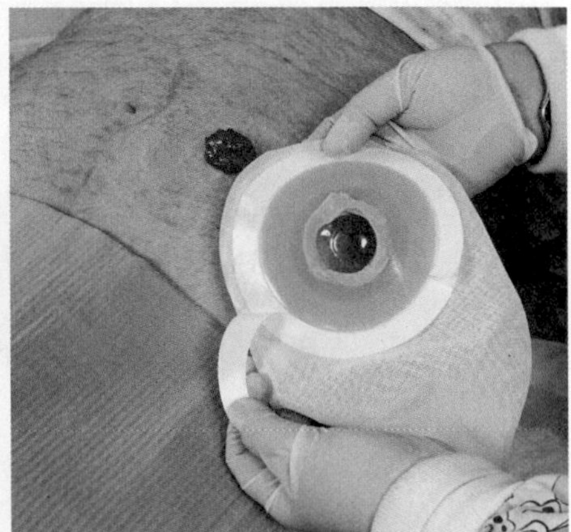

9 Remove paper from outer adhesive ring of pouch.

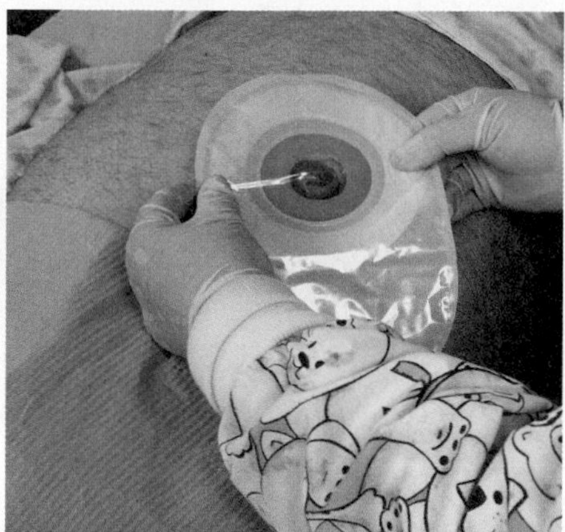

Center and apply pouch to clean, dry skin.

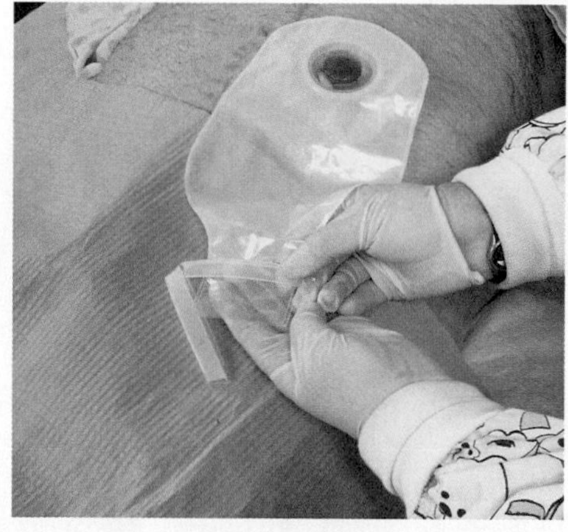

After applying one-piece pouch, clamp bottom of pouch.

Clinical Alert

To promote the client's self-esteem and body image, be aware of your own body language. Even subtle changes in the way you look at the stoma could indicate disgust or disapproval and an altered self-esteem could result.

5. Measure output, if ordered.
6. Clean skin and stoma gently with warm water and soft cloth. ▸ ***Rationale:*** Oily substances can interfere with pouch adhesive. If adhesive doesn't come off, leave it on the skin. If you pick at it, the peristomal skin can be damaged.
7. Dry skin well with soft cloth. Keep tissues available if stoma functions while pouch is off.
8. Observe skin; it should be free of erythema or excoriation. The stoma is assessed for changes in size, ulceration, and color (stoma should be moist, pink, or beefy red). Notify the physician if stoma is black, blue, or purple. This indicates a nonviable stoma.
9. Measure stoma at the base with measuring guide.
10. Trace measured pattern on pouch.
11. Cut pouch to pattern, making sure opening is large enough (at least 1/8 in.) to encircle stoma without pushing on edges. ▸ ***Rationale:*** No skin should appear between the pouch edge and the stoma.
12. If using a two-piece pouch, snap the wafer and pouch together. (See photo sequence for alternate method of using two-piece pouch.)
13. Remove paper from skin barrier on pouch and save it. ▸ ***Rationale:*** This may be used as a pattern for next pouch change.
14. Apply a ring of skin barrier paste to opening on pouch.
15. Apply Stomahesive powder to denuded skin only.
16. Remove paper from outer ring.
17. Center and apply pouch to clean and dry skin. Smooth edges of adhesive to skin. ▸ ***Rationale:*** If adhesive is wrinkled, it may result in leakage from pouch. To promote optimum wear of the pouch, warm the adhesive by placing your gloved hand over the adhesive and gently hold it over the site for 1/2 to 1 minute. *Rationale:* This will activate the adhesive in the skin barrier.
18. Pouches can be applied over an incision. ▸ ***Rationale:*** Incisions are sealed within 24 hr of surgery.
19. Close and secure end of pouch with tail closure.
    a. Ensure bowed end is next to body. ▸ ***Rationale:*** This provides a better fit to body, and prevents outpouching of clamp through clothing.
    b. Lay hook on top of bag and fold bag 1 in. over end of pouch.
    c. Squeeze clamp together to close.
20. Remove soiled pouch and tissues from bedside.
21. Remove gloves and perform hand hygiene.
22. Position client for comfort. Return bed to low position.
23. Put away supplies and reorder as necessary.

Clinical Alert

Clients with ostomies will need a nutritional consult and a written dietary guide. They need to limit the amount of hard-to-digest foods for at least the first 2–3 weeks post op. Also, limiting gas-producing foods will prevent gas-forming odors.

Applying Two-Piece Fecal Ostomy Pouch

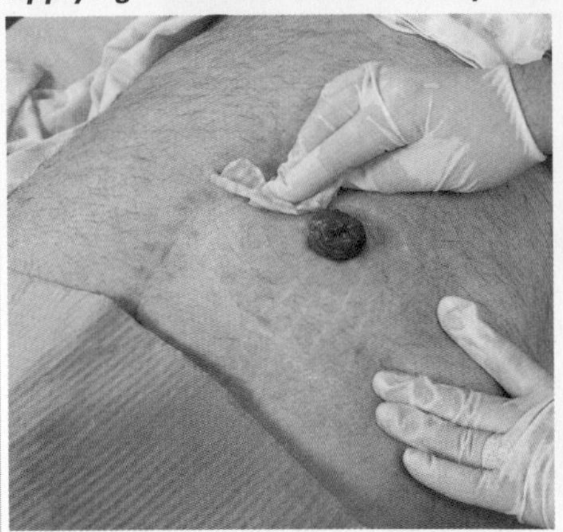

1 Clean and dry skin thoroughly before applying two-piece.

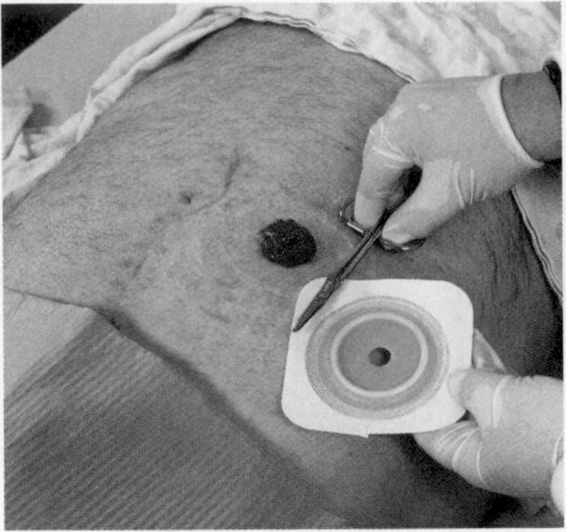

2 Cut opening of a two-piece pouch to exact size of stoma.

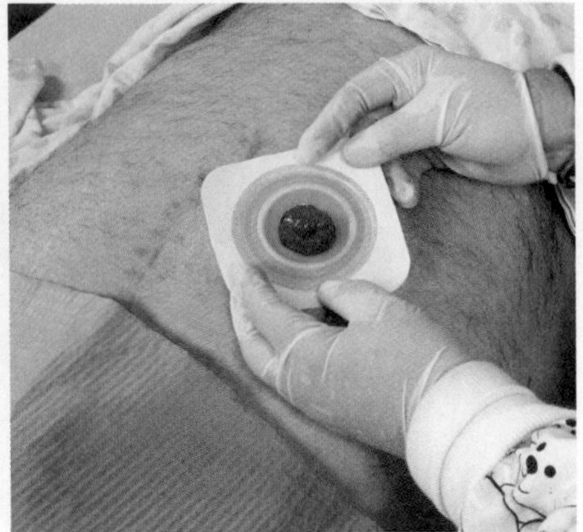

3 Check size of opening to ensure proper fit.

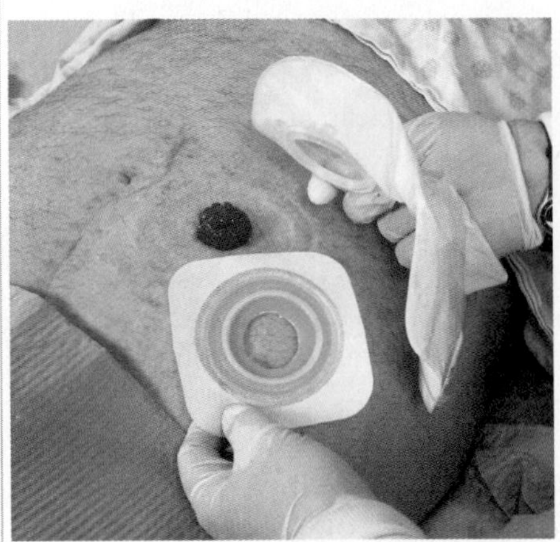

4 Snap pouch onto wafer when using a two-piece pouch.

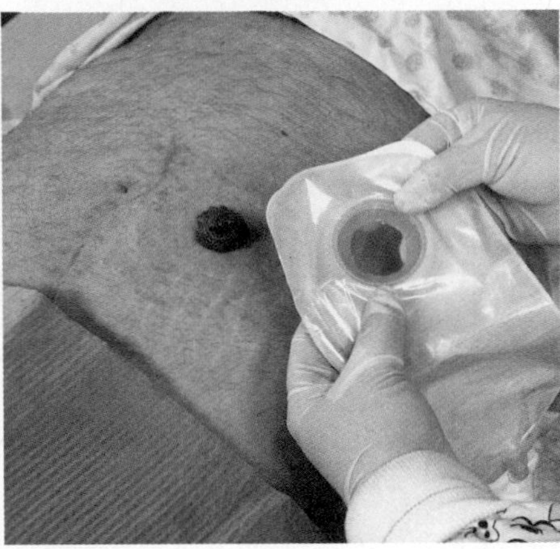

5 Check for secure fit by tugging at bottom of pouch.

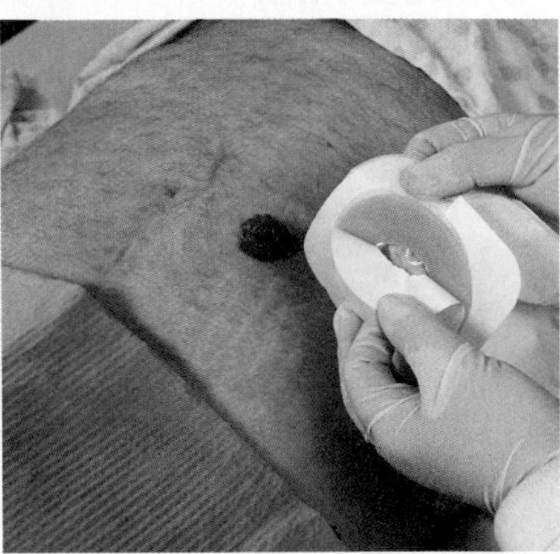

6 Remove paper from inner barrier.

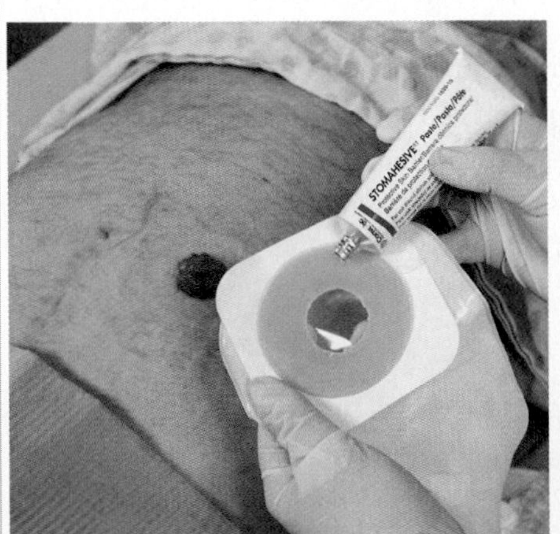

7 Apply paste to inner circle of wafer.

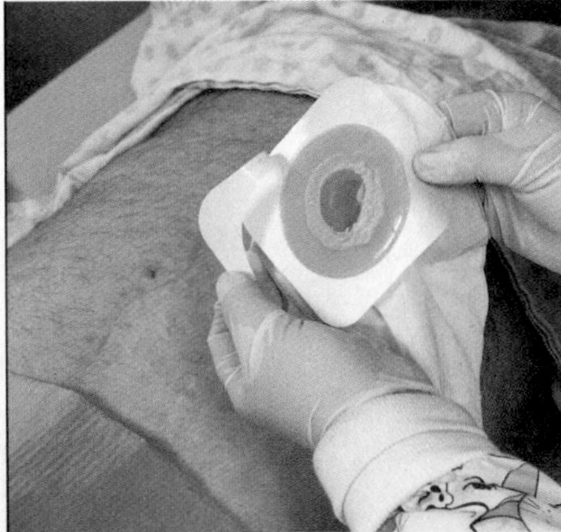

8 Remove paper from outer adhesive ring.

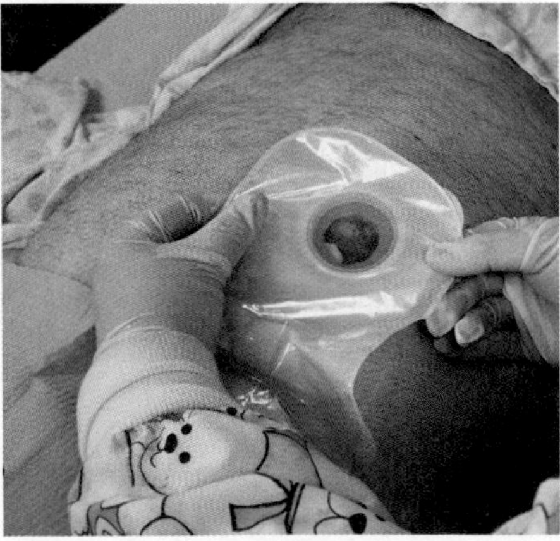

9 Center pouch over stoma and press onto skin.

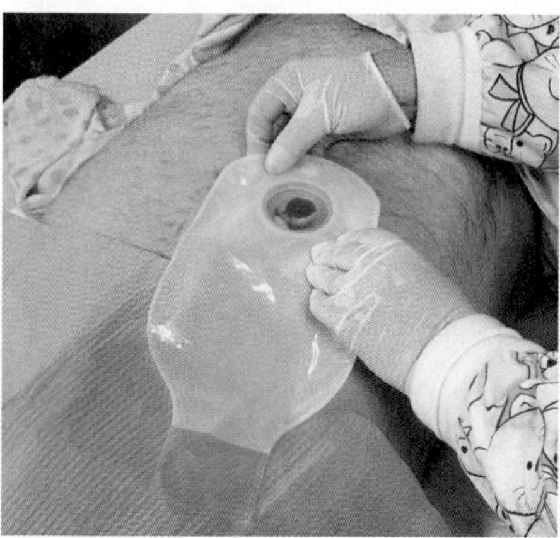
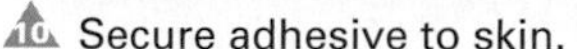
10 Secure adhesive to skin.

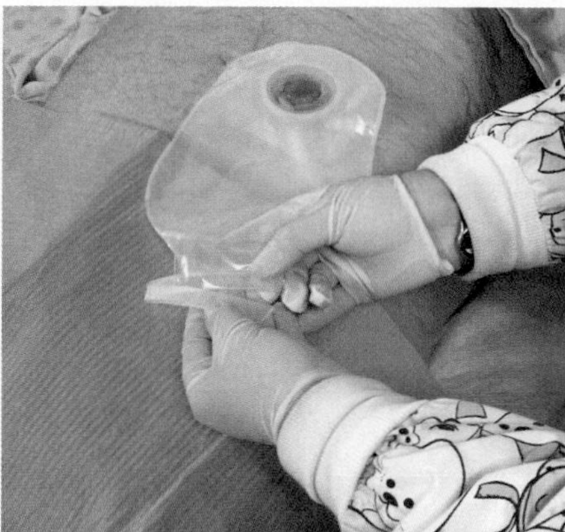
11 Clamp bottom of pouch.

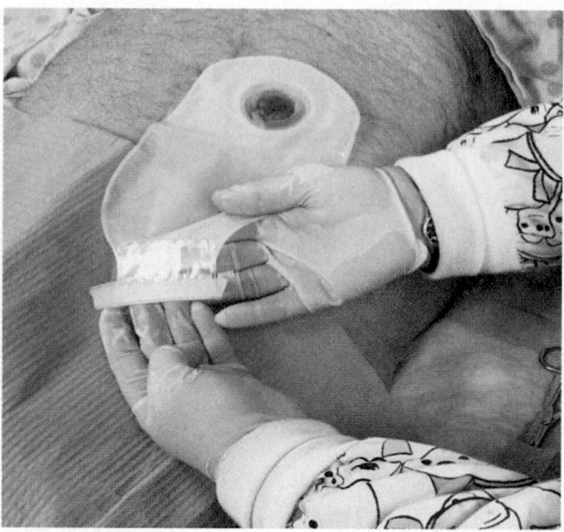
12 Check that clamp is secure.

Client Teaching

- Empty pouch when one-third full of stool or flatus.
  a. Empty into toilet.
  b. Pouch should last for 3–4 days.
- Rinse pouch using room temperature water and a rubber ear syringe (squirt into pouch).
- Use pouch deodorant if desired.
- Empty each morning and last thing at night even if not one-third full.
- Check seal on daily basis for tight fit; change if needed.
- Instruct client to always carry a supply of ostomy equipment for emergency use.
- Instruct client on emptying and cleaning pouch, opening and closing clamp, observing and cleaning peristomal area, and changing pouch.
- Have client return demonstration until able to perform activities correctly.

Loop Colostomy with Rod

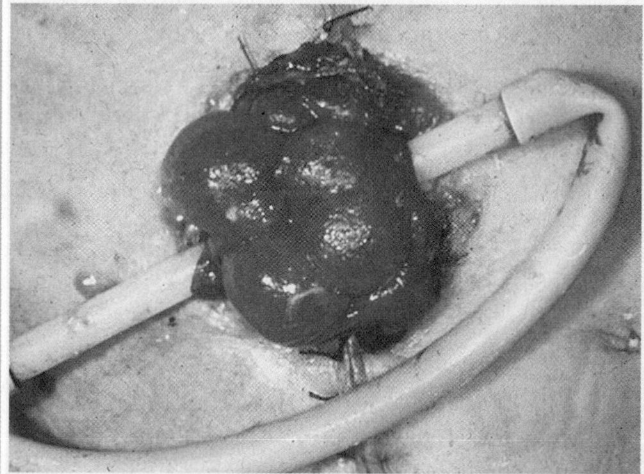

▲ A loop of bowel is brought onto abdomen and is supported by a plastic rod.

Loop Colostomy with Rod Removed

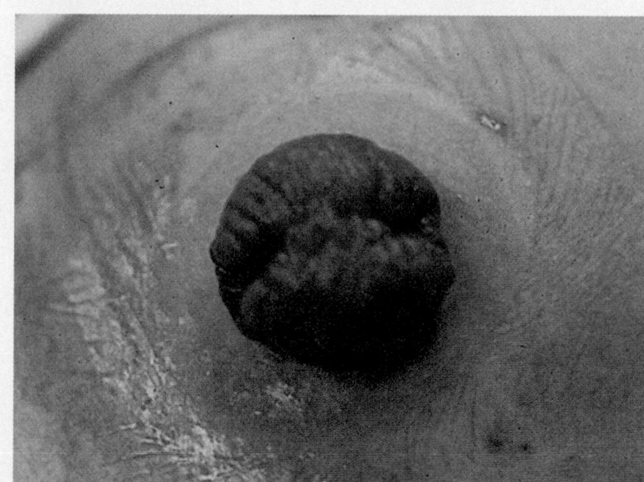

▲ Two openings are made in colostomy. Proximal loop is functional and discharges fecal material. Distal end is nonfunctional and discharge only mucus.

DOCUMENTATION for Fecal Ostomy Pouch Application

- Type of pouch and skin barrier used
- Time pouch applied
- Time pouch emptied
- Amount, color, and consistency of stool emptied from pouch
- Presence or absence of flatus through the stoma
- Location of stoma
- Client participation in and toleration of pouch application
- Condition of peristomal skin and stoma, including color and size
- Condition of incision line (i.e., any erythema or edema)
- Condition of abdomen (e.g., distention)
- Client teaching, which has been completed

CRITICAL THINKING Application

Expected Outcomes

- Pouch remains intact without leakage for 3–5 days.
- Pouching system provides maximal skin protection.
- Pouching system remains odor-proof for 3–5 days.
- Client gradually assumes an active role in applying the pouch.
- Client's skin remains free of erythema, excoriation, and infection.

Unexpected Outcomes	Alternative Actions
Stoma appears dark, dusky-colored, or black.	• Notify physician of findings, and document in chart. (Usually indicates stoma is ischemic.)
Stoma becomes ulcerated or cut.	• Examine pouching system to see if opening of pouch may be cutting into stoma. • Recut opening to exact size of stoma.
Stoma remains a persistent pale pink.	• Request physician to order Hgb, Hct (usually the result of low Hgb). • Instruct client to monitor effluent for constipation if iron preparation ordered.
Bleeding occurs when stoma is touched.	• Observe and note—usual occurrence postoperatively.
Erythematous rash at site of pouch.	• Assess for allergic reaction to product being used. • May need to change to different type of adhesive on pouch or change to a pouch with no adhesive.
Papular rash appears on peristomal skin.	• Assess for possible yeast sensitivity. • Be sure skin is clean and dry before applying pouch. • Do not rinse pouch with water because this traps water under wafer. • May need to use antifungal powder on skin with each pouch change until skin clears.
Peristomal skin complications occur.	• Evaluate cause of leakage. • Be sure pouch is cut to correct size. • Measure stoma at each pouch change for 4–6 weeks. Size will change as edema subsides. • Measure stoma at base. • May need to fill any creases around stoma with skin barrier paste. • Apply thin layer of ostomy powder over area and seal with an alcohol-free coating. • May need to use secondary skin barrier like Eakin seal. • May need to attach belt to minimize lateral leakage.

	• Change to a product like Durahesive that swells around stoma, preventing leakage, and holds up well to liquid output. • Be sure pouch is emptied before it is more than one-third full of stool or flatus, since an overfull pouch can break seal of pouch. • Pouches should not be changed more than once daily.
Ostomy is flush or below the surface.	• Apply convex pouch system to assist ostomy to protrude. • Apply ostomy belt.
Ostomy is in skin fold or crease.	• Apply a one-piece pouch for more flexibility. • Fill deep crevices with caulking material.
Client experiences itching or burning under appliance.	• May be a sign that stool is undermining seal of pouch.
Client not coping with altered body image.	• Refer to United Ostomy Associations of America, Inc., the Crohn's and Colitis Foundation of America, American Cancer Society or the local Enterostomal Therapy nurse.

GERONTOLOGIC Considerations

- Elderly clients frequently have concomitant cardiac problems, which can be affected by vagal stimulation during fecal removal or enema administration. Check with the physician before these skills are performed on elderly clients. Monitor the pulse carefully during the procedure.
- Fecal impaction is not uncommon with elderly clients due to decreased mobility and exercise, dietary habits, and tendency to overuse enemas and laxatives.
- Encourage clients to decrease use of laxatives and enemas, increase fluid intake and fiber in diet, and increase exercise. Dehydration resulting from inadequate fluid intake leads to constipation and fecal impaction.
- To select the proper ostomy appliance for an elderly client, the nurse must determine whether the client has any physical limitations that could influence the type of appliance needed. These limitations include poor vision, use of only one hand, arthritis, and inability to perform cleaning and pouching procedure.

MANAGEMENT Guidelines

Each state legislates a Nurse Practice Act for RNs and LVN/LPNs. Healthcare facilities are responsible for establishing and implementing policies and procedures that conform to their state's regulations. Verify the regulations and role parameters for each healthcare worker in your facility.

Delegation

- A CNA or unlicensed assistive personnel (UAP) may be assigned to administer a disposable enema or tap water enema in most facilities. This information is presented in the CNA curriculum. These personnel are not allowed to administer enemas with medications or a Harris flush.
- An LVN/LPN may be assigned to insert a rectal tube, administer enemas, and perform colostomy care.
- In some rehabilitation settings, aides may be instructed to administer glycerine suppositories. This requires additional training. Check facility policy and procedure manuals to determine which healthcare worker may be assigned to this task.
- A CNA *cannot be assigned to perform a fecal impaction removal because of the risk of a vagal response during the procedure*.

Communication Matrix

- Information relative to bowel elimination is provided both through report and written information on the Kardex card.
- Before delegating any of the tasks associated with bowel elimination to a CNA or UAP, determine their knowledge base to perform the task. Ask them to explain the procedure if you are unsure of their ability to perform the task.
- When an LVN/LPN or RN is assigned to perform colostomy care or assist a physician with an intestinal tube insertion, ensure he or she is familiar with the procedure. Review the procedure as needed.
- Clients who require a bowel program need instruction on the process so they may become independent in the skill. If someone else will be assisting them with this procedure, they should be included in the teaching process. The RN is

responsible for establishing the teaching program. An LVN/LPN may assist in carrying out the plan.

- When special steps or supplies are needed to perform a task (i.e., colostomy care), information should be written on the client care plan or clinical pathway. This allows all staff to perform the procedure the same way. Clients feel more secure when procedures are completed in a uniform method.

CRITICAL THINKING Strategies

Scenario 1

You are assigned to a 74-year-old man who had a transverse colostomy for cancer 4 days ago. During the night report, you heard the night nurse say his pouch is leaking and he is very angry with the staff for causing the mess. As you prepare to enter his room, you decide how to approach him.

1. Determine the most appropriate communication technique to use with the client. Provide rationale for your response.
2. As you observe the stoma and pouch, you determine the leak is at the bottom of the pouch.
   a. State two reasons the pouch may be leaking.
   b. Describe your initial nursing action after you assess the leaking pouch.
   c. What steps do you take to ensure the new pouch will not leak?
3. After removing the first pouch, you assess the skin and determine the peristomal skin to be erythematous and the stoma reddened and slightly edematous.
   a. What is your priority nursing intervention? Provide the rationale for your response.
   b. After completing the priority intervention, what is your next action?
4. After the application of the new pouch, you determine that a teaching plan needs to be developed for the client.
   a. Describe the method of developing a teaching plan for this client.
   b. After developing a plan, indicate the first step the nurse should incorporate to implement the plan.
   c. Describe your rationale for the first step of the teaching plan.
   d. List at least three nursing diagnoses that are appropriate for this client's care plan.
   e. Identify at least one community resource that is appropriate for a referral.

Scenario 2

You assess Mrs. Jacob, a 65-year-old who had a colostomy performed 6 days ago, for cancer of the descending colon. When you tell her you will be instructing her on how to apply a new pouch, she starts to cry and says, "No, I don't want to know how because all it does is leak everywhere."

1. Identify the initial nursing intervention and discuss additional actions you would take to resolve this problem.
2. Describe the assessment database that should be completed before a plan can be implemented.
3. Outline the steps in designing a client teaching plan for a client with an ostomy.

NCLEX® Review Questions

Unless otherwise specified, choose only one (1) answer.

1. The client is undergoing diagnostic tests for fecal incontinence. You would expect to prepare the client for which of the following tests?
   Select all that apply.
   1. Ultrasonography.
   2. Electromyography.
   3. MRI.
   4. Colonoscopy.
2. The client is scheduled for surgery in the morning for an ileostomy. He asks you what to expect when he returns from surgery. Your best response is
   1. "You will need to ask the physician, I can't tell you."
   2. "You will have an opening through the abdominal wall where the stool will pass into a bag."
   3. "You will have a drain in place from the abdominal incision until bowel function returns."
   4. "You will have a catheter inserted into the colon until the colon has healed."
3. One of the major differences in care of a client with a colostomy and one with an ileostomy is
   1. The stool of the ileostomy is liquid to semisoft, which requires increased fluid intake.
   2. Only the client with an ileostomy will require the use of a colostomy bag.
   3. The ileostomy is usually able to be reversed when the disease process heals.
   4. There are usually no dietary restrictions with either client.
4. Just before removing a fecal impaction, the nurse
   1. Obtains a consent form for the procedure.

2. Infuses at least 500 mL of fluid through a rectal tube into the lower colon.
3. Obtains baseline pulse and blood pressure.
4. Gives the client a laxative to assist with the fecal removal.

5. The client requires a rectal suppository. Which of the following actions is appropriate when inserting the suppository?
   1. Ask the client to bear down when you insert the suppository just beyond the external sphincter.
   2. Place the flat end of the suppository into the external sphincter.
   3. Insert the suppository into the fecal material if at all possible.
   4. Place the pointed end of the suppository 3–4 in. beyond the internal sphincter.

6. Contraindications for use of the Bowel Management System include

   Select all that apply.
   1. Recent sphincter reconstruction.
   2. Impacted or formed stool.
   3. Severe strictures of distal rectal or anal canal.
   4. History of severe diarrhea.

7. Place nursing actions in order they are to be carried out when inserting the BMS system.
   1. Gently tug and re-coil catheter to "seal" retention cuff.
   2. Fill syringe with 35–40 mL of lukewarm water and insert into retention cuff using blue connector.
   3. Confirm pilot balloon is fully collapsed.
   4. Hang collection bag on side of bed.

8. The client has an enema ordered before surgery. Which one of the following nursing actions will you perform when administering a large volume enema?
   1. Place client on right side in Sims' position.
   2. Instruct the client to take in a slow deep breath and insert tubing 3–4 in.
   3. Raise height of enema solution to the level of the client's shoulder.
   4. Instill solution over 5 to 10 minutes.

9. The student nurse has been instructed to teach the client and family the application procedure for a fecal ostomy pouch. In reviewing the skill, identify which action would not be considered appropriate for applying a pouch.
   1. Remove old pouch by pushing against skin as you pull backing from skin.
   2. Cleanse skin and stoma with warm water and generous amount of soap.
   3. Cut new pouch at least 1/8 in. larger than stoma without pushing on edges.
   4. Apply ring of skin barrier paste to opening on pouch.

10. The student nurse is preparing to begin the leadership component of the nursing program. The student remembers that the appropriate delegation of nursing skills includes
    1. Assigning the nursing assistant to complete a fecal impaction removal on an elderly client.
    2. Determining that the unlicensed assistive personnel cannot be assigned to care for a client requiring a tap water enema.
    3. Asking the RN team leader to administer a carminative enema to the client.
    4. Assigning the LVN to develop an ileostomy teaching plan for the client and family.

24

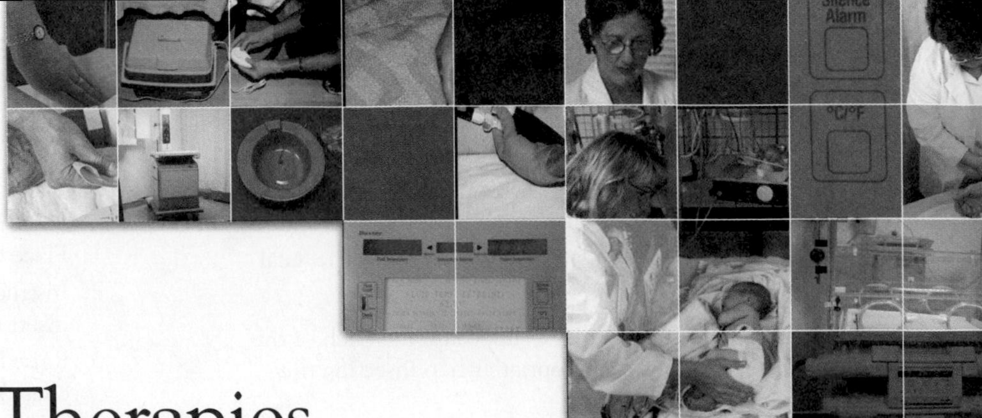

Heat and Cold Therapies

LEARNING OBJECTIVES

1. Describe the mechanisms responsible for the body's heat loss and heat production.
2. Discuss the role of the hypothalamus in thermoregulation.
3. List at least three adaptive processes that maintain the body temperature within a normal range.
4. Discuss how heat transfer occurs.
5. Identify various modes of heat therapy.
6. Describe the physiologic effects of local heat applications (thermotherapy).
7. Identify various modes of cold therapy (local cryotherapy and induced hypothermia).
8. Describe the physiologic effects of local cold applications (cryotherapy).
9. Identify indications and contraindications for various heat and cold therapies.
10. Predict the type of thermal agent that would be most therapeutic for a particular client's condition.
11. Discuss the rationale for induced hypothermia for special clients.
12. List four safety precautions to consider when applying heat and cold treatments.
13. State two nursing diagnoses related to thermal therapies.

CHAPTER OUTLINE

TERMINOLOGY

Afterdrop drop in core temperature upon discontinuation of rewarming therapy.

Ambient temperature temperature of the air surrounding a person.

Antipyretic an agent that reduces fever.

Compress a pad of cloth applied firmly to a part of the body; compress may be dry or wet, cold or warm.

Conduction heat transfer between materials of different temperatures that are in direct contact with each other (e.g., hot or cold pack).

Convection heat transfer by contact with circulating gas or fluid of a different temperature (e.g., whirlpool, wind).

Core temperature the temperature of internal sites; may be increased in rectum or tympanic membrane.

Cryotherapy transfer of heat from the client by use of a cooling agent.

Cyanosis bluish coloring of the skin and the mucous membrane due to decreased oxygenation.

Erythema reddish color of the skin due to dilation of capillaries.

Evaporation absorption of heat (energy) as a result of conversion of a material from a liquid to a vapor state (e.g., sweating, spraying).

Fever regulated rise in body temperature to a new hypothalamic "set point"; usually mediated by internal stimuli (e.g., pyrogenic cytokines), often caused by infection. Metabolic rate is increased; shivering and diaphoresis occur.

Hyperemia increased blood supply to an area.

Hyperthermia nonregulated rise in core body temperature exceeding 41.1°C; due to dysfunction of thermoregulation caused by injury to the hypothalamus (central fever), or failure of the body's ability to eliminate excess heat (e.g., environmental exposure, medications).

Hypothermia a reduction in core body temperature due to environmental exposure or thermoregulatory dysfunction: mild (33°–36°C) moderate (26°–32°C) deep (13°–25°C), profound (<12°C).

Insulator substance that is a poor conductor or a nonconductor of heat; a substance that helps prevent the escape or entrance of heat.

Mottling blue-gray to purplish blotches seen peripherally; usually the result of peripheral vasoconstriction.

Overshoot temperature over-compensation due to external temperature management therapy.

Pallor loss of reddish hue due to superficial vasoconstriction.

Radiation exchange of heat through the air without an intervening medium (e.g., heat lamp).

Shivering thermogenesis production of body heat by involuntary muscle activity, which increases metabolic rate and oxygen consumption and possible anaerobic metabolism with resulting acidosis.

Suppuration the process of pus formation.

Thermogenesis heat production by the body.

Thermotherapy transfer of heat to a client by use of a heating agent.

Vasoconstriction a narrowing of blood vessels.

Vasodilation expansion of blood vessels.

TEMPERATURE REGULATION

Body temperature is regulated and maintained by interrelated feedback systems, which can be altered by disease or environmental conditions. Temperature regulation is a homeostatic function that balances heat production and loss to maintain body temperature within a fairly constant range or "set point" (36.4°–37.3°C/97.5°–99°F), with temperature normally being lowest in the morning and highest in late afternoon. This function is controlled by the body's thermostat, the hypothalamus.

Twenty percent of the body's afferent temperature information reaches the hypothalamus indirectly through superficial thermal receptors in the skin and subcutaneous tissue by way of the spinal cord. Internal organs send core temperature information (80% of input) directly by circulating blood. The hypothalamus interprets information from both the superficial and internal (core) sources and triggers vasomotor responses to maintain a normal temperature through processes of conduction, convection, evaporation, and radiation.

As heat is gained through metabolism, exercise, or environmental factors, the body loses excess warmth through *convection, conduction, radiation, or evaporation.* In contrast, on sensing a loss of heat (cold), the body triggers one or more processes to produce heat (thermogenesis) or conserve it. Although these dynamic processes cannot be observed, their resulting effects, such as shivering, are readily evident. In addition, we consciously and unconsciously alter levels of activity in response to the physiologic stimulus from the body's thermostat, the hypothalamus. When we sense cold, we huddle or curl up and add clothing to decrease heat loss from the body

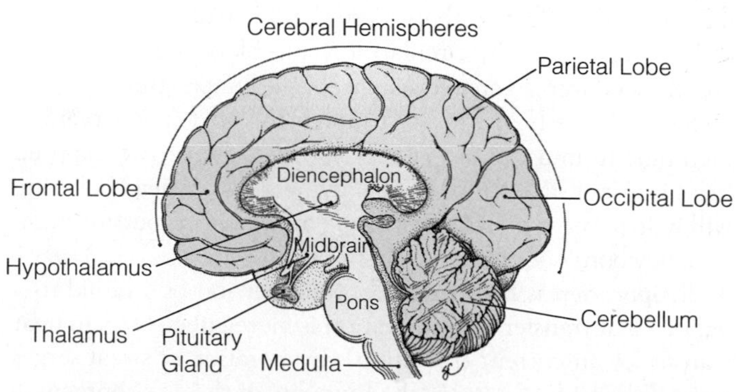

▲ The hypothalamus is located in the diencephalon portion of the brain. It controls the body's thermostat.

surface. When warm, we extend our bodies, separate our limbs, and shed our clothes.

When the hypothalamus perceives cooling, the sympathetic nervous system is activated to conserve and produce heat. Release of norepinephrine causes vessel constriction (a heat-conserving mechanism), which removes warm blood from the skin. This, along with piloerection (hair-raising), reduces conductive heat loss to the cooler environment. Increased muscle tension and shivering increase the metabolic rate, and heat is produced (thermogenesis). These responses continue until the temperature, as sensed by the hypothalamus, has reached its thermostat "set point." Extreme increases in tissue metabolism may result in metabolic acidosis.

In contrast, when the body perceives excess heat, opposite responses are activated. Peripheral vasodilation occurs and blood is brought to the surface, promoting radiation of heat away from the body. Behavioral responses (lighter clothing) expose the body for greater heat radiation into a cooler environment. A fan is used to assist heat convection.

Heat and cold therapies utilize physical principles/processes of conduction, convection, radiation, and evaporation to manipulate *heat transfer*.

Processes of Heat Transfer

Conduction is heat transfer when a warmer object is in direct contact with a cooler object (e.g., hot or cold pack, water-flow cooling blanket). The greater the temperature difference, the faster heat will transfer; however, very hot or very cold applications can cause tissue injury. Different objects have different heat conductivity. Metal conducts heat readily, but air has low conductivity. Therefore, metal objects should be removed from the treated area, and a towel may be placed under a hot or cold pack to trap air (insulate) and limit heat transfer in order to prevent tissue injury. The body's superficial tissues transfer (conduct) heat readily, but cooling or warming the surface has little impact on changing the temperature of deeper tissues. Therefore, surface measures to alter core temperature have limited effectiveness.

Convection is heat transfer by direct contact with a circulating medium (agent in motion) and another material of a different temperature. Therapeutic examples include whirlpool, aquathermic pad, air-flow cooling or warm air blanket, irrigations, or infusions. Heat transfer by convection is more rapid than heat transfer by conduction, and convection modalities that circulate fluid are more effective than those that circulate air. The body utilizes convection by circulating warm blood away from and cooler blood into an area to stabilize tissue temperature.

Radiation is heat transfer through the air (no intervening medium) from a *warmer* to a *cooler* area. Since the exposed head is responsible for 65% of body heat loss, a head covering will help prevent radiant heat loss. An example is putting a cap on a newborn's or operative client's head.

Evaporation is heat transfer by conversion of a liquid to a vapor. Heat transfer by evaporation is more effective than heat transfer by air current (radiation). Evaporation of sweat serves to cool the body as long as the humidity of the environment is low enough to support evaporation. Another example is a moist open body cavity that evaporates heat to the cooler environment of the surgical suite. Therapeutic examples of evaporation include tepid sponging or cold spraying.

CONDITIONS AFFECTING TEMPERATURE REGULATION

Fever

Fever, a temperature over 38.3°C, or 101°F is the most commonly encountered alteration of thermoregulation. Exogenous pathogens (viruses, bacteria) trigger the release of endogenous pyrogens or cytokines that cause the hypothalamus to reset its normal range (thermostat) higher. In response, the body perceives that it is cold and seeks to conserve and produce heat by peripheral vasoconstriction, piloerection, and shivering until the new set point is reached. Peripheral vasodilation follows as the thermostat is set to a lower temperature in response to a decrease in pyrogen concentration or antipyretic medication. This is accompanied by a feeling of warmth as the body cools by vasodilation and sweating until the lower set point is reached. Medications can lower hypothalamic set point as well as affect one's ability to shiver or to exert vasomotor control.

While fever increases metabolic rate, oxygen utilization, and heart and respiratory work and increases risk for dehydration, many studies substantiate that fever, as a natural defense, correlates positively with a quicker recovery and improved survival rates. Although antipyretic agents do reduce fever, their benefit has not been established beyond that of making clients feel more comfortable. *External* cooling measures (tepid sponging and the use of cooling blankets) are ineffective antipyretics because they only lower skin temperature. If the hypothalamic set point is high, external cooling can induce adverse counteractive mechanisms (shivering). Shivering imposes a tremendous metabolic burden by increasing metabolic rate and oxygen demand four- to fivefold.

Hyperthermia (Body Temperature Exceeding 41.1°C)

Hyperthermia, sometimes called *central fever*, is a heat-related emergency that can cause irreversible brain damage. Hyperthermia may be caused by strenuous exercise, environmental exposure (heat stroke), or central nervous system injury. It differs from fever because it is not mediated by pyrogenic cytokines but develops when the body's metabolic heat production or environmental heat load exceeds the body's ability to lose heat. The body's core temperature may exceed 41.1°C, even though the hypothalamic temperature set point is normal. No diurnal temperature variation, shivering, or sweating is observed.

In contrast to fever, which responds to antipyretic agents, hyperthermia ("central fever") tends to be refractory to treatment, requiring external cooling measures that combine evaporation and convection, such as water spraying and warm air fanning. More aggressive cooling measures (e.g., hypothermia garment) may induce shivering by creating a skin-to-core temperature gradient. The cool skin initiates shivering before the brain temperature cools. Vasoconstriction and risk of resultant shivering can be reduced by insulating the client's extremities and confining external cooling only to the torso. Additionally, the use of various sedating and analgesic medications can inhibit shivering and its resultant metabolic burden.

Hypothermia (Body Temperature <36°C Measured by Bladder Catheter, Pulmonary Artery Catheter, or an Esophageal or Rectal Probe)

Unintentional *hypothermia*, a potentially lethal condition, may be caused by loss of heat due to environmental exposure to cold or vasodilation (general anesthesia, cold IV fluids), decreased heat production (hypothyroidism, neuromuscular blockade), or loss of thermoregulation secondary to CNS pathology/injury or multiple trauma. Hypothermia decreases respiratory drive; slows peripheral nerve conduction, myocardial repolarization, and GI motility; and impairs coagulation. The skin is colder than core tissues, creating a skin-to-core temperature gradient that results in vasoconstriction to conserve heat and shivering to generate heat. Altered cognitive and cardiorespiratory function occur, followed by deterioration of all body functions as body temperature continues to drop (see Table 24-2).

THE INFLAMMATORY RESPONSE

Inflammation is the immediate local adaptive response of the body to tissue injury (external or internal). The response is the same regardless of the cause of injury: physical (e.g., burn), metabolic (e.g., ischemia), biologic (e.g., bacteria), or chemical (e.g., acid). The purpose of inflammation is to minimize injury, kill offending agents, and dispose of debris so healing can take place. The response may be acute, subacute, or chronic.

Cardinal signs of inflammation are redness, swelling, heat, pain, and loss of function. These are due to the action of chemical mediators (histamine, bradykinin, prostaglandins, and cytokines) activated at the time of the primary injury. Vasodilation, circulatory slowing, and increased vascular permeability allow the passage of protein-rich fluid (exudate) and white blood cells (neutrophils) into the site to initiate the process. These circulatory changes result in localized ischemia. Neutrophils destroy invaders by phagocytosis and enzymatic digestion, but this process results in production of oxygen free radicals and release of cytokines that may destroy other neutrophils and/or injure healthy adjacent tissue and perpetuate the inflammatory response (secondary injury). WBCs also initiate repair by inducing healthy cell division and new blood vessel growth.

Superficial heat and cold therapies are used to minimize or enhance the inflammatory response that accompanies acute tissue injury (e.g., musculoskeletal sprain, strain, fracture, or surgery). Cold (cryo) therapies reduce inflammation; heat (thermo) therapies enhance inflammation. For each degree centigrade increase or decrease in the injured site's temperature, the tissue metabolic rate is increased or decreased by 13%. The magnitude of this response is influenced by the temperature of the modality, duration of therapy, and surface area exposed to the treatment.

LOCAL HEAT THERAPIES (THERMOTHERAPY)

The physiologic effects of heat are generally opposite to those of cold. Heat applications are inappropriate during the acute inflammatory phase of musculoskeletal injury (with the exception of neck or back muscle strain), but are beneficial for subacute and chronic inflammation. Heat produces analgesia and sedation by promoting release of endorphins and by stimulating nerve endings to block pain transmission by the gate control theory of pain modulation. The benefits of heat therapy last only as long as the heat stimulus is applied. When removed, effects quickly disappear.

Heat facilitates soft tissue repair by increasing delivery of nutrients and oxygen and removal of cellular debris. Heat relaxes skeletal muscles, increases elasticity, and decreases

TABLE 24-1 Physiologic Effects of Heat and Cold Therapies

Thermotherapy	Cryotherapy
Increases superficial temperature	Reduces local tissue temperature
Increases local metabolic rate, oxygen consumption, may cause rewarming acidosis, arrhythmias	Decreases cellular metabolism and oxygen consumption
Dilates arterioles and capillaries, increases capillary permeability; may cause hypotension	Constricts arterioles, capillaries, reduces capillary permeability; may cause hypertension
Decreases blood viscosity; promotes bleeding Enhances blood flow to area (including nutrients and WBCs)	Increases blood viscosity; controls bleeding Decreases blood flow; reduces delivery of phagocytes Decreases secondary metabolic injury
Improves lymphatic and venous drainage of fluid and metabolites	Reduces venous and lymphatic drainage
Promotes inflammation	Blunts inflammatory response
Enhances flexibility of muscles, ligaments	Decreases muscle spasticity
Provides *analgesia* via gating mechanism; stimulates endorphin release	Has extreme *anesthetic* effect; slows nerve conduction via gating mechanism; stimulates endorphin release
Reduces edema *not* associated with acute inflammation	Reduces acute edema formation and accumulation

viscosity of connective tissue and thereby facilitates other treatments by producing relaxation.

Although tissue conduction of heat is limited to a depth of about 2 cm, burns can occur if heat application is too hot or prolonged or if the tissue is unable to mount the increased metabolic demand imposed. The body tends to acclimate to (annihilate) heat therapies; therefore, insulation is recommended with heat applications. Superficial heating therapies that get cooler during application (e.g., moist packs) are safer than therapies with a constant maintained temperature (e.g., heating pad).

A unique benefit of heat is its ability to inhibit sympathetic nervous system outflow. Heat promotes vasodilation both at the site of application and in distal cutaneous vessels (*consensual vasodilation*). By way of this spinal cord reflex, heat may be applied proximally (e.g., to low back) to increase peripheral circulation and facilitate healing in an area that lacks sufficient circulation or sensation to tolerate the direct application of heat.

LOCAL COLD THERAPIES (CRYOTHERAPY)

Cold therapies facilitate heat transfer from the body and are the treatment of choice immediately after local tissue injury and throughout the acute inflammatory phase. Cold applications are usually accompanied by compression and elevation of the affected area (see Orthopedic Interventions, Chapter 31).

The immediate benefit of cryotherapy is inhibition of local enzymatic/metabolic activity and limitation of secondary metabolic injury. Cold constricts vessels, controls bleeding, reduces edema formation, decreases nerve conduction velocity, increases the pain threshold, and decreases muscle spasticity. Paradoxically, cold-induced vasodilation may occur when applications to distal extremities (fingers, toes) exceed 15 minutes at temperatures below 1°C. The amount of vasodilation is usually small but should be avoided in

TABLE 24-2 Categories of Hypothermia and Heat Injuries

Categories of Hypothermia	Signs and Symptoms	Management
Mild (33°–36°C)	Tachycardia, tachypnea, hypertension, shivering	*Note: Rewarming the unintentionally hypothermic client should not exceed 2°C per hour.* Remove wet clothing, place in supine position, avoid excessive movement, monitor core temperature and cardiac rhythm *Passive rewarming* (blanket, head covering) *Active external rewarming* (heat pad to truncal areas only, forced air warmer, warmed blankets, radiant light, immersion in 40°C bath)
Moderate (26°–32°C)	Atrial arrhythmias, slow heart rate, hypotension, decreased reflexes	*Passive rewarming, plus active external rewarming* of truncal areas only *Active internal rewarming* (IV saline warmed to 40°–45°C/ 104°F–113°F, warm humid oxygen, 42°–46°C/ 107.6°F–114.8°F, endovascular warming device, extracorporeal blood warming, warm lavage of body cavities)
Severe (13°–25°C)	Oliguria, pulmonary edema, ventricular arrhythmias, nonreactive pupils coma, apnea Client appears to be dead; has no vital signs	Active rewarming, CPR, defibrillation/resuscitation until core temperature is at least 32°C
Categories of Heat Injury	**Signs and Symptoms**	**Management**
Dehydration	Sweating, ruddy appearance, signs of volume depletion	Rehydrate with caffeine-free or sugar-free beverages
Heat cramps	Painful leg or abdominal cramps associated with exercise in hot weather	Cease activity, move to cool location, rehydrate with cool fluids with electrolytes
Heat exhaustion (37°–40°C)	Tachycardia, normo- or hypotension, weakness, nausea, flushed skin, headache, concentrated or decreased urine output	Apply cool packs to neck, axilla, groin, or spray skin with cool water with warm fanning to speed evaporation. IV fluids may be necessary for rehydration
Heatstroke (>40°C)	Heatstroke is a medical emergency associated with hyperthermia and central nervous system dysfunction. Dizziness, delirium, confusion, seizures, coma, coagulopathies, and multisystem failure may develop	Seek emergency services. Provide oxygen, IV fluids, monitor core temperature, urine output, place NG tube. Immediate evaporative external cooling and internal cooling with chilled saline infusion, ice water lavage of body cavities to reduce body temperature to 38.3°–38.9°C in 1 hr

TABLE 24-3 Indications for Heat Therapies

Indications	Contraindications
Subacute or chronic inflammation Subacute edema Joint stiffness	Acute musculoskeletal injury Acute pain or inflammation Acute edema
Subacute or chronic pain	Impaired circulation (peripheral vascular disease)
Muscle soreness/spasm Postherpetic neuralgia Infection (supports suppuration) Consensual vasodilation Chronic ulcer	Sensory impairment Bruising or bleeding Malignancy Open wound

TABLE 24-4 Indications for Cold Therapies

Indications	Contraindications
Acute inflammation, acute or chronic pain	Impaired circulation (peripheral vascular disease)
Acute swelling or bleeding	Raynaud's disease/phenomenon
Muscle spasm	Hypersensitivity to cold/cold intolerance
Strain, sprain, or contusion Joint stiffness	Decreased sensation Open wound

certain situations, and therapy time should be limited to 15 minutes or less when treating fingers and toes. Longer treatment durations may be used for other areas of the body. With cold therapy, the area temperature remains lower than normal for 1 or 2 hr after removal of the cooling modality, so cold therapies are usually applied for 30–60 minutes, then repeated every 1–2 hr.

While cryotherapy prevents acute edema formation (swelling) during the first 24–48 hr after injury, it cannot remove swelling that has occurred. Swelling only decreases as inflammatory exudate (free protein) is removed from the area by lymph flow. Cryotherapy is beneficial in the rehabilitation period as it produces anesthesia and facilitates exercise, which stimulates lymph flow.

INDUCED HYPOTHERMIA

Hypothermia may be therapeutically induced in certain situations to protect vital organs because it provides metabolic quiescence. Central (internal) cooling, during cardiac or neurosurgery, can also induce postoperative shivering. Rewarming the blood or infusing warmed saline before terminating surgery helps to warm core tissues and a forced warm air blanket (e.g., Bair Hugger) may be used for active external rewarming. Peripheral vasculature, however, remains constricted for some time, unable to receive the warmed blood. Later, peripheral vessels dilate and hypotension may occur. As cool blood from the periphery moves to mix with warmer blood in the core, central temperature drops 2°–5°C (*afterdrop*). Acidosis may also occur as accumulated tissue acids enter the central circulation. Even a combination of measures may fail to promote homogeneous body rewarming; therefore, pharmacologic agents that blunt hypothalamic responses may be necessary adjuncts to suppress shivering in the centrally cooled client postoperatively.

Fever, irrespective of its cause, has a deleterious effect on neurologic outcome in various types of neurologic injury. An increase in core temperature of 1°C results in a 10% increase in energy expenditure. A growing number of studies demonstrate that induction of mild induced hypothermia (32°–35°C) for 24 hr provides neuroprotection and dramatically improves rates of survival with meaningful neurologic recovery if applied as soon as possible to victims of postanoxic brain injury (those with return of spontaneous circulation after cardiac arrest). Controlled hypothermia also shows promise as a treatment for severe traumatic brain injury (Glasgow Coma Score <8), stroke, myocardial infarction, refractory intracranial hypertension, bacterial meningitis, and hepatic encephalopathy.

For each degree centigrade reduction in body temperature, the cerebral metabolic rate is decreased by 6%–7%. Additional mechanisms of neuroprotection include decreased neutrophil infiltration with reduced cytokine, leukotriene, and oxygen free radical production (secondary injury); increased blood–brain barrier stability; and decreased intracranial pressure due to vasoconstriction.

The four modes of heat transfer are utilized in a variety of hypothermia techniques, including surface cooling with ice packs, body wraps (most effective), and an isolated head cooling helmet; vascular cooling using chilled crystalloid infusion, endovascular heat exchange via central venous catheter, and hemodialysis; and intracavitary cooling including chilled lavage (gastric, bladder) and delivery of a nasopharyngeal coolant.

CULTURAL AWARENESS

Determining the client's perspective about illness and treatment practices may provide a framework for developing a plan of care that is therapeutic and acceptable to both the client and the caregiver.

The application of heat and cold would seem to be concordant with beliefs and practices of several cultures that seek a harmonious balance of life forces. Hot-cold theories of health and disease and the opposing force of therapies, however, do not relate to temperature, but rather to a therapy's symbolic strength.

To regain balance, a "cold" disease is treated by eating or exposing oneself to "hot" therapies, such as acupuncture and cupping. For some cultures, an orange ("hot") medication may be more acceptable for a "cold" ailment than a blue ("cold") medication.

African-Americans shiver at lower temperatures than Caucasians. Their fingers cool faster in water and their temperatures fall more before they start to warm, and they do not rewarm as much. Caucasians and clients with type O blood are more susceptible to frostbite.

NURSING DIAGNOSES

The following nursing diagnoses are appropriate to use on client care plans when the components are related to heat and cold therapies.

NURSING DIAGNOSIS	RELATED FACTORS
Impaired Comfort	Environmental exposure, tissue injury, inflammatory process
Hyperthermia	CNS injury, strenuous exercise, environmental exposure, medications
Hypothermia	CNS injury, diabetes, hypothyroidism, environmental exposure, major trauma, surgery, alcoholism, medications
Deficient Knowledge (Specify)	*Lack of understanding* about inflammatory process; rationale for and hazards of heat/cold therapies
Peripheral Neurovascular Dysfunction, Risk for	Prolonged application of heat or cold therapy to joints or areas with impaired circulation
Impaired Skin Integrity, Risk for	Prolonged use of cold or heat therapy, excessive temperature of therapy, impaired sensation, impaired circulation
Ineffective Thermoregulation	Anesthesia, medications, alcoholism, infection, CNS injury, environmental exposure

CLEANSE HANDS The single most important nursing action to decrease the incidence of hospital-based infection is hand hygiene. *Remember to wash your hands or use antibacterial gel before and after each and every client contact.*

IDENTIFY CLIENT Before every procedure, introduce yourself and check two forms of client identification, not including room number. These actions prevent errors and conform to The Joint Commission standards.

Chapter 24

UNIT 1

Local Heat Therapies (Thermotherapy)

Nursing Process Data

ASSESSMENT Data Base

- Determine rationale for heat therapy.
- Review client's history for possible circulatory problems (peripheral vascular disease, diabetes).
- Environmental exposure, induced central cooling.
- Determine site, type, and duration of therapy to be applied.
- Assess area to be treated.
- Determine client's ability to sense temperature at site.
- Assess skin condition before and throughout therapy.

PLANNING Objectives

- To increase circulation to area
- To provide analgesia
- To promote inflammatory process
- To facilitate mobilization of interstitial fluid (noninflammatory edema)

IMPLEMENTATION Procedures

EVALUATION Expected Outcomes

- Circulation is increased to area.
- Client reports decrease in pain.
- Inflammation/suppuration is enhanced.
- Tissue fluid is mobilized/edema reduced.

Applying a Commercial Heat Pack

Equipment

Prepackaged heat pack
Tape

Preparation

1. Check physician's orders for type and duration of heat treatment.
2. Gather equipment.
3. Perform hand hygiene.

Procedure

1. Check two forms of client ID and introduce yourself.
2. Explain procedure to client.
3. Provide privacy.
4. Remove heat pack from outer wrapper.
5. Break inner seal by holding pack tightly in the center and in an upright position.
6. Squeeze firmly to break seal. ► ***Rationale:*** Breaking the seal activates the chemical ingredients and produces the heat.
7. Check for leakage from pack. Remove pack immediately if leakage occurs. ► ***Rationale:*** Chemicals from the pack may burn the skin.
8. Gently shake the pack, then apply to treatment area.
9. Remove pack after 5 minutes and assess skin for erythema.
10. Replace pack and secure with tape. Keep in place 15–30 minutes or as ordered by physician.
11. Place call bell in client's reach.
12. Remove pack and discard in appropriate container.
13. Perform hand hygiene.

Applying an Aquathermic Pad

Equipment

Aquathermic reservoir container with pump
Aquathermic pad (disposable)
Distilled water
Tape

Preparation

1. Review physician's orders to determine treatment area, type of application, and temperature of treatment.
2. Perform hand hygiene.
3. Gather equipment, and check it for safety factors (e.g., frayed cords, water leaks).
4. Take equipment to client's room.
5. Check two forms of client ID and introduce yourself.
6. Connect aquathermic pad to pump hoses (male and female fittings).
7. Snap locking rings into place to ensure hose fittings are snug, then open hose clamps.
8. Fill reservoir two-thirds full with *room temperature* distilled water.
9. Place pump on bedside stand or other surface at or above level of the pad. ► ***Rationale:*** If pump is placed below pad level, water will drain back into pump when it is shut off.
10. Use plastic key to set reservoir temperature as ordered, then remove key. ► ***Rationale:*** Temperature range is 30°–42°C. Removing key prevents tampering.

▲ Connect Aqua-K pad to pump hoses.

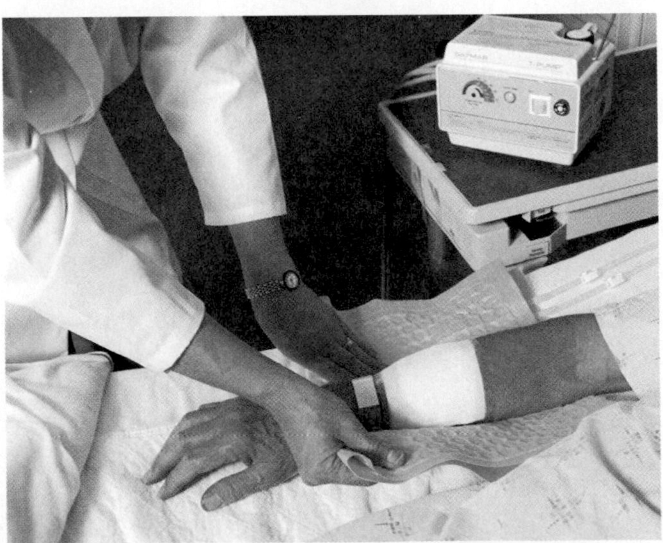

▲ Aquathermic pad is a form of local heat therapy.

11. Plug pump into grounded wall outlet.
12. Turn pump power switch "ON." Set temperature is reached in about 20 minutes.

Procedure

1. Explain procedure to client and provide privacy.
2. Apply aquathermic pad with its coiled surface against client's extremity or over moist pack that has been placed on area to be treated.
3. Secure pad with tape if necessary; *do not use safety pins.* ▸ ***Rationale:*** Pins can pierce coils in pad.
4. Check client's skin after 2–5 minutes. ▸ ***Rationale:*** To assess for possible skin reaction caused by a hot pad.
5. Instruct client to notify you if the pad feels too warm. ▸ ***Rationale:*** This prevents burning of skin.
6. Remove pad after 15–20 minutes. Observe area for redness, pain, or any untoward reaction.
7. When pad is used to keep dressings or soaks warm, continue treatment longer than 20 minutes if ordered. Treatment may be continuous when used for clients with subacute lower back or neck pain.
8. Turn pump "OFF." Close hose clamps; hold hose with connectors above pump and pad. ▸ ***Rationale:*** Prevents water spillage.

Clinical Alert
Heat transfers more quickly than cold therapy. Do not allow the client to lie on a "constant heat source" such as a heating pad or aquathermic pad.

Clinical Alert
Contraindications to heat therapies include acute injury or inflammation, recent or potential hemorrhage, deep-vein thrombophlebitis, impaired circulation, impaired sensation, and impaired mentation.

When treating an area where skin is not intact, cover lesion with sterile gauze and insulating barrier before applying heat (see Wound Care, Chapter 25).

9. Remove aquathermic pad and join male and female connectors.
10. Place pad on bedside stand until next treatment or place in appropriate disposal area.
11. Reposition client for comfort.
12. Perform hand hygiene.

Applying a Hot Moist Pack

Equipment

Box of 4 × 4 gauze sponges or other absorbent material necessary for size of area to be treated
Hot tap water or ordered solution and container
Plastic moisture barrier (plastic bag)
Or
Aquathermic pad (optional)
Tape
Bath thermometer
Gloves

Preparation

1. Check physician's order for type of hot moist treatment ordered, length of treatment, and time interval between treatments.
2. Gather specific equipment for type of hot moist pack ordered.
3. Place material in a warming solution (usually water).

Clinical Alert
Do not apply heat to an edematous area until the reason for edema has been determined.

4. Determine amount of time elapsed since last application.
5. Considering age of client, body part involved, and type of treatment, determine safe temperature of application to prevent burning. ▸ ***Rationale:*** Water temperature in hospitals is usually controlled at 43.3°C/110°F, but the individual client may require altered temperature.
6. Perform hand hygiene.

Procedure

1. Check two forms of client ID and introduce yourself.
2. Provide privacy.
3. Position client appropriately to expose and assess area to be treated. ▸ ***Rationale:*** Open wounds are generally *not* treated with heat application because heat increases the area's need for oxygen and may injure granulation tissue. Heat therapy to a recent bruise can restart bleeding.
4. Assess client's ability to sense touch and heat/cold at site to be treated. ▸ ***Rationale:*** Impaired skin sensation may contraindicate therapy.
5. Remove any jewelry from area to be treated. ▸ ***Rationale:*** Decreases risk of burn due to conductive potential of metal.
6. Open container of gauze sponges. Open ABD outer wrap if used.

7. Don gloves.
8. Saturate gauze sponges (or other selected material) with warm water (no greater than 43.3°C).

   NOTE: Water in hospitals is usually controlled at 43.3°C to prevent injury.

9. Pick up soaked sponges and wring out excess solution.
10. Place warm moist pack over area to be treated.
11. Use plastic barrier or aquathermic pad to mold and secure pack to site. ▸ ***Rationale:*** Barrier helps maintain heat by preventing evaporative cooling.
12. Set aquathermic pad temperature at 41°C. ▸ ***Rationale:*** While the warm moist pack will cool quickly, the aquathermic pad maintains heat—this also increases the risk of burns.
13. Use tape to secure the barrier. Do not allow client to lie on pack or pad.
14. Ensure that nurse call system is in client's reach. ▸ ***Rationale:*** Client should summon nurse if discomfort is felt.
15. Assess area in 5 minutes for signs of redness, mottling, or blistering. ▸ ***Rationale:*** These may be signs of burning. Thermotherapy should be discontinued and a cool pack should be applied.
16. Remove and dispose of pack after 20 minutes or as prescribed.
17. Assess and dry the treated area. ▸ ***Rationale:*** Slight redness and warmth are expected responses.
18. Document procedure and client's response to treatment.
19. Discard gloves and perform hand hygiene.

Assisting With a Sitz Bath

Equipment

Disposable sitz bath with tubing and bag

Warm water (40°–43°C)

NOTE: Cold temperature may be indicated for client's situation.

Towels for drying

Thermometer

Clean gloves

Preparation

1. Verify physician's order for sitz bath, duration and frequency of treatments.
2. Raise toilet seat and place sitz bath basin with "FRONT" facing the front of the toilet bowl.
3. Fill basin with warm water (40°–43°C) one half to two thirds full.
4. Close flow tubing clamp.

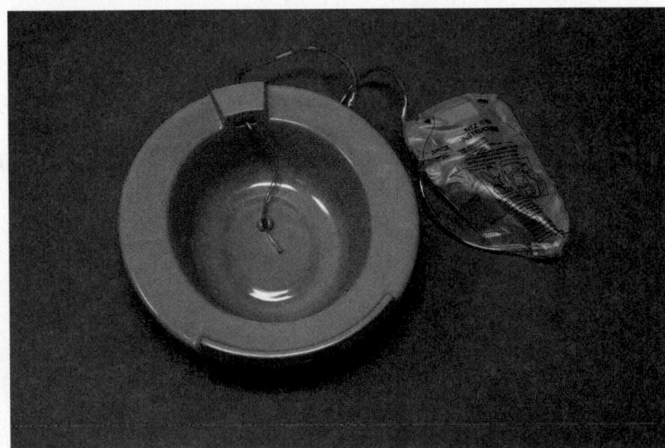

▲ Individual disposable sitz bath units are used for infection control purposes.

5. Open top of plastic bag and fill with hot water (40°–43°C).
6. Hang bag at a level higher than the sitz basin so that fluid will flow by gravity.
7. Insert tubing through front or rear entry hole in sitz bath, then snap or secure tubing into channel or "eye" in bottom of basin.
8. Perform hand hygiene.

Procedure

1. Identify client by checking Ident-A-Band and asking client to state name.
2. Explain procedure and rationale for sitz bath.
3. Assist client to treatment area with accessible call bell.
4. Provide privacy by placing sign on door.
5. Check to ensure that temperature is 40.5°–43.3°C.

   NOTE: Most hospitals control water temperature so that it will not exceed 110°F or 43.3°C.

6. Assist client to sit in sitz bath for 15–20 minutes.
7. Maintain water temperature by continually adding water of appropriate temperature to bag. ▸ ***Rationale:*** Overflow will drain into toilet through openings in back of basin.
8. Upon completion, assist client to dry area and allow client to sit briefly to allow normalization of blood pressure and to prevent hypotension upon standing. ▸ ***Rationale:*** Orthostatic hypotension may occur with rapid position change after warm sitz bath due to vasodilation.
9. Don clean gloves, empty and rinse client's sitz basin, and store in convenient location for future use.
10. Discard soiled linen.
11. Perform hand hygiene.

DOCUMENTATION for Local Heat Therapies

- Time of application
- Type of heat therapy applied
- Area of body treated
- Status of area pre- and post-treatment
- Positioning of area treated
- Duration of treatment
- Client's response to treatment

Legal Alert

Salter *v.* Deaconess Family Medicine Center, 1999

The nurse and hospital were found liable for injuries to an infant's foot after a nurse's application of a wet washcloth that had been heated for 1 full minute in a microwave oven, then applied to the infant's heel to facilitate drawing blood. Application of the hot cloth was the proximate cause of second-degree burns to the infant's heel.

Source: Westlaw.com

CRITICAL THINKING Application

Expected Outcomes

- Circulation is increased to area.
- Client reports decrease in pain.
- Inflammation is enhanced.
- Noninflammatory edema is reduced.

Unexpected Outcomes	Alternative Actions
Client experiences pain, asks about alternative measures for relief.	• Cold therapy may be an option, or heat/cold alternating therapy as counterirritants; these therapies alter nerve transmission. • Assess if application is too hot. • Ensure that temperature is not over 110°F (43.3°C) if heating pad is used.
Swelling is not reduced with heat therapy.	• Ensure that acute inflammation is not present, as heat therapy will not reduce swelling (exudate) due to acute tissue injury. • Support venous return by elevating the part.
Aquathermic pump signals "Over Temp."	• Check reservoir water level; it may be low or empty. • Be sure to use room temperature (not hot) distilled water in reservoir. Check that hoses are not kinked or hose clamps closed.
Pump continues to signal "Over Temp" after previous actions.	• Disconnect, label, and send to BioMed department. • Obtain a different pump.

Chapter 24

UNIT 2

Local Cold Therapies (Cryotherapy)

Nursing Process Data

ASSESSMENT Data Base

- Determine purpose for cryotherapy (acute injury, joint stiffness).
- Review client's history for possible circulatory problems (Raynaud's phenomenon, diabetes, peripheral vascular disease).
- Assess baseline data (peripheral circulation).
- Determine client's ability to sense temperature at site.
- Assess skin condition before and throughout cryotherapy.
- Assess for adverse responses to cryotherapy.

PLANNING Objectives

- To reduce local tissue metabolic/oxygen demand and prevent secondary metabolic injury
- To promote vasoconstriction and reduce bleeding
- To control the inflammatory response (edema formation)
- To achieve an anesthetic effect
- To reduce muscle spasticity and promote motion
- To facilitate rehabilitation exercise to stimulate lymph flow and reduce inflammatory edema

IMPLEMENTATION Procedures

EVALUATION Expected Outcomes

- Inflammatory response is controlled.
- Bleeding and edema formation are reduced/controlled.
- Local anesthetic response is achieved.
- Cryotherapy promotes rehabilitation exercise to reduce edema.
- Local cryotherapy causes no adverse effects.

Applying an Ice Pack/Commercial Cold Gel Pack

Equipment

Small plastic bag, ice bag, or glove (consider size to be treated and necessity to mold)
Flaked or crushed ice from an ice machine (−1°C)
Salt
Or
Reusable silicone gel cold pack that has been in freezer (−5°C) for at least 1.5 hr before initial use
Cloth or towel
Elastic bandage or towel
Tape (*do not use pins*)
Pillows

Preparation

1. Verify physician's order for type of cold pack, duration and frequency of therapy.
2. Fill ice bag one-half to two-thirds full. ▶ ***Rationale:*** Facilitates molding of pack to treatment area.
3. Remove excess air from bag. ▶ ***Rationale:*** Air interferes with cold conduction.
4. Add salt to ice if a colder slush mixture is needed.
5. Take equipment to client's room.
6. Perform hand hygiene.

Procedure

1. Check two forms of client ID and introduce yourself.
2. Provide privacy.
3. Explain procedure and rationale to client. Discuss sensory experiences to expect with cold therapy.
4. Position client to expose area to be treated and remove any jewelry if present.

Clinical Alert

- Frozen gel packs and crushed ice packs using ice frozen in a refrigerator or freezer (−16°C to −19°C) should not be applied directly to the skin.
- Packs with ice from an ice machine (−1°C) do not require insulation.
- During cryotherapy, erythema will occur.
- The client will experience four stages of cold progression: cold/stinging/burning/numbness.
- Discontinue therapy upon numbness.

5. Assess circulation and client's ability to sense touch and heat/cold at site to be treated. ▶ ***Rationale:*** Inadequate circulation or impaired sensory perception may contraindicate therapy.
6. Use pillows or other item to elevate area to be treated. ▶ ***Rationale:*** Elevation promotes venous return, reduces swelling and pain.

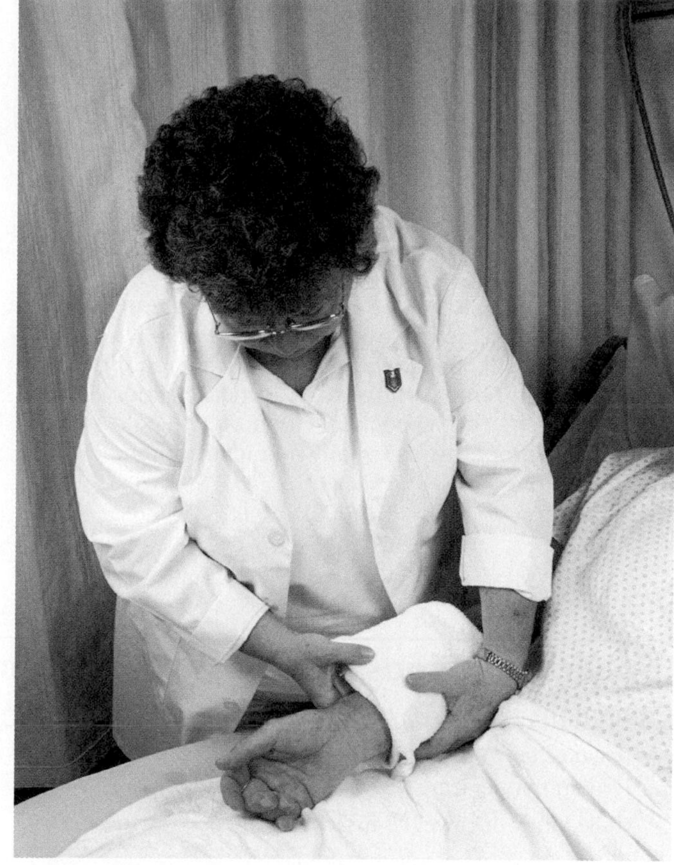

▲ Wrap and tape around pack to secure.

7. Place towel directly onto skin area. ▶ ***Rationale:*** Provides a barrier to protect the skin from extreme temperature.

   NOTE: Packs with crushed ice from an ice machine may be applied directly to the skin.

8. Place ice/cold gel pack atop towel and mold it to fit the treatment area. ▶ ***Rationale:*** Manufacturer's instructions vary among products and must be followed for safe use.
9. Secure pack in place with toweling or elastic wrap using tape. ▶ ***Rationale:*** Outer wrap decreases warming effect of environmental air.
10. Place call bell within client's reach.
11. Assess client and treatment site in 5 minutes. ▶ ***Rationale:*** If pallor, blanching, mottling, or blisters occur, or client reports increased pain, burning, or severe numbness, discontinue pack immediately.
12. Limit treatment time to 10–15 minutes or longer as prescribed. ▶ ***Rationale:*** A reusable cold pack usually loses its effectiveness after 15 minutes. Application time can be increased if cold is applied over bandages or against a cast.

13. Assess treatment area for adverse signs (wheals, cyanosis, pallor, pain, or tingling/numbness *distal* to treatment over a superficial nerve such as the radial nerve at the lateral elbow).
14. Discard used towels in linen hamper.
15. Return reusable ice bag or cold pack to freezer for at least 30 minutes before reusing.

Clinical Alert

Never apply a fully cooled *reusable cold pack* directly to the skin; also, do not overinsulate the area.

Bony areas (knee, ankle, elbow) usually require half the treatment time as fatty areas. Superficial nerves at these joint sites are especially vulnerable to cold-induced neuropathy, especially if cold is combined with compression.

EVIDENCE-BASED PRACTICE

Postoperative Cold Therapy

While several studies have demonstrated that the use of cold over compression reduces bleeding and swelling and improves return to motion, this research study concludes that compression is just as effective as cold after total knee surgery and is more cost-effective.

Source: Smith, J., Stevens, J., Taylor, M., & Tibbey, J. (2002). A randomized, controlled trial comparing compression bandaging and cold therapy in postoperative total knee replacement surgery. *Orthopaedic Nursing, 21(2)*, 61–66.

EVIDENCE-BASED PRACTICE

Clients receiving cold gel application four times a day for 14 days after soft tissue injury had less pain at rest and with movement and had less functional disability than those receiving a room temperature gel application.

Martin, S. N., Paulson, C. P., & Nichols, W. (2008). Clinical inquiries: Does heat or cold work better for acute muscle strain? *Journal of Family Practice*, 57(12), 820–821.

Applying a Disposable Instant (Chemical) Cold Pack

Equipment

One time only use instant chemical cold pack (kept at room temperature)

Moist cloth or towel (if indicated on pack instructions)

Elastic bandage or towel

Tape

Pillows for elevation of part treated

Preparation

1. Review physician's order for local cryotherapy.
2. Gather equipment.
3. Perform hand hygiene.
4. Identify client by checking Ident-A-Band and having client state name and birth date.
5. Explain procedure.
6. Provide privacy and position client.

Procedure

1. Grasp top of cold pack and shake contents to bottom of bag.

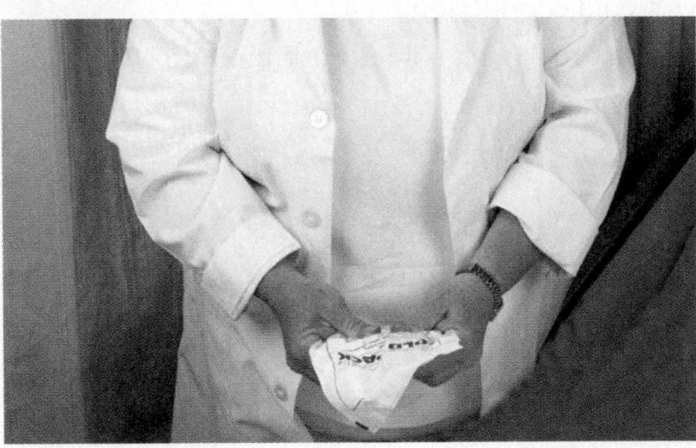

▲ Follow manufacturer's instructions to activate chemical cold pack.

2. Hold package in the middle with both hands, or follow manufacturer's directions on package.
3. Locate inner pouch and squeeze the package firmly to break the inner pouch.
4. Shake the package gently to mix the chemicals together.
5. Check that package is not punctured or opened. ▸ ***Rationale:*** If solution touches the skin, the chemicals can burn the skin.
6. Use pillows or other item to elevate part to be treated. ▸ ***Rationale:*** Elevation promotes venous return, reduces swelling and pain.
7. Apply pack directly to skin, or place disposable cold pack atop towel (according to instructions). ▸ ***Rationale:*** The degree of cold is not great with a chemical cold pack.
8. Mold pack to fit area and secure in place with toweling or elastic wrap and tape. ▸ ***Rationale:*** Outer wrap decreases warming effect of environmental air.
9. Place call bell within client's reach.

Clinical Alert

Crushable chemical packs should be used as last resort because they are not as cold nor do they last as long as crushed ice.

Do *not* apply an instant chemical pack to the face and never use pins to secure pack. Leakage of chemical contents can cause serious injury. If contents are exposed to skin, immediately flush with copious amounts of water and notify physician.

10. Assess client and treatment site in 5 minutes. ▸ ***Rationale:*** If mottling or blisters occur, or client reports numbness, discontinue pack immediately.
11. Limit treatment time to 30 minutes or as prescribed.
12. Dispose of "one time only use" pack. ▸ ***Rationale:*** Product cannot be reused by freezing as frostbite may result.
13. Perform hand hygiene.

Applying a Circulating Cold Therapy Pad

Equipment

Cold therapy system (e.g., EBIce) for single client use (cooler, site-specific disposable pad and straps, hose with connectors, pump with temperature control module)

Ice (4 quarts)

Cold water (2 quarts)

8-ply gauze or towel for insulation

Preparation

1. Review physician's order for application site.
2. Take cooler to client's room.
3. Check two forms of client ID and introduce yourself.
4. Explain purpose of cold therapy (to reduce pain, swelling).
5. Place 2 quarts cold water into cooler to reach water line marker.
6. Add ice to ice line marker (the pump inside cooler must be completely covered with ice/water).
7. Join short connectors on treatment pad to connectors on end of cooler system hose (disconnect these to discontinue treatment if, for instance, client gets out of bed).
8. Plug DC power cord into jack on side of cooler.
9. Plug wall mount adapter into wall electrical outlet.
10. Turn system to coldest setting to initiate circulating cold water into treatment pad.
11. Place cooler at or slightly *below* the level of the treatment site.
12. Perform hand hygiene.

Procedure

1. Place protective gauze or towel over area to be treated (e.g., knee). ▸ ***Rationale:*** Pad should not be placed directly on client's skin.
2. Place treatment pad over area to be treated.
3. Secure pad and hose in place with enclosed straps. ▸ ***Rationale:*** Tight securing may restrict water flow through the pad.
4. Turn temperature control knob to 12:00 midpoint position. ▸ ***Rationale:*** Cold water will circulate into pad for 30 seconds, then stop for 70 seconds. Intermittent cycling helps prevent treatment from being too cold.
5. After 10 minutes, assess color and sensation of site. ▸ ***Rationale:*** If site is discolored or numb, discontinue the treatment and notify physician.
6. Adjust cold water on/off cycling frequency according to client's comfort level. ▸ ***Rationale:*** Cycling periods may be 9, 30, or 52 seconds; off periods may be for 91, 70, or 48 seconds.
7. Periodically reassess client's response to cold treatment.
8. To refill ice and water, disconnect power cord from wall mount and cooler. ▸ ***Rationale:*** Cooler provides approximately 3 hr of treatment.
9. Discontinue treatment by unplugging power cord from wall and cooler, remove treatment pad; empty ice and water from cooler; place system in storage carton. ▸ ***Rationale:*** System belongs to the individual client.
10. Position client for comfort.
11. Perform hand hygiene.

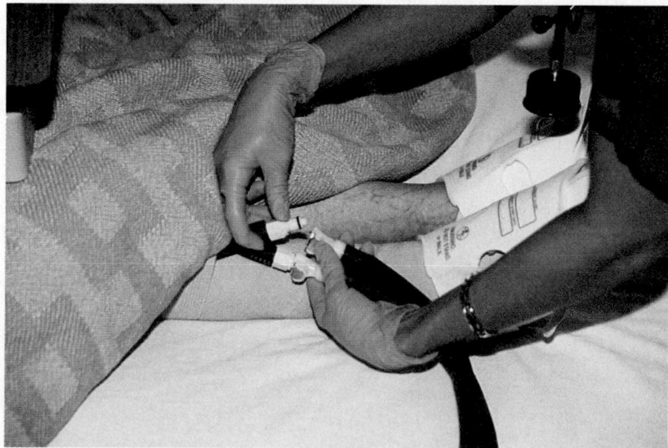

▲ Join connectors on treatment pad to connectors on end of cooler system hose.

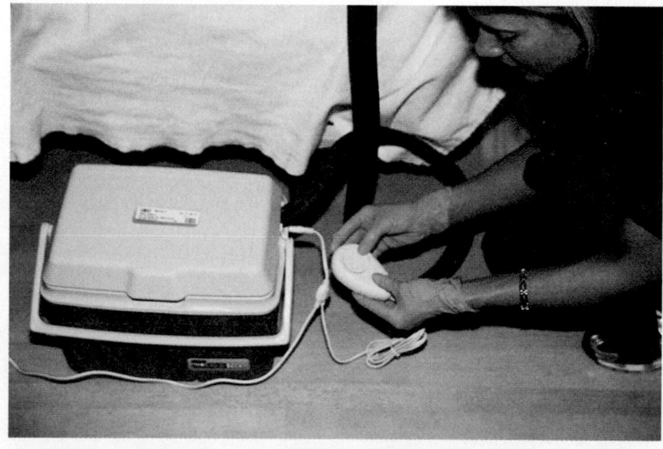

▲ Turn system to coldest setting to initiate treatment.

DOCUMENTATION for Local Cold Therapies

- Specific cold application used
- Area of body treated
- Positioning of area treated
- Duration and frequency of treatment
- Status of area pre- and post-treatment
- Client's response to therapy

CRITICAL THINKING Application

Expected Outcomes

- Inflammatory response is controlled.
- Bleeding and edema formation are minimized.
- Local anesthetic response is achieved.
- Local cryotherapy causes no adverse effects.
- Local cryotherapy facilitates rehabilitation therapies.

Unexpected Outcomes	Alternative Actions
Local edema is increasing.	• Elevate extremity above level of heart. • Ensure that area is sufficiently covered with cold application to cause vasoconstriction. Check that area is not overinsulated.
Bleeding/bruising continues in spite of local cold applications.	• Reassess area for possible "bleeders," which may require cautery or ligation by the physician. • Apply pressure to site to stop bleeding. • Assess pulse distal to bleed.
Area to be treated is near superficial nerve.	• Use caution: reduce time and duration of cold application. • Ask client to report any itching or tingling and discontinue therapy if these occur.
Hand develops waxy white sheen, mottling, and numbness during local cold therapy.	• Immerse part in moving water at 40°–42°C until area flushes (about 30 minutes). • Do not apply dry heat; keep area uncovered at room temperature. • Do not rub part; keep part elevated.
Cold cycling pad is not cooling properly.	• Examine if pad or hose is folded or kinked. • Determine whether securing straps are too tight and restricting flow of cold water. • Make sure pump inside cooler is completely covered with ice water. • Check all connections between hose and treatment pad. • If still not cooling properly, disconnect, label, and send to BioMed. • Obtain different machine.

Chapter 24

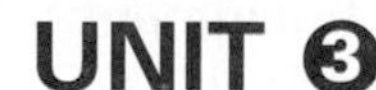

Temperature Management Therapies

Nursing Process Data

ASSESSMENT Data Base

- Determine purpose for ordered temperature management therapy.
- Assess medications client has received (e.g. sedative).
- Determine desired core temperature target.
- Assess client data (vital signs, neurologic status, cardiovascular status, CBC, serum chemistries, coagulation studies) before and throughout treatment (if indicated).
- Assess ECG tracings throughout treatment (if indicated).
- Assess that temperature management system is functioning properly.
- Assess for early signs of shivering.

PLANNING Objectives

- To maintain/restore normal body temperature
- To reduce body core temperature
- To reduce metabolic process/tissue oxygen demand
- To prevent secondary metabolic injury
- To improve neurologic outcomes after cardiac arrest and traumatic brain injury
- To ensure temperature management system functions properly
- To monitor for therapeutic or adverse responses to therapy

IMPLEMENTATION Procedures

EVALUATION Expected Outcomes

- Target core body temperature is achieved.
- Tissue oxygen demand is reduced.
- Secondary metabolic injury is minimized.
- Neurologic outcomes are optimized.
- Temperature management system functions properly.
- Client has no adverse responses to therapy (arrhythmias, bleeding, shivering, afterdrop, or rebound hyperthermia).

Pearson Nursing Student Resources

Find additional review materials at **nursing.pearsonhighered.com**

Prepare for success with NCLEX®-style practice questions and Skill Checklists

Using a Neonatal Incubator/Infant Radiant Warmer

Equipment

Radiant warmer with skin probe and temperature gel patch to secure probe to infant's skin

Bedding and positioning aids appropriate for bed and infant

Preparation

1. Follow manufacturer's operating instructions for safety. (Several different radiant warmers/infant care centers are available.)
2. Check caster locks to make certain that each is in locked position.
3. Adjust bed to desired position.
4. Plug cord into three-prong receptacle.
5. Turn power switch on; bed will take approximately 30 seconds to power up.
6. Set bed to manual control mode for desired temperature. ▶ ***Rationale:*** This allows bed to warm up prior to placing infant on bed.

Procedure

1. Plug temperature probe into bed. ▶ ***Rationale:*** To obtain a digital recording of the infant's skin temperature.
2. Place infant on bed, then set bed to skin control mode.
3. Attach skin probe with polished surface over a location of fatty tissue on infant's body, avoiding any bony prominence.
4. Attach temperature gel patch to secure probe to infant's skin; do not use adhesive tape. ▶ ***Rationale:*** To prevent skin irritation. The infant's skin is very thin and fragile.
5. Allow 3 to 5 minutes for probe to reach infant's temperature.
6. Monitor placement of skin probe:
   a. Validate appropriate skin temperature reading. ▶ ***Rationale:*** If reading is not at desired temperature, probe may need to be repositioned.
   b. Inspect infant's skin under probe at regular intervals. ▶ ***Rationale:*** Infant's skin is delicate and irritates easily.
   c. Change probe location if irritation begins to appear.

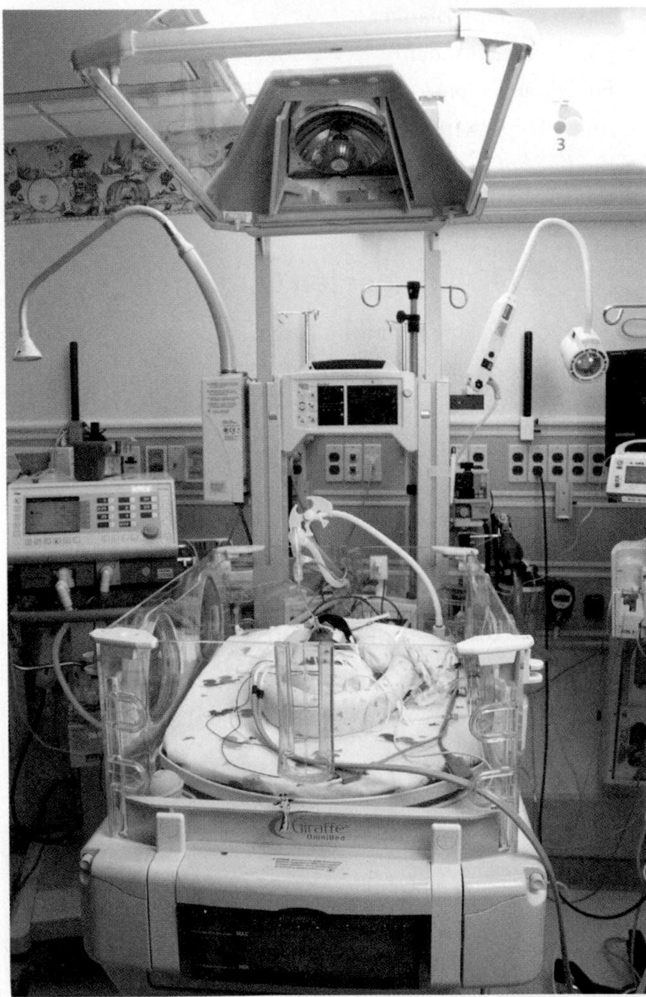

▲ Giraffe bed in radiant warmer mode, offering quick and easy access to the critically ill neonate.

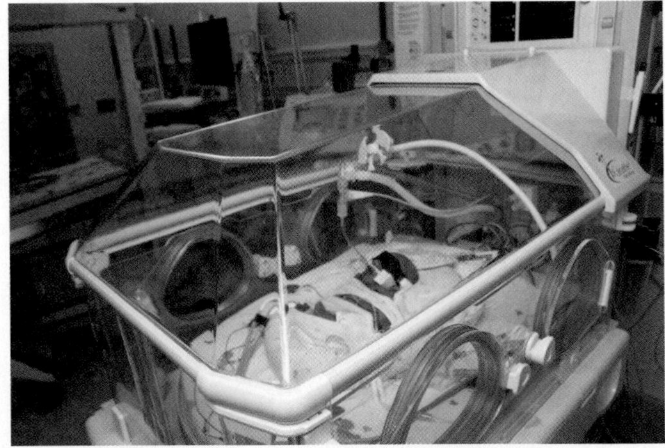

▲ Giraffe bed in incubator mode, offering a quiet, neutral thermal environment.

Using a Warm Air Blanket

Equipment

Means for continuous core body temperature monitoring (rectal, esophageal, bladder, pulmonary artery catheter), cable and module to monitor depending on thermometer used

Cardiac monitor

Automated blood pressure unit

Disposable warm air temperature management blanket with control unit and tubing

Gown or sheet and bath blanket

Preparation

1. Review order or agency protocol for client rewarming.
2. Obtain equipment and take to client's bedside.
3. Perform hand hygiene.
4. Check two forms of client ID and introduce self.

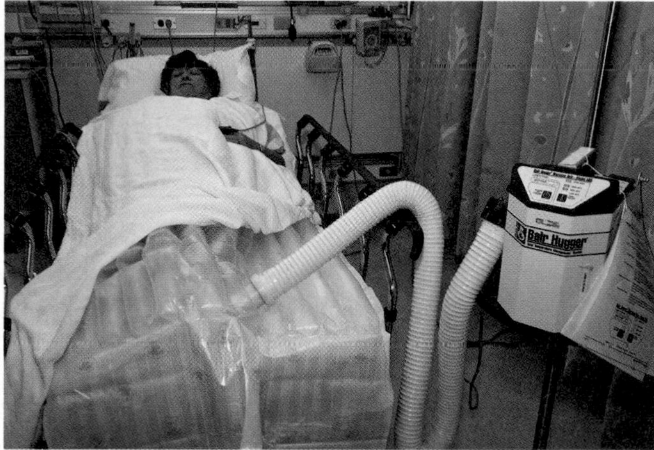

▲ A forced warm air convection blanket provides active rewarming. Client's temperature should increase gradually (2–3°C/hr).

5. Provide privacy and explain purpose of rewarming blanket and associated monitoring.
6. Establish continuous core body temperature, cardiac and blood pressure monitoring.
7. Obtain baseline vital signs.

Procedure

1. Remove seal from warm air blanket port and insert corrugated tubing connected to unit.
2. Remove all client covering or apply light gown or place sheet over client (not both). ▸ ***Rationale:*** Warm air must have close contact with client's skin.
3. Place warm air blanket (perforated side down) over client.
4. Apply bath blanket over warm air blanket. ▸ ***Rationale:*** To secure air blanket.
5. Clamp unit corrugated tubing to sheet or bed. ▸ ***Rationale:*** To prevent dislodgement and heat loss.
6. Set unit for overheat (rapid warming), high (43°C), medium (38°C), or low (32°C).
7. Turn system ON and reassure client that hum sound is due to air flow.
8. Monitor core temperature, cardiac rhythm, and blood pressure every 15 minutes. ▸ ***Rationale:*** Client's temperature should increase gradually (2°–3°C/hr). Hypotension may occur due to vasodilation with rewarming; arrhythmias may occur.
9. Discontinue procedure when client's core temperature is 37°C, but continue to monitor. ▸ ***Rationale:*** Afterdrop (drop in temperature) or overshoot (overcompensation) may occur.
10. Dispose of single-use warm air blanket and return reusable equipment to appropriate area for cleaning and storage.
11. Perform hand hygiene.

Providing Tepid Sponging

Equipment

Water or other coolant at prescribed temperature

Basin or tub

Washcloth and towels

Bath blanket

Electric fan

Automated blood pressure unit

Core temperature thermometer, cable and module to monitor

Preparation

1. Review order for cooling method.
2. Gather equipment and bring to client's room.
3. Check client's Ident-A-Band and have client state name and birth date.
4. Provide privacy and explain procedure.
5. Perform hand hygiene.
6. Establish continuous core temperature monitoring (rectal, esophageal, bladder, or pulmonary artery), if indicated.
7. Establish ongoing blood pressure and cardiac monitoring.

Procedure

1. Remove client's clothing to allow for cooling and observation. Use bath blanket for privacy.

2. Monitor skin color and vital signs every 15–30 minutes during cooling. Immerse washcloths or material for sponging in ordered solution, generally 21°–27°C. ▸ ***Rationale:*** Cool applications reduce heat by conduction.
3. Wring out excess solution and place cloths on neck, axillae, groin. ▸ ***Rationale:*** The vascularity of these areas promotes cooling.
4. Depending on type of bath, change cloths every 5 minutes. ▸ ***Rationale:*** This prevents cloths from warming and losing effectiveness.

Clinical Alert

Do not immerse the client in cold or ice slush. Resulting peripheral vasoconstriction will impair body cooling and induce shivering, which produces heat.

5. Cool the ambient temperature to 68°–72°F. ▸ ***Rationale:*** This enhances therapy by convection and evaporation.
6. Direct a warm fan onto client to promote evaporation. ▸ ***Rationale:*** This enhances cooling by evaporation.
7. Assess client for early signs of shivering (ECG tremor artifact, palpable jaw line "hum" or trapezius muscle tension).
8. Stop treatment if client has early signs of shivering and notify physician. ▸ ***Rationale:*** Shivering raises core temperature, defeating purpose of cooling intervention. The physician may order a narcotic or benzodiazepine for sedation.
9. Monitor client's temperature frequently. When temperature has decreased to desired level, dry skin and replace light covering over client and reposition for comfort. ▸ ***Rationale:*** A thin client will cool faster than one with more subcutaneous fat.
10. Continue to monitor vital signs, cardiac rhythm, I&O, electrolytes.
11. Provide fluids and a high-calorie diet. ▸ ***Rationale:*** Increased temperatures increase metabolic rate.
12. Place cloths in linen hamper and return equipment to storage area.
13. Perform hand hygiene.

Rapid Noninvasive Cooling

- Remove clothing.
- Place client in lateral recumbent position for maximal skin surface exposure.
- Spray entire body with water (20°C), direct a fan onto client to enhance evaporation.

Using a Cooling Blanket

Equipment

Thermal (heating/cooling) unit
Sterile or distilled water
Low reading (below 34.4°C) thermometer: Rectal probe and lubricant, esophageal probe, urinary retention catheter, or pulmonary artery catheter with cable and module for continuous core temperature monitoring, depending on thermometer used
Clean gloves
Disposable thermal (cooling) blanket
One sheet or thin blanket
Covering for client
Four towels to wrap client's lower arms and legs
Tape
Leg or foot compression wraps
Sphygmomanometer and stethoscope or automated BP monitoring equipment
Continuous ECG monitoring (See Circulatory Maintenance, Chapter 31)
Supplemental oxygen therapy equipment

Preparation

1. Check physician's orders for desired client temperature.
2. Identify medications client has received (narcotic, sedative).
3. Gather equipment and take to client's room.
4. Connect power cord to grounded outlet.
5. Ensure that reservoir (sterile or distilled water) level is adequate.
6. Perform hand hygiene.
7. Check client's Ident-A-Band and have client state name and birth date.
8. Provide privacy and explain procedure.
9. Obtain baseline vital signs.

Procedure

1. Place the cooling blanket on bed, and connect it to the Temperature Control Unit machine. ▸ ***Rationale:*** The cooling blanket increases heat transfer from client and reduces body temperature by conduction.
   a. Push the tubing tab to insert male tubing connector of the cooling pad into inlet opening. Release the tab.
   b. Repeat connection using the outlet opening.
   c. Turn the unit ON by pushing power switch.
   d. Enter client's target temperature set point
2. Place a sheet or a thin bath blanket over the cooling blanket.
3. Place client on the cooling blanket.
4. Apply leg or foot compression wraps. ▸ ***Rationale:*** To prevent thrombus formation and reduce edema.

5. Wrap client's lower arms and hands, lower legs, and feet (and scrotum, if indicated) in towels; tape to secure. ▸ ***Rationale:*** This prevents stimulation of skin thermoreceptors that initiate shivering.
6. Establish continuous core temperature monitoring.
7. Set the master temperature control to either automatic or manual operation. ▸ ***Rationale:*** There are two separate temperature controls, one for automatic and one for manual operation.

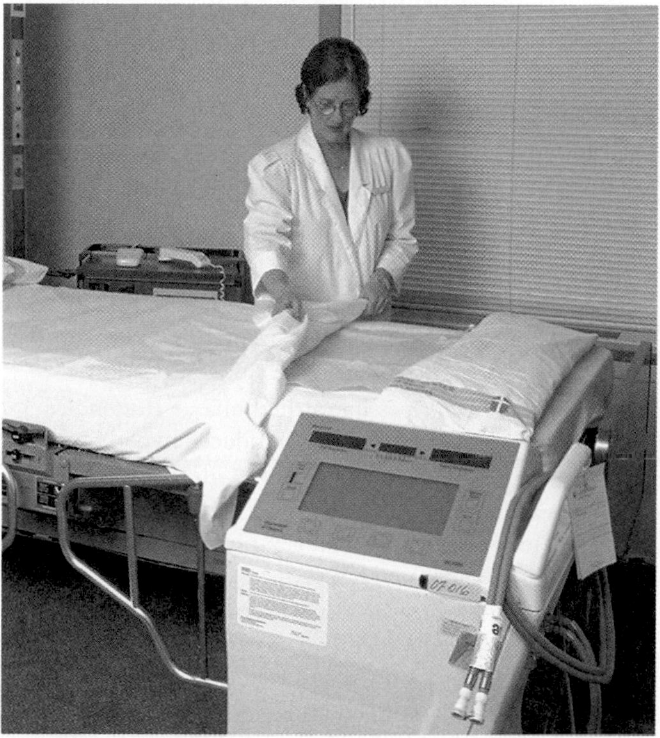

1 Disposable cooling blanket is covered by sheet to protect the client's skin.

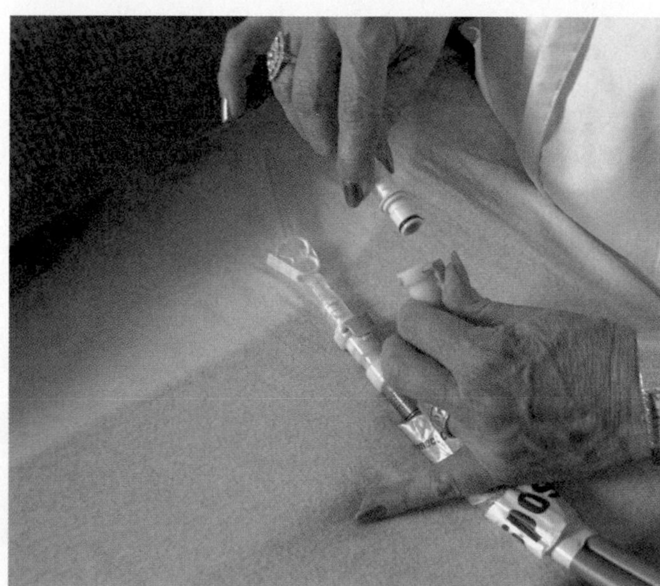

2 Connect two ends of tubing—one from blanket, the other from machine.

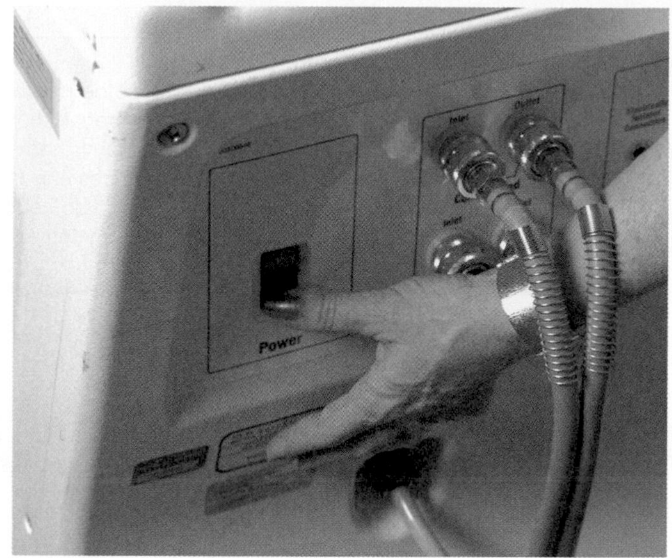

3 After machine is powered and connected to blanket, push unit ON button.

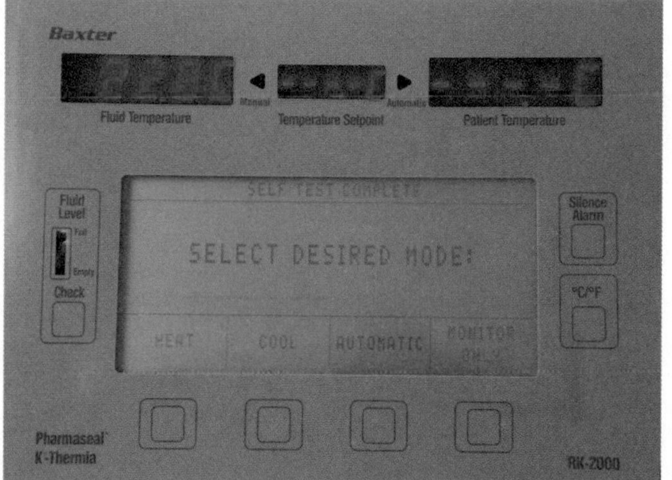

4 After checking fluid level, select desired mode: heat, cool, automatic, or monitor.

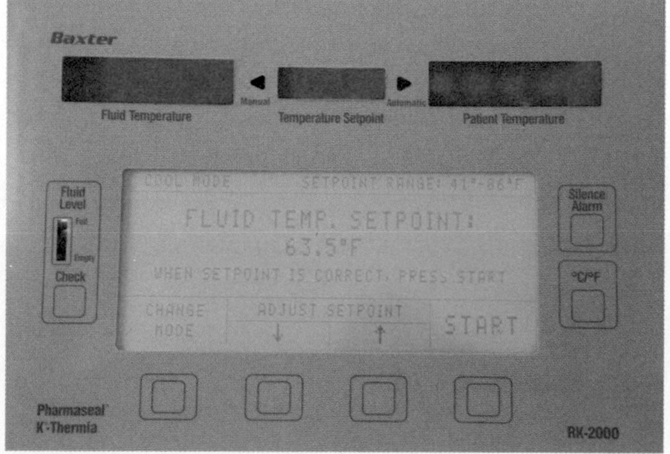

5 Set fluid temperature to ordered set point, and press START.

EVIDENCE-BASED PRACTICE

Hypothermia Improves Stroke Outcome

A study of stroke patients indicates that induced hypothermia to 32°C for a 3-hr period with cooling blankets and ice water/alcohol bath improved outcomes. Hypothermia reduces ischemic damage and reperfusion injury after thrombolysis and reduces bleeding risk associated with administration of tPA. It may also help prevent hyperthermia associated with shift of the third ventricle during an intracerebral hemorrhage.

Source: Mitka, M. (2001). Playing it cool in stroke research. *Journal of the American Medical Association, 285*(10), 1282.

Clinical Alert

Effectiveness and safety of cooling blankets for treatment of fever are poorly demonstrated. Use of a cooling blanket is discouraged except for environmental hyperthermia or cerebral damage.

For Automatic Control

a. Don clean gloves.
b. If using rectal thermometer probe, digitally examine client's rectum to determine it is empty of stool. ▸ ***Rationale:*** Rectal temperature probe must make contact with mucosa.
c. Insert lubricated temperature probe into client's rectum 2 inches.
d. If using bladder retention catheter with integrated temperature probe, determine that urine output is at least 20 mL/hr. ▸ ***Rationale:*** Probe actually measures urine temperature.
e. Set temperature control at the desired temperature (fluid temperature set point).
f. Turn automatic mode light on and press "START." ▸ ***Rationale:*** The pad fluid temperature will adjust automatically to bring client's temperature to a selected set point.
g. Check that the pad temperature limits are set as ordered.

For Manual Control

a. Observe that the *manual* mode light is on.
b. Monitor the fluid set point, which indicates temperature of pad. ▸ ***Rationale:*** This ensures pad temperature is maintained at desired level.

8. Set the temperature control to 37°C, and begin lowering temperature 1°C every 30 minutes to 1 hr as tolerated to prevent shivering, until 33° or 34°C or set temperature is reached. ▸ ***Rationale:*** Blanket will cool client to set temperature independent of client's temperature. Gradual cooling helps prevent shivering.
9. Monitor client's temperature. ▸ ***Rationale:*** To prevent excessive cooling.
10. Assess client every 15 minutes for early signs of shivering: ECG muscle tremor artifact, jaw line "hum," trapezius muscle tension.
11. If early signs of shivering occur, discontinue therapy and notify physician or refer to agency hypothermia protocol. ▸ ***Rationale:*** Shivering causes an increase in core temperature, thus defeating the purpose of treatment. Shivering imposes a heavy metabolic burden and increases oxygen demand.

Mild	32°–37°C	89.6°–98.6°F
Moderate	28°–32°C	82.4°–89.6°F
Severe	20°–28°C	68.0°–82.4°F

12. Monitor vital signs every 15–30 minutes during therapy. ▸ ***Rationale:*** Bradycardia may occur. Blood pressure usually remains elevated due to vasoconstriction.
13. Monitor ECG for possible arrhythmias. ▸ ***Rationale:*** Potassium shifts into cells with induced hypothermia.
14. Monitor client's serum glucose. ▸ ***Rationale:*** Insulin levels are decreased with induced hypothermia. Glucose levels may rise with shivering. An *insulin drip* may be necessary to maintain glucose at 80–130 mg/dL.
15. Turn and deep-breathe client every 1–2 hr. ▸ ***Rationale:*** Hypothermia reduces carbon dioxide production with possible resultant hypoventilation.
16. Monitor client's skin condition and bony prominences every 2 hr. ▸ ***Rationale:*** Client is at risk for pressure ulcers when skin temperature is lowered.
17. Turn off unit when client's temperature is 1°–3°C above desired temperature. ▸ ***Rationale:*** Cooling will continue upon discontinuation of therapy.
18. Monitor vital signs every 15 minutes during rewarming.
19. Observe for edema. ▸ ***Rationale:*** Hypothermia causes fluid shift into the interstitium.
20. Clean and return reusable equipment to appropriate area and dispose of blanket.
21. Monitor client's vital signs frequently after discontinuation of treatment. ▸ ***Rationale:*** Overshoot hypothermia may occur.
22. Make client comfortable.
23. Perform hand hygiene.

Using a Hypothermia Garment (Body Wraps)

Equipment

Water circulating vest and thigh wraps with temperature control console

Distilled water

Low-reading (below 34.4°C) thermometer: Rectal probe and lubricant, esophageal probe, urinary retention catheter, or pulmonary artery catheter with cable and module for continuous core temperature monitoring depending on thermometer used

Glucometer

Sequential compression devices (calf or foot)

Four towels for hands, feet, scrotum (if indicated)

Tape

Lubricating eye drops

Preparation

1. Review physician's order for induced hypothermia and target temperature.
2. Determine that client has ice packs to axillae, neck, and groin before initiating therapy.
3. Determine that client has infusion of refrigerated normal saline at a rate of 1 L/hr before initiating therapy.
4. Determine client specific rationale for temperature management (e.g., traumatic brain injury; comatose cardiac arrest client will be intubated and sedated and should be cooled within 4 hr of return of spontaneous circulation).
5. Determine whether client is intubated and receiving moderate sedation (see Diagnostic Procedures, Chapter 21).

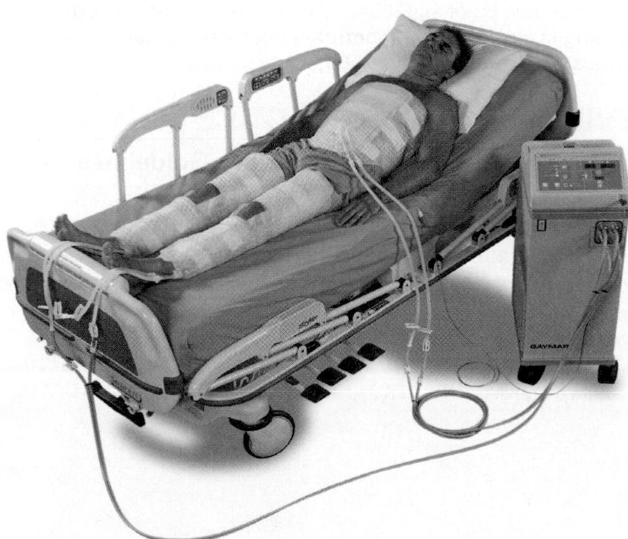

▲ Induced hypothermia system provides surface cooling to the torso and adjusts automatically to maintain client's target temperature.
Medi-Therm MTA7900 and Repround system. Courtesy of Stryker Medical (Gaymar Team).

6. Determine that essential continuous monitoring systems (ECG, arterial BP) have been established. (See Cardiovascular Maintenance, Chapter 31, and Advanced Skills, Chapter 33.)
7. Identify medications client has received (e.g., insulin drip).
8. Review client's recent lab results: INR/PTT, D-Dimer, fibrinogen, CBC, and complete metabolic panel (CMA chemistries).
9. Reduce room temperature and remove all sources of heat.
10. Fill water reservoir of temperature control console according to manufacturer's instructions.

Procedure

For Cooling

1. Identify client, introduce yourself, and briefly explain procedure and rationale, whether or not client is responsive.
2. Apply chest and thigh garments directly to client, fitting securely. ▸ ***Rationale:*** To maximize body surface contact.
3. Connect chest garment tubing to console.
4. Interconnect leg wraps' tubing; connect to single tubing, then connect to console.
5. Apply towel wraps to client's hands and feet and secure with tape. ▸ ***Rationale:*** Skin counter-warming prevents stimulation of skin thermoreceptors that initiate shivering and need for sedation.
6. Connect core temperature monitoring thermometer to console. ▸ ***Rationale:*** A consistent body site must be used for temperature monitoring.
7. Plug console into outlet and turn machine ON.
8. Set target temperature to 33°C. ▸ ***Rationale:*** Target temperature should be reached in <4 hr. Cool time should be 24 hr from start of cooling.
9. Establish "AUTO" rapid mode of operation. ▸ ***Rationale:*** Garment system automatically adjusts to maintain client's target temperature. When client's temperature is within 1°C of set point, machine will change to a slower mode to reduce "overshoot."
10. Obtain BMP and CBC every 12 hr during hypothermia. ▸ ***Rationale:*** Potassium levels decrease as potassium moves into cells with induction; a level of 2.5 is usually acceptable.
11. Monitor client's glucose per agency protocol. ▸ ***Rationale:*** Insulin levels decrease with hypothermia, and glucose levels may rise with shivering.
12. Adjust *insulin drip* to maintain glucose at 80–130 mg/dL.
13. Monitor client's BP, EKG, and temperature every 30–60 minutes for 6 hr or until goal temperature is reached,

then hourly. ▸ ***Rationale:*** BP may remain elevated due to vasoconstriction; bradycardia may occur; arrhythmias may occur as potassium moves into cells. Overshoot hypothermia may occur with cooling.

14. Assess client's neurologic status hourly. (For Glasgow Coma Scale, see Physical Assessment, Chapter 11; for the FOUR SCORE, see Neurological Management, Chapter 32.)
15. Monitor client every 15 minutes for early signs of shivering. ▸ ***Rationale:*** Shivering raises core temperature, fights the cooling process, and increases oxygen consumption.
16. Provide additional extremity and face counterwarming to help suppress shivering.
17. If shivering continues, medicate according to protocol (meperidine or benzodiazepine) or notify physician.
18. Monitor client's skin condition every 2 hr; skin should be kept dry. ▸ ***Rationale:*** Vasoconstriction increases risk for pressure ulcers.
19. Obtain blood cultures ×2, 12 hr after initiating hypothermia. ▸ ***Rationale:*** Hypothermia may cause neutropenia and may increase risk for aspiration pneumonia.
20. Provide frequent eye care using lubricating drops.
21. Assess client for signs of bleeding. ▸ ***Rationale:*** Hypothermia can prolong clotting time and decrease platelet count.
22. Monitor urine output hourly.

Hypothermia Toxicity: Related to Duration, Intensity of Therapy, and Rate of Rewarming

Cardiovascular – arrhythmias, bradycardia, reduced left ventricular function

Respiratory – hypoventilation with hypoxemia, atelectasis and pneumonia

Gastrointestinal – stress ulcer, ileus

Hematologic – platelet dysfunction, coagulopathy (prolonged PT/PTT)

Immunologic – impaired neutrophil function, risk for infection

Metabolic – hypokalemia, hyperglycemia due to decreased insulin release, possible systemic inflammatory response syndrome (SIRS) with rewarming.

For Rewarming

1. Stop all potassium administration 4 hr before rewarming. ▸ ***Rationale:*** Potassium level will increase with rewarming.
2. Enter target temperature to 36°C for rewarming.
3. Gradually rewarm client to normothermia over 12–24 hr or remove chest and leg garments and allow client to rewarm passively to normothermia. ▸ ***Rationale:*** Rewarming should be done slowly, no faster than 0.5°C/hr to prevent rewarming acidosis, shivering, or hypotension (due to vasodilation).
4. Continue to monitor client's temperature. ▸ ***Rationale:*** Rebound hyperthermia may occur with rewarming. Avoid temperature >37.5°C.
5. Monitor for hypoglycemia, especially if client has received continuous insulin infusion.
6. Obtain serum potassium level every 6 hr during rewarming. ▸ ***Rationale:*** Hyperkalemia may occur as potassium shifts out of cells with rewarming.
7. When client is stable, discontinue garment therapy and dispose of single-use body wraps.
8. Return reusable temperature control console to storage area.
9. Perform hand hygiene.

Clinical Alert

Fever should be aggressively controlled during the acute phase of brain injury. Fever occurs in 20%–50% of critically ill neurologic patients and is associated with increased morbidity and mortality after ischemic and hemorrhagic stroke and in subarachnoid hemorrhage. In traumatic brain injury patients, temperature elevation has been linked with increased intracranial pressure.

Mayer, S., Kowalksi, R., Presciutti, M., Ostapkovich, N., McGann, E., Fitzsimmons, B., et al. (2004). Clinical trial of a novel surface cooling system for fever control in neurocritical care patients. *Critical Care Med, 32(12)* p2508-2514.

EVIDENCE-BASED PRACTICE

2005 American Heart Association Guidelines for CPR and ECC

Unconscious adult patients with return of spontaneous circulation (ROSC) after out-of-hospital cardiac arrest should be cooled to 32°C to 34°C for 12 to 24 hr when the initial rhythm was ventricular fibrillation. Similar therapy may be beneficial for patients with non-VF arrest out of hospital or for in-hospital arrest.

2005 AHA Guidelines for CPR and ECC. *Circulation* 2005 112: IV-84-IV-88.

DOCUMENTATION for Temperature Management Therapies

- Specific type of temperature management therapy used
- Target temperature settings established
- Application of compression wraps
- Application of insulating towel wraps to extremities and scrotum
- Time of initiation and duration of therapy
- Baseline and vital signs trends, including monitored cardiac rhythm
- Serum glucose determinations
- Medications administered
- Client's response to temperature management therapy and any adverse effects
- Physician notification of client's response (if indicated)

CRITICAL THINKING Application

Expected Outcomes

- Target core body temperature is achieved.
- Tissue oxygen demand is reduced.
- Secondary metabolic injury is minimized.
- Neurologic outcomes are optimized.
- Temperature management system functions properly.
- Client has no adverse responses to therapy (arrhythmias, bleeding, shivering, afterdrop or rebound hyperthermia).

Unexpected Outcomes	Alternative Actions
Client's core temperature decreases rapidly to desired level.	• Turn off cooling blanket or discontinue tepid sponging. • Monitor temperature every 15 minutes to detect additional temperature decrease.
Cooling blanket does not function properly.	• Check that plug is connected to the outlet. • Check that the fluid level is sufficient and that unit freezing has not occurred. • Check that the thermistor probe is properly connected. • Check that the cool limit on the pad is not set too high.
Shows early signs of shivering.	• Adjust rate of cooling every 15 minutes to detect additional temperature decrease. • Cover client's face for additional counterwarming. • Contact physician for medication order (narcotic or sedative).
Hyperthermic client's core temperature is not reduced.	• Discuss need for cold water spray and warm air fan to reduce client's temperature. • Consider that cutaneous vasoconstriction due to external cooling may be conserving core body heat. • Discuss need for more aggressive internal cooling measures (e.g., endovascular cooling).
Rebound hyperthermia occurs after induced hypothermia cooling and rewarming.	• Provide supplemental oxygen therapy. • Leave the temperature management garment in place for up to 12 additional hr once goal temperature has been achieved. The garment can cool the client if rebound hyperthermia occurs.
Client shows early signs of skin breakdown with non-blanchable area noted.	• Loosen garment to remove direct cold and compression over area. • Apply a clear adhesive dressing over the area to add a layer of protection and help prevent shearing.

GERONTOLOGIC Considerations

Elderly clients are more susceptible to injury from heat and cold therapy as a result of physiologic changes or medical conditions

- The epidermal cells are replaced more slowly in the elderly.
- Skin in the elderly is thin and contains less moisture.
- The elderly have a reduced sensitivity to pain and therefore may not feel untoward effects of heat and cold treatment.
- Temperature should be reduced when using heat therapy because the elderly client's skin burns more easily.

Vital signs and frequent assessment may be necessary during heat and cold therapy, as vasodilation from heat or vasoconstriction from cold can cause changes in cardiac function and blood pressure

- Peripheral circulation may be compromised due to chronic volume depletion, atherosclerosis, or microvascular disease.
- Sensation in distal extremities may be impaired in elderly clients with neuropathy due to diabetes.
- The elderly may take medications that decrease sweating (anticholinergics for Parkinson's) or increase heat production (CNS stimulants or lithium).
- Serious infections may not elicit a febrile response.
- Temperature threshold for sweating is higher in the elder client and ability to mount a metabolic response to temperature loss is limited.
- Living conditions and financial limitations may not afford adequate environmental control.
- Hemodynamic responses to heat/cold therapies may be more unpredictable.

MANAGEMENT Guidelines

Each state legislates a Nurse Practice Act for RNs and LVN/LPNs. Healthcare facilities are responsible for establishing and implementing policies and procedures that conform to their state's regulations. Verify the regulations and role parameters for each healthcare worker in your facility.

Delegation

- RNs may assign LPN/LVNs to perform most of the skills covered in this chapter. For example, they may apply heat or ice to an extremity, set up a hypothermia blanket, or give a sitz bath.
- Assessment before delegation and evaluation of the client's response during and after therapy is required of licensed delegate.
- Systemic cooling or heating therapies are indicated for critically ill clients in special care settings who may be sedated. These clients are generally monitored and cared for exclusively by licensed personnel.
- CNAs and UAPs may be assigned to do many of the skills with supervision. They should not be assigned to use infant radiant warmers or cooling blankets without special guidance and supervision.

Communication Matrix

- Because many of the procedures in this chapter are performed by unlicensed personnel, there must be excellent reporting to the nurse responsible for client care. The treatment effect of these measures will influence client health, so outcomes of the procedures must be charted as well as orally reported to the nurse.
- Any adverse responses (local or systemic) should be reported to prescribing physician so that corrective measures can be provided.

CRITICAL THINKING Strategies

Scenario 1

Mrs. Moore is a 52-year-old client who has been admitted to your unit after a laparoscopic cholecystectomy. She has a peripheral IV infusion of 5% dextrose in 0.45% NS infusing at 120 mL/hr in the cephalic vein at the left wrist. She receives intermittent antibiotic therapy by IV piggyback.

One hour after the evening IV antibiotic administration, she calls the nurse and reports a discomfort in her left arm. Assessment findings include discomfort in the area, slight pallor, swelling (lower arm circumference 1.5 in. greater than contralateral arm), and coolness to touch.

1. Based on assessment findings, what is the probable complication and what are possible causes?
2. What should the nurse's first action be?
3. How should the area be treated?
4. When are heat or cold therapies indicated to manage IV complications?

Scenario 2

Mr. X, age 78, lives alone in a small urban dwelling. He has a history of heart failure and COPD, and was found unresponsive in his back yard by his neighbor at 2:00 PM He has been admitted to the ED with a temperature of 40°C. Additional findings include confusion, lack of perspiration, dizziness, blurred vision, tachycardia, and hyperventilation. His laboratory tests reflect dehydration; insertion of a Foley catheter reveals minimal urine output.

His diagnosis is heatstroke.

1. What causes hyperthermia and how does it differ from fever?
2. Why are the elderly at great risk for developing heat-related illness?
3. What is the immediate goal of treatment for Mr. X?
4. Why are external cooling measures the treatment of choice rather than the use of antipyretics?
5. What are the principles involved with application of external cooling measures?
6. Why should cooling therapy be discontinued if shivering occurs?
7. What other ongoing assessments are essential during the cooling process?
8. How can heat-related injuries be prevented?

NCLEX® Review Questions

Unless otherwise specified, choose only one (1) answer.

1. Fever is an elevation of body temperature due to
   1. Cytokine influence on the hypothalamus.
   2. Injury to the hypothalamus.
   3. Dehydration.
   4. Environmental extremes.
2. The most effective method to reduce fever is the use of
   1. Tepid sponging.
   2. A cooling blanket.
   3. Antipyretic medication.
   4. Cool packs to axillae and groin.
3. The effect of shivering in response to external cryotherapy used in the febrile client is
   1. Enhanced body temperature cooling.
   2. Reduced metabolic rate.
   3. Increased heat production.
   4. Increased pyrogen production.
4. Most hospitals control facility water to be a maximum temperature of
   1. 95°F.
   2. 100°F.
   3. 110°F.
   4. 120°F.
5. The surgical client wears a head covering to prevent heat loss by
   1. Radiation.
   2. Evaporation.
   3. Convection.
   4. Conduction.
6. Which of the following fluids is preferred to rehydrate an over-heated dehydrated client?
   1. Water.
   2. Intravenous dextrose in water.
   3. Sport drink.
   4. Sugared cola.
7. Expected effects of local cold (cryo) therapy include ***Select all that apply.***
   1. Pallor.
   2. Flushing.
   3. Blister formation.
   4. Anesthesia.
   5. Burning.
   6. Numbness.
8. After a sitz bath, the client should be monitored for possible
   1. Orthostatic hypotension.
   2. Perineal fungal infection.
   3. Increased vaginal bleeding.
   4. Exacerbation of hemorrhoid discomfort.
9. Cold applications to injured joints should be of short duration because
   1. Reactive vasodilation may occur.
   2. Joints become less flexible with cold application.
   3. Bleeding may be induced.
   4. Injury to superficial nerves can occur.
10. Heat therapies are contraindicated for areas with circulatory insufficiency because heat
    1. Increases tissue need for oxygen.
    2. Decreases metabolic rate thereby increasing ischemia.
    3. Promotes inflammation.
    4. Decreases sensation and increases risk for injury.

25

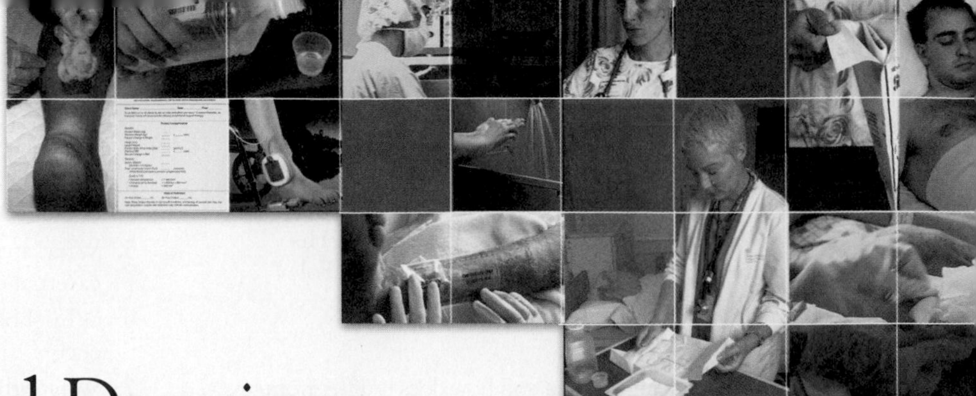

Wound Care and Dressings

LEARNING OBJECTIVES

1. Describe the three phases of wound healing.
2. Define the three types of wound healing.
3. Discuss three factors that affect wound healing.
4. State three complications associated with wound healing.
5. State criteria used to assess a wound.
6. Compare and contrast the four stages of pressure ulcers.
7. Write three nursing diagnoses for a client requiring wound care.
8. State three goals of wound care.
9. Discuss the effect of topical agents in wound healing.
10. Differentiate between clean, contaminated, and infected wounds.
11. Compare and contrast clean and sterile technique.
12. Describe dressing classification and indication for each type of dressing: gauze, transparent film, hydrogel, calcium alginate, foam, composite, hydrocolloid, and impregnated gauze.
13. Explain appropriate use of dressings: gauze, transparent adhesive film, hydrocolloid, and hydrogel.
14. Describe two methods to manage bacterial bioburden.
15. Outline the steps in irrigating a wound.
16. List steps to obtain a wound specimen for culture.
17. Perform the steps of a surgical hand scrub.
18. Prepare a sterile field for a dressing change.
19. Demonstrate the steps of putting on sterile gloves.
20. Describe the procedure for cleaning around a drain site.
21. List steps used to maintain a Hemovac or Jackson–Pratt suction drain.
22. Demonstrate changing a sterile dressing.
23. Outline the steps for removal of staples and sutures.
24. Outline the procedure for changing a wet-to-moist dressing.
25. Compare and contrast the three adjunctive wound care therapies.
26. Complete documentation on a wound assessment and wound care.
27. State five debridement methods.
28. Describe the term surgical site infection.

CHAPTER OUTLINE

TERMINOLOGY

Adhesions formation of fibrous scar tissue around the incision as a result of surgical intervention. Adhesions can cause obstruction or malfunction by distorting the organ.

Adjunctive wound care therapy wound treatments other than dressings and cleansing agents.

Aerobe a microorganism that lives and grows in the presence of free oxygen.

Anaerobe an organism that lives and grows in the absence of molecular oxygen.

Antimicrobial an agent that prevents the multiplication of microorganisms.

Asepsis prevention of contact with microorganisms.

Bacterial bioburden the number of contaminating bacteria present on an object.

Collagen formation formation of the protein substance of the white fibers of skin, bone, and cartilage.

Cytokines one or more than 100 distinct proteins produced primarily by WBCs. They regulate immunological aspects of cell growth and function during inflammation and immune response.

Debridement the removal of damaged tissue and cellular debris from a wound or burn to prevent infection and promote healing.

Debris remains of damaged or broken-down tissue or cells.

Decubitus ulcer see pressure ulcer.

Dehiscence a bursting open, as a graafian follicle or wound, especially abdominal wounds.

Dermis synonym for corium; the skin layer beneath the epidermis; contains vascular connective tissues.

Edematous the presence of abnormally large amounts of fluid in the intercellular tissue spaces of the body.

Electrical stimulation of wound transfer of electrical current through contact with moist wound bed.

Epidemiology division of medical science concerned with defining and explaining the interrelationships of the host, agent, and environment in causing disease.

Epidermis superficial avascular layers of skin.

Epithelium outer covering of the body; top layer of skin.

Erythema redness of the skin due to congestion of capillaries.

Eschar scabs or dry crust that result from trauma or infection.

Evisceration protrusion of the viscera; removal of the viscera.

Exudate fluid that filters from the circulatory system into areas of the body that are inflamed.

Gangrene death and putrefaction of body tissue precipitated by poor or absent blood supply to the tissue. Occurs as a result of infection, injury, or disease processes.

Granulation formation of granules; fleshy projections formed on the surface of a gaping wound that is not healing by the normal joining together of skin edges.

Hyperbaric oxygen therapy 100% oxygen administered at greater than one atmosphere pressure absolute.

Incision a cut made with a knife.

Infection morbid state caused by multiplication of pathogenic microorganisms within the body.

Inflammatory process localized response when injury or destruction of tissue has occurred; destroys, wards off, or dilutes the causative agent or the injured tissue.

Irrigate to rinse or wash out with a fluid.

Isolation limitation of movement and social contacts of a client; especially those having communicable diseases.

Keloid scar-like growth of collagen that results in a rounded, hard, shiny, white benign tumor.

Macrophage a large monocyte that has left the circulation and settled and matured in tissue and serves as scavenger of the blood, cleaning it of old cells and cellular debris.

Macration the softening and whitening of skin that is kept constantly wet.

Microorganism minute living body not perceptible to the naked eye.

Monocyte phagocytic white blood cell that matures into a macrophage.

Monokine chemical mediator released by monocytes and macrophages during the immune response. They affect growth and activity of other white blood cells.

Myofibroblast an atypical fibroblast with features of a fibroblast and a smooth muscle cell.

Necrotic death of a portion of tissue.

Negative pressure wound therapy negative pressure applied to wound to promote healing using an electrical pump.

Neutrophil white blood cells responsible for body's protection against infection. Plays a large role in the inflammatory process.

Occlusion the closure or state of being closed, of a passage.

Organism a living thing, either plant or animal.

Pathogen disease-producing organism.

Periwound area surrounding wound; healthy tissue around wound.

Phagocytosis ingestion and digestion of bacteria by phagocytes.

Pressure ulcer a break in the skin caused by pressure and restricted blood flow to the area. The ulcer generally occurs over bony prominences of the heels, sacrum, hip, and shoulder.

Primary intention healing minimal tissue loss and edges are closely approximated. Wound heals with minimal granulation tissue and scarring.

Purulent containing pus, or caused by pus.

Pus an inflammation containing leukocytes and exudate.

Secondary intention healing second stage in wound healing in which granulation occurs.

Semiocclusive dressing create and maintain a moist environment by holding liquid drainage from wound and moisture vapor at the wound surface.

Slough to shed or cast off dead tissue.

Surgical site infections (SSIs) an infection related to an operative procedure.

Tertiary intention healing using open method of wound healing; allow granulation to occur.

Warm-Up therapy heat therapy used to stimulate healing process.

Wound dehiscence the separation of layers of a surgical wound.

Wound evisceration protrusion of the internal viscera or organs through an opened incision site.

Wound healing three phases involved: inflammatory, proliferative, remodeling.

WOUND HEALING

The three major phases of wound healing are inflammation (or reaction), proliferation (or regeneration), and maturation (or wound remodeling).

Inflammatory Phase (Reaction)

The onset of the first phase of wound healing occurs immediately after an injury and lasts 2–5 days. After the injury, small blood vessels dilate and become more permeable and serous fluid leaks into the traumatized tissue as a result of histamine and prostaglandin release. Plasma and electrolytes leak into the interstitial spaces, causing edema. The edema leads to a reddened, swollen, and tender wound. Neutrophils reach the site in about 6 hr. Through the process of phagocytosis, they assist in preventing infection by ingesting and digesting bacteria. Oxygen is necessary for the neutrophils to destroy the bacteria. They survive only several hours after ingesting bacteria and necrotic tissue before releasing their intracellular contents, which forms part of the wound exudate. By the fourth day, monocytes enter the wound and differentiate into macrophages, which digest necrotic tissue, remove debris, and inhibit microbial growth. They also play a role in creating collagen synthesis. If macrophages are depleted, deposition of wound collagen decreases significantly. Macrophages direct healing through the release of monokines.

Proliferative, or Granulation, Phase (Regeneration)

This phase begins between about 2 days to 3 weeks after the injury and ends 14–24 days later. During granulation there is rapid growth of epithelial cells to produce a protective covering for the wound. The granulation tissue is formed from a rebuilding of the vascular capillary network and collagen tissue. The collagen fibers increase the tensile strength of the wound and provide wound integrity. Collagen fibers fill in the gaps and form the scar. Wound scar tissue is very fragile and susceptible to reinjury. In 6 weeks, the scar is only 10% of the tensile strength of normal skin. Large wounds may take months to build enough granulation tissue to close the wound. Healthy granulation tissue has a healthy reddish-pink color. The color results from increased blood flow that delivers oxygen and nutrients to the newly formed tissue.

Maturation, or Wound-Remodeling, Phase

Wound contraction begins between 14 and 21 days after the injury and can last up to 2 years. During this phase, the scar shrinks and thins. It becomes less red as the capillaries regress. Contraction of the wound occurs as a result of myofibroblasts, which assist in moving the wound edges toward the center of the wound. The skin and fascia of the healed wound achieve only about 70%–80% of the tensile strength of normal skin. Scar tissue has fewer melanocytes and thus has a lighter color than normal skin.

WOUND CLASSIFICATION

There are different wound classification systems used to describe wounds. These are useful when the nurse is planning for wound care management. The classification systems include categorizing the wound by cause: intentional or unintentional; cleanliness: clean, contaminated, or infected; depth: superficial, partial-thickness, or full-thickness; and by color. The RYB classification system has been used in wound care classification since the late 1980s. This system classifies open wounds that are healing by secondary or delayed primary intention in both acute and chronic wounds. It is used as an adjunct to other classification systems. It does not lend itself to an in-depth, comprehensive evaluation. It can be used to determine the state of healing. This system identifies what phase a wound is in on the continuum of the wound healing process. Red wounds (R) can be in the inflammatory, proliferative, or maturation phase of wound healing. Yellow wounds (Y) are infected or contain fibrinous slough and aren't ready to heal. Black wounds (B) contain necrotic tissue and aren't ready to heal. Treatment options are based on the color of the wound. Red wounds need to be kept clean and moist. Yellow wounds require the removal of slough or fibrinous tissue. Black wounds must have the eschar removed for healing to take place. If the wound has a combination of colors, the rule is that the most severe color treatment is completed.

Wounds are also classified in six main categories; surgical, trauma, diabetic, venous, arterial, and pressure. These categories can overlap.

TYPES OF WOUND HEALING

Primary Intention

This is the simplest form of healing. The skin is cleanly incised through a surgical incision or a traumatic laceration. The wound can be closed with sutures or staples, which approximates, or pulls together, the wound edges. These wounds close rapidly because there are no gaps in the tissue. The top layer of cells migrate, or epithelize, within 72 hr. The wound surface is "sealed," thus preventing bacteria from entering and fluid from escaping. The tensile strength of the wound is very weak at this stage of healing.

Secondary Intention

These wounds heal by granulation. As granulation tissue builds, it fills the gap under the skin and cells epithelize from the edge of the wound to create the closure. Burns, pressure ulcers, and wounds with large pieces of skin missing heal by this method. In these types of wounds, no edges are available to be approximated and sutured. These wounds are at risk for local and systemic infection due to the destruction of the dermis and the increased time necessary for healing to occur.

Tertiary Intention

Healing by tertiary intention is a method that leaves the wound open to heal. These wounds cannot be sutured or dehiscence occurs or the wounds are infected and need frequent irrigations and dressing changes to facilitate healing. Clients with peritonitis, a ruptured appendix, or diverticula frequently require this type of wound healing. After irrigations and dressing changes for approximately 10 days, the wound is sutured and allowed to heal by primary and secondary intention.

MAJOR FACTORS AFFECTING WOUND HEALING

In addition to proper wound care and generally good physical health, nutrition plays a major role in wound healing. Calories need to be increased to 30–35 cal/kg/day. Medication use may interfere with wound healing.

Nutrition

Low serum albumin levels slow the diffusion of oxygen and diminish the ability of neutrophils to kill bacteria. Low oxygen at the capillary level diminishes the proliferation of healthy granulation tissue. Zinc deficiency can slow the rate of epithelialization and decrease wound and collagen strength. Adequate amounts of vitamins A and C and of iron and copper are necessary for effective collagen formation. Collagen synthesis also depends on appropriate intake of protein, carbohydrates, and fats. Wound healing requires almost double the usual protein and carbohydrate requirements for age. For the scar to develop adequate tensile strength, the client's intake of vitamin C, iron, and zinc must be increased.

General Physical Health

The major obstacle to wound healing is infection. Infected wounds have friable tissue, bleed easily, and have delayed healing. Immunosuppressed clients have more difficulty healing wounds because the inflammatory phase is impaired. When the blood glucose level is consistently over 200 mg/dL or the hemoglobin is below 10 g/dL, wounds do not follow the usual phases of healing. Any condition that reduces the formation of adequate white blood cells, especially macrophages, adversely affects healing. Such conditions include diabetes mellitus, anemia, uremia, cancer, atherosclerosis, infection, and malnutrition. Older clients, clients who smoke or are obese, and those undergoing radiation or steroid therapy are also prone to delayed wound healing.

Medications

Any medication that reduces the inflammatory response, such as steroids and nonsteroidal medications used to treat arthritis or respiratory conditions, also impairs wound healing. Anti-inflammatories decrease epithelialization and wound contraction and may also affect fibroblast proliferation and collagen synthesis. Steroids decrease the tensile strength of a closed wound and cause inadequate deposits of collagen. Administration of vitamin A can reverse the processes associated with steroid use.

TABLE 25-1 Nutritional Support for Wound Healing

Nutrient	Food Sources
Protein	Meat, fish, poultry, milk, cheese, eggs, dried beans, peas, peanut butter
Carbohydrates	Legumes, fruits, vegetables, whole-grain cereal, bread, pasta
Vitamins	
Vitamin A	Dark green leafy vegetables, milk, eggs, carrots, liver, sweet potatoes
Vitamin C	Citrus fruits, vegetables, potatoes, tomatoes
Minerals	
Iron	Meat, eggs, cereal, vegetables
Copper	Seafood, nuts, seeds, organ meats
Zinc	Meat, liver, seafood, eggs, legumes
Calories	30–35 cal/kg/day

TABLE 25-2 RYB Wound Dressing Guidelines*

Dressings Most Commonly Used to Treat RYB Wounds	
Red Wounds	Yellow Wounds (fibrinous slough)
Biologicals	Alginate
Foams	Exudate absorbers
Gauze	Foams
Hydrocolloids	Hypertonic gauze
Hydrogels	Hydrocolloid
Moist gauze	Hydrogel
Nonadherent gauze	Transparent film
Transparent film	
Yellow Wounds (infected)	Black Wounds
Alginates	Alginate
Impregnated dressings	Hydrocolloid
Exudate absorbers	Hydrogel
Foams	Gauze
Hypertonic gauze	Transparent film
Wound pouches	

**See* Assessing a Wound, p. 905.

GOALS OF WOUND CARE

Wound assessment and measures to treat wounds have changed dramatically over the last 10 years. The major trend is to treat wounds using moisture-retentive dressing rather than drying the wound. Wound care specialists also diverge on the use of sterile versus clean technique during dressing changes.

Whatever plan is used in treating a wound, the goals remain the same:

- Remove necrotic tissue to promote wound healing.
- Prevent, eliminate, or control infection.
- Absorb drainage (exudate).
- Maintain a moist wound environment.
- Protect the wound from further injury.
- Protect the surrounding skin from infection and trauma.

To accomplish these goals, a moist wound environment must be maintained to allow tissue to granulate. A wound bed that is too moist or too dry kills healthy tissue and impairs healing. Drainage from the wound site needs to be contained to protect adjacent healthy skin from maceration. All wounds require a dressing that is dry on the air-exposed side to prevent bacterial invasion by downward capillary mobility of contaminants. The dressing should be secured over the wound and taped in place using the "window paning" method of taping if there is not an adhesive backing on the dressing. Using this method, the edges remain taped down and the dressing stays intact.

There are many types of wound care products available, including skin cleansers, skin barriers, irrigants, various types of dressings, gauze dressings, and enzymes. Physician and wound care specialist preferences, as well as type and extent of wound, determine wound care.

Complications Associated With Wound Healing

One complication that may occur after wound healing has seemed to progress satisfactorily is adhesions. Adhesions frequently form in the peritoneal cavity after abdominal surgery and can either constrict or fold around the intestines.

Frequently clients are admitted to the hospital with incisional strangulated internal hernias that may even be gangrenous. Other complications are surgical or incisional hernias that may occur when the intraperitoneal pressure pushes against the scar tissue, causing a hernia (or outpouching) through the incision.

Contractures, formed as a result of a shortening of scar tissue, can decrease mobility and joint movement. Contractures caused by incisional scars are far less common than those caused by scar tissue from burns.

Excessive collagen formation results in the formation of a keloid, a complication that does not present a serious problem with body function; however, it generally causes an altered self-image if the keloid is large or in a prominent place on the body.

WOUND INFECTIONS

Open wounds of any type provide an environment for bacterial invasion. All wounds may be considered contaminated but not necessarily infected. Wound care must include regular wound cleansing, the use of semiocclusive dressings, using Standard Precautions when providing care to the client, maintaining proper hand hygiene technique, and following dressing change protocols. Semiocclusive dressings in wound care have reduced the incidence of wound infections by more than 50% compared with gauze dressings. These dressings promote a moist environment, provide a mechanical barrier for bacterial invasion, and reduce airborne dispersal of bacteria during dressing changes.

The clinical symptoms of wound infection generally begin in 3–5 days postoperatively or after injury. When the client's temperature and pulse rate increase, an associated tachypnea occurs. As the inflammatory process occurs, the wound becomes progressively more tender, painful, and edematous. Erythema surrounds the edges of the wound unless the infection is in the deeper tissues. Abnormal firmness of the wound edge may be present. Usually, a persistent WBC count of 12,000/mm^3 or greater, lasting longer than 72 hr, accompanies the infection. Foul-smelling, purulent drainage may occur. An absence of local signs of infection does not necessarily mean that deep wound infections are absent.

Several microorganisms are responsible for the majority of wound infections. *Staphylococcus aureus* is still a major cause of postoperative infection. *Escherichia coli, Streptococcus faecalis, Proteus vulgaris, Klebsiella, Enterobacter*, and *Pseudomonas aeruginosa* are also closely associated with wound infection. Antimicrobial agents themselves can promote infection by increasing the susceptibility of clients to colonization with nosocomial microflora; these agents also select and concentrate antibiotic-resistant organisms on or in the host.

Maintaining asepsis during dressing changes assists in preventing wound infections. Using sterile equipment, including gloves, is the first barrier against infection. A mask and gown should be worn during dressing changes to prevent the spread of microorganisms to other clients and to the healthcare worker.

When wounds become grossly infected or are extensive in nature, the physician may order wound irrigations. Normal saline or Ringer's solution are the usual irrigating solutions used for wounds. Most of the agents used in the past have been identified as toxic to the cells generated in the inflammatory phase of healing.

Each hospital has its own protocol for wound irrigation, and you should become familiar with the institution's procedure. This chapter presents one method of wound irrigation that is helpful in most clinical situations.

Wound Specimens for Culture

Exudate, or purulent drainage, from infected wounds can contain a variety of aerobic and anaerobic microorganisms. In the majority of wound infections, the causative agent is usually found in the upper respiratory tract, gastrointestinal tract, and genitourinary tract. When these organisms invade other body parts, they can cause severe infections and sometimes death.

Before a wound can be cultured, it should be irrigated with normal saline to remove the surface bacteria. The best method of obtaining a culture specimen is to rotate a swab along the granulation tissue. Refer to Chapter 20, Specimen Collection, for the skill. For the most accurate results, the physician should take a biopsy of the tissue.

Surgical Site Infections

Surgical Site Infections (SSIs) are best described as an infection related to the operative procedure that occurs at or near the surgical incision within 30 days of a procedure or within 1 year of an implant left in place.

At the time of the incision, every surgical site becomes contaminated with bacteria inward from the skin or outward from the organs undergoing surgical intervention. The client's endogenous flora at the incisional site leads to the contamination. In addition to the skin, the mucosal membrane or viscera are also involved in the contamination process. The contamination does not cause the infection themselves; the virulence of the bacteria and local blood flow and nutritional components lead to the infection. The amount of bacteria in the wound at the end of the surgery is the major cause of the SSI.

SSIs account for more than 40% of all hospital-associated infections among surgical clients and 22% of all hospital associated infections. These clients are 60% more likely to be in an ICU, five times more likely to be readmitted to the hospital, and twice as likely to die as other postoperative clients. Seventy-five percent of surgical client deaths are related to a wound infection. As of October 2008, these SSI costs are not reimbursed by Medicare and Medicaid.

Wounds Caused by Vascular Insufficiency

There are three types of wounds caused by vascular insufficiency. These include venous insufficiency ulcers, arterial insufficiency ulcers, and pressure ulcers (capillary insufficiency ulcers). There are five major factors that contribute to ulcer formation in vascular insufficiency: poor nutrition and a lack of blood flow causing inability of nutrients to diffuse through the interstitial spaces; continuous pressure on certain areas of the body, such as bony prominences; mechanical, thermal, or chemical insults to limbs, resulting in lack of nutrients reaching the lower limbs; decreased sensation in the lower extremities; and excess moisture from incontinence.

Venous Ulcers

These are mistakenly termed venous stasis ulcers; however, they are not due to a lack of venous blood flow, but rather a diminished ability of nutrients to diffuse through the interstitial space from the capillaries. The usual etiology of this condition includes calf pump failure as a result of outflow tract obstruction, associated with pregnancy, obesity, tumor, or deep vein thrombosis. Insufficient valves, either deep venous valve incompetence or superficial vein incompetence (varicose veins), are causes as well. Peripheral neuropathy and musculoskeletal disorders may lead to venous ulcers as a result of calf muscle disuse.

Compression therapy is used to treat venous ulcers. This therapy includes the use of compression stockings, Unna's boot, or a compression dressing when wound care is included in the treatment. Compression therapy is contraindicated in clients with phlebitis, diminished sensation, and arterial insufficiency, as it will exacerbate the insufficiency.

Arterial Ulcers

Arterial ulcers are often seen in clients with diabetes mellitus and atherosclerosis. Clients with a history of smoking and who sustain mechanical trauma to the extremity are prone to arterial ulcers. In these situations, there is diminished oxygenation and thus, nutrients, to the periphery. Drug therapy with vasodilators, anticoagulants, or thrombolytic agents are part of the treatment plan for these clients. Surgical treatment may be necessary if drug therapy is insufficient to treat the ulcer. Sympathectomy, endarterectomy, or bypass surgery may be necessary treatment modalities.

Pressure Ulcers

Pressure ulcers are defined by the National Pressure Ulcer Advisory Panel as any lesion caused by unrelieved pressure resulting in damage to underlying tissue. Four mechanical factors contribute to the development of pressure ulcers: pressure, friction, shearing, and moisture. Pressure ulcers are usually located over a bony prominence, where normal tissue is squeezed between the bone and pressure or friction caused by the bed or chair. External pressure that lasts long enough to result in decreased blood flow causes altered oxygenation and nutrition to the tissue, resulting in a pressure ulcer. Immobility, especially associated with the elderly, is the primary cause of pressure ulcer formation. In addition to mechanical factors and immobility, aging skin and malnutrition increase the risk of skin breakdown.

Each year 1.5 million hospitalized clients develop pressure ulcers, resulting in 60,000 deaths. Data suggest that 25% of these clients develop the pressure ulcer in the operating room, especially when the surgery is prolonged beyond 3 hr. Surgical clients experience periods of prolonged immobility, resulting in unrelieved pressure and decreased blood flow to the skin. In addition to the 9% of hospitalized clients, 23% of all nursing home clients develop pressure ulcers. Elderly clients are affected most often and account for the highest number of cases. A large percentage of the clients who develop pressure ulcers while in a nursing home die as a result. These statistics are appalling when one considers that ulcers are usually preventable and treatable.

Pressure ulcers are classified in stages by the degree of tissue damage observed. See Unit 5 for illustration and description.

Management of pressure ulcers is best accomplished using a team of healthcare providers, including physicians, nurses, an enterostomal therapist, dietitian, physical therapist, family members, and the client.

Client education should include:

- Discussion of options for pressure ulcer treatment.
- Discussion of client's active participation in his or her own care.
- Developing a plan of care that is consistent with the client's goals and desires.

Client treatment plan should include:

- Assessment of the pressure ulcer.
- Managing tissue loads.
- Ulcer care.
- Managing bacterial bioburden and infection.
- Operative repair of the pressure ulcer.

Management and prevention of pressure ulcers should begin on hospital admission with a thorough assessment of the client's skin, especially over bony prominences. Preventive steps for high-risk clients include the following:

- Ensure that skin is kept clean, and prevent it from getting too dry by using moisturizing lotions.
- Provide a balanced diet high in protein, vitamins, and minerals for tissue repair.
- Ensure a fluid intake of 2000 mL/day for adequate hydration.
- Place clients on a pressure-reducing mattress or chair cushion.
- Use turning sheets to reposition.
- Avoid massaging over bony prominences.
- Do not elevate head of the bed more than 30°.
- Positioning is the basic standard of ulcer prevention.
- Reposition a bedridden client at least every 2 hr; reposition a chair-bound client every hour.
- Complete a risk assessment for the client, evaluating factors for developing pressure ulcers.

ADJUNCTIVE WOUND CARE THERAPY

Three of the more common types of adjunctive wound therapy include electrical stimulation, noncontact normothermic wound therapy, and the vacuum-assisted closure system.

Electrical stimulation uses transfer of an electric current through a surface electrode pad that is in contact with external skin surface or the wound bed itself. It influences wound healing by attracting cells of repair, changing cell membrane permeability, enhancing cellular secretion through cell membranes, and orienting cell structure. A moist wound environment must be maintained for this therapy to be successful in healing. Electrical stimulation increases blood flow, oxygen uptake, and DNA and protein synthesis. It can be used in a variety of wound problems, including burns, pressure ulcers, vascular ulcers, and surgical wounds.

Warm-up therapy stimulates the healing process through application of infrared heat to the wound. This system uses warmth to help the body heal itself. It also maintains humidity and absorbs exudates, and its transparent window allows the nurse to assess the wound without disrupting wound tissue. Wound cover allows clients more freedom in their movements, as well as an increased comfort level. The heat increases blood flow and oxygen to the wound. It is commonly used for clients with venous ulcers and pressure ulcers. It can also be used for clients with surgical or traumatic wounds and diabetic ulcers.

Negative pressure wound therapy uses a foam dressing applied directly to the wound. This system stimulates growth of granulation tissue while promoting a moist environment. Negative pressure is applied to foam through the use of tubing connected to a canister where exudate and wound fluids are collected. This system is used with infected wounds, as well as chronic wounds, acute and traumatic wounds, and dehiscence.

Hyperbaric oxygenation has been approved by Medicare and Medicaid for treatment of diabetic clients with leg ulcers. One hundred percent (100%) oxygen is delivered in a hyperbaric chamber. The oxygen is administered at greater than 1 atmospheric pressure absolute (ATA). This can only be accomplished in an environment of elevated atmospheric pressure, which is in the chamber.

The role of oxygen in wound healing takes on many roles. Disruption of microcirculation is the initial event leading to wound hypoxia. This hypoxia remains in chronic wound conditions. Cellular energy metabolism requires oxygen in the production of adenosine triphosphate (ATP). Without tissue oxygen at sufficient levels, acidosis occurs as a result of the hypoxia. Oxygen consumption is increased as leukocytes migrate to the wounded area, increasing the hypoxic state of the wound. An oxygen level of 40 mmHg is needed to sustain fibroblast activity that leads to collagen deposits for healing. Hyperbaric oxygen wound therapy has proven to be very effective in healing diabetic ulcers.

HOME CARE

Before discharge from the hospital, a multidisciplinary team meeting should be held with the client to review the care at home. The team should include the following: home care RN, dietician, wound care specialist, and mental health CNS, if appropriate. A home care plan needs to include a discussion of the wound care and dressing change; mobility and exercise routine, if appropriate; diet to promote wound healing; and discussions with the healthcare workers and family regarding wound care techniques, signs and symptoms of infection, and when to notify the physician or healthcare provider.

Wound assessments and dressing changes are the same as that in the hospital. The more advanced adjunctive wound therapy modalities are usually not done in the home. If a complicated dressing change is required, a wound care specialist should be assigned to the home care client.

NURSING DIAGNOSES

The following nursing diagnoses may be appropriate to use on client care plans when the components are related to the client requiring wound care.

NURSING DIAGNOSIS	RELATED FACTORS
Infection, Risk for	Altered circulation, invasive procedures, trauma Exposure to nosocomial agents, surgical incision, open wound
Impaired Physical Mobility	Bedrest, wounds, or pressure ulcers
Chronic Pain	Tissue injury, extensive dressing changes, recent surgery, vascular ulcers
Skin Integrity	Mechanical factors (shearing force, pressure), altered circulation due to pressure on a bony prominence, immobility, poor nutritional intake
Impaired Tissue Integrity	Interrupted blood supply to site depleting oxygen and nutrients

CLEANSE HANDS The single most important nursing action to decrease the incidence of hospital-based infections is hand hygiene. *Remember to wash your hands or use antibacterial gel before and after each and every client contact.*

IDENTIFY CLIENT Before every procedure, introduce yourself and check two forms of client identification, not including room number. These actions prevent errors and conform to The Joint Commission standards.

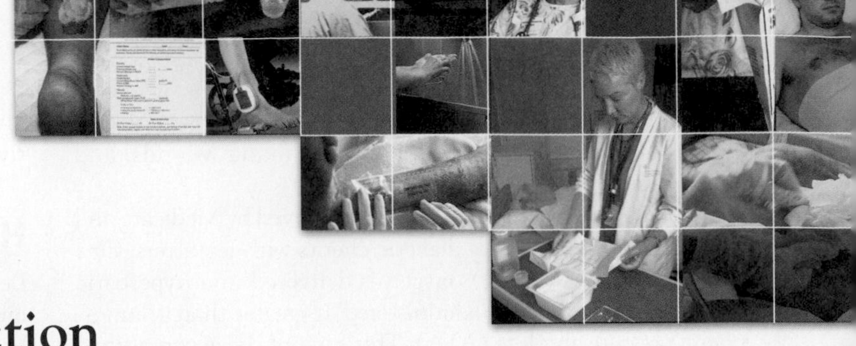

Chapter 25

UNIT 1

Measures to Prevent Infection

Nursing Process Data

ASSESSMENT Data Base

- Identify clients at risk for infection (i.e., diabetics, elderly, malnourished, obese, smokers, immunosuppressed).
- Identify length of time client remained in surgery (the more hours in surgery, the greater the risk for infection).
- Assess incision three times a day.
- Identify the components necessary to prevent infection for individual clients.
- Assess need for sterile technique compliance in client care.
- Assess lab results for abnormal values (i.e., WBC, Hgb, Hct).

PLANNING Objectives

- To remove transient microorganisms from nails, hands, and forearms
- To prevent clients with impaired resistance from becoming infected
- To prevent microorganisms from entering the wound
- To provide a sterile working field for dressing changes

IMPLEMENTATION Procedures

EVALUATION Expected Outcomes

- Infection is prevented in clients with impaired resistance.
- Sterile field is maintained when preparing for dressing changes.
- Sterile technique is maintained throughout wound care.

Pearson Nursing Student Resources

Find additional review materials at
nursing.pearsonhighered.com

Prepare for success with NCLEX®-style practice questions and Skill Checklists

Completing Surgical Hand Antisepsis

Equipment

Plastic or orangewood stick
Antimicrobial solution (soap)
Sterile towel

Procedure

1. Remove all jewelry: rings, watch, bracelets.
2. Turn on water using foot or knee pedal or hand lever. Water should be tepid. ▶ ***Rationale:*** Hot water dries skin and is uncomfortable. Cold water prevents soap from lathering and bacteria is not rinsed away.
3. Wet hands first with warm water. Apply 3–5 mL of antimicrobial soap to hands. Rub together for at least 15 seconds. Cover all surfaces of hands and fingers and 3 in. above wrists, keeping fingers pointing upward.
4. Scrub your hands for 10 strokes and nails for 15 strokes with an antimicrobial solution (time based on facility policy). Scrub each side of each finger for 2 minutes.
5. Scrub your hands using soap or alcohol-based hand rubs. When using antimicrobial soap, scrub hands and forearms up to 3 in. above elbows. This is done for length of time recommended by manufacturer (2–6 minutes) for each hand/arm. Most studies indicate this should be done for first OR scrub.
6. Rinse hands and arms by passing them through the water in one direction only, from finger tips to elbows. Do not move the hands and arms back and forth through the water.
7. When using alcohol solution, prewash hands and forearms with non-antimicrobial soap. Completely dry hands and forearms. Then use alcohol-based product according to manufacturer's directions, usually a vigorous 1-minute rub. Apply product to palm of one

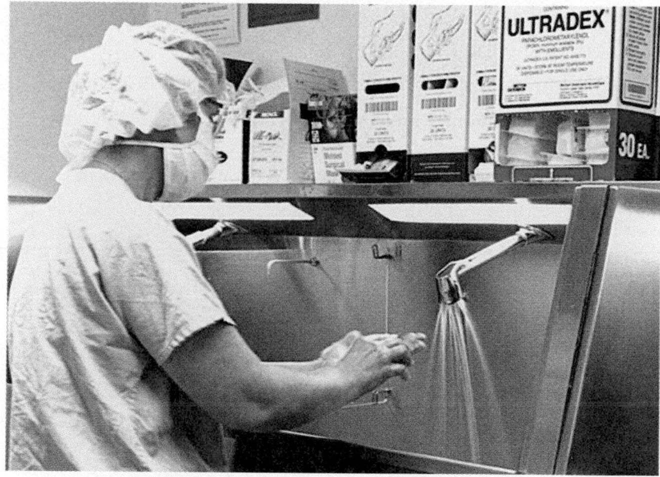

▲ Scrub hands with an antimicrobial solution.

Research Studies

1950s It was thought that administering antibiotics after surgery would prevent wound infections. This did not happen.

1960s Confirmed giving antibiotics within 3 hr of the incision was more effective in preventing wound infections. Studies confirmed that giving antibiotics more than 24 hr after incision closure was not effective in preventing infections. Even with these statistics, many physicians continued to order the antibiotics after surgery for 7–10 days, in 25%–50% of surgeries in U.S. hospitals.

2010 The Recommendations from the Surgical Care Improvement Project (SCIP) will include the following changes in antibiotic administration to reduce the incidence of surgical complications by 25%.

- Administering the antibiotic 1 hr before the incision is completed, or within 2 hr before the incision, is required for prophylaxis. Vancomycin is used when client has a documented beta-lactam allergy or has colonization with methicillin-resistant *S. aureus*.
- Discontinue the antibiotic within 24 hr after surgery, except in cardiothoracic surgeries, in which case the antibiotic should be continued for 48 hr.

Source: Surgical Care Improvement Project (SCIP). www.qualitynet.org or www.premiervine.com. Chettle, C. (2008, April 21). Shockingly high rates. *NurseWeek*, California.

Clinical Alert

Surgical site infection rates are the same in clients whose surgeon performed surgical hand antisepsis with either traditional antimicrobial scrub or an alcohol-based hand rub.

Decontaminating hands with alcohol-based hand rub:

- Apply 1.5–3 mL (size of a quarter) of alcohol gel or rinse to palm of one hand.
- Rub hands together, covering all surfaces of hands and fingers.
- Cover 3 in. above wrist with alcohol.
- Cover areas around and under fingernails.
- Continue to rub until alcohol dries (15–25 seconds).

Using soap and water for handwashing:

- Wet hand with water and place soap from dispenser on hands.
- Thoroughly spread soap on all surfaces of hands and fingers.
- Rub vigorously for 15 seconds, covering all surfaces.
- Rinse hands and dry thoroughly using single-use towel.
- Turn off faucet with towel if foot pedal not used.

Source: Baricenté, J. J., et al. (2002). *Journal of the American Medical Association*, 288. www.handhygiene.org.

hand and rub hands together covering all surfaces of hands and fingers until surfaces are dry.

8. Proceed to operative room and dry hands and arms thoroughly on sterile towel.
9. Dry hands and forearms thoroughly before donning sterile gloves.

Clinical Alert

Chlorhexidine added to alcohol-based preparations results in greater residual activity than alcohol alone. Minimal absorption, if any, occurs through the skin. Care should be taken to avoid contact with the eyes when using more than 1% chlorhexidine, as it causes conjunctivitis and severe corneal damage.

Donning Sterile Gloves

Equipment

Packaged sterile gloves

Procedure

1. Perform hand hygiene.
2. Place glove package on a clean, dry, firm surface that is at waist height (usually an overbed table). ▶ ***Rationale:*** Objects below waist level are considered to be out of the sterile field.
3. Remove outside wrapper of glove package by peeling the tabs apart where indicated on the wrapper. Pull edges laterally to expose glove package. Ensure that this step is accomplished over a firm surface. ▶ ***Rationale:*** This prevents the glove package from accidentally falling on a contaminated surface.
4. Place the glove package on the firm surface, maintaining sterility of gloves by touching only outside of wrapper.
5. Grasp two edges of wrapper and lift wrapper edges up and away from gloves, being careful to not touch gloves as you open the package. ▶ ***Rationale:*** Lifting the edges up and away as you open the package will prevent touching the gloves accidentally and causing contamination.
6. With your nondominant hand, pick up the opposite glove by grasping the section that has a folded edge (inside edge of the cuff). Lift the glove up and away from the wrapper. ▶ ***Rationale:*** This prevents accidental contamination of the glove or inside of glove package.
7. Holding your hands above waist level, insert your dominant hand into the glove opening. Gently pull the glove into place with your nondominant hand, touching only the inside of the cuff. Do not attempt to straighten out gloved fingers until both gloves have been put on. ▶ ***Rationale:*** It is easy to contaminate the glove when attempting to adjust the fingers in the glove.
8. With your dominant, gloved hand, remove the other glove from the package, making sure you touch only the inside of the folded cuff. Lift this glove up and away from the wrapper. ▶ ***Rationale:*** This prevents gloves from inadvertently touching wrapper and contaminating gloves.
9. Hold your gloved thumb away from your body to prevent touching your skin.
10. Place your ungloved fingers into the new glove opening. Gently pull the glove over your hand as before.
11. Keeping your hands above waist level, adjust both gloves by touching only your fingers, remembering to

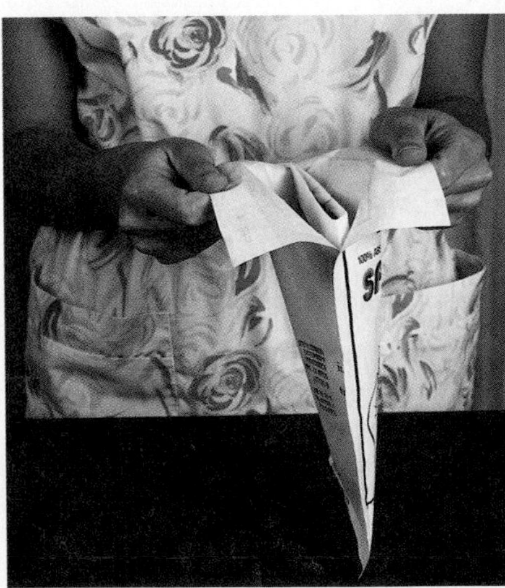

1 Grasp two upper edges of the glove package and pull laterally to open package.

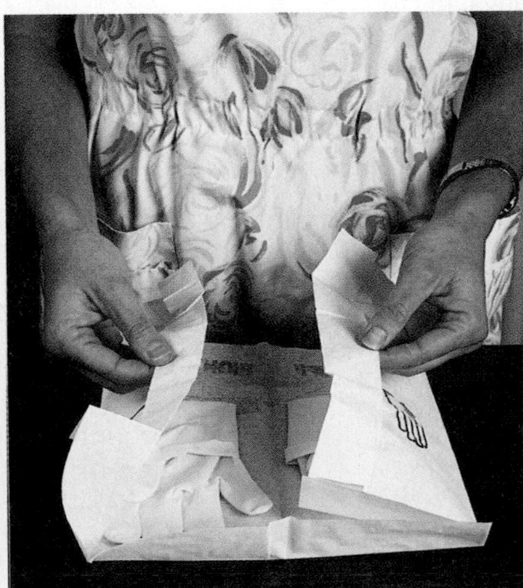

2 Place sterile glove wrapper on clean, flat surface and lift wrapper edges away from gloves.

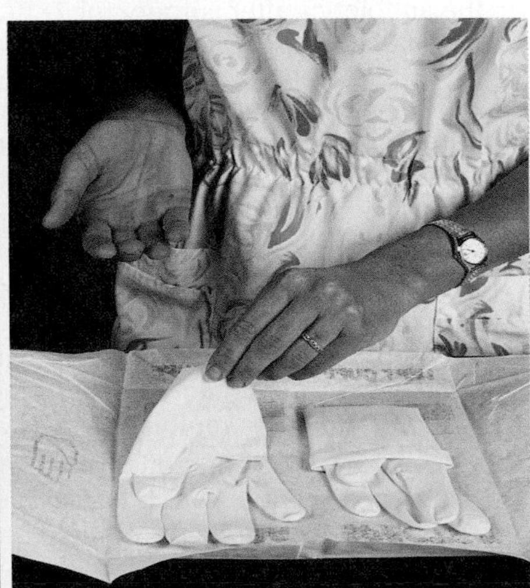

3 Grasp folded edge of glove with nondominant hand and lift glove away from wrapper.

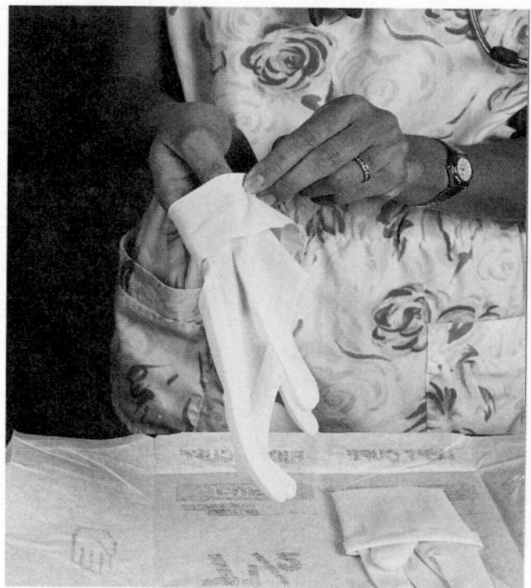
4 Slip dominant hand into glove opening without contaminating glove.

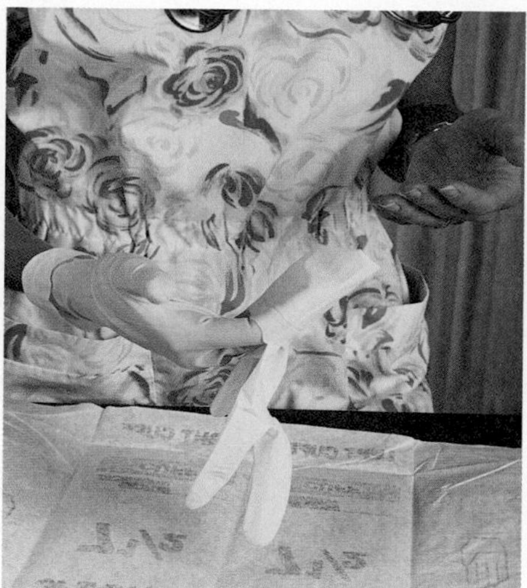
5 Remove second glove from wrapper by placing gloved fingers under cuff.

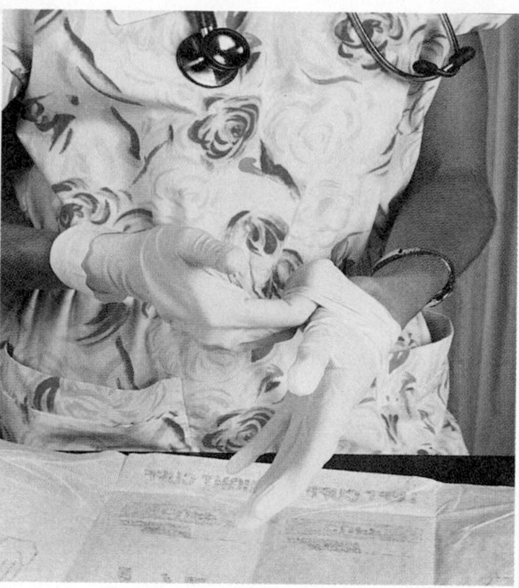
6 Continue to keep fingers under cuff of glove as the glove is pulled on.

touch sterile surfaces with sterile surfaces. ▸ ***Rationale:*** Fingers of gloves are considered sterile; cuff area is considered contaminated.

12. Keep both sterile gloves in front of you above your waist level. ▸ ***Rationale:*** Being able to see gloves at all times helps prevent potential contamination.

Pouring From a Sterile Container

Equipment

Sterile container
Nonsterile container
Sterile solution

Procedure

1. Perform hand hygiene.
2. Gather equipment.
3. Open sterile container according to procedure.
4. Place container on firm surface.
5. Take cap off the bottle and invert the cap before laying on firm surface. ▸ ***Rationale:*** This keeps the cap sterile.
6. Hold the bottle with the label facing up.
7. Pour a small amount of liquid into a nonsterile container. ▸ ***Rationale:*** This action cleans the lip of the bottle.
8. Pour the liquid into the sterile container while keeping the label facing up and not touching the container with the bottle. Do not reach over a sterile field if the container has been placed on one. ▸ ***Rationale:*** Crossing over a sterile field can lead to contamination of the field.
9. Replace the cap if liquid remains in the bottle. If total contents have been used, dispose of bottle in trash.
10. Date and initial bottle if reusing.
11. Replace partially filled bottle to storage area if it is to be reused.

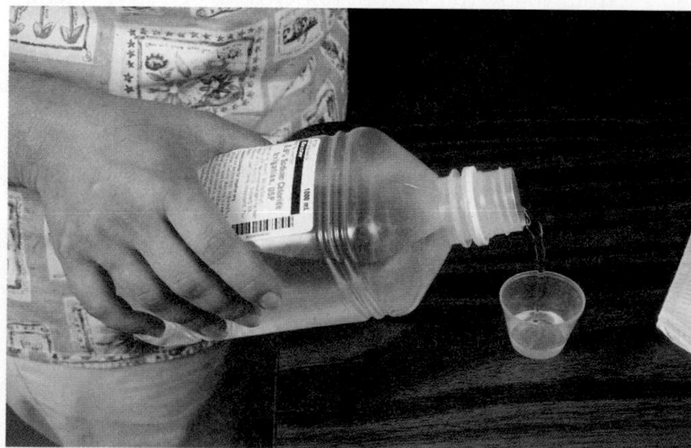
▲ First pour a small amount of liquid into nonsterile container.

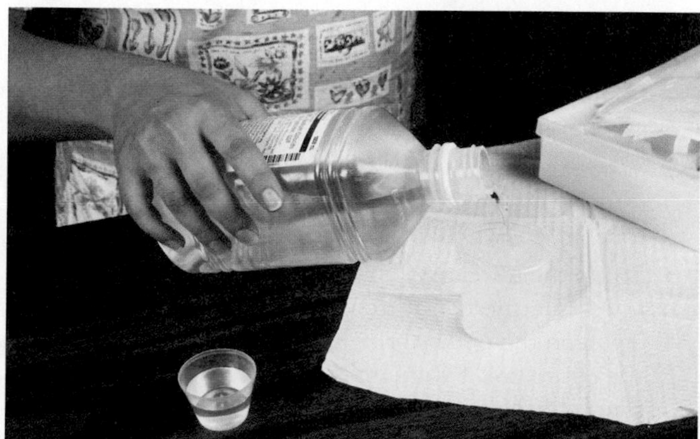
▲ Pour liquid by placing container close to edge of sterile area.

Preparing a Sterile Field

Equipment

Antiseptic cleansing solution, as ordered
Two packages of sterile towels
Number and type of dressings required for dressing change
Tape
Container for antiseptic solution
Paper bag for disposal of soiled dressings
Mask
Sterile gloves

Preparation

1. Check physician's orders and client care plan.
2. Gather equipment from supply area.
3. Clean off overbed table.

Clinical Alert
Preparing a sterile field is commonly used for burn dressings or large wound dressings. It is not used routinely for other dressings.

Procedure

1. Perform hand hygiene, using aseptic technique.
2. Place sterile towel packages on overbed table or on another surface close to the table. Place packages so that first wrapper edge can be opened away from the sterile area. ▸ ***Rationale:*** This prevents contamination when crossing over a sterile field.
3. Grasp far edge of the wrapper and open away from you. ▸ ***Rationale:*** This exposes the sterile part of package.
4. Don sterile gloves and mask according to hospital policy. Gloves and mask are usually used when preparing burn sterile field. This procedure may be performed without gloves, maintaining sterility.
5. Using both hands, pick up the two side edges of the first wrapper and open them away from the middle of the sterile field. Unfold the last edge toward you, without touching the wrapper.
6. Pick up one edge of the sterile towel and move away from the table. Gently shake the towel open, keeping it away from the sterile area.
7. When the towel is open, use your other hand to pick up the two edges that are away from you. Be careful to not touch towel with clothing.
8. Lower the towel onto the tray or bedside stand so the towel is farthest away from you. Then lay the towel down on the tray by bringing it toward you, covering the entire tray. ▸ ***Rationale:*** This prevents crossing over the sterile field.
9. Repeat the same steps with a second sterile towel.
10. If solutions for cleansing the skin are required, place sterile medicine cups near one side of the sterile towel.
11. Take the cap off the antiseptic bottle.
12. Pour a small amount of solution into a container, not on the sterile field, keeping the label in uppermost position. ▸ ***Rationale:*** This action rinses contaminated particles from the lip of the bottle.
13. Pour the antiseptic solution, from the side of the sterile field, directly into the medicine cup. ▸ ***Rationale:*** Pouring solution from the side prevents crossing over the sterile field.
14. Open sterile packages of dressings, and place on sterile surface.

For Commercially Prepared Packages

a. Open package at designated end by pulling edges apart and downward to expose contents.
b. Grasp the edges of the two sides of the package and invert the package over the edge of the sterile field. Allow the contents to drop onto the sterile field.
c. Repeat procedure for each item to be placed on the sterile field.

For Hospital-Wrapped Packages

a. Hold package in your hand and securely grasp one edge.
b. Open package wrapper by allowing edges to drop down, away from package.
c. Grasp the edges of the wrapper with your free hand and pull them toward your wrist, thus exposing the sterile contents.
d. Gently drop the contents on the sterile field. ▸ ***Rationale:*** Touching the sterile field with the wrapper contaminates it.
e. Repeat procedure for each item to be placed on the sterile field.

15. If sterile supplies are not to be used immediately, cover with sterile towels.
    a. Open sterile towel package by opening wrapper away from you so that you do not cross over a sterile field.

Guidelines for Sterile Field

- Never turn your back on a sterile field.
- Avoid talking, coughing, sneezing, or reaching across a sterile field.
- Keep sterile objects above waist level.
- Do not spill solutions on the sterile field.
- Open all sterile packages away from the sterile field to prevent crossover and contamination.
- One in. around edges is considered contaminated.

b. Pick up one towel at the edge and open towel by moving yourself away from the sterile field and allowing towel to fall open.
c. Grasp corner of towel opposite one you are holding. Keep towel from touching contaminated areas.
d. Place towel over sterile field starting at edge nearest you. Lay the towel down without touching the tray with your hand. Move the towel across the tray toward the opposite edge.
e. Repeat procedure with second sterile towel.

Preparing a Sterile Field Using Prepackaged Supplies

Equipment

Packaged supplies

Procedure

1. Perform hand hygiene.
2. Ensure working surface is clean and dry. Client's overbed table is frequently used as preparation area. ▸ ***Rationale:*** This prevents contamination of sterile package.
3. Remove outer plastic wrap.
4. Place package in center of work area and position so that you first open package flap away from you. ▸ ***Rationale:*** This prevents reaching across the sterile field as you continue to open package.
5. Grasp edge of the first flap of the wrapper, move it away from you, and place it on the working surface.
6. Grasp the first side flap, lift it up, grasp the second side flap, and together move both hands out toward the sides. Place the flaps down on the working surface.
7. Grasp the last flap of the wrapper and open it toward you, taking care not to touch the inside of the flap or any of the contents of the package. ▸ ***Rationale:*** This prevents contamination of the supplies.

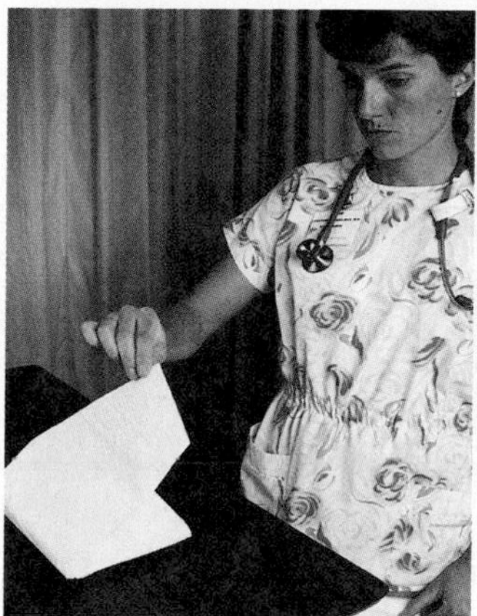

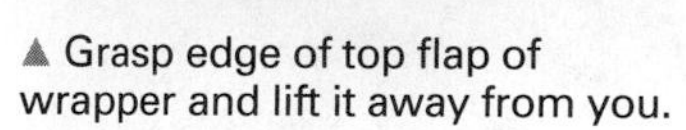

▲ Grasp edge of top flap of wrapper and lift it away from you.

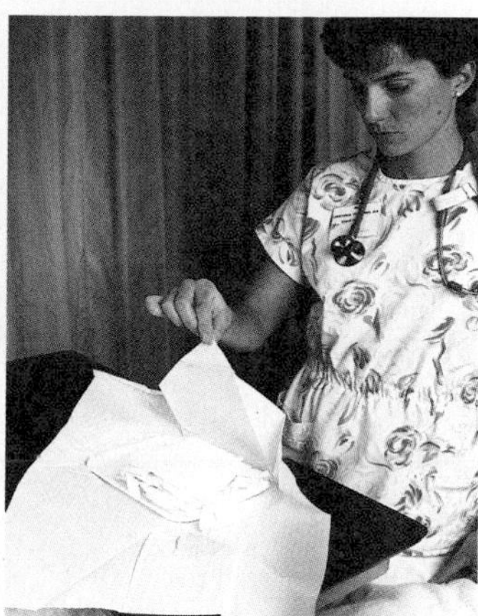

▲ Open last flap toward you—do not cross over sterile field.

Preparing for Dressing Change With Individual Supplies

Equipment

Antiseptic cleaner or cleaning solution
Number and type of dressings needed (i.e., 4 × 4 gauze pads, ABD pads, application sticks, transparent dressings)
Tape
Clean gloves
Sterile gloves
Disposal receptacle
Mask, if needed

Procedure

1. Perform hand hygiene.
2. Clean off bedside stand and wash thoroughly with antiseptic solution. Dry thoroughly.
3. Place supply packages on table in configuration that allows you to open packages without reaching over sterile field. ▸ ***Rationale:*** Reaching over sterile field will contaminate supplies.
4. Grasp cover of 4 × 4 pad plastic container and pull flap back and away from sterile area. Place cover in disposal bag.
5. Grasp edge of transparent dressings package, peel back top covering. Place open package on work surface. Do not cross over any open supply packages.
6. Continue to open all supplies using above steps.
7. Pour solution over pads in plastic container, if ordered.
8. Open sterile gloves. Place in position on table where you do not pass over a sterile field.

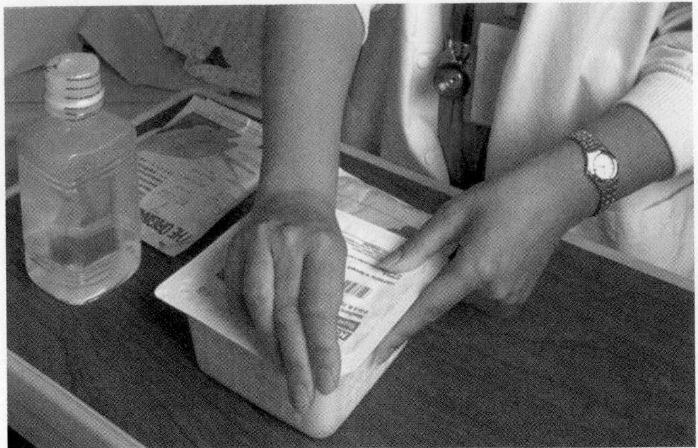

1 Open sterile 4 × 4 pads container by pulling back on flap.

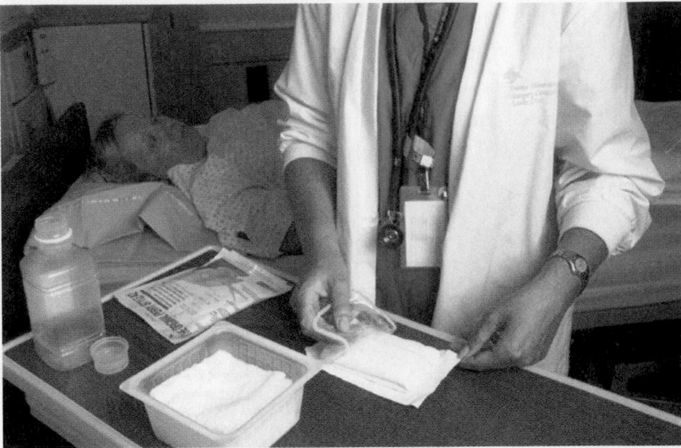

2 Open transparent dressing packet.

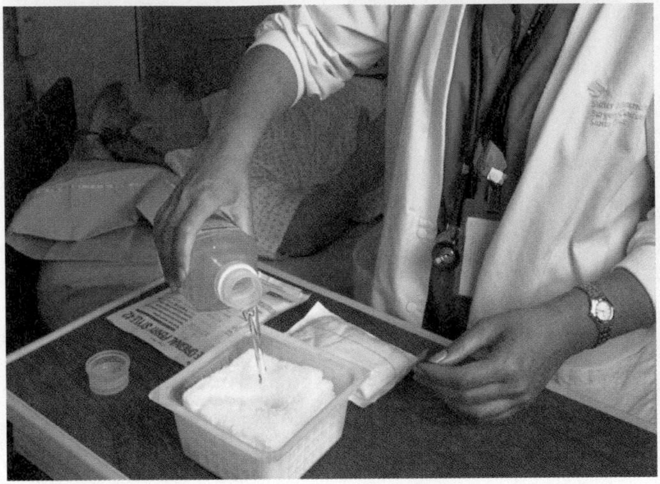

3 Pour cleaning solution over 4 × 4 pads.

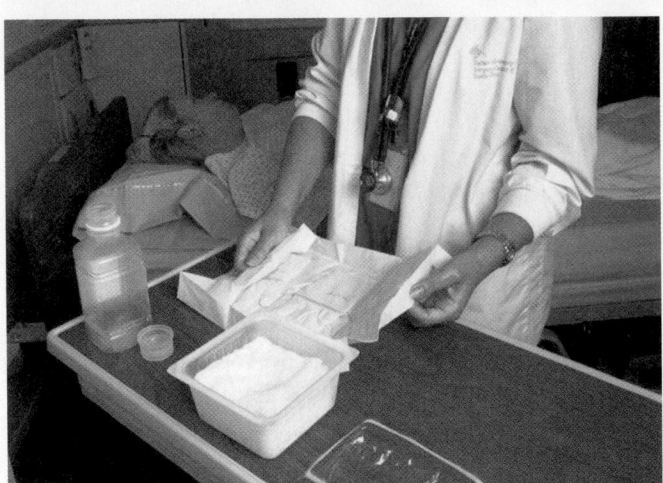

4 Open sterile glove packet on overbed table.

DOCUMENTATION for Measures to Prevent Infection

- Type and number of sterile dressings used
- Antiseptic solution used

CRITICAL THINKING Application

Expected Outcomes

- Infection is prevented in clients with impaired resistance.
- Sterile field is maintained when preparing for dressing change.
- Sterile field is maintained throughout wound care.

Unexpected Outcomes	Alternative Actions
Hole develops in glove while performing sterile technique.	• Discard gloves and replace with sterile gloves.
Sterile field becomes wet or damp.	• Examine hands for cuts if hole caused by sharp object. • If hands are cut, scrub hands and replace sterile gloves. • Discard supplies on sterile field. • Set up new sterile field.

Chapter 25

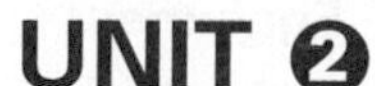

Dressing Change

Nursing Process Data

ASSESSMENT Data Base

- Identify type of dressing required.
- Determine if sutures or staples need to be removed.
- Assess incision for infection.
- Assess extent of healing.
- Assess nutritional status.

PLANNING Objectives

- To promote incision healing
- To prevent wound infection
- To maintain sterility during dressing change
- To remove sutures or staples using appropriate technique

IMPLEMENTATION Procedures

EVALUATION Expected Outcomes

- Client's wounds do not become infected.
- Client's sutures and staples are removed intact.
- Client's wound remains intact after staple and/or suture removal.

Pearson Nursing Student Resources

Find additional review materials at **nursing.pearsonhighered.com**

Prepare for success with NCLEX®-style practice questions and Skill Checklists

Changing a Dry Sterile Dressing

Equipment

Sterile gloves
Clean gloves
Mask
Gown
Disposal receptacle for used dressings
Dressing supplies, as needed
Micropore tape
Sterile normal saline, optional
Package sterile cotton swabs, or 4 × 4 pads
Bath blanket or sheet

Preparation

1. Check physician's orders and client care plan.
2. Perform hand hygiene.
3. Gather equipment.
4. Identify the client and explain procedure.
5. Provide privacy.
6. Clean off overbed table.
7. Place sterile supplies on overbed table.
8. Raise bed to HIGH position and lower side rails, if appropriate.
9. Place bag for soiled dressings near incision site.
10. Fanfold linen to expose incision area.
11. Cover client with bath blanket or sheet, leaving incision area exposed.
12. Open sterile packages and place on overbed table. Arrange packages to ensure you don't cross over the sterile field when reaching for dressings. ▸ ***Rationale:*** Commercially prepared sterile packages can be opened and used for the sterile field because the inside of the package is sterile.
13. Cut tape into appropriate length strips.

Procedure

1. Remove tape slowly by pulling tape toward the wound. ▸ ***Rationale:*** Pulling toward the wound decreases the pain of tape removal by not putting pressure on the incision line.
2. Don clean gloves.
3. Remove soiled dressings and dispose of in the proper receptacle. Wet dressing with sterile normal saline if it adheres to the suture line.
4. Assess incision area for erythema, edema, or drainage. ▸ ***Rationale:*** Persistent drainage, edema, or temperature above 100.4°F 2 days postop indicates a complication is occurring.
5. Assess color of incision. (A healing incision looks pink or red.) ▸ ***Rationale:*** Redness that does not fade 48 hr after surgery may indicate impaired healing.

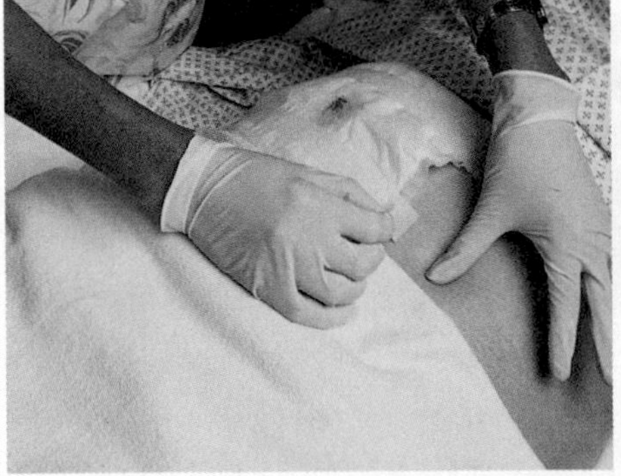
1 Remove tape by gently lifting toward wound.

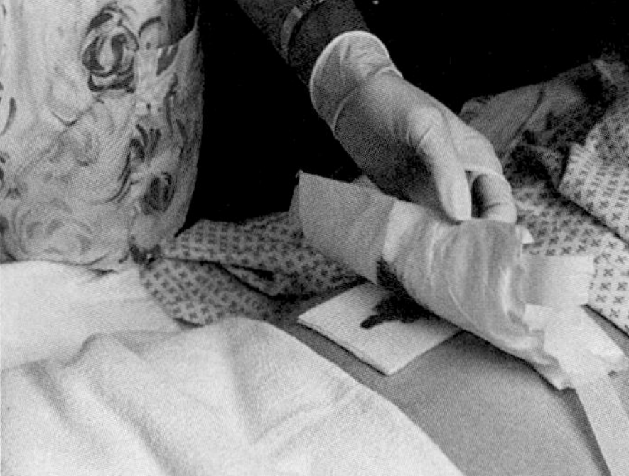
2 Remove soiled dressing carefully.

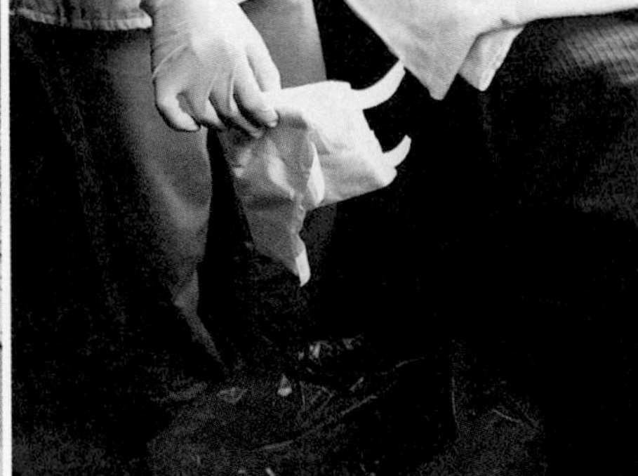
3 Dispose of dressing in appropriate container.

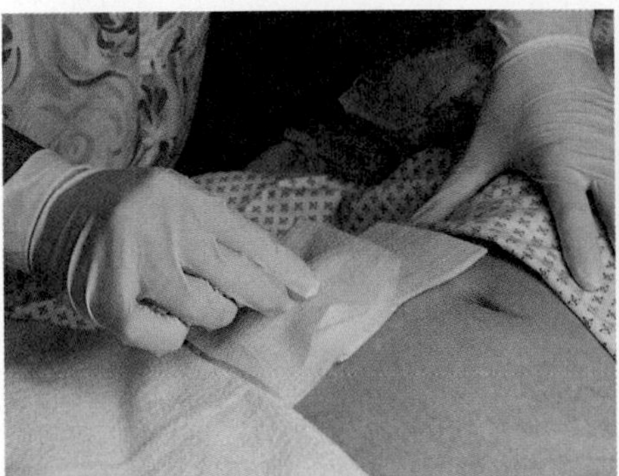
4 Do not touch incision when applying dressing.

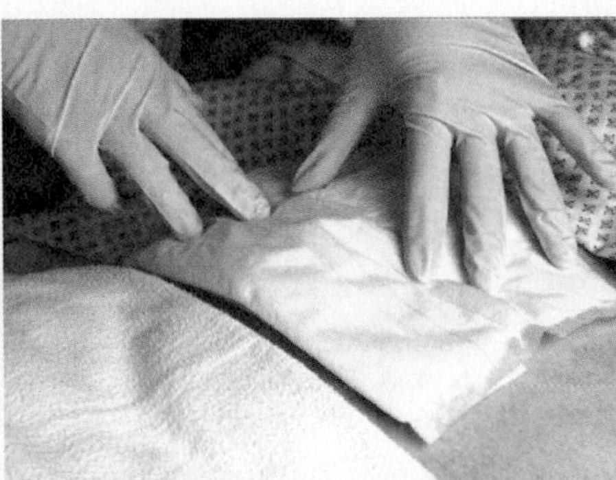
5 Place abdominal pad over center of incision.

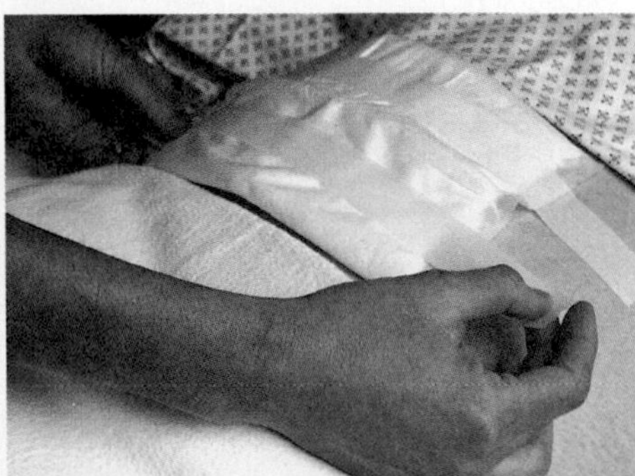
6 Tape dressing securely to prevent slipping.

6. Remove clean gloves, and discard.
7. Move overbed table next to working area.
8. Don sterile gloves.
9. Cleanse incision area with sterile swabs or 4 × 4 pads soaked in normal saline, according to hospital policy. Cleanse from incision line outward, cleaning from top to bottom, using the swab only once. Discard swabs or 4 × 4 pads in disposal bag. ▸ ***Rationale:*** Cleaning outward from incision cleans from least to most contaminated area. Cleaning from top to bottom prevents contamination from secretions that accumulate at the bottom of the wound.
10. Place 4 × 4 gauze pads over incision area, being careful not to touch incision or client with your gloves. ▸ ***Rationale:*** Touching the incision or client contaminates the gloves. You need to reglove if this occurs.
11. Place abdominal pad over incision, being careful not to contaminate the gloves.
12. Remove gloves and discard.
13. Tape dressing securely.
14. Discard trash in appropriate receptacle.
15. Lower bed and raise side rails. Position client for comfort.
16. Perform hand hygiene.

Removing Sutures

Equipment

Sterile suture removal set
Antiseptic solution
Tape
Butterfly tape
Paper bag for disposal of dressings
Two pair clean gloves (one pair optional)

Procedure

1. Gather equipment.
2. Perform hand hygiene and don clean gloves.
3. Remove dressing and discard in disposal bag. (Discard gloves only if soiled.)
4. Open suture removal set, and don gloves if second pair needed.
5. Pick up forceps with nondominant hand.
6. Grasp suture at the knot with forceps and lift away from skin.

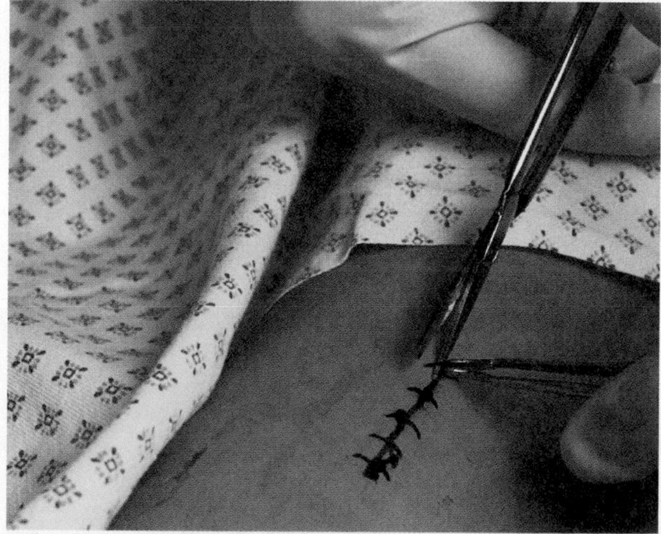

▲ Grasp suture at the knot with forceps and lift away from skin.

Topical Glue for Wound Closure

A new product to replace sutures and staples (estimated at 80–90 million procedures annually) was approved by the U.S. Food and Drug Administration after proving itself in clinical trials. This superglue is called *Dermabond.* It is a synthetic, noninvasive glue that mitigates trauma and post-procedure inflammation while providing a waterproof seal and protecting underlying tissue without the need for bandages. *Dermabond* is also painless, fast and simple to apply, and naturally sloughs off in 7–10 days.

7. Pick up suture scissors with dominant hand.
8. Place curved tip of suture scissors under suture, next to knot.
9. Cut suture, and with forceps, pull suture through skin with one movement.
10. Discard suture into disposal bag.
11. Check that entire suture is removed.

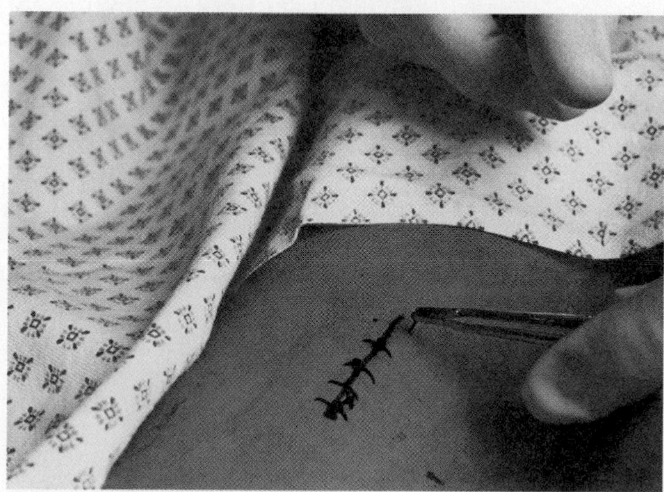

▲ After cutting suture, grasp suture at knot and pull through skin.

12. Continue to remove remaining sutures according to hospital policy. Some policies state that every other suture is removed and then remaining sutures are removed at a later time. ▶ ***Rationale:*** This prevents wound dehiscence.
13. Cleanse suture site with antiseptic solution.
14. Remove gloves and place in disposal bag.
15. Place dressing or butterfly tape over incision area, if ordered.
16. Discard disposal bag into contaminated waste container.
17. Perform hand hygiene.

Removing Staples

Equipment

Sterile staple remover
Disposal receptacle
Two pair clean gloves (one pair optional)
Dressings
Tape or butterfly tape
Antiseptic solution

Procedure

1. Gather equipment and open sterile staple remover.
2. Perform hand hygiene and don clean gloves.
3. Remove dressing and discard in disposal bag. (Discard gloves only if soiled.)
4. Don gloves if necessary.
5. Place lower tip of staple remover under staple.
6. Press handles together to depress center of staple.
7. Lift staple remover upward, away from incision site, when both ends of staple are visible.
8. Place staple removal device over disposal receptacle and release handles to release staple.
9. Remove all staples or as directed by hospital policy. Some policies indicate every other staple is removed

▲ Large abdominal wound with staples closing incision.

Clinical Alert

Steri-strips may be applied over incision to protect incision after staples are removed.

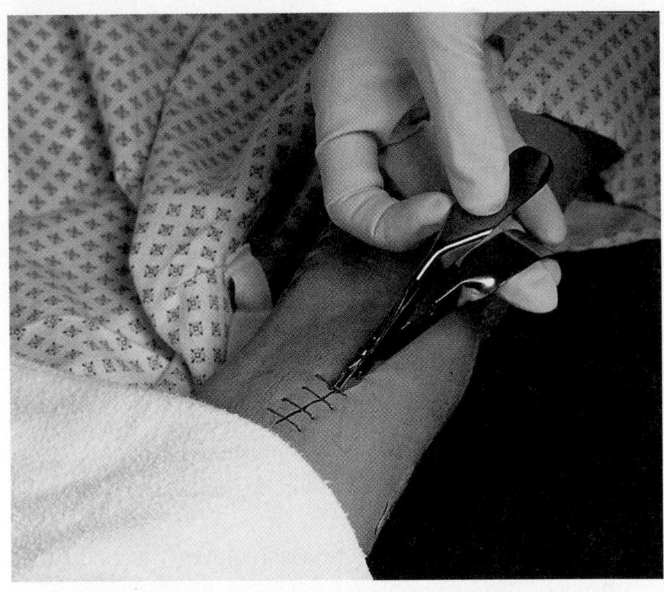

▲ Place lower tip of staple removal device under staple.

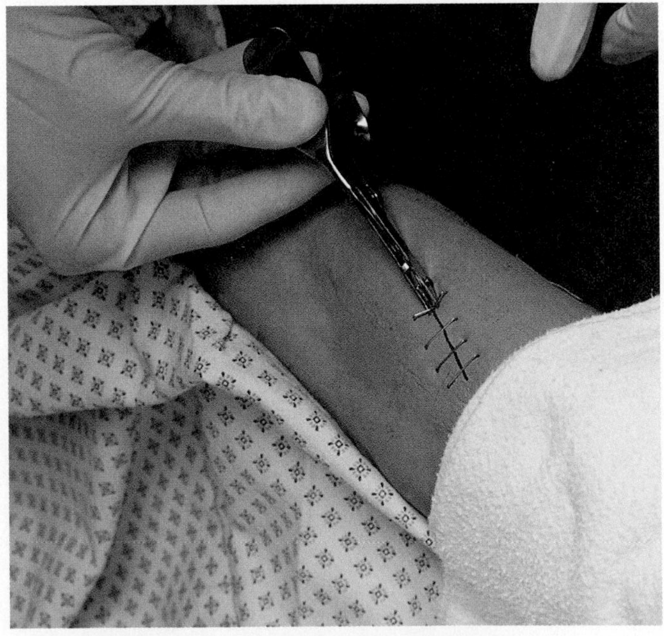

▲ Press handle together to depress center of staple.

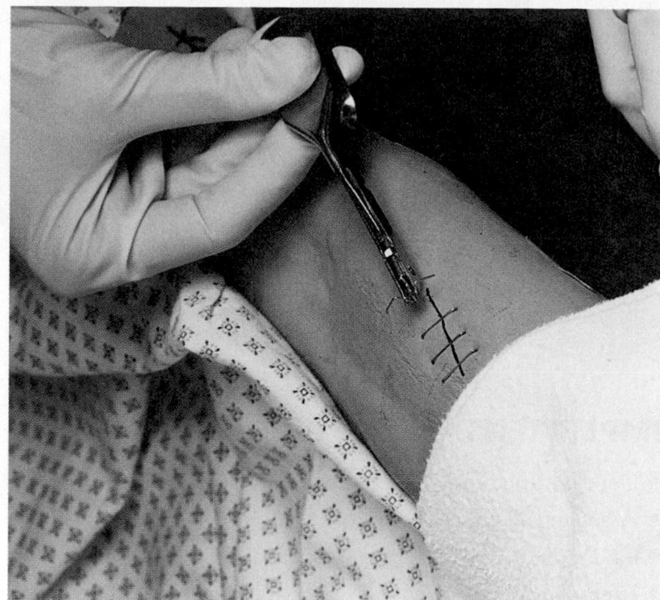

▲ Lift staple remover device upward and away from incision.

with remaining staples done at a later time. ▸ *Rationale:* To prevent wound dehiscence.

10. Cleanse incision area with antiseptic solution if ordered.
11. Remove gloves and place in disposal receptacle.
12. Place dressing over incision and secure with tape, or place butterfly tape over incision.
13. Perform hand hygiene.

Discharge Client Teaching

- Instruct client to eat foods high in protein, carbohydrates, vitamins, and minerals to promote wound healing.
- Splint wound when coughing or moving from chair or bed to prevent separation of wound edges.
- Provide list of signs and symptoms of wound infection or delayed healing. Include when to notify physician.
- Encourage use of daily showers; water may run over wound.
- Instruct not to use soap, lotions, or vitamin creams on incision.
- Instruct in dressing change procedure.
- Instruct to not lift heavy objects (anything over 10 lb).
- Instruct in measures to promote elimination.

DOCUMENTATION for Dressing Change, Removal of Sutures and Staples

- Conditions of suture line
- Presence of exudate or erythema
- Sutures removed
- Staples removed
- Dressing applied, if appropriate

CRITICAL THINKING Application

Expected Outcomes

- Client's wounds do not become infected.
- Client's staples or sutures are removed intact.
- Client's wound remains intact after staple and/or suture removal.

Unexpected Outcomes	Alternative Actions
Wound appears to be infected.	• Obtain order for wound culture. • Obtain order for different type of dressing. • Document observations.
Client complains of fever, pain in incisional area.	• Check incision for edema, erythema, or drainage; wound could be infected.
Wound edges separate when suture or staple is removed.	• Do not continue to remove sutures or staples. • Place Steri-strip over edges. • Notify physician.
Client complains of pain with dressing change.	• Lift small edge of tape or dressing. • Use alcohol pad, wipe area next to dressing with pad. • Remove dressing by wiping, with pad, each time the dressing is lifted up until entire dressing is removed.

Chapter 25

UNIT 3

Wound Care

Nursing Process Data

ASSESSMENT Data Base

- Identify type of dressing needed.
- Assess level of pain associated with wound care and dressing change.
- Assess wound for color, odor, drainage.
- Assess extent of wound.
- Assess type of wound.
- Assess for function of Hemovac or Jackson–Pratt suction.
- Assess for extent of wound healing.
- Assess wound.
- Assess for arterial insufficiency, claudication, pain, ischemic tissue loss, and functional limitations.
- Assess for suture site infections.

PLANNING Objectives

- To assess wound appropriately
- To assess for arterial sufficiency
- To promote wound healing by first or second intention
- To prevent microorganisms from entering the wound
- To decrease the presence of purulent wound drainage
- To maintain sterility during a dressing change
- To maintain patency of Hemovac or Jackson–Pratt suction
- To immobilize and support a wound
- To assist in removal of necrotic tissue
- To apply medication to wound
- To pack a wound to promote granulation of tissue
- To identify potential surgical site infections

IMPLEMENTATION Procedures

EVALUATION Expected Outcomes

- Wound care is provided for contaminated wound and healing occurs.
- Drainage system functions without obstructions.
- Wound irrigation is completed using sufficient pressure to cleanse wound bed.
- Abdominal binder supports client's abdominal wound.
- Compression dressing applied to vascular ulcer site.

Determining Surgical Site Infections (SSIs)

Procedure

1. Before surgery assess client for risk factors associated with surgical site infections (SSIs).
   a. Complete health history and physical assessment.
   b. Obtain information on all medications currently taking.
   c. Determine whether client is allergic to specific medications.
   d. Review lab values.
2. Determine whether client has a preexisting viral or bacterial infection. ▸ ***Rationale:*** If the answer is yes, the client is at an increased risk for SSI.
   a. Clients who must undergo surgery even with existing infections must be monitored closely postoperatively.
   b. Clients scheduled for routine surgery should be treated first and then rescheduled for surgery once the infection is cleared.
3. Check that client does not have nasal bacterial colonization. ▸ ***Rationale:*** Clients with positive anterior nares cultures of *S. aureus* should receive a topical antibiotic ointment mupirocin before surgical intervention. (More research is needed before this becomes a standard of practice).
4. Complete a nutritional assessment and review lab findings for serum albumin, prealbumin, serum transferring, and total lymphocyte levels. ▸ ***Rationale:*** Malnutrition in hospitalized adults is common and can prolong postoperative wound healing, increasing the risk of SSI. The client may need enteral or parenteral nutrition postoperatively.
5. Diabetic clients with an elevated fasting serum glucose are at higher risk than other diabetic clients for SSIs due to the high glucose levels. ▸ ***Rationale:*** High glucose levels impair phagocytosis, which affects the body's normal defense mechanisms. The client's serum glucose level must be kept below 200 mg/dL during and after surgery to prevent an SSI.

Advancing age does increase the risk of SSI. One study showed that elderly clients who developed SSIs after orthopedic surgery were at increased risk for death within the first year postoperatively. Clients with COPD and obesity were at higher risk for SSIs after cardiothoracic and neurologic surgery. Clients who used (or use) nicotine exhibit slow wound healing, leading to SSIs. Obese clients are at higher risk for SSIs due to their inability to ambulate, move in bed, and complete postoperative exercises. Obesity can lead to a disruption of sutures due to increased stress on the adipose tissue.

It is imperative that these clients be monitored closely for signs and symptoms indicating an SSI could be occurring.

6. Clients with chronic illnesses such as hypertension and other uncontrolled conditions are at high risk for SSIs and must be monitored carefully after surgery. It is preferable to get the conditions under control before surgery is considered.
7. Determine whether client was instructed to perform a preoperative skin cleansing at home. ▸ ***Rationale:*** The CDC strongly recommends a preventative home cleansing be done for high-risk clients for SSIs. Chlorhexidine gluconate is the most effective cleaning agent in decreasing the microbial count.
8. Check that client has not shaved the surgical site. The CDC recommends that hair be left on client's skin unless it interferes with the surgical procedure. If clipping of the hair is required, the OR staff will complete the clipping. ▸ ***Rationale:*** Shaving can lead to nicks in the surgical site, predisposing it to an SSI.
9. Check that the client has an antibiotic order for 1 hr before surgery or, if vancomycin is ordered 2 hr before surgery.

Assessing a Wound

Equipment

Pliable disposable measuring device/grid
Cotton-tipped applicator sticks
Saline-filled syringe
Plastic disposal bag or receptacle
Clean gloves
Sterile gloves if necessary

Preparation

1. Obtain health history, medical diagnosis, and physical examination data from chart or obtain missing information. The health history must include information on the following:
   a. Initialing event and duration of wound.
   b. Previous treatments, if any, and the outcome of treatments.
   c. Current medical diagnosis, including all disease processes. ▸ ***Rationale:*** Diseases that affect circulation and perfusion of blood can interfere with nutrition and oxygenation of cells. Infection and wounds can result from this pathology.
   d. Medications, both past and current, including anticoagulants, corticosteroids, immunosuppressives,

Nutrients for Wound Healing

- Protein
- Carbohydrates
- Fats
- Iron
- Zinc
- Copper
- Arginine
- Vitamin A
- Vitamin C
- Vitamin K
- Pyridoxine
- Riboflavin
- Thiamine
- Glutamine

and antineoplastics. ▶ ***Rationale:*** These drugs may adversely affect wound healing.

e. Nutrition and hydration status: Check for signs of malnutrition and assess hydration status of client. ▶ ***Rationale:*** Malnutrition leads to poor cell growth and repair. Both dehydration and overhydration lead to impaired oxygen and nutrient transportation.

f. Laboratory data evaluation: albumin, serum total protein, serum transferrin, and total lymphocyte count. ▶ ***Rationale:*** These lab values are used to determine nutritional status and potential for wound healing.

2. Determine type of wound (acute or chronic) and cause of wound. ▶ ***Rationale:*** This information is used to evaluate healing process.
3. Evaluate severity of pain.
4. Perform hand hygiene and don gloves.

NOTE: Acute wounds progress through normal process of wound healing in about 1 month. Chronic wounds do not go through normal wound healing phases. Wounds that do not heal within 1 month should be considered chronic.

Procedure

1. Assess location of wound. ▶ ***Rationale:*** Location influences rate of healing. Lower body heals more slowly.
2. Assess size of wound: length, width, and depth.
3. Observe color of wound: if using this classification.
   a. Black: necrotic tissue/black eschar (inhibits formation of granulation tissue)
   b. Yellow: presence of exudate or slough; pus, fibrin, debris (will advance to eschar), requires cleaning
   c. Red: indicates wound ready to heal (granulation tissue present)

Clinical Alert

Cephalosporins are the drug of choice as prophylaxis for most wound infections. First- or second-generation drugs such as cefazolin or cefoxitin are used for colon surgery clients. Cephalosporins have a broad spectrum of activity against both gram-positive (gram +) and gram-negative (gram –) bacteria and a wide ratio of therapeutic to toxic dosages. Allergic reactions are rare to these drugs.

4. Assess odor of wound.
   a. Foul: infected (necrotic tissue has an odor even if not infected)
   b. Sweet: *Pseudomonas* infection
5. Assess level of moisture in wound. (A moist environment allows wound to heal without forming a scab.)
6. Assess wound exudate.
   a. Type: dry or moist
   b. Amount: minimum, moderate, maximum (copious)
   c. Color of drainage: clear (serous), brown-brown/yellow (slough), yellow-yellow/green (pus from strep, staph), blue-green (*Pseudomonas*)
7. Assess tissue viability.
   a. Presence of granulation tissue; red, moist, beefy appearance.
   b. Presence of epithelialized tissue; new pink, shiny epidermis.
   c. Absence of necrotic tissue; slough of yellow, gray. Green and brown color or eschar of hard, black, leathery tissue.
8. Assess periwound condition.
   a. Skin nutrition: loss of hair, thickening of nails, atrophy.
   b. Edema of skin or scaly skin.
   c. Skin hydration: skin turgor indicates hydration or dehydration.
   d. Areas of inflammation surrounding wound.
   e. Skin integrity: maceration, induration, crepitus, hematoma, blisters.
   f. Color: red (inflammation), white (arterial insufficiency), blue (cyanosis, severe arterial insufficiency), black (necrosis), brown (venous insufficiency).
   g. Skin temperature: cool, cold, warm, normal temperature.
9. Assess extent of pain, if present.
   a. Determine whether pain is present during dressing change only or constant.
   b. Use pain scale to determine severity of pain.
   c. Observe for signs of infection.
   d. Arterial insufficiency wounds are very painful.
   e. Venous insufficiency wounds are relatively pain-free.
10. Measure the length and width of wound using a disposable measuring device/grid. Measure in centimeters (cm).
11. Measure depth of wound by placing a sterile cotton-tipped applicator stick into wound in several areas. Measure depth of each area using measuring device/grid. Measure in centimeters (cm).
12. Check for undermining and/or tunneling or sinus tracts by placing a sterile cotton-tipped applicator stick into

Clinical Alert

Moist wound environment is essential for healing without a scab. Epithelial tissue will not migrate into wounds with necrotic tissue or if deprived of oxygen.

suspected areas. Gently probe margins of lesion for extensions into surrounding tissue (undermining) and beyond wound base (sinus tract).

13. Evaluate laboratory values.
    a. Increased white blood cell count indicates infection, usually before other signs and symptoms are evident.
    b. Low hemoglobin and hematocrit indicates anemia, which can decrease oxygen transport to the wound.
    c. Altered serum glucose levels may indicate presence of diabetes mellitus, which interferes with normal wound healing.
14. Evaluate client's stress level. Increased stress leads to hypermetabolic states, which uses up oxygen and nutrients and affects wound healing.
15. Complete skill by following appropriate steps described in skill Changing a Wound Dressing.
16. Document findings and notify physician of any changes or unusual findings in the assessment.

TABLE 25-3 Moisture-Retentive Dressings

	Advantages	Disadvantages	Clinical Use
Transparent Adhesive Film	• Transparency allows wound visualization but is nonabsorptive • Conforms to area of application • Can reduce friction of area • Promotes autolysis of dry eschar • Semipermeable vapor can escape and environmental oxygen can enter to reduce chance of anaerobic bacterial growth • Barrier to bacterial invasion; can aspirate fluid and patch • Does not require secondary dressing	• Does *not* absorb exudate • Exudate may macerate skin around wound • Edges will roll in friction area • May be difficult to apply • May be too tightly applied • Removal may tear underlying skin • May increase bacterial growth in infected wounds	• Pressure ulcers, stage I and II • Donor sites • Abrasions • Partial-thickness wound with little or no exudate • Wound without necrotic tissue or slough • Extend edge to minimum $1^{1}/_{4}$ in. beyond wound; skin around wound must be dry for adhesion; apply without tension • Change when fluid buildup and leaking occurs and when edges are loosening to potentially expose wound
Hydrogel	• Comes in sheets or gel to conform to the wound • May have soothing and coating effect • Absorbs some exudate • Soften slough or eschar in necrotic wounds • Can be used when infection is present • Provides moist wound healing • Rehydrates dry wound beds	• Expensive • Held in place with gauze dressing or transparent film • May have transparent film on both sides (film next to wound must be removed)	• Wounds with necrosis and slough • Partial thickness (use sheets) • Gel can be used to fill wound cavity • Change every day or twice a day—based on wound exudate
Hydrocolloids	• Use on acute and chronic wounds • Absorbs exudate in limited capacity • Conforms to area • Prevents bacterial invasion • Occlusive or semiocclusive dressings	• Not transparent • Melts down with exudate • Characteristic drainage and odor • Edges may need to be taped to prevent rolling • Most do *not* allow environmental oxygen, so growth of anaerobic bacteria may be a problem • Cannot be used for infected wounds	• Noninfected dermal ulcers • May leave in place up to 7 days • Change if leaking • Change if clinical signs of infection • Cleanse wound before application • Roll dressing over wound • Do *not* stretch; press securely

Changing a Wound Dressing

Equipment

Sterile, prepackaged dressing(s) as needed
Tape; micropore, paper, or Montgomery tie tapes
Clean gloves
Sterile gloves
Sterile normal saline irrigation solution or commercially prepared cleansing spray
Wound culture media, as needed
Plastic bag
Bath blanket or sheet
Emesis basin

Preparation

1. Complete steps in Assessing a Wound.
2. Check physician's orders and client care plan.
3. Perform hand hygiene.
4. Gather equipment.
5. Identify the client, using two forms of identification, and explain procedure.
6. Provide privacy.
7. Clean off overbed table.

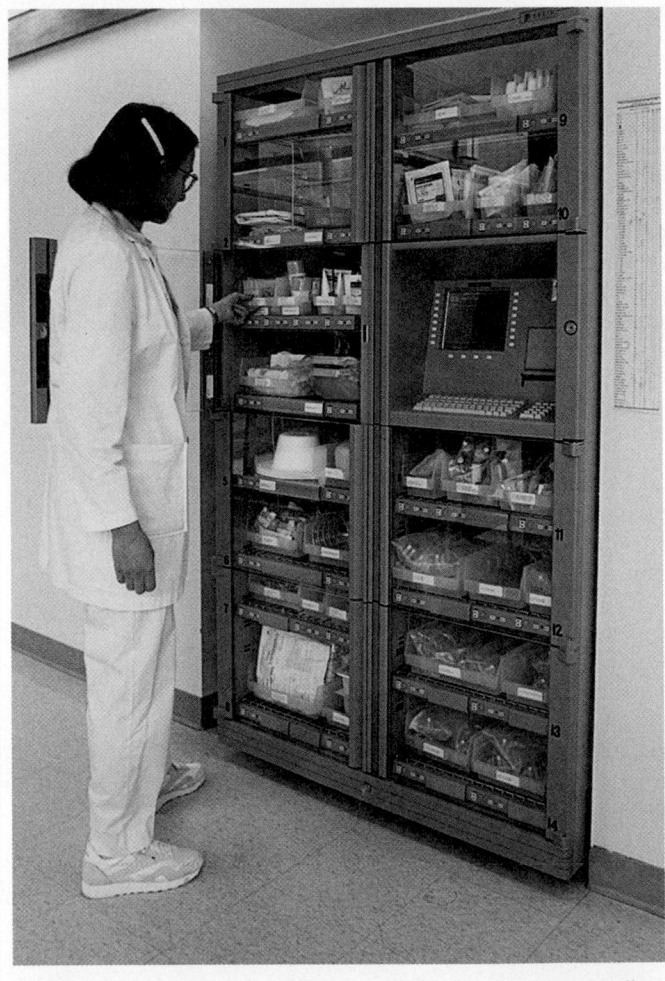

▲ PYXIS supply station provides easy access for dressing supplies.

> **Clinical Alert**
> Gauze dressings do not support healing or prevent entry of exogenous bacteria.

> **Clinical Alert**
> Normal saline or Ringer's solution are widely advocated as fluids of choice for cleansing and irrigating wounds. Iodine and chlorhexidine are cytotoxic, particularly to fibroblasts. In severely infected wounds, antimicrobial irrigations may be used.
>
> Povidone iodine, hydrogen peroxide, Dakin's solution, and other agents are not used on acute wounds. They are drying agents and as such, the wound bed is dried, and the exudate and all its beneficial cells are removed from the area. Wounds maintained in a moist environment have a lower infection rate than dry wounds.

8. Place sterile supplies on the over-bed table.
9. Raise bed to HIGH position, and lower side rails on working side of bed, if necessary.
10. Place bag for soiled dressings near wound site.
11. Open sterile packages and place on overbed table. Arrange packages to ensure that you don't cross over the sterile field when using dressings. ▸ ***Rationale:*** Commercially prepared sterile packages can be opened and used for the sterile field; the inside of the package is sterile.
12. Fanfold linens to expose wound site.
13. Cover client with bath blanket or sheet, leaving wound area exposed.
14. Cut tape into appropriate strips.

Procedure

1. Remove tape slowly by pulling tape toward the wound. ▸ ***Rationale:*** Pulling toward the wound decreases the pain of tape removal by not putting pressure on the incision line.
2. Don clean gloves.
3. Remove soiled dressings, and dispose of in bag. Soaking dressings that are dried to skin or incision with sterile normal saline prevents tissue damage and pain when dressings are removed.
4. Obtain wound specimen for culture if ordered.
5. Remove clean gloves and discard into plastic bag.
6. Bring overbed table close to working area.
7. Open sterile saline solution or commercially prepared cleansing spray and pour over wound. Place emesis basin next to skin surface to catch overflow.
8. Don sterile gloves.
9. Form a ball with gauze pads by tucking all four corners together. Use the center of gauze pads to cleanse the

How to Obtain a Wound Culture

- Rinse wound thoroughly with sterile saline.
- Use non–cotton-tipped swab.
- Rotate swab while obtaining specimen.
- Swab edges starting at top, crisscross wound to bottom.
- Do not take specimen from exudate or eschar.
- Place swab in culture medium and take to laboratory immediately.

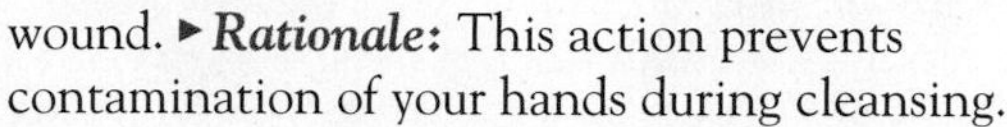

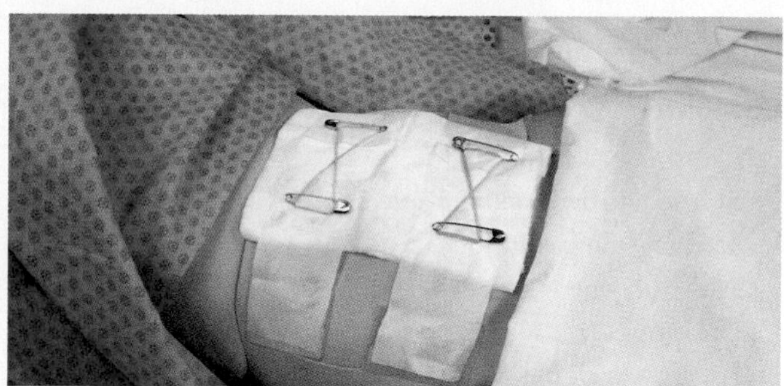

▲ Montgomery straps are used to prevent skin irritation when frequent dressing changes are required.

Use of Antimicrobial Agents in Wound Care

Antiseptics and antibiotics are two types of antimicrobial agents used in wound care management. Antiseptics, unlike antibiotics, cannot be used exclusively to kill bacteria. Systemic antibiotics should be used only to treat wound infections; however, wounds that have impaired blood flow will not receive the systemic antibiotics. Topical antibiotics are used only for a limited time with infected wounds. These agents are not used as preventative measures; they are used when infection is present.

Antiseptics return the wound back to bacterial balance, promoting wound healing. Cadexomer iodine gel is used to absorb wound exudates and assists in autolytic debridement. Silver nitrate and sulfadiazine are used against many antibiotic-resistant strains of bacteria, as they reduce the number of viable bacteria.

wound. ▸ ***Rationale:*** This action prevents contamination of your hands during cleansing.

10. Cleanse wound. When cleansing an area, always start at the cleanest area and work away from that area. Never return to an area you have previously cleaned. Usually start at top of wound and work toward bottom. ▸ ***Rationale:*** Prevents contamination of area.
11. Assess the wound, measure, identify type, and determine whether signs of infection are present. ▸ ***Rationale:*** This allows nurse to determine most effective treatment and type of dressing to be used.
12. Cleanse under the drain and around the site with a 4 × 4 gauze pad and cleansing solution if a drain is present. Do not use a cytotoxic or dangerous chemical. ▸ ***Rationale:*** These agents may harm granulating tissue.
13. Place several gauze pads under the drain.
14. Place several 4 × 4 gauze pads by placing at wound center, extending at least 1 in. (2.5 cm) beyond wound. Loosely pack a tunneling area of wound if present before filling the base of the wound. Cover with an ABD pad if necessary; remove gloves, and tape securely. Montgomery straps (tie tapes) may be used if frequent dressing changes are required or the client has sensitive skin. ▸ ***Rationale:*** Once a dressing has been placed over the wound, it is not to be moved and readjusted, as microorganisms from the skin could be introduced into the wound.
15. Use skin sealants or moisture barrier ointments on intact skin and moisture-retentive dressing over 4 × 4 gauze pad and even over ABD, if used. ▸ ***Rationale:*** Moisture-retentive dressings are flexible and water resistant, which allows clients to move freely and take showers without disturbing the dressing.
16. Cover client.
17. Close the plastic bag and dispose of bag as isolation material.
18. Remove gloves and perform hand hygiene thoroughly.
19. Check with client to see that he or she is comfortable before leaving room.
20. Lower the bed and raise the side rail, according to facility policy.

EVIDENCE-BASED PRACTICE

Maintaining a Moist Environment

Dressings that promote a moist wound environment stimulate rapid wound healing. Saline soaks are not as effective as moisture-retentive dressings. The type of dressing used is dependent on the type of wound, whether infected or if debris is present, amount of exudates, cost, and client comfort.

Source: The Joanna Briggs Institute. www.joannabriggs.edu.au.

Packing a Wound

Equipment

Dressing pack, optional
Sterile narrow packing gauze or 4 × 4 gauze pads
Normal saline solution
Alcohol wipe
Dressings
Forceps, optional
Sterile scissors
Paper tape
Montgomery tapes
Plastic bag or receptacle
Clean gloves
Sterile gloves

Procedure

1. Follow steps in Preparation for Changing a Wound Dressing.
2. Determine client's need for pain medication before beginning procedure. ▸ ***Rationale:*** Pain can be present particularly when removing old packing that may have become attached to the tissue.
3. Perform hand hygiene, don clean gloves, and place plastic bag near wound site.
4. Remove tape slowly by pulling tape toward wound.
5. Remove soiled dressings and dispose of dressings and packing into plastic bag. Moisten packing with sterile saline solution if dry.
6. Assess wound site.
   a. Identify location of wound.
   b. Observe wound bed and appearance.
   c. Check wound size, shape, depth, and margins.
   d. Observe exudates or drainage.
   e. Evaluate presence of pain.
7. Remove clean gloves and discard.
8. Don sterile gloves.
9. Clean wound with saline solution and pat wound dry with 4 × 4 gauze pads.
10. Place packing material in wound; pack lightly, filling tunneling or undermined areas. Forceps can be used to place packing material into corners and wound areas hard to reach. ▸ ***Rationale:*** Pack lightly to prevent wound margins from contracting. Wound packing is used to facilitate healing by secondary intention. Type of packing material is dependent on type of wound and material available. Gauze pads should be moistened before packing.
11. Cut ribbon gauze with sterile scissors and leave small wick exposed, if used for packing.
12. Cover packing with dressing and tape securely.
13. Dispose of used packing and gloves.
14. Perform hand hygiene.
15. Position client for comfort.

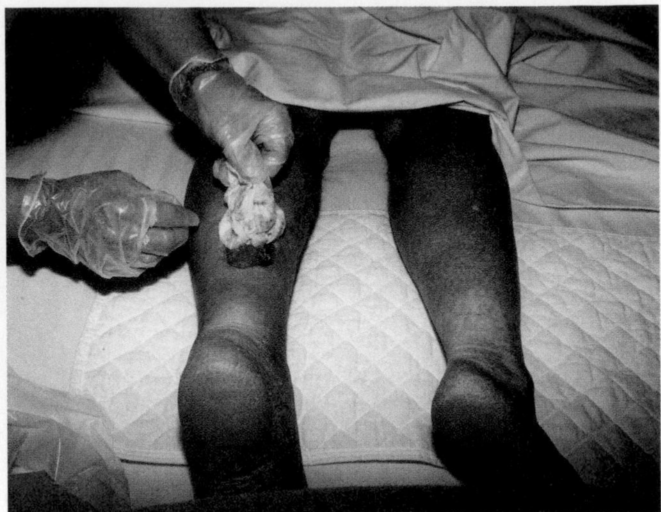

▲ Pack wound dressing in all tunneling and undermined areas.

EVIDENCE-BASED PRACTICE

Medieval Remedies

Medieval remedies, like maggots for bedsores, bee stings for MS, and leeches to improve blood flow after surgery, are enjoying a renaissance.

Leeches reemerged a while ago and now have a well-established role in plastic and reconstructive surgery. Maggots are being considered more often for treatment of chronic wounds that do not heal. Bee venom is also considered an alternative medicine.

Maggots do a better job than more conservative therapy for pressure ulcer treatment. Physicians who use maggots in their practice say they like them because they work.

Source: Graninger, M., Grassberger, M., Galehr, E., Huemer, F., Gruschina, E., Minar, E., & Graninger, W. (2002). Biosurgical debridement facilitates healing of chronic skin ulcers. (2002). *Archives of Internal Medicine, 162*(16), 1906–1907.

Assessing a Venous Ulcer

Equipment

Blood pressure cuff and stethoscope
Dressings
Chux
Clean gloves (two pair)
Sterile normal saline
Scissors, if needed

Procedure

1. Perform hand hygiene.
2. Don clean gloves.
3. Identify client using two forms of identification and explain procedure.
4. Place Chux under leg.
5. Remove dressings and discard into trash bag.
6. Cleanse site with normal saline as needed.
7. Remove gloves and don new gloves.
8. Observe lower leg. ▸ ***Rationale:*** The medial malleolus is the usual site for ulcer area.
9. Observe surrounding area of ulcer for:
   a. Dilated veins.
   b. Edema.
   c. Maceration.
   d. Hyperpigmentation.
   e. Eczematous skin change: scaling, pruritic, erythema, and vesicle.
   f. Atrophic blanch (white plaques with dot-like capillaries).
   g. Scarring from prior healed ulcers (lipodermatosclerosis).
10. Complete a pain assessment. ▸ ***Rationale:*** Deep ulcers are most painful.
11. Check wound bed for "ruddy" or "beefy-red" granular appearance.
12. Observe for flat, irregular wound margins without undermining.
13. Assess amount of drainage and exudates (may be heavy to moderate).
14. Complete an ankle–brachial index (ABI) to check for arterial insufficiency. See p. 915 for skill.

TABLE 25-4 Comparison of Arterial and Venous Ulcers

Differentiation	Arterial	Venous
Predisposing factors	Peripheral vascular disease Atherosclerosis Diabetes mellitus Advanced age Raynaud's syndrome	Valve incompetence in vein History of DVT Obesity Advanced age
Anatomic location	Between toes or tips of toes Over phalangeal heads Around lateral malleolus Area subjected to trauma	Medial distal lower leg and ankle Malleolar area
Wound characteristics	Even around margins Gangrene or necrosis Black eschar Deep, pale wound bed Blanched or purpuric periwound tissue Severe pain Cellulitis Minimal exudate	Irregular wound margins Superficial to deep wounds "Ruddy" granular tissue Minimal to moderate pain Minimal to moderate pain Moderate to heavy exudate

Changing a Dressing—Venous Ulcer

Equipment

Cleansing solution
Normal saline solution
Sterile 4 × 4 dressings
Moisture-retentive dressings (hydrocolloid, transparent film or foam for light-to-moderate drainage)
Absorbent dressings (foams, alginates, and absorptive dressings) for moderate to heavy exudate
Compression dressing
Clean gloves
Sterile gloves
Biohazard bag
Scissors
Absorbent pad

Preparation

1. Perform hand hygiene.
2. Gather equipment.
3. Explain procedure to client.
4. Provide privacy for client.
5. Raise bed to HIGH position and lower side rails.
6. Open sterile packages and arrange on overbed table.
7. Place absorbent pad under wound.

Procedure

1. Don clean gloves.
2. Remove compression bandage and old dressing and place in biohazard bag. Compression dressings may be left in place for 3–7 days depending on amount of drainage and type of dressing.

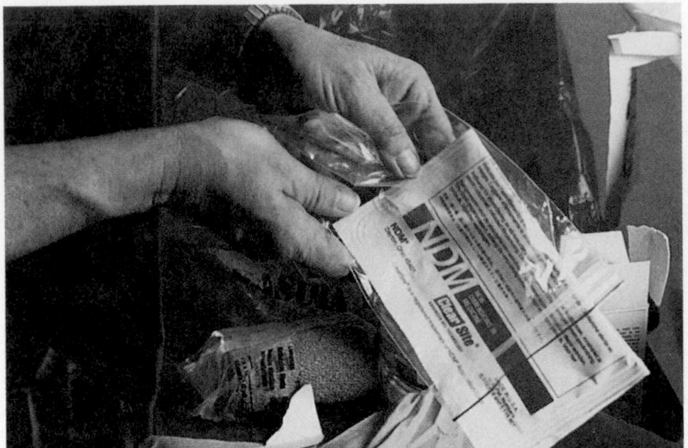

1 Obtain appropriate wound dressing kit, if available.

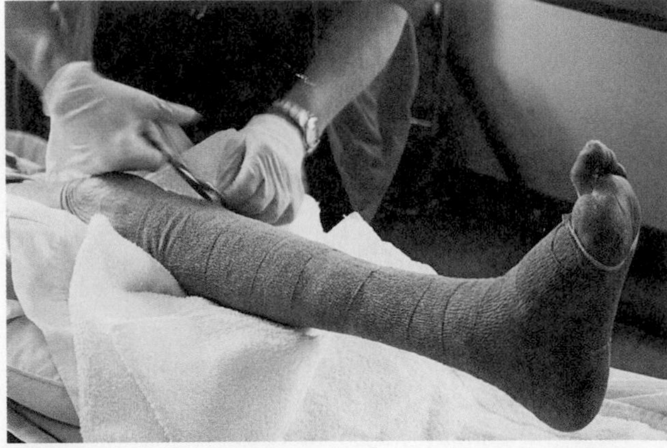
2 Remove compression dressing, being careful not to cut skin.

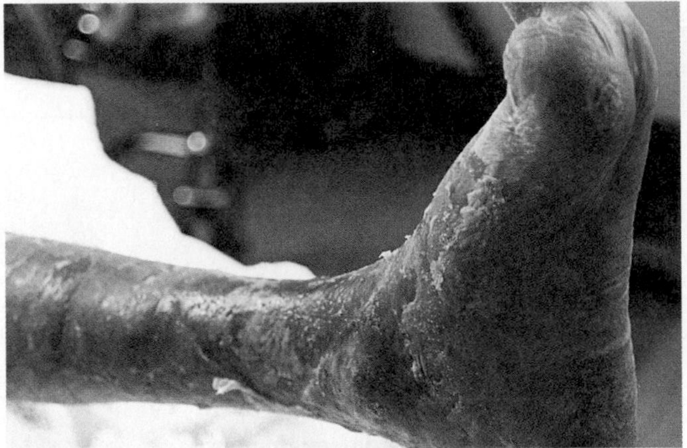
3 Assess wound healing and evaluate progress (stage II).

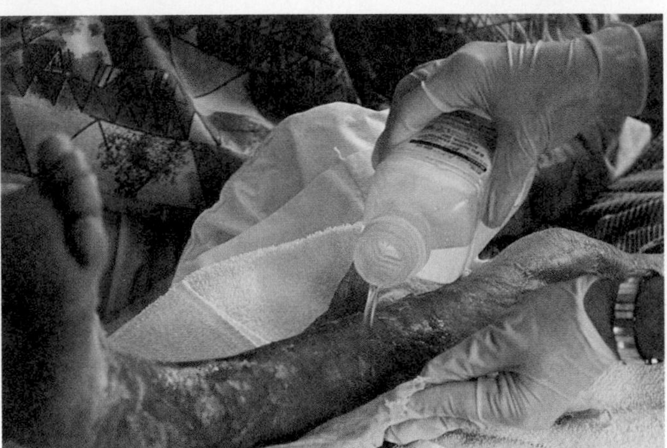
4 Pour normal saline solution over wound to clean off debris.

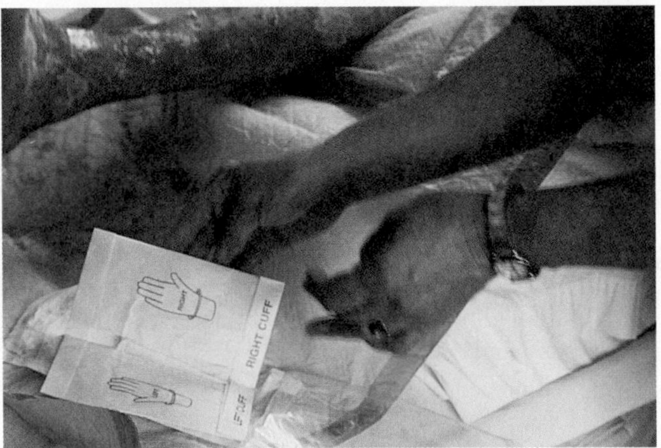

5 Don sterile gloves before cleaning wound with 4 × 4 gauze pads.

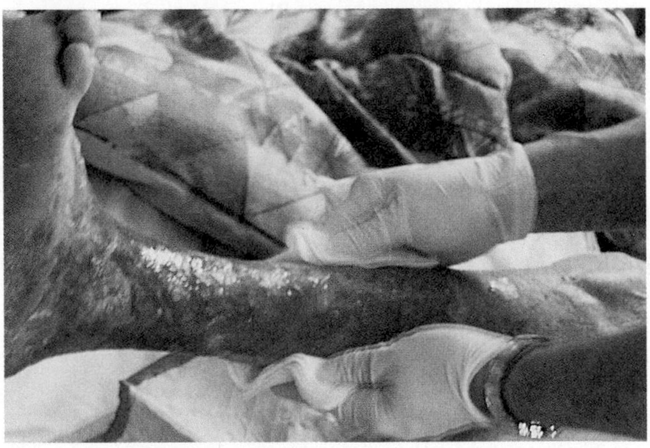
6 Dry with 4 × 4 gauze pad after cleansing.

3. Assess and measure wound. ▶ ***Rationale:*** This determines effectiveness of treatment.
4. Cleanse off debris by pouring cleansing solution over wound.
5. Rinse wound with sterile normal saline.
6. Debride wound, if ordered, using one of the following methods:
   a. Autolytic: Applying occlusive dressings that assist in maintaining a moist wound environment, therefore promoting reepithelialization. ▶ ***Rationale:*** Autolytic

uses body's own enzymes and moisture to rehydrate, moisten, and slough tissue.

b. Chemical: Apply enzyme debriding agents (Accuzyme, collagenase, papain, etc.).

NOTE: The major disadvantage of this method is that viable tissue is removed with necrotic tissue.

Clinical Alert

The wound bed should be kept moist to promote granulation and reepithelialization and to reduce pain. Ointments provide the most occlusive moisturizer because they contain oil and water.

c. Mechanical: Apply wet-to-dry dressings, use hydrotherapy, irrigation.

7. Dry wound using sterile 4 × 4 dressings. Place in biohazard bag.
8. Remove gloves, and don sterile gloves.
9. Apply medicated moisturizer over wound, if ordered.
   ▸ ***Rationale:*** This keeps wound area moist.

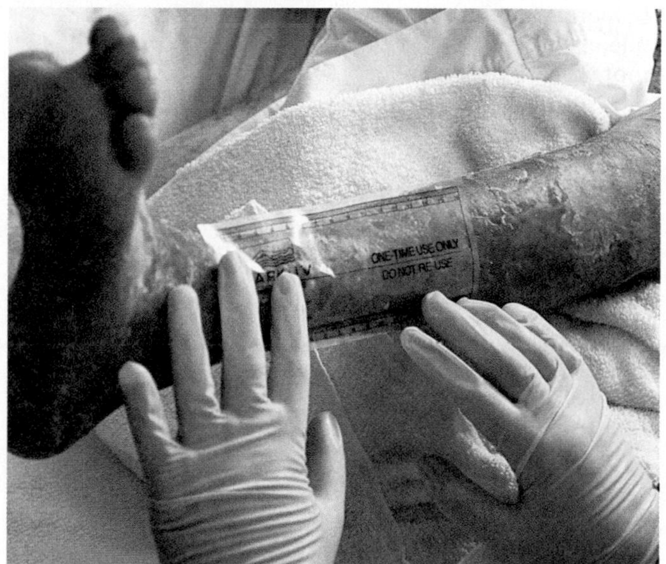

7 Measure wound to evaluate effectiveness of treatment.

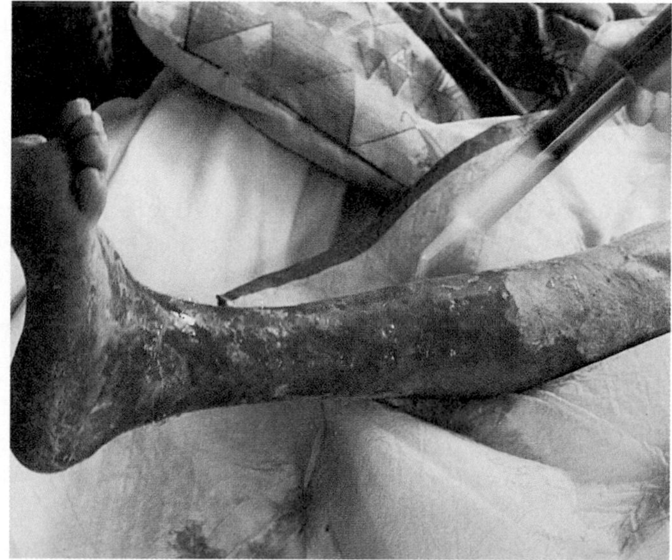
8 Apply medicated moisturizer on wound, if ordered.

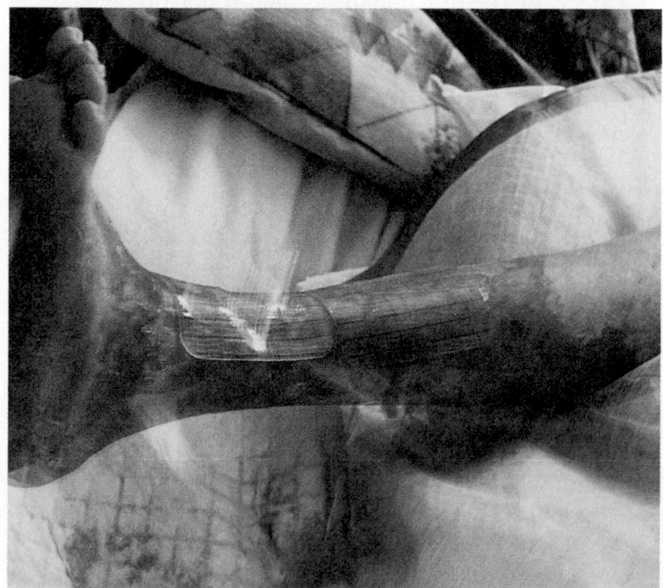
9 Apply moisture-retentive dressing over wound site.

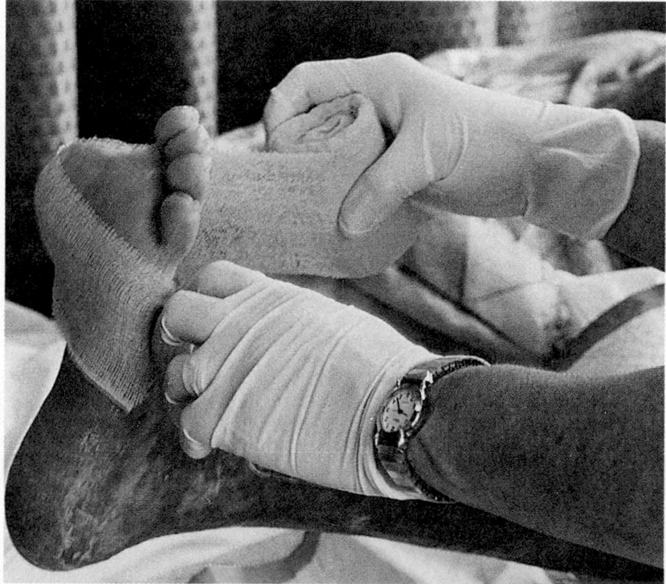
10 Apply compression dressing for venous or lymphatic conditions.

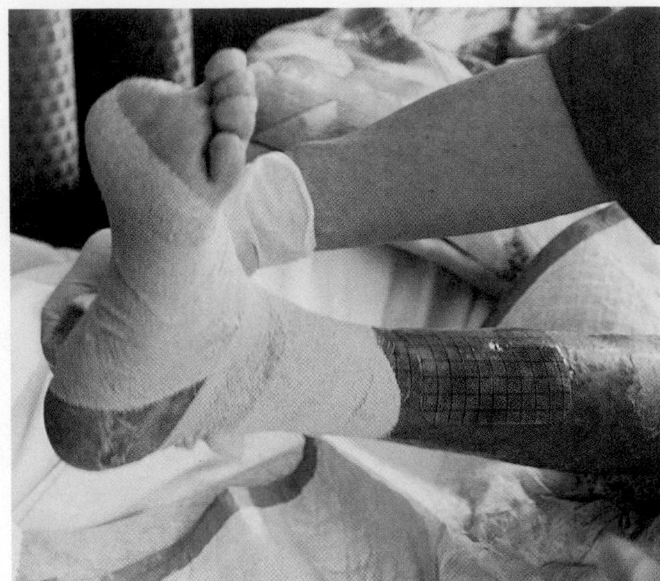

Cover entire area with compression dressing.

10. Remove backing on moisture-retentive dressing and place over open wound site. These dressings prevent entry of bacteria from surface of dressing.
11. Palpate arterial system; dorsalis pedis, posterior, or tibial pulse. If pulses are nonpalpable, obtain an Ankle-Brachial Index (ABI).
12. Apply compression dressing if ABI is greater than 0.6. ▸ ***Rationale:*** Effective compression bandages generate 40–70 mmHg of pressure. If arterial insufficiency is present, another ulcer can occur.

NOTE: Medicinal maggots were originally used in the 1930s. In the past 10 years they have been reintroduced, now used to debride or eliminate necrotic tissue and remove pathogenic bacteria. There is evidence from recent studies that they may accelerate wound healing by promoting the formation of granulation tissue. The larvae feed on dead tissue, cellular debris, and exudates from necrotic wounds through extracorporeal digestion. This treatment has proven to be effective in clients with venous ulcer, diabetic ulcers, and arterial ulcers.

13. Reposition leg in elevated position. Leg should be elevated 18 cm above heart for 2 to 4 hr during the day and night. ▸ ***Rationale:*** This prevents edema and venous stasis and promotes healing.
14. Remove gloves and place in biohazard bag. Place all used supplies in bag.
15. Place biohazard bag in appropriate receptacle.

Clinical Alert

Use of semiocclusive dressings reduces incidence of wound infections by more than 50%. They maintain a moist environment, reduce airborne bacteria, and provide a mechanical barrier for bacterial entry.

Clinical Alert

Compression Therapy

Inelastic System

An Unna boot is frequently used to control edema in lower extremities. An inelastic bandaging system is applied to the lower extremity. As it dries it becomes rigid, and when calf muscles press against the rigid bandage, it pumps blood more effectively. This system can be used for both mobile and immobile clients. As edema subsides, the boot becomes less effective.

Elastic Therapy

Graduated compression and multilayer compression stockings and compression pumps are more effective in increasing venous return. Both mobile and immobile clients can use these stockings, although it is more difficult for the client who is mobile. The stockings are available in different pressures.

16. Perform hand hygiene.
17. Lower bed and raise side rails.
18. Assess peripheral circulation every 4 hr. ▸ ***Rationale:*** This ensures compression dressing is not too tight.

Arterial Ulcers

Assessment

- Assess arterial flow; dorsalis pedis, femoral, popliteal, or posterior tibial.
- Use Doppler to assess pulses if necessary.
- Assess Ankle–Brachial Index; below 0.5 indicates severe arterial insufficiency.
- Assess temperature of skin.
- Observe color of extremities.
- Assess for presence of pain when client resting.

Treatment

- Debridement
- Pain control
- Occlusive dressings: reduce pain, protect the wound from infection, control exudates, enhance autolytic debridement, maintain moist wound environment.
- Secure dressing with gauze; do not use tape as skin is fragile and tears easily.
- Management of disease process, i.e. BP, eliminate smoking, control blood glucose
- Surgical intervention to improve circulation
- Vacuum compression therapy
- Hyperbaric oxygen therapy

EVIDENCE-BASED PRACTICE

Treatment of Ambulatory Venous Ulcer Patients and Warming Therapy

This was a limited study, but other studies indicate the same type of findings. Five clients with a mean age of 65 and pressure ulcers for more than 8 months were treated with warm-up therapy along with zippered compression stockings for 2 weeks. These clients were monitored for 12 weeks. The therapy consisted of warm therapy three times a day for 1 hr each at a temperature of 38°C. The results indicated that four of five clients increased granulation tissue and decreased pain. Four of five clients were completely healed during the 12-week follow-up.

Source: Cherry, G. C., & Wilson, J. (1999, September). The treatment of ambulatory venous ulcer patients and warming therapy. *Ostomy/Wound Management 45*(9), 65–70.

Assessing Ankle–Brachial Index (ABI)

Equipment

Sphygmomanometer (two cuffs, one arm and one leg)
Stethoscope
Doppler, handheld

Procedure

1. Review chart to determine whether client has diabetes. ▸ ***Rationale:*** The ABI may not be reliable in these clients because arterial calcification causes false readings (high). The ABI is used to indirectly assess lower-extremity peripheral blood flow.
2. Explain procedure to client.
3. Place client in supine position. Instruct to lie quietly for 5 minutes.
4. Place cuff above right or left elbow, apply ultrasound gel to brachial pulse area.
5. Hold ultrasound probe at 90° angle on top of gel. ▸ ***Rationale:*** This position opposes direction of brachial artery blood flow.
6. Inflate cuff pressure to the point that the "whooshing" sound of the brachial pulse stops and continue inflating at least 20 mmHg above that point.
7. Slowly deflate pressure until systolic pulse sound is heard (when "whooshing" sound restarts).
8. Obtain blood pressure readings in both arms. Use the higher systolic pressure as the brachial pressure for the ABI calculations.
9. Wrap leg cuff around leg 5 cm above ankle's medial malleolus. Place conductivity gel over posterior tibial or dorsalis pedis artery.
10. Place Doppler probe at a 90° angle to dorsalis pedis or posterior tibial artery.
11. Inflate cuff until Doppler sound stops.
12. Deflate cuff slowly while maintaining Doppler probe in place over artery.
13. Obtain two readings of posterior tibial or dorsalis pedis measurements and select highest value to be used in ABI calculation.
14. Divide ankle systolic pressure by brachial systolic pressure to obtain Ankle–Brachial Index (ABI). Normally, ankle pressure is equal to or slightly higher then brachial pressure.
15. Review ABI guidelines to determine severity of arterial insufficiency.
16. Document findings in nurses' notes and place note on chart for physician.

ABI Guidelines

1.0–1.2 ABI	Normal—No arterial insufficiency
0.8–1.0 ABI	Mild insufficiency
0.5–0.8 ABI	Moderate insufficiency
<0.5 ABI	Severe insufficiency
<0.3 ABI	Limb threatening

Caring for a Wound With a Drain

Equipment

Same items as for Changing a Wound Dressing
Sterile cotton applicators
Sterile safety pin
ABD dressings
Gauze pads
Sterile scissors
Sterile gloves
Clean gloves
Cleansing solution

Preparation

1. Check physician's orders.
2. Perform hand hygiene.
3. Gather equipment.
4. Provide privacy.
5. Identify client using two forms of identification and explain procedure.
6. Clean off overbed table.
7. Raise bed to HIGH position and lower side rails on working side of bed.

8. Place plastic bag for soiled dressings on bed near wound site.
9. Open sterile packages and place on overbed table.

Procedure

1. Remove tape from client's skin by pulling *toward* the incision. ▸ ***Rationale:*** This decreases pain and prevents damage to wound site by preventing a "pull" on the incision.
2. Don clean gloves.
3. Remove soiled dressing.
4. Discard gloves and dressings into plastic bag.
5. Observe wound closely for signs of infection or healing. Don sterile gloves.
6. If pin on the Penrose drain is crusted, replace it with a sterile pin. Be careful not to dislodge drain or suction tubing.
7. Using cotton applicators or gauze pads, cleanse drain site with cleansing solution and then saline.

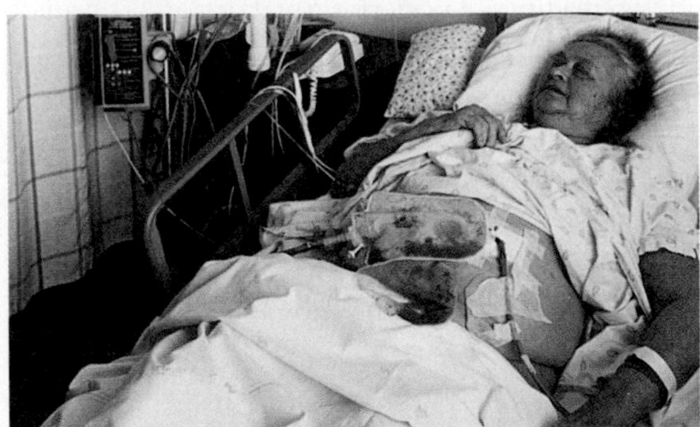

▲ Use drainage pouches for wounds with drains.

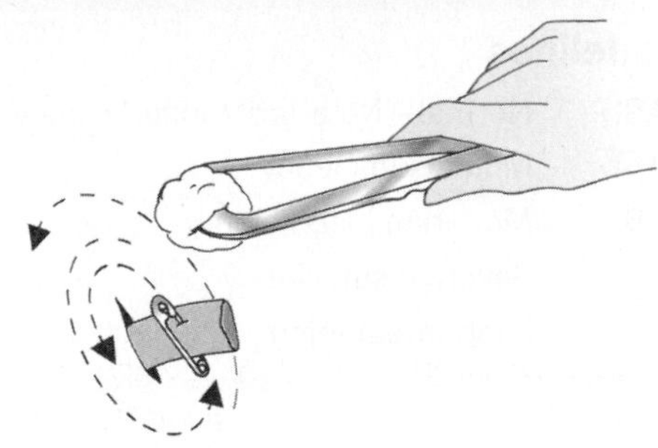

▲ Cleanse the drain site, using a circular motion (unless using chlorhexidine) from the inside to the periphery of the wound. With chlorhexidine, use a back and forth motion.

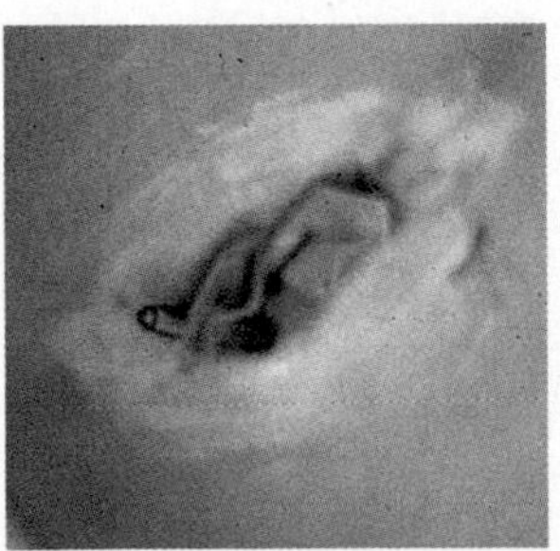

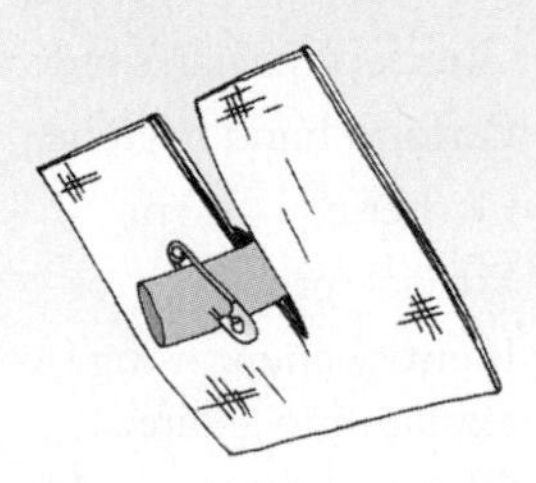

▲ Place a precut sterile 4 × 4 gauze dressing around the drain site to prevent skin excoriation.

8. Start cleansing at drain site, moving in a circular motion toward the periphery, unless using chlorhexidine swab; then use back-and-forth motion. Hold drain erect while cleaning around it. ▸ ***Rationale:*** This prevents contamination of the drain site area.
9. Dry the surrounding skin with gauze swab.
10. Discard applicators in plastic bag.
11. Advance drain if ordered:
    a. Using sterile forceps, pull drain out of wound the ordered number of centimeters. ▸ ***Rationale:*** To facilitate tissue healing.
    b. Reposition the safety pin so it is at the level of the skin. ▸ ***Rationale:*** The pin prevents the drain from slipping back into the wound.
    c. Cut off the excess tubing with sterile scissors. Leave at least 2 in. of tubing on the outside. ▸ ***Rationale:*** This prevents drain from being drawn up into the wound opening.

NOTE: Drains vary in length (25–35 cm or 10–14 in.) and width (1.2–4 cm or 0.5–1.5 in.).

12. Place several 4 × 4 dressings around the drain.
13. Apply gauze pad with a precut slit under the drain site.
14. Apply dry, sterile gauze pads over drain.
15. Apply ABD pads over sterile gauze.
16. Remove gloves and dispose of them in refuse bag.
17. Tape dressing or retie Montgomery straps (tie tapes).
18. Remove bag with soiled dressing from room.
19. Perform hand hygiene.
20. Position client for comfort.
21. Lower bed and raise side rail.

Drainage Pouches for Wounds

Apply a pouch to:

- Collect drainage
- Measure drainage
- Protect skin from drainage
- Contain drainage
- Contain microorganisms so spread is decreased
- Lessen frequency of care; dressing change is every 24–48 hr

Drainage Systems for Wounds

Open Drains: Discharge flows freely into an absorbent dressing or a drainage bag.

Closed Systems: Remove fluid and debris into a closed container (i.e., Hemovac or Jackson–Pratt). Fewer wound infections occur with this drainage system.

Applying an Abdominal Binder

Equipment

Abdominal binder: woven-cotton, synthetic, or elasticized material. Most facilities use commercial Velcro binders.

Safety pins for binders without Velcro closure

Procedure

1. Perform hand hygiene.
2. Explain use of binder to client.
3. Place client in supine position.
4. Ask client to raise hips, and then slide the binder under client's hips at level of gluteal fold. Place top of binder at client's waist.
5. Bring ends of binder around client, and secure by pressing Velcro surfaces together. If using non-Velcro binder, secure binder with safety pins placed vertically along edges. Start pinning at bottom of binder and pin toward waist. ▸ ***Rationale:*** Pinning binder from bottom to waist provides uplifting support for abdominal muscles.
6. Observe for wrinkles in binder. ▸ ***Rationale:*** Wrinkles can cause pressure areas, especially over iliac crest.
7. Assess client's ability to move freely, breathe deeply, and feel secure pressure over abdominal incision. ▸ ***Rationale:*** A binder that is too tight may compromise breathing or place pressure on incisional area.
8. Assess effectiveness of binder every 4 hr, and rewrap every 8 hr if non-Velcro binder is used. Many clients use this binder only when ambulating.

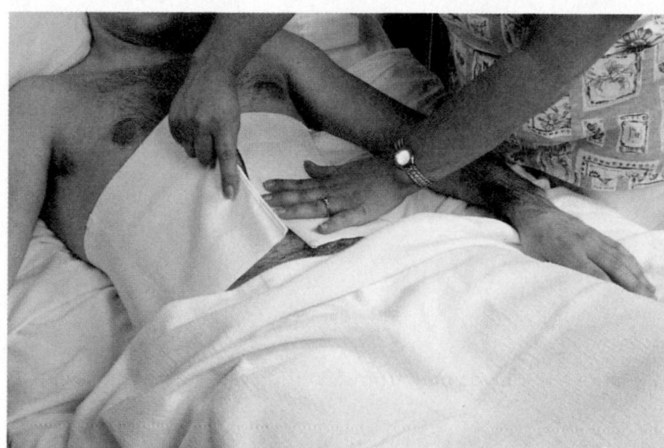

▲ Bring end of binder around client and secure Velcro surfaces.

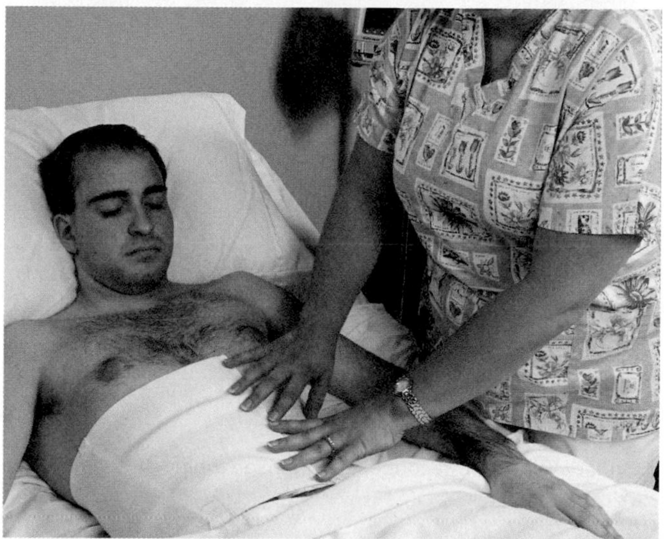

▲ Assess effectiveness of binder every 4 hr.

Maintaining Wound Drainage System

Equipment

Specimen cup for measuring drainage

I&O bedside record

Absorbent pad

Clean gloves

Hemovac suction or Jackson–Pratt suction drainage system

Preparation

1. Check physician's order and client care plan.
2. Bring specimen cup to bedside.
3. Identify client and explain procedure, giving client time to ask questions.
4. Provide for comfort and privacy.
5. Perform hand hygiene and don gloves.
6. Elevate bed to workable height.

Procedure

1. Expose catheter insertion site while keeping client draped. Place drainage system on absorbent pad.
2. Examine pump and catheter for patency, seal, and stability. If catheter is occluded, notify physician.
3. Remove Hemovac plug, which is labeled "Pouring Spout," or disconnect tubing from Jackson–Pratt system.
4. Pour drainage into specimen cup.
5. Compress the Hemovac by pushing the top and bottom together with your hands, or compress bulb on Jackson–Pratt.
6. Hold pump or bulb tightly compressed, and reinsert plug or connect tubing to Jackson–Pratt system. ▸ ***Rationale:*** This will reestablish closed drainage system.
7. Position suction devices on bed.
8. Measure and record amount of drainage.

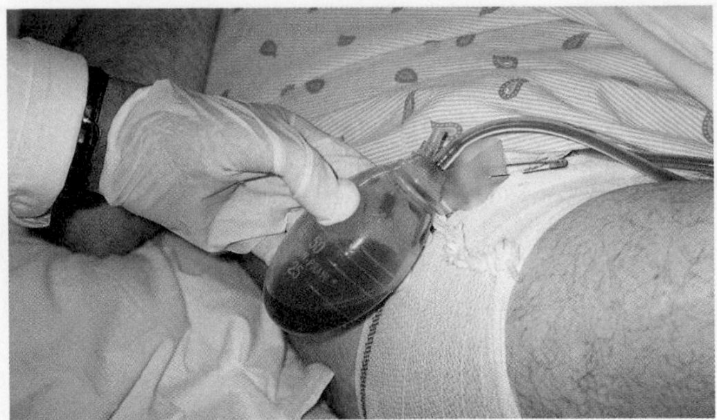
▲ Jackson–Pratt drainage system in place.

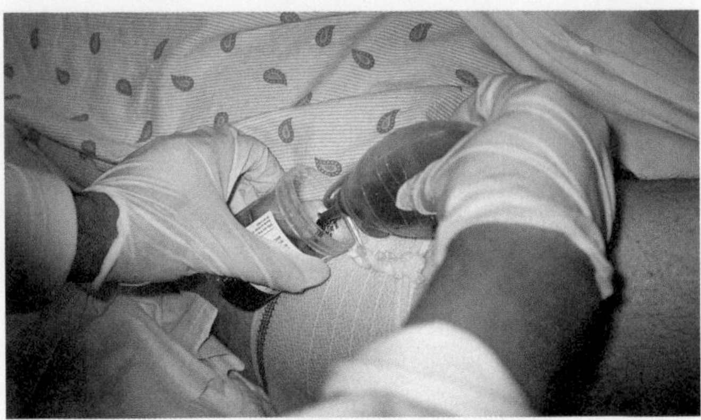
▲ Empty, measure, and record drainage every shift.

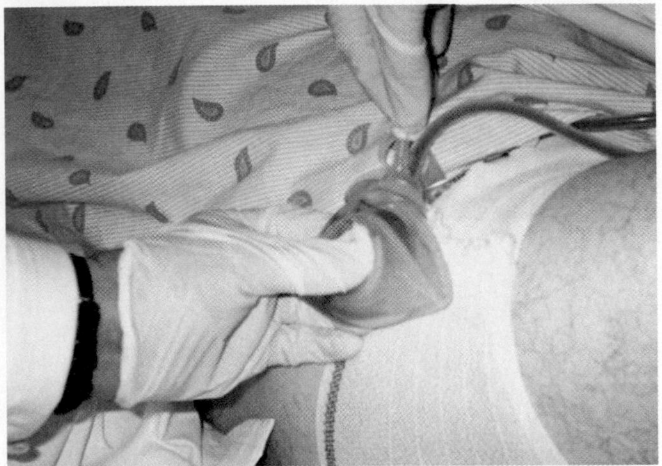
▲ Squeeze bulb and reconnect to drainage tubing after emptying.

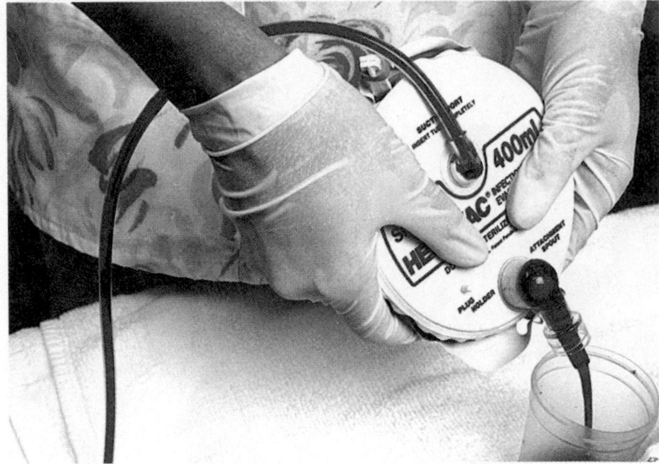

▲ Remove Hemovac plug from "Pouring Spout" for emptying.

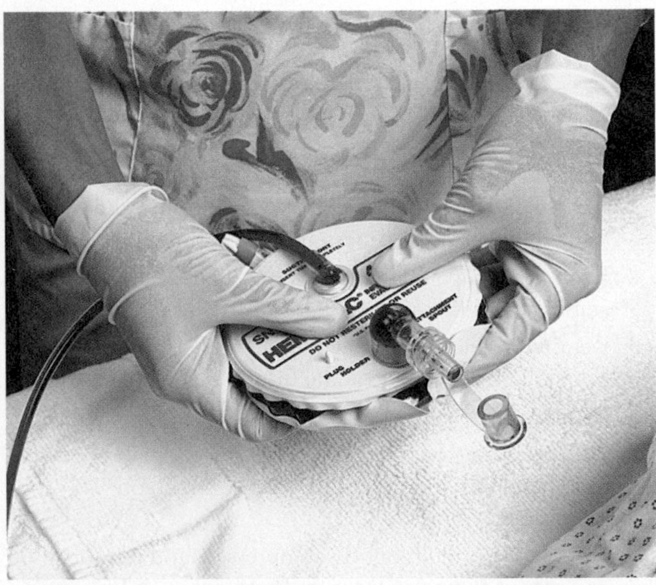
▲ Compress Hemovac by pushing top and bottom together.

9. Examine drainage for color, consistency, and odor.
10. Discard drainage and container; remove gloves, and wash hands.
11. Send culture specimen to laboratory if ordered.
12. Make client comfortable, and lower bed.
13. Compress evacuator at least every 4 hr to provide suction. Measure drainage at least every 8 hr.

Irrigating Wounds

Equipment

Sterile irrigation solution, preferably saline or Ringer's solution
Commercial wound cleaner container with nozzle
or
Sterile irrigating set with 35-mL syringe and 19-gauge Angiocath tip or 19-gauge needle
Absorbent pad
Sterile gloves
Equipment for dressing change

Preparation

1. Check physician's orders and client care plan.
2. Gather irrigation equipment and dressing material.
3. Identify client, using two identifiers.
4. Assemble equipment.
5. Explain procedure to client and answer any questions.
6. Raise bed and lower side rails.
7. Perform hand hygiene.
8. Open sterile packages on the overbed table as with dressing change.
9. Pour sterile irrigating solution into container.

Procedure

1. Place absorbent pads under the client. Place a bath blanket under absorbent pads when irrigating a large wound. ▸ ***Rationale:*** This will absorb any spilled irrigation solution.
2. Position client so that solution flows from wound to basin.
3. Don clean gloves.
4. Remove and discard used dressing.
5. Remove gloves and discard into plastic bag.
6. Place overbed table near working area with all packages open.
7. Don sterile gloves.
8. Inspect area surrounding wound for redness, tissue integrity, and signs of granulating tissue.
9. Place sterile basin under wound area.
10. Draw solution from sterile container into 35-mL syringe with syringe or Angiocath tip. Increasing syringe size decreases pressure of stream or increasing bore of catheter tip increases pressure.

NOTE: The goal of irrigation is to remove bacteria and debris without injury to normal tissue. Irrigation pressure of 5 to 15 pounds per square inch (psi) is required to accomplish the goal.

Clinical Alert

If wound has moderate to heavy drainage, alginate dressings should be used. Alginate forms a gel when it comes in contact with wound fluid. It absorbs up to 20 times its weight in fluid. It can be used in infected and noninfected wounds. It is not to be used in dry wounds, as it can dehydrate the wound.

11. Cleanse wound in the direction from least contaminated to most contaminated areas.
12. Open commercial cleaning solution package if using for irrigation.
    a. Read directions on commercial wound cleaner container to determine appropriate distance nozzle is positioned from wound during irrigation.
    b. If nozzle is too close to the wound, force may be higher than expected.
    c. If nozzle is too far from the wound, force may be lower than needed.
    d. If saline solution is used, deliver irrigant with 8 psi (pounds per square inch) pressure. The 35-mL syringe and 19-gauge Angiocath tip delivers this pressure. ▸ ***Rationale:*** Pressures effective in wound cleansing should be between 4 psi and 15 psi in order to effectively clean the wound surface by forcefully loosening foreign materials and nonattached bacteria.
    e. Repeat until all irrigation solution has been used.
13. After the irrigation, cleanse client's skin around wound and dry.
14. Apply sterile dressing.
15. Dispose of equipment properly.
16. Remove gloves. Check to see that client is comfortable before leaving the room.
17. Lower bed and raise side rails.
18. Perform hand hygiene.

Debridement

Physical removal of affected tissue by debridement is the most effective method of cleaning the wound. Infected tissue is best removed by surgical debridement. Other methods of debridement include chemical or enzymatic, mechanical, or autolytic. Stage II ulcers can be debrided by gentle mechanical debridement using mesh gauze moistened with saline, hydrocolloid dressings, or enzymatic debriding. Stage IV and large stage III ulcers require surgical debridement. Surgical debridement uses sterile instruments and requires local anesthesia. Only a qualified clinician can use this technique.

Chemical debridement is slower than surgical debridement but is able to be used in home care and long-term care settings. Proteolytic enzymes such as collagenase or papain-urea are commonly used chemical agents. Mechanical debridement is accomplished through whirlpool treatments. Autolytic debridement uses moisture-retentive or moisture-donating dressings to facilitate digestion of tissue by the client's own enzymes and phagocytes.

Biologic or larval debridement is currently being used for wounds that are difficult to heal.

Teaching Wound Care to Clients

Procedure

1. Begin client teaching as soon as client is able to participate in activity. ▸ ***Rationale:*** Client will need to care for wound at home for a period of time before sutures are removed and/or wound is healed.
2. Assess wound daily for any changes in color, odor, drainage.
3. Keep wound dry and clean.
4. Instruct client that he/she can take a shower, unless contraindicated by wound condition (i.e., dressing on wound, splint, etc.).
5. Do not remove dressing unless it is wet or soiled. If soiled or wet, change dressing according to directions. Wound or dressing can be covered by plastic when taking shower.
6. Report any signs of infection to healthcare provider: erythema, edema around incision site, warmth and/or tenderness surrounding incision site, discharge or foul odor from site, streaks on the skin running from wound, chills or temperature above 100° F: ▸ ***Rationale:*** These are signs and symptoms of SSIs or wounds.
7. After sutures are removed, instruct client to:
   a. Follow instructions from healthcare provider regarding activity level. ▸ ***Rationale:*** Even though sutures are removed, wound is not completely healed and will continue to strengthen over the next weeks.
   b. Keep suture line clean, cleansing it using soft strokes, and pat dry.
   c. Observe wound edges, they will appear red and slightly raised; this is normal.
   d. Observe suture site; if site continues to be reddened and painful to pressure beyond 8 weeks, notify healthcare provider. ▸ ***Rationale:*** This could indicate excessive collagen formation.

DOCUMENTATION for Wound Care

- Observation of wound site, including amount, color, and odor of drainage, as well as appearance of suture site
- Document color of wound: serous—clear, watery, plasma; serosanguineous—plasma and red blood cells; sanguinous—bloody; purulent—thick drainage
- Observation of granulating necrotic or epithelial tissue
- Observations pertinent to client's tolerance of procedure
- Observation of skin condition around incision site; erythema, maceration, induration, edema
- Changes in vital signs that indicate possible infection
- Client's activity level, any incontinence
- Compliance with prescribed treatment
- Type of dressing applied
- Material used in wound packing
- Observations on wound irrigation
- Type and amount of irrigation solutions used
- Unusual tension on sutures if present
- Amount and color of Hemovac or Jackson–Pratt drainage
- Document undermining using clock orientation; measure in centimeters (i.e., 2 to 5 o'clock)
- Tissue viability; percent healthy and necrotic tissue relative to entire wound
- Signs and symptoms indicating potential SSI
- Teaching information provided to client

CRITICAL THINKING Application

Expected Outcomes

- Wound care is provided for contaminated wound and healing occurs.
- Drainage system functions without obstructions.
- Wound irrigation is completed using sufficient pressure to cleanse wound bed.
- Abdominal binder supports client's abdominal wound.
- Compression dressing applied to vascular ulcer site.

Unexpected Outcomes	Alternative Actions
Wound becomes infected with multiple microorganisms.	• Notify physician about changes in color or odor of drainage. • Obtain culture and sensitivity if physician orders one. • Wash your hands thoroughly after caring for client to prevent the spread of infection. • Pay strict attention to changing dressings.
Wound does not heal.	• Evaluate use of dressing and perhaps choose a different type of dressing. • Assess nutritional status. Increase protein and carbohydrates if not contraindicated. • Determine availability of a vacuum-assisted closure machine.
Edges of wound split open (wound dehiscence).	• Place client in supine position. Apply butterfly tape to wound edges. Cover opening with sterile dressings. • Apply binder for abdominal incisions after obtaining order. • Notify physician if signs of infection are present. • Obtain culture of drainage if physician orders one. • Observe client for signs of shock. If client in shock, notify physician immediately. • Encourage high-protein diet.
Evisceration occurs (protrusion of bowel contents).	• Institute emergency measures. Place the client in supine position. Cover bowel with sterile gauze moistened with sterile saline. Have IV-certified nurse insert IV catheter and infuse normal saline. Reassure client. Obtain vital signs, and treat for shock if present. • After above measures are completed, notify physician, and prepare client for return to surgery. • After surgical repair, notify dietician for diet change to increase protein and vitamin C in diet. • Apply abdominal binder if ordered.
Wound hemorrhages.	• Outline area of blood on dressing with a pen and observe outline to see how quickly the bleeding spreads. • If bleeding is excessive, notify the physician immediately. • Apply pressure dressing to site if there is excessive bleeding.
Skin appears red and broken.	• Clean area with sterile saline and dry thoroughly with sterile 4 × 4 pads. • Apply moisture-retentive dressing.
Wound is too extensive for application of drainage.	• Obtain Stomahesive or Hollihesive 8 × 8 sheets and cut on diagonal 1/8 to 1/4 in. larger than wound.
ABD pads cannot contain drainage.	• If larger barrier needed, Stomahesive may be pieced together to form larger barrier, reinforcing juncture points with Karaya paste. • A superadhesive pouch may then be applied. • If dressings are used, they may be secured with Montgomery straps (tie tapes).
Abdominal binder is not effective in supporting incisional area.	• Evaluate the effectiveness of the abdominal binder. • Assess if the binder is properly positioned at the hip level and waist level to provide support. • Assess if the binder is too loose.
Client is too large for the abdominal binder.	• Fold a drawsheet in half lengthwise and place under client. Position the edges at the waist and pubic area. • Pull tightly on the drawsheet, and secure the edges with safety pins.

Drainage system expands quickly after being reconnected.	• Check all connections for an air leak because properly functioning reservoirs expand slowly.
Client is too large for bed.	• Request use of BariCare bed.
Client's assessment indicates he/she is at high risk for SSI	• Administer appropriate antibiotic 1 hr before surgery. • If client has a chronic illness, monitor carefully for signs and symptoms of SSIs postoperatively. • If client's surgery is not urgent, treat condition and then reschedule surgical intervention.

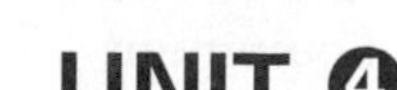

Chapter 25

UNIT 4

Promoting a Moist Environment

Nursing Process Data

ASSESSMENT Data Base

- Assess wound edges for presence of granulation tissue.
- Assess for changes in amount of drainage.
- Assess whether necrotic tissue is decreasing in amount.
- Identify whether appropriate dressing is used for wound care.

PLANNING Objectives

- To promote wound healing by secondary intention
- To maintain a moist environment conducive to wound healing
- To provide the most appropriate treatment for wound care
- To enhance local healing
- To maintain sterile technique throughout procedure
- To remove trapped exudate from wounds

IMPLEMENTATION Procedures

EVALUATION Expected Outcomes

- Wound heals without complications.
- Sterile technique is maintained throughout procedure.

Pearson Nursing Student Resources

Find additional review materials at **nursing.pearsonhighered.com**

Prepare for success with NCLEX®-style practice questions and Skill Checklists

Applying Wet-to-Moist Dressings

Equipment

Sterile 4 × 8 noncotton gauze dressings
Semiocclusive dressing, optional
Sterile gloves
Clean gloves
Tape
Plastic bag or receptacle for contaminated dressings
Sterile normal saline solution
Sterile receptacle (round basin or emesis basin) if dressing not in commercial pack
Montgomery straps, if desired

Clinical Alert

Wet-to-dry dressings are used only to debride wounds, as they cause tissue damage. Maceration of healthy tissue can occur with dressings that are always wet. Dry dressings cause damage to granulating tissue if removed without first soaking the gauze.

Preparation

1. Check physician's orders.
2. Perform hand hygiene and gather equipment.
3. Identify client using two forms of identification.
4. Explain procedure to client.
5. Provide privacy.
6. Raise bed to HIGH position, and lower side rail nearest you.
7. Remove tape by pulling it toward the wound. ▸ ***Rationale:*** This action prevents injury to newly formed tissue.
8. Don clean gloves.
9. Remove wound packing by gently grasping the gauze without touching the wound and tear it away at a right angle from the wound surface. ▸ ***Rationale:*** Touching only the gauze prevents contamination of the wound.
10. Place soiled dressings in disposable bag.
11. Remove gloves, and dispose of them in bag.
12. Perform hand hygiene.

Clinical Alert

Heat lamps should not be used to treat pressure ulcers. Preferred wound care is to promote a clean, moist environment.

Procedure

1. Open packages of dressings making sure sterility is maintained.
2. Pour normal saline solution over dressings.
3. Don sterile gloves.
4. Pick up sterile gauze dressings one at a time.
5. Fluff each dressing, and place over wound. ▸ ***Rationale:*** If packed tightly, dressing can prevent wound edges from contact with capillaries.
6. Place gauze in the wound, covering all exposed surfaces. Press gauze lightly into depressions or cracks. ▸ ***Rationale:*** Necrotic tissue is more prevalent in these areas.
7. Unfold a moist, sterile, 4 × 8 (ABD pad) dressing into a single layer and place it on top of wet dressings covering the wound area (not on skin).
8. Place a dry 4 × 8 pad over the dressing to hold it in place. Some protocols call for semiocclusive dressing in place of pad.
9. Remove gloves, and place in plastic bag.
10. Tape only the edges of the dressing. Montgomery tapes may be used to prevent excessive skin irritation and damage due to frequent dressing changes.
11. Position client for comfort. Lower bed and raise side rail to UP position, if appropriate.

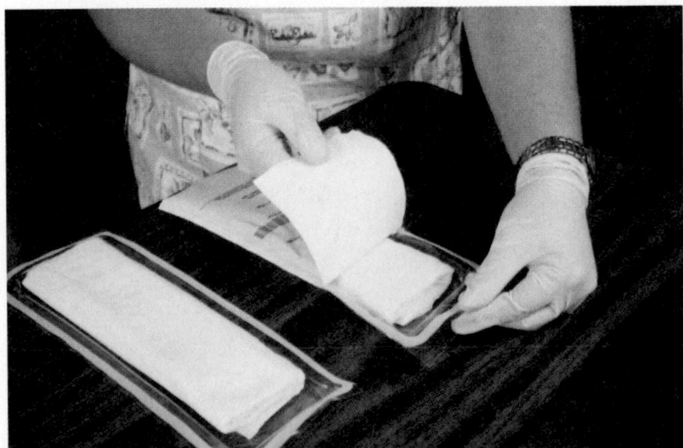

▲ Open sterile packages before beginning dressing change.

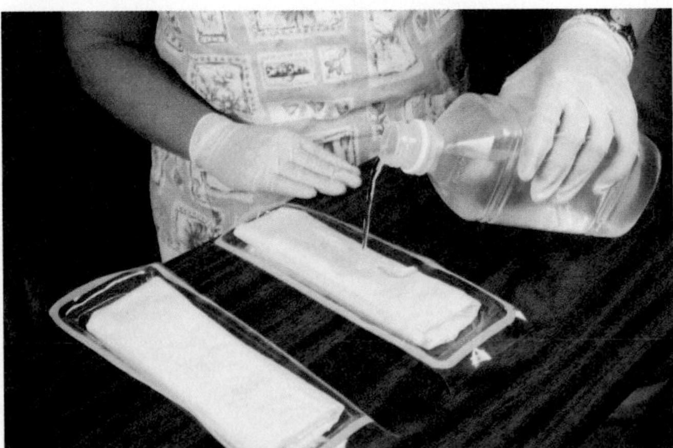

▲ Pour sterile saline solution over dressings to moisten.

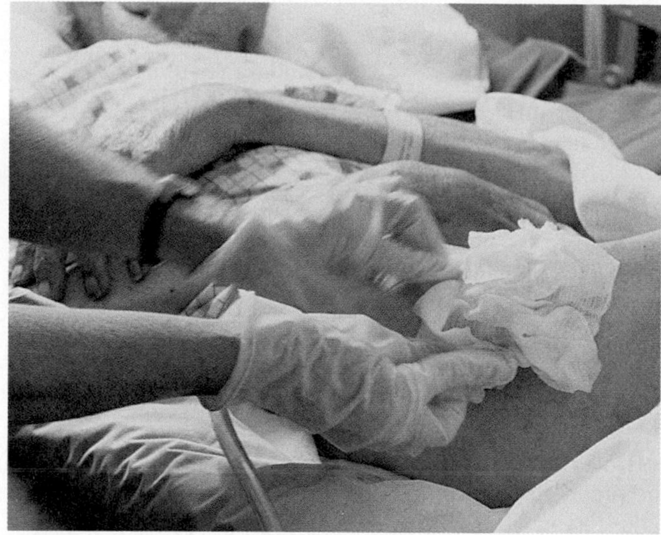
▲ Fluff dressings and apply over wound, covering all exposed surfaces.

12. Discard soiled material in appropriate container.
13. Perform hand hygiene.
14. Observe wound for excessive drainage or drying out of dressing between dressing changes. Remoisten dressing if dry. ▶ ***Rationale:*** Unless excessive drainage occurs, or dressing dries out, dressings are usually changed every 8 hr.

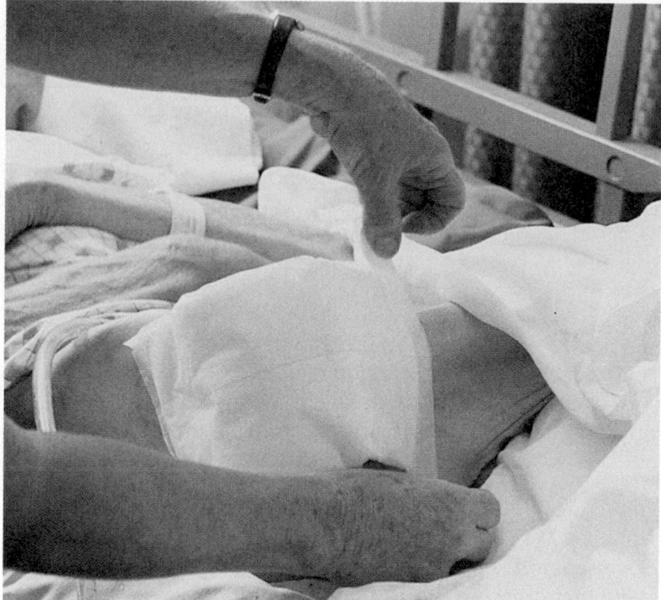
▲ Place moist ABD pad over dressings; then cover with dry pad.

15. Provide client or family teaching regarding wound care, if appropriate.

NOTE: These dressings function as an osmotic dressing. Normal saline is isotonic. As water evaporates from saline dressing, it becomes hypertonic and fluid from wound tissue is drained into dressing.

TABLE 25-5 Additional Moist Wound Dressings

Type of Alternative Use		Outcome of Treatment	Considerations
Hydrogel Sheet	• Interacts with aqueous solutions • Used with minor wounds with light to moderate drainage • Absorbs minimal to heavy exudates • Cannot be used with infected wound • Nonadherent	Softens necrotic tissue Creates moist environment	Use outer dressing to prevent wound from drying out Change dressing every 1–2 days
Impregnated Gauze Dressing	• Absorbs minimal to moderate exudates • Nonadherent	Conforms to irregular surfaces Eliminates dead space Creates moist environment	Requires outer dressing Change daily Non-absorptive
Alginate*	• Absorbs heavy exudates • Converts to gel when comes in contact with wound drainage • Easily removed from wound • Nonadherent • Absorbs up to 20 times its weight in fluid • Can be used in infected and non-infected wounds	Maintains moist environment Promotes fast healing of wound	Not to be used on dry wounds It dehydrates wound, delaying healing, eschar-covered wounds, third-degree burns or surgical wounds
Foams	• Absorbs minimal to heavy exudates • Highly absorbent • Used for deep cavity wounds	Maintains moist environment Decreases tissue trauma when removed Increases time between dressing changes (3–4 days)	Requires external dressing Can cause drying effect on wound

*Alginates are made from acids that are obtained from brown seaweed. The calcium salts of alginic, mannuronic, and gularonic acids are processed into nonwoven, biodegradable fibers. When the fibers come into contact with fluids, sodium, and calcium ions, it results in the formation of a soluble sodium gel.

Continued

TABLE 25-5 Additional Moist Wound Dressings *(Continued)*

Type of Alternative	Use	Outcome of Treatment	Considerations
Hydrophilic	• Type of foam dressing • Non-adherent • Very absorbent	Cushions wound Traps exudate	Used in wounds with moderate to heavy drainage
Hydrophobic	• Non-adherent flexible dressing • Minimal or no necrotic tissue • Used with lightly-to-moderately exudating wounds	Resists fluid penetration into wound Use on lightly draining wounds Provides cushion to irritated skin	
Medical Hydrolysate of Collagen	• Soluble and degrades in wound site • Absorbs wound exudates • Is interactive with wound site to provide mechanical protection against physical and bacterial insult	Absorbs up to 30 times own weight Used in stage I–IV pressure ulcers Accelerates tissue remodeling and reduces scarring	Cover with nonstick dressing Soak dressing in warm water before removing
Anticoat 7 Silver-coated contact dressing	• Used for wounds with moderate to heavy exudates • Has an antimicrobial barrier to protect against bacterial contamination and infection • Calcium in the dressing provides antimicrobial to protect against bacterial contamination and infection • Kills bacteria faster than any other forms of silver dressing	Used for leg ulcers Pressure ulcers Diabetic foot ulcers Burns	Stays in place for up to 3 days to provide moist environment

EVIDENCE-BASED PRACTICE

Silver-Eluting Antimicrobial Dressings Don't Help Leg Ulcers

Silver-eluting antimicrobial dressings have not been found to help heal leg ulcers to any greater extent that other dressings. A study conducted in the United Kingdon compared these dressings with standard low-adhesive bandages in 213 elderly clients. The results in 6 months indicated the wounds of the clients in the control group had healed 77% and those of the clients in the pilot group had healed 85%. By 1 year, the wounds of clients in both groups had healed by 96%. The silver dressing cost five times as much as the standard dressing. The cost of treating the client with the silver dressing was 30% more than the standard dressing. The study found there was little to support the use of silver or any other antimicrobial dressings in the treatment of venous leg ulcers.

Source: (2010, January). *The American Journal of Nursing* (News Caps) *110*(1), 20.

Using a Hydrocolloid Dressing

Equipment

Sterile normal saline
Hydrocolloid dressing (e.g., DuoDERM, Restore, Ultec, Comfeel Plus)
Hydrogel if needed (ClearSite, Aquasorb)
Sterile 4 × 4 gauze pads
Hypoallergenic tape
Clean gloves
Skin prep, optional

NOTE: These dressings are a combination of adhesive and gelling polymers that are impermeable to oxygen, water, and water vapor. They promote a moist wound environment, aid in autolytic debridement, and have no toxic components. They are waterproof and bacteria proof. These dressings are best used in clients who have partial- to full-thickness wounds with minimal to moderate exudates such as for pressure ulcers, skin tears, surgical wounds, and burns.

Procedure

1. Select dressing size to ensure coverage 1¼ in. beyond ulcer margin. (Dressing available in 4 × 4 to 8 × 8 sizes.) ▸ ***Rationale:*** This ensures complete covering of wound. Use for small ulcers and in stage II and III ulcers.

NOTE: These dressings can be used for dry wounds as they contain 95% water. They are occlusive and do not allow water or bacteria into the wound. Hydrocolloid causes the pH of the wound surface to drop, and this acidic environment can inhibit bacterial growth.

2. Perform hand hygiene and don clean gloves.
3. Cleanse skin with gauze pad moistened with sterile normal saline and pat dry with gauze pad.
4. Measure wound using pliable device.
5. Apply skin prep to surrounding skin to protect, if ordered.

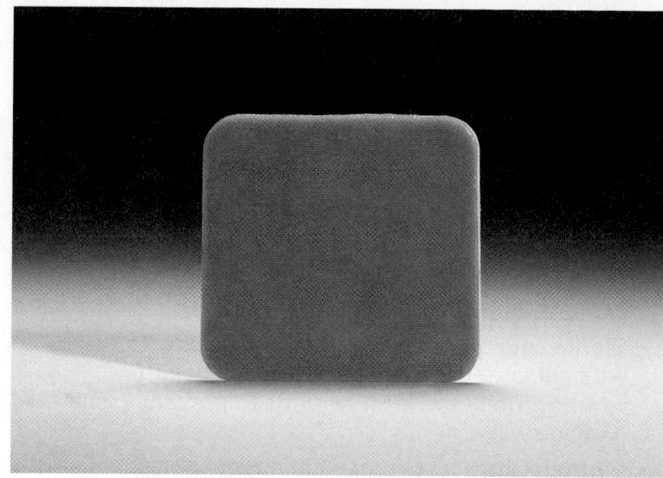

▲ Hydrocolloid dressing.

Clinical Alert

Hydrocolloids cannot be used if wound or surrounding skin is infected. The dressings are not used on wounds with heavy drainage or wounds with deep tunnels.

6. Fill ulcer area with Hydrogel if ordered—usually used with stage III or IV pressure ulcer of the hip when exudate is present. Do not overfill with gel. ▸ ***Rationale:*** Facilitates autolytic debridement of devitalized tissue.
7. Warm dressing by holding in hands. ▸ ***Rationale:*** To increase activity of adhesive, and it makes dressing more pliable.
8. Remove silicone release paper backing from dressing. Minimize finger contact with adhesive surface. ▸ ***Rationale:*** Dressing is sterile and contamination should be avoided.
9. Center dressing over affected area and extend at least 1 in. onto periwound skin. Gently roll dressing over pressure ulcer—do not stretch dressing. ▸ ***Rationale:*** Stretching the dressing may cause wrinkling of dressing, which allows air to enter wound.
10. Placing dressing one-third above wound and two-thirds below wound maximizes time between dressing changes. ▸ ***Rationale:*** Increases absorption capacity of dressing.
11. Mold the dressing gently to skin and hold down with hand for approximately 1 minute.
12. Apply skin prep to area that is to be covered by tape if ordered. Allow to dry. Do not apply skin prep under hydrocolloid dressing. ▸ ***Rationale:*** Hydrocolloid dressings are placed over broken skin; skin prep may cause damage to skin.
13. Picture-frame sides of hydrocolloid dressing with silk or hypoallergenic tape.
14. Check dressing each shift for impaired integrity.
15. Change dressing at first sign of impaired integrity. Dressings should not be left on longer than 7 days. Usually left in place for 3–4 days.

NOTE: DuoDERM is removed when exudate seeps from edges of dressing or white blister appears under dressing. Comfeel Plus is changed when dressing becomes transparent or there is leakage.

16. Remove dressing by pressing hand down on adjacent skin surface while carefully lifting edge of dressing from skin. Continue lifting dressing around periphery until all edges are released, then lift dressing carefully away from wound.
17. Remove gloves and perform hand hygiene.
18. Record stage, size, and appearance of ulcer; date; and reason for removal of hydrocolloid dressing.

NOTE: Although frequently listed as wound care alternatives, topical disinfectant agents such as iodine and silver sulfadiazine are very controversial in wound care. Iodine is cytotoxic to fibroblasts and can impair wound healing. Silver solutions are sometimes used to prevent bacterial colonization in infection-prone areas. They do not eliminate existing infections.

Using a Hydrocolloid Wafer Dressing

Procedure

1. Warm hydrocolloid sheet wafer between hands.
2. Apply wafer 1–2 in. larger than wound.
3. Monitor for periwound maceration.
4. Monitor dressing, as moisture from wound causes wafer to form a gel over wound.
5. Change every 3–7 days or as needed.
6. Secure edges with tape.
7. Remove dressing carefully. Residual may be noted on wound. Do not remove residual.

TABLE 25-6 Hydrocolloid Dressings

Dressing	Uses
Hydrocolloid dressing (2 mm thick) Exterior surface protects wound from contamination	On partial and full thickness wounds with exudate
Thin hydrocolloid dressing (less than 1 mm thick)	On superfluid wounds with minimal exudate and to protect areas at risk for skin breakdown
Hydrocolloid paste	To manage dermal wounds with light drainage
Hydrocolloid gel	On partial- and full-thickness wounds Fills dry wound cavities Promotes autolytes debridement

Hydrogel Dressings

- Hydrogel dressings contain 95% water; they are very absorbent and dehydrate easily when not covered with a secondary dressing.
- Dressings cannot absorb much exudate; they should be used for dry wounds such as skin tears, surgical wounds, and radiation therapy burns.
- Dressings are nonadhesive; can be transparent and conform to wound surfaces.
- Sterile aqueous hydrogen fiber is used to fill cavity with gel; also used to fill dead space in large wounds. Do not overfill wounds to prevent tissue damage.
- Hydrogel sheets are placed in direct contact with wound bed and margins; air bubbles and plastic covering on sheet must be removed. The unique cooling properties soothe painful wounds.

Applying a Foam Dressing

Equipment

Adhesive foam dressing

Receptacle for soiled dressing

Preparation

1. Identify client using two identifiers.
2. Perform hand hygiene.
3. Remove old dressing and discard in appropriate receptacle.
4. Clean wound according to policy.
5. Complete skin assessment and identify wounds that need dressings.
6. Measure wound and obtain dressing size: 1–2 in. larger than wound.

NOTE: Foam dressings are particularly useful for wounds with moderate to heavy exudate. The absorptive ability of the foam dressing must match the exudates property of the wound's exudate. Dry wounds with a scab or eschar are not candidates for foam dressing. They do not benefit from the foam dressing and the wound may dry out.

Procedure

1. Using foam dressing as primary dressing, measure wound and cut 1–2 in. larger than wound. ▸ ***Rationale:*** To protect periwound areas.
2. If wound is irregular, cut foam dressing to match shape of wound or specific part of body, such as toes.
3. If using foam under compression stockings, place foam in cavity of the wound. Leave space in cavity for expansion of dressing as exudates are absorbed.
4. Press down adhesive border to secure dressing.
5. Apply barrier cream to surrounding skin according to policy.
6. Perform hand hygiene.
7. Assess wound frequently if large volume of exudates in wound.
8. Change dressing every 3–5 days unless wet or soiled, then change as necessary

Foam dressings are useful in the following wounds:

- Wounds requiring negative pressure
- Minor burns
- Skin grafts and donor site
- Pressure ulcers
- Arterial and venous leg ulcers
- Sutured wounds

Foam can also be used around tracheostomy and gastrostomy tubes to absorb drainage and manage heavy exudate in wounds.

TABLE 25-7 Comparisons of Moisture-Retentive Dressings

	Transparent	Hydrocolloid
Common Brands	Tegaderm Op-Site Bioclusive	Tegasorb DuoDERM Comfeel Restore
Characteristics	Sterile Semipermeable membranes with hypoallergenic adhesive Permeable to oxygen and moisture vapor Allows oxygen exchange Impermeable to bacteria, prevents contamination	Impermeable to oxygen Dressing gel maintains moist environment that promotes autolysis Impermeable to external bacteria and contamination Minimally to moderately absorptive
Function	Provides moist environment Promotes autolysis and protects newly formed tissue Assists with debridement	Dressing contains hydroactive particles that absorb exudate to form a hydrated gel over wound When dressing removed, gel separates from dressing, which protects newly formed tissue
Use	Easy assessment of wound; dressing is transparent Nondraining or minimally draining wounds only, nonabsorbable Pressure ulcers, stage I and some stage II Minor burns, lacerations	Absorbs exudate while preserving moist environment needed for autolysis of slough Irrigate gel with saline to allow for assessing wound Pressure ulcers, some stage III and some clean stage IV Wounds with mild or moderate exudate Wounds with necrosis or slough
Contraindications	Infected wounds Wounds with fragile surrounding skin	Wounds that need frequent assessment, not transparent Wounds with heavy exudate

Applying a Transparent Film

Equipment

Sterile normal saline

Transparent dressing (e.g., Op-Site, Tegaderm, Bioclusive)

Sterile 4 × 4 gauze pads

Scissors

Hypoallergenic tape

Clean gloves

Plasticizing agent (e.g., skin prep [optional])

Syringe with 26 gauge needle, if needed

Preparation

1. Check physician's orders and client care plan.
2. Check type of dressing ordered. ▸ ***Rationale:*** These dressings are very important in preventing pressure ulcers; they prevent friction and shear over bony prominences when moving clients.
3. Gather supplies.
4. Obtain appropriately sized transparent dressing. Dressing can be applied to flat surface. (Coccyx area cannot be treated with this type of dressing.)
5. Perform hand hygiene.
6. Identify client using two types of identification and explain procedure to client.
7. Provide privacy.

Procedure

1. Raise bed to HIGH position, and lower side rail on working side of bed.
2. Don clean gloves.
3. Remove old dressing, "walk off" dressing from one edge to the other, and discard in appropriate receptacle.
4. Wash pressure ulcer with sterile gauze pads moistened with sterile normal saline.
5. Dry thoroughly with sterile gauze pad.
6. Measure wound using pliable device. ▸ ***Rationale:*** Comparison of measurement assists in determining effectiveness of treatment.
7. Apply plasticizing agent (skin prep, skin gel) over surrounding tissue if ordered. ▸ ***Rationale:*** Do not apply directly on ulcer area because the agent contains alcohol, which burns the ulcer area. *Alternate Treatment:* If skin is irritated, apply No Sting Barrier Film Spray to area surrounding tissue. ▸ ***Rationale:*** To protect/prevent skin breakdown.

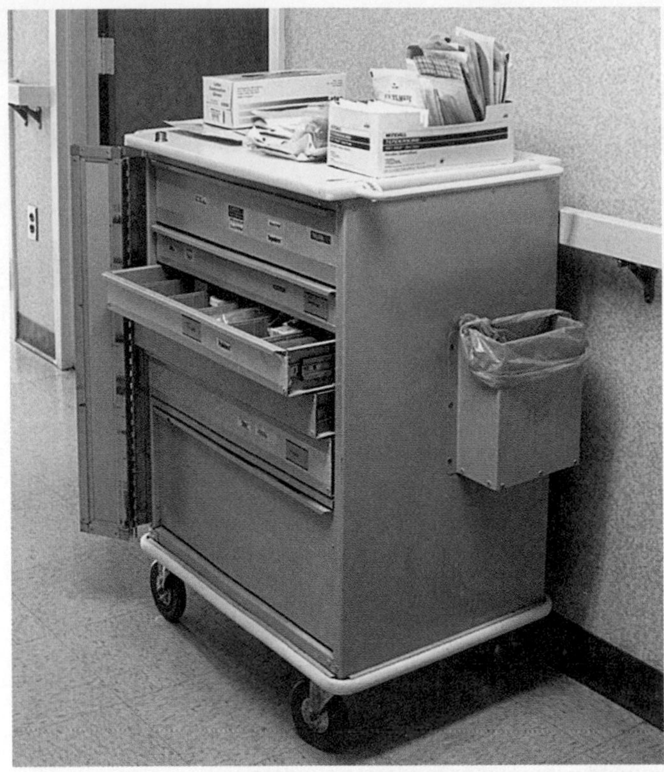

▲ Dressing carts may be used to keep supplies closer to client area.

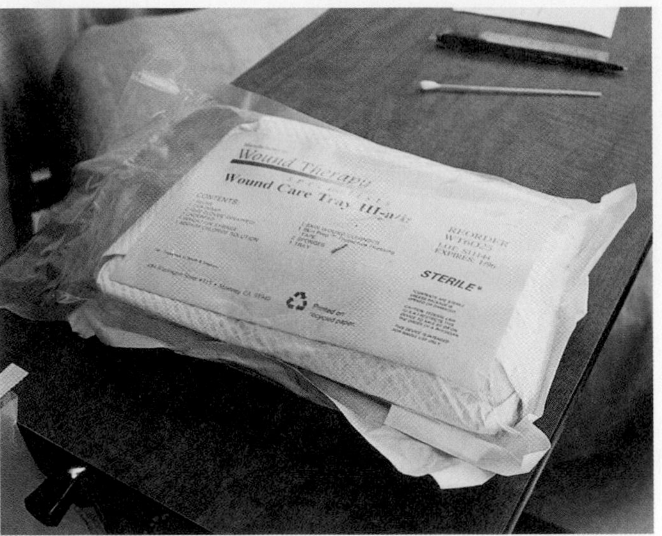

▲ Obtain specific dressing tray for ordered treatment.

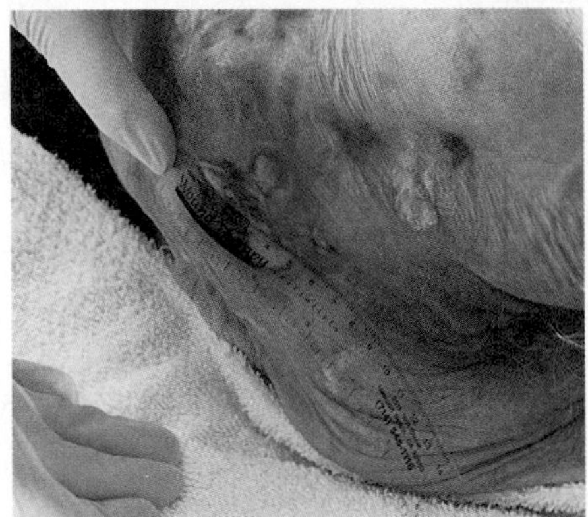

▲ Assess size of wound to determine appropriate size of transparent dressing.

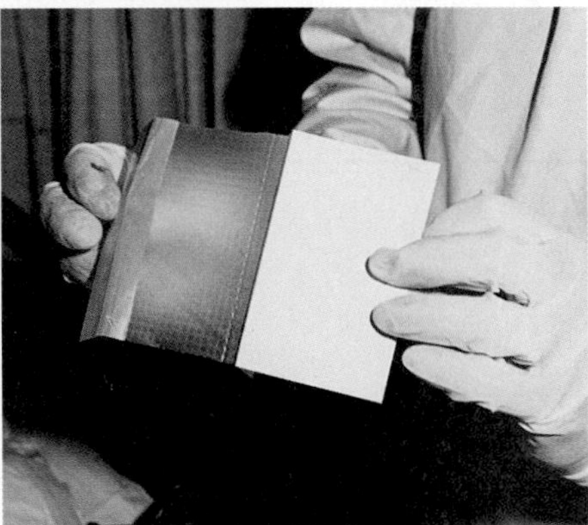

▲ Remove backing from Op-Site dressing before applying.

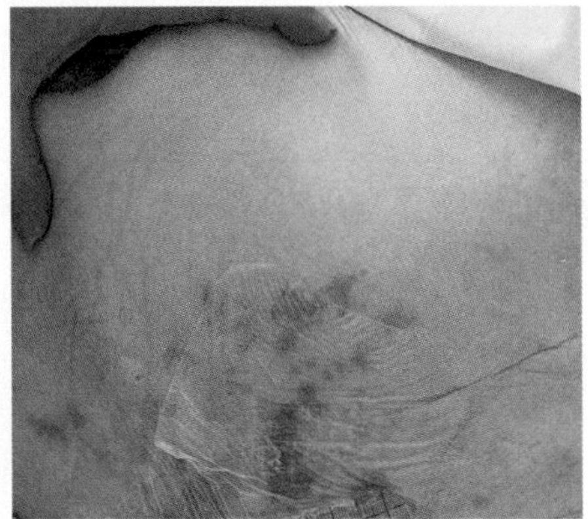

▲ Apply transparent adhesive dressing over wound.

Clinical Alert

Transparent film dressings remain in place for 5–7 days. These dressings are adhesive, permeable to moisture, vapor, and atmospheric gases. They are bacteria-proof and waterproof. It is imperative to observe the ulcer area daily to determine whether a large amount of secretions or serous fluid has accumulated under dressing. If fluid has increased, aspirate with a 26-gauge needle. These dressings are not used for infected areas.

8. Loosen transparent dressing from one side of backing paper.
9. "Walk on" dressing: Start at one edge of site and gently lay the dressing down, keeping it free of wrinkles. Allow at least a 1.5-in. margin of dressing beyond ulcer margin. ▸ ***Rationale:*** This ensures coverage of entire wound area.
10. Cut off tabs if using Op-Site after wound is completely covered.

11. Tape edges with hypoallergenic tape. ▸ ***Rationale:*** This assists in preventing frequent dressing changes due to loose dressings. These dressings can remain in place for 1 week.
12. Remove gloves and discard in appropriate receptacle.
13. Position client for comfort.
14. Lower bed and raise side rails.
15. Remove and discard equipment.
16. Perform hand hygiene.

DOCUMENTATION for Promoting a Moist Environment

- Condition of wound, location, size of wound
- Solution used
- Number and type of dressings used
- Signs and symptoms indicative of wound infection
- Color, consistency, presence of odor, amount of drainage on soiled dressings
- Presence of granular, necrotic, or epithelial tissue
- Condition of skin surrounding wound
- Client's reaction to procedure

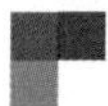

CRITICAL THINKING Application

Expected Outcomes

- Wound heals without complications.
- Sterile technique is maintained throughout procedure.

Unexpected Outcomes	Alternative Actions
Wound drainage increases.	• Decrease time between dressing changes. Change every 4 hr. • Obtain order for culture and sensitivity to determine whether different microorganisms are present or antibiotic medication is not sensitive to microorganism.
Dressings dry between dressing changes.	• Moisten dressing with sterile normal saline before removing to prevent debridement of granulation tissue. • Ensure that dressing is moist when applied to wound and cover with moist dressing. • Moisten and change dressing more frequently. • Semiocclusive dressing should be considered.

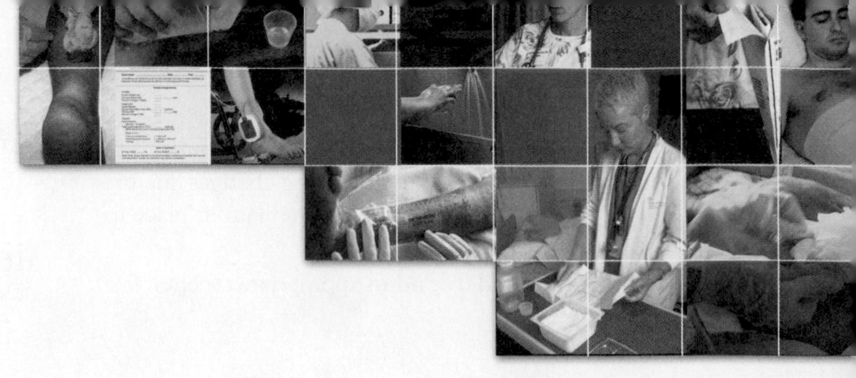

Chapter 25

UNIT ❺

Pressure Ulcers

Nursing Process Data

ASSESSMENT Data Base

- Assess stage of ulcer.
- Assess size and depth of pressure ulcer.
- Assess presence and location of undermining, tunneling, and sinus tracts.
- Identify if infection is associated with pressure ulcer.
- Assess wound exudate.
- Evaluate effectiveness of ulcer treatment.
- Assess healing process of the ulcer.
- Assess other bony prominences for potential formation of pressure ulcers.
- Assess for presence of conditions that inhibit wound healing.
- Assess wound size for changes.

PLANNING Objectives

- To identify the stage of the ulcer
- To provide appropriate treatment for specific ulcer stage
- To promote healing of established ulcer
- To prevent new ulcer formation
- To prevent spread of pathogens from ulcerated area

IMPLEMENTATION Procedures

EVALUATION Expected Outcomes

- Stage of pressure ulcer is accurately assessed.
- Pressure ulcer is treated effectively according to stage of ulcer formation.
- Pressure ulcer is healing within usual time frame.
- Skin remains free of breakdown in surrounding areas of pressure ulcer.
- Absence of additional pressure ulcer formation.

Nursing Guide for Assessment of Clients at Risk for Pressure Ulcers

Factors that contribute to development of pressure ulcers:

- Pressure
- Friction
- Shearing
- Moisture

Identify at-risk individuals needing preventative measures:

- Bed- and chair-bound individuals
- Clients with impaired ability to reposition themselves
- Clients who are immobilized
- Clients who are incontinent
- Clients with nutritional deficits, such as inadequate dietary intake, malnutrition
- Clients with altered level of consciousness
- Identification of stage I pressure ulcer may be difficult in a dark-skinned client.

A risk assessment tool should be used for all clients admitted to long-term care facilities, an acute care setting, or receiving home care (Braden scale or Norton scale). Systematic reassessments should be done at designated intervals.

- Nursing homes: Assess on admission and every week for 1 month, then every 3 months. Clients develop pressure ulcers within first month in nursing home.
- Home: Assess on admission and every visit. Instruct family to notify nurse if skin condition changes.
- Acute care: Assess on admission and every shift for at-risk clients in critical care units or daily to every other day for stable clients.

TABLE 25-8 Pressure Ulcer Staging and Treatment

Stage	Treatment Protocol for Pressure Ulcer Stages
Stage I: Intact skin with non-bleachable redness of a localized area usually over a bony prominence. Darkly pigmented skin may not have visible blanching; its color may differ from the surrounding area. The area may be painful, firm, soft, warmer or cooler as compared to adjacent tissue.	Unstageable Ulcers: Full thickness tissue loss in which the base of the ulcer is covered by slough (yellow, tan, gray, green, or brown) and/or eschar (tan, brown, or black) in the wound bed. Until enough slough and/or eschar is removed to expose the base of the wound, the true depth, and therefore stage, cannot be determined. National Pressure Ulcer Advisory Panel, February 2007

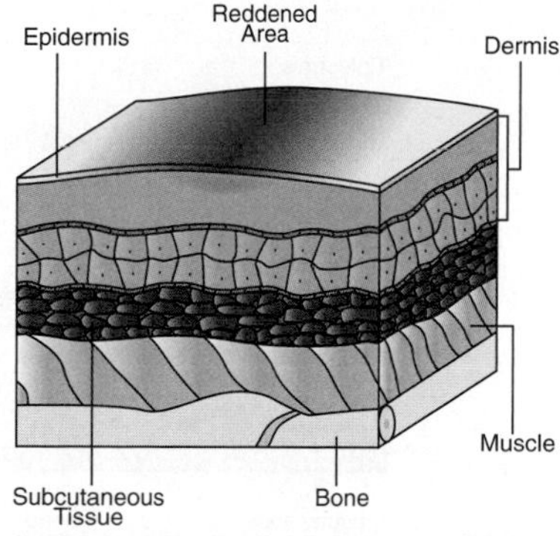

Stage I pressure ulcer. ▶

Continued

TABLE 25-8 Pressure Ulcer Staging and Treatment *(Continued)*

Stage	Treatment Protocol for Pressure Ulcer Stages
Stage II: Partial thickness loss of dermis presenting as a shallow open ulcer with a red pink wound bed, without slough. May also present as an intact or open/ruptured serum-filled blister. It presents as a shiny or dry shallow ulcer without slough or bruising. Bruising indicates suspected deep tissue injury.	

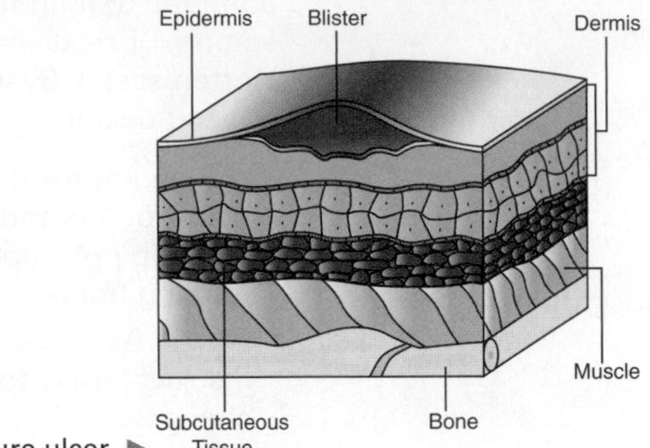

Stage II pressure ulcer. ▶

Stage	Treatment Protocol for Pressure Ulcer Stages
Stage III: Full thickness tissue loss. Subcutaneous fat may be visible but bone tendon or muscle are not exposed. Slough may be present but does not obscure the depth of tissue loss. It may include undermining and tunneling. The depth of this stage varies by the anatomical location. The bridge of the nose, ear, occiput and malleolus do not have subcutaneous tissue and therefore the ulcers can be shallow in contrast to areas of significant adipose tissue.	

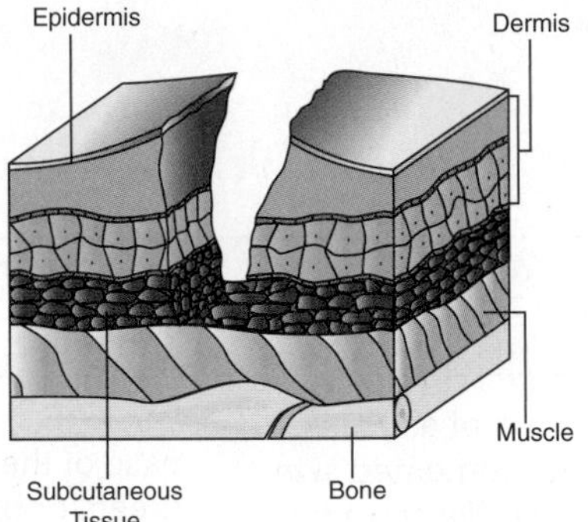

Stage III pressure ulcer. ▶

Stage	Treatment Protocol for Pressure Ulcer Stages
Stage IV: Full thickness tissue loss with exposed bone, tendon or muscle. Slough or eschar may be present on some parts of the wound bed. It often includes undermining and tunneling. The depth of this stage ulcer varies by anatomical location.	This stage can extend into muscle and/or supporting structures (fascia, tendon or joint capsule) making osteomyelitis possible. Other areas of the body without subcutaneous tissue will react the same as Stage III ulcers.

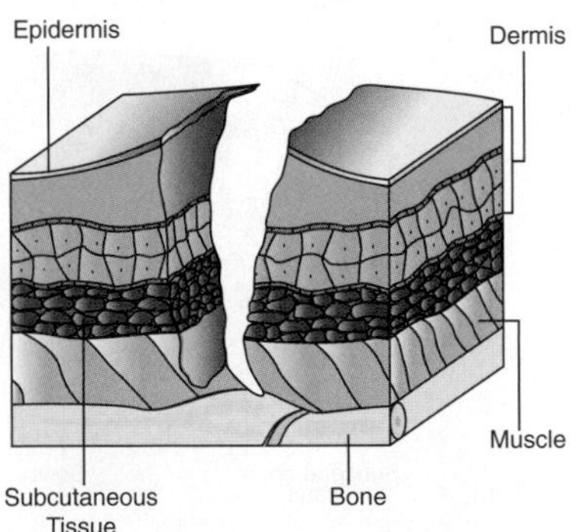

Stage IV pressure ulcer. ▶

Source: Wound Ostomy and Continence Nurses Society (WOLN) in the Standards of Care, 1992, the Agency for Healthcare Research and Quality (AHRQ), and the National Pressure Ulcer Advisory Panels (NPUAP). Guidelines published in *Advances in Wound Care* (1999, Nov.–Dec.), with update in revision of Stage 1 definitions by NPUAA.

Assessment for Dark-Skin-Tone Clients

Stage I. Ulcers appear with persistent red, blue, or purple hues. To assess darker skin tones that do not show erythema, shine a light at skin level to check for color change. Palpate area for induration or edema.

Stage II. Solid, smooth, dark pink tissue exposing basal membrane; exposed dermis epithelization.

TABLE 25-8 Pressure Ulcer Risk Assessment Scales

Norton Scale									
Physical Condition		**Mental Condition**		**Activity**		**Mobility**		**Continence**	
Good	−4	Alert	−4	Walks	−4	Full	−4	Good	−4
Fair	−3	Apathetic	−3	Walks with help	−3	Slightly limited	−3	Occasional incontinence	−3
Poor	−2	Confused	−2	Sits in chair	−2	Very limited	−2	Frequent incontinence	−2
Very poor	−1	Stuporous	−1	Remains in bed	−1	Immobile	−1	Urine and fecal incontinence	−1
Total ____		Total ____		Total ____		Total ____		Total ____	
Grand total = _____									
A score of 14 or less indicates risk of pressure ulcer; a score under 12 indicates high risk.									

Braden Scale											
Sensory Perception		**Moisture**		**Activity**		**Mobility**		**Nutrition**		**Friction and Shear**	
No impairment	−4	Rarely moist	−4	Walks frequently	−4	No limitations	−4	Excellent	−4		
Slightly limited	−3	Occasionally moist	−3	Walks occasionally	−3	Slightly limited	−3	Adequate	−3	No apparent problems	−3
Very limited	−2	Very moist	−2	Chairfast	−2	Very limited	−2	Probably inadequate	−2	Potential problem	−2
Completely limited	−1	Constantly moist	−1	Bedfast	−1	Completely immobile	−1	Very poor	−1	Problem	−1
Total ____		Total ____		Total ____		Total ____		Total ____		Total ____	
Grand total = _____											
Assign a score of 1 to 4 in each category. Total the score; no risk: 19–23; at risk: 15–18; moderate risk: 13–14; high risk: 10–12; very high risk: 9 or below.											

Norton Scale: Adapted from *Pressure Ulcers in Adults: Predictions and Prevention.* AHCRP Publication No. 92-0047 (May 1992), p. 15.
Braden Scale: Adapted from *Pressure Ulcers in Adults: Predictions and Prevention.* AHCRP Publication No. 92-0047 (May 1992), pp. 16–17.
Note: Refer to actual scales for detailed information about both scales.

Preventing Pressure Ulcers

Procedure

1. Inspect skin at least on admission and once a shift, particularly over bony prominences. Heels and sacrum are most common areas for skin breakdown. Use Braden or Norton scale for assessment. Document assessment findings. ▶***Rationale:*** If skin is red or skin breakdown is evident on admission, Medicare and other payers will reimburse for treatment. If not evident on admission, treatment costs will not be reimbursed.
2. Individualize client's bathing schedule. Daily baths are not essential. ▶***Rationale:*** Daily cleansing can destroy the skin's natural barrier, making it more susceptible to external irritants.
   a. Avoid hot bath water. ▶***Rationale:*** Tepid water prevents injury to skin.
   b. Use mild cleansing agents to minimize dryness.
   c. Cleanse skin immediately if urine, fecal incontinence, or wound drainage seeps onto skin.

   d. Provide humidity to prevent drying of skin.
   e. Use cream or thin layer of corn starch to protect skin.
3. Avoid massaging bony prominences. ▶ ***Rationale:*** Massaging can lead to deep tissue trauma.
   a. Keep bony prominences from direct contact with one another.
   b. Use pillow, foam wedges, or other positioning devices.
   c. Use elbow pads and heel elevators.
4. Promote adequate dietary intake of protein, calories, and nutrients. Protein should be approximately 1.2 to 1.5 g/kg body weight daily. ▶ ***Rationale:*** Adequate protein intake in addition to vitamins and minerals help prevent pressure ulcer formation.

Clinical Alert

Be alert to altered skin integrity when pressure is reduced in one anatomical area by turning and repositioning, as the newer location may be placed at risk for pressure ulcer formation.

5. Ensure adequate fluid intake. ▶ ***Rationale:*** Prevent dehydration which is a risk factor for pressure ulcer formation.
6. Reposition bedridden client every 1–2 hr.
   a. Do not position directly on trochanter.
   b. Do not turn more than 30° angle.

NUTRITIONAL ASSESSMENT OF CLIENT WITH PRESSURE ULCER(S)

Client Name: ______________ **Date:** __________ **Time** ________

To be filled out for all clients at risk on initial evaluation and every 12 weeks thereafter, as indicated. Trends will document the efficacy of nutritional support therapy.

Protein Compartments

Somatic:
Current Weight (kg) _____
Previous Weight (kg) _____ (_____date)
Percent Change in Weight _____

Height (cm) _____
Height/Weight _____
Current Body Mass Index (BM) _____ [wt/(ht)^2]
Previous BMI _____ (_____date)
Percent Change in BMI _____

Visceral:
Serum Albumin _____
(Normal ≥ 3.5 mg/dL)
Total Lymphocyte Count (TLC) _____ (optional)
(White Blood Cell count x percent Lymphocytes/100)

Guide to TLC:
- Immune competence ≥ 1,800 mm^3
- Immunity partly impaired < 1,800 but ≥ 900 mm^3
- Anergy < 900 mm^3

State of Hydration

24-Hour Intake _____ mL 24-Hour Output _____ mL

Note: Thirst, tongue dryness in non-mouth-breathers, and tenting of cervical skin may indicate dehydration. Jugular vein distention may indicate overhydration.

Estimated Nutritional Requirement

Estimated Nonprotein Calories (NPC) _____ /kg Estimated Protein _____ (g/kg)
Actual NPC _____ /kg Actual Protein _____ (g/kg)

Recommendations/Plan

1.
2.
3.
4.

SAMPLE PRESSURE ULCER ASSESSMENT GUIDE

Patient Name: ______________ Date: __________ Time: ________

Ulcer 1:			Ulcer 2:		
Site _____			Site _____		
Stage[a] _____			Stage[a] _____		
Size (cm)			Size (cm)		
Length _____			Length _____		
Width _____			Width _____		
Depth _____			Depth _____		
Sinus Tract	☐	☐	Sinus Tract	☐	☐
Tunneling	☐	☐	Tunneling	☐	☐
Undermining	☐	☐	Undermining	☐	☐
Necrotic Tissue	☐	☐	Necrotic Tissue	☐	☐
Slough	☐	☐	Slough	☐	☐
Eschar	☐	☐	Eschar	☐	☐
Exudate	☐	☐	Exudate	☐	☐
Serous	☐	☐	Serous	☐	☐
Serosanguineous	☐	☐	Serosanguineous	☐	☐
Purulent	☐	☐	Purulent	☐	☐
Granulation	☐	☐	Granulation	☐	☐
Epithelialization	☐	☐	Epithelialization	☐	☐
Pain	☐	☐	Pain	☐	☐
Surrounding Skin:					
Erythema	☐	☐	Erythema	☐	☐
Maceration	☐	☐	Maceration	☐	☐
Induration	☐	☐	Induration	☐	☐

Description of Ulcer(s): ______________________________

Indicate Ulcer Sites:

Anterior Posterior

(Attach a color photo of the pressure ulcer[s] [Optional])

[a]Classification of pressure ulcers:

Stage I: Nonblanchable erythema of intact skin, the heralding lesion of skin ulceration. In individuals with darker skin, discoloration of the skin, warmth, edema, induration, or hardness may also be indicators.

Stage II: Partial thickness skin loss involving epidermis, dermis, or both.

Stage III: Full thickness skin loss involving damage to or necrosis of subcutaneous tissue that may extend down to, but not through, underlying fascia. The ulcer presents clinically as a deep crater with or without undermining adjacent tissue.

Stage IV: Full thickness skin loss with extensive destruction, tissue necrosis, or damage to muscle, bone, or supporting structures (e.g., tendon or joint capsule).

▲ Nutritional assessment of client with pressure ulcer(s).

Source: Pressure Ulcer Treatment: Quick Reference Guide for Clinicians, No. 15. U.S. Department of Health and Human Services, AHCPR.

   c. Raise heels off bed by placing pillows under legs; allow heels to hang over edges.
   d. Use trapeze or turning sheet to reposition client.
7. Encourage mobility or range-of-motion exercises. ▶ ***Rationale:*** Range-of-motion exercises promote activity and reduce effects of pressure on tissue.
8. Minimize force and friction on skin when turning or moving client. Use turning sheets or Hoyer lift.
9. Maintain head of bed at lowest degree of elevation consistent with medical problem; below 30° if possible.
10. Place at-risk clients on pressure-reducing devices, in both bed and chair, such as foam, static-air, alternating gel, water mattress, or air-fluidized mattress.
11. Place client on specialty bed or mattress if highly at risk for pressure ulcer formation or has an ulcer.
12. Encourage chair-fast clients to shift position every 15 minutes.

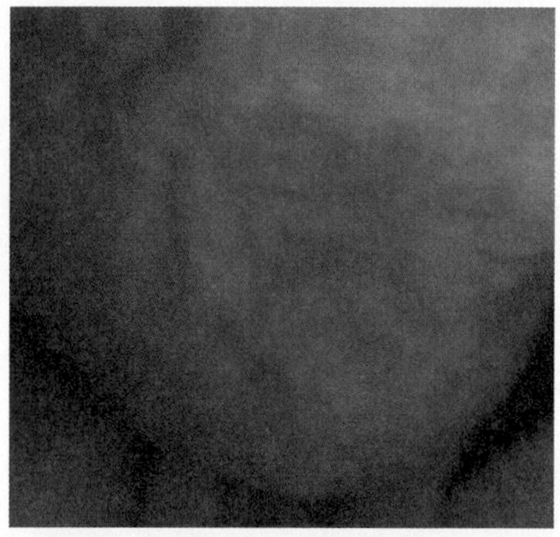

▲ Stage I pressure ulcer.

EVIDENCE-BASED PRACTICE

Pressure Relief in Surgical Clients

Pressure ulcers can begin in the operating room. The occurrence of ulcers can be as high as 45% of surgical clients. There are many risk factors leading to ulcer development in as few as 2.5 hr. Risk factors include position client is placed in during procedure and necessity of positioning devices that place pressure on bony prominences. Medications that constrict blood vessels or lower blood pressure can also lead to pressure ulcers.

Source: Armstrong, D., & Bortz, P. An integrative review of pressure relief in surgical patients. *American Organization of Operating Room Nurses Journal, 74*(3), 645-669 (2001).

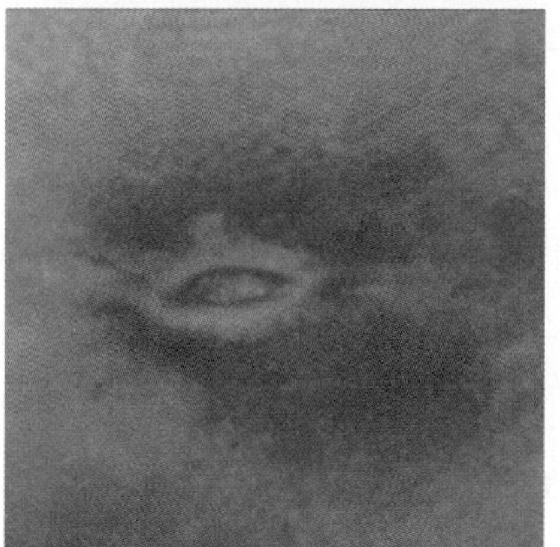

▲ Stage II pressure ulcer.

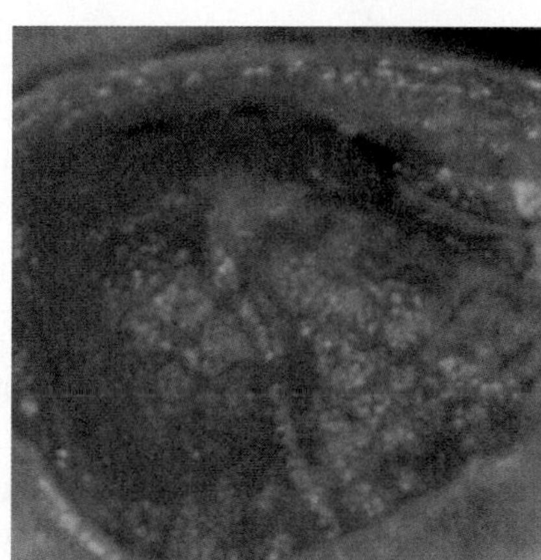

▲ Stage III pressure ulcer.

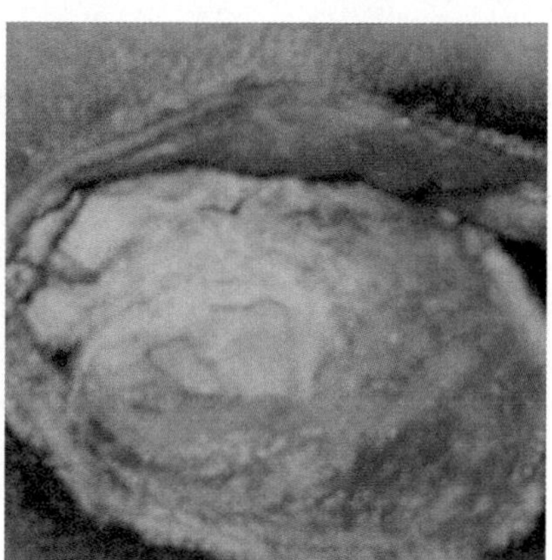

▲ Stage IV pressure ulcer.

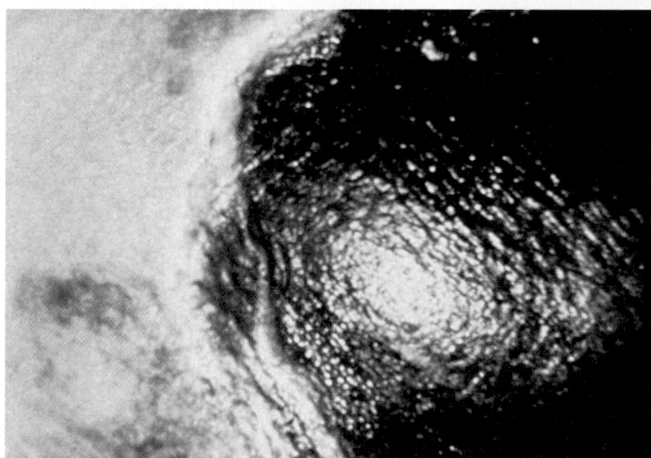

▲ Eschar must be removed by debridement before staging is done.

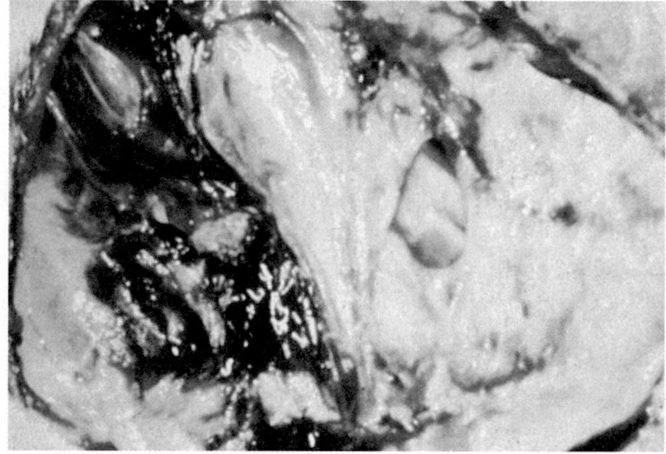

▲ Clinical signs of infection.

EVIDENCE-BASED PRACTICE

Pressure Ulcer Formation

There is an unresolved and inadequately explained issue of how a pressure ulcer progresses. Some clinicians believe the ulcer forms from top down, and other theories have indicated that the pressure ulcer progresses from bottom up. There is limited research on this theory. Current literature indicates that the bottom-up theory is more appropriate, as the deeper tissues are involved in pressure ulcer formation. Latest opinion is that true pressure ulcers are an injury to soft tissue and muscle that occurs from pressure over bony prominences. It is recommended that further research be done.

Source: WOCN Society Response to NPUAP White Papers: Deep Tissue Injury, Stage I Pressure Ulcers, and Stage II Pressure Ulcers: 9th National NPUAP Conference, February 2005. Phyllis Bonham, PhD, MSN, RN, CWOCN, and Janet Ramundo, MSN, RN, FNP, CWOCN.

Clinical Alert

Air-fluidized beds and low-air-loss beds are recommended to manage pressure ulcers, especially in clients with large or multiple ulcers.

Air-Fluidized

Warm, pressurized air circulates through beads in the bed and creates support surface.
Polyester sheet allows for moisture and air to pass through, keeping skin dry.
Treatment can take several months. Use of this bed is very expensive.

Low-Air-Loss

Head and foot of bed can be elevated. Bed is a modified standard bed frame, lighter and more portable than air-fluidized bed. Bed circulates cool air.
Urine and feces do not pass through fabric on the bed.
Bed is portable and lighter.

See also section on Special Beds in Chapter 8.

Providing Care for Clients With Pressure Ulcers

Procedure

1. Monitor client's overall condition daily. ▸ ***Rationale:*** Clients who are dying will have the tendency to develop new skin breakdown (skin failure) as other organs fail. Existing pressure ulcers of lesser staging (I and II) almost always worsen over time and become at least stage III.
2. Differentiate type of ulcer, pressure versus nonpressure.
3. Determine stage of ulcer.
4. Monitor and assess ulcer characteristics daily:
   a. Observe dressing to determine whether dry, intact, and not leaking.
   b. Observe ulcer bed, if appropriate, and document findings.
5. Assess pain level of client and provide adequate pain relief.
6. Photograph ulcer according to facility policy. ▸ ***Rationale:*** To determine progress of ulcer healing.
7. Monitor progress toward healing and for potential complications.
   a. Measure pressure ulcer size weekly using a Pressure Ulcer Scale. Usual healing time is 2 to 4 weeks.
   b. If healing is not progressing or has not healed in usual time frame, reevaluate treatment plan and client's condition.
8. Maintain turning and positioning schedule to promote healing and prevent additional ulcer formation.
9. Complete a nutritional assessment. Positive nitrogen balance and protein intake are necessary for healing.
10. Complete a psychosocial assessment to determine client's adherence to pressure ulcer treatment regimens.

Clinical Alert

Clients near the end of life have the right to refuse ulcer care. However, "Do Not Resuscitate" orders do not relieve the staff from providing quality pressure ulcer prevention or treatment.

11. Complete dressing change according to facility policy and type of dressing used. Follow manufacturer's guidelines for dressing change. ▸ ***Rationale:*** Dressing changes are based on a combination of factors, such as manufacturer suggested use, pressure ulcer characteristics, and goals for healing.

Clinical Alert

Centers for Medicare and Medicaid Services have indicated that long-term care facilities must implement evidence-based protocols of prevention and care for pressure ulcers.

DOCUMENTATION for Pressure Ulcers

- Client's general skin condition
- Periwound assessment
- Assessment of wound (i.e., size, presence of tunneling drainage, evidence of tissue granulation)
- Color, volume, type of exudate
- Type of ulcer care provided
- Type of pressure reducing/relieving device used
- Results of Braden or Norton pressure ulcer assessment scale
- Pressure ulcer record completed
- State the exact location of pressure ulcer; if bony prominence involved, use an anatomic name. Turning surface involved. (RI, LI, post., ant., medial, lateral)

- Size: Indicate size in centimeters
- Identify ulcers by number. Use chart
- Measure depth of ulcer
- Identify and measure undermining and tunneling location
- Stage: Write the number of the stage that corresponds to the description of the pressure ulcer (stage I–IV)
- Treatment: Chart treatment used (e.g., hydrocolloid dressing applied, transparent adhesive film applied, etc.)
- Position: Indicate time client's position was changed

CRITICAL THINKING Application

Expected Outcomes

- Stage of pressure ulcer is accurately assessed.
- Pressure ulcer is treated effectively according to stage of ulcer formation.
- Pressure ulcer is healing within usual time frame.
- Skin remains free of breakdown in surrounding areas of pressure ulcer.
- Absence of additional pressure ulcer formation.

Unexpected Outcomes	Alternative Actions
Client does not have sufficient exercise; appetite decreased.	• Encourage small, frequent feedings. • Offer high-calorie drinks like eggnog or Isocal.

Client's wound does not heal with traditional types of treatments	• In client care conference discuss the following:
	  • Is everyone following same treatment?
	  • Are causative agents preventing healing?
	  • Should treatment be adjusted or changed?
	  • Would use of a support surface be effective?
	  • Is surgical debridement and grafting necessary for healing?

Skin is exposed to moisture.	• Establish bowel or bladder program and select absorbent products for wound care that wick the moisture from skin. • Cleanse skin with pH-balanced cleansers, avoiding friction and dry skin after each incontinence and dry thoroughly. • Apply skin barrier product. • Consider use of fecal management system or urinary catheter.
Nutritional or hydration deficit occurs.	• Monitor nutritional and fluid intake accurately. • Obtain order for vitamin supplements if client is not already on vitamins. • Increase protein intake by supplementing with high protein drinks.
Shearing and friction secondarily related to immobility or reduced activity.	• Keep head of bed in lowest position possible to prevent client from sliding down in bed. • Use lifting devices to move client up in bed or out of bed to prevent friction on skin. • Instruct client on use of trapeze to assist in repositioning.

Chapter 25

UNIT 6

Adjunctive Wound Care Therapy

Nursing Process Data

ASSESSMENT Data Base

- Identify why usual wound therapy treatments are ineffective.
- Identify most effective adjunctive treatment for client.
- Assess wound for baseline data before initiating treatment.
- Determine if wound is healing using adjunctive therapy.
- Assess if client is good candidate for adjunctive therapy.
- Assess client's nutritional status to ensure best results from V.A.C. therapy.
- Determine if wound is maintaining a moist environment with adjunctive therapy.
- Assess periwound area for signs of maceration.
- Assess for adverse reactions during hyperbaric oxygenation therapy (HBO).

PLANNING Objectives

- To assess if adjunctive therapy is providing adequate wound healing
- To place client on pressure relief surface if wound is over bony prominence
- To determine if client is able to participate in specific therapy
- To select appropriate type of dressing for adjunctive therapy
- To determine if client is a good candidate for HBO

IMPLEMENTATION Procedures

EVALUATION Expected Outcomes

- Granulation tissue is evident using adjunctive therapy.
- Periwound area remains healthy without evidence of maceration.
- Moist wound environment is maintained.
- Pain is reduced with adjunctive therapy.
- Wound progresses through usual phases with electrical stimulation.
- Wound healing occurs faster with radiant heat dressing.
- Exudate is removed and wound healing occurs with negative pressure wound therapy.
- Hyperbaric oxygen therapy is effective in treating diabetic leg ulcers.

Using Electrical Stimulation

Equipment

Normal saline solution
Bag for soiled dressings
Gauze pads
Two sterile basins
Hydrogel sheets
Electrode
Bandage tape
Alligator clip
Stimulator
Two pair clean gloves
Sterile gloves

Preparation

1. Determine whether client is candidate for electrical stimulation.
2. Determine phase of wound healing. ▸ ***Rationale:*** This determines the correct treatment protocol.
3. Set the stimulator settings according to manufacturer's directions, based on client's phase in wound healing. The settings include polarity, pulse rate, intensity, duration, and frequency.
4. Explain procedure to client.
5. Gather equipment.
6. Perform hand hygiene.
7. Provide privacy.

Procedure

1. Raise bed to high position, lower side rails as needed.
2. Place client in position to enable staff to work with wound area and equipment. (Placement depends on wound site.)
3. Place supplies on overbed table, near working area.
4. Open all supply packages, maintaining sterility.
5. Pour sterile normal saline into one basin.
6. Don clean gloves.
7. Place disposal bag near wound. ▸ ***Rationale:*** For ease in disposing of soiled dressings.
8. Remove dressing carefully to avoid interfering with granulation tissue.
9. Remove clean gloves; place in disposal bag. Don sterile gloves.
10. Place sterile basin next to wound to catch irrigation solution as wound is cleansed.
11. Pour sterile normal saline into wound to cleanse wound. ▸ ***Rationale:*** To remove exudates, slough, and petrolatum products. Current will not be conducted into wound tissue if petrolatum products remain in the wound.
12. Remove excess irrigation solution using sterile gauze pads.
13. Place fluffed gauze pads into normal saline solution, squeeze out excess liquid.
14. Fill wound cavity with gauze, including any undermined/tunneled spaces. Pack gently.
15. Place surface (active) electrode in wound bed, over gauze packing. ▸ ***Rationale:*** This transfers electrical energy into wound bed, producing positive effects on necessary components for wound healing (i.e., blood flow, oxygen uptake, DNA, and protein synthesis).
16. Cover with dry gauze pad.
17. Tape dry pad securely.
18. Connect alligator clip to foil.
19. Connect to stimulator lead.
20. Place a wet washcloth over area where dispersive electrode will be placed.
21. Select a dispersive pad that is larger than the sum of areas of active electrodes and wound packing.
22. Place dispersive electrode proximal to wound, over soft tissue, avoiding bony prominences.

    NOTE: The greater the separation between two electrodes, the deeper the current path. Larger separation space is used to treat deep and undermined wounds. Closer separation space is used for shallow or partial thickness wounds. Ensure electrodes do not touch.

23. Ensure all edges of electrode are in good contact with skin. Hold electrode in place with nylon elasticized strap.
24. Place client in position of comfort. Electrical stimulation treatments usually last 60 minutes.
25. Remove gloves and discard.
26. Perform hand hygiene.
27. Don clean gloves.
28. Remove electrode from wound after treatment.
29. Remove saline-soaked gauze and cover wound with occlusive dressing.

    NOTE: Hydrogel sheets or amorphous hydrogel-impregnated gauze can be used to conduct current. If hydrogel gauze is the conductor, it is changed BID.

Candidates for Electrical Stimulation

- Pressure ulcers, stage I–IV.
- Diabetic ulcers
- Venous ulcers, ischemic ulcer
- Traumatic wounds
- Surgical wounds
- Wound flap
- Donor site, burn wound

Using Noncontact Normothermic Wound Therapy

Equipment

Warming cover (latex free)
Warming card
Temperature control unit (TCU)
AC adapter
Wound measuring guide
Sterile normal saline solution
Skin sealant
Carrying pouch
Sterile normal saline
Gauze pads
Moisture-proof pad
Sterile basin and irrigating syringe
Sterile gloves
Clean gloves
Disposable bag

The wound cover is sterile and protects wound from contamination and trauma. The cover maintains a moist and warm wound, which creates a healing environment. The cover is a thin shell with a window and a foam frame. The shell has an adhesive border, is water resistant, and can be cleaned. It is flexible and moves with the client. The foam cover absorbs excess exudates to protect periwound area from maceration. The foam frame keeps the pocket above the wound surface, so warming card is not in contact with the wound. The window is in the center of the cover and contains a pocket for the warming card.

Preparation

1. Check physician's orders and client care plan.
2. Gather equipment. Select appropriate-size wound cover and warming card after measuring wound.
3. Check that temperature control unit's battery is charged; if not, recharge with battery pack or wall outlet power source.
4. Explain procedure to client.
5. Provide privacy for client.
6. Perform hand hygiene.

Procedure

1. Place equipment on overbed table.
2. Open sterile normal saline bottle, gauze pads, and basin with irrigating syringe.
3. Place disposable bag near wound site.
4. Position client for easy access to wound.
5. Remove compression stockings, if used.
6. Don clean gloves.
7. Remove old dressing and place in disposal bag.
8. Remove clean gloves and discard into disposal bag. Don sterile gloves.
9. Fill irrigating syringe with normal saline. ▸ ***Rationale:*** Using the syringe will increase pressure in wound to assist with removing debris and slough.
10. Place moisture-proof pad or sterile basin under wound site.
11. Irrigate wound using the prescribed amount of irrigating solution.
12. Cleanse the surrounding skin with normal saline.
13. Dry periwound skin area.
14. Apply sealant to periwound area. ▸ ***Rationale:*** This protects periwound area from exudates.
15. Select wound cover size that is appropriate size for wound. ▸ ***Rationale:*** To ensure that there is adequate healthy periwound skin between edge of foam and wound.
16. Hold wound cover near edges only. Pull away half of wound cover liner.
17. Place wound cover over wound, so wound can be seen through window. Do not stretch wound cover over skin while applying. ▸ ***Rationale:*** Damage can occur to skin.
18. Check for holes in wound cover, wrinkling, and folding of its edges. ▸ ***Rationale:*** Wound cover will not be a barrier if this occurs.
19. Press adhesive portion of cover to skin.
20. Pull away other half of wound cover liner and press adhesive portion to skin.
21. Gently smooth adhesive portion of wound cover with your finger tips to ensure adhesive sticks to skin.
22. Instruct the client that wound cover is worn 24 hr per day and requires no additional dressing.
23. Attach wound cover to Warm-Up therapy system.
24. Remove gloves and discard into disposal bag.
25. Perform hand hygiene.

For Using Warm-Up Therapy® System

1. Select appropriate-size warming card based on size of wound cover.
2. Plug warming card into gray socket on temperature control unit (TCU).

Clinical Alert

This warming treatment is done three times a day for 1 hr each treatment. Ensure that there is at least 1 hr between treatments. You can expect a significant increase in exudate for at least 7–10 days. This is considered a normal consequence of wound healing process.

TABLE 25-9 Adjunctive Therapies in Wound Care

Therapy	Outcomes
Hydrotherapy	Promotes debridement and cleans wound.
Electrical Stimulation	Increases oxygen and nutrients to tissues, reduces pain and edema, improves scar tissue elasticity.
Ultrasound	Increases collagen elasticity, decreases pain and muscle spasms. Increases oxygen, decreases edema, and accelerates wound recovery.
Hyperbaric Oxygen	Increases tissue oxygenation and promotes wound healing.
Compression	Promotes venous blood return, prevents pooling of blood and edema formation.
Nutritional Support	Decreases susceptibility of soft tissue breakdown.
Support Surfaces	Distributes body weight and reduces tissue pressure. Controls shear forces on skin surfaces and provides stability for client's torso.
Biological Products	Increases wound healing by increasing wound strength, increasing cellular content, and controlling collagen deposition.

3. Insert warming card into wound cover pocket. (Warming card is used throughout warming therapy and is only for one client; it can be cleaned with damp cloth and clean water, if needed.) Do not apply the warming card directly to the periwound area. Always cover the card with the wound cover. ▸ ***Rationale:*** Thermal injury can occur.
4. Turn off TCU.
5. Select mode of power (can use battery or AC adapter wall outlet).
6. Check that battery has sufficient charge for therapy session, usually 1 hr.
   a. If battery needs charging; plug AC adapter into TCU, then plug the AC adapter into wall outlet.
   b. Charge TCU until amber light on AC adapter flashes rapidly. It takes up to 2 hr to fully charge battery.
7. Plug AC adapter into black socket on the TCU if using the TUC with the AC adapter. Plug AC adapter into wall outlet.
8. Position TCU and warming card cable to allow client some movement. Instruct client not to lie on any electronic component, cable, cord, or wound cover.
9. Press the ON button to begin therapy. Follow physician orders for length of time for therapy. The unit will automatically turn off after 2 hr of continuous use.
10. Shut off TCU and remove warming card by grasping edge of card and sliding it out of wound cover pocket. Place card in plastic pouch for storage between treatments. DO NOT REMOVE WOUND COVER. ▸ ***Rationale:*** Wound cover is replaced if drainage occurs, the cover comes loose, the periwound area becomes macerated, or it has been in place 72 hr.
11. Replace compression therapy if ordered.

Clinical Alert

Do not use compression therapy while warming card and TCU are in place. Client injury could occur.

For Changing Wound Cover

1. Check wound cover to ensure it needs to be changed.
2. Gather equipment for new wound cover.
3. Explain procedure to client.
4. Perform hand hygiene.

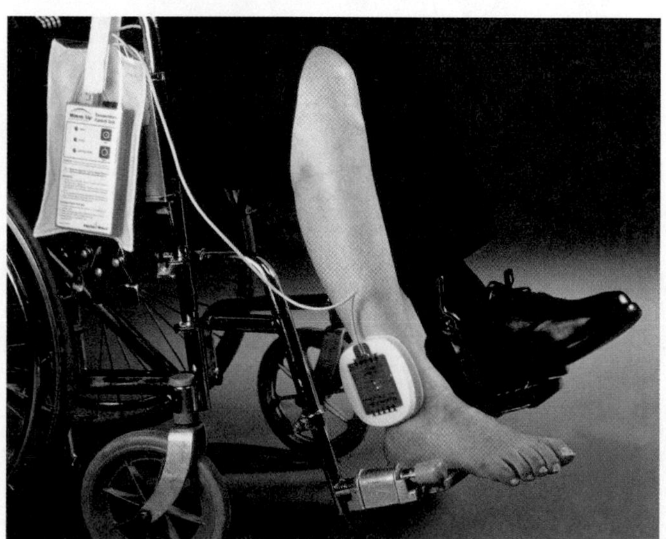

▲ Warm-Up Therapy® unit. (Courtesy of Augustine Medical, Inc., Eden Prairie, MN.)

5. Follow steps in skill Using Noncontact Normothermic Wound Therapy, Preparation.
6. Don clean gloves.
7. Place disposal bag near wound.
8. Gently press down on skin along one edge of wound cover.
9. Carefully lift edge of wound cover.
10. Slowly peel away wound cover until all edges are loose.
11. Discard wound cover in disposal bag.
12. Remove gloves, discard, and wash hands.
13. Reapply new wound cover following steps in skill Using Noncontact Normothermic Wound Therapy.

For Charging Batteries

1. Plug AC adapter connector into black socket on temperature control unit.
2. Plug AC adapter power cord into AC adapter inlet.
3. Plug AC adapter power cord into properly grounded wall outlet.
4. Observe that green light and a steady amber light on AC adapter panel are on.
5. Charge until amber light is flashing rapidly on AC adapter. Full charge takes 2 hr.

EVIDENCE-BASED PRACTICE

Radiant Heat Therapy and Chronic Wound Healing

A prospective, randomized, controlled study of 41 clients with stage III or IV pressure ulcers on the trunk explored effects of radiant heat therapy (RHT) versus a hydrocolloid dressing on full-thickness pressure ulcers in various settings, including clinics, long-term care, and a rehabilitation center. The clients were managed for up to 12 weeks or healing, whichever came first.

The results indicated that eight clients healed in the RHT group, and seven clients healed in the hydrocolloid dressing group. Therefore, no statistical significance was found between the two groups.

Source: Thomas, D. R., Diebold, M. R., & Eggemeyer, L. M. (2005). A controlled, randomized, comparative study of a radiant heat bandage on the healing of stage 3–4 pressure ulcers: A pilot study. *Journal of American Medical Directors Association*, 6(1), 46–49.

EVIDENCE-BASED PRACTICE

Effects of a Normothermic Dressing on Pressure Ulcer Healing

Twenty clients with stage III and IV ulcers were studied to determine the effects of wound healing when heat was applied. Three groups were treated using three different methods; one group used heating therapy for 4.5 hr each day Monday–Friday for 4 weeks. One group had wounds warmed for two 60-minute periods daily. One group received no heat therapy. Results of the study indicated that the clients who received the most heat therapy healed significantly faster than the others. There were no adverse affects from the heat therapy.

Source: Kloth, L. C., Berman, J. E., Dumit-Minkel, S., Sutton, C. H., Papanek, P. E., & Wurzel, J. (2000, March/April). Effects of a normothermic dressing on pressure ulcer healing. *Advances in Skin & Wound Care*, *13*(2), 69–74.

Using Negative Pressure Wound Therapy

Equipment

- Foam, Black or White V.A.C.® kit
- Gauze pads
- Sterile normal saline
- Irrigating syringe
- Moisture proof pad or sterile basin
- Skin prep agent, optional
- Razor, optional
- Clean gloves
- Sterile gloves
- V.A.C. device
- Disposal bag
- Sterile scissor

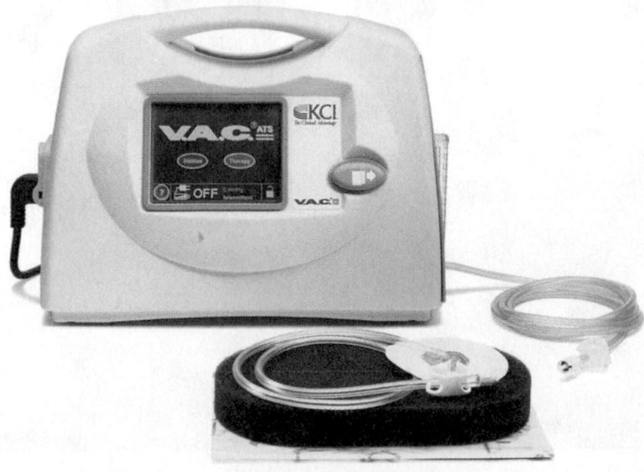

1 V.A.C.® unit.

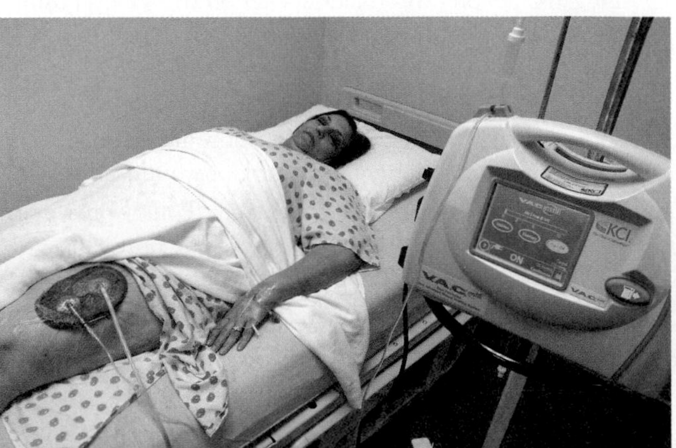

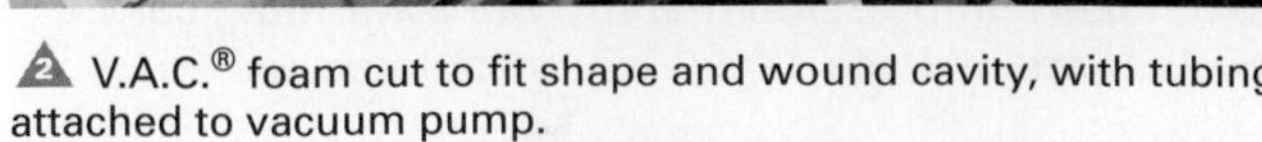

2 V.A.C.® foam cut to fit shape and wound cavity, with tubing attached to vacuum pump.

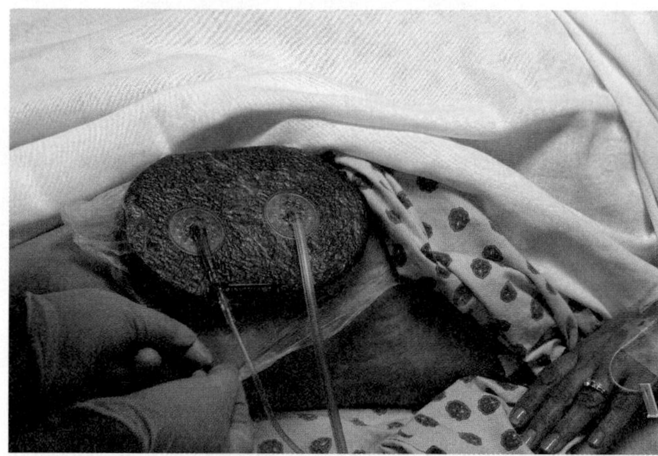

Remove adhesive drape by gently pulling away from skin.

Negative Pressure Wound Therapy

Uses	Contraindications
Acute and chronic wounds	Malignancy in wound
Traumatic	Untreated osteomyelitis
Partial-thickness burns	Nonenteric and unexplored fistula
Dehisced wounds	Necrotic tissue with presence of diabetic ulcers eschar
Pressure ulcers	Directly over exposed blood flaps vessel or organ
Grafts	When using hydrogen peroxide and alcohol-based solutions
	Clients who cannot tolerate temperature of fluid

Preparation

1. Evaluate whether client is candidate for V.A.C. therapy: nutritionally stable, able to use device 22 hr each day, uses a pressure support surface if wound is over bony prominence. ▶ ***Rationale:*** If therapy turned off longer than 2 hr, dressing must be removed and replaced with traditional dressing.
2. Assess wound to determine whether therapy can be implemented.
   a. Wound surrounded by at least 2 cm of intact periwound tissue to maintain airtight seal.
   b. Wound open enough to insert foam dressing that touches all edges.
   c. Wound debrided.
   d. Sufficient circulation to assist in healing process.
3. Select correct foam dressing according to size and type of wound. Black foam has larger pores and is used to stimulate granulation tissue and wound contraction. White (soft) foam is used when granulation tissue needs to be restricted or client cannot tolerate pain associated with black foam. White foam is used with superficial wounds, shallow chronic ulcers, and tunneling or undermining wounds.
4. Gather equipment and supplies.
5. Provide privacy.
6. Explain procedure to client and determine his willingness to use this therapy.
7. Perform hand hygiene.

Procedure

1. Place disposal bag near wound.
2. Open supplies and place on overbed table. Open kit maintaining sterility.
3. Draw up normal saline irrigating solution in syringe.
4. Don clean gloves.
5. Place moisture-proof pad or sterile basin under wound. ▶ ***Rationale:*** Protects skin and bed during irrigation.
6. Clean wound using aggressive irrigation. If debridement is to be done, only a trained professional can perform the skill. Notify the appropriate person. ▶ ***Rationale:*** Devitalized tissue should be removed as areas of soft or stringy slough delays the healing process.
7. Remove gloves and place in disposal bag.
8. Don sterile gloves.
9. Dry wound and prepare periwound tissue with skin preparation agent if necessary. ▶ ***Rationale:*** To promote an airtight seal.
10. Cut the V.A.C. foam to fit the shape and entire wound cavity, including tunneling or undermined areas. White foam is used for tunneled wounds.
11. Size and trim drape to cover foam dressing, leaving a 3.5-cm border per wound area.
12. Gently place the foam into wound, ensuring entire wound is covered.
13. Apply tubing to foam. Tubing can be laid on top of foam or placed inside foam dressing. Keep tubing away from bony prominences.
14. Cover foam and 3.5 cm per wound area with drape. Do not stretch drape or compress foam with drape. ▶ ***Rationale:*** This ensures a tight seal without causing tension or a shearing force on periwound tissue.
15. Lift tubing and place on drape that has been bunched up to protect skin from pressure of tube.

Clinical Alert

Do not pack foam into any areas of the wound. Forcing foam dressings in a compressed manner into any wound may lead to risk of adverse health issues.

16. Secure tubing with additional piece of drape or tape several centimeters away from dressing. ▸ ***Rationale:*** This prevents pulling on the dressing, leading to a leak.
17. Remove gloves and discard.
18. Remove canister from sterile package and push it into the V.A.C. unit until you hear it click in place. Alarm will sound if canister is not properly inserted into unit.
19. Connect dressing tubing to canister tubing.
20. Open both clamps, one on dressing tubing and one on canister tubing.
21. Place V.A.C. unit on level surface or hang from footboard.
22. Press power button ON.
23. Adjust V.A.C. unit settings according to physician's orders or Guidelines for Treating Wound Types in the Reference Manual. Target pressure should be set for 5 minutes on and 2 minutes off (intermittent therapies on machine). Intensity of setting sets the negative pressure.
24. Assess dressing in 1 minute. ▸ ***Rationale:*** The dressing should collapse unless air leak is present.
25. Dressing changes must be completed every 48 hr unless wound is infected, then change every 12–24 hr.

For Removing Dressing

1. Perform hand hygiene.
2. Don clean gloves.
3. Raise tube connector above level of pump unit.
4. Tighten clamp on dressing tube.
5. Separate canister tube and dressing tubes by disconnecting the connector.
6. Allow pump unit to pull exudates in canister tube into canister; then tighten clamps on canister tube.
7. Press Therapy ON/OFF to deactivate pump.
8. Stretch drape horizontally and slowly pull up from skin. Gently remove it from skin. Do not peel it off skin.
9. Discard disposable equipment including gloves in appropriate bag or container.
10. Perform hand hygiene.

NOTE: Dressing changes are completed every 48 hr; if infected, every 12 hr.

For Disconnecting V.A.C.® Unit

1. Turn the unit to OFF.
2. Clamp both clamps on tubing.
3. Press quick-release connector to separate dressing tubing from canister tubing.
4. Cover ends of tubing with gauze and secure.

For Reconnecting V.A.C.® Unit

1. Remove gauze from ends of tubing.
2. Connect tubing.
3. Unclamp clamps
4. Press V.A.C. green power button to ON.
5. Select NO at new client prompt. Unit will resume previous settings.
6. Press therapy to ON.

V.A.C.® GranuFoam Silver

- Provides continuous delivery of silver directly to wound bed.
- Provides a protective barrier to reduce aerobic, gram-negative, and gram-positive bacteria, yeast, and fungi, and it may reduce infections in wounds.
- Indicated for client with chronic, acute, traumatic, and dehisced wounds, partial thickness burns, and pressure ulcers.

Clinical Alert

For deep wound, reposition tubing to minimize pressure on wound edges every 2 hr. Excess foam can be used to cushion skin under tubing.

EVIDENCE-BASED PRACTICE

Vacuum-Assisted Closure (V.A.C.®) for Sternal Wounds: A First-Line Therapeutic Management Approach

A retrospective review of 103 clients was completed at one institution. The clients underwent vacuum-assisted closure therapy after median sternotomy between June 1999 and March 2004. The clients' wounds were classified as sterile wounds, superficial sternal infections, and mediastinitis. The wound closure device was applied sterilely to all wounds over a layer of Acticoat. The results indicated that vacuum-assisted closure was utilized in the treatment of 103 clients with sternal wounds (67 males and 36 females). The median age was 52 years (3 months to 91 years). Client comorbidities included diabetes, chronic obstructive pulmonary disease, end-stage renal disease, immunosuppression, and other conditions. The therapy was utilized for 11 days per client. Sixty-eight of the clients had definitive chest closure with open reduction internal fixation and/or flap closure. The remaining 32% of the clients had no definitive closure method. The overall mortality rate was 28%, although none of the four deaths were directly related to the use of the therapy. The conclusion indicated that vacuum-assisted closure therapy has been shown to decrease wound edema, decrease time to definitive closure, and reduce wound bacterial colony counts.

Source: Agarwal, J. P., Ogilvie, M., Wu, L. C., Lohman, R. F., Gottlieb, L. J., Franczyk, M., & Song, D. H. (2005). Vacuum-assisted closure for sternal wounds: A first-line therapeutic management approach. *Plastic Reconstructive Surgery, 116*(4), 1035–1040.

Safety Tips for Negative Pressure Therapy

- Maintain therapy 22 hr per day.
- Perform wound cleansing and dressing changes every 48 hr unless wound infected, then change to every 12 hr.
- Monitor wound and dressing at least every 4 hr to ensure foam is collapsed and for signs of infection or other complications.
- Change type of wound system or medicate if client complains of pain or discomfort during treatment.
- Use continuous therapy (24 hr) to minimize movement and help stabilize wound bed over unstable body structures such as chest wall.
- Change canister when full or at least weekly. Use Standard Precautions.

For Changing Canister

1. Don clean gloves.
2. Assess that canister unit is full. Unit will alarm when full.
3. Tighten clamps on canister tubing from dressing tubing.
4. Pull back on release knob on V.A.C. unit at same time as you pull canister from slot.
5. Put canister in biohazard disposable bag and place in designated area for disposal.
6. Dispose of gloves.
7. Perform hand hygiene.

NOTE: Average length of treatment is 4–6 weeks. Home systems are available as well.

Using Hyperbaric Oxygenation for Diabetic Ulcers

Equipment

Hyperbaric chamber
Compressed air mask (optional)

Preparation

1. Identify client using two forms of identification. Introduce yourself.
2. Explain the procedure to client.

Procedure

1. Perform hand hygiene.
2. Ensure client is wearing 100% cotton fabrics only. ▸ ***Rationale:*** to prevent spark potential.
3. Ensure client does not have petroleum-based and alcohol-based products on hair or cosmetics. ▸ ***Rationale:*** Vapors from sprays, cosmetics, and Vaseline can spontaneously combust in an increased atmospheric environment of 100% oxygen.
4. Check that topical wound and skin care products with petroleum base are not present on client.
5. Take client to treatment area.
6. Once client is placed in chamber, the following observations must be observed constantly during compression and during entire treatment.
   a. Assess client for ability to equalize pressure changes in ear. Client will complain of ear pain. Instruct client to yawn, swallow, or perform Valsalva maneuver.
   b. Determine if client has sensation of warmth as the pressure increases, temperature increases, and decreasing rate of compression of the chamber.
   c. Check for confinement anxiety. Minimize this potential adverse effect through orientation to the

HBO Therapy

Two types of chambers are used in HBO therapy: multiplace chamber and monoplace chamber.

Multiplace chamber

- Compressed with 100% oxygen administered through direct piped-in gas.
- Multiple clients treated at one time (1–12 clients can be done at the same time).
- Nurse is in chamber to provide care.
- Critically ill client can be more readily treated.

Monoplace chamber

- Single client therapy.
- Uses 100% O_2 to compress chamber.
- Client can breathe compressed air by mask during treatment.
- For clients with claustrophobia or who can't tolerate mask, alterations in treatment protocols may be required.

Risk to nurse is minimized by strict adherence to diving protocols that allows for period of decompression of the nerve. See also Chapter 30, page 1187.

process of decompression. Anxiolytic therapy using benzodiazepines may be ordered.

d. Determine potential for hypoglycemia with diabetic client. Assess client during decompression for loss of consciousness, disorientation, and seizures. Preventive measures include maintaining blood glucose levels by adequate nutrition and timing of insulin injections in relationship to treatment. Peak insulin levels should not occur during treatment.

7. Observe client continuously while in chamber and when decompression is reversed.
8. Evaluate client for signs of oxygen toxicity or other potential adverse reactions. Report adverse findings to physician.

DOCUMENTATION for Adjunctive Wound Care Therapy

- Wound assessment including location, measurement of wound, presence of tunneling or undermining
- Color of wound, presence of exudates, color, and odor
- Wound stage, if appropriate
- Eschar description if present
- Presence of pain in periwound area
- Type, frequency, and duration of adjunctive therapy
- Date and time of wound cover change in Warm-Up Therapy
- Client's response to therapy
- Length of time negative pressure therapy treatment is off
- Client's reaction to HBO and any adverse effects

Legal Alert

Wound care practitioners are at risk for litigation. Clients who experience wounds frequently believe it is because of neglect by healthcare workers. Wound care practitioners may face liability for:

- Negligence
- Violations of Medicare and Medicaid fraud and abuse prohibitions
- Abandonment for terminating services to clients

To prove negligence, a client must show that the provider owed the client a duty and breached the duty owed the client, and the breach of duty must result in injury or damage to the client. Owing a duty of reasonable care to a client incorporates the standards of wound care. Breaching a duty occurs when the healthcare practitioner does something that should not have been done. To be charged with causing injury, the client would need to prove that injuries occurred as a result of practitioner error.

Source: Hess, C. T. (2002). *Clinical guide to wound care* (4th ed., pp. 109–114). Springhouse, PA: Springhouse.

CRITICAL THINKING Application

Expected Outcomes

- Granulation tissue is evident using adjunctive therapy.
- Periwound area remains healthy without evidence of maceration.
- Moist wound environment is maintained.
- Pain is reduced with adjunctive therapy.
- Wound progresses through usual phases with electrical stimulation.
- Wound healing occurs faster with radiant heat dressing.
- Exudate is removed and wound healing occurs using negative pressure wound therapy.
- Client's diabetic wound heals with hyperbaric oxygen therapy.

Unexpected Outcomes	Alternative Actions
Warm-Up Therapy® system shows heat light is on and low battery light is flashing.	• Charge battery. • Use TCU and AC adapter together.
Fault light is flashing and an alarm is sounding on TCU.	• Reconnect warming card, it may be disconnected. • Warming card or cable could be bent or damaged. Replace warming card. • TCU is broken. Turn TCU on and off. If light continues and alarm continues, turn off TCU and obtain new unit.
Nothing lights up on TCU panel.	• TCU is not on or battery is low. Turn unit ON or charge battery.

Wound is too large for V.A.C.® kit.	• Use more than one foam piece. • Place pieces so they touch each other. • Use only one tubing to one of the pieces.
Periwound skin is fragile.	• Use skin prep before applying drape. • Frame wound with skin barrier or DuoDERM. • Cut drape large enough to enclose foam dressing and skin barrier layer.
Dressing does not collapse following V.A.C.® application.	• Listen for whistling sound indicating a leak in the system. • Gently press around tubing, check for wrinkles or drape not covering correctly. • Most leaks occur around tubing. • Use excess drape to patch over leak.
Foam is not collapsed in wound bed.	• Ensure therapy is ON. Ensure clamps are open and tubing is not kinked. • Check for leaks and patch.
Audible alarm sounds on V.A.C.® system and therapy is stopped.	• Check for blockage in tubing and replace as needed. • If problem continues after tubing is replaced, notify company that produces the system.
Dressing adheres to wound with negative pressure system.	• Instill sterile water or normal saline into dressing, let sit for 15–20 minutes, then gently remove dressing from wound.
Client exhibits signs of anxiety when providing education regarding use of hyperbaric chamber.	• Place client in multichamber where a nurse is present to assist client with anxiety-reducing interventions.

GERONTOLOGIC Considerations

As clients grow older, the usual function of the skin declines, leading to major complications. Nearly 40% of clients aged 65–75 have at least one significant problem related to the skin.

- Dry skin is present in 77% of clients over 64.
- Vitamin D deficiency.
- Decrease in sebum production.
- Decrease in sweat production.
- Decrease in thermoregulation.
- Basal cell carcinoma is most common skin malignancy.
- Decrease in sensory perception.
- Decrease in adequate oxygen or nutrition occurs when issue is subjected to excessive pressure.

The inflammatory and proliferation phases of wound healing are often defective with elderly clients who have chronic diseases.

- A hemoglobin below 10 g/dL increases susceptibility.
- Uncontrolled diabetes mellitus or a blood glucose level that exceeds 200 mg/dL presents a risk.
- Hyperglycemia retards neutrophil production.
- T and B cells diminish in function and number, indicating a reduced inflammatory response. Elderly clients are at risk for cutaneous viral and fungal infections.
- Clients with rheumatoid arthritis who take steroids or nonsteroidal anti-inflammatory medications are at risk for decreased wound healing. There is a slower rate of epithelialization and severely inhibited contraction.
- Ischemia, anemia, and edema from vascular insufficiency or pressure leads to lack of blood flow to a wound area. Lower oxygen-carrying capacity results from anemia. Edema makes it difficult to transport oxygen and cellular wastes to and from cells. Ischemia leads to diminished oxygen necessary for wound healing.

Nursing actions to counteract risks against wound healing

- All at-risk elderly clients should have a pressure ulcer risk assessment completed at the time of admission and at regular intervals thereafter.
- Use of compression stockings assists in treating both the edema and ultimately the ischemia, therefore increasing blood flow to wound area.
- Turning frequently, at least every 2 hr, for clients free of pressure ulcers and every 1 hr for those at high risk, should be a priority.
- Use of pressure-relieving mattresses decreases risk potential.
- Wound care, including irrigation, use of appropriate dressings, and maintaining aseptic technique with dressing changes, should be priority care for clients with any type of wound.

MANAGEMENT Guidelines

Each state legislates a Nurse Practice Act for RNs and LVN/LPNs. Healthcare facilities are responsible for establishing and implementing policies and procedures that conform to their state's regulations. Verify the regulations and role parameters for each healthcare worker in your facility. Nurses working in a hyperbaric chamber must be trained in how to work with the clients and how to protect themselves when in the chamber. Before being assigned to this activity, ensure they have had the education necessary to work in this environment.

Delegation

- Assessment and evaluation of wounds and their management modalities are only RN functions and may not be delegated to other healthcare workers. The RN in collaboration with the physician develops a plan of care for clients requiring wound management.
- An LVN/LPN may be assigned to complete a sterile dressing change following instructions from the RN and in accordance with the wound care protocol established for the individual client.
- An LVN/LPN may remove staples and sutures after instruction and return demonstrations have been documented. (Most nursing programs include this information in the curriculum.)
- A CNA may apply a dry dressing, but may not perform a sterile procedure.

Communication Matrix

- Information regarding assessment of the wound should be reported to all staff caring for the client. This can be accomplished during report or documented on the nurses' notes and on client care plans or clinical (critical) pathway documents, or electronic forms.
- Wound care procedures (i.e., dressing changes) should be outlined or special wound care steps inserted into computer record. Specific instructions regarding type and amount of dressing material needed and specific directions in the application of the dressings must be written clearly so all nurses may follow appropriate directions.
- Specific directions for wound management and use of specialized equipment must be given to the nurse during report from the RN team leader or manager.
- Reports outlining specifics of the wound, such as color, odor, and amount of drainage, must be provided to the RN manager after the dressing change has been completed.
- Any change in wound appearance must be immediately reported to the RN team leader or manager before the dressing change has been completed.

CRITICAL THINKING Strategies

Scenario 1

Mrs. Johnson is an 84-year-old retired school teacher who was widowed 10 years ago and now lives alone. She developed diabetes mellitus at the age of 58. She has been in failing health for the last 3 years and has been at home with the assistance of home health aides and weekly visits by the RN. Her coccyx area has had frequent skin breakdown. The Homecare RN determined she now has a stage III pressure ulcer as a result of her being on bedrest the past week. She is being admitted to the hospital for treatment of the ulcer.

1. Identify risk factors for Mrs. Johnson developing pressure ulcers.
2. Describe the stage III pressure ulcer.
3. Identify the most effective treatment for the stage III pressure ulcer.
4. Compare and contrast the two Pressure Ulcer Assessment Scales and identify the score indicating that Mrs. Johnson is a high risk for pressure ulcer formation on one of the scales.
5. In addition to dressing changes, identify a preventative therapy that should be used for clients at high risk for pressure ulcers.
6. Explain why massaging bony prominences should be avoided for clients at risk for pressure ulcer formation.
7. Briefly describe the application of a hydrocolloid dressing.
8. Identify and briefly explain the use of one new advance in the treatment of pressure ulcers.

Scenario 2

A young client was in a motor vehicle accident and has numerous wounds on his buttocks, back, and both legs. He is in extreme pain and is on a PCA pump with morphine sulfate for pain control. He is able to respond to questions. His vital signs are BP 140/88, P. 110, R. 26, O2 Sat 96% on room air.

1. When assessing the client's wounds, what questions will you need to ask to determine the client's history and physical findings that contribute to his treatment?
2. Describe how you would determine the extent of the wounds.
3. The physician has determined that the negative pressure wound therapy protocol would be the most beneficial treatment for the leg wounds. This decision is based on what criteria?
4. Compare and contrast the use of white foam and black foam for the leg wounds.
5. Describe the method you will use to prepare the wound for the V.A.C. system.
6. Provide the rationale for using GranuFoam silver dressings for wound care.

NCLEX® Review Questions

Unless otherwise specified, choose only one (1) answer.

1. The phase of wound healing which begins about 2 days to 3 weeks after injury is termed
   1. Maturation.
   2. Inflammatory.
   3. Regeneration.
   4. Wound remodeling.
2. Tertiary intention in wound healing is described as
   1. A wound that heals by granulation.
   2. The simplest form of wound healing.
   3. The skin is cleanly incised through a surgical incision.
   4. A wound that heals by leaving it open.
3. Instructing clients in measures to increase wound healing should include increasing the client's daily intake of calories to
   1. 20–25 Cal/kg/day.
   2. 30–35 Cal/kg/day.
   3. 35–45 Cal/kg/day.
   4. 45–50 Cal/kg/day.
4. Instructing student nurses in the use of alcohol-based hand rub to decontaminate hands includes instructions to
   1. Apply 1.5–3 mL of alcohol in palm of hand and begin to rub hands together.
   2. Vigorously rub hands for 10 seconds, covering all hand surfaces.
   3. Scrub hands for 3 minutes.
   4. Rinse hands and dry using a single-use towel.
5. To maintain a sterile field, the nurse needs to
   1. Place the sterile package near the edge of the overbed table on the opposite side of the bed.
   2. Open the package by placing it directly in front of you and grasping the wrapper.
   3. Open the last flap of the wrapper toward you.
   4. Move the sterile dressing tray toward you after opening the last flap of the wrapper.
6. The physician asks you to remove the sutures on a client with an abdominal incision. Which one of the following steps is appropriate to carry out?
   1. Don sterile gloves before removing sutures.
   2. Grasp suture at knot with forceps and lift away from skin.
   3. Place straight tip of suture scissors over knot and cut knot.
   4. Begin to remove sutures in the middle of the incision to ensure it is healed.
7. Advantages to using transparent adhesive film dressing for wound care include

   Select all that apply.
   1. Allows visualization of wound.
   2. Promotes autolysis of dry eschar.
   3. Does not require secondary dressing.
   4. May be soothing by having a cooling effect.
8. A wound culture has been ordered for a client with a leg wound. You remember that the appropriate method for obtaining the culture includes
   1. Cleaning the wound area with hydrogen peroxide before swabbing the wound.
   2. Swabbing the wound using a single straight motion with the swab down the middle of the wound.
   3. Swabbing the edges of the wound starting at the top and crisscrossing the wound to the bottom.
   4. Cleaning the edge of the wound with saline and then swabbing inner aspects of wound.
9. The client requires a wet-to-moist dressing change daily. When placing the dressing in the wound, the most appropriate method is to
   1. Pack several flat sterile 4×4 dressings into the wound bed.
   2. Fluff each sterile dressing and place over the wound.
   3. Place a moist dressing on top of the sterile dry dressings in the wound.
   4. Unfold a dry dressing and place on top of moistened dressings in the wound.
10. The physician has ordered negative pressure wound therapy. The nurse needs to evaluate the wound before this therapy can be initiated to ensure it can be effective. If the wound can accommodate the therapy, it will

    Select all that apply.
    1. Be surrounded by at least 2 cm of intact periwound tissue.
    2. Open enough to insert the foam dressing that must touch all edges.
    3. Be debrided.
    4. Be on the extremities.

26

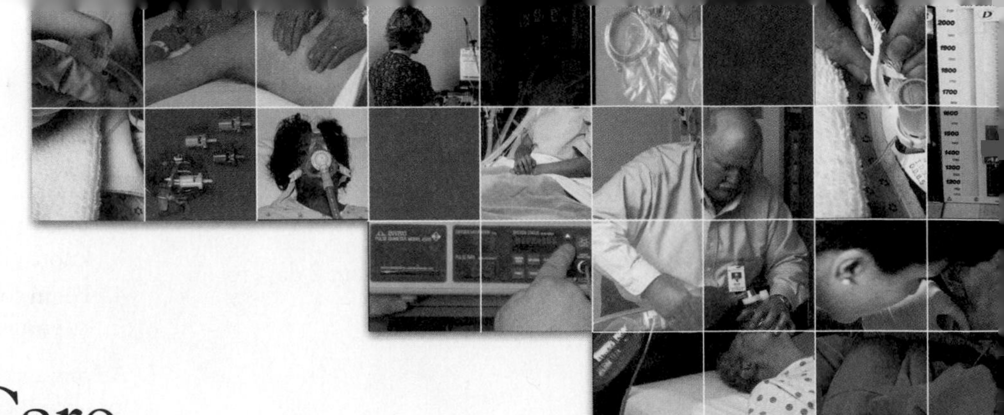

Perioperative Care

LEARNING OBJECTIVES

1. Define the word *perioperative*.
2. Discuss the nursing care focus in each of the three stages of the perioperative period.
3. Identify at least three factors that influence the surgical client's degree of stress.
4. Explain why postoperative complications are reduced by decreasing the stress level.
5. Describe at least one potential problem and the suggested solution for clients demonstrating high stress levels in the preoperative period.
6. State the primary purpose of providing preoperative care for clients.
7. Discuss how preoperative teaching can reduce the surgical client's stress.
8. Describe the information contained in the surgical permit.
9. Outline the essential steps in physically preparing a client for surgery.
10. Describe information contained in the surgical safety checklist.
11. Explain the purpose for administering the three classifications of drugs used for preoperative medications.
12. Describe the nurses' role in caring for a client with moderate (conscious) sedation.
13. Outline the essential postoperative nursing interventions completed in the surgical unit.
14. Summarize the major categories of postoperative pain medications and describe the general side effects of each category.
15. Discuss at least three major postoperative complications and the nursing interventions to prevent and treat the complications.
16. Describe the process of "Hand Off" communication.
17. Discuss the differences in procedure when a client is discharged to home after outpatient surgery.

CHAPTER OUTLINE

TERMINOLOGY

Adaptation ability of an organism to adjust to a change in environment.

Analgesia absence of the sense of pain.

Analgesic a drug that relieves pain without altering the conscious state.

Anesthesia partial or complete loss of sensation by administration of a drug or gas.

Anxiety experiencing a sense of dread or fear without a known stimulus. A condition associated with physiologic changes.

Arthrogram a diagnostic radiological test involving use of dye, which is injected into a joint to visualize tears in ligaments and surrounding tissue.

Arthroscopy using a scope to visualize, diagnose, or treat problems inside a joint.

Asepsis sterile; a condition free from germs.

Atelectasis a collapsed or airless section of the lungs.

Bronchitis inflammation of the bronchial mucous membrane.

Bronchoscopy examination of the bronchi with a scope.

Capnography indicator of respiratory depression because it measures $ETCO_2$ (end-tidal carbon dioxide).

Conscious (Moderate) Sedation a medically controlled state of depressed consciousness that allows protective reflexes to be maintained.

Contamination the introduction of disease, germs, or infectious materials into or on normally sterile objects.

Dehydration loss of water to the body or tissues due to low intake or high output of fluid.

Diplopia double vision.

Egophony a nasal sound heard while auscultating the lungs of a person as he speaks; a sound heard in pleural effusion.

Emesis vomiting.

Emphysema a condition in which the alveoli of the lungs become distended or ruptured.

Enema injection of water or fluid into rectum and colon to empty the lower intestine or to introduce medicine or food for therapeutic purposes.

Euphoria an exaggerated feeling of well-being.

Exudate fluid, cells, or other substances that have been slowly discharged from cells or blood vessels through small pores or breaks in cell membranes.

"Hand Off" communication method of reporting off from one nursing staff to another nursing staff or between nursing units.

Hernia the protrusion or projection of an organ or part of an organ through the wall of the cavity that normally contains it.

Hypertension higher blood pressure than normal; usually above 140 mmHg/90 mmHg.

Hypnotic drugs that cause insensibility to pain or partial to complete unconsciousness; includes sedatives, analgesics, anesthetics, and intoxicants.

Hypothermia the state of low body temperature.

Hypovolemia diminished intravascular volume.

Immunosuppressive acting to suppress the body's natural immune response to an antigen.

Induction the process of causing or producing; in anesthesia, the period from the initial inhalation or injection until optimum level of anesthesia is reached, including airway competency intubation.

Intervention the act of coming in or between so as to modify.

Laparoscopy a scope is inserted into the abdominal cavity to perform diagnostic and/or surgical procedures.

Laser surgery procedure used to divide or cause adhesions or to destroy or fix tissues in place.

Lethargy a condition of sluggishness; stupor.

Lithotripsy procedure for eliminating a calculus in the renal pelvis, ureter, bladder, or gall bladder.

Magnetic resonance imaging (MRI) use of electromagnetic energy in radiography to provide soft tissue images, especially of the musculoskeletal and central nervous system.

Maladaptive poorly adjusted; inability to adapt.

Mesentery a peritoneal fold connecting the intestine with the back of the abdominal (postabdominal) wall.

Narcotic producing stupor or sleep; a drug that depresses the central nervous system.

Neurohormonal concerning the interaction between nerves and hormones.

Orthopedic concerning the prevention or correction of deformities of the musculoskeletal system, especially bones, tendons, and ligaments.

Palpitation rapid, violent, or throbbing pulsation, as an abnormally rapid, throbbing, or fluttering heart.

Perioperative refers to the three phases of the surgical experience: preoperative, intraoperative, and postoperative.

Peritonitis inflammation of the peritoneum.

Pneumonia inflammation of the lungs caused primarily by bacteria, viruses, and chemical agents; can be characterized by chills, high fever, pain in the chest, cough, and purulent and often bloody sputum.

Stress a mentally or emotionally disruptive or disquieting influence; distress.

Surgical site infection (SSI) the infections that result from the surgical procedure.

Therapeutic having medicinal or healing properties.

Thrombophlebitis inflammation of a vein associated with thrombus.

Topical pertinent to a particular area; local.

Trauma a physical injury or wound caused by external force or violence; an emotional or psychologic shock that may produce disordered feelings or behavior.

Vasoconstriction constriction of a blood vessel.

THE SURGICAL EXPERIENCE

Just a few years ago, the surgical experience involved 3 to 10 days in a hospital setting; now it is often a short hospital stay or an outpatient experience. Many procedures are now performed safely in an outpatient setting and may consist of a same-day surgical procedure lasting a few hours. The short-stay procedure involves an observation period during an overnight stay in the facility, usually less than 24 hr. In these situations, much of the postoperative period is managed at home. Depending on the protocol, if necessary a home health nurse may visit, or some outpatient facilities provide a postoperative follow-up visit by the nursing staff. In all cases where outpatient procedures are performed, the nurse does phone follow-up within the first 1 to 3 postoperative days.

Surgical procedures are classified as either emergency or elective procedures. Elective procedures can be scheduled in advance. This allows the client time to plan for child care arrangements and employment responsibilities, as well as prepare psychologically for the experience. Emergency procedures usually are a result of a life-threatening situation such as hemorrhage, obstruction, malignancy, or body system disruption. Procedures are also termed major or minor according to the degree of risk to the client. Major surgical procedures involve a risk of bleeding and loss of organs or bodily parts. Minor surgical procedures usually involve less risk of bleeding and fewer complications. Examples of these procedures include arthroscopic procedures of the knee, rhinoplasty, and eye surgeries.

Nurse's Role Nurses take an active role in the psychologic and physiologic preparation of the surgical client. Nurses instruct the preoperative client in stress-reduction techniques, explanations of the operating room experience, expectations for the postoperative period, and use of special postoperative equipment. In fact, many hospitals provide time for the operating room nurse to make postoperative visits to clients to assess the client's evaluation of the surgical intervention.

PERIOPERATIVE CARE

Perioperative Areas There are specific physical areas of the hospital where client care takes place during the operative experience.

Personnel working in these areas must adhere to regulations regarding appropriate attire with personal protective equipment identified for each specific area. Personnel must also follow standard precautions and are not permitted to work if they have open lesions on the hands or arms, eye infections, diarrhea, or respiratory infections.

Preoperative Area Preoperative care can take place in a holding area for invasive procedures and/or the preoperative area of the operating room. Care can also take place in a central testing area, an inpatient room, or clinic examination or treatment room. During this stage the client must be identified by at least two identifiers (i.e., medical record number, birth date, name, charge number).

The operative site needs to be verified, both to site and side, and then marked by two parties (ideally the client and the physician).

If a female client is of childbearing age, a pregnancy test is usually done. The potassium levels are checked if the client is on diuretics.

Intraoperative Area This includes the operating room suite or a procedure room where invasive surgical procedures occur. The intraoperative area of the operating room suite includes the area surrounding the operating room and the actual operating room suite. Intraoperative care begins when the client enters the invasive procedure area or the operating room suite.

Postoperative Area Care can commence in the operating room suite, the procedure room, a recovery room/postoperative area, a client room (ICU), or a treatment room. The postoperative care begins immediately after the completion of the surgical procedure.

Preoperative Stage The first stage of the perioperative period is the *preoperative stage*. During this stage, a health history, including identification of all allergies (including latex allergies and Betadine/prep solutions), medical concerns in other systems, identification of side and site of procedure, and verification of a client's understanding of the procedure including side and site, a thorough physical assessment, and review of all laboratory tests ordered is completed. Some clients will require an ECG, chest x-ray, pregnancy test, or blood type and screen. The registered nurse completes the operative check list and notifies the surgeon and anesthesiologist of any abnormal findings according to facility policy and procedures. Infections such as urinary tract infections must be treated before any surgical procedure is done. Not all infections such as urinary tract or respiratory are obliterated before surgery, but must be identified and reported to the surgeon and anesthesiologist to determine whether surgery can proceed. Some clients receive preoperative IV antibiotic therapy before surgery. The nurse must ensure that these orders have been completed before surgery. If clients are to receive preoperative antibiotics, they should be administered before the beginning of surgery to maximize the effects. The antibiotics are frequently administered in the holding area.

Admission to the hospital or outpatient surgery facility and anticipation of surgery result in some degree of anxiety and stress. Stress is a physiologic and psychologic response to a stressor. Anxiety is one of the manifestations of stress. The degree of anxiety and stress depends on many factors:

- The client's likelihood of reacting to anticipated stressors with high anxiety
- The number of stress-producing events that have occurred recently in the client's life or within the client's family
- The client's perceptions of the hospitalization and surgical experience
- The significance of the surgery to the client and how life will be altered
- The number of unknowns that confront the client on admission
- The client's degree of self-esteem and self-image and perception of how surgery will impact body image
- The client's belief system and religious conviction

The body responds physiologically to an actual or perceived threat. The hypothalamus controls a neurohormonal response. The heart rate is increased, and the heart contracts more forcefully. Blood volume is redistributed by vasoconstriction of the vessels in the skin, stomach, mesentery, and kidneys. Increased blood volume increases cardiac output. Increased blood flow to the skeletal muscles results in the muscles becoming tensed for action. The bronchi dilate, and the increased respiratory rate increases oxygenation. Mechanisms that provide energy include increased glucose release and decreased insulin production. The effects of these mechanisms make it important to know the blood glucose status of a diabetic client; a higher blood glucose level immediately preceding the procedure is better than one that is too low.

Behavioral responses to stress or anxiety can be adaptive or maladaptive (Table 26-1). Adaptive behaviors are purposeful. The client adapts to a stressful situation by preparing to face it or by removing the threat. Maladaptive behaviors result from the inability to adapt to a stressful situation.

One of the objectives of providing preoperative care is to identify the level of stress present in the client. If nursing interventions can be planned that reduce high anxiety levels, the result is a safer intraoperative period. High levels of anxiety can prevent successful preoperative adaptation and can negatively influence postoperative recovery. Mild anxiety, on the other hand, increases alertness, increases the ability to learn, and increases the ability to assess and to adjust to one's environment. Mild anxiety also increases the ability to adjust to several simultaneous stressors. In the preoperative client this level of anxiety is adaptive in nature, while a high level is maladaptive. When levels of anxiety or stress become intolerably high, defense mechanisms are unconsciously implemented to reduce the distress by concealing, falsifying, or distorting reality.

Preoperative anxiety is increased by ambiguity, conflicting perceptions, misconceptions, fears of the unknown, and bombardment by many simultaneous stressors. Ambiguity occurs from uncertainty or vagueness concerning the hospital environment, preoperative procedures, intraoperative procedures, or postoperative events.

Conflicting perceptions occur when preconceived notions about the operative experience are different from those actually encountered. A client may not have comprehended the pertinent facts about the procedure (i.e., incision site and how the procedure is going to be done). The client who thought that a herniorrhaphy would be a quick, safe cure can become quite anxious after the anesthesiologist informs him or her of potential complications.

Misconceptions arise when inaccurate information is given, or accurate information is misinterpreted, when terminology is not understood, and when events are not explained clearly. A client who is scheduled for a bronchoscopy in the morning, and whose nurse silently places an NPO sign over the bed, may believe that he is destined for the same hospital regimen as his roommate, who had a gastrectomy.

Stress responses are cumulative. An increasing number of stressors can eventually drain adaptive energy. The newly admitted surgical client who has been confronted with many stressors before admission is more likely to respond with a higher level of stress as each new stressor is encountered.

Preoperative teaching is essential for clients undergoing any surgical procedure. Research studies have repeatedly identified the positive outcomes of client teaching as decreased perception of pain, increased compliance with treatments, decreased

TABLE 26-1 Responses to Anxiety States

Low Anxiety	High Anxiety
Less likely to react with high anxiety to stressors	Likely to react with high anxiety to stressors
Few changes in personal situation in recent past	Many changes in personal situation in recent past
Perceives hospital and surgical experience as beneficial	Perceives hospital and surgical experience as threatening
Believes surgery will end chronic problem	Fears that surgery may lead to pain, disability, and possibly death
Regards admission procedures as friendly and supportive	Regards admission procedures as strange and frightening
Finds hospital conditions comfortable and the nursing staff supportive and informative	Finds hospital conditions unbearable and the nursing staff nonsupportive

See also Chapter 17, Alternative Therapies and Stress Management.

TABLE 26-2 Managing Surgical Clients

Conscientious Preoperative Care of Clients Prevents Postoperative Complications

- Preparing the client psychologically reduces the client's stress level and helps to prevent postoperative complications.
- Teaching coughing and deep breathing exercises, procedures for getting out of bed, and uses of specialized equipment enhances the client's cooperation and prevents postoperative complications.

Scrupulous Asepsis Throughout the Perioperative Period Reduces Complications

- Maintaining strict asepsis reduces cross-contamination.
- Completing the surgical scrub reduces microorganisms on the body surface and the possibility of wound infections postoperatively.
- Identifying breaks in sterile technique and taking appropriate actions decrease the risk of postoperative complications.

Accurate Identification of Client and Surgical Site Prevents Surgical Errors

- Marking of correct site and side by client, nurse, and surgeon reduces errors.
- Time to reconfirm client identifiers and correct procedure should involve the entire surgical team.

postoperative complications, and decreased duration of hospitalization. Of course, fear and anxiety are greatly reduced when explanations are complete and time is allowed during the teaching session to answer questions by both the client and family. The client has the right to know what to expect during the surgical procedure and the postoperative period as set forth in The Client's Bill of Rights. Informing the client to expect postoperative presence of a urinary catheter, drainage tubes, central/arterial IV lines, cast, etc., while awake before anesthesia, promotes postoperative cooperation.

The teaching plan needs to include the preoperative preparation, time of surgery, and postoperative activities. A tour of the postoperative unit is also an important aspect of the teaching, particularly if the client will be going to a critical care or special care unit. Clients should also know what to expect about invasive tubes (i.e., Foley catheter, drains, chest tube) and monitoring lines (i.e., arterial and central venous pressure), which will help to decrease their anxiety postoperatively. A demonstration of specific equipment such as incentive spirometer, PCA pumps, cardiac monitors, and immobilizers should be presented to increase compliance with the equipment postoperatively. Information regarding time of arrival to the hospital and fluid and food restrictions should be provided before hospitalization, whether it is for outpatient or inpatient surgery.

Other areas covered in the preoperative stage are the type of anesthesia (usually described by the anesthesiologist) and the physical preparation of the client, which includes preoperative skin preparation, identifying the correct client in the operating room, and in some cases, the preoperative scrub. This may include the surgical cleansing prep and hair removal. Cutting excessive hair has replaced shaving, which produces minute dermal cuts and increased risk of infection. If it must be completed in the intraoperative area, a method that controls aerosolization of hair and epithelium is utilized.

Intraoperative Stage

This stage includes the time the client arrives in the preinduction or holding room until he or she arrives in the recovery room. The client may well complain of being cold. The operating room is kept cool, so offering a warm blanket will make the client more comfortable. The use of the Bair Paws Warming System provides heat more effectively than a blanket. Nurses complete an assessment, and may insert IVs and Foley catheters.

Once the client is moved to the operating room itself, a "Time Out" is called before anything transpires. The Time Out is a formal verbalization and checking of "Correct Client, Correct Procedure, Correct Site." All members of the OR team must participate in the process, including surgeon, anesthesiologist, surgical assistant, circulating RN, surgical scrub nurse, or technician. The process includes verification of antibiotic administration, allergies, presence of appropriate prosthesis/implants, and correct client positioning. The process is an Association of Perioperative Registered Nurses (AORN) Standard of Practice and a mandate of The Joint Commission. The anesthesiologist prepares the client for and administers the anesthesia while monitoring the client throughout the procedure. The operating room nurses, circulating and scrub, prepare the operating room and provide for client safety. Operating room technicians are used in many facilities in place of scrub nurses.

AORN has developed a position statement regarding the role of the scrub nurse to achieve optimal client outcomes (AORN, Inc., 2004, "Perioperative Patient-focused Model: Standards Recommendations, Practices, and Guidelines"). An RN must be assigned to the operating room when an OR technician is used as a member of the team. In this case, the OR nurse functions as the circulating nurse. The circulating nurse must always be an RN. The nurse assists in the preparation of the client, positions the client on the operating room table, and ensures that a grounding pad (if electrocautery is used) is securely attached to the client. To maintain client safety, the role of the circulating nurse is highly complex due to the mandates, technical innovations, client advocacy issues, interactions with physicians, operating room personnel, and scheduling/timing of cases. Critical responsibilities of the circulating RN include ensuring sterile technique, correct counts of instruments and sponges, and availability of correct instrumentation. The circulating nurse must be an RN as he/she supports the anesthesiologist during the procedure. The assistance includes starting and monitoring venous lines, administering IV medications when necessary, verifying and hanging blood, and assisting in monitoring the condition of the client. The circulating nurse also assists the team in gowning and gloving for the procedure.

Moderate (Conscious) Sedation Conscious sedation is used for some surgical procedures and for invasive procedures or tests. Procedures once performed only in an operating room can now be safely done in outpatient settings and special procedures rooms. Conscious sedation may be used in critical care units when clients are restless and anxious and this proves detrimental to treatment. Conscious sedation requires a signed permit, the same as when using general anesthesia. Conscious sedation is the administration of an IV sedative, opioid, or hypnotic drug that produces sedation, analgesia, and amnesia. Clients receiving conscious sedation can respond to commands and maintain their own airway. Clients under light sedation are able to maintain normal respiration, eye movements, and protective reflexes. They usually do not remember the procedure or even the environment. After the use of conscious sedation, the client may have slurred speech and nystagmus at the end point of the sedation.

Moderate sedation occurs on a continuum from the state of being alert to being in deep sedation. When the client is in a minimum sedation state, he or she can still be anxious. In deep sedation, the client is in a controlled state of depressed consciousness or unconsciousness and is not easily aroused and does not respond to command. Moderate sedation is considered to be safer than general anesthesia; however, there are risks involved with the use of conscious sedation. As the level of sedation increases, the risk of complications increases as well. Clients can become too deeply sedated and require intervention to maintain a patent airway and breathing. Unlike general anesthesia, conscious sedation allows clients to maintain a patent airway and respond appropriately to physical stimulation and verbal commands. Another benefit of conscious sedation includes a quicker return to baseline neurologic status.

A qualified anesthesia provider must give orders for administration of conscious sedation. Some states and institutional guidelines allow qualified registered nurses to administer sedating drugs. The American Nurses Association (ANA) and other nursing organizations have written position papers relative to the practice of administering and monitoring clients undergoing conscious sedation. Nurses must be familiar with the state nurse practice act as well as the institutional policies regarding their role in this procedure. Nurses allowed to administer conscious sedation must meet additional criteria and demonstrate proficiency in the skill. The nurses are working under *standard procedures* in this situation. Nursing students are not allowed to administer conscious sedation or monitor clients while they are receiving conscious sedation.

During the entire procedure the safety of the client is the priority goal for the entire staff assigned to the procedure. All staff assist in monitoring the client, ensure that sterile technique is maintained throughout the procedure, and maintain accurate and complete documentation, including sponge and instrument counts. OSHA guidelines are followed by the staff to protect both the client and the staff from exposure to bloodborne pathogens.

Surgical Safety Checklist

The surgical safety checklist was established in 2008 as a result of the World Health Organization (WHO) published guidelines, with recommended practices to ensure the safety of surgical clients worldwide. The guidelines were developed to reduce the rate of major surgical complications. A worldwide study was completed to determine whether complications could be reduced by following the surgical checklist before each surgical procedure. There are an estimated 234 million surgical procedures performed annually. Perioperative death rate in inpatient surgery is 0.4%–0.8%, and there is a 3%–17% rate of major complications. Data have suggested that at least half of all surgical complications are avoidable. The checklist was used to collect data on 500 consecutively enrolled clients in eight cities throughout the world. Clients were followed from surgery to 30 days postoperative. A 20% reduction in complications occurred in study participants after the checklist was implemented.

Surgical Safety Checklist

Before Induction of Anesthesia
(with at least nurse and anesthetist)

Has the patient confirmed his/her identity, site, procedure, and consent?

[ ] Yes

Is the site marked?

[ ] Yes
[ ] Not applicable

Is the anesthesia machine and medication check complete?

[ ] Yes

Is the pulse oximeter on the patient and functioning?

[ ] Yes

Does the patient have a: Known allergy?

[ ] No
[ ] Yes

Difficult airway or aspiration risk?

[ ] No
[ ] Yes, and equipment/assistance available

Risk of >500 mL blood loss (7 mL/kg in children)?

[ ] No
[ ] Yes, and two IVs/central access and fluids planned

Risk of hypothermia (operation >1 hr)?

[ ] No
[ ] Yes, and warmer in place

BEFORE INDUCTION check complete

Before Skin Incision
(with nurse, anesthetist, and surgeon)

Confirm all team members have introduced themselves by name and role.

[ ] Yes

To surgeon, anesthetist and nurse:

[ ] What is this patient's name?
[ ] What procedure is planned?
[ ] Where will the incision be made?

Has the antibiotic prophylaxis been given within the last 60 minutes?

[ ] Yes
[ ] Not applicable

Is venous thromboembolism prophylaxis needed?

[ ] Yes, and boots/anticoagulants in place
[ ] Not applicable

Anticipated Critical Events to Surgeon:

[ ] What are the critical or non-routine steps?
[ ] How long will the case take?
[ ] What is the anticipated blood loss?
[ ] What implants/equipment issues or any concerns?

To Anesthetist:

[ ] Are there any patient-specific concerns?

To Nursing Team:

[ ] Has sterility (including indicator results) been confirmed?
[ ] Are there equipment issues or any concerns?

Is essential imaging displayed?

[ ] Yes
[ ] Not applicable

BEFORE SKIN INCISION check complete

Before Patient Leaves Operating Room
(nurse or anesthetist reads out load)

Nurse verbally requests from the team:

[ ] How shall I record the name of the procedure?
[ ] Are the instrument, sponge, and needle counts complete?
[ ] How shall I label the specimens (including patient name)?
[ ] Are there any equipment problems to be addressed?

To Surgeon, Anesthetist, and Nurse:

[ ] What are the key concerns for recovery and management of this patient?

BEFORE LEAVING ROOM check complete

Source: World Health Organization. (2008). Based on the WHO Surgical Safety Checklist. Available at: http://whqlibdoc.who.int/publications/2009/9789241598590_eng_Checklist.pdf.

After the procedure the client is transferred to the postanesthesia room by the anesthesiologist and/or surgeon and, in some facilities, the circulating nurse. A complete report of the client's status is provided to the postanesthesia staff.

Postoperative Stage The *postoperative stage* can be divided into three segments. The immediate postoperative period includes the care given to the client in the postanesthesia room and in the first few hours on the surgical floor. The intermediate period usually involves the care given during the course of surgical convalescence to the time of discharge. The third segment in the postoperative stage is discharge planning, teaching, and referral. Discharge planning and teaching begin during the preoperative period and are reinforced and continued in the postoperative period.

Universal Protocol for Preventing Wrong Site, Wrong Procedure, Wrong Person Surgery

The implementation of the universal protocol is required by all hospitals accredited by The Joint Commission. The protocol is based on the consensus of experts from clinical specialties and professional disciplines and more than 40 professional medical associations and organizations (The Joint Commission: Effective July 1, 2004).

The protocol identifies the principles necessary to eliminate a surgical client's injury from a wrong procedure, wrong site, wrong person. It includes the method of marking the operative site and active communication amongst all surgical team members to ensure that procedures are carried out to prevent these tragedies. Markings are required whenever there is a procedure involving right/left distinction, multiple structures such as toes and fingers, or levels such as spinal procedures. These markings are placed at the operative site indicating the exact surgical site. This is critical when it involves limbs to ensure the surgical procedure is performed on the correct limb. The person performing the surgical procedure should do the marking. If the surgeon is unable to perform the markings, a surgical team member can be designated to mark the site. In most states, nurses on the surgical team may be delegated to mark the surgical site.

Source: The Joint Commission. http://www.thejointcommission.org.

Besides nursing care, nursing management during the postoperative period centers on assessing the client's postoperative condition and monitoring for complications. It also includes client teaching, pain control, and psychologic support of both the client and family.

When the client is deemed stable, he or she is transferred to the nursing unit, critical care unit, and in the case of an outpatient client, to home. The nursing care provided in the postoperative period is well described in the chapter.

CULTURAL AWARENESS

Most religions and cultures allow the administration of blood and blood products. The exception is Jehovah's Witnesses, who forbid the use of blood and blood products. Christian Science followers ordinarily do not allow blood and blood products either. Surgical procedures are accepted by all religions and cultures with some modification. Buddhists permit surgery, but will avoid extremes in surgical procedures. Roman Catholics do not allow abortion or sterilization procedures.

NURSING DIAGNOSES

The following nursing diagnoses are appropriate to include in a client care plan when the components are related to a surgical experience.

NURSING DIAGNOSIS	RELATED FACTORS
Ineffective Airway Clearance	Pulmonary secretions, allergic response, medications, suppressed cough reflex, decreased oxygen intake, pain, mechanical obstruction
Anxiety	Actual or perceived threat to body image, ability to maintain independence, long-term effects of surgical procedure
Ineffective Coping	Inadequate support system, change in body integrity, unrealistic expectations regarding surgical outcome, stress from surgery
Infection, Risk for	Impaired wound healing, nutritional deficits, inadequate acquired immunity
Deficient Knowledge	Inadequate understanding of surgical procedure, language barrier, incomplete client teaching, lack of motivation, cognitive limitation
Latex Allergy Response, Risk for	Clients at risk have allergies to bananas, tropical fruit, poinsettia plants; clients with multiple surgical procedures who have repeated contact with natural latex rubber
Acute Pain	Tissue damage resulting from surgical intervention, ineffective pain relief, psychological factors
Perioperative Positioning Injury, Risk for	Joints and extremities malpositioned or maintained in one position for long period of time
Impaired Skin Integrity, Risk for	Excessive hours on operating table, operative table drapes wrinkled, excessive fluid accumulation on drapes
Delayed Surgical Recovery	Evidence of interrupted healing of surgical area; difficulty in ambulation, pain, fatigue

CLEANSE HANDS The single most important nursing action to decrease the incidence of hospital-based infections is hand hygiene. *Remember to wash your hands or use antibacterial gel before and after each and every client contact.*

IDENTIFY CLIENT Before every procedure, introduce yourself and check two forms of client identification, not including room number. These actions prevent errors and conform to The Joint Commission standards.

Chapter 26

UNIT ❶

Stress in Preoperative Clients

Nursing Process Data

ASSESSMENT Data Base

- Identify if high level of stress exists.
- Assess exaggerated anxiety or stress behaviors.
- Assess client's use of defensive behaviors.
- Assess client's vulnerability to number and significance of changes in life before admission.
- Assess client's level of knowledge and perceptions of the impending surgery and perioperative period.

PLANNING Objectives

- To identify the level of stress and anxiety present in preoperative clients
- To provide interventions that decrease stress levels and promote optimal preoperative behavioral and physiologic responses
- To observe for use of defensive behaviors that mask a failure to adapt appropriately in stressful situations
- To prepare the client for a smooth preoperative and postoperative period
- To prevent postoperative complications

IMPLEMENTATION Procedures

EVALUATION Expected Outcomes

- Client's level of stress and anxiety is identified.
- Nursing interventions are provided that decrease stress levels and promote optimal preoperative responses.
- Denial, as a defense mechanism, is identified in the client and therapeutic interventions are made.
- Client identifies stressors and own stress response.
- Client demonstrates coping strategies to control stress and anxiety.
- Client and family state expectations for perioperative experience.
- Client demonstrates activities that will be performed postoperatively.

Preventing Anxiety and Stress

Procedure

1. Establish a trusting relationship.
2. Encourage verbalization of feelings.
3. Listen attentively.
4. Communicate acceptance of the client as an individual.
5. Identify the client's needs (Table 26-3) and keep the charge nurse informed of them.
6. Give adequate information regarding hospital procedures.
   a. Hospital environment, including sights, sounds, and equipment.
   b. Hospital personnel and routine procedures: mealtimes, telephone usage, call light.
   c. Ordered preoperative procedures: lab tests, diagnostic procedures (explain the sensory experiences that will be encountered).
   d. Scheduled time of surgery.
   e. Hospital regulations: visiting hours, children's age for visiting.
   f. Preoperative procedures: skin preparation, NPO, medications, side rails, dentures, nail polish.
   g. Anticipated intraoperative events: monitors, oxygen mask, intravenous line, etc.
   h. Anticipated postoperative events: recovery room, pain and pain medications, coughing and deep breathing exercises, dressings, IVs, Foley catheter.

TABLE 26-3 Preoperative Stress Assessment

Physiologic Responses	Emotional and Defensive Responses	Anxiety and Activity Responses
Heart rate: rate increases 10 beats/min over baseline during three observations	Withdrawal: daydreaming, increased time in sleep, unwillingness to talk, disinterest	Hyperactivity: pacing, hand-wringing, lip or nail biting, finger-tapping, impatience, irritability, insomnia
Presence of palpitations	Anger: resentment, aggressiveness, noncompliance, swearing, boasting, attempts to gain control, and independence	Disorganization of thought: repetitive speech, constant conversation, difficulty concentrating
Blood pressure: increases more than 10 mmHg over baseline during three observations	Denial: joking, carefree attitude, inappropriate laughter, refusal to discuss impending surgery	Increased sensitivity to environmental noise, light, temperature, activity
Respiratory rate: increases more than five per minute over baseline during three observations		Increased muscle tensing: furrowed eyebrows, facial tics, clenched jaws, loud or high-pitched voice, stammering, rapid speech, elevated shoulders, clenched fists, urinary frequency, tension, or inability to relax
Vasoconstriction of blood vessels near the skin: cool, pale fingers and toes; increased capillary filling time of more than 3 seconds		Increased energy and preparedness: restlessness, easily startled, increased activity level
Vasoconstriction of renal vessels: decreased urine output compared with baseline and fluid intake		
Vasoconstriction of gastric and mesenteric vessels: anorexia, nausea, vomiting, abdominal distention with flatus, decreased bowel sounds, hyperactivity, diarrhea		

Reducing Anxiety and Stress

Equipment

CD player or Ipod

Appropriate relaxation tape

Procedure

1. Establish a trusting relationship.
2. Encourage verbalization of feelings.
3. Use touch to communicate caring and genuine interest, if culturally appropriate.
4. Avoid false reassurance.
5. Use realistic outcomes.
6. Assist client in exploring effective coping methods to reduce anxiety and/or stress.
   a. Ask the client or the family what method the client normally uses to successfully reduce stress.
   b. Provide activity: walking, range of motion.
   c. Provide a back rub to loosen tense muscles.
   ▸ ***Rationale:*** Physical relaxation will often lead to mental relaxation.
   d. Teach client relaxation techniques. One technique is to ask the client to picture a blue sky that is clear except for one white, fluffy cloud. Tell client to concentrate on this scene for 10 minutes. This often relaxes the mind and body.
   e. An alternative is to ask the client to picture a favorite place (e.g., a warm, sunny beach with sand and a clear, blue lake).
7. As the client begins to relax, reinforce success. Assist client in recognizing his or her strengths.
8. Encourage self-awareness of increasing tension and immediate reversal of escalation.

Assisting the Client Who Uses Denial

Procedure

1. Establish a trusting relationship.
2. Encourage verbalization of feelings and use an interpreter if necessary.
3. Use touch to communicate caring and genuine interest if acceptable to client (i.e., some cultures prefer not to be touched).
4. Do not attempt to enforce reality. The client is denying reality to prevent outright panic. Allow use of this defense.
5. Use techniques to reduce anxiety and stress to manageable proportions.
6. Attempt to determine the cause of the need for denial.
7. Listen for cues that indicate readiness to discuss the stressors causing the need for denial.
8. Notify physician of your findings.

DOCUMENTATION for Preoperative Stress

- Objective and subjective indications of anxiety or stress levels
- Nursing interventions used to decrease stress and the results of the intervention
- Changes that occurred as a result of the nursing interventions
- Specific fears verbalized by the client
- Nonverbal indications of stress or anxiety

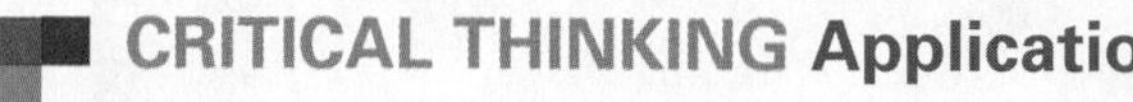

CRITICAL THINKING Application

Expected Outcomes

- Client's level of stress and anxiety is identified.
- Nursing interventions are provided that decrease stress levels and promote optimal preoperative responses.
- Denial, as a defense mechanism, is identified in the client and therapeutic interventions are made.
- Client identifies stressors and own stress response.
- Client demonstrates coping strategies to control stress anxiety.
- Client and family state expectations for perioperative experience.
- Client demonstrates activities that will be performed postoperatively.

Unexpected Outcomes	Alternative Actions
Anxiety level increases rapidly.	• Maintain calm composure and speak in a soft, caring manner. • Use touch to communicate caring and peacefulness, if culturally appropriate. • Reinforce client self-acceptance as an individual. • If unable to achieve success with stress-reducing techniques, notify physician.
Client becomes angry or hostile.	• Maintain calm composure. • Accept anger, but place limits on how it may be expressed (e.g., no destructive behavior). Understand that anger is usually the result of feeling helpless and powerless to change an intolerable situation. • Do not reward this behavior, but explore other means of meeting client's needs. • Do not isolate client, but continue to respond to needs. • Notify physician of client's behaviors and the actions you used to decrease anger or hostility.
Client becomes depressed because of overwhelming anxiety and feelings of helplessness or hopelessness.	• Convey respect and belief that the client is worthwhile. Question the client's appraisal of reality and provide support while the client works through his or her feelings. • Provide positive feedback and recognition of strengths, progress, and improved self-esteem. • Spend additional time with the client to allow time to verbalize fears.

Chapter 26

UNIT 2

Preoperative Teaching

Nursing Process Data

ASSESSMENT Data Base

- Identify type of surgical procedure planned.
- Determine whether client understands type of anesthesia planned.
- Assess client's sociocultural needs.
- Assess client's learning needs.
- Determine most appropriate method of client teaching.
- Assess client's willingness and ability to learn.
- Determine availability of prepared audiovisual material or printed information regarding surgical procedure.

PLANNING Objectives

- To reinforce physician's explanation of surgical procedure and answer questions regarding treatment
- To identify client's readiness to learn about surgical treatment
- To select appropriate time and place for client instruction regarding surgery
- To provide instruction in measures to prevent postoperative complications
- To provide a time for client to ask questions regarding surgical procedure
- To instruct client in use of special equipment required during the postoperative period
- To provide tour of specialty units, such as critical care unit, lithotripsy, or laser rooms

IMPLEMENTATION Procedures

EVALUATION Expected Outcomes

- Client is psychologically and physically prepared for surgery.
- Client demonstrates deep breathing, coughing, turning, and leg exercises accurately.
- Client verbalizes knowledge of operative procedure, potential problems, and expected nursing actions postoperatively.
- Client's family states what they expect during perioperative period.
- Client uses appropriate audiovisual and written materials to increase understanding of perioperative experience.
- Client reports decreased fear regarding special equipment used during perioperative experience.
- Client states safety precautions used with laser and lithotripsy surgery.

Providing Surgical Information

Equipment

Quiet room for client and family where there will be no interruptions during the teaching program

Equipment that may be used postoperatively by the client (e.g., IV solution, drainage tubes, nasogastric tube, suction equipment, cardiac monitor, and electrodes)

Procedure

For the Preoperative Client in the Hospital

1. Explain necessity for blood work, ECG, urinalysis, chest x-ray.
2. Describe preoperative skin preparation.
3. Discuss placement of nasogastric tube, Foley catheter, as indicated.
4. Describe enema or special bowel preparation as ordered.
5. Explain use of ongoing medications preoperatively and postoperatively.
6. Demonstrate deep breathing and coughing exercises (use of incentive spirometer if indicated).
7. Assess alcohol use and smoking habits. Emphasize smoking cessation techniques.
8. Assess and document medications used at home, including prescribed, OTC, and herbal remedies; verify that medications related to clotting have been discontinued for an adequate amount of time, usually 1 week before surgery.
9. Demonstrate leg exercises, antiembolic stockings, and sequential compression device.
10. Demonstrate turning and moving in bed.
11. Explain use of postoperative medications for pain control; PCA.
12. Discuss reason for NPO, when it begins, and medication schedule.
13. Explain alterations in diet preoperatively or postoperatively.
14. Describe activities and preparation the morning of surgery, including their participation in the "Time Out" process.
15. State need for quiet environment after medications have been given.
16. State time of surgery to client and family.
17. Describe and reinforce information usually provided by anesthesiologist and surgeon.
18. Offer tour of procedure room, PACU, or ICU that would be used with client and explain monitoring devices and special equipment used there.

For the Preoperative Client in an Outpatient Setting

1. Check two forms of client ID.
2. Verify accurate consent form has been signed by the client.
3. Call the client several days in advance if long-duration surgical preparations need to be completed before the procedure. If short-duration preparations are required, call the client in the afternoon before the procedure. It is best if the nurse who will care for the client during the surgery calls the client. ▸ ***Rationale:*** The call begins the nurse–client relationship and helps decrease anxiety.
4. Assess client's ability to understand instructions. If necessary, ask to speak to someone else in the home. ▸ ***Rationale:*** If instructions are not followed, it could result in unsafe canceled surgery.
5. Review any lab work that needs to be completed before the scheduled surgery. Explain where the lab work is to be done.
6. Answer the client's questions regarding the surgery and the procedures carried out by the staff during the surgery, including "Time Out" process.
7. Arrange for preadmission as needed.
8. Discuss the procedure for admission to the facility; when to check in at the facility (usually 1.5–2 hr before the scheduled surgery), and what documents need to be available at the time of registration (e.g., insurance card and possibly deductible payment).
9. Determine whether client has an advance directive available or explain what it is and how to obtain a temporary advance directive.
10. Discuss procedure-appropriate clothing to be worn to the setting. For example, clients having knee surgery should wear loose-fitting sweatpants or shorts.
11. Explain that all jewelry and valuables should be left at home for safekeeping.
12. Explain that someone needs to be with the client to take him/her home.
13. Instruct client to not shave surgical site at home. ▸ ***Rationale:*** Skin nicks increase the risk of infection.

For the Intraoperative Client

1. Describe mode of transportation to operating room.
2. Discuss procedure in preinduction room or operating room suite in relationship to anesthesia.
3. Reinforce physician's explanation of surgery.
4. Describe dressings, tubes, or equipment that will be used postoperatively.
5. Verify side of body and site involved. See pages for "Time Out" process.

Clinical Alert

All herbal medications must be stopped at least 2 weeks before surgery. Side effects vary depending on type of herbal remedy, ranging from sympathomimetic effects, tachycardia, and hypertension to inhibition of platelet activity.

6. Describe postanesthesia room physical environment and procedures.
7. Explain administration of oxygen.
8. Explain administration of medications.

For the Postoperative Client

1. Describe assessment procedures.
2. Provide overview of routine procedures of vital signs.
3. Demonstrate deep breathing, turning, and coughing exercises.
4. Describe IV therapy if indicated.
5. Explain irrigation of tubes when indicated.
6. Discuss Foley catheter care if indicated.
7. Review dietary alterations.
8. Describe observation and changes of dressing.
9. State ambulation or restrictions in ambulation.
10. Define type of medications used postoperatively.
11. Provide anticipated discharge and plans for assisted care if needed.

Providing Client Teaching

Equipment

Prepare teaching aids when available: audiovisual, videos, interactive computer programs, pamphlets, pictures, posters, programmed learning modules, cassette tapes, overhead transparencies, equipment used with client.

NOTE: Ask client about the best way they learn (auditory, kinesthetic, visual). This will determine the best method for teaching.

Procedure

1. Assess client's knowledge base and readiness to learn. ▸ ***Rationale:*** This provides framework for client education at the level client can understand.
   a. Determine the information provided to client by physician by reading physician's progress notes and asking client specific questions.
   b. Identify client's psychosocial and cultural background and ability to listen to teaching by communicating with client and asking direct questions.
   c. Be alert for cultural or religious beliefs that may influence client's surgical experience.
   d. Identify client's perceptions of expected surgical experience and preferences for learning.
2. Develop individualized teaching plan based on client's needs.
   a. Choose appropriate equipment for teaching, based on client's level of understanding, knowledge base, and language of preference.
   b. Review information previously provided. ▸ ***Rationale:*** To determine retention of information and needless repetition of information already mastered.
   c. Choose a quiet environment, and provide for sufficient time to allow client to ask questions. ▸ ***Rationale:*** To ensure client understands planned surgical experience.
   d. Be alert for clues indicating client confusion or misunderstanding of information. Clients may be nodding "yes" even though they do not understand, especially non–English-speaking clients. ▸ ***Rationale:*** Misunderstanding information can be detrimental to the client's sense of well-being.
3. Select appropriate audiovisual materials to assist with teaching.
4. Demonstrate use of special equipment or devices (e.g., incentive spirometer, chest tubes, suction equipment).
5. Evaluate client teaching by assessing client's ability to return demonstration of exercises and verbally answer specific questions. Reinforce information or provide additional data as needed.

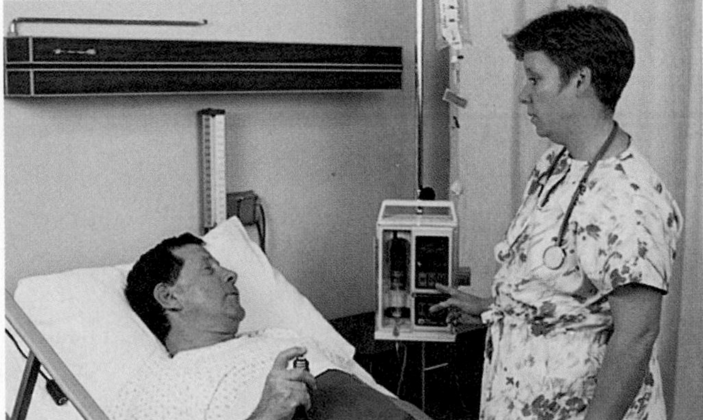

▲ Demonstrate use of special equipment in prospective teaching plan.

Providing Family Teaching

Procedure

1. Include family in teaching provided to client.
2. Instructions to family members should include:
   a. Visiting hours.
   b. Where to wait during surgery.
   c. Where the surgeon will meet with them and when.
   d. Where they can find bathrooms, telephones, and food and beverage service.
   e. When they can see the client after surgery.
   f. How to contact a spiritual or religious resource person.
   g. How they can best get information regarding the client's condition while they are at home or in the hospital.
   h. Whether they will be called if there is a change in the client's condition.
   i. What to expect: client's behavior, which may be regressive; attitude, which may be depressed or angry; physical condition, which may appear worse than it is; and postrecovery period. ▸ ***Rationale:*** Some medications may impair client's memory of events.
   j. If parents are allowed in recovery room, remind them child will still be under effects of anesthesia. Child may cry, be combative, or agitated. Child may be held down by nurses to prevent injury.
   k. Instruct parent they should touch and speak to child to promote reassurance until medications and anesthesia effects are diminished.

Teaching for Laser Therapy

Procedure

1. Determine type of laser (Table 26-4) to be used for surgery.
2. Check two forms of client ID and introduce yourself.
3. Determine client's willingness to accept instruction.
4. Determine most appropriate time and place for instruction.
5. Identify client's level of understanding of surgical procedure and what information physician has provided (Table 26-5).
6. Reinforce explanation of surgical procedure by physician as needed.
7. Describe operating room setting or outpatient setting, including the environment.
8. Explain that client and operating room staff will wear goggles. ▸ ***Rationale:*** Goggles protect eyes from the laser beam.
9. Explain the use of wet drapes placed over client's skin if required. ▸ ***Rationale:*** Wet drapes protect skin from burns when some types of laser therapy are used.
10. Describe that laser machine may be very noisy.
11. Describe physician's actions during laser therapy. Physician will discharge laser by using a foot pedal while at the same time issuing instructions to nurses using terms such as *fire*, *watt seconds*, and *standby*. ▸ ***Rationale:*** Describing these words to client allays fear of unfamiliar terms or actual fire. It also describes nurses' role of regulating power and duration of laser beam use.
12. Caution client, if under local anesthesia, he or she may feel heat and smell smoke and a burning odor from tissue being lased.
13. Instruct client to tell physician if pain occurs. ▸ ***Rationale:*** Additional anesthetic may need to be administered as client should not feel pain.

TABLE 26-4 Types of Laser*

Types	Uses
Carbon dioxide	High-precision cutting instrument used in areas where function must be preserved (e.g., vocal cords, brain, GYN procedures). Also used to treat snoring and for dermatology procedures (e.g., removal of scars and skin cancers).
Holmium	Combines the cutting properties of the CO_2 laser with the coagulation properties of the YAG laser. It is used in targeted tissue affecting adjacent, healthy tissue. Can be used with dense or hard tissue. Used in urology procedures (e.g., laser ablation of the prostate [TLAP, HOLAP], stone fragmentation [lithotripsy], strictures, obstructions, condylomata, bladder and ureteral tumors and contractures)
Nd: YAG	Laser made of a neodymium alloy, yttrium, aluminum, and garnet crystals. Beam penetrates deeply; can be passed through flexible fibers for cardiovascular laser therapy and scopes (e.g., cystoscope, bronchoscope, and endoscope to treat bladder, prostate, and lung tumors and coagulate esophageal varices; also used for eye surgery)
Argon	Used for ophthalmic and dermatologic procedures (e.g., treating glaucoma, cataract, retinal detachment, and removing birthmarks, hemangiomas)
Liquid dye	Used for diagnostic procedures and in conjunction with drugs for photodynamic treatment (e.g., lithotripsy)

*Light amplification by the stimulated emission of radiation. Choice of laser type is determined by procedure required for treatment.

TABLE 26-5 Common Types of Laser Surgical Procedures and Complications

Procedure	Client Teaching	Assessment Findings for Potential Complications
Pulmonary	Gag reflex returns in 2–4 hr Begin taking fluids when gag reflex returns Expect hoarseness, dyspnea, sore throat, difficulty swallowing for 48–72 hr	Bright red blood expectorated related to hemorrhage Fever, shortness of breath Use of accessory muscles for breathing related to tracheal edema Wheezing related to airway obstruction Pneumonia and respiratory insufficiency related to aspiration of secretions Altered arterial blood gases and sudden pain causing altered vital signs related to pneumothorax
Upper GI	May experience burning sensation in esophagus May experience difficulty swallowing Heartburn present for 3 days	Poor skin turgor and decreased urine output related to dehydration that may be caused by dysphagia Vomiting bright red blood related to perforation Abdominal pain related to perforated bowel Vomiting and abdominal distention related to obstruction of GI tract due to edema
Urology	May experience traces of blood, small blood clots, or traces of tissue in urine for 24 hr Catheter may be left in place temporarily for up to 1 week Urinary frequency and urgency may occur for 1 week	Bright red urine related to hemorrhage Abdominal pain related to perforated bladder Fever, increased pulse, malaise related to infection Inability to void related to blood clots
Cardiovascular	May experience slight burning or chest pain over coronary vessels	Arrhythmias related to hypoxia or laser treatment Bleeding at site of percutaneous laser angioplasty; related to catheter insertion Intake and output values altered related to osmotic contrast media used for laser treatment Changes in vital signs (i.e., may become hypotensive with cardiac tamponade)
Eye	Most clients feel no pain because local or topical anesthesia is used Need to remain quiet during procedure	Corneal injury can occur if eye is rubbed or bumped Increased intraocular pressure is unusual but can occur

14. Instruct client to maintain NPO status 6–8 hr before surgery.
15. Instruct client in postoperative care specific to procedure performed.
16. Instruct client to notify physician if temperature is above 100°F for more than 24 hr after laser therapy. ▶ ***Rationale:*** Infections are unlikely but can occur; therefore, client needs to monitor for presence of symptoms.

Teaching for Lithotripsy

Preparation

1. Identify type of extracorporeal shock wave lithotripsy (ESWL) used for kidney stones and occasionally for gallstones.
2. Identify type of anesthesia that will be used: local, epidural, spinal, or general. General anesthesia is usually used to prevent pain as stones are fragmented.
3. Identify whether client will have a ureteral stent or Foley catheter inserted after the procedure. A string may be visible at the end of the penis and is attached to a stent; this will aid in the removal of the stent at a later time.

Procedure

1. Check two forms of client ID and introduce yourself.
2. Determine client's knowledge base and information provided by physician.
3. Reinforce physician's description of procedure, as needed.
4. Answer client's questions regarding procedure.
5. Explain that lithotriptor discharges a series of shock waves through water or water-filled cushion.
6. Describe to client that he or she may feel fluttering or mild blows where shock waves are beamed. From 500 to 2,400 shocks are required to disintegrate stones.
7. Discuss use of specialized equipment that will be used. Client may sit in tank of water or lie with water-filled cushion pressed against area of back or abdomen where stones are present.
8. Describe use of monitoring equipment throughout procedure. ▶ ***Rationale:*** The heart rate and rhythm are monitored throughout procedure and shocks may be synchronized with the rhythm to prevent arrhythmias.

9. Explain that the procedure takes 20 minutes to 2 hr, depending on type of procedure.
10. Describe postlithotripsy care.
    a. After procedure, client is removed from tub, covered with warm blanket, and taken to recovery room.
    b. Vital signs are monitored as with any surgical client.
    c. Urine output is monitored for hematuria. ▸ ***Rationale:*** To determine kidney damage from procedure.
    d. Strain all urine at the facility and at home. ▸ ***Rationale:*** To obtain fragments of the stones in order to send them for analysis. Knowing composition of the stone is essential for altering dietary habits in some cases.
    e. Liver function studies are performed after lithotripsy for gallstones. ▸ ***Rationale:*** To assess whether shock waves have damaged liver.
    f. Pain management is monitored and maintained as gravel is passed after disintegration of stones.
    g. Medication is provided for nausea and vomiting. ▸ ***Rationale:*** Nausea and vomiting often accompany pain and postanesthesia.
    h. Intake and output measurements are taken. ▸ ***Rationale:*** Fluids are encouraged to hydrate clients with kidney stones to assist in the excretion of gravel.
    i. Catheter care is provided for clients having kidney procedure requiring indwelling catheters. If a stent is used, it may cause urgency, dysuria, frequency, and bleeding. ▸ ***Rationale:*** Indwelling catheters and ureteral stents, if used, are left in place for 24 hr to assist with passage of gravel or if second ESWL treatment is required.
    j. Exercise is encouraged to assist with passing of gravel.
    k. Ecchymoses and discomfort may be felt over area of the body that experienced shock waves.
11. Provide tour of lithotriptor room, if possible.

Teaching for Laparoscopy

Preparation

1. Identify purpose of laparoscopy.
2. Identify type of anesthesia that will be used. Usually, it is done under general anesthesia.
3. Determine whether ultrasound, CT scan, and/or MRI was done; if so, have results available for physician.
4. Obtain results of standard blood tests and urine tests if done.

Procedure

1. Check two forms of client ID and introduce yourself.
2. Determine client's knowledge base and information provided by physician.
3. Reinforce physician's description of procedure: as needed.
4. Describe equipment used for procedure: instrument used in procedure is a medical telescope with a light and high-resolution television camera so physician can see what is in the abdomen.
5. Describe procedure to client: incision is made into umbilicus; CO_2 gas is infused into abdomen to insert a small air pocket; a small camera and instruments are inserted through incision.
6. Instruct client that procedure is usually done in a same-day surgery setting. Client will go home the same day. More major procedures require overnight stay for observation and pain management.
7. Instruct client to not eat or drink for 6–8 hr before procedure.
8. Explain that client should shower evening before or day of surgery with chlorhexidine or agent prescribed by physician. The umbilicus is cleaned with soap, water, and a Q-tip. ▸ ***Rationale:*** Chlorhexidine is well tolerated and does not leave discoloration on skin as a povidone–iodine preparation does.
9. Instruct client to be at the hospital 1–2 hr before the scheduled surgery, according to hospital policy. Tell client to bring someone to drive home.
10. Have client discuss with the surgeon whether to take routine medications the morning of surgery. If medications are taken, only a sip of water is used to swallow pills. Medications causing increased risk for bleeding need to be discontinued before surgery, such as

Therapeutic procedures commonly include:

- Cholecystectomy
- Bowel resection
- Nephrectomy
- Adrenalectomy
- Radical prostatectomy
- Tubal ligation
- Hysterectomy
- Repair of pelvic prolapsed
- Appendectomy
- Hernia repair
- Pulmonary resection
- Nissen procedure
- Urethral repair

A diagnostic laparoscopy is used for the following purposes:

- Diagnose causes of abdominal pain
- Obtain tissue from an abdominal mass to determine diagnosis
- Determine cause of ascites
- Obtain liver tissue for diagnosis
- Assist in cancer staging or for a "second look" procedure

those prescribed for arthritis, anticoagulants, OTC (i.e., aspirin), or certain alternative herbal medications, according to physician's orders.

11. Instruct client to follow specific orders from physician's office regarding other preoperative directions.
12. Explain setting where surgery will be performed. If possible, allow client to visit the area if he or she is anxious.
13. Describe postlaparoscopy care to client:
    a. After surgery, client will go to the recovery room.
    b. Vital signs are monitored, dressing will be observed for signs of bleeding, and medication for pain may be administered. IV fluids will be infused and monitored until effects of anesthesia have dissipated.
    c. Client is discharged home as soon as he or she is fully awake and able to get out of bed unassisted. Many facilities require the client to urinate and manage nausea without emesis after light intake of crackers and soda or juice before discharge.
    Client must be accompanied by someone who can drive him or her home. ▶ ***Rationale:*** The effects of anesthesia may persist for several hours or as long as a day, even if the client feels fully awake.
    d. Instruct client that some soreness around incision is normal. Take pain medications as prescribed by physician. It is important to take pain medication on time or at the beginning of pain cycle for first 24–48 hr.
    e. Notify physician if chills, vomiting, redness at incision site, or worsening pain is not controlled by medication, or if unable to urinate. ▶ ***Rationale:*** These are signs of infection.
    f. Instruct client there may be a sharp pain under the scapula up to 24–48 hr postop and that changing positions may relocate "gas" bubble. ▶ ***Rationale:*** Retained carbon dioxide irritates the phrenic nerve in the diaphragm, causing referred pain. Carbon dioxide is used to distend the abdominal cavity to aid in visualization and provide working space during a laparoscopy.
    g. Instruct client to schedule a follow-up appointment with physician within 2 weeks.

Teaching for Arthroscopy

Preparation

1. Determine joint on which arthroscopy will be performed. Most common joints: knee, shoulder, elbow, ankle, hip, and wrist.
2. Identify type of anesthesia that will be used. General, spinal, or local anesthetic is used, depending on specific joint involved and suspected problem.
3. Determine whether diagnostic tests were done, i.e., MRI, x-rays, or arthrogram. Obtain results for physician.

Procedure

1. Check two forms of client ID and introduce yourself.
2. Determine client's knowledge base and information provided by physician.
3. Reinforce physician's description of procedure, as needed.
4. Describe equipment used for the procedure: pencil-sized instruments (arthroscope) that contain small lens and lighting system to magnify and illuminate structures inside the joint are inserted through incision.
5. Describe procedure to client: a small incision is made in client's skin to allow instruments to be inserted into the joint so that physician can see the interior of the joint. Several small incisions may be made to see other parts of the joint if needed. The image is projected on a television screen. The surgeon can then determine the amount or type of injury and repair or correct the problem.
6. Instruct client that procedure is done in an outpatient setting and he or she will go home the same day.

Conditions usually found and corrected by arthroscopy include:

- **Inflammation:** Synovitis
- **Injury:** acute and chronic:

  Shoulder—rotator cuff tendon tears, dislocation, and impingement syndrome

  Knee—meniscal tears, chondromalacia, and anterior cruciate ligament (ACL) tears and instability

  Wrist—carpal tunnel syndrome
- **Loose bodies of bone and/or cartilage:** knee, shoulder, elbow, ankle, or wrist

7. Explain preoperative preparation that is completed before the day of surgery:
   a. Diagnostic tests completed.
   b. Operative permit signed.
   c. Physical examination and health history completed.
   d. Physician informed of routine medications and any allergies.
   e. Procedure discussed with physician and anesthesiologist.
   f. Client meets with physical therapist to be fitted with crutches and/or knee brace, if lower extremity affected.
8. Instruct client to not eat or drink anything after midnight unless otherwise instructed by physician.
9. Explain skin prep that is to be completed the night before surgery. A 5-minute scrub with an antiseptic is usually ordered. Follow facility policy for specifics—some physicians order a full shower and some concentrate on the surgical site.
10. Instruct client to follow surgeon or anesthesiologist instructions regarding taking routine medications.
11. Instructions to client before admission:
    a. Remove all nail polish and make-up according to hospital policy. (This may not be necessary as newer oxygen saturation monitors use laser light that are not affected by nail polish.) ▶ ***Rationale:*** Capillary refill and skin coloration is assessed on all clients receiving anesthesia.
    b. Do not bring jewelry, money, or other valuables to facility. ▶ ***Rationale:*** Facility is not responsible for client's valuables.
    c. Wear comfortable, loose-fitting clothes such as loose-fitting button-down shirts or blouses, drawstring shorts, sweatpants, and boxer-style shorts. ▶ ***Rationale:*** This is to make it easier to dress after surgery, especially if a brace or sling has been applied.
    d. Bring crutches, brace, sling, or immobilizer to facility, if available.
    e. An adult must accompany client to facility to provide transportation home. ▶ ***Rationale:*** Even if client feels alert and awake, effects of anesthesia can last up to a day or two.
    f. Arrive at the facility 1.5 to 2 hr before scheduled surgery, according to facility policy.
12. Describe post-arthroscopy care to client:
    a. After surgery he/she will go to recovery room.
    b. Vital signs, circulatory assessments, pain management, IV fluid infusion will continue until client is fully awake and ready for discharge.
    c. A pressure dressing, brace, and/or ice may be applied to joint.
    d. Discharge instructions are based on joint involved with arthroscopy. Most common joint is knee. Client is to use crutches for short time. Weight bearing is allowed according to physician orders. Brace is worn when walking. Physical therapy will begin within a day or two of surgery.
13. Repeat instructions for home care.
    a. Explain to client that wound and dressing is to be kept clean and dry and changed if it becomes soiled.
    b. Instruct client to place a plastic bag over brace and tape it securely when showering.
    c. Instruct client to apply ice to joint for 24–48 hr after surgery. ▶ ***Rationale:*** To reduce pain and edema.
    d. Demonstrate how to elevate joint (leg, ankle, wrist) to reduce pain and edema.
    e. Explain how pain medication is to be taken: 30 minutes before exercises; tell client to not drink alcohol when on medications.
    f. Discuss symptoms that indicate complications and should be reported immediately to physician: swelling; tingling; pain or numbness in extremities; drainage that is yellow, green, or foul-smelling; chills or temperature above 38.5°C (101.3°F).

Instructing in Deep Breathing Exercises

Procedure

1. Check two forms of client ID and introduce yourself.
2. Explain procedure and purpose of exercises. ▶ ***Rationale:*** Deep breathing and coughing exercises promote lung expansion; lower the risk of pneumonia, atelectasis, and pulmonary emboli.
3. Instruct and have client demonstrate deep breathing exercises. ▶ ***Rationale:*** Encouraging the client to practice and return the demonstration before surgery assists him or her to deep breathe more effectively after surgery.
4. Have client sit in upright position.
5. Place client's hands along lower borders of rib cage. Client should feel rib cage expand when breathing in. ▶ ***Rationale:*** This assists client to feel adequate chest movement.
6. Instruct client to breathe through nose slowly, take a deep breath, hold 1–2 seconds, then exhale through mouth. ▶ ***Rationale:*** This expands alveoli and prevents hyperventilation if client is breathing too quickly.
7. Repeat exercise sequence 3–4 times, at least every 2 hr when awake.

NOTE: Incentive spirometry is preferred by most facilities. Refer to respiratory chapter for incentive spirometry instructions.

Instructing in Coughing Exercises

Procedure

1. Check two forms of client ID and introduce yourself.
2. Explain procedure and purpose of exercises.
3. Instruct and have client demonstrate coughing exercises.
4. Have client sit in upright position.
5. Instruct client to splint incision when deep breathing and coughing.
6. Demonstrate placement of hands on either side of incision. Instruct client to press hands firmly toward incision during exercises. ▸ ***Rationale:*** This prevents tension on the suture line and diminishes pain.
7. Instruct in use of cough pillow. Place folded bath towel in pillowcase. Hold pillow directly over incision and press on pillow when performing exercises. ▸ ***Rationale:*** This prevents pain and discomfort by splinting the incision and reducing stress on suture line.
8. Demonstrate technique for inhaling deeply and holding breath for 1–2 seconds.
9. Instruct client to take 2–3 breaths slowly and exhale passively; on third breath, hold for 2–3 seconds.
10. Encourage client to cough forcefully 2–3 times by using abdominal and other respiratory muscles to assist with coughing. ▸ ***Rationale:*** This extra force provides a more effective cough.

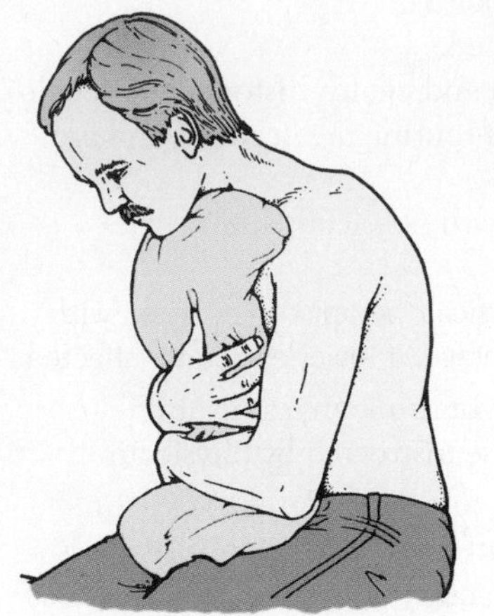
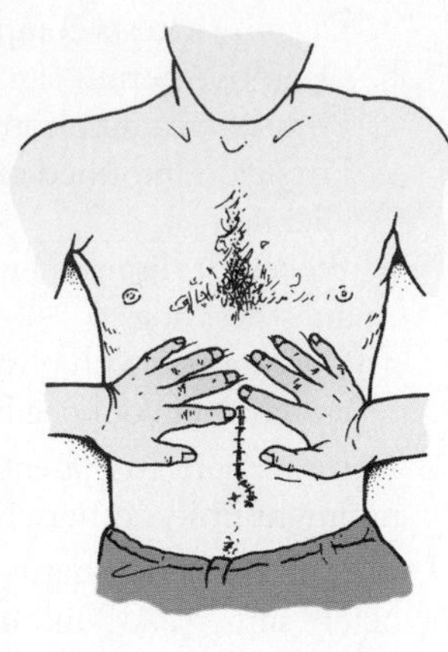

▲ Instruct client in coughing exercises using cough pillow or demonstrate placement of hands on either side of incision for support during coughing.

11. Have client cough a second time.
12. Instruct client to do coughing exercises after deep breathing exercises at least every 2 hr when awake.
13. Have tissue available for secretions if client has a productive cough.

Providing Instruction to Turn in Bed

Procedure

1. Check two forms of client ID and introduce yourself.
2. Explain turning procedure and purpose. ▸ ***Rationale:*** Turning assists in the prevention of thrombophlebitis, pressure ulcer formation, and respiratory complications.
3. Instruct and demonstrate turning procedure.
4. Instruct client to splint incision whenever turning.
5. Have client move to far side of bed with side rails up. ▸ ***Rationale:*** This position allows client to turn without rolling to edge of bed.
6. Instruct client to splint incision with hand on side toward which he or she will be turning. ▸ ***Rationale:*** This leaves the uppermost hand available to grasp side rail or trapeze to assist with turning.
7. Instruct client to keep leg straight on side to which he or she will turn.
8. Flex other leg over straight lower leg. ▸ ***Rationale:*** Flexing the leg assists in shifting the weight when turning to opposite side.
9. Instruct client to turn on side and grasp side rail.
10. Instruct client to move pillow into comfortable position under head or place pillow under top leg and place arm into comfortable position.

Instructing in Leg Exercises

Procedure

1. Check two forms of client ID and introduce yourself.
2. Explain exercise and purpose. ▸ ***Rationale:*** These exercises assist in preventing stasis of blood in lower extremities and thus thrombophlebitis.
3. Place client in supine or semi-Fowler's position.
4. Instruct client to bend knee, raise foot in air, and hold this position for 2–3 seconds.
5. Have client extend the leg and lower it to bed.
6. Repeat procedure with other leg.

NOTE: Inhale when extending leg and exhale slowly when lowering leg. This prevents back strain and strengthens abdominal muscles.

7. Complete sequence 5–10 times each hour while awake.
8. Have client extend toes (plantar flexion) toward bottom of bed, then flex (dorsiflexion) toward head of bed.
9. Repeat foot extension and flexion with other side.
10. Repeat sequence five times each hour while awake.
11. Instruct client to make circles with the ankle moving first to the left and then to the right.
12. Repeat sequence five times each hour while awake.

NOTE: Sequential compression devices are more commonly used during the postoperative period.

DOCUMENTATION for Preoperative Teaching

- Type of instruction provided
- Amount of time provided for instruction
- Type of audiovisual materials or written information used
- Client's response to teaching
- Accuracy and participation in return demonstration exercises
- Areas of instruction that need to be reinforced
- Psychological response to preoperative teaching and impending surgery
- Preop teaching form if available

CRITICAL THINKING Application

Expected Outcomes

- Client is psychologically and physically prepared for surgery.
- Client demonstrates deep breathing, coughing, turning, and leg exercises accurately.
- Client verbalizes knowledge of operative procedure, potential problems, and expected nursing actions postoperatively.
- Client's family states what they expect during perioperative period.
- Client uses appropriate audiovisual and written materials to increase understanding of perioperative experience.
- Client reports decreased fear regarding special equipment used during perioperative experience.
- Client states safety precautions used with laser and lithotripsy surgery.

Unexpected Outcomes	Alternative Actions
Client refuses to participate in preoperative teaching.	• Encourage client to state reasons for refusal. • Encourage client to discuss knowledge of surgery. • Assess whether client is experiencing fear or denial regarding impending surgery. • Ask client to provide a time frame more acceptable for teaching. • Notify physician of client's refusal if facility policy.
Client unable to understand directions.	• Identify client's learning capabilities. • Determine whether a language barrier exists. If so, find person who speaks client's primary language and ask for assistance with teaching. • Use different words to explain information. • Determine a different teaching strategy that the client can understand, or involve family members who can assist with explanations to client. • Evaluate client's stress level to determine whether it is interfering with learning. • Establish a new time for teaching when client may be able to concentrate on teaching. • Develop a slower pace for instruction and present less information at one time.

Client not adequately prepared for surgery.	• Ascertain where data are insufficient or unclear and provide additional instruction in that area. • Use a different approach or teaching style to provide information. • Select different teaching materials that may explain information in a more useful way.
Client becomes angry or hostile.	• Maintain calm composure. • Acknowledge anger, but place limits on how it may be expressed (e.g., destructive behavior). Understand that anger is usually the result of feeling helpless and powerless to change an intolerable situation. • Do not reward this behavior, but explore other means of meeting client's needs. • Do not isolate client; continue to respond to needs. • Try to defuse anger, but if safety is threatened, call for assistance.
Client becomes depressed because of overwhelming anxiety and feelings of helplessness or hopelessness.	• Convey respect and belief that client is worthwhile. Question client's appraisal of reality; provide support while client works through feelings. • Provide positive feedback and recognition of strengths, progress, and improved self-esteem. • Spend additional time with the client to allow time to verbalize fears.

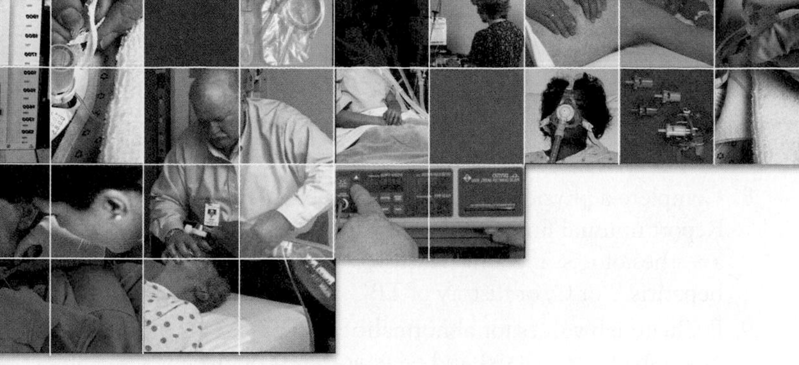

Chapter 26

UNIT 3

Preoperative Care

Nursing Process Data

ASSESSMENT Data Base

- Assess type of surgical procedure to be carried out and extent of data base needed.
- Evaluate the client's ability to provide accurate information.
- Assess level of anxiety present that may interfere in the transmission of information at that moment.
- Identify the appropriate physical care needed for the specific surgical intervention.
- Assess special needs for the surgical shave.
- Check hospital protocol for shaving surgical site or if a special permit is needed for shaving, such as the head for neurosurgical clients, extremities for orthopedic clients, or children.
- Check for need for special soap or antiseptic scrub before shave.
- Check if a policy exists in the hospital for disposing or handling of scalp hair.
- Assess surgical site before preparing; observe for unusual cuts, abrasions, or markings, and report findings to charge nurse.
- Assess client's knowledge of side and site of surgical procedure.

PLANNING Objectives

- To assist with monitoring the client's progress through the operative experience
- To assist in identifying deviations from the client's baseline data that may occur as a result of anxiety or stress of admission, preoperative events, diagnostic procedures, the surgical trauma, postoperative complications, responses to and side effects of drugs
- To provide appropriate preoperative physical care to enable the client to have a safe intraoperative and postoperative period
- To report client's statements about allergies or chronic problems that could affect postoperative nursing care
- To complete a surgical prep correctly

IMPLEMENTATION Procedures

EVALUATION Expected Outcomes

- Client's physical or emotional deviations from normal are identified preoperatively.
- Preoperative baseline data are obtained.
- Surgical site is marked and prepared correctly.
- Client states expectations regarding intraoperative and postoperative course.

Pearson Nursing Student Resources

Find additional review materials at **nursing.pearsonhighered.com**

Prepare for success with NCLEX®-style practice questions and Skill Checklists

Obtaining Baseline Data

Equipment

Thermometer
Sphygmomanometer and stethoscope
O_2 saturation probe
Chart or computer for documenting findings

Procedure

1. Check two forms of client ID and introduce yourself.
2. Ask about allergies to drugs, food, or latex.
3. Assess for surgical risk: nutritional status, fluid and electrolyte balance, use of prescribed medications, over-the-counter complementary medications (i.e., herbs), and illicit drugs. ▸ ***Rationale:*** Medications such as anticoagulants, tranquilizers, or CNS depressants can adversely affect surgical experience.
4. Assess for alcohol use and smoking habits. ▸ ***Rationale:*** Complications can arise in clients using these substances, particularly with anesthesia.
5. Take and record vital signs and weight of client. Obtain oxygen saturation levels.
6. Check if client wears dentures, hearing aid, glasses, has an artificial eye, or body piercing jewelry. Check for toe rings. If body piercing jewelry cannot be removed, cover with tape to protect skin from electrical arcing from the electrical surgical unit, which could cause skin burns.
7. Assess mental attitude; record any unusual stress or anxiety exhibited by the client.
8. Complete a physical assessment and health history. Report unusual findings to physician, OR staff, and anesthesiologist if client has history of MRSA, VRE, hepatitis B or C, or history of TBC.
9. Evaluate lab values for abnormalities (ECG, x-rays, blood work, urinalysis) and pregnancy test on age-appropriate client if she has an intact uterus. ▸ ***Rationale:*** To detect potential sources for complications (e.g., low Hct, Hgb, urine glucose, lung or cardiac abnormalities).
10. Determine whether skin preparation was completed either evening before or morning of surgery. Check if shower or bath with designated antiseptic was completed.
11. Assess for fall potential (unsteady gait, use of assistive devices).
12. Identify topics requiring client teaching.
13. Identify discharge plans.
14. Determine religious or cultural beliefs that may affect surgical experience.

Clinical Alert

It is imperative that nurses on the surgical floor check documentation carefully to find any abnormalities in the H&P, lab results, or assessment indicating potential complications during procedure. This information must be reported to the anesthesiologist and OR staff.

Preparing the Surgical Site

Equipment

Washcloth and towels
Absorbent pad
Bath blanket or drape
Scissors or electric clippers (optional)
Disposable prep kit (for shaving)
If kit not available:
- Disposable razor (number according to area to be shaved)
- Two sterile bowls
- 4 × 4 gauze pads
- Emesis basin
- Applicator sticks
- Cleansing solution
- Sterile water

Clean gloves
Depilatory
Antiseptic solution
Tongue blade
4 × 4 gauze pad

Procedure

1. Refer to physician's orders for specific operative site or area to be prepared. If orders do not state preference for site, refer to procedure manual for appropriate area to be prepared, based on surgical procedure.

NOTE: Many surgeons do not require hair to be shaved for a surgical site unless it interferes with the surgical procedure or wound closure. Based on clinical research, it has been found that shaving the hair does not prevent surgical site infections, but it does interfere with the client's psychological status. Client's body image can be impaired and he or she senses a loss of control with shaving of the hair, particularly of the head or pubic area.

2. Determine type of preparation to be done: clipping of hair, shaving site, or hair removal using depilatory. Gather equipment.
3. Check two forms of client ID and introduce yourself.

4. Explain procedure to client and provide privacy.
5. Adjust light to ensure good visualization.
6. Perform hand hygiene.
7. Position client for maximum comfort and site exposure.
8. Drape client for comfort and to prevent undue exposure.
9. Protect bed with absorbent pad.
10. Arrange equipment for your convenience.
11. Put on clean gloves.
12. Assess surgical site before skin preparation for moles, warts, rash, and other skin conditions. ▶ ***Rationale:*** Inadvertent removal of lesions traumatizes skin and may contribute to infection.

NOTE: CDC standards indicate that clients are to shower or bathe with an antiseptic agent at least the night before surgery. The FDA has also shown that antimicrobial activity of the antiseptic agent prevents skin infections.

13. Prepare site using scissors or clippers according to facility policy/procedures.
    a. Use scissors or electric clippers and cut hair 1 cm above surgical site or according to facility policies.
    b. Clip small amount of hair each time.
    c. Cut in direction hair grows.
    d. Remove all hair from site and discard.
14. Prepare site using depilatory.
    a. Clip hair before applying cream.
    b. Apply cream to designated area using tongue blade or gloved hand.
    c. Leave on skin for designated time, according to directions on package, usually 10 minutes.
    d. Remove cream by rubbing off with tongue blade or moistened 4 × 4 gauze pads.
    e. Wash skin with antiseptic soap; dry area thoroughly.
    f. Remove all hair with washing. ▶ ***Rationale:*** This provides clean, smooth skin, free of abrasions and cuts.
15. Prepare site using razor.
    a. Lather skin with antiseptic soap and 4 × 4 gauze pads. ▶ ***Rationale:*** Wet shave results in fewer microabrasions to the skin. Shaving should be done in direction of hair growth.
    b. Discard soiled sponges frequently.
    c. Using sharp razor, shave hair moving away from incision site. With free hand, stretch skin taut and shave, following the hair growth pattern and using firm, steady strokes. Shave small area at one time. ▶ ***Rationale:*** Shave is closer and nicks are prevented.
    d. Change razor as often as necessary. Avoid nicking the skin. Report if skin is nicked. ▶ ***Rationale:*** Nicks, if severe, can cause infection by bacteria normally found on the skin.
    e. Wash all hair off site with 4 × 4 gauze pads or use sticky mitt or tape to remove hair.
    f. The shave should be completed close to the time of surgery. The shave prep is completed before the client enters the operating room. ▶ ***Rationale:*** Shaving and clipping hair immediately before surgery is associated with a lower risk of infection than if done the night before.
16. After removing hair, apply antiseptic solution with 4 × 4 pads or use disposable prep kit.

Clinical Alert

If hair must be removed, scissors or clippers should be used and procedure completed before the client reaches the operating room suite. Many hospitals use the minimal shave and scrub preparation approach. The shaved area may be as small as 2 cm surrounding the surgical incision site. Refer to the policy and procedure manual and physician's orders before beginning the surgical prep.

Clinical Alert

Electric or battery-powered clippers are preferred to razors to prevent skin irritation and microscopic cuts to the skin. Clippers must have a disposable head that is changed between clients. Handles should be disinfected.

EVIDENCE-BASED PRACTICE

Surgical Site Infection (SSI)

A preoperative antiseptic shower or bath decreases skin microbial colony count. In a study of more than 700 clients who received two preoperative antiseptic showers, chlorhexidine reduced bacterial colony counts nine fold. Iodine or triclocarban-medicated soap reduced colony counts 1.3- to 1.9-fold, respectively.

Chlorhexidine gluconate–containing products require several applications to obtain maximum antimicrobial benefit, so repeated antiseptic showers are indicated. Even though these showers reduce the colony count, they have not definitively shown a reduction in SSI rate.

Source: Mangram, A. J., Horan, T. C., Pearson, M. L., Silver, L. C., & Jarvis, W. R. (1999). Guideline for prevention of surgical site infection, 1999. The Hospital Infection Control Practices Advisory Committee. *Infection Control and Hospital Epidemiology*, 20(4), 250–278.

EVIDENCE-BASED PRACTICE

Skin Preparation and Surgical Site Infections

Many studies show that hair removal with a razor or clippers can cause skin abrasion or even nicks in the skin. This can lead to subsequent surgical site infections (SSIs). In a study discussed in the *CDC Guideline for Prevention of Surgical Site Infection*, it was identified that SSIs occurred in 5.6% of clients who had their hair removed by razor shave, compared with an 0.6% rate among those who had hair removed by depilatory or had no hair removed at all. The CDC advises that if hair is to be removed, it should be done so immediately before surgery, and preferably with electric hair clippers.

Source: Mangram, A. J., Horan, T. C., Pearson, M. L., Silver, L. C., & Jarvis, W. R. (1999). Guideline for prevention of surgical site infection, 1999. The Hospital Infection Control Practices Advisory Committee. *Infection Control and Hospital Epidemiology*, 20(4), 250–278.

17. Begin at incision site and, with light friction, make ever-widening circles, moving outward from the center to the most distant line of area. ▶ ***Rationale:*** Working from most clean to least clean area prevents contamination. Scrub area for 2–3 minutes.
18. Rinse area with warm water and blot dry with 4 × 4 gauze pads.
19. Remove and dispose of equipment; scissors and razors are disposed of in sharps container.
20. Remove gloves and discard.
21. Perform hand hygiene.
22. Assist client to put on clean gown.
23. Position the client for comfort.

Preparing the Client for Surgery

Equipment

Preoperative checklist
Operative permit
Specific equipment needed to provide physical care as ordered, such as enema equipment, nasogastric tube, Foley catheter
Antiseptic agent for shower

Procedure

1. Check two forms of client ID and introduce yourself.
2. Obtain client's signature on surgical consent form and check agency policy. Ensure all preoperative forms are complete, with no blank areas.
3. Assist client to complete anesthesia questionnaire if required.
4. Assess whether bowel prep was completed at home. ▶ ***Rationale:*** Most clients complete bowel prep before admission to facility. Administer an enema if ordered.
5. Assist client to shower if not completed at home. Instruct on how to shower and specific time guidelines according to facility guidelines.
6. Complete skin prep, if ordered. Follow facility guidelines for skin prep.
7. Assess for latex allergy. If present, ensure allergy band is applied, physician is notified, and OR staff are notified. ▶ ***Rationale:*** All latex products must be removed from OR and client must be scheduled for first case in morning.

COMMUNITY HOSPITAL

Client Information

AUTHORIZATION FOR AND CONSENT TO SURGERY, ADMINISTRATION OF ANESTHETICS, SPECIAL DIAGNOSTIC OR THERAPEUTIC PROCEDURES

Date ____________ Time ____________

Your admitting physician is ______________________________, M. D.

Your surgeon is ______________________________, M. D.

1. The hospital staff and facilities assist your physicians and surgeons in the performance of various surgical operations and other diagnostic and therapeutic procedures. These surgical operations and special diagnostic or therapeutic procedures all may involve calculated risks of complications, injury or even death, from both known and unknown causes and no warranty or guarantee has been made as to result or cure. Except in a case of emergency or exceptional circumstances, these operations and procedures are not performed upon clients unless and until the client has had an opportunity to discuss them with his/her physician. Each client has the right to consent to or refuse any proposed operation or special procedure (based upon the description or explanation received).
2. Your physicians and surgeons have determined that the operations or special procedures listed below may be beneficial in the diagnosis or treatment of your condition. Upon your authorization and consent, the operations or special procedures will be performed by your physicians and surgeons and their staff. The persons in attendance for the purpose of administering anesthesia or performing other specialized professional services, such as radiology, pathology and the like, are not the agents, servants or employees of the hospital or your physician or surgeon, but are independent contractors performing specialized services on your behalf and, as such, are your agents, servants, or employees. Any tissue or member severed in any operation will be disposed of in the discretion of the pathologist, except ______________ and those body parts specified as donor organs.
3. Your signature opposite the operations or special procedures listed below constitutes your acknowledgement (a) that you have read and agreed to the foregoing, (b) that the operations or special procedures have been adequately explained to you by your attending physicians or surgeons and that you have all of the information that you desire, and (c) that you authorize and consent to the performance of the operations or special procedures.

Operation or Procedure

____

____

Signature ______________ Signature ______________
Client Witness

(If client is a minor or unable to sign, complete the following): Client is a minor, is unable to sign because

____

____
Father Guardian

____
Mother Other person and relationship

▲ Surgical consent form.

COMMUNITY HOSPITAL

SURGICAL CHECKLIST PLEASE PRINT

1. Surgical Procedure scheduled: ______________ Rt. Lt. (circle)
2. Surgeon ______________

SURGICAL REQUIREMENTS		
NPO SINCE: DATE:	TIME:	
RECORDS	YES	NO
HISTORY & PHYSICAL		
SIGNED INFORMED CONSENT		
STERILIZATION: SIGNED CONSENT FOR		
PREVIOUS RECORDS		
ANESTHESIA EVALUATION		
REPORTS	ORDERED	ON CHART
CBC		
URINALYSIS		
CHEST X-RAY		
EKG		
OTHER		
BLOOD ORDERED	☐ YES	☐ NO
BLOOD CONFIRMED # UNITS		

CLIENT PREPARATION				
15. Prosthesis	None	Removed	Disposition	Left in
a. Bridge				
b. Partial				
c. Plates				
d. Artificial limbs				
e. Artificial eyes				
f. Contact lenses				
g. Hearing aid				
h. Pacemaker				
i. Hairpieces, Hairpins, Eyelashes				

16. Valuables	Removed Yes or No	Disposition, if yes
a. Rings		
b. Watch		
c. Medal and chain		
d. Glasses		
e. Radio		
f. Wallet		
g. Other		

17. Identification band checked with chart ______________ Yes or No

PRE-OP CHECK SIGNATURE ______________ R.N.

TIME TO OR ______________

RELEASE SIGNATURE ______________

CLIENT ASSESSMENT

LANGUAGE SPOKEN

PHYSICAL DISABILITIES

CHRONIC ILLNESS

TEACHING NEEDS ☐ Pre-op ☐ Post-op
☐ Medications ☐ Treatment ☐ Equipment
☐ Other

COMMENTS

DISCHARGE PLANNING NEEDS

TRANSPORTATION HOME BY

AVAILABLE AT:

CLIENT PREPARATION

BATH/SHOWER ☐ YES ☐ NO

SHAVE/PREP ☐ YES ☐ NO

SKIN CONDITION

VITAL SIGNS

TEMP	PULSE	RESP	B/P
HEIGHT		WEIGHT	

MEDS TAKEN AT HOME	LAST DOSE	AMT.

PARENTERAL FLUIDS		
TYPE	AMT.	TIME STARTED

PRE-OP MEDICATIONS			
DRUG	AMT	ROUTE/SITE	TIME

ALLERGIES	ALLERGY BAND

▲ Surgical preoperative checklist.

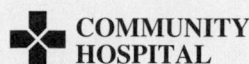

PRE-ANESTHESIA EVALUATION

1. Proposed Procedure

2. Present Illness (diagnosis)

3. Current H&P ○ **In progress notes reviewed/approved** (Skip sections **4, 5, 6** and **7** then *Complete only sections* ***8, 9, 10, 11, 12 and 13***)

4. Pertinent Past Medical History ***If no H & P in chart complete sections 4, 5, 6, 7, 8, 9, 10, 11b, 12 and 13 below*** *on this page*

	Y	N	Describe any "Yes" responses
Cardiac events			
Arrhythmia			
Pulmonary disease			
Liver disease			
Renal insufficiency			
Diabetes/Metabolic disease			
Seizures/CNS events			
Bleeding disorder			
Possible Pregnancy			
Pt./Family hx anesth problem			
Alcohol use			
Tobacco use			
IV Drug abuse			

5. Allergies & Sensitivities ○ NKDA

6. Current Medications

7. Pertinent Physical Exam: (check all responses that apply. Circle WNL as appropriate) **O2 Sat.**_____ %

○ **Airway – WNL Class** ___ ○ **Dental – WNL** or ○ poor dentition ○ dentures ○ obese ○ **Pulmonary – WNL** ○ **Cardiac/B/P – WNL** ○ **Neuro Status – WNL**

Describe any "Abnormal" responses

8. Pertinent Investigations: (Check all responses that apply. Circle WNL as appropriate) HT_____ Ft/cm WT _____ Lb/kg

○ Hgb/Hct – WNL ○ Labs – WNL ○ EKG – WNL ○ CXR – WNL ○ Other Imaging – WNL

"Comments"

9. Assessment **ASA Scoring System** (circle appropriate one)

1........Normal patient; elective surgery/procedure
2........Mild systemic disease, not activity-limiting
3........Severe systemic disease
4........Severe systemic disease; constant threat to life
5........Moribund patient; not expected to survive without surgery
6........Brain dead; organ donation
E........Emergency

10. Hours Since Last Oral Intake: NPO___ hours Liquids ___ hours Solids ___ hours ☐ Unknown

11. Plan .....Patient is an appropriate candidate for:

11a. Anesthesia
○ General ○ Spinal/epidural ○ Regional ○ Monitored Anesthesia Care
Surgeon
☐ Informed consent is documented in the progress notes
Anesthesiologist
☐ Anesthetic alternatives/risks/benefits discussed with patient including but not limited to: tooth damage, nerve damage, life threatening events (i.e. MI, CVA, Death) and has been explained and accepted by patient/family. Questions answered

11b.
○ **Procedure Sedation**
Procedure Sedation ***only:***
☐ Risks, benefits and alternatives for the procedure and sedation have been discussed with the patient.

12. Completed by: **Date:** **Time:**

13. Reassessment (complete if over 30 Minutes has elapsed from Initial Assessment) ASA 1 2 3 4 5 6 E NPO Status_____ hours

○ Patient's status unchanged—appropriate candidate Other: (following changes has occurred)

Completed by: **Date:** **Time:**

White Copy -- Medical Record
Yellow Copy -- Anesthesia Office (for Anesthesia) or QM Office (for Procedure Sedation)

▲ Preanesthesia evaluation form.

Clinical Alert

The Association of PeriOperative Registered Nurses (AORN) recommends preop skin prep should be an antimicrobial agent that has a broad germicidal range and is nontoxic.

The most common antiseptic agents used for preoperative skin preparation and surgical scrubs include alcohol, chlorhexidine, iodine/iodophors, and Triclosan.

Alcohol has the most rapid microbial action, which denatures proteins and is effective against both gram-positive (gram +) and gram-negative (gram −) bacteria, viruses, and fungi.

Chlorhexidine has an intermediate rapidity of action, disrupting the cell membrane. It should not be used on mucous membranes, eyes, or brain tissue (neurotoxic). It works well against gram-positive bacteria, and less well against gram-negative bacteria.

Iodine/iodophors has an intermediate action and is acceptable for use against a wide range of bacteria, fungi, and viruses.

Triclosan disrupts the cell wall and has an acceptable kill rate against bacteria. Even though alcohol has microbial action, it is not often used as a surgical skin prep because it does not stay on the skin.

8. Enquire for symptoms and observe for signs of cold or upper respiratory infection.
9. Explain need for client to be NPO for 8–10 hr preoperatively.
10. Remove lipstick and nail polish if required by hospital policy.
11. Insert Foley catheter if ordered.
12. Take and record vital signs.
13. Remove earrings, necklaces, medals, watch, rings (ring may be taped to finger or toe in some facilities). If possible, remove body piercing jewelry. Cover with tape if not possible to remove. ▸ ***Rationale:*** Protect skin from possible burns from electrical arcing generated by electrical cautery machines.
14. Remove contact lenses, glasses, hairpieces, and dentures. Some hospitals/anesthesiologists allow full dentures to remain if using a mask.
15. Assist client to void if catheter not inserted, and record time and amount.
16. Check Ident-A-Band, blood band, and allergy bracelet. During this stage the client must be identified by at least two identifiers (i.e., medical record number, birth date, name, charge number).
17. Put antiembolic stockings on client as ordered.
18. Administer preoperative medications.
19. The operative site needs to be verified and marked, both site and side, by the physician while the client is awake.
20. Place side rails in UP position and bed in low position after administration of medications.
21. Darken room and provide quiet environment after administration of medications.
22. Check client 15 minutes after medication administered to observe for possible side effects.

EVIDENCE-BASED PRACTICE

Surgical Checklist May Improve Outcomes for Noncardiac Surgery

Surgical procedures are estimated at 234 million operations performed yearly throughout the world. A longitudinal study over 1 year utilizing eight participating hospitals representing a diverse group of socioeconomic environments within the World Health Organization regions from Amman, Jordan, to Seattle, Washington, and Toronto, Canada, were utilized in the study of 3,733 consecutive inpatient noncardiac surgery clients 16 years or older. The objective of the study was to evaluate the effect on rates of mortality and major complications with implementing the surgical checklist in inpatient surgical units. Data were first prospectively collected regarding clinical processes and outcomes. Then after implementing the Surgical Safety Checklist, data were collected from 3,955 consecutive inpatient noncardiac surgery clients.

Death rates during hospitalization decreased from 1.5% in the initial cohort to 0.8% after implementation of the checklist. This represents a decline in the rate of inpatient complications from 11.0% to 7.0%.

Source: Barclay, L. (2009). Surgical Checklist May Improve Outcomes for Noncardiac Surgery. *New England Journal of Medicine*, 360, 491–499.

Administering Preoperative Medications

Equipment

Preoperative checklist
Preoperative medications

Procedure

1. Check two forms of client ID and introduce yourself.
2. Complete preoperative checklist.
3. Check orders for medication, dosage, route, and time.
4. Verify that surgical consent is accurate, understood by client, and properly signed before giving any preop sedation.
5. Check history for allergy to ordered medication.
6. Explain purpose of medication to client.
7. Warn client that injection may sting or burn.
8. Follow procedure for administration of injections.
9. Administer medications 30 minutes before beginning of surgery.
10. Raise side rails to UP position and put bed in low position.
11. Explain why client should not get out of bed after medications have been given. ▶ ***Rationale:*** Medication makes client drowsy and affects equilibrium.
12. Place call light within reach and encourage client to use it.
13. Ask if there are any questions or assistance you can offer before leaving the room. Darken room or close curtains.
14. Inform client of the estimated time he or she will be going to surgery.

Preoperative Medications: Type and Action

Hypnotic or Antianxiolytic—Given Night Before Surgery

Decreases anxiety
Promotes good night's sleep

Hypnotic or Opiate—Preoperative Medication

Decreases anxiety
Allows smooth anesthetic induction
Provides amnesia for immediate perioperative period

Anticholinergic—Preoperative Medication

Decreases secretions
Counteracts vagal effects during anesthesia

Clinical Alert

Universal Protocol for Preventing Wrong Site, Wrong Procedure, and Wrong Person Surgery

- Preoperative validation of the right client, procedure, and site should occur when the client is awake, aware, and before he/she leaves the preoperative area or enters the surgical suite.
- Person performing the procedure must do the marking.
- Incision site must be marked, using a marker that is not easily removed, at or near the incision site.
- DO NOT MARK any nonoperative site(s) unless necessary for some other aspect of care.
- Use initials, word "yes," or a line indicating proposed incision site to prevent ambiguous marks.
- Mark must be visible after client is prepped and draped.
- Final verification of site mark must take place in the location where the procedure will take place. This time is identified as the "Time Out" period. Nothing happens until this has occurred. The entire team must be present during this check.
- Verification must include:
  a. Correct client identity.
  b. Correct site and side.
  c. Agreement on procedure to be done.
  d. Correct client position.
  e. Availability of any special equipment or implants needed for procedure.

Exemptions From the Marking Procedure

Single organ cases (e.g., C-section, cardiac surgery).
Interventional cases: insertion site of instrument/catheter not predetermined.
Premature infants: for whom the mark may cause permanent mark.

Source: The Joint Commission. http://www.jointcommission.org/PatientSafety/UniversalProtocol/.

DOCUMENTATION for Preoperative Care

- Safety measures carried out preoperatively
- Completion of preoperative site preparation and area involved
- Antiseptic solution used and length of time of scrub
- Operative checklist completed
- Review physician's explanation of potential surgical complications
- Physical care completed before surgery

- Surgical site marking procedure (site, individual who marked site, persons present during "Time Out" step in procedure)
- Preoperative medications given and effects of medications
- Time and method of transportation to operating room
- Preoperative teaching completed

Legal Alert

In 2001, The Joint Commission reported surgical mistakes were on the rise. After this report a study was completed. The study analyzed 126 cases involving surgical mistakes and found that 76% of the cases involved operating on the wrong body part, 13% involved the wrong client, and 11% involved the wrong surgical procedure.

Source: http://MedicalMalpracticeLawyers.us.

CRITICAL THINKING Application

Expected Outcomes

- Client's physical or emotional deviations from normal are identified preoperatively.
- Preoperative baseline data are obtained.
- Surgical site is marked and prepared correctly.
- Client states expectations regarding intraoperative and postoperative course.

Unexpected Outcomes	Alternative Actions
Factors that can affect the postoperative course are identified during the preoperative care (e.g., arthritic changes in client's back, history of thrombophlebitis).	• Place information in client's care plan and inform charge nurse and surgeon about findings. • Write a note in client's chart and alert the operating room and recovery room staff of the findings so that they can assess for the problems.
Client refuses to go to operating room without dentures.	• Explain to client that dentures are likely to be lost, broken, or inadvertently pushed to back of mouth if not removed. • If client refuses to remove dentures, alert anesthesiologist that dentures are in place.
Client's skin is cut during shave.	• Notify MD and OR staff of client's condition. • Follow specific directions; surgery may be canceled as infection could occur as result of break in skin integrity.
Client unable to void before surgery.	• Run water so client can hear trickling sound to stimulate voiding. • Run warm water over perineum. • Place ammonia or oil of wintergreen on a cotton ball in urinal or bedpan. • Help male to stand or sit at edge of bed with urinal positioned. • Help female to commode if urinating into bedpan is difficult. • Notify MD and OR staff. Record in chart.
Client appears to be abnormally stressed.	• Explore feelings and reasons for client's or family's stressed behaviors. • Explore more effective methods to reduce stress for client and family. • Provide additional stress reduction exercises. • Clarify misconceptions and inappropriate perceptions. • Introduce client to another client who has had similar surgery. • Have physician speak to client and answer questions.

Client's preoperative laboratory findings are abnormal.	• Check with laboratory to have them reevaluate if lab results are accurate. • Have laboratory redo tests if extremely abnormal. • Notify physician of abnormal findings. • Notify surgeon and anesthesiologist.
Client is unable to participate in marking surgical site.	• If client is comatose, non–English speaking, or incompetent, follow protocol as with informed consent. • Guardian or individual with power of attorney should be involved with marking, if possible.
Client refuses site marking.	• Client has right to refuse; document client refusal on appropriate forms. • Procedure may be performed without marking. • Provide client with information regarding safety aspects for marking procedure. • Discuss rationale for client's refusal to determine whether insufficient information was provided regarding marking procedure.

Chapter 26

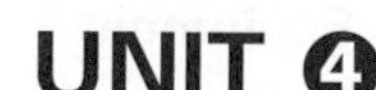

Moderate (Conscious) Sedation

Nursing Process Data

ASSESSMENT Data Base

- Assess type of procedure to be done and determine whether moderate (conscious) sedation is appropriate.
- Assess type of sedation to be used for procedure.
- Determine whether medication can be administered by nurse or only by physician.
- Check whether physician has ordered medication for moderate (conscious) sedation and whether nurse is approved to administer medication.
- Determine whether history and physical is in client's chart.
- Check that signed consent form is in chart.
- Assess client according to American Society of Anesthesiologists (ASA) Classification of Physical Status.

PLANNING Objectives

- To determine whether client is to receive moderate (conscious) sedation from nurse or physician
- To establish venous access before sedation administration
- To monitor vital signs throughout procedure
- To continuously assess for changes in client's condition and/or untoward responses or effects of medication
- To immediately notify physician of changes in client's condition

IMPLEMENTATION Procedures

EVALUATION Expected Outcomes

- Client maintains airway and respiratory status throughout procedure.
- Client does not experience anxiety or pain during procedure.

Pearson Nursing Student Resources

Find additional review materials at **nursing.pearsonhighered.com**

Prepare for success with NCLEX®-style practice questions and Skill Checklists

Preparing Client for Moderate (Conscious) Sedation

Equipment

Consent form
History and physical
Lab test results, if necessary
Sedation Scale

Procedure

1. Ensure that client is candidate for conscious sedation. Use ASA Classification of Physical Status. ▸ ***Rationale:*** Clients in ASA categories 1 and 2 may receive conscious sedation by qualified physicians and nurses. Clients in category 3 or 4 are referred to anesthesia provider for further evaluation because their condition puts them at risk for complications. Further evaluation of elderly, pregnant, or obese clients, and those with a history of substance abuse, sleep apnea, or severe cardiac, respiratory, hepatic, renal or central nervous system diseases is necessary because these clients are placed at higher risk during the use of conscious sedation.
2. Determine whether client has any contraindications for conscious sedation:
   a. Recent ingestion of large food or fluid volumes (in past 2 hr).
   b. Physical status IV or greater.
   c. Lack of support staff or monitoring equipment.
   d. Lack of experience on part of clinician.
3. Determine whether nurse or physician will administer medication.
4. Check that qualified anesthesia provider has written order for conscious sedation.
5. Check two forms of client ID and introduce yourself.
6. Check that client has been informed about procedure and use of conscious sedation.
7. Ensure that history and physical has been completed and on client's chart.
8. Obtain height and weight. ▸ ***Rationale:*** To use for drug calculation when administering conscious sedation.
9. Ask about allergies, particularly sedatives.
10. Ensure client has been NPO for at least 2 hr.

ASA Classification of Physical Status

Class	*Definition*
P1	A normal healthy client
P2	A client with mild systemic disease
P3	A client with severe systemic disease
P4	A client with severe systemic disease that is a constant threat to life
P5	A moribund client who is not expected to survive without surgery
P6	A declared brain-dead client whose organs are being removed for donor

Source: Adapted from the American Society of Anesthesiologists. (1999). ASA Physical Classification System. Available at: http://www.asahq.org/clinical/physicalstatus.htm

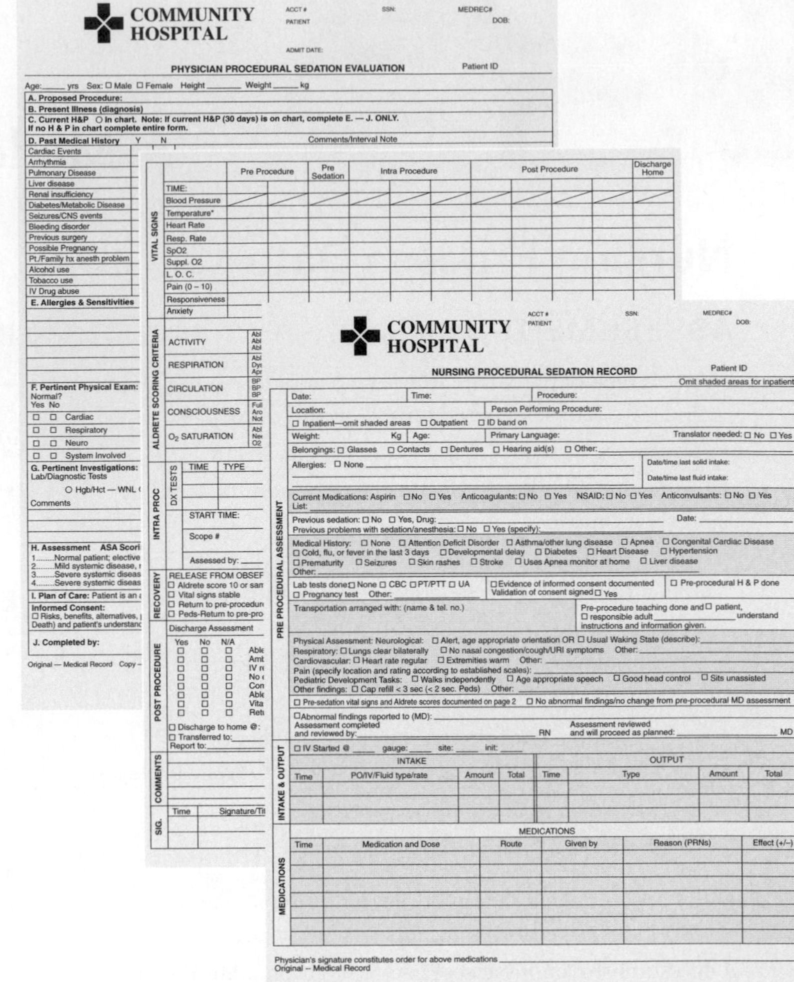

COMMUNITY HOSPITAL
ACCT # SSN: MEDREC#
PATIENT DOB:
ADMIT DATE:
PHYSICIAN PROCEDURAL SEDATION EVALUATION Patient ID
Age:____ yrs Sex: ☐ Male ☐ Female Height ____ Weight ____ kg
A. Proposed Procedure:
B. Present Illness (diagnosis)
C. Current H&P ○ In chart. Note: If current H&P (30 days) is on chart, complete E. — J. ONLY. If no H & P in chart complete entire form.
D. Past Medical History Y N Comments/Interval Note
Cardiac Events
Arrhythmia
Pulmonary Disease
Liver disease
Renal insufficiency
Diabetes/Metabolic Disease
Seizures/CNS events
Bleeding disorder
Previous surgery
Possible Pregnancy
Pt./Family hx anesth problem
Alcohol use
Tobacco use
IV Drug abuse
E. Allergies & Sensitivities
F. Pertinent Physical Exam: Normal? Yes No
☐ ☐ Cardiac
☐ ☐ Respiratory
☐ ☐ Neuro
☐ ☐ System Involved
G. Pertinent Investigations: Lab/Diagnostic Tests
○ Hgb/Hct — WNL
Comments
H. Assessment ASA Scori
1.........Normal patient; elective
2.........Mild systemic disease,
3.........Severe systemic diseas
4.........Severe systemic diseas
I. Plan of Care: Patient is an
Informed Consent:
☐ Risks, benefits, alternatives, Death) and patient's understanc
J. Completed by:
Original — Medical Record Copy –

		Pre Procedure		Pre Sedation	Intra Procedure			Post Procedure			Discharge Home
VITAL SIGNS	TIME:										
	Blood Pressure										
	Temperature*										
	Heart Rate										
	Resp. Rate										
	SpO2										
	Suppl. O2										
	L. O. C.										
	Pain (0 – 10)										
	Responsiveness										
	Anxiety										

ALDRETE SCORING CRITERIA
ACTIVITY
RESPIRATION
CIRCULATION
CONSCIOUSNESS
O_2 SATURATION
INTRA PROC
DX TESTS TIME TYPE
START TIME:
Scope #
Assessed by:
RECOVERY
RELEASE FROM OBSERV
☐ Aldrete score 10 or sam
☐ Vital signs stable
☐ Return to pre-procedur
☐ Peds-Return to pre-pro
POST PROCEDURE
Discharge Assessment
Yes No N/A
☐ Discharge to home @:
☐ Transferred to:
Report to:
COMMENTS
SIG. Time Signature/Ti

COMMUNITY HOSPITAL
ACCT # SSN: MEDREC#
PATIENT DOB:
NURSING PROCEDURAL SEDATION RECORD Patient ID
Omit shaded areas for inpatients
PRE PROCEDURAL ASSESSMENT
Date: Time: Procedure:
Location: Person Performing Procedure:
☐ Inpatient—omit shaded areas ☐ Outpatient ☐ ID band on
Weight: Kg Age: Primary Language: Translator needed: ☐ No ☐ Yes
Belongings: ☐ Glasses ☐ Contacts ☐ Dentures ☐ Hearing aid(s) ☐ Other:
Allergies: ☐ None
Date/time last solid intake:
Date/time last fluid intake:
Current Medications: Aspirin ☐ No ☐ Yes Anticoagulants: ☐ No ☐ Yes NSAID: ☐ No ☐ Yes Anticonvulsants: ☐ No ☐ Yes
List:
Previous sedation: ☐ No ☐ Yes, Drug: Date:
Previous problems with sedation/anesthesia: ☐ No ☐ Yes (specify):
Medical History: ☐ None ☐ Attention Deficit Disorder ☐ Asthma/other lung disease ☐ Apnea ☐ Congenital Cardiac Disease ☐ Cold, flu, or fever in the last 3 days ☐ Developmental delay ☐ Diabetes ☐ Heart Disease ☐ Hypertension ☐ Prematurity ☐ Seizures ☐ Skin rashes ☐ Stroke ☐ Uses Apnea monitor at home ☐ Liver disease
Other:
Lab tests done: ☐ None ☐ CBC ☐ PT/PTT ☐ UA ☐ Pregnancy test Other:
☐ Evidence of informed consent documented Validation of consent signed ☐ Yes
☐ Pre-procedural H & P done
Transportation arranged with: (name & tel. no.)
Pre-procedure teaching done and ☐ patient, ☐ responsible adult ____ understand instructions and information given.
Physical Assessment: Neurological: ☐ Alert, age appropriate orientation OR ☐ Usual Waking State (describe):
Respiratory: ☐ Lungs clear bilaterally ☐ No nasal congestion/cough/URI symptoms Other:
Cardiovascular: ☐ Heart rate regular ☐ Extremities warm Other:
Pain (specify location and rating according to established scales):
Pediatric Development Tasks: ☐ Walks independently ☐ Age appropriate speech ☐ Good head control ☐ Sits unassisted
Other findings: ☐ Cap refill < 3 sec (< 2 sec. Peds) Other:
☐ Pre-sedation vital signs and Aldrete scores documented on page 2 ☐ No abnormal findings/no change from pre-procedural MD assessment
☐ Abnormal findings reported to (MD):
Assessment completed and reviewed by: ____ RN Assessment reviewed and will proceed as planned: ____ MD
INTAKE & OUTPUT
☐ IV Started @ ____ gauge: ____ site: ____ init: ____

INTAKE				OUTPUT			
Time	PO/IV/Fluid type/rate	Amount	Total	Time	Type	Amount	Total

MEDICATIONS

Time	Medication and Dose	Route	Given by	Reason (PRNs)	Effect (+/–)

Physician's signature constitutes order for above medications
Original – Medical Record

▲ Moderate (Conscious) sedation record samples.

11. Explain that the medication will relax him or her during procedure, client will feel sleepy but will not be asleep, and will be able to communicate during procedure. ▸ ***Rationale:*** This is necessary to determine comfort and level of sedation during procedure.
12. Discuss the possibility of unpleasant sensations of pain, nausea, vertigo.
13. Determine gestures that will be used during procedure to indicate whether client is having pain.
14. Ensure that someone is with the client to take him or her home if discharge is anticipated after the procedure. ▸ ***Rationale:*** Residual effects of sedation can last for several hours. Driving can be impaired and thus it is unsafe for the client to drive home.

NOTE: The American Nurses Association and other nursing organizations allow nurses to administer sedating drugs, assess client responses, and monitor vital signs during the use of conscious sedation. Nurses who administer conscious sedation must function within the standard of practice and be allowed to administer conscious sedation according to the nurse practice act in the state in which they are practicing. They must also administer conscious sedation according to policies and procedures of the facility in which they are working. At no time will student nurses be allowed to administer conscious sedation.

Capnography

Capnography has been shown to be effective in detecting hypoventilation during procedural sedation. The traditional PCA pump now has built in sensors that monitor ventilation and oxygenation. It is also used to monitor clients on PCA pumps using narcotics.

A capnography monitor is a device that measures carbon dioxide. The monitor is attached to tubing at the end of the tracheostomy or endotracheal tube. The Alaris PCA pump with capnography/pulse oximetry has a module that measures CO_2. CO_2 can also be measured by attaching a tube to an oxygen mask or nasal cannula. The mask or nasal cannula contains a sensor that measures the CO_2. The results are reported on a hand-held device rather than the monitor.

Monitoring Client During Procedure

Equipment

Crash cart or following list of equipment:
- Suction equipment; machine, tubing, and suction catheter (tonsil tip)
- Oxygen supply and appropriate delivery system
- Laryngoscope handle and blades of appropriate size
- Endotracheal tubes and stylets in various sizes
- Oral and nasal cannulas
- 3-mL and 10-mL syringes
- Needles, if not using needless system
- IV solution bags
- Reversal drug agents (i.e., Narcan, Romazicon)

Pulse oximeter (optional with capnography)
ECG machine and defibrillator, cardiac monitor
Intubation tray and bag–valve–mask device
Vital sign portable machine
Client's chart
Procedural sedation record
Conscious sedation medications; usually benzodiazepines and opioids
Emergency cardiac drugs, naloxone, flumazenil

Procedure

1. Ensure that backup personnel skilled in ACLS are available if needed.
2. Verify correct client by using two identifiers.
3. Evaluate ASA Classification of Physical Status again.
4. Check that chart contains appropriate documents.
5. Check that preprocedural assessment is completed on sedation record.
6. Check that consent form was signed.
7. Gather emergency equipment and place near client.
8. Determine whether premedication was ordered and given.
9. Obtain vital signs and document findings on procedural sedation record.
10. Start peripheral IV with ordered solution.
11. Determine gesture to be used for communication regarding pain and sedation.
12. Place ECG leads on, if appropriate.
13. Administer oxygen via nasal cannula at 2 L/min.
14. Monitor end-tidal CO_2 with capnography.
15. Begin administration of medication as ordered.
16. Monitor vital signs, oxygen saturation, sedation level, pain level, ECG rate, and rhythm every 1 to 5 minutes according to facility policy and client condition.
    ▸ ***Rationale:*** Close monitoring of these values identifies potential complication such as respiratory depression, oversedation, hypoxia, and hypotension.
17. Continue to monitor client every 15 minutes until stable after completion of procedure using conscious sedation.

TABLE 26-6 Levels of Sedation/Analgesia

Level	Description
Minimal (Anxiolysis)	Client is relaxed but able to respond to verbal commands. Cognitive function and coordination may be impaired; ventilatory and cardiovascular functions are not affected.
Moderate (Conscious Sedation)	Client is drowsy and may sleep throughout procedure, responds purposefully to verbal commands. Airway remains patent with spontaneous ventilation and cardiovascular status is maintained.
Deep	Client will sleep through procedure with little or no memory of the procedure. Airway intervention may be required (supplemental oxygen or ventilatory support); cardiovascular status is maintained.

Source: American Society of Anesthesiologists. http://www.asahq.org/publicationsandservices/standards/20pdf

TABLE 26-7 Moderate (Conscious) Sedation Medications

	Benzodiazepines	Opioids
Drugs	Midazolam (Versed), diazepam, lorazepam*	Fentanyl, morphine, meperidine
Action	Produce anxiolysis and amnesia	Produce sedation, euphoria, pain relief
Disadvantages	Lack of analgesic properties	Can cause respiratory depression and decreased level of consciousness
Side Effects	Decreased blood pressure Increased heart rate	Apnea, hypotension, vertigo, nausea
Reversal Agent	Flumazenil	Naloxone

Note: The most common drugs used for conscious sedation are the benzodiazepines and opioids.

*Frequently administered with narcotics.

Clinical Alert

The sedation assessment parameters that need to be observed during the procedure include responsiveness, speech, facial expressions, and eyes. Scales available that provide a scoring system are the Ramsay Sedation Scale and the Riker Sedation–Agitation Scale.

EVIDENCE-BASED PRACTICE

Over- and Under-Sedation

A survey of critical care nurses and physicians revealed they felt that their critically ill clients were receiving adequate sedation only 50% of the time. Interestingly enough, physicians felt their clients were over-sedated and nurses felt clients were under-sedated.

Source: McGaffigan, P. A. (2000, February). Advancing sedation assessment to promote patient comfort. *Critical Care Nurse Supplement*, 29–36.

Caring for Client After Moderate (Conscious) Sedation

Equipment

Electronic vital sign machine
Oxygen supply
Oxygen nasal cannula
Procedural sedation record
Aldrete scale
Pulse oximeter
ECG monitor and leads
Emergency equipment
Naloxone

Procedure

1. Check two forms of client ID and introduce yourself.
2. Observe vital signs, oxygen saturation, respiratory rate and rhythm, and ECG rate and rhythm every 15 minutes unless more frequent monitoring is required according to client condition. ▸ ***Rationale:*** Major complications during the use of conscious sedation and immediately after include respiratory depression, oversedation, hypoxia, and hypotension. Assess need for naloxone, an antagonist of the opioids, to reverse narcotic analgesic (rarely needed).
3. Observe client for patent airway if he or she was intubated during procedure and ensure oxygen cannula is in place immediately after extubation.
4. Assess client for pain and medicate accordingly.
5. Monitor client and obtain sedation scale score in preparation for discharge. Client must attain specified score within 1 hour of completion of procedure. ▸ ***Rationale:*** If using Aldrete Scale, client must attain Aldrete score of ±1 point of preprocedure score before discharge. This score should be achieved within 1 hour of the procedure. A potential complication is occurring if this score is not attained within the specified time.
6. Provide instructions as needed before client is discharged.
7. Ensure client has someone with him or her if discharged to home.
8. Complete documentation on Procedural Sedation Record.

DOCUMENTATION for Moderate (Conscious) Sedation

- Preprocedural assessment: past medical history, drug allergies, anesthetic history
- Consent form signed
- Baseline vital signs, particularly respiratory and cardiac findings, ECG findings
- Height and weight

- Teaching provided regarding medication and procedure
- ASA rating
- Continuous documentation of level of consciousness, speech, facial expression, agitation level, pupils, respiratory rate and rhythm, ECG findings if appropriate during procedure
- Score on a sedation scale (Aldrete, Ramsay, or Riker)
- Oxygen saturation levels during and after procedure
- Amount and type of medication administered
- Supplemental oxygen, liter flow, and system used
- Aldrete score before discharge
- Complications that occurred during the procedure and actions taken
- Complete Procedural Sedation Record

CRITICAL THINKING Application

Expected Outcomes

- Client maintains airway and respiratory status throughout procedure.
- Client does not experience anxiety or pain during procedure.

Unexpected Outcomes	Alternative Actions
Client is scheduled to have conscious sedation for procedure but scores above P2 on ASA scale.	• Notify anesthesiologist and physician; nurses may not administer conscious sedation if the client scores above P2 on the scale. • Client is physically compromised and could be unstable during use of conscious sedation medications.
Client does not respond to verbal commands during procedure when using minimal or moderate sedation.	• Notify physician of change in client's status. • Notify anesthesiologist immediately and prepare for intubation. • Have reversal drug available to administer if directed by physician. • Continue to monitor client every 1 minute for changes in status. • Administer oxygen via nasal cannula if not already in place.
Client experiences airway obstruction or respiratory depression.	• Reposition client's head, lifting jaw and tipping back the head. • Suction client or insert oral airway. • Be prepared to bag client with bag–valve–mask device.
Client experiences hypoxemia.	• Ensure pulse oximeter is on client. • Check respiratory rate, pattern, and effort. • Increase amount of oxygen delivered. May need to change delivery system to oxygen mask. • Use Capnography to evaluate CO_2 level.
Client experiences a 20% drop in blood pressure during procedure.	• Inform physician. • Assess client for potential complications leading to decrease in blood pressure. • Check for presence of hypovolemia. Administer 200 mL bolus of fluid and monitor for response.
Client experiences pain during procedure.	• Dosage of amnesia or analgesic agents needs to be reviewed. • Ensure client's weight was calculated correctly. • Allow sufficient time for agents to work. • Allow time to titrate effect of medication.

Chapter 26

UNIT 5

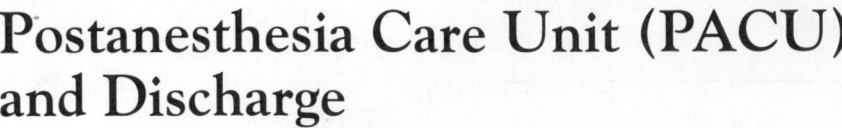

Postanesthesia Care Unit (PACU) and Discharge

Nursing Process Data

ASSESSMENT Data Base

- Assess for patent airway.
- Assess for order and type of oxygen administration set.
- Check gag reflex and remove endotracheal tube as ordered.
- Assess vital signs and appropriate pulses.
- Assess body temperature.
- Check all IVs for type, amount of fluid, and infusion rate.
- Observe all dressings, tubes, and drains.
- Monitor urine output, color, and consistency.
- Assess color, skin temperature, and condition.
- Assess monitor findings if ordered.
- Assess neurologic status if necessary.
- Assess heart and lung sounds.
- Assess bowel sounds.
- Assess residual anesthetic effect.
- Assess for postoperative bleeding.

PLANNING Objectives

- To provide safe, effective nursing care during the immediate postoperative period for clients in the recovery room
- To promote and maintain adequate airway function
- To monitor and maintain adequate circulatory status
- To identify potential postanesthesia complications and initiate nursing interventions to prevent complications
- To identify client's readiness to return to nursing unit or to be discharged if an outpatient
- To use "Hand Off" communication process when discharging client to surgical unit

IMPLEMENTATION Procedures

EVALUATION Expected Outcomes

- Client has an uneventful experience in the recovery period.
- Potential postoperative complications are identified early and corrective interventions prevent occurrence of complications.
- Client is discharged to home or nursing unit within prescribed time frame.
- Client reports pain: < 4 on a scale of 0–10.
- Client does not experience nausea or vomiting.

"Hand Off" Communication

- Report focuses on client safety.
- Report is coordinated effort among healthcare professionals involved in changeover of client.
- Communication must be accurate, clear, specific, and allow time for questions and concerns.
- Communication occurs in all areas of surgical care.

SBAR—Approach to "Hand Off" Communication

S - Situation—Identify yourself and the client. State what is happening with the client.

B - Background—Review chart. Provide the client's background. Anticipate other caregiver's questions.

A - Assessment—Provide your observations and evaluation of client's current state. Be accurate and complete.

R - Recommendations—Make informal suggestions based on correct information for continued care of client.

Source: Standardized Approach to Hand-Off Communications is part of National Patient Safety Goals from The Joint Commission.

Providing Postanesthesia Care

Equipment

Blood pressure cuff and stethoscope
Pulse oximeter
Oxygen administration device: nasal cannula or mask
Cardiac monitor and leads
IV pole
Suction catheters
Gloves
Special equipment needed—based on surgical procedure

Procedure

1. Check two forms of client ID, introduce yourself, and determine surgical procedure performed.
2. Complete Hand-Off Communication process.
3. Connect client to monitoring systems.
4. Assess for patent airway. Leave airway in place until gag reflex returns and client attempts to remove it. ▸ ***Rationale:*** This promotes adequate airway exchange and prevents tongue from falling back and occluding airway.
5. Administer humidified SpO_2 by mask or nasal cannula at 6 L/min or as ordered. ▸ ***Rationale:*** Humidified oxygen prevents drying of the tracheobronchial tree and liquifies secretions to facilitate expectoration.
6. Monitor oxygen saturation using pulse oximetry (SpO_2).
7. Monitor carbon dioxide levels in client's expiration, using capnography.
8. Encourage client to cough and deep breathe when awake.
9. Suction client as needed.
10. Position client to ensure adequate ventilation. Side-lying position is best if not contraindicated. Turn every hour if not contraindicated. ▸ ***Rationale:*** This prevents pooling of secretions in lungs and assists with ventilation.
11. Monitor vital signs every 5–15 minutes as condition warrants. Vital signs are sometimes difficult to obtain due to hypothermia and movement from operating room to postanesthesia care unit.
    a. Check pulse rate, quality, and rhythm; include pulse distal to surgical site.
    b. Check blood pressure, pulse pressure, and quality.
    c. Check respiratory rate, rhythm, depth, and pattern.
    d. Assess pain level, determine cause, and medicate as needed.

Clinical Alert

- Ineffective communication is the most frequently cited root cause of sentinel events.
- Adverse events occur more often for surgical clients than clients in other clinical specialties.

12. Maintain body temperature by applying warm blankets or use Bair Paws Warming System. ▸ ***Rationale:*** Operating rooms are cold, which promotes vasoconstriction and increases risk of infection.
13. Observe for adverse signs of general or spinal anesthesia:
    a. Level of consciousness.
    b. Movement of extremities.

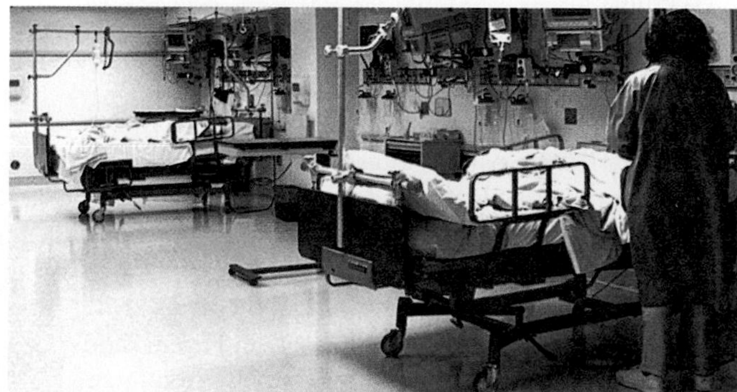

▲ Recovery room is usually an open space for easy observation of all clients.

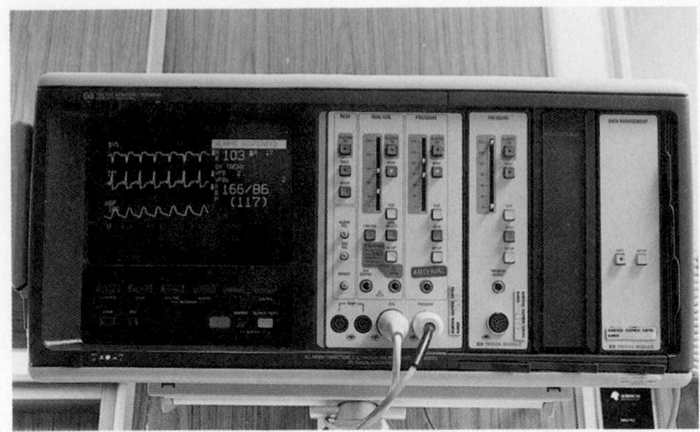

▲ Clients are connected to monitoring system for cardiac surveillance.

14. Monitor IV fluids.
    a. Verify correct type and amount of solution being administered.
    b. Set appropriate flow rate using IV pump or controller if needed.
    c. Observe IV site for signs of infiltration.
    d. Maintain accurate IV intake record.
15. Monitor blood or blood component infusions.
    a. Identify appropriate replacement fluid.
    b. Check client's name and identification number with fluid.
    c. Check blood type, blood bank number, and expiration date.
    d. Check time infusion initiated.
    e. Observe and record amount of fluid remaining in bag when admitted to recovery room.
    f. Determine time frame for completion of fluid.
16. Monitor and measure urine output hourly if indwelling catheter is in place or before client leaves recovery room.
17. Observe surgical dressings and drains hourly.
    a. Follow hospital policy for marking drainage on dressings.
    b. Note color and amount of drainage on dressings and from drains or tubes.
    c. Check that dressings are secure.
    d. Reinforce dressings as needed.
    e. Empty drainage collection device as needed.
    f. Report unusual amount or type of drainage to physician before client leaves recovery room.
18. Monitor skin for warmth, color, and moisture.
19. Check nail beds and mucous membranes for color and blanching. Report unusual findings or signs of cyanosis to physician immediately.
20. Orient client to surroundings and relieve anxiety and fear.
21. Observe for return of movement, especially if client received spinal or epidural anesthesia.
22. Monitor for muscle strength/movement.
23. Administer all STAT drugs.
24. Provide pain medication as needed.
25. Complete PAR record.
26. Assess parameters for discharge from postanesthesia room.

Discharging Client From Postanesthesia Unit to Nursing Unit

Procedure

1. Assess that lung sounds are clear to auscultation and airway is maintained without artificial measures (unless client is to remain on mechanical assistance).
2. Assess that vital signs are within normal range for at least 1 hr and appropriate for client's condition.
3. Observe that client is awake, alert, and responds to commands.
4. Assess that reflexes are present (including gag, swallowing) and that client can move all extremities.
5. Assess skin color and nail beds for signs of cyanosis.
6. Ensure IVs are patent, infusing with correct solution and at prescribed rate. Record total amount of IV fluid infused and amount remaining in bags. Ensure all IVs and irrigating solutions are in sufficient quantity for transfer and immediate continuity of care.
7. Check that all dressings are intact, and there is no excessive drainage from drains or tubes. Reinforce dressings if needed and empty all drainage collection receptacles before returning to nursing unit.
8. Ensure urinary output is adequate. Record all urine output and empty drainage bag before transporting to nursing unit.
9. Record all medications administered in recovery room.
10. Medicate client one half hour before transport if vital signs are stable and client requires pain medication. ▸ ***Rationale:*** Transporting clients from postanesthesia room can increase pain due to moving and transfer from gurney to bed.
11. Call anesthesiologist for discharge orders or use Aldrete Postanesthesia Recovery Scoring System if used by facility.
12. Call for transport assistance if available. Postanesthesia room nurse accompanies client to nursing unit.
13. Call nursing unit and provide information on equipment needs for client (e.g., oxygen, IVs).
14. Document all findings in computer or in chart before discharge.
15. Prepare data for "Hand Off" communication with Surgical floor RN.

Data to Include In "Hand Off" Communication Process (SBAR)

- Situation.
  1. Client's name and date of birth.
  2. Procedure completed with site identified.
- Background.
  1. Type of anesthesia and name of anesthesia care provider.
  2. Intraoperative PACU medications; dose and time.
  3. IV fluids administered in OR and PACU.
  4. Estimated blood loss.
  5. Data regarding dressings, tubes, drains, or packing.
  6. Significant OR events and PACU events.
- Assessment.
  1. Hemodynamic stability.
  2. Airway and oxygenation status.
  3. Temperature.
  4. Urine output.
  5. Surgical complications if present.
  6. Pain level.
  7. Type of pain management.
- Recommendations.
  1. Ensure PACU MD orders were completed.
  2. Surgeon's plan of care has been implemented.
  3. Identify educational needs for client and family.
  4. Provide discharge instructions.
  5. Discharge within 2 hr or when stable.

Source: Amato-Vealey, E. J., Barba, M. P., & Vealey, R. J. (2008, November). Hand-off communication: A requisite for perioperative patient safety. *AORN Journal*, 88(5), 763–770. http://www.aorn-greaterhouston.org/files/Nov_08_handoff.pdf.

TABLE 26-8 Aldrete Postanesthesia Recovery Scoring System

Activity
2 = moves all four extremities voluntarily or on command
1 = moves two extremities voluntarily or on command
0 = unable to move any extremity voluntarily or on command
Respiration
2 = able to breathe, cough freely
1 = requires assistance, shallow or limited breathing
0 = apneic
Circulation
2 = BP+20 mmHg of preanesthetic level
1 = BP+20 to +50 mmHg of preanesthetic level
0 = BP+50 mmHg of preanesthetic level
Consciousness
2 = fully awake
1 = arousable on calling
0 = not responding
Oxygen saturation
2 = SpO_2 >92% on room air
1 = Supplemental O_2 required to maintain SpO_2 >90%
0 = SpO_2 supplementation
10 = Total score >9 for PACU discharge

This is one method for determining whether postanesthesia room discharge criteria have been met. In addition to stable vital signs, a total score of 10 for the five assessed areas must be achieved for nurses to discharge clients without a physician's order.

Discharging Client From Phase II Unit to Home

Procedure

1. Follow all actions for Discharging a Client From Postanesthesia Unit to Nursing Unit.
2. Assess for nausea or light-headedness. ▸ ***Rationale:*** These symptoms may be a result of anesthesia or hypovolemia. The client is not discharged until these symptoms have abated or are medically treated.
3. Provide discharge teaching regarding medications, activity, dressing changes, physician office visit, etc. If client is unable to understand instructions, provide information to person taking client home. Send written instructions home with client as well.
4. Assist client to side of bed, feet on floor, and allow to sit for a few minutes. ▸ ***Rationale:*** To prevent a fall when standing as a result of postural hypotension.
5. Assess client's ability to dress self or identify what assistance is needed.
6. Ensure client has urinated, ambulated to bathroom, and is not vomiting before discharge.
7. Obtain prescriptions from pharmacy if needed.
8. Place client's equipment, supplies, and medications in a plastic bag and hand to person taking client home.
9. Transfer client to wheelchair.
10. Take client to car and assist with transfer.
11. Document all activity related to discharge, including person taking client home and method of transport.

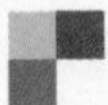

DOCUMENTATION for Postanesthesia Care

For Nursing Unit

- Assessment findings—follow SBAR
- Effects of anesthesia
- Status of airway management
- Need for oxygen administration
- Status of neurologic signs and reflexes
- Fluid replacement—type and amount
- Blood and blood product replacement
- Medications administered
- Condition of dressings, drains, and tubes
- Intake and output from all sources: urine, drains, tubes, IVs
- Vital signs: T, P, R, BP, and pain
- Description of pain and interventions for relief of pain
- Response to postanesthesia room activities
- Discharged to room (number) and transporter
- "Hand Off" Communication Data

For Discharge Home

- Additional charting includes ability to stand or transfer to wheelchair and having urinated
- Discharge teaching completed
- Signs or symptoms of nausea, light-headedness
- Discharged to care at home
- Discharged via automobile or other means of transportation.

Legal Alert

Operating Room Negligence

The nurse's responsibility is to accurately count and monitor the sponge count and equipment. A common litigation against operating room nurses involves sponges or instruments left in a client after a surgical procedure.

After a hysterectomy, three different sponge counts were completed (before, during, and after the procedure) and confirmed by the nurse. Two years later, when the client had a second surgery for bowel obstruction, a sponge was found in the site. A suit was filed against the physician and the hospital (which included the nurse) for negligent acts by the nurse who had made an inaccurate sponge count. Both were found negligent by the jury.

Source: Truhitte v. French Hospital (1982).

CRITICAL THINKING Application

Expected Outcomes

- Client experiences no untoward effects during recovery period.
- Potential postanesthesia complications are identified early, and appropriate nursing actions are taken to prevent occurrence of complications.
- Client is discharged from postanesthesia unit at appropriate time.

Unexpected Outcomes	Alternative Actions
Client experiences untoward effects in postanesthesia room.	• Contact physician for additional orders. • Complete physical assessment. • Identify and initiate appropriate nursing interventions within allowed guidelines and parameters of the facility.
Client does not awaken easily.	• Retain client in postanesthesia room; check Glasgow scale. • Continue to provide oxygen. • Arouse every 15 minutes. • Check pain medication (may need Narcan).
Client has postoperative hemorrhage.	• Apply direct pressure. • Notify physician immediately. • Assess for signs of hypovolemia. • Assess for signs of overt bleeding (i.e., saturated dressings, large amount of drainage in drainage collection devices, increase in girth of affected surgical area). • Check lab values for hematocrit, hemoglobin, and coagulation levels. • Check records for estimated blood loss during surgery.

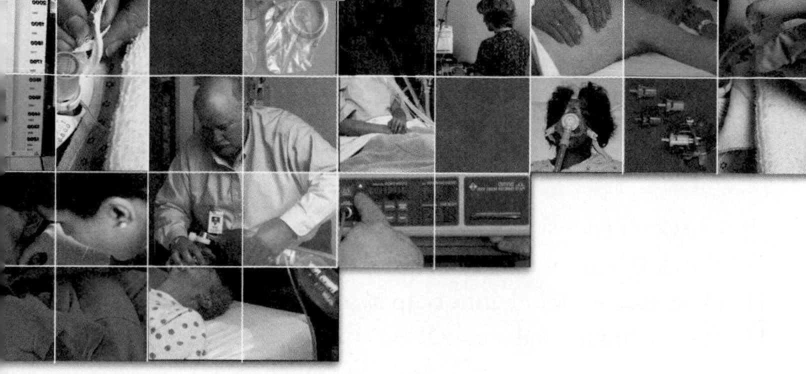

Chapter 26

UNIT 6

Postoperative Care

Nursing Process Data

ASSESSMENT Data Base

- Assess for patent airway.
- Check if oxygen is ordered.
- Auscultate lungs.
- Observe for adverse signs of general anesthesia or spinal anesthesia.
- Take vital signs (T, P, R, BP, and pain).
- Check client's temperature for heat control.
- Observe dressings and surgical drains.
- Check IVs for type and amount of fluid to be infused.
- Observe color and amount of urine.
- Auscultate bowel sounds and verify bowel movement and flatus.
- Observe client's overall condition.

PLANNING Objectives

- To ensure that the client experiences an uneventful postoperative course
- To provide safe, effective nursing care in the immediate postoperative period
- To ensure that postoperative pain is relieved promptly
- To be aware of the common postoperative drugs for pain control

IMPLEMENTATION Procedures

EVALUATION Expected Outcomes

- Client experiences an uneventful postoperative course.
- Postoperative nursing interventions are carried out effectively and in a timely manner.
- Client reports pain levels: <4 on scale of 0–10.
- Client is free of nausea and vomiting.

Providing Postoperative Care

Equipment

Absorbent pads
Warm blankets or Bair Paws Warming System
IV pole
Oxygen source, tubing, and equipment
Emesis basin and tissues
Sphygmomanometer and stethoscope
Thermometer (tympanic, oral, or rectal)
Nurses' notes
Intake and output record
Special equipment depending on type of surgery
Pulse oximeter
Sterile dressings

Procedure

1. Perform hand hygiene before each client contact.
2. Check two forms of client ID and introduce self to client.
3. Orient client to time, person, and place. Reorient as needed.
4. Assess for patent airway and level of consciousness; administer oxygen if ordered. Attach pulse oximeter if ordered.
5. Assess for effects of anesthesia including general, regional, or local.
6. Take vital signs, including pain assessment: usual orders are every 15 minutes until stable; then every half hour for 2 hr; every hour for 4 hr; then every 4 hr for 24–48 hr, or according to hospital policy.
7. Check pulse oximetry every hour for 4 hr, then every 4 hr. ▸ ***Rationale:*** To detect early signs of hypoxemia.
8. Check ETCO2 using capnography monitoring, if available.

COMMUNITY HOSPITAL

PAR Record

ADMITTED TO PAR AM PM | AWAKE ON ARRIVAL ☐ | TIME AWAKE AM PM | RELEASED AM PM | OPERATION

APPARENT CONDITION ON ARRIVAL: GOOD FAIR POOR | APPARENT CONDITION ON RELEASE: GOOD FAIR POOR | SURGEON

ALLERGIES: | ANESTHEOLOGIST

INTAKE
ADMITTED TO PAR WITH: | RELEASED FROM PAR WITH: | ANESTHESIA: GENERAL REGIONAL SPINAL CAUDAL
IV | IV | OXYGEN: NASAL MASK TRACHAEL TENT
AIRWAY: ORAL NASAL TRACHEAL
BLOOD | BLOOD | MONITORING:
TOTAL IV FLUIDS OR | TOTAL BLOOD OR | TIME: ON OFF
TOTAL IV FLUIDS PAR | TOTAL BLOOD PAR | EKG

OUTPUT
TOTAL FLUID LOSS OR | PAR: | CVP
EBL: | ART
URINE: | VENTILATOR
DRAINAGE:
NG: | OTHER:
HEMOVAC:
CHEST:

ALDRETE SCORING CRITERIA	Post Anesthetic Recovery Score		TIME	ADM	15'	30'	45'	1'	15'	30'	45'	2'	15'	30'
	ACTIVITY	Able to move 4 extremities voluntarily or on command	2											
		Able to move 2 extremities voluntarily or on command	1											
		Able to move 0 extremities voluntarily or on command	0											
	RESPIRATION	Able to breathe deeply and cough freely	2											
		Dyspnea or limited breathing	1											
		Apneic (needs ventilator or assistance)	0											
	CIRCULATION	BP ± 20% of pre-anesthetic level	2											
		BP ± 20–49% of pre-anesthetic level	1											
		BP ± 50% of pre-anesthetic level	0											
	CONSCIOUSNESS	Fully awake	2											
		Arousable on calling	1											
		Not responding	0											
	O2 SATURATION	Able to maintain O_2 saturation > 92% on room air	2											
		Needs O_2 inhalation to maintain O_2 saturation > 90%	1											
		O_2 saturation < 90% even with O_2 supplement	0											
			TOTAL SCORE											

▲ PAR record.

9. Check for nausea and vomiting.
10. Check IV site and patency frequently.
11. Observe, and record urine output, amount, and color.
12. Measure intake and output.
13. Observe skin color and moisture and nail beds. ▸ ***Rationale:*** To determine adequacy of tissue perfusion.
14. Position client for comfort and maximum airway ventilation according to orders.
15. Turn every 2 hr and PRN.
16. Give back care at least every 4 hr.
17. Encourage coughing and deep breathing every 2 hr (may use spirometer or Tri-flow if ordered).
18. Keep client comfortable with medications.
19. Monitor for side effects of medications.
20. Check dressings and drainage tubes every 2–4 hr; if abnormal amount of drainage, check more frequently. Empty drainage system when needed
21. Assess for signs and symptoms of Surgical Site infections (SSIs).
    a. Superficial incisional:
       - Purulent drainage with or without elevated white blood cell count
       - Pain or tenderness at the site
       - Localized swelling, heat, or redness
       - Positive wound culture
    b. Deep incisional:
       - Purulent drainage
       - Temperature above 100.4°F (38°C)
       - Leukocytosis
       - Localized pain or tenderness
    c. Organ/space:
       - Purulent drainage from a drain placed in an organ or space
       - Positive culture from fluid or tissue in the organ or space

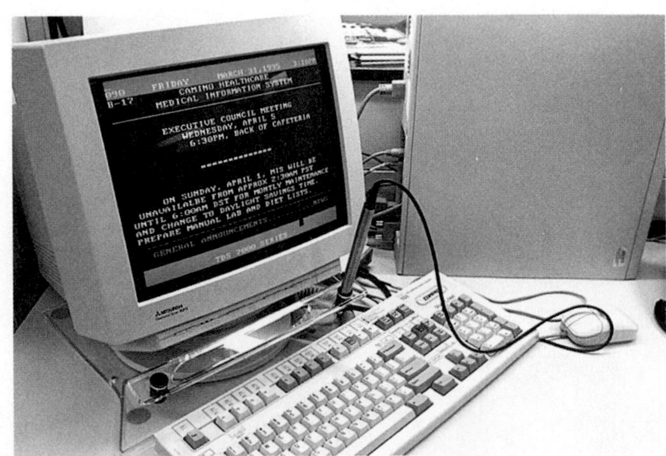

▲ Recovery room documentation is accomplished using computerized system.

- Temperature above 100.4°F
- Leukocytosis
- Pain
- Abscess formation or other evidence of infection in the organ or space

NOTE: See Wound Care, *Chapter 25*, for further information.

22. Provide oral hygiene at least every 4 hr; if nasogastric tube or nasal oxygen is inserted, give oral hygiene every 2 hr. ▶ ***Rationale:*** To decrease risk of infection from presence of oral bacteria.
23. Bathe client when temperature can be maintained. ▶ ***Rationale:*** Bathing removes the antiseptic solution and stimulates circulation.
24. Keep client warm and avoid chilling, but do not increase temperature above normal. Use of Bair Paws Warming System allows client to maintain warmth and provides comfort. (See Chapter 24.) ▶ ***Rationale:*** Increased temperature increases metabolic rate and need for oxygen. Excessive perspiration causes fluid and electrolyte loss.
25. Irrigate nasogastric tube every 4 hr and PRN, as ordered, with normal saline to keep patent and to prevent electrolyte imbalance.
26. Maintain dietary intake: type of diet depends on type and extent of surgical procedure.
    a. Minor surgical conditions: Client may drink or eat as soon as he or she is awake, desires food or drink, and has gag reflex present.
    b. Major surgical conditions: NPO until bowel sounds return. Clear liquid advanced to full diet as tolerated.

Use of Spirometry for High-Risk Clients After Coronary Artery Bypass Surgery

A study was conducted to determine whether the addition of incentive spirometry to postoperative pulmonary physical therapy is more effective than physical therapy alone in reducing postoperative pulmonary complications in high-risk clients after coronary artery bypass grafting. One group received pulmonary physical therapy combined with the spirometry and the other did not receive the spirometry. The results indicated that no difference was found between the two groups in atelectasis, oxygen saturation, or pulmonary infection. Use of the spirometer was not monitored; therefore, the effectiveness of the spirometer could not be fully evaluated.

Source: Crowe, I.M. (1997). Physical Therapy, 77(3), 260–268.

Conditions That Place Clients at Risk for Postoperative Infection

- Uncontrolled diabetes
- Renal failure
- Obesity; advanced age
- Receiving corticosteroids
- Receiving immunosuppressive agents or are immunosuppressed
- Prolonged antibiotic therapy
- Protein or ascorbic acid deficiencies
- Marked dehydration and hypovolemia
- Decreased cardiac output
- Edema and fluid and electrolyte imbalances
- Anemia
- Preoperative infection

27. Place client on bedpan 2–4 hr postoperatively if catheter not inserted.
28. Check physician's orders when to begin the client's postoperative activity. Most clients are ambulated within first 24 hr.
29. Observe for signs and symptoms of possible postoperative complications, particularly postoperative bleeding and infection.
30. Dangle or position client in chair as ordered.

Surgical Site Infections

Prevention

- Appropriate use of prophylactic antibiotics
- Appropriate hair removal
- Maintenance of perioperative glucose control
- Maintenance of perioperative normothermia

Bacterial Causes of SSIs

Common battery

- *Staphylococcus*
- *Enterococcus*
- *Pseudomonas*
- *Streptococcus*

Newer causes (due to antibiotic resistance)

- *Escherichia coli*
- Methicillin-resistance *staphylococcus aureus*
- *Candida*

Administering Postoperative Medications*

Equipment

Medication as ordered

Appropriate syringe and needle for parenteral medications

*See Chapter 16, Pain Management, for PCA and epidural.

Procedure

1. Check two forms of client ID and introduce self to client.

TABLE 26-9 Postoperative Complications

Potential Complication	Clients at Risk	Indicative Findings	Prevention	Intervention	Drug Therapy
Atelectasis: Collapse of alveoli; may be diffuse and involve a segment, lobe, or entire lung *Potential Onset:* First 48 hours	All with general anesthesia *Special risk clients:* Smokers Chronic bronchitis Emphysema Obesity Elderly Upper abdominal surgery Chest surgery Abdominal distention	Fever to 102°F Tachycardia Restlessness Tachypnea 24–30 minutes Altered breath sounds Dullness to percussion Diminished or absent breath sounds Crackles ABGs: decreased PaO_2	*Preoperative:* Have client practice turning, coughing, and deep breathing Discuss importance of exercises *Postoperative clients at risk:* Turn every 30 minutes Deep breathe and cough *Other clients:* Initiate turning and deep breathing exercises every 1–2 hr Ambulate as soon as possible Medicate to reduce pain, splinting, and resistance to treatment	Deep breathing and incentive spirometry Administer supplemental oxygen as ordered Monitor response to treatment Monitor for onset of pneumonia If entire lobe of lung is involved, prepare for bronchoscopy to remove plug Change position every 2 hr	Analgesics: pain control Bronchodilators (nebulized through IPPB); liquefy secretions Water or saline (nebulized through IPPB); liquefy secretions
Pneumonia: Inflammatory process in which alveoli are filled with exudate *Potential onset:* First 36–48 hr	Clients with unresolved atelectasis Following aspiration Smokers Elderly Chronic bronchitis Emphysema Heart failure Debilitated Alcoholic Immobile Cough suppressant medications Respiratory depressant medications	Client complains of dyspnea, tachycardia, increasing temperature, productive cough, and increasing amount of sputum becoming tenacious, rusty, or purulent Tactile fremitus Dullness to percussion Bronchial breath sounds Increased crackles or rhonchi Voice sounds present ABGs: decreased PaO_2	Provide vigorous treatment of atelectasis Prevent aspiration Ambulate as soon as possible	Turn, cough, and deep breathe every 1 hr May need to stimulate cough with nasotracheal suctioning Send sputum for culture and sensitivity Frequent mouth care for comfort Administer oxygen as ordered Increase fluid intake Monitor for response to treatment	Antibiotics: Cephalosporin or ampicillin prophylactically for 48 hr for high-risk clients Cephalosporin IV or parenteral for infections Antipyretics: decrease temperature
Pulmonary embolism: Foreign object has migrated to branch of pulmonary artery *Potential onset:* Seventh to tenth day	Superficial vein thrombosis: rare Deep vein thrombosis: 40% to 60% Air emboli: intraperitoneal surgery Fat emboli: long bone fracture, split sternum	Only 10% recognized clinically Pain sharp and stabbing, occurs with breathing, localized (right lower lobe most frequent) Marked shortness of breath Increased heart rate—tachycardia Restlessness and other symptoms of hypoxia (severe anxiety)	Provide range of motion Encourage early ambulation Prevent thrombophlebitis Do not massage an area with potential for or suspected thrombus Elastic stockings or leg compression devices	Administer oxygen to relieve hypoxia Reduce anxiety Position client on left side with head dependent to prevent air embolus Prevent recurrent embolization; prepare for fibrinolysis; prepare for anticoagulation	Anticoagulation therapy: IV heparin to maintain therapeutic APTT Sodium prophylactically for high-risk clients Urokinase, t-PA, streptokinase: thrombolytic effect (24 hr) Analgesics: pleuritic pain control Prepare for x-ray or scan Adequate hydration

Thrombophlebitis: Inflammation of vein with clot formation *Potential onset:* Seventh to fourteenth day	*Abnormal vein walls:* Varicose veins Previous thrombophlebitis Trauma to vein wall Tight strap on operating room table Surgery on hips or in pelvis Age over 60 years (arteriosclerosis) *Venous stasis:* Immobility, long duration surgery Casts, restrictive dressings Constant Fowler's position Prolonged dependent lower extremities Knee gatch elevated Pillows under knees, calves Obesity Abdominal distention Shock Heart failure *Hypercoagulability:* Surgical stress response Anesthesia Decreased circulation Hypovolemia, dehydration Malignant neoplasms Postpartum Oral contraceptives Insert rectal tube	*Superficial vein thrombophlebitis:* Pain, redness, tenderness, and induration along course of vein Palpable "cord" corresponding to course of vein History of trauma including IV site *Deep small vein thrombophlebitis:* Increased muscle turgor and tenderness over affected vein Deep muscle tenderness Most frequent site: vessels at call Affected limb warm to touch with occasional swelling Client complains of tightness or stiffness in affected leg Positive Homan's sign (dorsiflexion of foot leads to calf pain) Fever rarely more than 101°F *Major deep vein thrombophlebitis:* No superficial signs of inflammation Homan's sign unreliable *Femoral vein thrombosis:* Pain and tenderness in distal thigh and popliteal region Swelling extends to level of knee	*Avoid injury to vein wall:* Use care when strapping to operating room table Avoid IVs in lower extremities Pad siderails for restless, convulsive, and/or combative client Avoid restraints *Avoid venous stasis:* Encourage early ambulation Provide feet and leg exercises Elastic stockings; sequential-compression devices Increase frequency of exercise for client at risk Prevent client's sitting with legs in dependent position Place pillow between legs while client is lying on side to prevent pressure from upper leg on lower Provide deep breathing exercises Provide range of motion Increase velocity of blood flow: No standing Steady IV flow Antiembolic stockings (controversial) Decrease hypercoagulability: Provide adequate hydration Prevent infections Maintain circulation Decrease stress/anxiety	*Superficial vein thrombophlebitis:* Treat symptoms Continue ambulation unless accompanied by deep venous involvement Monitor for progression toward saphenofemoral junction (may need ligation) *Deep vein thrombophlebitis:* Provide adequate bedrest Elastic stockings Sequential-compression devices Elevate foot of bed with 6–8-in. blocks Administer warm moist compresses to relieve venospasm and help resolve inflammation Monitor for pulmonary embolism	Streptokinase: thrombolytic effect (24 hr) Heparin IV or subcutaneous: decrease clotting time (short-term) Nonorthopedic surgery—low-dose subcutaneous heparin (or low molecular-weight heparin) Coumadin PO: decrease clotting time (long term) Analgesics: pain control Low-molecular-weight dextran IV on operative day and 2 days postoperative Aspirin 1.2 g/day in divided doses
Ileus: Failure of peristalsis *Potential onset:* First 24–36 hr	All surgical clients Stress response to surgical trauma	No bowel sounds or fewer than 5/min (normal; 5–35 clicks or gurgles/min) Vomiting Abdominal distention	Do not feed until bowel sounds return Offer only sips of water until return of bowel sounds Maintain normal serum potassium level	Monitor for return of normal bowel sounds (enteral feeding following non-GI surgeries will resolve ileus faster) Monitor for distention Monitor for passage of flatus signaling return of peristalsis Monitor signs of hypokalemia	Switch to nonopioid analgesic (opioids slow GI motility), NSAIDs, and acetaminophen

Continued

TABLE 26-9 Postoperative Complications (*Continued*)

Potential Complication	Clients at Risk	Indicative Findings	Prevention	Intervention	Drug Therapy
Paralytic ileus: Paralysis of intestinal peristalsis *Potential onset:* First 3–4 days	Intraperitoneal surgery Peritonitis Kidney surgery Decreased cardiac output Pneumonia Electrolyte imbalance Wound infection	No bowel sounds Abdominal distention No passage of flatus or feces Nasogastric drainage green to yellow, 1–2 L in 24 hr Anorexia, nausea Complaints of fullness and diffuse pain	Maintain electrolyte balance, especially potassium Maintain cardiac output Prevent pneumonia Provide early ambulation	Treat cause Maintain nasogastric suction until peristalsis returns Monitor for intestinal obstruction	Potassium chloride if serum level is low Dexpanthenol (Ilopan) to stimulate return of peristalsis total parenteral nutrition (TPN) if indicated
Urinary tract infection *Potential onset*: Third to fifth day or 48 hr after removal of catheter	*Decreased resistance*: History of bladder distention History of urinary retention Previous urinary tract infection History of prostatic hypertrophy History of catheterization Diabetic Debilitated Immobile	Dysuria Frequency Urgency High fever: up to 104°F with fewer systemic toxic symptoms than would be expected Change in urine odor Pus in urine Sediment May be asymptomatic	Maintain sterile technique with catheterization and catheter removal Provide competent indwelling catheter care Encourage early ambulation to decrease retention and stasis	Encourage fluid intake; cranberry juice to decrease urine pH Increase activity to enhance bladder emptying Encourage voiding every 2 hr while awake Send specimen for culture and sensitivity Monitor for residual urine of more than 100 mL	Urinary antiseptics (sulfonamicles); bacterial suppression Antibiotics (ampicillin, tetracycline); bacterial suppression Anticholinergics; antispasmodic Topical urinary analgesic; pain relief
Wound infection *Potential onset* Streptococcal: 24–48 hr after contamination *Staphylococcus* gram-negative rods, etc.: 5–7 days postoperatively	*Slow to heal:* Obese Diabetic *Poor nutrition:* Debilitated Elderly Ulcerative colitis *Poor circulation*: Elderly Hypovolemic Heart failure *Lack of oxygen to wound:* Vasoconstriction Severe anemia Depressed immunity Cancer Renal failure Preoperative steroid therapy Prolonged complex surgery (stress response leading to increased ACTH) Malnutrition Elderly *At risk for transmission* Proximity of another client with infection Transmission by hands of personnel	Initial inflammation: 36–48 hr Wound tender, swollen, warm, increased redness Increasing heart rate Increasing temperature (100.4°F or more) Increasing or recurring serous drainage; drainage becomes purulent, foul odor There may be no local signs if infection is deep Elevated WBC Malaise	Practice meticulous hand hygiene and gloving Practice aseptic technique in wound care Separate from infected clients Use special caution for a new wound, easily contaminated Maintain nutrition Provide frequent turning Ambulate as soon as possible Maintain PaO_2 Increase attention to prevention for clients with depressed immunity Operative site: clip excess hair and cleanse with chlorhexidine (reduces bacterial counts)	Maintain nutrition Maintain oxygenation Maintain circulation and blood volume Maintain pulmonary toilet Cleanse wound or irrigate as ordered Apply wet-to-moist dressings Monitor for systemic response to infection, fever, malaise, headache, anorexia, nausea Treat symptoms	Administer antibiotics as ordered New cyanoacrylate adhesives (Dermabond, Indermil) close wounds and promote healing Send wound drainage specimen for culture and sensitivity

Source: Smith, S. F. (2009). *Sandra Smith's review for NCLEX-RN* (12th ed.). Sudbury, MA: Jones and Bartlett.

2. Evaluate client's need for pain relief.
3. Provide nonmedication measures for relief of pain, such as relaxation techniques, back care, positioning.
4. Identify the pharmacologic action of the ordered medication.
5. Review the general side effects of the medication.
   a. Drowsiness
   b. Euphoria
   c. Sleep
   d. Respiratory depression
   e. Nausea and vomiting
6. Administer medications as ordered, usually at 3- to 4-hr intervals for first 24–48 hr for better action and pain relief. Assess for pain relief.
7. Instruct in use of PCA pump, if ordered.
8. Know the action of the following drugs:
   a. Opiates.
   b. Synthetic opiate-like drugs.
   c. Nonnarcotic pain relievers.
   d. Narcotic antagonists.
   e. Antiemetics.

DOCUMENTATION for Postoperative Care

- Postoperative nursing interventions
- Fluid replacement—type and amount of solution
- Condition of dressings and drains
- Urine output, fluid intake
- Orientation to place, person, time
- Vital signs
- Signs and symptoms of potential complications
- Preventive nursing measures
- Client's activity level
- Clinical manifestations indicating pain
- Type, time, and amount of pain medication administered
- Site of injection
- Any side effects of medications observed
- Effectiveness of pain medication

CRITICAL THINKING Application

Expected Outcomes

- Client has an uneventful experience in the recovery period.
- Potential postoperative complications are identified early and corrective interventions prevent occurrence of complications.
- Client is discharged to home or nursing unit within prescribed time frame.
- Client reports pain: < 4 on scale of 1–10.
- Client does not experience nausea or vomiting.

Unexpected Outcomes	Alternative Actions
Client develops abnormal breath sounds.	• Increase deep breathing and coughing exercises to every 2 hr. • Medicate for pain before coughing or ambulating. • Encourage use of incentive spirometer. • Turn every 1–2 hr and ambulate if allowed. • Place client in Fowler's position to expand lungs. • Increase fluid intake to liquify secretions if not contraindicated. • Obtain physician's order for nebulizer treatments if indicated.
Bowel sounds are absent.	• Do not give ice chips or fluids; keep on NPO status until discussed with physician. • Notify physician if client is experiencing nausea and vomiting or if abdomen is distended and bowel sounds remain absent. It may be necessary to insert an NG tube. • Auscultate bowel sounds every 4 hr. • Encourage frequent turning and ambulation, if allowed.

Deep vein thrombosis (DVT) occurs.	• Place on bedrest. • Remove antiembolic stockings or compression devices on affected leg. • Check for calf pain, discoloration, or Homan's sign. • Do not massage legs. • Monitor clotting times and titrate anticoagulants if using heparin, according to physician's orders. • Measure circumference of both legs each shift to determine effectiveness of treatment. • Encourage leg exercises on unaffected leg.
Temperature increases.	• Day of surgery—check for dehydration. • Days 1 and 2—check breath sounds for potential atelectasis. • Fever in first 24 hr is most commonly from atelectasis. • Days 2—check for urinary tract infection. • Days 3–10—check for possible wound infection or pneumonia. • Check breath sounds for adventitious sounds or diminished breath sounds. • Increase fluids if not contraindicated. • Monitor temperature frequently until it returns to normal.
Blood pressure decreases; pulse and respirations increase.	• Check for IV access. • Check skin turgor and urine output and hypovolemia. • Observe dressings and drains for signs of bleeding. • Check intake and output values to determine hydration status.
Urinary retention occurs.	• Check bladder using bladder scanner. • Assist to commode or bathroom if possible. • Increase fluid intake if appropriate. • Review I&O record to determine findings. • Assess for signs and symptoms of dehydration. • Obtain order for catheter if necessary.

GERONTOLOGIC Considerations

Statistics for elderly clients requiring surgery are important to consider when providing care.

- Fifty percent of clients over 60 years of age require surgery before they die.
- Forty percent of elderly clients admitted to hospitals undergo a surgical procedure before discharge.
- The most common surgical procedures for elderly clients involve tissue biopsy and pacemaker insertion. Fractures comprise a large percentage of surgical interventions, particularly hip fractures.

Elderly clients are more prone to fluid and electrolyte imbalance.

- Dehydration is the most common cause of fluid and electrolyte imbalance.
- Check IV fluid type and amount to ensure adequate hydration.
- Elderly clients require 1.5–2.5 L of fluid every 24 hr.
- Monitor intake and output carefully to ensure adequate hydration.
- Monitor neurologic status for possible electrolyte imbalance.
- Fluid loss occurs with nasogastric tube placement and preop bowel preparation; clients requiring either of these interventions should be observed for dehydration.
- Evaluate electrolyte lab values for abnormal levels. (Hyperkalemia is common as a response to age-related alterations in the renin–aldosterone system.)

Elderly clients are at risk for complications associated with immobility after surgical interventions.

- Turn client frequently, at least every 2 hr.
- Ambulate as soon as possible postoperatively.
- Evaluate skin for early signs of breakdown (nonblanching erythema).
- Encourage deep breathing and coughing exercises every 1–2 hr. Instruct in use of incentive spirometer if ordered.
- Encourage leg exercises every hour when awake.

Preoperative teaching should be individualized, keeping in mind the following:

- Elderly clients may have chronic conditions that make movement difficult, altering preventative measures such as turning.
- Clients may have visual or auditory alterations requiring a quiet environment for teaching.
- Larger print or brochures with photos and large print should be used when teaching elderly clients.

Chronic conditions may alter normal vital signs, which may be misinterpreted during the perioperative phases.

- Document abnormalities in vital signs on client care plan so that all healthcare workers are alerted to client's usual values. Blood pressure and pulse alterations can be different for this age group.
- Monitor peripheral pulses to ensure adequate circulation.

Altered physiologic states need to be communicated to all healthcare workers.

- Document if client has an artificial eye or other prosthesis.
- Document client's visual or auditory alterations. If hearing aid is necessary for client to hear, indicate clearly on care plan.
- Identify if client has any condition that can interfere with postoperative care.

Elderly clients may not be candidates for conscious sedation.

- Many elderly clients have an ASA reading above 3. This would be considered a contraindication for this sedation.
- Anesthesiologists would most likely have to administer the medication.

Consent forms must be signed by legally competent client.

- Signing of consent form can only be done if client is considered competent to understand directions given and explanation of procedure.
- Signing of consent form must be voluntary.
- Client must be informed about procedure and must understand what he or she is signing.
- A court-appointed conservator may need to be obtained for clients not considered mentally competent to sign for themselves.
- Family members may not sign for client unless they are legally considered the client's guardian or advance directive provides instructions.
- In emergency situations, permission may be obtained from family members, but not for routine procedures.
- Two physicians can sign for emergency surgery; however, the surgeon performing the surgery should not sign the permit.

MANAGEMENT Guidelines

Each state legislates a Nurse Practice Act for RNs and LVN/LPNs. Healthcare facilities are responsible for establishing and implementing policies and procedures that conform to their state's regulations. Verify the regulations and role parameters for each healthcare worker in your facility.

Delegation

- RNs and LVN/LPNs can complete routine preoperative teaching and care. Anything out of the ordinary would be the responsibility of the RN.
- Postanesthesia room staff are usually RNs because they need to make quick decisions and use nursing judgment in times of crisis.
- Postoperative care of clients may be provided by both RNs and LVN/LPNs.
- Clients undergoing conscious sedation may be monitored by RNs if their State Nurse Practice Act and hospital policy allows it and the clients are in ASA categories 1 and 2 (see section on conscious sedation).
- CNAs can be delegated to take vital signs and do routine hygienic care for clients once they are stable.
- Many facilities use "scrub techs" or OR techs to perform routine duties such as the preoperative scrub. OR techs are also assigned to assist the physician during surgery.

Communication Matrix

- It is very important that all preoperative forms be completed in a timely manner. If data are missing, the client's surgery may be delayed while laboratory tests are taken, history and physical examination reports are found and placed in the chart, or chest x-ray results are placed in the chart. History and physical provide information to ensure continuity of care.
- Notify OR staff and physician if client indicates he or she has a known latex allergy or does not know of a latex allergy. All latex supplies and equipment must be removed from the OR suite before surgery can commence.
- When the phone call is received from the operating room indicating the nurse should give the preoperative medications or that the OR is ready for the client, ensure the message is relayed immediately to the staff caring for the client. This will allow the nurse to give the medication or complete any last-minute charting and have the client ready for the transporter.
- If there are any client issues or problems that directly affect the surgical procedure, contact the operating room or physician immediately. Surgery may need to be delayed or canceled. Examples of issues that could impact the surgery include an overly anxious client, if the client has a temperature, symptoms indicating an upper respiratory or

urinary tract infection, labs that are abnormal (bleeding time, cardiac enzymes, electrolytes), or new abnormal ECG changes.

- Specific report regarding the client's condition will be completed upon admission to the postanesthesia room and again when the client is returned to the nursing unit. The report is given by the RN in the operating room to the RN in the postanesthesia room. The postanesthesia room nurse accompanies the client to the nursing unit and gives report to the RN. The report is outlined as Step 15 of the skill Discharging Client From Postanesthesia Room to Nursing Unit.

CRITICAL THINKING Strategies

Scenario 1

You are assigned to the postanesthesia room on the day shift. You have just arrived on the unit to begin the shift. There are two clients assigned to your care:

- Mrs. Cohen, a 54-year-old client, had an exploratory laparoscopy with general anesthesia and is just arriving in the recovery room.
- Mr. Brewer is a 24-year-old client who had local anesthesia for an arthroscopy of the right knee. He has been in the recovery room for 1 hr.

1. Which client will you see first? Provide rationale for your response.
2. Identify the first action you will take when first seeing each of the two clients. Provide rationale for your response.
3. Identify the priority assessment for Mrs. Cohen and state your rationale.
4. Identify the priority assessment for Mr. Brewer and state your rationale.
5. State nursing interventions that will be provided for all clients in the postanesthesia room.
6. Before discharge from the recovery room, you assess Mr. Brewer on the Aldrete Recovery Scoring System and his score is 7. What is your next action?
7. Mr. Brewer is being discharged home. He tells you he is concerned about going home because he has a dry mouth and is thirsty. What would be an appropriate response to him?
8. Write the SBAR "Hand Off" communication you will prepare for transfer of Mr. Brown to the surgical floor.

Scenario 2

You assess that Mr. Marconi is very anxious while you are admitting him for a surgical procedure.

1. List four priority components of baseline data you need to obtain before surgery. Provide a rationale to support this data.
2. What factors might contribute to preoperative stress?
3. Identify a priority intervention to use after assessing that Mr. Marconi is in high-level stress.
4. Mr. Marconi becomes angry and hostile when you attempt to provide preoperative teaching. Describe three possible actions you could take, and state the priority intervention and the rationale for selecting this intervention.

NCLEX® Review Questions

Unless otherwise specified, choose only one (1) answer.

1. During the preoperative stage, the client activity not completed is
   1. Obtaining a health history.
   2. Identifying a client's allergies.
   3. Beginning the infusion of a moderate sedative drug.
   4. Identifying the side and site of the surgical procedure.
2. The role of the circulating nurse in the operating room is to
   1. Mark the operative site with a felt pen.
   2. Insert the IV and begin infusing fluids.
   3. Assist the physician during the operative procedure.
   4. Position the client on the operative table and attach grounding pad.
3. The most common malpractice action against operating room nurses is
   1. Sponges and instruments left in the surgical site accidentally.
   2. Surgical procedure performed on wrong site or side.
   3. Burns from electrical grounding pad not placed correctly on client.
   4. Infection at surgical site after surgical procedure.
4. The student's client assignment includes a preoperative client scheduled for surgery in 3 hours. The initial

intervention is to reduce anxiety and stress for this client. This can best be accomplished by _____________.
Select all that apply.

1. Discussing realistic outcomes with the client.
2. Avoiding promoting false reassurances.
3. Using touch to communicate caring.
4. Encouraging range of motion and walking activities.

5. As a student nurse working in the outpatient setting, you are asked to provide postoperative instructions to a client after a laparoscopy. The most appropriate instructions should be to
   1. Instruct the client that he/she may experience a sharp pain under the scapula up to 24–48 hr after surgery.
   2. Inform the client he/she will be hospitalized for a minimum of 24 hr to monitor for pain.
   3. Inform the client that this type of surgery usually requires very little pain medication; Tylenol is sufficient to control the pain.
   4. Explain that the client can return to work the next day, as long as they do not lift anything over 50 pounds.

6. While you are working on a surgical unit, you are preparing the client for a surgical procedure. Your responsibilities in this preparation include
   1. Asking the client if he/she has made arrangements for home care after discharge.
   2. Instructing the client to sign the surgical consent form at the time the OR transporter arrives in the room.
   3. Administering the preoperative medication at least 2 hr before the surgery is scheduled.
   4. Checking for allergies to latex, food, and medications.

7. The Joint Commission standards regarding Universal Protocols for preventing wrong site, wrong procedure, and wrong person surgery includes _____________.
   Select all that apply.
   1. Marking the surgical site by the preoperative nurse.
   2. Validating the correct surgical site by the surgeon before beginning the procedure.
   3. Writing the word "yes" on the surgical check list line indicating the correct incision site.
   4. Completing a final verification of the site in the location where the procedure takes place.

8. You are caring for a client after a procedure where moderate (conscious) sedation was used. You understand the client will not be discharged until the
   1. Ramsay Sedation Scale is normal.
   2. Riker Sedation-Agitation Scale is -1 to $+1$.
   3. Aldrete score is ± 1 point of preprocedure score.
   4. Glasgow Coma scale is more than 9.

9. A client is returning to the nursing unit after an abdominal surgical procedure. The priority nursing intervention is to
   1. Take and record vital signs.
   2. Assess type of IV solution and amount of IV solution remaining in bag.
   3. Check pulse oximeter reading.
   4. Assess for patent airway.

10. Pneumonia is a major postoperative complication related to inactivity and decreased pulmonary ventilation. As you are assessing the client postoperatively, you recall the usual onset of signs and symptoms is _____________
    1. Within 24 hr.
    2. 24–36 hr.
    3. 36–48 hr.
    4. More than 72 hr.

27

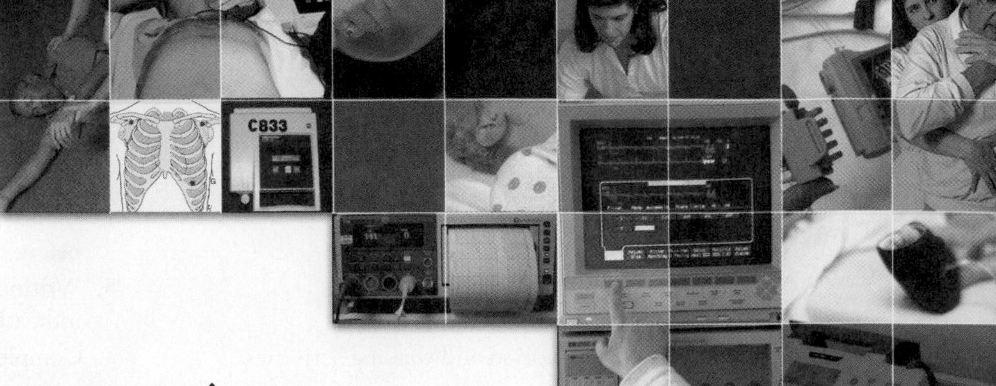

Orthopedic Interventions

LEARNING OBJECTIVES

1. Identify nursing diagnoses that apply to care of clients with orthopedic conditions.
2. Outline emergency measures for an injured extremity.
3. Describe different ways to classify fractures.
4. Assess circulation, motion, and sensation in an injured limb.
5. Recognize indicators of circulatory compromise in an injured or immobilized extremity.
6. Apply a variety of immobilizing devices (sling, bandage, splint, brace).
7. Describe differences between plaster of Paris and synthetic casts.
8. Explain the purpose for skin versus skeletal traction.
9. Identify types of skin and skeletal traction.
10. Develop a teaching plan for the client with a cast.
11. Outline the nursing care needs of the client in traction.
12. Outline the teaching needs of a client with an amputation.
13. Develop a teaching plan for a client undergoing joint replacement (arthroplasty).
14. Discuss the advantages of autologous reinfusion after joint replacement surgery.

CHAPTER OUTLINE

TERMINOLOGY

Abduction movement away from the midline of the body or body part, as in raising the arm or spreading the fingers.

Adduction movement toward the midline of the body.

AKA above-the-knee amputation.

Alignment arranged in a straight line.

Amputation traumatic or surgical removal of a diseased limb or part.

Arthroplasty repair/replacement of a joint.

Autologous reinfusion involves collection of shed blood through suction into a reservoir and reinfusion through the client's venous access.

Balanced suspension use of a sling or splint to elevate and support an extremity that is in traction.

BKA below-the-knee amputation.

Bryant's traction a type of skin traction used to treat fracture of the femur in a small child.

Buck's traction a type of skin traction applied to the lower leg to reduce muscle spasm and immobilize hip fracture.

Callus fibrous matrix of protein that bonds a fracture site, but has not ossified and cannot support weight bearing.

Cast circumferential immobilizer generally reserved for short-term fracture management.

Comminuted broken in pieces; usually occurs in spongy bone areas.

Contusion soft tissue injury.

Diaphysis the part of the long bone between the ends, also known as the shaft.

Edema excess fluid in the interstitial space.

Epiphysis the wide spongy end of a long bone.

Extension a movement that increases the angle between two bones, straightening a joint.

External fixation device a metal frame of telescoping rods with attached metal percutaneous pins inserted into or through a bone to maintain alignment.

External rotation turning an extremity away from the midline.

Exudate inflammatory response: migration of plasma fluid and circulating components to an injury site.

Flexion a movement that decreases a joint angle.

Hyperextension continuation of extension beyond the anatomic position, as in bending the neck backward.

Internal rotation turning an extremity toward the midline.

Intracapsular within the joint capsule (e.g., head and neck of the femur).

Metaphysis wide part of bone at end of shaft adjacent to the epiphysis.

Mobility state or quality of being mobile; facility of movement.

Musculoskeletal pertaining to the muscles and bones.

Osteoblasts immature cell, which on maturation plays a role in bone production.

Orthostatic concerning an erect or standing position.

Orthostatic hypotension drop in blood pressure upon standing.

Osteoclast cell that resorbs bone.

Paralysis loss of voluntary motion.

Paresthesia abnormal sensation of tingling or numbness.

Pearson attachment an attachment to Thomas splint that supports lower leg. Used in balanced suspension traction. Allows continuous traction in line with the femur by the use of cords and weights.

Periosteum connective tissue that covers the bone; contains proliferating cells.

Prosthesis artificial replacement for a body part.

Prosthetist specialist who provides preoperative training, prosthetic fabrication, prosthetic training, and follow-up assessments of fit, alignment, and appearance of prostheses.

Restorative promoting a return to health.

Russell's traction type of skin traction used to treat fracture of the shaft of the femur.

Shrinker A rigid or sock device suspended by a strap; worn to reduce edema and protect the stump of an amputated extremity.

Spica figure-eight bandage with one of the two loops larger than the other (used for ankle or stump).

Spiral bandage used to cover a cylindrical part.

Splint Noncircumferential immobilizer used for management of a variety of musculoskeletal conditions in which swelling is anticipated (sprain, acute fracture period).

Sprain injury caused by wrenching or twisting of a joint that results in tearing or stretching of the associated ligaments.

Strain injury caused by excessive force or stretching of muscles or tendons around the joint.

Stryker frame a special bed used to treat clients with spinal cord injuries.

Syncope a transient loss of consciousness due to inadequate blood flow to the brain.

Thomas splint used for balanced suspension along with skeletal traction for fracture of the femur.

Torque a rotary force.

Traction application of a mechanical pulling force applied to soft tissue.

RESTORING FUNCTION

Orthopedic nursing involves the prevention and correction of alterations in the musculoskeletal system. To help clients achieve and maintain optimal mobility, nurses use preventative, restorative, and rehabilitative methods. Preventative and restorative measures include the use of bandages, positioning, splints, casts, and traction.

The most common cause of injury to the musculoskeletal system is trauma, which results in soft tissue injuries, fractures, and dislocations. Injuries occurring from falls in the home account for many admissions to healthcare facilities.

Sprains and strains are common musculoskeletal injuries. The usual initial treatment is "RICE." "R" stands for resting the injured part, "I" refers to application of ice, "C" stands for compression such as with a bandage, and "E" stands for elevating the part 6 in. above the heart. These early interventions help to minimize pain, muscle spasm, edema formation, and secondary injury (review Inflammatory Response in Chapter 24).

Bandages are used for applying pressure over an area, immobilizing a body part, preventing or reducing edema formation, correcting a deformity, and securing splints in place. Several types of material are used as bandages: woven cotton, elastic webbing, and gauze.

Fractures

A fracture is a break in the continuity of a bone that occurs when the bone is subjected to stress forces greater than ordinary. No two fractures are alike since forces occur from different directions and in different amounts and muscle pulls differ in response to injury.

Long bones, most commonly involved in fractures, are composed of the shaft, or diaphysis, and the flared end of the bone, termed the metaphysis. In children the metaphysis consists of two segments: the growth plate, and the epiphysis, which is directly adjacent to joints. The epiphysis fuses to the metaphysis when long bone growth has ceased. Mid-shaft injuries to long bones in childhood can result in excessive growth of the extremity, while intra-articular fractures involving the growth plate can cause retardation or arrest in the longitudinal growth of the limb.

Bone healing is similar to soft tissue healing except that bones heal by limited regeneration rather than by scar formation. When a bone is fractured, a specific repair process takes place, beginning with formation of a blood clot at the fracture site. Osteoblasts and fibroblasts then converge on the site and start laying down an organic matrix or "callus," which bonds the fracture site and is similar to cartilage. Immobilization is an important factor during these critical phases. This callus is then mineralized by calcium deposition and thus converted into bone. In the final stage of the repair, osteoblasts and osteoclasts remodel the bone so that it is suited to perform its intended function (Wolff's Law).

When a fracture occurs, deformity is noted because bone fragments override due to spasm of surrounding muscles. In order to align ("reduce") fracture components, muscle spasm must be overcome. This can be accomplished by closed reduction (without surgery) or by open reduction (with surgery). Open reduction (ORIF) incorporates a form of internal fixation of fracture fragments with screws, plates, nails, etc. External immobilization with a cast or splint may be used along with either method of fracture reduction. An external fixator apparatus is used to reduce and immobilize fractures often associated with soft tissue injury. The fixator stabilizes fractured parts by the use of percutaneous pins.

Fractures are classified in a variety of ways. One classification is by fracture configuration. Examples include a transverse fracture, which breaks directly across the bone; an oblique fracture, which breaks at an angle across the bone; and a comminuted

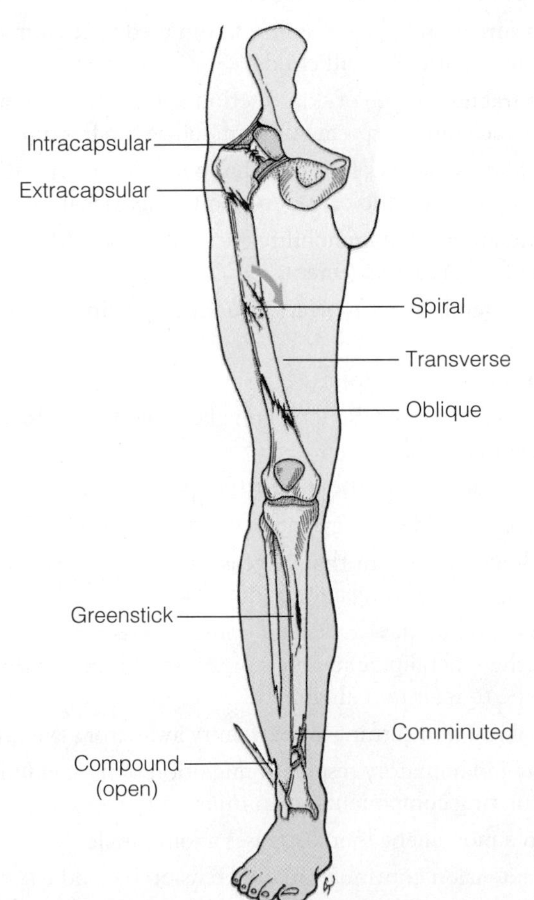

▲ Types of fractures.

Classification of Fractures

Greenstick

- A crack; the bending of a bone with incomplete fracture. Only affects one side of the periosteum.
- Common in children when bones are pliable.

Comminuted

- Bone broken into several fragments.
- Common in long bone ends (spongy bone).

Open (Compound)

- Bone is exposed to the external environment through a break in the skin.
- Can be associated with soft tissue injury.
- Infection is common complication.

Closed (Simple)

- Skin remains intact.
- Has reduced risk for infection.

Compression

- Frequently seen with vertebral fractures.
- Fractured bone has been compressed by other bones.

Impacted

- One part of fractured bone is driven into another.

Depressed

- Usually seen in skull or facial fractures.
- Bone or fragments of bone are driven inward.

Pathologic

- Break associated with a disease process (e.g., osteoporosis, cancer).

fracture, which results in more than two fragments of bone. Fractures can also be classified as open or closed. A closed fracture occurs with no break in the skin and is usually reduced without surgery, then immobilized with a cast. An open fracture is one in which the skin has been broken due to penetration of a bone fragment or external trauma. An open fracture requires additional treatment to prevent infection as a result of tissue exposure to the external environment. Surgical debridement and irrigation must be completed within hours of the fracture.

Casts and Splints

Casts are rigid cylinders applied to maintain the reduced (realigned) fracture in proper alignment and usually include the joint adjacent to the fracture. Casts are made from plaster of Paris or synthetic materials, such as polyester, polyurethane, fiberglass, or plastic. Synthetic casts dry faster, weigh less, and can get wet without fear of cracking or disintegration. Splints are not circumferential or as constrictive as casts and may be applied temporarily until swelling in the injured extremity has resolved. Frequent ongoing assessment of circulation, motion, and sensation in parts distal to the cast is essential for early recognition of neurovascular complications. Splitting or windowing the cast may be necessary to release pressure over a specific area, particularly a bony prominence.

Traction

Skin Traction Traction is the application of a mechanical pulling force. Skin traction can be applied to immobilize an injured site and to relieve pain. A rope, pulley, and weight system (5–10 lb) is attached to the device to provide pulling force to skin and soft tissues.

There are many types of skin traction. Buck's traction consists of a foam boot with Velcro straps applied to the lower leg to help immobilize and may relieve pain in clients with fractured hip before surgery. Superficial peroneal nerve compression can result if the straps are too tight. Frequent release of the straps prevents this complication. Bryant's traction, another type of skin traction, is used primarily for children under 3 years of age who have sustained a fractured femur. The cervical halter and pelvic girdle are also used in skin traction.

Skin traction for acute muscle spasm (fracture of the femur) should be continuous, but skin traction for chronic problems such as muscle strain is *intermittent*, removed and reapplied as specified by the physician. Complications of skin traction relate to skin integrity and neurovascular impairment.

Skeletal Traction Skeletal traction is applied directly to bone to reduce a fracture or to maintain a surgically manipulated bone alignment. Significantly greater weight is used with this mode of traction. Pins or wires are inserted through the skin and soft tissue and into bone, then the desired weight is applied to maintain bone alignment. This type of traction is *continuous;* removing or lifting weights displaces fragments and can cause neurovascular damage. Balanced suspension uses splints and slings to support the extremity and weights applied for countertraction (e.g., Thomas splint with Pearson attachment). Suspended support allows greater mobility for the client with skeletal traction.

External Fixation Device External fixation devices have a rigid metal frame of telescoping rods with attached percutaneous pins or wires. They are used to align and immobilize complex fractures with extensive soft tissue injury or may be used to stabilize a closed fracture that will not remain in position otherwise. These self-contained devices provide traction without the use of ropes and weights and therefore allow client mobility. Similarly, a client with fracture or dislocation of cervical or high thoracic vertebrae can mobilize with a halo ring and vest.

Complications include neurovascular compromise, inadequate bone alignment, skin or soft tissue injury, pin tract infection, and osteomyelitis. Neurovascular function must be assessed every 4 hr because clients requiring these devices usually have extensive soft tissue, nerve, and vessel damage. Extensive client teaching is necessary since these clients go home with the devices in place.

To be effective, any mode of traction must include *countertraction*. This might be provided by the client's body weight, by the pull of weights in the opposite direction, or by elevating the bed under the part in traction. The line of pull must be maintained, weights must hang freely, ropes must be intact and glide freely in the pulley, and knots must be secure. Weights and knots should hang far from the pulleys. The system should be free of any impingement such as linens. It is essential that the nurse have a clear understanding of the traction type and purpose, prescribed amount of weight, and client positioning.

Acute Compartment Syndrome

Since muscle groups are bound in a nonyielding fascia and injury causes swelling due to bleeding, edema, and the like, increased pressure within the "compartment" can compromise circulation to involved tissues. Similarly, external pressure (e.g., a cast) can compromise circulation and cause muscle ischemia and necrosis. As pressure increases within the site, venous return is compressed, leading to increased interstitial fluid (edema), then compression of arterioles and eventual ischemic myositis (necrosis) and contracture formation. The client can nevertheless have intact distal pulses.

To prevent this complication and ultimate loss of limb, immediate fasciotomy is necessary to release the unyielding fascial boundaries. The nurse must be vigilant to early signs and symptoms of acute compartment syndrome:

- Pain on *passive* stretching of the muscle (or distal digits)
- Pain out of proportion to the injury
- Pain that is unrelieved by pain medication
- Pain that increases with *elevation* of the part
- Pain when pressure is applied over the compartment
- Weak active movement of distal digits

Diminished or absent pulses, coolness, and pallor are late signs and unreliable indicators of acute compartment syndrome.

Joint Replacement (Arthroplasty)

Degenerative joint disease of the hip and knee is the number one cause of disability among the elderly. This chronic disease, sometimes called osteoarthritis, has an insidious onset that may progress to pain and stiffness, which impact the client's activities of daily living and role functioning. Elective total joint replacement (arthroplasty) has become increasingly popular because it restores mobility and relieves pain for clients who cannot be managed by medication or physical therapy.

Total hip arthroplasty includes replacement of both the femoral and acetabular components of the hip joint. The components are usually implanted with cement. Cementless components are also available and are preferred for younger clients who may require implant revision over time. These are textured prostheses that "cement" themselves by bony ingrowth.

After total hip arthroplasty or hemiarthroplasty (femoral prosthesis only), the client must adhere to precautions to prevent prosthesis dislocation and infection in remote sites that may spread by blood to the implanted component's site. Additionally, clients may be on long-term anticoagulant therapy and must understand the need for follow-up laboratory appointments.

Discharge planning begins before admission for elective joint arthroplasty. The client receives education about the perioperative process and "clinical path" expectations, including essentials of self-care rehabilitation. The home is typically equipped with adaptive and safety features before the planned surgery. Prepared clients experience less anxiety, fewer postoperative complications, shorter length of hospital stay, and reduced incidence of hospital readmissions.

Hip Fracture

Hip surgery for the fracture client presents a different challenge. The fracture client is not undergoing *elective* surgery, has had no preoperative preparation, and is frequently ill prepared for hospitalization. The emergent hip fracture client may not have the physical health enjoyed by the elective client. The trauma client is more apt to experience serious adverse consequences of emergent hospitalization and surgery, including delirium, and requires vigilant monitoring. Care and teaching for the client with prosthetic replacement for intracapsular hip fracture is identical to care and teaching for the client with total hip replacement.

Hip fracture involving the head or neck of the femur is classified as *intracapsular* (within the joint capsule). Since intracapsular bone lacks periosteum, fracture healing is limited. A hemiarthroplasty is performed whereby the head and neck of the femur are surgically removed and replaced with a *prosthesis*. The client is weight bearing with an assistive device soon after surgery. Because the joint capsule has been surgically disrupted, the hip prosthesis is at risk for dislocation until healing is complete. Specific rehabilitative adherence promotes healing and prevents dislocation of the prosthesis. If the fracture is *extracapsular* (involving the intertrochanteric region), internal fixation with nail, plate, and screws is performed. There is no disruption of the joint capsule, no prosthetic implant, and therefore no risk of femoral head dislocation, and dislocation precautions are not necessary. On the other hand, a repaired fracture site must heal, so total weight bearing is usually delayed.

Amputation

Amputation of a limb may be due to trauma, in which case the psychological ramifications can be very complex, or it can be a planned reconstructive procedure and a welcome source of relief for the client who has suffered painful vascular insufficiency and tissue necrosis (80% of cases). Regardless, the client who has lost a limb must regain psychological equilibrium and learn new skills. A supportive nurse–client relationship can assist the client to cope with grieving and body image reintegration. A rehabilitation team approach addresses goals to reduce stump edema, promote healing, prevent contractures, increase strength, and facilitate adjustment to loss by maximizing fractional independence.

It is normal for amputees to experience *phantom sensation*, a feeling that the amputated part is still there. This occurs early postamputation and goes away over time. Clients should be informed of this before amputation, if possible. *Phantom pain*, however, appears later (after 2–3 months) and is more likely to occur in above-the-knee amputees. The client experiences knife-like pain, squeezing, or burning sensations triggered by a number of stimuli (urination, defecation, cigarette smoking, and others). This complication is thought to be due to signals generated by intact nerves previously associated with the amputated part and relayed to the cerebral cortex as originating in the phantom limb, or there may be a response by the central nervous system to a stimulus that seems to come from an intact body or a response to stored pain sensations from the previously intact limb. Analgesics are effective in managing postoperative stump pain, but have no effect on phantom pain. Unfortunately, there is no treatment that is consistently effective. Interventions to reduce phantom pain include:

- Intense preoperative pain management
- Use of opioids, ketamine
- Use of anticonvulsants, antidepressants, TENS
- Stump desensitization with massage and transdermal anesthetics
- Early prosthetic use

Orthopedic Assessment

All orthopedic clients must be vigilantly monitored for skin and neurovascular status (circulation, motion, and sensation) of the affected part. Assessments should be conducted before, during, and frequently after application of any immobilizing modality. The contralateral extremity and documented baseline findings should be used for comparison.

TABLE 27-1 Neurologic Assessment

	Motion	Sensation
Upper Extremity		
Radial nerve	Hyperextends wrist Hyperextends thumb and four fingers	Web space between thumb and index finger
Ulnar nerve	Abducts (spreads) fingers	Lateral aspect of hand and distal end of little finger
Median nerve	Flexes wrist Opposes thumb and little finger	Distal end of index finger
Lower Extremity		
Peroneal nerve	Dorsiflexes ankle Flexes toes	Web space between great and second toe
Tibial nerve	Plantar flexes ankle and toes	Medial and lateral surfaces on sole of foot

NURSING DIAGNOSES

The following nursing diagnoses may be appropriate to include in a client care plan when the components are related to a client who requires special orthopedic procedures.

NURSING DIAGNOSIS	RELATED FACTORS
Disturbed Body Image	Trauma or injury, illness, chronic pain, situational crisis, treatments
Acute Confusion	Delirium
Ineffective Health Maintenance	Motor impairment
Injury, Risk for	Altered mobility, risk for falls or trauma, physical environmental factors, impaired balance, gait difficulties
Impaired Physical Mobility	Loss of integrity of bone structures, musculoskeletal impairment, neuromuscular impairment, pain, prescribed movement restrictions
Acute Pain	Physical injury
Chronic Pain	Arthritis, neurologic injury
Disturbed Sensory Perception	Amputation, nerve impingement
Impaired Tissue Integrity	Altered circulation, impaired physical mobility, mechanical factors
Ineffective Peripheral Tissue Perfusion	Interruption of arterial flow, interruption of venous flow, mechanical reduction of venous or arterial blood flow

CLEANSE HANDS The single most important nursing action to decrease the incidence of hospital-based infections is hand hygiene. *Remember to wash your hands or use antibacterial gel before and after each and every client contact.*

IDENTIFY CLIENT Before every procedure, introduce yourself and check two forms of client identification, not including room number. These actions prevent errors and conform to The Joint Commission standards.

Chapter 27

UNIT ❶

Application of Immobilizing Devices

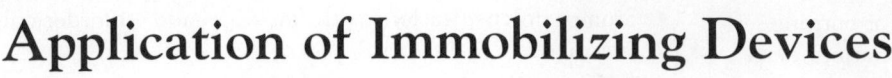

Nursing Process Data

ASSESSMENT Data Base

- Recognize need for site immobilization.
- Determine type of immobilization required.
- Select appropriate immobilizing equipment.
- Assess status of surrounding tissue.
- Assess affected extremity for circulation, motion, and sensation (CMS) before and after applying modality.

PLANNING Objectives

- To immobilize an extremity or body part
- To maintain functional alignment
- To limit harmful movement
- To reduce or prevent pain
- To prevent further soft tissue injury and complications
- To preserve neurovascular function
- To promote healing

IMPLEMENTATION Procedures

EVALUATION Expected Outcomes

- Treated part is effectively immobilized.
- Pain is reduced.
- Edema and bleeding are controlled.
- Further injury is prevented.

Pearson Nursing Student Resources

Find additional review materials at
nursing.pearsonhighered.com

Prepare for success with NCLEX®-style practice questions and Skill Checklists

Applying a Sling

Equipment

Commercial sling or
Triangular cloth or bandage
Safety pins

Clinical Alert

Never move an extremity yourself to see if it is fractured. Ask if the client is able to move the limb instead. Always splint the extremity as found.

Preparation

1. Check physician's orders for a sling.
2. Do not remove clothing or shoes.
3. Assess injured extremity circulation, motion, and sensation (CMS) before sling application.
4. Explain procedure and purpose of immobilization.
5. Remove any circumferential jewelry (ring, bracelet).
6. Have client sit or stand with forearm across chest.

Procedure

1. Place one end of triangular cloth against the chest on the affected side and over the shoulder of the unaffected arm.
2. Place the apex (point) of the triangle toward the elbow of the affected extremity.

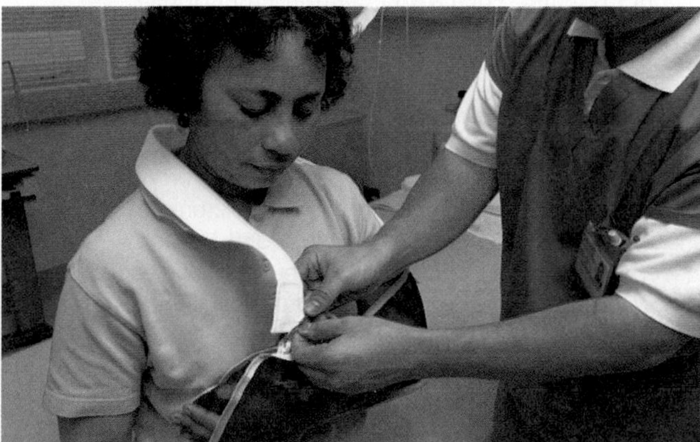

▲ Bring strap over shoulder and pull strap through metal hoops on sling.

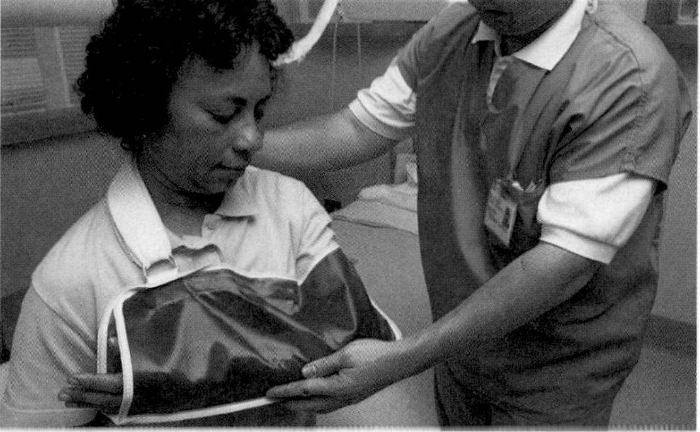

▲ Hand should be supported at a level slightly higher than the elbow to prevent edema.

3. Bring the opposite end of the triangle over the affected arm and over the affected shoulder.
4. Tie the sling at the side of the neck.
5. Fold the apex of the triangle over the elbow in the front, and secure with a safety pin or twist end and tie a square knot.
6. Assess client for comfort and for support of the affected arm.
7. Assess for neck pressure and peripheral CMS after 30 minutes and then every 2 to 4 hr.

NOTE: If using commercial sling, check directions on package for proper application.

Clinical Alert

If greater immobilization is indicated (e.g., for shoulder dislocation or fracture), a swathe can be applied over the sling, circling and securing the upper arm to the thorax.

8. Check that hand is supported at a level higher than elbow to prevent dependent edema.
9. Teach client to support the arm higher than heart level and to perform external rotation shoulder exercises to prevent shoulder joint stiffness.

Applying a Spiral Bandage

Equipment

Elastic or gauze roller bandages (width and number required to treat site)
Safety pins or tape
Supplies for wound care if indicated

Preparation

1. Check physician's orders, identify client, and explain procedure and purpose of immobilization.
2. Assess CMS of extremity before bandage application.
3. Remove any circumferential jewelry (ring, bracelet).
4. Have client sit or lie with part elevated.

Procedure

1. Remove existing elastic bandage or use bandage scissors to remove previously applied gauze bandage.
   ▸ ***Rationale:*** To prevent further injury and allow direct observation of site and wound care if indicated.
2. Remove dressing and redress wound if indicated (see Chapter 25).
3. Place part to be bandaged in an elevated position.
   ▸ ***Rationale:*** This promotes venous return and facilitates bandage compression to control edema and bleeding.
4. If area is functional or to be exercised, apply bandage with muscle in full contraction. ▸ ***Rationale:*** This prevents bandage constriction with future muscle activity.
5. Hold gauze or elastic roll with loose end of outer part of bandage facing client's skin several inches below the site of injury.
6. Unroll bandage twice around extremity to anchor bandage.
7. Continue wrapping extremity upward, using a moderate amount of tension to stretch and apply bandage uniformly. ▸ ***Rationale:*** Unequal pressure can adversely affect circulation.
8. Wrap the extremity *proximally* with spiral or angled turns. ▸ ***Rationale:*** Circular turns create a tourniquet effect. Proximal wrapping promotes venous return.
9. Make bandage turns that overlap by at least one half the previous wrap to prevent bandage separation. ▸ ***Rationale:*** Bandage turn separation tends to pinch the skin.

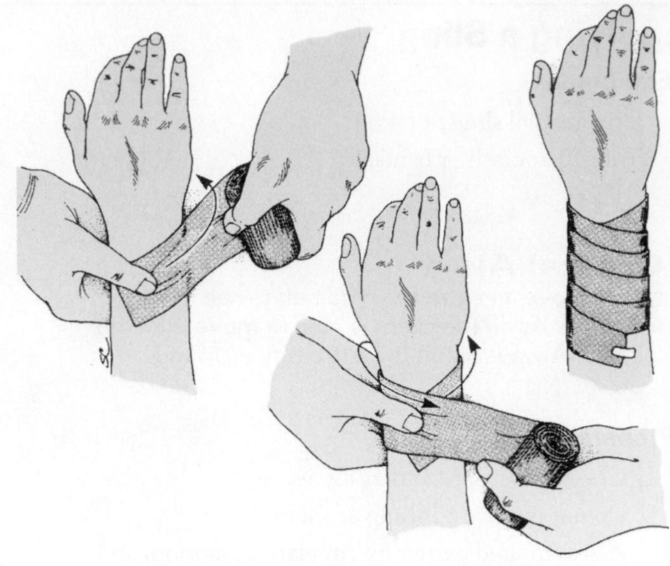

▲ Spiral bandage may be used to secure a wound dressing.

10. Finish wrap with a couple of wraps directly overlying each other.
11. Secure the bandage by tying or using tape or safety pin.
12. Observe that bandage is snug but not tight, is free of wrinkles, and is not occluding distal circulation.
13. Assess distal digits for CMS in 30 minutes and every 2–4 hr initially.
14. Maintain elevation of involved extremity and encourage active motion of digits. ▸ ***Rationale:*** This helps reduce edema and maintain function.
15. Rewrap bandage at least every 8 hr.

Cryotherapy Limits Injury

Application of ice (cryotherapy) causes vasoconstriction, reduces capillary permeability, and decreases tissue metabolism. The decreased metabolism results in decreased secondary metabolic injury and thus less tissue debris (free tissue protein). Cryotherapy used as soon as possible limits the extent of the injury, but once secondary metabolic injury has occurred, cryotherapy has no value in removing edema that has formed. The only way to relieve the edema is by removing excess free protein in the tissue by way of the lymphatic system. This generally requires intermittent compression as occurs with active exercise. (see Chapter 24, Heat and Cold Therapies).

EVIDENCE-BASED PRACTICE

Rest vs. Early Mobilization

Rest seems to be overused as a treatment. Forty-nine trials of immobilization for soft tissue injuries and fractures of both upper and lower extremities were reviewed (3,366 clients). All the studies reported either no difference between rest and early mobilization or found in favor of early mobilization. Benefits of earlier mobilization included return to work; decreased pain, swelling, and stiffness; and more preserved range of joint motion. Early mobilization caused no increased complications, deformity, or residual symptoms.

Source: Nash, C., Mickan, S. M., Del Mar, C. B., & Glasziou, P. P. (2004). Resting injured limbs delays recovery: A systematic review. *The Journal of Family Practice*, *53*(9), 706–712.

Applying a Figure-Eight Bandage

Equipment

Roller bandage
Safety pin or tape

Preparation

1. Identify client and explain procedure and rationale.
2. Provide privacy.
3. Position ankle in neutral alignment, neither overflexed nor overextended.

Procedure

1. Gather necessary bandages. The number and width of the bandage depends on the extent and area of the extremity to be bandaged.
2. Hold roll with outer part next to client's skin over instep.
3. Anchor bandage by making an angled turn around instep.
4. Make a circular turn around heel and return to starting point.

5. Make a spiral turn down over the ankle and around the foot.
6. Continue to make alternate turns around the ankle and foot. Overlap the preceding turn by at least two-thirds over the preceding layer.
7. Wrap the entire area below and above the involved joint. ▸ ***Rationale:*** This immobilizes the affected area.

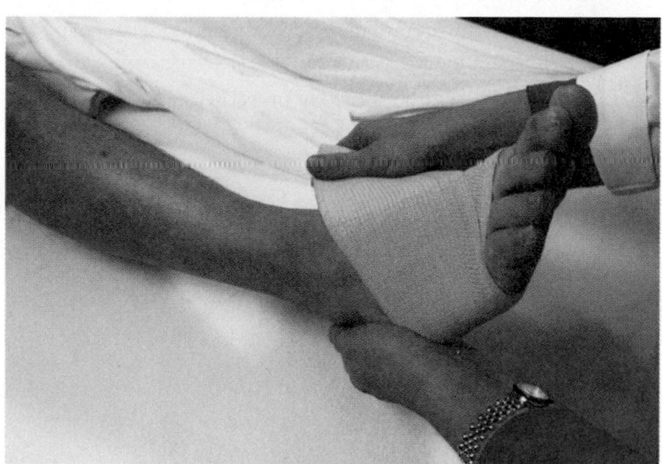

▲ Make an angled turn around instep.

8. Assess extremity (exposed digits) for CMS and evenness of pressure as well as comfort of client.
9. Assess extremity after 20 minutes and then every 2 to 4 hr, and rewrap every 8 hr.
10. Maintain elevation of extremity.

NOTE: Edema can result if the heel is not enclosed within bandage.

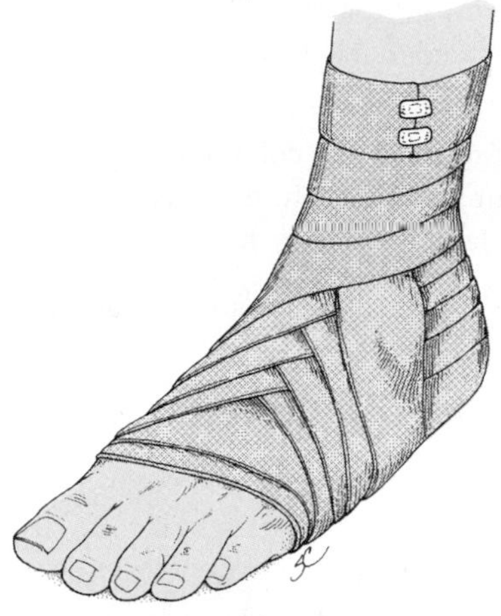

▲ A figure-eight turn is used to support and limit joint movement.

Applying a Splint

Equipment

Splint materials: pieces of wood or pillows, magazines, blankets

Padding materials: pieces of cloth or towel

Wrapping materials: strips of cloth, rope, tape, elastic bandage

Preparation

1. Assess involved extremity for deformity or soft tissue injury.
2. Do not remove clothing or shoes (except with scissors). ▸ ***Rationale:*** To prevent excessive manipulation of the injured part.
3. Remove any jewelry from extremity to prevent circulatory compromise with swelling.
4. Assess neurovascular status of distal digits.
5. Explain need for and purpose of splint to client.

Procedure

1. Gather needed supplies.
2. Control bleeding by applying direct pressure and by using pressure dressings; apply clean covering to any wound.
3. Explain the rationale for the intervention to client.
4. Move injured extremity as little as possible and splint as it lies.

Clinical Alert

Never straighten an injured extremity or push bone or tissue back into place. Splint a deformed extremity in its deformed shape using a soft support such as a pillow.

5. Pad joints, bony prominences, and between digits. ▸ ***Rationale:*** This prevents skin damage. Also make sure that the padding does not affect the client's circulation (e.g., don't put padding in axilla).
6. If splint material is not available, use the client's body for support.
   a. Splint the legs together.
   b. Splint an arm to the torso.
   c. Splint toes or fingers together.
7. Use a spiral (not circular) technique to wrap splint.
8. Strap the splint and extremity together securely so that the extremity is immobile. Try to include the proximal and distal points in the splint.
9. Check the client's distal circulation by assessing pulse, capillary refill, color, and temperature.
10. Elevate part to reduce edema formation.
11. Arrange to transport client to medical facility as soon as possible.
12. Report specifics to transport personnel.

Applying a Cervical Collar

Equipment

Sizing chart

Two collars of appropriate size (a spare for alternate use), each with an additional removable pad

Assistant, if client has known or suspected cervical injury

Preparation

1. Explain procedure to the client.
2. Place client flat supine.
3. Select appropriate size collar based on length of neck from client's mandible to the clavicle (the longer the neck, the larger the collar).

NOTE: Some collars allow for anterior and posterior vertical height adjustment.

4. Select appropriate size collar.

Procedure

1. Perform hand hygiene.
2. Obtain assistance if client has known or suspected cervical injury. One maintains neck alignment while the collar is applied.
3. Follow manufacturer's instructions to apply collar. Save instructions and container for later use.
4. Place back half of collar on client's neck, centering with the spine, arrow pointing up.
5. Center front half of collar on front of client's neck, using a scooping motion upward from the chest, so that chin fits into the indentation. ▶ ***Rationale:*** This ensures neutral alignment.
6. Lap back half over front half of collar.
7. Adjust velcro straps, to ensure a secure fit. ▶ ***Rationale:*** Collar should be snug enough to prevent movement, but not interfere with client's ability to breathe, swallow, or speak.
8. Inspect skin under collar regularly, and cleanse with soap and water.
9. Assess neurovascular status of upper and lower extremities every 4–8 hr, if indicated.
10. Clean collar and removable pads as needed with soap and water and allow to dry naturally; do not use a hair dryer.
11. Maintain collar use 24 hr/day or as ordered, using alternate collar when necessary.
12. Caution the ambulatory client that without neck flexion, visibility of stairs or objects on the floor is limited.

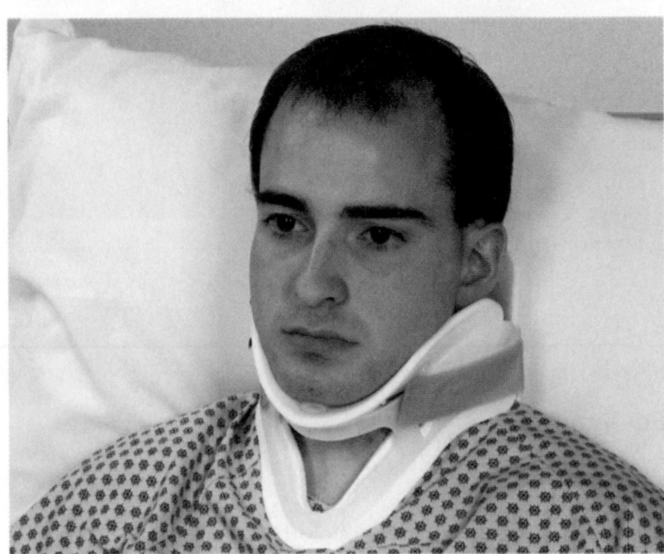

▲ Ensure side straps of collar are properly adjusted for a secure fit.

Applying a Jewett–Taylor Back Brace

Equipment

Front and back brace with Velcro straps

T-shirt

Preparation

1. Check physician's order and determine rationale for brace application.
2. Determine that client's brace has been fitted by an orthotist (brace fitter).
3. Identify client, explain procedure, or supervise client's application and reinforce previous teaching.
4. Provide privacy.
5. Change wound dressing, if indicated, before applying brace.

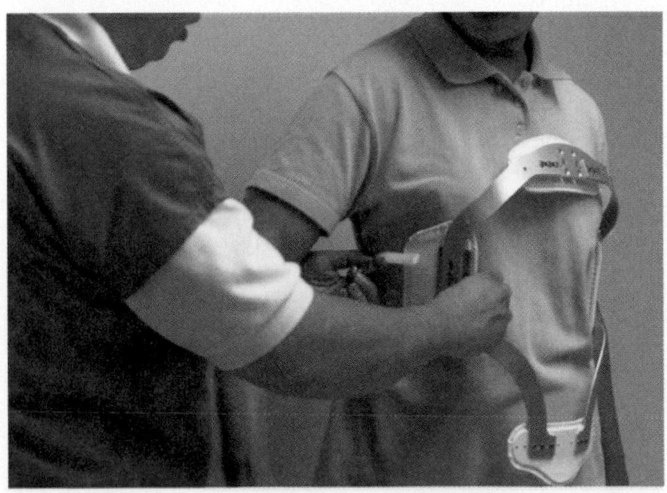

▲ Jewett-Taylor brace is applied to client while lying supine. This photo is for demonstration.

Procedure

1. Perform hand hygiene.
2. Put T-shirt on client.▸ ***Rationale:*** This protects the skin from the brace rubbing on bare skin.
3. Place bed in a flat position. Keep side rail in UP position on side of bed opposite from you.
4. Log-roll or ask client to roll to side away from you. ▸ ***Rationale:*** This position prevents torque on the spine.
5. Position brace on back so that struts fit on either side of spine and it fits the natural contour of the back. ▸ ***Rationale:*** Struts provide an open space along the spine so pressure is not exerted on a surgical site or on vertebrae.
6. Log-roll the client back onto brace to a supine position.
7. Place front section of brace over the iliac crest and position iliac wings (made of plastic material). Adjust triangular sternum piece; metal struts will fall into place.
8. Secure brace with Velcro straps.
9. Check under brace for pressure areas. If pressure areas are present, report to orthotist.
10. Provide client with adaptive aids (i.e., reacher). ▸ ***Rationale:*** Client cannot bend forward while wearing brace.

DOCUMENTATION for Applying Immobilizing Modalities

- Time of application
- Site involved
- Skin integrity or wound status
- Type of immobilizing modality applied
- Circulatory and neurologic status of distal parts before and after modality application
- Site positioning or alignment
- Subjective statements of client

CRITICAL THINKING Application

Expected Outcomes

- Treated part is effectively immobilized.
- Pain is reduced.
- Edema and bleeding are controlled.
- Further injury is prevented.

Unexpected Outcomes	Alternative Actions
Bandage securing wound dressing continues to fall off.	• Avoid tape if skin is fragile or area has impaired circulation. • Use expanding "turkey skin" wrap to secure dressing. • Consult wound care specialist for alternative suggestions.
Client with back brace refuses to eat.	• Loosen brace before and for a while after meals. • Encourage small, frequent meals. • Reduce intake of gas-forming foods (cabbage, beans, corn). • Suggest intake of liquid nutritional supplement.
Client with brace expresses feelings of "being trapped."	• Allow client to voice concerns and explore options for self-control, such as access to telephone, call bell.
Elevation of extremity and passive stretching of digits increase pain, pain medications are ineffective, and pressure applied to injured site produces severe pain.	• Suspect acute compartment syndrome and notify physician immediately. Fasciotomy may be indicated if tissue swelling compromises circulation within a muscle compartment. • Loosen external immobilizing device. • Maintain extremity in *dependent* position.
Client experiences pain while wearing back brace.	• Encourage the client to not sit for longer than 30 minutes after back surgery. This increases pain due to spinal alignment in this position.

Distal edema is noted in bandaged extremity and client is unable to move digits and states sensation is altered.	• Remove bandage and check distal circulation, motion, and sensation. • Keep extremity elevated. • Rewrap bandage with extremity in elevated position. • If edema persists, notify physician for possible addition of cold therapy, anti-inflammatory medication, or further evaluation.
Toes become edematous after ankle bandaging.	• Do *not* apply ice to extremity since this reduces blood flow to area. • Elevate extremity and encourage active exercise of toes to promote venous return. • If area feels warm to touch, consider application of ice to help reduce inflammation. • Loosen bandage.
Client with neck brace expresses fear of falling.	• Suggest removal of scatter rugs, other obstacles that might cause tripping. • Have client view environment from a distance before advancing into it. • Suggest use of a "blind" cane to scan or tap the area in front of client to warn of potential obstacles or steps.

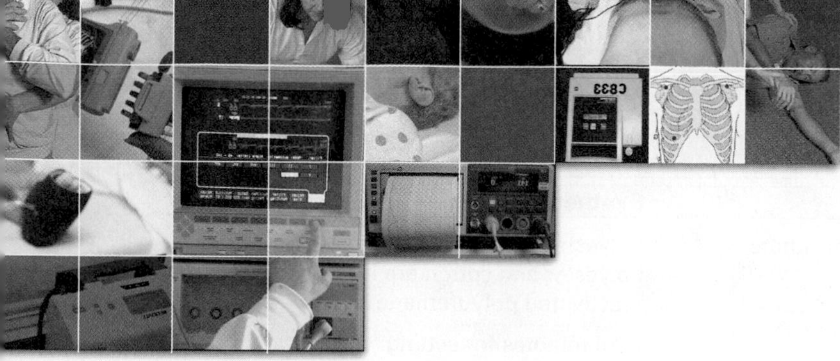

Chapter 27

UNIT 2

Cast Care

Nursing Process Data

ASSESSMENT Data Base

- Identify type of cast applied and rationale for application.
- Note condition for which the cast was applied.
- Observe condition of the cast.
- Assess neurovascular status of involved extremity.
- Assess client's understanding of and adherence to care instructions.

PLANNING Objectives

- To immobilize a fracture site
- To maintain normal sensation, movement, and circulation in a casted extremity
- To improve muscle tone and joint flexibility
- To promote bone healing
- To facilitate self-care after cast application and removal

IMPLEMENTATION Procedures

EVALUATION Expected Outcomes

- Cast integrity is maintained to provide adequate site immobilization.
- Client experiences minimal swelling.
- Neurovascular complications do not occur.

Pearson Nursing Student Resources

Find additional review materials at **nursing.pearsonhighered.com**

Prepare for success with NCLEX®-style practice questions and Skill Checklists

TABLE 27-2 Comparison of Cast Types

	Plaster	Synthetic
Material	Plaster of Paris, comprised of powdered calcium sulfate crystals impregnated into the bandages	Polyester and cotton, fiberglass, or plastic. Polyester and cotton are impregnated with water-activated polyurethane resin.
Drying time	24–48 hr No weight bearing until dry, 48–72 hr	7–15 minutes for setting 60 minutes for weight bearing
Advantages	Less costly More effective for immobilizing fracture site Smooth surface Doesn't require expensive equipment for application	Less likely to indent into skin Lighter in weight Less restrictive Doesn't crumble Nonabsorbent

Caring for a Wet Cast

Equipment

Pillows for support

Pen to mark drainage

Preparation

1. Note physician's orders for any client-specific instructions about positioning or cast handling.
2. Identify client and explain all procedures.
3. Recruit assistant(s) to help turn client.
4. Consider client's need for an analgesic.

Procedure

1. Explain that the cast feels warm as plaster dries, but urge client to report undue warmth or a burning sensation. ▸ ***Rationale:*** Cast burns can cause serious tissue injury.
2. Until the cast is dry, use *only* the palms of your hands to handle cast when turning and positioning. ▸ ***Rationale:*** Fingers can indent cast and create pressure areas on underlying tissue.
3. Avoid handling over joints where nerves and blood vessels are superficial.
4. Support cast with pillows, with extremity elevated above heart level. ▸ ***Rationale:*** This promotes venous return and reduces edema formation.
5. Maintain contours built into the cast; support leg so that heel is free of pressure. ▸ ***Rationale:*** To prevent flattening.
6. Keep wet cast uncovered and turn client to both sides, prone, and supine to expose all surfaces, allowing cast to dry by natural evaporation from the inside out.

NOTE: The wet plaster of Paris cast is dry when musty odor is gone, the cast is white and shiny, and it sounds resonant when tapped.

7. Do not try to hasten drying by using artificial measures such as a hair dryer. ▸ ***Rationale:*** Outer layer may dry before inner aspect, resulting in cast weakening.

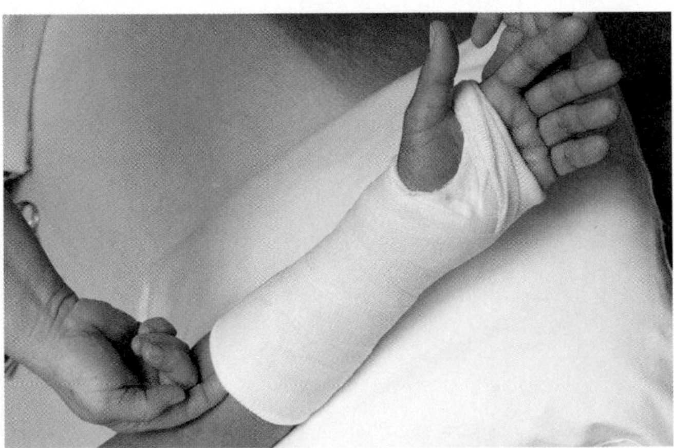

▲ Position extremity above heart level to reduce edema formation. Check cast for tightness. The nurse should be able to insert one or two fingers between cast and skin.

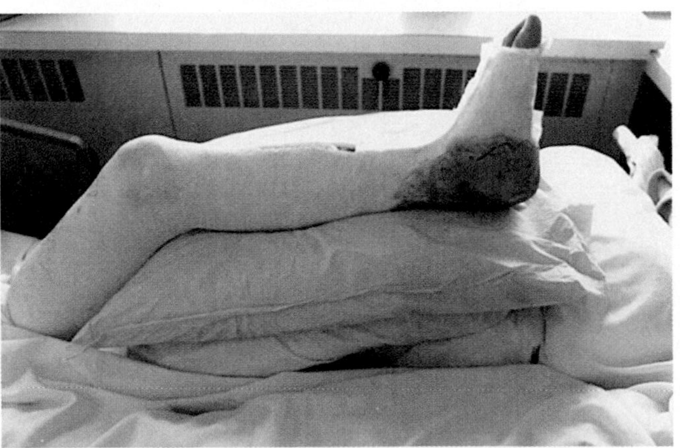

▲ Plaster casts are still being used, especially in disaster situations. Position casted extremity above level of heart to reduce edema formation.

8. If ice pack is ordered to reduce edema, place it alongside of cast, not on cast. ▶ ***Rationale:*** Placing ice pack on the cast can cause flattening.
9. If cast edges are rough or crumbly, pull inner stockinette out and over the edge and secure with tape.

Clinical Alert
Injured tissues swell, but encircling therapies do not expand. For any encircling modality, assess distal digits for circulation, motion, and sensation. Assessment is ongoing and continues after discharge.

Assessing a Casted Extremity

Equipment

Pen to mark drainage on cast

Procedure

1. Explain rationale for the procedure to client.
2. Encourage client to notify you of any change in sensation, mobility, or color/temperature in the casted extremity.
   a. Circulation
      - Report if digits are swollen despite elevation and active exercise.
      - Report if digits are pale, blue, or cold to touch.
      - Report delayed (>2 seconds) capillary refill (pinch finger to blanch and determine length of time required for color to return)
   b. Motion
      - *Immediately* report pain on passive movement of digits.
      - Report inability to actively move digits (see Table 27-1).
      - Compare strength of action with uninvolved extremity.
   c. Sensation
      - *Immediately* report increasing or unrelieved pain, pain with passive motion of digits, or pain that increases when the extremity is elevated.
      - Report numbness or paresthesia (pins-and-needles feeling).
      - Assess involved nerve sites for sensation (see Table 27-1).
3. Emphasize that a fine margin exists between reversible and irreversible damage to neurovascular structures.

Clinical Alert
Do not use abductor bars (incorporated into cast) for moving the client. Move the client as a unit instead.

Clinical Alert
When casting material inhibits palpation of peripheral pulses, assess capillary refill, assess for edema, comfort level, and other parameters of CMS as an indication of neurovascular status.

4. Assess for capillary refill by applying pressure to one of the client's digits. After you stop the pressure, observe the area to see how rapidly the color returns.
5. Ask the client to move the fingers or toes distal to the cast. The client should be able to move them without difficulty.
6. Check for any drainage on cast. Note color and size of drainage and mark cast with time.

Clinical Alert
Casted extremity should be assessed every half hour for 4 hr, then every 4 hr.

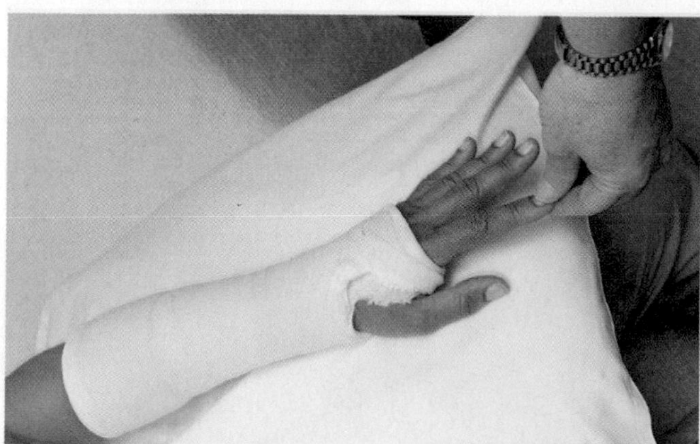

▲ Check fingers or toes for color, temperature, capillary refill, sensation, and motion.

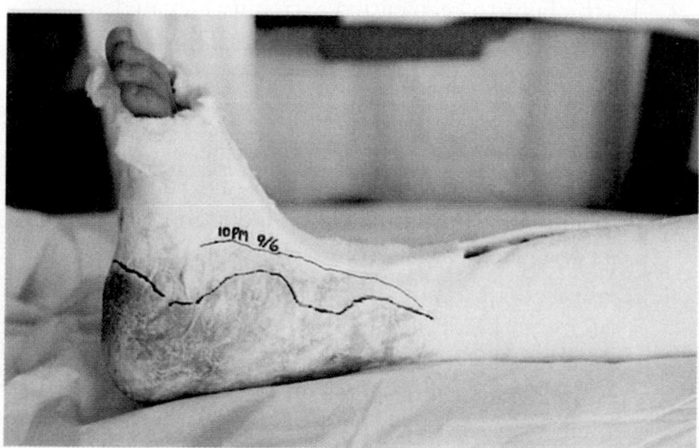

▲ Observe casted extremity frequently to monitor and mark drainage. Assess dependent area for drainage as well.

7. Report any unusual odor or increase in drainage. ▸ ***Rationale:*** Active bleeding should cease. Stain should turn brown after 24 hr.
8. Check for redness around casted area.
9. Cover rough edges of cast with stockinette or smooth tape "petals." ▸ ***Rationale:*** Prevent skin irritation, which can lead to skin breakdown.
10. Massage area under cast, but avoid lotions and powders.

Clinical Alert

If the client has had open reduction, wound drainage will be absorbed and spread rapidly or seep down to back of cast. The visible drainage does not necessarily indicate the amount of actual drainage.

Inspect all cast surfaces and mark drainage regularly if it is increasing. Bleeding should not persist after 24 hr.

11. Remind client to not stick objects inside the cast to scratch skin. ▸ ***Rationale:*** Skin breakdown can occur, leading to infection.
12. Suggest use of an aseptic syringe or hair dryer (cool setting) to blow under cast to relieve itching or to apply pressure over the area.

Clinical Alert

Diminished or absent pulses, coolness, and pallor are late signs and unreliable indicators of acute compartment syndrome. Always assess active extension, flexion, adduction, and abduction of the fingers, flexion and extension of the toes, and inversion and dorsiflexion of the foot. Pain on passive stretching of the muscle or distal digits is an *early* indicator of circulatory compromise.

Instructing Client in Self-Care

Equipment

Instructions pamphlet

Relevant telephone numbers

Preparation

1. Review client's chart for type of reduction performed (open or closed).
2. Identify client and explain importance of self-care to prevent complications.
3. Provide written instructions that reinforce teaching.
4. Provide telephone number of patient care coordinator if relevant for follow-up concerns.

Procedure

1. Demonstrate and teach importance of regular neurovascular checks, comparing with contralateral extremity. (*See* Assessing a Casted Extremity.)
2. Teach client to keep casted extremity elevated and to actively exercise digits. ▸ ***Rationale:*** This reduces edema formation, pain, and stiffness; stimulates lymph flow; and reduces risk of thrombus formation.
3. Report any unusual odor, new drainage, or fever. ▸ ***Rationale:*** These are signs of possible infection, especially if client has had open reduction or an object has been placed or fallen into the cast.
4. Remind client to not stick objects into the cast to scratch the skin. Encourage client to blow cool air (hair dryer on cool setting or Asepto bulb syringe) or to apply pressure over the area to relieve itching. ▸ ***Rationale:*** Scratching the area abrades the skin and can cause infection.
5. Teach cast protection.
   a. Remove stains with nonabrasive powder cleanser and damp cloth.
   b. Do not shellac or varnish to waterproof the cast. It must "breathe."
   c. Use plastic covering (garbage bag) for showering. Do not cover for prolonged periods as this will cause condensation and weaken the cast.
   d. Report any cracking or softening of cast and redness of skin at cast edges.
   e. Protect cast from urine or stool by covering edge with plastic wrap as odor can't be removed.
   f. Sleep with casted lower extremity next to wall, if possible. ▸ ***Rationale:*** If the casted extremity falls off the bed, the client will go with it.
6. Cast removal.
   a. Inform client that cast saw blade is safe. It does not cut through material, but vibrates.

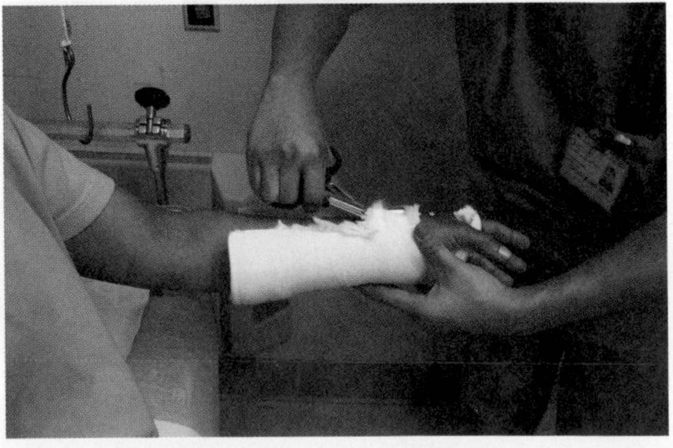

▲ Cast is split with a vibrating blade. Underlying padding is cut with bandage scissors.

b. Prepare client that muscle will have atrophied with disuse, joints will be stiff, and bone is vulnerable to refracture.
c. Teach client to continue to protect, support, and elevate the extremity after cast removal.
d. Teach client that skin will be caked with adherent exudate and not to forcibly remove this. Soften exudate with olive oil or use full-strength cold water wash (e.g., Woolite, Delicare), leave on 20 minutes, then rinse in warm water. ▶ ***Rationale:*** Aggressive removal of exudate can cause bleeding. Enzymes in special cleansers will loosen dead cells and fatty or crusty lesions without injuring underlying cells.

DOCUMENTATION for Cast Care

- Type of cast applied
- Positioning of cast
- Client's complaints and nursing responses
- Color, warmth, movement, and sensation in casted extremity
- Presence, location, and amount of drainage from wound
- Client's acceptance of the cast

Legal Considerations

Collins v. Westlake Community Hospital (1974)

In this case a client treated for a fractured leg developed ischemia within 3 days, necessitating amputation. The physician had written an order for the nurses to monitor peripheral CMS, and although the standard of nursing care required frequent monitoring of the client's circulation, the nurses' notes failed to show that the client's circulation had been monitored at any time during the crucial 7-hr period when the client's condition became critical. Nursing negligence was upheld by the court.

Standard nursing practice dictates that clients with casts be monitored frequently to detect and prevent complications. Additionally, clients discharged post-cast application must receive discharge instructions including self-care, cast care, and adverse signs/symptoms to be reported.

NOTE: Monitoring the client's condition and reporting changes are primary nursing responsibilities. Nurses who fail to record their observations run the risk of being unable to convince a jury that such observations actually were made. Failure to report the client's worsening condition is also another source of litigation.

Source: Bernzweig, E. (1996). *The Nurse's Liability for Malpractice* (6th ed.). St. Louis: Mosby.

CRITICAL THINKING Application

Expected Outcomes

- Cast integrity is maintained to provide adequate site immobilization.
- Client experiences minimal swelling.
- Neurovascular complications do not occur.

Unexpected Outcomes	Alternative Actions
Cast cracks from improper drying or stress.	• Notify physician immediately. • Reassure client. • Do not reposition client until physician assesses.
Synthetic cast has rough edges.	• Smooth edges by filing with nail file if necessary. • Make sure furniture and clothing are protected from scratches and snags by covering cast with stockinette.
Cast edges begin to crumble.	• "Petal" edges of cast with 1- to 2-in. strips of tape. • Place half of tape inside cast, pull tape over cast, and anchor on outside of cast. • Continue to petal cast until all edges are covered.
Client develops itching and burning under synthetic cast after swimming.	• Immersion should be avoided. • Flush skin under cast with plain water if it has been exposed to chlorine. • Dry skin under cast thoroughly with hair dryer on LOW. This may require several hours!

Fingers swell after application of arm cast.	• Assess that there is room for two fingers to be slipped under cast. • Apply ice along side of cast and maintain elevation after cast application. • Maintain arm positioning with hand higher than elbow. • Encourage client to exercise fingers to help reduce edema. • Monitor neurovascular status frequently.
Client develops pain not relieved by analgesics, pain that worsens with extremity elevation and passive stretching of digits.	• Maintain extremity in dependent position. • Notify orthopedic technician immediately: windowing or bivalving cast may be indicated. • Suspect acute compartment syndrome and notify physician immediately to obtain measurement of compartment pressure. • Fasciotomy may be indicated if tissue swelling or external device compromises circulation within a muscle compartment.

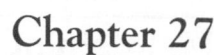

Chapter 27

UNIT 3

Traction

Nursing Process Data

ASSESSMENT Data Base

- Determine type and purpose of traction used.
- Note the amount of weight ordered.
- Note any conditions requiring special treatment (i.e., continuous or intermittent traction).
- Assess circulation, motion, and sensation of affected extremity.
- Assess pin site for drainage and signs of infection.
- Assess neurovascular status of clients with external fixation devices.

PLANNING Objectives

- To relieve muscle spasm
- To maintain alignment of fracture site
- To prevent unnecessary injury to soft tissue
- To prevent neurovascular complications
- To use for temporary management of fractures in adults
- To maintain pin site free of infection

IMPLEMENTATION Procedures

EVALUATION Expected Outcomes

- Extremity is maintained in correct alignment.
- Neurovascular status is within normal limits.
- Pin site remains free of infection.

Pearson Nursing Student Resources

Find additional review materials at **nursing.pearsonhighered.com**

Prepare for success with NCLEX®-style practice questions and Skill Checklists

Maintaining Skin Traction

Preparation

1. Determine whether client is preoperative. If so, do not manipulate the extremity.
2. Determine whether client has condition (diabetes, peripheral vascular disease) that predisposes to skin damage with traction.
3. Determine whether traction is continuous or intermittent.
4. Recruit an assistant to apply manual traction when removing and replacing traction.
5. Explain purpose of traction to client and family.

Procedure

1. Examine type of traction used that attaches weights to the extremity.
   a. Material should be held firmly in place.
   b. Material should fit comfortably, neither too loose nor too tight.
   c. Client should be in functional alignment.
2. Examine all bony prominences of the involved extremity for abrasions or pressure areas.
   a. Traction should be released at least every 8 hr for skin inspection.
   b. Have an assistant apply manual traction when discontinuing for assessment.
   c. Check for redness, which, if present, indicates excessive pressure on site.
3. Examine extremity distal to the traction.
   a. Note any presence of edema.
   b. Palpate peripheral pulses.
   c. Check temperature and color contralaterally to see if both extremities are normal.
   d. Check capillary refill time.
4. Assess for possible neurologic impediment from traction slings encroaching on popliteal space, peroneal nerve, or axilla. ▶ ***Rationale:*** Numbness or tingling, if present, indicates possible neurologic involvement.

Clinical Alert

Unless ordered otherwise, the client with Buck's extension should have the knee gatch of the bed elevated 20°–30° to flex the hip in a neutral position.

▲ Remove straps on Buck's traction every 8 hr to maintain function and allow inspection.

EVIDENCE-BASED PRACTICE

Traction vs. No Traction for Hip Fracture

Trials of traction versus no traction for patients with hip fracture have found no significant differences in pain, operative blood loss, ease of fracture reduction, or length of hospitalization. It seems that providing adequate intravenous analgesia and placing the extremity in a comfortable position are the best measures for reducing preoperative pain.

Source: Gregory W. Hendy, MD, FACEP (2005). 7 myths of orthopedic emergencies. *Emergency Medicine* 7: 38–43.

Clinical Alert

Do not apply Buck's traction over or under a calf compression device. Foot pumps (only around the foot) are acceptable for deep-vein thrombosis prophylaxis.

Principles of Traction Maintenance

- Maintain traction pull by ensuring weights are hanging freely, off the floor or bed frame.
- Ensure knots are secure in all ropes.
- Maintain ropes in pulley system and ensure rope moves freely through system and knots do not interfere with movement.
- Maintain prescribed amount of traction (5–10 lb for adult clients).
- Maintain countertraction, with client aligned in center of bed.
- Maintain traction, either continuous or intermittent, according to physician's orders.

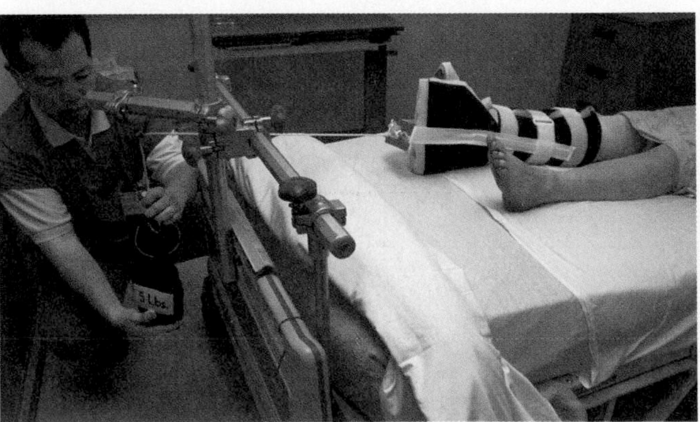

▲ Maintain traction by ensuring that weights hang freely.

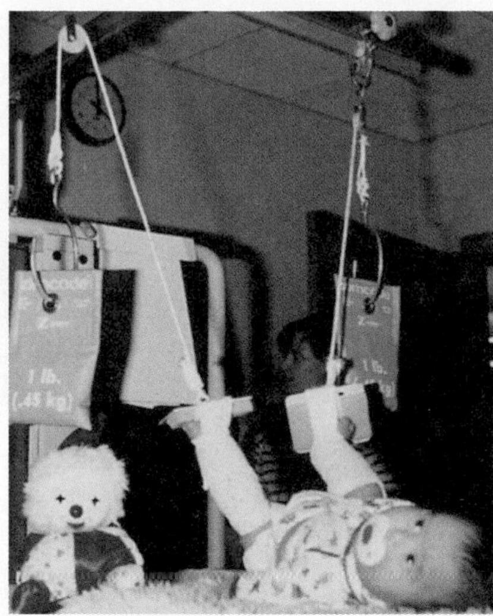

▲ Bryant's traction is used to reduce fractured femur or treat hip dislocation in a small child.

5. Examine traction system to see that the pull aligns with the long axis of the fractured bone.
6. Check the traction mechanism.
   a. Weights should hang freely, off the floor and bed.
   b. Weights are 5–10 lb for adult clients.

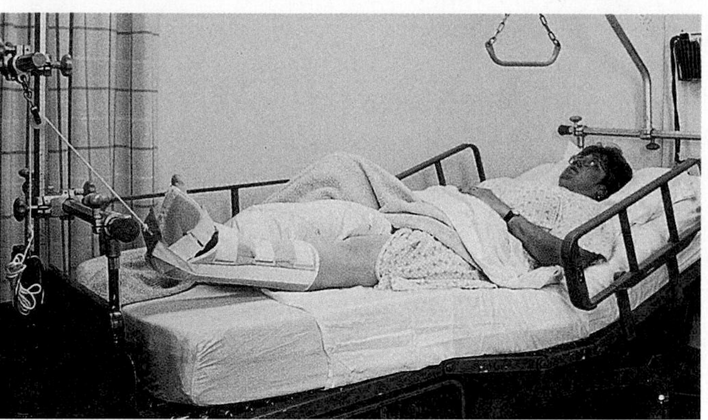

▲ Ensure client is positioned correctly in bed.

   c. Knots should be secure in all ropes.
   d. Ropes should move freely through pulleys.
   e. Pulleys should not be constrained by knots.
7. Position correctly in bed: The client should be positioned in the center of the bed. Affected leg or arm should be aligned with trunk of body. ▶ ***Rationale:*** Misalignment is the leading cause of pain for traction clients. The client should not migrate or be pulled down to the end of the bed because this negates the traction.

TABLE 27-3 Skin Traction

Type	Purpose	Bed Position
Buck's extension	Short-term immobilization of a hip fracture before surgical intervention	Head elevated 10°–20° for ADLs, knee flexed 20°–30°
Cervical	Degenerative or arthritic conditions of cervical vertebrae, neck strain	Flat in bed or head can be elevated 15°–20°
Dunlop	Either skin or skeletal, used for fractured humerus	Flat in bed; arm suspended and flexed
Pelvic girdle	Low back pain, muscle spasm, or herniated disc	Head of bed and knee gatch raised so hips flexed 45° angle (William's position)
Russell's	Used for fractured shaft of femur or lower leg and some knee injuries	Head of bed elevated 30°–45°
Bryant's	Used specifically for child weighing less than 30 lb for fractured femur or hip dysplasia	Flat in bed with both hips flexed at 45°–90°, legs extended and buttocks raised 1 in. from mattress

Maintaining Skeletal Traction

Equipment

Sterile cotton-tipped applicators
Prescribed cleansing agent
Sterile cup for solution
Sterile gloves
Sterile gauze sponges (as ordered)

Preparation

1. Check physician's orders regarding pin site care and client positioning.
2. Check client using two forms of ID.
3. Gather necessary equipment.
4. Perform hand hygiene.
5. Provide privacy and explain procedure to client.

Procedure

1. Check pin and site surrounding the pin.
   a. Pin should be immobile.
   b. Pin site should be clean and dry.

2. Assess for infection at the pin site. Note any local pain, redness, heat, or drainage.
3. Provide pin site care if ordered.
   a. Open applicator sticks and gauze package.
   b. Open prescribed cleansing agent and pour into cup.
   c. Don sterile gloves.
   d. Clean area with prescribed cleansing agent. Soak cotton-tipped applicators. Dip stick into solution bottle, or pour solution over sticks.
   e. Clean pin site starting at insertion area and working outward (away from pin site). ▸ ***Rationale:*** To cleanse site from cleanest to dirtiest area.
   f. Use new applicator stick for cleaning each pin site. ▸ ***Rationale:*** This prevents cross-contamination of sites.
   g. Loosely dress site with separate gauze sponge.
   h. Remove gloves and discard sticks.
   i. Perform hand hygiene.
4. Examine all bony prominences for signs of pressure areas or abrasions.
5. Check for circulation, motion, and sensation in the affected extremity.
6. Assess distal extremity for color and edema.
7. Check ropes and weights to make sure pull goes directly through long axis of the fractured bone. ▸ ***Rationale:*** This pull maintains fracture in alignment.
8. Check traction mechanism.
   a. Weights should hang freely, off the floor and bed.
   b. Knots should be secure in all ropes.
   c. Rope should move freely through pulleys.
   d. Pulleys should not be constrained by knots.

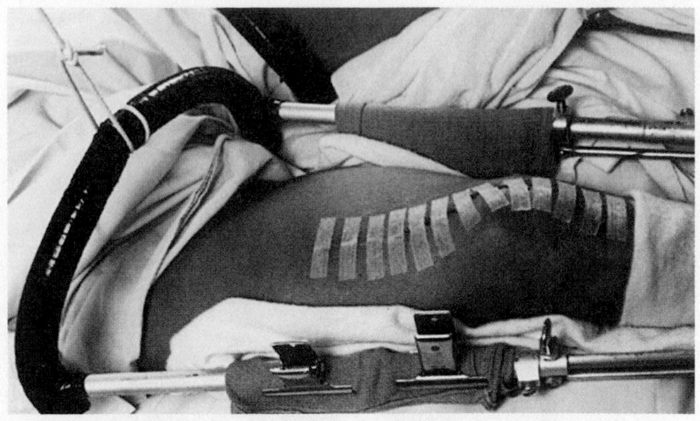

▲ A Thomas splint supports the thigh. It is used for balanced suspension along with skeletal traction for fracture of the femur. A Pearson attachment supports the lower leg.

9. Instruct client to use trapeze correctly to assist in moving in bed and during linen change and back care. ▸ ***Rationale:*** Use of the heel of the unaffected foot for repositioning can cause pressure ulceration. The foot should be placed flat on the bed for assistance in using the trapeze.
10. Make sure client is positioned correctly in bed. ▸ ***Rationale:*** If the client is pulled down to the foot of bed, the traction is negated.
11. Check placement of the foot rest. The client's foot should be correctly positioned to prevent footdrop.
12. Check if client has migrated to foot of bed—pull client up using turn sheet. Do *not* release traction during repositioning.
13. Change bed linen in a top-to-bottom manner while client uses trapeze to lift buttocks.

TABLE 27-4 Skeletal Traction

Type	Purpose	Bed Position
External fixation devices Hoffman Synthes	Manage complex fractures with soft tissue damage; provide stability for severe comminuted fractures	Allows client mobility and active exercise of uninvolved joints
Cervical tongs Crutchfield Gardner–Wells Vinke	Used to immobilize and reduce cervical fractures Tongs maintain alignment of cervical spine	Bedrest, supine position; may be log-rolled
Balanced suspension with Thomas splint and Pearson attachment	Align bone and promote effective line of pull	Bedrest in supine position; may turn side to side for care; knee is flexed

EVIDENCE-BASED PRACTICE

This study examined six randomized controlled trials (349 participants) to assess the effect on infection of different methods of cleansing and dressing pin sites. Three trials compared a cleansing regimen with no cleansing, two trials compared cleansing solutions, one trial compared identical pin site care performed daily or weekly, and four trials compared dressings. One trial reported infection rates were lower (9%) with a regimen that included cleansing with 1/2 strength hydrogen peroxide and application of Xeroform dressing when compared with other regimens (rates >26%). There was no evidence of a difference between groups in any of the other trials.

Authors concluded that there is insufficient evidence for a particular strategy of pin site care that minimizes infection rates.

Lethaby, A., Temple, J., & Santy, J. (2008). Pin site care for preventing infections associated with external bone fixators and pins. *Cochrane Database of Systematic Reviews*, (4), CD004551.

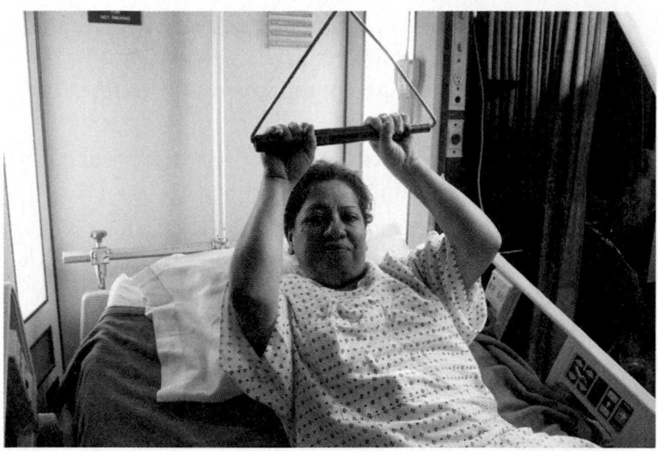

▲ A trapeze attached to an overhead frame facilitates client mobility and nursing care. Client uses both hands for repositioning to avoid twisting and back strain.

Clinical Alert

Skeletal traction is never released without a physician's order.

Stages of Pin-Site Reaction

	Findings	Treatment
Stage I	Copious serous drainage in first 72 hr	Absorbent dressing
Stage II	Superficial cellulitis: erythema, tenderness, swelling around pin	Oral antibiotics
Stage III	Deep infection: purulent drainage, swelling erythema over several pins, loose pins	IV antibiotics Pin removal
Stage IV	Osteomyelitis: loose pin, ring sequestrum on x-ray, persistent drainage	Debridement Long-term IV antibiotics

Source: Patterson, M. (2005). Multicenter pin care study. *Orthopaedic Nursing, 24*(5), 349–360.

Maintaining an External Fixator Device

Equipment

Sterile cotton-tipped applicators
Prescribed cleansing solution
Sterile gloves
Sterile gauze sponges (as ordered)

Procedure

1. Follow steps 1–5 of previous skill.
2. Assess neurovascular status of affected part every 4 hr. ▸ ***Rationale:*** Clients with external fixation devices usually have extensive soft tissue, nerve, and vessel damage.
3. Provide client teaching before discharge.
   a. Instruct client on the importance of, and how to perform, neurovascular checks and when to call the physician.
   b. Demonstrate pin site care. Have client return the demonstration. ▸ ***Rationale:*** To ensure he or she is using appropriate technique.

Clinical Alert

The fixator–fat tissue interface may show fatty drainage that appears with movement of the tissue at the pin site. This should not be confused with purulent drainage.

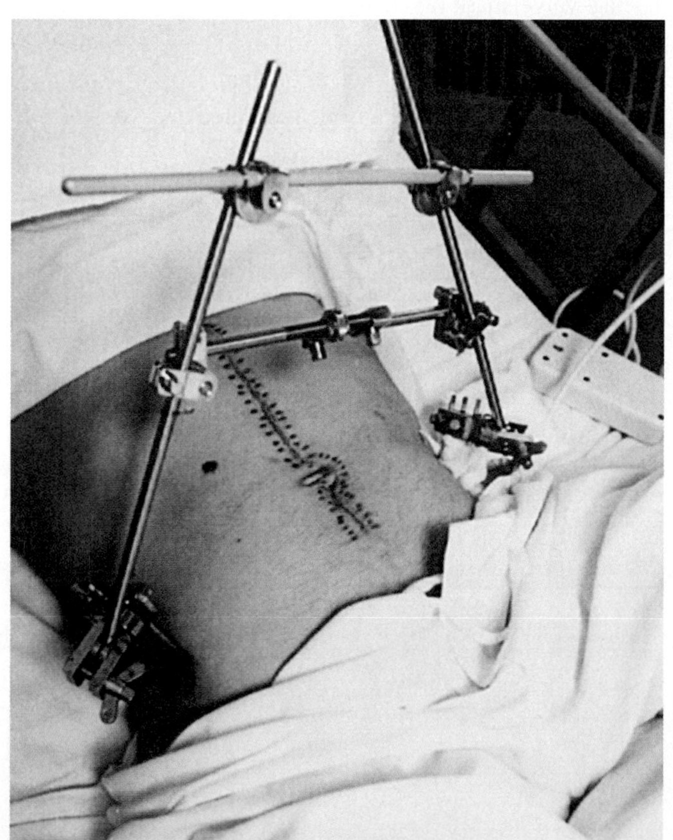

▲ Hoffman frame, external fixator is used for complex fractures and to allow early mobility.

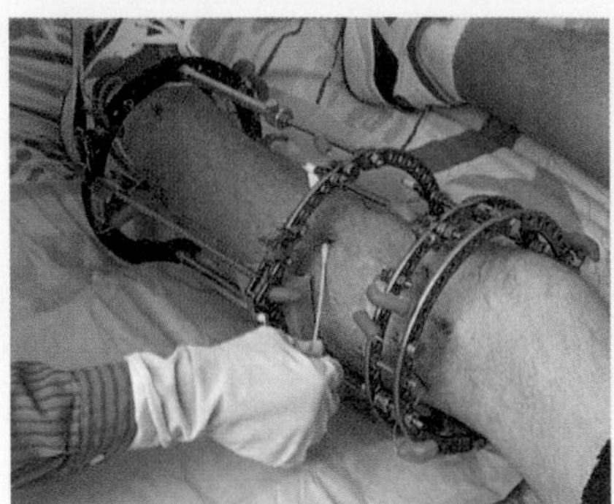

▲ Pin site care for external fixator.

NOTE: Clean technique is used after discharge.

c. Reinforce physician's instructions regarding activity level. Discuss weight bearing on affected limb, if appropriate.

d. Explain that fixator device is not to be used as a handle.

4. Demonstrate range-of-motion exercises, if appropriate, and have client perform return demonstration.
   ▸ ***Rationale:*** To ensure appropriate exercises are being performed correctly.
5. Instruct client to continue to elevate extremity if edema occurs in affected limb.
6. Teach appropriate use of assistive devices as necessary.
   ▸ ***Rationale:*** To prevent falls or inappropriate use of the device, which could cause accidents. Lower-extremity fixators particularly alter the client's balance.

Clinical Alert

The extremity and the external fixator should be moved as a unit, supporting the joint above and below the frame. Repeated lifting and manipulation of the frame itself can lead to pin loosening and fracture malalignment.

Maintaining Halo Traction

Equipment

Allen wrench
Emergency tracheostomy set (available)
Bag–valve–mask (available)
Bright nail polish
Equipment for pin site care, as ordered
Prescribed cleansing solution, as ordered
Sterile cup for solution
Sterile cotton-tipped applicators
Clean gloves

Preparation

1. Review client's history to determine level and type of spinal injury and purpose of halo brace immobilization.

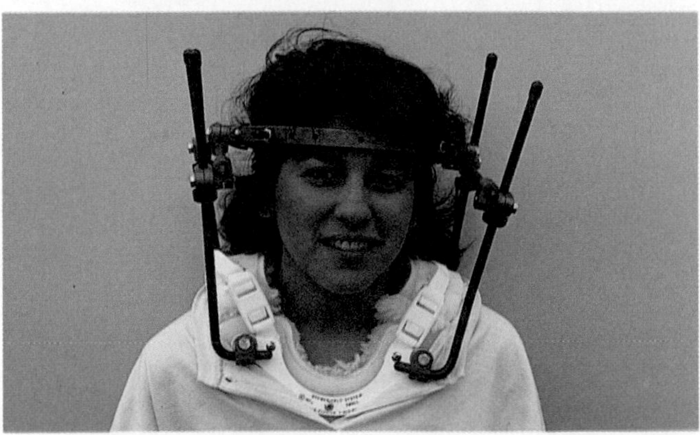

▲ Halo brace traction provides immobilization after cervical or upper thoracic vertebral injury.

2. Determine specific assessment required for the particular client (depends on the level of client's spinal injury). Cervical injury at C3–C5 may compromise ventilation.
3. Gather necessary equipment.
4. Perform hand hygiene.

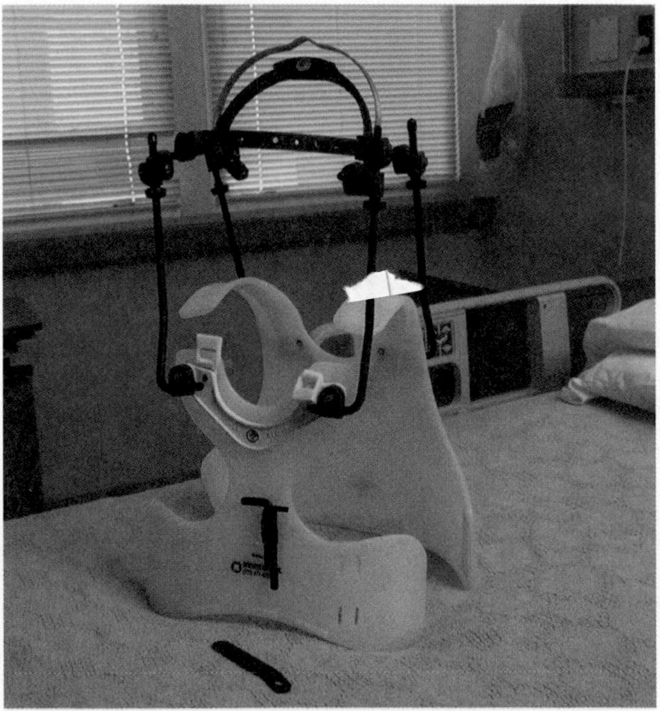

▲ The halo ring is attached to the vest by vertical bars (two in front and two in back). The ring is attached to the skull by two anterior and two posterior pins. Wrench on vest is for emergency release.

Procedure

1. Evaluate client's understanding of halo traction and its purpose.
2. Assess client's respiratory status regularly.
3. Perform complete neurologic assessment (peripheral nerves, motion, and sensation). ***Rationale:*** Because of their location, these nerves are prone to injury or excessive stretching with halo traction.
4. Check alignment of traction–brace system. Client's neck should not be flexed or extended.
5. Discuss safety issues. Halo alters client's center of gravity and balance.
   a. Client has a limited view of the surrounding environment. Pathways for walking must be clear of obstacles.
   b. Consult PT and OT for adaptive aids and tips for ADLs. ▸ ***Rationale:*** Client should anticipate situations and problems that may occur at home such as sleeping position, bathing, and getting in and out of a car.
   c. Keep Allen wrench taped to front of vest. Mark anterior screws that attach vertical bars to brace with bright nail polish. ▸ ***Rationale:*** When marked they are easy to locate. The anterior vest is removed for emergency measures such as CPR.

Clinical Alert
Never use the bars of a halo brace to move the client.

Clinical Alert
If skull pins are loose, apply manual traction and keep client immobilized. Notify physician immediately.

6. Have emergency equipment available for establishing an airway and maintaining ventilation.
7. Suggest that client cover bolts/screws with moleskin or tape to protect clothing.
8. Inspect anterior (above eyebrows) and posterior (above and behind ears) pin sites for signs of drainage, crusting, or inflammation.
9. Provide skin care under vest:
   a. Open vest at both sides during bath.
   b. Check skin at vest edges and where vest overlaps.
   c. Wash and dry skin thoroughly.
   d. Do not use lotion or powder under brace. ▸ ***Rationale:*** They combine with perspiration and irritate the skin.
   e. Replace vest liner if it becomes wet or dirty.
10. Provide pin site care as prescribed. See steps in previous skill for skeletal traction.

DOCUMENTATION for Traction

- Type and location of traction, intermittent, or continuous
- Alignment of traction, client's positioning
- Integrity of the skin
- Circulation, motion, and sensation in extremity
- Specific client concerns and nursing actions taken to solve problems
- Client's comfort and overall feelings
- Pin site, assessment, and care
- Client and family teaching including written materials provided
- Client's progress in self-care

CRITICAL THINKING Application

Expected Outcomes

- Extremity is maintained in correct alignment.
- Neurovascular status is within normal limits.
- Pin site remains free of infection.

Unexpected Outcomes	Alternative Actions
Client in skeletal traction keeps migrating to foot of bed.	• Without releasing traction, use pull sheet and an assistant to reposition client up in bed. • Elevate lower part of bed to provide countertraction. • Increase weight of countertraction at head of bed.
Bone in skeletal traction has migrated to end of Kirschner wire.	• Notify orthopedic surgeon. • Pin will be sterilized and moved so that bone centers on wire. • Review ordered mobility restrictions with client.

Client experiences "tightness" in thigh after fracture of the femur.	• Measure thigh circumference and compare with contralateral thigh. • Assess for presence of ecchymosis. • Monitor vital signs closely for hypovolemia (several units of blood may be sequestered in the thigh after fracture of the femur) • Notify physician for significant changes.
Client in Buck's traction is unable to dorsiflex the foot.	• Release proximal strap as it may be compressing peroneal nerve over head of fibula. • Assess sensation over dorsum of foot and between big and second toes. • Notify physician.
Halo pin site appears to be infected.	• Notify physician. • Obtain culture of drainage for antibiotic sensitivity studies. • Cleanse pin site as prescribed, using aseptic technique, separate applicator for each site. • Remove crusts to allow drainage. • Monitor for systemic signs of infection.

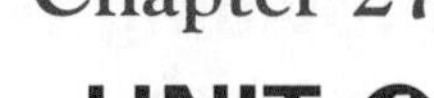

Chapter 27
UNIT 4

Client With Joint Replacement

Nursing Process Data

ASSESSMENT Data Base

- Determine type of joint replacement performed (hemiarthroplasty, total joint arthroplasty).
- Determine surgical approach to total hip arthroplasty (anterolateral or posterolateral)
- Determine whether client has had elective surgery with preoperative preparation.
- Review client's understanding of protective and preventive self-care measures.
- Assess client's progress with clinical path (pain management, activity, client's understanding of expected progress toward discharge).
- Assess that leg position is abducted with pillows or splint.
- Determine whether client uses assistive devices appropriately.

PLANNING Objectives

- To assist the client to progress with self-care after elective joint replacement surgery
- To promote activities that prevent hip dislocation
- To determine that client understands joint motions that could cause joint dislocation
- To encourage use of safety and assistive devices in performing activities of daily living

IMPLEMENTATION Procedures

EVALUATION Expected Outcomes

- Client benefits from autologous reinfusion of wound drainage.
- Client actively participates in elective arthroplasty experience.
- Client describes positions and activities to avoid in order to prevent hip prosthesis dislocation.
- Client voices understanding and demonstrates correct use of assistive devices for ADLs.

Pearson Nursing Student Resources

Find additional review materials at
nursing.pearsonhighered.com

Prepare for success with NCLEX®-style practice questions and Skill Checklists

Providing Wound Suction/Autologous Reinfusion

Equipment

Auto-transfusion reservoir ready for second collection/reinfusion
Standard blood transfusion tube set with 40- or 20-micron filter
200 mL of normal saline for IV tubing and filter prime and flush post reinfusion
Blood (IV therapy) transfusion documentation form
Clean gloves

NOTE: A complete collection reinfusion and wound drainage system accompanies the client from PACU, consisting of a drain tube leading from the client's wound to a suction system (e.g., Hemovac). The suction collection unit is attached to the wound drainage evacuator to produce a vacuum.

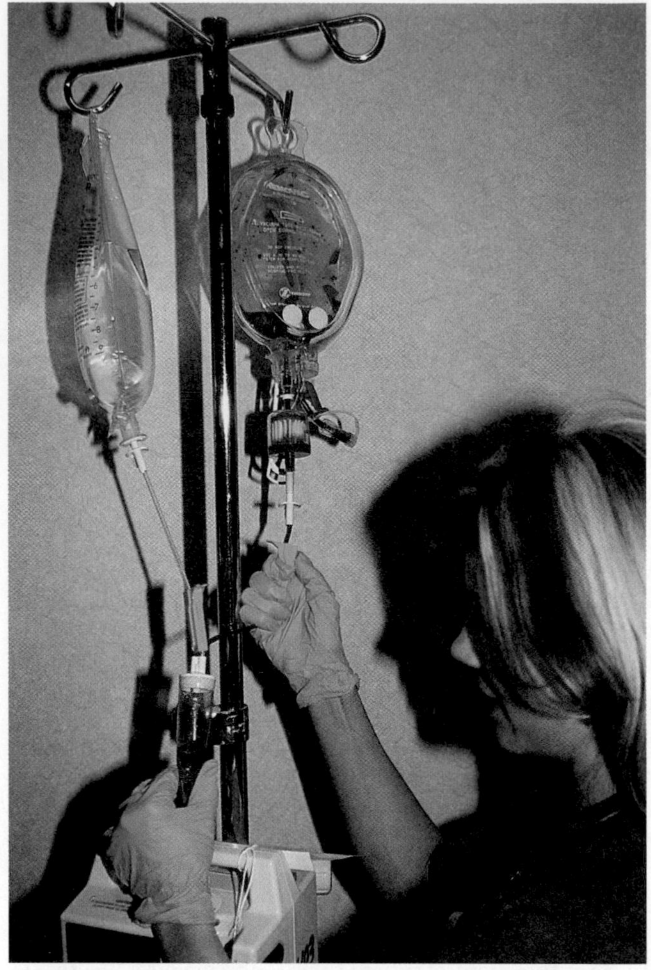

▲ Auto-reinfusion system with filter provides gravity infusion of autologous blood obtained within 6 hr of wound suction activation in the OR.

Preparation

Upon client's return from PACU

1. Review physician's order for reinfusion.
2. Identify time reinfusion system was activated in the OR.
3. Mark time reinfusion should be completed.
4. Identify client using two forms of ID.
5. Ensure that collection reservoir is connected to the wound tubing (done in OR).
6. Ensure that evacuator suction tubing is connected to drainage reservoir and evacuator is compressed for suction.
7. Monitor drainage collection, allowing 4 hr to drain, then 2 hr for reinfusion. ▸ ***Rationale:*** Total reinfusion of blood should be completed within 6 hr of system activation in the OR.

Procedure

For Reinfusion/Establishing New Collection System

NOTE: If physician has ordered to reinfuse a second time, check the reservoir 4 hr after the first reinfusion was started. If greater than 100 mL has been collected, repeat the above Preparation.

1. Don clean gloves.
2. Place new (empty) collection system in a convenient location.
3. Detach the Hemovac evacuator (secured by clip or Velcro) and remove it from the wound drainage collection reservoir.
4. Close both drain clamps on the evacuator tubing.
5. Unscrew the wound drainage tubing clamps on the evacuator tube.
6. Cap the full wound drainage collection reservoir and set it aside.
7. Connect the evacuator tube to new (empty) reinfusion reservoir.
8. Unscrew tubing connecting Hemovac evacuator to full reservoir to be reinfused.
9. Connect Hemovac evacuator tube onto new (empty) collection reservoir.
10. Uncap the Hemovac attachment spout and activate the evacuator, then open the client's wound drain clamp.
11. Mark start time on new collection system.
12. Hang new collection unit on client's bed frame.

For Reinfusion

1. Remove the spike port cap on full reservoir.
2. Insert the filter spike and begin reinfusion.
3. Gravity reinfuse autologous blood within 6 hr of system activation (in OR).
4. Dispose of equipment in biohazard receptacle.
5. Remove gloves and perform hand hygiene.

For Continued Wound Drainage

1. Connect client's wound drainage tubing to Hemovac evacuator and activate to initiate suction.
2. Empty evacuator every 8 hr.
3. Remove gloves and perform hand hygiene.

Caring for a Client With Posterolateral Approach Hip Arthroplasty

Equipment

Abductor pillow ("wedge") or pillows (posterolateral approach)
Non-rotation boot (if ordered)
Bath blanket
Poster reminder for exercises
Walker
Toilet seat extender
Adaptive aids

Preparation

1. Identify client and assess client's understanding of postoperative expectations.
2. Determine what instructions client has received. ▸ ***Rationale:*** To reinforce and not contradict previous teaching. The client may be included in an acute care group exercise program.

Procedure

For Bed Positioning

1. Maintain body in alignment using abductor pillow or wedge. ▸ ***Rationale:*** The abductor serves as a reminder to keep legs in abduction to prevent dislocation of the prosthesis.
   a. Place narrow end of wedge between the thighs, above the knees, as high as possible.
   b. Place legs flush with sides of wedge and strap into place above the knee and above the ankle. ▸ ***Rationale:*** Avoid pressure over joints where nerves and vessels are superficial.

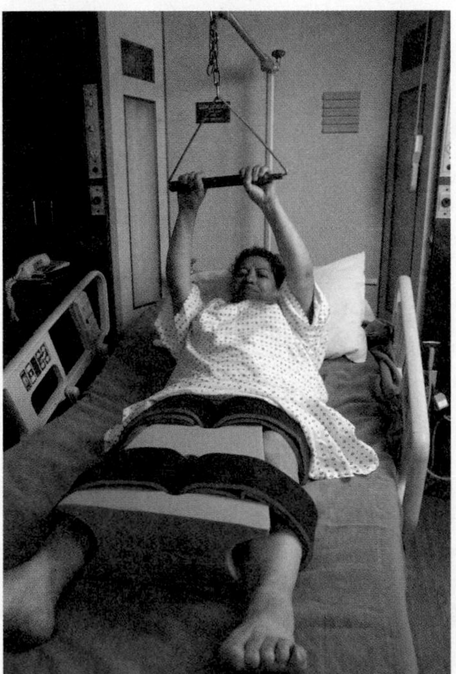

▲ The abduction wedge or pillow prevents hip adduction and internal rotation to prevent dislocation after hemiarthroplasty or posterolateral approach total hip arthroplasty.

   c. If abductor has separate leg straps, the *unoperated* side may be loosened for comfort and to allow range of motion while client is supine.
2. Place rolled soft blanket or towel under ankles to free heels from the mattress. ▸ ***Rationale:*** To prevent skin breakdown.
3. Turn client every 2 hr, keeping legs abducted with both legs strapped. *Although not generally contraindicated, review surgeon's orders before turning client to operated side.*
4. Maintain non-rotation boot (if indicated) while client is supine, but remove when client is turned. ▸ ***Rationale:*** This boot with bar prevents hip rotation.
5. Encourage standard postoperative preventive measures such as deep breathing, foot pumps, and ankle rotations.
6. Encourage strengthening exercises such as gluteal sets and quadriceps sets.
7. Assess CMS and skin integrity at least every 4 hr.

For Strengthening Exercises

1. Place an exercise reminder sign at foot of bed. Have client hold muscle contraction for a count of 5 and repeat 10 times, then increase hold and number of repetitions each day (may do during commercials if watching TV).
2. Quadriceps strengthening:
   Have client push back of the knee into bed. ▸ ***Rationale:*** This contracts muscle on top of the thigh. The quadriceps muscle is used to rise to a standing position, to climb stairs, and to walk.
3. Gluteal strengthening:
   a. Have client squeeze buttocks together tightly and hold for a count of 5 and repeat 10 times. ▸ ***Rationale:*** These exercises help strengthen muscles surrounding the hip.
   b. While standing, move operated leg backward, placing one hand on lower back to prevent arching, then return leg to starting position.
   c. While standing, move operated leg laterally (out to the side), keeping foot and knee pointing straight forward, then return to starting position.

EVIDENCE-BASED PRACTICE

Preparing for Total Hip/Knee Arthroplasty

Preoperative exercise has been shown to reduce postoperative complications and length of stay for cardiac and abdominal surgery patients. This review of research literature from 1998–2008 (three studies met inclusion) found that evidence is inconclusive regarding preoperative exercise benefits for patients having THA or TKA. This was due to lack of functional measurements and small sample size in two of the studies. One of the studies did show that the exercise group had more patients discharged to home rather than to a rehabilitation unit. Additional research is needed.

Barbay, K. (2009). Research evidence for the use of preoperative exercise in patients preparing for total hip or total knee arthroplasty. *Orthopaedic Nursing, 28*(3), 127–133.

For Mobility and Dislocation Prevention

1. Assist client to get out of bed.

NOTE: A physical therapist usually supervises and assists with the first time out of bed.

a. Raise bed to high position. ▸ ***Rationale:*** This allows client to exit bed without acute hip flexion.
b. Elevate head of bed and instruct client to exit bed from unoperated side. ▸ ***Rationale:*** The stronger side should lead a transfer.
c. Have client pivot on hips, while keeping legs abducted, and sit on edge of bed with operated leg out in front. Do not allow client to bend forward and push down to stand. ▸ ***Rationale:*** Bending forward may cause prosthesis dislocation.
d. Assist client by supporting operative leg.
e. Have client push down with hands on mattress to rise to a standing position. Walker should not be used for support when rising to a standing position.
f. Walk client first postoperative day (as ordered) with an assistant and a walker with weight bearing as tolerated.

2. Instruct client about positions to avoid.

NOTE: Gluteal isometrics strengthen muscles that surround the joint capsule and decrease the risk of dislocation.

a. Do not cross the legs at ankle or knee. Keep knees apart at all times. ▸ ***Rationale:*** Adduction can cause prosthesis dislocation.
b. Do not stand with toes turned in. ▸ ***Rationale:*** Internal rotation can cause prosthesis dislocation.
c. Do not flex hips greater than 90°. Always sit with knees lower than hips. Avoid low chairs and do not bend over. Use toilet seat extender (elevator). ▸ ***Rationale:*** Flexion beyond 90° can cause prosthesis dislocation.
d. Do not sit in bathtub. Use a standing shower or shower/tub chair.
e. When standing and turning is necessary, turn toward unoperated side. ▸ ***Rationale:*** Turning toward operated hip can cause hip dislocation due to internal rotation.

For Assistive Devices and Adaptive Aids

1. Consult physical therapy and occupational therapist to obtain a walker, client instruction, and supervised ambulation and activity precautions.

Clinical Alert

Hip prosthesis dislocation usually requires a simultaneous combination of contraindicated hip positions, such as crossing the legs and acutely flexing at the same time. Dislocation precautions are continued until the joint capsule has healed. Only the orthopedic surgeon should advise clients when and if precautions are no longer necessary.

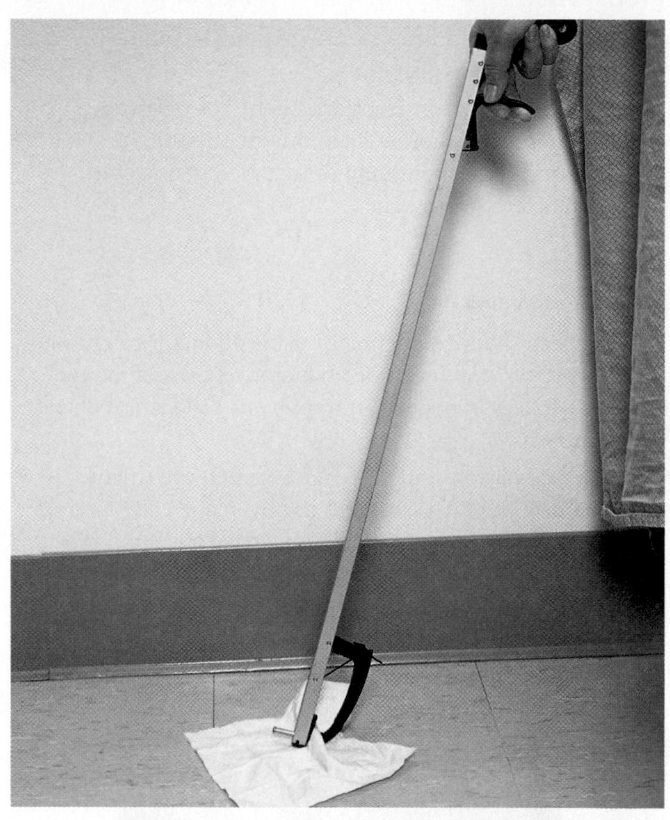

▲ Adaptive aids, such as a reacher, facilitate independence in ADLs.

TABLE 27-5 Total Hip Arthroplasty Precautions Differ with Surgical Approach

Posterolateral Approach	Anterolateral Approach
Keep leg in abduction and extension (pillow or wedge often used).	Sitting at 90° is allowed. Avoid active abduction.
Avoid flexion of the hip beyond 90° angle. If while sitting you can put your hands on your legs below your knees, that's too much flexion.	Keep legs side by side without a wedge or pillow between them.
Do not bend at the waist to put on shoes.	Avoid turning toes and knee outward. Do not extend the leg backward.
Keep needed items on the nonoperative side. Use a toilet elevator (21 in.) and shower chair. Do not cross the operative leg past the body's midline. Do not inwardly rotate the operative leg.	Place needed items on operative side.
To turn while standing, turn away from the operative side.	To turn while standing, turn toward the operative side.

2. Consult occupational therapy for provision and instruction in use of adaptive aids such as toilet seat extender, reachers, sock aid, long-handled sponge, and shoehorn. Instruct client to avoid wearing shoes with laces that must be tied.

Clinical Alert

The client undergoing hemiarthroplasty (replacement of the femoral head and neck) for fracture of the femur must adhere to the same precautions as the elective total hip replacement client to prevent prosthesis dislocation.

3. Discuss home safety adaptations which client may have already installed in preparation for *elective* surgery: toilet extender (21 in.), elevated chair seats, shower or tub chair, safety rails, removal of loose rugs and electrical cords, placement of frequently used items within easy reach.

Clinical Alert

Because of changes in the skin that occur with aging, older clients are at increased risk for blistering and accidental removal of the epidermis by mechanical means such as tape removal. Tape should be applied vertically only, and without tension.

Caring for a Client With Knee Arthroplasty

Equipment

Knee splint immobilizer

CPM device or rocking glider chair

Preparation

See previous skill.

Procedure

For Continuous Passive Motion

1. Assist client to comfortable position. Client may turn from side to side and may have head of bed up or down. There is little risk of dislocation of knee prosthesis.
2. Place pillows lengthwise under lower leg, but not under knee.
3. Apply soft foam knee immobilizer or brace (if ordered).
   a. Place wide strap over knee.
   b. Allow client to direct tightness of fit.
   c. Monitor surgical wound drainage output frequently for the first 48 hr postoperatively.
   d. Assess CMS and skin integrity at least every 4 hr while splint is in place.

▲ CPM (continuous passive motion) device may be used to increase joint mobility after knee surgery.

For Postoperative Exercises

1. Maintain accurate positioning of continuous *passive* motion device, if ordered, to gently flex knee by adjusted increments. Settings start at 10°–30° and are gradually increased until 90° of flexion is achieved.
   ▸ ***Rationale:*** CPM may prevent adhesion formation and improve range of joint motion during early postoperative period.
2. *Alternate:* Client may use a rocking glider chair.
   ▸ ***Rationale:*** This encourages independent *active knee flexion and extension*, which has added benefit of getting the client out of bed, improving venous return, reducing edema formation, and preventing clot formation and other complications of bedrest.
3. Encourage foot pumps, straight leg raising, ankle rotations, quadriceps, and gluteal sets as for client with a total hip replacement.

For Getting Out of Bed

1. Assist client to pivot and sit on side of the bed, supporting the leg.
2. Unless brace is worn, encourage client to alternate bending and straightening the knee. Flex unaffected leg to support weight to a standing position while keeping operative leg extended.
3. Weight bearing as tolerated with an assistant and use of a walker is usually allowed first postoperative day.
4. A raised seat will assist client to get in and out of a chair.

Clinical Alert

There may be an increase in wound bleeding when initiating knee flexion exercises (CPM or mobilizing client).

Clinical Alert

Infection is a grave complication with joint replacement surgery. It may occur during the first 3 months postoperatively or even after a year. Late infection is usually due to hematogenous spread from a distant site (teeth, GI, or urinary tract).

Clients should remind their physicians and dentists about their prosthesis; antibiotics may be prescribed before dental work or other invasive procedure to prevent infection.

EVIDENCE-BASED PRACTICE

Continuous Passive Motion

Studies on the use of continuous passive motion (CPM) have not clearly identified its use as best practice. There are no differences in range of motion, edema, drainage, and the amount of pain experienced in clients who use and those who do not use CPM. Differences may relate to initiation of therapy, hours of use, length of time used, use of a knee immobilizer.

Source: Roberts, D. (2002). Degenerative disorders. In A.B. Maher, S. W. Salmond, & T.A. Pellino (Eds), *Orthopaedic Nursing*. Philadelphia: Saunders.

DOCUMENTATION for Client With Joint Replacement

- Character and amount of wound drainage
- Auto-reinfusion times and amounts on I&O record as output from a drainage system and intake as a blood product
- Wound assessment findings
- Character and amount of wound drainage
- Client positioning and frequency of turning
- Neurovascular and skin status of involved extremity
- Placement of abductor splint or brace
- Use of continuous passive motion or rocking glider chair
- Exercises performed: type, duration, and client's tolerance
- Client and family teaching and teaching materials aids provided
- Client's understanding of teaching (return demonstration of preventive measures), use of assistive devices and other aids

CRITICAL THINKING Application

Expected Outcomes

- Client benefits from autologous reinfusion of wound drainage.
- Client actively participates in elective arthroplasty experience.
- Client describes positions and activities to avoid in order to prevent hip prosthesis dislocation.
- Client voices understanding and demonstrates correct use of assistive devices for ADLs.

Unexpected Outcomes	Alternative Actions
Client's hemoglobin lab result remains less than 10 g/dL after reinfusion.	• Notify physician of lab results. • Obtain order for type and cross and type for possible allogenic blood transfusion.
Client with knee arthroplasty is fearful of dislocation.	• Assure client that, in contrast to hip arthroplasty, knee dislocation rarely occurs. • Encourage client to continue quadriceps and gluteal setting and knee flexion/ extension exercises. • Consult with physical therapist regarding client's concerns/need for reassurance and encouragement.
Client is unable to remember instructions for hip precautions.	• Provide written instructions with pictures of positions to avoid. • Request occupational therapist to work with client and caregiver to reinforce instructions/precautions. • Request Social Service consult for postoperative rehabilitation living needs. • Request OT consult for individualized assessment and recommendations/teaching.

Client with hip arthroplasty asks about adapting ADLs to accommodate hip precautions.	• Suggest purchasing a raised toilet seat before leaving hospital (many agencies sell these). • Use a standing shower or tub with shower chair for bathing. • Wear lace-up shoes with elastic laces so tying is not required and the foot can be slipped in with a long-handled shoe horn. • Purchase reachers or long barbecue tongs to retrieve things from the floor. • Place frequently used items at arm level so bending is not required. • Remove scatter rugs, electric cords, and small objects from the floor. • Move car seat back as far as possible. Keep operated leg out in front, slide back into seat, then semi-recline and pivot to face front of car.

Chapter 27

UNIT 5

Client With an Amputation

Nursing Process Data

ASSESSMENT Data Base

- Determine whether amputation was therapeutic or traumatic.
- Determine rationale for therapeutic amputation (tumor, peripheral vascular disease, diabetes).
- Assess status of stump wound.
- Assess stump positioning.
- Inspect stump for presence of edema.
- Assess for phantom sensation or phantom pain.
- Assess client's acceptance of amputation.

PLANNING Objectives

- To promote wound healing
- To reduce edema and discomfort
- To prevent contracture development
- To mold and prepare stump for prosthesis use
- To assist the client in acceptance and self-care

IMPLEMENTATION Procedures

EVALUATION Expected Outcomes

- Stump wound heals without complication.
- Stump maintains functional alignment.
- Stump is prepared for prosthesis use.

Positioning and Exercising the Stump

Equipment

Pillows

Preparation

1. Check chart for physician's orders.
2. Identify client and explain purpose of positioning and exercising.
3. Provide privacy.
4. Perform hand hygiene.

Procedure

For Preoperative Care

1. Evaluate nutritional status and request nutritional consult if indicated. ▸ ***Rationale:*** Adequate protein is necessary to promote wound healing.
2. Recruit assistance of OT, PT, and social worker for early multidisciplinary care planning. A prosthetist explains future prosthetic care to the client and possibly organizes amputee peer visit, as this helps lessen anxiety about living with an amputation.
3. Explain importance of exercises to client. Tell client that because flexor muscles are stronger than extensors, stump will be permanently flexed and abducted unless the client practices extension and adduction exercises. ▸ ***Rationale:*** Exercises increase muscle strength and improve mobility of amputated extremity. Both are necessary for optimal ambulation with a prosthesis.
4. Teach client quadriceps-setting exercises with a below-the-knee amputation.
   a. Extend leg and try to push back of knee into bed; try to move patella proximally.
   b. Contract quadriceps and hold contraction for 10 seconds.
   c. Repeat this procedure four or five times.
   d. Repeat the exercise at least four times a day.
5. Teach use of ambulatory aids. ▸ ***Rationale:*** Prepares client for post-surgery mobility.
6. Explain phantom limb sensation; the client may continue to "feel" the lost limb after surgery.

Clinical Alert
Adequate pain management in the preoperative period can reduce the occurrence of phantom limb pain postoperatively.

Clinical Alert
Keep a tourniquet nearby in the event of excessive stump incision bleeding.

7. Counsel families, for they also mourn the loss of a visible body part. ▸ ***Rationale:*** They too need psychological support and education about rehabilitation and necessary skills for self-care.

For Postoperative Care

1. Monitor for complications: hemorrhage, infection, unrelieved pain, wound that will not heal.
2. Assess for excessive wound drainage. Keep tourniquet at bedside. ▸ ***Rationale:*** If excessive bleeding occurs, tourniquet must be applied, as hemorrhage is a potentially life-threatening complication.
3. Administer ordered pain medication and continually assess to determine whether pain is controlled.
4. Do not place stump on pillow, but elevate foot of bed for first 24 hr ONLY to reduce stump edema and pain. ▸ ***Rationale:*** Elevation on a pillow can promote flexion contracture of stump.
5. Turn client to prone or supine position for at least 1 hr every 4 hr. ▸ ***Rationale:*** This promotes hip extension and helps counteract possible flexion contracture formation.
6. Avoid dependent positioning of stump. ▸ ***Rationale:*** To prevent edema and discomfort. Edema may be present for up to 4 months after amputation.
7. While washing the stump, tap and massage the stump skin toward the incision line. ▸ ***Rationale:*** To prevent development of painful adhesions.
8. Teach stump extension exercises.
   a. Lie in a prone position with foot hanging over the end of the bed.
   b. Keep stump next to intact leg to extend stump and to contract gluteal muscles.
   c. Hold the contraction for 10 seconds.
   d. Repeat this exercise at least four times a day.
9. Teach adduction exercise.
   a. Place a pillow between the client's thighs.
   b. Squeeze the pillow for 10 seconds and then relax for 10 seconds.
   c. Repeat this exercise at least four times a day.
10. Have the client keep track of time spent with the stump flexed and then spend an equal amount of time with the stump extended.
11. Encourage appropriate use of trapeze: Use both hands to pull up with trapeze; place foot flat on mattress to lift body. Do not use heel to push in the mattress. ▸ ***Rationale:*** Pushing with the heel can lead to pressure ulcers.
12. After stump incision heals, have client begin to bear weight on stump, initially pressing into padded surface (pillow on chair seat). ▸ ***Rationale:*** To reduce pain and help prepare the stump for prosthesis.

Shrinking/Molding the Stump

Equipment

Two elastic bandages: 4 in. for below-the-knee amputation (BKA), 6 in. for above-the-knee amputation (AKA)

Tape or safety pins

Commercial stump shrinker (sheath)

Preparation

1. Review client's chart to determine date and type of amputation.
2. Gather equipment.
3. Identify client using two forms of ID and explain rationale for procedure.
4. Perform hand hygiene.
5. Provide privacy.

Procedure

1. Wash stump with soap and water and allow to dry for at least 10 minutes before bandaging. Do not use lotions, powders, or alcohol.
2. Inspect and encourage client to assess stump for circulatory status, pressure areas, wound healing, and edema.
3. Explain that purpose of wrap is to form a conical AKA stump to prepare for prosthesis use.
4. Explain that wrap is to be worn at all times except during bathing or when wearing a prosthesis.
5. Start by placing bandage end outer surface on distal stump. ▸ ***Rationale:*** The pressure gradient of the bandage should be greatest at the distal stump.
6. Wrap bandage medially and diagonally around stump. Have client assist by holding turns. Stretch bandages to two-thirds of the limit of the elastic.
7. Continue to wrap smoothly up the stump with medially directed spirals or figure eight turns (not circular). Progress up the stump and well into groin area. ▸ ***Rationale:*** Circular turns constrict circulation. Medial turns help correct stump tendency toward abduction.
8. Finish bandaging with a "spica" turn over and around the client's pelvis, then back down to stump. ▸ ***Rationale:*** Large "spica" turn prevents bandage slipping.
9. Secure the bandage with tape or (*cautiously*) with safety pins. Do not use bandage clips. ▸ ***Rationale:*** Clips can pierce the skin or easily come loose.
10. Reapply elastic bandage every 4–6 hr or when loose. ▸ ***Rationale:*** It must never be in place for more than 12 hr without being rewrapped.
11. If client has a stump "shrinker sheath," roll down and stretch the sheath using plastic ring. Fit onto stump end and apply, making sure there are no wrinkles.
12. Teach client home care of residual limb and prosthesis (washing; assessing for redness, pressure points, irritation, swelling skin breakdown; socket, stump, socks, liners, mechanical parts, etc.).

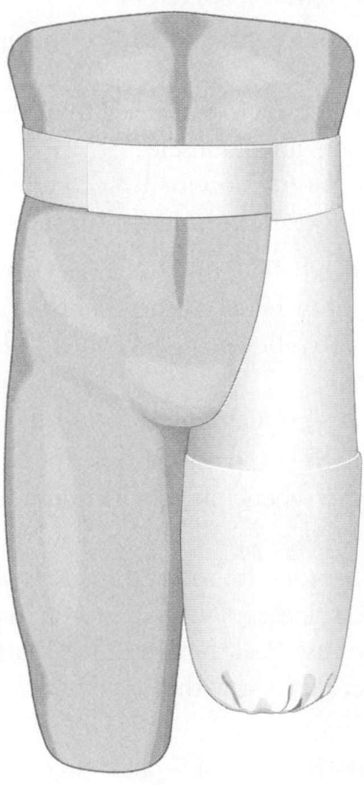

▲ "Commercial shrinkers" may be used for above-the-knee amputations (AKA).

Clinical Alert

Amputees use more energy in ambulation than nonamputees. The elderly with an AKA must put forth an effort 100% above normal to walk at a slow rate. The longer the residual limb, the less energy the client must expend for ambulation.

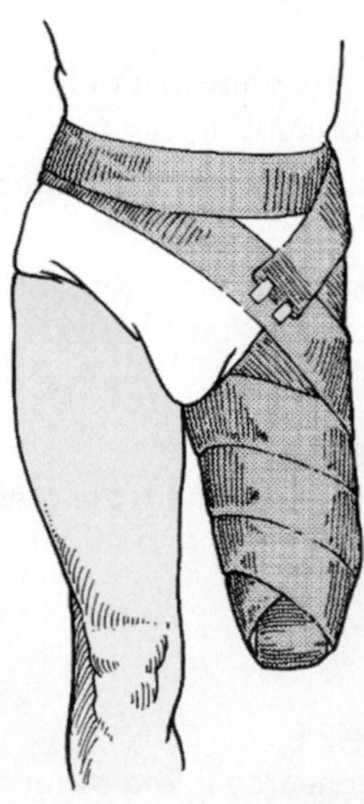

▲ Compression bandage may be used after amputation to mold and shrink stump in preparation for prosthesis.

DOCUMENTATION for Client With an Amputation

- Time, type, and site of bandage application
- Stump positioning
- Stump and wound assessment
- Exercises performed
- Client teaching
- Client's response to stump and participation in self-care

CRITICAL THINKING Application

Expected Outcomes

- Stump wound heals without complications.
- Stump maintains functional alignment.
- Stump is prepared for prosthesis use.

Unexpected Problems	Alternative Actions
Client sits in chair most of the day and keeps stump elevated on a pillow while in bed.	• Discuss hip and knee contracture complications that occur with prolonged flexion positioning of the stump. • Review and reinforce exercises that promote stump adduction and extension to prevent contractures and facilitate prosthesis use.
Stump edema occurs in spite of compression bandage application.	• Evaluate wrapping procedure. • Ensure that wraps are applied with pressure greater at distal stump and reapplied several times a day. • Instruct client to avoid prolonged dependent positioning of stump. • Consult prosthetist for possible rigid shrinker use. • Apply shrinker before client gets out of bed.
Client expresses fear of losing other leg.	• Teach client to care for the remaining extremity. • Inspect for lesions; wash and dry daily; use lotion for dry skin (not between toes); keep nails trimmed straight across; avoid mechanical, chemical, or thermal injury; wear shoes that are wide and deep enough for toes. • Avoid smoking; exercise daily. • Consult podiatrist for individual foot care or shoe orthotic adaptations, especially if diabetic. • Consult physician for management of diabetes or atherosclerosis.

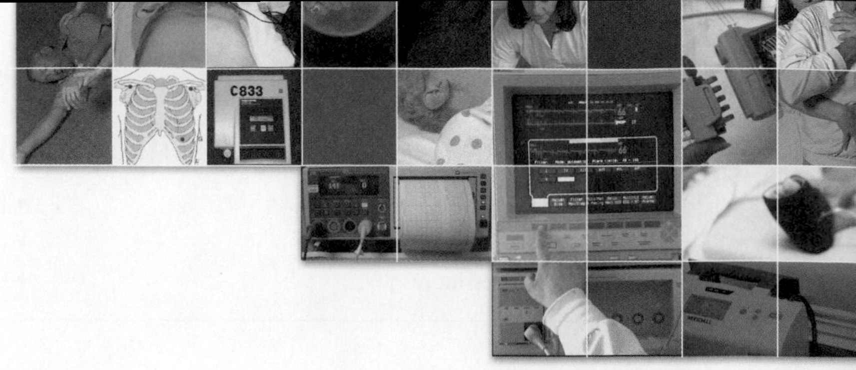

Chapter 27

UNIT 6

Stryker Frame

Nursing Process Data

ASSESSMENT Data Base

- Determine client's musculoskeletal and neurologic status.
- Evaluate client's understanding of turning procedure.
- Assess client alignment and security of device.
- Evaluate client's ability to assist with turning.

PLANNING Objectives

- To turn client horizontally from supine to prone to supine positions
- To provide optimal skin care for immobilized clients
- To prevent pressure areas and pressure ulcers
- To provide optimal nursing care to clients with skin grafts or other conditions that require minimum client movement

IMPLEMENTATION Procedures

EVALUATION Expected Outcomes

- Client turns horizontally without torsion or abnormal flexion/extension of the spine.
- Client receives optimal skin care without developing pressure ulcers.
- Client receives optimal nursing care for skin grafts or neurologic condition.

Using a Stryker Wedge Turning Frame

Equipment

Stryker wedge turning frame
Armrests and footboard
Software: mattress, canvases, linen, straps
Safety straps
Pillows and sheepskin (if used)

Procedure

1. Explain procedure to client.
2. Show client the Stryker frame before placing on the frame.
3. Position the posterior frame at the bottom of the turning circle.
4. Place client supine on the posterior frame (using the three-man carry transfer method, if necessary).
5. If client is on a backboard, place client and board on the posterior frame.
6. Attach the anterior frame.
7. Turn client and remove the backboard.
8. Reverse the procedure, and turn client to his or her back.

NOTE: The Stryker frame has been infrequently used for the past 10 years. However, due to increased numbers of spinal instrumentation procedures, the new Stryker wedge turning frame is again being used after surgery in many parts of the country.

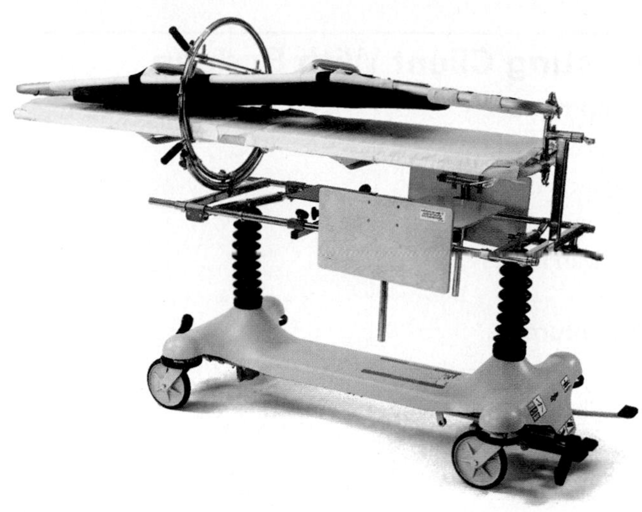

▲ Stryker wedge turning frame.

Turning From Supine to Prone

Procedure

1. Explain procedure to client. This procedure requires only one person; however, it is advisable to have two people when possible.
2. Position sheepskin, pillows, or comfort aids on top of client.
3. With client on posterior frame, open the turning circle and put head end of anterior frame on the securing bolt and fasten it with the nut.
4. Fasten the foot end of the anterior frame with the nut, making sure that client's legs and feet are correctly positioned.
5. Have client clasp hands around anterior frame. If client is unable to do this, put a safety strap around the whole frame at elbow level to keep arms contained.
6. Close the turning circle until it locks.
7. Move the armrests down out of the way of the turn.
8. Pull out the bed-turning lock.
9. Turn the frame toward the client's right until it locks automatically. The narrow side of the wedge (at the client's right) always turns down. The frame automatically locks when the bottom frame is horizontal.
10. Open the turning circle, unscrew the nuts, and remove the upper posterior frame. Relock the turning circle for safety.
11. To turn the client on the Stryker wedge from prone to supine, reverse procedure for turning from supine to prone. Remember that the narrow side of the wedge (on client's right) always turns down so client cannot slip out.

Using a Stryker Parallel Frame

Equipment

Stryker parallel frame
Armrests and footboard
Software: mattress, canvases, linen, straps
Safety straps
Pillows and sheepskins

Procedure

1. Place a pillow lengthwise over the client's legs to prevent moving during turning.
2. Attach the anterior frame to the main frame using the two nuts on the turning circle. Make sure the client is held firmly between the frames.

3. Put three safety straps around the frame at level of knees, waist, and elbows. Tighten securely.
4. With a person at each end of the frame, pull out the locking pins at the center of each end, turn the frame slightly to hold the lock open, and then quickly finish turning the client. The bed automatically locks when the bottom frame is horizontal.
5. Remove the top frame and reposition the client for comfort.

Assisting Client With Bedpan

Equipment

Special bedpan
Plastic drape
Towels
Clean gloves

Procedure

1. Explain procedure to client.
2. Place client in a supine position.
3. Don clean gloves.
4. Drop the center section of the posterior frame by releasing the hooks or rubber bands from the sides of the frame.
5. Protect the linen by putting plastic or towels around the edges.
6. Insert the bedpan into the opening and hold securely with hands or with the arm supports.
7. Remove the bedpan, clean the client, and reattach the center section of the frame.
8. Clean bedpan and replace in storage area.
9. Remove gloves and discard.
10. Perform hand hygiene.

DOCUMENTATION for Stryker Frame

- Time and frequency of turning
- How client tolerates turning procedure
- Neuro assessment findings
- Neurovascular status
- Status of the traction apparatus, if indicated
- Vital signs
- Skin assessment

CRITICAL THINKING Application

Expected Outcomes

- Client turns horizontally without torsion or abnormal flexion/extension of the spine.
- Client receives optimal skin care without developing pressure ulcers.
- Client receives optimal nursing care for skin grafts or neurologic condition.

Unexpected Outcomes	Alternative Actions
The client expresses fear of being turned.	• Encourage client to be on frame and be turned before surgery. • Explain each step of the turning process and the use of each piece of equipment. • Allow client to express fears and concerns. • Carefully answer all questions in a way that the client can understand.
The client experiences unusual pain or discomfort when turned.	• Have the client describe details of pain. • Assess the client's neurologic status and compare it with the client's status before turning. • Ensure that the traction apparatus is intact. • Notify physician if pain persists or if there is a change in neurologic status.

GERONTOLOGIC Considerations

Musculoskeletal integrity can be enhanced and therapeutic goals reached if the aging effect on the musculoskeletal system is appreciated and incorporated into individualized care planning.

Elderly clients generally experience:

- Decreased height
- More brittle bones, decreased density
- Reduced muscle mass
- Diminished strength
- Joint stiffening
- Weakness and slowed movement
- Thinning of the dermis and structures supporting the junction of the epidermis and dermis weaken. Older clients are at increased risk for blistering and epidermal stripping.
- Slower and less effective healing, which may result in greater incidence of malunion and nonunion after fracture

Elderly clients are at high risk for falls and musculoskeletal injury as a result of:

- Weakness and being easily fatigued
- Unsteady balance, gait, and alterations in posture
- Poor eyesight
- Altered mobility resulting from medications or use of assistive device
- Increased time on bedrest, leading to muscle weakness
- Presence of chronic disease

Active elderly clients may seek joint replacement surgery to:

- Decrease pain
- Increase mobility
- Continue an active life

MANAGEMENT Guidelines

Each state legislates a Nurse Practice Act for RNs and LVN/LPNs. Healthcare facilities are responsible for establishing and implementing policies and procedures that conform to their state's regulations. Verify the regulations and role parameters for each healthcare worker in your facility.

Delegation

- All healthcare workers can be assigned to clients with orthopedic conditions for nursing tasks associated with activities of daily living. Occupational and Physical Therapists are assigned to the more complex tasks of ambulating and teaching clients with hip replacements, clients requiring assistive devices to ambulate, etc.
- Some facilities employ orthopedic technicians who set up and monitor traction, assist with cast application, bivalve or removal and help with transfer.

Communication Matrix

- The RN needs to assess the skill level of all staff assigned to clients requiring assistive devices or special equipment. Documentation of the skill level for the staff should be available on the unit. This is a major safety factor for all staff assigned to orthopedic clients.
- When new equipment is purchased, and before it is put into service, the manufacturer should provide in-service education to all staff to prevent damage to the equipment and promote safety in client care.
- Most orthopedic clients are followed by a multidisciplinary care team, which includes physicians, nurses, physical and occupational therapists, and social workers. The team use the client's DRG related "clinical path" as an action plan for coordinating hospital, discharge, and subacute setting or home care services. Variances can be identified as the client moves through the sequences of specific interventions that promote timely discharge. Such collaboration requires open and ongoing communication among all members of the team. Special documentation forms may be used to facilitate this process.
- The nurse "Patient Care Coordinator" oversees the client's progress and brings multidisciplinary issues to the physician's attention so that the "path" can be individualized to reflect the client's unique needs.
- Assistive personnel (aides, orthopedic technicians) must be informed of any restriction in client positioning or mobility. They should report any noted changes in the client's condition or problem with any immobilizing device or equipment to the RN so that further assessment and problem solving can be conducted.
- On-coming staff should receive information about the client's progress toward satisfaction of expected outcomes, any unexpected variance that impedes the client's progress toward discharge, and any change in the medical plan of care.

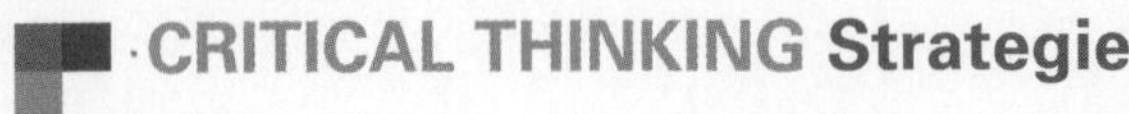

CRITICAL THINKING Strategies

Scenario 1

Your orthopedic unit has just admitted an 84-year-old female, Nora James. She was brought to the ED after a fall in the grocery store. Her admitting diagnosis is "intertrochanteric fracture of the left hip." She is scheduled for hip "nailing" surgery as soon as she is cleared by her primary physician, cardiologist, and anesthesiologist.

1. What behaviors would you expect to see upon initial assessment of Miss James?
2. What are the priorities of care in the preoperative period?
3. How will this client's care plan differ from that of the client with hemiarthroplasty replacement of the femoral head and neck?

Scenario 2

Mrs. Jacobson, a 73-year-old retired school teacher, has been admitted to the hospital for a right total hip replacement as a result of osteoarthritis. She has been very active her entire life, playing golf three times a week, bowling on a team, hiking, and gardening. She is very concerned that she will be unable to continue with these activities if she doesn't have surgery. Her lab work was completed before her admission. She did give 2 units of autologous blood in case she needs it for surgery. Her vital signs are: BP 148/80, P 88, R 26. She uses a cane, which she says is "for balance."

1. Identify the priority preoperative intervention for Mrs. Jacobson. Provide a rationale for your choice.
2. Develop a client care plan: identify short- and long-term goals, state three nursing diagnoses in priority order, and provide the rationale for your choices. Describe at least two priority nursing interventions for each nursing diagnosis.
3. Identify two safety issues related to Mrs. Jacobson's care.
4. Describe at least three procedures that need to be discussed before her discharge.

NCLEX® Review Questions

Unless otherwise specified, choose only one (1) answer.

1. Appropriate application of a sling to the upper arm includes
   1. Positioning so that hand is higher than elbow.
   2. Positioning so that hand is lower than elbow.
   3. Teaching client to avoid any shoulder joint motion.
   4. Teaching client to avoid any movement of distal digits.
2. Wet plaster casts are best dried by
   1. Using a hair dryer.
   2. Covering with blankets.
   3. Using a heat lamp.
   4. Natural evaporation.
3. A synthetic cast, compared with a plaster cast
   Select all that apply.
   1. Is more expensive.
   2. Dries more quickly.
   3. Is heavier.
   4. Provides greater stability.
   5. Will not cause skin burns.
   6. Is nonabsorbent.
4. The following are early indications of acute compartment syndrome in a casted extremity
   Select all that apply.
   1. Weak or absent distal pulses.
   2. Pain with passive extension of distal digits.
   3. Pain relieved with extremity elevation.
   4. Pain worsens with extremity elevation.
   5. Pain worsens when extremity is dependent.
   6. Pain unrelieved by analgesics.
5. Injury to the peroneal nerve can result in permanent
   1. Urinary incontinence.
   2. Inability to plantarflex the foot.
   3. Inability to dorsiflex the foot.
   4. Anesthesia on sole of the foot.
6. The client with posterolateral approach total hip replacement surgery should be kept in this position postoperatively
   1. Legs adducted.
   2. Legs abducted.
   3. Operative leg in external rotation.
   4. Operative leg in internal rotation.
7. Adaptive aids for the client with total hip replacement primarily help the client avoid
   1. Hip flexion.
   2. Falls.
   3. Hip extension.
   4. Pain.
8. Studies show that clients receiving CPM (continuous passive motion) versus those who do not receive CPM after total knee replacement surgery have
   1. Better joint range of motion.

2. Less venous thrombosis.
3. Less edema.
4. Less wound drainage.
5. None of the above.

9. Phantom pain in the amputated extremity is most apt to occur in clients with
   1. Drug dependency.
   2. Inadequate stump shrinkage/shaping.
   3. Traumatic limb amputation.
   4. Limb pain preoperatively.

10. The client with above-the-knee amputation should be encouraged to perform exercises that promote stump
    1. Adduction and hip flexion.
    2. Abduction and hip flexion.
    3. Adduction and hip extension.
    4. Abduction and hip extension.

28

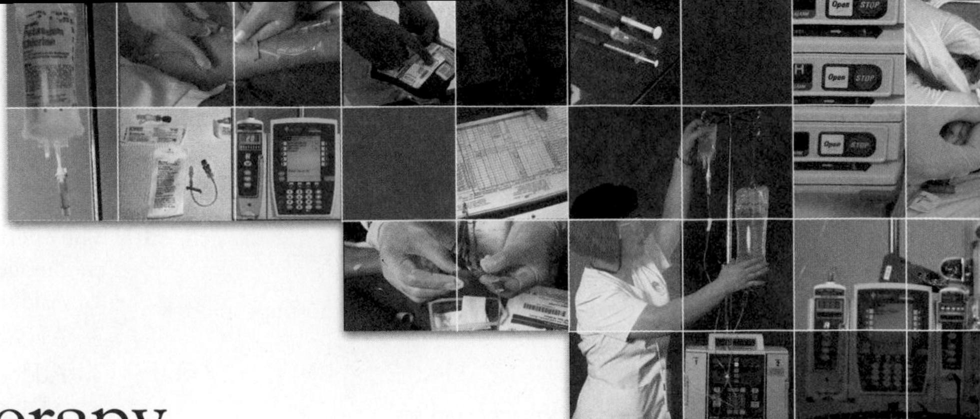

Intravenous Therapy

LEARNING OBJECTIVES

1. Describe the role the kidneys play in maintaining fluid and electrolyte balance.
2. Discuss the two hormonal regulatory systems that influence urinary excretion by the kidneys.
3. State the major cations and anions in the body.
4. Identify the assessment data to determine a client's fluid status.
5. Compare and contrast the client assessment data associated with fluid volume excess or deficit.
6. Describe the steps for performing venipuncture using a winged needle or over-the-needle catheter.
7. State at least two potential problems that can occur with venipuncture and one suggested solution for each problem.
8. Describe the steps for performing vein cannulation.
9. Outline the steps in preparing the IV bag for fluid administration.
10. Describe the steps for hanging a secondary IV bag.
11. Calculate an IV flow rate using a standard formula.
12. Describe the procedure for administering an intravenous push medication.
13. Discuss client safety and the use of infusion control pumps.
14. Describe the proper use of chlorhexidine gluconate as a skin preparation for intravenous access.
15. Discuss the nursing interventions required for each type of venous access connectors.
16. Describe safety checks utilized to ensure proper blood administration.
17. Differentiate signs and symptoms of hemolytic and allergic blood transfusion reactions.

CHAPTER OUTLINE

TERMINOLOGY

Anaphylaxis a hypersensitive state of the body to a foreign protein or drug.

Antiarrhythmic an agent used to regulate heart rhythm.

Antidiuretic hormone that decreases urine production.

Antimicrobic preventing the development or pathogenic action of microbes.

Ascites the excessive accumulation of serous fluid in the peritoneal cavity.

Aspirate to remove material by suction.

Autologous blood transfusion client's own blood is collected before a surgical procedure or future need for transfusion.

Bolus direct injection of a medication intravenously in order to achieve rapid serum concentrations.

BSI bloodstream infection.

Cardio pertaining to the heart.

Cardiovascular pertaining to the heart and blood vessels.

Catheter-related bloodstream infection the same organism is found in the blood and catheter segment with clinical symptoms of BSI and no other sources of infection present.

Central line bundle a bundle is a collection of interventions delivered as a group to improve outcomes for catheter-related bloodstream infections.

Colonization growth of an organism from the proximal or distal catheter segment or catheter lumen in conjunction with signs of infection at catheter site.

Cyanosis slightly bluish, grayish, slate-like, or dark purple discoloration of the skin/mucous membranes.

Diarrhea frequent passage of watery stool.

Diffusion passive movement of molecules from an area of high concentration to one of lower concentration.

Directed donation of blood friends or relatives donate blood for a specific client.

Diuretic a chemical agent that increases the production of urine.

Dyspnea a subjective feeling of difficulty breathing.

Edema an excessive amount of extracellular fluid.

Electrolyte substance that develops an electrical charge when dissolved in water.

Evaporation change from liquid to vapor.

Extracellular outside the cell.

Girth the distance around something; circumference, as in measuring abdominal circumference.

Granulocytes a granular leukocyte (e.g., neutrophil).

Hematoma a collection of blood confined in a space.

Hematuria blood in the urine.

Hemo- prefix meaning blood.

Hemolytic pertinent to the breaking down of red blood cells.

Homeostasis state of equilibrium of the internal environment.

Homologous blood transfusion blood from another individual is used for transfusion.

Hydration the chemical combination of a substance with water.

Hydrostatic pressure the pressure of liquids during equilibrium.

Hypersecretion abnormally large amount of secretion.

Hypertonic solution having greater than 340 mOsm, increased amount of solutes in relationship to plasma.

Hypotonic solution having less than 240 mOsm, decreased amount of solutes in relationship to plasma.

Hypovolemia diminished circulating blood volume.

Infiltration blood leaks into surrounding tissue when IV fluids are infusing.

Infusion-related bloodstream infection the same organism found in the infusion and separate percutaneous blood cultures without an identified source of infection.

Infusion introduction of a liquid into a vein or other body part.

Interstitial extracellular fluid found between the cells.

Intracellular inside the cell.

Intravascular within blood vessels.

Isotonic having the same tonicity as plasma, 240–340 mOsm.

Local-catheter-related infection growth of an organism from the proximal or distal catheter or lumen with accompanying signs of inflammation at the catheter site.

Metabolism the sum of all physical and chemical changes that take place within an organism.

Nephro prefix meaning kidney.

Nephrotoxic damaging to renal cells.

Osmolality concentration of osmotically active particles per Kg of body water (tonicity).

Osmosis transmission of water across a semipermeable membrane from an area of low solute concentration to one of higher solute concentration.

Osmotic pressure pressure exerted on a semipermeable membrane separating a solution from a solvent, the membrane being impermeable to solutes in solution and permeable only to solvent.

Palpate to examine by touch; to feel.

Pruritus severe itching.

Purulent containing pus.

Skin turgor elastic property of the skin reflecting body fluid status.

Smart pumps computerized IV pumps.

Specific gravity weight of a substance compared with an equal volume of water.

Transfusion injection of blood or a blood component of one person into the blood vessels of another.

Urticaria a vascular reaction of the skin characterized by the eruption of pale raised wheals, which are associated with severe itching.

Valsalva's maneuver attempt to forcibly exhale against a closed glottis.

Venipuncture puncture of a vein with a needle.

Vesicant blistering; causing or forming blisters, irritant to blood vessels.

Viscosity resistance offered by a fluid; property of a substance that is dependent on the friction of its component molecules as they slide by each other.

FLUID AND ELECTROLYTE BALANCE

The body's internal environment is made up of fluids and dissolved substances including electrolytes. Fluids and electrolytes are in a constant state of dynamic equilibrium in order to maintain the delicate balance essential for all the physiologic processes that support life.

Fluids

Body fluid is primarily water. Depending on the amount of body fat, a person's total body weight is usually 50%–70% water. Since fat is essentially water-free, an obese adult's body weight is 50% water. In a leaner individual, the percentage of body weight due to body water is closer to 70%. With aging, there is a decrease in lean body mass; therefore, the elderly may have only 46%–52% of body weight as water.

Body water is divided into two main compartments: intracellular and extracellular. The majority of body water (64%) is located inside the cells. The remaining 36% of body fluid is extracellular. Three-fourths of this extracellular fluid is interstitial (surrounding cells), and the remaining one-fourth is intravascular plasma.

Communication between these fluid compartments varies. Intracellular water does not move readily out of the cell. In contrast, in the capillary beds there is constant movement of fluids between the extracellular fluid (interstitial and intravascular) compartments. The movement of body fluid between the intravascular and interstitial space is controlled by two opposing forces: *osmotic pressure* (holding fluid in the vessels) and *hydrostatic pressure* (forcing fluid into tissue spaces). Interstitial and intravascular fluid are similar in composition except for the presence of plasma proteins (which provide osmotic pressure) in the intravascular space.

Body water balance is the result of physiologic homeostatic responses to the fluid gains (intake) and losses (output) that occur on a daily basis. The major sources of intake and output are shown in Table 28-1.

The primary organ of fluid balance is the kidney. The kidneys excrete the end products of cellular metabolism, as well as eliminate excess fluids. In order to clear the blood of wastes, they must produce a minimum of 500–600 mL of urine every 24 hr. To balance a typical amount of fluid intake, however, the usual amount of urine produced on a daily basis varies from 1 to 2 L.

Regulation of the volume, composition, and osmolality of body fluid is controlled by homeostatic mechanisms. A major regulator of intake is thirst. Thirst is stimulated by receptors in the central nervous system. Under normal circumstances, an individual ingests fluids when these receptors are activated. During illness or an altered level of consciousness, and in the aged, the thirst response may be depressed, resulting in hypovolemia and increased tonicity or concentration of the extracellular fluids (Deficient Fluid Volume).

Urine production by the kidneys is influenced by two hormonal regulatory systems, one of which is the antidiuretic hormone (ADH). When extracellular body fluids become concentrated, osmoreceptors located in the hypothalamus stimulate the release of ADH, which stimulates the kidneys to retain more water. As this retained water circulates through the extracellular fluid compartment, the concentration of body fluid is reduced. The osmoreceptors sense this change, slow the secretion of ADH, and the kidneys stop retaining water (negative feedback).

TABLE 28-1 Average Daily Fluid Gain and Loss

Intake (mL)		Output (mL)	
Oral intake (liquid and food)	2300	Urine	1500
Cellular catabolism		Skin	600 (insensible loss by evaporation)
of proteins, carbohydrates, and fats	300	Lung	300 (insensible loss by vapor)
		Feces	200
	2600		2600

Other conditions that can stimulate the secretion of ADH and lead to increased water retention by the kidneys include hemorrhage, decreased cardiac output, trauma, pain, fear, surgery, and dehydration. Drugs such as morphine, barbiturates, nicotine, and some anesthetics and tranquilizers also increase the secretion of ADH. The secretion of ADH can be inhibited by alcohol, decreased concentration of body fluids, and hypervolemic states.

Another major regulatory hormone is aldosterone, which is secreted by the adrenal cortex. Aldosterone regulates fluid volume by stimulating the kidneys to reabsorb sodium and water (an isotonic gain). During this process, sodium is exchanged for potassium or hydrogen; therefore, aldosterone also affects levels of these electrolytes. Secretion of aldosterone is increased in response to several stimuli, which include decreased sodium and increased extracellular potassium, hypovolemia, and stress states.

When blood flow to the kidneys is decreased, a receptor-like area in the glomerulus of the nephron releases an enzyme called renin. As renin circulates in the body, it converts a plasma protein in the liver into a vasoconstrictor substance called angiotensin I. When this substance enters the lungs, it is converted into angiotensin II. Angiotensin II acts directly on the adrenal cortex to increase aldosterone secretion. This then leads to extracellular volume expansion and even possible fluid volume excess if the cause of decreased renal blood flow was due to heart or liver failure.

Electrolytes

In partnership with body fluids are substances called electrolytes. These substances, mostly minerals, contribute to body function in many ways and are essential to life (Table 28-2). Electrolytes are important components of intracellular and extracellular fluids. The major intracellular electrolytes are potassium, magnesium, phosphate, and sulfate. Major extracellular electrolytes are sodium, chloride, and bicarbonate.

Electrolytes are distributed throughout the body, both intracellularly and extracellularly. In the extracellular compartment, the main electrolytes are sodium, chloride, and bicarbonate. Intracellular electrolytes are potassium, magnesium, phosphate, and sulfate.

Electrolytes develop an electric charge when dissolved in water. Electrolytes with a positive charge are called cations. Negatively charged electrolytes are called anions. Positive cations and negative anions are attracted to each other because of their opposite electric charges. When they combine with each other, they form neutral compounds that either remain in body fluids or dissociate and regain their electric charges. When they dissociate, or ionize, they are referred to as ions.

TABLE 28-2 Major Electrolytes

Cations		Anions	
Na^+	Sodium	Cl^-	Chloride
K^+	Potassium	HCO_3^-	Bicarbonate
Ca^{2+}	Calcium	HPO_4^{2-}	Phosphate
Mg^{2+}	Magnesium		

FLUID AND ELECTROLYTE IMBALANCE

Alterations in fluid and electrolytes may occur as a primary event or as a secondary response to a preexisting disease state or to a sudden, unexpected traumatic event. When alterations of fluid and electrolytes exceed the narrow limits consistent with health, the body needs to adjust quickly.

Changes in the composition of body fluid and electrolytes may be relative or absolute. Relative losses or gains can occur when fluids or electrolytes shift from one body space to another. Absolute losses or gains occur when fluids and electrolytes are lost outside the body or added to the overall body stores by IV fluid.

The kidney has an obligatory urine output, and the body has an insensible water loss. A minimum fluid intake of 1500 mL is essential to balance these losses. If the loss of body water is greater than fluid intake (fluid volume deficit), weight loss results. If the gain of body water is greater than output, weight gain results. One kilogram of body weight gain or loss is equal to 1000 mL (1 L) of fluid.

In addition to methods of assessing fluid balance, this chapter discusses interventions for providing fluid and electrolytes to clients who have experienced alterations in their homeostasis. The rationale for interventions associated with alterations in either fluids or electrolytes is to maintain homeostasis.

Clients undergoing major surgery or trauma may be subjected to blood loss necessitating fluid replacement therapy. Clients requiring prolonged intravenous therapy may have associated nutritional losses. Support for these clients must be considered.

IV ADMINISTRATION

Initiating, monitoring, and providing care for clients with IV therapy consumes a large portion of the nurses' time each shift, and requires safe nursing practice to protect the client from complications. Up to 90% of hospitalized clients require some form of IV therapy. *Source: (Hanchett, 2004)*.

Administering IV drugs can lead to medication errors, even if the nurse does not mix the medication, but hangs and monitors the IV. Whenever the nurse administers an IV, both the hospital and federal guidelines must be followed. Guidelines include being properly educated in the use of IV equipment, understanding venous anatomy to ensure proper IV selection sites, and knowing the appropriate catheter gauge and length for the vein selected. In addition, it is imperative that the nurse is knowledgeable about drugs and solutions being administered, the side effects, and treatment if a side effect occurs.

Frequent monitoring of IV infusions is a requisite for safe nursing practice. Knowing the solution infusing, medications added to the solution, and rate of infusion promotes safe care. Maintaining the IV site and following guidelines established by the Intravenous Nurses Society, The Joint Commission, and the CDC are critical to prevent complications associated with the IV site and cannula.

The CDC Guidelines for Prevention of Catheter-Related Infections state that skin should be disinfected before catheter placement and that chlorhexidine gluconate is preferred. Use of chlorhexidine gluconate has demonstrated superiority to povidone–iodine in decreasing infections at the site of IV catheter insertion. In addition to the use of chlorhexidine gluconate, the CDC recommends the use of a sterile catheter securement device such as the Statlock. This device protects the client's skin from damage and prevents movement of the IV catheter. Movement can damage the vessel and lead to infection. Another recommendation is the use of semipermeable transparent film dressings to prevent the passage of liquids, bacteria, and viruses to the IV site. The use of this type of dressing allows easy observation and monitoring of the IV site without removing the dressing. It is recommended that tape not be used to secure the IV site. Tape used to stabilize IVs has historically been unsterile, leading to infections at the IV site. In addition, tape not only allows movement of the catheter, but also has been shown to be the cause of infiltration, phlebitis, occlusion/thrombosis, and other device-related complications. If the tape is necessary, it is highly recommended that sterile tape be utilized to prevent infection.

Intravenous devices are an important part of hospital practice for the administration of fluid, nutrients, medications, blood products, and to hemodynamically monitor unstable clients. These devices are not without problems. Catheter-related bloodstream infections can be associated with increased hospital stays, even life-threatening events or death. Peripheral venous catheters are usually not associated with these infections, whereas central vascular devices are the most problematic devices. Phlebitis and infiltration are the most common complications associated with peripheral vein catheters. The risk of phlebitis differs between sites. It is much higher if the lower limb is used as the IV site. Catheters inserted in the hand carry a lower risk of phlebitis than those inserted higher up on the wrist and arm. Providing intravenous therapy for clients is one of the main skills provided by nurses.

Most medication errors resulting in client deaths occurred with IV infusions. To meet the need for improved medication safety at the point of care, "smart technology" was developed to standardize IV infusion administration, reduce IV programming errors, and streamline IV administration processes. The infusion pumps are programmed with a database of information about medications and parameters for correct dosage and infusion rate. The pump can alert the nurse if it is not programmed correctly for a given drug. The pharmacy alters the provided database from the company to meet the specifications of the hospital and formulary that goes into the pump. There are two levels of alerts in the pump: a soft stop and a hard stop. When a minor error is detected, the pump warns the user, but will allow the user to override the alert. When a more serious problem occurs, the pump shuts down and does not allow an override.

A point-of-care "smart pump" consists of the computer (brain) that programs the infusions and contains the safety software. Lightweight, large-volume infusion modules, as well as a syringe, client-controlled analgesia (PCA), capnography ($EtCO_2$), and pulse oximetry (SpO_2) modules, can be attached to or removed from the "smart pump" (brain) as needed for each client.

The safety software can also be added to some traditional infusion pumps. The hospital can configure up to 10 profiles for specific client care areas such as ICU and Medical–Surgical units. These profiles include customized operating parameters and drug libraries. Each drug library contains institution-specific parameters for up to 1000 drugs, all of which can be customized. The drug library provides the best-practice guidelines for each medication. If programmed parameters are outside of pre-established limits, the software provides an alert that must be addressed before the infusion can begin.

An IV Medication Harm Index monitors the number of potential errors that were avoided through the use of the system. Potential errors that can be detected are overdose of drugs and adverse events. Having these data available allows the hospital to identify practice issues that were difficult to identify with earlier IV pumps. Several studies have been conducted to determine the extent of the error prevention when using the "smart technology." One of the studies indicated a 350-bed hospital averted potentially life-threatening IV programming overdoses every 2.6 days and additional potentially significant IV errors every 3.6 days (Cardinal Health, 2003). Examples of potentially significant IV administration errors included morphine sulfate reprogrammed from 100 mg to 5 mg; heparin errors with extra zeros; and 705 units insulin reprogrammed to 7.5 units (Brigham and Women's Case Report, 2004).

This chapter presents skills for providing fluids and electrolytes, blood, and blood components, as well as pharmacologic therapy through the intravenous route. Methods for assessing baseline data and evaluating fluid and electrolyte gains or losses are included in this chapter.

CULTURAL AWARENESS

Religion and Use of Blood and Blood Products

It is important to know clients' religious beliefs about the use of blood and blood products in order to understand their preferences in choosing to allow or not allow transfusions.

- Clients who practice Christian Science (Church of Christ, Scientist) usually do not accept use of blood or blood products in their medical care.
- Clients who are Jehovah's Witnesses believe blood in any form and agents in which blood is an ingredient are not acceptable. Blood volume expanders are acceptable if they are not derived from blood. Mechanical devices for circulating blood are acceptable as long as they are not primed with blood initially. Their religious belief is based on scripture references and precedents in the history of Christianity. There are times when court orders are obtained for children in life-threatening situations so they may receive blood or blood products.

NURSING DIAGNOSES

The following nursing diagnoses are appropriate to include in a client care plan when the components are related to intravenous therapy.

Nursing Diagnosis	Related Factors
Deficient Fluid Volume	Excess fluid loss secondary to vomiting, increased temperature, blood loss, drainage sites or tubes, diarrhea, and diuretics
Excess Fluid Volume	Excessive fluid accumulation secondary to excess sodium intake, medications, renal or cardiac failure; inaccurate IV infusion rate
Infection, Risk for	Chronic diseases, invasive procedures, immunodeficiency, tissue destruction and increased environmental exposure
Noncompliance	Inaccurate I&O records, denial, lack of instruction regarding I&O, fluid restriction, care of IV site
Impaired Skin Integrity	Alterations in skin turgor, edema, tissue damage, IV infiltration, infection, immobilization
Ineffective Peripheral Tissue Perfusion	Loss of blood related to hemorrhage or loss related to hemodialysis

CLEANSE HANDS The single most important nursing action to decrease the incidence of hospital-based infections is hand hygiene. *Remember to wash your hands or use antibacterial gel before and after each and every client contact.*

IDENTIFY CLIENT Before every procedure, introduce yourself and check two forms of client identification, not including room number. These actions prevent errors and conform to The Joint Commission standards.

Chapter 28

UNIT 1

Initiating Intravenous Therapy

Nursing Process Data

ASSESSMENT Data Base

- Validate physician's order for IV therapy.
- Assess need for client teaching about IV therapy.
- Evaluate client for IV site selection.
- Select appropriate vessel for venipuncture.
- Determine appropriate type and size of cannulation device for client.
- Determine IV equipment needed.

PLANNING Objectives

- To maintain fluid and electrolyte balance
- To aseptically prepare infusion system
- To identify and prepare the appropriate site for venipuncture
- To perform successful venipuncture using appropriate equipment

IMPLEMENTATION Procedures

EVALUATION Expected Outcomes

- Fluid and electrolyte needs are met.
- Appropriate IV site is selected and IV inserted without difficulty.
- IV fluids infuse at prescribed rate without complications.
- IV equipment is appropriate for client.
- IV site is maintained using sterile technique.

Pearson Nursing Student Resources

Find additional review materials at **nursing.pearsonhighered.com**

Prepare for success with NCLEX®-style practice questions and Skill Checklists

Preparing the Infusion System

Equipment

IV solution in bag

NOTE: The only glass bottles used today are for infusions of certain medications (e.g., nitroglycerin amiodarone and lipids). Check facility procedures for correct infusion of these medications using the glass bottle.

Primary administration tubing set (compatible with infusion pump)

Add-on particulate filter (according to agency policy) compatible with infusion pump psi

Electronic infusion device or free pole for bag suspension and gravity infusion

Except when infusing TPN, TPN with lipids, or certain IV medications, PCAs, continuous epidurals, and blood products, in-line filters are not recommended. There is no evidence to suggest that in-line filters prevent infections associated with intravascular devices and infusion systems. Some studies do suggest that they may reduce the incidence of infusion-related phlebitis; however, it has not been proven. Because studies do not justify the cost of the in-line filters, the CDC does not recommend them for infection control purposes. Before hanging drugs, check the drug formulary to determine the need for an in-line filter.

Clinical Alert

Take IV solutions out of refrigerator (if stored in refrigerator) and allow to warm to room temperature. This will reduce the number of air bubbles in the IV solution.

It is difficult to detect air bubbles because gas is well assimilated into liquid at low temperatures; thus air bubbles are fully assimilated into the IV solution when kept in refrigerator. Once solution warms to room temperature, air bubbles appear.

Preparation

1. Verify the type and amount of solution with physician's order.
2. Perform hand hygiene.
3. Check pharmacy label for client's identification, solution type, additives, and expiration date.
4. Select IV tubing appropriate for infusion device.
5. Select add-on filter if indicated.

Procedure

1. Remove outer wrap around IV bag if necessary. (It may be wet due to condensation.)
2. Inspect bag carefully for tears or leaks by applying gentle pressure to bag.
3. Hold bag up against both a dark and light background to examine for discoloration, cloudiness, or particulate matter. ▸ ***Rationale:*** Any evidence of change may indicate contamination, and bag should be discarded.
4. Hang the IV bag on the IV pole. Close tubing roller clamp. (Affix time strip on bag according to facility policy.)
5. Remove plastic protector from tubing spike (end of tubing with drip chamber).

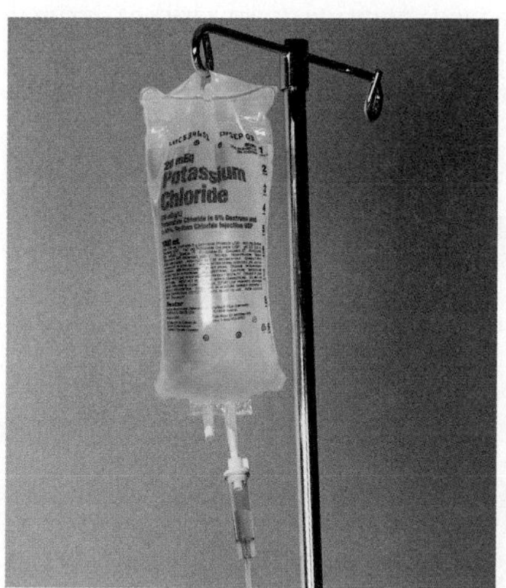

1 Most hospitals require a "Red Label" if potassium or other drugs are pre-added to the solution.

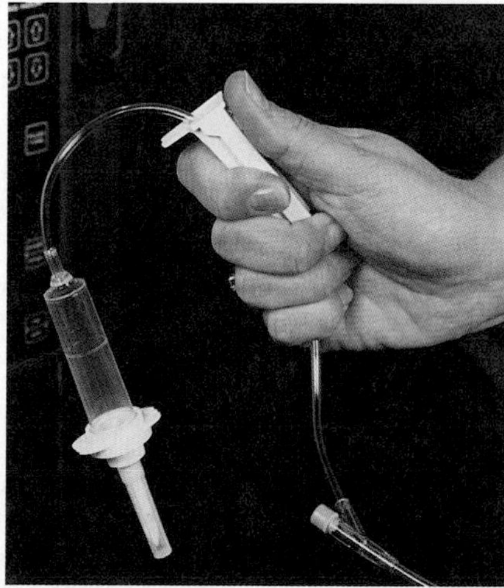

2 Clamp tubing before spiking IV fluid bag.

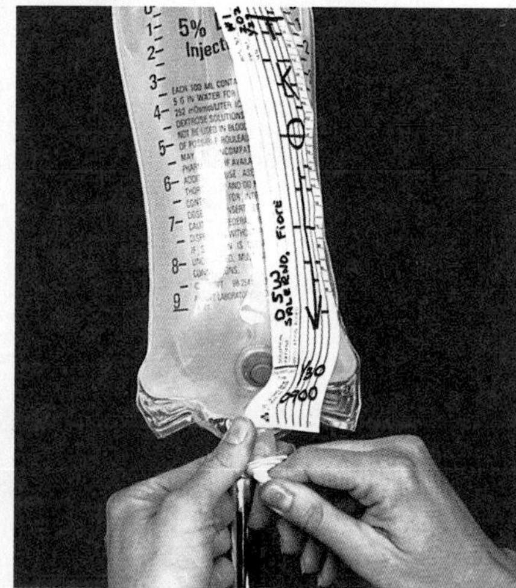

3 Pull to remove port cap on IV bag.

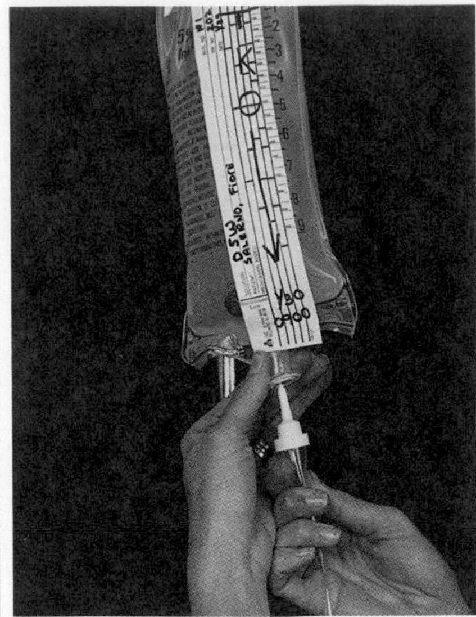

4 Squeeze drip chamber while spiking bag port, maintaining sterility.

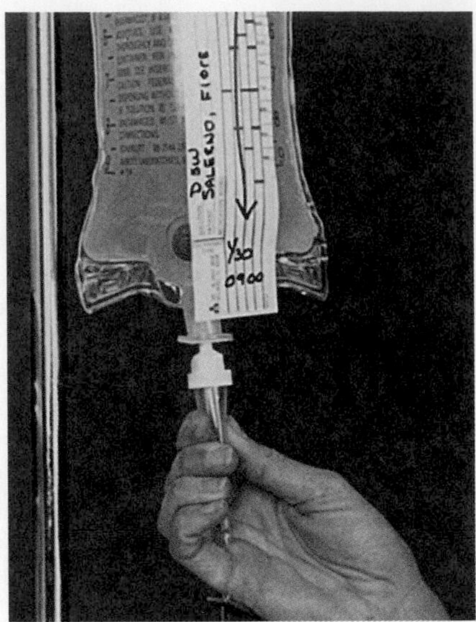

5 Squeeze and release drip chamber to fill.

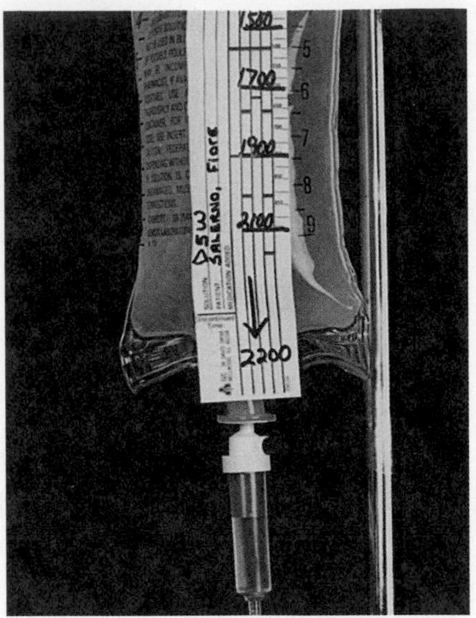

6 Fill drip chamber one-half full of fluid.

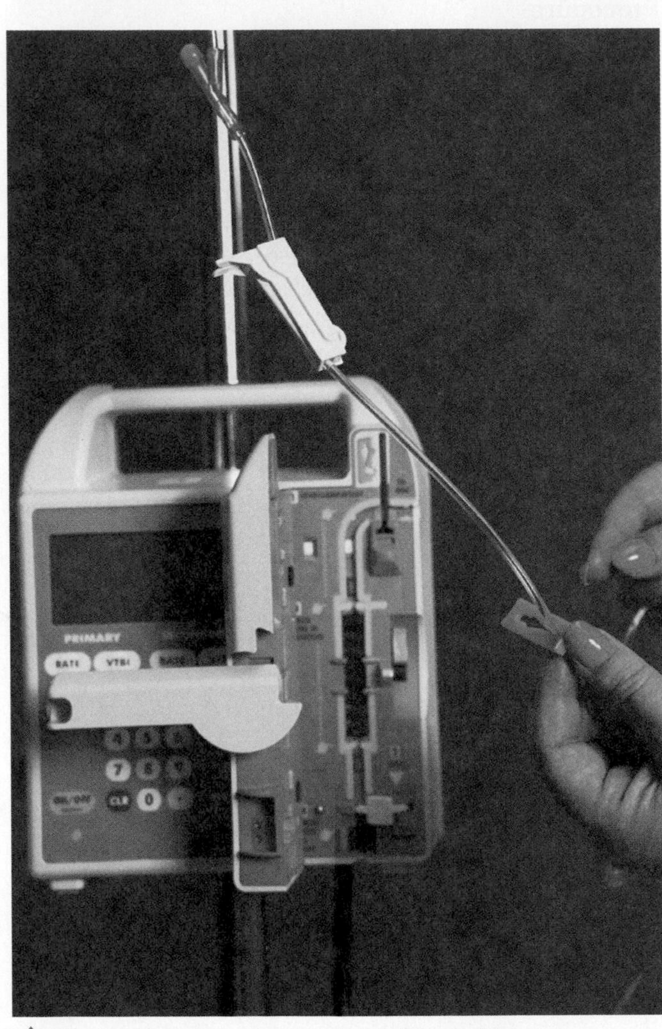

7 Close tubing clamp when priming is complete.

6. Squeeze drip chamber while inserting tubing spike into bag port, holding port securely to prevent contamination. ▶ ***Rationale:*** Squeezing chamber during insertion prevents air entry into bag.
7. Release pressure on the drip chamber until chamber is partially full.
8. Attach add-on terminal filter (if indicated).
9. Remove protective cap at end of tubing.
10. Open clamp on line to prime tubing and filter.
11. Hold tubing tip higher than tubing-dependent loop while priming. ▶ ***Rationale:*** Air rises and passes out as fluid primes tubing.
12. Invert and tap Y injection sites to remove air as tubing primes.
13. Hold filter (if attached) pointing downward so proximal (closest to client) half of filter fills with fluid first, then invert to complete filter priming, tapping air out as filter primes.
14. Close tubing clamp when primed.
15. Load administration set into electronic pump according to manufacturer's instructions. Most pumps require dedicated tubing and specific loading format.

Clinical Alert

Do not use felt-tip pens to mark directly on IV plastic bag. ▶ ***Rationale:*** The ink may leach through the plastic and contaminate the solution.

Adding Extension Tubing

Equipment

Extension tubing
2% Chlorhexidine gluconate
Injection cap with Luer-Lok adapter, if necessary
Syringe cannula
Two syringes of 0.9% preservative-free normal saline (NS) in volume at least twice the volume capacity of the catheter and any add-on devices

Procedure

1. Gather equipment and determine type of cap, if needed. Extension tubing may be attached directly to IV catheter.
2. Swab tubing's terminal injection cap and insert syringe cannula.
3. Remove protector at opposite end and prime extension tubing with 1 mL of NS solution.
4. Add needleless IV access device to tubing or use Luer-Lok with attached extension tubing.

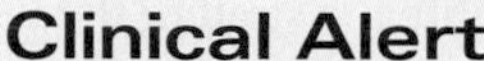

Clinical Alert
Peripheral IVs should be started using aseptic technique. IVs started without proper asepsis, for example, in an emergency or outside the hospital, should be replaced at the earliest opportunity, and within 24 hr.

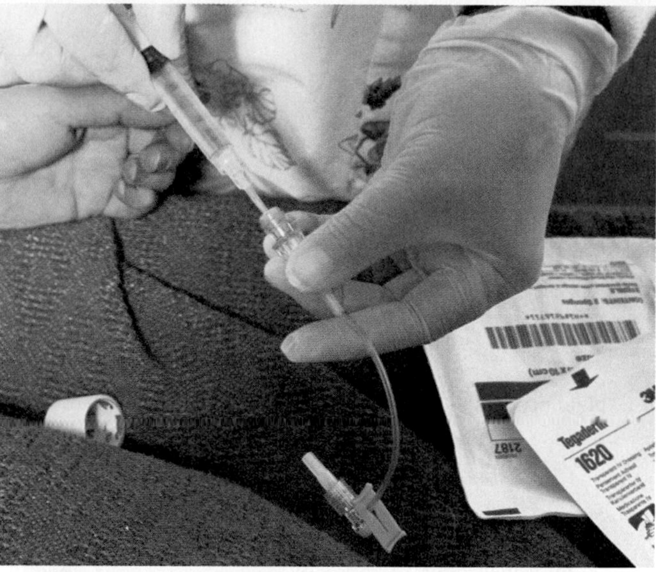

▲ Swab injection cap and insert syringe cannula.

5. Swab client's established IV cannula resealable cap and connect extension tubing or insert primed extension tubing directly into client's IV catheter.
6. Flush with 0.9% NS at twice the volume (capacity) of the catheter and any add-on devices.

NOTE: INS standards discourage the use of additional routine extension tubing. ▶ ***Rationale:*** This adds additional potential source of IV contamination.

Preparing the Venipuncture Site

Equipment

Prepared IV administration setup or sterile needleless access device
Single-use, latex-free tourniquet (constricting band)
Chlorhexidine gluconate swab (not used on infants under 1000 grams)
Sterile needle or catheter for venipuncture
Half-inch wide sterile tape
Transparent semipermeable dressing
Securement device
Gloves (clean or sterile depending on facility policy)
Electronic infusion pump

Preparation

1. Check physician's orders and MAR.
2. Identify client using two forms of identification.
3. Assemble equipment.

Procedure

1. Explain procedure.
2. Provide privacy.
3. Hang solution bag and primed administration set within easy reach.
4. Position client and adjust lighting as necessary. Explain procedure to client.
5. Perform hand hygiene and don gloves.
6. Select appropriate IV device. Catheter gauge should be smallest size that allows greatest flow, without occluding vessel lumen.

NOTE: Over-the-needle catheters are used most commonly for IV fluid/blood administration. A smaller catheter (22 gauge) may be used for routine antibiotics or maintenance fluids, but a larger catheter (20 gauge) is needed for blood products. For irritating medications, a small-bore catheter is preferable.

7. If possible, select a vein on client's nondominant arm. Also consider client's activity level and expected duration of IV therapy.
   a. Inspect both of client's arms, palpating and visualizing the course of the veins.
   b. Vein should be superficial, easily palpated, and large enough for needle insertion and advancement.
   c. Area should be free of lesions or scars and away from joints and areas of frequent motion. ▶ ***Rationale:***

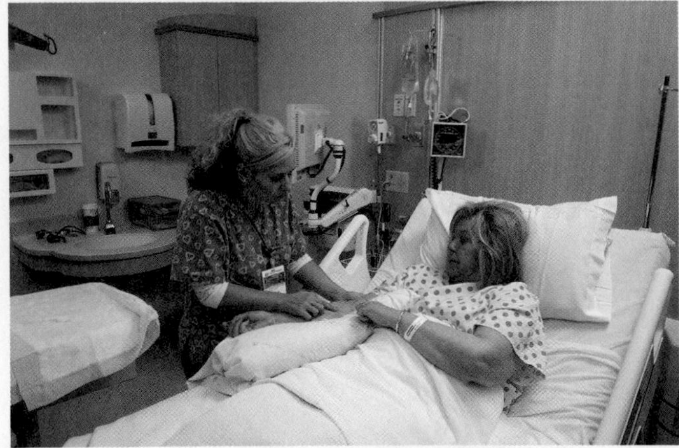

▲ Explain procedure to client.

Motion frequency increases the risk of mechanical phlebitis.

d. Do not use the antecubital fossa except in atypical circumstances.

e. Do not use the same vein below a site where infiltration or phlebitis has occurred.

f. Select shortest and smallest cannula that will be sufficient to deliver fluids/medications. ▸ ***Rationale:*** The longer the catheter, the greater the risk of infiltration, infection, and thrombus formation. A catheter that is too large does not allow for adequate blood flow around catheter, and this can lead to phlebitis.

g. Distal end of vein should be selected first, reserving more proximal sites for future IV therapy.

h. Select larger veins for hypertonic solutions, blood, and viscous fluids.

Clinical Alert

Do not shave the venipuncture site. Shaving can facilitate the development of infection through the multiplication of organisms in resulting microabrasions. Hairy sites can be clipped with scissors.

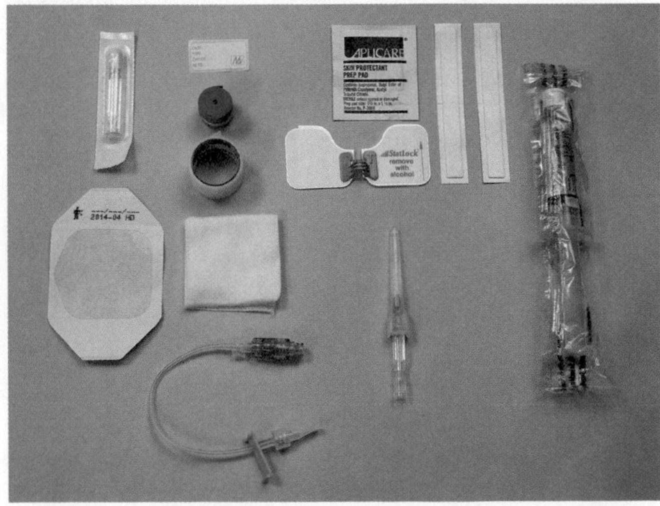

▲ Equipment for IV start for over-the-needle.

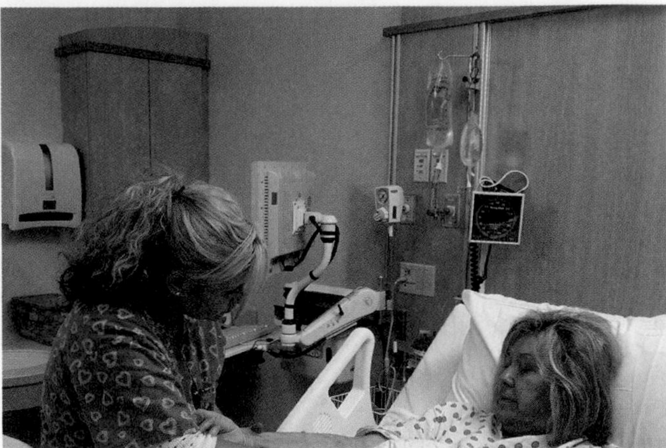

▲ Hang IV bag and primed administration set within easy reach.

i. Avoid using veins in affected arm after mastectomy.

j. Lower extremity sites are associated with complications (e.g., thrombosis) and should be used ONLY if necessary. The legs and feet of diabetic clients and those with peripheral vascular disease should never be used. Check the facility policies to determine if a physician's order is needed when using lower extremity for IV site.

8. Apply tourniquet 6 in. above the selected site to distend vein. Overlap ends of tourniquet, lift and stretch, then tuck top end under bottom; keep ends pointing away from puncture site. ▸ ***Rationale:*** Tourniquet traps blood and engorges vein for better visibility.

9. Prepare vein for venipuncture.

Clinical Alert

Some agencies allow only certified IV therapists to perform venipuncture.

a. Place arm in dependent position. ▸ ***Rationale:*** This position increases capillary refill and venous distension to increase chance of successful venipuncture.

b. Lightly tap vein. ▸ ***Rationale:*** To distend vein in preparation for venipuncture.

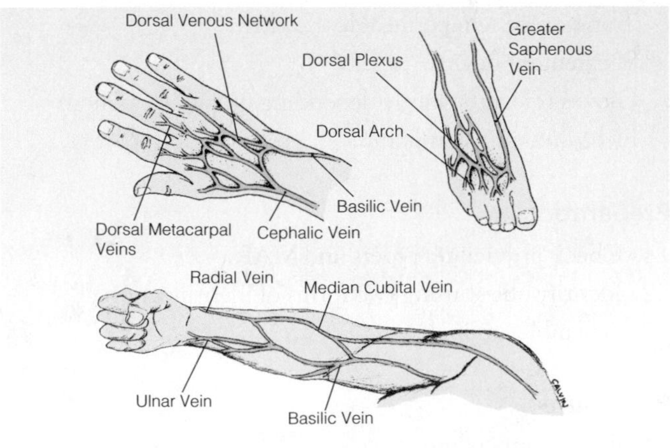

▲ Anatomical sites used for venipuncture.

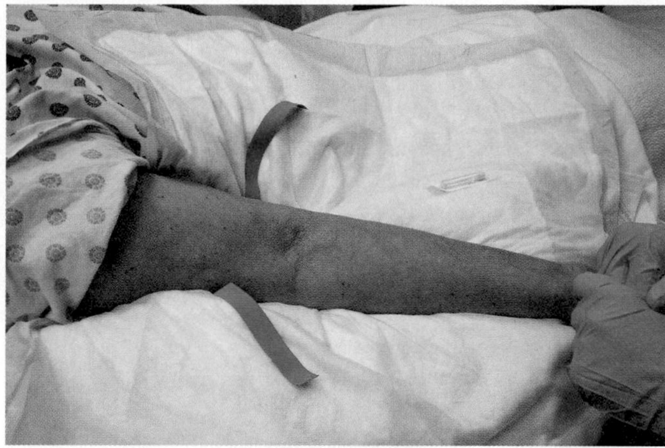

▲ Apply tourniquet 6 in. above insertion site.

c. Ask client to open and close fist several times to help distend selected vein.

d. If vein is difficult to palpate, release tourniquet and apply warm, moist compresses to arm for 10–20 minutes before reapplying tourniquet.

10. Prep site with chlorhexidine gluconate swab. Cleanse area using back-and-forth motion, 2–4 in. in diameter. ▸ *Rationale:* Vigorous skin preparation decreases organisms at the venipuncture site.

Clinical Alert

Latex-free tourniquets should be used and disposed of after each use.

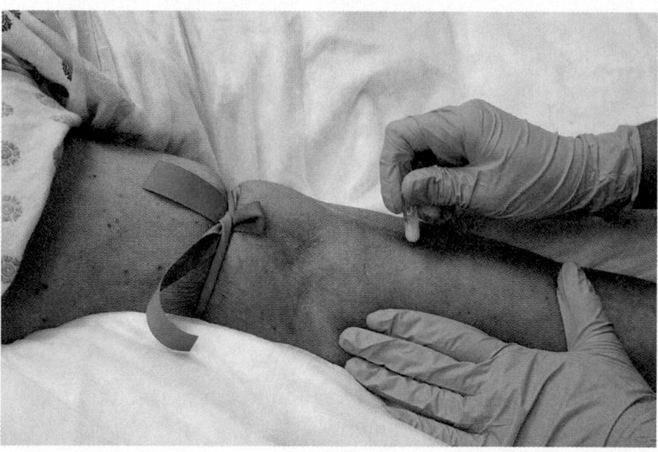

▲ Use back-and forth-movement to cleanse site with chlorhexidine gluconate.

11. Let prep solution air dry for a minimum of 30 seconds or until skin is dry. ▸ *Rationale:* Area must be dry for antimicrobial action before continuing with venipuncture. Do not fan to dry skin.
12. Do not touch selected insertion site after prepping.
13. Proceed to appropriate procedure for inserting the needle.

Clinical Alert

When repetitive peripheral IV access fails and IV medication doses and fluids are missed, many facilities are now inserting PICC lines or implantable ports. Use of PICC lines decreases incidence of phlebitis as little as 2% to 22%.

Using a Vascular Imaging Device

Equipment

Infrared or transillumination device

Specific type of IV equipment

NOTE: The infrared device projects invisible infrared or near-infrared light waves onto the client's skin. The light is reflected off tissue surrounding vein, but not off blood inside the veins so it can differentiate between tissue and veins. The transillumination device is applied to the client's skin by focusing bright visible light onto the skin; it illuminates the tissue under the skin and helps locate superficial veins.

Procedure

1. Obtain all IV equipment necessary for specific type of infusion and IV infrared machine.
2. Identify client using two identifiers.
3. Explain procedure to client. The vascular imaging device can highlight vein location. It determines sites for placement of IV. Identifying sites can minimize pain and provide more options where sites may be secured. It will not come in contact with client, nor will they experience heat at the site.
4. Instruct client to take off all jewelry in the area that will be assessed. ▸ *Rationale:* Metal reflects light and can interfere with the projected image, causing blank or distorted images in some instances.
5. Plug in device and lock wheels.
6. Turn on device and calibrate. Place the calibration card on a horizontal surface and position the device head perpendicular over it, approximately 2 feet away. Check the card to ensure the device was successfully calibrated. It will indicate when it is calibrated.
7. Place the device head perpendicular to the area and 2 feet from where the IV is to be inserted. ▸ *Rationale:* An inaccurate focus can cause a shift from the projected image away from the vein location, cast shadows, and decrease image quality.
8. Check the focus by making sure the text around the image border is clean and legible.
9. Using the projected image, identify a vein site suitable for IV access.

10. Move the imaging modes and contrast levels to determine the view that is most useful to assist with the venipuncture.

NOTE: If the site has excessive hair, select the Hair Reduction Mode.▸ ***Rationale:*** This mode highlights the veins and minimizes the shadowing caused by the hair.

11. Perform the venipuncture. Insert the needle just outside the lighted area to prevent reflection from the metal of the light. Another option is to turn off the light after marking the IV site with a surgical skin marker and access the vein at the mark.

Inserting a Winged Needle

Equipment

- Prescribed solution, infusion administration set, and electronic infusion pump
- Protective resealable injection cap (if indicated)
- Syringe with 0.9% preservative free NS, 2–3 times the volume of catheter and all connecting devices, for locking resealable injection cap
- Tourniquet or blood pressure cuff
- Sterile winged (small vein) needle (typical hub replaced by two flexible wings) with attached tubing and resealable injection cap or short tubing to affix to infusion administration tubing. (Used for IV push medication lasting only 24 hr.)

NOTE: Winged needles are available as steel needles or flexible over-the-needle catheter types. The hub is replaced by flexible wings for easier insertion and taping.

- Scalp vein needle: Stainless steel—gauge 17–25; or
- Siliconized—gauge 18–25 if using scalp site (usually for infants).
- Chlorhexidine gluconate swab
- Sterile tape
- Transparent dressing
- Gloves

Procedure

1. Follow steps in Preparing the Venipuncture Site.
2. Select a winged needle for adults and for children, infants, and elderly clients who have small or fragile veins. Winged-needle access is only used for intermittent infusion access or access needed for less than 24 hr.

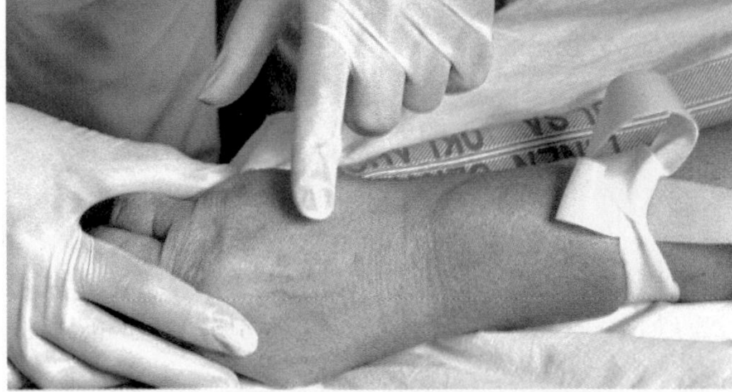

▲ Select site at distal end of vein to preserve future proximal IV sites.

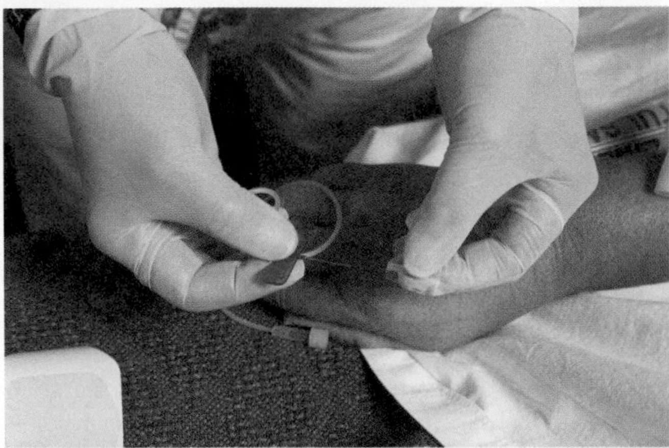

▲ Remove protective cap from winged needle.

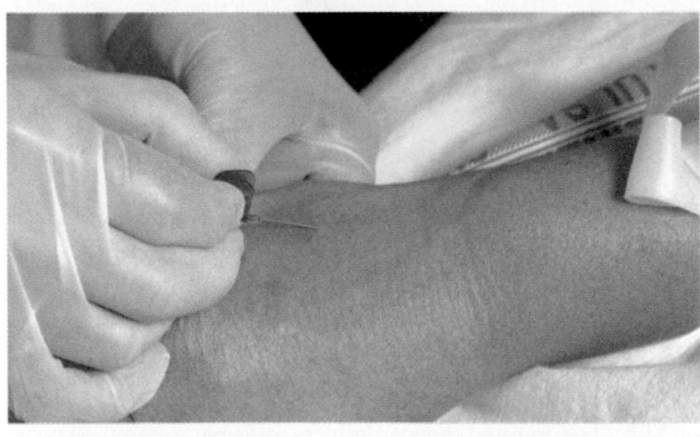

▲ Insert needle at 30° angle through skin below selected vein.

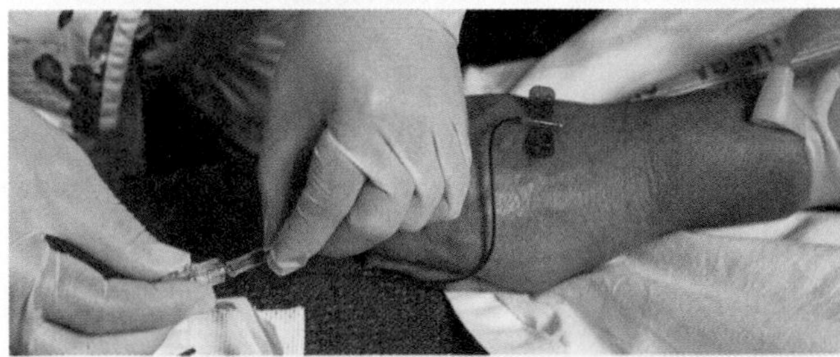

▲ Attach sterile resealable injection cap to end of winged needle tubing.

3. Carefully affix end of IV infusion tubing to end of winged needle tubing. Remove sterile cover from needle and run fluid through needle to prime tubing, then clamp it, and replace needle cover.
4. Apply tourniquet to distend selected vein.

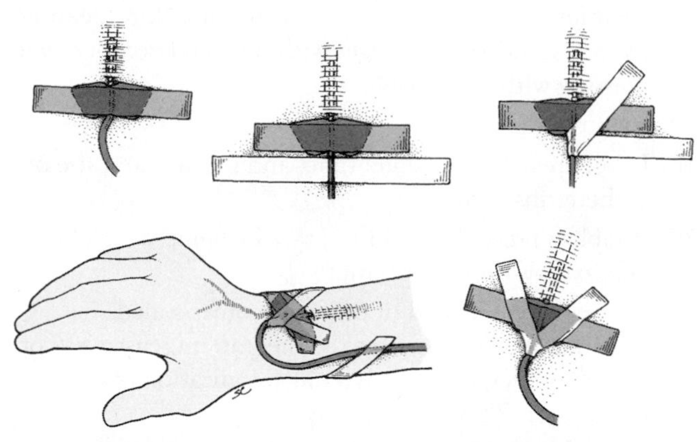

▲ Use chevron method to secure winged small vein needle; then apply occlusive transparent dressing over infusion site

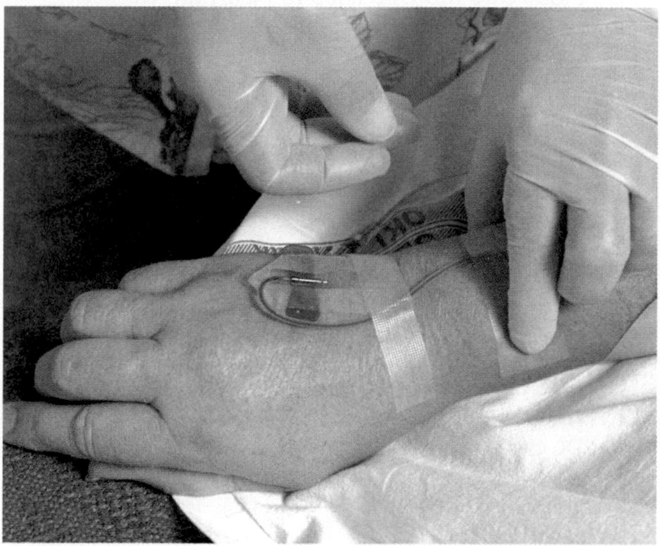

▲ After chevron method secure needle, loop, and tape tubing.

5. Prep the selected site with chlorhexidine gluconate; it should be applied with back-and-forth motion for a minimum of 30 seconds. Allow to air dry.
6. Remove protective cap from winged needle and hold needle by its wings, anchor vein by placing thumb below client's vein.
7. Place thumb of nondominant hand below selected site and pull skin taut. With needle bevel up, enter client's skin at a 30° angle. You may use either of these methods:
   a. Enter skin next to or alongside vein. Flatten angle to 15° once needle is under skin and then enter vein from side.
   b. Insert needle through skin below intended puncture site, then enter vein. ▶ ***Rationale:*** Inserting needle through skin and into small vein with one thrust will result in hematoma formation.
8. Follow course of vein. Sudden "pop" and lack of resistance is felt when vein is entered.
9. Observe for flashback of blood in needle tubing.
10. Carefully advance needle up course of the vein until it reaches hub.

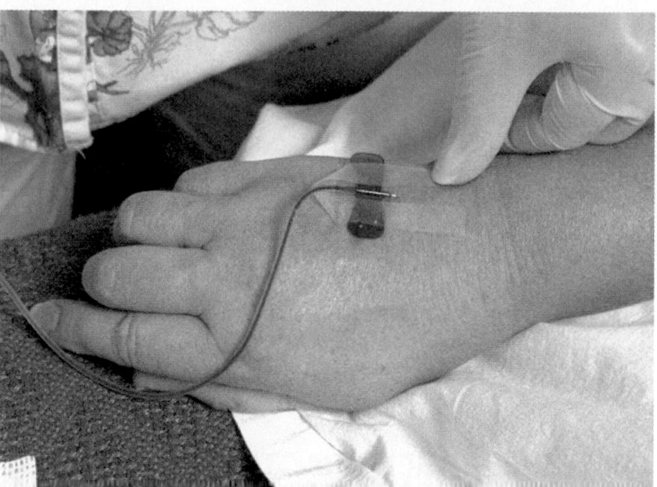

▲ Bring sterile tape over needle and secure needle and wings with chevron method.

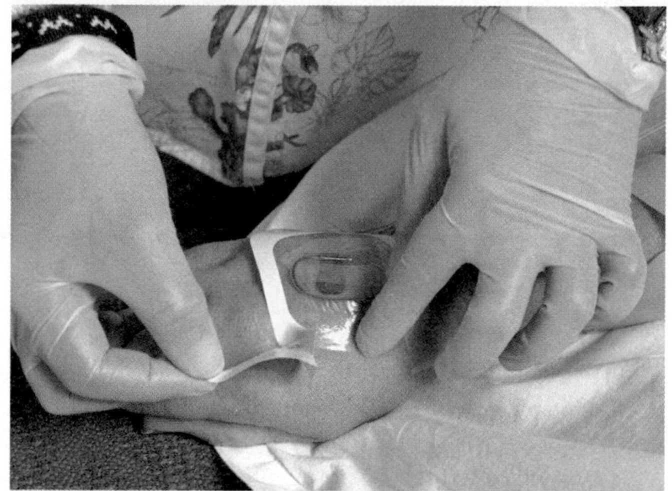

▲ Cover site with transparent dressing: date, time, initials, and size of catheter.

11. Release tourniquet.
12. Inject normal saline for lock, or affix IV tubing, open clamp, and observe drip chamber. ▶ ***Rationale:*** Fluid should flow easily, and there should be no sudden swelling at the IV site.
13. Reduce flow rate to keep open until you have secured needle in place.

General Time Frame for Tubing Changes

- Primary and secondary tubing— 72 hr
- Primary intermittent tubing—24 hr
- Extension tubing—replace when vascular device is replaced (it is considered part of the IV system)
- TPN and lipids—every 24 hr
- Blood or blood products tubing—every 4 hr or after 2 units of blood
- Always check facility policies and procedures and follow their regulations.

IV Insertion Sites

Select	Avoid
Use vein in nondominant arm	Antecubital fossa
Use smallest catheter for site	Lower extremities
Use most distal sites first. Save antecubital site for emergencies.	Previously used veins and injured or sclerotic veins
Assess client's condition; vein condition, size, location; type and duration of therapy	Veins in affected arm with dialysis fistula or axillary dissection

EVIDENCE-BASED PRACTICE

Needle Sticks Related to IV Devices

In a 2002 study of 47 facilities, 1,693 needle-stick injuries were reported. One-half of all documented injuries were caused by devices used by nurses throughout their daily practice. The number one injury was the disposable syringe (35%). The second most common injury was the use of a winged steel needle (7%). Most injuries occurred after use, when the devices were being discarded. Most facilities have converted to needleless IV systems for connecting IV lines.

Source: Perry, I., & Metules, T. (2004, November). How to avoid needlesticks. *RN*, 28ns2–28ns7 (supplement).

14. Secure needle with half-inch wide sterile tape and place over the hub or attach a securement device according to manufacturers' directions.
15. Loop and tape IV tubing a short distance from needle.
16. Apply occlusive transparent dressing over infusion site. Gently smooth dressing from center to edges.
    ▸ ***Rationale:*** Excessive tension can cause skin shearing. Do not seal dressing's edges with tape and do not cover dressing with roller gauge.
17. Remove gloves.
18. Label dressing with date, time, and initials, and size of catheter inserted.
19. Establish prescribed infusion rate by pump or calculated gravity flow drops per minute.
20. Change site every 48 hr or if it becomes soiled.
    ▸ ***Rationale:*** According to studies, an increased risk of thrombophlebitis and bacterial colonization of catheters occurs after 72 hr.

Clinical Alert

Meticulous care must be used to insert the winged-tipped needle because these needles lead to the majority of reported needle-stick injuries.

Clinical Alert

All tape placed under transparent dressings should be sterile. Check facility policy before securing IV site. Some hospitals do not allow tape under the transparent dressing.

Source: Intravenous Nurses Society, Standard 49, 2006.

Clinical Alert

The CDC has not established a recommendation for hang time of IV fluids. Follow hospital policy and change fluids accordingly.

Inserting an Over-the-Needle Catheter

Equipment

- Tourniquet (constrictive band)
- 2% Chlorhexidine swab
- Sterile over-the-needle catheter sizes 12–24 gauge, ½–2 in. long

NOTE: Some winged devices are over-the-needle catheters.

- Optional: EMLA cream (lidocaine and prilocaine) cream or syringe with local anesthetic (lidocaine) and 25–26-gauge needle (check agency policy or physician's orders and client sensitivity before using)
- Prepared administration set and infusion solution if ordered
- Electronic infusion device
- Protective needleless cap if required
- Syringe with at least 2–3 times the volume capacity of the catheter and add-on devices with preservative-free normal saline for lock (if indicated)
- Sterile half-inch tape
- Sterile gloves

Procedure

1. Prepare IV system and follow steps in Preparing the Venipuncture Site.
2. Select appropriate size over-the-needle catheter.
3. Perform hand hygiene and don gloves.
4. Position extremity for venipuncture.

NOTE: Apply EMLA cream or inject site (intradermally) with small wheal of local anesthetic, according to hospital policy. (Allow 60 minutes for cream and 90 seconds for anesthetic to take effect.)

5. Place extremity flat on bed or place in a dependent position. ▸ ***Rationale:*** Gravity will slow venous return and thus dilate the vein. If vein is not distended sufficiently for easy venipuncture, ask client to make a fist or lightly tap on the vein with your fingertips.
6. Hold catheter with bevel up and examine the integrity of end of catheter.
7. Apply traction to stabilize vein.

8. With bevel of needle up, insert needle/catheter unit at a 45° angle into client's skin either:
   a. Alongside of vein, or
   b. About a half-inch distal to selected puncture site.
9. Revisualize vein; reduce angle of cannula to 30°, pierce vein. A "pop" will frequently be felt. Observe for backflow of blood in plastic hub. Slide needle into vein about 1/4 in. after backflow observed. Continue to apply traction. ▶ ***Rationale:*** This indicates you are in the vein. If vein is hard to find, use the vascular imaging device if the facility has one.
10. Hold needle and gently advance plastic catheter hub over needle and up vein no more than halfway.

NOTE: Maintain aseptic technique throughout procedure and prevent trauma to site and vein. These catheters are associated with a very high rate of phlebitis—80% in one study.

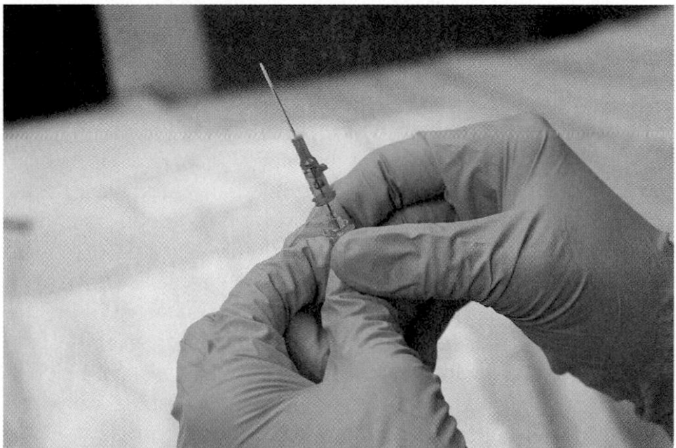

1 Inspect integrity of needle tip.

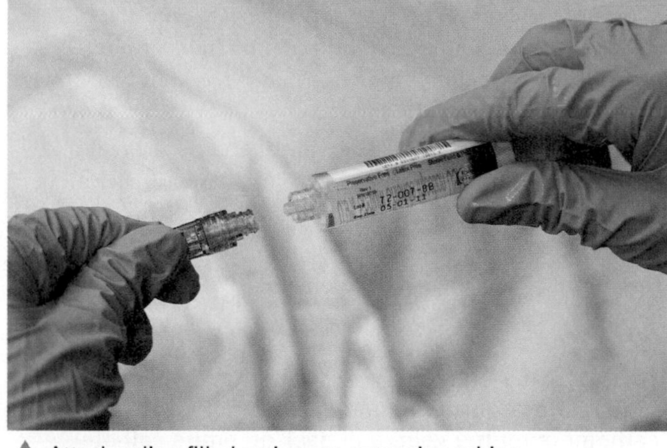

2 Attach saline-filled syringe to extension tubing.

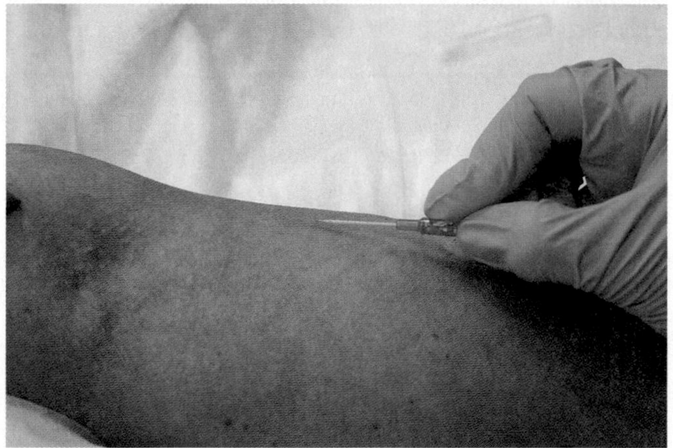

3 Insert needle, with bevel up, at 30° angle.

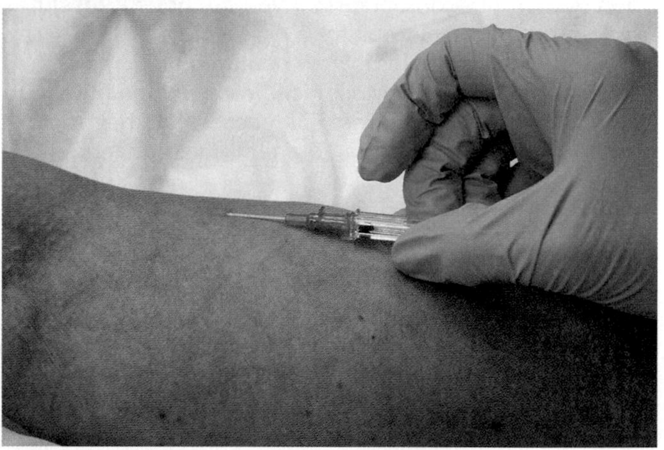

4 Check for blood return or check the flashback.

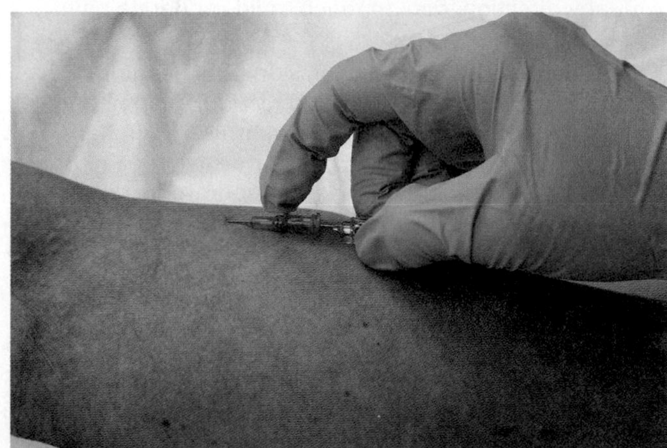

5 Pick up protective covering.

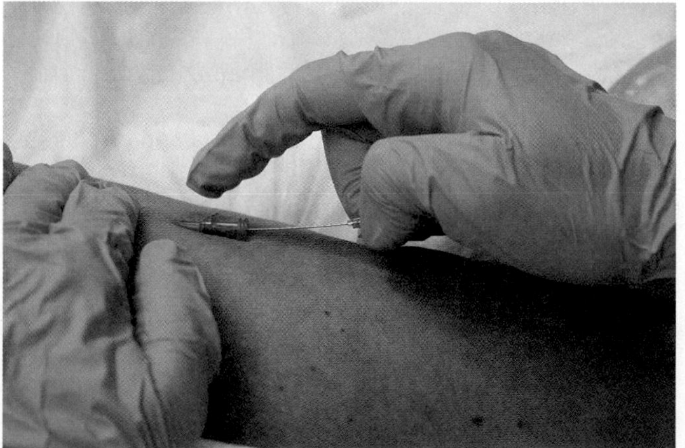

6 Separate, but do not completely remove, the stylette.

11. Stop and separate, but do not completely remove, the stylet from catheter.
12. Advance only the catheter until catheter hub meets the skin. The catheter moves over the stylet. If the hub is against the vein valve, you will need to initiate the infusion of IV fluids in order to float catheter to the middle of the vein.
13. Release tourniquet. Leave stylet in catheter while you tape catheter to the skin. ▶ ***Rationale:*** Stylet acts like a plug, and leaving it partially in place you don't have to hurry to tape catheter to the skin.
14. Tape catheter under hub of needle, without touching puncture site, and without touching hub/catheter juncture. Securement device may be used in place of taping procedure.
15. Place digital pressure above distal end of catheter and carefully remove stylet. Maintaining aseptic technique, connect catheter to IV tubing or place a saline lock on catheter.
16. Connect catheter to needleless cap or insert IV tubing into catheter.

Clinical Alert

If no blood is observed and you did not feel the catheter enter the vein, pull back on entire catheter apparatus without exiting skin. Reassess vein position, then reattempt venipuncture. If you are not successful, remove catheter and look for a different site. Remember the catheter is now contaminated and cannot be used again. Most facilities allow the nurse to attempt two venipunctures; if unsuccessful, they must notify another professional to attempt venipuncture.

EVIDENCE-BASED PRACTICE

Flushing With Low-Dose Heparin

There are many conflicting studies indicating outcomes that are both pro and con for using low-dose heparin with peripheral venous catheters. In one study, low-dose heparin infused continuously through peripheral venous catheters required further study to determine effectiveness in prolonging catheter life. Studies have proven that using heparin in arterial catheters is of benefit. Using intermittent heparin flushes for peripheral IV catheters also requires further validation, as it seems to be no more effective than using NS flushes.

Source: Randolph, A., Cook, D. J., Gonzales, C. A., & Andrew, M. (1998, March 28). Benefit of heparin in peripheral venous and arterial catheters: Systematic review and meta-analysis of randomized controlled trials. *British Medical Journal, 316*(7136), 969–975.

Flushing Using Saline or Heparin

In a second study completed at the Mayo Clinic, Rochester, MN, a prospective, randomized, and double-blind study was completed on 73 hospitalized pregnant women between 24 and 42 weeks gestation. The clients were randomly assigned to receive a peripheral intermittent IV lock flush of either saline or heparin after each medication administration, or at least every 24 hr. The IV sites were assessed every 12 hr for signs of phlebitis. The results of the study indicated there were no statistically significant differences in IV lock patency or in phlebitis between heparin or normal saline flushes. The conclusion was that the study provides support for both normal saline and heparin in the doses studied as being equally effective in the maintenance of peripheral IV locks. With the small number of participants, the authors suggest additional studies are needed to determine optimal therapy over time.

Source: Niesen, K. M., Harris, D. Y., Parkin, I. S., & Henn, L. T. (2003). The effects of heparin versus normal saline for maintenance of peripheral intravenous locks in pregnant women. *Journal of Obstetric, Gynecologic, Neonatal Nursing, 32*(4), 503–508.

Evaluation Criteria

Catheter sites are evaluated at least each shift for both phlebitis and infiltration using evaluation criteria established by the Intravenous Nurses' Society (standards were revised in 2000).

Phlebitis

0 = no clinical symptoms
1+ = erythema at access site with or without pain
2+ = pain at access site with erythema and/or edema
3+ = pain at access site with erythema and/or edema, streak formation
4+ = pain at access site with erythema and/or edema, streak formation, palpable venous cord >1 in. in length, purulent discharge

Note: No catheter should remain in place with signs of phlebitis, even with good blood flow and IV infusion rate.

Infiltrations

0 = no symptoms
1 = skin blanched, edema
2 = skin blanched, edema 1–6 in. in any direction, cool to touch, with or without pain
3 = skin blanched, translucent, gross edema >6 in. in any direction, cool to touch, mild-moderate pain, possible numbness
4 = skin blanched, translucent, skin tight, leading, gross edema >6 in. in any direction, deep pitting tissue edema, skin discolored, bruised, swollen, circulatory impairment moderate-severe pain, infiltration of any amount of blood product, irritant, or vesicant.

Note: Infiltrations should be diagnosed well before obvious swelling occurs. Most infiltrations should be warm packed to promote reabsorption of fluid into vascular bed and out of tissues, except in case of infiltration by a vesicant drug, then follow facility policy or drug manufacturer's directions.

EVIDENCE BASED PRACTICE

Heparin Flush vs. Saline Flush for Maintaining CVC

Two studies completed at the University of Pennsylvania and Seattle's Children's Hospital suggested there was insufficient evidence to conclude that a heparin flush is more effective than a saline flush. Flushing CVCs with heparin poses a risk of heparin induced thrombophlebitis. In the University of Pennsylvania study, the evidence for using heparin to flush CVCs is small, and the published studies reviewed by the committee were of low quality, therefore the nursing policy for maintaining CVCs was changed to flushing catheters with saline only.

In the first 18 months after the change in policy there was a reduction in catheter-assisted blood stream infections, no increase in catheter or vein occlusion, and a reduction in nursing workload without compromising patient safety.

In a study conducted at Seattle's Children Hospital and reported in *Nursing Times*, February 12, 2010, there was no evidence to support a difference between normal saline and heparin for patency of locked peripheral IVs. Seattle elected to conform to the Infusion Nurses Society (INS) standards published in late 2008. It recommends the use of NS for flushing peripheral IVs.

Source: Anderson, Barbara: Abstract (2010, February 12). A comparison of heparin and saline flush to maintain patency in central venous catheters. *Nursing Times*.
Source: Seattle Children's Clinical Effectiveness Program. Executive Summary NS Flush PIV. December 12, 2009. www.seattlechildrens.org/doc/executive-summary.

17. Open clamp and observe drip chamber for fluid flow (or preserve patency of system by injecting 2–3 times the amount of volume of the catheter and connecting devices using 0.9% preservative free normal saline through access site). There should not be any sudden swelling at IV site.
18. Observe for signs of infiltration.
19. Reduce flow and proceed with stabilizing the catheter. ▸ ***Rationale:*** Stabilizing the catheter reduces the need for unscheduled restarts and risks for health workers from unnecessary exposure to needles.
20. Prep site with skin protectant and place catheter in securement device.
21. If using sterile tape, do not tape over connectors. ▸ ***Rationale:*** Taping impedes access to the IV site in emergencies. Cover insertion site with sterile transparent dressing.
22. Loop IV tubing only once to prevent decreasing length of tubing. ▸ ***Rationale:*** Too many loops in tubing reduce distance from IV solution container to client's IV site.

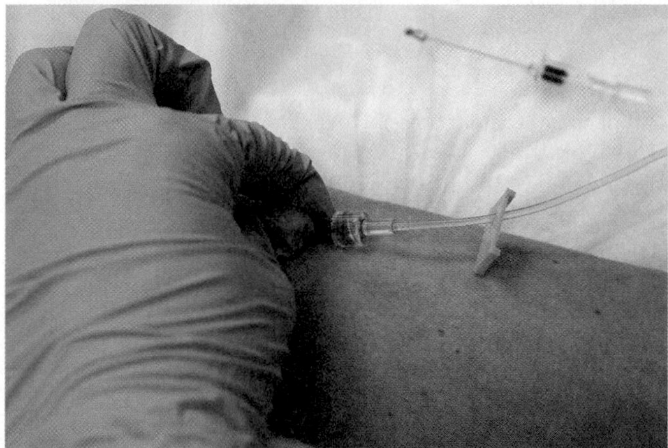

7 Attach extension tubing.

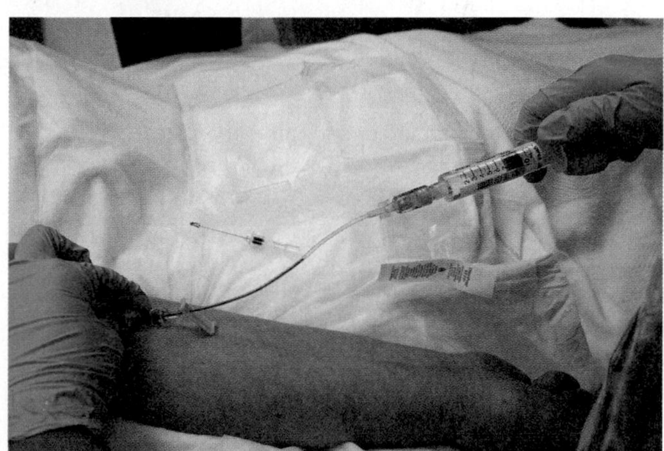

8 Backflush and instill 3 mL of normal saline.

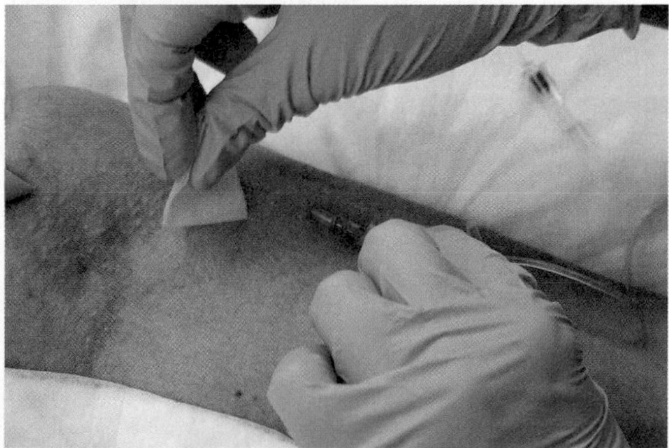

9 Prep site with skin protective for Statlock device.

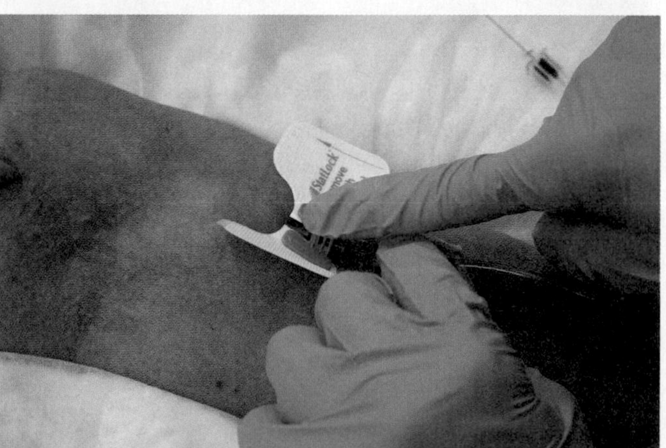

10 Place Statlock under cannula with arrows pointing up.

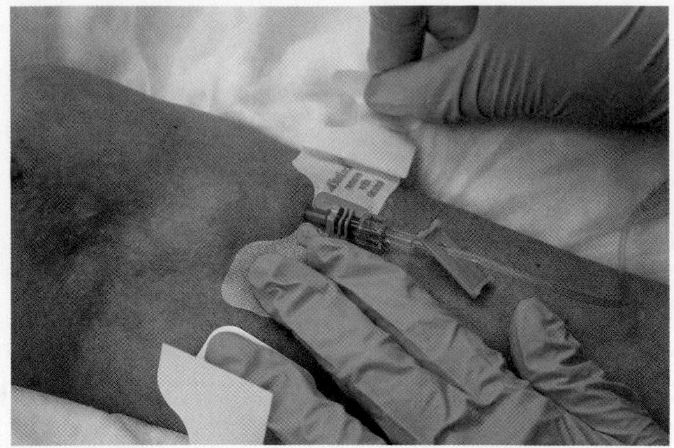

11 Remove cover carefully and press down on skin.

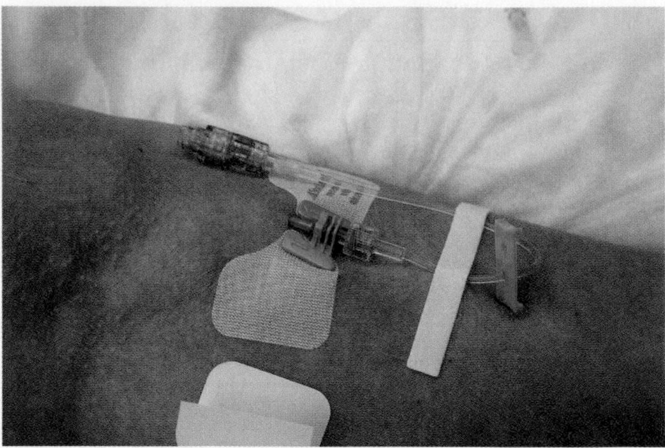

12 Anchor tubing with tape.

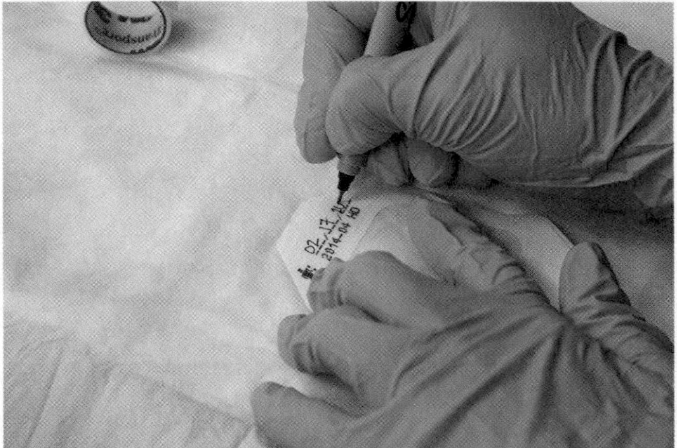

13 Place date, initials, and size of catheter on dressing tab.

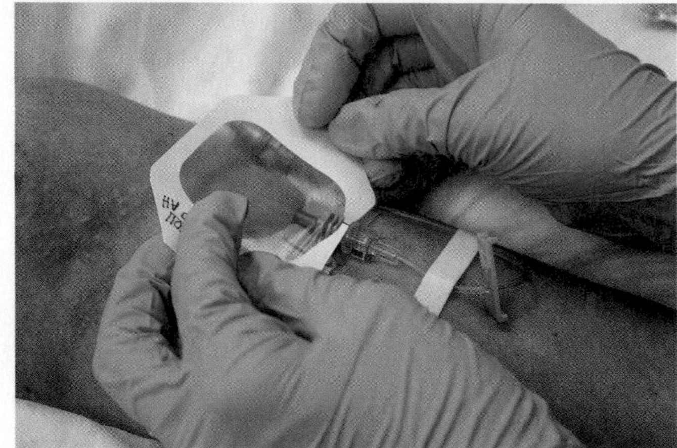

14 Place transparent dressing over site.

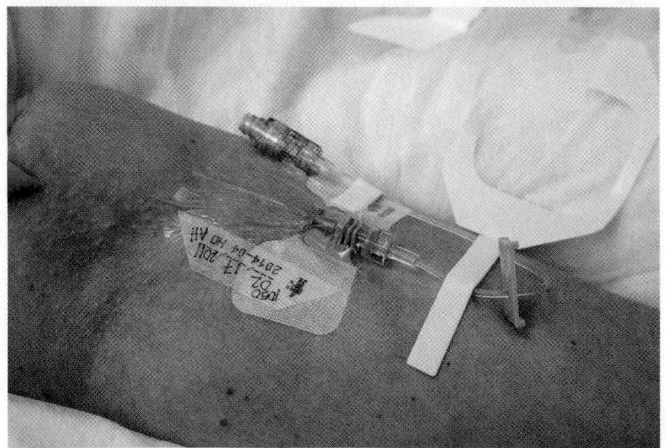

15 Secure dressing and place tab on dressing.

This can put excess pressure on IV site and potentially cause catheter to dislodge from vein or infiltration to occur.

23. Loop and tape tubing to client's arm a short distance from site.
24. Set drip rate according to physician's order.
25. Label IV site with date, time, initials, and size of catheter.
26. Remove gloves and perform hand hygiene.
27. Change cannula and infusion site every 72 hr unless infiltrated, site shows evidence of phlebitis, or cannula comprised.

IV catheter stabilization devices should include manufactured catheter stabilization devices, sterile tape, and surgical strips. The INS promotes the use of manufactured catheter stabilization devices such as the StatLock IV catheter securement device.

Source: (2006). Catheter stabilization. In *Infusion nursing: Standards of practice* (chapter 43). Hagerstown, MD: Lippincott Williams & Wilkins.

Clinical Alert

If using needleless Angiocath system, once the "flash" is noted and catheter is advanced, the retract button is pushed and the needle automatically shielded.

DOCUMENTATION for IV Therapy

- Time and date of insertion
- Location of insertion site, name of vein cannulated
- Gauge length and type of needle/catheter inserted
- Number of attempts (if more than one)
- Type of dressing applied
- Flush administered for cannula patency
- Type, amount, and rate of solution infused
- Status of IV site
- Client response to procedure

CRITICAL THINKING Application

Expected Outcomes

- Fluid and electrolyte needs are met.
- Appropriate IV site is selected and IV inserted without difficulty.
- IV fluids infuse at prescribed rate without complications.
- Appropriate IV equipment for client.
- IV site is maintained using sterile technique.

Unexpected Outcomes	Alternative Actions
Venipuncture is unsuccessful for needle/catheter insertion.	• Remove needle/catheter, apply pressure at insertion site until bleeding stops. (This prevents ecchymosis at site.) Apply Band-Aid. • Apply small pressure dressing if client on anticoagulant therapy. • Select another site more proximal in vein or use another extremity. • Avoid the one-step entry method since this frequently results in a through-and-through vein puncture. • After two failed attempts, seek a more experienced person to perform venipuncture. • Place extremity in dependent position before placing tourniquet. Allows vein to fill. • Place warm compress on extremity to increase vasodilation before placing tourniquet.
Vein rolls and is difficult to enter.	• Apply traction with thumb and index finger to stabilize skin and vein; maintain traction until venipuncture complete. • Select a smaller gauge catheter. • Advance catheter slowly.
Vein is fragile and "balloons" around needle on vein entry.	• Release tourniquet as soon as vein entry is evident. • Avoid use of tourniquet if veins are very fragile or client is taking an anticoagulant. • Enter vein with needle bevel down.
Infiltration occurs.	• Place warm moist pack, using warm towel, enclose area from fingertips to elbow. Place extremity in plastic bag with open end at elbow. Leave in place no more than 10 minutes.
Vesicant drug infuses into tissue.	• Clamp IV tubing. • Infuse antidote for specific medication, according to physician orders.

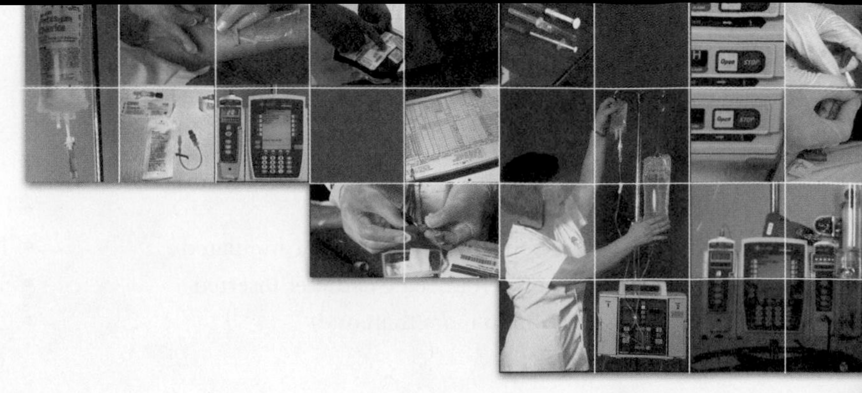

Chapter 28

UNIT ❷

Intravenous Management

Nursing Process Data

ASSESSMENT Data Base

- Assess site for erythema, swelling, or pain.
- Assess infusion for correct solution, amount, and flow rate.
- Assess need to change IV to saline lock.
- Assess need to change client's gown while IV is infusing.
- Assess need to change IV solution/administration set and infusion site.

PLANNING Objectives

- To maintain the IV site free from erythema, swelling, or pain
- To monitor the IV infusion rate accurately
- To change a gown while maintaining the IV site
- To discontinue IV therapy without complication
- To convert IV to saline lock

IMPLEMENTATION Procedures

EVALUATION Expected Outcomes

- Fluids are administered without adverse effects.
- IV site remains clean without signs of infection or filtration.
- IV is converted to a saline lock and is functioning properly.
- Client's gown is changed while maintaining IV placement.
- IV is discontinued intact; site remains free of infection or bleeding.

Pearson Nursing Student Resources

Find additional review materials at **nursing.pearsonhighered.com**

Prepare for success with NCLEX®-style practice questions and Skill Checklists

Regulating Infusion Flow Rate

Procedure

1. Check manufacturer's drip-rate calibration on administration set package. Macrodrip sets vary from 10 to 15 gtt per 1 mL. Microdrip factor is 60 drops/mL.
2. Check physician's order for amount of fluid to be delivered per unit of time (e.g., 1 L every 8 hr, or hourly flow rate such as 100 mL/hr).
3. Calculate flow rate.
   a. To find the number of milliliters to be given per hour:

$$\frac{\text{Total solution}}{\text{No. of hours to run}} = \text{mL/hour}$$

   b. To find drops per minute:

$$\frac{\text{mL/hr} \times \text{drop factor}}{\text{60 minutes}} = \text{gtts/minute}$$

4. Note drip chamber; count the drops in 1 minute (or in 15 seconds and multiply by 4).
5. Adjust tubing clamp until the chamber drips the desired number of drops per minute (or 15-second increment).
6. Monitor flow rate frequently—adjustments to maintain desired delivery are often necessary.

IV Calorie Calculation

- 1000 mL of D_5W provides 50 g of dextrose.
- 50 g of dextrose provides 4 Cal/g; therefore, multiply 50 g × 4 Cal.
- 1000 of mL D_5W provides 200 Cal.
- Usual IV fluid maintenance is 2000–3000 mL/day (400–600 Cal/day).
- 4 cal/g is used in calculation; however, it is actually 3.4 cal/g.

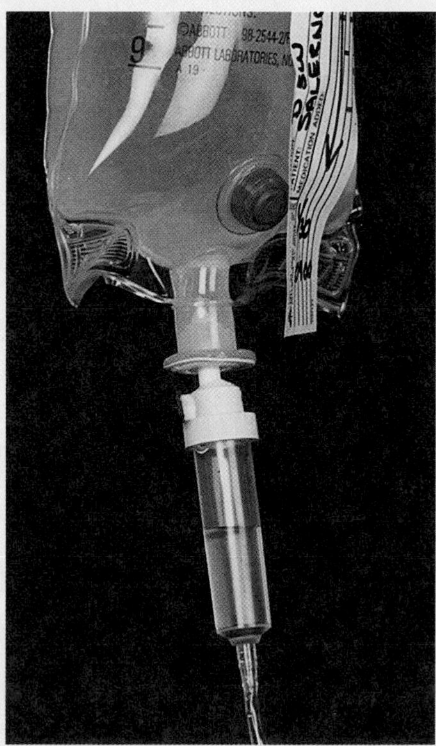

▲ Count drops per minute to check accuracy of drip rate.

Factors That Influence IV Flow Rates When Using Gravity for Infusion

- Warm fluids drip faster than cold fluids.
- The higher the bag is above insertion site, the faster the infusion.
- The more IV administration is tilted, the larger each drop from drip chamber.
- The larger the catheter diameter, the faster the flow rate.
- The longer the catheter, the slower the flow rate because of resistance.
- Increased blood pressure or coughing will slow the flow rate (this is a temporary situation usually).

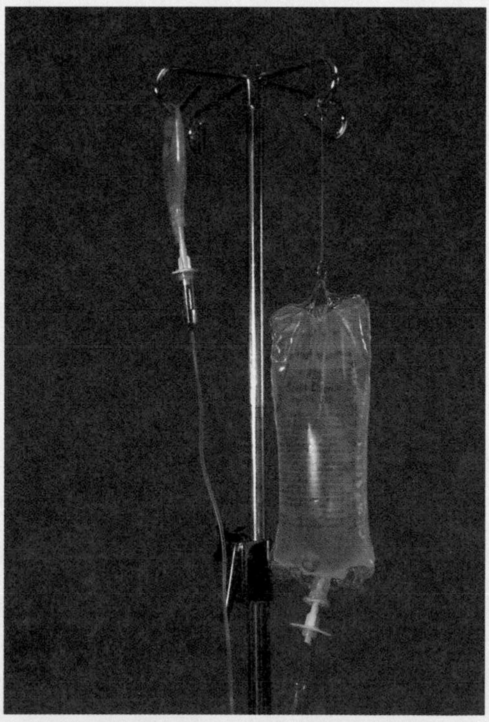

Note: Because of these variables, manual control of IVs is not recommended. IV pumps are the most predictable method of infusing fluids.

Using an Electronic Flow-Control Device

Equipment

Electronic infusion device (pump)
Device-compatible IV administration set
Needleless access device
Gloves

Preparation

1. Verify client using two identifiers.
2. Attach controller to IV pole.
   a. Attach controller to the IV pole so it is below and in-line with IV container.
   b. Plug machine into electric outlet (unless using battery-operated).

NOTE: Batteries last up to 6 hours. Keep device plugged into electric outlet unless it is necessary to move device.

Procedure

1. Explain procedure to client and discuss the various sounds that can be heard during the use of the equipment.
2. Perform hand hygiene.

Clinical Alert

Observe IV site frequently when pumps are used. IV pumps do not normally detect infiltration at the IV site. Infiltration does not produce enough pressure to trigger an alarm. Check for edema, cool skin, discomfort, and tenderness at the IV site.

IF Alarm Sounds, Check the Following

Most devices have a message system that specifies the exact problem. You should be prepared to troubleshoot various components of the system.

- *Infusion Complete:* When the exact volume to be delivered is set and the volume limit has been reached, an alarm sounds and the machine goes to a KVO "keep-open" mode. Establish if the total volume of the container has been delivered; change the solution container if needed, and reset the volume to be infused.
- *Occlusion:* All devices sound an alarm when they cannot maintain delivery in the face of increasing resistance. In this instance, check the insertion site for infiltration and look for position problems, pinched tubing, closed clamp, turned stopcock, or clogged filter.
- *Other Problems:* Other messages may indicate "air in the line," "low battery," "cassette" (improperly loaded), or "free flow."
- *Nursing Action:* Check trouble spot carefully, readjust, and restart the infusion.

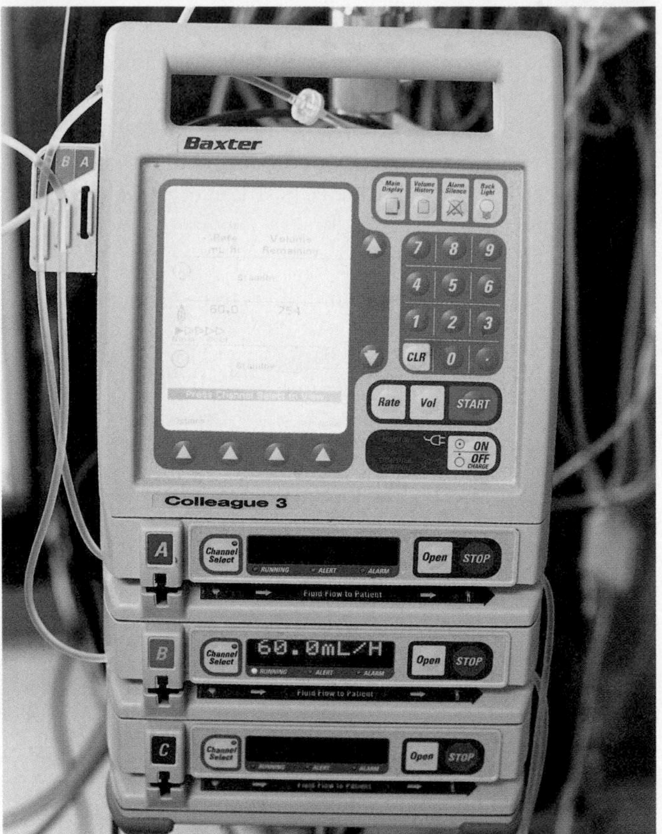

▲ Baxter: Multiple Channel Pump.

3. Close regulating clamp on the set tubing before hanging bag.
4. Spike IV solution bag.
5. Fill drip chamber to minimum one-third full. ▶ ***Rationale:*** This amount allows sufficient air space in drip chamber.
6. Prime tubing by opening regulating clamp slowly and allowing tubing to fill with IV solution. If using a cassette-type tubing, follow package instructions to correctly prime the cassette portion of the tubing that engages into the control device.

NOTE: Check if tubing has anti–free-flow device that must be opened before primary tubing.

7. Follow manufacturer's instructions to load administration set into device, taking care to fit tubing and cassette into appropriate receptor sites. (One type of pump is a multiple-channel pump that can infuse three different IV solutions at one time.)
8. Close device door and latch.
9. Perform hand hygiene and don gloves.
10. Check that client's venipuncture site is free from signs of vein irritation or infiltration.
11. Connect administration set tubing to established infusion site.
12. Open regulating clamp on administration set.
13. Turn device ON.

14. Set device parameters for operation, again following manufacturer's instructions or machine's setup prompts. Parameters may include:
    a. Infusion (e.g., primary)
    b. Volume to be infused
    c. Rate (mL/hr)
    d. Pressure (measure can vary; e.g., mmHg, cm H_2O, or psi)
15. START device when parameters are set.
16. Observe that infusion is running properly.
17. Remove gloves and perform hand hygiene.
18. Check client's infusion site frequently.

Infusion Pump

In contrast to gravity flow devices, positive-pressure infusion pumps are more accurate in the preselected volume delivery by adding pressure to overcome resistance to fluid flow produced by tubing diameter, filter, viscosity of infusing fluid, cannula, etc. Pumps usually require use of specially designed administration sets. When the system is working with normal resistance, delivery pressure is minimal. When resistance (5 psi over baseline) develops in the catheter or tubing, the pump adds pressure (within limits) to maintain infusion. Changes in resistance at an insertion site due to infiltration or thrombosis may not set off the system's alarm, and site problems could become serious. When the pump's maximum pressure limit is reached, an occlusion pressure alarm sounds. The nurse must become familiar with infusion devices by reading the manufacturer's literature and adhering to all instructions to ensure safe, efficient operation.

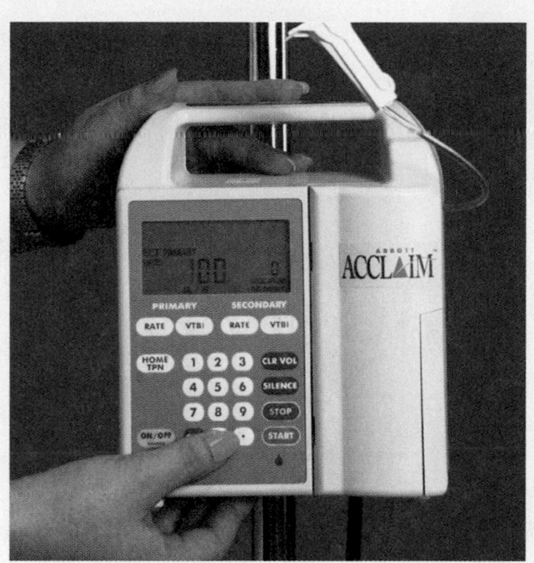

Smart IV Pumps

- Smart pumps have a "brain" (computer).
- Nurses are alerted when a pump setting does not match the facility's drug administration guidelines.
- Data is logged from pump to pharmacy computer: time, date, drug that was infused, concentration, programmed rate, and volume infused are recorded.
- Individual facility pharmacists create the data base of information for their own facility, and then the information is programmed into the pump.
- Facilities program pumps with specific data sets or "profiles." Each area of the facility develops their own drug library, i.e., OB, Peds, ICU.
- Manufacturers of smart pumps offer different features:
    - Add-on syringe pumps for small-volume IV push or bolus infusions.
    - Multiple infusions through one pump.
    - Administration of patient-controlled analgesia (PCA).

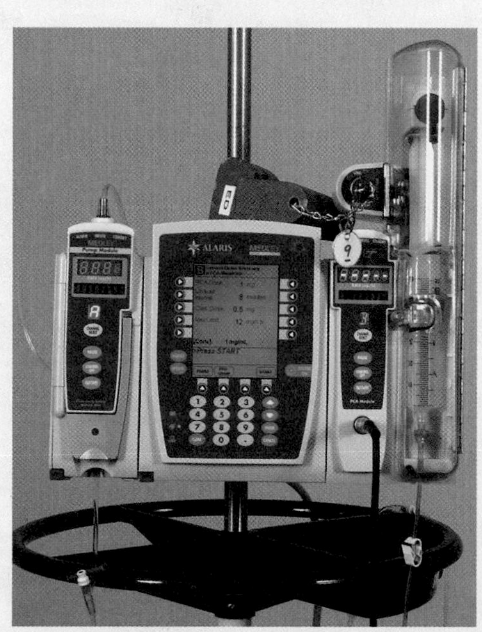

Using a "Smart" Pump

Equipment

Point-of-care computer specific to nursing unit
IV tubing
IV fluids and/or IV medications

Procedure

1. Identify client using two identifiers and explain pump's function.
2. Assemble equipment and bring to client's bedside.

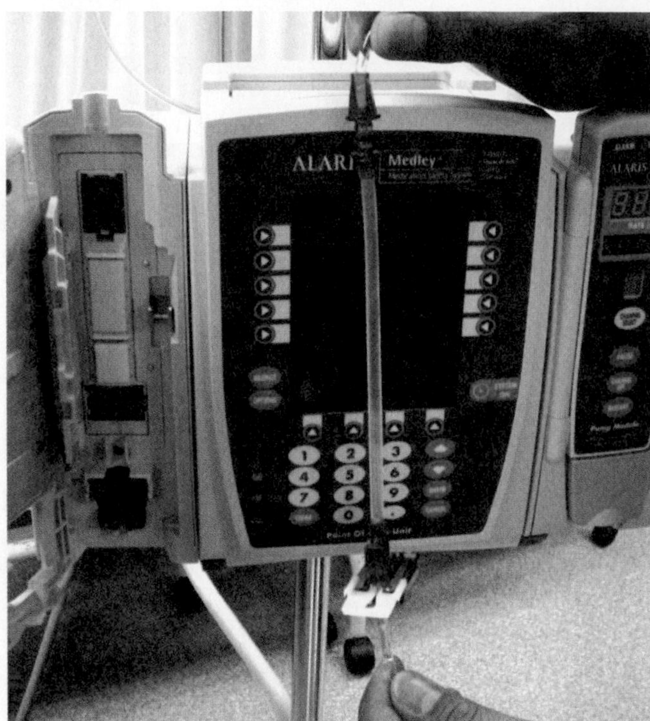

▲ Hang IV on pole. Prime tubing and insert into pump module cassette.

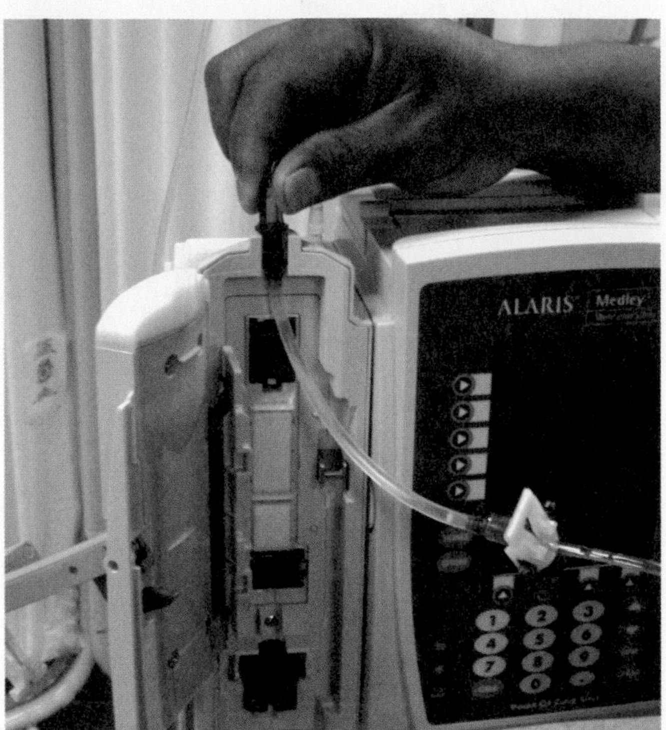

▲ Place top of IV tubing into top of cassette and listen for click indicating it is seated.

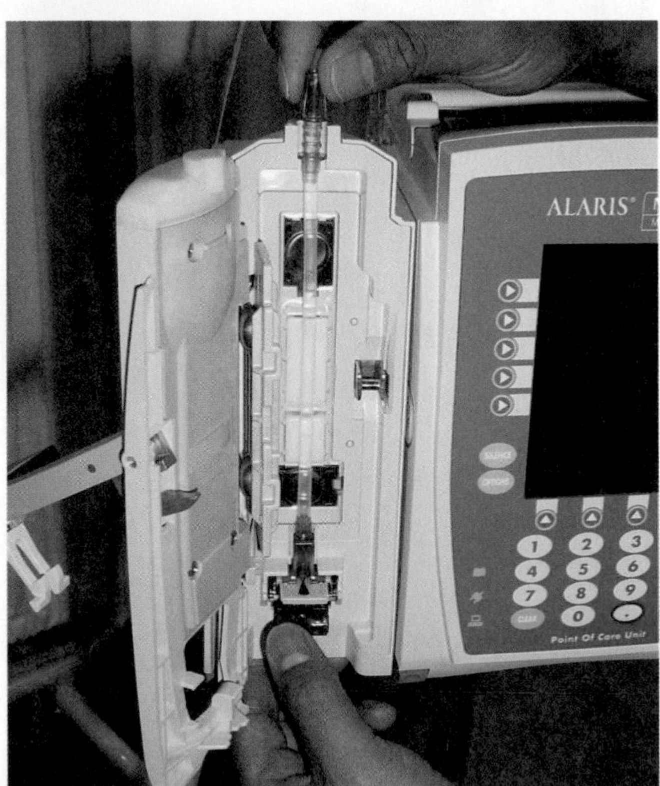

▲ Insert white slide clamp into cassette and listen for click.

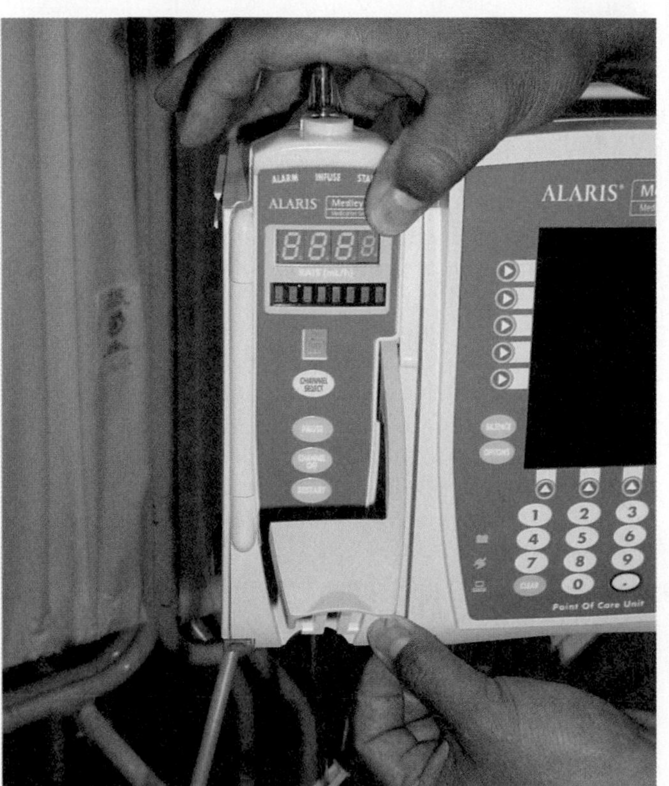

▲ Close pump module door and lower locking level.

3. Perform hand hygiene.
4. Verify IV site is patent and without signs of infiltration.
5. Plug pump into electrical outlet.
6. Insert the pump module into the point-of-care computer ("brain").
7. Spike IV fluid bag.
8. Prime IV tubing with appropriate solution.
9. Insert the IV tubing into the pump module and close the door to the pump. (Follow photos for inserting tubing into cassette.)
10. View screen will ask which client care area is being used. ▸ ***Rationale:*** The pump automatically configures itself to provide the infusion parameters for that area.
11. Choose the intended drug and concentration from the list outlined on the screen.
12. Enter the ordered dose and infusion rate; the pump checks this information against the drug library. If what was programmed matches the pump's drug library, the pump allows the infusion to begin. Follow manufacturer's directions on how to program the pump. Each manufacturer's equipment is somewhat different.

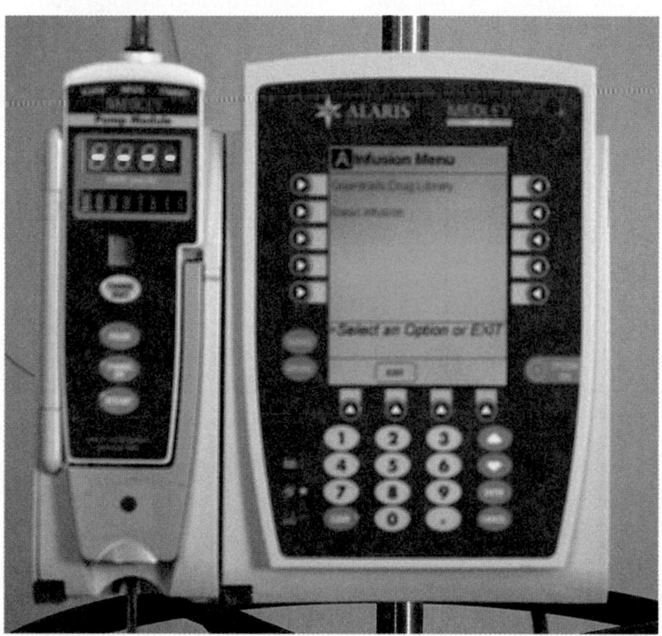

▲ Select medication to be infused.

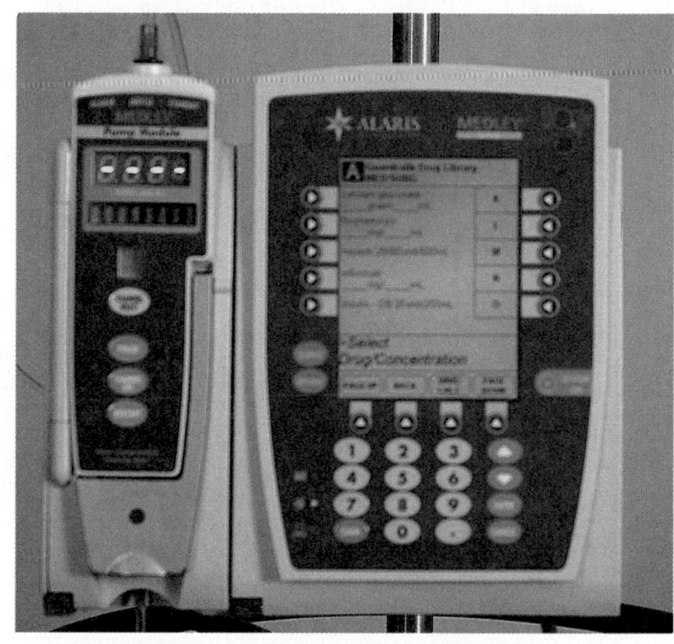

▲ Check screen for drug name and infusion rate.

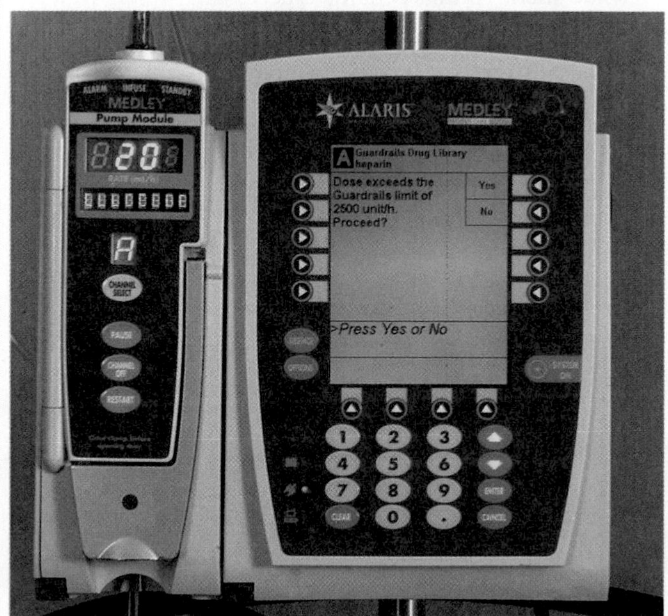

▲ Check screen when "soft alert" sounds to determine problem.

Using a Bar Code Medication Administration System

- If the facility uses a bar code medication administration (BCMA) system, a computerized prescriber order entry (CPOE), automatic medication dispensing, and electronic medication records, smart pumps can provide a very high level of client safety. The system will tell you which IV medications were ordered via a CPOE for your client and when the medication is due.
- When the nurse enters the client's room with the scanning device, she/he scans the bar-code labels on the medication, the client's ID band. and the nurse's ID badge. The information from the bar-code label attached to the medication IV bag will be transmitted wirelessly to and programmed into the infusion pump.
- The pump will begin infusing only when scanning of all pieces of information is completed.
- The pump automatically communicates with a computer in the pharmacy, providing the status of the infusion.

13. If an audible and visual alert occurs, the programmed data are outside the specified limits. The alert informs you about which parameter is out of the recommended range.
14. Depending on the medication or client care area, the pump will sound a "soft" alarm or a "hard" alarm. Some facilities allow a "soft" alarm to be overridden. If you override the alarm, the infusion will begin. This alarm is considered a minor error.
15. When "hard" alarm occurs, the pump shuts down. It cannot be overridden. Reprogram the pump with settings that are within your facility's specified limits to begin infusing when a "hard" alarm sounds.

NOTE: The smart pump's software logs and tracks all alerts, recording the time, date, drug, concentration, and infusion rate, as well as any action taken, whether the pump is overridden or not.

Clinical Alert

Check the facility's policies and procedures to determine whether the pump can be run with the override or whether a verbal verification of the order with a physician or pharmacist must be obtained before proceeding.

16. Observe the screen to ensure medication is infusing at prescribed rate.

EVIDENCE-BASED PRACTICE

Smart Pump Technology Reduces Errors

There has been little IV error-prevention data published that documents the actual frequency of IV medication errors with infusion devices.

In a study conducted in the intensive care unit and operating room areas at Massachusetts General Hospital where use of an electronic drug library was implemented, a 50% reduction in the number of drug administration errors involving syringe pumps occurred over a 3-month period using the smart pump. The study indicated that logs from the 135 smart pumps showed:

- 40,644 infusion starts (potential for error)
- 693 alert messages (1.7% of start-ups)
- 158 programming changes (0.4% of start-ups, 22.8% of alert messages).

Source: Reves, J. (2003). "Smart pump" technology reduces errors. Anesthesia Patient Safety Foundation: (2003). 18: 1–10. www.apsf.org/resource_center, 2003. Information was based on a study by Ellen Kinnealey, BSN, Infusion pumps with "drug libraries" at the point of care: A solution for safer drug delivery.

Using a Syringe Pump

Equipment

Battery or electronic operated syringe infusion pump

Pharmacy-prepared and labeled syringe with prescribed medication

Microbore tubing with needleless access device

Chlorhexidine gluconate

Procedure

1. Check syringe label with physician's order for drug, dosage, and amount of drug to be delivered over specified time.
2. Assure that medication is compatible with primary infusing solution.
3. Calculate amount of medication to be delivered per minute.
4. Attach microbore tubing to syringe, and holding syringe upright, expel air from medication syringe before priming tubing.
5. Holding syringe downward, carefully prime microbore tubing with medication (about 0.5 mL).
6. Insert syringe into cradle of pump, squeezing clamp around designated parts of syringe; attach pusher to plunger.
7. Verify that IV site is free from infiltration or vein irrigation.
8. Swab primary IV tubing port closest to client.
9. Insert microbore cannula into port.
10. Set rate for drug delivery according to pharmacy specifications on syringe label, or as prescribed. Drug will be infused *independent* of the primary infusion rate.
11. Start syringe pump.
12. Check infusion indicator to verify pump is infusing.
13. Monitor site and pump function frequently.
14. For subsequent doses, pharmacy dispenses a new syringe, but microbore tubing may be reused for 48–72 hr (according to agency policy). A sterile cap is used each time client's primary tubing is accessed.

NOTE: For other brands of syringe pumps, follow directions for setup and delivery of meds with their product.

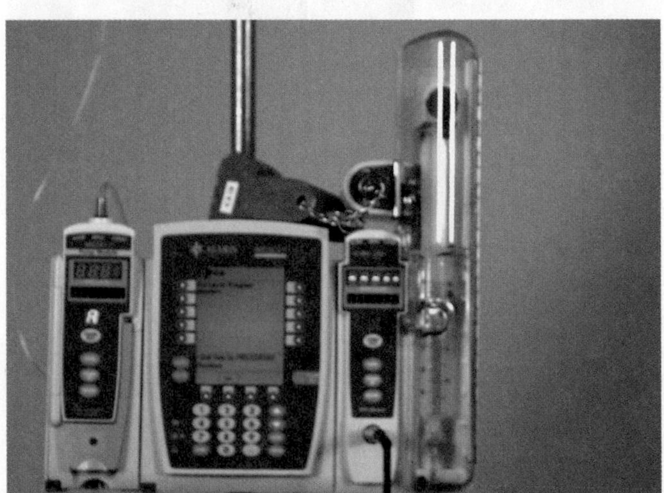

▲ Smart Pumps have syringe modules available to be attached to the point-of-care computers. To attach module, follow manufacturer's directions.

Managing the IV Site

Equipment

Appropriate tubing for IV site
IV cap (according to hospital policy)
Clean gloves
Transparent dressing
Sterile tape
Stabilizing device

> **Clinical Alert**
> Clients receiving hypertonic, acidic, or irritating agents; geriatric clients with fragile veins; and pediatric clients who are active are at particular risk for IV site problems.

Procedure

1. Evaluate every 2 hr for site-related complications (Table 28-3).
2. Identify client using two forms of ID and perform hand hygiene.
3. Include gentle palpation through an intact transparent dressing.
4. Remove IV cannula in the periphery, and change to a new more proximal site every 72–96 hr. (CDC recommends 72–96 hr; INS Standards of Practice recommend 72 hr.)

> **Clinical Alert**
> To check for extravasation, place constrictive band proximal to infusion site tight enough to restrict blood flow through the vein. Set tubing roller clamp to a "keep open" (or slow) rate, and remove tubing from infusion pump. If the infusion continues to drip, fluid is extravasating into the surrounding tissue.

TABLE 28-3 Complications of IV Therapy

Assessment: Signs and Symptoms	Implementation: Nursing Action
Phlebitis	
Pain along the vein, tenderness	Discontinue infusion, and remove needle
Erythema—red streak at vein site	Apply warm compresses
Edema at insertion site	Start IV at another site
	Select a large vein when administering irritating agents
	Anchor cannula to prevent movement in vein
Sluggish flow rate	Do not use positive irrigation with sluggish flow rate—there may be a clot at the end of the needle and it could be flushed into bloodstream
	Reposition extremity. Note where the IV catheter is in relationship to joint, such as wrist, antecubital
Area is warm to touch	Document description and location of site
Infiltration of fluid	
Edema around insertion site—swelling of cannulated extremity	Discontinue infusion and remove needle
Blanching of infusion site	Apply warm compresses to encourage absorption
Coolness of skin around site	Notify physician if solution contains potassium or other irritating component (e.g., 10% dextrose)
	Do not rely on backflash of blood to determine location of catheter/needle in vein
No backflow of blood when tubing is pinched or fluid container lowered below IV site (tubing must be removed from infusion device)	Lower container below IV site—if blood returns, needle is in vein, *but* fluid may be leaking into tissue if bevel has pierced posterior wall of vein
	Restart IV at another site
Extravasation of medication	
Pain, stinging, or burning at site	Discontinue infusion; attempt to aspirate the drug
Redness and swelling	Apply ice compress to area
	Research the medication—some agents have specific antidotes for extravasation injury
	Notify physician
	Administer irritating or vesicant medications through a central venous device

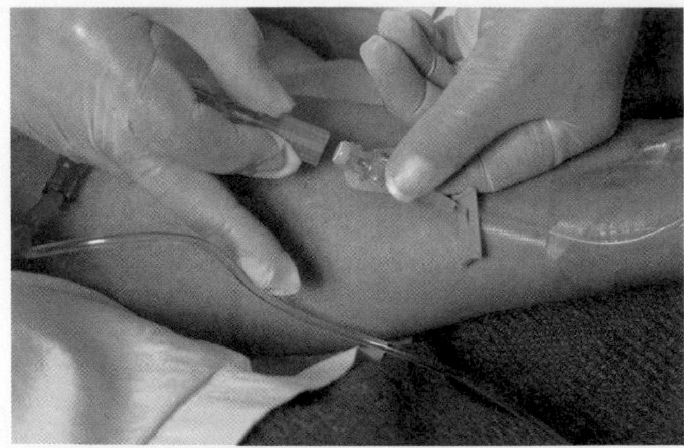

▲ Flush site, then attach needleless cannula into needleless cap.

5. Assess IV site every 4 hr if client's status prohibits changing IV site.

For IV Administration Sets

1. Change administration sets, including all stopcocks, access devices, and extension tubings, every 72 hr (according to agency policy). This can be done routinely at the same time a new container of IV solution is started.
2. Change IV tubing according to use.
   a. Primary intermittent tubing, every 24 hr.
   b. Hyperalimentation, every 24 hr.
   c. Secondary infusion tubing, every 24 hr. ▸ ***Rationale:*** Once a secondary tubing is disconnected, it must be treated as a primary tubing according to INS Standard 54.
   d. Blood and blood component tubing, every 4 hr or after 2 units of blood.
   e. Hemodynamic and arterial pressure monitoring tubing, every 96 hr.
3. Use separate secondary tubing for each "piggy-backed" agent if agents are incompatible.

For Converting From Continuous IV to a "Lock"

1. Ensure site is patent and functional.
2. Perform hand hygiene and don clean gloves.
3. Clamp infusion tubing.
4. Disconnect IV tubing from catheter.
5. Attach needleless injection cap or primed T connector extension tubing with needleless injection cap to catheter hub.
6. Prep, then inject port with 1 mL of sterile normal saline to maintain patency.

Clinical Alert

Some facilities use a single secondary tubing for all agents. The tubing is back-flushed with the primary solution before administering a new agent, providing the agents are compatible.

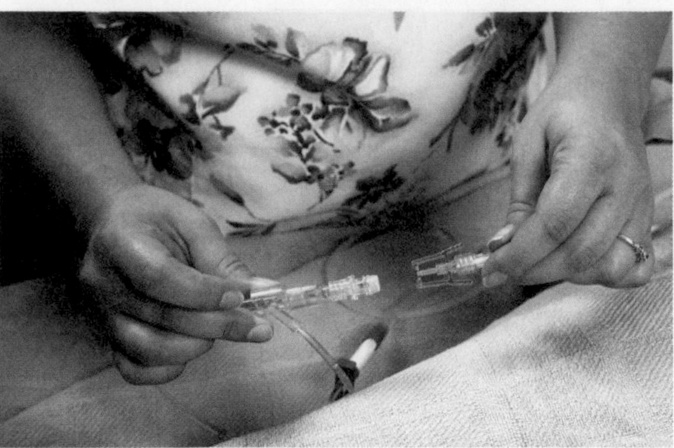

▲ Using the needleless cannula reduces risk of needle sticks during IV procedures.

For Applying a Securement Device

1. Prepare skin area according to facility policy—chlorhexidine recommended.
2. Apply skin prep provided with device. ▸ ***Rationale:*** To increase adhesion of device and protect skin.
3. Place IV catheter into device before adhering anchor pad to skin.
4. Assess site daily. ▸ ***Rationale:*** To ensure placement of device on skin.
5. Assess skin under device for skin tears.
6. Change device every 7 days by gently stroking under device surface with alcohol swab while continuing to lift pad off skin.

For Applying a Transparent Dressing

1. Cover IV insertion site with transparent dressing.
   a. Line up slit in the frame with the catheter hub.
   b. Apply the dressing over insertion site just to top edge of the hub.
   c. Do not stretch the dressing during application.
   d. Firmly smooth down the dressing edges as the frame is slowly removed.
   e. Gently pinch and seal the dressing around the catheter hub.
   f. Smooth down the entire dressing from the center out to the edges, using firm pressure to enhance adhesion.
   g. Label dressing with date of insertion, date of change, gauge used and initials of nurse.
2. Document catheter insertion and dressing information.

Clinical Alert

Regard IV systems as closed sterile systems and maintain as such. All entries into the tubing should be made through injection ports that are disinfected just before entry.

Needleless IV Access Devices

Split Septum Technology-Needleless Access System

The system consists of a pre-split injection cap that requires a blunt cannula to access the fluid path. One new version of the split septum is accessed with a standard male Luer syringe or administration set.

Luer Access Mechanical Valve

A needleless access device that consists of a valve that is opened by the insertion of a standard male Luer syringe or administration set to access the fluid path. There are two types:

1. Compression seal that is depressed by male Luer, opening the fluid path.
2. Open Luer that houses a valve that is activated by the male Luer; it requires a new cap on the Luer after each use.

Luer Access Mechanical Valve With Positive Displacement-Needleless Access Device

The system consists of a valve and a fluid reservoir. The valve is opened by the insertion of a standard male Luer syringe tip or administration, accessing the fluid path. When the male Luer is disconnected, the compression seal reseats, causing the reservoir to empty and creating positive displacement of fluid into the catheter lumen.

Source: Hadaway, Lynn, RN, RNC. (2006). Principles of flushing vascular access devices. In: *Becton Dickinson (BD) Medical Clinical Resource*, Service Department CD, Franklin Lakes, NJ.

Converting IV to Saline Lock

Equipment

Extension tubing with needleless connector

Needleless syringe

Clean gloves

Saline flush syringes with 0.9% preservative-free normal saline

2 × 2 sterile gauze

Procedure

1. Gather equipment and perform hand hygiene.
2. Assess that IV is infusing and there are no signs of phlebitis or infiltration.
3. Don gloves.
4. Prime extension tubing with normal saline syringes
5. Turn off IV and disconnect from pump if necessary.
6. Disconnect IV tubing and attach extension tubing. A 2 × 2 gauze can be placed under IV site to catch drops from IV tubing disconnect.

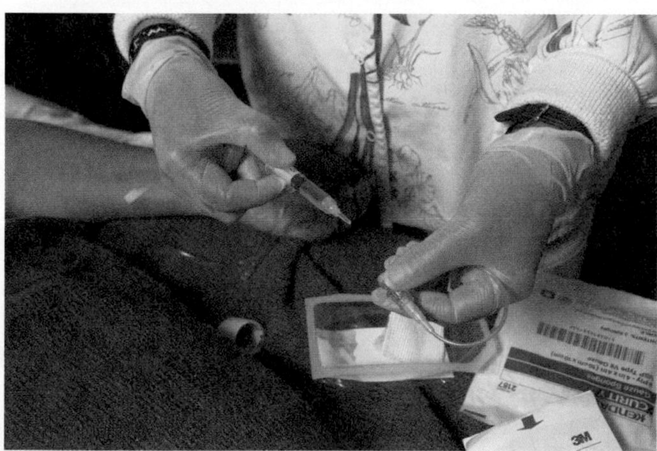

▲ Prime extension tubing.

7. Redress IV site.
8. Discard equipment.
9 Remove gloves and perform hand hygiene.

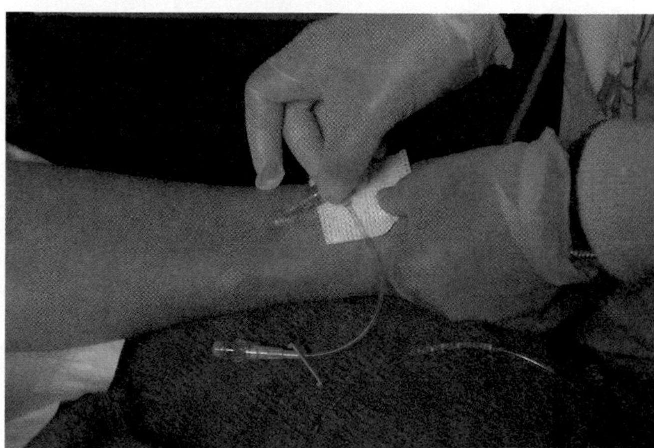

▲ Attach extension tubing to IV catheter.

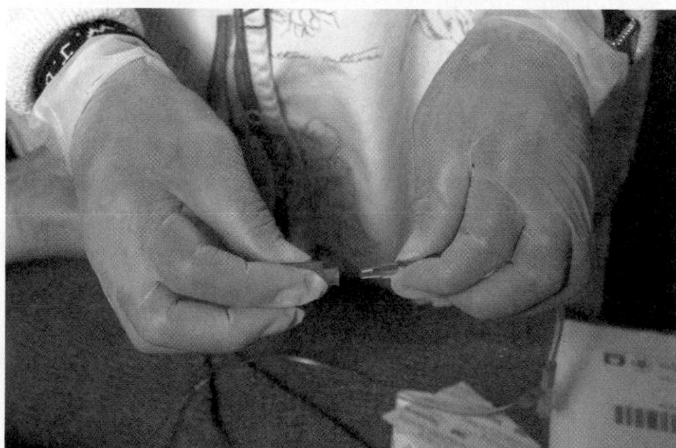

▲ Attach IV tubing to threaded lock cannula.

Changing Gown for Client With IV

Equipment

Clean gown
Bathing supplies, if needed

Procedure

1. Check client care plan for infusion drip rate, type of solution, and any special considerations.
2. Perform hand hygiene.
3. Identify client using two descriptors.
4. Take equipment to client's room and explain procedure to client.
5. Untie back of gown and remove gown from unaffected arm.
6. Support arm with IV and slip gown down arm to IV tubing.
7. Place clean gown over client's chest and abdomen.
8. Use tubing clamp to slow infusion to "keep open" rate and remove tubing from infusion pump if in use.
9. Remove IV bag from hook and slip sleeve over bag, keeping bag above client's arm. ▶ ***Rationale:*** This prevents backflow of blood into tubing. Do not jar or pull tubing. ▶ ***Rationale:*** IV tubing may become dislodged and infiltrate into surrounding tissue.
10. Place your hand up through distal end of clean gown sleeve and grasp IV bag. Pull bag and tubing out through clean gown sleeve.
11. Rehang bag on hook and check to see that infusion is running according to ordered drip rate.
12. Replace tubing into infusion pump, unclamp, and reestablish prescribed infusion flow rate.
13. Guide sleeve of gown up client's arm to shoulder.
14. Assist client to put other arm through remaining sleeve.
15. Tie gown at the back.
16. Check IV infusion rate and IV tubing to determine that solution is flowing unimpeded into client's vein. ▶ ***Rationale:*** Kinks in tubing impede solution flow.
17. Return bed to comfortable position for client.
18. Remove dirty linen from room.
19. Perform hand hygiene.

NOTE: Most facilities provide "IV gowns" that snap from the shoulder down the sleeve of the gown for ease in removal without disturbing the IV.

Discontinuing an IV

Equipment

Sterile 2 × 2 gauze pads (3–4)
Sterile tape
Clean gloves

Procedure

1. Gather equipment.
2. Perform hand hygiene and don gloves.
3. Identify client using two descriptors and explain procedure to client.
4. Turn off infusion.
5. Loosen transparent dressing and securement device. Alcohol swabs can be used to loosen dressing and devices to prevent skin tears.
6. Stabilize catheter while removing dressing and securement device. ▶ ***Rationale:*** Stabilizing site prevents unnecessary movement that could injure the vein.
7. Hold sterile gauze over site and remove catheter carefully and smoothly, keeping it almost flush with skin. Observe catheter for breakage and ensure it is intact.
8. Quickly press sterile pad over venipuncture site and hold firmly until bleeding stops.
9. Hold pressure for several minutes if client's drug therapy prolongs bleeding.
10. Apply sterile pad and tape in place.

Clinical Alert

Assess whether client has been receiving antithrombotic (aspirin) or anticoagulant (Coumadin, heparin) therapy. Hold pressure for several minutes if client has prolonged bleeding caused by drug therapy.

11. Elevate arm to reduce venous pressure and help collapse vein to facilitate clot formation. Do not bend arm at elbow. ▶ ***Rationale:*** Bending elbow causes hematoma formation.

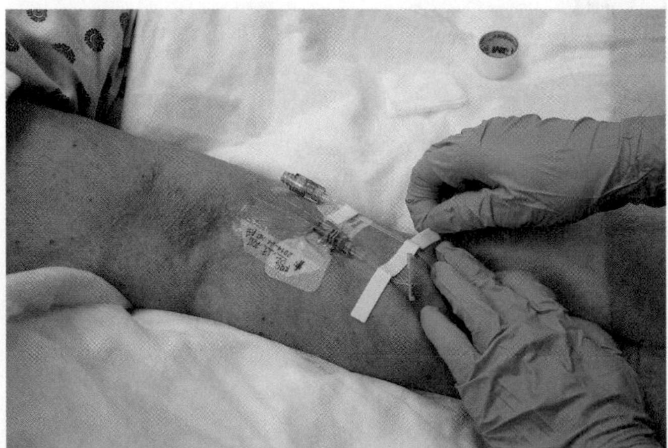

⚠ Remove tape carefully from tubing site.

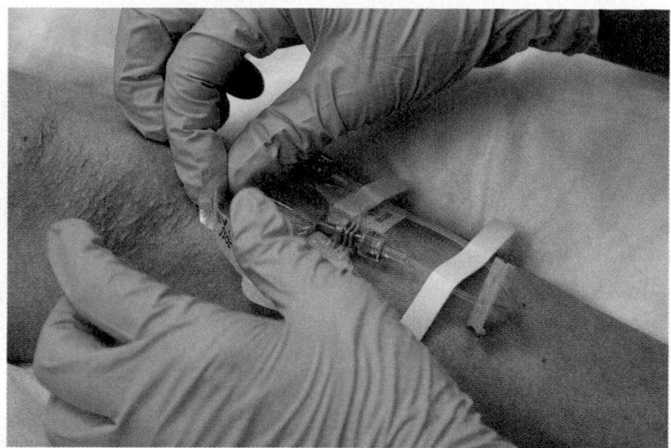

2 Remove occlusive dressing, starting at top and pulling down toward IV site.

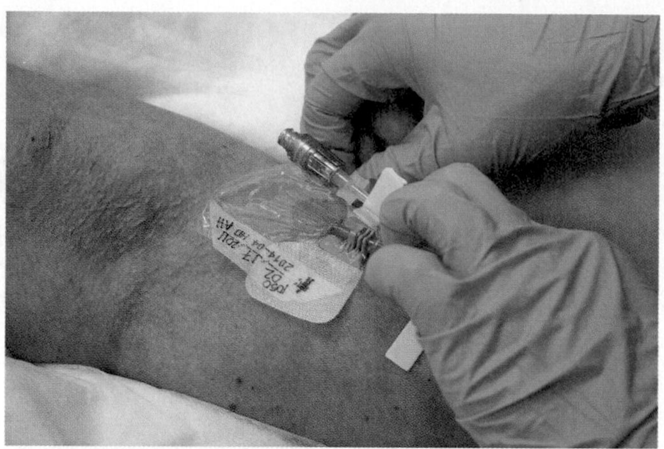

3 Holding cannula in place, continue to pull dressing toward IV site.

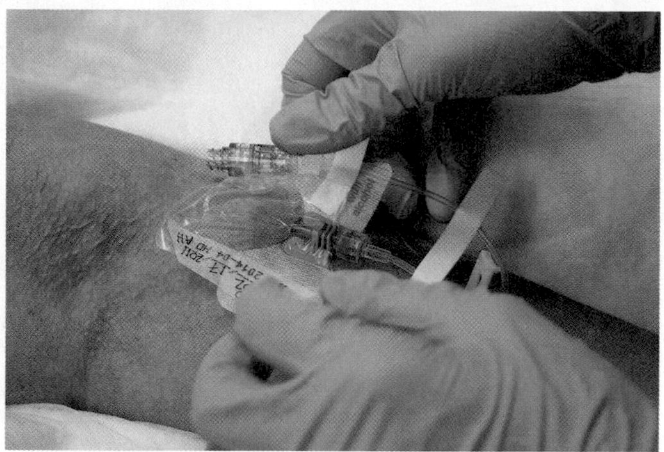

4 Lift dressing off skin.

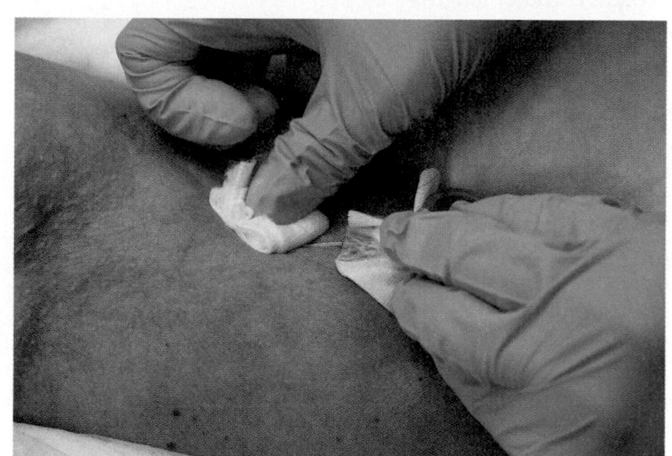

5 Remove IV cannula carefully.

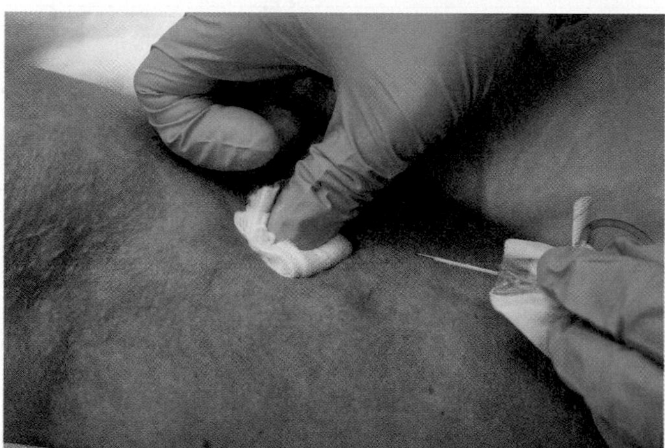

6 Place sterile gauze directly over IV site and press firmly until bleeding stops.

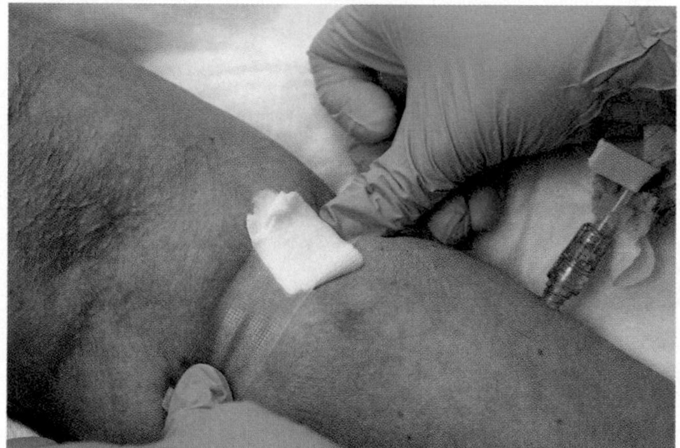

7 Tape gauze dressing in place.

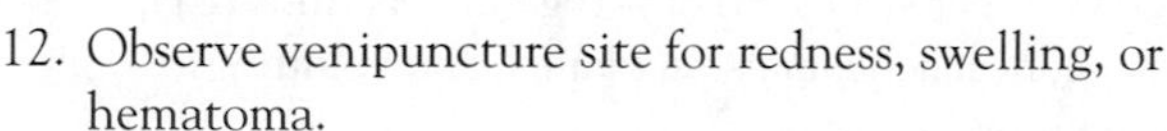

12. Observe venipuncture site for redness, swelling, or hematoma.
13. Dispose of equipment and gloves.
14. Perform hand hygiene.
15. Check site again in 15 minutes.
16. Record volume infused on I&O sheet.

NOTE: If there are signs of infection or inflammation at catheter site or client complains of symptoms related to infection, cut tip of catheter with sterile scissors, place in sterile container, and send to lab for culture.

DOCUMENTATION for Intravenous Management

IV Insertion

- Date and time
- Location of insertion site
- Gauge and length of catheter inserted
- IV solution and flow rate
- Site care given
- Condition of site
- Client response to procedure

IV Discontinued

- Date and time
- Note condition of the catheter—"intact"
- Assess catheter length
- Condition of site
- Client response to procedure
- Catheter tip to lab if appropriate

Legal Alert

By 2006, the FDA mandated that all drug manufacturers must label most prescription medications and certain over-the-counter drugs with machine-readable bar codes, using the National Drug Code number that uniquely identifies each drug, its dosage form, and strength. The FDA predicts that using bar codes will prevent up to 500,000 adverse drug events and transfusion errors over the next 20 years.

Source: U.S. Food and Drug Administration. (2005, September). *FDA issues bar code regulation, 2004*. www.fda.gov/oc/initiatives/barcode.

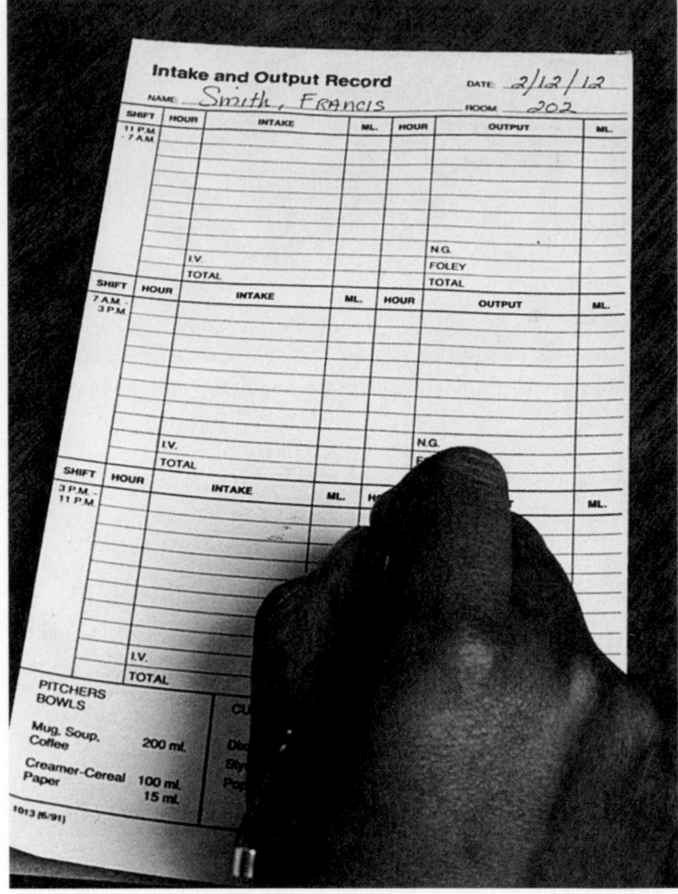

▲ Example of Intake and Output Record.

CRITICAL THINKING Application

Excepted Outcomes

- Fluids are administered without adverse effects.
- IV site remains clean, without signs of infection or infiltration.
- IV is converted to a saline lock and is functioning properly.
- Client's gown is changed while maintaining IV placement.
- IV is discontinued intact and site remains free of infection or bleeding.

Unexpected Outcomes

Client develops unexplained fever with chills and rising pulse rate.

Alternative Actions

- Unexplained fever may be associated with catheter-related sepsis. Report to physician.
- Assess IV site for signs of infection.
- Ensure that IV solutions hang for no more than 24 hr.
- Check client's vital signs: temperature usually above 100°F when caused by IV-related sepsis.
- Check for other symptoms of pyrogenic reactions (e.g., backache, headache, malaise, nausea, and vomiting).
- Stop the infusion.
- Obtain blood specimens, if ordered.

IV solution does not flow properly.	• Ensure that the control clamp is open. • Check that blood pressure readings are not taken on arm in which IV is running, as flow is impeded and a clot can form on the end of the catheter. • Ensure that IV administration set is properly loaded. Check pump for flow problem indicator (e.g., cassette seating, air in line). • Check IV tubing from insertion site to IV solution for kinks/obstructions. • Check for extremity causing positional obstruction to flow (e.g., elbow bent, arm rotated).
IV solution appears to be infiltrating, resulting in tissue swelling.	• Decrease the flow rate. (Remove from pump for "keep open" rate.) • Lower bag of IV solution; if blood returns, cannula may be in the vein but fluid may be leaking into surrounding tissue via existing puncture in vein wall. • Discontinue infusion and establish a new site.
Phlebitis is suspected at infusion site (tenderness, warmth, erythema, and pain).	• Check infusion solution and medications being administered. (Potassium chloride and hypertonic solutions are particularly irritating to veins.) • Discontinue IV. • Apply warm compress per hospital policy.
Postinfusion phlebitis may also occur after the IV has been discontinued in response to either chemical or mechanical factors of the preexisting IV.	• Check IV solution; hypertonic solution causes irritation necessitating use of large veins and changing IV sites more frequently. • Follow hospital policy for treatment. Warm compresses to the site are generally recommended. • Elevate extremity.

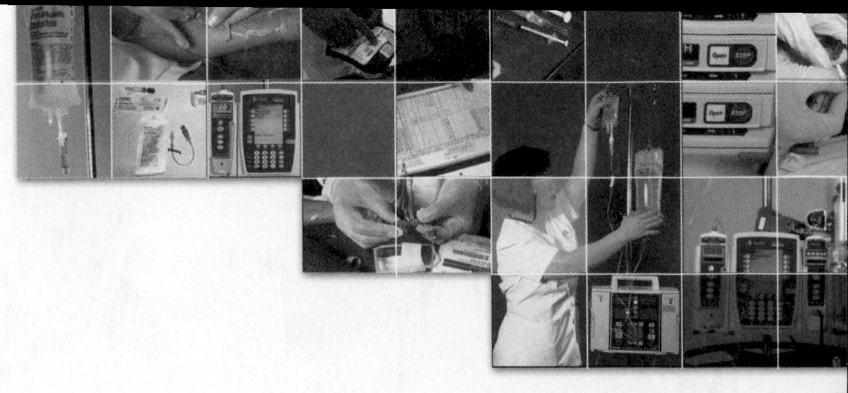

Chapter 28

UNIT ❸

Monitoring Fluid Balance

Nursing Process Data

ASSESSMENT Data Base

- Assess client's need for intake and output recording.
- Assess client's ability to keep intake and output fluid records.
- Evaluate client for any factors that might affect his or her intake and output (e.g., preexisting disease states, concurrent disease, drug therapies, and current physical status).
- Determine all measurable sources of fluid intake: fluids with and between meals, tube feeding, liquid medications, IV fluids, and IV medications.
- Determine all measurable sources of fluid output: urine, emesis, diarrhea, and drainage sites.
- Determine alterations in nonmeasurable sources of fluid intake and loss: food, increased metabolism (e.g., fever), rapid respirations, and perspiration.
- Determine balance of daily intake and output.

PLANNING Objectives

- To establish a written record of the client's total fluid intake (oral, parenteral, and feeding tubes) and fluid output (urine, wound/tube drainage, diarrhea, and vomiting)
- To plan fluid replacement or appropriate therapy by assessing deficits or excesses of fluid and electrolytes
- To ensure a fluid intake of at least 2000–2600 mL unless contraindicated by diagnosis
- To monitor the client's fluid status, vital signs, and mental state to determine homeostasis

IMPLEMENTATION Procedures

EVALUATION Expected Outcomes

- Client's intake and output are maintained within expected parameters of 200–300 mL of each other.
- Fluid intake is at least 2600 mL unless contraindicated by diagnosis.
- Client's fluid status, vital signs, and mental status are within normal range.
- Output is maintained at more than 30 mL/hr.
- IV flow rate is maintained at prescribed rate.

Monitoring Intake and Output

Equipment

- Graduated container in client's bathroom
- I&O bedside record sheet and PDA for recording in computer
- Urinal or bedpan; bedside commode or underseat basin for toilet
- Hourly in-line urine measurement device for clients requiring frequent monitoring
- Posted measurement standards for commonly used drinking and eating utensils (e.g., glasses, mugs, bowls)
- Posted signs, dietary slips, and other communication devices to notify hospital personnel about how client's I&O is to be measured

Procedure

1. Determine whether client needs I&O measurements by checking client's chart or care plan. All clients with an IV need I&O measurement.
2. Instruct client and/or family about the need to measure all intake and output. Keep I&O sheet at bedside for the family to record I&O.
3. Measure intake from all sources.
   a. Oral fluids.
   b. IV fluids.
   c. Fluid medications (oral, enteral, or IV).
   d. Tube feedings and water used to clear tubing.

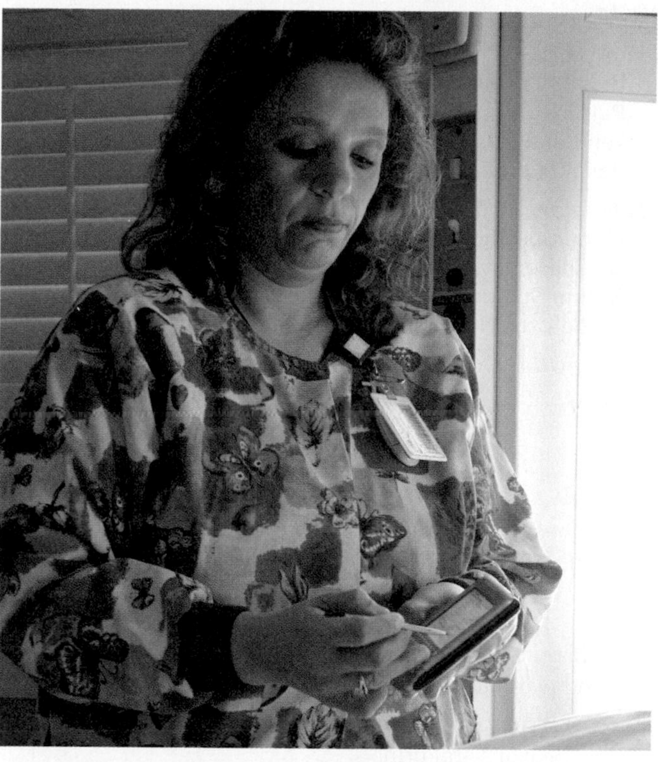

▲ The trend in most facilities is to eliminate paper records. Electronic recording through Palm Pilots is now frequently utilized.

Clinical Alert
Measurement of all fluids is done in milliliters (mLs).

TABLE 28-4 Body Sites for Assessment of Fluid Status

Site	Fluid Excess	Fluid Deficit
Head and Neck		
Face	Eyeballs firm or protruding Edema, especially around eyes	Eyeballs soft or sunken Decreased skin turgor over forehead
Mucous Membranes	Excessive salivation Swollen tongue	Dry or sticky mucosa with thick mucous secretions Shrunken tongue with multiple longitudinal furrows Crusted lips
Neck	Jugular vein distention	
Trunk		
Chest	Crackles in lung bases	Decreased skin turgor over sternum Dry, flaking skin
Abdomen	Ascites (measure girth at umbilicus)	
Sacrum	Edema	
Extremities		
Arms	Distended veins Edema, particularly of the hands Delayed capillary refill Pulse bounding	Flattened veins Delayed capillary refill Dry, flaking skin Pulse weak and thready
Legs	Edema Taut shiny skin Peripheral cyanosis	Poor skin turgor, especially across shins Dry, flaky skin, especially on feet Weak pedal pulse or decreased capillary refill

TABLE 28-5 Objective Data Associated With Fluid Status

Data	Fluid Excess	Fluid Deficit
Vital Signs		
Blood Pressure	Increased*	Decreased (especially on standing)
Pulse	Increased rate	Increased rate
Temperature	Unchanged	Elevated
Respirations	Increased rate	Unchanged or increased
Laboratory Findings		
Urine-Specific Gravity	Decreased, approaching 1.003	Increased, approaching 1.025 or greater
Blood Hematocrit	Less than three times the hemoglobin	Greater than three times the hemoglobin
Serum Sodium (Na)	Less than 135 mEq/L or normal	Greater than 145 mEq/L or normal
Blood Urea Nitrogen (BUN)	Decreased (except in heart or renal failure)	Proportionately greater than the serum creatinine
Hourly Urine Output	More than 60 mL/hr	Less than 30–60 mL/hr
Weight	A 5% or greater gain	Mild: 2% loss Moderate: 3%–5% loss Severe: 6% or greater loss

*If the heart is unable to pump the increased blood volume, the blood pressure (reflecting cardiac output) may decrease. Polyuria can also be seen with fluid volume deficit (FVD) as in diabetic states.

4. Measure output from all sources to establish a record and plan fluid therapy.
   a. Urinary catheters
   b. Bedpans and urinals
   c. Nasogastric drainage
   d. Drainage tubing (e.g., T-tubes, wound, or chest tube)
   e. Diarrheal stools
   f. Draining wounds
   g. Emesis
5. Record I&O on bedside record each time you check on client's intake or measure output, or enter data into computer.
6. Correlate intake and output with daily weight. Weight is measured in kilograms (1 kg = 2.2 lb).
7. Record 24-hr totals of I&O on bedside record and place in client's chart, or enter data into computer.
8. Notify physician of any significant imbalance; more intensive monitoring may be indicated. ▸ ***Rationale:*** Hourly urine output less than 25–30 mL/hr for 2 consecutive hours or 24-hr urine output less than 500 mL can indicate dehydration or internal bleeding and can result in acute renal failure.

Clinical Alert

Check all drainage receptacles such as Foley bag and NG canister at the beginning of each shift to ensure they were emptied from the previous shift and that there has not been excessive drainage.

Fluid Replacement Solutions

Hypertonic Solutions—a solution with higher osmolality than blood serum

- Solution causes cells to shrink
- Used in severe salt depletion (very rare)
- Used as nutrient source (10% dextrose)
- Examples of solutions: 5% dextrose in 0.45% normal saline; 10% dextrose in water; 3% normal saline

Hypotonic Solutions—a solution with lower osmolality than blood serum

- Hydrates cells, causes them to expand
- Used to correct dehydration
- Examples of solutions: 0.45% normal saline; 0.2% normal saline; 2.5% dextrose

Isotonic Solutions—a solution with the same osmolality as blood serum

- Cells remain unchanged
- Used for replacement or maintenance (expands extracellular volume). Especially used to expand circulating (intravascular) volume.
- Examples of solutions: 5% dextrose in water; 0.9% normal saline (NS); Lactated Ringer's

NOTE: One liter of normal saline (0.9% NaCl) meets the usual daily requirement of these electrolytes in an adult.

TABLE 28-6 Intake and Output Flow Sheet (Sample)

		Intake							
Date	**Time**	**IV No.**	**IV Started**	**Description**	**IV Intake**	**Oral Intake**	**Urine Output**	**Other**	**N/G**
1/9/12	9 A			Full liquid breakfast		620			
	9:45 A			Vomitus				400	
	10:30 A	#1	1000						
	12 N						500		
	2:30 P						400		
				7–3 Total	600	620	900	400	100
	6:30 P	#2	1000						
	9 P						500		
				3–11 Total	1000	NPO	500		350
1/10/12	2:30 A	#3	1000		450				
	5 A				550		350		
				11–7 Total	1000	NPO	350		375
				24-hr Total	2600	620	1750	400	825

Monitoring IV Intake

Equipment

Electronic infusion device
I&O record
Graphic sheet
IV container marked with timed intervals
IV flow sheet or PDA

Procedure

1. Place I&O worksheet at bedside unless using PDA to record I&O.
2. Determine time interval required for monitoring IV intake.
3. Mark time intervals on IV container according to facility policy (use tape to mark, or use preprinted time strips).
4. Set IV drip rate according to physician's orders.
5. Observe IV container and read IV solution level.
6. Record amount of IV solution infused at prescribed time (e.g., every hour, every shift).
7. If using electronic infusion device, push "total volume infused" for shift amount, then "clear."
8. Record total IV intake on I&O record at end of each shift or record in electronic PDA.
9. Record 24-hr IV total at midnight. Take into account all sources of IV fluid (all IV sites, IV medications).

DOCUMENTATION for Monitoring Fluid Balance

- Amount and description of all measurable I&O
- Approximate volume of loss when unable to measure contents (e.g., incontinent of urine in bed)
- Dietary intake (food that liquefies at room temperature, as well as liquids)
- 8-hr and 24-hr totals
- Signs and symptoms of client's fluid status, including vital signs, mucous membranes, daily weight, etc.

NOTE: I&O records are frequently inaccurate due to numerous possibilities for error, estimation being a common source of inaccuracy. It is important to maintain these records accurately.

CRITICAL THINKING Application

Expected Outcomes

- Client's intake and output are maintained within expected parameters of 200–300 mL of each other.
- Fluid intake is at least 2600 mL unless contraindicated by diagnosis.
- Client's fluid status, vital signs, and mental status are within normal range.
- Output is maintained at more than 30 mL/hr.
- IV flow rate is maintained at prescribed rate.

Unexpected Outcomes	Alternative Actions
Recorded I&O do not balance.	• Correlate I&O imbalance with weight changes. • Emphasize importance of accurate measures to client and family. • Check that entries into computer are accurate (i.e., entering 100 mL instead of 1000 mL). • Identify possible nonmeasurable sources of I or O. • Report to charge nurse so she can ensure that all nurses are keeping accurate records. • Check if client or family can help with keeping the I&O record. • Check the addition on the I&O record to see if an error was made.
Client unable to maintain an intake of at least 1500 mL/day.	• Ensure that fluid restriction is not ordered. • Offer fluids in small amounts more frequently. • Determine client's fluid preferences. • Determine client preference for fluid to be hot, cold, or room temperature. • Consider "other" fluids such as Jell-O, Popsicles. • Assess client's ability to use a straw (hemiplegic client is often unable to suck through a straw). • Check if client is able to drink fluids independently or if assistance is needed. • Ensure that adequate fluids are accessible at the bedside for the client. • Do not administer fluids with a bulb syringe. • Address client's toileting needs every 2 hr—some clients restrict their fluid intake for fear of incontinence. • Use a thickening additive to liquids to facilitate swallowing for the client with aspiration precautions.
IV flow not maintained at appropriate rate.	• Monitor IV fluid intake hourly. • Observe IV site for complications. • Restart IV immediately when infiltrated to ensure continuous IV fluid intake. • Document IV fluid intake every shift. • Account for interruption of primary infusion and the delivery of intermittent infusions of medications. • Check accuracy of IV administration equipment: electronic device, dial-a-flow, etc. • Inform physician of alterations in fluid received from what was ordered.

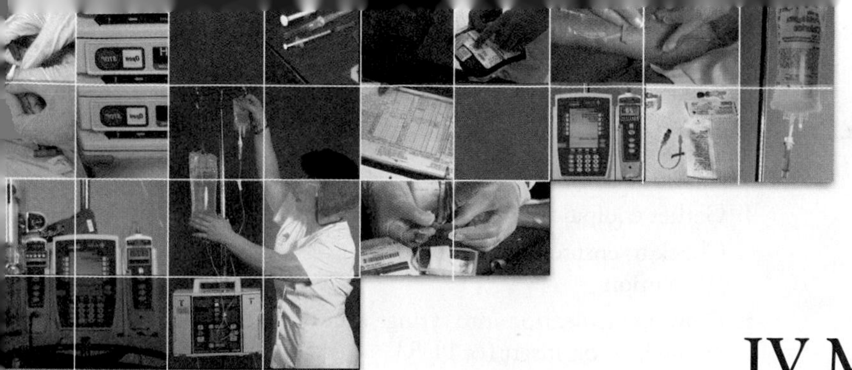

Chapter 28

UNIT 4

IV Medication Administration

Nursing Process Data

ASSESSMENT Data Base

- Note client's allergies.
- Note any drug or solution incompatibilities.
- Assess amount and type of diluent needed to prepare medications.
- Assess client's general status to establish a baseline.
- Assess patency of infusion set and condition of IV insertion site.
- Assess physical parameters as indicated such as blood pressure, heart rate.

PLANNING Objectives

- To maintain a therapeutic level of medication in the client's bloodstream
- To administer medication safely over a specific period of time
- To prevent complications associated with medication administration

IMPLEMENTATION Procedures

EVALUATION Expected Outcomes

- Solutions from secondary IV bags infuse without difficulty.
- Therapeutic blood levels of medication are maintained.
- Complications of medication administration are prevented.
- Medication is infused over appropriate time span using volume control set.
- Saline lock inserted for medication administration without complications.

Pearson Nursing Student Resources

Find additional review materials at **nursing.pearsonhighered.com**

Prepare for success with NCLEX®-style practice questions and Skill Checklists

Adding Medication to IV Solution

Equipment

IV solution bag
Syringe with medication
Antimicrobial swab
Label with medication dosage, date, time, and initials

Clinical Alert

Only under unusual circumstances will the nurse be asked to add medications to parenteral solution. Refer to the facility's policy and procedure manual to determine which medications can be added by the nurse.

Procedure

1. Check physician's orders, MAR, and agency policy.

NOTE: The addition (admixture) of medication to an IV solution for continuous administration is usually performed by the pharmacist, according to standards established by the American Society of Health System Pharmacists (ASHP) and Occupational Safety and Health Administration (OSHA). Special precautions for this procedure include preparation in a laminar airflow environment, strict adherence to requirements of asepsis, safety regarding components' stability and compatibility, proper dilution of agents, and control of extraneous particle addition to the admixture.

2. Perform hand hygiene.
3. Gather equipment.
4. Check to ensure that prescribed drug is compatible with IV solution.
5. Draw up medication into syringe according to directions on medication insert (or PDR).
6. Check all medications to be added to IV solutions with a second RN before injecting into the IV solution.
7. Wipe injection port on IV bag with antimicrobial swab.
8. Inject medication into bag while maintaining aseptic technique.
9. Mix IV solution and medication by gently agitating bag to mix thoroughly.
10. Affix medication label to IV bag.
11. Hold bag against both dark and light backgrounds to inspect for any precipitate.
12. Insert IV tubing into bag, and proceed with appropriate method of administration as ordered.

Clinical Alert

Some drugs are incompatible with saline solution; these include diazepam (Valium), chlordiazepoxide hydrochloride (Librium), and amphotericin B. Check compatibility of all IV drugs with solutions infusing.

Using a Secondary ("Piggyback") Bag

Equipment

Primary IV set, consisting of compatible IV solution bag and IV administration set with injection port
Short secondary administration set with needleless cannula and extension hook or lowering hanger for primary bag (if indicated)
Pharmacy-prepared medication bag with label, including name of medication, date, time, rate for infusion, and client's name
2% Chlorhexidine gluconate swab

Preparation

1. Check medication with physician's orders and MAR.
2. Perform hand hygiene.
3. Gather equipment.
4. Identify client using two forms of identification.

Procedure

1. Ensure medication compatibility with primary infusing solution.

NOTE: If medication is incompatible with primary IV solution, temporarily discontinue primary infusion. Flush client's injection port, initiate a normal saline (or other compatible) solution as the primary, then proceed with "piggyback" into the "new" compatible primary. When complete, restart original primary solution (use new needleless cannula to access client's injection site).

2. Spike bag with secondary administration set.
3. Cleanse injection port of primary tubing with chlorhexidine gluconate swab.
4. Insert needleless connector of secondary "piggyback" tubing into primary tubing port (port above pump).

NOTE: If using the same tubing from a previous administration, change needleless connector before inserting into primary tubing.

5. Hang the secondary bag on the IV pole.
6. Use extension hook to lower primary bag below secondary bag if indicated (some infusion devices do not require this). ▶ ***Rationale:*** Primary solution ceases flow because of increased hydrostatic pressure in higher secondary bag.
7. Clear tubing of medication bag by opening clamp, temporarily placing secondary bag lower than the primary solution bag, and allowing primary solution to flow retrograde into secondary bag tubing (back-priming).
8. Backfill until secondary tubing chamber is one-third full. Clamp secondary tubing. ▶ ***Rationale:*** This ensures that no medication is lost during priming.

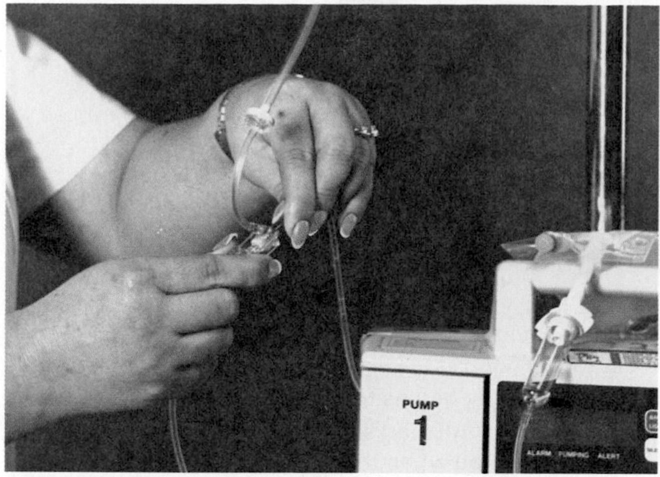

▲ Insert needleless cannula of secondary tubing into distal primary tubing port.

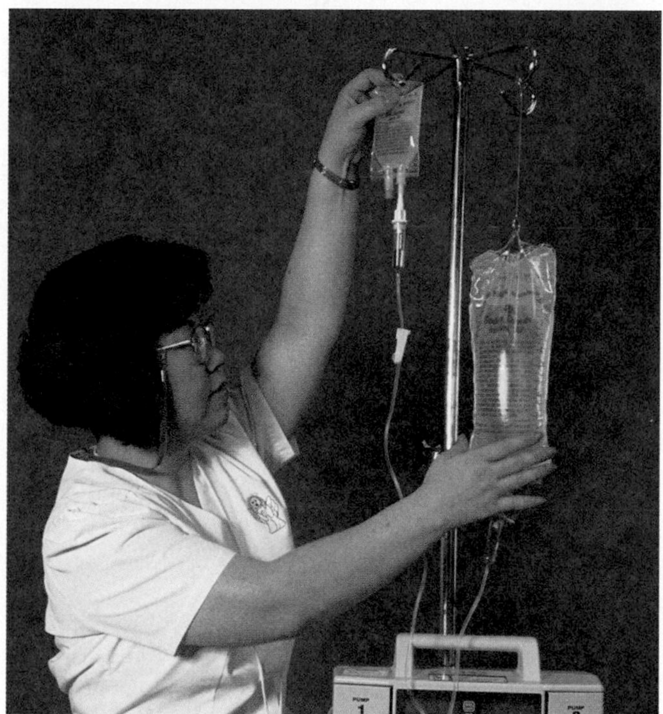
▲ Hang secondary bag on IV pole; lower primary bag.

9. Program secondary settings into infusion device if used.
10. Open clamp on secondary bag tubing. The secondary solution should begin to flow.
11. Check that primary infusion resumes at its "set" rate when secondary volume has been infused.

NOTE: Some infusion devices control secondary infusions without necessitating bag height differentials.

12. When secondary bag is empty, readjust rate of administration in primary solution to desired flow (unless infusion device controls this).
13. To add a new secondary bag, ensure that medication is the same as previously administered since some drug remains in the secondary tubing. A *different* medication requires its own secondary tubing. ▸ ***Rationale:*** This prevents admixture of potentially incompatible drugs.

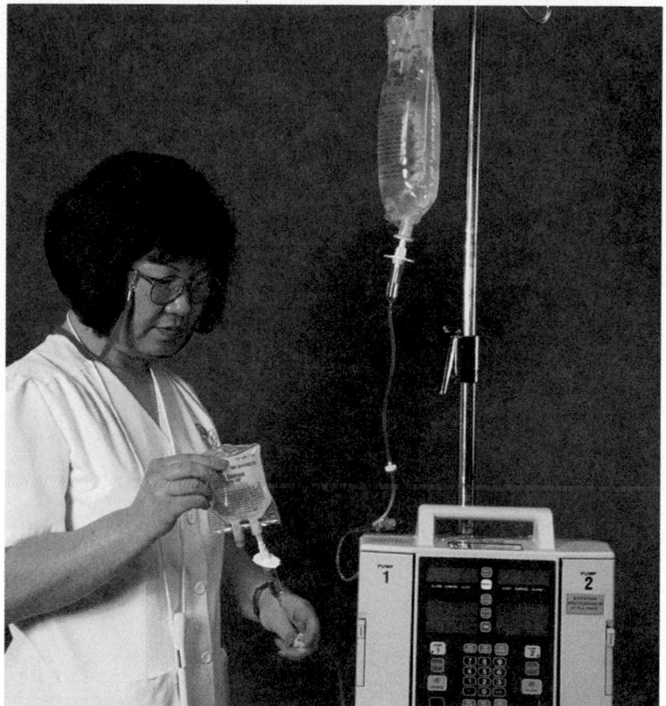
▲ Lower medication bag to clear tubing and back-prime tubing.

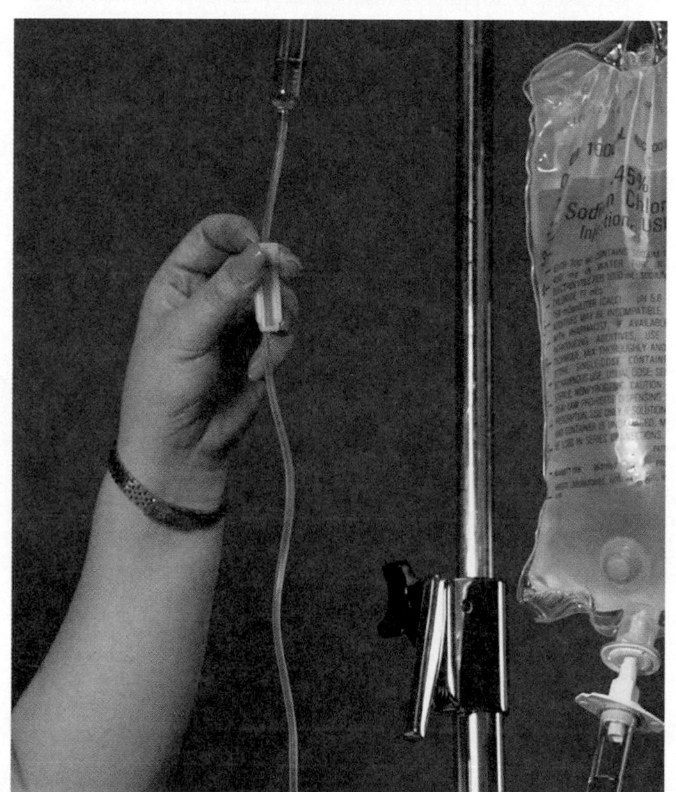
▲ Unclamp secondary tubing.

14. Remove old secondary bag, and spike new "piggyback" medication bag.

15. Lower partial-fill bag below injection port of primary IV.
16. Open clamp on secondary tubing and allow solution from primary IV set to enter tubing, backfilling the tubing to drip chamber. ▸ ***Rationale:*** This procedure displaces air in the secondary tubing.
17. Replace new secondary bag on IV pole and proceed with administration.
18. Change secondary tubing every 24 hr.

Clinical Alert

Always document all fluids as intake used for administering medications in piggyback or volume control sets.

Using a Mini-Infuser Pump

A mini-infuser pump is a tandem device that allows a small amount of medication to be given (5–60 mL) as a controlled infusion.

- The prefilled syringe is added to the battery-operated mini-infuser and connected to the main IV line.
- A needleless system is connected to the primary IV line.
- The infusion pump is hung with the primary IV bag and activated by an ON button.
- After infusion of medication, the primary infusion automatically begins to flow as the pump stops.
- The primary infusion should be checked and the flow regulated when the mini-infusion pump stops.

Using a Volume Control Set

Equipment

Primary IV set (IV solution bag and IV administration set)
Calibrated volume control set
Medication prepared in syringe
2% Chlorhexidine gluconate swab
Label with medication, date, time, and nurse's initials

▲ Add extension tubing, if necessary.

Preparation

1. Check physician's orders and MAR.
2. Identify client using two descriptors.
3. Determine compatibility of medication with primary infusion.
4. Perform hand hygiene.

Procedure

1. Add extension tubing to volume control set if needed and close clamps on volume control set, both above and below volume chamber.
2. Open air vent by turning clamp located on top of volume chamber.
3. Spike IV bag with volume control set and then hang bag. Attach IV tubing to volume control set.
4. Open upper clamp (between the bag and volume chamber) and fill chamber with IV solution so that chamber is one-third full.
5. Close upper clamp.
6. Open lower clamp and squeeze drip chamber (located underneath the volume chamber) until it is one-half full.
7. Allow solution to flow down tubing.
8. Prime tubing and cannula affixed to end of tubing. If volume control set has membrane filter instead of floating valve filter, follow manufacturer's instructions for priming so that you do not damage the filter.

Clinical Alert

New guidelines from The Joint Commission require that all syringes with medication must be labeled with client's name, drug, and time syringe was prepared.

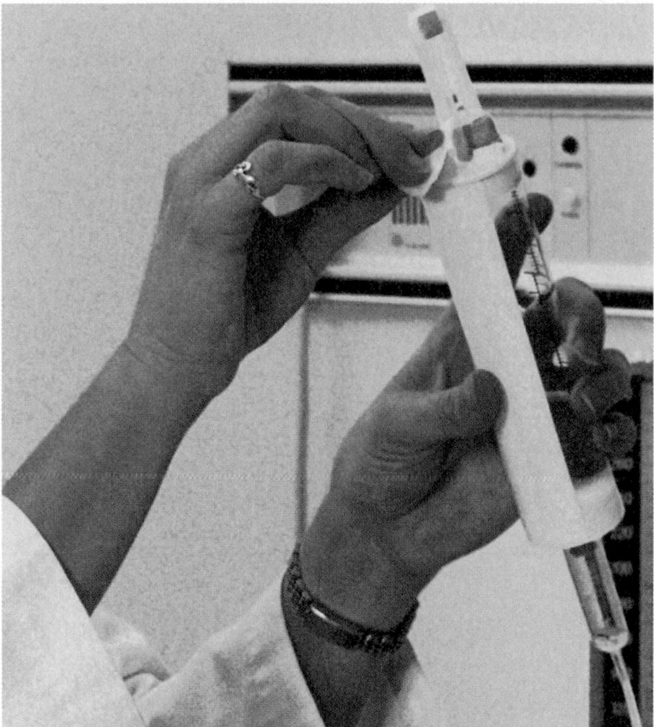

▲ Swab injection port before infusing medication.

9. Close clamp.
10. Swab off injection port (located on top of the volume chamber) with antimicrobial swab.

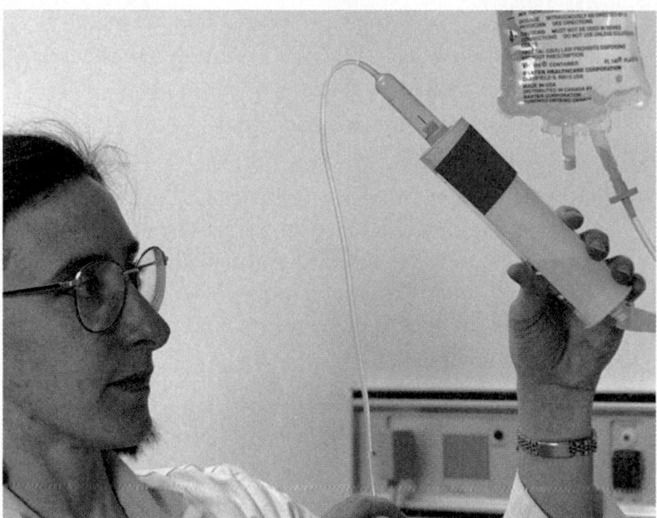

▲ After instilling medication, gently mix with solution in volume control chamber.

11. Inject prepared medication into chamber and agitate gently to mix medication with solution in chamber.
12. Dilute medication, if necessary, by opening upper clamp and adding additional fluid from the IV bag.
13. Open clamp on volume control set and adjust drip rate to desired rate of administration.
14. Place medication label on volume control set. Include client's name, medication, dose, and time medication infusion began.

Using a Peripheral Saline Lock

Equipment

Needleless injection cap with primed extension tubing and port (if one is not in place)
Needleless access device
Syringe for medication and diluent (if indicated)
Two 0.9% preservative-free normal saline prefilled syringes (3–5 mL each) (preferred method)
2% Chlorhexidine gluconate swab
Clean gloves
Stethoscope and sphygmomanometer (if indicated)

Preparation

1. Check physician's orders and MAR.
2. Gather equipment.
3. Perform hand hygiene and don gloves.
4. Identify client using two descriptors.
5. If client does not have peripheral lock in place, proceed with venipuncture, selecting veins that are both large enough to receive the medication and away from areas of movement (e.g., the elbows and wrists).

Procedure

1. Prepare medication with appropriate diluent according to manufacturer's instruction for IV injection and draw it up into syringe. (See drug insert or PDR.)
2. Fill two syringes, each with 1 mL of 0.9% preservative-free normal saline.
3. Explain procedure to client.
4. Check client's vital signs if agent to be given has hemodynamic effects.
5. Prep needleless injection port with antimicrobial swab.
6. Insert *first* saline syringe into port, briefly aspirate to check patency, then flush system and observe for site swelling. ► ***Rationale:*** Presence of blood and absence of swelling at site indicate that needle is probably in vein, not in surrounding tissue.

7. Insert medication syringe into port and inject medication into vein, timing injection administration rate according to drug manufacturer's instruction (see insert or PDR).
8. Observe client for any adverse reactions.
9. Remove medication syringe.
10. Flush with *second* saline syringe to clear line and maintain patency of lock. Administration of saline should take same time period as the medication administration. ▸ ***Rationale:*** This prevents a bolus of medication or "speed shock" when fluid is administered.
11. Dispose of equipment and gloves and perform hand hygiene.
12. Recheck client's vital signs if indicated.

Clinical Alert

Studies indicate that there is no significant difference in the use of saline or heparin to maintain catheter patency, maintain dwell time, and avoid phlebitis. Some hospitals still use a small amount of dilute heparin for flushing peripheral locks; it is usually prepared with 1 mL of heparin (1000 units/mL) added to 9 mL of normal saline to produce 100 units/mL solution. Prefilled syringes of heparin and saline for infusion come in 10 units of heparin/mL. Caution should be exercised because heparin-induced thrombocytopenia can occur with as little as 500 units of heparin/day.

Flushing a Peripheral Saline Lock

Equipment

Two prefilled syringes with 0.9% preservative-free normal saline
2% Chlorhexidine gluconate swab
Clean gloves

Preparation

1. Check physician's order and MAR including allergies.
2. Gather equipment.
3. Perform hand hygiene.
4. Identify client using two descriptors.

Procedure

1. Explain procedure to the client.
2. Don clean gloves.
3. Prep injection port with chlorhexidine gluconate swab. ▸ ***Rationale:*** When prepping with an antimicrobial swab, it is the pressure and friction applied that produce the antimicrobial effect.

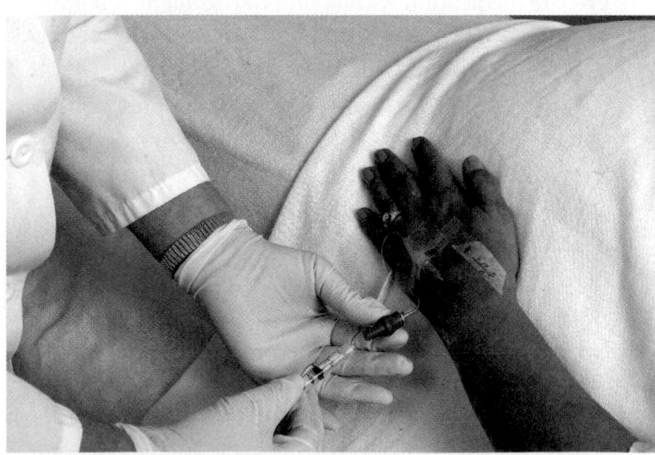

▲ After swabbing injection port, attach syringe with normal saline.

4. Insert/connect first saline syringe into injection port and gently aspirate for blood.
5. Observe for blood in syringe. ▸ ***Rationale:*** Blood will indicate catheter is not occluded (see Clinical Alert).
6. Remove and discard used syringe in appropriate trash/sharps container. Be careful not to contaminate

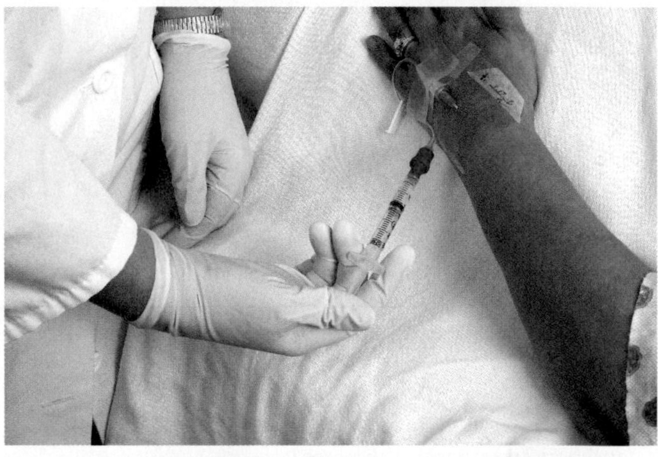

▲ After checking for blood return, discard syringe and attach second syringe with saline into port and gently irrigate lock.

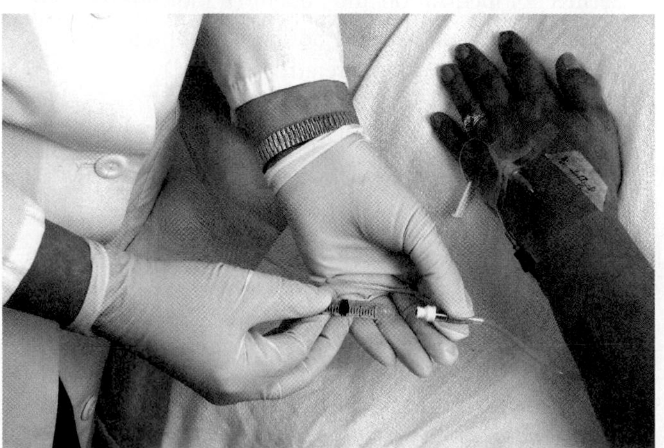

▲ Remove syringe and discard in sharps container.

the injection port. If the port is contaminated, prep again with an antimicrobial swab.

7. Insert/connect second syringe into injection port and gently flush with saline. Assess IV insertion site for tissue swelling or pain when injecting saline. ▸ ***Rationale:*** This could be a sign of infiltration.
8. Disconnect syringe and discard in appropriate trash/sharps container.
9. Remove and discard gloves.
10. Perform hand hygiene.
11. Document flush on MAR.

Clinical Alert

If the gauge of the catheter is small, i.e., 22 gauge or smaller, it is possible that you may not get a blood return. This can be due to the collapse of the tip of the catheter as negative pressure is applied when attempting to aspirate blood. This does not always mean that the catheter is occluded. You may attempt to gently inject the saline while feeling for resistance. If any resistance is felt, it is possible that the catheter is occluded and needs to be removed and a new catheter inserted.

Administering Medications by Peripheral IV Line Injection "Push"

Equipment

Medication prepared in syringe with needleless access device, according to pharmaceutical instruction for IV administration

2% Chlorhexidine gluconate swab

Clean gloves

Stethoscope and sphygmomanometer (if indicated by drug action)

Two prefilled 0.9% normal saline solution syringes

Preparation

1. Check physician's orders and MAR.
2. Gather equipment.
3. Perform hand hygiene.
4. Prepare medication according to pharmaceutical company's instructions for IV administration according to drug insert or PDR.
5. Check package insert or other references for drug's compatibility with primary infusing solution. ▸ ***Rationale:*** Flushing the primary infusion tubing will be necessary both before and after administering the drug if incompatibility exists. Alternatively, a secondary "piggyback" bag of normal saline can be hung and used for flushing the primary line during the drug injection.
6. Check medication according to the *Six Rights*.
7. Take medication to client's bedside.
8. Check that client is not allergic to the drug.
9. Don clean gloves.

Procedure

1. Identify client using two descriptors.
2. Obtain vital signs if agent to be given has hemodynamic effects.
3. Don gloves.
4. Validate placement using first prefilled syringe.
5. Prep primary tubing injection port closest to client.
6. Insert medication syringe cannula into line port.
7. Pinch primary tubing between port and infusion bag while injecting medication slowly in calculated increments (e.g., inject one-fourth of medication over a 20-second period). Always check literature to determine injection times for specific medication.
8. After injecting small increments, unpinch primary tubing to allow flushing of medication.
9. Observe client for any adverse effects.
10. Deliver next increment, using your watch and timing drug injection according to the drug insert instructions.
11. Withdraw syringe when medication injection is complete.
12. Prep primary tubing injection port again.
13. Insert second saline syringe to flush all medication from IV tubing. Use same time rate as medication administration. ▸ ***Rationale:*** To prevent adverse reactions.
14. Discard equipment.
15. Remove gloves and perform hand hygiene.
16. Recheck client's vital signs and document if indicated.

Clinical Alert

Before any IV push or if drug is irritating, validate intravenous line placement. Place a tourniquet proximal to primary infusion; slow drip rate and remove tubing from pump. Ensure that infusion slows or stops before injecting the IV medication. This action validates intravenous status of infusion. Blood flashback is not a reliable indicator of such.

Clinical Alert

In contrast to IV "push," an IV bolus of a drug is rapidly injected in order to achieve an immediate desired drug level—usually for emergency situations. Always refer to pharmaceutical company's instructions for *IV drug injection* before administering.

DOCUMENTATION for IV Medications

- Amount of medication administered
- Method of drug administration
- Flush (e.g., NS) if indicated for compatibility
- Document flush solutions on I&O flow sheet
- IV site status
- Client's response to medication
- Parameters such as vital signs, as indicated

Legal Alert

Up to 90% of all clients receiving healthcare services require some form of IV therapy. As a nurse, you will most likely be involved in starting, monitoring, and discontinuing IV therapy.

Administering drugs is a major problem related to IV therapy. Medication errors account for 2 in 1,000 hospital deaths and are frequent causes of malpractice actions. The most frequent errors are incorrect dose, wrong drug, and improper technique (such as infusing the medication too quickly).

Ensure that you administer IV therapy according to the acceptable nursing standards established by your facility, as well as state and federal guidelines. Keeping up with new standards and reading journal articles will assist you in keeping current. In order to accomplish this, you will need to update your skills yearly.

Documentation must be appropriate, accurate, and concise in case of lawsuits regarding client injuries.

Documentation: "Do and Don't"

- Document only what you observed firsthand, what the client stated, and what was done. Do not offer opinions.
- Use the word "observed," not "noted." This could mean something was written in the medical record.
- Do write "no IV-related complications observed." If you document only parts of the assessment, such as "no redness noted," it could be taken that you didn't observe for any other signs of infection.
- Document details about complications: nursing interventions, physician orders, client's comments regarding complications or responses to treatments.
- Document catheter length when removing a peripheral venous access device or PICC line.
- Do not write "client tolerated procedure well." Provide statement from client as to how he/she felt.
- DO NOT rely solely on charting by exception or check-off flow sheets to document. They do not prove proper client assessment and may or may not hold up in court.

Source: Satarawala, R. (2000, August). Confronting the legal perils of i.v. therapy. *Nursing*, *30*(8), 44–47.

CRITICAL THINKING Application

Expected Outcomes

- IV solutions from secondary IV bags infused without difficulty.
- Therapeutic blood levels of medication are maintained.
- Complications of medication administration are prevented.
- Medication is infused over appropriate time span using volume control set.
- Saline lock inserted for medication administration without complications.

Unexpected Outcomes	Alternative Actions
Secondary bag solution does not infuse adequately.	• Check that primary IV bag is lower than secondary bag (if infusion device requires). • Ensure that secondary needleless connector is properly attached in the primary injection port and secondary bag is sufficiently spiked. • Check that the roller clamp of the secondary tubing is open fully.

Solution in primary IV tubing is incompatible with medication to be administered via secondary "piggyback."	• Turn primary infusion off. • Before administering medication, flush primary tubing with solution compatible with medication (e.g., normal saline, 5% D/W). • Hang a separate solution compatible with medication and run through line to flush during drug administration.
Solution does not infuse through peripheral lock.	• Gently turn lock to establish flow. • Reposition client's extremity. • Initiate a new IV site.

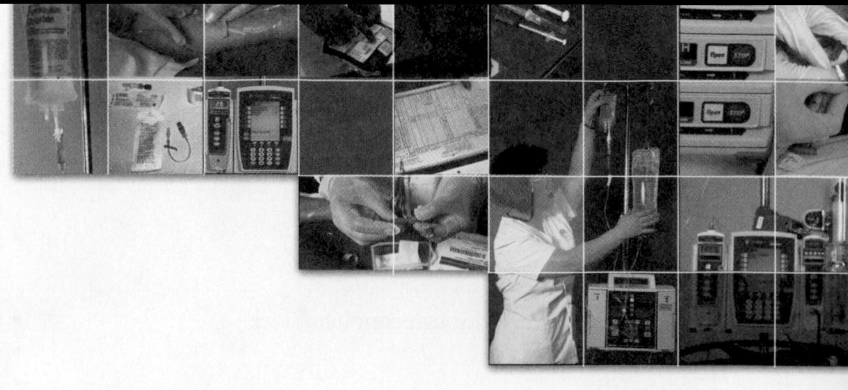

Chapter 28

UNIT 5

Blood Transfusions

Nursing Process Data

ASSESSMENT Data Base

- Assess that client has signed informed consent for transfusion.
- Assess if client has an established IV site.
- Assess client's vital signs, especially temperature, for baseline data.
- Ensure that client's number and blood type on unit match client's blood ID bracelet name and number before administration to ensure compatibility. (Validate consistency with another nurse.)

PLANNING Objectives

- To provide blood or blood components (e.g., platelets, fresh-frozen plasma) for clients with a demonstrated deficiency
- To ensure compatibility between client's blood and the blood or blood component to be transfused
- To prevent the infusion of microaggregates or leukocytes
- To prevent febrile reaction to the transfusion
- To monitor and ensure a timely transfusion
- To monitor for potential complications during and after the blood transfusion

IMPLEMENTATION Procedures

EVALUATION Expected Outcomes

- Transfusion of blood is performed in a timely manner.
- Client's blood deficiency is corrected.
- Transfusion reaction does not occur.

Pearson Nursing Student Resources

Find additional review materials at **nursing.pearsonhighered.com**

Prepare for success with NCLEX®-style practice questions and Skill Checklists

Administering Blood Through a Y-Set

Equipment

Blood unit (packed RBCs)

NOTE: Few conditions require the transfusion of whole blood. Most whole blood is used to prepare separate components to meet specific client needs (e.g., RBCs, plasma, platelets).

250-mL bag of normal saline
Y-set blood tubing with filter
Venipuncture supplies if client does not have established site, at least an 18- or 20-gauge needle or catheter
Needleless injection cap (if not in place)
2% Chlorhexidine gluconate swabs
Tape
Clean gloves

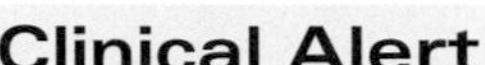

Clinical Alert
In emergency situations, when time does not allow ABO determination, group O red blood cells may be given. Whole blood, however, *must* be administered ABO identical.

Preparation

1. Check physician's order for number and type of transfusion units (order must dictate "transfusion").
2. Identify client using two descriptors.
3. Explain procedure to client and confirm that client has signed consent form for transfusion.
4. Check that type and crossmatch have been completed and that blood is ready in blood bank.
5. Determine patency of client's IV and needle or catheter gauge. Begin infusion of NS with appropriate blood tubing.
6. Obtain client's pretransfusion vital signs. ▸ ***Rationale:*** If client has temperature above 100°F (37.8°C), physician must be notified before proceeding.
7. Obtain ordered typed and matched blood component bag from blood bank, or notify blood bank to deliver unit (according to agency policy). Both nurse and lab tech check transfusion number and sign transfusion form.

If transfusion requires electronic monitoring device to control blood flow, only pumps designed for the infusion of whole blood and RBCs may be used. These pumps require the use of special tubing and filter. Other types of pumps may cause hemolysis of RBCs.

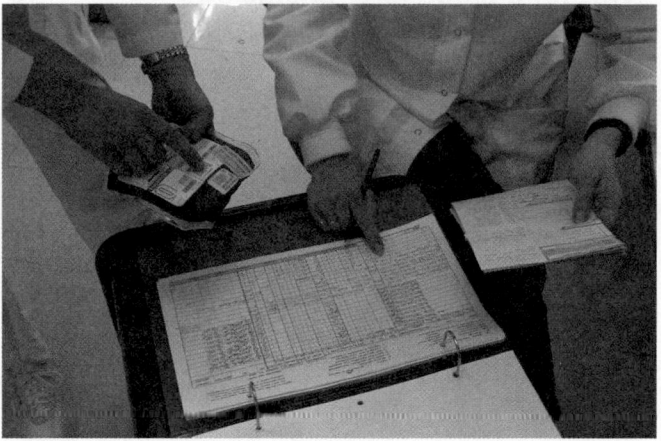

▲ Obtain ordered typed and matched blood/component bag from blood bank.

Clinical Alert
Always determine patency of the IV line before obtaining blood from the blood bank.

8. With another nurse, validate that client's ID bracelet number matches blood bank number on unit of blood to be transfused.
9. Validate client's name, ID number, blood group/Rh, blood product, unit number, and expiration date.
10. Take and record client's vital signs on transfusion record 5 minutes before starting, 5 minutes after starting infusion, 15 minutes, and then every 30 minutes until transfusion is completed (1–1.5 hr), and immediately after the transfusion.
11. Remember that blood cannot be returned to the blood bank after it has been checked out for 20 minutes.

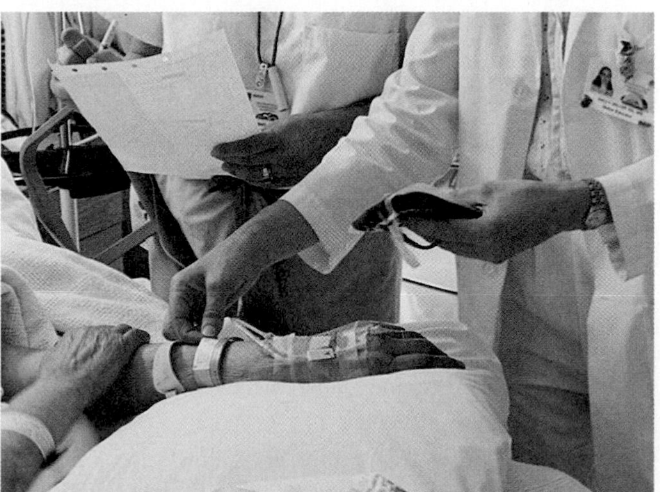

▲ Ascertain that client's name, ID number, blood group, number/Rh, unit expiration date, and hospital number match number on record on the blood bag.

Warming Blood for Transfusion

Routine transfusions are not usually warmed. Warming is required in massive transfusions or, more commonly, may be ordered in maternity or the postanesthesia care unit. A blood warming device is used. Never warm blood bag in hot water or microwave. Once blood is warmed, it must be used or disposed of, as it cannot be returned to the blood bank. Hemolysis of the blood occurs at temperatures above 104°F.

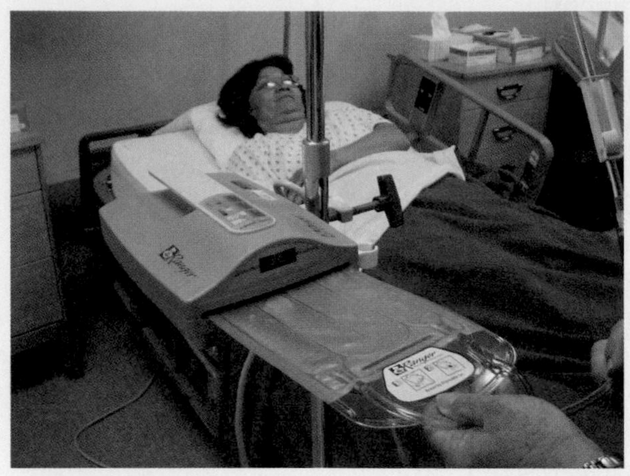

Clinical Alert

Most clients can tolerate a flow rate of one unit of packed cells in 1.5–2 hr. For elderly clients or those with respiratory or cardiac conditions, nurse may need to adjust flow rate according to client's status.

12. Check blood bag for bubbles, cloudiness, dark color, or sediment. ▸ ***Rationale:*** These signs indicate bacterial contamination.
13. Perform hand hygiene and don clean gloves.

Procedure

1. Close all clamps on the Y-set tubing.
2. Spike bag of normal saline with one arm of the Y-tubing.
3. Open clamps on both arms of the Y-tubing to flush.
4. Close clamp on free arm of Y-set (blood side) and open clamp below tubing filter to prime main tubing.
5. Close main clamp when tubing is primed.
6. Close clamps.
7. Gently agitate blood unit bag. ▸ ***Rationale:*** Agitation suspends the red cells in the anticoagulant.
8. Pull back tabs on blood unit bag, and expose port.
9. Spike blood bag port with free arm of Y-tubing, then hang unit.
10. Prep client's injection port.
11. Connect blood tubing via needleless connection.
12. Open clamp to blood bag.
13. Start blood infusion, administering slowly at 5 mL/min for first 15 minutes. ▸ ***Rationale:*** Slow administration allows time to observe for adverse reactions. Most reactions occur in the first 15 minutes.

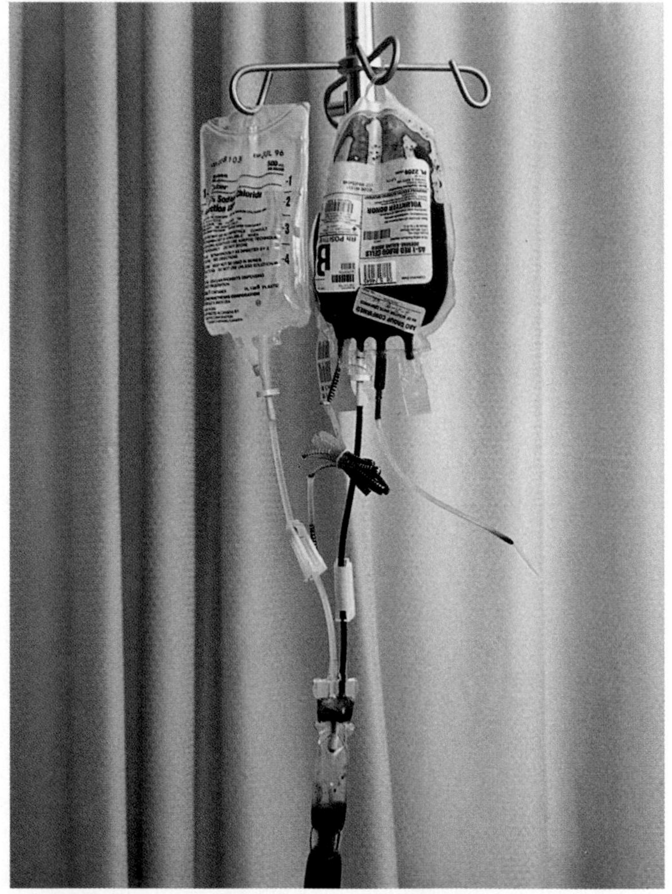

▲ Prime blood administration Y-set tubing with sterile normal saline before starting infusion.

Clinical Alert

Blood must be hung within 30 minutes after taking it from blood bank. Usually only 1 unit of blood is dispensed at a time.

NOTE: According to American Association of Blood Banking (AABB) Technical Manual, 14th ed., 2002.

14. Take vital signs 5 minutes *before*, and 5 minutes, 15 minutes, and every 30 minutes *after* starting transfusion and record on Transfusion Record. Check hospital policy and procedures.
15. Observe client closely for adverse signs: chilling, backache, headache, nausea or vomiting, tachycardia, tachypnea, respiratory distress, skin rash, itching, or hypotension.
16. Agitate blood bag each time the client is checked.
17. If venous spasm occurs with cold blood infusion, apply warm pack to site to improve flow rate.
18. Complete the blood transfusion in less than 4 hr. ▸ ***Rationale:*** Blood deteriorates rapidly after a 2-hr exposure to room temperature and increases risk of bacterial infection.
19. Check that transfusion is completed, then flush line with normal saline.
20. Obtain posttransfusion vital signs.
21. Report a 1°C (2°F) rise in temperature to the physician. ▸ ***Rationale:*** This could be indicative of a transfusion reaction.
22. Complete documentation on the Transfusion Record: place one copy on client's chart and send remaining copy of the Transfusion Record to the Blood Bank as soon as transfusion is completed.
23. Discard administration set within 4 hr of use.

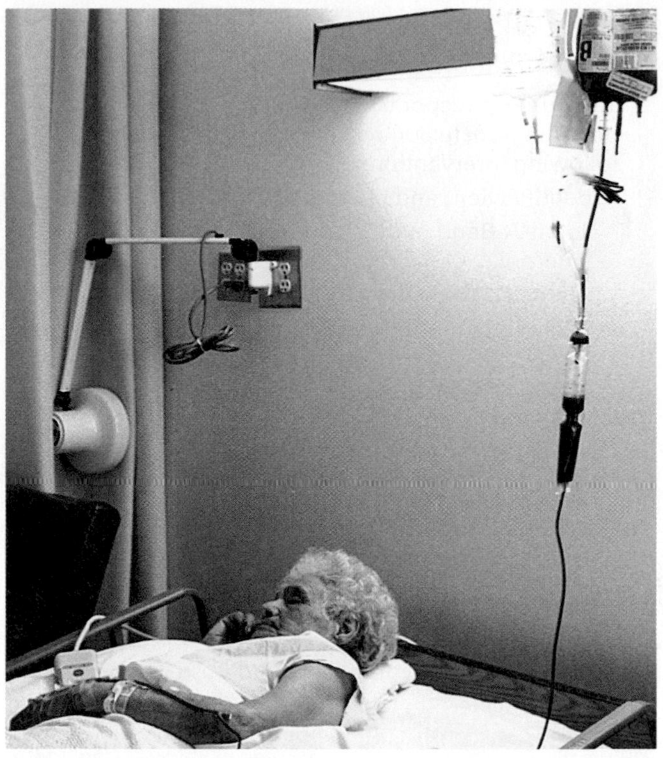

▲ Observe client carefully for first 15 minutes and frequently throughout the blood transfusion.

24. Place all transfusion-related equipment in a biohazard waste receptacle.
25. Remove gloves and perform hand hygiene.
26. Continue to observe client.

Administering Blood Through a Straight Line

Equipment

Blood unit
Blood administration straight-line set with 170-micron filter microaggregate or leukocyte-depleting filter
Needleless cannula
Electronic infusion device (optional)
Clean gloves

Procedure

1. Obtain and check blood as stated in Preparation for Administering Blood through a Y-Set.
2. Perform hand hygiene and don gloves.
3. Spike blood bag port carefully and hang unit.
4. Gently agitate unit, and suspend on IV pole.
5. Open clamp and fill drip chamber, making sure filter is totally submerged in the blood.
6. Open clamp on tubing and run blood through tubing, then clamp.
7. Load tubing into infusion pump if used.
8. Carefully connect blood tubing to client's IV site catheter or lock.
9. Begin blood transfusion.
10. Observe client closely and obtain vital signs 5 minutes before, 5 minutes after start, then after 15 minutes, then every 30 minutes or per hospital policy and procedures.

Blood Transfusion Protocol

The nurse is responsible for early assessment of possible transfusion reactions by completing the following interventions.

- Identify client and blood bag.
  - Ident-A-Band number matches transfusion record number.
  - Name spelled correctly on transfusion record.
  - Blood bag number and pilot tube number are the same.
  - Blood type matches on transfusion record and blood bag.
- Double-check blood with another RN before infusing; record on transfusion record.
- Determine client allergy history and previous blood reactions.
- Establish baseline vital sign data.
- Start transfusion slowly to observe for severe reactions.
- Maintain aseptic technique during procedure.
- Observe time rules for administering blood. (Hang no longer than 4 hr.)
- Observe blood bag for bubbles, cloudiness, dark color, or black sediment, which is indicative of bacterial invasion.

11. When blood bag is empty, close all clamps and remove blood tubing cannula from IV site.
12. Dispose of equipment in biohazard waste receptacle.
13. Remove gloves and perform hand hygiene.
14. Continue to observe client.

Administering Blood Components

Equipment

Blood component
Appropriate IV administration set
Filter, if indicated
Clean gloves

Procedure

1. Check physician's orders and client's signed consent for transfusion.
2. Obtain blood component from blood bank.
3. Obtain appropriate administration set.
4. Perform hand hygiene and don gloves.
5. Read directions for proper administration of the solution.
6. Identify rate at which blood component should infuse.
7. Check Table 28-8 for appropriate rate, risk factors, and possible complications.

Modified Blood Products

In addition to the usual blood components such as platelets and cryoprecipitate, modified blood products are becoming more popular. Washed, irradiated, or leukocyte-removed blood is being used for clients at risk because of multiple transfusions or a weakened immune system. Testing for cytomegalovirus and matching RBC or human leukocyte antigens is also done to ensure safe transfusions.

Clinical Alert

When infusing a blood product that has undergone leukocyte reduction, it still must be filtered again through a standard blood administration set in order to trap cellular debris that may have accumulated since the original filtration.

Monitoring for Potential Complications

Equipment

Sphygmomanometer
Stethoscope
Thermometer

Procedure

1. Check temperature, blood pressure, pulse, and respiration before transfusion is started.

2. Check vital signs 5 minutes before, then 5 and 15 minutes and every 30 minutes for the first 100 mL after transfusion has started. ▸ ***Rationale:*** Most blood transfusion reactions occur during this time.
3. Maintain vital sign assessment throughout blood infusion according to hospital policy.
4. Monitor client for possible transfusion reactions.
   a. Hemolytic or incompatibility reaction—most severe reaction
   b. Bacterial contamination
   c. Allergic reaction
5. If any severe untoward sign occurs (increase in temperature, pain in kidney region), STOP transfusion immediately.
6. Remove blood and any blood-filled tubing and replace with saline bag and new tubing to keep line open. Return blood bag and administration set to blood bank or laboratory.
7. Notify physician immediately after stopping IV for signs of transfusion reaction. Also notify physician if any unusual sign (itching or hives) occurs.

TABLE 28-7 Transfusion Reactions

Type	Clinical Manifestations	Nursing Interventions
Bacterial	Sudden increase in temperature Hypotension Dry, flushed skin Abdominal pain Headache Lumbar pain Sudden chill	Stop transfusion immediately and remove blood tubing. Maintain IV site; change tubing and start infusion of normal saline. Observe for shock. Monitor vital signs every 5 minutes. Insert Foley catheter and monitor urine output hourly. Notify physician and obtain order for antibiotic and steroids/shock management. Draw blood cultures before antibiotic administration. Send remaining blood and tubing to laboratory for culture and sensitivity.
Allergic	Mild: urticaria and hives, pruritus Severe: respiratory distress, wheezing Anaphylactic reaction: shock, loss of consciousness	Stop transfusion immediately if symptoms are severe—immediate resuscitation may be necessary. Monitor vital signs for possible anaphylactic shock. If symptoms are mild, stop transfusion or follow hospital policy and obtain physician's orders. Monitor for signs of progressive allergic reaction as transfusion continues.
Hemolytic	Severe pain in kidney region and chest Pain at needle insertion site Fever (may reach 105°F), chills, flushing Dyspnea and cyanosis Oozing of blood at IV site Headache Hypotension Hematuria Nausea	Stop transfusion immediately and remove blood tubing. Start normal saline infusion at "keep open" rate with a new IV tubing. Obtain vital signs. Notify blood bank STAT. Administer oxygen. Notify physician. Obtain orders for IV volume expansion and diuretic or vasopressor to dilate renal blood vessels to prevent acute renal tubular necrosis. Complete transfusion reaction form. Send two blood samples (from different sites), urine specimen, remaining blood and tubing, and transfusion record to laboratory. Monitor vital signs every 15 minutes for shock. Monitor urine output hourly for possible acute renal failure.

TABLE 28-8 Blood Component Therapy

Type	Use	Alerts	Administration Equipment
Fresh plasma	To replace deficient coagulation factors To increase intravascular compartment	Hepatitis is a risk Administer as rapidly as possible Use within 6 hr	Any straight-line administration set
Platelets	To prevent or treat bleeding problems, especially in surgical clients To replace platelets in clients with acquired or inherited deficiencies (thrombo cytopenia, aplastic anemia) To replace when platelets drop below 20,000 mL/mm (normal 150,000–350,000 mL/mm)	Administer at rate of 10 minutes a unit (usually comes in multiple platelet packs)	Platelet transfusion set with special filter to allow platelets to infuse through filter
Granulocytes	To treat oncology clients with severe bone marrow depression and progressive infections To treat granulocytopenic clients with infections that are unresponsive to antibiotics To treat clients with gram-negative bacteremia or infections where marrow recovery does not develop	Administer slowly, over 2–4 hr Give one transfusion daily until granulocytes increase or infection clears Use within 48 hr after drawn Observe for shaking, fever, chills Observe for hives and laryngeal edema (treat with antihistamines)	Use Y-type blood filters and prime with physiologic saline. A microaggregate filter is not used as it filters out platelets
Serum albumin	To treat shock To treat hypoproteinemia	Available as 5% or 25% solution Infuse 25% solution slowly 1 mL/minute to prevent circulatory overload Administer 100–200 mL (25% solution) for shock clients and 200–300 mL for hypoproteinemia	Special tubing accompanies albumin solution in individual boxes
Gamma globulin	To treat agammaglobulinemia To act as a prophylaxis for hepatitis exposure	Pooled plasma contains antibodies to infectious agents Administer 0.25–0.50 mL of immune serum globulin/kg of body weight every 2–4 weeks	Given IM
Coagulation factors	To treat clients with von Willebrand's disease	Made from fresh-frozen plasma	Standard syringe or component drip set only
Factor VIII (cryoprecipitate)	To treat clients with factor VIII, hemophilia A	Administer one unit cryoprecipitate for each 6 kg of body weight initially, followed by 1 unit/3 kg of body weight at 6–12-hr intervals until treatment discontinued Administer 1 unit/5 minutes Observe for febrile reactions	

TABLE 28-8 Blood Component Therapy *(Continued)*

Type	Use	Alerts	Administration Equipment
Factor IX	To treat clients with factor IX, hemophilia B	Administer in 12–24-hr cycle Preparation for administration is 400–500 units/vial. Must reconstitute in 10–20 mL diluent One unit/pound of body weight increases the circulating factor activity by 5% Serum hepatitis can be transmitted	Any straight-line set—drip or by IV push—not to exceed 10 mL/min

DOCUMENTATION for Blood Transfusions

- Type, unit number, and amount of blood product administered
- Name of healthcare provider who verified information with nurse
- Amount of normal saline used
- Type and gauge of catheter or needleless access device
- Time transfusion began and ended
- Vital signs 5 minutes before transfusion begins; 5, 15, 30, and 60 minutes after infusion begins; and then hourly until infusion completed (check hospital blood administration policy and procedure for vital sign frequency)
- Document on I&O record
- Transfusion tag may have space for vital sign information as well
- Client's response to procedure
- Any unusual clinical manifestations; any nursing interventions
- Warning device if used
- Infusion device used and flow rate setting
- Filter if used

CRITICAL THINKING Application

Expected Outcomes

- Transfusion of blood is performed in a timely manner.
- Client's blood deficiency is corrected.
- Transfusion reaction does not occur

Unexpected Outcomes	Alternative Actions
Transfusion reaction occurs.	• Stop blood administration and begin infusion of normal saline or ordered solution to keep IV open. • Check transfusion reaction form for appropriate nursing intervention. • Complete all relevant nursing actions.
Blood does not flow through tubing.	• Check client's IV site and gauge of needle or catheter (at least 18 or 20 gauge). • Gently agitate blood bag to mix blood cells with the anticoagulant. • Raise blood bag higher on IV pole. Squeeze flexible tubing to promote blood flow. • Adjust clamp on tubing. As the blood passes over the filter, more blood microaggregates clog the filter and slow drip rate. • Replace tubing. • Utilize an infusion pump, especially if administering blood through a small catheter or lock. • Consider using blood warmer.

Blood has been hanging for more than 4 hr.	• Take down blood bag and send to laboratory. • Document amount of blood administered. • Maintain IV with normal saline or ordered IV solution. • Monitor vital signs for complications. • Notify physician.
Potential circulatory overload occurs.	• Monitor symptoms: sudden dyspnea, tachypnea, tachycardia, chest discomfort, distended neck veins, moist crackles and rales, restlessness, sudden increase in blood pressure. • Stop transfusion and place client in Fowler's position. • Start oxygen at 2 L/min per nasal cannula. • Be prepared for ECG and chest x-ray. • Be prepared to administer Lasix and morphine sulfate.

GERONTOLOGIC Considerations

Elderly Clients' Veins Are Fragile and Roll Easily, and Frequently the Needle Punctures the Wall of the Vessel

- Insert small-gauge winged catheter in distal vein first to preserve proximal vessel.
- Tourniquet (constricting band) may not be necessary for venipuncture. If used, it should be applied loosely.
- If used, release tourniquet as soon as venipuncture yields blood return to prevent excessive pressure in vein.
- Maintain close assessment of IV sites to promote long-term use of vessel.

Elderly Clients Are Prone to Fluid and Electrolyte Disorders as a Result of the Normal Aging Process

- Thirst mechanism is decreased.
- Renal threshold is altered.
- Total body fluid is less due to decreased lean muscle mass.
- Fluid replacement therapy requires close monitoring to prevent fluid overload, leading to pulmonary edema and electrolyte imbalance.
- Dehydration is a common reason for IV therapy.
- When infusing IV fluids, monitor closely for signs of fluid volume overload.
- Monitor BUN and electrolytes regularly for signs of overload.
- Use IV pump whenever infusing fluids into elderly clients. If dextrose solution is being infused, IV pumps *must* be used. Dextrose overload can lead to cerebral edema if infused too rapidly.

Stabilizing IV Catheter and Dressing Is Problematic Due to Client's Fragile Skin

- Avoid excessive use of tape.
- Apply skin protector solution before dressing site.
- Use stretch mesh gauze to cover site and tubing to prevent catching on bed (avoid roll-type gauze).

Protect Fragile Skin That Is More Susceptible to Injury, Infiltration, and Discomfort From Irritating Drugs

- Observe IV site carefully for signs of infiltration. Because of skin's loose folds and decreased tactile sensation, a large amount of fluid can sequester in subcutaneous tissue and go unnoticed before client complains of pain.
- Check IV site frequently when client is receiving drugs that can cause irritation and even necrosis if they infiltrate.
- At first sign of phlebitis or infiltration, remove IV and restart in a new site.
- If client complains of discomfort during IV therapy, apply a moist and warm pack to site, decrease rate of fluid infusion.

MANAGEMENT Guidelines

Each state legislates a Nurse Practice Act for RNs and LVN/LPNs. Healthcare facilities are responsible for establishing and implementing policies and procedures that conform to their state's regulations. Verify the regulations and role parameters for each healthcare worker in your facility.

Delegation

- Each state identifies the scope of practice for RNs and LPN/LVNs. Several states have identified that the LPN/LVN has a specific role in IV therapy, but the scope of practice is always dictated by each agency (e.g., initiating, regulating, discontinuing IVs).
- Daily weighing of clients is usually assigned to the CNA or UAP. The RN should verify that weights are taken in the morning before breakfast, using the same scale each time. The client should urinate before weighing for accuracy. Since a client's weight changes are frequently taken into consideration for prescribing fluid allowances or

medication adjustments, accuracy in measurement and documentation is imperative.

- All care providers must be aware of clients whose intake and output are monitored and must conscientiously participate in accurate measurement.
- All care providers must be aware of clients for whom fluid restriction is ordered and carefully adhere to designated allowances.
- CNAs and UAPs report vital data to the professional nurse by monitoring vital signs. This skill can be delegated for the pre-, intra-, and post-blood transfusion, and results should be given immediately to the nurse. The professional nurse then validates and acts upon any abnormal findings accordingly.
- The CNA/UAP providing personal hygiene must understand that the IV system is a closed one and must be able to give care without disrupting this system. The components of the system must never be disconnected for the convenience of care (e.g., changing gown). The CNA/UAP should receive training in changing the client's gown without disrupting the IV system.
- It is the nurse's responsibility to monitor and document intravenous fluid volume administered.
- It is the nurse's responsibility to evaluate the client's total balance of intake and output and to investigate significant imbalances for further decision making.
- While the professional nurse monitors the IV infusion site regularly, the CNA/UAP must communicate observations of swelling, client reports of concern (e.g., pain), and infusion device signals that prompt the professional to further assess the client.

Communication Matrix

- All care providers participate in accurate recording of the client's intake and output. Records are usually kept at the bedside. All must be familiar with the standard capacities for frequently used vessels (bowls, cups) to facilitate accurate recording of intake.
- Likewise, careful recording of measurable output and best estimation of unmeasurable losses (e.g., incontinence) will facilitate care decisions.
- The nurse must ensure that CNA/UAPs know to report any unusual fluid loss the client is experiencing (e.g., vomiting). It is the nurse's responsibility to evaluate alterations in fluid loss (e.g., vomiting, scant urine output) and act upon these findings accordingly. Knowledge and judgment cannot be delegated.
- It is the nurse's responsibility to document vital client information on the Transfusion Record, which is placed into the client's hospital chart.

CRITICAL THINKING Strategies

Scenario 1

Mrs. Beatty is a 40-year-old client, 5′1″ tall and weighing 300 lb. She had emergency abdominal surgery for lysis of adhesions. You are assigned to care for her on her first postoperative day. As you begin your assessment, you note she has an NG tube that is draining bile-colored return. Her IV is D5% in 0.45NS infusing at 125 mL/hr. The IV is on a pump. As you observe the IV site, you find it difficult to determine whether the site is edematous or it is just her normal appearance. It seems like the area surrounding the site is cooler to the touch than the remaining part of the arm. Mrs. Beatty states the IV area is sore. A gauze dressing is placed directly over the IV site, making it difficult to visualize it. The IV fluid seems to be infusing at the prescribed amount and the IV pump alarm is not ringing.

1. What is your priority action in this situation?
2. After completing the first priority, what is your second priority?
3. While assessing the IV site, what would you look for if you suspect phlebitis or infiltration? With the initial information provided in the scenario, which of these potential complications do you suspect? Provide rationale for your answer.
4. How will you check the IV to determine whether the client does have an infiltration?
5. Indicate your priority intervention if you determine the client has an IV that has infiltrated.
6. Indicate your priority intervention if you determine the client has beginning signs of phlebitis.

Scenario 2

The head nurse comes to you, a new RN, and tells you that Mr. Jones' physician has ordered whole blood for his client, to be given immediately, and hands you a unit of blood.

1. What is your first action after this interaction with the head nurse?
2. What additional data should be collected before implementing this order?
3. After starting the transfusion, the client develops urticaria, hives, and slight respiratory distress. From these symptoms, what would you conclude about the client's status and what intervention would you make?

NCLEX® Review Questions

Unless otherwise specified, choose only one (1) answer.

1. In-line filters are not recommended for which one of the following IV infusions?
   1. Ringer's Lactate.
   2. TPN.
   3. PCA.
   4. Blood platelets.
2. The nurse begins to assess the client's arms to determine the most appropriate site for the venipuncture. Which of the following principles should be kept in mind when determining this site?
   1. The veins that are deeper in the forearm should be assessed first.
   2. The antecubital fossa is a primary site.
   3. The most appropriate site is below an infiltrated area to save the vein.
   4. The distal end of the vein should be selected first.
3. Nursing actions that are completed when preparing for a venipuncture include
   Select all that apply.
   1. Lightly tap the vein to distend it.
   2. Instruct the client to open and close fist to distend vein.
   3. Apply cool cloth to arm for 10 minutes before attempting venipuncture.
   4. Position arm on pillow to increase blood flow to area.
4. It is recommended that the skin prep used before attempting the venipuncture is
   1. Alcohol swab.
   2. Betadine swab.
   3. Iodine swab.
   4. Chlorhexidine glucontate swab.
5. You are preparing to change IV tubing as required during your shift. You recall that
   1. Primary and secondary tubing is changed every 24 hr.
   2. Primary intermittent tubing is changed every 96 hr.
   3. TPN and lipids are changed with each bottle.
   4. Blood or blood products tubing is changed every 4 hr or 2 units.
6. As you review the steps of inserting an over-the-needle catheter, you recall that the steps include the following
   1. Check catheter with the bevel in a "downward" position to examine the integrity of the end of the catheter.
   2. Place the bevel of the needle in the "up" position and insert the catheter at the 45° angle into the skin.
   3. Insert the needle into the anterior surface of the vein.
   4. After hearing the "pop" sound in the vein, remove the plastic catheter hub.
7. The client's IV order is: Administer 2500 mL of normal saline in 24 hr. The administration set delivers 10 gtt/mL. The IV will deliver ____ mL/hr
   1. 10.
   2. 15.
   3. 60.
   4. 104.
8. You walk into the room of a client whose Smart Pump is sounding a "hard" alarm. Your initial action is to
   1. Reset the pump after checking for possible air in tubing.
   2. Reset the rate of the medication infusion on the pump.
   3. Notify the client's nurse.
   4. Reprogram the pump after scanning your badge into the system.
9. The client has an isotonic IV solution ordered for the next 24 hr. The faculty asks you to explain the rationale for this solution. Your answer is that it
   1. Hydrates the cells, causing them to expand.
   2. Corrects dehydration.
   3. Is used as a nutrient source.
   4. Is used to expand intravascular volume.
10. One of your clients has a medication ordered to be infused through the primary tubing injection port. Which of the following safety issues must be considered when administering IV drugs through this method?
    1. Administer the medication over 20 seconds.
    2. Flush the primary infusion tubing before and after administering any drug.
    3. After injecting a small amount of drug, unpinch primary tubing and flush medication.
    4. Administer IV drugs using only a dextrose solution to ensure drug compatibility.

29

Central Vascular Access Devices

LEARNING OBJECTIVES

1. Identify the common types of central vascular access devices (CVADs).
2. Discuss the rationale for using central vascular catheters for long-term IV therapy.
3. Discuss the special needs of clients with central vascular catheters (prevention of infection, air embolism).
4. Describe the role of the nurse in the insertion of CVADs.
5. Explain the nurse's responsibility for assisting the physician with a percutaneous central vascular catheter insertion.
6. Compare and contrast features of various central vascular access devices.
7. Describe initiation and discontinuation of infusions via CVADs.
8. Differentiate protocols for maintaining patency of intermittently used CVADs.
9. Outline steps for dressing and protecting the CVAD insertion site.
10. Discuss the advantage of using a BIOPATCH at the catheter insertion site.
11. Outline the steps in changing an access cap.
12. Discuss the data that is included in client education for the care and maintenance of vascular access devices.

CHAPTER OUTLINE

TERMINOLOGY

Antimicrobic preventing the development of pathogenic action of microbes.

Aspirate application of negative pressure to check for blood return.

Calorie the amount of heat necessary to raise the temperature of 1 kilogram of water 1°C. One thousand (1 kcal) of these calories equals 1 dietary calorie (or calorie).

Carbohydrates a group of chemical substances, including sugars, glycogen, starches, dextrins, and cellulose, that contain only carbon, oxygen, and hydrogen.

Cardio word part that pertains to the heart.

Cardiovascular term that pertains to the heart and blood vessels, as cardiovascular system.

Central vascular access device (CVAD) catheter, centrally placed in the superior vena cava, to provide medication, fluid, and nutrition.

Central venous pressure (CVP) measurement monitors central venous return (volume) and right ventricular function.

Catheter-related bloodstream infection (CRBSI) fourth most common hospital-acquired infection with central line catheter placement.

Cyanosis slightly bluish, grayish, slate-like, or dark purple discoloration due to desaturation of hemoglobin.

Digestion the process by which food is broken down mechanically and chemically in the gastrointestinal tract.

Dyspnea a subjective feeling of difficulty breathing.

Electrolyte substance that develops an electrical charge when dissolved in water.

Erythema redness of the skin produced by capillary congestion as in a sunburn.

Extracellular fluid outside the cell (interstitial and intravascular fluid).

Fat substance made up of carbon, hydrogen, and oxygen, occurring naturally in most foods but especially in meats and dairy products.

Gastrointestinal term that pertains to the stomach and intestines.

Hemo prefix meaning blood.

Hemodynamic study of circulation of blood.

Hemolytic pertinent to the breaking down of red blood cells.

Huber needle a right-angled (90°) or straight, noncoring needle.

Hydrostatic the pressure exerted on liquids.

Hyperalimentation the process of nourishing the body through parenteral means.

Hyperglycemia condition characterized by an increase in blood glucose levels.

Hypertonic solution having a higher osmotic pressure or tonicity than a solution with which it is compared.

Hypovolemia diminished circulating fluid volume.

Implanted inserted under the skin.

Implanted infusion port device placed in subcutaneous tissue with a tunneled catheter that goes into the central venous system.

Infusion a liquid substance introduced into the body via a vein for therapeutic purposes.

Intracellular fluid inside the cell.

Intravascular within blood vessels.

Irrigate to rinse or wash out with a fluid.

Isotonic a solution that has the same concentration of salts, or tonicity, as another solution with which it is compared.

Lipids emulsion containing fats used to correct fatty acid deficiencies via parenteral nutrition.

Lumen the inner open space of a tube or blood vessel.

Malnutrition a condition characterized by a lack of essential food substances or improper absorption and distribution of food substances in the body.

Minerals inorganic elements or compounds.

Nutrient nourishing food item that supplies the body with necessary elements.

Obstruction blocking of a structure that prevents it from functioning normally; obstacle.

Osmosis transmission of water across a semipermeable membrane from an area of low solute concentration to one of higher solute concentration.

Palpate to examine by touch; to feel.

Peripherally inserted central catheter (PICC) long, soft, flexible catheter placed through an arm vein to the superior vena cava.

Phlebitis inflammation of a vein.

Polyunsaturate a long chain of carbon compounds with more than one double bond between the carbons; especially refers to fats.

Port subcutaneously implanted plastic or metal case that provides access to the venous system.

Protein substance that contains amino acids essential for growth and repair of tissues.

Sepsis pathologic state, usually febrile, resulting from the presence of microorganisms or their poisonous products in the bloodstream.

Thrombo a clot of blood; a thrombus.

Thrombophlebitis an inflammation of a vein due to the presence of a thrombus.

Transfusion injection of blood or blood component of one person into the blood vessels of another.

Tunneled catheter a long single or multi-lumen catheter inserted into a central vein, the remainder tunneled subcutaneously to a distant exit site on the chest or abdomen.

Valsalva's maneuver attempt to forcibly exhale with the glottis closed.

Venipuncture puncture of a vein with a needle.

Viscosity resistance offered by a fluid; property of a substance that is dependent on the friction of its component molecules as they slide by each other.

Vitamins a group of organic substances essential for life.

VENOUS ACCESS DEVICES

Peripheral Catheters

Intravenous therapy is administered through a variety of catheters and devices. Several factors are considered when selecting the proper catheter: duration of therapy, pH, and osmolarity of solution to be infused. The most common type of venous access device is the peripheral catheter, inserted into veins of the hands, arms, and antecubital area. These are short catheters, less than 3 in. length, (7.5 cm), intended for short-term IV therapy, usually no more than 7 days. The insertion site needs to be changed frequently, usually every 48–72 hr, according to facility policy. Therapies not appropriate for short catheters include continuous solutions with pH less than 5 or greater than 9, and osmolarity greater than 600 mOsm/L. Medication that cannot be infused in short catheters include vancomycin, penicillin, ganciclovir, dilantin, and Phenergan due to their pH.

Short catheters are used for one-time infusions of less than 7 days. They are used frequently in emergency situations where medications must be administered quickly. They are not recommended for blood draws. If used, they should only be in place for 48 hr.

Site selection is based on four factors: condition of selected vein, type of infusate, rate of infusion, and duration of infusion. When considering the vein, keep in mind that if it has been used previously, you must select a site above the previously used site, especially if there was an infection. It is best to place the first catheter at the lowest point on the upper extremity: this allows for further catheter placement, if needed.

Areas above the flexion of a joint, such as wrist and elbow, should be avoided. These sites can result in mobility problems and catheter dislodgement due to movement of the extremity.

Lower extremities are used only if necessary and require a physician's order in most facilities due to the risk of deep vein thrombosis and pulmonary embolism. (See Chapter 28 for more details on these IV devices.)

Midline Catheters

Midline catheters are 3 to 8 in. (7.5–20 cm) in length and are inserted 1.5 in. (2.5–3.8 cm) above or below the antecubital fossa and terminate in one of the client's arms in a proximal vein. The basilic, cephalic, or median antecubital sites are also used. They are similar to the peripherally inserted central catheter (PICC) but shorter in length. Both catheters are used for long-term IV therapy. Midline catheters are used only for administering nonirritating, normal pH solutions or medications, whereas the PICC can be used to infuse vesicants, hyperosmolar solutions, and TPN. Clients with midline catheters should not receive any medications or IV fluids where the pH is below 5 or above 10, and osmolarity greater than 600 mOsm/L. Damage to the vessel walls can lead to phlebitis or thrombosis.

Midline catheters, because they are placed in larger veins, can be left in place for up to 2–4 weeks. Because of the longer dwell time as compared with the peripheral catheter, complications such as thrombosis at the catheter site can occur. Phlebitis, infection, occlusion, clotting, breakage, and leakage at the insertion site of the catheter are also associated with use of the midline catheter. Unfortunately, complications are not as easy to assess in clients with midline catheters, as opposed to clients with peripheral lines. For example, it takes longer for symptoms of phlebitis to occur in the client with a midline catheter. The short peripheral or midline catheters are not checked by x-ray for placement because they do not enter the superior vena cava as do the central vascular catheters.

Central Vascular Access Devices

Long-term intravascular therapy is best accomplished through use of medically placed central vascular access devices

(CVADs), which include subcutaneous ports and catheters as well as central venous catheters. The specific type of device used depends on the type and duration of treatment, as well as client variables. CVADs are placed in clients who are actively involved and at home, as well as critically ill hospitalized clients. Clients requiring chemotherapy, nutritional supplements, blood products, and fluids can benefit from CVADs. These devices allow repeated access to the vascular system without venipuncture.

Central vascular catheters are categorized into three types: central catheters, PICC lines, and subcutaneously implanted ports. Central catheters are further classified as tunneled or nontunneled catheters. Nontunneled catheters are large-bore catheters that vary in length from 6 to 8 in. (15 to 20 cm) and have one to four lumens. The catheters are made of soft silicone or a polyurethane material. Some of the newer catheters are impregnated with heparin, chlorhexidine, or an antibiotic. In most cases, physicians insert these catheters. Inaccurate placement of any central vascular catheter that is threaded to the superior vena cava can present a potential life-threatening arrhythmia if the catheter lodges against the myocardium.

Central Venous Catheters Central venous catheters are medically placed percutaneously through the chest wall into the jugular or subclavian vein and are used for fluid or blood administration, obtaining blood specimens, and administering medications and parenteral nutrition. Catheter extension into the superior vena cava minimizes vessel irritation and sclerosis of the vessel due to infusion. Because of the high volume of blood that normally flows through this portion of the superior vena cava (2000 mL/min) the risk of complications is lessened. Central catheters can be single or multi-lumen catheters.

Tunneled Catheters Hickman, Broviac, and Groshong catheters are tunneled catheters. The closed-ended or Groshong-type catheter is designed to prevent backflow into the catheter when it is not in use. The Groshong catheter is used when low flow rates will be infused. In the Groshong, fluids infuse through a slit valve on the side of the tip; when there is not an infusion of fluids into the catheter, the slit valve remains in a closed position. These catheters are never clamped due to this design factor. Pressure related to clamping the catheter or extension tubing can force the slit valve to open, allowing a blood leak back into the lumen. Heparin flushing is not routinely done because of the design of the catheter tip.

The Hickman catheter is open-ended with a silver ion impregnated cuff in the subcutaneous tract. This promotes growth of a connective tissue seal, reducing the risk of microbial immigration from the exit site along the catheter tract. The catheter has a reinforced sleeve of silicone on which the catheter clamp is used.

Hickman catheters are flushed with heparin. The client may shower and swim once the exit site has healed, but the hub of the catheter must be covered.

Tunneled catheters are used for long-term replacement therapy, medication administration, nutritional supplementation, and blood specimen withdrawal. These catheters can remain in place from months to years. The catheter's tip is inserted into a central vein (e.g., subclavian or internal jugular vein) and advanced to the distal area of the superior vena cava. The remaining portion of the catheter is threaded subcutaneously to exit at a convenient distal site (chest, abdomen). A Dacron cuff on the catheter promotes scar formation to seal the tract to prevent ascending tract infection. Only physicians may discontinue a tunneled catheter.

Client Selection for CVADS

- Long-term intravenous therapy
- Need for frequent venous access
- CVP monitoring
- Administration of total parenteral nutrition (TPN)
- Self-administration of intravenous therapies
- Sclerosed peripheral veins
- Limited peripheral venous access
- Irritating IV solutions

Subcutaneously Implanted Ports

These implanted ports are surgically placed under the skin in a subcutaneous pocket in the chest, arm, abdomen, and occasionally, the back. The newer ports are MRI compatible and available as a titanium port or titanium dome. Implanted ports are used for long-term and complex IV therapy such as chemotherapy. The septum of the port is made of silicon or polyurethane rubber latex, allowing more than 2,000 punctures with a 19-gauge noncoring needle. The attached catheter enters the superior vena cava. Single and dual septal ports are available with open end or closed catheter endings.

Access to the port is by placement of a noncoring needle through the skin, into the self-sealing injection port housed in a plastic or metal case. This needle can remain in place for 7 days, then be replaced. Since the entire unit is implanted subcutaneously, risk for infection and maintenance requirements are greatly reduced.

Peripheral Insertion of a Central Catheter (PICC)

Peripheral (antecubital) insertion of a central vascular catheter (PICC) to the superior vena cava is easier and less risky than entering the central vein through the chest wall or neck. The basilic vein is the usual choice for catheter insertion due to the blood flow rate of 95 mL/min. and it provides the straightest pathway to the superior vena cava. The tip of the catheter resides in the lower third of the superior vena cava, not in the right atrium. The usual length of the catheter is 40–60 cm. The PICC lines result in fewer problems than other types of access devices; however, common problems associated with PICC lines include phlebitis and infection. One common problem is that they tend to occlude frequently due to their small diameter. They need to be assessed thoroughly for breakage and phlebitis. Using a PICC line is the most appropriate method for infusing vesicants such as dopamine HCL, hyperosmolar solutions such as TPN or blood products, and antibiotics that are potentially irritating drugs. These drugs and solutions can be infused through the PICC line because the superior vena cava is large and has a large volume of blood by which these medications are diluted before they enter the systemic circulation. Studies have indicated that PICC lines have been in place for up to 1 year. Current research is looking at the exact time frame for PICC line placement, so this time frame may change. These access devices may be inserted by specially trained nurses who complete a certification process. The PICC line is inserted at the bedside using a bedside ultrasound, which makes it possible to accurately visualize and access the veins in the upper arm. The PICC line is inserted in the upper arm 95% of the time. Upper arm insertion has a lower rate of thrombosis, phlebitis, and catheter migration. A small gauge (21–22 gauge) needle can be used that reduces the incidence of hematomas and damage to the vein. Most facilities use PICC-certified nurses to insert the line. As with all centrally placed catheters, a chest x-ray is taken to verify placement of the radiopaque catheter to validate that the tip is in the superior vena cava. The catheter must not be used until IV placement is verified. Trained healthcare workers may discontinue the line when no longer needed.

StatLock securement devices are routinely used to prevent complications and restarts in hospitalized clients. Documentation indicates there is a 45% decrease in these problems since the securement device has been instituted. When compared with suture securement, these devices have eliminated the sharps injuries when securing the central catheter lines. Arterial catheter restarts have been decreased by 49%. Using the StatLock device has lowered the rate of total IV complications by approximately 67%, decreased IV total complications from 48% to 16%, decreased phlebitis rate by approximately 80%, and decreased the rate of tape-related skin damage, which is documented to be as high as 54%. *Source:* www.bardaccess.com.

Sterile technique must be maintained throughout all procedures associated with CVADs and PICC lines. Infection may occur if contamination results from poor technique in maintaining insertion sites, flushing catheters, or inserting the noncoring needle. Transparent dressings are placed over the insertion site for better stabilization and easy assessment and monitoring.

Catheter-Related Bloodstream Infections

Catheter-related bloodstream infections (CRBSIs) are the fourth most common hospital-acquired infections with central line catheter placement. Approximately 80,000 CRBSIs occur yearly in U.S. ICUs with central lines, with 25% of the cases resulting in death. As of October 2008, the Center for Medicare and Medicaid Services (CMS) stopped reimbursing hospitals for these costs. Hospitals have been developing central line bundle procedures to reduce the rates of infection, usually following the Institute for Healthcare Improvement (IHI) guidelines.

Source: Martin, Walter MD, Harnage, Sophie RN. (May-June 2008.) A new bundle of preventing CRBSIs. Patient safety and quality healthcare. www.psqh.com.

Use of Antimicrobial Central Venous Catheters

Antimicrobial central venous catheters (CVCs) have been recommended for clients at risk for CRBSIs and for whom the expected duration of use is between 1 and 3 weeks. There are several types of antimicrobial CVCs. There is concern that the use of these catheters may encourage the emergence of resistant microorganisms; however, there is no evidence to support this at this time.

The most common type of antimicrobial CVC is coated with chlorhexidine and silver sulfadiazine. The newest available catheter has three times the concentration of chlorhexidine, with silver sulfadiazine on the external CVC surface. It has a coating of chlorhexidine on the internal surface of the CVC lumen. The results of a meta-analysis have demonstrated that the earlier type of CVC shows a significant reduction in CVC colonization and a trend toward a reduction in CRBSIs. There have been insufficient numbers of studies to form a conclusion on their effectiveness.

Total Parenteral Nutrition

Parenteral nutrition is a method whereby nutrients are introduced intravenously. Bypassing the normal gastrointestinal system, this route provides a nitrogen source for those with a nonfunctional gastrointestinal tract (enteral starvation) or those with high caloric requirements (burn client), or acute hypoalbuminemia.

Balanced blends of nutrients, including vitamins and minerals, can be administered both by central line and peripherally using isotonic concentrations of glucose (no greater than 10% dextrose). In contrast, hypertonic solutions that are irritating to veins are administered through a central, high-flow vein. Rapid dilution of the solution decreases risk of phlebitis, clot formation, and hemolysis. This technique requires special handling and management, presents greater risk for complications, and is the most expensive method of feeding.

Central Line Bundle

These are groupings of best practices that individually improve care, but when used together, greatly increase the outcome or prevention of CRBSIs. The central line bundle has five key components (www.ihi/IH1program):

- Hand hygiene
- Maximal barrier precautions
- Chlorhexidine gluconate skin antisepsis
- Optimal catheter site selection, with preferred site, the subclavian vein for nontunneled catheters
- Daily assessment of skin and lines

NURSING DIAGNOSES

The following nursing diagnoses may be appropriate to include in a client care plan when the components are related to intravascular therapy.

NURSING DIAGNOSIS	RELATED FACTORS
Activity Intolerance	Change in setting—intensive care, catabolic state Compromised cardiac reserve
Anxiety	Lifestyle modification, pain, chronic condition Uncertainty related to illness and diagnosis, placement of a CVAD
Decreased Cardiac Output	Impaired myocardial function, hypovolemia
Excess Fluid Volume	Excess fluid replacement, medications, renal and cardiac dysfunction
Infection, Risk for	Invasive procedures, inadequate site care, use of hypertonic glucose solutions
Deficient Knowledge	Ability to care for intravenous catheter or administer TPN
Imbalanced Nutrition: Less Than Body Requirements	Chronic fatigue states, nausea and vomiting, inadequate absorption, faulty metabolism, eating disorders, side effects of chemotherapy
Ineffective Peripheral Tissue Perfusion	Altered blood supply, arterial or venous, impaired myocardial contractility, hypovolemia

CLEANSE HANDS The single most important nursing action to decrease the incidence of hospital-based infections is hand hygiene. *Remember to wash your hands or use antibacterial gel before and after each and every client contact.*

IDENTIFY CLIENT Before every procedure, introduce yourself and check two forms of client identification, not including room number. These actions prevent errors and conform to The Joint Commission standards.

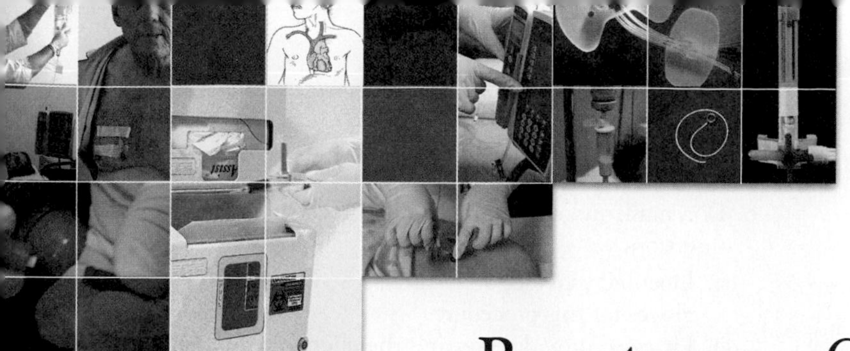

Chapter 29

UNIT 1

Percutaneous Central Vascular Catheters

Nursing Process Data

ASSESSMENT Data Base

- Determine client's level of consciousness so explanation of procedure can be done to allay anxiety.
- Assess level of anxiety to determine need for possible premedication.
- Assess skin and surrounding tissue for erythema, edema, and warmth.
- Assess circulating volume status and right heart function.
- Assess StatLock® site for potential complications.

PLANNING Objectives

- To assist the licensed practitioner with percutaneous central vascular catheter insertion
- To maintain patency of central vascular catheter
- To change central venous catheter dressing without complications
- To maintain the insertion site free of infection
- To prevent air embolism
- To monitor central venous pressure

IMPLEMENTATION Procedures

EVALUATION Expected Outcomes

- Central vascular line is properly placed without complication.
- Central vascular line remains patent and free of infection.
- CVP monitoring guides fluid management.
- Central vascular catheter dressing is changed without complications.
- BIOPATCH is applied and potential infection prevented.
- Access cap replaced, maintaining sterile technique.
- StatLock® prevents catheter displacement.

Pearson Nursing Student Resources

Find additional review materials at **nursing.pearsonhighered.com**

Prepare for success with NCLEX®-style practice questions and Skill Checklists

Assisting With Percutaneous Central Vascular Catheterization

Equipment

Specific nontunneled catheter
Routine IV setup (tubing and solution)
Through-the-needle radiopaque central catheter
Local anesthetic, syringes, and needles
Sterile gloves, sterile gown, masks, drapes, and sutures
Antimicrobial 2% chlorhexidine gluconate swabs
Intermittent infusion caps or positive pressure device
Prefilled syringes with preservative-free normal saline
Transparent semipermeable dressing
Securement device

Procedure

1. Identify client using two descriptors and validate signed consent for catheter insertion.
2. Perform hand hygiene and explain procedure to client, including rationale for mask, positioning, and Valsalva's maneuver.
3. Place client in Trendelenburg position. ▶ ***Rationale:*** This position prevents air embolism and helps distend subclavian and jugular veins.
4. According to licensed practitioner's preference, extend client's neck and upper chest by placing a rolled pillow or blanket between shoulder blades. ▶ ***Rationale:*** Usual insertion sites are either subclavian or right jugular vein.
5. Place mask on client and turn client's head away from side of venipuncture. ▶ ***Rationale:*** This facilitates filling the vessel with blood and prevents contamination.
6. Maintain sterility while opening glove packet and sterile drape pack.
7. Open antimicrobial prep pads.

NOTE: New guidelines to prevent catheter-related bloodstream infection recommend that licensed provider dons cap and sterile gown in addition to mask and sterile gloves (Institute for Healthcare Improvement).

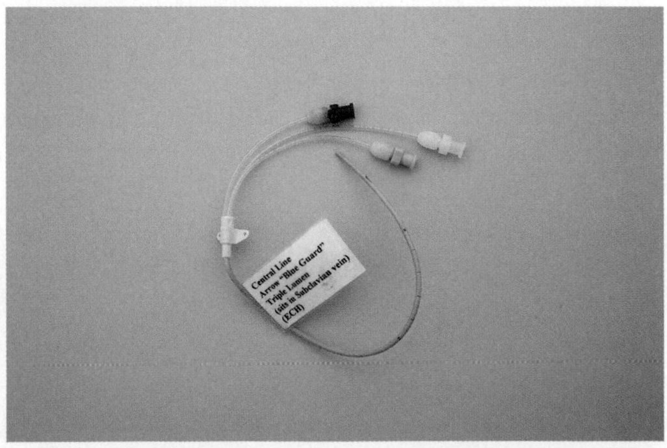

▲ Central line "Blue Guard." Triple lumen catheter—subclavian vein.

8. Don mask and gloves and assist with central catheter insertion.
   a. Licensed provider dons mask, gown, and sterile gloves for this procedure.
   b. Licensed provider prepares the client's skin, drapes area, and, using a sterile syringe and needle, draws up anesthetic to infiltrate the site.
   c. As licensed provider inserts catheter, client is instructed to perform Valsalva's maneuver to prevent air embolism.
      (1) Instruct client to exhale against a closed glottis or to hum.
      (2) If client is unable to do this, compress client's abdomen. ▶ ***Rationale:*** Both these procedures help to decrease chances of air embolism.

NOTE: A 14-gauge needle is inserted into the subclavian vein, using the clavicle as a guide. When blood returns in syringe, the syringe is removed from the needle and a wire is threaded through the needle into the subclavian vein. The needle is removed and the catheter is fed over the wire into the subclavian and brachiocephalic vein. The wire is removed when the tip of the catheter rests in superior vena cava.

9. When catheterization is complete, insert injection cap, flush with 5 mL of normal saline, and then heparinize with 3 mL of dilute heparin (according to agency policy).
10. Apply securement device to skin and place catheter in clamp.
11. Cover securement device and catheter with sterile transparent dressing (according to hospital policy).
12. Label insertion site dressing with date, nurse's initials, and time of insertion.
13. Obtain x-ray for validation of placement into superior vena cava before initiating infusion (unless emergency placement performed).
14. Monitor client's vital signs. ▶ ***Rationale:*** Bleeding or pneumothorax may occur.

Clinical Alert

Required drying time needed in order to prevent skin breakdown as a result of chemical reaction between solutions and dressings is as follows:

Solutions	Required Drying Time
Chlorhexidine gluconate 2% with alcohol	30 seconds
Chlorhexidine gluconate without alcohol	2 minutes
Povidone–iodine	2 minutes
70% isopropyl alcohol	Dries quickly, kills bacteria only when first applied. No lasting bactericidal effect; can excessively dry the skin.

Source: Hadaway, L. C. (2002). I.V. infiltration: Not just a peripheral problem. *Nursing, 32*(9), 36–48; Hadaway, L. C. (2003). Skin flora and infection. *Journal of Infusion Nursing, 26*(1), 44–48.

Guidelines to Prevent Catheter-Related Blood Stream Infections

Hand Hygiene

- Decontaminate hands with alcohol-based hand cleaner; if hands are visibly contaminated with blood or body fluids, use antimicrobial soap and water.
- Use hospital-provided hand lotions compatible with antiseptic agents to maintain integrity of skin. Home lotions may neutralize antibacterial agents in antiseptic agents used in hospitals.
- Decontaminate hands before and after putting on or removing gloves, providing direct client care, assisting with insertion of central venous catheter, inserting peripheral catheter, changing central venous dressing, or accessing catheter to administer medication or flush.
- Do not use artificial nails when working in the healthcare facility.

Barrier Precautions

- Use maximum barrier precautions when inserting or assisting with insertion of central venous catheters, including PICC lines. Include: cap that covers all hair, mask covering mouth and nose, sterile gown, and sterile gloves.
- Cover client from head to toe with large sterile drape leaving small opening for insertion of catheter.
- Place mask on client when PICC insertion is done, and cover face if subclavian or jugular vein placement site for central venous catheters.
- Keep all supplies together on nursing unit to prevent need to look for additional supplies after CVC insertion is begun.

Site Preparation Using Chlorhexidine Gluconate

- Prepare site using 2% chlorhexidine gluconate.
- Pinch wings on chlorhexidine applicator to break open ampule. Hold applicator down to allow solution to saturate pad.
- Press sponge against skin.
- Swab with applicator using a gentle back-and-forth motion. This motion creates friction and lets solution more effectively penetrate epidermal layers.
- Swab site for 30 seconds and then allow to dry thoroughly, approximately 2 minutes. Do not wipe or blot area.

Catheter Site Selection

- Use central venous catheters (CVCs) impregnated with antimicrobial agents, if available.
- Nontunneled percutaneously inserted CVCs are available with three different agents: chlorhexidine/silver sulfadiazine; rifampin/minocycline; and silver/platinum ionic metals. PICC brand uses rifampin/minocycline agents.
- Catheter should be inserted in the subclavian vein for nontunneled catheter.
- These catheters should be used for clients with dwell time of more than 5 days and in healthcare facilities where catheter-related bloodstream infection rates are high.
- There is inconclusive evidence that multiple-lumen catheters should not be used; even though they have higher infection rates, they also have fewer mechanical complications than single-lumen catheters.

Daily Assessment

- Evaluate need to determine when lines are no longer necessary and should be removed.
- Provide site care when needed.

Source: Institute for Healthcare Improvement, http://www.ihi.org/IHI.

EVIDENCE-BASED PRACTICE

Antimicrobial Swabs

Studies have shown that 2% chlorhexidine gluconate solution significantly lowers catheter-related bloodstream infection rates when compared with 70% povidone–iodine and 70% isopropyl alcohol.

Sources: LeBlanc, A., & Cobbett, S. (2000). Traditional practice versus evidence-based practice for IV skin preparation. *Canadian Journal of Infection Control, 15*(1), 9–14, Ringer, M., & Alvarado, C. J. (1991). Prospective randomized trial of povidone–iodine, and chlorhexidine for prevention of infection associated with central venous and arterial catheters. *The Lancet, 338*, 339–343; Rosenthal, K. (2003). Pinpointing intravascular device infections. *Nursing Management, 34*(6), 35–43.

Other studies revealed that chlorhexidine gluconate offered a broad spectrum of antimicrobial activity and long-term microbactericidal action after application.

Source: Hadaway, L. C. (2003). Infusing without infecting. *Nursing, 33*(10), 58–64; Chaiyakunapruk, N., Veenstra, D. L., Lipsky, B.A, & Saint, S. (2002). Chlorhexidine compared with povidone-iodine solution for vascular catheter site care: A meta-analysis. *Annals of Internal Medicine, 136*(11), 792–801.

Source: Chaiyakunapruk, N. et al. Vascular catheter site care: The clinical and economic benefits of chlorhexidine gluconate compared with povidone iodine. Clinical infectious diseases. (2003). 362, 18-26 (Abstract).

Clinical Alert

To decrease pressure in the catheter, use a 10-mL syringe.

Clinical Alert

All continuous IV infusions administered via a central line must have an electric infusion controller device in place.

EVIDENCE-BASED PRACTICE

Chlorhexidine gluconate-impregnated sponges reduced rate of catherter-related infections in ICU

Using chlorhexidine-impregnated sponge dressings with intravascular catheters reduced the risk for major catheter-related infections by 60% among patients treated in the ICU. Changing unsoiled, adherent dressings weekly was not inferior to a three-day changing schedule, according to data from the randomized controlled trial.

A randomly assigned study consisted of 1,636 patients over the age of 18 in an ICU setting. The patients were expected to need an arterial catheter, central vein catheter, or both for 48 hours or longer. Some of the patients received chlorhexidine-impregnated sponges and some the standard dressings, scheduled for change either once every seven days or once every three days. The rate for major catheter-related infection decreased from 1.40 per 1,000 catheter days to 0.60 per 1,000 catheter days with the use of the chlorhexidine-impregnated sponge. The three-day group had a 7.8% rate of catheter colonization vs. 8.6% for the seven-day group, which proves noninferiority for the seven-day dressing schedule compared with the three-day dressing schedule. Use of chlorhexidine gluconate-impregnated dressings decreases the rate of major catheter-related infection when the baseline rate is lower than two per 1,000 catheter days.

Source: Timsit, J F (2009: April 14). Chlorhexidine gluconate-impregnated sponges reduced rate of catheter-related infections in ICU,. JAMA 2009:301: 1231-1241.

Changing a Central Line Catheter Dressing

Equipment

2% chlorhexidine gluconate or according to facility policy
Antimicrobial hand soap
Tape or transparent dressing
Needleless access caps
Receptacle for soiled dressing
Clean gloves
Sterile gloves
Mask
Sterile long-sleeved gown, according to facility policy

Preparation

1. Review facility policy and procedure manual to determine protocol for skin prep.
2. Check Medication Administration Record and client chart for last dressing change (usually changed every 96 hr or per agency protocol), unless site is oozing.
3. Gather equipment.
4. Identify client using two descriptors and explain procedure to client.
5. Perform hand hygiene.
6. Position client flat on back. ▸ ***Rationale:*** Reduces risk of air embolism.
7. Turn client's head away from the insertion site and mask the client's nose and mouth. ▸ ***Rationale:*** Decreases exposure to microorganisms at site.
8. Make sure that all personnel don masks and/or gloves according to hospital policy.

Procedure

1. Don clean gloves and gown, according to facility policy.
2. Carefully remove old dressing or tape without pulling on catheter. Remove edges toward insertion site. ▸ ***Rationale:*** This prevents stress on insertion site.
3. Discard old dressing and gloves in proper receptacle.
4. Inspect site for loose sutures, signs of infection, inflammation, or infiltration, and check length of exposed catheter.
5. Remove clean gloves, perform hand hygiene and don sterile gloves.
6. Cleanse insertion site, sutures, and catheter with 2% chlorhexidine in 70% alcohol or according to facility policy.
7. Cleanse site using back-and-forth scrubbing motion for 30 seconds.
8. Cover site with a sterile transparent dressing.
9. Change IV tubing according to hospital policy.
   a. Clamp central catheter using on-line slide or squeeze clamp.
   b. Use aseptic technique to change needleless access cap.
   c. Prepare cap with antimicrobial swab.
   d. Insert new tubing with needleless connector.

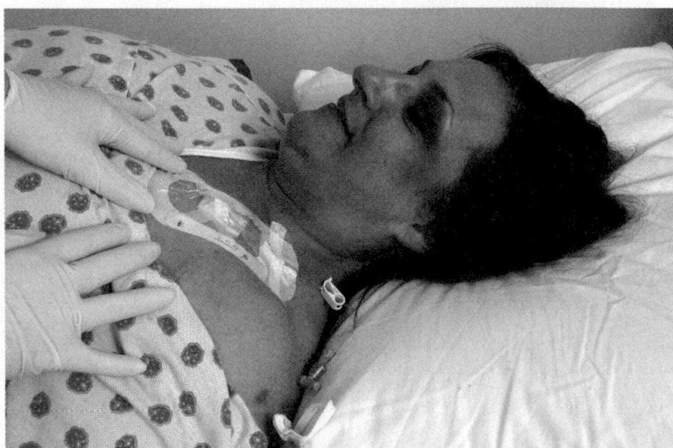

▲ Gauze dressings are used only if the catheter insertion site is oozing. The dressing should be changed every 48 hr or if soiled.

10. Label dressing and tubing with date and your initials.
11. Change dressing if it becomes loose, wet, or soiled or according to facility policy. ▶ *Rationale:* If it is wet, soiled, or loose, it is considered contaminated.
12. Discard equipment, gown, and gloves, and perform hand hygiene.

Clinical Alert

All primary and secondary continuous IV administration sets should be replaced at least every 96 hr (according to facility policy) or immediately if signs/symptoms of infection are present.

Intermittent sets should be changed every 24 hr.

TABLE 29-1 Administration Set Change According to Solution Type

Solution Type	Set Change Frequency
Parenteral Nutrition (Amino Acids)	q 72 hr or when integrity compromised
Lipids, Parenteral Nutrition Solutions containing Lipids	q 24 hr or when integrity compromised
Whole blood and components (platelets, red blood cell concentrate, plasma, cryoprecipitate)	4 hr or 2 units or immediately upon suspected contamination
Fractionated products (IVIG, Clotting factors, Albumin)	Upon completion of infusion

Source: U.S. Centers for Disease Control and Prevention, 2002.

Prevention of Air Embolism in Clients With Central Lines

1. Clear central line of air before insertion.
2. Use IV pumps with in-line air detectors.
3. Use the head-down position and Valsalva's maneuver during both insertion and removal.
4. Use screw-on connections and secure with tape. ▶ *Rationale:* Hemostats or other clamps can crack hub and open system.
5. Use transparent dressing during the time the catheter is in place and after removal of a central catheter. Leave in place for at least 24 hr.

TABLE 29-2 Infusion Site Complications

Signs and Symptoms	Possible Indications
• Redness, swelling at CVAD infusion site	• Infiltration, hematoma, or sepsis
• Crepitus on chest	• Subcutaneous emphysema that can lead to respiratory distress
• Respiratory distress with recent placement of a central line	• Pneumothorax
• Arm, shoulder, or neck pain	• Infiltration or thrombosis
• Temperature elevation	• Catheter-related infection
• Fluid leaks from IV site	• Hole or break in catheter

Infusing IV Fluids Through a Central Line

Equipment

Primed IV fluid administration set with needleless Luer-Lok connector

Infusion delivery pump

Antimicrobial swabs

10-mL needleless syringe with 5 mL of preservative-free 0.9% normal saline solution

CLC 2000 Positive Pressure Cap (or another brand)

Clean gloves

Preparation

1. Check physician's order sheet and client's Medication Record for IV order.
2. Check IV order with IV solution bag.
3. Take equipment to client's room.
4. Identify client using two descriptors.
5. Explain procedure to client and provide privacy.

Procedure

1. Perform hand hygiene and don gloves.
2. Hang IV solution on IV stand.
3. Wipe access port with antimicrobial swab and allow to dry.
4. Insert needleless cannula from saline flush syringe and unclamp lumen. (Clamp is not found on PICC lines or Groshong valve catheter.)
5. Aspirate for blood return, using very little force, to check for lumen patency and placement.
6. Instill saline solution slowly. The CVD and tubing has a volume of 1–3 mL; therefore, about 5 mL solution in 10 mL syringe should be used to thoroughly flush the catheter. ▶ *Rationale:* To clear lumen of in-line dilute heparin.
7. Maintain positive pressure when withdrawing syringe by clamping catheter before removing syringe or by maintaining pressure on syringe plunger before you

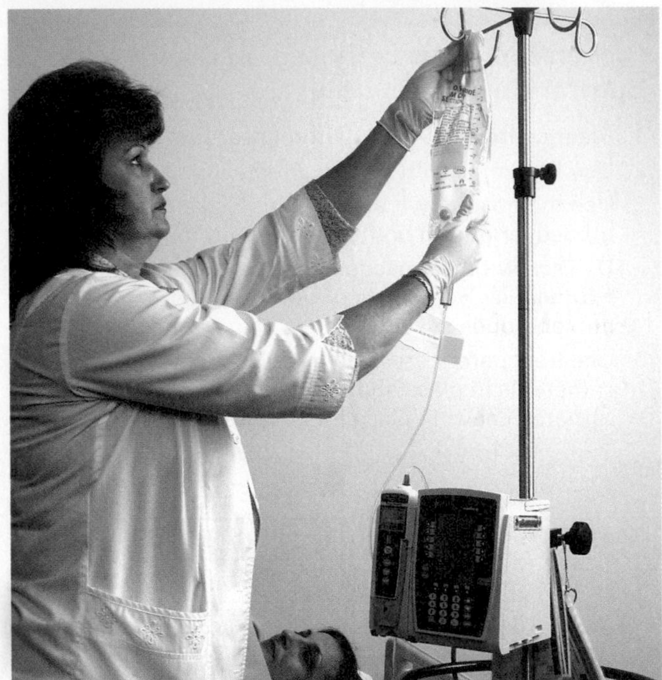

1 Hang IV solution on IV stand.

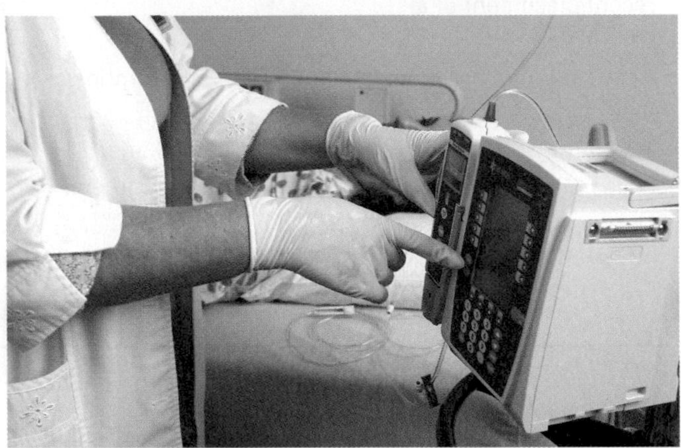

2 Attach point-of-care module and program.

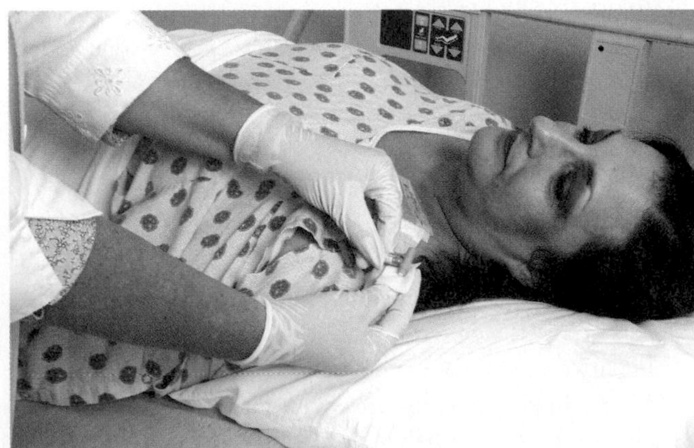

3 Wipe access cap or positive pressure clamp with antimicrobial swab and allow to dry.

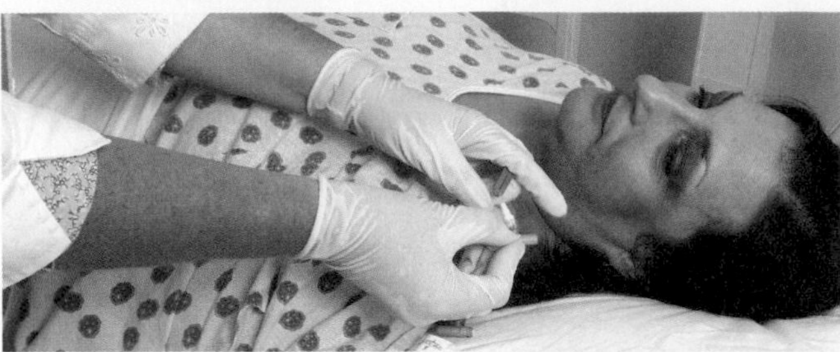

4 Ensure clamp is open before attaching syringe.

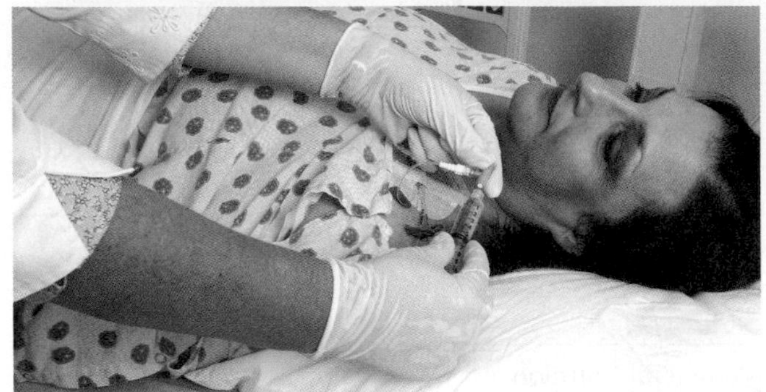

4 Attach 10-mL needleless syringe with saline to pressure valve.

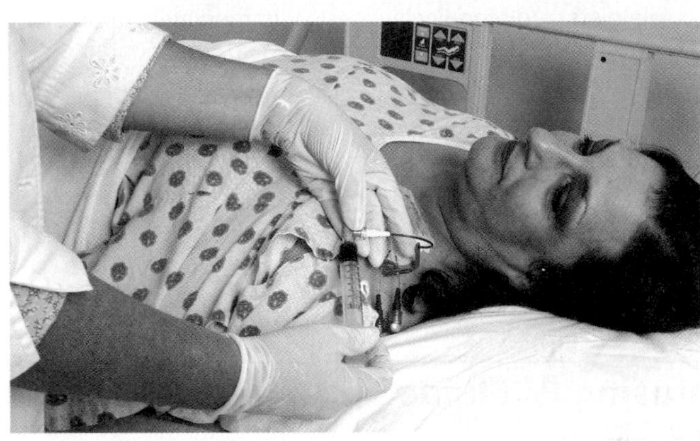

5 Aspirate and check for blood return before infusing saline solution.

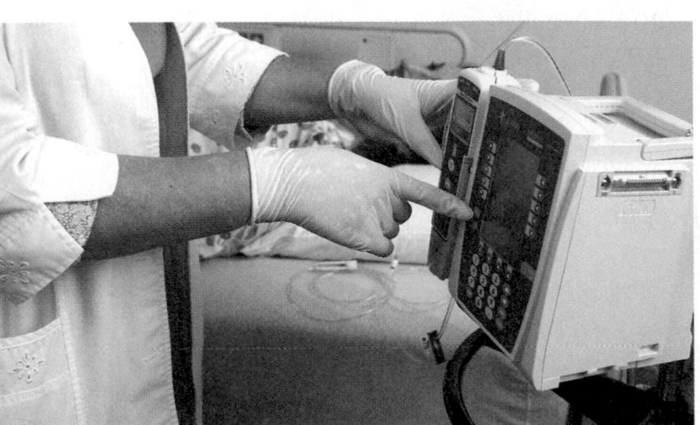

6 After connecting IV to catheter, turn on electronic device to prescribed rate.

clamp or use the CLC 2000 Positive Pressure Cap. ▸ ***Rationale:*** This prevents aspiration of blood into lumen and decreases risk of catheter occlusion.

8. Swab access port again with antimicrobial swabs.
9. Insert IV tubing with Luer-Lok connector into access port. Unclamp lumen.
10. Set electronic device to prescribed rate and begin infusing IV fluids.
11. Ensure central line dressing is clean and intact.
12. Remove gloves and perform hand hygiene.

Positive fluid displacement and positive end-pressure prevent blood reflux into catheter lumen. The device provides the saline flush to prevent clotting of catheter. (See Skill, Using a Positive Pressure Device, page 1141.)

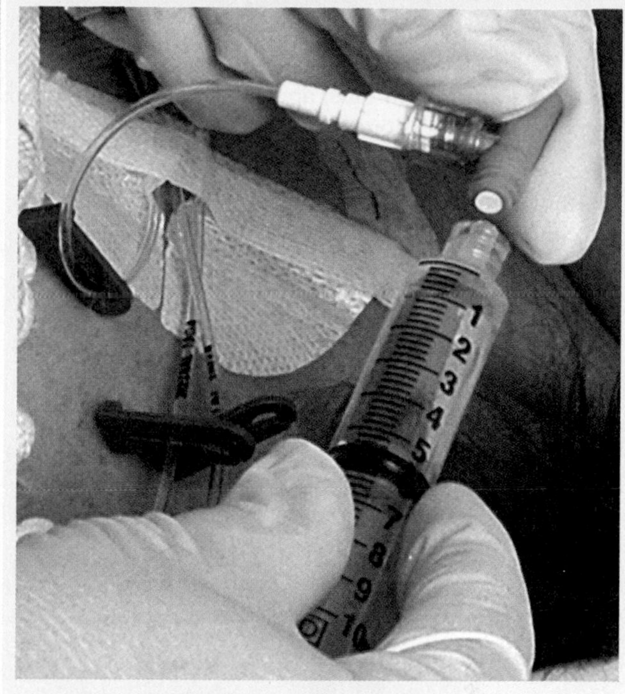

Clinical Alert

To minimize pressure on the catheter during injection NEVER use less than a 10-mL syringe for central lines. Smaller syringes increase pressure within the catheter.

Clinical Alert

Nontunneled central vascular access devices have the highest infection rate of all types of CVADs; therefore, it is crucial that aseptic techniques be used in all aspects of catheter care.

Drawing Blood From Central Venous Access Device

Equipment

2 × 10-mL Luer-Lok syringes filled with sterile preservative-free normal saline

3-mL Luer-Lok syringe with 3 mL of heparinized saline (10 units/mL heparin) **ONLY** if policy of facility

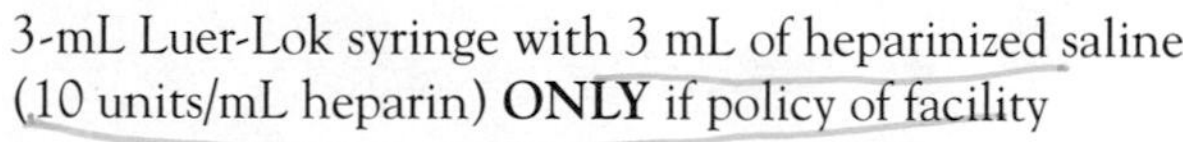

Two 10-mL syringes (or larger if needed)

Antimicrobial swabs

Blood tubes appropriate for tests ordered

Sterile injection cap

Clean gloves

Preparation

1. Check physician's orders and MAR.
2. Identify client using two descriptors.

Procedure

1. Explain procedure to client.

Clinical Alert

Some facilities do not allow Vacutainers to be used for blood draws from central lines because of increased pressure buildup in catheter.

2. Perform hand hygiene and don gloves and mask.
3. If fluids are infusing through catheter, turn off infusion for at least 1 minute before drawing blood specimen.
4. Swab cap and hub with antimicrobial swabs for 30 seconds and allow to dry. Use most distal lumen of catheter for blood draw. ▸ ***Rationale:*** Proximal port specimen will not be contaminated if fluids are infusing distally.
5. Remove cap from syringe, insert 10-mL saline-filled syringe, and unclamp catheter.
6. Flush catheter with 3–5 mL of normal saline. ▸ ***Rationale:*** To determine patency of catheter.

Using the Vacutainer Method

a. Clamp catheter
b. Attach needleless connector to Vacutainer barrel holder.
c. Place blood tube into Vacutainer holder.
d. Disinfect injection or access cap with alcohol.
e. Remove needle cover and insert Vacutainer needleless connector into injection or access cap.
f. Unclamp catheter.
g. Advance blood tube inside Vacutainer holder to activate retrograde blood flow.

h. Hold tube in place until blood flow ceases; this is considered the "discard." The volume should be 1.5–2 times the fill volume of the CVAD.
i. Clamp catheter and remove blood tube from Vacutainer holder, leaving needles and holder connected to injection or access cap.
j. Discard blood tube immediately into appropriate container.
k. Insert another blood tube, unclamp catheter, and obtain blood specimens as ordered.
l. After all specimens are collected, clamp catheter.
m. Remove Vacutainer holder and needleless connector from injection or access cap.
n. Disinfect injection or access cap with alcohol.
o. Flush catheter using 5 to 10 mL of preservative-free 0.9% sodium chloride.
p. Change injection or access cap and extension set, if needed.

Source: Alexander, M., Corrigan, A., Gorski, L., et al. (2010). *Infusion nursing: An evidenced-based approach*. 3rd ed. St. Louis, MO: Saunders/Elsevier, Chapter 25, p. 503.

Using the Syringe Method

a. Clamp catheter.
b. Remove injection or access cap and discard.
c. Disinfect catheter hub with alcohol.
d. Attach empty 10-mL syringe to catheter hub.
e. Unclamp catheter.
f. Withdraw 1.5–2 times the fill volume of the CVAD of blood and discard.
g. Reclamp catheter.
h. Remove and discard syringe into biohazard container.
i. Attach second syringe to catheter hub and unclamp catheter. Withdraw blood into syringe.
j. Reclamp catheter. Remove syringe.
k. Cleanse catheter hub with alcohol.
l. Attach prefilled injection or access cap attached to 10mL syringe with 5–10mL of preservative-free 0.9% sodium chloride.
m. Unclamp catheter and flush with sodium chloride solution.
n. Transfer blood from syringe into collection tube using needleless transfer device.

Source: Alexander, M., Corrigan, A., Gorski, L., et al. (2010). (2010). *Infusion nursing: An evidenced-based approach*. 3rd ed. St. Louis, MO: Saunders/Elsevier.

7. Clamp catheter, remove syringe and attach new 10-mL empty syringe. Unclamp catheter.

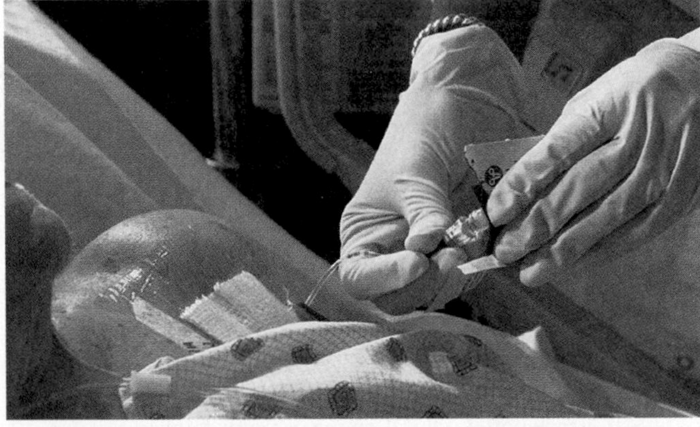

1 Unclamp catheter; clean cap and hub with antimicrobial swab, and allow to dry.

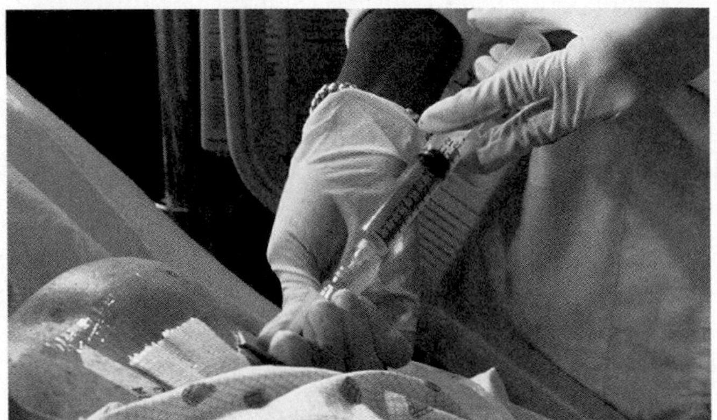

2 Insert 10-mL needleless syringe into cap and unclamp catheter.

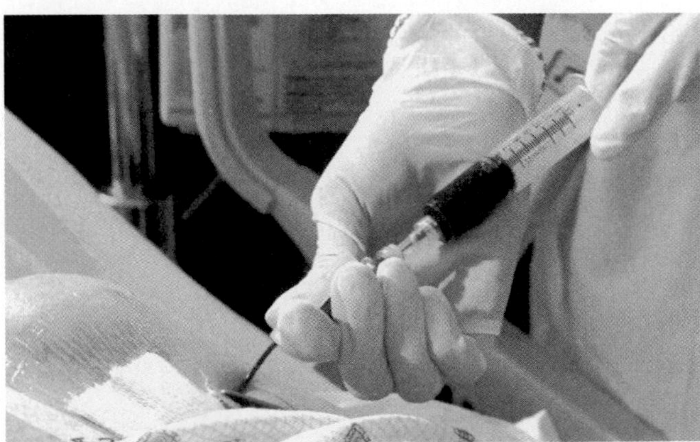

3 Withdraw 5 mL of blood for discard before drawing blood sample unless specimen is for culture.

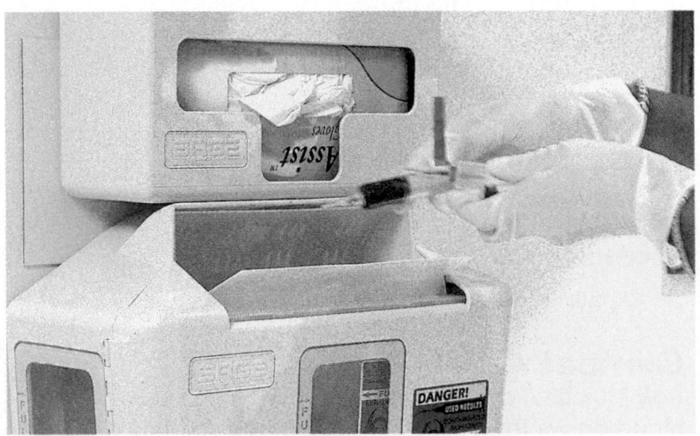

4 Dispose of blood waste in biohazard container.

8. Withdraw 1.5–2 times fill volume of the CVAD; discard volume of blood from catheter slowly and then clamp catheter. Discard syringe. ▸ ***Rationale:*** To clear the catheter of fluids or medications, particularly heparin, before blood samples are obtained.

NOTE: Withdraw 8–10 mL of blood if coagulation studies have been ordered.

Clinical Alert
Do not discard any blood if drawing blood for cultures. Blood from the first draw is always used for blood cultures.

9. Discard syringe in biohazard box.
10. Remove gloves and discard.
11. Perform hand hygiene.

Clinical Alert
Specimens obtained from central catheter lines have been reported as inaccurate in some studies, especially coagulation studies. Heparin molecules can bind within the catheter to cause abnormal results. If lab values are significantly different from earlier values or from the normal range, assess client to determine whether additional lab tests need to be drawn. In this case, draw specimens from a direct vein, if possible.

Applying a BIOPATCH

Equipment

BIOPATCH Antimicrobial Dressing with Chlorhexidine Gluconate
BIOCLUSIVE Transparent Dressing or other similar dressings
Sterile gloves
Clean gloves
Mask

Procedure

1. Check the client chart to determine last dressing change.
2. Gather equipment.
3. Identify client using two descriptors and explain procedure to client.
4. Remove dressing using clean gloves.
5. Perform hand hygiene and don sterile gloves.
6. Prepare skin surrounding percutaneous device according to hospital protocol. Ensure sufficient space is left between hub of catheter and insertion site for placement of dressing.
7. Remove dressing from sterile package using aseptic technique.
8. Place the BIOPATCH dressing around catheter so catheter rests on slit portion of patch. Ensure GRID side of patch is facing upward. The smooth foam side of patch is next to the skin.
9. Ensure edges of slit approximate each other to ensure efficacy of patch.

Clinical Alert
The patch is made of a hydrophilic polyurethane absorptive foam with chlorhexidine gluconate (CHG). The patch absorbs up to eight times its own weight in fluid and the CHG inhibits bacterial growth under dressing.

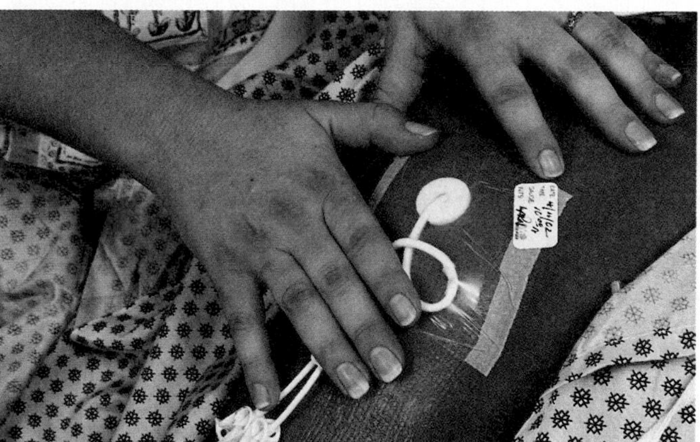

▲ BIOPATCH with transparent dressing over insertion stie.

10. Apply transparent dressing over patch and catheter insertion site. Ensure complete contact between skin and transparent dressing.
11. Discard equipment packages.
12. Remove gloves and place in receptacle.
13. Perform hand hygiene.
14. Change BIOPATCH as necessary. Follow facility policy; however, dressing change should be at a minimum of every 7 days.
    a. Don clean gloves.
    b. Remove patch by picking up corner of dressing and stretching dressing away from catheter while holding catheter in place. Dressing should partially lift off skin when stretching dressing.
    c. Peel back dressing until resistance is felt.
    d. Repeat stretch and peel action until dressing is removed. Both the dressing and the patch will be removed together with this action.
    e. Discard old dressing in biohazard container.
    f. Discard gloves in appropriate receptacle and perform hand hygiene.

EVIDENCE-BASED PRACTICE

Evaluation of BIOPATCH Antimicrobial Dressing

A controlled, randomized study of 687 clients with 1,699 central venous or arterial catheter insertion sites was conducted in two centers. Results indicated a 44% reduction in local infections and a 60% reduction in catheter-related bloodstream infections. There were no serious device-related adverse events during the study. Data regarding use of patch on children under 16 is limited. Patch should not be used on premature infants as hypersensitivity reactions and necrosis of the skin have occurred.

Source: Maki, D. G., Genihner, D., Hua, S., Chiacchierini, R. P. (2000). An evaluation of Biopatch Antimicrobial Dressing compared to routine standard of care in the prevention of catheter-related bloodstream infection. www.ethicon.com. Johnson & Johnson Medical Division of ETHICON, Inc.

Applying a StatLock® Securement Device

Equipment

Securement device
Sterile gloves
Antimicrobial skin prep, according to facility policy
Transparent dressing

Procedure

1. Identify client using two identifiers.
2. Introduce yourself to client and explain procedure.
3. Open device package, sterile skin prep, and gloves.
4. Perform hand hygiene and don gloves.
5. Cleanse insertion and securement site with antimicrobial skin prep according to directions. Allow to completely dry.
6. Apply protectant (in package) to securement site. Allow to dry completely, about 10–15 seconds.
7. Align anchor pad so directional arrow points toward insertion site.
   a. *Using Post Version:* Place suture hole in catheter wing over first post, then slide catheter to capture second post.
   b. *Using Fixed Version:* Place suture holes in catheter wings over fixed posts.
8. Support undersurface of anchor pad and catheter while closing retainer doors.
9. Peel away paper backing from anchor pad, one side at a time, then place on skin.
10. Apply transparent dressing per facility policy.
11. Apply both provided dressing change labels.
12. Discard equipment in appropriate receptacle.
13. Perform hand hygiene.

NOTE: Monitor the device daily, and replace when clinically indicated, at least every 7 days. Treat insertion site according to facility policy. This device is sterile and latex-free; however, clients with known adhesive allergies should not use the device.

Removing a StatLock® Securement Device

Equipment

Sterile gloves
New StatLock device
3–4 alcohol pads

Procedure

1. Open new device package.
2. Don gloves.
3. Remove transparent dressing using the "stretch technique." Lift edge of anchor pad using three to four alcohol pads. Fold alcohol pad to squeeze out alcohol. ▸ ***Rationale:*** This will dissolve undersurface of pad away from skin. Do not pull or force pad to remove.
4. Fold adhesive anchor pad underneath.
5. Stabilize catheter while holding the StatLock device.
6. Use thumb of opposite hand to gently lift retainer door from behind, while pressing down with index finger.
7. Reposition hands and repeat process to open second door.
8. Remove PICC from retainer and carefully reapply new device or discontinue line.

EVIDENCE-BASED PRACTICE

Peripheral Intravenous Catheter Dwell Times

This prospective, sequential clinical trial evaluated the survival time of IV catheters using three methods: nonsterile tape, StatLock, and the Hub-Guard. The use of nonsterile tape securement resulted in an 8% peripheral IV catheter (PVI) survival rate, the Hub-Guard result was 9%, and the StatLock had a survival rate of 52%. The study was completed in an effort to determine the best method to assist in prolonging the 96-hr PIV change protocol. This study strongly suggests that a mechanical catheter securement device allows the implementation of the 96-hr IV change protocol that was sanctioned by the CDC.

Source: Smith, B. (2006). Peripheral intravenous catheter dwell times: A comparison of 3 securement methods for implementation of a 96-hour scheduled change protocol. *Journal of Infusion Nursing, 29*(1), 14–17.

Changing an Access Cap

Equipment

Antimicrobial swabs

Sterile resealable injection cap

10-mL syringe with 5–10 mL of preservative-free 9% normal saline for flush

10-mL syringe with 2–3 mL of heparin solution for maintenance according to agency policy

Clean gloves

Procedure

1. Check client's chart to determine time of last access cap change.
2. Identify client using two descriptors.
3. Explain procedure to client, and provide privacy.

> **Clinical Alert**
>
> The exact time interval is not scientifically known at this time, but it is suggested that the access cap be changed at least every 7 days, when the cap has been accessed more than the manufacturer's recommendations, if the integrity of the port is compromised, if residual blood remains within the port, or after blood draw or blood administration. Positive Pressure Caps (such as the CLC 2000) are changed after blood draws.

4. Gather equipment.
5. Perform hand hygiene and don gloves.
6. Open access cap package maintaining sterility and place near working area.
7. Assess access cap to determine whether cap should be changed even if time frame is not met.
8. Place client in supine position. Clamp catheter using on-line slide or squeeze clamp. ▸ ***Rationale:*** To prevent air embolism during cap change. Client can be instructed to perform Valsalva's maneuver during cap change as an alternative to lying supine.
9. Stop any IV infusion and disconnect IV tubing from access cap.
10. Remove existing cap using aseptic technique.
11. Take new access cap out of package, flush access cap with saline to prime, maintaining sterility, and place on catheter hub.
12. Cleanse injection cap with antimicrobial swab.
13. Flush catheter using 10-mL syringe with normal saline or insert new IV fluid tubing and begin infusion at prescribed rate.
14. Infuse heparin solution if central line is used for intermittent infusions ONLY if agency policy.
15. Remove gloves and perform hand hygiene.

TABLE 29-3 Maintaining CVADS: General Guidelines

CVAD	Frequency of Irrigation	Flush Solution
Single or multi-lumen	q 12 hr to daily, after each use	10–20 mL of normal saline
Percutaneous Catheter short-term long-term	 daily to weekly and after each use	 2–5 mL of dilute heparin (10 units) per lumen
Implanted Port	weekly and after each use	10 mL of normal saline after each infusion 3–5 mL of dilute heparin in 10-mL syringe monthly (100 units/mL)
Groshong Valve Device	weekly and after each use	10–20 mL of normal saline ONLY in 10-mL syringe
PICC	q 4–12 hr and after each use	Normal saline (twice the normal volume of the catheter and access device) followed by 5 mL of dilute heparin (10 units/mL)

Note: Check frequency and flush solutions according to agency protocols.

Measuring and Monitoring Central Venous Pressure (CVP)

Equipment

Disposable CVP manometer with stopcock

IV solution according to facility policy.

Extension tubing with needleless Luer connector

IV pole

Carpenter's level, laser

Antimicrobial swabs

Prefilled 10-mL syringe with 5 mL of preservative-free 9% normal saline

Marker

Preparation

1. Check physician's order.
2. Identify client using two descriptors.
3. Explain procedure to client.
4. Provide privacy.
5. Determine client's previous CVP parameters. ▸ ***Rationale:*** Trends are more relevant than isolated pressure readings.

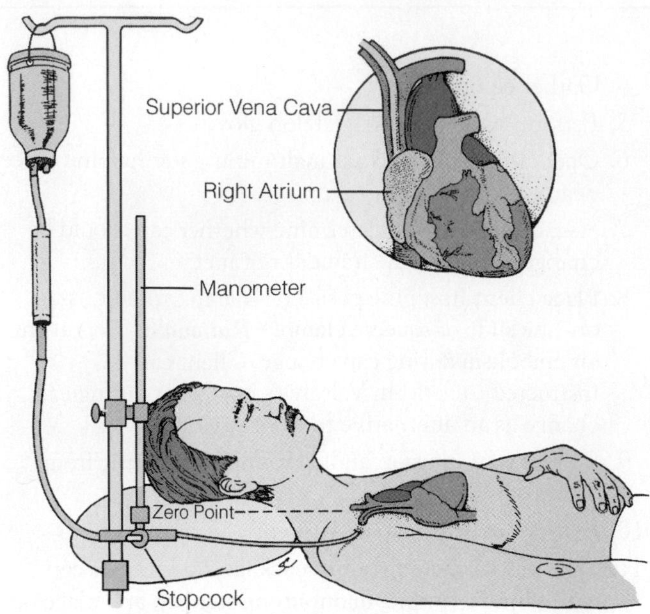

▲ When a CVP reading is taken, the zero of the manometer must be level with client's right atrium, regardless of his position.

Procedure

1. Perform hand hygiene.
2. Spike IV solution bag with IV administration set using sterile technique.
3. Prime tubing with solution.
4. Close clamp on tubing.
5. If you are using a one-piece disposable manometer and stopcock, affix unit to IV pole.
6. Push male end of IV administration set into female end of stopcock, connecting the IV set to stopcock.
7. Turning stopcock so that manometer and IV solution are open to each other, open clamp on IV tubing and fill manometer with IV solution to between 18 and 20 cm. ▸ ***Rationale:*** Overfilling the manometer may expose the client to contamination resulting from overflow.
8. Close clamp and rotate stopcock so that IV solution is open to client.

Clinical Alert

Central venous pressure (CVP) is a measure of venous return or the pressure of blood in the right atrium. Used to guide fluid administration, it is measured in centimeters of water pressure (normal is 5–10 cm H_2O).

9. Prime the rest of IV tubing that extends from stopcock to client's central line.
10. Place client flat in bed, without a pillow, if client can tolerate this position. If not, place client in position of comfort (e.g., head of bed at 15°–30°).
11. Record position so that same position can be used each time a CVP reading is made. ▸ ***Rationale:*** This allows accurate CVP trending.
12. Locate client's right atrium (midaxillary at fourth intercostal space). Mark this location on client's skin using marking pen.
13. Adjust level of CVP manometer (using carpenter's level) so that zero on manometer is at the same level as client's right atrium, 5 cm on manometer level to sternal notch. ▸ ***Rationale:*** Using level at right atrium reflects blood volume and cardiac function of client.
14. Turn stopcock to open position for manometer, filling manometer with additional solution if needed.
15. Turn stopcock to the manometer→client position and watch level of the solution in the manometer fall to the pressure level existing in the right atrium. ▸ ***Rationale:*** Normally this pressure should be between 5 and 10 cm. Remember, however, there are no absolute values and trends—the rise and fall of CVP readings are more important than one isolated pressure reading.
16. Observe meniscus at eye level and watch rise (with exhalation) and fall (with inhalation) of fluid column in response to client's breathing. ▸ ***Rationale:*** Fluctuations reflect changes in intrathoracic pressures during respiratory cycle and indicate that manometer is functioning properly.
17. Take reading at end of exhalation (rise of fluid in manometer).
18. Turn off stopcock to manometer, and adjust rate of infusion to reestablish IV solution flow to client.
19. Return client to desired position and record CVP reading.

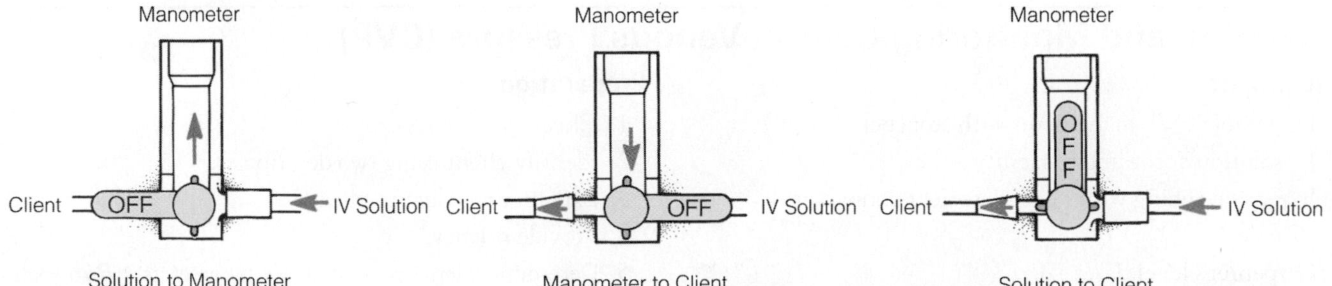

▲ Left stopcock: Fill the manometer by turning stopcock OFF to the client. This allows solution to flow from the container to the manometer. Middle stopcock: Measure CVP by turning stopcock OFF to the IV solution, allowing fluid to flow from manometer to client. Right stopcock: Reinstitute flow from IV container to the client by turning stopcock OFF to the manometer.

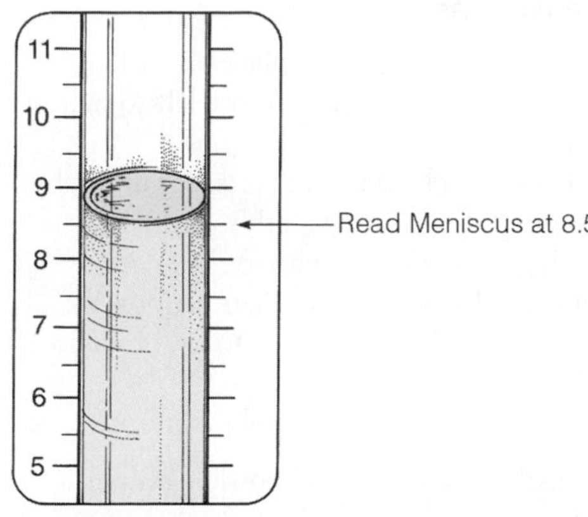

▲ Take CVP reading.

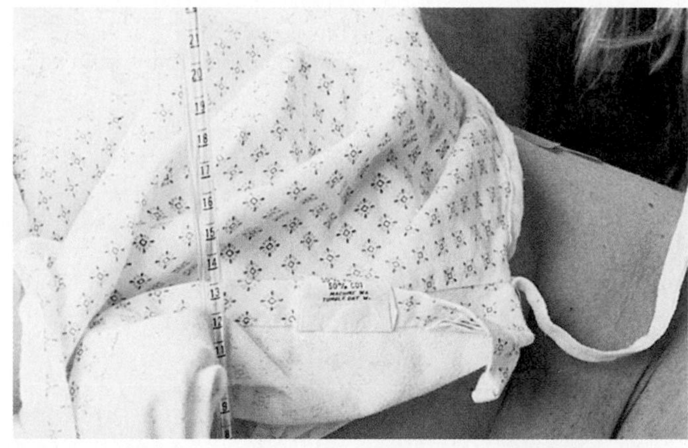
▲ CVP reading is taken with manometer zeroed at client's maxillary fourth space

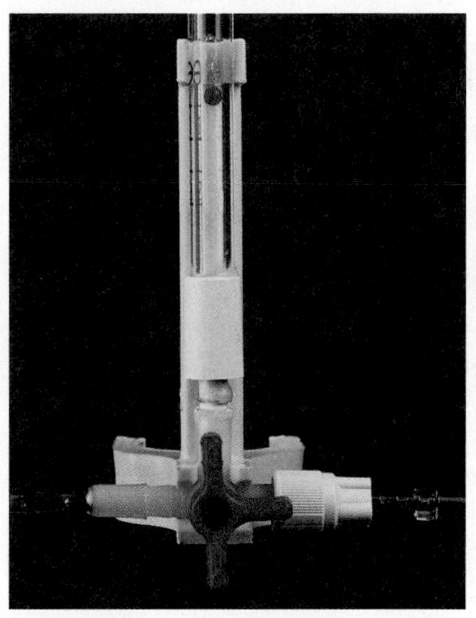
▲ Solution to manometer.

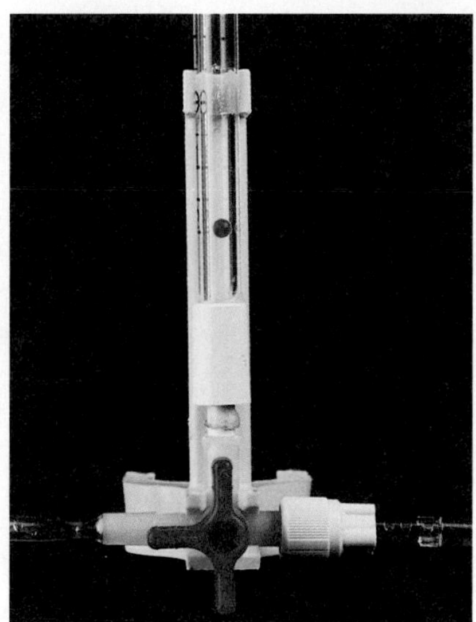
▲ Manometer to client.

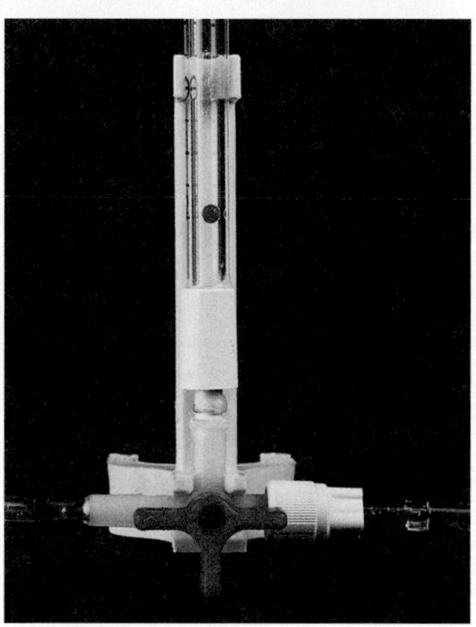
▲ Solution to client.

DOCUMENTATION for Central Vascular Catheterization

- Location of insertion site
- Type and size of cannula used for insertion
- Time of insertion
- Assessment of site and dressing every 8 hr
- Name of physician performing catheterization
- Types of solutions infused
- Amount of solution infused
- Time x-ray was performed to check position of catheter
- Time, initials, date dressing and tubing changed
- Date and time of CVP reading (record subsequent CVP readings on appropriate flow sheets)
- Client's response to treatment
- Any unusual conditions or reactions

CRITICAL THINKING Application

Expected Outcomes

- Central vascular line is properly placed without complication.
- Central vascular line remains patent and free of infection.
- CVP monitoring guides fluid management.
- Central vascular catheter dressing is changed without complications.
- BIOPATCH is applied and potential infection prevented.
- Access cap replaced, maintaining sterile technique.
- StatLock prevents catheter displacement.

Unexpected Outcomes	Alternative Actions
Air enters central vein, producing air embolism from system being open to atmosphere.	• Immediately clamp catheter and place client in Trendelenburg's position (turned to the left so right ventricle is uppermost). • Immediately inform physician and monitor until physician arrives. Assess vital signs and breath sounds. • Administer high-flow O_2 as necessary. • Prevent air embolism by having client perform Valsalva's maneuver any time catheter is open to air, or use in-line catheter clamp. • Ensure client has a patent peripheral IV line.
Infection at insertion site.	• Prepare for catheter removal and possible reinsertion at another site. • If catheter is removed, cut off catheter tip with sterile scissors and place in sterile container; send tip to laboratory for culture. • Administer antibiotics as ordered. • Observe client carefully for signs of systemic infection.
Dysrhythmia detected.	• Change client's position. • Notify physician. • Verify catheter position on chest x-ray (right atrium placement causes dysrhythmias). • Prepare for catheter repositioning or removal of catheter by physician.
Catheter becomes dislodged.	• Check the exact length of catheter to determine extent of problem. • Secure catheter and extension tubing with securement device to prevent further migration of tube. • Notify physician immediately.
Catheter appears to be or becomes occluded.	• Reposition client. • Ask client to raise arms overhead. • Follow facility policy and procedure • Assess mechanical problem: tubing, pumps, catheter, clamps, insertion site, or securement device. • Assess nonthrombotic problem: medications infused, fluids, or withdrawal of blood. Use of precipitate clearance agent is established by individual facility policies and procedures. • Assess thrombotic problem: use of thrombolytic clearance agents is established by individual facility policy and procedures. • Perform Valsalva's maneuver. Turn head to one side. • Attempt to flush catheter with normal saline, using gentle pressure. • Notify physician for order to administer fibrinolytic agent or other agents.
CVP system does not infuse.	• Check line for kinks. Change client's position. Check to make sure the manometer stopcock is in the IV→client position. • Obtain order for placing heparin in IV bag to maintain patency. • Notify physician and prepare for possible reinsertion.

CVP readings vary greatly.	• Assess patency of setup. • Assess client's level of pain; pain increases the CVP reading. • Assess if position of client has been changed; raising the head of the bed alters the reading unless setup is adjusted. • Check that the marked area at midaxillary level is at the level of the client's right atrium (4th ICS). • If client has COPD, heart failure, or hypovolemia, expect readings to differ from normal range. However, once baseline is established for individual client, trends should be watched and evaluated against goals of therapy.

Chapter 29

UNIT ❷

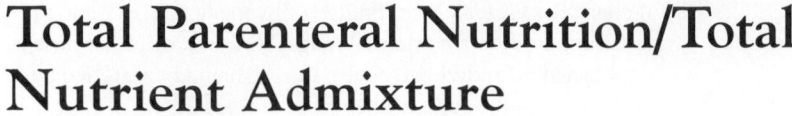

Total Parenteral Nutrition/Total Nutrient Admixture

Nursing Process Data

ASSESSMENT Data Base

- Complete a physical assessment and client history.
- Assess client's nutrition status.
- Identify any condition that would affect TPN (renal or cardiac disease).
- Assess nutritional needs of clients who are unable to process nutrients normally (gastrointestinally).
- Observe for correct additives in each hyperalimentation bag or container.
- Check rate of infusion on physician's orders.
- Monitor catheter insertion site for signs of infection or possible infiltration.
- Monitor regularly client's blood sugar response to hyperalimentation.

PLANNING Objectives

- To provide a nutrition source for clients unable to process nutrients normally
- To provide nutrients for clients requiring bypass of the gastrointestinal tract (bowel rest)
- To provide increased calories for clients in a catabolic state
- To prevent or correct a deficiency of essential fatty acids
- To provide a contamination-free mode of delivering parenteral nutrition
- To regularly administer sliding scale insulin according to client's glucose level

IMPLEMENTATION Procedures

EVALUATION Expected Outcomes

- Catheter is placed correctly.
- Dressing remains dry and intact.
- Catheter insertion site remains free of infection and inflammation; sepsis does not occur.
- TPN infuses at prescribed rate and client receives nutrients necessary for tissue repair.
- Client's blood glucose is maintained within normal parameters.
- Client's electrolytes, protein, renal, and liver function maintained within normal parameters.

NOTE: Total Nutrient Admixture (TNA) is being used more frequently in healthcare facilities. Skills are the same as for TPN, only the solution composition is different.

Pearson Nursing Student Resources

Find additional review materials at **nursing.pearsonhighered.com**

Prepare for success with NCLEX®-style practice questions and Skill Checklists

Assisting With Catheter Insertion

Equipment

Multi-lumen catheter
Antimicrobial swabs, 2% chlorhexidine gluconate
Transparent dressing
Sterile 4 × 4 gauze pads
Sterile gloves
Sterile drapes
Sterile gown
Two masks
3-mL syringe with 25-gauge needle
Lidocaine (Xylocaine—local anesthetic agent)
Suture material, only if securement device not used
Syringe with 5 mL of normal saline
Syringe with 2 mL of dilute heparin
IV administration set with appropriate filter
Hyperalimentation solution
Blanket or pillow to provide roll under shoulders

Preparation

1. Identify client using two descriptors and validate signed consent for catheter insertion.
2. Reinforce procedure explanation to client to allay anxiety.
3. Teach Valsalva's maneuver for use during catheter insertion procedure. ▶ ***Rationale:*** This maneuver prevents air from entering the catheter during catheter insertion or tubing changes.
    a. Ask client to take a deep breath and bear down without exhaling.
    b. This action produces increased intrathoracic pressure.
4. Review physician's orders for correct hyperalimentation solution.
5. Inspect TPN container for layering, turbidity, or precipitates. If there are layers, return to pharmacy.
6. Assemble IV system with in-line filter. Tubing with a 1.2 micron filter is used for TPN with lipids; a 0.2 micron filter is used for TPN without lipids.

NOTE: Many facilities use interventional radiology to insert central venous catheters.

Composition of TPN Solutions

- Amino acid
- Carbohydrates—10%–35% glucose
- Vitamins (become inactive when exposed to light)
- Minerals and trace elements
- Electrolytes (individualized)
- Water
- Hyperalimentation solution is prepared aseptically in the pharmacy under a laminar flow hood

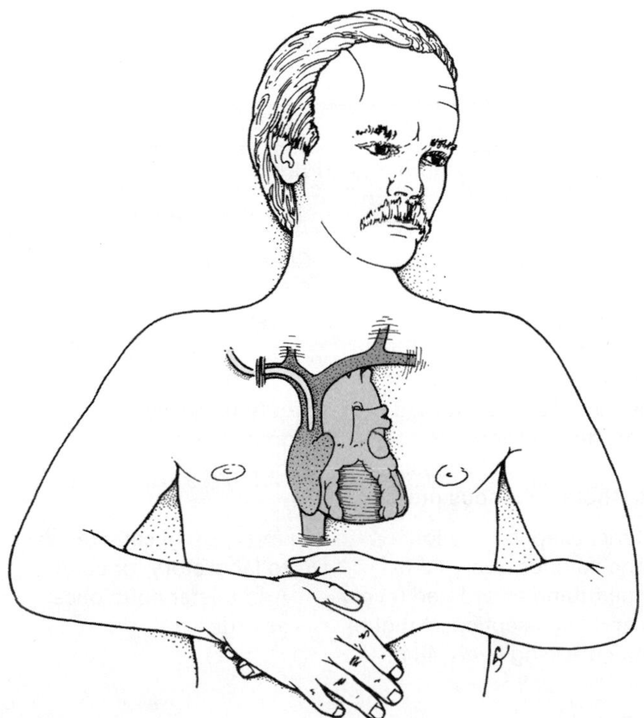

▲ Right subclavian vein is preferred access to right atrium.

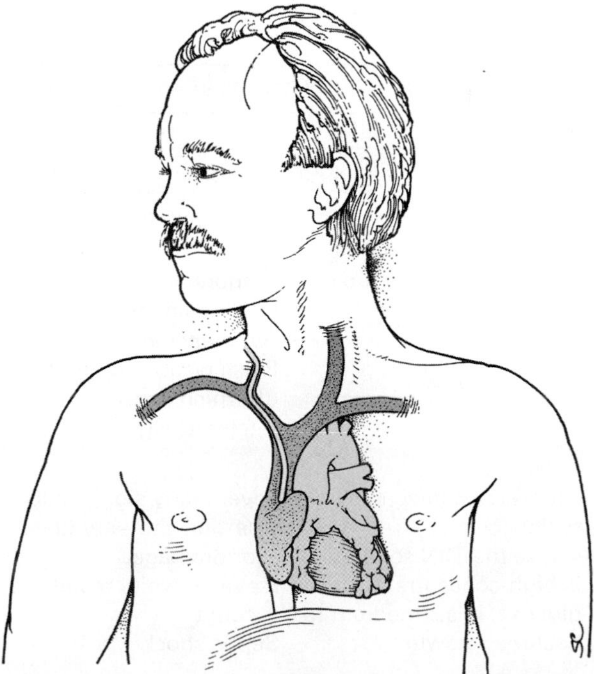

▲ Central venous catheter inserted via right jugular vein.

7. Perform hand hygiene.
8. Prime IV tubing and filter with solution.
9. Insert IV tubing into infusion pump.

Procedure

1. Position client in head-down position with head turned to opposite direction of catheter insertion site. Place a small roll between client's shoulders to expose insertion site. ▶ ***Rationale:*** This position increases intrathoracic venous pressure and reduces risk of air embolism.
2. Assist physician to put on gown, mask, and gloves before beginning procedure.
3. Don mask and sterile gloves.
4. Cleanse insertion area with antimicrobial swab.
   a. Cleanse a large area around insertion site.
   b. Use a scrubbing back-and-forth motion.
   c. Scrub for 30 seconds.
5. Assist physician as needed during catheter insertion.
6. Instruct client in Valsalva's maneuver when stylet is removed from catheter and injection cap is connected to catheter.
   a. Instruct client to exhale against a closed glottis.
   b. If client is unable to do this, compress client's abdomen. ▶ ***Rationale:*** Both these procedures help decrease possibility of air embolism.
7. After cap is connected, instruct client to breathe normally.
8. Flush catheter with saline, then heparinize with dilute heparin according to agency policy.
9. Apply transparent dressing over insertion site.
10. Obtain portable chest x-ray to verify correct catheter placement.
11. After confirmation of catheter placement, initiate hyperalimentation solution and adjust flow rate as ordered.
12. Observe for signs of complications.
13. Take vital signs every 4 hr. ▶ ***Rationale:*** If signs change or temperature rises significantly, the client may be developing complications.

Clinical Alert

TPN and lipids are frequently infused together in the same bottle to prevent microorganism growth from lipid emulsion.

Monitoring Guidelines for TPN

- Monitor for signs of infection or sepsis at the insertion site—the most common complication of TPN.
- Weigh client daily—observe for fluid gain or loss (0.5–1.5 kilograms or 1–3 pounds per week). Weight gain may indicate fluid overload rather than nutritional gain.
- Monitor electrolyte and protein levels. Electrolyte imbalances may occur.
- Regularly monitor blood glucose levels observing for hyperglycemia (thirst, polyuria).
- Assess blood urea nitrogen and creatinine levels—increases may indicate excess amino acid intake.
- Check liver function test results—abnormal values may indicate an excess of lipids or problems in protein or glucose metabolism.

TABLE 29-4 Complications With Total Parenteral Nutrition

		Implementation	
Complication	**Symptoms**	**Prevention**	**Nursing Action**
Air embolism Air enters catheter during catheter insertion or tubing changes	Potentially fatal Respiratory distress, apprehension Chest pain, dyspnea Hypotension Pulse weak and rapid Churning heart murmur (classic sign)	Instruct client in Valsalva's maneuver for tubing and cap changes Check all catheter connections Place client in head-down position with head turned opposite direction of insertion site (increases intrathoracic venous pressure)	Clamp catheter Place client in left Trendelenburg position (to trap air in right side of heart) Notify physician Administer oxygen as ordered
Catheter-related infection (sepsis) Because the TPN solution is high-concentrate glucose, it is a medium for bacterial growth	Fever (early sign), chills Insertion site—erythema or drainage Elevated white blood cell count Septic shock	Use strict aseptic technique Change solution every 12 hr Change tubing as ordered (every 24 hr using aseptic technique) Change dressing every 48 hr	Remove tip of catheter, send to laboratory for culture Administer antibiotics as ordered

TABLE 29-4 Complications With Total Parenteral Nutrition *(Continued)*

		Implementation	
Complication	**Symptoms**	**Prevention**	**Nursing Action**
Hyperglycemia Increased blood glucose level due to infusion, stress, medications, diabetes	Elevated glucose levels (more than 200 mg/dL) Excessive thirst, fatigue, restlessness, confusion, weakness, diuresis When severe—coma	Check history for glucose intolerance; frequent glucose monitoring—check medications (e.g., steroids) Begin infusion at slow rate (usually 40 mL/hour) Increase proportion of calories as lipids Do not "catch-up" if infusion rate falls behind	Start sliding-scale insulin therapy as ordered Monitor blood glucose levels every 4–6 hr Maintain blood glucose <200 mg/dL
Hypoglycemia TPN is discontinued abruptly or client is receiving too much insulin	Client is shaky, weak, anxious, diaphoretic May be hungry Decreased blood glucose (less than 70 mg/dL)	Continue blood glucose monitoring Gradually decrease infusion when discontinuing TPN Use infusion pump	Infuse 10% dextrose in water (50% may be needed) (Restart IV if necessary) Assess blood glucose 1 hr after discontinuing TPN

Maintaining Total Parenteral Nutrition (TPN) Infusions

Equipment

Parenteral nutrition solution (TPN) (refrigerated)
IV tubing, filter, and infusion pump
Extension tubing
Glucometer
I&O record
Securement device

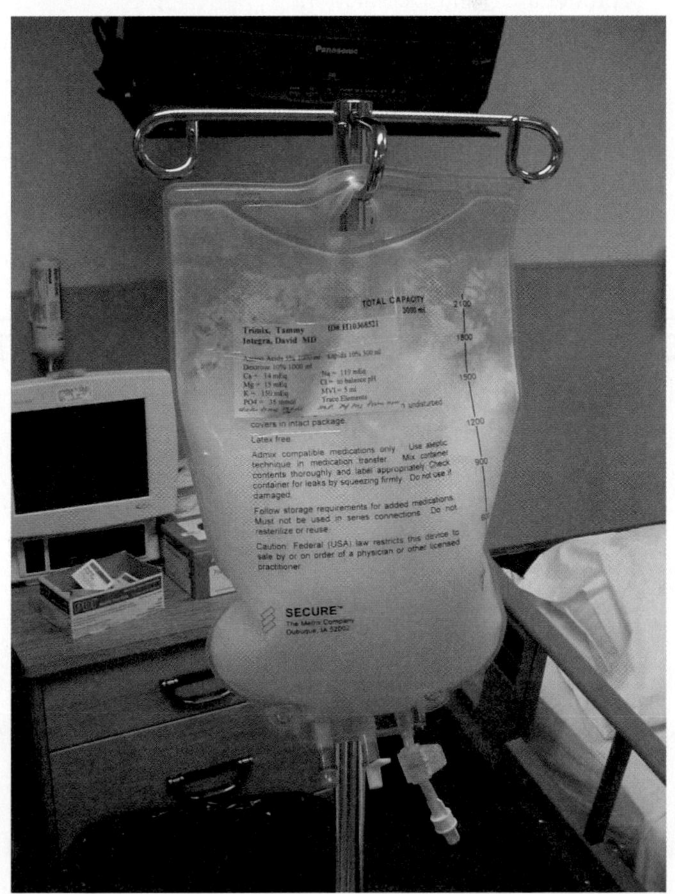

▲ Total parenteral nuitrition.

Procedure

1. Store TPN solution in refrigerator until 30 minutes before use. (Some pharmacies deliver the solution before each infusion.) ▶ ***Rationale:*** Solution is refrigerated to prevent growth of organisms, but should be left at room temperature 1 hr before use.
2. Ensure central line is patent when infusing TPN. Check for patency according to facility policy.
3. Change IV tubing and filter every 24 hr. This is completed when entire system is changed. ▶ ***Rationale:*** This is recommended for TPN infusions to prevent infection.
4. Maintain IV flow rate as prescribed. Use infusion pump for infusion.
   a. If rate is too rapid, hyperosmolar diuresis occurs (excess glucose and water is excreted); if severe enough, intractable seizures, coma, and death can occur.
   b. If rate is too slow, little benefit is derived from the calories and nitrogen.

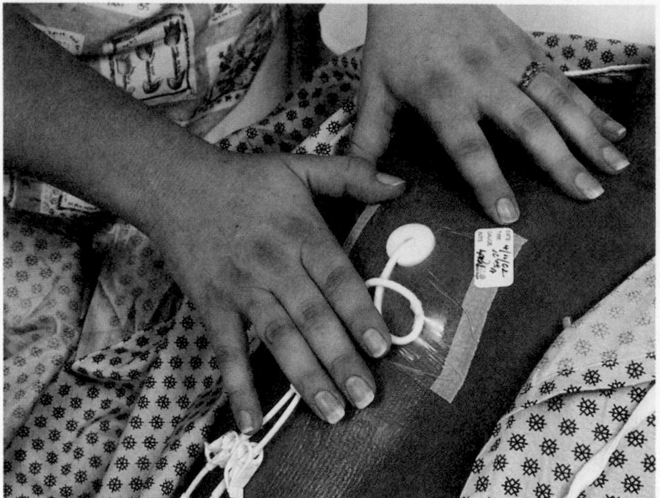

▲ Nontunneled catheter used to deliver parenteral nutrition.

Clinical Alert

Do not "catch up" a deficit in infused volume, as doing so could result in complications for the client. To ensure constant flow rate, check rate every 2 hr.

5. Change solution every 24 hr. ▸ ***Rationale:*** Changing the solution prevents growth of bacterial organisms that proliferate in glucose solution.
6. Monitor client's blood glucose regularly (e.g., every 6 hr).
7. If necessary, administer Regular insulin according to prescribed "sliding scale."

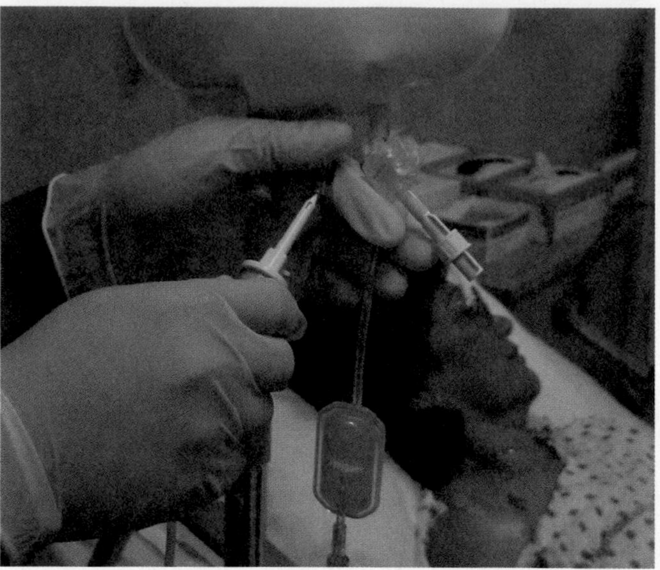

▲ In-line filter used when administering TPN solution.

8. Maintain accurate I&O.
9. Observe for complications, such as air embolus, hyperglycemia, osmotic diuresis, infiltration, or sepsis.

Clinical Alert

No medication or blood products are to be added or piggybacked into TPN line.
No blood specimen should be withdrawn from an IV line infusing TPN.
TPN is never stopped abruptly. It should be tapered off.

Changing Total Parenteral Nutrition (TPN) Dressing and Tubing

Equipment

Clean and sterile gloves
Mask
IV tubing and filter (0.22 micron)
TPN solution
2 × 2 sterile gauze pads and tape
Antimicrobial swabs, 2% chlorhexidine gluconate
Transparent semipermeable dressing
Securement device

Preparation

1. Check to determine when tubing was last changed.
2. Gather equipment and perform hand hygiene.
3. Verify client ID using two descriptors and explain procedure to client.
4. Connect IV tubing and filter to parenteral hyperalimentation (TPN) solution container.
5. Flush tubing to clear air.
6. Place IV tubing through infusion pump.
7. Prepare dressing: antimicrobial swabs, sterile 2 × 2 gauze pads and tape, or sterile transparent dressing.
8. Place client supine with head turned in opposite direction of insertion site. Instruct client not to talk or cough. (Place mask on client if client cannot cooperate.) ▸ ***Rationale:*** These instructions reduce risk of contamination.

Procedure

1. Don mask (according to institutional policy) and clean gloves.
2. Remove old dressing and discard both dressing and gloves in appropriate receptacle.
3. Don sterile gloves.
4. Observe insertion site for signs of erythema, drainage, or swelling.

Clinical Alert
When central-line dressings are loose, wet, or soiled, they are considered contaminated and must be changed. Dressings are routinely changed every 72 hr.

5. Cleanse insertion site with antimicrobial swabs, using back-and-forth motion for 30 seconds.
6. Allow 30 seconds for drying.
7. Apply securement device following package instructions and according to agency policy.
8. Place sterile transparent dressing over insertion site.
9. Change IV tubing.
   a. Clamp catheter using slide clamp.
   b. Loosen tubing in catheter hub.
   c. Insert new primed tubing *or*
   d. Cap catheter and insert new IV tubing using needleless connector or use positive pressure device.
10. Remove gloves and perform hand hygiene.
11. Label dressing with date and your initials.

Clinical Alert
Transparent dressings are changed every 72–96 hr. Transparent dressings are preferred unless site is draining.

Maintaining Total Parenteral Nutrition (TPN) for Children

Equipment

Same as for adult Parenteral Nutrition with these additions:

Intracath, 22-gauge needle
Microdrip IV tubing administration set
0.22 micron in-line filter
Restraints, only if necessary and ordered

Preparation

1. Identify client using two descriptors.
2. Gather equipment for blood glucose monitoring and dressing change.
3. Perform hand hygiene.

Procedure

1. Verify solution with physician's orders.
2. Examine solution. Generally, there is a higher concentration of calcium, phosphorus, magnesium, and vitamins. Either a 10% dextrose/2% amino acids or 5% dextrose/4% amino acids solution can be infused peripherally. Higher concentrations are infused centrally, as is long-term therapy.
3. Monitor patency of catheter. Stopcocks are never used. Monitor infusion pump and filter.
4. Obtain finger stick or urine glucose samples every 8 hr. Glucose level rises, but usually exogenous insulin is not required as the pancreas adapts to high glucose loads.
5. Monitor intake and output and daily weight.
6. Change the dressing every 96 hr and the tubing every 24 hr using aseptic technique. Stockinette can be used to keep scalp dressing secure. Tight-fitting T-shirt can keep chest site secure.
7. Monitor for accurate rate of infusion. Do not "catch up" if infusion is behind. Pumps can be used to maintain infusion rates, particularly when small amounts of solution are being infused.
8. Observe the child when ambulating for twisting or kinking of tubing, getting the tubing caught in the crib, or stepping on it.
9. Instruct parents on rationale for treatment and methods to prevent accidental dislodging of the tubing.
10. Provide play therapy and sources of stimulation to distract the child from the catheter.
11. If discontinuing TPN, taper infusion for 1 hr (decrease rate every 30 min). ▶ ***Rationale:*** Abrupt discontinuation may cause a hypoglycemic reaction since insulin production is increased.

DOCUMENTATION for Total Parenteral Nutrition

- Special TPN sheet may be used; if so, charting is done directly on the sheet or computer
- Catheter type, insertion site, physician's name
- X-ray, following insertion
- Type of parenteral nutrition solution and flow rate
- Results of blood glucose monitoring
- If insulin administered, type, amount, and site
- Date and time of dressing and tubing change with name or initials of person who did the change
- Condition of insertion site
- Client's tolerance of procedure
- Daily weights
- Intake and output

CRITICAL THINKING Application

Expected Outcomes

- Catheter is placed correctly.
- TPN infuses at prescribed rate and client receives necessary nutrients for tissue repair.
- Dressing remains clean, dry, and intact.
- Catheter insertion site remains free of infection and inflammation; sepsis does not occur.
- Client's blood glucose remains within normal parameters.
- Client's electrolytes, protein, renal, and liver function maintained within normal parameters.

Unexpected Outcomes	Alternative Actions
Parenteral nutrition solution is not infused at the prescribed rate.	• Observe filter to ensure patency. A plugged filter is the most common cause of infusion failure. Change the filter and tubing. • Ensure that the next parenteral nutrition bag is ready to be superimposed. • Observe for signs of hypoglycemia caused by sudden change in dextrose concentration—weakness, trembling, sweating, hunger. Check blood glucose. • Adjust flow rate to that which was ordered. Do not attempt to "catch up" the amount not infused as this action could lead to osmotic diuresis from hyperglycemia.
Catheter insertion site becomes inflamed.	• Notify physician immediately so catheter can be discontinued if catheter-related sepsis is suspected. • Cut tip of catheter off with sterile scissors and place in sterile container. Send to laboratory for culture and sensitivity for specific causative organism. • Cleanse site of catheter insertion with antimicrobial swab and place sterile dressing over site. • Obtain order for and administer antibiotics as needed.
The dressing becomes wet or loose.	• Change the dressing as soon as moisture is observed, using aseptic technique. • If the dressing is exposed to moisture or secretions, cover with transparent dressing (e.g., showering).
TPN solution temporarily unavailable.	• Infuse D10W IV solution at prescribed rate until TPN solution is available.

Chapter 29

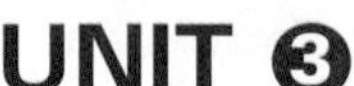

UNIT 3

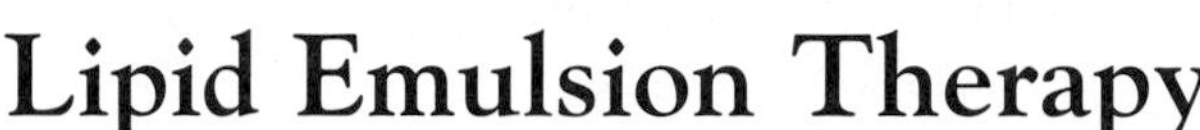

Lipid Emulsion Therapy

Nursing Process Data

ASSESSMENT Data Base

- Observe for signs of essential fatty acid deficits: rash; eczema; dry, scaly skin; poor wound healing; sparse hair.
- Assess pancreatic function.
- Assess client for predisposing factors that could promote fat emboli, such as anemia, coagulation disorders, abnormal liver or pulmonary function.
- Check IV site for patency, erythema, and edema before infusing solution.
- Assess vital signs to establish baseline.

PLANNING Objectives

- To spare protein in critically ill client
- To provide a source of energy for clients with deficient protein intake
- To provide essential fatty acids

IMPLEMENTATION Procedures

EVALUATION Expected Outcomes

- Lipids infused within time frame.
- Adequate calories and essential fatty acids are provided to clients unable to ingest orally.
- Parenteral nutrients are provided without complications or adverse effects.
- Normal pancreatic function is maintained.

Infusing IV Lipids

Equipment

IV lipid solution in container

Non-phthalate vented IV tubing infusion set (to prevent pooling of fat in IV tubing)

Needleless cannula

2% chlorhexidine gluconate swabs

Volume control device

NOTE: Many facilities do not infuse lipids alone but combine with TPN.

Preparation

1. Review physician's orders and MAR.
2. Obtain lipid emulsion (refrigerated) from the pharmacy and allow to warm to room temperature (may take 1 to 2 hr).
3. Examine solution for separation of emulsion into layers or fat globules or for accumulation of froth. Do not use if any of these appear.
4. Label bottle/bag with client name, medical record number, room number, date, time, flow rate, bottle number, and start and stop times.
5. Identify client using two forms of identification.
6. Explain procedure to client.

Procedure

1. Take vital signs for baseline assessment. ▸ ***Rationale:*** Baseline information is needed because an immediate reaction can occur.
2. Perform hand hygiene and then swab stopper on IV bottle with antimicrobial swab and allow to dry.
3. Attach vented non-PVC infusion set to bottle, twisting the spike to prevent particles from stopper falling into the emulsion, or spike bag with regular IV tubing.
4. Hang IV bottle at least 30 in. above IV site. ▸ ***Rationale:*** Due to solution viscosity, lipid emulsion needs to be at this height to prevent backing up into infusion tubing.
5. Fill drip chamber two-thirds full, slightly open clamp on the tubing, and prime the tubing slowly. ▸ ***Rationale:*** Priming more slowly reduces chance of air bubbles with this solution.
6. Attach the tubing to the IV site.
7. If piggybacking lipids into hyperalimentation, use port closest to client, below tubing filter.

Clinical Alert

Administration sets that contain di-(2-ethylhexyl)phthalate (DEHP) plasticizers extract lipids from infusion set. It is recommended to use a separate administration set, glass infusate containers, or special non–polyvinyl chloride (non-PVC) IV bags.

Clinical Alert

Lipid emulsions alone promote growth of specific bacteria and yeasts as soon as 6 hr after the infusion. When lipids are combined with TPN (solution of amino acids, lipid emulsion, and glucose) in the same bag, it doesn't appear to support any greater microbial growth than non–lipid-containing TPN fluids. Thus TPN solution can hang safely for 24 hr.

Clinical Alert

In-line filters are not recommended by CDC as a routine infection control measure; however, the Infusion Nurses Society favors the filters. Always check hospital policies and procedures to determine use of filters.

8. Infuse lipid solutions initially at 1 mL/min for adults and 0.1 mL/min for children for first 15–30 minutes. Then increase rate to 2 mL/min for adults and 0.2 mL/min for children.
9. Monitor vital signs according to facility policy and observe for side effects during first 30 minutes of the infusion. If side effects occur, stop the infusion and notify the physician.

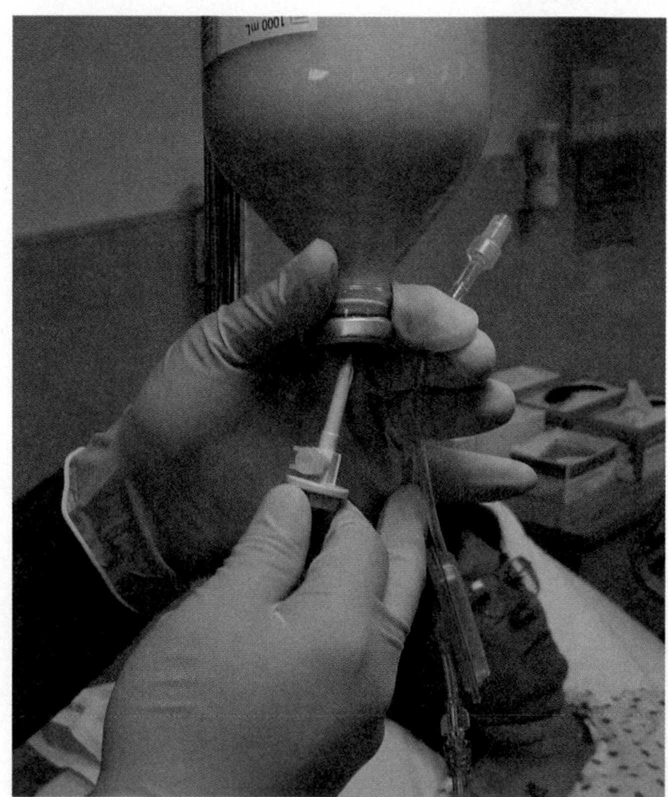

▲ Lipids are administered from glass container or non-PVC infusion sets.

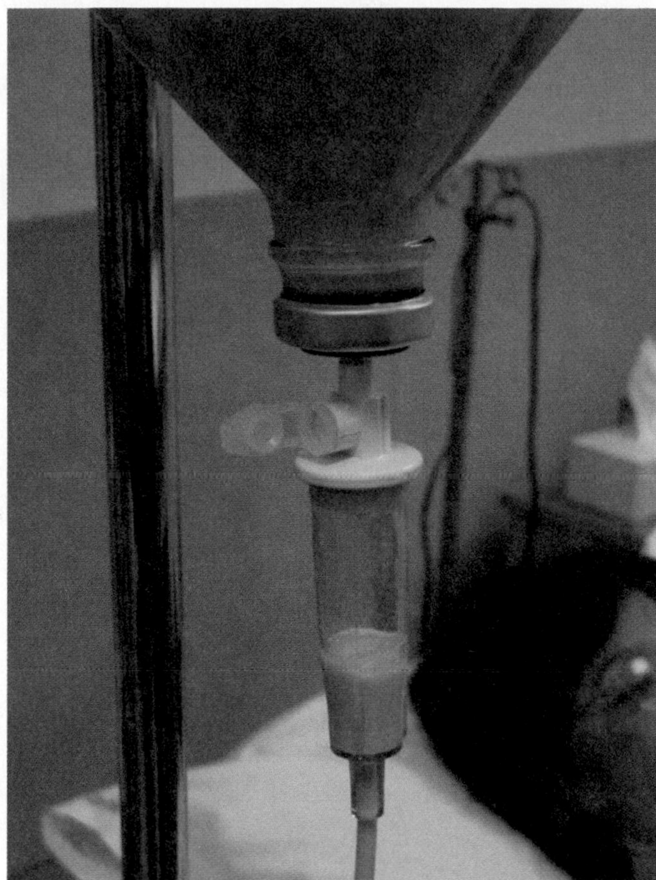

▲ Vented tubing is required for lipid infusion.

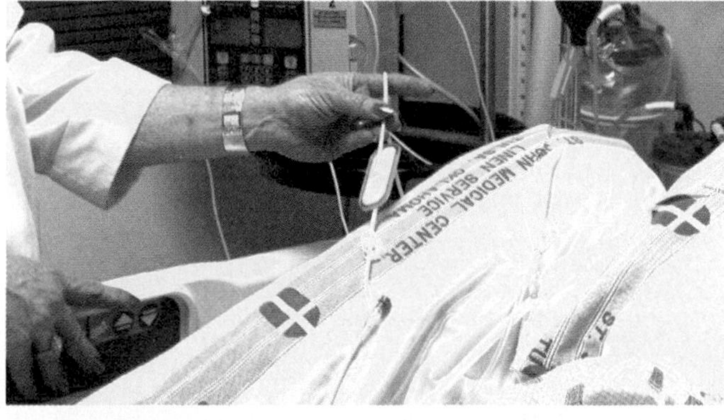

▲ Check facility policy regarding use of in-line filters for lipid administration. Filters are not recommended by CDC but Infusion Nurses use them.

10. Adjust flow to prescribed IV rate if no adverse reactions occur.
11. Monitor and maintain the infusion at the ordered rate.

Guidelines for IV Lipid Infusion

- IV lipid solutions are isotonic and provide 1.1 kcal/mL of solution in a 10% solution or 2.0 kcal/mL in a 20% solution.
- Do not put additives into IV lipid bottle.
- Do not use an IV filter because the particles are large and cannot pass through.

For Adults

- Lipid 10%: Up to 500 mL 4–6 hr on first day to maximum of 2.5 g/kg body weight per day. Do not exceed 60% of client's total caloric intake per day.
- Liposyn 10%: No more than 500 mL/day in 4–6 hr.

For Children

- Lipid 10%: Up to 1 g/kg in 4 hr. Do not exceed 60% of total caloric intake.

12. Monitor serum lipids 4 hr after discontinuing infusion. ▶ ***Rationale:*** If you draw blood too soon after infusion is completed, incorrect blood values result.
13. Monitor liver function tests for evidence of impaired liver function. ▶ ***Rationale:*** These tests indicate the liver's ability to metabolize the lipids.
14. Discard partially used bottles/bags. ▶ ***Rationale:*** This action prevents contamination.
15. Discard administration set after each unit unless additional units are administered consecutively.
16. Continue to monitor vital signs and observe client for adverse reactions during the entire process of infusion.
17. Answer any questions the client may have about the procedure and make client comfortable before leaving room.

Clinical Alert

Observe for IV lipid side effects after starting lipid infusion:

chills	chest and back pain
fever	nausea and vomiting
flushing	headache
diaphoresis	pressure over the eyes
dyspnea	vertigo
cyanosis	sleepiness
allergic reactions	thrombophlebitis

DOCUMENTATION for Lipid Emulsion Therapy

- Type of solution infused
- Rate of infusion
- Site of infusion
- Vital signs monitored
- Adverse clinical manifestations and appropriate nursing intervention

CRITICAL THINKING Application

Expected Outcomes

- Lipids infuse within time frame.
- Adequate calories and essential fatty acids are provided to clients unable to ingest orally.
- Parenteral nutrients provided without complications or adverse effects.
- Normal pancreatic function is maintained.

Unexpected Outcomes	Alternative Actions
Client experiences side effects and cannot continue with lipid infusion.	• Reassess client's ability to tolerate fat solution. • Notify physician for order to discontinue fat solution, and administer hyperalimentation solution. • Monitor liver function test results.
Client develops dyspnea, cyanosis, or allergic reaction, such as nausea, vomiting, increased temperature, or headache.	• Stop infusion immediately and notify physician.
Client's serum triglyceride and liver function test results remain elevated.	• Continue IV lipid infusion. • Begin the feeding with a weaker concentration of formula and increase the concentration slowly as ordered. • Repeat lab values.
Client develops hyperlipemia or hypercoagulability.	• Monitor laboratory results, particularly liver function tests, and notify physician when any abnormality occurs.

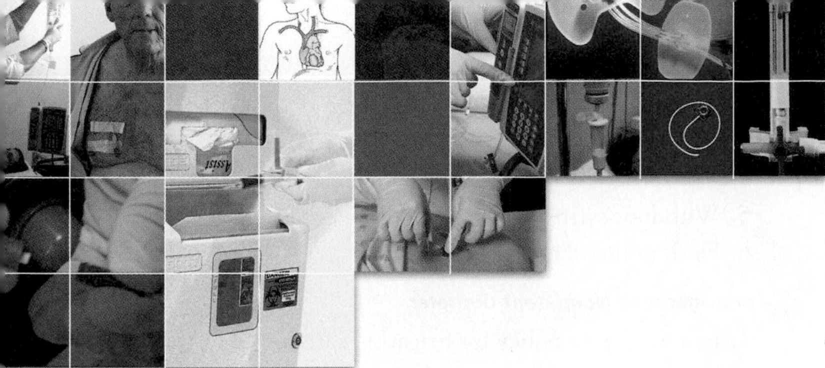

Chapter 29

UNIT 4

Tunneled Central Vascular Access Devices (CVADs)

Nursing Process Data

ASSESSMENT Data Base

- Assess patency of catheter.
- Assess insertion site for signs of infection.
- Assess the tubing for accidental breaks.
- Assess injection cap at the end of catheter to ensure tightness.

PLANNING Objectives

- To provide a patent catheter
- To clear a nonpatent catheter
- To provide an access for blood drawing
- To provide an access for infusions

IMPLEMENTATION Procedures

EVALUATION Expected Outcomes

- IV catheter remains patent using CLC 2000 device.
- The catheter site remains infection-free.
- Blood samples are obtained without difficulty.
- Infusions of medications or fluids are accomplished without difficulty.

Maintaining the Hickman or Broviac CV Catheter

Equipment

10-mL Luer-Lok syringe with 3 mL of dilute heparin (100 units/mL solution or 10 units/mL) or tissue plasminogen activator (t-PA) 2 mg/2 mL (Anteplase).

2% chlorhexidine gluconate swab

Clean gloves

Syringes (size per facility policy)

10-mL syringe prefilled with preservative-free 9% sodium chloride

CLC 2000 (or other brand) positive pressure device

Preparation

1. Check client care plan.
2. Identify client using two forms of identification and explain procedure to client.
3. Provide privacy for client.
4. Perform hand hygiene and don gloves.

Procedure

For Flushing Intermittently Used Line

1. Wipe catheter cap with antimicrobial swab.
2. Insert syringe cannula into needleless access cap or CLC 2000 device and unsnap catheter squeeze clamp.
3. Inject heparin solution slowly through catheter until almost empty.
4. Remove syringe while still moving plunger forward or clamp catheter before removing syringe if not using positive pressure device (see page 1141 for skill).
   ▸ ***Rationale:*** This maintains positive pressure in the catheter and prevents clotting by preventing backflow of blood into catheter.
5. Withdraw syringe.
6. Flush nonused capped lines daily.

For Irrigating a Nonpatent Catheter

1. Follow facility policy for irrigating catheter.
2. Prepare 10-mL syringes with dilute heparin.
   ▸ ***Rationale:*** The size of this syringe decreases pressure exerted in the system.
3. Swab catheter cap with antimicrobial swab.
4. Insert syringe with Luer-Lok and unclamp catheter.
5. Inject heparin from syringes, 1 mL at a time or per facility policy.
6. Leave heparin in catheter tubing for prescribed time.
7. Check that dwell time is completed, then use a 10-mL syringe to aspirate solution from catheter by gently pulling back on plunger.
8. Follow with an irrigation of 5–10 mL of heparinized solution if aspiration is successful. Use same solution for irrigation as with maintenance solution.
9. Repeat procedure once. If unsuccessful, notify physician and be prepared to instill thrombolytic agent, t-PA (t-PA is infused at 2 mg/2 mL). Alteplase is the only approved thrombolytic agent for treatment of catheter occlusion.
10. Discard equipment and gloves and perform hand hygiene.

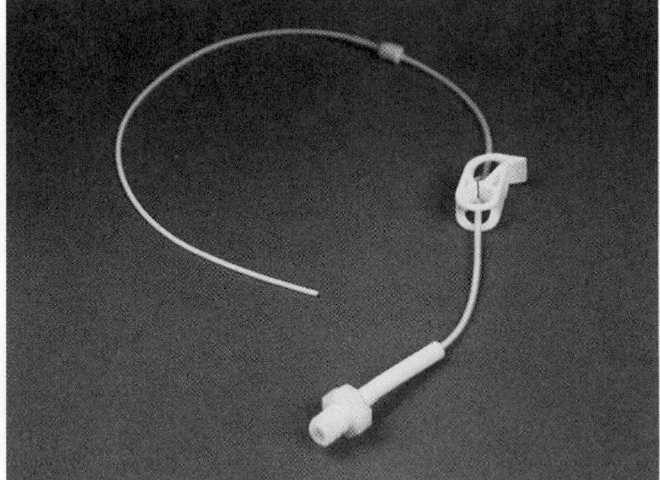

▲ The tunneled Broviac catheter (single, double, or triple lumen) is commonly used for children.

Tunneled Central Vascular Access Devices (CVADS)

- Tunneled central vascular access devices (CVADs) provide long-term access to a central vein for the purpose of drawing blood, administering drugs (chemotherapy, antibiotics), administering total parenteral nutrition (TPN), or administering blood and blood products.
- Catheters are soft, silicone elastomers, thermoplastic polyurethane, or PVC. Used because of tensile strength and biocompatibility.
- Long-term catheters have one, two, or three lumens.
- The tip is inserted into a central vein and advanced to the superior vena cava. The remainder of the catheter passes through a subcutaneous track and exits on the chest wall or abdomen for easy access. A Dacron cuff on the catheter elicits scar formation that prevents ascending tract infection.
- Three common tunneled CVADs are the Hickman, Broviac, and Groshong.
- Clients with tunneled CVADs are advised to display medical-alert information.

Using a Positive Pressure Device

Equipment

Positive Pressure Device; CLC2000 or FloStar, or SmartSite
Antimicrobial swab
Gloves
10-mL prefilled saline syringe

Procedure

1. Assess peripheral or central venous access site for signs of infection.
2. Perform hand hygiene and don gloves.
3. Use aseptic technique to open package, remove device, and remove cap without contaminating.
4. Prepare positive pressure device by attaching prefilled saline syringe and priming through device with saline. Leave syringe attached.
5. Attach the syringe to the female Luer and prime the CLC2000 device according to facility policies and procedures. Invert the device to expel air.
6. Attach the male spin lock to the venous access device. Push and twist the male spin lock of the CLC2000 into the VAD until it is tight.
7. Cleanse the female Luer vigorously with an antimicrobial swab for 5–10 seconds.
8. Attach the prefilled saline syringe; push and twist the Luer into the CLC2000 until there is a tight fit; unclamp catheter.
9. Irrigate with saline as ordered.
10. Remove the syringe and dispose of it in the sharps container.
11. Remove gloves and discard.
12. Perform hand hygiene.

NOTE: If using device for IV fluid infusion, cleanse female Luer and attach IV tubing. Open clamp on catheter and begin IV flow.

The positive pressure device (CLC2000) creates positive pressure within the central venous access device, preventing blood from being drawn back into the catheter when the flush syringe is removed. The CLC2000 is a Luer-Lok that replaces the other needleless caps and should be used when a CVAD cannot be flushed with heparin. The device is only flushed with saline, and the line must not be clamped, nor should extension sets be added as these actions negate the antireflux action of the device.

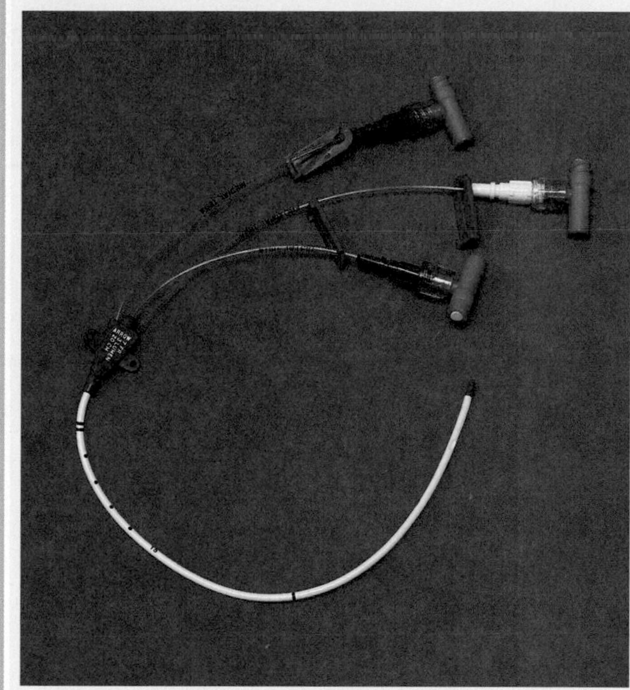

▲ CLC2000 devices are applied to PICC line.

Attach Positive Pressure Device

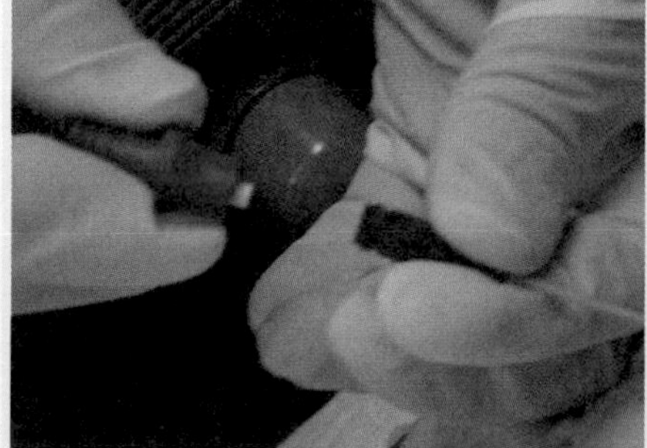

1 Clamp catheter and remove cap from line, maintaining sterility of device.

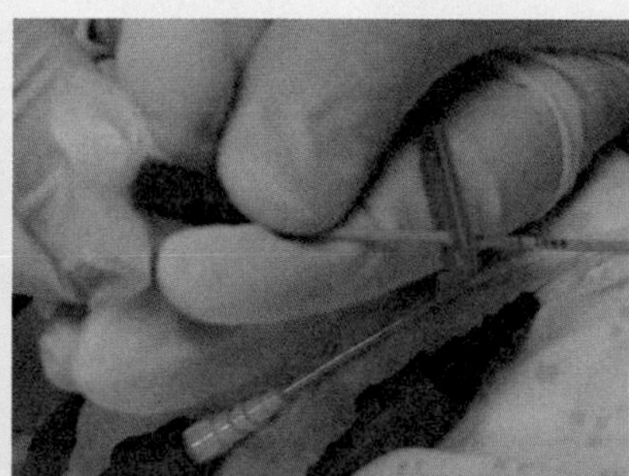

2 Cleanse proximal adapter tip with chlorhexidine before attaching device.

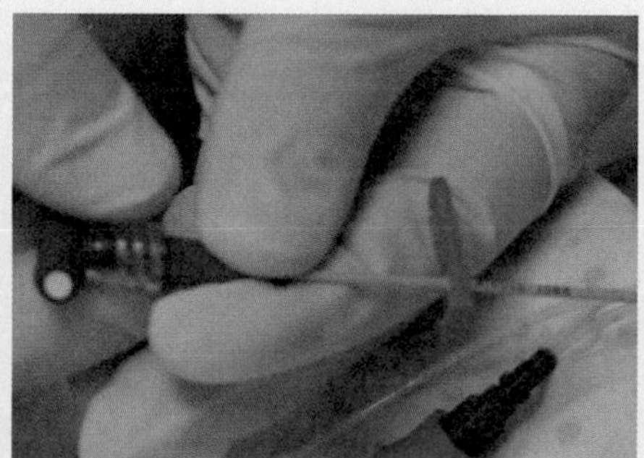

3 Attach male spin lock to venous access device by screwing device into catheter.

Irrigating Catheter Using Positive Pressure Device

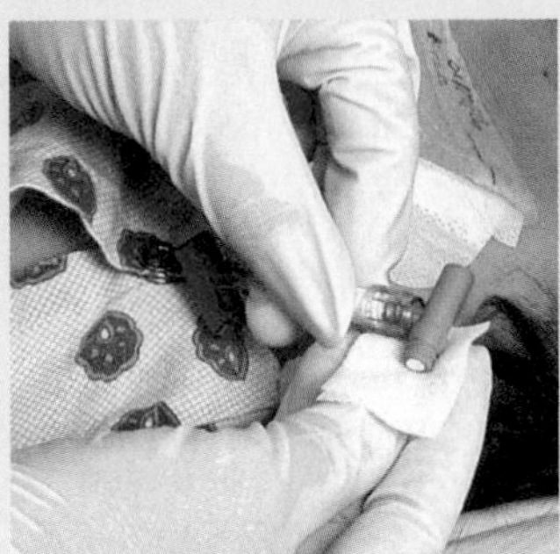
1 Cleanse female Luer vigorously.

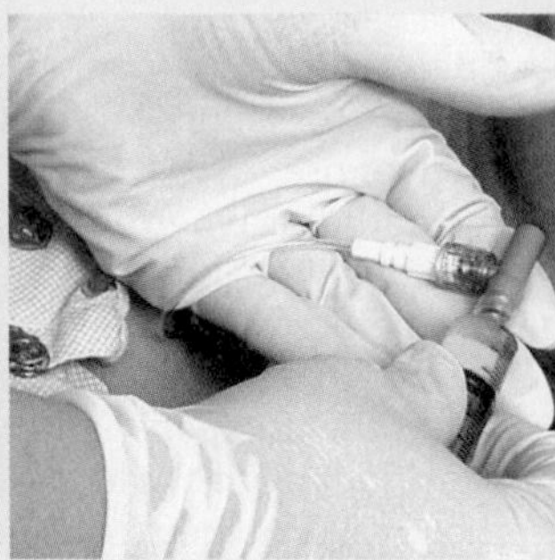
2 Attach 10-mL prefilled saline syringe, infuse saline, and aspirate for blood return.

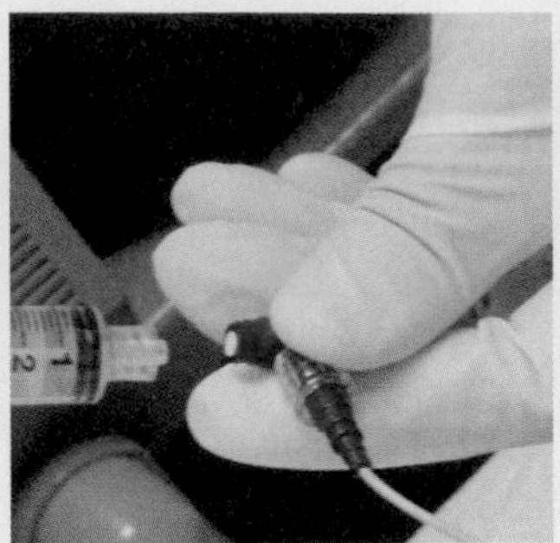
3 Remove syringe from device and cleanse Luer.

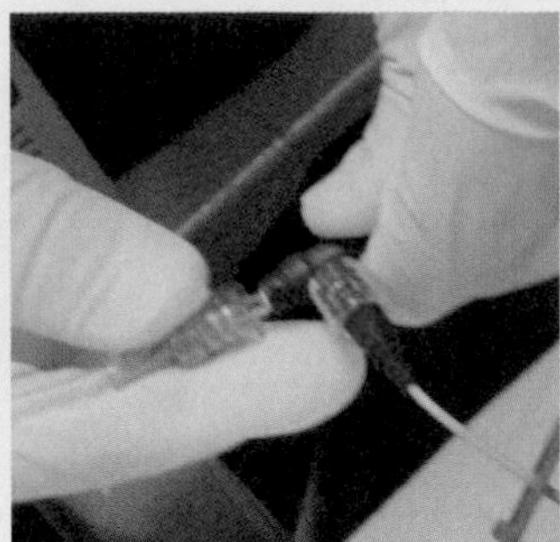
4 Attach IV tubing to device.

Changing the Hickman or Broviac CV Catheter Dressing

Equipment

Antimicrobial swabs, 2% chlorhexidine gluconate
Transparent, semipermeable dressing
Clean gloves
Sterile gloves
Mask (if client is neutropenic and per agency policy)

Procedure

1. Identify client using two descriptors.
2. Apply mask as needed.
3. Perform hand hygiene and don gloves.
4. Remove old dressing and place in appropriate receptacle.
5. Observe for signs and symptoms of infection and crepitus at insertion site. ▸ ***Rationale:*** Signs most frequently observed are erythema, edema, and drainage for infection; crackling under the skin denotes crepitus due to air in the subcutaneous tissue—this finding should be reported to physician.
6. Remove and discard gloves.
7. Set up supplies on a sterile field and don sterile gloves.
8. Clean exit site using antimicrobial swabs. Swab with back-and-forth movement for 30 seconds.
9. Clean catheter tubing at exit site. Allow to dry.
10. Apply sterile transparent dressing; change weekly or if soiled. When cuff heals into place, dressings are not necessary.
11. Remove gloves and discard.
12. Sign and date dressing.
13. Secure catheter to prevent dislodging; tape to chest.
14. Perform hand hygiene.

NOTE: Nonhospitalized clients who are not immunosuppressed may protect exit site with a Band-Aid or leave the site undressed. They should cleanse daily with antibacterial soap and water, palpate site daily to check for signs of infection, and tape catheter to chest to prevent accidental dislodgement.

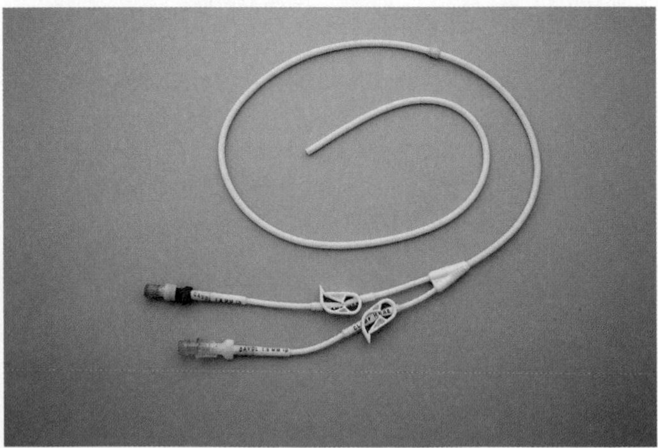
▲ Hickman catheter.

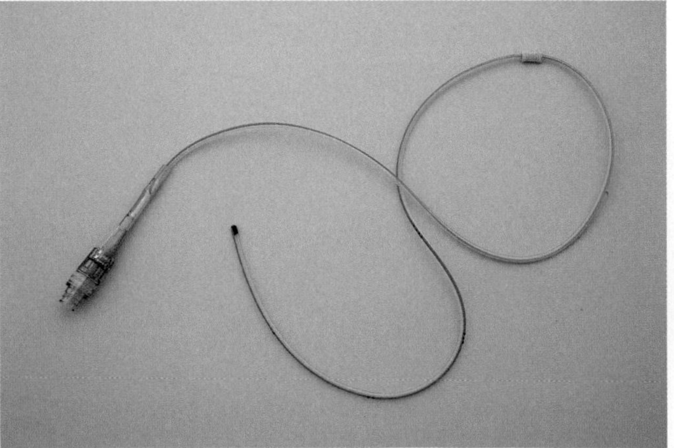
▲ The tunneled CV catheter with Groshong valve is ideal for long-term therapy.

Clinical Alert

To prevent a potentially life-threatening mistake, never use scissors near central venous catheters.

Flushing Tunneled Catheters

Flush catheter with 3–5 mL of heparin (10 units/mL) daily when catheter is not used and before and after each use. The SASH protocol is used (saline, administer drug or withdraw blood, saline, and heparin). This type of flushing is not done with a closed-ended (Groshong) catheter, as its internal valve is designed to prevent blood reflux into the catheter.

Irrigation Protocols

Using 10 mL of Saline

- Irrigate catheter weekly when not in use.
- Irrigate catheter after every use.

Using 20 mL of Saline

- Irrigate catheter before and after any aspiration of blood, after transfusion of blood, or when blood is seen in the catheter (client straining or lifting may cause blood to back up into catheter).
- Irrigate catheter after infusion of lipids or hyperalimentation solutions.

NOTE: Regardless of the volume of saline used, ALWAYS irrigate in a stop–start action. ▸ ***Rationale:*** This creates a swirling effect at the distal end of the catheter.

Maintaining the CV Catheter With Groshong Valve

NOTE: The Groshong valve is available in a variety of CVADs, including ports and PICCs. The Groshong allows infusion, but prevents backflow of blood unless negative pressure is applied. There is no need for heparin flush, and external clamps are not used. Clamping could force the slit valve open, allowing blood to leak into the lumen.

Equipment

Normal saline, preservative-free
Antimicrobial swab, 2% chlorhexidine gluconate
Sterile injection cap
Appropriate syringe: 10 mL or 20 mL
Clean gloves
Sterile gloves
Positive pressure device

Preparation

1. Check physician's orders.
2. Gather equipment.
3. Identify client using two descriptors.
4. Perform hand hygiene and don gloves.

Procedure

1. For non–positive pressure device, wipe injection cap and catheter connection with antimicrobial swab.
2. While holding catheter, remove catheter cap and attach hub of syringe directly to catheter hub.
3. Inject normal saline rapidly into lumen.
4. Maintain positive pressure on syringe plunger as last 0.5 mL is injected and syringe is withdrawn. ▸ ***Rationale:*** Keeping pressure on the plunger prevents backup of blood into catheter.
5. Remove cap by holding catheter connector between thumb and forefinger of one hand and grasping barrel of cap with other hand.
6. Twist and pull counterclockwise to separate cap from connector.
7. Continue to hold connector with one hand. ▸ ***Rationale:*** Holding connector prevents inadvertent contamination by placing connector on dirty surface.
8. Discard old cap.
9. Clean liberally around connector using antimicrobial swab.
10. Holding new sterile injection cap, twist clockwise and insert into connector.

For 10- or 20-mL Irrigation

1. Remove syringe from package.
2. Remove injection cap carefully from connector and discard.
3. Clean connector with chlorhexidine gluconate wipe. DO NOT let go of connector. ▸ ***Rationale:*** Holding connector prevents inadvertent contamination.
4. Insert syringe barrel directly into catheter connector, twisting slightly to ensure good connection.
5. Irrigate lumen with preservative-free normal saline using stop–start action. ▸ ***Rationale:*** Heparin is not used

Clinical Alert

Nursing attention to the catheter during dressing change is important to ensure catheter is not pinched, kinked, occluded, cut, or dislodged. It is recommended that the external portion of catheter be coiled and taped to avoid a straight pull on catheter insertion site.

because clotting is not a factor with catheter tip design of the Groshong.

6. Maintain positive pressure on syringe barrel as syringe is removed from connector. DO NOT clamp the catheter after irrigation. ▸ ***Rationale:*** The Groshong CV catheter does not require clamping to keep blood from entering the lumen. Clamping the catheter damages it.
7. Change injection cap.
8. Remove gloves and perform hand hygiene.

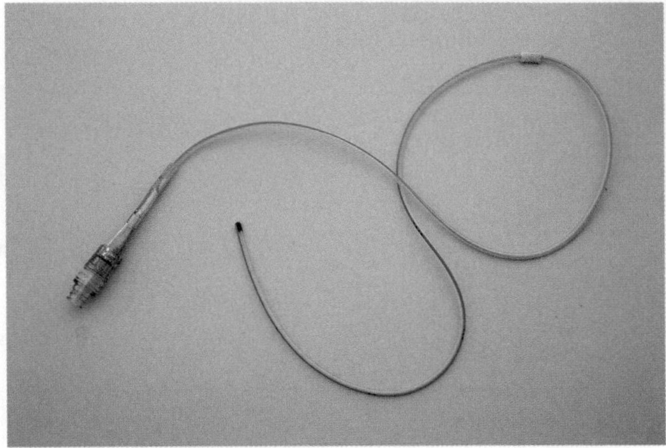

▲ The tunneled CV catheter with Groshong valve is ideal for long-term therapy.

The Groshong Catheter

The Groshong catheter offers an alternative to the Hickman and Broviac catheters. It is distinguished by a rounded, blunt catheter tip with a three-way pressure-sensitive valve that remains closed at normal vena caval pressure. When closed, it restricts air from entering the venous system or a backflow of blood from the catheter. When a syringe is inserted to create a vacuum, it allows the valve to open inward for blood aspiration. Positive pressure into the catheter by infusion forces the valve to open outward. The primary advantages of this type of catheter are:

- Decreased risk of air emboli or bleeding
- Elimination of heparin to flush the catheter
- Elimination of catheter clamping
- Reduced flushing protocols between use

NOTE: It is recommended that a positive pressure device be used for irrigating CVADs. See page 1141 for skill.

Drawing Blood From the CV Catheter With Groshong Valve

Equipment

Sterile injection cap.

Three 10-mL Luer-Lok syringes for drawing blood

One 20-mL Luer-Lok syringe filled with preservative-free normal saline

Blood tubes appropriate for tests ordered

Antimicrobial swabs, 2% chlorhexidine gluconate

Clean gloves

NOTE: Vacuum tubes should not be used with the Groshong valve.

Procedure

1. Perform hand hygiene and don gloves.
2. Clean cap and outside of connector with swabs and allow to dry.
3. Remove and discard injection cap while holding connector so that it does not make contact with any surface.
4. Insert first 10-mL syringe with saline directly into catheter, twisting slightly to ensure connection.
5. Irrigate with stop-start action. Groshong catheter must be irrigated with stop–start action with at least 10 mL of normal saline before blood sample removal.
6. Pull back plunger 0.5 mL, pause 2 seconds, and then continue aspirating until 5 mL of blood is in syringe.
7. Remove syringe, set aside; continue to hold connector.
8. Connect second 10-mL syringe directly to catheter connector, twisting slightly to ensure connection.
9. Proceed to aspirate blood volume needed for sample after same aspiration procedure of pulling 0.5 mL and waiting for 2 seconds.
10. Remove syringe and continue to hold connector.
11. Flush catheter briskly with 20 mL of preservative-free normal saline and attach new sterile injection cap.
12. Transfer blood sample from second syringe into appropriate tube(s), and label. Do not hold receiving tube during transfer.
13. Discard syringe containing first aspirated blood into biohazard container.
14. Remove gloves and perform hand hygiene.

DOCUMENTATION for CVADs

- Flush frequency and solution used
- Dressing changes and type applied
- Site condition
- Condition and patency of catheter
- Medications or solutions administered through catheter
- Amount of blood withdrawn for testing and the amount discarded.
- Infusion cap change
- Positive pressure device in place

CRITICAL THINKING Application

Expected Outcomes

- IV catheter maintains patency with use of CLC2000 device.
- Catheter site remains free of infection.
- Blood samples are obtained without difficulty.
- Infusions of medications or fluids are accomplished without difficulty.

Unexpected Outcomes	Alternative Actions
CV Catheter:	
Unable to aspirate blood even though solution flows through the catheter.	• Use less negative pressure on syringe when aspirating blood. Tip of catheter may be sucking against wall of vessel. • Have client raise arms above head. This can alter position of catheter. • Have client perform Valsalva's maneuver. • Change client's position.
Clotting of catheter occurs (client develops arm or neck swelling on catheter side of body).	• Do not force plunger with Groshong; this may rupture catheter. • Make sure clamps are open and tubing is not kinked. • Use irrigating procedure for catheter with a recently developed clot. Instill 1 mL of normal saline. • Allow 15 minutes before aspirating to see if declotting occurs. Repeat if necessary. • Prevent occlusion due to drug sludge by flushing carefully after administration. • Thrombolytic agent is required for fibrinous clot. • FDA approved use of t-PA (tissue plasminogen activator) for thrombolytic protocol. Follow facility policy regarding instillation of drug. • Instill 2 mg of t-PA in a 10-mL syringe. Wait 60 minutes. Aspirate; if unable to obtain blood flow, instill a second dose of t-PA. If this does not produce blood flow, notify physician.
Catheter breaks or is pierced by clamp.	• Immediately clamp catheter proximal to break site, if necessary (Groshong may be clamped using rubber band). • Obtain repair kit for catheter.
Air enters catheter when open to atmosphere; client experiences chest pain, shortness of breath, or coughing.	• Clamp catheter (use rubber band if Groshong device). • Turn client on left side with head lower than rest of body to trap air in right heart. • Notify physician immediately. • Administer oxygen.
Signs of infection develop at exit site (redness, pain, fever, chills).	• Notify physician immediately. • Catheter will have to be removed and cultures taken.

Chapter 29

UNIT 5

Implanted Subcutaneous Port

Nursing Process Data

ASSESSMENT Data Base

- Assess site.
- Assess patency of port.

PLANNING Objectives

- To provide an access for blood withdrawal
- To provide an access for drug or blood/fluid administration

IMPLEMENTATION Procedures

EVALUATION Expected Outcomes

- Subcutaneous implanted port remains patent to facilitate medication administration.
- Implantation site remains infection-free.
- Blood samples are obtained without difficulty.

Accessing and Flushing an Implanted Port Using a Huber Needle

NOTE: Implanted venous access ports, such as Port-a-Cath, are usually placed in a subcutaneous pocket on the chest wall, require minimal maintenance, and may be used for months to years before the maximum 2,000 punctures are achieved. Ports are best utilized for cyclic therapies like chemotherapy or antibiotic therapy. They are well suited for care of clients with cancer or others with long-term illnesses requiring IV medications. Ports can be used for either bolus or continuous infusions.

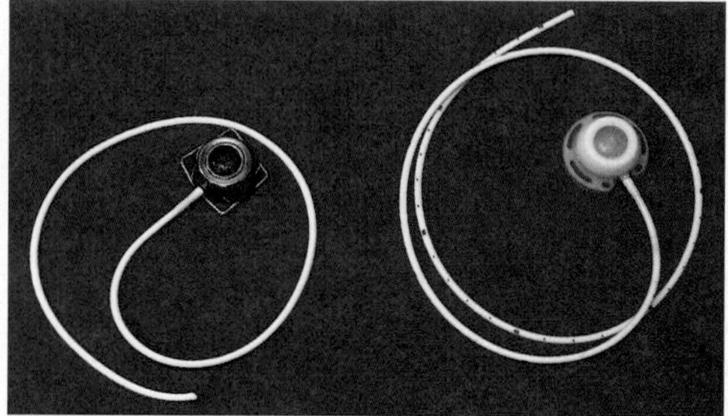

▲ Implanted subcutaneous port.

Equipment

Noncoring needle (Huber) with attached extension tubing and clamp
Intermittent infusion cap or CLC 2000
Two 10-mL Luer-Lok syringes
Preservative-free normal saline or prefilled syringes
Heparin (100 or 10 units/mL) according to facility policy
Antimicrobial swabs, 2% chlorhexidine gluconate
Sterile gloves
Clean gloves
Mask

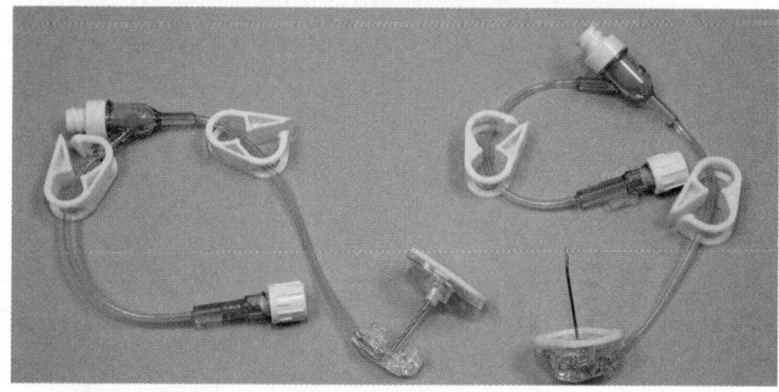

▲ Huber needle.

Preparation

1. Check physician's orders and client care plan. Review specific hospital policy and procedure for care of implanted port.
2. Gather equipment.
3. Perform hand hygiene.
4. Draw up 10 mL of normal saline into 10-mL syringe, or use prefilled syringes.
5. Draw up 5 mL of dilute heparin (10 mL or 100 units/mL according to facility policy) into 10-mL syringe.
6. Identify client using two forms of identification.
7. Explain procedure to client.
8. Don clean gloves.

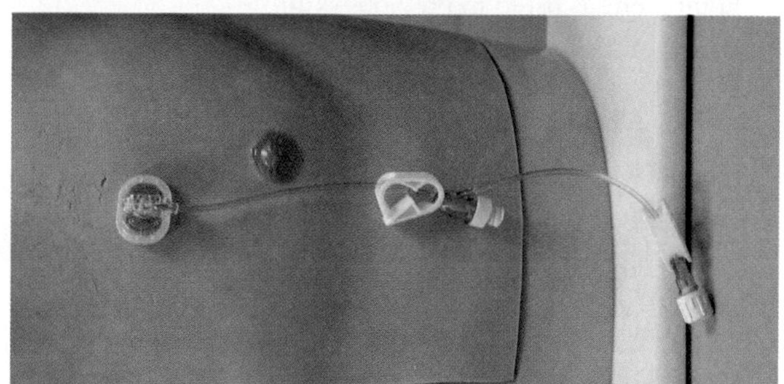

▲ Placement of Huber needle.

Procedure

1. Palpate skin over subcutaneous infusion port. ▶ ***Rationale:*** This identifies location and contours of the device.

- Noncoring needles, such as the Huber needle, are the only ones used to access the port.
- Huber needle and tubing are changed every 7 days.
- This specially designed needles (bent at 90° angle to its hub or wings) has a sharp-angled bevel and attached extension tubing with clamp and needleless cap. Huber needles can also be straight.
- Inserted through skin and into rubber septum for central venous access.
- Prevents coring of the port.
- Produces insertion tract that seals itself when it is removed.

2. Place thumb and forefinger of left hand on port (right hand if left-handed) and feel for septum with right hand. ▶ ***Rationale:*** This position stabilizes the port.
3. Numb the area with a topical anesthetic cream or ice, according to facility policy. Depending on the product used, the time for effective anesthesia may vary from a few minutes to 1 hr.
4. Clean skin with antimicrobial swab using a back-and-forth movement. Scrub for 30 seconds.
5. Allow site to air dry for 30 seconds. ▶ ***Rationale:*** Drying permits solution to work best against bacteria, fungi, and spores.
6. Affix syringe with 10 mL of normal saline into Huber needle extension tubing cap and prime tubing; leave syringe attached.
7. Remove clean gloves and dispose in appropriate container.
8. Apply mask according to facility policy, perform hand hygiene, and don sterile gloves.

9. Stabilize port using thumb and index finger or index finger and middle finger.
10. Insert needle into port at a 90° angle until it meets resistance from the stainless steel back of the port.
11. Check for correct placement by aspirating for blood return.
    a. Withdraw flash of blood to check needle position. If no blood is obtained, try repositioning client (sit up, raise arms, cough.)
    b. If still unable to obtain blood, try flushing port with small amount (2–3 mL) of normal saline.
    c. If no blood return, remove noncoring needle and reaccess port.
    d. If still unable to obtain blood, call the physician (x-ray for placement may be required.)
12. If placement is correct, stabilize needle and inject remaining normal saline. There should be no sign of infiltration into surrounding tissue.
13. Close clamp of needle extension tubing.
14. Exchange syringe of normal saline for syringe filled with dilute heparin flush, then open clamp.
15. Instill 5 mL (in 10 mL syringe) of heparin flush (100 units/mL).
16. Clamp extension tubing before removing syringe.
17. Remove needle by pulling straight out from port while stabilizing port with free hand.
18. If needle is to be left in place for intermittent use, secure wings with tape for hub (chevron style) and apply sterile transparent dressing over all.
19. Dispose of equipment.
20. Remove gloves and perform hand hygiene.

NOTE: If CLC2000 device is used, follow directions for use on page 1141.

Clinical Alert

Implanted ports have the lowest risk of infection of all chest-accessed central lines.

Administering Drugs via a Subcutaneous Implanted Port

Equipment

Syringe filled with medication
Equipment as listed in previous skill
Syringe filled with 10 mL of saline
Syringe with 10 mL of dilute heparin solution

Procedure

1. Follow procedure listed in previous skill. (Using sterile gloves, access port verifying correct placement, i.e., blood return on aspiration, ability to infuse normal saline flush, and no infiltration.)
2. Clamp short needle extension tubing.
3. Exchange saline syringe for syringe filled with ordered medication.
4. Unclamp tubing.
5. Administer medication at prescribed rate.
6. Flush port between drugs with 5 mL of saline if giving more than one drug. ▶ ***Rationale:*** This prevents the possibility of drug–drug interactions.
7. Flush system with saline, then with dilute heparin.
8. Inject last 0.5 mL of heparin flush while simultaneously withdrawing needle and stabilizing port.
9. Wipe skin gently with dry swab to remove any solution.
10. If client is to receive intermittent IV drugs or solution, the Huber needle may remain in place for 1 week. After intermittent administration, clamp tubing, insert new sterile protective cap into extension tubing, open clamp to flush and heparinize, then reclamp tubing.
11. Flush used port with 5 mL heparin (100 units/mL) daily; if unused, flush monthly.
12. Dispose of equipment (including gloves) and perform hand hygiene.

NOTE: Change port dressing weekly or when wet or soiled.

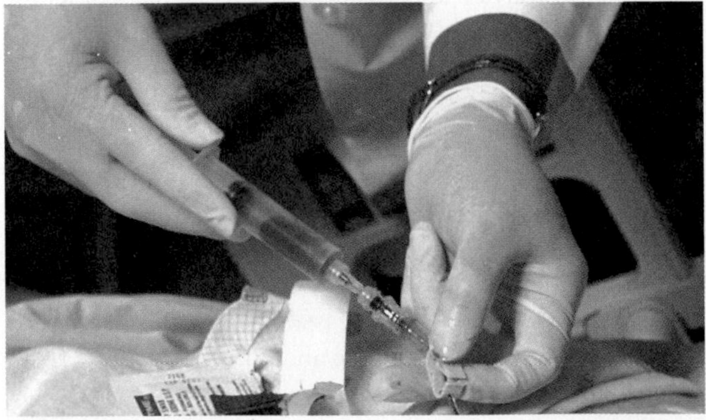

▲ Check for blood flashback when flushing CVAD (unless Groshong valve present).

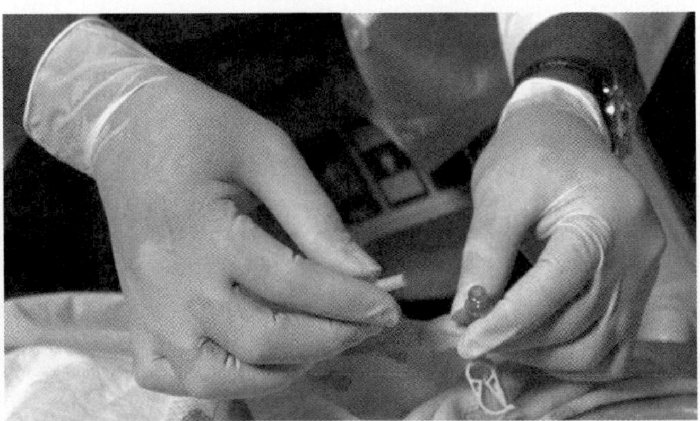

▲ Always have CVAD clamped when changing infusion cap (Groshong valve does not require).

Administering Infusions via a Subcutaneous Port

Equipment

Huber needle with attached extension tubing and in-line clamp
Intermittent infusion cap
5-mL syringe with needleless cannula
Two 10-mL syringes with needleless connector
Normal saline
Heparin (10 units/mL or100 units/mL according to facility policy) or normal saline
Antimicrobial swabs, 2% chlorhexidine gluconate
Sterile and clean gloves
Mask
Sterile gauze squares
Transparent dressing
Sterile tape
Prescribed IV solutions, drugs, or blood products

Preparation

1. Check physician's orders.
2. Gather equipment.
3. Identify client using two descriptors.
4. Explain procedure to client.
5. Provide privacy.
6. Raise bed to comfortable working position.
7. Perform hand hygiene.
8. Don clean gloves.

Procedure

1. Remove dressing, prepare site, and access port using sterile technique (sterile gloves and mask) as previously described.
2. Secure needle hub with sterile tape, or wings with tape or Steri-strips.
3. Place transparent dressing over insertion site, needle, and proximal IV tubing; date and initial.
4. Flush port with 10 mL of saline solution.
5. Proceed with administration of ordered solution, drug, or blood.
6. Upon completion, flush with 10 mL of normal saline, followed by 5 mL of dilute heparin flush.
7. Clamp tubing before removing syringe to maintain positive pressure; cap tubing.
8. For continuous infusion, change tubing daily and dressing every 96 hr.
9. Dispose of equipment (including gloves) and perform hand hygiene.

NOTE: If using CLC2000 device, refer to page 1141 for directions.

Clinical Alert

Electrical controller device (pump) should be used for continuous IV infusion via CVAD.

Drawing Blood From an Implanted Subcutaneous Port

Equipment

Huber 19-gauge needle with short extension tubing
Needleless injection cap or CLC2000 device
Two 10-mL syringes
Blood collection tubes
Heparin 3-mL and normal saline 10-mL flush solutions
Antimicrobial swabs, chlorhexidine gluconate
Sterile tape
Sterile gloves

Procedure

1. Gather equipment.
2. Check physician's orders for type of blood test.
3. Identify client using two descriptors and explain procedure to client.
4. Perform hand hygiene and don sterile gloves.
5. Access implanted port using Huber needle with capped extension tubing as discussed previously.
   a. Prep tubing cap or CLC2000 device with antimicrobial swab.
   b. Clean around junction of cap and hub with antimicrobial swab before removing cap or before inserting syringe into CLC2000 device.
6. Insert syringe into hub of extension tubing.
7. Unclamp tubing.
8. Withdraw 5–10 mL blood, remove syringe, and discard. ▸ ***Rationale:*** This discards the filling volume of the catheter.
9. Maintain aseptic technique—attach new syringe to hub of extension tubing or insert into CLC2000 device.

Clinical Alert

When drawing blood, attach syringe directly to hub of extension tubing. Never draw through an older type cap as hemolysis can occur. Always place a new cap on extension tubing after withdrawing blood samples. Check the newer caps to determine if blood can be drawn through the cap.

Withdraw appropriate amount of blood for tests and remove syringe.

10. Fill appropriate type of blood tubes with specified amount of blood according to tests ordered.
11. Flush catheter with 10 mL of saline solution after obtaining blood specimens.
12. Place new cap on extension tubing. CLC2000 device is changed every 24 hr.
13. Discard equipment.
14. Remove gloves and perform hand hygiene.

DOCUMENTATION for Implanted Subcutaneous Port

- Condition of port implantation site
- Frequency and type of flushes
- Name and dosage of drugs or solutions administered
- Presence of Huber needle, if left in place
- Document gauge and length of Huber needle
- Dressing type
- Amount of blood withdrawn
- CLC2000 device if used

CRITICAL THINKING Application

Expected Outcomes

- Subcutaneous implanted port remains patent to facilitate medication administration.
- Client's subcutaneous port implantation site remains infection-free.
- Blood samples are obtained without difficulty.

Unexpected Outcomes	Alternative Actions
Needle entry is painful.	• Use topical anesthetic or apply ice before accessing. • Use local anesthetic injected intradermally before inserting needle (check client sensitivity and agency policy).
Occluded catheter.	• Change needle. If no improvement, suspect occluded catheter. • Try gentle aspiration to dislodge clot. • Never try to forcefully flush system—clot may mobilize; catheter may rupture. • Thrombolytic agent may be required to lyse fibrin clot (specialty nurse skill). • Transfuse packed red blood cells along with continuous infusion of normal saline; use an infusion pump; flush catheter well with 20 mL of normal saline after infusion to prevent occluded catheter.
Inability to aspirate blood when checking placement.	• Needle may not be in port reservoir. • Tip of catheter may be against vessel wall. Try changing client's position from sitting up to lying or ask client to raise one or both arms. If appropriate, have client bear down or cough using Valsalva's maneuver while irrigating with normal saline. • Heparinize catheter and return in 40 minutes to aspirate. • Removal of a fibrin clot, thrombolysis, is done by a certified IV nurse (according to agency policy).
Pain, swelling at site.	• Suspect catheter rupture. Report to physician. • Suspect port migration and infusion infiltrating subcutaneously.
Port becomes movable.	• Port may not be anchored securely. Port could be flipped under skin. • Silicone tubing has separated from port. • Always check for blood return to ensure accurate needle placement, before injecting medications. • Notify physician and prepare for removing port.

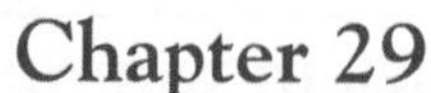

Chapter 29

UNIT 6

Peripherally Inserted Central Catheter (PICC)

Nursing Process Data

ASSESSMENT Data Base

- Assess length of exposed catheter.
- Assess that catheter is secure.
- Assess insertion site.
- Assess catheter patency.

PLANNING Objectives

- To provide access for infusion, parenteral nutrition, or drugs
- To provide access for blood sampling
- To provide patent access

IMPLEMENTATION Procedures

EVALUATION Expected Outcomes

- PICC remains patent without sign of infection.
- Catheter is irrigated at designated time frames.
- Transparent dressing remains intact for 7 days.

Pearson Nursing Student Resources

Find additional review materials at **nursing.pearsonhighered.com**

Prepare for success with NCLEX®-style practice questions and Skill Checklists

Maintaining the PICC

Equipment

Pre-filled syringe with 10 mL of preservative-free normal saline (0.9%)
Pre-filled syringe with 20 mL of preservative-free normal saline
Pre-filled syringe with 3–5 mL of dilute heparin (10 units/mL) solution (per hospital policy)
Optional CLC2000
Sterile gloves
Antimicrobial swabs, 2% chlorhexidine gluconate
Transparent dressing
StatLock Securement device

For Medication Administration

Medication IV bag
Two 10-mL syringes pre-filled with preservative-free 0.9% normal saline
Heparin flush according to facility policy
2% Chlorhexidine gluconate swabs

NOTE: Midline catheters are very similar to PICC lines, except they are shorter. The same policy and procedures apply to the care and maintenance of these lines.

Preparation

1. Check client care plan and MAR.
2. Identify client using two descriptors.
3. Explain procedure to client.
4. Provide privacy for client.

Procedure

1. Perform hand hygiene and don gloves.
2. Assess IV site and surrounding area for signs of infection (i.e., erythema, tenderness, edema, and drainage).
3. Assess securement device site for stability, cleanliness, and intact dressing.

Clinical Alert

If catheter tip is resting in the right atrium or pericardium instead of the superior vena cava, the tip can move across the muscle to the sinoatrial node (SA node) and can cause cardiac arrhythmias, cardiac rupture, or other associated conditions. The PICC catheter must be withdrawn 1 in. (2.5 cm) and a repeat x-ray taken to check for catheter placement.

Clinical Alert

All continuous infusions using a PICC line should be connected to an electric infusion device to maintain infusion and patency of line.

4. Swab catheter port with chlorhexidine swab. Allow to dry for 30 seconds.
5. Inject pre-filled syringe with preservative-free 0.9% normal saline into catheter hub and aspirate.
   ▸ ***Rationale:*** Check for patency.
6. Inject solution of 0.9% preservative-free sodium chloride (twice the internal volume of the CVD and injection cap) slowly; flush with minimal force using a pulsatile motion until syringe is almost empty.
   ▸ ***Rationale:*** This action creates turbulence for catheter cleansing.
7. Continue to inject flush while removing syringe from catheter port.
8. For medication administration:
   a. Perform hand hygiene.
   b. Check client using two identifiers.
   c. Don gloves, if facility policy.
   d. Remove protective tab from both the PICC tubing and the IV bag. (The tabs are usually in bright colors so you can easily identify them.)
   e. Push the pointed end of the tubing into the opening on the IV bag. Hold the bag up high and squeeze the drip chamber until it is half full.

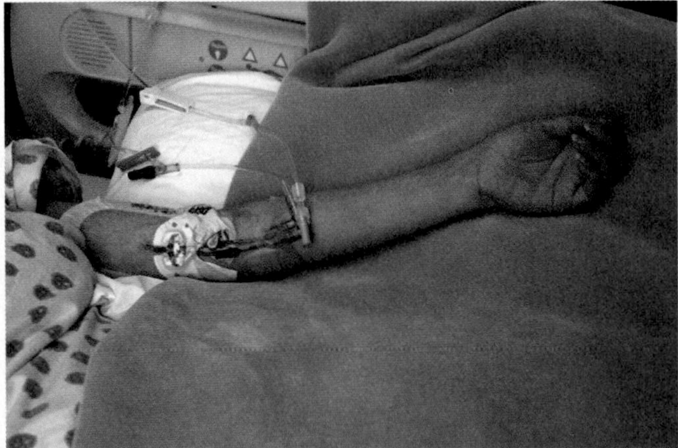

▲ Maintain PICC line with cleaning and irrigation.

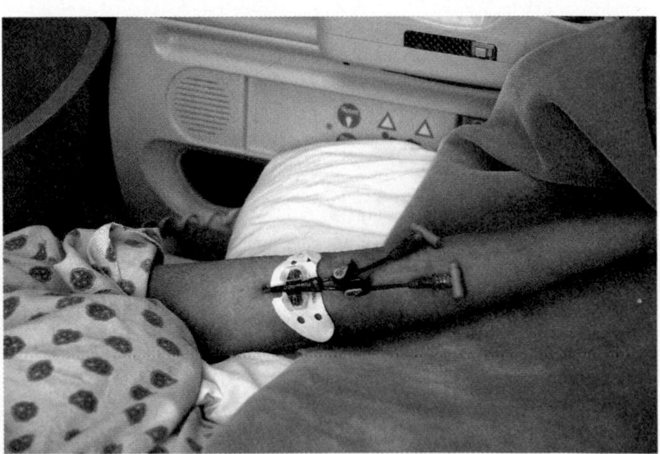

▲ Double-lumen PICC with CLC 2000 positive pressure device.

f. Open roller clamp and observe fluid run through tubing until all air is removed from tubing. Close roller clamp.
g. Flush PICC line using saline solution and a push–pause technique.
h. Attach needleless connector on PICC tubing to rubber cap of IV catheter. Unclamp catheter and adjust the roller clamp to prescribed rate.
i. When IV bag is empty, clamp PICC tubing and remove tubing from rubber cap.
j. Clean lumen with 2% chlorhexidine gluconate swab by vigorously rubbing port.
k. Flush PICC line with saline using push–pause technique. ▶ ***Rationale:*** Avoids buildup of precipitates, which can occur in catheter occlusions.
l. Flush PICC line with heparin according to facility policy.
m. Clamp IV catheter.

9. Flush nonused catheter at least every 12 hr using push–pause technique.
10. Place discarded equipment in appropriate receptacle. Place syringe in sharps container.
11. Remove gloves and perform hand hygiene.

NOTE: The use of positive pressure devices is now suggested for catheter care.

Recommendations for Use of Catheter Securement Devices

Infusion Nurses Society

The Infusion Nurses Society has published major guidelines that state a preference for using a securement device such as the StatLock for stabilizing catheters.

Centers for Disease Control and Prevention (CDC)

The CDC states that sutureless securement devices are an advantage over sutures in preventing bloodstream infections and complications.

The Joint Commission and National Patient Safety Foundation

The Joint Commission and the National Patient Safety Foundation identify securement devices as a major contributor to client safety because they reduce catheter-related infections and overall complications. This is in addition to improving safety for healthcare providers.

Occupational Safety and Health Administration (OSHA)

OSHA has issued directives that instruct healthcare employers to consider using securement devices to reduce needle-stick injuries in healthcare providers.

Source: Dowling, L. (2006, February). To save lives, guidelines recommend safer catheter securement. Dowling & Dennis Public Relations. www.nappsi.org/news.php.

Flushing Procedure

Frequency

1. Check facility policy and follow protocol.
2. Suggested recommendations:
   a. Every 4–6 hr for no. 2 French or smaller catheters and after each use.
   b. Every 8–12 hr for larger size catheters and after each use.

Other Times

1. When LOCK is applied.
2. After blood draws.
3. After intermittent medication administration.
4. After blood or blood component administration.
5. After administration of TPN.

Pulsatile (Push–Pause) Flushing

Use a rapid succession of push–pause–push–pause movements exerted on the plunger of the syringe barrel. This motion creates a turbulence within the catheter lumen causing a swirling effect to move fibrin, lipids, medications, or other adherents attached to catheter lumen and prevents occlusions to the catheter.

Peripherally Inserted Central Catheter

PICCs are long, soft, flexible, single or multi-lumen catheters placed in basilic, cephalic, or brachial vein and advanced into the superior vena cava for central venous access. The length of catheter is documented. Placement is less invasive and less expensive than other CVADs since they can be inserted by specially educated certified IV nurses. As with tunneled catheters, exit site below heart level decreases risk of air embolism when system is open to the atmosphere. PICC lines need to be checked by x-ray to verify tip placement if inserted into a proximal arm. Clients receiving TPN or vesicants should have tip inserted into SVC, and x-ray should be done to confirm position. Research has shown that PICC lines inserted into SVC have fewer complications such as inflammation or thrombosis.

Securement devices are now recommended to prevent catheter migration. These catheters may be used for long-term therapy if changed every 6 weeks. PICC lines can be left in place for at least 1 year.

Preservative-free 0.9% saline is recommended for flushing. Heparin is usually not recommended. You will need to check facility policy regarding heparin usage and dosage.

Prevention of Catheter-Related Bloodstream Infections

- Hand hygiene
- 2% chlorhexidine gluconate skin antisepsis
- Optimal catheter site selection; subclavian vein preferred route
- Maximal barrier protection
- Daily monitoring of IV site
- Dressing change every 7 days unless soiled or loose.

Source: 100,000 Lives Campaign. (2006). How-to guide: Preventing catheter-related bloodstream infections—Five components of care. Retrieved June 14, 2006, from www.ihi.org/IHI/Programs/campaign.

EVIDENCE-BASED PRACTICE

Peripheral Intravenous Catheter Dwell Times

This prospective, sequential clinical trial evaluated the survival time of IV catheters using three methods: nonsterile tape, StatLock, and the Hub-Guard. The use of nonsterile tape securement resulted in an 8% peripheral IV catheter (PVI) survival rate, the Hub-Guard result was 9%, and the StatLock had a survival rate of 52%. The study was completed in an effort to determine the best method to assist in prolonging the 96-hr PIV change protocol. This study strongly suggests that a mechanical catheter securement device allows the implementation of the 96-hr IV change protocol that was sanctioned by the CDC.

Source: Smith, B. (2006). Peripheral intravenous catheter dwell times: A comparison of 3 securement methods for implementation of a 96-hour scheduled change protocol. *Journal of Infusion Nursing, 29*(1), 14–17.

EVIDENCE-BASED PRACTICE

Complication Rates for Valved Versus Nonvalved PICCs

In a randomized study, 362 clients (233 men, 129 women; mean age, 44) were given PICC catheters; half of the clients received clamped catheters and half received valved catheters. The complication rate for the clamped PICC clients was double that of clients with valved catheters as a result of occlusions or infections (26 for clamped and 12 for valved catheters).

Source: Hoffer, E. K., J. Borsa, P. Santulli, R. Bloch, A. B. Fontaine. (2005). Comparisons of valved versus nonvalved PICC catheters. http://www.ajronline.org/cgi/content

EVIDENCE-BASED PACTICE

It has been found that the use of a single-lumen CVC is recommended to reduce the risk of catheter-related bloodstream infections. Studies evaluating this issue have produced variable results, with some studies indicating multi-lumen CVCs are significantly more at risk to develop infections, whereas other studies indicated no increased risks with multi-lumen CVCs. It is well recognized that intraluminal migration from hubs and ports is a major source of microorganisms; therefore, keeping the number of ports or lumen to a minimum is preferred.

(O'Grady, et al. 2002, DH 2007, Pratt 2007, Zurcher) (Dezfulian, et al. 2003).

Changing the PICC Dressing

Equipment

- Antimicrobial swabs, 2% chlorhexidine gluconate
- Securement device
- Transparent semipermeable dressing
- BioPatch disc (optional)
- Clean gloves
- Sterile gloves
- Mask

Procedure

1. Identify client using two descriptors and check electronic medical record and client care plan for last dressing change (review facility policy and procedure).
2. Explain procedure to client.
3. Perform hand hygiene and don mask and clean gloves.
4. Remove old transparent dressing by gently pulling in an upward direction. ▸ ***Rationale:*** Prevents dislodgement of catheter.
5. Check site for bleeding, infection, or signs of phlebitis. ▸ ***Rationale:*** Bleeding may occur with arm use. Phlebitis is the most common complication.
6. Discard old dressing and gloves. Perform hand hygiene.

Clinical Alert

Unless absolutely necessary, avoid blood pressure measurement in the arm with a PICC and avoid venipunctures on the extremity with a PICC line.

7. Prepare sterile supplies.
8. Don sterile gloves.
9. Clean exit site and catheter with antimicrobial swabs using back-and-forth movement.

NOTE: The catheter is anchored by a securement device, which does not require suturing of PICC line. Approximately 1 in. of catheter extends from the insertion site.

10. Allow time for antimicrobial solution to dry. Do not blow on arm or wave hand to hasten drying. ▸ ***Rationale:*** Waving hand or blowing may contaminate site—antibacterial action does not take effect until solution is dry.
11. Place securement device over catheter. ▸ ***Rationale:*** Catheter is not sutured in place, so securement device is used to prevent catheter migration. (Refer to skill in Unit 1, page 1122, Applying a StatLock Securement Device.)

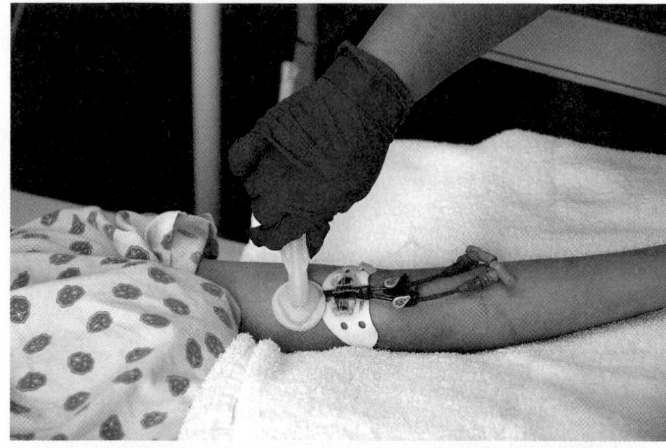

▲ Cleanse site with chlorhexidine gluconate swab using back-and forth motion.

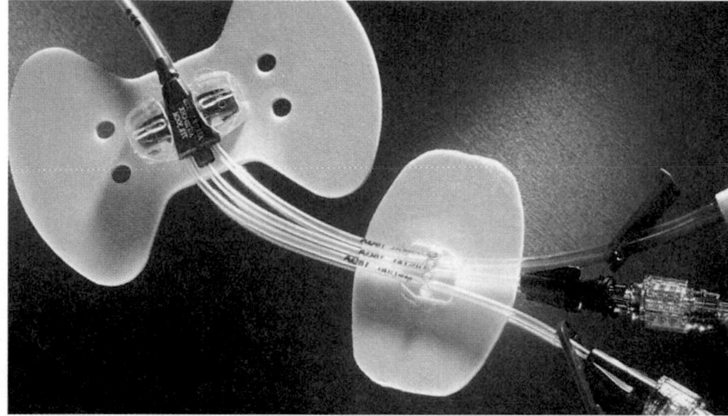

▲ StatLock device, the only evidence-based catheter stabilization device that meets national standards. (Courtesy of Venetec, Intl.)

12. Cover exit site with transparent semipermeable dressing. Avoid stretching the dressing. Press down on dressing to seal catheter site. No part of actual catheter should be outside transparent dressing.

NOTE: Transparent dressings are not occlusive; they allow air to circulate through the semipermeable dressing and thus prevent perspiration from collecting under the dressing.

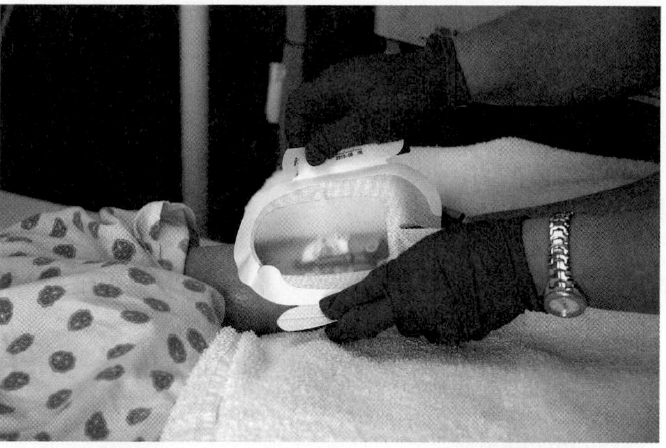

▲ Allow site to dry before applying dressing. Place transparent dressing over site.

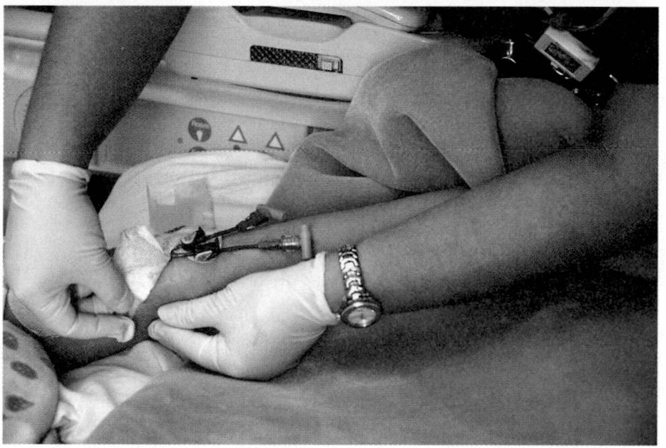

▲ Remove dressing by gently pulling in an upward direction.

13. Remove gloves, mask, and perform hand hygiene.
14. Initial and date dressing.
15. Change initial transparent dressing in 24 hr and then every 7 days or whenever it is soiled or loose. ▸ ***Rationale:*** First dressing change is done to check insertion site.

Drawing Blood From the PICC

Equipment

Antimicrobial swabs—2% chlorhexidine gluconate
Two 10-mL syringes with needleless connector
20-mL syringe with needleless connector filled with saline
Syringe with 3–5 mL of dilute heparin (per hospital policy) and needleless connector
Clean gloves

Preparation

1. Check physician orders.
2. Identify client using two descriptors.
3. Perform hand hygiene and don gloves.
4. Explain procedure to client.

Procedure

1. Stop all infusing fluids for at least 1 minute before drawing a specimen.
2. Swab catheter cap with antimicrobial swab and allow to dry.
3. Use 10-mL syringe and withdraw 5 mL of blood and discard appropriately in biohazard container. Check facility policy and procedure for amount to discard.
4. Use 10-mL syringe with needleless connector and withdraw required amount of blood for laboratory tests. Do not use Vacutainer. ▸ ***Rationale:*** Catheter will collapse with intense vacuum.
5. Change cap after all blood draws and transfusions. Flush with 20 mL of saline solution to clear catheter.

6. Complete procedure with dilute heparin flush (unless Groshong valve present).
7. Discard equipment and gloves; perform hand hygiene.
8. Handle blood sample appropriately. Transfer to collection tube.

Removing the PICC

Equipment

Gloves

10-mL syringe pre-filled with 0.9% preservative-free sodium chloride

Sterile 2 × 2 gauze

Tape

Procedure

1. Check physician's order.
2. Identify client using two descriptors.
3. Explain the procedure to the client. Client may be in bed or sitting in a chair.
4. Perform hand hygiene and don gloves.
5. Flush catheter with 0.9% sodium chloride.
6. Carefully remove dressing, loosening edges toward insertion site. Remove Steri-strip on securement device.
7. Grasp catheter at insertion site.
8. Gradually pull catheter parallel to skin 1 in. at a time.
9. Continue inching catheter out—if resistance is felt, stop and reposition arm, wait 15 seconds.
10. After removal, measure length of catheter and compare to documented length on chart.
11. Culture tip according to facility policy. Cut tip with sterile scissor and place in sterile container. Be careful not to contaminate tip when withdrawing blood from vein.
12. Hold gauze at exit site for hemostasis.
13. Apply tape to gauze securely. Leave in place for 24 hr.
14. Dispose of catheter in biohazard container.
15. Document length of catheter removed.

NOTE: Certified infusion nurses only remove the PICC.

Clinical Alert

NEVER FORCE catheter removal (apply warm moist pack to upper arm to relax vein for approximately 15 minutes).

Notify Physician or IV Therapist if There Is:

- Infusion leaking from insertion site
- Inconsistent flow rates
- Inability to infuse fluids
- Excessive bleeding or drainage at insertion site
- Chest, neck, ear pain, numbness, tingling of affected arm
- Swelling, pain, redness, palpable cord at or above insertion site

DOCUMENTATION for the Peripherally Inserted Central Catheter

- Label site "PICC" to ensure proper use of line
- Frequency of flush and type of solution
- Type of dressing applied. Label date, time, initials, and "PICC."
- Site assessment
- Length of exposed catheter
- Amount of blood withdrawn for specimen
- Solutions or drugs administered including flow rate
- Electronic infusion device utilized

For Discontinuing PICC

- Note condition and length of catheter
- Document site assessment
- Client's response to treatment and procedure
- Catheter tip sent to lab for culture, if appropriate

CRITICAL THINKING Application

Expected Outcomes

- PICC remains patent without signs of infection or migration
- Catheter is irrigated at designated time.
- StatLock remains in place.
- Transparent dressing remains intact for 7 days.

Unexpected Outcomes	Alternative Actions
Mechanical phlebitis (pain, redness spreading to surrounding tissue).	• Apply warm moist compresses for 20 minutes 4 times a day. • Elevate the arm and encourage mild exercise. • Report problem—antiinflammatory drugs may correct problem and prevent PICC removal.
Bleeding occurs at insertion site.	• Apply direct pressure on insertion site. • Check client's coagulation profile (bleeding time, platelet count, PT, PTT) for coagulation problem. • Consider removal if excessive bleeding persists after using pressure.
Exudate occurs at insertion site.	• Notify physician or IV therapist. • Send specimen to lab for culture. • Maintain aseptic technique during site care.
Solution does not infuse.	• Increase volume of flush solution. • Utilize infusion pump or elevate infusion bag for gravity pressure. • Flush with a push–pull motion and clamp catheter before removing syringe. • Report problem—thrombolytic declotting may be necessary.
Pain in shoulder or neck occurs during infusion—or client hears gurgling sound with flush.	• Report so x-ray can validate catheter placement (catheter may have migrated with client maneuvers).
Sepsis occurs (rare).	• Monitor client for fever and assess insertion site for drainage, tenderness, redness. • PICC may be removed—send tip to lab for culture.

GERONTOLOGIC Considerations

Elderly Clients Requiring Chemotherapy or Parenteral Nutrition Are Good Candidates for Implanted Vascular Access Devices.

- Decreased amounts of fluids can be administered to prevent fluid overload.
- Risk of infection is decreased, and in the elderly infection is a concern. Frequency and severity of infection tend to increase with age due to a decline in the immune response.
- Repeated IV punctures are not necessary so veins are preserved and discomfort minimized.
- Greater client mobility is achieved.

With Aging, Epidermal Turnover Decreases and Skin Fragility Increases. Even Minimal Trauma May Result in Serious Erosion.

Healthcare Providers or Family Members Can Be Instructed to Provide Medication Administration, Fluid Therapy, or Parenteral Nutrition at Home.

MANAGEMENT Guidelines

Each state legislates a Nurse Practice Act for RNs and LVN/LPNs. Healthcare facilities are responsible for establishing and implementing policies and procedures that conform to their state's regulations. Verify the regulations and role parameters for each healthcare worker in your facility.

Delegation

- Each state identifies the scope of practice for RNs and LVN/LPNs. Several states have identified that the LVN/LPN has a specific role in IV therapy, but the scope of practice is always dictated by each agency (e.g., initiating, regulating, discontinuing IVs). The LPN/LVN educated in IV therapy is the minimum level practitioner to assist in tasks delegated by the RN for the delivery of IV therapy. The RN may be assisted by an LVN/LPN educated in IV therapy, but the RN remains responsible for the care given.
- Policies outlining the responsibility of the IV nurse vary significantly among agencies. A written policy should clearly outline all aspects of this role, and all staff should be familiar with its scope. Policies and procedures should follow national guidelines and standards of practice established by the Centers for Disease Control and Prevention, the American Association of Blood Banks, and the IV Nurses Society. All nurses must be aware of the many physical hazards associated with IV therapy and related OSHA rules to be observed.
- Central line catheter management must be done by an RN.
- The nurse who delivers IV therapy must be qualified by specific knowledge and experience to perform such highly specialized skills. Many agencies utilize a team of specialty educated and experienced certified IV nurses who focus their attention solely on aspects of IV therapy (initiation, drug preparation, fluid/blood/drug administration, regular client assessment and site care, as well as monitoring product integrity). While these nurses are freed from other care responsibilities, the professional nurse must provide for ongoing client care and ensure client safety.
- TPN and lipids may be administered only by an RN according to specific physician orders.
- The CNA/UAP providing personal hygiene must understand that the IV system is a closed one and must be able to give care without disrupting the system. The components of the CVAD system must never be disconnected. Doing so places the client at risk for infection and air embolism. The CNA/UAP should receive training in changing the client's gown without disrupting the CVAD system.
- For the client with a CVAD allowed to shower, the RN should disconnect infusion lines, place a dry sterile gauze (4 × 4) over the dressed site and exposed tubing(s), then cover all with a large transparent dressing for waterproofing. Post-shower removal of the covering and inspection of the dressing should also be performed by the RN.

Communication Matrix

While the professional monitors the IV infusion site regularly, the CNA/UAP provides vital data to the professional nurse by immediately reporting:

- Observations of redness or swelling around the CVAD insertion site (signs of possible infiltration, hematoma, sepsis).
- Presence of crepitus (bubble-wrap feeling) on the client's chest (sign of possible subcutaneous emphysema that can lead to respiratory distress).
- Observations of respiratory distress in any client with recent (24 hr) placement of a central line (symptoms of possible pneumothorax).
- Any client complaint of arm, shoulder, or neck pain (symptom of possible thrombosis or infiltration).
- Temperature elevation (fever—sign of possible catheter-related infection if otherwise unexplainable).
- Infusion device alarms to prompt the professional to further assess the client.
- Presence of blood backup in the catheter.
- A loose or soiled/wet dressing.

CRITICAL THINKING Strategies

Scenario 1

Mr. John Baker is a 68-year-old retired pharmacist who has just returned from surgery after placement of a tunneled CVAD with a Groshong valve. He will be started on a long-term intermittent chemotherapy regimen for acute lymphocytic leukemia. His wife is a retired RN who worked in the operating room for many years.

1. Identify at least three advantages for inserting the tunneled catheter for his treatment.
2. His wife is very concerned about the initial care of the catheter. What explanation will you give her?
3. After the explanation regarding the care of the catheter, Mrs. Baker asks you how they can prevent an infection of the catheter.
4. The client needs to be instructed on how to flush the catheter. What are the most important directions you should provide to him?
5. Mrs. Baker asks you to describe what symptoms require reporting to the physician. What is your best response to this question?

Scenario 2

Seth Eley, age 24, has been admitted to your unit with the diagnosis of inflammatory bowel disease (Crohn's disease) with exacerbation of fever, severe diarrhea, right lower quadrant pain, weight loss, and anemia. Short-term total parenteral nutrition and bowel rest are planned. A triple-lumen central venous catheter has been placed for these purposes.

1. Based on these data, what generalizations can you make about the purpose of hyperalimentation for this client?
2. Why is central venous access necessary?
3. Develop several scenarios about the most common complications of central catheter placement.
4. How does TPN affect fluid and electrolyte balance?

NCLEX® Review Questions

Unless otherwise specified, choose only one (1) answer.

1. The best device for long-term IV therapy is a
   1. Peripherally inserted central vascular catheter.
   2. Midline catheter placed in the basilic vein.
   3. Peripheral catheter placed in the antecubital vein.
   4. Long-line catheter threaded into the right atrium.
2. Guidelines to prevent catheter-related bloodstream infections include
   Select all that apply.
   1. Using good hygiene principles.
   2. Using a catheter impregnated with an antibiotic agent.
   3. Preparing the IV site with Betadine or alcohol swabs.
   4. Placing a mask on the client when inserting a PICC line.
3. You are preparing the site for an IV insertion of a PICC line. Which one of the following drying times is required when using chlorhexidine gluconate 2% with alcohol?
   1. 30 seconds.
   2. 1 minute.
   3. 2 minutes.
   4. 3 minutes.
4. Primary and secondary continuous IV administration sets should be replaced at least every ________ hours, or immediately if signs and symptoms of infection occur.
   1. 24.
   2. 48.
   3. 72.
   4. 96.
5. When assessing the client's IV that is infusing a parenteral nutrition solution, you find it not infusing at the prescribed rate. Your priority intervention is to
   1. Recalculate the amount of solution and time remaining for the infusion and set the flow rate at that newly calculated rate.
   2. Notify the physician immediately and have a new IV catheter available for insertion by the physician.
   3. Change the dressing to ensure it was not too tight, causing the change in IV flow rate.
   4. Observe the filter because a plugged filter is the most common cause of infusion failure.
6. Place in sequence the steps in obtaining a central venous pressure reading.
   1. Turn stopcock so manometer and IV solution are open to each other.
   2. Close clamp and rotate stopcock so IV solution is open to client.
   3. Open clamp on IV tubing and fill manometer to 18–20 cm.
   4. Turn stopcock to the manometer-client position and obtain reading.
7. A client is admitted to the healthcare facility and has an implanted port in place for chemotherapy. Instructions for care of the port include irrigating the port
   1. Weekly with heparin.
   2. Daily with normal saline.
   3. Monthly and after each use.
   4. Every 12 hr.

8. The physician has ordered a blood sample using a central line catheter. Which one of the following steps will be implemented after turning off the IV flush infusion for one minute?
   1. Flush the catheter with normal saline.
   2. Swab cap and hub with antimicrobial swabs.
   3. Remove cap from syringe.
   4. Flush catheter with 10 mL of normal saline.
9. The client has a medication order to be administered through a subcutaneous implanted port. Which one of the steps is appropriate for this procedure?
   1. Scrub the site over the port using a Betadine solution for 1 minute.
   2. Insert a 10-mL syringe with a large-bore needle and withdraw 10 mL of blood and discard the sample.
   3. Insert a Huber needle into the port at a 90-degree angle until it meets resistance.
   4. After infusion is completed, irrigate port with normal saline and remove needle by pulling it out at a 60-degree angle.
10. The major advantage of using a positive pressure device, such as a CLC2000, is to
    1. Ensure ease of obtaining blood samples from the IV site.
    2. Maintain an accurate IV solution at the prescribed rate.
    3. Maintain sterility at the junction of the IV tubing and the cap.
    4. Prevent blood from being drawn back into the catheter when the flush syringe is removed.

30

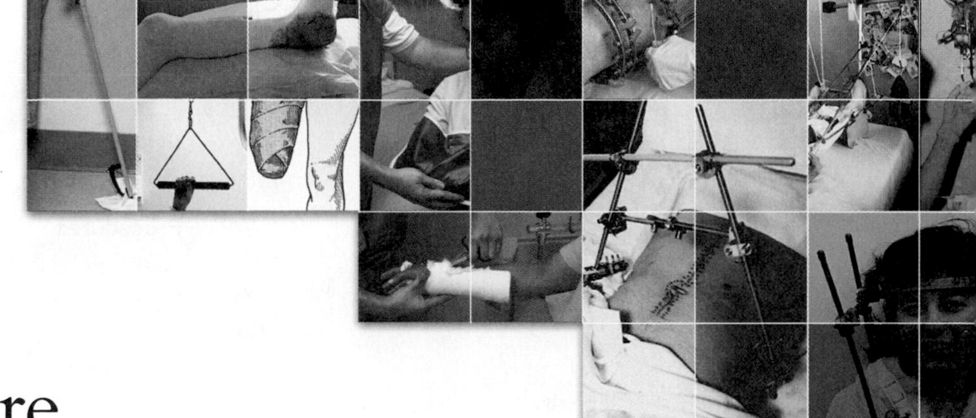

Respiratory Care

LEARNING OBJECTIVES

1. Outline the three processes of respiration.
2. Identify three nursing diagnoses for clients with ventilatory dysfunction.
3. Describe the steps for teaching a client deep breathing and coughing exercises.
4. Discuss the purpose of using an incentive spirometer.
5. Describe the steps for peak flow measurement.
6. Describe positions for postural drainage and chest percussion and vibration.
7. Differentiate modes of oxygen delivery and describe nursing care relevant to each mode.
8. Differentiate various modes of airway maintenance.
9. Outline the care needs of the intubated client.
10. Describe the nursing actions included in tracheostomy care.
11. Explain the procedure for inflating a tracheal tube cuff.
12. Describe safety measures used when suctioning clients.
13. List measures to promote safe, effective care for clients with chest tubes.

CHAPTER OUTLINE

TERMINOLOGY

Acidosis accumulation of acids (metabolic or respiratory), potentially disturbing acid–base balance and causing acidemia (low pH).

Adventitious abnormal extra sounds (crackles, wheezes) superimposed on breath sounds.

Alkalosis condition in which the alkalinity of the body tends to increase beyond normal, potentially resulting in alkalemia (high blood pH).

Apnea cessation of breathing, usually of a temporary nature.

Atelectasis collapse of alveoli, which may lead to hypoxemia, increased PCO_2, and pneumonia.

Auscultation process of listening for sounds produced by body organs.

Bradycardia slow heart rate (below 60 beats/min).

Bronchiectasis dilation of a bronchus or bronchi with production of large amounts of malodorous secretions.

Crackles discontinuous popping (opening) sounds indicative of hypoventilation of alveoli, usually auscultated at end of inspiration in dependent lung areas.

Cyanosis bluish or grayish discoloration of the skin resulting from significant reduction of oxygen saturation of hemoglobin.

Diaphoresis profuse sweating.

Dyspnea a subjective feeling of having difficulty breathing.

Expectorant an agent that facilitates the removal of airway secretions.

Hemothorax blood in the pleural space resulting in compression of normal lung tissue.

Hyperventilation abnormally deep breathing that results in a decrease in PCO_2 (respiratory alkalosis).

Hypoventilation reduced rate and depth of breathing resulting in retention of carbon dioxide (respiratory acidosis).

Hypoxemia insufficient oxygenation of the blood (decreased PO_2).

Hypoxia lack of adequate amount of oxygen transported to the tissues.

Intubation insertion of a tube into a body opening, as into the trachea.

Narcosis unconscious state due to narcotics or other depressing agent (e.g., elevated PCO_2).

Nares the nostrils.

PEP An abbreviation that means positive expiratory pressure.

Percussion rhythmic striking of the thorax to loosen pulmonary secretions.

Pneumothorax presence of air in the intrapleural space resulting in lung collapse.

Polycythemia excess number of red blood cells.

Postural drainage the use of gravity to drain secretions from the airways.

Spirometer device used for measuring inhalation and exhalation volumes.

Sputum substance expelled by coughing.

Tachypnea increased rate of breathing (over 24 breaths/min).

Tension pneumothorax lung collapse with potential contralateral shift of mediastinal structures resulting from accumulation of air or fluid in the intrapleural space.

Tracheostomy surgical opening into the trachea, usually for insertion of a tube to provide airway patency.

Ventilation the acts of inspiration and exhalation for the exchange of oxygen and carbon dioxide between the lungs and the atmosphere.

Vibration therapeutic high-frequency shaking of a body part.

Wheezes musical adventitious sounds heard on inspiration and/or expiration due to airway spasm, retained secretions, or other obstruction.

THE RESPIRATORY SYSTEM

The respiratory system provides for the exchange of gases between the blood and the external environment so that cellular respiration can occur. The respiratory structures involved include the nose, pharynx, larynx, trachea, bronchi, lungs, diaphragm, intercostal muscles, and ribs.

The upper respiratory tract includes the nose, pharynx, and larynx. These structures filter, warm, and humidify the air before it passes into the lower airways. When the upper respiratory tract is bypassed by intubation or tracheostomy, these protective processes are lost.

The lower respiratory tract is considered a sterile environment. It begins below the larynx. The trachea is composed of smooth muscle reinforced by C-shaped rings of cartilage lined with a membranous sheath. It branches into the right and left mainstream bronchi. The right bronchus extends vertically from the trachea, whereas the left bronchus branches from the trachea at an angle. The right and left bronchi divide further and further into terminal bronchioles and finally into respiratory bronchioles, alveolar ducts, and alveoli.

Because of the anatomical difference of the bronchi, migration of an endotracheal tube (ET) into the right bronchus occurs more frequently. Such a migration would result in ventilation of only the right lung. Chest x-rays are taken to ensure proper placement of ET tubes in the trachea. Auscultation of *bilateral* breath sounds also helps to verify optimal ventilation of intubated clients.

Protective processes of the lower airway include mucus secretion and the presence of special hairlike cells (cilia). This "mucociliary escalator" continuously traps and moves inhaled irritants up toward the pharynx to be removed by swallowing or coughing. Drying pharmacologic agents and pathophysiologic states (e.g., immobility) interfere with these protective processes and place the client at risk for pulmonary complications.

PROCESSES OF RESPIRATION

Cellular respiration occurs when oxygen is transported from the atmosphere to tissue cells, and carbon dioxide is removed and carried from the cells to the atmosphere. RBC hemoglobin is the carrier for these gases. Three processes—ventilation, diffusion, and perfusion—are essential for this to occur.

Ventilation is the mechanical exchange of air between the lungs and the atmosphere. *Inspiration* is the *active* phase of ventilation. It requires contraction of the diaphragm and external intercostal muscles to expand the thorax. When thoracic expansion occurs, intrapulmonic pressure becomes negative compared with atmospheric pressure, and air flows into the lungs. *Exhalation* is the *passive* phase of ventilation. It occurs when alveolar pressure increases due to elastic recoil of lung tissue and relaxation of the respiratory muscles, and air flows out of the lungs back into the atmosphere.

Ventilation is controlled by the brainstem, which responds to a rise in blood carbon dioxide level ($P{CO_2}$). As breathing eliminates CO_2, there is a negative feedback to the brain. Through exhalation of carbon dioxide (which with water forms the volatile acid carbonic acid in the bloodstream) the lungs play a vital role in maintaining the normal alkaline pH of the blood (7.35–7.45). Conditions that result in metabolic acidosis (e.g., diabetic ketoacidosis) make the blood more acidic, also stimulating the brainstem to increase the rate and depth of breathing. The resultant lowering of $P{CO_2}$ (exhalation of volatile acid or respiratory alkalosis) helps return the

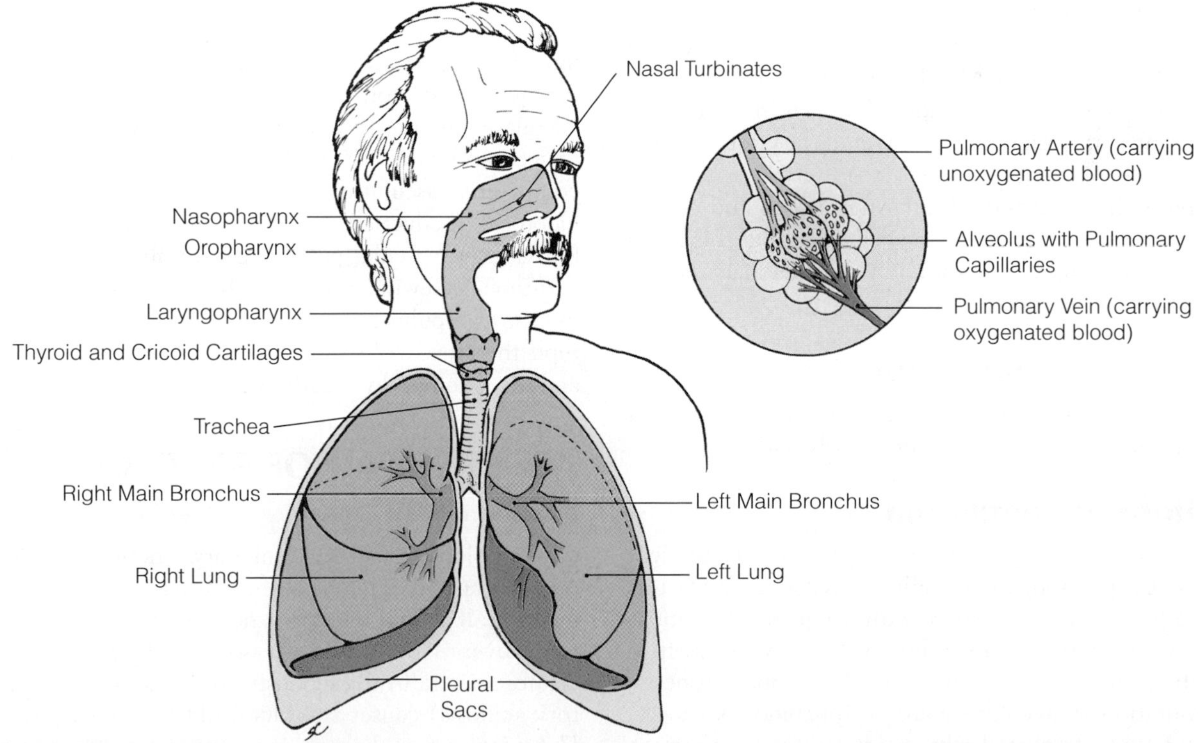

▲ Anatomy of the respiratory system.

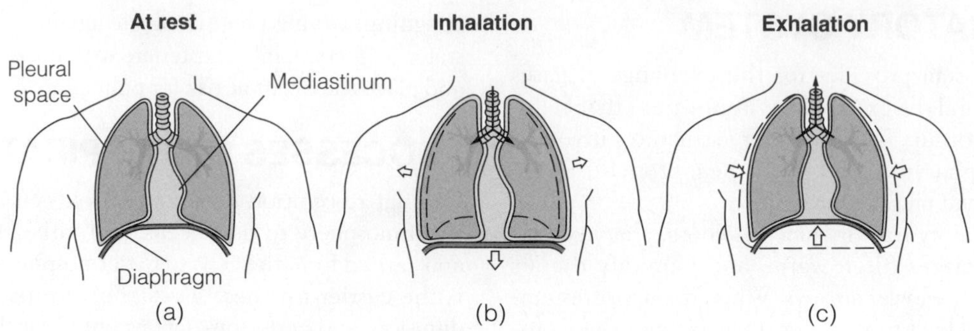

▲ Diaphragm contracts and descends on inspiration. Diaphragm relaxes and ascends on expiration.

blood pH to an alkaline state. This process is called respiratory compensation for metabolic acidosis.

Although CO_2 is the major stimulus for breathing, high sustained levels of carbonic acid depress the respiratory center, and respiratory arrest can occur. Individuals who have chronically elevated PCO_2 levels due to chronic obstructive pulmonary disease (COPD) may become insensitive to PCO_2 as a stimulus for breathing. Instead, their brain responds to a lower than normal PO_2 (less than 60 mmHg) to stimulate breathing. The administration of high flows of oxygen to such "hypoxic-dependent breathers" can eliminate their stimulus to breathe. Such individuals are at high risk for CO_2 narcosis.

Diffusion is the process of gas exchange between the alveolar air and the blood. The respiratory unit (respiratory bronchiole, alveolar ducts, and alveoli) is surrounded by capillaries, which allow for this exchange of oxygen and carbon dioxide. Alveoli must be ventilated and must remain diffusable for gas exchange to prevent respiratory failure. Oxygen tension in blood flowing through alveolar capillaries is *lower* than the oxygen tension in the alveoli. This pressure gradient causes oxygen to pass from the alveoli to the blood, thus increasing the PO_2 and "arterializing" the blood. Conversely, carbon dioxide tension is *higher* in the capillary blood than it is in the alveoli, thus promoting its diffusion into alveoli and the elimination of carbon dioxide on exhalation.

Perfusion is the process of circulating oxygen and carbon dioxide between the lungs and tissue cells. Without this blood transport and exchange of gases at both the pulmonary and tissue capillary levels, survival is impossible.

Alterations in Respiration

Alterations in tissue respiration can result from dysfunction of any of the three essential processes previously outlined.

Alterations in Ventilation

Ventilation depends on patent airways, the ability to clear airways, chest expansion, and compliant alveoli. Many factors and disease processes can interfere with adequate ventilation, including (1) any limitation in ability to clear airways (ineffective cough, intubation, decreased level of consciousness); (2) any limitation of alveolar expansion (pneumonia, congestive heart failure, fractured ribs, pain, thoracic deformity, neurologic disease, respiratory depressants, immobility); and (3) factors that interfere with surfactant activity, which is essential for alveolar inflation (narcotics, anesthetics, hypoventilation, high oxygen flow rates). Inadequate ventilation results in abnormal arterial blood gases (low PO_2 and low SaO_2, and eventually, an increase in PCO_2).

Pathologic processes that cause ineffective exhalation due to loss of elasticity (overcompliance) of small airways and alveoli also result in an increased PCO_2 (respiratory acidosis). Chronic obstructive pulmonary disease is an example.

Alterations in Diffusion

Diffusion is dependent on a partial pressure difference in gases and an adequate amount of permeable alveolar surface area. Any disease that thickens the alveolar membrane (fibrosis, congestive heart failure) reduces alveolar permeability and leads to a reduced PO_2 (hypoxemia). Alveolar surface area can be reduced by lobectomy or pneumonectomy.

Alterations in Perfusion

For cells to receive oxygen and give off their wastes, blood must flow at both the pulmonary and tissue capillary levels. Adequate perfusion depends on a normal blood volume, an adequate amount of hemoglobin capable of combining with oxygen and carbon dioxide, effective cardiac function, and competent vasculature. Any pathology that interferes with blood cell production, maintenance of blood volume, cardiac function, or vascular patency can result in inadequate tissue perfusion. Likewise, any factor that prevents blood from flowing through pulmonary capillaries (pulmonary embolism) disrupts the process of gas exchange for replenishment of oxygen and the elimination of carbon dioxide.

ASSESSMENT OF RESPIRATORY FUNCTION

Arterial blood gases and pulmonary function tests reflect pulmonary capacity. The pH of the blood is affected by pulmonary function. If carbon dioxide is not eliminated by the lungs due to hypoventilation for any reason, the PCO_2 rises. Since CO_2 creates an acid in the bloodstream, its accumulation (respiratory acidosis) causes the blood pH to decrease (acidemia). *Hypoventilation* is the only mechanism for PCO_2 accumulation and is encountered when factors depress the respiratory center, inhibit breathing, or a client has a disease, such as COPD, that prevents efficient exhalation. The peak flow meter measures maximum expiratory flow rates. These units are used by asthma clients to regularly self-assess. A declining flow rate (by 20%) may indicate a worsening condition. Serial measurements help the physician to adjust the client's medical regimen. *Hyperventilation* (due to anxiety, neurologic dysfunction, or iatrogenic overventilation) causes the PCO_2 to fall below normal (respiratory alkalosis) and the blood pH to rise above normal (alkalemia).

Arterial blood gas (ABG) studies also evaluate diffusion and perfusion as reflected by the PO_2 and SaO_2. Pulse oximetry is often preferred over ABGs as a cost-effective laboratory test of SaO_2.

It is essential that ventilation of alveoli is matched with blood flowing through alveolar capillaries. If alveolar ventilation occurs without matched perfusion (e.g., pulmonary embolism), the PO_2 falls, but the PCO_2 remains normal because of the greater solubility of CO_2; the PCO_2 may even decrease due to hyperventilation (respiratory alkalosis). Conversely, if the alveoli are perfused but not ventilated (as in atelectasis), the blood is not adequately oxygenated. This condition results in a low PO_2 and a normal PCO_2, because carbon dioxide is highly diffusible. Continued hypoventilation, however, eventually results in an increased PCO_2 (respiratory acidosis).

Normal pulmonary ventilation and perfusion are reflected by *normal blood gas values*: *Note*: Pulse oximetry (SPO_2) allows noninvasive estimation of SaO_2.

pH	7.35–7.45
PCO_2	35–45 mmHg
HCO_3	22–26 mEq/L
PO_2	80–100 mmHg (breathing room air)
SaO_2	90%–100%

Pulmonary function (spirometry) tests measure lung volumes and capacity and help differentiate restrictive and obstructive defects of ventilation.

VC (vital capacity)	75%–80% of that predicted by age, sex, and height (decreased in restrictive disease)
FEV (forced expiratory volume)	65%–85% of VC in 1 second and 95% in 3 seconds (decreased in obstructive disease)
FEV_1 (forced expiratory volume in 1 sec)	Normal = 75% VC (decreased in obstructive disease)
FEV 25–75	Measures expiratory flow capacity of small airways; most sensitive measure of small airway disease

Nursing Interventions

The goal of respiratory nursing interventions is to maintain, restore, or to artificially provide the vital functions of the respiratory system.

Nursing interventions are used routinely to help prevent pulmonary complications for clients with known pulmonary problems, for clients at risk for pulmonary complications (e.g., immobility), or for surgical clients who have undergone general anesthesia and who experience pain.

These interventions include pain management; maintaining adequate hydration (2–3 L of water/day unless contraindicated); turning to help ventilate dependent lung areas; deep breathing to stimulate surfactant and inflate hypoventilated alveoli; coughing to remove retained secretions; airway suctioning to assist ineffective airway clearance; and early ambulation. Protective splinting of operative sites promotes client comfort, adherence, and prevents wound strain.

Continuous positive airway pressure (CPAP)/bilevel positive airway pressure (BiPAP) is the noninvasive application of positive pressure to upper airways to prevent their obstruction by the soft tissues that surround them. This mode improves alveolar ventilation and decreases PCO_2, respiratory rate, and the work of breathing. Clients with obstructive sleep apnea (OSA), central sleep apnea, or respiratory insufficiency may benefit from this therapy. It can also provide life support for clients who have decided to forego endotracheal intubation.

Similarly, oscillating positive expiratory pressure devices function as a cough support to assist COPD clients to clear their airways.

Techniques such as postural drainage, chest percussion, and vibration (CPT) utilize gravity and mechanical energy to help mobilize secretions. These measures are reserved for the client who produces excessive amounts (>25 mL/day) of thick secretions that are difficult to mobilize.

A variety of devices are used to deliver supplemental oxygen to the hypoxic client (SaO_2 under 90%). These devices differ in the degree that they control the client's inspired air.

The most common clinical manifestations indicative of inadequate ventilation are:

- Tachycardia (heart rate over 100/min)
- Tachypnea (breathing rate over 24/min)
- Anxiety reflected in facial expression
- Restlessness or confusion
- Use of accessory muscles for breathing
- Change in cognition or level of response
- Increased blood pressure

Early recognition of these indicators of possible hypoxemia should prompt further investigation and appropriate intervention

Artificial means to establish and maintain patent airways include oral/pharyngeal and endotracheal devices. Bypassing the body's natural protective airway and communication processes, these devices render the client dependent and at risk for serious respiratory complications. Clients with artificial airways require additional nursing measures to ensure ventilation and to protect the respiratory system. Such skills include suctioning, tracheostomy care, providing a means for communication, and regular oral hygiene.

If air or fluid accumulates in the intrapleural or mediastinal space due to trauma, disease, or surgery, the lung cannot expand. Cardiac tamponade with decreased cardiac output can occur due to decreased venous return secondary to compression of mediastinal structures. Chest tubes are placed to evacuate air and fluid from the pleural or mediastinal space to facilitate lung re-expansion and prevent increased mediastinal pressure. In certain postoperative settings, chest drainage may be reinfused to replace blood lost.

NURSING DIAGNOSES

The following nursing diagnoses may be appropriate to use on client care plans when the components are related to respiratory conditions.

NURSING DIAGNOSIS	RELATED FACTORS
Activity Intolerance	Imbalance between oxygen supply and demand
Ineffective Airway Clearance	Fatigue; excessive secretions; pain; immobility; neuromuscular disease; chronic obstructive pulmonary disease
Aspiration, Risk for	Depressed airway protective mechanisms; presence of artificial airway; enteral feeding, neuromuscular disease
Ineffective Breathing Patterns	Immobility; fatigue, pain; neuromuscular impairment; chronic respiratory disease; pharmacologic agents
Impaired Gas Exchange	Ventilation/perfusion imbalance; hypoventilation, chronic obstructive pulmonary disease, airway obstruction, heart failure, pulmonary edema
Disturbed Sleep Pattern	Obstructive airway (sleep apnea)

CLEANSE HANDS The single most important nursing action to decrease the incidence of hospital-based infection is hand hygiene. *Remember to wash your hands or use antibacterial gel before and after each client contact.*

IDENTIFY CLIENT Before every procedure, introduce yourself and check two forms of client identification, not including room number. These actions prevent errors and conform to The Joint Commission standards.

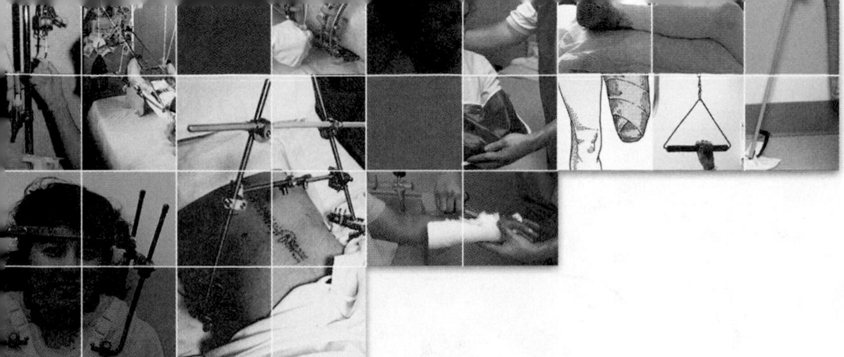

Chapter 30

UNIT 1

Respiratory Preventive and Maintenance Measures

Nursing Process Data

ASSESSMENT Data Base

- Observe client's physical ability to perform exercise (e.g., to assume Fowler's position, energy level, degree of pain experienced, and need for pain medication).
- Observe rhythm, rate, and depth of breathing.
- Auscultate breath sounds.
- Note client's report of dyspnea or signs of increased work of breathing.
- Note presence of adventitious sounds.
- Note proximity of incision to muscles necessary for breathing and coughing.
- Assess need for supported ventilation/resuscitation.

PLANNING Objectives

- To improve pulmonary ventilation.
- To conserve energy and decrease the work of breathing.
- To loosen secretions and promote clear airways.
- To prevent hypoventilation and hypoxemia.

IMPLEMENTATION Procedures

EVALUATION Expected Outcomes

- Breath sounds are normal; adventitious sounds are cleared.
- Vital capacity, pulmonary ventilation, and gas exchange are improved/supported.
- Client reaches predetermined tidal volume level when using incentive spirometer.
- Client's energy is conserved and work of breathing is eased.
- Secretions are loosened and airways are clear.
- Client monitors peak-flow appropriately.
- Client experiences an improved sleep pattern.

Pearson Nursing Student Resources

Find additional review materials at **nursing.pearsonhighered.com**

Prepare for success with NCLEX®-style practice questions and Skill Checklists

Instructing Client to Deep Breathe

Equipment

Straight chair or hospital bed at 90° elevation

Preparation

1. Perform hand hygiene.
2. Provide privacy.
3. Explain the rationale for the procedure.
4. Help client to sit straight up in bed with knees slightly flexed or on side of bed. ▸ ***Rationale:*** This position promotes maximum lung expansion.

Procedure

1. Demonstrate the deep breathing steps, allowing time for client to practice each step.
2. Place your hand or have client place hands palm down around the sides of client's lower ribs. ▸ ***Rationale:*** This action supports deep breathing and assists you to evaluate depth of inspiration.
3. Tell client to breathe in slowly through nose until chest expands and abdomen rises visibly.
4. Have client hold a sustained maximal inspiration 3–5 seconds, then exhale slowly through the mouth.
5. Evaluate client's response to determine how often exercise should be performed—diminished breath sounds or presence of crackles indicates need for frequent deep breathing, turning, and early ambulation.

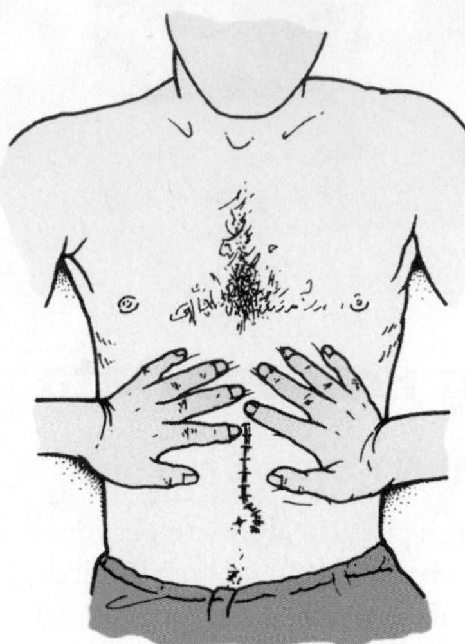

▲ Nurse demonstrates placement of hands on either side of incision for support.

EVIDENCE-BASED PRACTICE

Improving Oxygenation

Studies show that the Po_2 is lower when the client with unilateral lung disease is positioned on the diseased side. Since the dependent lung has greater blood flow, placing the healthy lung down improves oxygenation.

Source: Bridges, E. (2001). Ask the experts. *Critical Care Nurse, 21*(6), 66.

Instructing Client to Cough

Equipment

Straight chair or hospital bed at 90° elevation
Pillows for positioning and incisional support
Tissues for secretions
Protective gear (gloves, gown, goggles, mask) as indicated

Preparation

1. Premedicate client if indicated for pain relief.
2. Perform hand hygiene.
3. Provide privacy.
4. Explain procedure to client.
5. Don protective gear if indicated.
6. Provide client with tissues.

Procedure

1. Place client in upright position, upper body positioned slightly forward. ▸ ***Rationale:*** This position assists client to cough more effectively.
2. Ask client to slowly take two or three deep breaths through the nose and exhale through the mouth.
3. Instruct client to inhale deeply, hold breath for several seconds, lean forward, and cough, using abdominal, thigh, and buttock muscles. ▸ ***Rationale:*** This promotes a more effective cough.
4. Instruct client with pulmonary condition to exhale through pursed lips and to "huff" while coughing in mid-exhalation (not at end of deep inspiration). ▸ ***Rationale:*** The "huff cough" maintains an open glottis; helps prevent high expiratory pressures that collapse diseased airways, thus facilitating movement of secretions along the tracheobronchial tree; and reduces fatigue.

Clinical Alert

Deep breathing is indicated, but coughing is *contraindicated* for the client post-eye, -ear, -brain, or -neck surgery, or if efforts are nonproductive.

5. Support any incision with the palms of your or client's hands, or place a rolled pillow firmly against the incision. ▶ ***Rationale:*** This prevents incisional strain and encourages client to cough more effectively.
6. Encourage client to deep breathe and cough more frequently if cough is productive. Explain why coughing is beneficial and keep tissues and disposal receptacle handy. ▶ ***Rationale:*** Accumulated secretions in airways promote bacterial growth and interfere with ventilation.

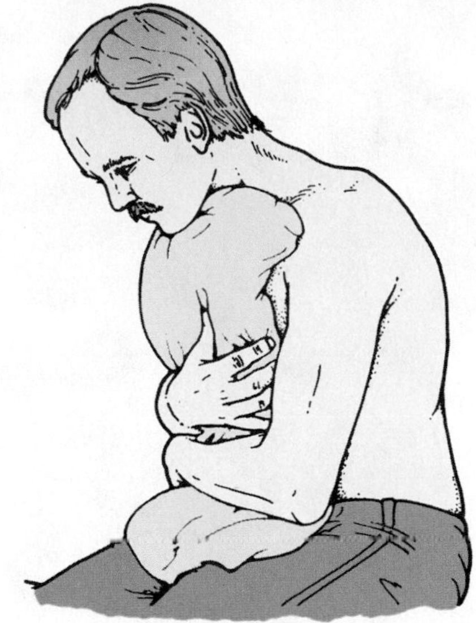

▲ Holding pillow against incision when coughing prevents incision strain.

Teaching Diaphragmatic Breathing

Equipment

Hospital bed in flat position

Preparation

1. Check physician's orders and client care plan.
2. Perform hand hygiene.
3. Provide privacy.
4. Inform client that the purpose of this exercise is to learn how to breathe by using abdominal muscles.

NOTE: Clients with COPD tend to overwork the upper chest muscles and suck in the abdomen on inspiration, making it difficult for the diaphragm to descend. This exercise improves breathing efficiency.

Procedure

1. Place your hands on client's abdomen, below ribs.
2. Have client breathe in through the nose and try to push stomach outward against your hands.
3. Instruct client to hold breath for 3–5 seconds to keep alveoli open.
4. Have client breathe out slowly through the mouth as you apply slight pressure at the base of the ribs.
5. Encourage client to practice diaphragmatic breathing frequently, using own hands to feel the abdomen rise.
6. Placing progressive increments of weight on the abdomen (recumbent position) strengthens the diaphragm, while practice improves neuromuscular coordination of diaphragmatic breathing.

Teaching Use of Incentive Spirometer (IS)

Equipment

Hospital bed or straight chair

Incentive spirometer with flow rate indicator (save bag for storage of device)

Tissues for secretions

Preparation

1. Check physician's orders and client care plan.
2. Gather equipment.
3. Perform hand hygiene.
4. Explain purpose and procedure to client.
5. If preoperative measurement was not done, use guide in spirometer package to determine client's volume goal, and set marker at this goal.
6. Attach open end of tubing to stem on front of exerciser.
7. Auscultate lungs before and after using IS. ▶ ***Rationale:*** This evaluates effectiveness of spirometry.

Procedure

1. Instruct client to hold exerciser, place mouth tightly around mouthpiece, and breathe in a trial breath through the mouth. ▶ ***Rationale:*** Client can see the flow rate indicator on side of unit to visualize appropriate *rate* for inhalation.

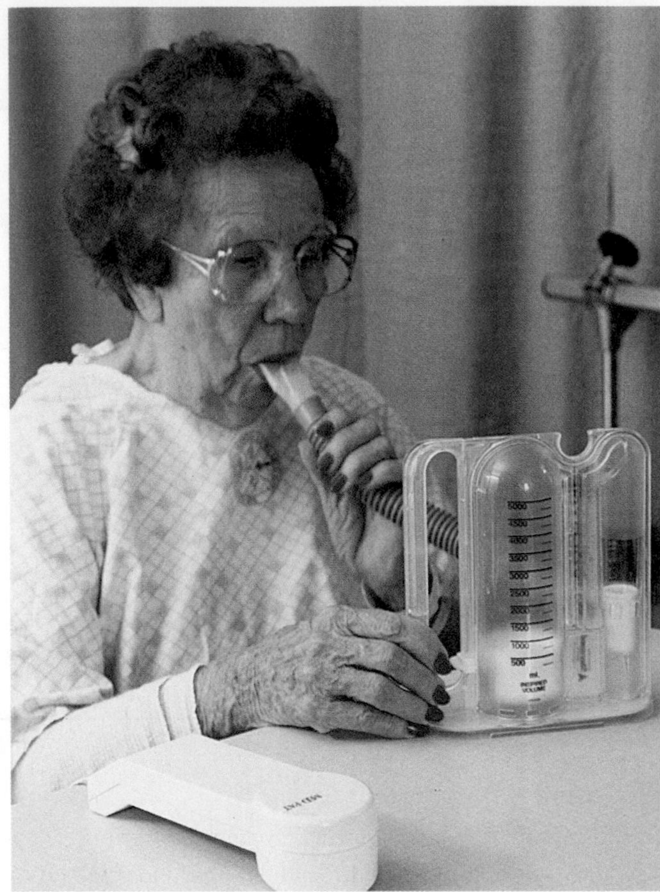

▲ Client places mouth tightly around mouthpiece and inhales slowly, while watching yellow flow rate indicator, to promote lung expansion.

2. Explain that a slow deep breath is better than a fast breath.
3. Instruct client to exhale completely, then place mouth tightly around mouthpiece.
4. Instruct client to inhale slowly to raise and maintain yellow flow rate indicator at the "best" flow rate range, and continue inhaling to try to raise piston to prescribed (or preoperative measured) volume level.
5. Instruct client to remove mouthpiece but hold breath at maximum inspiration 3–5 seconds, then exhale through pursed lips. Repeat a few times, then cough.
6. Encourage client to use spirometer hourly, coordinating use with TV program breaks, for instance, as a reminder.
7. Provide positive feedback as client uses IS to reattain predetermined inspiratory capacity, using marked goal as an incentive.
8. Replace unit in bag when not in use and keep in accessible place for client.

EVIDENCE-BASED PRACTICE

In patients undergoing coronary artery bypass grafting, there is no evidence of benefit from incentive spirometry compared with preoperative education or standard postsurgical PT for preventing postoperative pulmonary complication, improving pulmonary function and oxygenation, and reducing length of hospital stay. There is evidence that IS may have some drawbacks compared with positive airway pressure techniques.

Source: Freitas, E. R., Soares, B. G., Cardoso, J. R., & Atallah, A. N. (2007). Incentive spirometry for preventing pulmonary complications after coronary artery bypass graft. *Cochrane Database of Systematic Reviews*, (3), CD004466.

Teaching Peak Flow Measurement

Equipment

Peak flow meter with instructions for client

Preparation

1. Check physician's orders or client care plan.
2. Gather equipment.
3. Perform hand hygiene.
4. Explain purpose of procedure and provide instruction sheet to client.

Procedure

1. Assist client to follow product instructions to assemble meter.
2. Instruct client to attach mouthpiece to peak flow meter, if desired. ▶ ***Rationale:*** Most meters can be used with or without mouthpiece.
3. Slide indicator to bottom of meter scale to zero position.
4. Instruct client to inhale as deeply as possible, then place mouth around mouthpiece, forming a tight seal. If possible, client should be standing.

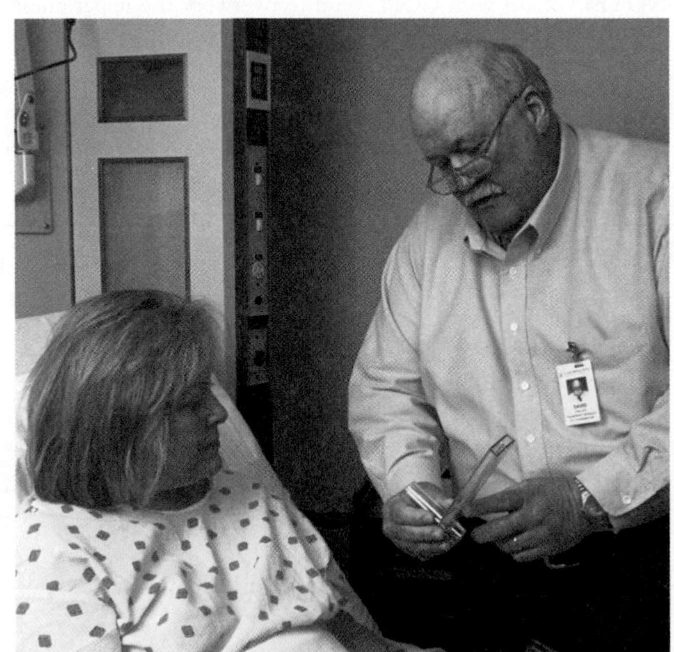

▲ Slide indicator to bottom of meter scale to bring indicator to zero point.

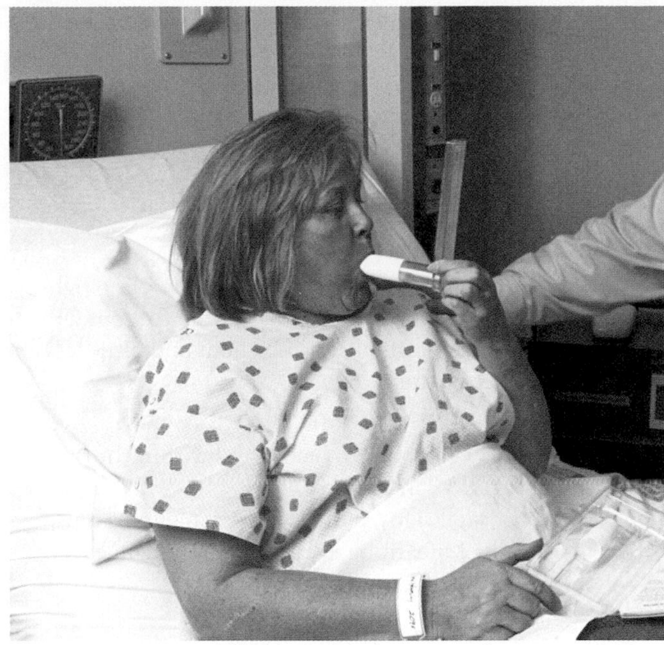

▲ Have client blow out through mouth as hard and fast as possible—indicator moves up scale to record peak expiratory flow (L/min).

5. Have client blow out through mouth as hard and fast as possible. ▸ ***Rationale:*** As client forcefully exhales, indicator moves up scale to record client's peak expiratory flow (liters per minute).
6. Repeat peak flow measurement three times and record highest value. ▸ ***Rationale:*** Client may keep daily record of peak flow values and report significant changes.
7. Instruct client to clean unit weekly, following manufacturer's instructions.

EVIDENCE-BASED PRACTICE

Peak Flow Monitoring

Color-coded zones indicate forced expiratory volume. The green zone indicates 80–100% of the individual's best, yellow zone indicates 60–80%, red zone is less than 60%. Client should take appropriate actions prescribed by the healthcare provider if peak flow is below the red zone.

National Heart, Lung, and Blood Institute Expert panel report 3: Guidelines for diagnosis and management of asthma (2007). http://www.nhibi.nih.gov/guidelines/asthma/asthgdln.pdf

Teaching Use of Oscillating Positive Expiratory Pressure (PEP) Cough Support Device

Equipment

"Flutter valve system" with adjustment dial, one-way inspiratory valve, and detachable mouthpiece

Preparation

1. Identify client.
2. Explain use and purpose of device. ▸ ***Rationale:*** The device functions to maintain positive pressure throughout exhalation to facilitate pulmonary secretion removal—cough support device.
3. Open packet and save for device storage.
4. Secure all device connections.
5. Adjust vibration frequency dial clockwise to low resistance setting when initiating therapy. ▸ ***Rationale:*** Higher frequency of vibrating pressure waves and higher resistance of opening changes produce higher resistance to exhalation.
6. Position client sitting with elbows resting on table.

Procedure

1. Instruct client to place mouthpiece in mouth with tight seal during exhalation.
2. Have client take a deep breath in and hold it for 2–3 seconds.
3. Instruct client to exhale through the device, prolonging exhalation actively (not forcefully, but three to four times longer than inhalation) as the device vibrates.
4. If client cannot maintain exhalation for 3–4 seconds, adjust dial clockwise to increase resistance and allow client to exhale at a lower flow rate. ▸ ***Rationale:*** Proper resistance range produces inspiratory to expiratory (I:E) ratio of 1:3 or 1:4.
5. Once a proper range is determined, the client may change adjustments for harder or softer exhalation to meet a subjective comfort with the device. ▸ ***Rationale:*** Adjustments may be necessary to meet client needs.
6. Clean mouthpiece and return device to storage bag.
7. Encourage client to use the "PEP" device for 10–20 minutes, four times a day.

NOTE: This device directs exhaled air through an opening that alternately closes and opens the path of air flow. This maintains a vibratory positive pressure through exhalation (common lay term is "flutter valve").

Providing CPAP/BiPAP

Equipment

Nasal mask, full face mask, or nasal pillows of proper size (S, M, L)
Indelible marker
Airflow generator
Delivery tubing
If ordered:
  Oxygen source
  Oxygen tubing
  Pulse oximetry

Preparation

1. Check physician's orders or client's care plan.
2. Gather equipment.
3. Perform hand hygiene.

Clinical Alert

Clients with obstructive sleep apnea (OSA) are at risk for cardiovascular complications including hypertension, stroke, arrhythmias, heart failure, and myocardial infarction.

4. Explain purpose of procedure to client and provide written instructions for home use.
5. Have client wash face.

Procedure

1. Connect CPAP/BiPAP device delivery tubing to pressure generator.
2. Plug pressure generator into grounded outlet.
3. Connect oxygen delivery tubing into device tubing adapter port (if ordered).
4. Turn on pressure generator.

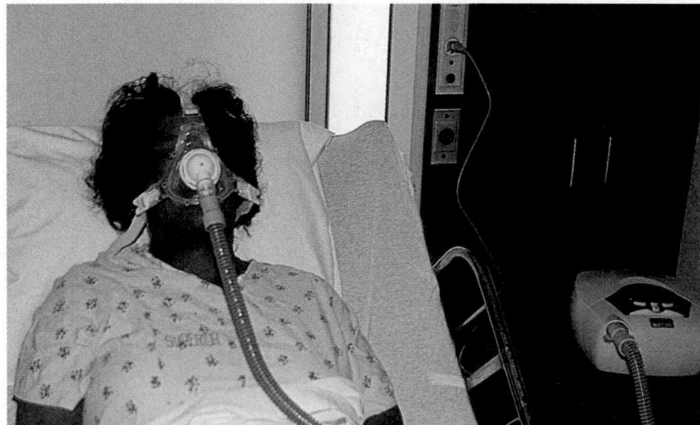

▲ Client receiving CPAP via face mask. Machine is capable of CPAP and BiPAP.

5. Establish CPAP/BiPAP parameters:
   a. RAMP: time frame for pressure achievement, usually 5–15 minutes.
   b. CPAP or BiPAP setting.
   c. Respiratory rate if applicable.
   d. FIO_2 if applicable.
6. Apply device over client's nose or face, avoiding tight fit, and mark straps for future proper fit. ▶ ***Rationale:*** Tight fit is uncomfortable for the client and unnecessary for device functioning.
7. Establish continuous pulse oximetry if ordered.
   a. ABGs may be obtained before and within the first hour of BiPAP initiation.
   b. Monitor vital signs, pulse oximetry, mental status, and work of breathing every 30 minutes X2, every hour X6, and every 2 hours X8.

Clinical Alert

Respiratory therapy and biomedical engineering departments must check to ensure proper functioning and electrical safety of outside equipment (e.g., CPAP) brought from home to be used in an agency.

- CPAP provides single positive pressure to establish minimal airway value (e.g., 5 mmHg) at end of exhalation.
- BiPAP provides two positive airway pressures, one to assist peak pressure on inhalation (e.g., 10 cm H_2O) and a lower one (e.g., 5 cm H_2O) to establish minimal airway value at end of exhalation.
- BiPAP with Rate Set provides two positive airway pressures and a set respiratory rate to augment breathing for the client with respiratory insufficiency. This capability qualifies this unit as a "noninvasive mechanical ventilator." The client is spared intubation.
- BiPAP Autotitration Device senses and measures the client's airflow and adjusts its pressure setting automatically to maintain airway patency.

Clinical Alert

Clients using CPAP/BiPAP are constantly at risk for aspiration and subsequent respiratory complications. The candidate must be alert and responsive orally, must demonstrate airway protective measures (cough and swallow), and must not be restrained or sedated. Opioids relax the pharynx and contribute further to airway obstruction.

CPAP/BiPAP should never be used on a sedated client. There is great danger of aspiration should the client vomit.

8. Tell client to detach tubing from face device if getting up during the night.
9. Monitor client periodically.
10. Teach client to clean device according to manufacturer's instructions.

Providing Bag–Valve–Mask Ventilation

Equipment

Manual resuscitator bag with nonrebreathing valve
Oxygen source and tubing
Airway adapter or face mask

Preparation

1. Determine that client's breathing is absent or inadequate.
2. Summon an assistant if client is not intubated. ▸ ***Rationale:*** If no artificial airway present, two responders are preferred. Assistant holds mask while nurse compresses resuscitator bag.
3. Gather equipment.
4. Place client in supine position.
5. Connect mask or airway adapter to bag.
6. Connect oxygen tubing and oxygen flow meter to bag inlet.

Procedure

1. Turn oxygen flow meter wide open to 15 L/min ("flush").
2. Stand at client's head and hyperextend client's neck.
3. Place apex of mask over client's nose and place base of mask between client's lower lip and chin. ▸ ***Rationale:*** This ensures a tight seal.
4. Use dominant hand to compress central portion of resuscitator bag until client's chest rises (1–2 seconds), then allow exhalation. ▸ ***Rationale:*** Overinflation may result in gastric distention.
5. Provide ventilations every 5 seconds for an apneic adult, noting that client's chest rises and falls with each compression.
6. Check to see if client breathes spontaneously; if so, give compressions in synchrony to support ventilation.
7. Observe for possible gastric distention. ▸ ***Rationale:*** Gastric insufflation may result in regurgitation and aspiration.
8. Reposition client's head if gastric distention is present and reduce compression volume, noting that client's chest rises.
9. Notify physician or respiratory care practitioner for further client evaluation.

▲ The BiPAP Vision noninvasive ventilator support system has most features of any standard mechanical ventilator.

Clinical Alert

If client's chest does not rise with ventilations, suspect foreign body airway obstruction. See Chapter 31 for Abdominal Thrust maneuver.

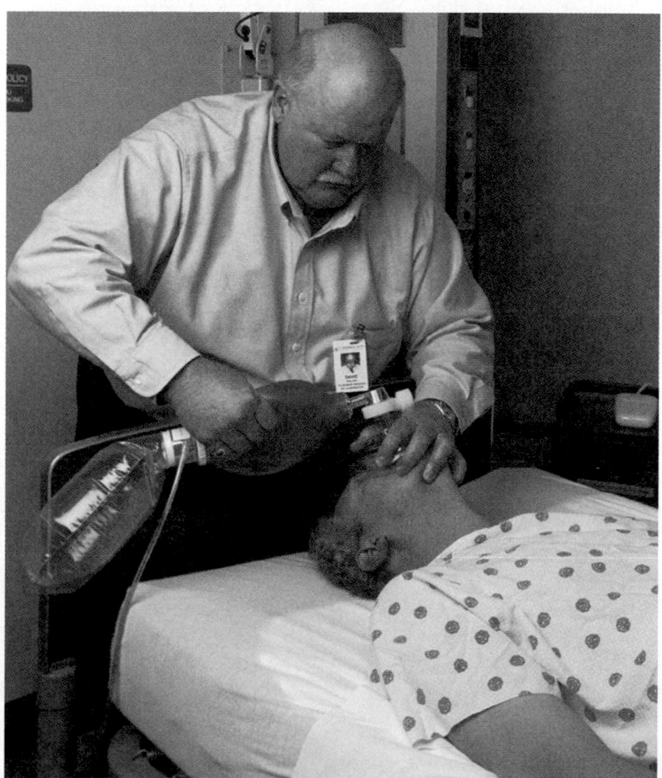

▲ Compress central portion of resuscitator bag until client's chest rises, then allow exhalation.

Bag-Valve-Mask With Rescue Pod

The bag-valve-mask with Rescue Pod (circulatory enhancer) is used only for clients who are *unable to breathe spontaneously* (e.g., during CPR). This device with one-way valve is attached between the resuscitator bag and mask or airway tube. It allows the rescuer to deliver air to the client.

The system accepts attachment of an expiratory filter for epidemiologic considerations and an external PEEP device for maintaining positive expiratory pressure to enhance diffusion (PO_2) during its use. A pressure manometer indicates pressure from resuscitator bag compression. Desired pressure is sufficient to achieve adequate chest wall movement (normally 15–25 cm H_2O). Maintaining minimal necessary ventilation pressure helps prevent barotraumas to lung tissue and/or gastric air insufflation. The Rescue Pod device must be removed *immediately* if the client is able to resume spontaneous breathing.

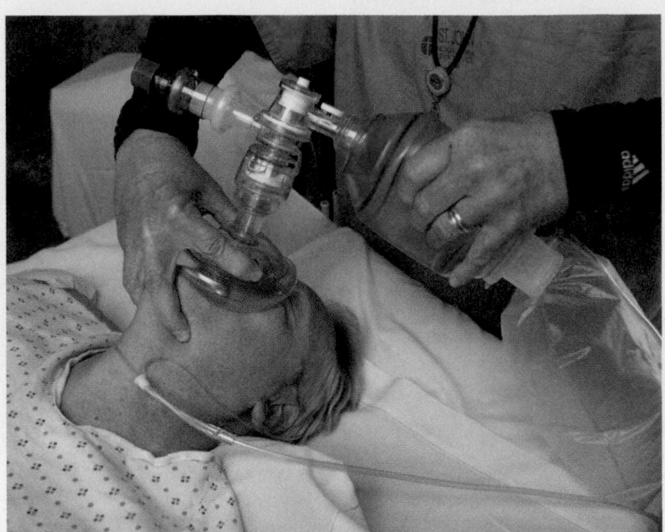

DOCUMENTATION for Respiratory Preventive and Maintenance Measures

- Pre- and post-intervention breath sounds and adventitious sounds
- Frequency of deep breathing exercises or use of IS
- Whether cough is productive or not
- Amount and character of secretions expectorated
- Changes in vital signs, SpO_2, or other client responses
- Inspiratory capacity attained with IS
- Circumstances necessitating use of mask and bag resuscitator
- Client outcome after manual breathing
- Peak flow measurement: highest of three therapy sequential measures
- Client teaching and return demonstration

For CPAP/BiPAP

- Type of CPAP/BiPAP device used
- Established parameters
- Respiratory rate if programmed
- FIO_2 if ordered
- SpO_2 findings pre- and post- therapy
- Client's tolerance of therapy

CRITICAL THINKING Application

Expected Outcomes

- Client coughs effectively, supporting incision to prevent strain.
- Client is able to breathe through nose without distress.
- Client demonstrates appropriate use of incentive spirometer.
- Client experiences benefits of CPAP/BiPAP with undisturbed sleep.

Unexpected Outcomes	Alternative Actions
Client is unwilling to complete exercise because of misunderstanding or fear of pain or wound dehiscence.	• Inform client that fresh incision is secure. • Instruct again on rationale and necessity for procedure. • Support incision area more fully, using the palms of your hands or a firmly rolled pillow to allay fears of dehiscence. • Medicate 30–60 minutes before using spirometer and coughing.
Nasal congestion inhibits client's breathing capability.	• Ask client to blow nose before the breathing exercise. • Check with physician to prescribe medications, such as saline spray to open nasal passages.

Client is unable to master use of incentive spirometer device.	• Instruct client to start slowly and increase volume over several exercise sessions. • Supervise practice with encouragement. • Provide positive reinforcement with increments in volume. • Ensure that client does regular deep breathing if device interferes with client adherence. • Turn client every 2 hr and encourage ROM and early ambulation to help stimulate deep breathing and secretion mobilization. • Instruct client to deep breathe effectively without using the spirometer: to inhale slowly and deeply through the nose, hold the breath several seconds, then exhale.
Client doesn't tolerate BiPAP therapy.	• Loosen the appliance since some leakage is acceptable and does not compromise function of the device. • Increase RAMP time to improve tolerance/increase comfort. • Use nasal spray (saline solution) to reduce nasal congestion. • Find a more individually suited device. • Reassess true need for BiPAP.

Chapter 30

UNIT 2

Chest Physiotherapy (CPT)

Nursing Process Data

ASSESSMENT Data Base

- Note any contraindicating conditions for CPT: acute exacerbation of COPD, pneumonia *without* evidence of significant sputum production, osteoporosis, lung cancer, cerebral edema.
- Determine rate and depth of breathing and heart rate/rhythm.
- Auscultate breath sounds and check for adventitious sounds or excessive sputum production (over 25 mL/day).
- Note time elapsed since eating (perform CPT between meals to prevent regurgitation).
- Observe quality of secretions. Thick, tenacious secretions may require aerosol therapy before treatment.
- Note client's ABGs/SpO_2 and changes on chest x-ray report.

PLANNING Objectives

- To decrease respiratory rate and improve ventilation and gas exchange
- To reduce client's feeling of shortness of breath
- To facilitate clearance of retained secretions
- To assist client to cough more productively and effectively
- To decrease adventitious lung sounds
- To decrease risk of infection due to stasis of secretions

IMPLEMENTATION Procedures

EVALUATION Expected Outcomes

- Chest x-ray shows improvement.
- Breath sounds and adventitious sounds improve on auscultation.
- Shortness of breath is reduced.
- Sputum production is over 25 mL/day (to justify continuation of CPT).
- ABGs/SpO_2 values are improved.

Preparing Client for CPT

Equipment

Hospital bed or other surface to place client in head-down position
Gown or towel (optional)
Tissues
Container for sputum
Clean gloves
Stethoscope
Pulse oximeter (if indicated)
Mouthwash/oral hygiene product

Procedure

1. Validate physician's order for CPT. ▸ ***Rationale:*** These procedures are tiring to clients, time-consuming, and contraindicated in cases of osteoporosis, pulmonary embolism, cardiac conditions, lung cancer, or other conditions not associated with excessive sputum production.
2. Perform hand hygiene.
3. Administer CPT before or at least 2 hr after meals to prevent vomiting.
4. Establish the location of lung segments if the entire lung field is to undergo CPT; the affected segment should be drained first. ▸ ***Rationale:*** Usually, the lower areas are the most affected.
5. Provide privacy.
6. Prepare client by explaining CPT and purpose.
7. Auscultate chest for breath sounds and adventitious sounds before therapy.
8. Obtain pulse oximetry (SpO_2) if indicated before therapy.
9. Place towel over skin when performing CPT (optional).

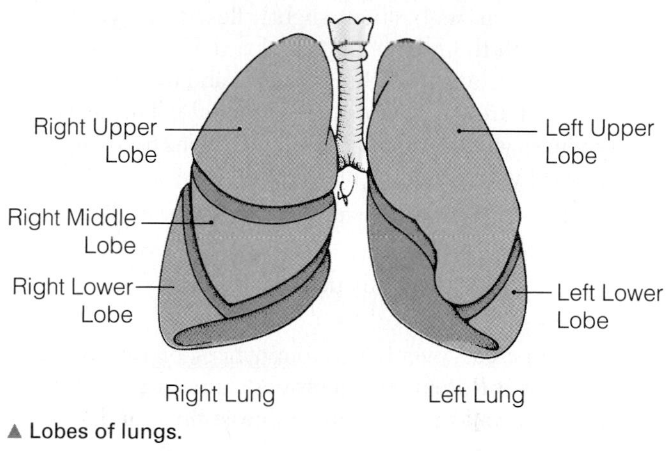

▲ **Lobes of lungs.**

Performing Postural Drainage

Equipment

See Preparing Client for CPT.

Preparation

1. See Preparing Client for CPT.
2. Perform hand hygiene.

Procedure

1. Loosen any tight clothing.
2. Lower head of bed slowly so that client's head is positioned at no greater than a 25° downward angle. ▸ ***Rationale:*** Gravity helps mobilize secretions.
3. Place sputum container and tissues in client's reach.
4. Tell client to remain in position for 3–15 minutes. ▸ ***Rationale:*** Percussion and vibration may be added to help mobilize secretions (*skills to follow*).
5. Instruct client to expectorate secretions.
6. Instruct client to turn to other side, then to supine position, then repeat procedure.

NOTE: Clients should deep breathe between position changes.

7. Assist client to slowly return to normal sitting position after coughing in dependent positions.
8. Determine pulse oximetry if ordered.
9. Auscultate chest areas for improved breath sounds.
10. Note character and measure sputum, then discard.
11. Remove gloves and perform hand hygiene.
12. Offer oral hygiene after secretion expectoration.

EVIDENCE-BASED PRACTICE

Bronchial Hygiene Therapy

There is no firm scientific evidence that CPT measures are effective in preventing pulmonary complications. In order to justify continuation of postural drainage, the client must demonstrate one or more of the expected outcomes listed on unit opening page.

Source: Goodfellow, L., & Jones, M. (2002). Bronchial hygiene therapy. *American Journal of Nursing 102*(1), 38.

Performing Chest Percussion

Equipment

See Preparing Client for CPT.

Preparation

1. See Preparing Client for CPT.
2. Perform hand hygiene.

Procedure

1. Cover area to be percussed with gown or cloth towel (optional).
2. Holding arms with elbows slightly flexed, cup your hands with thumbs and fingers closed. Keeping wrists loose and relaxed, rhythmically flex and extend wrists to clap over area to be drained. ▸ ***Rationale:*** This motion produces vibrations that loosen secretions for easier removal with coughing or suctioning.
3. Percuss by alternating hands and listen for hollow sound with strikes.
4. Slowly and rhythmically percuss each area for 3–5 minutes.
5. Do not percuss over bony prominences, breasts, or tender areas. ▸ ***Rationale:*** Vibrations are not transmitted to the chest wall through bone or breast tissue and percussion in these areas can cause discomfort.
6. Encourage client to "huff" cough after percussion of lung areas.
7. Auscultate all lung areas for changes in breath sounds.
8. Don gloves, note character and measure quantity of sputum, and discard.
9. Remove gloves and perform hand hygiene.
10. Offer oral hygiene.
11. Document procedure and client's response.

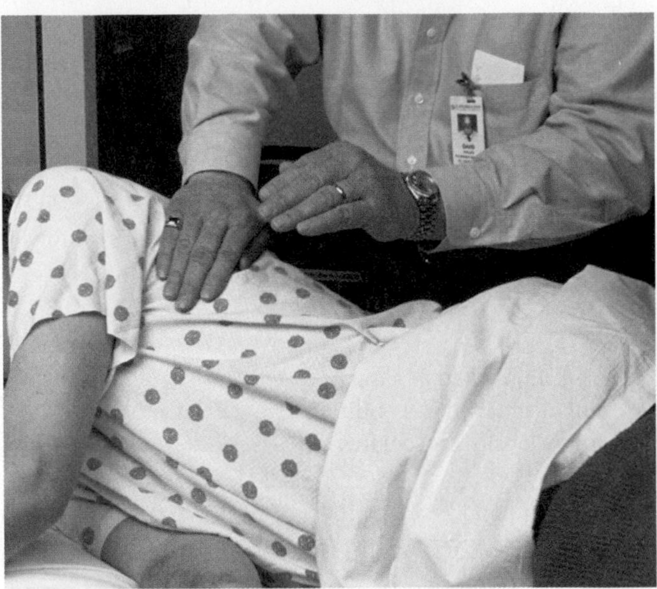

▲ Perform percussion and vibration with each position change.

Clinical Alert

Since chest percussion is taxing and time-consuming for both client and nurse, it is indicated only in clients with serious secretion retention (e.g., client with cystic fibrosis).

Performing Chest Vibration

Equipment

See Preparing Client for CPT.

Preparation

1. See Preparing Client for CPT.
2. Perform hand hygiene.

Procedure

1. Perform vibration after postural drainage and percussion in each position.
2. Cover area to be vibrated with gown or towel (optional).
3. Instruct client to breathe in through nose and exhale slowly through pursed lips.
4. Place your hands flat over area to be vibrated or place one hand on top of the other. Keep your arms and shoulders straight and wrists stiff.
5. Have client inhale deeply.
6. As client exhales through pursed lips, use moderate pressure to vibrate chest by quickly contracting and

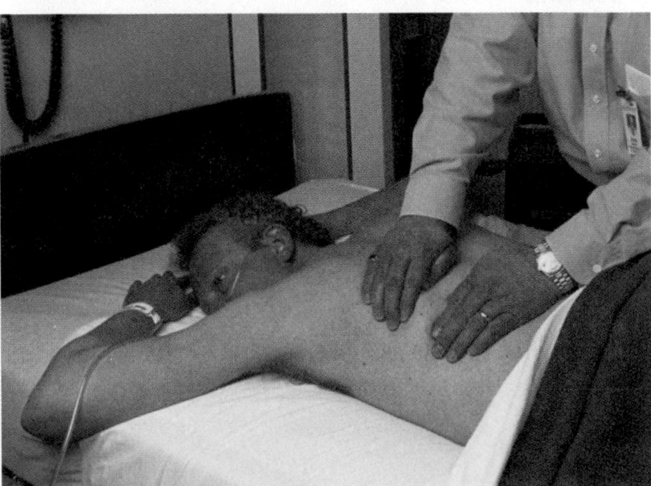

▲ Place hands flat over area to be vibrated, keeping wrists stiff.

relaxing your arms and shoulders. ▶ ***Rationale:*** This increases the turbulence and velocity of exhaled air and loosens and mobilizes secretions from peripheral airways.

7. Vibrate for three or four exhalations over the area.
8. Encourage clients to "huff" cough before changing positions.
9. Assess vital signs, pulse oximetry, and auscultate breath sounds.
10. Don gloves.
11. Measure and note character of expectorated secretions, then discard.
12. Remove gloves and perform hand hygiene.
13. Provide oral hygiene.
14. Document procedure and client's response.

Using an Airway Clearance System (Wrap)

Equipment

See Preparing Client for CPT

Disposable inflatable chest wrap of appropriate size (small, medium, large, or extra large)

Air pulse generator with connecting tubes

Preparation

1. Validate physician's order for high-frequency chest wall oscillation therapy, frequency, and duration of therapy.
2. Perform hand hygiene.
3. Identify client by name and birth date.
4. Provide privacy.
5. Explain function and purpose of vest/wrap.
6. Assess lung sounds before therapy.

Procedure

1. Elevate head of bed or have client sit in chair. *Alternately*, place wrap on bed and roll client onto wrap.
2. Apply wrap over single layer of clothing, wrapping deflated vest around client's chest, just beneath axillae; have client inhale deeply; and secure with Velcro fasteners. ▶ ***Rationale:*** Wrap should fit snugly, but not be uncomfortable.

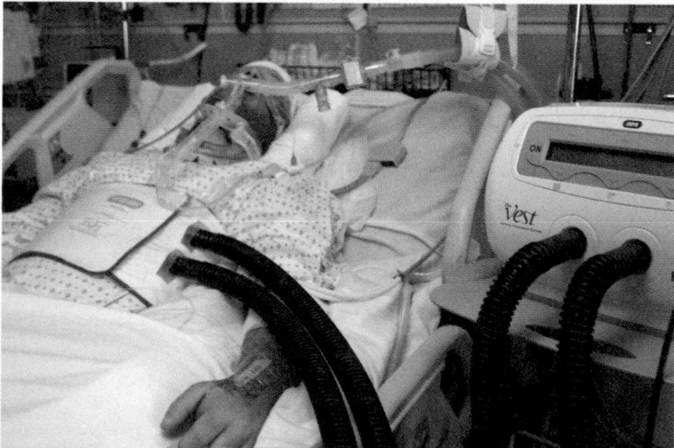

▲ Vest/wrap high-frequency chest wall oscillation therapy increases mobilization and clearance of airway secretions.

3. Adjust generator to a comfortable working height.
4. Lock generator castors. ▶ ***Rationale:*** To prevent movement.
5. Slide air hose into connector port on front of generator using a twist and push motion.
6. Slide other end of hose into disposable vest slits.
7. Fasten Velcro loops to secure air hoses in position.
8. Plug the power cord into the power inlet on back of air pulse generator.
9. Plug power cord into grounded outlet.
10. Adjust arrows up or down to set frequency, pressure, and treatment time, confirming that setting on screen matches those prescribed.
11. Press "ON" button to inflate disposable vest. ▶ ***Rationale:*** Air pulsation provides vibration to client's chest. Treatment will last 10 minutes, but then must be restarted if indicated. Usual treatments are 10–20 minutes qid.
12. Press "OFF" button to end treatment before set time and wrap will deflate.
13. "Session complete" message will show on screen when treatment set time is complete and wrap will deflate.
14. Unplug system and remove disposable air hoses and vest from client.
15. Store vest and air hoses in client's area and return generator to storage for future use.
16. Reassess client's breath sounds; note character and amount of coughed/suctioned secretions.
17. Assist client to a comfortable position.
18. Perform hand hygiene.

EVIDENCE-BASED PRACTICE

Vest/Wrap Therapy Causes Compromized Monitoring

EKG and hemodynamic monitoring are distorted with artifact during airway clearance with vest/wrap therapy. The respiratory care practitioner should notify the nurse before initiating therapy to determine that it is safe to have monitoring compromised for the time period of therapy.

Adams, M. et al., 2005: Beside monitoring of spinal cord injuries, AJCC, Vol. 14, #1

Vest/wrap high-frequency chest wall oscillation therapy increases mobilization of secretions while requiring no caregiver skill and no special positioning, and many clients require no assistance.

Clinical Alert
Strenuous coughing should be avoided with head-down position since it raises intracranial pressure.

DOCUMENTATION for CPT

- Time, specific treatment, and duration of therapy
- Pre- and post-therapy vital signs, breath sounds, and pulse oximetry
- Quantity and character of sputum produced
- Client's physical tolerance of procedures

CRITICAL THINKING Application

Expected Outcomes

- Client tolerates postural drainage.
- CPT facilitates expectoration of secretions.

Unexpected Outcomes	Alternative Actions
Client experiences dyspnea during postural drainage.	• Change client's position so head is no lower than 25° below horizontal.
Client vomits with CPT treatment and coughing.	• Perform treatments between or before meals.
Client tires with manual chest vibration.	• Notify physician to alter therapy with a mechanical device for chest vibration. • Limit total CPT time.
Slapping sounds produced with percussion.	• Cup hands more and ensure that clapping is with wrist flexion and extension only.

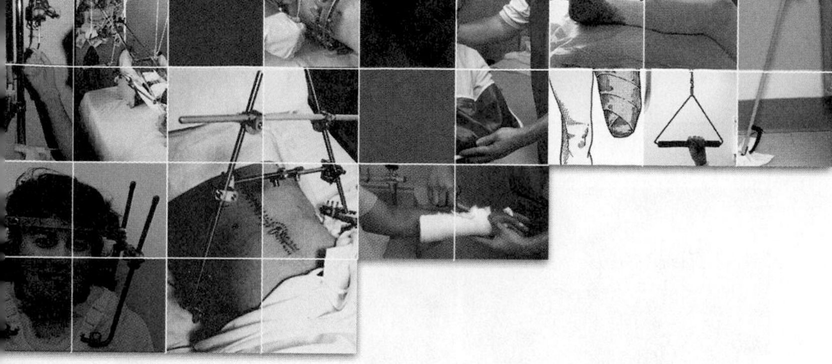

Chapter 30

UNIT 3

Oxygen Administration

Nursing Process Data

ASSESSMENT Data Base

- Review client's ABG or pulse oximetry values.
- Assess client's vital signs.
- Observe client for signs of increased work of breathing.
- Assess skin under oxygen mask for irritation.
- Assess for signs of carbon dioxide narcosis.

PLANNING Objectives

- To return arterial PO_2 or SPO_2 values to normal or acceptable range
- To correct hypoxic condition
- To assist breathing to return to normal rate and effort
- To increase client's comfort, breathing efficiency, and activity tolerance

IMPLEMENTATION Procedures

EVALUATION Expected Outcomes

- Arterial PO_2 and SPO_2 values return to normal or acceptable range.
- Signs and symptoms of hypoxia are relieved.
- Comfort, breathing efficiency, and activity tolerance increased.
- Complications of oxygen use do not occur.

Pearson Nursing Student Resources

Find additional review materials at
nursing.pearsonhighered.com

Prepare for success with NCLEX®-style practice questions and Skill Checklists

Monitoring Clients Receiving Oxygen

Equipment

Oxygen supply source
Oxygen delivery device

Procedure

1. Check physician's orders for mode of oxygen delivery and prescribed oxygen liter flow.
2. Perform hand hygiene.
3. Employ safety precautions for oxygen administration.
4. Place client in semi- or high-Fowler's position to facilitate lung expansion.
5. Turn and reposition client frequently to promote ventilation.
6. Encourage deep breathing and coughing exercises unless directed otherwise.
7. Ensure adequate fluid intake, especially if secretions are thick.
8. If ordered, humidify oxygen.
9. Assess client's progress by frequently checking vital signs, color, level of consciousness, and presence of hypoxia—the best indicator of oxygen delivery problems.

Clinical Alert

Oxygen is indicated for clients with COPD, but is used conservatively. High levels of oxygen may suppress breathing stimulus, cause hypoventilation and CO_2 retention, and lead to respiratory arrest due to CO_2 narcosis.

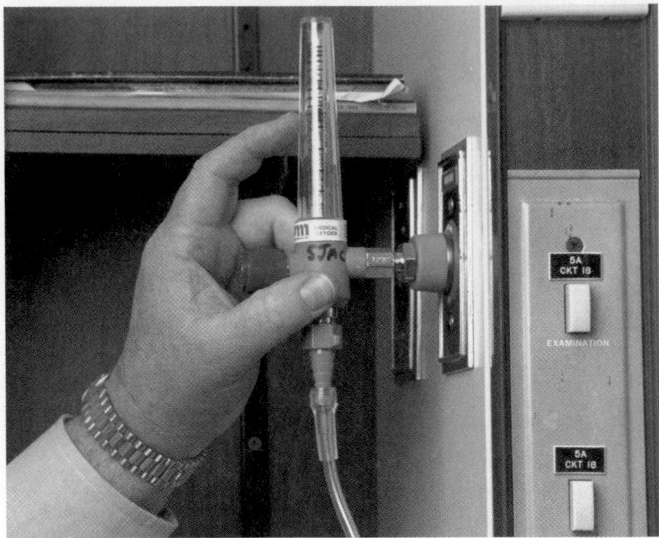

▲ Oxygen flow meter indicates liters per minute delivered to administration setup.

10. Assess clients with COPD frequently for signs of carbon dioxide narcosis:
    a. Bounding peripheral pulses
    b. High blood pressure
    c. Altered sensorium
    d. Increased pulse pressure
    e. Warm, clammy skin
11. Evaluate SpO_2 30 minutes after any change in oxygen flow rate.

Using Pulse Oximetry

Equipment

Oximeter (battery or line power operated)
Sensor (clip-on or disposable adhesive sensor)

Preparation

1. Evaluate client's health status before using oximetry. ▸ ***Rationale:*** Inaccurate oximetry readings can be found in clients with:
    a. Alkalosis, acidosis
    b. Fever, hypothermia
    c. Poor peripheral blood flow
    d. Carbon monoxide poisoning
    e. Recent dye injection studies
    f. Shivering or excessive movement
2. Remove dark nail polish or artificial nails, if using finger for sensor placement. ▸ ***Rationale:*** These substances can distort readings.
3. Obtain appropriate sensor. ▸ ***Rationale:*** Sensor probes are designated for specific sites (clips for finger or earlobe, wraps for toes or across the nose).

Procedure

1. Identify client and explain purpose and procedure for pulse oximetry.
2. Plug unit into electric outlet.
3. Turn on power.
4. Apply sensor probe to selected site flush with skin and secure. Make sure both sensor probes are aligned directly opposite each other. ▸ ***Rationale:*** Oximeter sensors contain both red and infrared light-emitting diodes (LEDs) and a photo detector. The photo detector registers light passing through vascular bed, the basis for microprocessor determination of oxygen-saturation.

Clinical Alert

- Avoid placing SpO_2 clip sensor on the thumb or edematous site. Wrap sensors can be used on the thumb or great toe.
- Avoid extremity with an intra-arterial catheter or noninvasive automatic BP cuff.

5. Set alarms to predetermined saturation levels or pulse rate.

NOTE: New motion-tolerant pulse oximeters are associated with fewer false alarms.

6. Read oxygen saturation level on digital readout monitor.
7. Evaluate findings with previous saturation levels and changes in oxygen therapy.
8. Rotate site of clip-on probes every 4 hr. Replace disposable probes every 24 hr. ▶ ***Rationale:*** Skin irritation can occur with continuous usage.
9. Validate that oximeter pulse rate is consistent with manually assessed pulse rate.
10. Document findings on appropriate hospital record.

▲ Sensor probe placed on finger with continuous oximeter unit display of hemoglobin oxygen saturation (SpO2) and pulse rate. Alarms are set at predetermined limits.

Pulse Oximetry SpO_2

Arterial blood gas (ABG) analysis has been used for decades to determine a client's gas exchange and oxygenation transport ability. Pulse oximetry technology allows for more cost- and time-efficient PRN or continuous monitoring of arterial oxygen saturation (SaO_2). The primary advantages of this method are:

- It is cost-effective.
- It is a noninvasive evaluation tool.
- Minute-to-minute changes in saturation can be assessed and timely intervention made to meet client needs.
- The client's response to treatment can be evaluated immediately and ongoing.

EVIDENCE-BASED PRACTICE

Pulse oximetry measures the arterial saturation of available hemoglobin. The anemic patient may have a normal SpO_2 and not have adequate tissue oxygenation because available hemoglobin is maximally saturated with oxygen.

Source: Bridget, P. (2009). Pulse points. *Nursing 2009, 39*(2), 8.

Safety Precautions for Oxygen Administration

- Set up "No Smoking" and "Oxygen in Use" signs at the site of administration and at the door, according to agency policy.
- Provide cotton gown—synthetics and wool may generate sparks of static electricity.
- Remove matches, lighters, and ashtrays from bedside (these items should NOT be present as hospitals are smoke-free facilities).
- Remove any friction-type or battery-operated toys/devices.
- Disconnect ungrounded electric equipment.
- Remove all volatile or flammable materials (alcohol, oils, petroleum products).
- Make sure that all electrical monitoring equipment is *properly* grounded.
- Locate fire extinguishers and unit/area oxygen meter turn-off lever.

Using an Oxygen Cylinder

Equipment

Steel cylinder portable oxygen tank

Regulator/flow meter

Oxygen delivery tubing

Procedure

1. Place oxygen cylinder in carrier in secure upright position. ▶ ***Rationale:*** If cylinder of compressed air falls accidentally, unit becomes a missile with uncontrollable force and direction.
2. Using hexagon key, slowly turn cylinder release valve clockwise (left is loose) to crack tank open for a brief period, then close (right to tighten). ▶ ***Rationale:*** This action removes lint from system.
3. Check pressure gauge on front of tank to determine amount of oxygen pressure in tank. ▶ ***Rationale:*** Full status is 2,200 PSI.
4. Attach flow meter regulator unit over neck of cylinder, aligning pins with green "O" ring openings.
5. Use turn key to tighten regulator to cylinder neck.

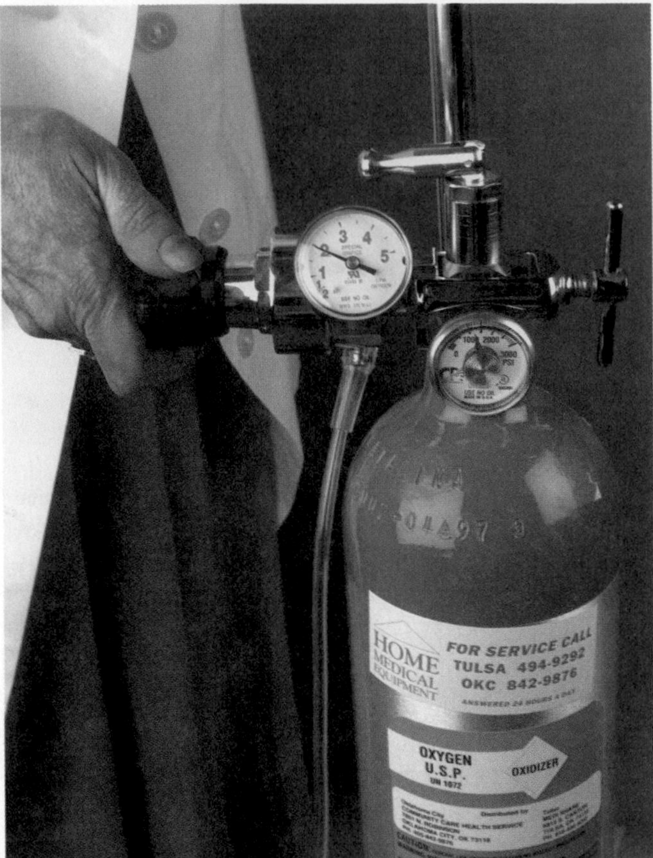

▲ Attach regulator to cylinder neck, attach tubing, open cylinder release valve, and adjust oxygen flow rate (L/min) as prescribed.

6. Connect delivery tubing to "Christmas tree" adapter on regulator unit.
7. Open cylinder release valve using hexagon key on top of cylinder. ▸ ***Rationale:*** This allows oxygen flow.
8. Slowly open regulator/flow meter and adjust to prescribed rate of oxygen delivery in liters per minute.

Clinical Alert

Oxygen cylinders are mandated by the Compressed Gas Association to be green or incorporate a green collar at the gauge and flowmeter mechanism. Wall outlets are also green for oxygen, yellow for air, and white for suction.

Signs and Symptoms of Hypoxia ($SaO_2 < 90\%$ or below desired range for client's situation)

Early Symptoms
- Restlessness
- Headache
- Visual disturbances
- Confusion or change in behavior
- Tachypnea
- Tachycardia
- Hypertension
- Dyspnea
- Anxious face

Advanced Symptoms
- Hypotension
- Bradycardia
- Metabolic acidosis (production of lactic acid)
- Cyanosis

Chronic Hypoxia
- Polycythemia
- Clubbing of fingers and toes
- Peripheral edema
- Right-sided heart failure
- Chronic PO_2 less than 55 mmHg; O_2 saturation less than 87%
- Elevated PCO_2 (respiratory acidosis)

Using Nasal Cannula

Equipment

Oxygen source
Oxygen flow meter
Disposable humidifier if ordered (flow rate over 4 L/min or per agency policy)
Nasal cannula and tubing

Preparation

1. Check physician's order for oxygen prescription (flow rate).
2. Gather equipment.
3. Insert oxygen flow meter into wall outlet.
4. Connect cannula tubing to flow meter.
5. Place disposable humidifier unit between flow meter and cannula tubing if humidification is ordered.
6. Perform hand hygiene.

Procedure

1. Explain purpose and procedure of oxygen use to client.
2. Place nasal prongs of cannula into client's nares.
3. Fit cannula tubing around client's ears and adjust tubing slide under client's chin.
4. Adjust flow of oxygen. Should be limited to 6 L/min or less, FIO_2: 24%–44%, flow: 1–6 L. ▸ ***Rationale:*** Since atmospheric air mixes with prescribed oxygen

concentration as client inhales, the FIO_2 varies depending on the flow and nature of client's breathing. Deep breathing dilutes rather than enhances the FIO_2 because more room air is inhaled.

NOTE: Oxygen therapy is not corrective for hypoxia caused by anemia, abnormal hemoglobin, or vascular insufficiency.

5. Monitor vital signs and check client's condition regularly.
6. Provide nares care every 4 hr—use ONLY water-soluble products and avoid petroleum products. ▸ ***Rationale:*** Petroleum products are combustible, not absorbed by the body, and difficult to clear from the mucosa.
7. Monitor for pressure around ears and pad cannula tubing for comfort if indicated.

Clinical Alert

Humidification of low-flow oxygen through nasal cannulae is not considered essential and is contraindicated because it supports bacterial growth.

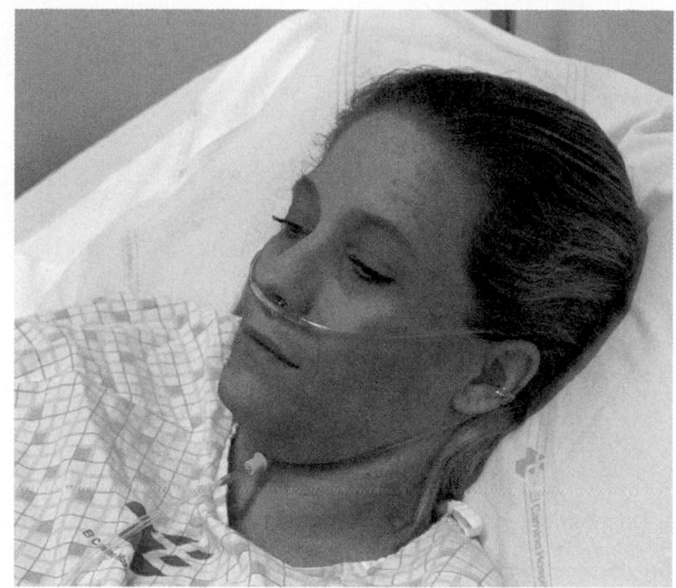

▲ Oxygen administration by nasal cannula.

Using an Oxygen Face Mask

Equipment

- Oxygen mask
- Four types of masks:
  - Simple face mask
  - Partial rebreather mask with reservoir bag
  - Nonrebreather mask with reservoir bag
  - Venturi mask used to specifically control oxygen concentration
- Oxygen source
- Oxygen flowmeter
- Disposable humidifier (if indicated)

Preparation

1. Check physician's orders for oxygen.
2. Gather equipment.
3. Perform hand hygiene.

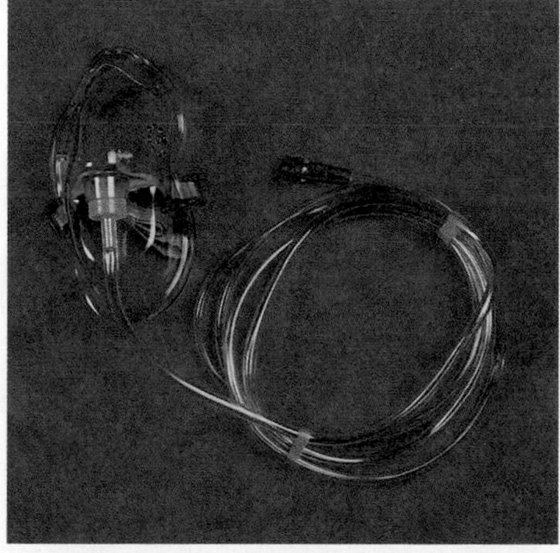

▲ Simple face mask delivers moderately high flow of oxygen.

Procedure

1. Explain procedure and rationale for administration of oxygen to client.
2. Check size of face mask to make sure it fits client.
3. Turn on oxygen flow to liters prescribed. If reservoir bag is attached, partially inflate it with oxygen.
4. Place client in semi- or high-Fowler's position.
5. Fit mask to client's face from nose downward during expiration. If reservoir bag is attached, oxygen flow must be at a level to prevent bag from collapsing. ▸ ***Rationale:*** A tight fit prevents oxygen from escaping around eyes or nose.

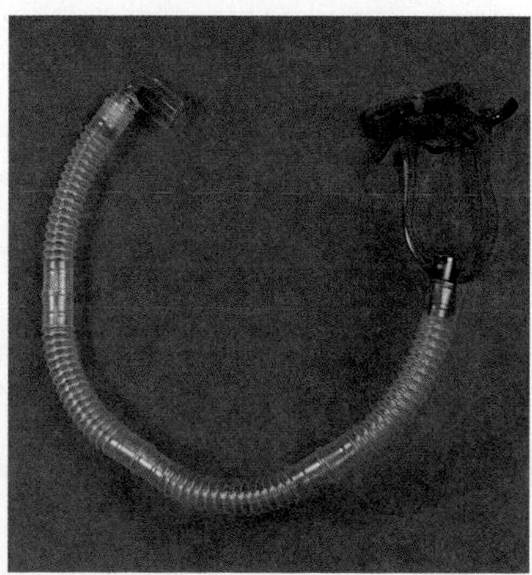

▲ Oxygen face tent delivers unpredictable oxygen flow with high humidity.

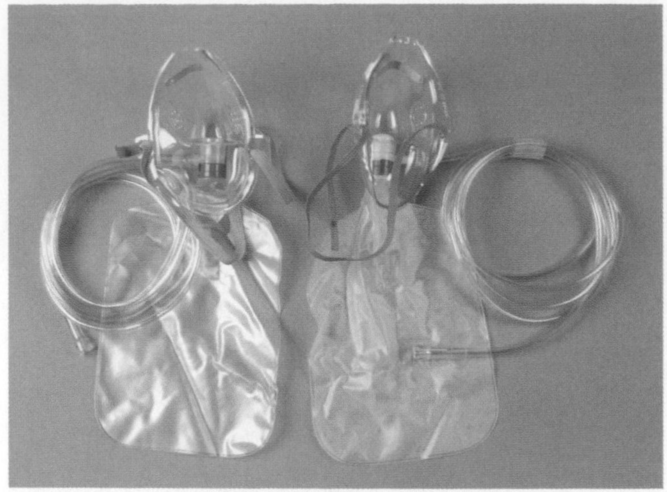

▲ Left: Partial rebreather mask provides higher FIO_2 than a simple mask, but is seldom used. Right: Nonrebreather mask provides highest FIO_2.

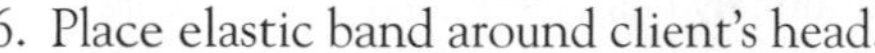

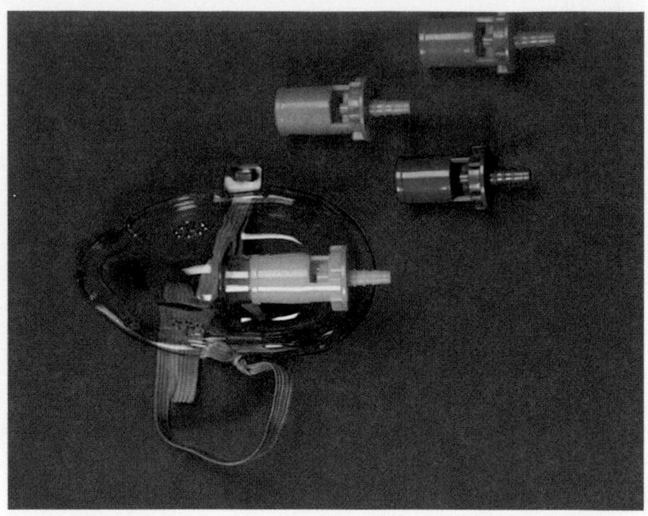

▲ Venturi mask with oxygen percent control pieces.

6. Place elastic band around client's head.
7. Stay with client until client feels at ease with mask. ▸ ***Rationale:*** Clients may be afraid of suffocating.
8. Assess client's condition by checking vital signs and oxygenation status.
9. Change mask and tubing according to agency policy and provide skin care to face.
10. Check equipment frequently. If humidifier is attached, check water level, dispose, and change PRN.

TABLE 30-1 Oxygen Delivery Devices (FIO_2 Numbers Are Approximate)

Nasal Cannula

This equipment is easily tolerated by most clients. It is also simpler than a mask. The fraction of inspired oxygen (FIO_2) varies depending on the oxygen liter flow and the rate and depth of client breathing.

FIO_2:	24%–38%	Flow:	1–2 L
FIO_2:	30%–35%	Flow:	3–4 L
FIO_2:	38%–44%	Flow:	5–6 L

Simple Face Mask

This equipment requires fairly high oxygen flow to prevent rebreathing of carbon dioxide. About 75% of the inspired volume is room air drawn in through side holes in the mask. Accurate FIO_2 is difficult to estimate.

FIO_2	35%–65%	Flow:	8–12 L

Mask With Reservoir Bag

The reservoir allows higher FIO_2 to be delivered. At flows of less than 6 L/min the risk of rebreathing carbon dioxide increases. Two types are available:

Partial rebreather mask: No inspiratory valve so that the beginning portion of exhaled air returns to the bag and mixes with the inspired air. Ports are present so that most expired air escapes. The reservoir bag remains one- third to one-half inflated.

FIO_2	40%–60%	Flow:	6–10 L

Nonrebreather: Valve closes during expiration so that exhaled air does not enter reservoir and is not rebreathed. Valves on mask side ports allow exhalation but close on inspiration to prevent inhalation of room air.

FIO_2	60%–100%	Flow:	6–15 L

Venturi Mask

This system utilizes different-sized adapters to deliver a fixed or predicted FIO_2. The FIO_2 is dependent on liter flow and/or entrainment port size. It is used effectively on clients with COPD when accurate FIO_2 is necessary. Carbon dioxide buildup is kept at a minimum. Humidifiers usually are not used. FIO_2 is dependent on liter flow and/or entrainment port size.

FIO_2	24%–50%

Face Tent

This soft aerosol mask fits loosely around the face and neck. It is an alternative to an aerosol mask for clients who feel claustrophobic, but it is sometimes difficult to keep in place. It is convenient for providing humidification and oxygenation; however, oxygen concentration cannot be controlled.

FIO_2:	28%–100%	Flow:	8–12 L

TABLE 30-1 Oxygen Delivery Devices (FIO_2 Numbers Are Approximate) *(Continued)*

Oxygen Hood
This disposable vinyl box fits over a child's head to provide warm humidified oxygen at a controlled temperature. FIO_2: 28%–40% Flow: 5–8 L FIO_2: 40%–85% Flow: 8–12 L *Less than 5 L flow may lead to carbon dioxide narcosis.*
Oxygen Tent
This canopy encloses the child and is used to provide oxygen, humidification, and/or a cool environment to control temperature. FIO_2: Up to 50% Flow: 10–15 L

Using an Oxygen Hood

Equipment

Disposable oxygen hood
Oxygen source
Oxygen analyzer
Flexible oxygen tubing

Procedure

1. Check physician orders for oxygen level.
2. Perform hand hygiene.
3. Place hood around child's head and/or upper body and attach tubing to oxygen supply.
4. Close ports and lid, but do not obstruct neck opening. ▸ ***Rationale:*** Obstructing neck opening can lead to carbon dioxide accumulation.
5. Infants are cared for through portholes or lid. ▸ ***Rationale:*** This prevents excessive oxygen leakage.
6. Maintain oxygen levels at 40%–50%, and check for moisture that accumulates inside hood.
7. Observe usual oxygen administration precautions.

New Trends Hyperbaric Oxygen Therapy (HBOT)

Intermittent HBOT supports healing and alleviates symptoms in a number of acute and chronic health problems where blood flow and tissue oxygenation are reduced. This modality:

- Increases oxygen concentration in body tissues, even those with inadequate blood flow
- Reduces local tissue edema
- Stimulates growth of new blood vessels
- Causes rebound vasodilation after therapy
- Stimulates the body's immune response, production of antioxidants, and free radical scavengers
- Enhances WBC activity and potentiates effects of antibiotics

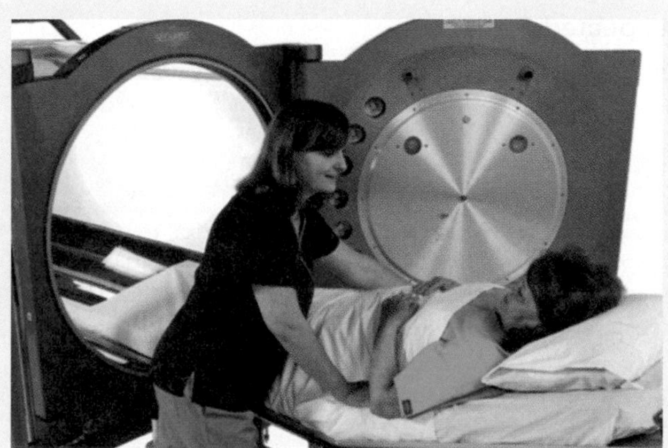

▲ Delivery of 100% oxygen at greater than atmospheric pressure is used for a number of acute and chronic health problems where blood flow and tissue oxygenation are reduced. (Courtesy: Sechrist Industries, Inc.)

HBOT is used intermittently to deliver 100% oxygen at greater than normal atmospheric pressure (1 atmosphere absolute). The client reclines on a cot in a transparent cylinder ("chamber") with room air and breathes 100% O_2 through a hood or mask while pressure in the chamber is increased 1.5 to 2 times atmospheric pressure. Treatments usually last 1 hr, during which the client can watch TV, read, sleep, or converse with others outside of the chamber. At completion of treatment the client is gradually decompressed to normal atmospheric pressure. Studies regarding the usefulness of HBOT are ongoing.

Source: Lyon, K. (2008.) The case for evidence in wound care: Investigating advanced treatment modalities in healing chronic diabetic lower extremity wounds. *Journal of Wound, Ostomy, and Continence Nursing, 35*(6), 585–590.

DOCUMENTATION for Oxygen Administration

- Type of equipment used for oxygen administration, liter flow, FIO_2
- Arterial PO_2 and SaO_2 or pulse oximetry results
- Vital signs
- Client's tolerance of device
- Client and family teaching and indication of understanding

Legal Considerations

Gordon v. Presbyterian Hospital: In this case a patient was being received for emergency surgery. Available oxygen tanks were empty in the holding area, so the nurse obtained a tank from one of the surgical suites. The room was dark, color of the tank was not appreciated, and the patient received CO_2 (gray tank) rather than O_2 (green tank). When discovered, a CODE BLUE was called. The patient remained comatose for several weeks before her death.

Manning v. Twin Falls Clinic & Hospital, Inc.: There was substantial evidence in medical malpractice action against a nurse to support award of punitive damages where the plaintiff's expert witness concluded that the nurse's conduct in disconnecting supplemental oxygen to the client during the client's transfer to another room was extreme deviation from the standard of care. Evidence was also present that the nurse disconnected oxygen despite pleadings from family members present who claimed that the client could not survive without his oxygen and who requested that he be provided with a portable oxygen unit preparatory to the move. From this evidence, the jury could have found that the nurse's conduct was grossly negligent and that she acted with disregard for consequences that were likely to follow.

CRITICAL THINKING Application

Expected Outcomes

- Client breathes without distress.
- Oxygen administration does not have adverse effects.
- Breath sounds are normal in all lung fields.
- Client's respiratory rate remains within normal limits.
- SPO_2 values do not vary significantly.
- SPO_2 false alarms do not occur.
- Client remains comfortable with oxygen therapy delivery.

Unexpected Outcomes	Alternative Actions
Client reports having difficulty breathing (dyspnea).	• Check SPO_2 and compare with previous findings. • Encourage client to describe what he or she is experiencing. • Place client in Fowler's position. • Assist with all ADLs to conserve client's energy. • Employ measures to alleviate pain or anxiety.
Client shows these abnormal signs and symptoms: changes in blood pressure, tachycardia, tachypnea, abnormal color, restlessness, or altered sensorium.	• Check ABGs for drop in blood pH (acidemia) or rise in PCO_2 (respiratory acidosis) and report if found. These conditions can occur if hypoxic drive is blunted by the administration of high oxygen concentration. a. Check oxygen delivery setting. b. Reduce oxygen concentration as ordered. • Clients who chronically retain carbon dioxide may require controlled oxygen concentration delivery device (e.g., Venturi mask).
Client develops atelectasis.	• Encourage deep breathing, range of motion, frequent position changes, and early ambulation if possible. • Use sedatives or other respiratory depressants carefully. • CPT may be ordered. • Check breath sounds. (They are usually decreased with this condition and crackles are frequently heard at the end of inspiration in dependent lung areas and may clear after client coughs.)

Client develops tachypnea.	• Report change and check SPO_2 immediately, since inadequate flow rates may be causing the problem. • Increase flow rate as ordered and monitor. • Monitor vital signs and correlate with client findings as pulmonary embolus may be the cause. • Check client's breathing pattern and breath sounds and report significant change.
Oxygen toxicity occurs.	• Toxicity occurs soon after initiation of oxygen use and is directly related to the FIO_2. • Monitor closely for nausea, restlessness, pallor, lethargy, weakness, and dyspnea. • Validate that sensor and oximeter are from the same manufacturer. • Do not exceed 40% oxygen concentration (FIO_2) unless using continuous monitoring of SpO_2.
Oxygen saturation (SpO_2) findings are erratic.	• Check that sensor probes are aligned to prevent photodetector picking up light from sources other than sensor. • Check that appropriate sensor site was selected for specific probes (e.g., finger site for finger sensor).
Pulse oximeter alarm sounds frequently.	• Do not disarm the system. • Encourage client to immobilize sensor site. Movement scrambles signals from photodetector, interfering with readings. • Obtain wrap sensor if thumb or toe is used. • Place sensor on different site. • Avoid placing sensor on hand of arm used for continuous blood pressure monitoring.
Client experiences discomfort with nasal prongs.	• Obtain smaller-gauge pediatric cannula. • Obtain mustache pad or foam wrap for easing tube pressure behind ears.

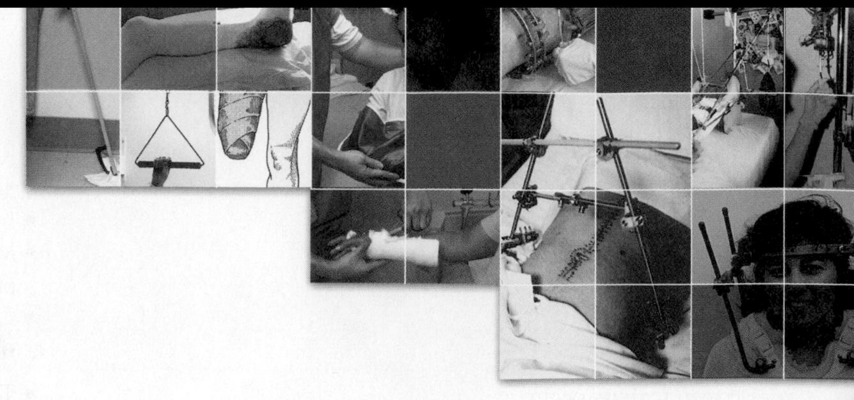

Chapter 30

UNIT 4

Intubated Airways

Nursing Process Data

ASSESSMENT Data Base

- Assess client's level of consciousness.
- Determine whether gag/swallow reflex is present.
- Assess breath sounds in all lung fields, SpO_2, ABGs.
- Observe for shortness of breath, labored breathing, tachypnea, or tachycardia.
- Note presence of adventitious sounds.
- Note character of secretions.

PLANNING Objectives

- Oropharyngeal or nasopharyngeal intubation:
  - To provide patent airway
- Endotracheal intubation:
  - To provide patent airway
  - To provide route for mechanical ventilation
  - To facilitate removal of airway secretions
  - To improve gas exchange

IMPLEMENTATION Procedures

EVALUATION Expected Outcomes

- Patent airway is established.
- Intubation assessment parameters indicate correct placement.
- Accidental extubation does not occur.

Pearson Nursing Student Resources

Find additional review materials at **nursing.pearsonhighered.com**

Prepare for success with NCLEX®-style practice questions and Skill Checklists

Inserting an Oropharyngeal Airway

Equipment

Oropharyngeal tube
Tongue depressor
Clean gloves
Suction catheter
Suction source

Procedure

1. Ensure that client is unresponsive and has NO gag reflex. ▸ ***Rationale:*** Conscious client may vomit and aspirate or develop laryngospasm during tube insertion.
2. Select appropriate size airway—length should be from corner of mouth to corner of ear tragus.
3. Perform hand hygiene; don gloves.
4. Gently open client's mouth with crossed finger technique, placing your thumb on client's lower teeth and index finger on the upper teeth and gently pushing them apart. You may need to use modified jaw thrust to insert tube.
5. Perform oral suctioning.
6. Hold tongue down with tongue depressor and advance airway to back of tongue OR advance airway upside down (curved upward) and, as airway passes uvula, rotate the airway 180°.
7. Check that concave curve fits over tongue. It should extend from the lips to the pharynx, displacing the tongue anteriorly. ▸ ***Rationale:*** Proper positioning helps prevent injury to lips, teeth, tongue, and posterior pharynx.

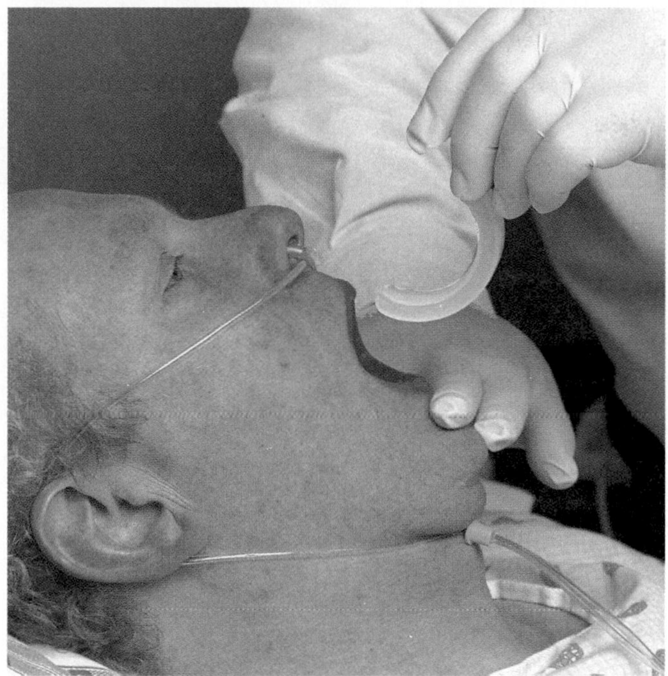

▲ Orophaxyngeal airway is initially inserted upside down (curved upward), then rotated 180°.

8. Tape top and bottom of airway in position. ▸ ***Rationale:*** Stabilization of the tube prevents injuries.
9. Position client on side to facilitate drainage.
10. Remove gloves, discard, and perform hand hygiene.
11. Observe position of airway and evaluate quality of client's spontaneous breathing.

Inserting a Nasopharyngeal Airway (Nasal Trumpet)

Equipment

Flexible nasopharyngeal airway
Water-soluble lubricant
Clean gloves

Procedure

1. Select appropriate size tube (length from tip of nose to earlobe and lumen slightly narrower than client's naris).
2. Perform hand hygiene; don gloves.
3. Lubricate entire length of tube.
4. Explain procedure to client.
5. Insert entire tube gently through naris, following anatomic line of nasal passage. If obstructed, try other naris.
6. Validate position by:
   a. feeling exhaled air through tube opening

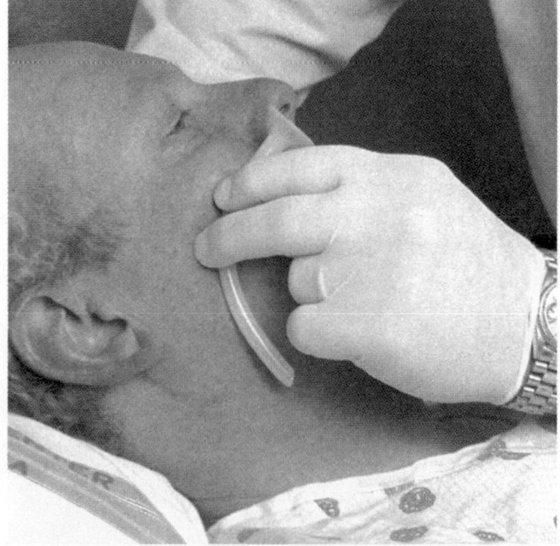

▲ Nasal trumpet protects airway from repeated trauma with upper airway (nasopharyngeal) suctioning.

b. Inspecting for tube tip behind uvula.
7. Position client on side to facilitate drainage of secretions.
8. Remove gloves, discard, and perform hand hygiene.
9. Continue to monitor position of airway and client's response.
10. Suction upper airway PRN using clean technique.

Assisting With Endotracheal Intubation

Equipment

"Crash cart" (contains most needed supplies)
Laryngoscope with several blade sizes
Stylet to guide endotracheal tube (*ONLY for oral intubation*)
Endotracheal tubes
Water-soluble lubricant
McGill forceps
Suction source
Oxygen source
Bag–valve–mask
Twill, adhesive tape, or Velcro holder
10-mL syringe for cuff inflation
Stethoscope
CO_2 detector (for airway placement validation)
Oral airway or bite block
Clean gloves and personal protective equipment including face shield
Established pulse oximetry and cardiac monitoring if available
Wrist restraints (if ordered by physician)
Prepared sedative as ordered
Labeled container for client's dentures

NOTE: Noninvasive positive pressure ventilation methods (CPAP, BiPAP) provide an appropriate alternative to intubation for many clients with ventilatory insufficiency.

Clinical Alert

The presence of an endotracheal tube bypasses defenses that normally protect the lower airways (filtration, humidification, and hydration of inspired air and epiglottal closure). In addition, mucociliary transport of secretions and trapped pathogens is impaired. These alterations place intubated clients at risk for aspiration pneumonia.

Preparation

1. Determine that client has *no protective airway reflexes*.
2. Bring crash cart to client's doorway.
3. Check that all necessary equipment is functioning (oxygen/suction source and delivery systems, laryngoscope batteries).
4. Inflate and deflate airway cuff to determine whether it is intact.
5. Perform hand hygiene and don gloves. Don personal protective equipment.
6. Insert stylet into tube (only for oral intubation); ensure that stylus does not extend beyond tube tip.
7. Lubricate tube.
8. Administer medication as ordered.
9. Remove client's dentures/bridgework and place in labeled container.
10. Review Procedure for Bag–Valve–Mask Ventilation.

Procedure

1. Don clean gloves and personal protective gear.
2. Place client in flat supine position with pillow under shoulders to hyperextend neck and help open airway. Position so that mouth, pharynx, and trachea are aligned. ▸ ***Rationale:*** Proper positioning facilitates intubation.
3. Restrain client's wrists only if necessary.
4. Premedicate client as ordered.
5. Preoxygenate client for several minutes, using bag–valve–mask. ▸ ***Rationale:*** To create an "oxygen reserve."

Clinical Alert

While cuff pressures are typically maintained at 20–25 mmHg, an individual client's tracheal capillary pressure cannot be determined and excessive cuff pressure is the best predictor of tracheo-laryngeal injury.

Clinical Alert

Even if spontaneously breathing, the client should be preoxygenated with 100% O_2 for endotracheal tube placement. Ventilation must not be interrupted for over 30 seconds.

6. Using thumb and index finger, apply cricoid pressure during tube insertion. ▸ ***Rationale:*** This facilitates tracheal placement and protects against aspiration of gastric contents.
7. Maintain cricoid pressure while inflating cuff to "minimal leak" inflation by placing stethoscope at client's suprasternal notch and noting a slight hissing sound at peak of inspiration.
8. Attach bag–valve–mask, provide ventilation, and look for chest to rise. ▸ ***Rationale:*** If chest does not rise, esophageal intubation is likely.
9. Check tube placement using CO_2 detector. ▸ ***Rationale:*** Presence of CO_2 indicates tracheal intubation.

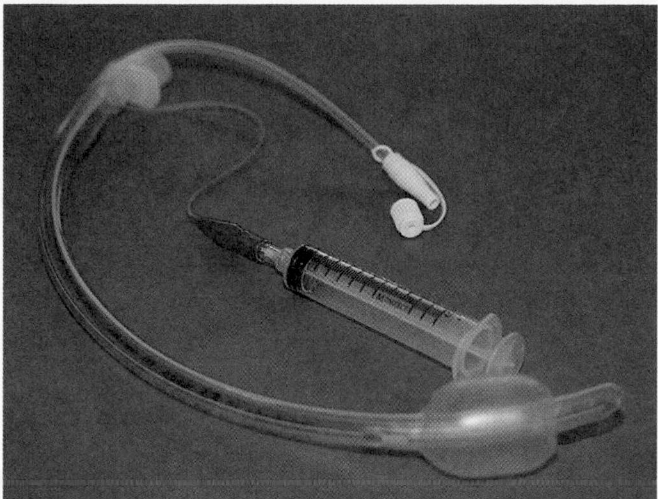

▲ CASS-ETT ® has a lumen that opens above the tube cuff. Lumen (white tip) is connected to continuous suction to remove subglottic secretions that accumulate above the cuff in order to prevent pneumonia due to aspiration of these secretions.

10. Place stethoscope over epigastrium. ▸ ***Rationale:*** If gurgling is heard and abdominal distention noted, esophageal placement is likely.
11. Auscultate lung fields for bilateral breath sounds. ▸ ***Rationale:*** This ensures that accidental right main stem intubation has not occurred.

Clinical Alert

Cricoid pressure may be used only if the client:

- Is nonresponsive
- Is not vomiting
- Does not have a cuffed tracheal tube in place

Clinical Alert

CDC guidelines recommend orotracheal over nasotracheal intubation to reduce the incidence of sinus infection.

12. Mark tube at level of client's front teeth and tape securely with twill or adhesive tape or Endotube stabilizer. ▸ ***Rationale:*** Securement prevents tube displacement.
13. Recheck tube placement with the previous measures (steps 9–11).

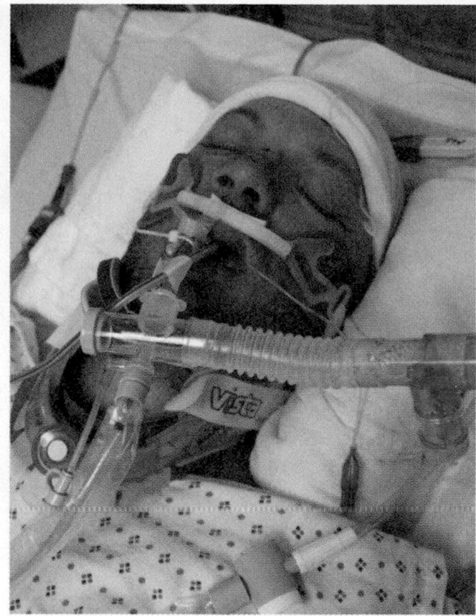

▲ Endotube stabilizer distributes equipment weight and pressure evenly on the client's face and facilitates easy periodic relocation of tube from side-to-side to prevent oral tissue trauma.

14. Place bite block or oral airway if ET tube has been positioned orally.
15. Attach O_2 source to ET tube.
16. Discard disposable equipment, remove protective gear and gloves, and perform hand hygiene.
17. Position client in position as ordered.
18. Obtain chest x-ray to confirm tracheal placement of ET tube.
19. Place call bell and writing material within client's reach (as indicated).
20. Reposition right, center, left, then repeat (using velcro or Endotube stabilizer.) ET tube every 4 hours.

Clinical Alert

Low-pressure tracheal tube cuffs provide adequate blood flow to trachea, thus decreasing potential of tracheal tissue necrosis. These cuffs do not need periodic deflation.

Inflating a Tracheal Tube Cuff

Equipment

10-mL syringe
Suction equipment
Stethoscope
Clean gloves

NOTE: The tracheostomy tube with foam cuff (Binova) does not require injected air. Air enters the balloon when port is open.

Procedure

1. Don clean gloves.
2. Attach 10-mL syringe to distal end of inflatable cuff port, making sure seal is tight.

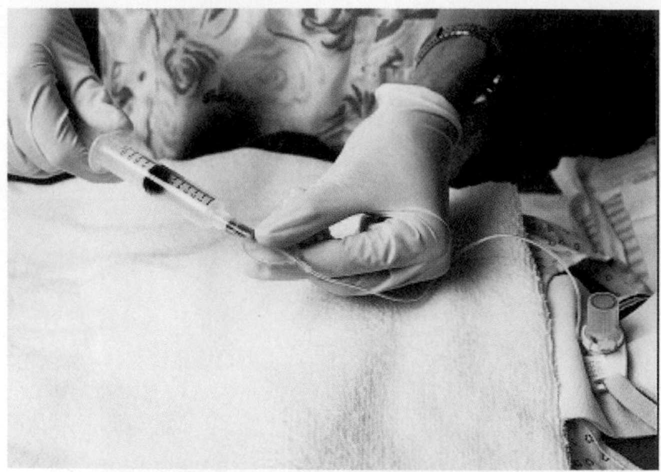

▲ Attach 10-mL syringe to inflate tube cuff.

3. Inflate cuff for a minimal leak or minimal occlusive volume detected by auscultating over the suprasternal notch for a hissing sound at peak of inspiration. ▸ ***Rationale:*** This provides an adequate seal without risking tracheal pressure necrosis.
4. Ask client to speak—if voice is heard, inflation is inadequate for mechanical ventilation.
5. Connect ventilator or T-piece to tracheal tube opening if indicated.
6. Assess breath sounds every 2 hr. ▸ ***Rationale:*** Presence of bilateral breath sounds indicates proper tube position in trachea.

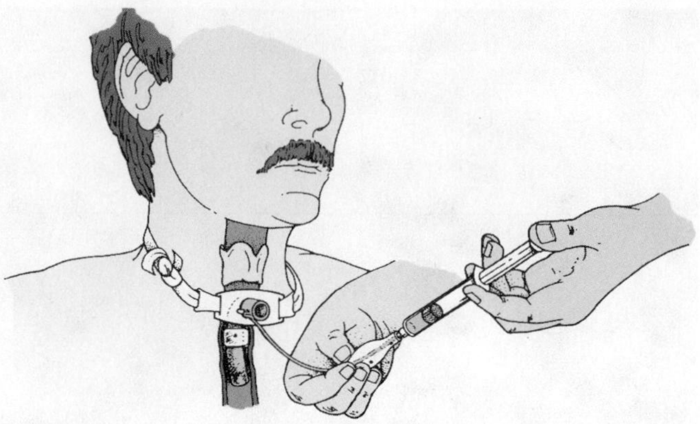

▲ Inflate endotracheal or tracheostomy tube cuff to minimal occlusive volume.

7. Monitor cuff pressure regularly. ▸ ***Rationale:*** This may detect inadvertent cuff overinflation and prevent potential necrosis of tracheal tissue. Pressure is usually maintained at 20 to 25 mmHg to prevent tracheal necrosis. However, an individual client's tracheal capillary pressure cannot be determined.

Clinical Alert

Tracheal tube cuff inflation is essential for mechanically ventilated clients. Without cuff inflation, delivered air diverts out through the nose and mouth, and lungs are not ventilated.

Providing Care for Client With Endotracheal Tube

Procedure

1. Monitor breath sounds every 4 hr. Breath sounds should be heard equally throughout lung fields bilaterally.
2. Check marked points on tube at insertion level. ▸ ***Rationale:*** This determines whether tube has moved.
3. Inspect positioning and stabilization of tube. ▸ ***Rationale:*** A change of position can obstruct airway or cause erosion and necrosis of tissues.
4. Inspect and clean mouth and nose. Observe for pressure areas or ulceration.
5. Reposition ET tube every 4 hours (right, center, left) noting tube depth each time.
6. Support client's head and tube when turning. ▸ ***Rationale:*** This prevents tube from becoming dislodged or airway from becoming obstructed.
7. Place call bell within reach and provide alternative means of communication when cuffed tube is in place. ▸ ***Rationale:*** No air passes over larynx, so client is not able to summon help or communicate.
8. Support client by spending extra time, using touch, and anticipating client's needs.
9. Ensure adequate hydration. ▸ ***Rationale:*** Artificial airways bypass the humidifying process of normal breathing.
10. Provide suction toothbrushing every 12 hr, oral swabbing every 2 hr, and oropharyngeal subglottal suctioning every 6 hr. ▸ ***Rationale:*** This reduces oropharyngeal bacteria and helps prevent pulmonary infection.

Clinical Alert

Even with appropriate cuff inflation, intubated clients receiving gastric/enteral tube feedings are at high risk for aspiration.

Extubating an Endotracheal Tube

Equipment

Suction source
Oral suction catheter (or Yankauer)
Sterile suction catheter set
Clean gloves
Sterile gloves
Personal protective equipment
Oxygen source
Postextubation oxygen delivery device
Syringe for cuff deflation

Preparation

1. Assess client's readiness for extubation.
2. Obtain vital signs.
3. Explain procedure to client.
4. Prepare postextubation oxygen administration device.
5. Place client in Fowler's position.

Procedure

1. Perform hand hygiene and don clean gloves and personal protective equipment.
2. Perform oral or nasopharyngeal suctioning.
3. Have client take several slow deep breaths. ▶ ***Rationale:*** This hyperoxygenates client in preparation for extubation.
4. *Deflate* tube cuff using syringe.
5. *Untie* the endotracheal tube.
6. Remove gloves, perform hand hygiene, and don sterile gloves.
7. Connect sterile catheter to suction source.
8. Insert sterile suction catheter into airway until resistance is met, then retract slightly.
9. Leave suction catheter in place.
10. Have client take a deep breath. ▶ ***Rationale:*** This dilates the vocal cords and makes removal easier and less traumatic.
11. Apply suction while removing catheter and airway at the same time.
12. Immediately apply supplementary oxygen device.
13. Monitor client frequently at first, then regularly.
14. Dispose of equipment, remove gloves, protective gear, and perform hand hygiene.

Clinical Alert

Do not feed client orally immediately after extubation. Seek consult for a feeding trial for clients at risk for aspiration.

DOCUMENTATION for Intubation

- Clinical manifestations indicating need for intubation
- Specific reason for intubation
- Premedication administered
- Size and type of inserted endotracheal, nasopharyngeal, or oropharyngeal tube
- Minimal occlusive pressure for cuff inflation or measured mmHg pressure
- Preoxygenation and postoxygenation when suctioning
- Quantity and character of secretions
- Pre- and post-procedure vital signs
- Client's tolerance of procedure
- Settings of ventilator or other oxygen mode

CRITICAL THINKING Application

Expected Outcomes

- Patent airway is established.
- Intubation assessment parameters indicate correct placement.
- Accidental extubation does not occur.

Unexpected Outcomes	Alternative Actions
Naso/oropharyngeal airway cannot be placed.	• Change size of tube; change naris; do not force insertion. • Hyperextend client's neck. • Direct insertion of nasopharyngeal tube more medially. • Insert oropharyngeal rather than nasopharyngeal airway. • Use tongue depressor to facilitate insertion of oropharyngeal tube. • Relubricate airway and attempt to reinsert. • Call Rapid Response Team if indicated.
Laryngospasm occurs when endotracheal tube is inserted.	• Remove tube and wait a few minutes. • If severe, administer sedation per physician order. • Possibly prepare for immediate cricothyroidotomy or tracheotomy.
Tube placement is incorrect: air movement heard over epigastrium; bilateral breath sounds not heard; CO_2 indicator does not register.	• Withdraw tube and assist with reintubation. • Verify tube placement with x-ray (tube tip should be between larynx and carina). • Recheck CO_2 indicator for correct placement. • Recheck for bilateral breath sounds and SpO_2 status. • Ensure that mark is visible at insertion level for monitoring ETT placement.
Accidental extubation occurs.	• Immediately call a CODE or Rapid Response Team for airway replacement. • Call for crash cart/emergency supplies. • Immediately seek assist to provide bag–valve–mask ventilations. • Assess marker on tube frequently to ensure proper placement.

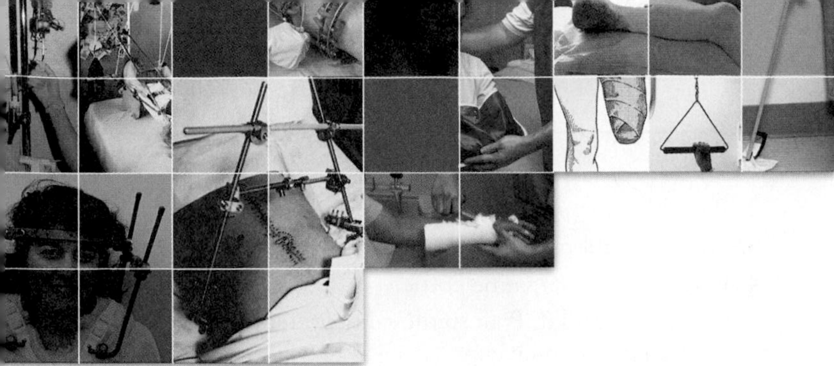

Chapter 30

UNIT 5

Suctioning

Nursing Process Data

ASSESSMENT Data Base

- Assess client's need for suctioning.
- Observe vital signs for increases in pulse and respiration.
- Auscultate breath sounds and for presence of adventitious sounds.
- Observe respiratory status for tachypnea, shortness of breath, and restlessness.
- Observe for signs of hypoxia.

PLANNING Objectives

- To provide patent airway
- To remove secretions
- To improve ventilation
- To decrease breathing rate
- To increase tissue oxygenation

IMPLEMENTATION Procedures

EVALUATION Expected Outcomes

- Secretions removed without complication.
- Tube-fed client does not aspirate feeding.

Pearson Nursing Student Resources

Find additional review materials at **nursing.pearsonhighered.com**

Prepare for success with NCLEX®-style practice questions and Skill Checklists

Suctioning With Multi-Use Catheter in Sleeve

NOTE: For Suctioning Using Single-Use Catheter for Tracheostomy, see Unit 6.

Equipment

Portable suction machine or wall suction unit with receptacle and tubing

Appropriate length suction catheter in protective sleeve packet (with pop-up cup)

Clean gloves

Sterile saline/water

Receptacle for used equipment

Oxygen source and administration device (e.g., bag–valve device with tube adapter)

Personal protective equipment—gown, goggles, mask if splash anticipated

Stethoscope

Preparation

1. Check physician's orders.
2. Gather equipment.
3. Recruit an assistant for manual ventilation, if indicated.
4. Attach resuscitator bag to oxygen tubing, if indicated.
5. Perform hand hygiene.
6. Assess lung sounds and heart rate and rhythm.
7. Open saline flush solution bottle.
8. Set suction control regulator at 100–120 mmHg vacuum.
9. Don protective gown, mask, and goggles. ▸ ***Rationale:*** For self-protection if splash anticipated.

Procedure

1. Explain procedure and rationale to client regardless of client's level of consciousness.
2. Place client in semi-Fowler's or Fowler's position.
3. Turn on suction.
4. Remove cap from saline bottle.
5. Open catheter kit. Pour sterile saline/water flush solution into pop-up cup.
6. Don gloves.
7. Administer 100% oxygen (oxygen flowmeter to maximum "flush") for 1–2 minutes. Use resuscitator bag with tracheal tube adapter to hyperoxygenate client. ▸ ***Rationale:*** Suction removes residual lung volume, resulting in hypoxemia and potential cardiac arrest. Hyperoxygenation prevents these complications.
8. Hold catheter in protective covering and attach end to suction tubing.
9. Retract sleeve enough to lubricate sterile catheter tip by dipping it into cup with sterile saline/water.
10. Advance catheter into client's artificial airway approximately 28 cm (11 in.), or 1 cm beyond tip of ET tube or trach tube, while retracting protective sleeve before applying suction. ▸ ***Rationale:*** Suctioning during insertion deprives client of oxygen and inhibits catheter advancement. Deep suctioning traumatizes tissue.
11. Apply suction and withdraw catheter using a rotating motion as the catheter is retracted back into protective sleeve.
12. Suction intermittently by placing and releasing thumb over catheter suction port. ▸ ***Rationale:*** Intermittent versus continuous application of suction may help to reduce airway injury.
13. Limit suction to no more than 10 seconds. ▸ ***Rationale:*** This prevents hypoxemic complications induced by suctioning.
14. Reattach oxygen delivery device to artificial airway and have client take several deep breaths, or hyperoxygenate client's lungs with resuscitator bag for 30 seconds.
15. Flush suction catheter and tubing with sterile saline/water and retract back into protective sleeve.

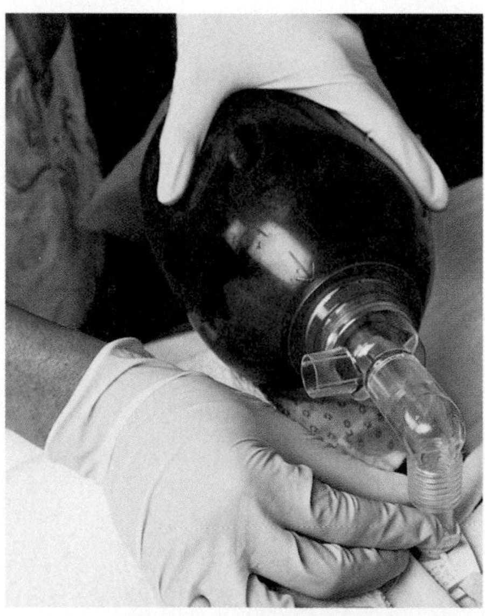

▲ Connect resuscitator bag to hyperoxygenate before and after suctioning.

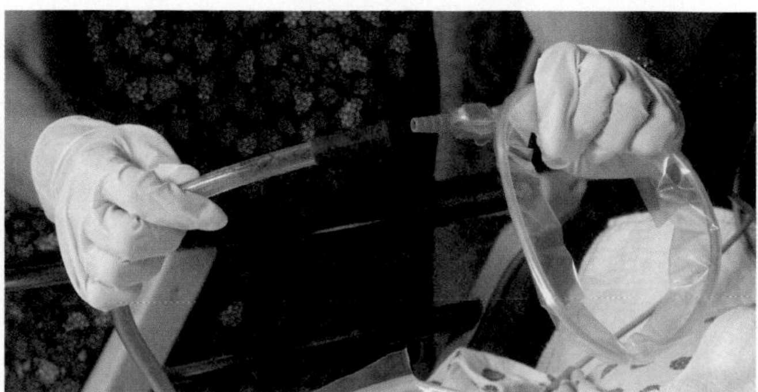

▲ Hold catheter in protective covering and attach to suction tubing.

16. Catheter remains in sleeve and attached to suction tubing. ▶ ***Rationale:*** To allow PRN use. Reuse same catheter (according to agency policy).
17. Replace catheter in sleeve packet at time interval according to agency policy (e.g., 24 hr).

NOTE: A separate catheter must be used for pharyngeal suctioning.

18. Perform hand hygiene.
19. Assess lung sounds and heart rate and rhythm for changes. ▶ ***Rationale:*** Suctioning usually causes tachycardia, but hypoxemia and vagal response may cause serious bradycardia/cardiac arrest.
20. Don clean gloves to empty suction receptacle PRN or at end of every shift, noting character of secretions.
21. Ensure call bell is within client's reach.

EVIDENCE-BASED PRACTICE

Instillation of normal saline should not be performed with endotracheal suctioning. No studies have found this practice to be beneficial; it places patients at risk for hospital-acquired pneumonia. Saline does not liquefy or mobilize secretions; it acts as a vehicle to wash bacteria that normally cling to the inner aspects of the artificial airway into the lung. Instillation of saline also adversely affects arterial oxygenation.

Source: Halm, M. A., & Krisko-Hagel, K. (2008). Instilling normal saline with suctioning: beneficial technique or potentially harmful sacred cow? *American Journal of Critical Care, 17*(5), 469–472.

EVIDENCE-BASED PRACTICE

Nasotracheal suctioning is a blind procedure that should not be used except in an emergency/resuscitation situation. It is probable that the catheter does not enter the airway and that nasopharyngeal suctioning is actually performed.

Repeatedly injuring an unprotected airway must be avoided. The presence of an artificial airway reduces the risk of mechanical trauma.

NTS has many contraindications and complications in addition to those for any type of suctioning (hypoxemia, arrhythmia, changes in blood pressure), including sinusitis, laceration of nasal turbinates, perforation of the pharynx, uvular edema, and gagging/vomiting. Passing a catheter through the nose into the lower airway may lead to bacterial (Methicillin-resistant *Staphylococcus aureus*) colonization, resulting in healthcare-associated pneumonia.

Source: (2004). Nasotracheal suctioning: 2004 revision & update. *Respiratory Care, 49*(9), 1080–1082.

Suctioning With Closed Suction System

Equipment

In-line closed system (ET or tracheostomy connected) suction unit with catheter enclosed by plastic sleeve

10 mL of normal saline in unit dose vial

Suction source

Connecting tubing

Oxygen source and side-arm connector (e.g., bag–valve device or ventilator)

Clean gloves

NOTE: In-line closed system suctioning allows rapid suctioning for intubated clients and does not interrupt ventilator/client interface.

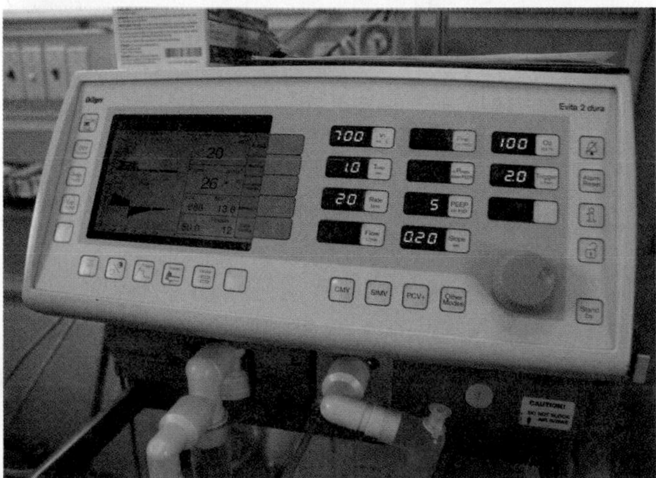

▲ Mechanical ventilator provides 100% oxygen for hyperoxygenation.

Procedure

1. Explain procedure and rationale to client regardless of client's level of consciousness.
2. Perform hand hygiene and don gloves.
3. Place client in semi-Fowler's or Fowler's position.
4. Turn on suction source.
5. Connect oxygen source to side arm of tube connector.
6. Hyperoxygenate client with 100% oxygen, using manual bag or mechanical ventilator (100% oxygen source with several manual sighs, if indicated.)
7. Open access valve and advance catheter within plastic sleeve into client's artificial airway using your dominant hand. ▶ ***Rationale:*** Sterility is maintained because catheter is enclosed by plastic cover and slides within it.
8. With nondominant hand, activate suction valve. Intermittently apply suction (for no more than 5 to 10 seconds) while rotating and withdrawing catheter *completely* back into plastic sheath. ▶ ***Rationale:*** If not totally out of the airway, the catheter impairs client ventilation.

9. Repeat steps 4–6 as necessary to clear secretions; allow time between suctioning for hyperoxygenation. ▶ ***Rationale:*** Repeated suctioning without hyperoxygenation causes complications such as hypoxemia and cardiac dysrhythmias.
10. Attach saline vial to catheter irrigation port; inject saline while applying suction to rinse catheter and tubing, then close irrigation port and suction valve. ▶ ***Rationale:*** Rinsing prevents catheter occlusion by dried secretions.
11. Remove syringe, release suction, and lock mechanism. ▶ ***Rationale:*** Locking catheter prevents inadvertent catheter advancement and occlusion of client's airway.
12. Remove gloves and perform hand hygiene.
13. Ensure that call bell is within client's reach.

Clinical Alert

Monitor client closely and suction PRN, as coughed secretions may accumulate at the suction catheter/client's airway interface and obstruct airflow to client's lungs.

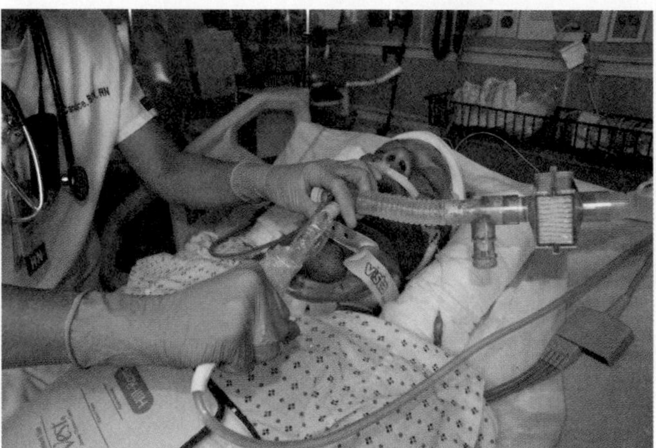

▲ Intubated client with in-line closed suction catheter being advanced.

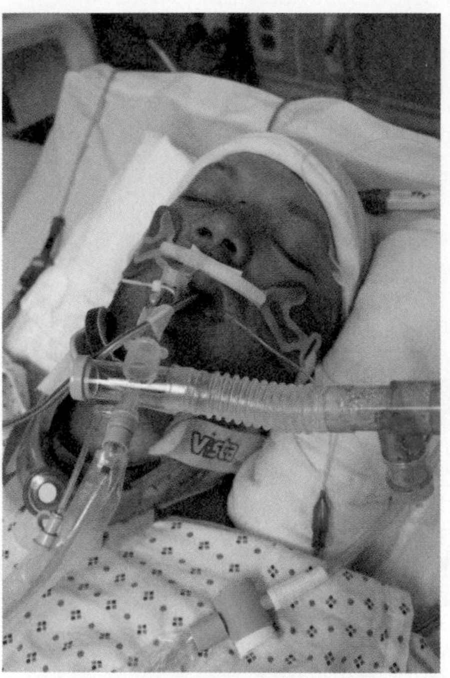

▲ Note black indicator to ensure that catheter is completely withdrawn.

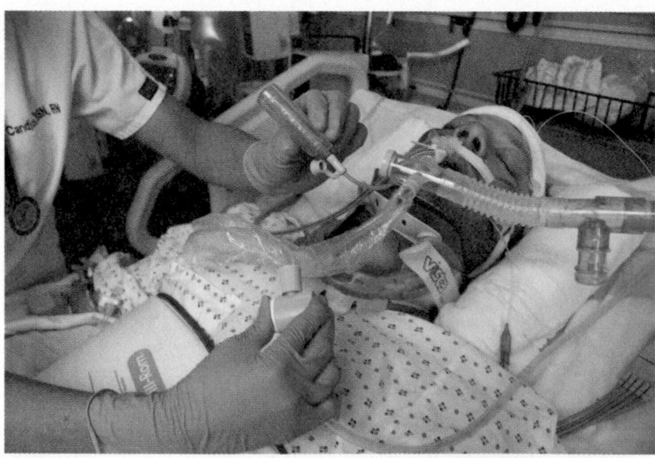

▲ Apply suction while instilling saline to flush catheter and tubing.

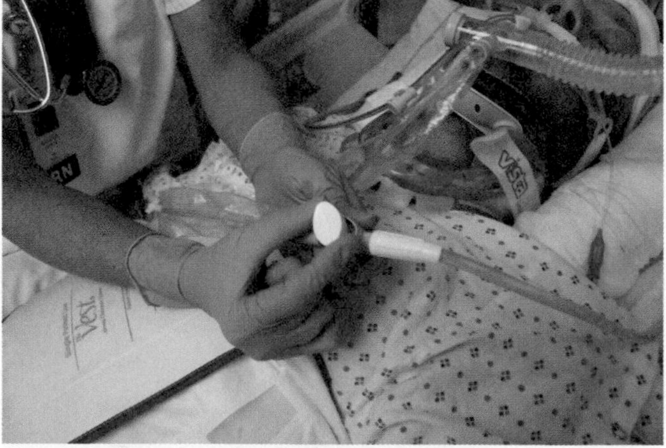

▲ Lock access valve when suctioning is complete.

DOCUMENTATION for Suctioning

- Frequency of suctioning
- Amount and character of secretions
- Pre- and postsuctioning hyperoxygenation
- Breath sounds, respiratory rate, heart rate and rhythm, and SpO_2
- Client's tolerance of procedure
- Reestablishment of oxygen therapy and L/minute

CRITICAL THINKING Application

Expected Outcomes

- Secretions are removed without complication.
- Tube-fed client does not aspirate feeding.

Unexpected Outcomes	Alternative Actions
Hypoxemia and tachycardia or bradycardia occur with suctioning.	• Suction only as needed. • Preoxygenate before and postoxygenate after suctioning, seeking assistance if necessary. • Limit suctioning time to no more than 10 seconds. • Ensure that catheter diameter is no larger than half the inner diameter of the airway it enters.
Excessive secretions necessitate frequent suctioning.	• Suction more frequently but administer 100% oxygen before and after suctioning. • Establish in-line catheter in sleeve, check frequently and suction secretions PRN. • Allow rest period before suctioning again. • Turn client regularly to mobilize secretions. • Notify physician for CPT or other therapy. • Maintain adequate hydration.
Aspiration is suspected in enterally tube-fed intubated client.	• Check suctioned secretions for presence of glucose. (Secretions should not contain blood for accurate determination.) • Recommend use of continuous aspiration of subglottic secretions ET tube. • Maintain 30°–45° elevation of HOB at all times if feeding is continuous. • Monitor gastric residuals regularly. • Advocate small-bore enteral versus gastric tube feeding.

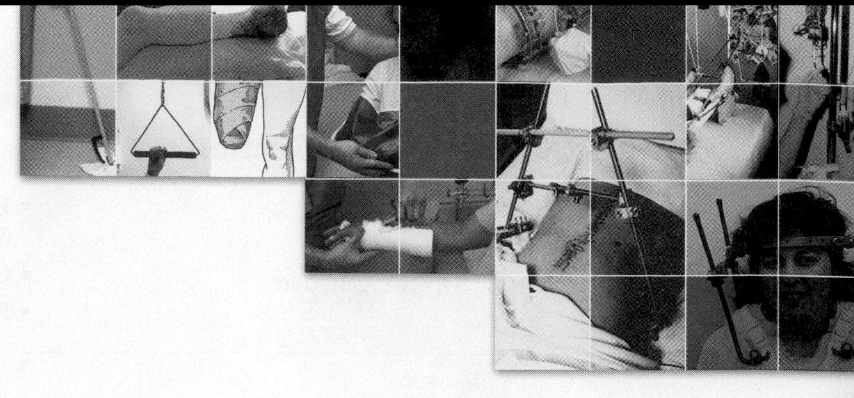

Chapter 30

UNIT ❻

Tracheostomy Care

Nursing Process Data

ASSESSMENT Data Base

- Note presence of dried or moist secretions surrounding cannula or on tracheal dressing.
- Note excessive coughing or expectoration of secretions.
- Assess whether routine tracheal care is adequate for this client.
- Assess respiratory status: breath sounds, respiratory rate, use of accessory muscles for breathing.
- Observe for signs of respiratory distress while tracheal tube is capped: labored breathing, anxious face, flaring of nares, tachypnea, tachycardia.
- Monitor pulse oximetry (SpO_2).
- Auscultate for minimal occlusive cuff inflation pressure.

PLANNING Objectives

- To ensure a patent airway
- To suction secretions more easily
- To improve ventilation
- To prevent infection
- To prevent aspiration while feeding

IMPLEMENTATION Procedures

EVALUATION Expected Outcomes

- Tracheostomy tube remains stable.
- Tracheostomy tube provides a patent airway.
- Client is able to communicate with speaking valve placement.

Assisting With Tracheostomy

Equipment

Sterile tracheostomy tray
Antimicrobial solution
Lidocaine for local anesthesia
Two sterile tracheal tubes
Sterile gloves
Clean gloves
Personal protective equipment
Suction equipment
Oxygen source
Manual resuscitator bag with adapter
Mechanical ventilator if indicated
Sterile normal saline
Sterile preslit 4 × 4 dressing
Twill (or commercial holder)
Prescribed premedication
Stethoscope
Soft wrist restraints (if indicated)

Preparation

1. Explain procedure and rationale to client.
2. If not an emergency situation, obtain permission from client or other legally responsible individual before tracheostomy.
3. Perform hand hygiene.
4. Don personal protective equipment.
5. Assemble all necessary equipment.
6. Set up tracheostomy tray where sterile field can be maintained; open tray when physician is ready.

Procedure

1. Explain procedure as it is being done.
2. Medicate or restrain client, if necessary, with soft wrist restraints. ▸ ***Rationale:*** Interference during insertion can result in injury to client.

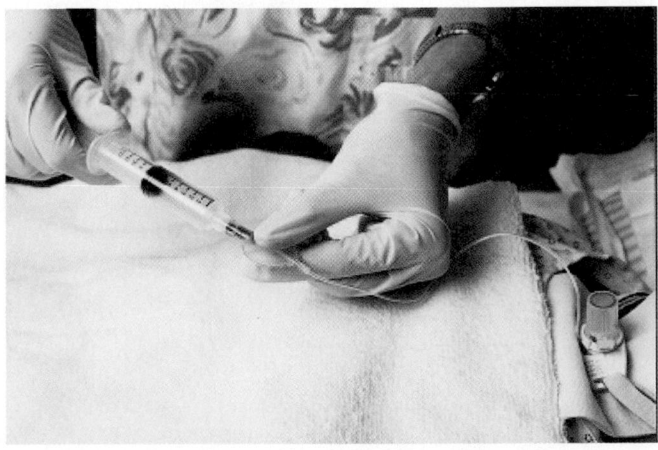

▲ Attach 10-mL syringe to distal end of inflatable cuff.

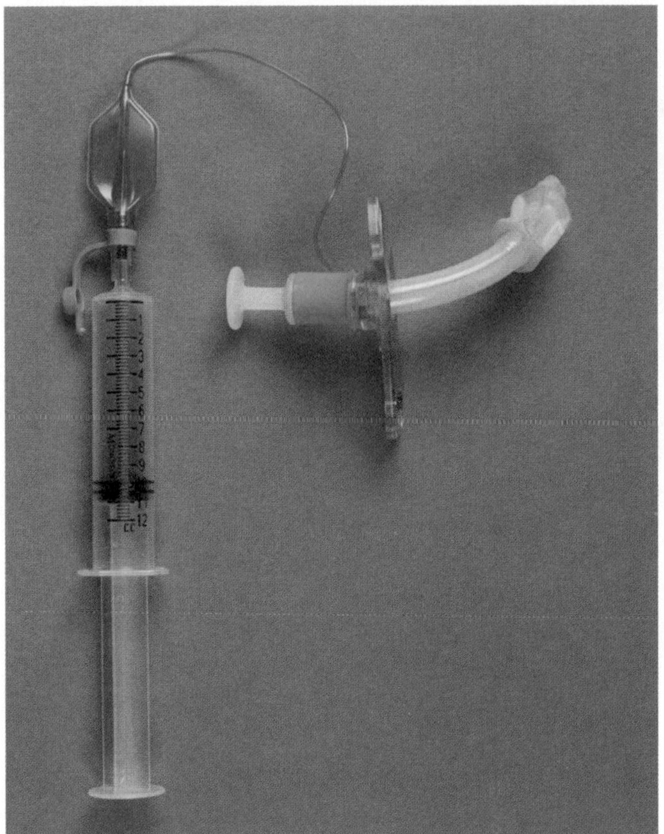

▲ Attach 10-mL syringe to distal end of inflatable cuff. (Tracheostomy tube shown.)

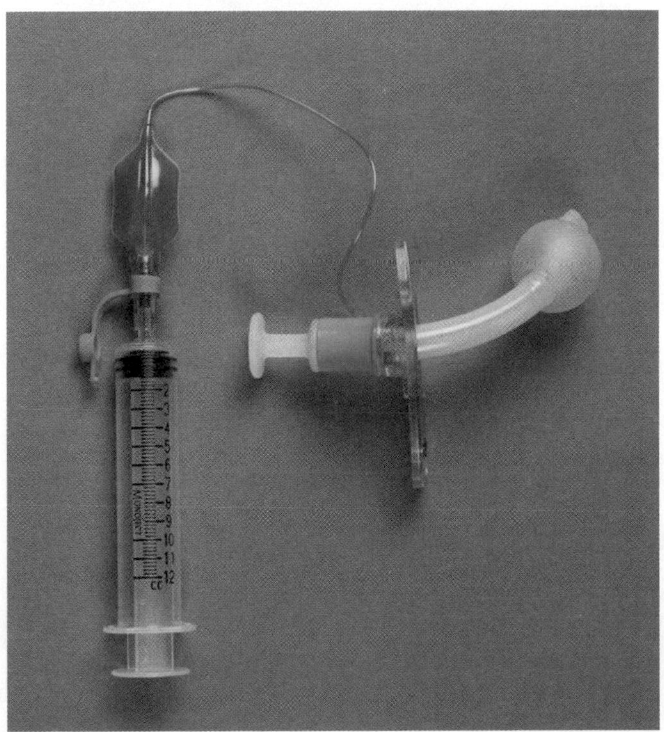

▲ Inflate cuff for minimal leak using minimal occlusive pressure. (Tracheostomy tube shown.)

3. Open sterile gloves for physician. Don clean gloves.
4. Assist physician by pouring antimicrobial solution into sterile containers on tray. To maintain sterile technique, lidocaine is usually held by the nurse while the physician draws it out of vial.
5. Have suction and oxygen administration equipment ready when trach tube is inserted. (Use suction catheter with diameter half the inner diameter of the tracheostomy tube.) ▸ ***Rationale:*** Introduction of a foreign body increases secretion production. In addition, tube presence hinders effective coughing.
6. Inflate tube cuff. (See Inflating a Tracheal Tube Cuff on page 1193.)
7. Hyperoxygenate client, then don sterile gloves and, *using sterile technique*, suction when tube is in place. Hyperoxygenate after suctioning.
8. Attach tracheostomy tube with adapter to mechanical ventilator if indicated.

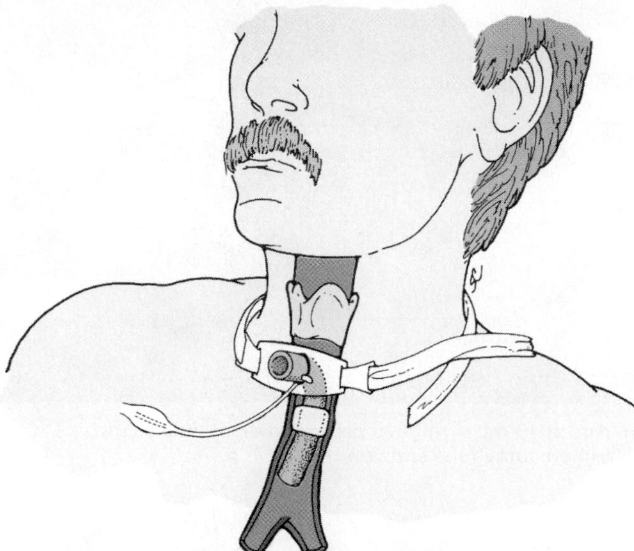

▲ Anatomic placement of a tracheostomy tube.

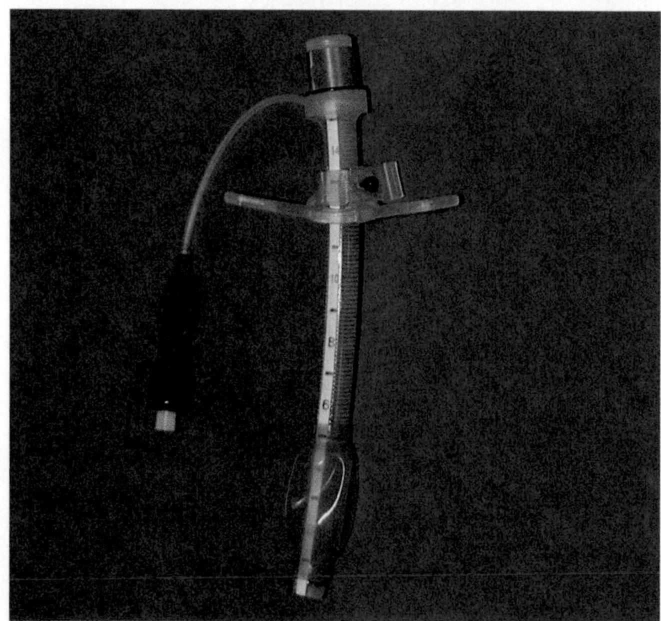

▲ Tracheal flex-tube of various lengths has adjustable neck flange and flexible wire reinforced shaft that can be adjusted to accommodate diverse neck shapes.

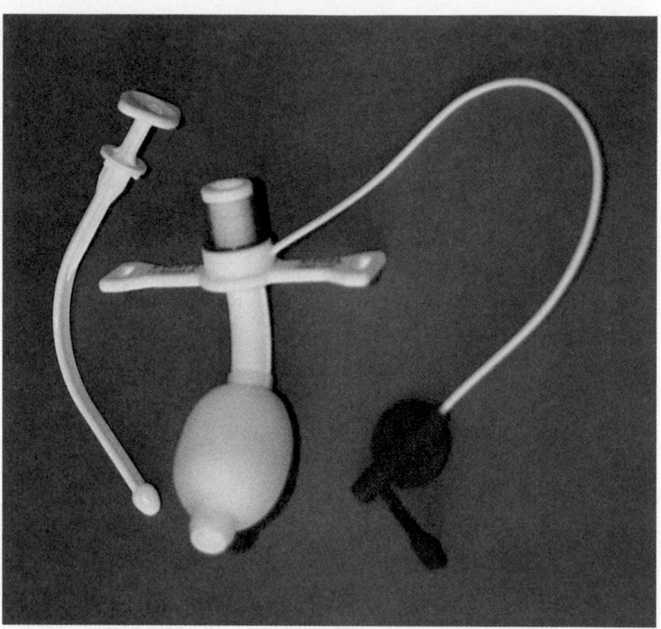

▲ Bivona Fome-Cuf® tube with obturator. Tube cuff expands passively and is evacuated with special device to collapse the Fome-Cuf®.

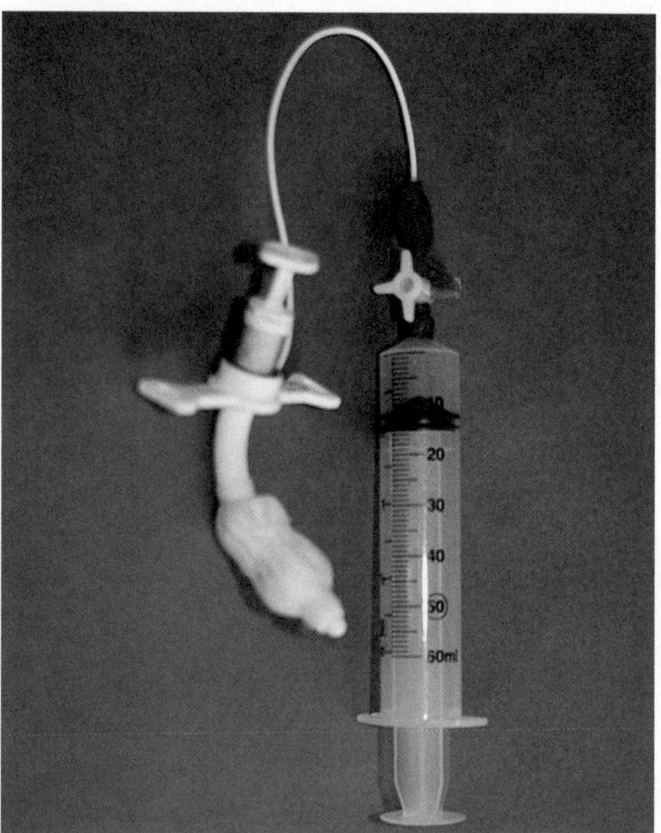

▲ Fome-Cuf® is actively deflated with special syringe device.

Preventing Infection

- Maintain sterile technique during suctioning.
- Maintain good hand hygiene.
- Change gloves when providing respiratory care to prevent cross-contamination from another part of the client's body.
- Administer oral care routinely per protocol.
- Avoid instillation of saline into airways.
- Change ventilatory equipment only when visibly soiled or malfunctioning.
- Do not allow condensation in circuit to drain toward client.

Clinical Alert

Suction client's airway PRN. Secretions are usually more copious after the irritation of intubation.

9. Cleanse tracheostomy site with sterile normal saline, secure tube with twill (or commercial holder), and dress site with presplit 4×4.
10. Position client for comfort. Semi-Fowler's position makes breathing easier.
11. Tape trach tube obturator to head of bed and place second sterile tracheostomy tube at client's bedside. ▶ ***Rationale:*** If tube inadvertently decannulates, a replacement will be available.
12. Discard used disposable equipment and remove gloves. Perform hand hygiene.
13. Place *call bell* where client can reach it and provide a means of *communication* (e.g., paper and pencil). ▶ ***Rationale:*** Tracheostomy tube bypasses the upper airway and prevents ability to vocalize.
14. Perform tracheostomy care every 8 hr and PRN.
15. Provide oral care and oropharyngeal suctioning per protocol and PRN.

Suctioning Using Single-Use Catheter for Tracheostomy

Equipment

Portable suction machine or wall suction unit with receptacle and tubing

Oral suction catheter (e.g., Yankauer)

Suction catheter set with: suction catheter, sterile gloves, container (or pop-open cup) for sterile saline

Select catheter of appropriate length—6–8 in. (15–20 cm)

Sterile saline or sterile water (mark time and date bottle is opened and discard in 24 hr)

Receptacle for used equipment

Oxygen source and administration device (e.g., bag–valve device with tracheal tube adapter)

Personal protective equipment—gown, goggles, mask if splash anticipated

Stethoscope

Preparation

1. Check physician's orders and client care plan.
2. Gather equipment.
3. Recruit an assistant for manual ventilation if indicated.
4. Attach resuscitator bag to oxygen tubing, if indicated.
5. Perform hand hygiene.
6. Assess lung sounds and heart rate and rhythm.
7. Set suction control regulator at 100–120 mmHg vacuum.
8. Don protective gown, mask, and goggles. ▶ ***Rationale:*** For self-protection if splash anticipated.

NOTE: This skill is more safely performed with an assistant who manages the resuscitator bag for hyperoxygenation while the nurse performs suctioning.

Clinical Alert

Suction catheter diameter should be no larger than one-half the inner diameter of the artificial airway. To determine catheter diameter size, multiply the artificial airway's diameter times 2 (e.g., for 8-mm tube, use a 16-French suction catheter).

Indications for Suctioning

- Ineffective cough
- Client with depressed level of consciousness
- Thick, tenacious mucus
- Impaired pulmonary function

Procedure

1. Explain procedure and rationale to client regardless of client's level of consciousness.
2. Place client in semi-Fowler's or Fowler's position.
3. Turn on suction (100–120 mmHg vacuum).
4. Remove cap from saline bottle.
5. Open catheter kit using wrapper as sterile field.
6. Carefully open container (pop open cup) and fill with sterile saline/water.
7. Administer 100% oxygen (oxygen flowmeter to maximum "flush") for 1 minute, or have assistant use resuscitator bag with adapter to hyperoxygenate client. ▶ ***Rationale:*** Suction removes oxygen, resulting in hypoxemia and potential cardiac arrest. Hyperoxygenation prevents these complications.
8. Don sterile gloves. *Dominant* hand will remain sterile, *nondominant* hand becomes "clean."
9. Holding catheter connecting end with *dominant* (sterile) hand, attach to suction tubing held with *nondominant* hand (nondominant hand is no longer sterile at this point).

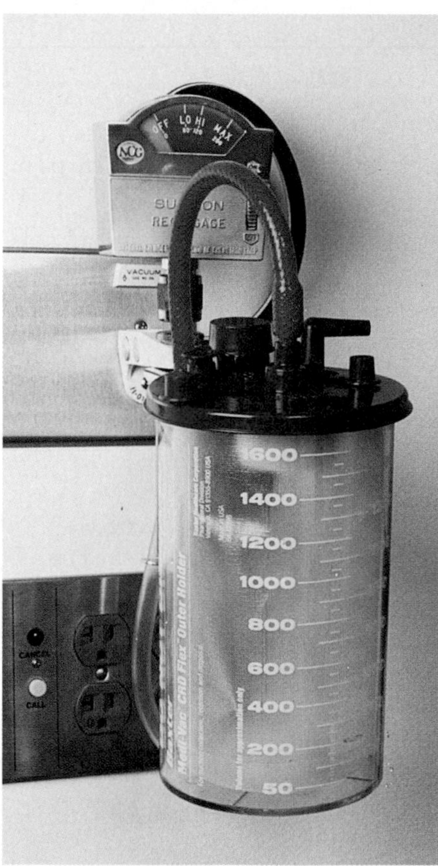

▲ Turn wall suction or other source to 100–120 mmHg vacuum.

> **Clinical Alert**
> Hyperoxygenate the client before and after each time the airway is entered for suctioning, and wait 1 minute before suctioning again to prevent severe hypoxemia.

10. Lubricate sterile catheter tip by dipping it into cup with sterile normal saline/water.
11. Using *dominant* (sterile gloved) hand, insert catheter into tracheostomy without applying suction. ▶ ***Rationale:*** Suctioning during insertion deprives client of oxygen and inhibits catheter advancement.
12. Advance catheter quickly 1–2 cm beyond end of trach tube until resistance is felt, even if client coughs. ▶ ***Rationale:*** Deep suctioning traumatizes tracheal mucosa.
13. Suction intermittently by placing and releasing *nondominant* thumb over catheter suction port while withdrawing catheter using a rotating motion. ▶ ***Rationale:*** Intermittent versus continuous application of suction may help to reduce airway injury.
14. Limit suction to no more than 10 seconds. ▶ ***Rationale:*** This prevents hypoxemic complications induced by suctioning.
15. Reattach oxygen delivery device and have client take several deep breaths, or hyperoxygenate client's lungs with resuscitator bag.
16. Flush suction catheter and tubing with sterile saline/water.
17. Use same catheter (according to agency policy) and repeat suctioning procedure one time, if necessary. Allow 1 minute between suctioning attempts for hyperoxygenation.
18. After lower airway suctioning, use the same catheter to suction client's oropharyngeal secretions. ▶ ***Rationale:*** Lower airway is sterile; upper airway is not.
19. Coil suction catheter around hand and deglove over it to discard.
20. Discard gloves and catheter and remove personal protective equipment.
21. Turn off suction source.
22. Assess lung sounds and heart rate and rhythm for changes. ▶ ***Rationale:*** Suctioning usually causes tachycardia, but hypoxemia and vagal response may cause serious bradycardia/cardiac arrest.
23. Perform hand hygiene.
24. Empty suction receptacle PRN or at end of every shift, noting character of secretions.
25. Ensure call bell is within client's reach.

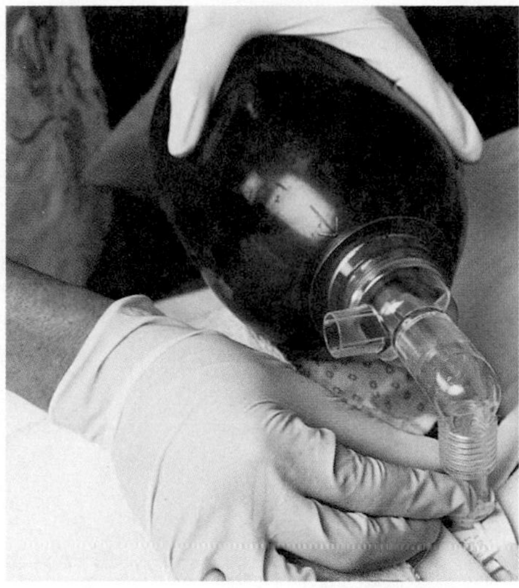

1. Connect resuscitator bag to hyperoxygenate before and after suctioning.

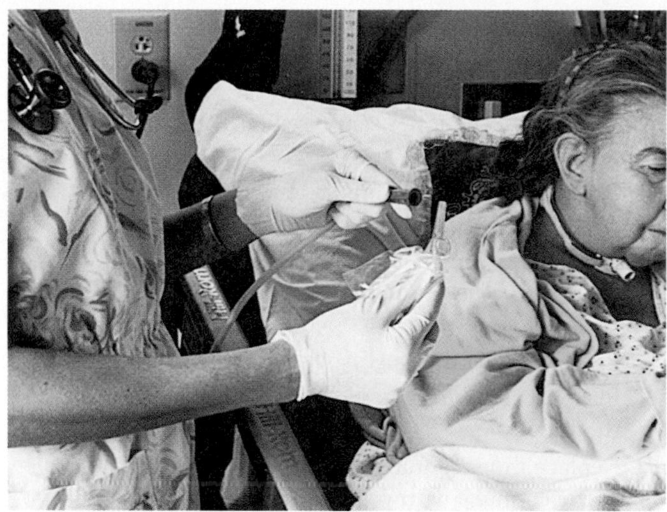

2. Hold sterile catheter with dominant (sterile) hand and connect suction tubing to catheter.

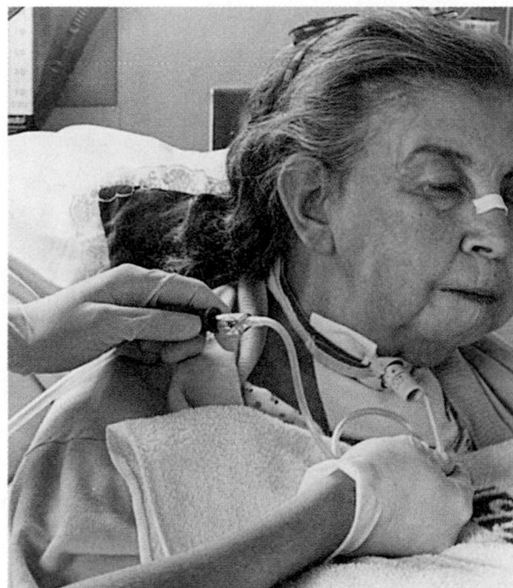

3. Guide catheter into tracheostomy tube using sterile hand.

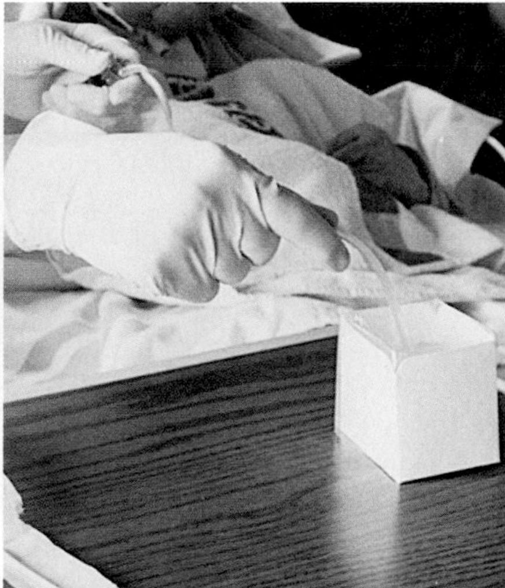

4. Rinse catheter and connecting tubing to clear.

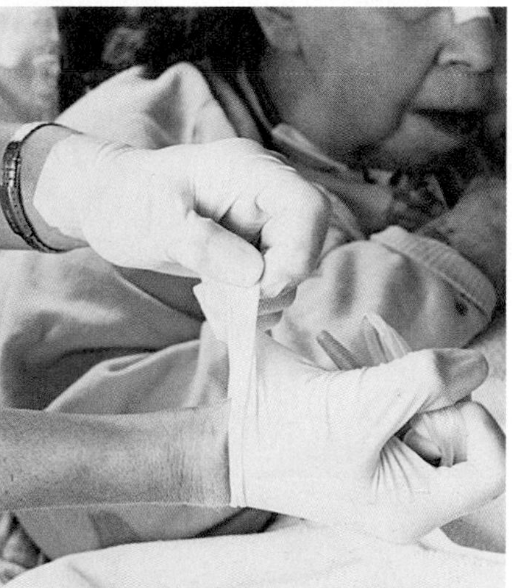

5. Coil catheter around fingers and pull glove over it for disposal.

Cleaning the Inner Cannula and Ostomy

Equipment

NOTE: Most agencies use disposable inner cannulas that eliminate the need for cleaning.

- Tracheal cleaning tray (includes two sterile basins, pipe cleaners, 4 × 4 gauze pad)
- Sterile gloves
- Suction equipment
- Complete tracheal tube set for emergency use
- Disposable inner cannula of same size
- Sterile normal saline
- Sterile nonraveling presplit dressings
- Clean tracheal ties or commercial tube holder

Preparation

1. Check physician's orders.
2. Assemble equipment.
3. Make sure suction equipment and additional tracheal tubes are available. Suction trach tube before cleaning if indicated.
4. Perform hand hygiene.

Procedure

1. Explain procedure and rationale to client.
2. Open trach tray and put on one sterile glove.
3. With gloved hand, separate basins; with ungloved hand, pour saline into basin.

4. Don second sterile glove. Secure outer cannula neck plate with index finger and thumb. Unlock inner cannula by turning left about 90°.
5. Gently pull the inner cannula slightly upward and out toward you.
6. Soak nondisposable cannula in sterile basin with saline to remove dried secretions.
7. Cleanse the lumen and outer surface of the cannula with pipe cleaners moistened with saline.
   ▶ ***Rationale:*** To remove dried secretions.
8. Rinse cannula thoroughly with saline.
9. Place clean tube on sterile 4 × 4 gauze pad and dry tube thoroughly.
10. Replace inner cannula carefully, stabilizing outer flange of the cannula, with your other hand.
11. Lock the inner cannula by turning the lock to the right so that it is in an upright position.

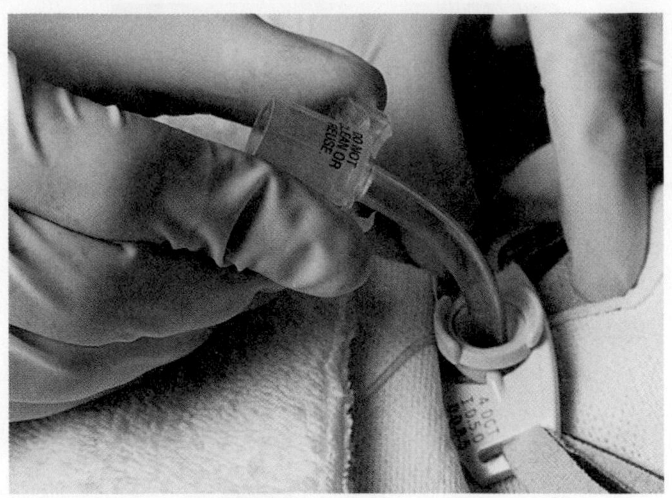
▲ Gently pull inner cannula upward and outward to remove.

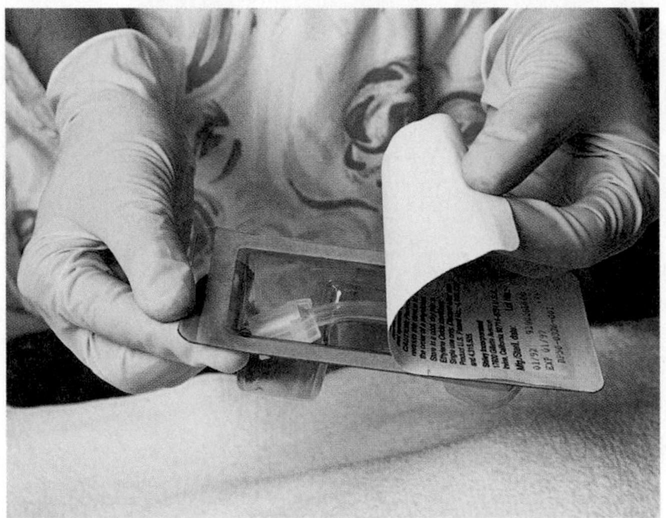
▲ Disposable inner cannula eliminates need for cannula cleaning.

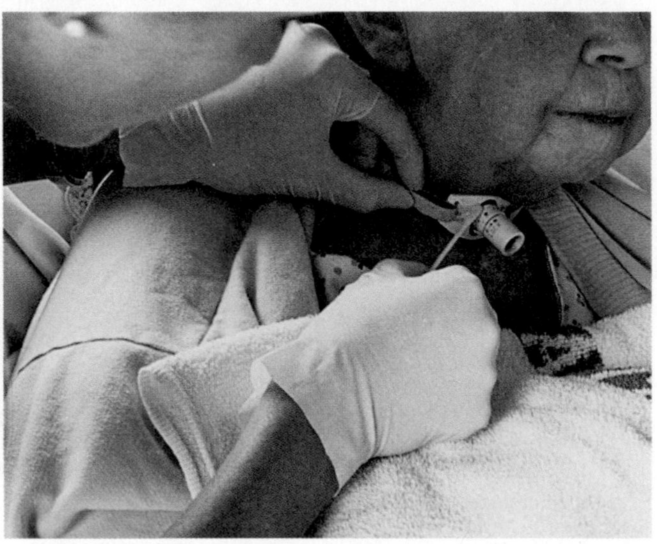
▲ Clean around tracheostomy site and outer cannula.

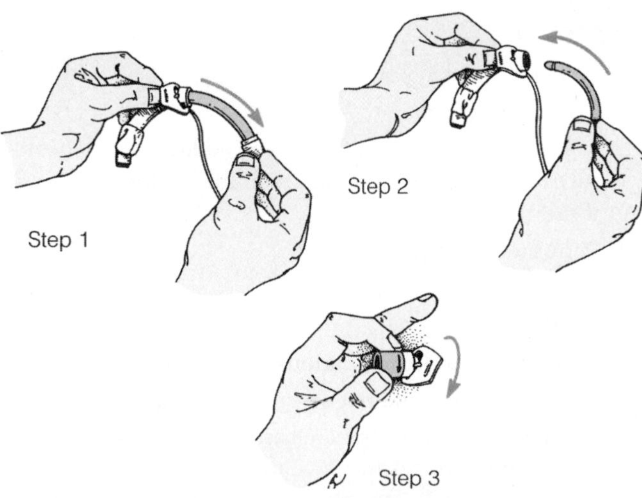

▲ Inner cannula is removed for cleaning. Outer cannula is not.

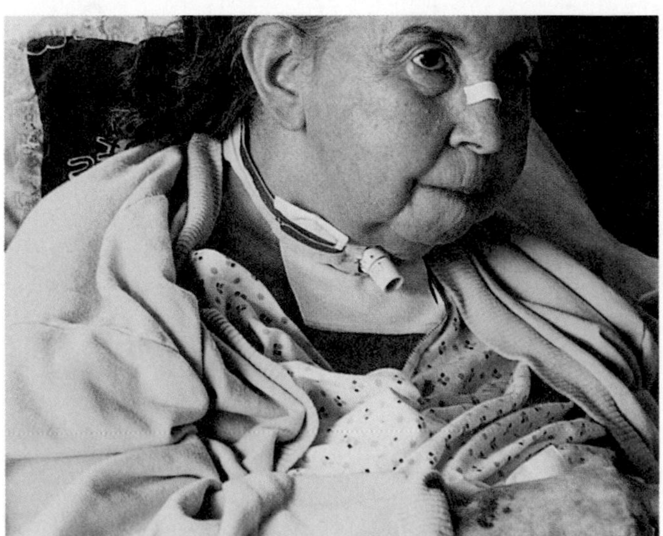
▲ Apply precut nonraveling dressing around tracheostomy.

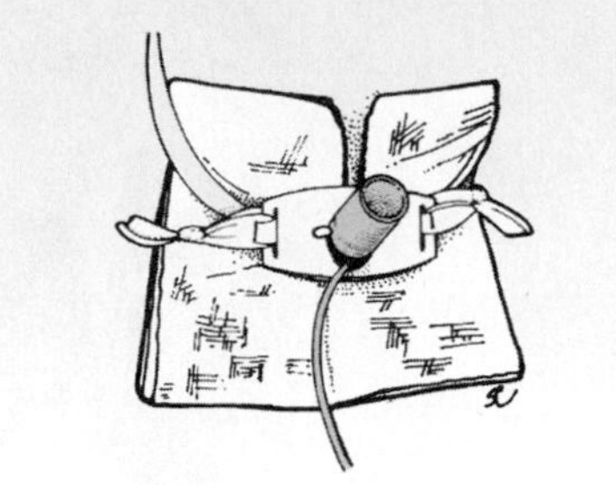

▲ A precut nonraveling sponge is used for the trach dressing to prevent fibers from entering trach site.

12. Cleanse around tracheostomy site with applicator soaked in normal saline.
13. Cleanse outer cannula with separate applicator.
14. Apply precut, nonraveling trach dressing around insertion site (flaps pointing up), and change tracheal ties if needed. ▸ ***Rationale:*** Nonraveling dressing prevents fibers from entering trach tube.
15. Discard soiled dressings, tapes, cleaning equipment, and gloves.
16. Perform hand hygiene.
17. Ensure call bell is within client's reach.

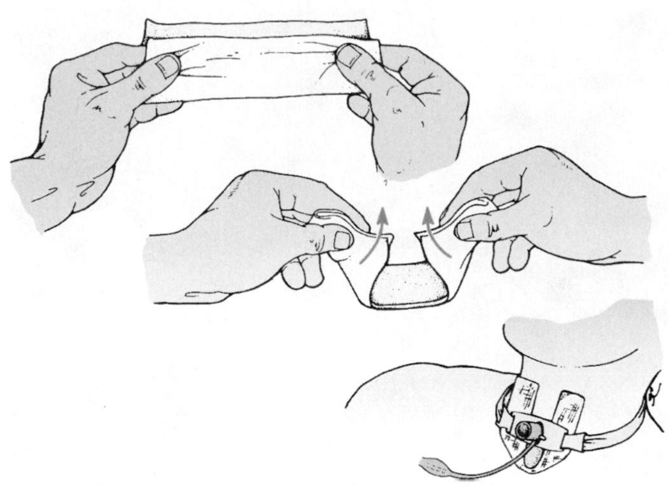

▲ Folded 4 × 4 trach dressing for use if presplit dressing is not available.

Clinical Alert

An obturator is kept at the bedside for emergency use. If the tracheostomy tube is inadvertently dislodged, it can be reinserted immediately using the obturator.

Changing Tracheostomy Tube Ties

Equipment

Scissors

Forceps

Twill tape or commercial tracheostomy tube holder.

Preparation

1. Seek assistance from another person. ▸ ***Rationale:*** It is safer to have someone hold the trach tube in place when changing ties.
2. Explain procedure to client.
3. Perform hand hygiene.
4. Gather equipment.
5. Place client in semi- to high-Fowler's position.

Procedure

For Twill Tape Ties

1. Cut trach ties length you desire, if not precut.
2. Fold ends of the trach ties over 1½ in., and cut a slit in the piece starting at the folded edge.
3. If available, have assistant hold the trach tube in place. Cut the old trach ties, remove, and discard. ▸ ***Rationale:*** Securing tube helps prevent accidental extubation if client coughs.
4. Pass the slit end of the ties through the flange loop of the trach tube about 2–3 in. (you may use Kelly forceps to grab tie). ▸ ***Rationale:*** Leave the old trach tie in place if you are changing the ties without assistance. This prevents accidental dislodging of the trach tube.
5. Thread the other end of the tie all the way through the slit. Pull it firmly in place. ▸ ***Rationale:*** This action anchors the tie around the flange loop.
6. Repeat steps 4 and 5 on other flange loop.
7. Bring ties around client's neck and tie in a square knot to one side of neck, leaving one finger-breadth slack under tie. ▸ ***Rationale:*** Slack prevents pressure on the neck and jugular vein.
8. Cut off soiled trach ties if not already done and discard.
9. Position client for comfort.
10. Perform hand hygiene.

Clinical Alert

Some agencies recommend that tracheostomy tube and ties not be changed for the first 72 hr because of risk for stoma closure.

Alternate Method

1. Using a long piece of twill, pull end of tape through flange slit.
2. Double tape around back of neck.
3. Thread one end through other flange slit and tie to other end.
4. Apply new tape before old one is cut off and removed (doesn't require an assistant).

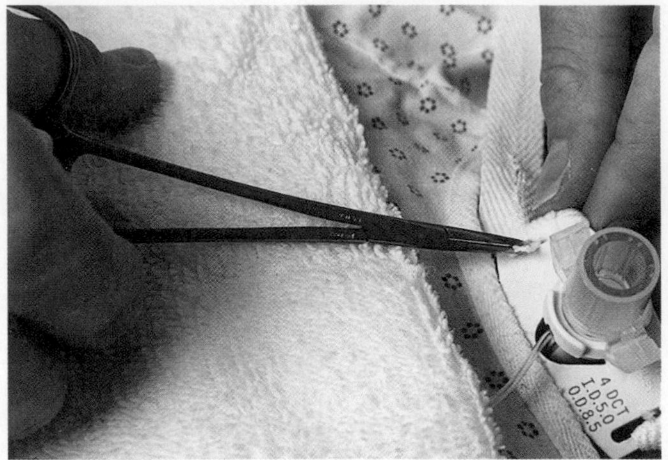

▲ Use forceps to thread tape through tracheostomy neck plate flanges.

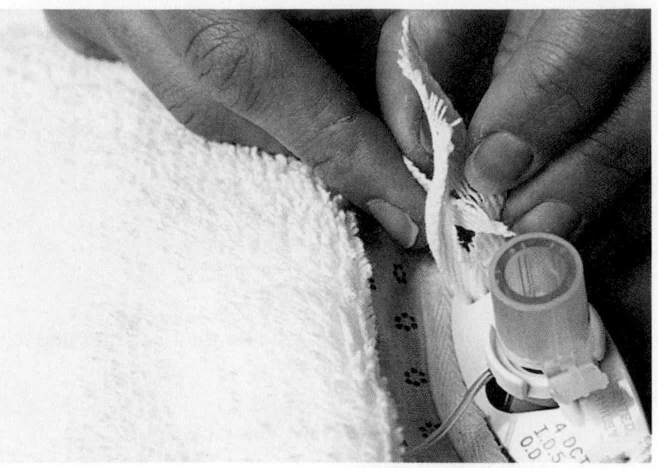

▲ Thread other end of tie through slit and pull in place.

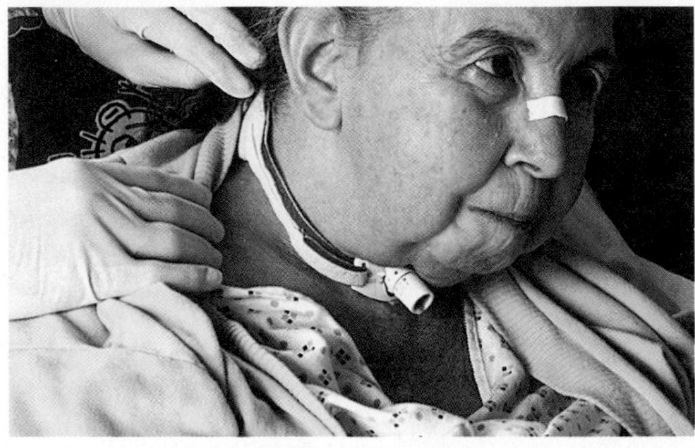

▲ Allow one finger-breadth slack under trach ties to prevent pressure on neck and jugular vein. Note: Velcro is frequently used for track ties in place of twill tape.

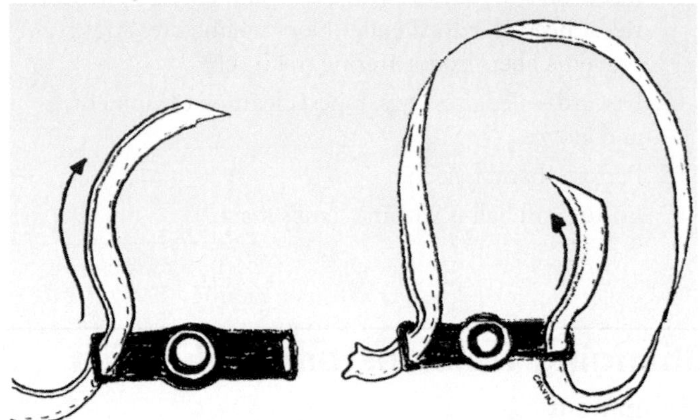

▲ (a) Use a long piece of twill. Pull end through flange slit and double tape around back of neck. (b) Thread one end through other flange slit and tie to other end of twill in square knot.

Capping With a Passey–Muir Speaking Valve

Equipment

Passey–Muir speaking valve and storage container

Fenestrated uncuffed tracheostomy tube (preferred)

Suction source

Two suction catheters

Clean gloves

10 mL syringe

NOTE: A fenestrated uncuffed tracheostomy tube has openings that allow the client's exhaled air to flow through the upper airway as well as the tracheostomy opening. When the outer cannula is capped with a one-way valve, exhaled air flows over the vocal cords for speech production.

Preparation

1. Check physician's orders and client care plan.
2. Determine that client has been screened with trial for candidacy by a speech pathologist and respiratory care practitioner.
3. Determine type of tracheostomy tube present. ▸ ***Rationale:*** A fenestrated uncuffed tube is preferred. The valve is *not* used with endotracheal tube.
4. Review client's vital signs, SpO_2, breath sounds, work of breathing.
5. Perform hand hygiene.
6. Gather equipment.
7. Explain procedure to client.
8. Place client in Fowler's position. ▸ ***Rationale:*** This assists with lung expansion and helps to maintain a patent airway.
9. Don clean gloves.

Clinical Alert

The speaking valve should be removed during sleep.

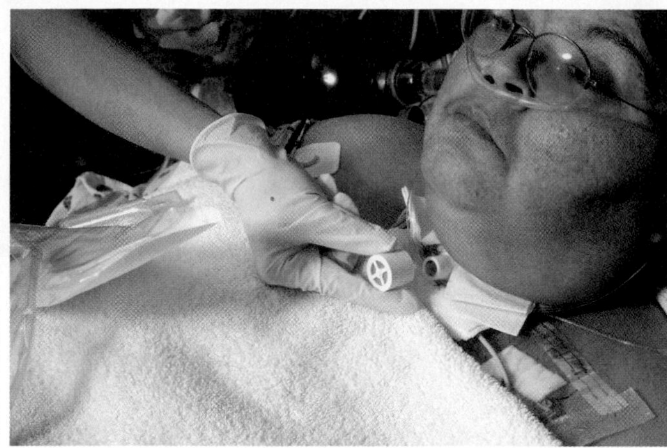

▲ Tracheostomy tube is capped with a one-way valve to allow client to speak.

Passey–Muir Speaking Valve

The Passey–Muir Speaking Valve can be used on or off a ventilator and is safe for infants and adults in acute or home care. The valve expedites mechanical ventilation weaning and reduces decannulation time.

The speaking valve opens only during inspiration and closes automatically before the beginning of the expiratory cycle, restoring exhaled airflow through the oronasopharynx. The valve restores a more normal "closed respiratory system," resulting in many benefits including hands-free, clear, uninterrupted speech production; improved swallowing; reduced aspiration; and stronger, more effective cough. Additionally, use of the valve restores the sense of smell and taste, thus improving appetite and promoting nutritional intake.

EVIDENCE-BASED PRACTICE

Use of a One-Way Speaking Valve

Subglottal air pressure is lost when a tracheostomy tube is in place. This reduction in air pressure is thought to be the primary mechanism responsible for aspiration in tracheostomized clients. Placement of a one-way speaking valve may restore this air pressure as well as improve laryngeal and pharyngeal sensation, may improve ability to expel material from the laryngeal vestibule either through throat clearing or coughing, and may improve swallow safety.

Source: Suiter, D. M., McCullough, G. H., & Powell, P. W. (2003). Effects of cuff deflation and one-way tracheostomy speaking valve placement on swallow physiology. *Dysphagia, 18*(4), 284–292.

Clinical Alert

If a cuffed tracheostomy tube is capped and cuff is not deflated, client has no airway. Place notice: *"Do not inflate cuff with cap in place"* on pilot balloon, over bed, and on client's chart. An uncuffed fenestrated tube is preferred when speaking valve is used.

Procedure

1. Using clean technique, suction nasopharynx *if cuffed tube in place.* ▸ ***Rationale:*** This removes secretions that have pooled above cuff and prevents their mobilization into lower airways upon cuff deflation.
2. Attach syringe and **DEFLATE TRACHEAL CUFF** if present. ▸ ***Rationale:*** If tracheostomy tube is capped and cuff is not deflated, client has no airway.
3. Allow the client to adjust to cuff deflation. ▸ ***Rationale:*** Initiation of upper airway breathing increases resistance to airflow.
4. Place speaking valve over opening of tracheostomy tube.
5. Place notice: "Do not inflate cuff with speaking valve in place" on pilot balloon, over bed, and on client's chart.
6. Gently stabilize the tracheostomy tube to remove the valve and place in container.
7. When the valve is removed, reinflate tube cuff (if indicated).
8. Discard gloves and perform hand hygiene.

DOCUMENTATION for Tracheostomy Care

Tracheostomy Procedure

- Name of physician performing procedure
- Size and type of tube inserted
- Respiratory status before and after procedure
- Client's tolerance of procedure
- Amount and character of secretions
- Any equipment attached to tracheal tube (ventilator or other oxygen delivery device and percent oxygen delivered)
- Provision of means to communicate and summon help.

Tracheostomy Tube Suctioning

- Frequency of client suctioning
- Before and after suctioning hyperoxygenation
- Amount, color, and consistency of secretions
- Client's tolerance to procedure
- Unanticipated problems and client's response

Cleaning the Inner Cannula and Ostomy

- Time and date of care
- Ostomy site status
- Cannula cleaning or disposable cannula replacement
- Tracheostomy ties or holder replacement

Capping Tracheostomy Tube

- Type of tracheostomy tube in place
- Type of speaking valve utilized
- Tracheal tube DEFLATION status
- Baseline data before procedure
- Client's tolerance of valve placement
- Respiratory/O_2 status during valve use
- Client's ability to speak and swallow

Tracheal Tube Cuff Inflation

- Cuff inflation auscultated for minimal occlusive pressure.
- Bilateral breath sounds present on auscultation.

CRITICAL THINKING Application

Expected Outcomes

- Tracheostomy tube remains stable.
- Tracheostomy tube provides a patent airway.
- Client is able to communicate with speaking valve placement.

Unexpected Outcomes	Alternative Actions

Client experiences tracheostomy tube decannulation.	• Call a "CODE" immediately.
	• For new stoma:
	  • If present, pull tracheal retention sutures apart to lift the trachea and hold the stoma open.
	  • *Or*: Cover stoma and have assistant provide bag–mask ventilations.
	  • Or: Obtain new tracheostomy tube, place obturator and insert tube into client's stoma, then remove obturator.

Client experiences distress—tracheostomy tube is obstructed; breath sounds not heard.	• Call Rapid Response Team or "CODE" or immediately. • Deflate cuff. • Cut tracheostomy ties. • Remove tube. • See above options.
Client experiences distress with speaking valve placement.	• Request repeat assessment by speech pathologist and respiratory care practitioner. • Monitor client's SpO_2. • Downsize tracheostomy tube. • Reduce time of valve use. • Remove speaking valve if respiratory distress occurs. • Administer O_2 per nasal cannula if desaturation occurs. • Obtain Passey–Muir valve with oxygen adapter to administer O_2 if indicated. • Remind client that use of the speaking valve is a step toward trach tube removal.

Chapter 30

UNIT 7

Chest Drainage Systems

Nursing Process Data

ASSESSMENT Data Base

- Assess client's respiratory status, vital signs.
- Note placement site of chest tube (intrapleural or mediastinal).
- Assess that all drainage system connections are securely taped.
- Note prescribed amount of negative pressure to be established.
- Check patency of chest drainage system.
- Assess for signs of mediastinal shift.
- Note character and amount of chest drainage.

PLANNING Objectives

- To evacuate air and/or fluid from intrapleural space to promote lung re-expansion
- To reestablish negative intrapleural pressure
- To facilitate drainage of fluid from the mediastinum after cardiac surgery
- To administer autotransfusion after cardiac surgery

IMPLEMENTATION Procedures

EVALUATION Expected Outcomes

- Chest drainage system is patent.
- Mediastinal shift does not occur.
- Chest tube remains securely placed.

Pearson Nursing Student Resources

Find additional review materials at
nursing.pearsonhighered.com

Prepare for success with NCLEX®-style practice questions and Skill Checklists

Maintaining Chest Gravity Drainage/Suction Bottle System

Equipment

Three-bottle chest drainage system in holder with manufacturer's instructions for use

Tape

Suction source, if indicated (e.g., wall suction or Emerson pump)

Clean gloves and personal protective equipment

Procedure

For Underwater Seal (One-Bottle System)

1. Don gloves and personal protective equipment.
2. Fill water seal bottle with 300 mL of water to submerge water seal tube.

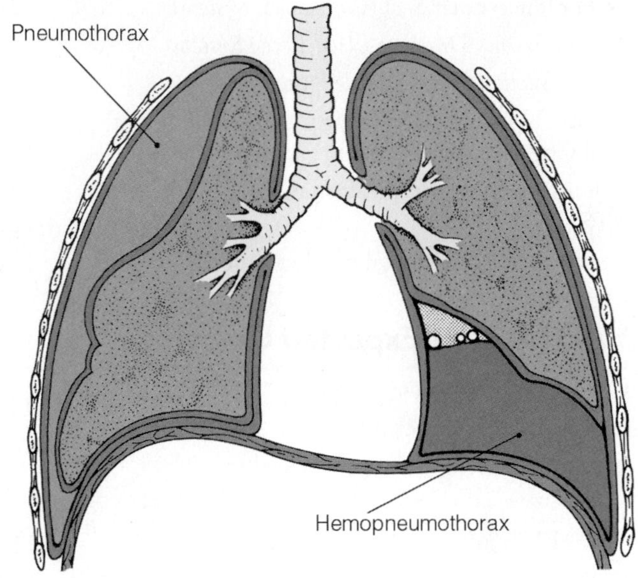

▲ Pneumothorax refers to air in the intrapleural space and hemothorax to blood in the intrapleural space around the lung; both conditions lead to buildup of positive pressure, compression of lung tissue, and possible compression of mediastinal structures with decreased venous return and decreased cardiac output.

3. Attach client's chest tube drainage tubing to water seal tube to prevent atmospheric air from entering client's pleural space.
4. Check that water seal bottle air vent is open to atmosphere. ▸ ***Rationale:*** The bottle stopper has two openings, one for inlet from the client, one for outlet to the atmosphere. Air vent allows air from client's intrapleural space to escape and to maintain negative pressure relative to client's intrapleural pressure.
5. Coil drainage tubing from client's chest tube to water seal bottle so that there are no dependent loops. ▸ ***Rationale:*** Dependent loops will inhibit air removal.
6. Make sure all tubing and bottle connections are sealed to ensure system is airtight.
7. Ensure patency of system by noting "tidaling" in underwater tube. Fluid should rise on inhalation and descend on exhalation.
8. Note occasional bubbling of air from the water seal tube. ▸ ***Rationale:*** This is sign that air is being evacuated from the client's intrapleural space.
9. Check tubing for obstruction. ▸ ***Rationale:*** Tidaling ceases when lung has re-expanded or tube system is obstructed.
10. Report event of continuous bubbling in the water seal bottle. ▸ ***Rationale:*** This is indicative of an air leak. See steps for locating air leak, page 1216.
11. Assess for return of breath sounds or obtain chest x-ray to determine re-expansion.

Clinical Alert

Chest tubes should not be clamped except briefly while checking for an air leak or for changing a disposable collection system.

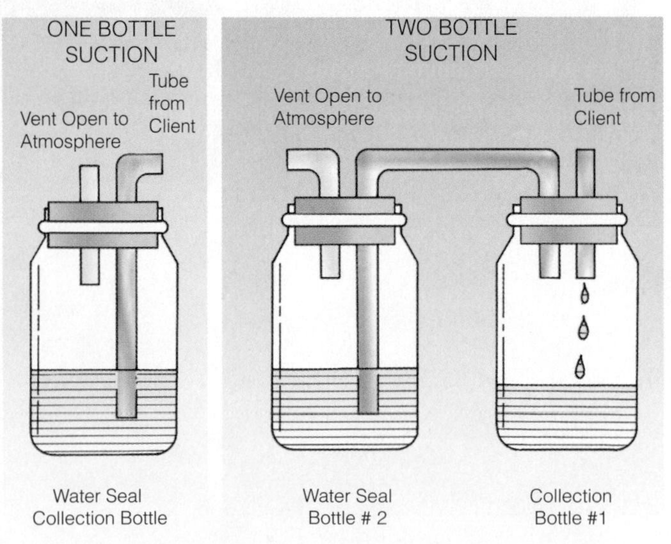

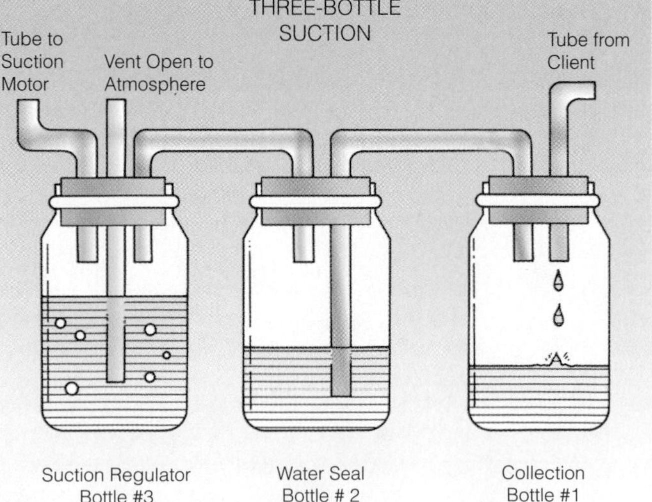

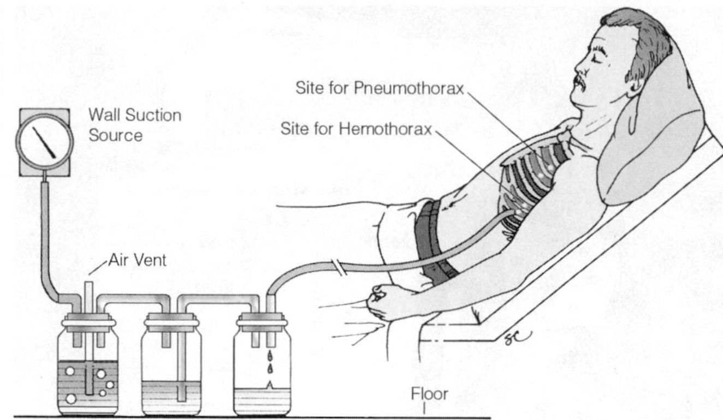

▲ Keep collection system at least 12 in. below client's chest. Coil tubing to prevent dependent loops.

For Gravity Drainage (Two-Bottle System)

1. Don gloves and personal protective equipment.
2. Attach client's chest tube drainage tubing to collection bottle. ▸ ***Rationale:*** Chest tube drainage is monitored in this bottle.
3. Attach drainage bottle outlet tube to submerged inlet tube of underwater seal bottle.
4. Follow steps 4–10 in previous skill for underwater seal system.

For Suction (Three-Bottle System)

1. Follow steps 1–6 in previous skill for gravity drainage.
2. Submerge suction control tube of third bottle under prescribed amount of water. ▸ ***Rationale:*** The third bottle stopper has three openings, one for inlet from the second bottle, one for suction control and air venting, and one for connection to a suction source. Depth of immersion of the suction control tube dictates the amount of suction applied to the three-bottle system (20 cm of water produces −20 cm of water suction).
3. Connect water seal (second) bottle outlet tube to stopper of third bottle.
4. Leave suction control tube open to atmosphere. ▸ ***Rationale:*** This provides the outlet for air from client's intrapleural space.
5. Connect suction source tubing to wall suction.
6. Regulate wall suction to a point where water in the second bottle just bubbles. ▸ ***Rationale:*** This indicates that desired suction has been reached.
7. Note *occasional* bubbling of air in the water seal bottle. ▸ ***Rationale:*** This indicates that air is being evacuated from client's intrapleural space. *Continuous* bubbling in water seal bottle should not occur.
8. Note *continuous* bubbling of air through open end of control tube in the suction bottle.
9. Monitor fluid levels in water seal and suction control bottles.
10. Note and mark chest tube drainage on drainage bottle. Notify physician if there is more than 100 mL of drainage per hour. ▸ ***Rationale:*** This amount represents excessive bleeding requiring medical management; however, drainage of old blood may increase with position change.
11. Continue to monitor client's SPO_2 and vital signs.

Using Chest Drainage/Suction Bottle Systems

One-Bottle System

One bottle functions as a drainage collection bottle as well as water seal. Used mainly to reestablish negative intrapleural pressure to reinflate lung from pneumothorax.

Two-Bottle System

Water-seal bottle and drainage collection bottle are separate. System not usually connected to suction source. Used after thoracic or cardiac surgery.

Three-Bottle System

Third bottle is connected to an external suction source. The other two bottles are the same as for two-bottle system. Used after thoracic or cardiac surgery.

Small Mobile Chest Drains Allow Mobility and Early Discharge From the Hospital. Examples Include:

Heimlich one-way valve, which, attached to the client's chest tube, allows *air* to escape, but not enter; the distal end of the valve remains open. It, and the chest tube, should be taped to the client's chest. The Heimlich valve is not used for chest tube drainage.

Pneumostat is a plastic device that has a one-way valve and a gravity drainage collection chamber. The unit can be clipped to the client's clothing.

Setting Up and Maintaining a Disposable Water Seal Chest Drainage System

Equipment

- Disposable water seal chest drainage system and stand
- Suction source
- Connecting tubing and adapter
- 60-mL sterile syringe with catheter tip
- Sterile water in pouring bottle
- Tape
- Gloves
- Personal protective equipment

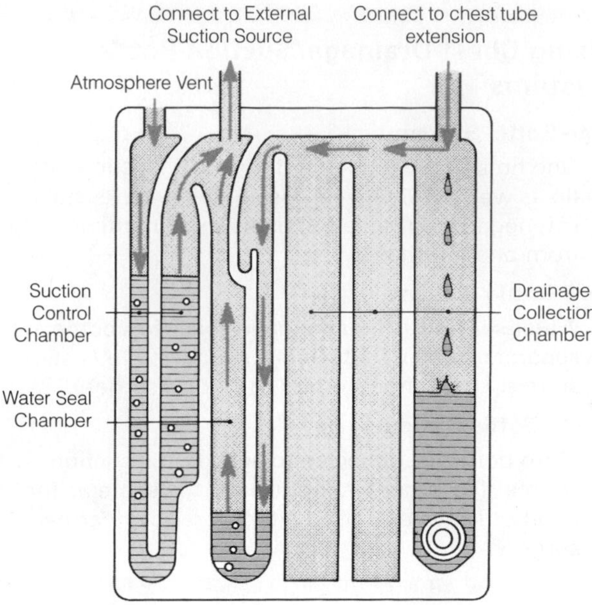

▲ Disposable water-seal chest drainage system principles correspond to the three-bottle drainage system.

NOTE: Placement of chest tubes in the mediastinum for drainage after cardiac surgery is common. Intrapleural pressure is not affected.

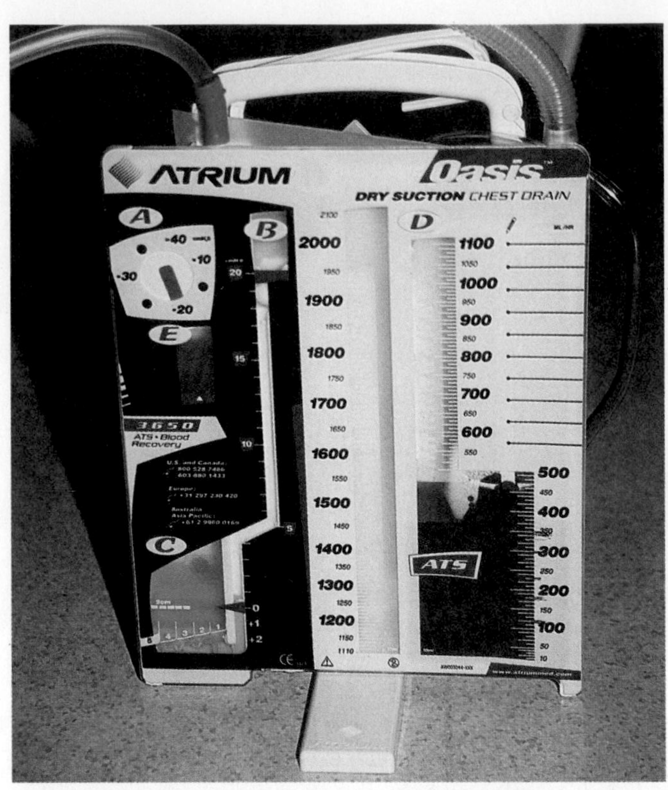

▲ This dry suction system (OASIS) requires that water be added to the water seal, but does not require water in the suction chamber. The suction is wall regulated. These systems are quieter and easier to use.

Procedure

1. Gather equipment.
2. Perform hand hygiene; don gloves and personal protective equipment.
3. Unwrap water seal chest drainage system.
4. Place unit in stand on floor at bedside or hang from foot of bed frame.

Check Points for Chest Tube Air Leaks

Check Insertion Site

- Pinch or briefly clamp with padded hemostat tube at chest insertion site. Bubbling stops in the water seal chamber if there is an air leak at insertion site.

Check Tubing

- Pinch rubber connecting tubing. Bubbling stops if there is a leak at chest tube connector site.

Check Water Seal Drainage System

- Pinch rubber connecting tubing. Bubbling continues if there is a leak in water seal connection.

Observe water seal chamber. There should not be excessive continuous bubbling. A small amount of bubbling is seen in the water seal:

- When suction is first initiated.
- As air is displaced by drainage in the collection chambers.
- As client exhales and coughs and air is forced out of intrapleural space.

When lung has re-expanded, the bubbles cease.

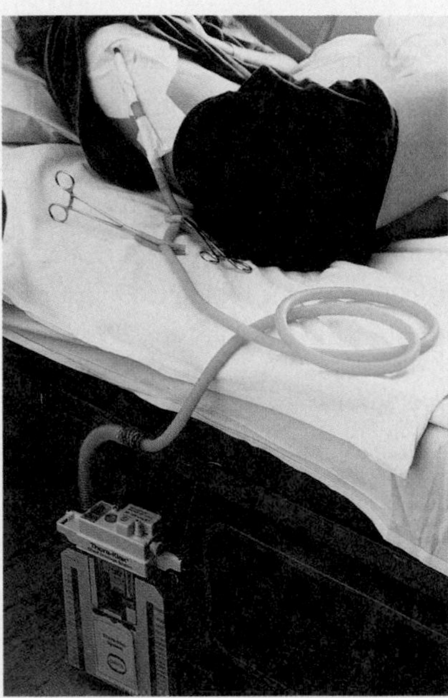

▲ Padded hemostat or plastic tube clamp is used for clamping chest tube. Tube clamped only if ordered.

5. Remove plastic connector on short tube attached to water-seal chamber.
6. Remove plunger from 60-mL syringe and attach barrel of syringe to short tube.
7. Pour specified amount of sterile water into barrel of syringe, filling water seal chamber to 2-cm level (according to package directions). ▸ ***Rationale:*** This level provides sufficient fluid to create a one-way valve to prevent atmospheric air from entering client's intrapleural space.
8. For gravity drainage: leave suction control source tubing open to air.
9. For suction drainage: remove plastic plug from atmosphere vent to suction control chamber.
10. Attach 60-mL syringe barrel to atmosphere vent and pour sterile water into suction control chamber.
11. Fill suction control chamber to 20-cm level. ▸ ***Rationale:*** Fluid level controls amount of negative pressure created throughout system.

NOTE: Some chest drainage systems do not require water in either chamber, or only the suction control chamber. See manufacturer's instruction for waterless system use. Dry suction is quieter and capable of achieving greater degrees of negative pressure (up to –40 cm H_2O). These units may have a "dry suction control" dial usually set at –10 to –20 cm H_2O. Turn on suction source until orange bellows appears in indicator window to establish suction.

Clinical Alert

Subcutaneous emphysema (air in tissue) may be felt around the chest tube insertion site, but should be reported if it extends beyond this.

12. Remove long tube adapter from collection chamber and connect it to client's chest tubing.
13. Tape connection.
14. Coil tubing loosely on the bed, but provide a straight line of tubing from bed to collection system. ▸ ***Rationale:*** Straight-line tubing prevents pooling of fluid pressure alterations and system obstruction.
15. Make sure tubing is free and not kinked. Do not use pins or restrain tubing. ▸ ***Rationale:*** Pins could puncture tubing, causing an air leak.
16. Attach short rubber tube on water-seal chamber to wall suction tubing using an adapter.
17. Turn suction device on slowly until bubbling occurs in suction control chamber.
18. Monitor water levels daily in both water seal chamber and suction control chamber.
19. Maintain pressure.
    a. Keep drainage system at least 12 in. below client's chest level. ▸ ***Rationale:*** Raising the unit can cause backflow of drainage into client's intrapleural space.
    b. Maintain wall suction to create gentle bubbling in suction control chamber.
    c. Maintain water seal level (2 cm). ▸ ***Rationale:*** Water seal prevents room air from entering pleural space.
    d. Maintain suction control chamber water level at 20 cm or as ordered.

Clinical Alert

Strip and milk chest tubes *only* with physician's orders. Excessive negative pressure created by stripping and milking increases negative pressure in intrapleural space.

20. Maintain chest tube patency. Only if physician orders, milk chest tubes to maintain drainage and tube patency.
    a. If ordered, milk tube by alternately folding or squeezing and then releasing drainage tubing. ▸ ***Rationale:*** This provides intermittent suction to the chest tube but generates extreme negative pressure in intrapleural space.
    b. Milk tube away from client toward the drainage receptacle (disposable system or bottles).
21. Strip chest tubes *only* if physician orders.
    a. To strip chest tube, pinch tubing close to client's chest with one hand and, using a lubricated thumb and forefinger, compress and slide fingers down tube toward drainage chamber/bottle. (Lubricant material is usually petrolatum or alcohol swab.)
    b. Release pressure on tube and repeat stripping action until reaching receptacle. Increased negative pressure can occur.
22. Keep rubber-tipped hemostat at the client's bedside. ▸ ***Rationale:*** In emergency, tube can be clamped nearest to chest insertion site.
23. Keep collection system at least 12 in. below client's chest level. ▸ ***Rationale:*** This enables fluid to flow by gravity.
24. Mark drainage on disposable system collection chamber hourly, or every shift. Drainage should be measured at eye level. Report drainage exceeding 100 mL/hr.
25. Assess client's status.
    a. Instruct client to deep breathe and cough at frequent intervals. ▸ ***Rationale:*** Frequent deep breathing helps to expand the lungs. Coughing helps evacuate air from intrapleural space.
    b. Encourage client to change positions frequently. Chest tube drainage does not limit client activity.
    c. Observe and report any adverse change in SPO_2, vital signs, or client's tolerance.

Administering Autotransfusion Using Pleur-evac ATS

Equipment

- Sterile disposable Pleur-evac ATS including blood collection bag
- Replacement bag
- Microaggregate filter
- Clean gloves
- Sterile saline or water in parking bottle

NOTE: A variety of sterile chest drainage systems provide evacuation of air and/or fluid from the chest or mediastinum. Evacuated blood may be simultaneously reinfused or collected and reinfused in postoperative or trauma cases.

Procedure

1. Perform hand hygiene and don gloves.
2. Connect client's pleural or mediastinal chest tube by following steps 1 through 3 printed on Pleur-evac unit. ▸ ***Rationale:*** Tight connection establishes water-seal drainage system.
3. Check that ALL clamps are open on blood collection bag and drainage tubing and that connections are airtight.
4. Check that blood begins collecting in bag.
5. Mark time and amount of drainage on bag.
6. Close clamp on chest drainage tubing and collection bag and connect new bag to drainage system. Make sure all connections are tight.
7. Depress button on high-negativity relief valve and release it when negativity drops to desired level. ▸ ***Rationale:*** This reduces excess negativity before removing first collection bag.

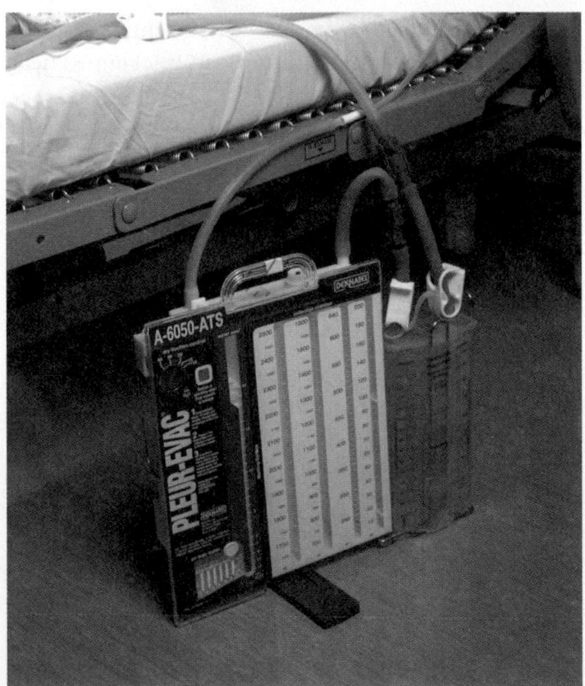

▲ Pleur-evac autotransfusion system (ATS) frequently placed in cardiac surgery.

8. Close white clamp on client tubing, then close two white clamps on top of collection bag, and disconnect all connectors on first bag.
9. Remove protective cap from collection tubing on replacement bag. Maintain aseptic technique when changing tubing.
10. Use red connectors to connect unit's collection tubing to client's chest drainage tube.
11. Remove protective cap from replacement bag's suction tube.
12. Use blue connectors to attach replacement bag's suction tube to Pleur-evac unit.
13. Open all clamps, and check that system is airtight.
14. Attach red (female) and blue (male) connector sections on top of autotransfusion bag.
15. Move out and disconnect metal support arms, and disconnect foot hook. ▸ ***Rationale:*** Releasing these connections allows you to remove bag from drainage unit.
16. Attach replacement bag by using foot hook and support arm.
17. Slide bag off support frame and invert bag with spike port pointing up. ▸ ***Rationale:*** This position allows blood to be reinfused from original collection bag.
18. Remove protective cap from spike port, and insert a microaggregate filter. Twist filter into position. ▸ ***Rationale:*** Filter is essential for reinfusion.
19. Prime filter by gently squeezing inverted bag until drip chamber is half full.
20. Close clamp on reinfusion line, and remove residual air from bag.
21. Invert bag on IV pole.
22. Flush IV tubing to remove air, then reinfuse blood by gravity or pump according to hospital policy. Blood should be totally reinfused within 6 hr from *start of collection*.
23. Remove gloves and perform hand hygiene.
24. Assess neurologic signs and pulmonary status every 4 hr. ▸ ***Rationale:*** Microemboli can occur with autotransfusion.

Clinical Alert

Reinfusion is not indicated unless system is primed with drainage and an additional 50 mL of drainage has been collected for reinfusion.

No more than 6 hr should elapse from time of *beginning* collection to *completion* of reinfusion.

Refer to evacuation/reinfusion system manufacturer's package insert for indications, contraindications, and instructions for use.

Assisting With Removal of Chest Tube

Equipment

Suture removal set
Rubber-tipped hemostat
Disposable underpad
Sterile 4 × 4 gauze for mediastinal tube
Or
Sterile petrolatum gauze dressings for intrapleural tube
Tape (elasticized foam tape for intrapleural tube)
Sterile gloves
Personal protective equipment (face mask/shield)
Prescribed premedication

Preparation

1. Identify client using two forms of identification and introduce self.
2. Gather equipment and prepare client for procedure, including instruction to take a deep breath and hold it or to hum during tube removal.
3. Premedicate client (as ordered), allowing time for peak effect upon tube removal.

Procedure

1. Perform hand hygiene and don personal protective equipment.
2. Place client in semi-Fowler's position.
3. Don sterile gloves.

Clinical Alert

The chest tube can be removed when drainage is less than 50–100 mL in 24 hr, or, if inserted for blood removal, drainage has become serous or sero serosanguineous and less than 100 mL in the past 8 hr.

4. Assist physician to remove dressing, clip suture securing chest tube, and clamp chest tube.
5. Instruct client to take a deep breath or hum during tube removal.
6. Hold sterile dressing in place while chest tube is being removed.
7. Dispose of chest tube and drainage equipment.
8. Remove personal protective gear, gloves, and discard.
9. Perform hand hygiene.
10. Reevaluate client's status regularly. ▸ ***Rationale:*** Client should be assessed for unstable vital signs, diminished or absent breath sounds, or respiratory distress (pneumothorax, mediastinal shift) after removal of chest tube.

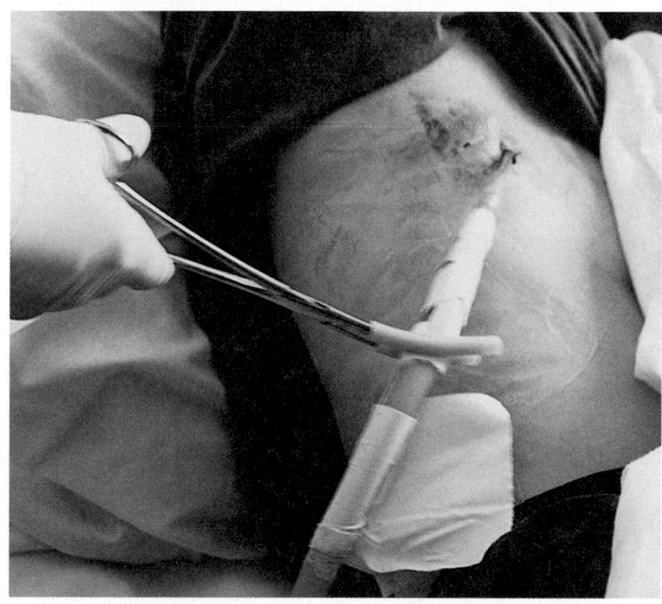

▲ Chest tube is clamped in preparation for removal.

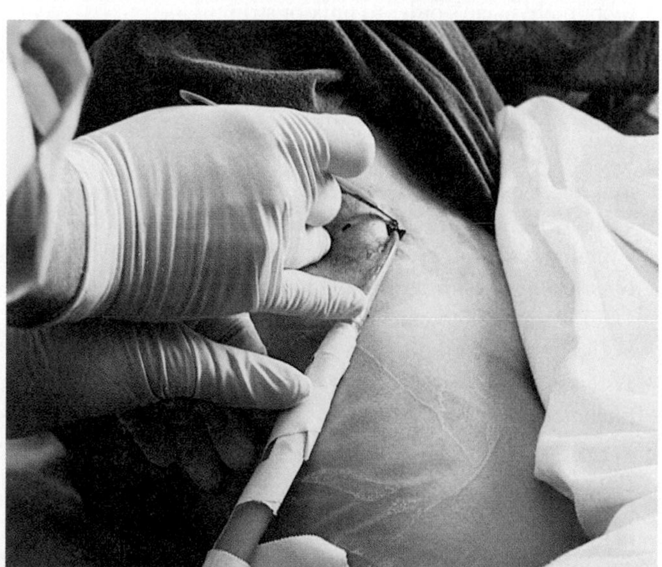

▲ Sutures anchoring chest tube are cut.

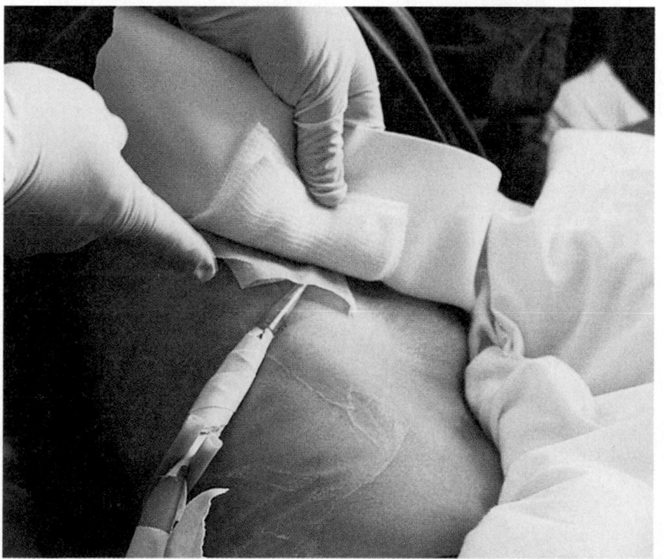

▲ Dressing is applied immediately upon tube removal.

DOCUMENTATION for Chest Drainage Systems

Chest Drainage System

- Site and size of chest tubes inserted and drainage system established
- Negative pressure established
- Client's tolerance of procedure
- Vital signs
- Breath sounds
- Drainage—amount, color
- Any problem with the system and its management
- Client activity (turning, ambulation)
- Chest-tube milking/stripping if performed

Autotransfusion

- Amount of blood reinfused
- Time collection started to completion of reinfusion
- Signs and symptoms of any complications encountered
- Changes in coagulation times or hemoglobin, hematocrit
- Client's response to treatment

Chest Tube Removal

- Breath sounds
- Premedication administered
- Name of physician removing tube
- Status of insertion site and dressing applied
- Client's tolerance of procedure

CRITICAL THINKING Application

Expected Outcomes

- Chest drainage system is patent.
- Mediastinal shift does not occur.
- Chest tube remains securely placed.

Unexpected Outcomes	Alternative Actions
Air leak is present.	• Check for specific leak area by briefly clamping chest drainage tube between client and bottle closest to client. a. If water-seal bottle continues to bubble, the leak is in the tubing. b. If water-seal bottle stops bubbling, the leak is in the client's chest tube at insertion site. • Secure all connections with tape. • Change tubing if necessary (obtain physician's order). • Apply sterile petrolatum gauze around chest tube insertion site if leak is at that site.
Drainage system is obstructed.	• Assess tubing for kinks or clots. • Loop tubing on bed to allow straight drainage to collection system. • Obtain physician's order to milk or strip tubing.
Client develops signs of mediastinal shift (trachea deviated to unaffected side, paradoxical pulse develops, jugular veins distend, cardiac output decreases).	• Note signs of respiratory distress and call Rapid Response Team or "CODE" immediately. Check drainage tube for patency. Prepare to assist with thoracentesis.
Chest tube becomes disconnected from drainage system.	• Clamp chest tube near chest insertion site. **a.** Replace extension tubing leading from chest tube and submerge into open bottle of sterile water to create underwater seal. **b.** Unclamp chest tube as soon as extension tubing is placed underwater or connected to new system. • Secure connecting sites with tape to prevent disconnection. • Assess client for signs of respiratory distress due to pneumothorax and report.
Chest tube becomes dislodged.	• Notify physician. • Instruct client with external chest disruption to exhale and apply sterile nonporous 4 ×4 gauze dressing with tape on three sides to allow air to escape on exhalation but inhibit air intake on inspiration.

GERONTOLOGIC Considerations

The Physiologic Age Changes That Occur in the Elderly Affect the Respiratory System.

- The respiratory muscles lose their strength and the rib cage becomes more rigid.
- The alveoli increase in size and decrease in number as well as become less elastic and more dilated.
- Gas exchange is reduced; the PaO_2 decreases 1 mm/year after age 60, so a reading of 77 mmHg is not unusual in an elderly client.
- Skeletal alterations affect posture and may restrict lung expansion.

Pulmonary Disorders Occur More Frequently in the Elderly. COPD is the Fourth Leading Cause of Death.

- Respiratory reserves are reduced with aging; the elderly are at greater risk for respiratory failure.
- Pneumonia may develop primarily or secondary to other conditions. Because it is a major cause of death in the elderly, pneumonia vaccine, influenza vaccine, and other preventive measures should be employed.
- Asthma may occur as a problem in the elderly who have never had the disease.
- Cancer of the lung is the leading cause of cancer death in the elderly.

It Is Important to Implement Nursing Actions That Support the Respiratory System in the Elderly.

- Deep breathing and exercise help promote ventilation.
- Hydration helps to liquefy secretions and reduce risk for infection.
- Monitor oxygen therapy closely with the elderly—note signs of hypoxia and decreased responsiveness due to possible carbon dioxide narcosis.
- The elderly are at risk for hypoxemia with bedrest (PO_2 may drop to 40 mmHg even with a night's sleep). Position change, range of motion, and early mobilization all stimulate ventilation and must be encouraged in all clients.

MANAGEMENT Guidelines

Each state legislates a Nurse Practice Act for RNs and LVN/LPNs. Healthcare facilities are responsible for establishing and implementing policies and procedures that conform to their state's regulations. Verify the regulations and role parameters for each healthcare worker in your facility.

Delegation

- Each state identifies the scope of practice for RNs, LVN/LPNs, and Respiratory Care Practitioners. States may differ in defining responsibilities of respiratory care by these practitioners. Usually, the respiratory care practitioner is licensed to perform invasive procedures such as suctioning, changing tracheostomy inner cannulas, and administering medication by aerosol. The initiation of oxygen administration by various modes and utilization of biophysical parameters (ABGs, etc.) and standard protocols in decision making and management of the mechanically ventilated client are also within the scope of respiratory care practice.
- All professionals collaborate in the care planning and evaluation of client responses to respiratory care interventions. The nurse must be aware of the unique role competencies, responsibilities, and accountabilities of specialty personnel when a variety of care providers are involved.
- The nurse should ensure that regular turning and deep breathing are encouraged by the CNA/UAP to promote ventilation and prevent complications of immobility in bedfast clients.
- The CNA/UAP should be familiar with appropriate client positioning to promote airway patency and reduce risk for aspiration of oral intake.
- Even though hospitals are "smoke free" today, all personnel must take precautions when oxygen is in use: No petrolatum products around nose or mouth; no battery-operated equipment or friction-type toys to be used. The area surrounding the client is oxygen-rich and can support combustion.
- All personnel should be able to locate the main oxygen supply valve to the area for discontinuation of oxygen flow in case of fire.
- The nurse must verify that the CNA/UAP understands the importance of oxygen administration so that it is appropriately maintained. The nurse ensures that the CNA/UAP seeks assistance so portable oxygen can be provided if it is required during client ambulation.
- Unlicensed personnel should be informed that aspiration is an ever-present danger for the client with a tracheostomy tube.
- Clients who require oxygen administration may be unable to perform activities of daily living independently. The CNA/UAP providing basic care should be *instructed to assist* the client with these activities (e.g., set up food tray, provide bed or partial bath).
- All care providers must be familiar with the location of emergency supplies and should be prepared to retrieve equipment and assist with manual respiratory resuscitation if necessary.

Communication Matrix

- The CNA/UAP usually performs routine vital signs assessment and documentation (including respiratory rate).

The nurse should request that respiratory rates less than 12 or greater than 20 be reported immediately, as more specific assessment may be indicated.

- The CNA/UAP should know to *report* any change in the client's breathing status or tolerance of activity. The character and amount of sputum production should also be reported and saved for the nurse's inspection and documentation.
- While the nurse or respiratory care practitioner is responsible for suctioning clients, the CNA/UAP must recognize the client's need for such and *report* it immediately.
- The PO status of intubated clients must be clearly communicated to all personnel. NPO status should be clearly posted at the bedside.
- All care providers must ensure that the intubated client has nonvocal means for summoning help (call bell) and communicating (paper and pencil).
- There should be clear postings at the bedside of the client for swallowing precautions, oxygen precautions, communication through nonvocal means, intubation precautions.

CRITICAL THINKING Strategies

Scenario 1

Mrs. Harvey, age 72, has a history of chronic obstructive pulmonary disease (COPD) with components of emphysema and chronic bronchitis. She has frequent recurrence of respiratory infection requiring hospitalization. With her most recent hospitalization, she has developed pulmonary hypertension and right-sided heart failure with weight gain and systemic edema. After treatment with IV antibiotics, she is ready for discharge, but will be sent home with continuous low-flow (1.5 L) oxygen therapy. Her ABGs at the time of discharge shows elevated P_{CO_2} (respiratory acidosis), elevated bicarbonate level (metabolic alkalosis), P_{O_2} of 60 mmHg, and O_2 saturation of 90% on oxygen. Her blood pH is low normal due to the *compensated* respiratory acidosis.

1. What is the rationale for home oxygen therapy for Mrs. Harvey?
2. What are the hazards that accompany home oxygen therapy?
3. What should the client know about home oxygen therapy?
4. What are the expected outcomes of home oxygen therapy (ABGs)?

Scenario 2

Joe Snodgrass has been referred to the sleep laboratory for an overnight polysomnogram (sleep study) due to his complaints of excessive fatigue, daytime sleepiness, awakening with a headache, and his heart racing. In addition, his wife reports that he snores a lot and has breathing pauses when he's sleeping that frighten her.

Outcomes of his study reveal that Mr. Snodgrass has obstructive sleep apnea (OSA). His physician has prescribed nasal continuous positive airway pressure (nCPAP) for night-time use. As his nurse, you are to obtain follow-up assessment data regarding your client's tolerance, adherence, and response to this therapy.

1. What is obstructive sleep apnea?
2. What are the risk factors for developing obstructive sleep apnea?
3. What are potential complications of untreated OSA?
4. How does CPAP benefit the client with OSA?
5. Why do many clients fail to adhere to CPAP therapy?
6. Are there other treatment options available for the client who cannot tolerate CPAP?

NCLEX® Review Questions

Unless otherwise specified, choose only one (1) answer.

1. Instructions for use of an incentive spirometer device should include to inhale through the mouthpiece
   1. Quickly to maximum level, then exhale slowly through the nose.
   2. Slowly to maximum level, hold several seconds, then exhale forcefully.
   3. Quickly to maximum level, hold for several seconds, then exhale slowly with mouth open.
   4. Slowly to maximum level, hold for several seconds, then exhale through pursed lips.

2. Chest Physical Therapy (CPT) only benefits
   1. Clients with pneumonia.
   2. Clients with retained secretions.
   3. COPD clients with acute exacerbation.
   4. Mechanically ventilated clients.

3. CPAP/BiPAP mask application should not be used for clients who are
   1. Allergic to latex.
   2. Sedated.
   3. Asleep.
   4. Claustrophobic.

4. The greatest oxygen delivery (FIO_2) is provided by
   1. Nasal cannula.
   2. Face mask.
   3. Venturi mask.
   4. Nonrebreathing mask with reservoir bag.
5. Hemoglobin saturation measurement by pulse oxymetry (SPO_2) is less reliable in ____________.
   Select all that apply.
   1. Anemic clients.
   2. Black clients.
   3. Hypovolemic clients.
   4. Hypertensive clients.
   5. Clients post dye injection.
6. The purpose of tracheal intubation/tracheostomy tube placement is to
   1. Provide mechanical ventilation.
   2. Establish a patent airway.
   3. Prevent aspiration.
   4. Provide oxygenation.
7. Inflation of an endotracheal or tracheostomy tube cuff
   1. Allows the client to eat.
   2. Prevents aspiration of pharyngeal secretions.
   3. Prevents tube migration.
   4. Allows mechanical ventilation.
8. The Bivona Fome Cuff differs from other tracheostomy tubes in which of the following ways?
   1. The cuff is inflated with sterile water.
   2. It does not require an obturator for insertion.
   3. Air must be withdrawn to deflate the cuff.
   4. Decannulation cannot occur.
9. The client with a tracheostomy tube that is capped with a speaking valve must have
   1. Mechanical ventilation.
   2. Tube cuff deflated.
   3. Tube cuff inflated.
   4. A Bivona Fome Cuff tube.
10. Place the following steps in correct sequence for suctioning a client's airway with a single-use catheter: ____________.
    1. Hyperoxygenate client.
    2. Suction client's oropharynx.
    3. Pour catheter flush solution into container.
    4. Attach catheter to end of suction tubing.
    5. Set suction source to 100 mmHg.
    6. Don sterile gloves.
    7. Apply suction.
    8. Advance catheter into client's airway.

31

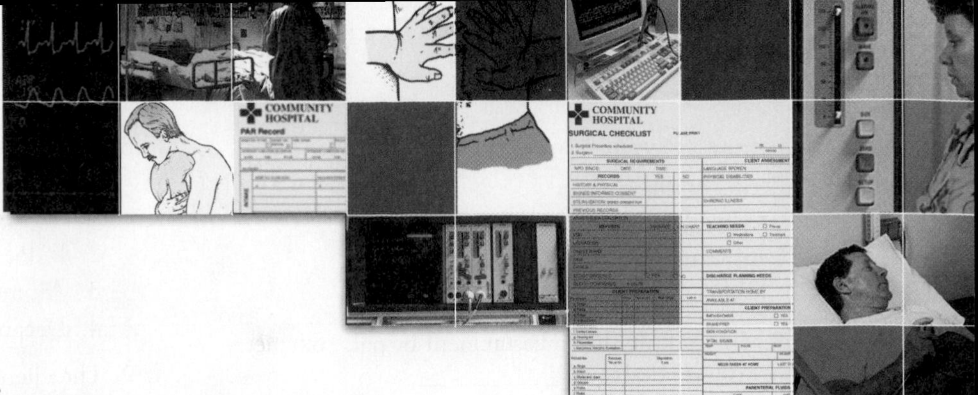

Circulatory Maintenance

LEARNING OBJECTIVES

1. Identify four properties of the cardiac muscle and define cardiac output.
2. Define the words *inotropic* and *chronotropic*.
3. Locate the following sites to palpate the pulse: temporal, carotid, brachial, radial, femoral, popliteal, posterior tibial, and dorsalis pedis.
4. Outline the assessment actions for a client who is hemorrhaging.
5. Identify two interventions for treating heart failure.
6. Define the term *ischemia*.
7. List the nine pressure points in the body that can be used to control bleeding if hemorrhage occurs.
8. Identify two potential problems that could occur in clients who are bleeding, and state one suggested intervention for each problem.
9. Describe how to measure for appropriate-size graduated compression stockings.
10. List at least four potential problems for clients requiring CPR and two suggested interventions for each problem.
11. Outline the steps in administering CPR with one rescuer and with two rescuers.
12. Demonstrate performing the Heimlich maneuver.
13. Describe four steps in using the automatic external defibrillator (AED).
14. State two nursing diagnoses relevant to clients with alterations in circulation.
15. Differentiate between a normal and abnormal ECG pattern.
16. Describe lead placement for a 12-lead ECG.
17. Describe the rationale for use of a permanent pacemaker versus a temporary pacemaker.
18. Compare and contrast the various types of pacemakers.
19. Identify three benefits of internal cardiac defibrillator (ICD).
20. Discuss teaching for home care clients with cardiac pacemakers.
21. Determine symptoms requiring physician notification when reviewing the diary of a client using a Holter monitor.

CHAPTER OUTLINE

TERMINOLOGY

Aberrancy abnormally conducted beat or cardiac rhythm.

Afterload resistance or impedance to blood flow during ventricular systole.

Antiembolic a preventive measure used to help prevent the formation of an embolism, such as elastic hosiery.

Atherosclerosis accumulations of lipid-containing material within inner and middle layers of the arterial wall forming a fixed atheromatous plaque.

Cardiovascular pertaining to the heart and blood vessels.

Chronotropic factors known to alter the heart rate through external causes (e.g., medication).

Conductivity the electrical conducting capability of a substance.

Congestion excessive accumulation of blood or fluid within a blood vessel, tissue, or organ.

Contractility having the ability to contract or shorten.

Cyanosis bluish, purplish, discoloration of the skin resulting from reduced hemoglobin or oxygen in the blood.

Diastole relaxation filling phase of the cardiac cycle.

Dilatation expansion of an organ or vessel.

Dorsiflexion flexion of the foot in an upward direction so as to bend the joint toward the dorsum.

Dysrhythmia an abnormality in cardiac rhythm.

Ecchymosis escape of blood into the tissues from a ruptured blood vessel causing a discoloration of the skin; color is blue-black, changing to greenish brown or yellow.

Ectopy beat originating in the heart other than from the sinoatrial node.

Edema an excessive accumulation of fluid within tissue or bodily cavity.

Embolism sudden obstruction of a blood vessel by debris (e.g., a blood clot, plaque).

Endocardial arising from the endocardium.

Endocardium serous lining membrane of the inner surface and cavities of the heart.

Endotracheal within the trachea.

Epistaxis hemorrhage from the nose.

Heart failure a condition whereby the heart is unable to pump sufficient blood at either an adequate rate or volume to meet the metabolic demands of the body.

Hematemesis vomiting of blood.

Hematoma a swelling or mass of blood, usually clotted, confined to a specific space and caused by a break in a blood vessel.

Hemodynamic the study of blood flow within the systemic circulation.

Hemoptysis expectoration of blood from the larynx, trachea, bronchi, or lungs.

Hemorrhage abnormal internal or external bleeding.

Homan's sign pain in the calf when the foot is dorsiflexed.

Hydrostatic is a pressure of liquids in equilibrium and to the pressure exerted by the liquids.

Hypotension a low systolic blood pressure that is insufficient to maintain adequate tissues and/or organ perfusion.

Immobilize to fix a body part to reduce or eliminate motion.

Inotropic influencing the contractibility of muscle tissue.

Ischemia a decrease in circulation to tissue, organ, or limb due to obstruction of the inflow of arterial blood, which is reversible if blood flow is reestablished promptly.

Manubrium the sternum articulating with the clavicle and first pair of costal cartilages.

Pacemaker a device that provides electrical stimulation to the heart muscle.

Perfusion passing of fluid through spaces; the circulation of blood through tissues.

Petechiae small, purplish, hemorrhagic spots on the skin.

Phlebitis inflammation of a vein.

Precordial pertaining to the precordium or occurring in front of the heart.

Preload length or stretch of the cardiac muscle fiber imposed by the volume of blood in the ventricles at the end of diastole.

Purpura hemorrhage into the skin, mucous membranes, internal organs, and other tissues.

Resuscitation act of bringing one back to consciousness.

Sclerosis hardening or induration of an organ or tissue due to excessive growth of fibrous tissue.

Shock term used to designate a clinical syndrome with varying degrees of disturbances of reduced blood flow and oxygen supply to the tissues.

Stasis standing still; stagnation of normal flow of fluids.

Syncope fainting, transient loss of consciousness due to inadequate blood flow to the brain.

Thrombosis formation of a blood clot.

Vertigo sensation of moving or having objects moving around when they are actually still.

THE CIRCULATORY SYSTEM

The heart is a three-layered organ, approximately the size of an adult fist, weighing approximately 250–350 g. The pericardium is a double-walled, strong nondistensible sac that encloses the heart, the aorta, and the other great vessels attached to the heart. The pericardium contains a fibrous and a serous layer, the function of which is to restrict excessive movement of the heart and act as a lubricated container during cardiac contraction. The pericardium protects the heart from positional changes and infection and prevents friction between the heart and other organs. There are two layers of the serous pericardium, the parietal and visceral layers. These two layers are separated by a thin fluid-containing cavity, the pericardial sac, which contains 50 mL of pericardial fluid that lubricates and facilitates the movement of the heart. The fibrous pericardium and parietal layer of the serous pericardium are supplied by the phrenic nerve, whereas the visceral layer of the serous pericardium is innervated by the sympathetic nervous system and the vagus nerve. Both influence reflex changes in the heart rate and blood pressure. The myocardium is the thickest layer of the heart and is composed of cardiac muscle cells. Cardiac muscle cells are unique and possess four properties: (1) automaticity—ability of some cardiac cells to initiate an impulse spontaneously and repetitively; (2) conductivity—cells can transmit the electrical impulses; (3) contractility—which characterizes all muscle; however, a cardiac contraction is an all-or-nothing response to an impulse as opposed to partial contractions in skeletal muscles; and (4) excitability—the ability to respond to an external stimuli, resulting in a contraction. The endocardium is the innermost lining of the heart and is continuous with the endothelium that lines arteries, veins, and capillaries.

The heart serves as a pump and is made up of four chambers: the right atrium, right ventricle, left atrium, and left ventricle. Unidirectional blood flow is regulated through the heart by four valves: the tricuspid, pulmonary, mitral, and aortic valves. Venous blood enters into the right atrium of the heart from the

▲ Blood flow pattern through the right and left side of the heart.

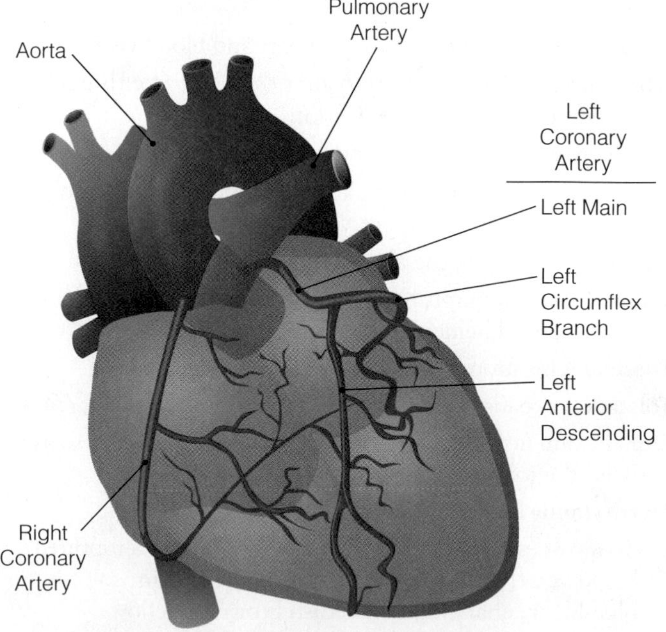

▲ Blood flow in coronary arteries.

superior and inferior vena cava. Blood flows from the right atrium into the right ventricle via the tricuspid valve, then into the lungs for oxygenation via the pulmonic valve. After gases exchange in the pulmonary system, the blood enters the left atrium, left side of the heart, by way of four pulmonary veins. These are the only veins within the body that carry oxygenated blood. From the left atrium, blood flows into the left ventricle via the mitral valve, then out into the aorta via the aortic valve. Blood flows to all parts of the body through the systemic circulation system. The heart pumps the entire circulating volume each minute (4–7 L of blood).

Superior / Inferior Vena Cava → Right Atrium → Tricuspid Valve → Right Ventricle → Pulmonary Valve → Pulmonary Artery → LUNGS (oxygenation)

LUNGS → Pulmonary veins → Left Atrium → Mitral Valve → Left Ventricle → Aortic Valve → Aorta – BODY

Arteries carry oxygenated blood from the heart throughout the body from the largest vessel, the aorta, to the smallest, arterioles. Arteries have three layers: endothelium, smooth muscle, and connective tissue. Capillaries join the arterial system to the venous system and are a single cell layer that allows for the exchange of gases, nutrients, and waste material.

Arteries → Arterioles → Capillaries → Venules → Veins

Capillaries are also known as capacitance vessels, which serve to regulate blood flow within the venous system by returning it to the right side of the heart.

Cardiac Output

Cardiac output (CO) is the amount of blood flow ejected by the heart within 1 minute and is measured in liters per minute. Heart rate and stroke volume determine cardiac output. Cardiac output (CO) is determined by multiplying the amount of volume ejected from the heart with each contraction, or stroke volume (SV), by the heart rate (HR).

$$CO = SV \times HR$$

(Cardiac Output = Stroke Volume × Heart Rate)

In order to maintain its continuous pumping activity, the heart muscle must receive oxygen and nutrients. Approximately 5% of blood leaving the heart and pumped into the aorta enters the coronary circulation for oxygenation and waste removal from cardiac tissue. The coronary arteries branch from the aorta, extend over the surface of the heart, supply blood to all areas of the heart muscle, and fill during diastole. The major coronary arteries are the right coronary artery and the left coronary artery, which divides into two branches, the anterior descending artery and the circumflex artery.

If the blood flow in the coronary arteries to the heart muscle is severely reduced, ischemia or injury can occur, but it is reversible. If the flow is blocked completely for a prolonged

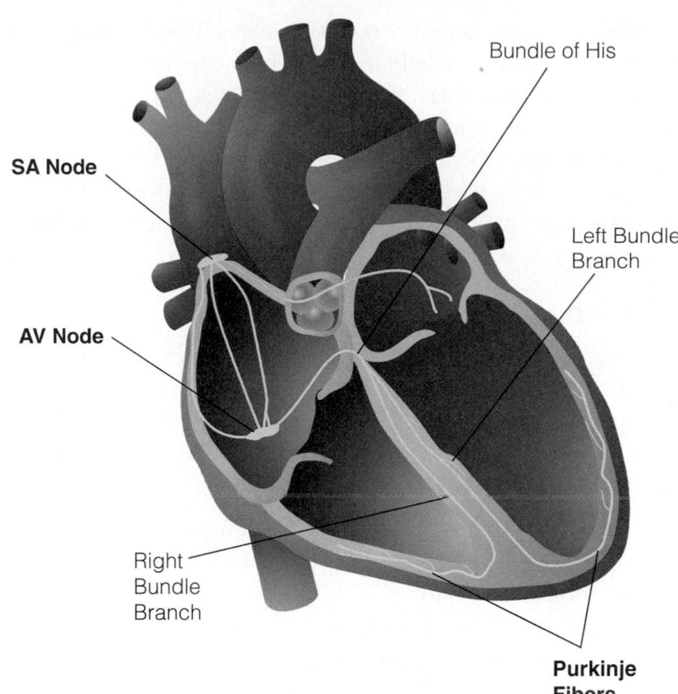

▲ Intrinsic conduction system of the heart.

period, necrosis will occur; necrosis is irreversible. This is referred to as a myocardial infarction or "heart attack."

After supplying the heart muscle, 15% of the cardiac output (600–500 mL) travels to the brain, 25% (1000–1750 mL) goes to the kidneys, and another 25% to the other viscera. The extremities and skin normally receive approximately 30% of the cardiac output.

ELECTRICAL CONDUCTION

Cardiac muscle cells have the ability to generate their own rate and rhythm that allows for their spontaneous, repetitive self-stimulation, previously mentioned as automaticity. The rate and rhythm of cardiac contractions are primarily determined by this self-generated impulse. The autonomic nervous system influences the heart rate. Sympathetic stimulation increases heart rate, speeds the conduction through the atrioventricular (AV) node, and increases force of contraction. Parasympathetic stimulation slows the heart rate by decreasing the firing rate of the sinoatrial (SA) node and decreasing the speed of conduction through the AV node.

Normally, the electrical impulse originates within specialized cells within the SA node located on the posterior wall of the right atrium, just right of the opening of the superior vena cava. It functions as the pacemaker for the heart. The SA node initiates approximately 60–100 impulses each minute. The impulse travels to the AV node, located in the right atrial wall near the tricuspid valve. If there is a problem with the impulse being generated in the SA node, the AV node can actually take over as the pacemaker. Over the long term, this may present a problem because the intrinsic rate of the AV node is only 40–60 impulses per minute. The AV node coordinates the incoming electrical impulse from the atria and relays an impulse to the ventricles, via the septum and through the bundle of His specialized conduction fibers, which divide into the right and left bundle branches. Then, the impulse continues to the Purkinje fibers, where it terminates. Further depolarization of the myocardium takes place by conduction through the muscle fibers themselves. If both the SA and AV node are dysfunctional, or there is blockage in the bundle of His, the Purkinje fibers are capable of maintaining their own intrinsic rate, but the rate is less than 40 beats/min.

Electrocardiogram (ECG)

The electrocardiogram (ECG) is used to detect abnormalities associated with the conduction system of the heart. The waveforms, which indicate the electrical activity of the myocardium, are analyzed using the ECG tracing. (See page 1251 for illustration.)

P wave—represents atrial depolarization, indicating the contraction of both atria. The P wave is usually smooth and upright or "positive."

PR interval—is measured from the beginning of the P wave (onset of atrial depolarization) to the R wave. It represents the time required for atrial depolarization and for the impulse to travel through the entire conduction system, including the Purkinje fiber network. Normal PR interval is 0.12 to 0.20 seconds.

QRS complex—represents depolarization of the ventricles, which causes the ventricular contraction. It is measured from the beginning of the Q wave (or R) to the end of the S wave. Not all leads have a Q wave. The normal QRS interval duration is 0.06–0.12 seconds and represents the time required for depolarization of both ventricles.

ST segment—represents the period of early ventricular repolarization. The ST segment is normally isoelectric (line is flat). The segment normally is not elevated >1 mm or depressed >0.5 mm from the isoelectric line.

QT interval—represents the total time required for ventricular depolarization and repolarization. It is measured from the beginning of the QRS complex to the end of the T wave and represents ventricular systole (contraction). The normal QT interval is 0.34–0.43 seconds.

T wave—represents ventricular repolarization or the return of the ventricles to a resting state. The wave is normally asymmetrically rounded and upright or "positive." The end of the T wave marks the end of systole.

Segments and waves are measured for duration (time) and configuration. Abnormalities in duration or configuration may indicate a problem is occurring in that specific area of the heart.

Any disturbance in the rate or rhythm of the heartbeat is termed *dysrhythmia*. Historically, the term *arrhythmia* has been used in the literature. Although the terms are often used interchangeably, dysrhythmia, which means a disturbance in cardiac rhythm, is more accurate. Dysrhythmias are classified according to their site of origin. The sites include sinus, atrial, junctional, ventricular, and AV nodal tissue. A sinus dysrhythmia usually reflects a change in rate or rhythm. An atrial dysrhythmia results from a disturbance with the SA node or atria indicated by an abnormality in the P wave configuration.

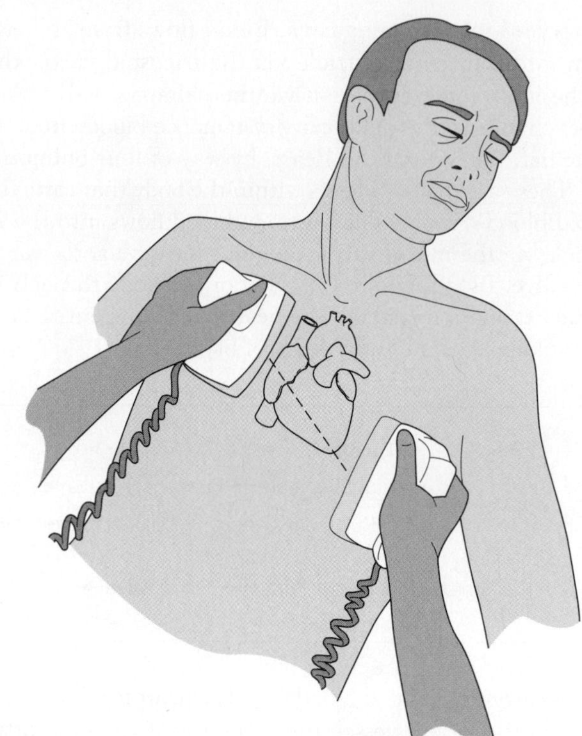

▲ Defibrillation pads applied to chest wall.

A junctional dysrhythmia occurs when there is a problem associated with the AV node as indicated by a change in the PR interval. A ventricular dysrhythmia results from a problem with the ventricle and is indicated by an abnormality in the configuration of the QRS complex. Although many dysrhythmias have no clinical manifestations, many others have serious consequences. A ventricular dysrhythmia is the most life-threatening because it compromises cardiac output.

Cardiac Monitoring

The choice of monitoring is dependent on the client's clinical condition and determined by the arrhythmias most likely to occur and the potential severity of the arrhythmia. Any lead that displays a clear P wave and QRS complex can identify premature atrial complexes, abnormal sinus rhythms, and most heart blocks. Most leads recognize atrial fibrillation by the irregular R-R intervals and chaotic atrial activity. When the QRS complex becomes wide, as it does when the client is in bundle branch block or has ventricular rhythms, the lead that best differentiates these findings is selected. The V1 and V6 leads (equivalent to MCL1 and MCL6) are the best leads to differentiate the wide QRS rhythms. Multiple lead monitoring is best for observing and detecting these arrhythmias. The newer bedside monitors allow monitoring of two leads simultaneously, but only allow monitoring of one precordial (V) lead at a time. Most bedside monitoring is now done using the five-lead system. The three-lead system is still used in the emergency rooms and when monitoring clients during procedures.

ST-segment monitoring is now being used in clients with a potential for ischemia (clients admitted with chest pain or unstable angina or clients having a surgical procedure who have a history of cardiac disease). This monitoring identifies any reocclusion to the affected heart vessels. If the 12-lead

ECG is not available, the American Association of Critical-Care Nurses recommends leads III and V3 for monitoring clients with acute coronary syndrome.

If the client has had a previous episode of ischemia, an ischemic fingerprint can be obtained. It is the unique pattern of ST-segment changes noted during a period of ischemia. This pattern is observed during an episode of chest pain or if the client undergoes balloon inflation during angioplasty. If the fingerprint is unknown, the best leads to use are III and V3 for the monitoring.

Refer to Chapter 33: Advanced Nursing Skills for life-threatening dysrhythmias.

Pacemakers

Pacemakers are electronic devices that stimulate the heart with electrical impulses to produce a heartbeat or to override an abnormally fast rhythm. Most commonly, a pacemaker is used for a slow heart rate (bradycardia) or when the conduction system within the heart is diseased and unable to maintain effective cardiac output due to conduction disturbances such as heart block. The use of a temporary or permanent pacemaker may be necessary to provide an electrical impulse to pace the heart when the inherent electrical system fails.

Temporary pacemaker A temporary pacemaker is inserted invasively to stimulate cardiac contraction until the underlying pathology is treated or a permanent pacemaker can be placed. Clients with temporary pacemakers require hospitalization with continuous monitoring. The pulse generator of the temporary pacemaker is located outside the body, and the leads are positioned to provide low-voltage electrical stimuli to the myocardium. The leads are positioned in one of several ways:

- The pacemaker wires are threaded percutaneously through the subclavian, external jugular, or femoral vein or through a cutdown in the brachial vein. The lead is advanced through the vena cava, to the right atrium, or advanced through the tricuspid valve and positioned in the right ventricle on the endocardial surface. The lead is then attached to the external pulse generator.
- During cardiac surgery, the pacing leads are attached to the outer surface of the heart (epicardially). This type has wires (electrodes) located in the lower chest and can be attached to an external pulse generator if pacing the heart postoperatively is necessary.

In emergency situations, such as in cases of symptomatic bradycardia, these external pacing pads are applied to the chest wall (transcutaneously), according to the manufacturer guidelines. The machine delivers approximately 25 joules of electricity through the pads to the heart, via the chest wall. These pacing pads resemble defibrillator pads.

Permanent pacemaker The decision to place a permanent pacemaker and the type of pacemaker selected depends on multiple factors, including:

- The exact nature and underlying cause of the conduction disturbance
- Whether the condition is temporary or permanent
- The presence or absence of symptoms and the impact on activities of daily living
- The potential risk for life-threatening dysrhythmias

Permanent pacemakers are intended for long-term use. The pulse generator is implanted into the subcutaneous tissue of the upper chest. The pacemaker leads are typically inserted into a major vein in the neck or shoulder (transvenously) and advanced into the right side of the heart until they are secured within the intended region(s) of the myocardium. The other ends of the leads are attached to the implanted pulse generator.

The pacemaker continuously monitors the heart's electrical activity and the type of pacemaker selected is designed to meet different needs. The three basic types of permanent pacemakers include:

- *Demand Pacemaker*—monitors the heart's natural rate and discharges an electrical impulse only when the rate falls below a programmed minimum rate.
- *Fixed-rate Pacemaker*—discharges a steady electrical impulse at a programmed rate, regardless of the underlying heart rate.
- *Rate-responsive Pacemaker*—increases or decreases the discharge electrical impulse rate (pacing rate) to meet the body's demands. The pacemaker monitors various physical changes in the body and alters the rate of discharge according to changes in the client's activity and rest.

Pacemakers can send electrical impulses to one or more chambers of the heart. These signals stimulate the heart to contract in a regular rhythm.

Types of Pacemakers

Types of pacemakers include atrial, ventricular, or dual-chamber pacemakers.

Single-chamber In a single-chamber pacemaker, one lead is located in either the right atrium or right ventricle. Atrial pacemakers are indicated when the SA node is diseased or damaged but the remaining conduction system through the heart is normal. A pacemaker spike precedes the P wave because the pacing electrode is placed within the atria. Ventricular pacemakers are indicated when conduction abnormalities occur above the ventricles. The pacing lead is located in the ventricle and when discharged results in a pacemaker spike before the QRS complex, producing a wide QRS complex because of the abnormal conduction pathway.

Dual-chamber In a dual-chamber pacemaker, two leads, one in the right atrium and one in the right ventricle, can monitor and initiate impulses to one or both chambers. The dual-chambered pacemaker can produce an atrial contraction followed closely by a ventricular contraction, thereby mimicking the normal cardiac cycle while preserving atrial contraction and thus ventricular filling.

Triple-chamber or biventricular pacing With this type of pacemaker, one lead in the right atrium, one in the right

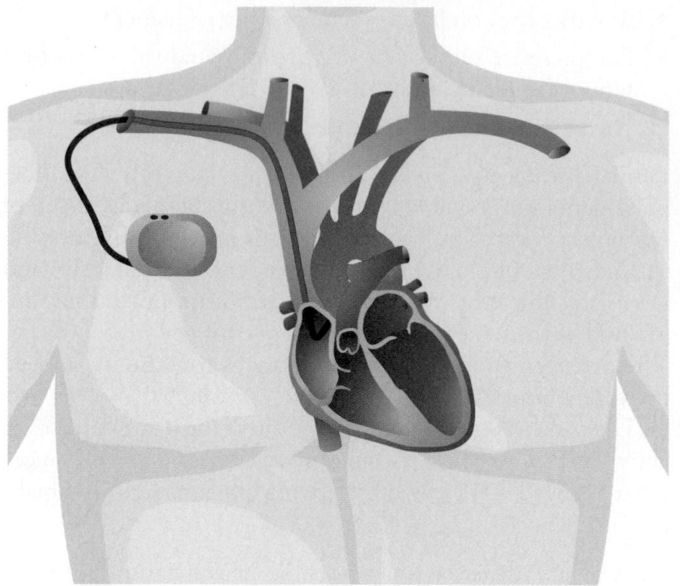

▲ Permanent pacemaker: single chamber.

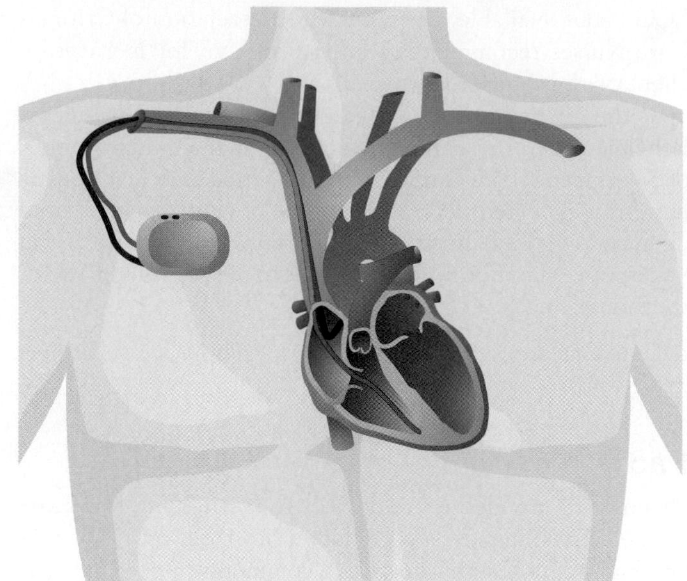

▲ Permanent pacemaker: double chamber.

ventricle, and one in the coronary sinus stimulate the lateral wall of the left ventricle. These pacemakers are inserted in clients who have a weakened myocardium (heart muscle) or a severely depressed myocardial function, causing problems with shortness of breath and inability to tolerate physical activity. With left ventricle enlargement, the wave of depolarization and repolarization is prolonged. Placing a third lead in the coronary sinus facilitates a coordinated wave of depolarization and repolarization simultaneously within the myocardium, allowing for the heart to contract in a more unified manner, thus improving the cardiac output.

ALTERATIONS IN CIRCULATION

The closed circulatory system is made up of the heart, arteries, veins, and capillaries. Alteration in the structure or function of any part of the system will result in impaired circulation. There are many ways to categorize circulatory disorders. For the purposes of this chapter, alterations in circulation will include hemorrhage, shock, pump failure, ischemia, thrombosis, and embolism.

Hemorrhage

Hemorrhage may occur when trauma or disease disrupts the closed circulatory system. Normally, when a blood vessel ruptures or is severed, compensatory mechanisms protect the body from significant blood loss. The wall of the injured vessel contracts immediately. A platelet plug forms at the site, blood clots, and new connective tissue penetrates the clot for permanent closure of the injured site.

For the client with hemorrhage, the nurse assesses the nature of the bleeding as external, internal, or both. An assessment is made to determine the body's response and establish baseline data, including vital signs and urinary output (see Table 31-1, Assessment Guide for Hemorrhaging). A priority of care is to monitor the client frequently and regularly and minimize the client's stress, thus decreasing the sympathetic response. Sympathetic nervous system stimulation will increase heart rate (chronotropic effect) and force of contraction (inotropic effect), thereby increasing bleeding.

Interventions for clients who are hemorrhaging include restricting activity, elevating involved body areas above the heart if possible, applying direct pressure, and replacing lost fluid volume. A tourniquet is generally not used unless there has been a traumatic amputation, because a tourniquet crushes the underlying tissues and results in ischemia to the affected limb. But, if used, it is placed proximal to the site of the traumatic limb amputation.

Shock

Hemorrhage is the most common cause of hypovolemic shock, a potentially life-threatening condition, which is the most common cause of preventable post-injury deaths. Hypovolemic (hemorrhagic) shock means there is insufficient intravascular volume (insufficient venous return) to maintain adequate tissue perfusion. Rapid assessment of the client's hemodynamic status is mandatory. Level of consciousness (LOC), skin color, pulse, and urinary output are four elements that can be determined rapidly during clinical observation. LOC is impaired when blood flow to the brain is reduced because of lack of circulating blood volume. The earliest signs include anxiety, agitation, and dizziness coupled with orthostatic hypotension. Skin color is important to immediately assess because clients with pink skin are rarely critical, whereas clients with ashen gray facial color and/or a white exsanguinate extremity are ominous hypovolemic signs of shock. Pulse is determined by accessing central pulse, either the carotid or femoral artery, and assessing the quality, rate, and rhythm. If the client's pulse is slow, regular, and full, these are indications that the client is normovolemic, whereas if the pulse is rapid (tachycardic) and thready, then the client is hypovolemic, although other factors may also contribute to this sign. If the pulse is rapid and irregular, then cardiac dysfunction is occurring. This sign is a signal for rapid assessment, immediate resuscitation measures, and rapid replacement of volume. Urinary output is a good indicator for kidney perfusion. If blood flow is normal to the kidneys, then hourly urine output is maintained greater than 30 mL/hr. However, if blood flow to the kidneys is compromised, the first indication is decreased urinary output less than 30 mL/hr.

Children, because of their remarkable physiologic reserve, display very minimal early signs of hypovolemic shock even after severe volume depletion. However, when symptoms are manifested in a child, these symptoms are precipitous and may be catastrophic.

Hemorrhagic shock occurs on a continuum. In the initial phases, there are subtle changes in the hemodynamic status of the client. However, as blood loss continues and the intravascular blood volume continues to decrease, organ involvement worsens because of lack of perfusion. For example, in the kidneys, the client initially becomes oliguric, but as the blood flow continues to be reduced to the kidneys, the client becomes anuric. The pulse gradually increases, whereas the blood pressure continues to drop precipitously. Eventually, if rapid interventions are not implemented immediately to stop this downward spiral of events, then death will be the eventual outcome.

TABLE 31-1 Assessment Guide for Hemorrhaging

1. Observable bleeding from skin, mucous membranes. Check under the person's clothing, dressing, casts.
2. Observable bleeding into the skin, mucous membranes. Check for petechiae, ecchymosis, hematomas, purpura.
3. Observable bleeding from body orifice. Check for epistaxis, hematemesis, hemoptysis.
4. Observable bleeding from tubes. Check drainage tubes, endotracheal tubes, suction drainage, urinary catheters.
5. Generalized signs and symptoms of bleeding.
   a. Thirst.
   b. Narrow pulse pressure.
   c. Positional vital sign changes.
   d. Low blood pressure (systolic below 90 mm-Hg and diastolic below 50 mm-Hg).
   e. Tachycardia.
   f. Weak pulses or absence of pulses.
   g. Clammy skin and central cyanosis.
   h. Deep, rapid respirations (above 24/min).
   i. Low body temperature (one or more degrees below 98.6°F, or 37°C, oral temperature).
   j. Reduced urine output (less than 30 mL/hr).
   k. Behavioral changes.
   l. Syncope and visual disturbance.
   m. Loss of consciousness.

Interventions for Hypovolemic Shock

- Maintain airway.
- Place client in supine position.
- Administer supplemental oxygen.
- Keep client warm.
- Immediately establish two large-bore intravenous catheters—the loss of significant blood volume requires rapid infusion of at least 2–3 L of warmed intravenous solution.
- Fluid and blood replacement: isotonic crystalloids, such as Ringer's solution, are preferred over 0.9% normal saline to replace extracellular volume. Colloid solutions, such as blood transfusions or serum albumin, may also be given to expand intravascular space. Packed RBCs are used for acute blood loss.
- Drug administration: only occurs after adequate fluid replacement. Vasopressor agents, such as vasopressin, norepinephrine, or dopamine, may be given, if volume replacement is unsuccessful.

Heart Failure

Heart failure results from any condition that reduces the ability of the heart to effectively pump blood. When this occurs, the cardiac output is decreased, which impedes adequate blood flow to all tissues. Causes of heart failure are numerous, with coronary artery disease being the most common cause. Other causes of heart failure include valvular heart disease, myocardial infarctions, myocardial infections, and/or toxin.

Heart failure may involve either right, left ventricle, or both ventricles. Although most heart failure begins on the left side, as the disease process progresses, the right ventricle may become involved; this is known as *bi-ventricular failure*.

Do Not Use Trendelenburg Position

Placing shock clients in Trendelenburg position or a modified Trendelenburg position (client lying flat with the lower extremities raised) has not been proven to significantly raise the systolic pressure in prehospital hypotensive clients. Of the 30 articles written on Trendelenburg positioning, only 9 articles were peer reviewed. Trendelenburg or modified Trendelenburg did increase the risk of aspiration, and in cardiogenic shock clients, pulmonary edema worsened.

Additionally, although CVP and PAP pressures increase with Trendelenburg position, intrathoracic blood volume and cardiac function do not increase.

Source: Wesley, K. (2009). The myth of Trendelenburg position. *JEMS: A Journal of Emergency Medical Services*. April 5, 2009.

Source: Reuter, D. A., Felbinger, T. W., Schmidt, C., Moerstedt, K., Kilger, E., Lamm, P., & Goetz, A. E. (2003). Trendelenburg positioning after cardiac surgery: Effects on intrathoracic blood volume index and cardiac performance. *European Journal of Anaesthesiology*, *20*(1), 17–20.

Cardinal manifestations of heart failure are dyspnea and fatigue, with limited activity tolerance. When the heart is unable to adequately pump, the blood begins to back up. In left-sided failure, the left ventricle is unable to pump effectively, which leads to the buildup of fluid in pulmonary capillaries, termed *pulmonary edema*. Pulmonary edema is the most common result of left ventricle pump failure and is a life-threatening condition. As fluids accumulate in alveoli of the lungs, gas exchange is impaired. Clinical manifestations of left-sided failure include dyspnea; moist, hacking cough; bibasilar crackles; distended neck veins; and orthopnea. Increased pulmonary vascular pressure may cause right-sided heart failure with resultant reduction of circulation into the pulmonary artery, causing a backup of fluid in the systemic venous circulation. Clinical manifestations of right-sided heart failure include weight gain, peripheral edema, oliguria, hepatomegaly, ascites, and fatigue.

The goal of treatment for heart failure is to reduce workload on the heart, increase efficiency of contractions, and reduce fluid retention. Both physiological and pharmacological interventions are necessary to meet this goal. Bedrest during the most critical time may be ordered to reduce the workload on the heart. Oxygen therapy is essential to maximize the oxygen available to the tissues, as well as both reduced sodium intake and restricted fluid intake to decrease fluid volume and edema. Pharmacological interventions include:

- Diuretics—furosemide, spironolactone
- Nitrates—nitroglycerine because of vasodilating properties
- Antihypertensive agents
- Angiotensin-converting enzyme (ACE) inhibitors
- Antidysrhythmics, if needed
- Inotropic medications—digitalis
- Beta-blockers
- Potassium chloride (KCl)—client cannot be on potassium-sparing diuretics, such as spironolactone

Ischemia

Tissue ischemia results when blood flow is reduced to a critical level. Hypotension can cause relative ischemia because blood flow is insufficient to meet the metabolic demands. Absolute ischemia is usually due to a sudden, complete occlusion of a blood vessel, resulting in tissue necrosis. Leaving a tourniquet on an extremity for more than 15 minutes may cause tissue necrosis. Other causes of ischemia due to decreased blood flow include Raynaud's disease, Buerger's disease, thromboembolism, mechanical obstruction, arteriosclerosis, and atherosclerosis.

Deep Vein Thrombosis (DVT)

Venous thromboembolism is a frequent cause of preventable illness and death in hospitalized clients. The incidence of DVT in clients without DVT prophylaxis is unacceptably high in both surgical and medical hospitalized clients. As a result, this is considered a high client safety indicator by The Joint Commission, the Agency for Healthcare Research and Quality (AHRQ), and the Center for Medicare and Medicaid Services because of the underutilization of simple, cost-effective prophylactic measures.

Most hospitalized clients, whether medical or surgical, have multiple risk factors for developing deep vein thrombosis. Risk factors include thrombophilia; hypercoagulability states regarding clotting factors; cancer; obesity; pregnancy; smoking; surgery; trauma; head injury; medications (birth control pills, hormone replacement therapy, tamoxifen); surgical conditions involving the hip, pelvis, or knee; prolonged sitting for more than 6 hr in aircraft; or when on bedrest.

The exact incidence of deep vein thrombosis is unknown because most studies are limited by the inaccuracy of clinical diagnosis. The known data probably underestimate the true incidence of DVT and suggest that about 80 cases per 100,000 population occur annually. Approximately 1 person in 20 will develop a DVT during their lifetime. Approximately 600,000 hospitalizations per year in the United States occur from DVTs. The incidence of hospitalized clients experiencing DVTs varies from 20%–70%.

The classic symptoms of a DVT, if present, include swelling, pain, warmth, and redness in the involved extremity. Some may experience a dull ache or tightness in the calf upon walking, and may show slight edema, a palpable cord, venous collateral distention, low-grade fever, cyanosis, and a positive Homan's sign. Homan's sign, which was previously a mainstay for the diagnosis of DVT, is no longer considered accurate. It is present in less than one-third of clients with confirmed DVTs and is found in more than half of clients without DVTs.

Hypercoagulable state, thrombophilia, venous stasis, and vascular (endothelial) injury are factors that may lead to platelet aggregation, fibrin, WBC and RBC deposition, and eventual formation of a free-floating clot. In 80% of cases clots begin in deep veins of the calf. Within 7 to 10 days, the clot adheres to the vein wall, phlebitis develops, the clot is invaded by fibroblasts, scar is formed, and blood flow is restored, but the vein valves are usually permanently damaged. The clot propagates proximally; pieces can break off and embolize to the heart and obstruct the pulmonary circulation, with resultant right heart failure, atelectasis, hypoxemia, decreased cardiac output, or cardiac arrest.

DVT prophylaxis is indicated for all moderate- to high-risk medical and surgical clients. Low-molecular-weight heparin and unfractionated heparin decrease incidence of asymptomatic or symptomatic DVT and pulmonary emboli by 50%–65%.

Compression stockings, also known as TED hose, reduce venous stasis and reduce the incidence of postoperative venous thrombosis in low-risk surgical patients and moderate-risk neurosurgical clients. Mechanical devices (sequential compression devices [SCDs]) prevent venous thrombosis by improving blood flow through the deep leg veins, which prevents venous

DVT Statistics for Hospitalized Clients

50–70% of clients hospitalized with venous thromboembolism occur on the medical services. In hospitalized, high-risk clients not receiving prophylaxis, DVT was diagnosed by means of a venography in 10.5 to 14.9% of patients. Additionally, in high-risk surgical clients, without DVT prophylaxis, 20% of patients undergoing hip or knee arthroplasty or hip surgery developed proximal DVT. Proximal DVT, meaning proximal in a limb, is the most life threatening as this frequently leads to pulmonary embolism.

Source: Francis, CW. (2007). Prophylaxis for thromboembolism in hospitalized medical patients. *NEJM*, 356(14): 1438–1444.

stasis. Additionally, SCDs reduce plasminogen activator inhibitor, which increases fibrinolytic activity, although the exact mechanism is not known. SCDs are effective in reducing the incidence of DVT in moderate-risk surgical clients, including neurosurgical and coronary artery bypass clients. They are not as effective in calf vein thrombosis in orthopedic surgical clients. SCDs are beneficial when used in conjunction with anticoagulant therapy. Other interventions to prevent development of DVT in bedrest clients include:

- Assessment of risk factors
- Early ambulation
- Adequate hydration
- Foot and leg exercises while in bed
- Minimal interruptions during application
- Accurate assessment, measurement, and application of devices

NOTE: These measures help venous flow, but do not decrease the incidence of pulmonary embolism.

The goal of treatment for *existing* thrombophlebitis is to prevent clot propagation, pulmonary emboli, and thrombus recurrence. Care interventions include early ambulation, avoidance of rubbing or massaging the affected extremity, and adequate hydration. Pharmacological (systemic) intervention includes anticoagulation with heparin drip to a goal of 1.5 to 2 times normal PTT, or use of low-molecular-weight heparin to stop propagation of the clot. This is followed by oral warfarin therapy for 3 or 6 months or longer, with a therapeutic international normalized ratio goal of 2.0 to 3.0.

ALTERED CIRCULATION

Assessment

Alterations in circulation are indicated by a variety of signs and symptoms. If bleeding exists, external and/or internal sites must be identified. Attention is given to disease conditions of major organs or coagulation and the family history. Although a variety of sophisticated devices are available to monitor the client's circulatory status, direct observation is also reliable. Baseline data are obtained for vital signs and arterial blood pressure. Note the color, temperature, and condition of the skin. Abnormalities of superficial veins often indicate obstruction or pooling. Additional assessment data include:

- Vein distention
- Edema (fluid retention)
- Petechiae (platelet abnormalities)
- Homan's sign (calf tenderness with dorsiflexion); positive in less than 50% of cases; therefore, not frequently used

Information obtained from the client's medical history, medications, and lifestyle influences selection of nursing interventions. Trauma victims require especially close inspection since more overt signs and symptoms may not appear until days later. Table 31-1 illustrates an assessment of a hemorrhaging client.

Emergency Life Support Measures

The 2010 American Heart Association Guidelines for Cardiopulmonary Resuscitation (CPR) and emergency cardiovascular care (ECC) are recommendations designed to improve survival from sudden cardiac arrest and acute life-threatening cardiopulmonary incidents. According to the AHA, *basic life support* includes recognition of signs of sudden cardiac arrest (SCA), myocardial infarction (heart attack), cerebral vascular accident (stroke), and foreign-body airway obstruction (FBAO); cardiopulmonary resuscitation (CPR); and defibrillation with an automated external defibrillator (AED).

The 2010 Guidelines focus on giving chest compression first to keep the blood and the oxygen in the blood flowing to the heart and brain. Chest compressions act like an artificial heart by pumping blood to the heart and brain.

There is a significant amount of oxygen in the bloodstream capable of sustaining brain tissue for several minutes even without breathing. Many who believe doing only chest compressions is sufficient for adequate blood flow feel that interrupting compressions with rescue breathing doesn't allow oxygen to reach vital organs.

Studies published in the American Journal of Medicine and The Lancet have shown that there is a better outcome of victims who had only chest compressions. Not all cardiac arrests are from heart disease. Victims of drowning, drug overdose, or respiratory problems that lead to cardiac arrest will need rescue breathing.

To provide the victim with the best chance of survival these actions must occur within the first moments of a cardiac arrest.

a. Activate the EMS System (Emergency Medical Services) by calling 911.
b. Begin chest compressions at 100 compressions/minute with a depth of at least 2 inches in the adult client.
c. Send for and initiate the Automated External Defibrillator.

The new CPR Guidelines are termed CAB: compression, airway, breathing. This replaces the ABCs of CPR.

Use of airway devices by trained medical personnel will deliver air to the lungs rather than the stomach, greatly reducing complications such as aspiration and pneumonia. Mouth-to-mouth resuscitation is not done with the new guidelines if the rescuer is not trained in CPR, or they do not want to do it.

After 30 compressions, the trained CPR individual will open the victim's airway using the head-tilt, chin lift method. After pinching the nose and making a seal over the victim's mouth give the victim a breath big enough to make the chest rise. It is recommended that the rescuer use a CRP mask when performing rescue breathing.

Infants and children may still require mouth-to-mouth resuscitation by a trained CPR individual as breathing issues are more common in this age group. Lay personnel are now trained to do compression only CPR.

The American Heart Association guidelines place priority on caring for victims of stroke as well as those with an acute myocardial infarction (MI). Early fibrinolytic treatment for the MI client is necessary; also, clients with a stroke require treatment within 3 hr of onset of symptoms for a quality outcome. EMS personnel are trained to provide stroke screening tools and then rapidly transport stroke clients to the nearest hospital where fibrinolytic therapy can be administered within 1 hr of arrival at the facility.

The *Automated External Defibrillator* (AED) is a battery-operated computerized defibrillator that analyzes the heart rhythm, recognizes a shockable rhythm, and advises the operator when

TABLE 31-2 Summary of Basic Life Support ABCD Maneuvers for Infants, Children, and Adults (Newborn Information Not Included)

Maneuver	*Adult* *8 Years and older*	*Child* *1 Year to 8 Years*	*Infant* *Under 1 Year of Age*
Compression landmarks	Lower half of sternum (center between the nipples to prevent compression over the xiphoid)		Just below nipple line (lower half of sternum)
Compression method Push hard and fast Allow complete recoil	Heel of one hand, other hand on top	Heel of one hand or as for adults	2 or 3 fingers (2 rescuers): 2 thumb-encircling hands
Compression depth	2 in.	2 in.	1.5 in.
Compression rate	Approximately 100/min		
Compression-ventilation ratio	30:2	30:2	
Airway	Head tilt–chin lift (suspected trauma, use jaw thrust)		
BREATHING Initial	2 breaths at 1 second/ breath, after 30 compressions Use CPR mask	2 effective breaths at 1 second/breath, after 30 compressions	
HCP: Rescue breathing without chest compressions	10 to 12 breaths/min (approximate)	12 to 20 breaths/min (approximate)	
HCP: Rescue breaths and CPR with advanced airway	30 compressions, 2 breaths	1 breath every 3–5 seconds	
Foreign-body airway obstruction	Abdominal thrusts		5 Back blows 5 chest thrusts
Defibrillation AED	Use adult pads Witnessed: Use AED, shock as indicated Unwitnessed: AED after 5 cycles of CPR	Use AED after 5 cycles of CPR (out of hospital) Use child pads for child 1 to 8 years if available **HCP: For sudden collapse (out of hospital) or in-hospital arrest use AED as soon as available.**	No recommendation for infants

Note: Maneuvers used by only healthcare providers are indicated by "HCP."

Source: Field, J. M., Hazinski, M. F., & Gilmore, D. (2006). *Handbook of Emergency Cardiovascular Care for Healthcare Providers*, Guidelines CPR/ECC, p. 1. Dallas, TX: American Heart Association.

Note: The American Heart Association (2010) announces new CPR sequence in 2010 AHA Guidelines for CPR and Emergency Cardiovascular Care: No more A-B-Cs, now C-A-B.

the victim should be shocked. Outside the hospital facility, AEDs should be accessible in areas where there is a high probability of cardiac arrest situations and when EMS is 5 minutes or more away from the location. Laypersons, properly trained, can recognize signs of cardiac arrest and apply and operate the AED.

Early Defibrillation Programs in Hospitals

The American Heart Association standard-of-care recommendation is that the collapse-to-shock interval be less than 3 minutes in all areas of the hospital and ambulatory care facilities. Even though emergency (crash) carts with defibrillators are available in hospitals, Automated External Defibrillators (AEDs) should be available on the nursing units if the cart is more than 3 minutes away. It is estimated that time from collapse to first defibrillation in hospitals can be 5 to 10 minutes.

The major benefit for AED usage throughout noncritical care units within the hospital is that other healthcare providers and noncritical care nurses can easily provide defibrillation within the AHA standard of 3 minutes. Every minute is crucial if the person is in ventricular fibrillation, the most common cause of sudden death in adults. Survival decreases 7%–10% for each minute that defibrillation is not completed.

Planning and Intervention

Once an initial assessment of a client for alterations in circulation has been made, the nurse develops a plan of care and prioritizes interventions. Interventions for circulatory problems usually fall into three broad categories: inputs, outputs, and pressure supports. Inputs include arterial lines, venous lines, fluids, drug regimens, transfusions, and blood component therapies. Outputs include suctioning with specialized equipment such as

Hemovacs and chest tubes and procedures such as thoracentesis. Pressure supports include dressings, direct compression, tourniquets, and cardiopulmonary resuscitation. An evaluation of the planned actions, based on the client's response, should be continuous and modified as the client's condition dictates.

In coping with alterations in circulation, care should be directed toward promoting, maintaining, or regaining the best possible cardiopulmonary function. The design for nursing action is to assess the situation and client for stressors. The client should be interviewed if possible, observed, and examined to identify actual and/or potential circulatory problems. The client's responses are appropriate, deficient, or excessive, and interventions should be planned accordingly. The nurse attempts to reduce client stress, supports adaptive behaviors, replaces deficiencies, modifies or removes excessive responses, and prevents injury and complications. The nurse should always assist in the evaluation of planned actions, report client responses, and assist in modifying the interventions as indicated.

Adaptations to Home Care

Circulatory skills performed in the home setting are similar to those in the hospital. Vital signs are taken using the same equipment and procedures. CPR and Heimlich maneuver are performed exactly the same way. Care of the pacemaker client, however, is somewhat different.

Clients with permanent pacemakers are expected to monitor pacemaker function on a daily basis. While in the hospital, the client is taught how to monitor pulse, vital signs, symptoms of pacemaker failure, and indications of infection at the pacemaker insertion site. When the client returns home, the home health nurse needs to reinforce the teaching that was initiated in the hospital.

The client should be taught to monitor the pulse daily on awakening to identify altered pacemaker function. This may indicate a need for a battery change earlier than scheduled. Normally, lithium batteries last 6 years or more, whereas mercury-zinc batteries last 5 years. Nuclear-powered pacemakers (plutonium-238) can last 20 years or more. Some batteries can be recharged externally.

The generator is usually placed in the abdominal subcutaneous tissue or under the clavicle on the left side where the outline of the generator can be easily observed. The client must be taught to assess the site during the postoperative period for erythema, edema, and warmth, which may indicate the presence of infection.

A periodic telephone pacemaker check may be used for clients living in rural settings or in areas where a cardiologist is not easily available with the longer lasting batteries. The client usually does not need to check the pacemaker unless there are indications that alterations in the pulse or other symptoms are occurring. Heart sounds can be transmitted via telephone signals and recorded on an ECG strip. The technician at the clinic compares a baseline ECG strip that is on file with that of the newly recorded ECG. If there are any alterations from normal, the client is asked to call his or her physician, and the technician also notifies the physician. This procedure identifies early pacemaker dysfunction and aids in preventing complications. New pacemakers usually do not need to be checked except with routine physician visits.

For client safety, it is imperative to stress the importance of having someone present while checking for pacemaker malfunction when a magnet is used. The telephone number of the pacemaker clinic should be kept readily accessible in case of an emergency situation, particularly when testing the magnet.

New "wireless pacemakers" are available. It has a small radio transmitter inside the pacemaker that talks to a base station attached to a phone. The physician can more easily and quickly evaluate the pacemaker function in his office. Most clients do not use this system; they are checked during a routine physician's office visit.

A Holter monitor, also called an ambulatory electrocardiology (ECG) monitor, is a small battery-operated device that the client wears. The monitor shows the heart's electrical activity while the client performs usual activities. The monitor will show how fast a heart beats, and if it beats in a regular pattern. If the client has a heart problem, the signals in the heart may not function properly, resulting in vertigo, chest pain, or death. As with the pacemaker, the Holter monitor is now being replaced by Event Monitoring and Signal-Averaged ECG monitoring. These monitors can measure the heart function periodically and do not necessarily measure only for 24–36 hr.

NURSING DIAGNOSES

The following nursing diagnoses may be appropriate to use on a client care plan when the components are related to circulation.

NURSING DIAGNOSIS	RELATED FACTORS
Decreased Cardiac Output	Cardiac disease states, altered electrical conduction, altered contractility, altered preload and afterload drug side effects, hypovolemia
Deficient Fluid Volume	Blood loss from hemorrhage, dehydration
Ineffective Peripheral Tissue Perfusion	Altered blood supply, arterial or venous, hypovolemia, shock
Impaired Gas Exchange	Ventilation–perfusion imbalance, abnormal blood gases, tachycardia
Excess Fluid Volume	Compromised regulatory mechanism, heart failure
Deficient Knowledge	Understanding pacemaker function, corrective lifestyle habits for heart failure

CLEANSE HANDS The single most important nursing action to decrease the incidence of hospital-based infections is hand hygiene. Remember to perform hand hygiene or use antibacterial gel before and after each and every client contact.

IDENTIFY CLIENT Before every procedure, check two forms of client identification, not including room number. These actions prevent errors and conform to The Joint Commission standards.

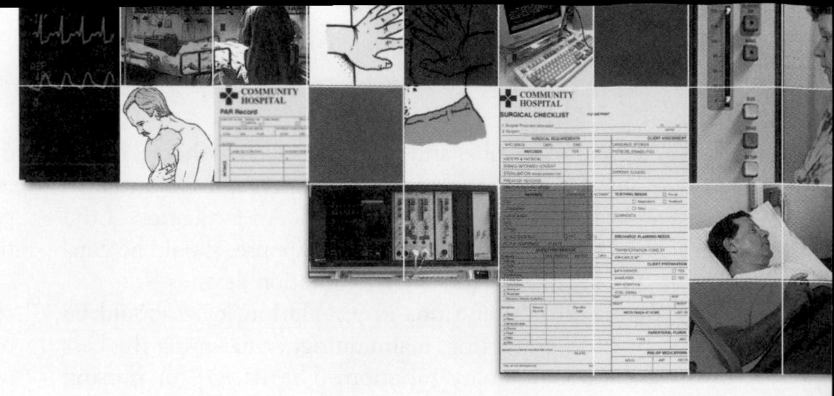

Chapter 31

UNIT 1

Control of Bleeding

Nursing Process Data

ASSESSMENT Data Base

- Observe the amount of bleeding.
- Check for the source of bleeding.
- Observe the extent of the wound.
- Identify familial history of bleeding disorders.
- Assess baseline vital signs and blood pressure readings.
- Observe color, temperature, and condition of the skin.
- Current medications taken by client.

PLANNING Objectives

- To detect source of bleeding
- To stop or control bleeding or hemorrhage before large blood loss occurs
- To provide pressure as an assist (adjunct) to stop bleeding
- To minimize capillary seepage, hematoma, and serum accumulation

IMPLEMENTATION Procedures

EVALUATION Expected Outcomes

- Early detection of bleeding occurs and loss of blood is minimized.
- Pressure dressing is applied and bleeding is controlled.
- Peripheral circulation is preserved.
- Vital signs are within normal limits.

Pearson Nursing Student Resources

Find additional review materials at **nursing.pearsonhighered.com**

Prepare for success with NCLEX®-style practice questions and Skill Checklists

Using Digital Pressure

Equipment

Towels or gauze dressing if available

Gloves

Procedure

1. Perform hand hygiene and don gloves (sterile preferred).
2. Identify the closest artery proximal to the bleeding site. ▸ ***Rationale:*** The rapid loss of more than 40% of the total blood volume will lead to death if rapid aggressive intervention is not implemented.
3. Apply direct pressure to artery using your gloved finger.
4. If towels or 4 × 4 gauze pads are available, apply direct pressure to site if wound does not contain glass particles. ▸ ***Rationale:*** If pressure is placed on wound when glass is present, additional tissue damage can occur.
5. Raise the affected limb above the level of the heart about 30°. ▸ ***Rationale:*** This decreases arterial blood flow to area and promotes venous return.
6. Maintain direct pressure on site for 5 minutes. ▸ ***Rationale:*** This action promotes clot formation.
7. When bleeding has subsided, proceed to gently clean and dress the wound.
8. To control nose bleeds (epistaxis), place client in sitting position, with head tilted forward. Pinch nose for 5 minutes. Apply ice pack to back of neck. ▸ ***Rationale:*** This assists in vasoconstriction.
9. Remove gloves when bleeding subsides.
10. Perform hand hygiene immediately. ▸ ***Rationale:*** To protect yourself from possible contamination should any leakage have occurred through the gloves.

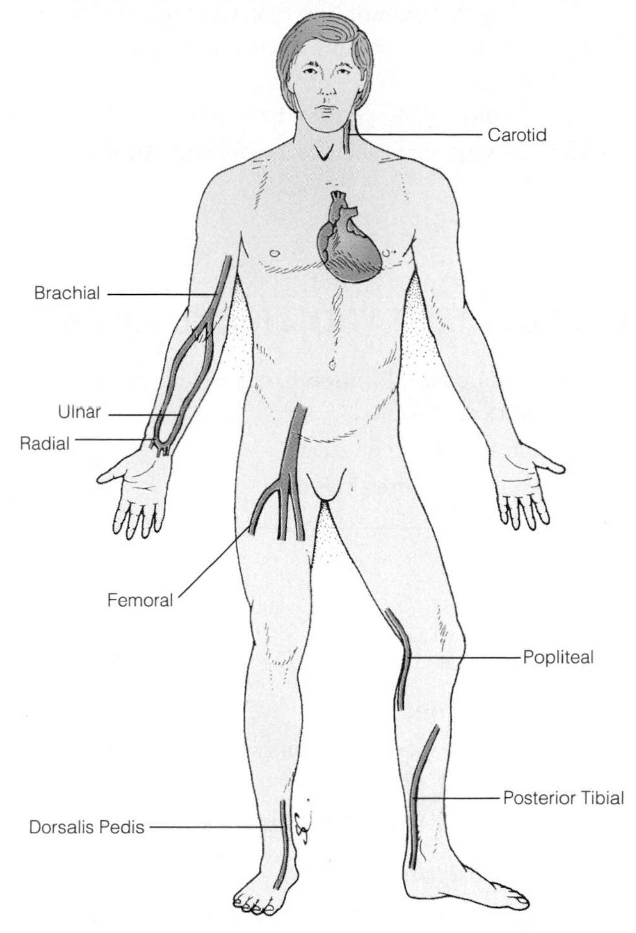

▲ Pulse sites that may be used to control bleeding.

Clinical Alert

Determine whether individual is receiving medications or herbal therapies which affect blood coagulation (e.g., Coumadin). If so, increase time of applying pressure.

Using Pressure Dressing

Equipment

4 × 4 gauze pad

Sterile dressings—number and size depend on wound

Sterile gloves

Cleansing solution

Tape

Preparation

1. Check physician's orders.
2. Assemble necessary supplies according to extent of wound.
3. If time permits, explain procedure to client and provide light and privacy.
4. Perform hand hygiene thoroughly if time permits.
5. Set up sterile field and prepare cleansing solution if time permits.

Procedure

1. Put on sterile gloves.
2. Cleanse wound and apply dressing. Use several layers of 4 × 4 gauze pads.
3. Place tape tightly over entire dressing to provide an occlusive dressing. Do not completely circle an extremity or the body. ▸ ***Rationale:*** Encircling an extremity with a bandage acts like a tourniquet and may prevent blood flow.

4. Check for pulses distal to pressure site. ▸ ***Rationale:*** To ensure that collateral blood flow is maintained.
5. Place all soiled materials in biohazard bag. ▸ ***Rationale:*** To prevent cross-contamination and ensure proper disposal.
6. Remove gloves and perform hand hygiene.
7. Monitor vital signs and observe for signs of shock.
8. Continue to monitor extremity distal to pressure dressing. ▸ ***Rationale:*** Ensures adequate circulation.
9. Position client for comfort.
10. Elevate extremity ▸ ***Rationale:*** To minimize bleeding.
11. Monitor frequently for signs of bleeding and hematoma.

NOTE: Hematomas feel spongy even under bandages.

DOCUMENTATION for Control of Bleeding

- Size (in centimeters), location based on anatomical landmark, condition of wound
- Color, odor, amount of drainage
- Type and number of dressings used
- Approximate amount of blood loss
- Condition of dressing when removed (e.g., saturated with drainage)

CRITICAL THINKING Application

Expected Outcomes

- Early detection of bleeding occurs and loss of blood is minimized.
- Pressure dressing is applied and bleeding is controlled.
- Peripheral circulation is preserved.
- Vital signs are within normal limits.

Unexpected Outcomes	Alternative Actions
Even with direct pressure and application of pressure dressing, bleeding continues.	• Reinforce pressure dressing. • Maintain IV infusion. • Notify physician and be prepared to send client to surgery for wound closure. • Monitor closely for signs of shock (LOC, vital signs, oliguria or anuria, tachycardia, narrow pulse pressure, hypotension). • Apply pressure directly or proximal to wound. • Place tourniquets proximal to site of hemorrhage to control bleeding if all other actions are unsuccessful, notify physician immediately, and prepare for surgery.
Wound edges do not approximate.	• Notify physician. • Be prepared to assist with wound closure or to send client to surgery.
Glass particles are evident in wound.	• Irrigate wound profusely with sterile saline solution as ordered. • If large amount of glass or if glass is difficult to extract, notify physician, and be prepared to send client to surgery for wound cleansing and debridement. • Do not apply direct pressure or pressure dressing to wound containing glass.

Chapter 31

UNIT 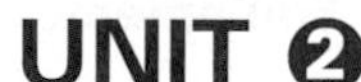

Circulatory Maintenance

Nursing Process Data

ASSESSMENT Data Base

- Evaluate client's overall physical status, particularly client's risk for venous thrombus formation.
- Assess baseline vital signs before procedures are initiated.
- Determine whether client is at risk for pooling of blood in extremities or decreased venous return. Clients who require use of graduated stockings or sequential compression devices are postoperative clients, those who are immobile, and those with a history of venous insufficiency.
- Assess peripheral pulses, observing skin color and temperature, and fluid accumulation or edema.
- Compare findings with contralateral extremity.

PLANNING Objectives

- To prevent venous stasis
- To prevent thrombus formation and subsequent emboli
- To use compression stockings or sequential compression devices to prevent venous stasis

IMPLEMENTATION Procedures

EVALUATION Expected Outcomes

- Compression stockings remain wrinkle-free and pressure is evenly distributed.
- Peripheral pulses are present during use of sequential stockings and elastic hosiery.
- Compression devices function properly.
- Client's skin remains intact while using compression stockings.

Pearson Nursing Student Resources

Find additional review materials at **nursing.pearsonhighered.com**

Prepare for success with NCLEX®-style practice questions and Skill Checklists

Applying Graduated Compression Stockings (Elastic Hosiery)

Equipment

Tape measure

Specific type of hosiery (e.g., below-the-knee or above-the-knee)

Preparation

1. Check physician's orders for type and specifications.
2. Gather supplies, identify client, and explain procedure.
3. Perform hand hygiene, and provide for client's privacy and comfort.
4. Apply drape as top linens are removed. Bathe and ensure legs are dry before applying stockings.
5. Assess lower extremities for edema, dry skin, and palpable pulses.
6. Position client in dorsal recumbent position, and elevate bed to working height.
7. Measure client for hosiery size (Table 31-3). Length is determined by measuring distance from gluteal fold to bottom of the heel.
    a. For thigh-high stockings, measure midcalf and midthigh circumference to determine size.
    b. For below-the-knee stockings, measure from the Achilles tendon to the popliteal fold, and measure the midcalf circumference.
8. Compare your measurements with manufacturer's chart to obtain correct hose size.

Procedure

1. Invert foot of stocking back to heel area.
2. Holding both sides of hose at inverted foot area, pull hose over toes and ease gently toward top of foot.
3. Gather top of hose down to heel area, and with curving motion, cover heel. Pull hose up leg, positioning support section on inner thigh.
4. Reposition client, lower bed, and perform hand hygiene.
5. Observe that stockings are wrinkle-free and correctly placed on extremity. ▸ ***Rationale:*** Stockings tend to roll down and create a tourniquet effect that inhibits venous return.

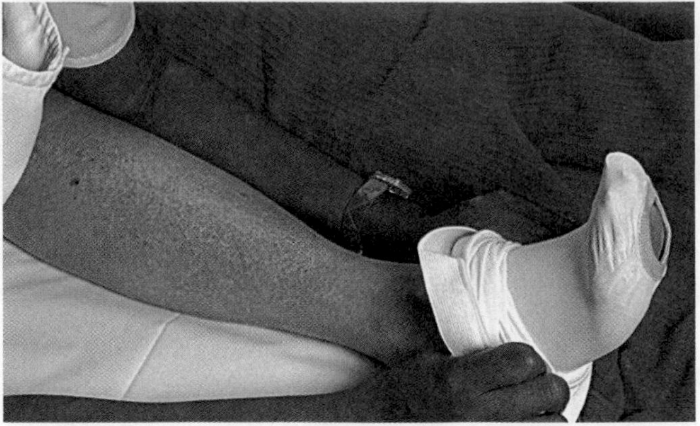

▲ Gather elastic hose and pull over toes and then to top of foot.

6. Check client in 30 minutes for adequate circulation, assessing for warmth, color of feet, blanching of nail beds, and edema above level of stockings.
7. Remove hose two to three times daily for 30 minutes. Assess skin integrity and peripheral circulation and perform neurovascular checks (CMS).
8. Wash hose in mild detergent and warm water daily and hang to dry.

NOTE: A second pair of hose should be available to use when hose are drying.

Effectiveness of Graduated Compression Stockings

Compression stockings, whether alone or in combination with anticoagulation, are beneficial for the reduction of post-thrombotic syndrome (PTS), a sequelae of events that occur after a DVT. The research supporting the use of compression stockings in the prevention of DVT in moderate- to high-risk clients is variable and inconclusive. The data do not support the use of compression stockings for DVT reduction, only for reduction of PTS. In low- or moderate-risk clients, compressive stockings may be of benefit. Stockings reduce stasis and PTS. They are inexpensive and have minimal side effects if applied properly.

TABLE 31-3 Measuring for Graduated Compression Stockings (Elastic Hosiery)

Thigh-High Measuring		Knee-High Measuring	
Circumference	**Length**	**Circumference**	**Length**
Measure mid-thigh circumference	Measure leg from bottom of heel to fold of buttocks	Measure calf at largest circumference	Measure leg from Achilles tendon to popliteal fold

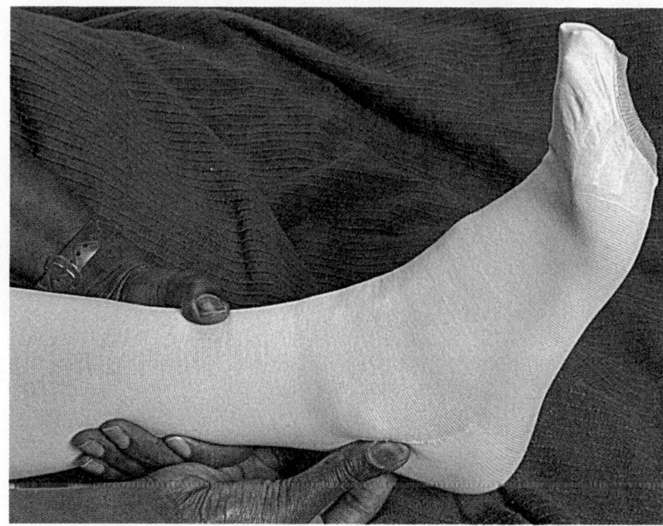

▲ Ensure hose fits properly without wrinkles over toe or heel.

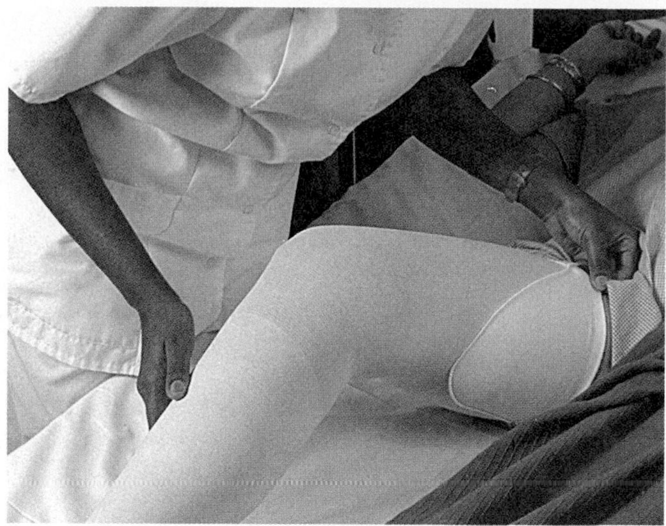

▲ Position support section on inner thigh.

EVIDENCE-BASED PRACTICE

Compression Stockings—Safe Practice Issues

This study explored the use of graduated compression stockings and found that poorly fitting hose can be a direct cause of DVT and of pressure ulcers on heels and the top of foot due to tourniquet effect. Thigh-length hose are more difficult to apply and more apt to wrinkle and are less comfortable. Clients often complain of stockings being painful, hot, and itchy. It is important that nurses measure the client's legs for correct fit, assess extremities regularly, and encourage compliance through client education.

Source: Hayes, J., Lehman, C., & Castoguay, P. (2002). Graduated compression stockings: Updating practice, improving compliance. *MEDSURG Nursing, 11*(4), 163.

In a randomized controlled clinical study, 180 clients, after their first episode of asymptomatic proximal DVT, received conventional therapy and were randomly assigned to wear or not to wear knee-high compressive stockings for 2 years after the initial DVT event. The results revealed that PTS was reduced by 50% when below-the-knee compressive stockings were worn as compared with the control group.

Source: Prandoni, P., Lensing, A. W., Prins, M. H., Frulla, M., Marchiori, A., Bernardi, E.,... & Girolami, A. (2004). Below the knee elastic compression stockings to prevent post-thrombotic syndrome: A randomized, control trial. *Annals of Internal Medicine, 141*(4), 249–256.

Applying Pneumatic Compression Devices

Equipment

Disposable leg sleeve(s): knee length or thigh length
Tubing assembly
Compression controller (motor)
Measuring tape

Preparation

1. Review physician's orders for type of disposable leg sleeve needed.
2. Identify client and explain that this device decreases the risk of developing deep-vein thrombosis (DVT) for clients after surgery or those on long-term bedrest. ▸ ***Rationale:*** This device counteracts blood stasis by increasing peak blood flow velocity. It helps to carry pooled blood from vein.
3. Assess client for potential problems and contraindications for use of these devices. ▸ ***Rationale:*** Clients with ischemic conditions, massive edema of the leg, dermatitis, gangrene, on long-term bedrest, or with preexisting DVT within last 6 months are not candidates for these devices.
4. Complete a neurovascular assessment. Include an evaluation of skin color, temperature, sensation,

Clinical Alert

Postoperative deep vein thrombosis of the lower extremity is often asymptomatic, and in many clients a fatal pulmonary embolism is the first clinical sign of postoperative venous thromboembolism.

Source: Agnelli, G. (2004). Prevention of venous thromboembolism in surgical patients. *Circulation, 110*(24 Suppl 1), IV4–IV12.

Clinical Alert

In hospitalized high-risk clients not receiving prophylaxis, DVT was diagnosed by means of venography in 10.5% to 14.9% of clients. Additionally, in high-risk surgical clients without DVT prophylaxis, 20% undergoing hip or knee arthroplasty or hip surgery developed proximal DVT. If DVT occurs at the proximal end of a limb, it is more life-threatening, as this frequently leads to pulmonary embolism.

Source: Francis, C. W. (2007). Prophylaxis for thromboembolism in hospitalized medical patients. *New England Journal of Medicine*, 356(14):1438–1444.

capillary refill, and presence and quality of pedal pulses. Document findings. ▶ ***Rationale:*** This assessment provides baseline data for evaluating neurovascular changes while devices are used.

5. Assemble equipment. Read manufacturer's directions for connecting and operating compression controller.
6. Read directions for setting sleeve pressure (between 35 and 45 mmHg). Maximum pressure should not exceed client's diastolic pressure.
7. Locate and identify the indicator lights on the controller for the ankle, calf, and thigh pressure. ▶ ***Rationale:*** Light is on when the pressure is applied to the three leg sleeves.

Procedure

1. Remove sleeve from plastic bag.
2. Unfold sleeve and follow directions to fit sleeve to client's leg. Leg is placed on white side (lining) of sleeve. Markings on the lining indicate the ankle and popliteal area.
3. Place client's leg on sleeve. Position back of knee over popliteal opening.
4. Starting at the side, wrap sleeve securely around client's leg.
5. Attach Velcro straps securely.
6. Check the fit by placing two fingers between client's leg and sleeve to determine whether sleeve fits properly. Readjust Velcro as needed. ▶ ***Rationale:*** To ensure sleeve does not constrict circulation.
7. Attach tubing and connect to plugs on leg sleeve by pushing ends firmly together.
8. Connect tubing assembly plug to controller at the tubing assembly connector site.
9. Ensure tubing is free of kinks or twists. ▶ ***Rationale:*** Kinks and twists can restrict airflow through system.
10. Plug controller power cable into grounded electric outlet and attach unit to bed frame.
11. Turn controller power switch to ON. Monitor that alarms are audible.
12. Check that pressure indicator lights are functioning properly.
13. Monitor that compression cycles are correct.
14. Monitor neurovascular checks every 2–4 hr. Turn machine off immediately if the client complains of numbness or other signs of DVT.
15. Monitor client's tolerance of device.
16. Turn off machine at prescribed time intervals to assess skin and to provide skin care.
17. To remove sleeve, turn power switch OFF, and disconnect tubing assembly from sleeve at connection site. Unwrap sleeve from leg.

Clinical Alert

Follow hospital policy for amount of time alternating pneumatic compression devices are removed during the day. The effectiveness of the mechanical device is dependent on appropriate fitting and being consistently applied, with minimal interruptions, in order to prevent clot formation.

Applying Sequential Compression Devices (SCDs)

Equipment

Disposable leg wraps (knee- or thigh-length) or foot wraps
Tubing set
Pump controller

Preparation

1. Review physician's order for type/length of SCD.
2. Determine that device is not contraindicated for client (see box on page 1244).
3. Review product information for application and use.
4. Gather equipment.
5. Perform hand hygiene.

Procedure

1. Introduce yourself and identify client.
2. Provide privacy.
3. Perform neurovascular assessment noting circulation, motion, and sensation in lower extremities. ▶ ***Rationale:*** To provide a baseline of ongoing assessment of neurovascular status after devices are in place.

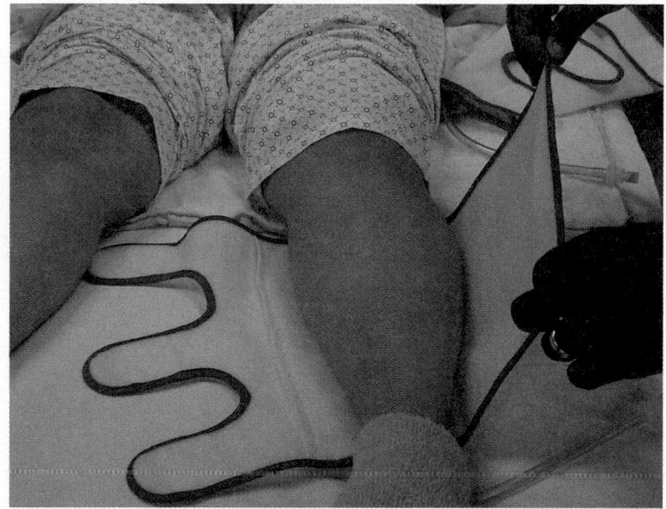

▲ Place inflatable bladder directly behind client's calf.

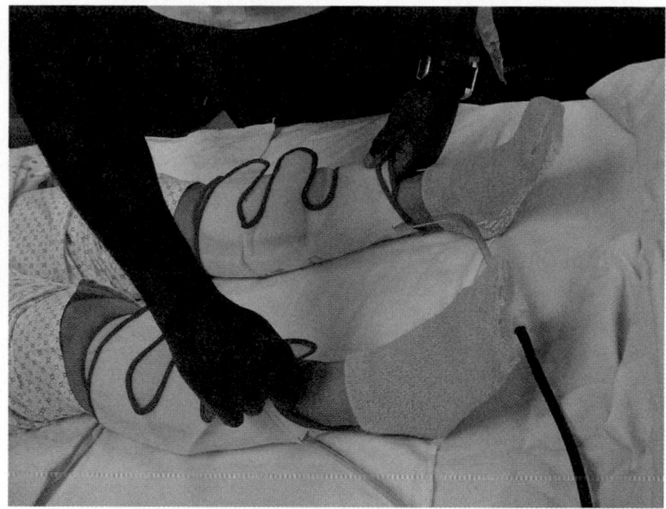

▲ Slip two fingers under wrap to ensure that it is not too tight.

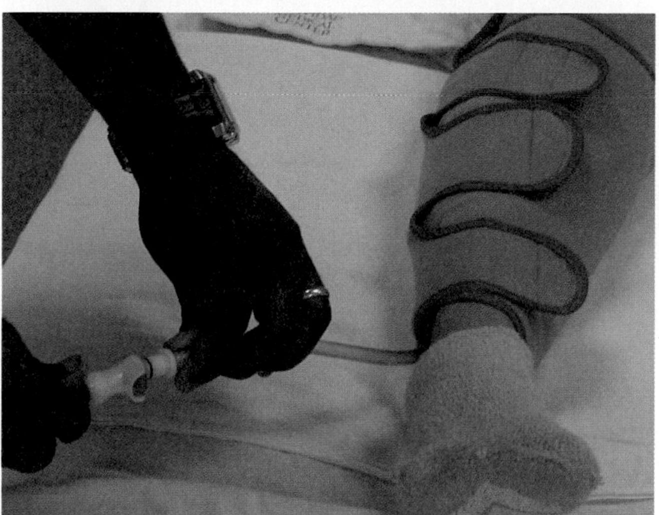

▲ Attach tubing from wrap to tubing connected to pump.

Compression Pattern

Each sleeve in the sequential devices is inflated in sequence. The inflation begins at the ankle and progresses to the knee or mid-thigh. Pressures range from a maximum pressure in the ankle of 45–50 mmHg, 35 mmHg at the calf, and 30 mmHg at the thigh. Compression duration is 11 seconds, with a 60-second relaxation time between compressions.

For intermittent devices, sleeve inflates, then deflates, alternating from one leg to the other.

4. Explain the purpose of the sequential compression device:
   a. They are used to reduce risk of developing deep vein thrombosis by improving blood flow through the leg veins.
   b. The wraps must be used continuously (unless ambulating) in order to be effective.
5. Plug the pump into the electrical wall outlet but leave unit turned *off*.
6. Remove wraps from plastic bag (leg wraps and foot wraps can be used on either leg).
7. Connect tubing set to the pump, making certain a connecting click is heard.
8. Unfold wrap and place the inflatable bladder directly behind client's calf.
9. Wrap the device around client's leg and secure the fastener tabs. Repeat process on other leg.
10. For foot (venous plexus) wraps (see photo of foot pump):
    a. Place foot in center of wrap with back of wrap in line with client's heel.
    b. Bring large wrap over top of foot, holding it in place.
    c. Bring the two narrower wraps over foot and secure.
    d. Bring the heel strap around back of heel and fix in place to secure wrap.
11. Check that wrap is not too tight by slipping two fingers underneath. ▶ ***Rationale:*** To validate that wraps do not constrict circulation distally.
12. Attach the wraps to the tubing set, making certain a connecting click is heard.
13. Adjust pump pressure regulator to product-recommended pressure (130 mmHg pressure, with 3 seconds inflation phase and 30 seconds cycle time), or as physician has ordered. ▶ ***Rationale:*** Intermittent compression and relaxation reduces venous stasis and thus improves the body's natural fibrinolytic activity.
14. Ensure that tubing is free of kinks. ▶ ***Rationale:*** Kinks can restrict airflow through the system.
15. Turn the pump on, noting that green light illuminates.
16. Place client in position of comfort; place call bell in reach.
17. Inform client to notify nurse if tingling, numbness, or discomfort develops. ▶ ***Rationale:*** Wraps should be removed should any of these occur.
18. Perform hand hygiene.
19. Regularly remove wraps for skin inspection and neurovascular assessment.

Clinical Alert

Contraindications to Use of Sequential Compression Devices

- Known or suspected acute DVT, phlebitis, severe atherosclerosis, or ischemic peripheral vascular disease.
- DVT within last 6 months.
- Pulmonary embolism.
- Any condition where an increase in venous return to the heart might be detrimental.
- Local conditions such as dermatitis, gangrene, recent skin graft, infected leg wound, or ulcer.

EVIDENCE-BASED PRACTICE

Recommend Bedrest for DVT?

Recent prospective studies show that routine bedrest should not be recommended as part of standard care for clients with DVT. While elevation and rest of a swollen extremity provide some symptomatic relief, bedrest has been shown to increase the risk of clot propagation and does not decrease the rate of pulmonary embolism. Early ambulation may provide more rapid relief of pain and swelling.

Source: McRae, S., & Ginsberg, J. (2004). Initial treatment of venous thromboembolism. *Circulation, 110*(9 Suppl), 1–3.

Foot Pumps

Foot pumps gently squeeze the sole of the foot to mimic circulatory effects of walking. The plexus of veins in the foot act as a powerful venous pump in the weight-bearing phase of ambulation. The foot pump is designed to mimic natural effects of walking on blood circulation in feet and legs. These pumps increase circulation and decrease edema and pain to the lower extremities in clients who are not ambulatory.

Example shown is the Kendall Sequential Compression Device (SCD) Foot Pump.

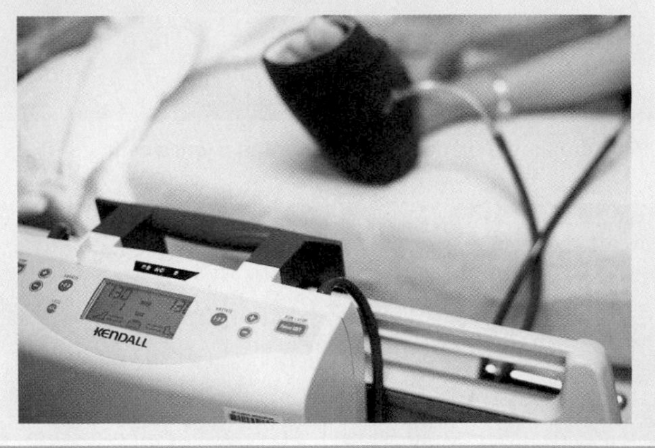

DOCUMENTATION for Circulatory Maintenance

Elastic Hosiery

- Size and type of elastic hose applied
- Condition of skin
- Presence of pulses
- Capillary refill time
- Edema formation below or above hose
- Time and length of time hose removed

Compression Devices

- Neurovascular assessment baseline data
- Neurovascular assessment after application
- Condition of skin
- Presence of SCDs
- Type of sleeve used; thigh high, knee high

CRITICAL THINKING Application

Expected Outcomes

- Compression stockings remain wrinkle-free, and pressure is evenly distributed.
- Peripheral pulses are present during use of sequential stockings and elastic hosiery.
- Compression devices function properly.
- Client's skin remains intact while using compression stockings.

Unexpected Outcomes	Alternative Actions
For Graduated Compression Stockings	
Graduated compression stockings are not available.	• If ordered, use elastic (Ace) bandages. Anchor bandages on top of the foot and proceed up the leg. Bandage should overlap one-third of bandage width; for a 4-in. width each turn overlaps by 1.5 in. Ensure pressure is evenly distributed throughout bandage application.

	• Assess that elastic bandages are tight enough for support but do not obstruct arterial flow. Assess neurovascular status 20 minutes after bandages applied and every 2–4 hr thereafter. • While making each turn, place a finger between the bandage and skin with rotation to prevent bandage from becoming too tight.
Graduated compression stockings are loose and don't provide support	• Remeasure legs and compare with chart to determine correct size. • Hosiery may be old with no elasticity and should be discarded; ensure line drying rather than with electric dryer.
Graduated compression stockings do not provide support.	• Need to order different knit design and elastomeric yarn denier that will increase pressure. Pressure ranges from less than 15 mmHg to 30–40 mmHg at the ankle. Check physician's order for appropriate order.
For Compression Devices Client complains of numbness or tingling in leg.	• Remove devices immediately. • Suggest use of foot pulse device as alternate. • Complete neurovascular assessment. • Notify physician of assessment findings.
Buildup of excess sleeve pressure (above 80 mmHg).	• Check tubing for kinks or twists. • Turn power switch to OFF position and then ON to restart system.

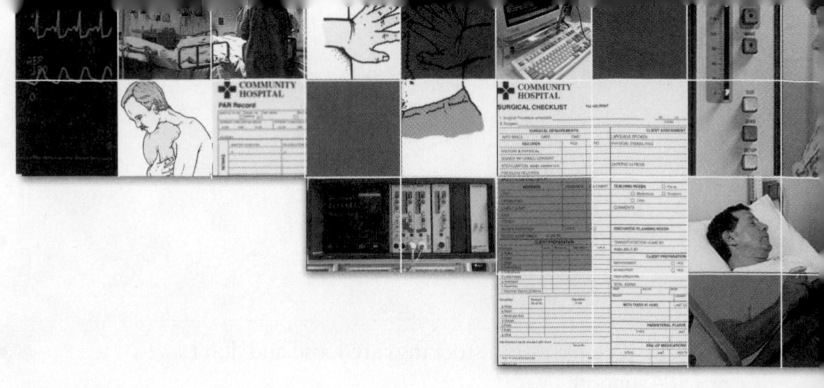

Chapter 31

UNIT 3

Electrocardiogram (ECG)

Nursing Process Data

ASSESSMENT Data Base

- Determine whether there is preexisting cardiac disease or chest pain.
- Assess client's level of understanding and cooperation with procedure.
- Determine client's fear or anxiety regarding diagnosis, procedure, or outcome.
- Identify pharmacologic agents currently prescribed.
- Determine other factors that may precipitate conditions, such as fever, anxiety, alcohol, tobacco, or caffeine ingestion.
- Determine subjective complaints of diaphoresis, palpitations, dizziness, or fainting.
- Identify electrolyte abnormalities affecting the electrocardiogram, particularly potassium and calcium deficiencies or excesses.

PLANNING Objectives

- To obtain 12-lead ECG
- To continuously monitor a client on telemetry
- To identify ECG changes
- To determine cardiac dysrhythmias
- To identify and treat potentially dangerous rhythms accordingly

IMPLEMENTATION Procedures

EVALUATION Expected Outcomes

- ECG leads applied appropriately and without difficulty.
- Abnormal ECG findings interpreted accurately.
- Heart rate calculated correctly.
- Monitor wave forms are distinct and readable.

Pearson Nursing Student Resources

Find additional review materials at **nursing.pearsonhighered.com**

Prepare for success with NCLEX®-style practice questions and Skill Checklists

Monitoring Clients on Telemetry

Equipment

Telemetry transmitter box with 9-volt battery
Electrode pouch or gown with transmitter pocket
5-lead electrode cable and wires
Electrodes
Skin prep pad or alcohol swab

Preparation

1. Review the client's cardiac assessment. ▶ ***Rationale:*** The choice of monitoring lead is based on the client's assessment and potential arrhythmias that could occur.

- **Abnormal sinus rhythms**, premature atrial complexes, and most heart blocks can be recognized in any lead that displays a clear P wave and QRS complexes.
- **Atrial fibrillation** can be recognized in most leads by the irregular R-R intervals and chaotic atrial activity.
- **Bundle branch block** and ventricular rhythms are depicted by a widened QRS complex. Leads V_1 and V_6 (or MCL_1 and MCL_6) are the best leads for differentiating a widened QRS rhythm. These leads aide in differentiating ventricular tachycardia from supraventricular tachycardia with aberrant conduction. It is best to monitor the client with multiple leads or a 12-lead ECG.
  i. The V_1 and V_6 leads are obtained by using the 5-lead bedside monitoring cable and limb electrodes. Arm electrodes are placed on the shoulders as close as possible to where the arms join the torso. Leg electrodes are placed at the level of the lowest ribs on the thorax or on the hips.
  ii. To monitor lead V_1, place the chest electrode in the 4th intercostal space (ICS) at the right sternal border and select "V" on the bedside monitor.
  iii. To monitor lead V_6, place the chest electrode in the 5th ICS at the left midaxillary line and select "V" on the bedside monitor.
- A second method used to diagnose the widened QRS complex is to use the V_1 and the bipolar lead MCL_6 together by placing the electrodes accordingly:
  i. Arm electrodes placed on shoulders.
  ii. Right leg electrode placed on right thorax or right hip.
  iii. Left leg electrode placed in the V_6 position (5th ICS, left midaxillary line).
  iv With the electrodes in place, select "V" on the first channel of the monitor to display "v1" and select lead III on the second channel to display MCL_6.

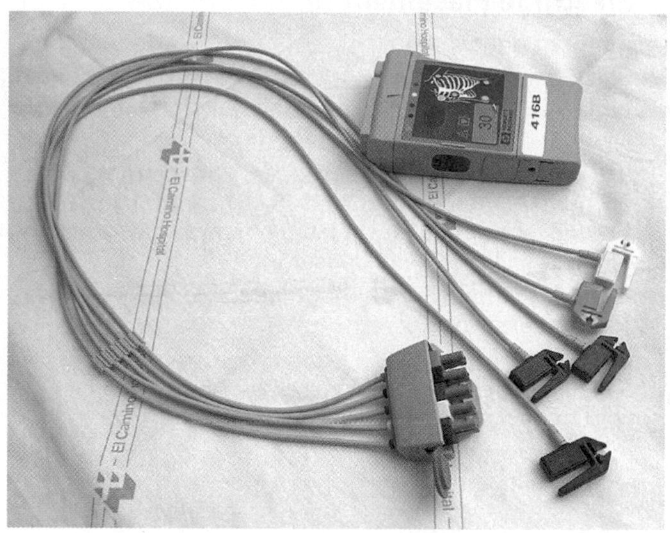

▲ Transmitter box, cable, and lead wires for telemetry.

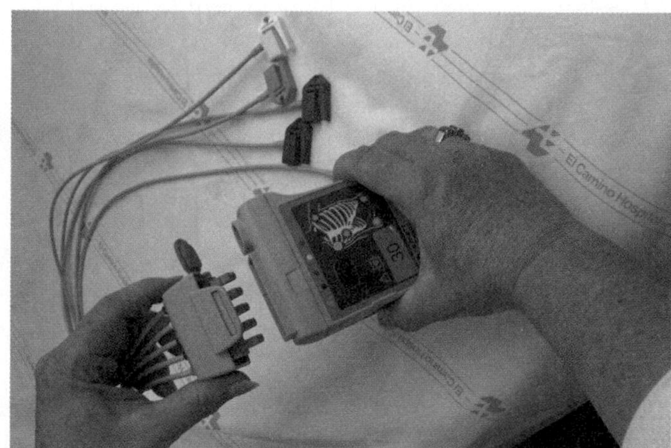

▲ Insert electrode cable into transmitter box.

2. Gather equipment and perform hand hygiene.
3. Place a fresh 9-volt battery in the telemetry transmitter box, if needed.
4. Attach lead wire securely into color-coded transmitter box, ensuring colors match.
5. Explain procedure to client. Radio waves transmit the heart's electrical activity to a central monitoring station. This system allows the client to move around while his/her heart is constantly being monitored. Explain that the telemetry range is limited; therefore, client cannot wander out of the range, which is usually the nursing unit. If client goes off the unit, nurse must be notified.
6. Instruct the client to notify the nurse if the electrode falls off.

Electrode Placement

White to right shoulder

Black to left shoulder

Red to left midclavicular upper abdominal area (lead II positive electrode)

Brown to fourth intercostal space, right sternal border (MCL_1 or precordial lead V1), or left sternal border, or alternatively at left 5th intercostal space, anterior axillary line (V_5 position)

Green to right abdomen or other convenient area (ground electrode)

NOTE: Limb leads and any one chest lead can be monitored using these electrode positions.

Procedure

1. Check the expiration date on the electrode packet. ▶ ***Rationale:*** To ensure electrode gel is moist.
2. Select electrode sites according to leads to be used for monitoring. Ensure they are not over bony prominence, muscular area, joints, breasts, or skin creases.▶ ***Rationale:*** Placing electrodes on these areas can lead to artifact on the monitor screen. See diagrams for lead placements.

NOTE: If client is overly obese, electrodes may have to be placed on the bones, since a large amount of adipose tissue results in poor image on the oscilloscope.

3. Assess skin site before placing electrode. Wipe skin areas using alcohol swab. Allow site to dry thoroughly before affixing electrode. ▶ ***Rationale:*** This removes oily substances and dead skin for better adherence of electrodes. Rub skin until slightly red. If client's chest is hairy, then clip hair. ▶ ***Rationale:*** This enables electrode to adhere well to skin and minimizes artifact.

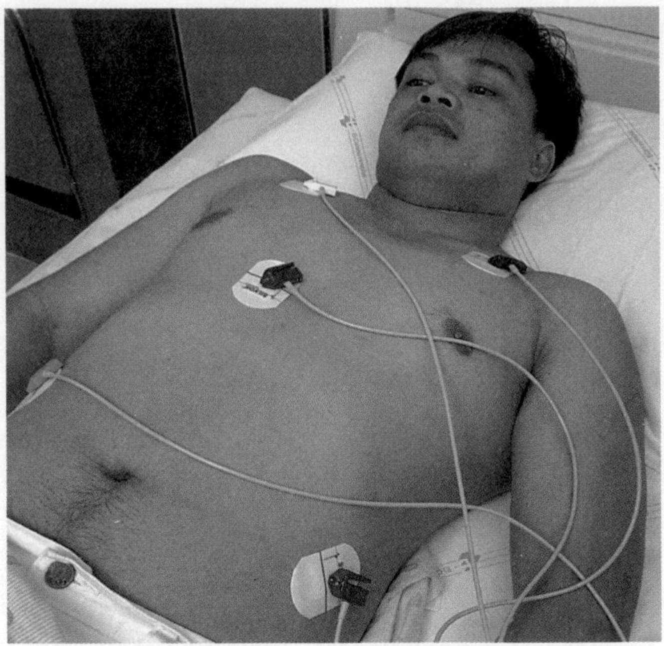

▲ Color-coded lead wires and placement of electrodes for ECG monitoring.

4. Attach lead wires to chest electrodes.
5. Apply electrodes to client's chest: peel off paper backing on electrode disc. Check that sponge pad in center of

TABLE 31-4 Telemetry Electrode Placement

• **Lead I:** Records activity between a negative electrode (below right clavicle) and a positive electrode (below left clavicle). This lead looks at the heart's left lateral wall. Atrial arrhythmic activity is poorly identified.	• **Lead II:** * Records activity between a negative electrode (below right clavicle) and a positive electrode (midclavicular line on left flank). This lead looks **at left** inferior wall. It is used to diagnose supraventricular rhythms which arise from the atrial and junctional nodes. It best detects atrial activity.
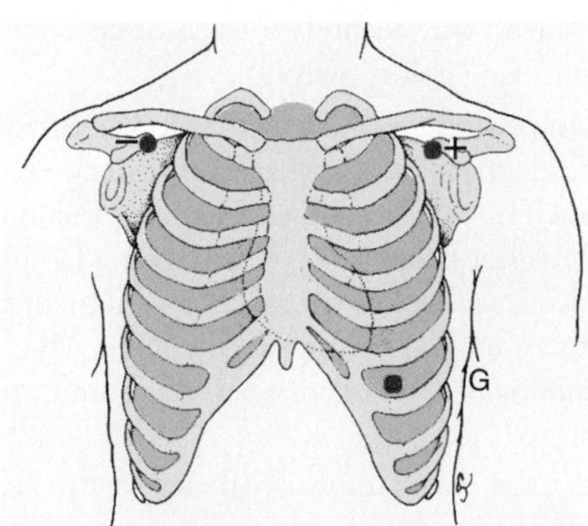	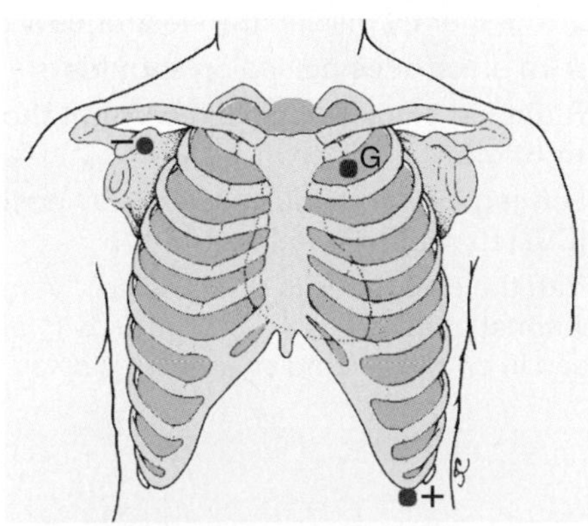

TABLE 31-4 Telemetry Electrode Placement *(Continued)*

- **Lead III**: Records activity between a negative electrode (below left clavicle) and a positive electrode (lowest rib, left midclavicular line). It looks at left inferior wall.

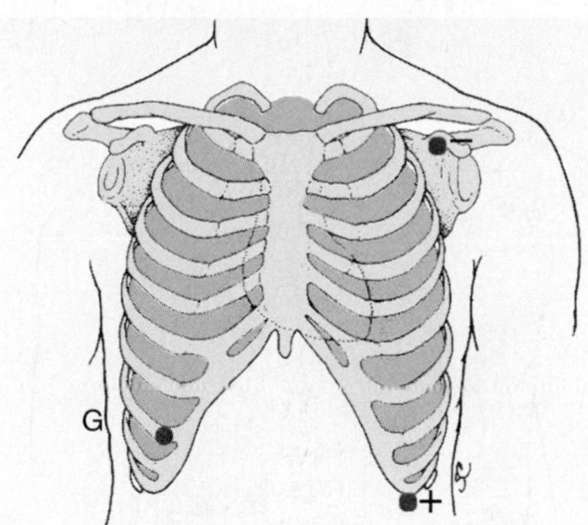

- **Lead MCL_1**: * Records activity between a negative electrode (below left clavicle) and a positive electrode (fourth intercostal space, right of sternum). **It is used to differentiate between ectopy versus abnormally conducted beats such as supraventricular tachycardia with aberrancy versus ventricular tachycardia.**

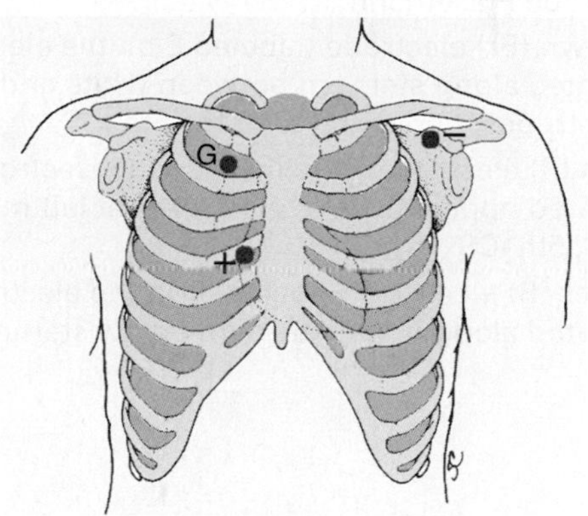

- **Lead MCL_6**: Records activity between a negative electrode (below left clavicle) and a positive electrode (fifth intercostal space, left midaxillary line). It monitors ventricular conduction changes much like MCL_1. Not as frequently used.

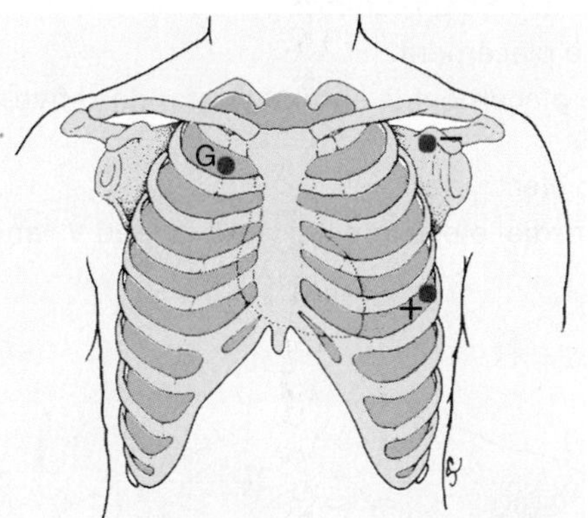

*Most popular leads for telemetry.

Note: Check frequency and flush solutions according to agency protocols.

electrode is moist with conductive jelly. Place electrode on skin with adhesive side down. Press edges down to secure.

6. Attach wire into transmitter box, matching the color codes of the cable wires to the telemetry box.
   ▸ ***Rationale:*** Mismatch of the colors will cause the client's rhythm pattern to appear inverted.
7. Have base station run an ECG strip to check clarity of transmission.
8. Set HIGH and LOW alarm limits on the monitor. Turn alarm buttons to ON per agency/unit protocol (e.g., 50 low, 100 high).
9. Assess skin surrounding electrode for signs of irritation regularly.
10. Check lead placement at least once a shift unless notified by client or monitoring station that electrodes are not functioning properly.
11. Change electrodes at least every 3 days or if ECG strip indicates poor conduction of wave form.

Two New Systems for Monitoring 12-Lead ECGs Using Smaller Cable Systems

EASI™ (Philips Medical Systems)

The electrode configuration is very similar to the standard five-lead system with four limb electrodes, but with two precordial electrodes located at lead V1 and lead V5. This system simulates a 12-lead ECG reading.

Electrode Placement:

- Brown (Br) electrode (labeled E on the electrode) is located along sternum between white and red electrodes, horizontal with the 5th ICS.
- Red (R) electrode (labeled A on the electrode) is located opposite white electrode, at left mid-axillary line, 5th ICS
- Black (B) electrode (labeled S on the electrode) is located along upper sternum below sternal angle.
- White (W) electrode (labeled I on the electrode) is located at right mid-axillary line, 5th ICS.
- Green (G) or ground electrode can be positioned in convenient site on torso.

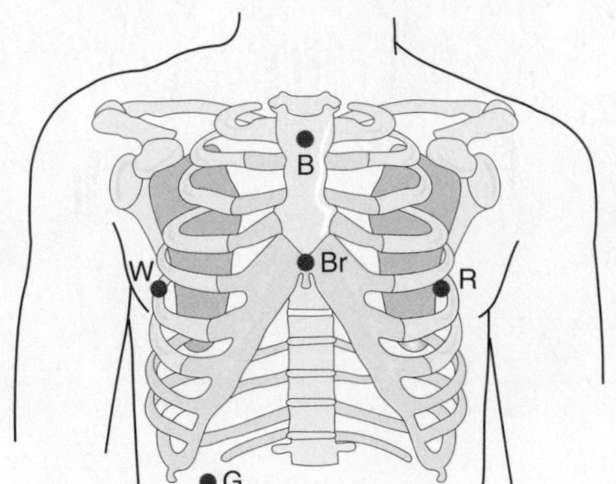

▲ EASI™ Lead System.

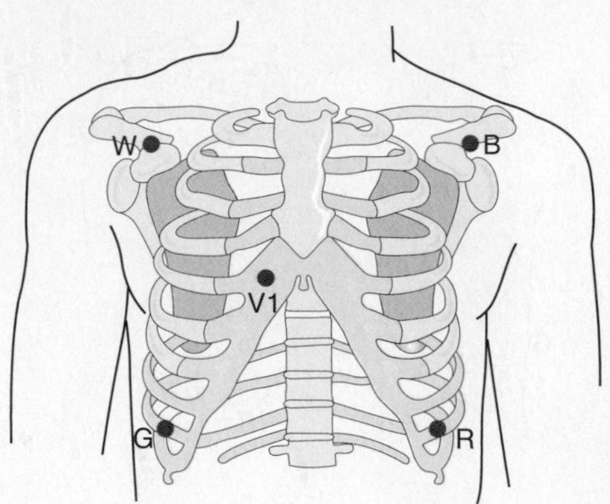

▲ Five-lead wire ECG system using lead V_1.

Interpolated 12-Lead System Using a Six-Cable System (General Electric Medical Systems)

The electrode system uses six-wire ECG system to produce 12-lead ECG reading.

Electrode placement:

- Electrode placement is similar to standard five-lead wire ECG.
- Four limb electrodes.
- Two precordial electrodes located at lead V_1 and lead V_5.

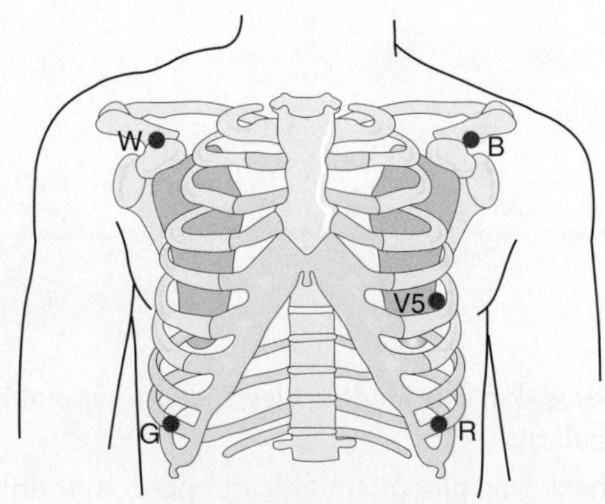

▲ Five-lead wire ECG system using lead V5.

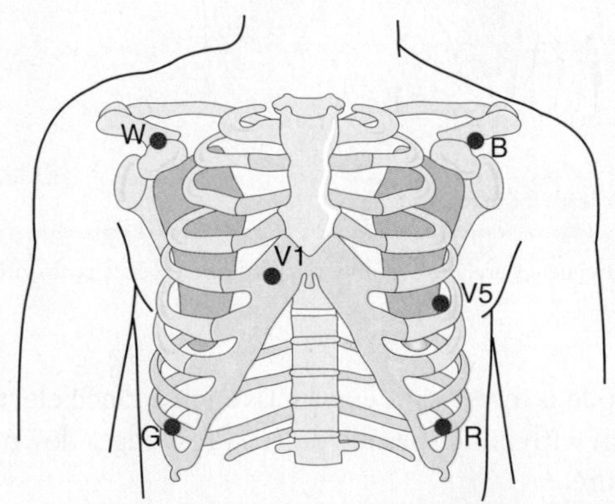

▲ Interpolated 12-lead system using 6-cable system.

Source: Nursecom Educational Technologies, 2003.

Interpreting an ECG Strip

Equipment

Calipers (optional)
ECG rhythm strip

Procedure

1. Assess ECG grid.
   a. Each small square represents 0.04 seconds (horizontal measurement).
   b. Each large block (five small squares) represents 0.20 seconds.
   c. 15 large blocks represent 3 seconds.
2. Determine heart rate by calculating ventricular rate; normal is 60–100 per minute.
   a. Count the number of R waves in a 6-second period (30 large blocks) and multiply this by 10 to obtain the heart rate.
   b. For true accuracy, count client's apical heart rate for 1 full minute.
3. Determine the regularity of ventricular rhythm (R waves should be equally spaced).
4. Determine the P wave rate (atrial depolarizations).
   a. There should be one P wave in front of each QRS complex.
   b. Note if there are more P waves or fewer P waves than QRS complexes.

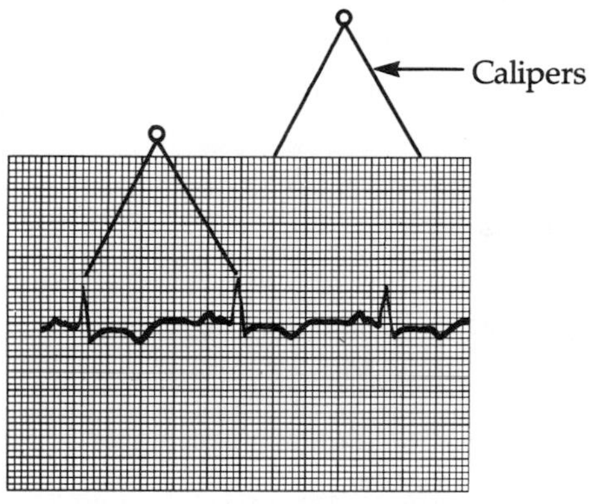

▲ Use calipers to measure heart rate.

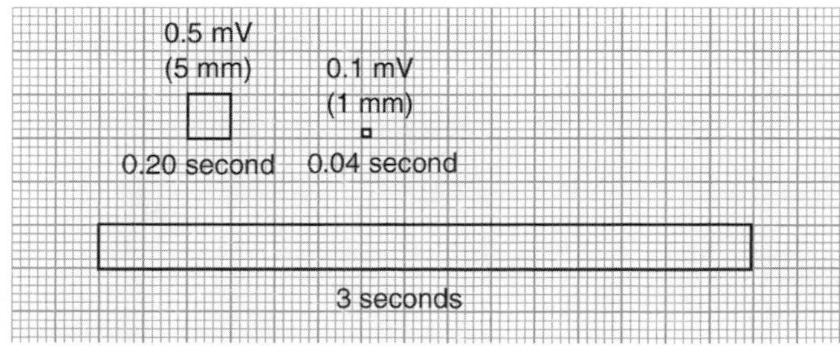

▲ ECG grid.

5. Determine the regularity of the P waves; are they all equally spaced?
6. Measure the PR interval (beginning of the P wave to the beginning of the QRS complex); represents conduction time through the electrical tissue to the ventricles (from the SA node, through the AV Node, bundle of His, bundle branches, and Purkinje fibers); normal is 0.12 to 0.20 seconds. Normally shortens as the heart rate increases.

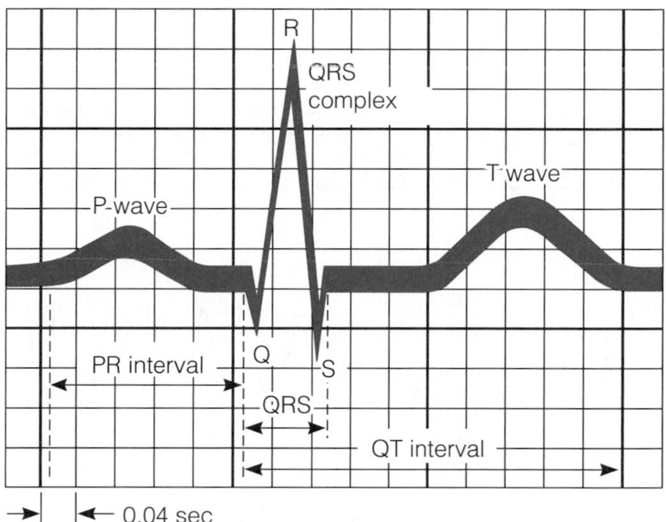

▲ It is important to determine configuration and location of wave pattern to interpret an ECG accurately.

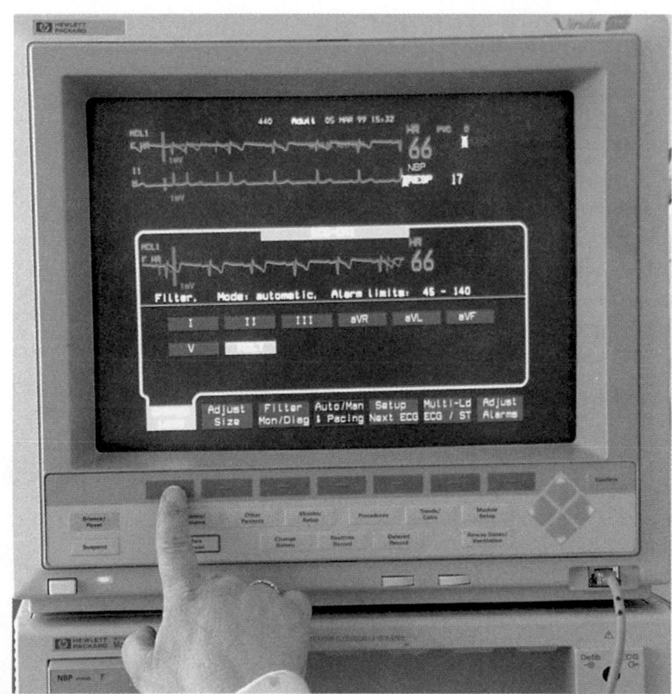

▲ ECG pattern and lead placement are depicted on oscilloscope.

7. Measure the QRS duration from beginning of the Q wave, if present, to end of the S wave (normal is less than 0.12 seconds).
8. Interpret the client's cardiac rhythm and place ECG rhythm sample strip in client's chart, according to hospital policy.

TABLE 31-5 Normal Sinus Rhythm

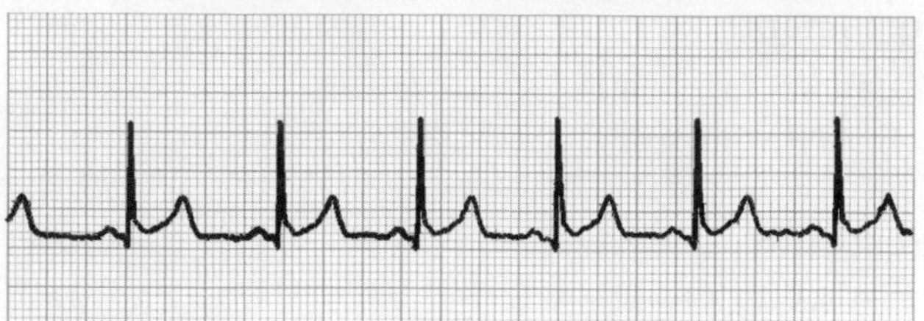

Regular configuration, uniform P wave precedes each QRS

Atrial rate 60–100

PR interval 0.12–0.2 seconds

QRS width < 0.12 seconds

Ventricular rate 60–100

TABLE 31-6 Selected Cardiac Rhythms and Dysrhythmias

Sinus Tachycardia

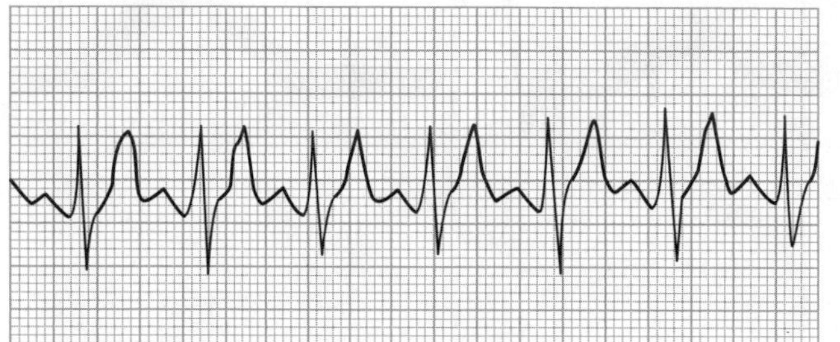

Regular rhythm >100/min
P waves—normal
Atrial rate—>100/min
PR interval—0.12–2.0 seconds
QRS complex width—0.06–0.08 seconds usually normal

Note: A moderately faster heart rate can be a physiological normal variant.

Etiology
Underlying causes such as anxiety, fever, shock, drugs, exercise, electrolyte disturbances

Initial Treatment
Immediately initiate cardioversion if unstable
Treatment dependent on elimination of cause
Decreasing anxiety
Pain relief
Antipyretics
O_2
Medications (sedatives, tranquilizers, anti-anxiety, etc.)
Calcium channel blockers and beta-blockers

Sinus Bradycardia

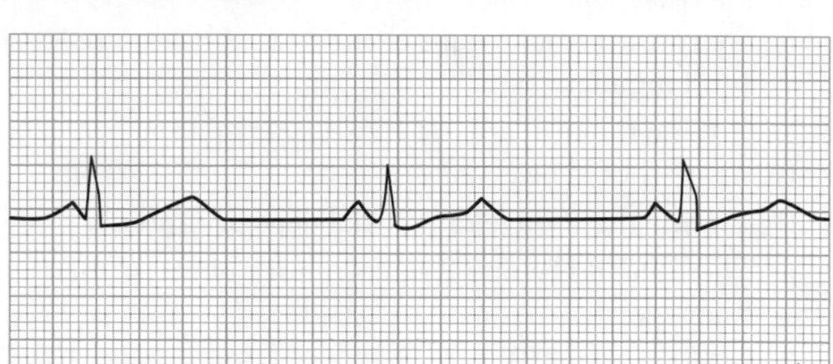

Regular rhythm <60/min
P waves—normal
Atrial rate—<60/minute
PR interval—0.20 seconds
QRS complex width—0.08 seconds usually normal

Note: A slow heart rate can be physiologically normal for some clients.

Etiology
Drugs, hypoxia, altered metabolic states (hypothyroidism), cardiac diseases, athletes

Initial Treatment
Maintain patent airway; assist breathing as needed
Oxygen
IV
Atropine 0.5–1 mg bolus IV while awaiting pacemaker
May repeat to a total dose of 3 mg
Then, epinephrine (2–10 mg/min) or dopamine (2–10 mg/kg/min) infusion while awaiting pacer
Transcutaneous pacing

Multifocal Premature Ventricular Contraction (PVCs)

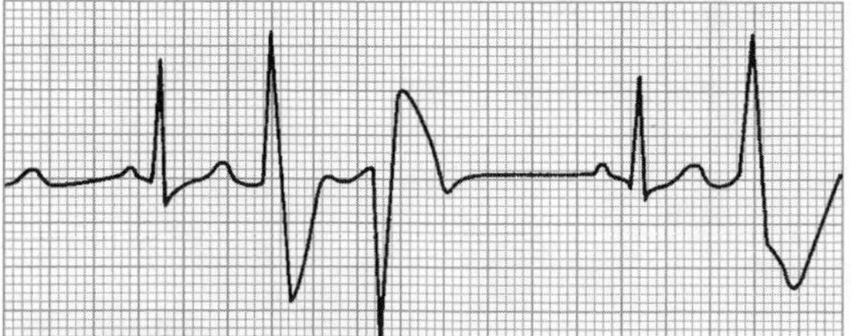

Ventricular Tachycardia

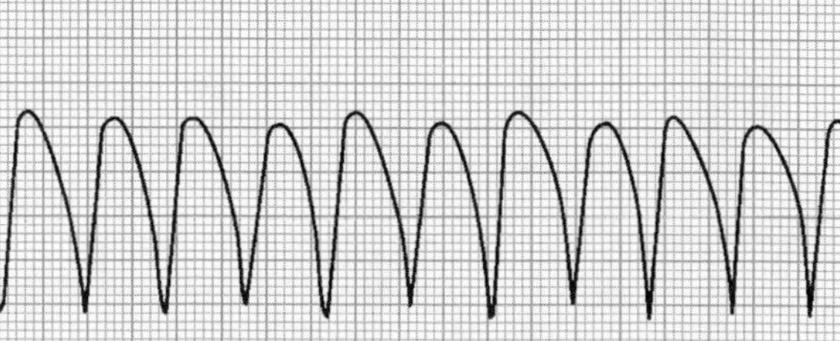

TABLE 31-6 Selected Cardiac Rhythms and Dysrhythmias *(Continued)*

Multifocal Premature Ventricular Contraction (PVCs) *(Continued)*	Ventricular Tachycardia *(Continued)*
Irregular rhythm P waves—none with premature beat, impulse originates in ventricle Atrial rate—undetermined PR interval—none with premature beat QRS width—greater than 0.12 seconds for premature beat Ventricular rate—varies *Note: Each PVC has different configuration as foci are from different areas of heart.* PVCs may be the result of an imbalance between oxygen demand versus supply, thereby making the myocardium irritable.	Regular rhythm Atrial rate—cannot differentiate PR interval—none QRS width—greater than 0.12 seconds Ventricular rate—130–250 *Note: Ventricular tachycardia is a result of myocardial irritability and is life-threatening.*
Etiology • Heart disease, MI • Hypoxia • Acidosis • Electrolyte imbalances • Myocardial ischemia • Drug toxicity (especially digitalis)	**Etiology** • Acute MI • Coronary artery disease, cardiomyopathy • Electrolyte imbalance • Drug intoxication (digitalis)
Initial Treatment • Oxygen • Potassium or magnesium if electrolytes dictate • Lidocaine bolus—1–1.5 mg/kg; may repeat doses of 0.5–0.75 mg/kg every 5–10 minutes up to 3 mg/kg • Refractory to lidocaine: amiodarone or procainamide • Continuous IV drip may be started • Correct underlying cause	**Initial Treatment** • Lidocaine 1.5 mg/kg bolus; may repeat in 3–5 minutes to maximum dose of 3 mg/kg • Amiodarone 300 mg IV/IO can be followed by 150 mg IV/IO • Cardioversion if cardiac output is compromised • Pulseless ventricular tachycardia—follow treatment for ventricular fibrillation (epinephrine)
Atrial Fibrillation	**Atrial Flutter**
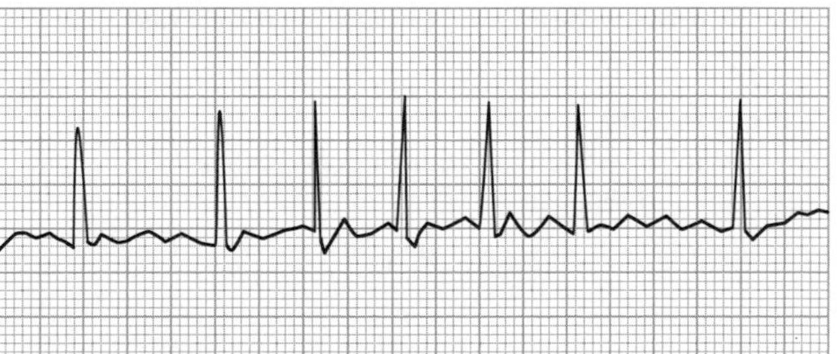	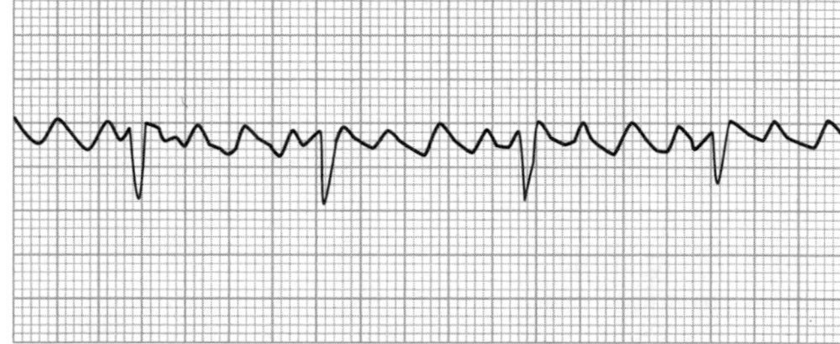
Irregularly irregular rhythm Disorganized atrial activity—greater than 350 BPM P waves—none identifiable PR interval—not measured QRS—variable QRS complex: irregular	Regular or irregular rhythm (depending on block) Atrial rate greater than 250 beats/min P wave usually sawtooth pattern; PR interval cannot calculate PR interval—regular Ventricular rate can be irregular QRS complex—0.6 to 0.10 seconds
Etiology Heart failure Rheumatoid heart disease Coronary heart disease Hypertension Hyperthyroidism	**Etiology** Sympathetic nervous system stimulation (i.e., anxiety), caffeine, and alcohol intake Thyrotoxins Coronary heart disease; MI; pulmonary embolism
Initial Treatment Cardioversion	**Initial Treatment** Cardioversion—if symptomatic

Continued

TABLE 31-6 Selected Cardiac Rhythms and Dysrhythmias (*Continued*)

Atrial Fibrillation (*Continued*)

Diltiazem

Beta-blocker: Carvedilol or Toprol Xl
Digoxin
Quinidine
Procainamide

Amiodarone or Dronedarone
Ibutilide
Anticoagulant to reduce risk of clot formation and stroke, if atrial fibrillation duration new in onset but older than > 48 hr

Atrial Flutter (*Continued*)

Diltiazem
Calcium channel blocker (Cardizem) or beta-blocking agents to slow ventricular response
Followed by ibutilide, quinidine, procainamide

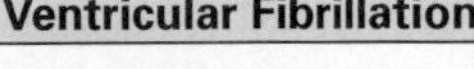

Ventricular Fibrillation

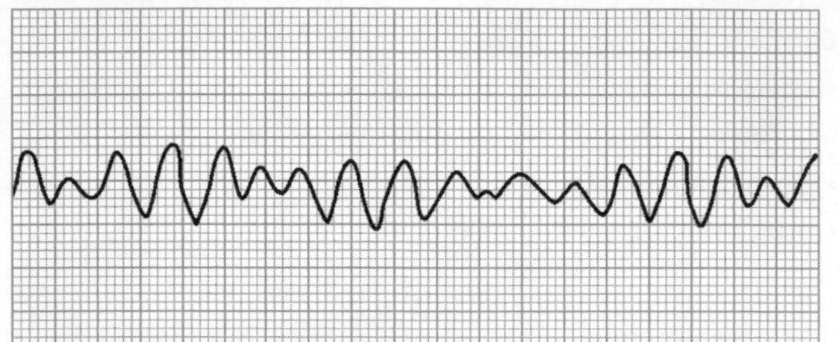

Irregular, totally chaotic rhythm
Atrial rate—cannot differentiate
PR interval—none
QRS width—fibrillating waves only

Ventricular rate—cannot differentiate

Note: Ineffective quivering of ventricles with no audible heartbeat, pulse, or respirations.

Etiology

- Myocardial ischemia, Acute MI
- Coronary artery disease
- Cardiomyopathy
- Acid-base imbalance
- Severe hypothermia
- Electrolyte imbalance

Initial Treatment

- Immediately defibrillate, shock
- CPR—100 chest compressions/minutes—no cycles
- Ventricular fibrillation continues—give a vasopressor (epinephrine 1 mg IV push), repeat 3–5 minutes
- Defibrillate again and continue CPR
- Second-line drugs may be used, such as amiodarone (300 mg IV), lidocaine

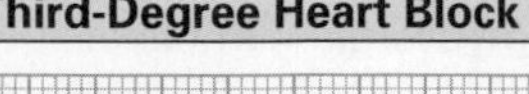

Third-Degree Heart Block

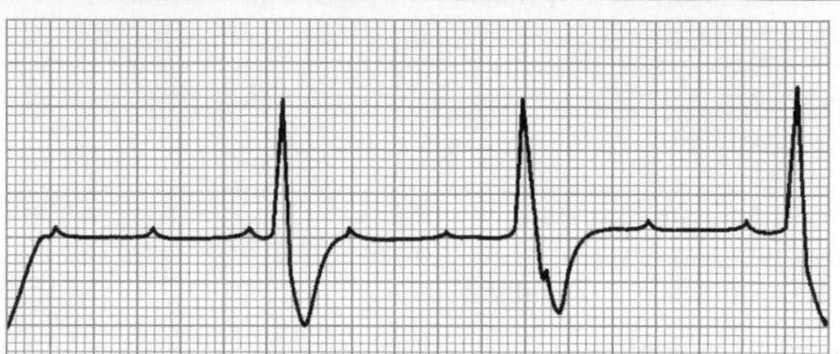

Regular atrial and ventricular rhythm
Atrial rate—greater than ventricular rate
PR interval—varies
QRS width—less than 0.12 seconds if pacemaker cell in junction; greater than 0.12 seconds if cell in ventricle
Ventricular rate—40–60 beats/min if pacemaker from bundle of His; < 40 if from Purkinje fibers in ventricle.

Note: Electrical impulse originates in SA node but is blocked in either the AV node, the bundle of His, or Purkinje fibers. There is no correlation between the atrial rate and the ventricular rate.

Etiology

- Digitalis toxicity
- Myocardial infarction: inferior or anterior wall
- Organic heart disease

Initial Treatment

- Atropine bolus
- Transcutaneous pacing
- Dopamine or epinephrine
- Prepare for pacemaker insertion

Clinical Alert

Always assess client to determine whether the abnormal rhythm is potentially life-threatening and emergency measures should be taken. Signs of hemodynamic instability include:

- Ongoing chest pain
- Shortness of breath
- Change in mental status
- Systolic blood pressure (SBP) <90 mmHg
- Heart rate <150 per minute.

Recording a 12-Lead ECG

Equipment

Electrodes
Skin prep pad or alcohol swab
ECG machine
Cable

Preparation

1. Review physician's order for ECG and perform hand hygiene.
2. Identify client using two forms of ID and explain procedure. Reassure client that machine will not cause discomfort or electrocution.
3. Assess chest for placement of electrodes.
4. Determine whether skin site care is necessary. If so, cleanse areas with skin prep pad, alcohol swab, or clip hair if needed. Allow area to dry thoroughly before placing electrodes. ▶ ***Rationale:*** This will ensure a more secure fit for the electrodes and provide a better ECG tracing.
5. Attach wires to electrodes before pressing onto client's chest. ▶ ***Rationale:*** This prevents pressure being applied to chest area. This is particularly necessary after open heart surgery or chest trauma.
6. Check the color coding on the manufacturer's directions before placing electrodes to ensure they are correct.

Procedure

1. When placing electrodes, ensure lead wires are all going in the same direction.
2. Place electrodes on fleshy areas, avoiding bone and muscle. ▶ ***Rationale:*** To ensure good electrical conduction and clear ECG tracings.
3. Place the four limb leads, one on each limb, according to the color coding. Three standard leads will be recorded on the 12-lead ECG.
   a. **Lead I:** Right arm wrist (negative electrode) white; and left arm (positive electrode) black. Records activity between the two arms.
   b. **Lead II:** Right arm (negative electrode) and left leg ankle (positive electrode) red. Records activity between arm and leg.
   c. **Lead III:** Left arm (negative electrode) black and left leg (positive electrode) green. Records activity between arm and leg.
4. Three augmented limb lead tracings are obtained on the ECG as follows.
   a. **aVR:** Records activity between the center of the heart and right arm.
   b. **aVL:** Records activity between the center of the heart and left arm.
   c. **aVF:** Records activity between the center of the heart and the left leg or foot.
5. Place the chest leads as follows. (See photo below.)
   a. **V_1:** Fourth intercostal space, right sternal border. Records activity between the center of the heart and the fourth intercostal space; P wave is shown best here.
      i. Palpate the jugular notch above sternum (feels like a depression).

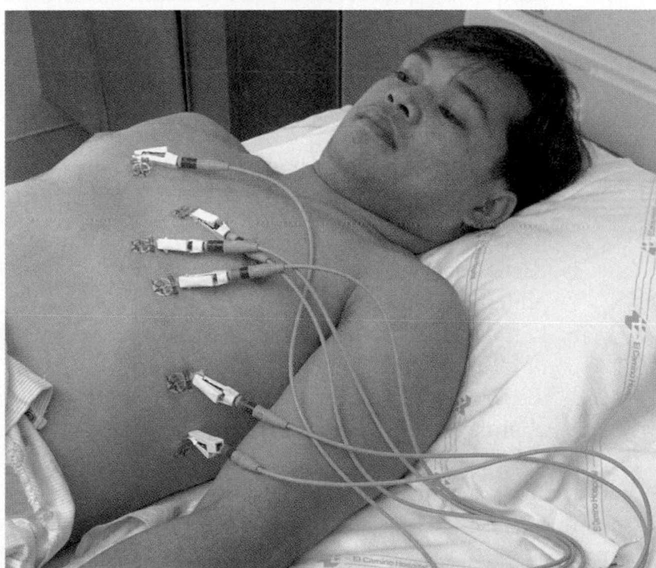

▲ Electrode placement for chest leads V_1–V_6.

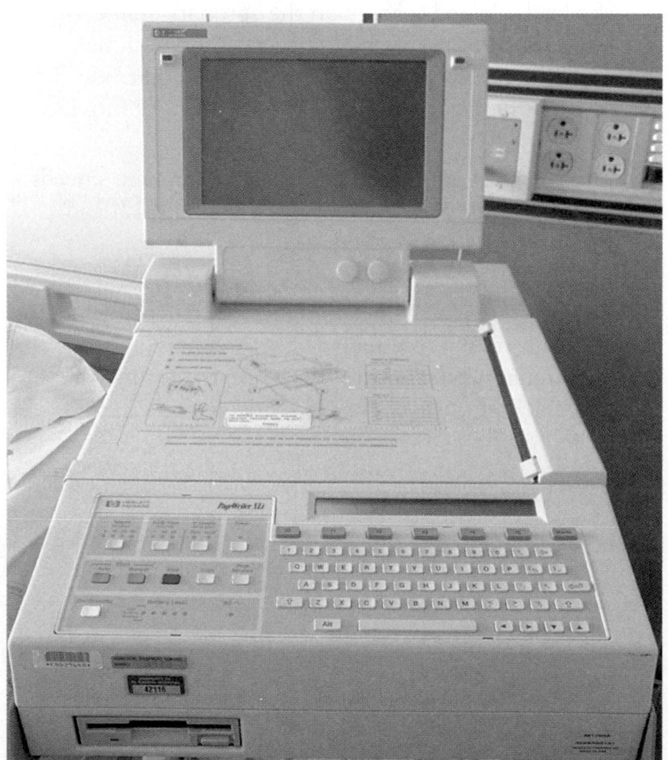

▲ Portable ECG machine for taking 12-lead ECG tracing.

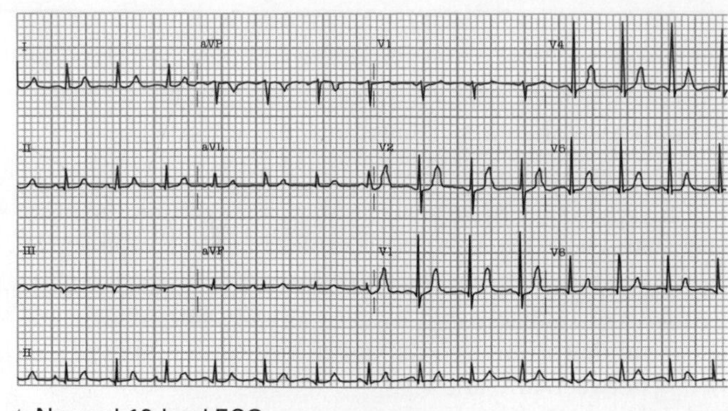
▲ Normal 12-lead ECG.

ii. Move finger down and palpate the manubrium of sternum (feels solid).

iii. Continue to move finger down to the angle of Louis, which is at the top of the sternal body.

iv. Move finger to the right of the angle of Louis to the second right rib.

v. Below the rib is the second intercostal space.

vi. Move fingers down, palpating the next two ribs. Below the fourth rib and to the right of the sternal body is the fourth intercostal space. Place electrode in this area.

b. **V_2:** Fourth intercostal space, left sternal border.

c. **V_3:** Midway between V_2 and V_4, between 4th and 5th ICS.

d. **V_4:** Fifth intercostal space, left midclavicular line.

e. **V_5:** Fifth intercostal space, anterior axillary line.

f. **V_6:** Fifth intercostal space, left midaxillary line.

6. Begin taking the ECG according to manufacturer's directions on machine.
7. Place tracing copy on client's chart.
8. Remove electrodes; perform hand hygiene.

ST-Segment Monitoring

Equipment

12-Lead ECG machine
Electrodes
Cable
Skin Prep

Procedure

1. Check physician's orders for type of ST-segment monitoring. If the 12-lead ECG is not available, then the lead selected is based on the coronary artery involved in the acute infarction or interventional procedure being performed. ▸ ***Rationale:*** The best ST-segment monitoring is using the 12 lead as it provides a global view of the heart.
2. Use the most appropriate leads based on client's needs and risk for ischemia and/or dysrhythmia if 12-lead monitoring is not available.

   a. Acute coronary syndromes (ACS) with a known "ST fingerprint," obtained during ST-Segment Elevation, myocardial infarction (STEMI), or percutaneous coronary intervention (PCI), use the lead(s) that best display the client's "ST fingerprint" when monitoring.

      i. If the "ST fingerprint" is not known in ACS, use leads III and V_3.

      ii. If the client's diagnosis is not confirmed as ACS, but it is being ruledout, use leads III and V_5.

      iii. In noncardiac clients undergoing surgical procedures or admitted to the ICU, lead V_5 is the best lead to identify demand-related ischemia, which appears to be more common in these clients.

   b. Use the lead selection for ST-segment monitoring if specific coronary artery injury is known.

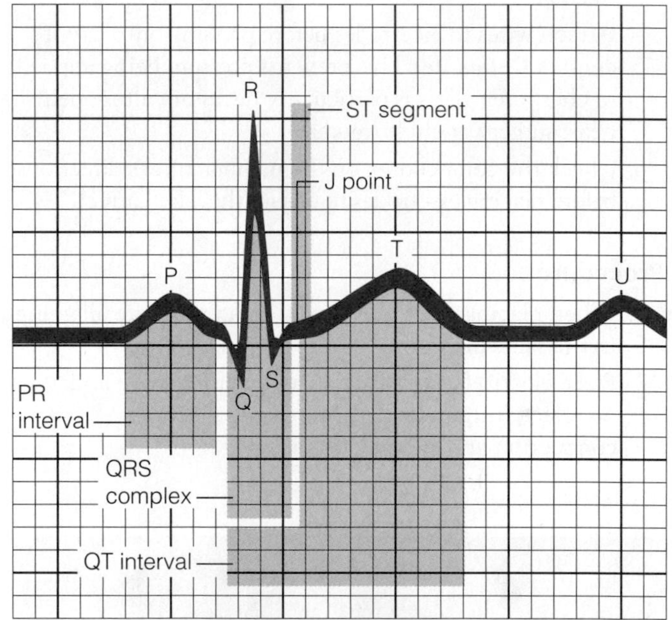

▲ ST-segment and J point ECG waveform.

      i. Circumflex (lateral wall injury): use lead I, aVL, V_5, or V_6. V_5 is preferred for noncardiac clients undergoing surgery.

      ii. Right coronary (inferior wall): lead III is preferred, then a VF or II.

      iii. Left anterior descending (anterior wall): lead V_2 or V_3 preferred, then V_4. V_1 and V_2 are associated with the septal wall. V_3 is preferred for clients with ACS who do not have an ST fingerprint.

3. Introduce yourself and identify client using two forms of identification.
4. Explain the monitoring procedure to the client.
5. Perform hand hygiene.

ST-Segment Monitoring

This monitoring is used to detect myocardial ischemia, electrode imbalance, and coronary artery reocclusion in clients who have received thrombolytic therapy or interventional cardiology procedures such as atherectomy, stents, or rotablation. It is also used to detect silent ischemia and in evaluating chest pain in clients presenting with atypical pain and nondiagnostic ECGs.

6. Connect cable to ECG machine and turn on the machine.
7. Clean skin before applying electrodes to skin. Cleanse skin with alcohol and clip hair where electrodes are placed, if needed. ▸ ***Rationale:*** To rid skin of oil and hair to provide a secure adherence of the electrodes to the skin.
8. Attach lead wires in chest electrodes.
9. Place electrodes in appropriate area of the chest with the adhesive side down. Ensure the electrodes are placed on the site for leads being used in ST-segment monitoring. ▸ ***Rationale:*** Appropriate placement is imperative as just a 1 cm change in the placement of the lead can interfere with the waveform patterns. This is particularly a problem when the precordial leads are not properly positioned.
10. Press edges of electrode pad down on skin. ▸ ***Rationale:*** To secure the electrode to the skin to provide a good ECG waveform.
11. Attach wire into transmitter box.
12. Check the clarity of the waveform transmission.

Clinical Alert

Ischemia can be easily detected by observing the T wave. If it is inverted and/or the ST segment is depressed, it indicates ischemia has occurred. The ST segment depression is often seen in combination with a sharp angle at the junction of the ST segment and the T wave.

Evaluate ST segment with the client in the supine position, set the ST alarm parameter 1–2 mm above and below the client's baseline ST segment, and measure ST segment changes 60 ms beyond the J point of the ECG complex. ST depression or elevation of 1–2 mm that lasts for at least 1 minute can be clinically significant, and further assessment is necessary.

DOCUMENTATION for ECG Monitoring

- 12-lead ECG taken
- Telemetry initiated
  - ST-segment monitoring initiated and monitoring leads used
  - Findings based on the interpretation of the ECG strip
- Nursing interventions carried out, based on the ECG findings
- Rhythm strips entered into client's record at least once each shift
- Telemetry strip documentation:
  - Lead monitored
- Interpretation of ECG strip to include:
  - Rate
  - Rhythm
  - PR interval
  - QRS complex
  - Q-T interval
- Document a telemetry strip for:
  - Any change in client condition
  - Client symptoms during procedures as appropriate
  - Administration of medications as appropriate (i.e., lidocaine)
- Health teaching completed
- Physician notification of abnormal findings

CRITICAL THINKING Application

Expected Outcomes

- ECG leads applied appropriately and without difficulty.
- Abnormal ECG findings interpreted accurately.
- Heart rate calculated correctly.
- Monitor wave forms are distinct and readable.

Unexpected Outcomes	**Alternative Actions**
For ECG Interpretation	
ECG is not clearly displayed on monitor.	• Ensure that electrodes are applied in correct position and are securely attached. • Observe for electrical interference resulting in a 60-cycle interference on oscilloscope. • Observe for excessive client activity resulting in artifact display on oscilloscope.
Electrodes do not adhere to skin and interference appears on oscilloscope.	• Change placement of electrodes to another area. Clip hair if needed for improved skin contact. • Recleanse skin thoroughly using skin prep or alcohol and allow to dry.
Alarms ring without change in pattern.	• Check HIGH and LOW parameters. They may need to be changed. • Check GAIN. It may be too low to sense pattern.
ECG pattern is abnormal.	• If client is asymptomatic, recheck lead placement and ensure cables are attached properly. • Check if pattern is a life-threatening arrhythmia (for ventricular tachycardia, call rapid response team; for ventricular fibrillation, call code). • Increasing PVCs—notify Rapid Response Team. • Notify physician immediately.
Electrical interference appears on monitor.	• Check all other electric equipment in the immediate environment. • Check for proper grounding of monitor. • Change electrodes and cable; poor conduction may cause 60-cycle interference. • Check that monitor is calibrated.
Electrodes cause skin irritation.	• Remove electrodes, cleanse site, and reapply electrodes on new site.
Chaotic rhythm appears on monitor.	• Assess client's vital signs and level of consciousness. • Check electrode contact on skin, and ensure that wires are in contact with cable.
High or low alarms on monitor continue to sound.	• Check for loose electrodes or try a different lead. • Observe activity level of client. • Check that alarm parameters on monitor are not set too close to client's pulse. • Check client's position. • Reposition electrodes, avoiding large muscle masses or bone.
Electrodes conduct poorly on diaphoretic client.	• Clean skin sites as usual; apply benzoin to the skin and let dry and apply electrodes. • Clean skin sites as usual; apply spray deodorant to the skin, allow skin to dry, and apply electrodes.
Asystole displays on monitor.	• Check client's LOC and electrodes, wires, and cable connection. • If the client has an arterial line, check for an arterial waveform in the absence of an ECG waveform.
For Telemetry	
ECG only provides partial information on heart activity.	• Obtain 12-lead ECG. It portrays activity in all areas of heart except posterior aspect—monitor different lead (i.e., MCL).

Client experiences life-threatening arrhythmia.	• Begin treatment for arrhythmia. Notify Rapid Response Team. Obtain 12-lead ECG when client is stable.
Telemetry signal not picked up at base station.	• Check that client hasn't wandered to an area where transmission is not available. • Check that transmitter battery is functioning. • Check that transmitter is ON. • Change wires. • Usual cause is a dry electrode. Replace electrodes.
For 12-Lead ECG	
Interference apparent on ECG tracing.	• Ensure that lead wires are hanging in same direction on corresponding extremities. • Assess chest to determine whether chest dressing is interfering with ECG electrode placement or signal. • Breast tissue may be interfering with ECG signal. Reapply electrodes under the breast as close to the heart as possible. • Instruct client to remain still.

Chapter 31

UNIT 4

Emergency Life Support Measures

Nursing Process Data

ASSESSMENT Data Base

- Assess client for signs of cardiac or respiratory arrest (responsiveness, breathing, circulation, etc.).
- Know emergency number to summon help and identify location of AED.
- Identify location of emergency cart.
- Identify procedure for activation of Rapid Response Team.

PLANNING Objectives

- To provide adequate oxygenation of lungs through mechanical support
- To support ventilation and circulation
- To reestablish a patent airway for client with foreign body airway obstruction

IMPLEMENTATION Procedures

EVALUATION Expected Outcomes

- Basic life-support measures established within 3 minutes after arrest.
- Emergency measures performed according to established protocol.
- Client is stabilized/resuscitated with basic life support measures.
- No permanent neurologic damage is sustained.
- Obstructed airway is reestablished.

Pearson Nursing Student Resources

Find additional review materials at **nursing.pearsonhighered.com**

Prepare for success with NCLEX®-style practice questions and Skill Checklists

Administering Basic Life Support to an Adult/Child

Equipment

Cardiac board
AED
CPR mask or Ambu bag

Procedure

For Unresponsiveness

1. Quickly approach client.
2. Check responsiveness. Tap shoulders. Shout, "Are you OK?" ▶ ***Rationale:*** To determine responsiveness of client.

> **Clinical Alert**
> Institute CPR within 3 minutes. Cardiopulmonary resuscitation is usually not effective in preventing brain damage unless initiated within 4 minutes of an arrest.

3. Call out or phone for help. Get AED (should be stored by telephone).
4. Move victim to flat, firm surface and position yourself next to victim, left side near head of victim. ▶ ***Rationale:*** Left side is preferred when using AED. A firm surface enhances effective compression between chest wall and sternum.
5. Place heel of hand in middle of chest. Place other hand on top of first with fingers interlaced.
6. Start chest compressions at 100/min with a depth of 2 in. for adults.

For Airway

1. The old guidelines were A, B, C: airway, breathing, and compressions. The new guidelines (2010) are C, A, B: compressions, airway, and breathing.
2. Press backward on forehead, if no suspected head or neck injury. ▶ ***Rationale:*** This causes head to tilt back and open airway.
3. Lift chin by placing two fingers under chin. Lift chin up and forward until teeth are nearly closed.
4. Pinch nose and make a seal over victim's mouth, either with your mouth or, preferably, a CPR mask or Ambu bag.

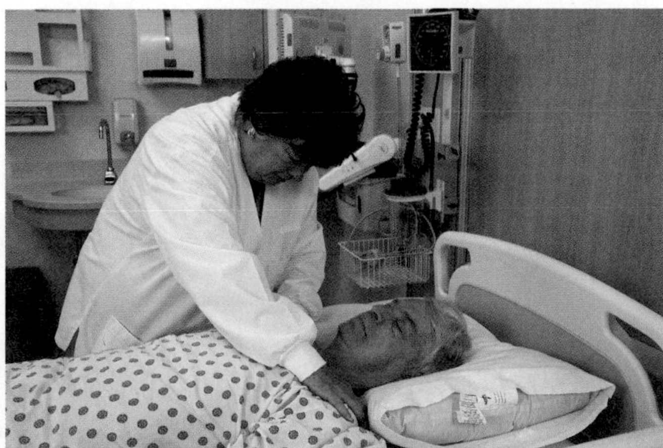

▲ Check for response: tap victim, speak loudly and clearly.

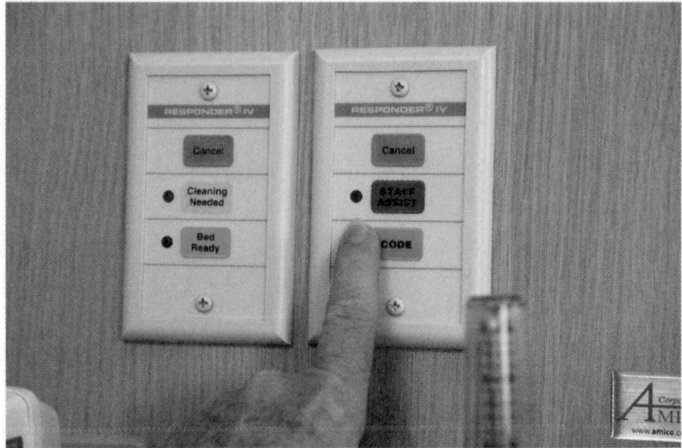

▲ Call for help and retrieve AED before starting CPR.

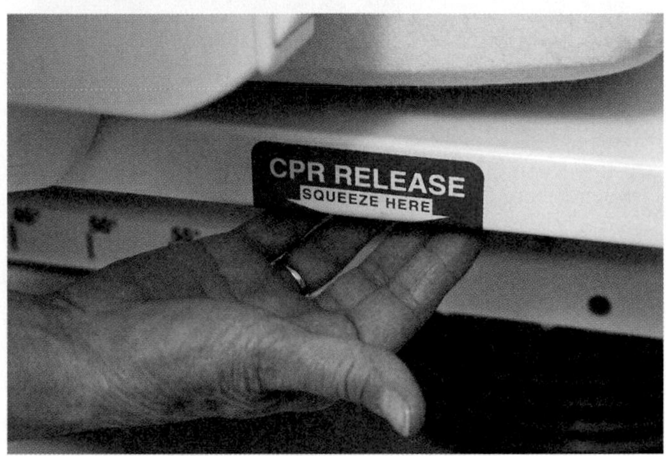

▲ Pull CPR release to place bed in flat position for CPR.

5. Perform 30 compressions; open airway if trained in CPR. Otherwise, continue chest compressions.
6. Apply AED immediately if witnessed collapse, or attach after 1 minute of CPR if collapse was not observed.

> **Clinical Alert the New CPR (2010)**
> 1. Check for response: "Are you all right?" Tap shoulder. If person does not respond, roll client on back.
> 2. Start chest compression: "Push hard, push fast" at a rate of 100/minute, allowing chest to recoil compress chest at least 2 inches in adults and children (new CPR guidelines as of Oct. 2010).
> 3. Activate the EMS system and send someone for the AED, or call 911.
> 4. If you have been trained in CPR, open the airway and check for adequate breathing: head tilt–chin lift.
> 5. Give rescue breath: 2 rescue breaths, each 1 second with enough volume to produce visible chest rise.
> 6. Continue compressions and breaths—30 compressions, two breathless until keep arrives.

For Rescue Breathing

1. Evaluate respiratory function:
   a. Check for rise and fall of chest. ▶ ***Rationale:*** If chest movement occurs but you cannot feel or hear air, then airway is obstructed.
   b. Repeat rescue breath.
2. Reposition head and try again if chest does not rise. Give 2 more breaths.
3. Repeat 30 compressions and 2 breaths for 5 cycles.
4. Stop compressions after 2 minutes and check for breathing. If not breathing, continue compressions and breathing until help arrives or AED is activated.

NOTE: It is recommended that a barrier device be used when performing rescue breathing.

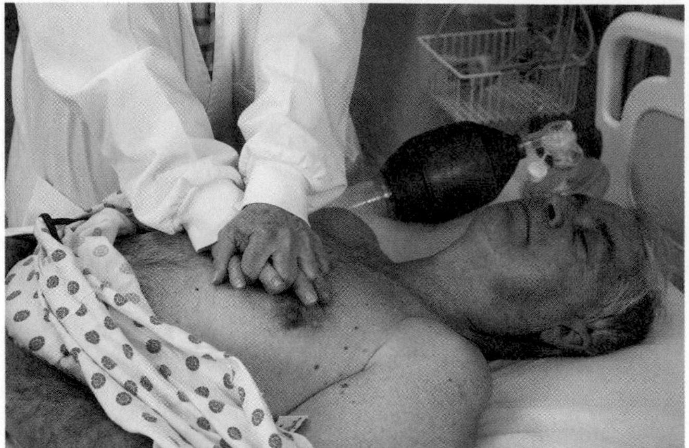

1 Begin compressions at 100 per minute, unless other instructions are provided.

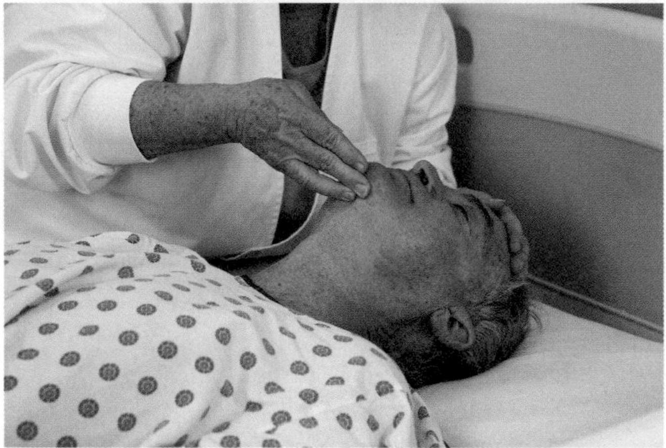

2 Open airway by tilting client's head back and lifting chin after 30 compressions.

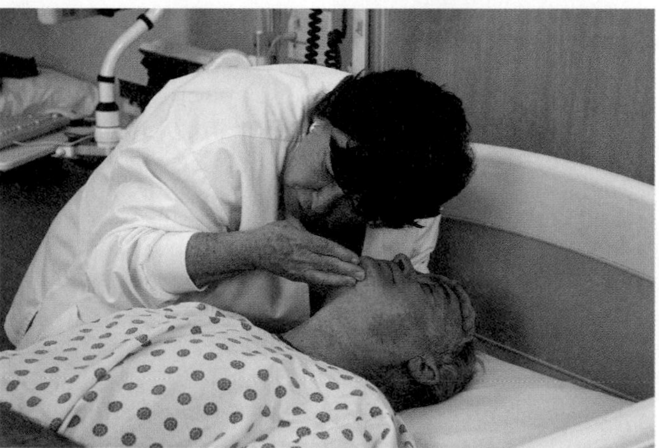

3 Reposition head and try ventilation again, if chest does not rise.

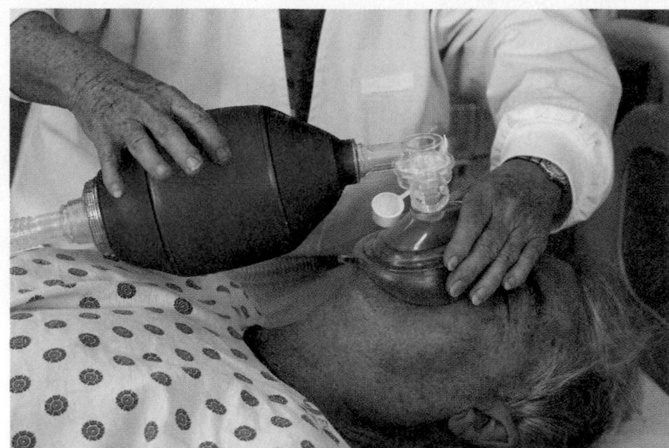

4 Ventilate with two rescue breaths using bag–valve–mask or CPR mask.

EVIDENCE-BASED PRACTICE

Chest Compressions for CPR

An observational study concluded that chest compressions are the most important aspect of CPR. The chest is able to fully recoil during each compression, thereby lowering intrathoracic pressures, which promotes improved cardiac preload and improved filling of the coronary arteries. Interruptions in chest compressions, even if brief, produce a dramatic decline in coronary perfusion pressures and worsens outcomes. For a single rescuer, it is believed that continuous cardiac compression will improve outcomes. Chest compressions first has now been approved by the AHA and released October, 2010.

Source: SOS-KANTO Study Group. (2007). Cardiopulmonary resuscitation by bystanders with chest compression only (SOS-KANTO): An observational study. *The Lancet*, 369(9565), 920–926.

Clinical Alert

There have been no documented cases of transmission of HIV, hepatitis, or tuberculosis during mouth-to-mouth or mouth-to-mask ventilation.

Source: American Heart Association.

Clinical Alert

If victim has been nonresponsive for more than 4 minutes, provide five cycles of CPR before applying AED.

CPR Guidelines—2010

The most significant new recommendations (changes) in the guidelines are as follows:

- Compressions, Airway, Breathing (CAB) rather than previous guidelines Airway, Breathing, Compressions (ABC).
- Chest Compressions first: "push hard and push fast, allow full chest recoil after each compression," about 100 compressions/minute for all victims. Minimize interruptions in chest compressions. Mouth to mouth breathing is only done if client's condition warrants, and a CPR mask is used, unless an Ambu bag is available (AHA, 2008).
- Universal Compression-to-Ventilation Ratio: 30:2 for all victims (except newborns)
- Rescue Breathing: Each breath (2) should last for 1 second and should result in a visible rise of the chest. 12–20 breaths/minute or 1 breath every 3–5 seconds.
- Defibrillation: In witnessed arrests, use AED. Single shock followed by immediate CPR. In unwitnessed arrest, first five cycles CPR then use AED.
- Rhythm check: After about five cycles or approximately 2 minutes.
- AEDs: Use in children beginning at age 1 through adult only.

The AHA guidelines emphasize the need to use bag–mask ventilations or other airway devices such as the Combitube if the BLS rescuer is trained in the use of these devices.

Barrier Devices

Face Shield: Clear plastic or silicon sheet placed over victim's face to prevent direct contact with victim during rescue breathing. Face shields are small, flexible, and portable.

Face Mask: Hard plastic device that fits over mouth and nose. They cost more than face shields and are bulkier, preventing people from carrying them on their person.

New Trends

CPR in a Box

The American Heart Association has designed a $30 instructional kit that teaches CPR in 20 minutes. The purpose of the kit is to raise cardiac survival rates by having community teachers share the CPR information. In one situation an instructor, in 2 hours, trained 96 school students and they went home and trained their families. The kit includes a mini-inflatable manikin, booklet, and DVD. The principles include starting cardiac compressions immediately. Kits can be ordered at 877-242-4277 or www.cpranytime.org.

Administering Basic Life Support to an Infant (under 12 months)

NOTE: Basic Life Support guidelines for Healthcare Providers defines "infant victims" as less than 12 months old, whereas "pediatric victims" are defined as victims from about 1 year of age to the onset of adolescence or puberty, as defined by the presence of secondary sex characteristics.

Procedure

1. Try to wake the infant by gently tapping infant. Small infants respond to rubbing and tapping the soles of their feet.
2. If infant does not wake up have someone call 911. If no one is available, call 911 and then begin CPR.
3. Begin chest compressions, place two fingers on the breastbone directly between the baby's nipples. Push straight down an 1 ½ inches and 13 depth of baby's chest.
4. Allow chest to rise back to usual position. Complete 30 compressions, about 2 compressions per second.
5. Trained CPR rescuers begin rescue breathing. If not trained, continue compressions until help arrives.
6. Cover the baby's entire mouth an nose with your mouth and gently blow until you see the hest rise. Let the air escape and the chest go back to normal. Give a second breath
7. If chest does not rise and fall, adjust the baby's head and try again. If chest still does not rise and fall, continue with 30 chest compressions and try rescue breathing again.
8. Continue to give 2 minutes of CPR, if no help has arrived, call 911 again.
9. Continue CPR until help arrives.

For Foreign Body

1. If foreign body or aspiration is suspected:
   a. *Infant:* clear airway by administering back and chest thrusts.
   b. *Conscious Infant*
   (1) Position infant over your forearm, head lower than trunk. Support the head by holding it firmly while resting your arm on your thigh.

Clinical Alert

AEDs are not used in infants; only in clients older than 1 year.

Use adult pads if child is 8 years or older—child pads are preferred if available for 1 to 8 years.

(2) With free hand, deliver five sharp blows to infant's back, over spine and between shoulder blades. If object is not expelled, then:

(3) Turn infant as a unit to supine position, maintaining head support. Deliver five chest thrusts by placing two fingers over sternum and providing thrusts.

c. *Unconscious Infant*

(1) Attempt to ventilate. If unable, reposition head and try again. Lift chin. ▸ ***Rationale:*** Trachea can collapse if neck is hyperextended.

(2) Form tight seal by encircling mouth of child and mouth and nose of infant. ▸ ***Rationale:*** Maintain tight seal.

(3) If unable to ventilate, then commence CPR.

2. Administer two breaths.
   a. Give breaths slowly—1 second/breath.
   b. Fill cheeks with air and use short puffing breaths for infants. Do not use full breaths for children or infants. ▸ ***Rationale:*** Small breaths prevent overinflation of the lungs and abdominal distention.
3. Between breaths, release seal for exhalation, and turn your head to side.
4. Administer one breath every 3 to 5 seconds.
5. Continue ventilations until infant is intubated or Ambu bag is available.

Placing Victim in Recovery Position

Procedure

1. Assess for potential head or neck trauma; if you suspect injury, do not tilt or turn client's head. If no trauma and client has a pulse and is breathing adequately, place in recovery position.
2. Straighten victim's legs.
3. Place victim's arm nearest to you at right angles to his/her body with elbow bent and palm upward.
4. Place other arm across chest and place hand near his/her cheek.
5. Grasp victim's far-side thigh above knee; pull thigh up toward his/her body.
6. Roll victim toward you onto his/her side.
7. Ensure upper leg (including knee and hip) is bent at right angles over the lower leg.
8. Tilt head back to maintain open airway, place hand under cheek to maintain head tilt, if necessary. (This is hand that was placed near cheek.)
9. Monitor victim closely until transported to facility.

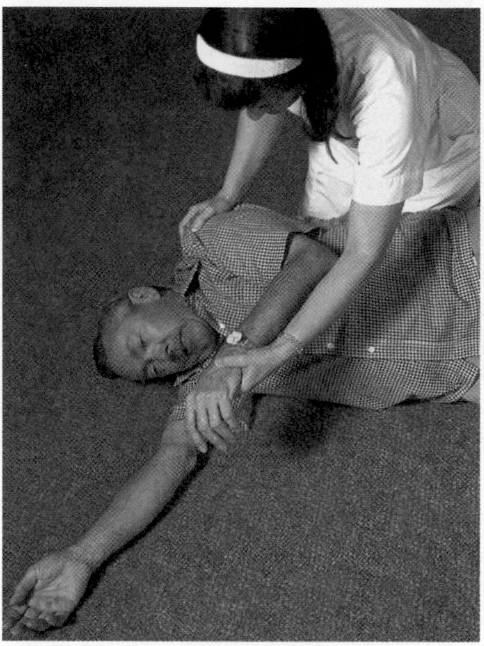

▲ Place on side to assume recovery position.

Providing Bag–Valve–Mask (BVM) Ventilation

Equipment

Manual resuscitator bag with non-rebreathing valve, clear face mask, and reservoir bag

Oxygen source and tubing

Airway adapter

Preparation

1. Determine that client's breathing is absent or inadequate.
2. Summon an assistant if client is not intubated. ▸ ***Rationale:*** If no artificial airway present, two responders are essential. Assistant holds mask while nurse compresses resuscitator bag.
3. Gather equipment.
4. Place client in supine position.

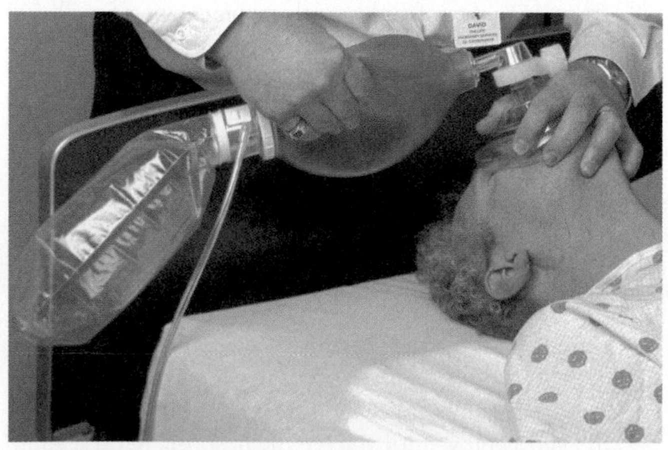

▲ Compress central portion of resuscitation bag.

5. Connect mask, airway adapter to bag, attach reservoir bag if not attached.
6. Connect oxygen tubing and oxygen flowmeter to bag inlet.

Procedure

1. Turn oxygen flowmeter wide open to 15 L/minute ("flush") and ensure reservoir bag is filled with oxygen. ▸ ***Rationale:*** reservoir bag delivers 90%–100% concentration of oxygen at 15 L/min.
2. Standing at client's head, hyperextend client's neck, if no suspected trauma.
3. Clear airway of any secretions or vomitus, then place apex of mask over client's nose and place base of mask between client's lower lip and chin.

Clinical Alert

Cricoid pressure may be used only if the client:

- Is nonresponsive—deeply unconscious (no cough or gag reflex)
- Is not vomiting
- Does not have a cuffed tracheal tube

▸ ***Rationale:*** Reduces incidence of aspiration, improves oxygenation, and provides for tight seal.

4. Using dominant hand, compress central portion of resuscitator bag just until client's chest rises, then allow exhalation. ▸ ***Rationale:*** Overinflation may result in gastric distention.
5. Provide ventilations every 5–6 seconds for an apneic adult, noting that client's chest rises and falls with each compression.
6. If client breathes spontaneously, give compressions in synchrony to support ventilation.
7. Observe for possible gastric distention. ▸ ***Rationale:*** Gastric insufflation may result in regurgitation and aspiration.
8. If gastric distention is suspected in the unresponsive client, have assistant apply pressure to the cricoid cartilage in the trachea. ▸ ***Rationale:*** Protect airway from aspiration of client's gastric secretions. Anticipate insertion of Naso/oro gastric tube to remove gastric secretions.
9. Notify physician or respiratory care practitioner for further client evaluation.

NOTE: Refer to respiratory chapter for similar skill.

Using an Automated External Defibrillator (AED)

Equipment

AED unit

Procedure

1. Place AED near head on left side of victim. ▸ ***Rationale:*** This placement facilitates easy use of machine by rescuer.
2. Open AED. This automatically turns on power in some devices.
3. Press power button on, if not automatically part of opening AED. Sound alerts, lights, and voice prompts will tell you that power is on and will direct you in use of the AED.
4. Remove victim's clothing on torso.
5. Ensure chest is dry. ▸ ***Rationale:*** To ensure electrode pads will stick to chest.
6. Open package of adhesive electrode pads. Most defibrillation electrode pads are preconnected to cables. If pads are dry, then discard and obtain new adhesive electrode pads. ▸ ***Rationale:*** Dry pads will prevent accurate rhythm analysis and conduction.
7. Peel off protective plastic backing from pads to expose adhesive surface.
8. Place two adhesive electrode pads directly on chest skin following pictures on pads.
    a. First pad goes on upper right side of victim's chest, with top edge touching bottom of clavicle.
    b. Second pad (marked with a ♥) goes to outside of left nipple, with top margin of pad at anterior axillary line, or may be placed posteriorly between the two scapulas.
    c. Do not place pads directly over nitroglycerin patches.
    d. Do not place pads within 1 in. of implanted devices such as pacemakers or ICD. If ICD is in process of delivering a shock and the rescuer is in contact with the client, he/she will feel the shock. Wait for 30–60 seconds for device to complete the shock cycle. ▸ ***Rationale:*** ICD are designed to shock the client's lethal rhythm back into their normal rhythm. If effective, then AED shock may not be required.
9. Stop CPR if CPR is being performed. Instruct everyone to not touch the victim, in order for AED to analyze rhythm. You may need to push ANALYZE button to start the analysis. Some machines begin analyzing rhythm as soon as pads are applied.

10. If analysis indicates and commands a shock, push SHOCK on AED. (It may automatically charge when the rhythm indicates the need to shock. A voice message will inform everyone to "stay clear.")

NOTE: A voice prompt will inform you if electrode pads are not securely attached to chest.

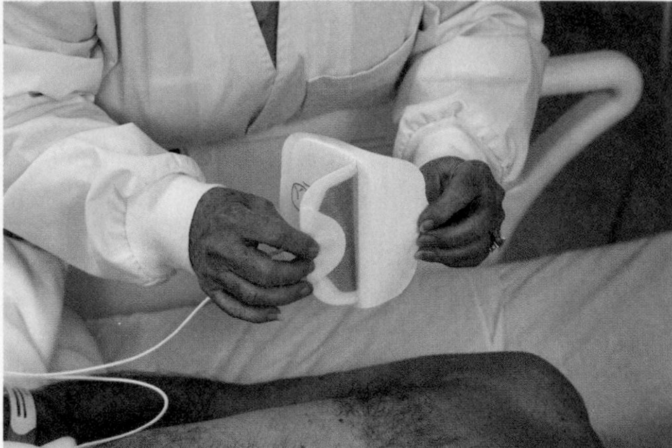

▲ After connecting defibrillator pad to AED unit, remove backing and apply pads to victim's chest.

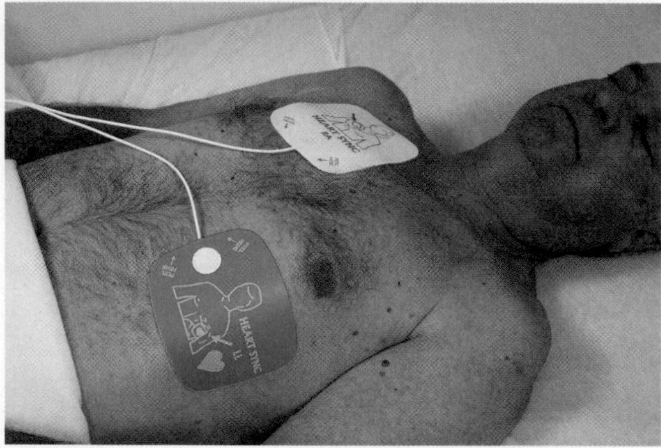

▲ Apply pads to chest, one below right clavicle, one below and lateral to heart.

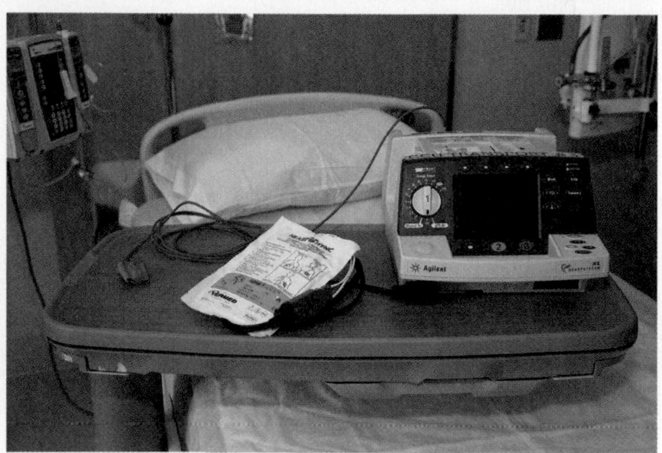

▲ If AED indicates need for shock, push SHOCK on AED.

11. Give one shock, then immediately begin CPR for five cycles or 2 minutes. Press ANALYZE button on AED. Repeat this procedure.
12. If victim is not in need of shock, rescuer immediately checks for pulse and begins CPR, beginning with chest compressions (30:2 ventilations).
13. When shockable rhythm is not present, AED will signal "*no shock indicated*" or "*no shock advised.*"
14. Check for presence of pulse—if none found, resume CPR.
15. Leave AED electrodes attached to victim's chest and leave AED in ON position.
16. Follow protocol for rescue breathing or CPR as victim's condition warrants.

Clinical Alert

AEDs should be used as soon as possible in the hospital setting. However, if 4 or 5 minutes have passed, the rescuer should provide five cycles of CPR (about 2 minutes) before attempting defibrillation in an unwitnessed collapse. The ventricular fibrillation waveform deteriorates rapidly within a few minutes of cardiac arrest as the heart consumes all available oxygen. Providing CPR initially will make the shock more likely to eliminate the ventricular fibrillation, and the heart more likely to function after defibrillation.

Source: American Heart Association. (2005–2006, Winter). Healthcare provider basic and advanced life support. *Currents in Emergency Cardiovascular Care*, 16(4), 16.

Pediatric adhesive electrode pads are available for children. The AED machine automatically converts the pediatric defibrillation threshold. Currently, there are no recommendations to use AED in infants.

Source: Aehlert, B. (2007). *ACLS Study Guide* (3rd ed.). Toronto, Canada: Elsevier.

Clinical Alert

The AutoPulse, an automated, noninvasive cardiac support pump, delivers chest compressions using a "hands-free" approach to restore blood flow faster and at a higher rate than manual resuscitation after a cardiac arrest.

The number of shocks an AED delivers and the energy level for each shock are preset by the manufacturer. Follow the AED voice and visual prompts. The shock sequence is usually completed three times if the client remains in fibrillation.

Administering the Abdominal Thrust (Heimlich) Maneuver to Adult or Child

Procedure

1. Be familiar with choking signs:
   a. Ask client if he or she can speak.
   b. Ask client to hold hand on neck if choking.
      ▸ ***Rationale:*** This is the universal sign for choking.
2. If unable to talk or coughing becomes ineffective, begin abdominal thrusts.
3. Stand behind client. Place your arms around the client's waist.
4. Position hands halfway between xiphoid process and umbilicus. (Identify area by placing thumb near xiphoid and index finger on umbilicus.)

NOTE: For pregnant or obese client, chest thrusts rather than abdominal thrusts are used.

5. Make a fist with one hand and press thumb side of fist into victim's abdomen above umbilicus. Place other hand over the fist.
6. Press your fist into client's abdomen.
7. Using a rotating motion of the hands, forcefully thrust your hands in an upward direction to assist in expelling the foreign body. (Client will probably fall over your arms.)
8. Repeat measures until foreign body is expelled or the client becomes unconscious.

Clinical Alert
Foreign bodies may partially block airway but still allow good air movement. When victim remains conscious and can forcefully cough and speak—do nothing!

Airway Obstruction Signs
- Poor air exchange
- Weak, ineffective cough
- Inability to speak
- High-pitched noise with inhalation
- Cyanosis

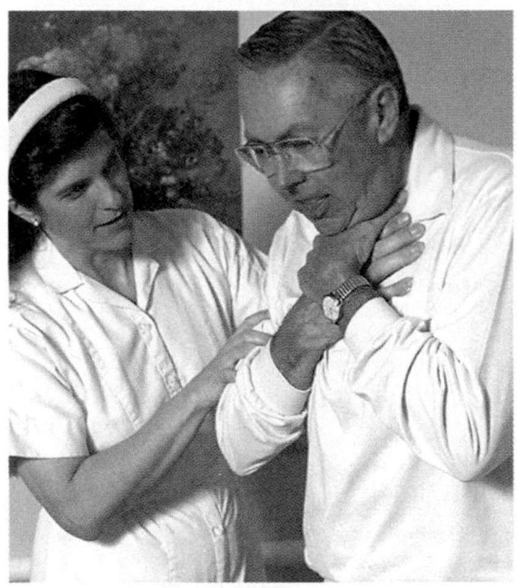
▲ Determine whether client is choking.

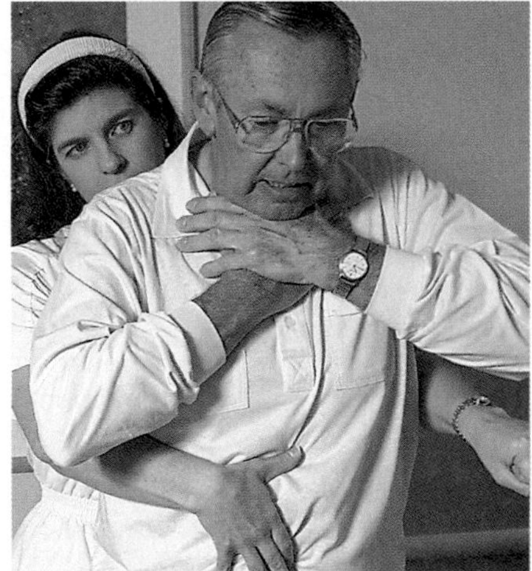
▲ Position hands to perform Heimlich.

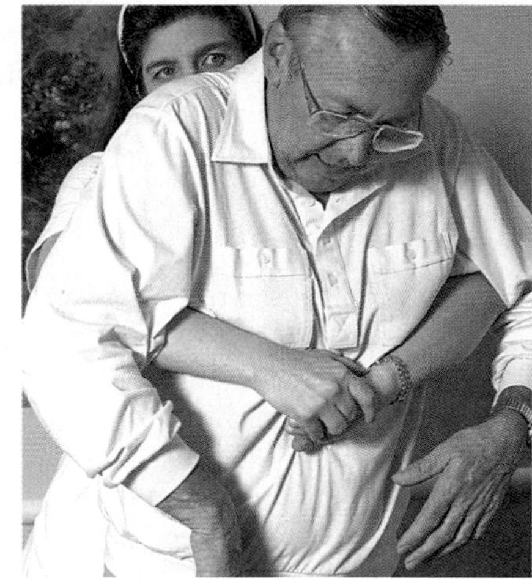
▲ Make fist and place other hand on top.

Administering the Abdominal Thrust (Heimlich) for Unresponsive Client

Procedure

For Unresponsive Adult

1. Immediately activate EMS system.
2. Open mouth and use finger sweep to remove visible foreign object.
3. Begin cardiac compressions at 100/minute until foreign object is ejected. ▸ ***Rationale:*** Chest compressions have been shown to increase intrathoracic pressure higher than abdominal thrusts. Attempt 2 rescue breaths. Check if chest rises.
4. Look in mouth for foreign body each time the airway is opened for rescue breath.
5. Use finger sweep only to remove a visible foreign body.
6. Continue compressions and rescue breaths.

For Unresponsive Child

1. Begin cardiac compressions at 60/minute. continuing for five cycles (2 minutes) *before* summoning EMS (unless another rescuer is available to do so immediately).
2. Activate EMS after five cycles, then return to child to continue CPR until EMS arrives.

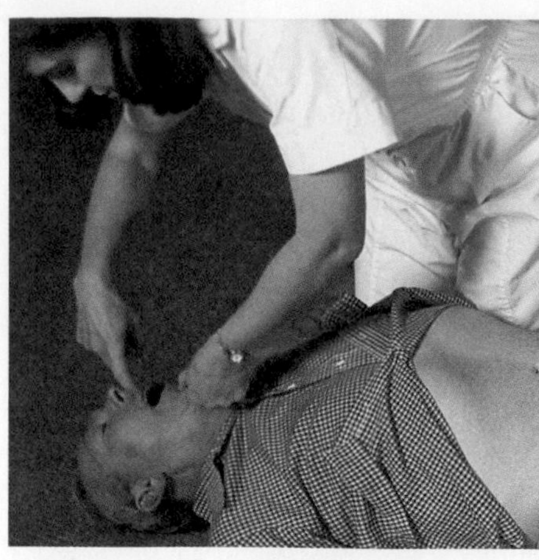

▲ Open mouth and use finger sweep only to remove visible foreign object.

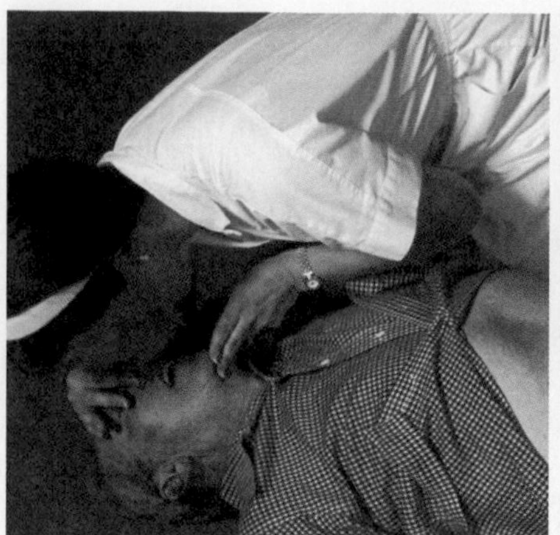

▲ If client is unresponsive, begin CPR.

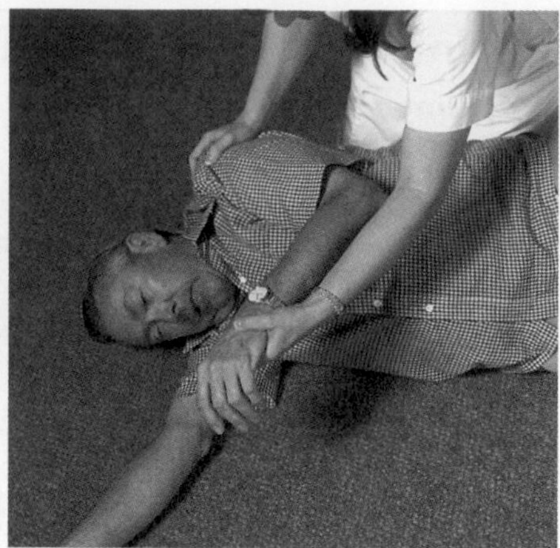

▲ Place on side to assume recovery position.

Calling for Rapid Response Support

Preparation

1. Be familiar with facility's pre-arrest response team policy ("Condition C," Rapid Response Team, "Light Code"). ▸ ***Rationale:*** This team is summoned to assist in *preventing* avoidable deaths. The facility's team may consist of a bedside nurse, ICU nurses, respiratory therapists, physician, physician assistant, and pharamacists have been added to many teams.
2. Identify location of emergency equipment and medications.

Procedure

1. Identify clients at risk for pre-arrest at the beginning of each shift.
2. Monitor client frequently and closely for signs of a potentially serious complication. ▸ ***Rationale:*** Most in-hospital arrests are preceded by a change in the client's physiological/mental responses.
3. Establish a flow sheet for more intensive monitoring of client's vital signs, neurological assessment, urinary output, etc., as indicated.
4. Anticipate need for emergency equipment (e.g., bag–valve–mask, oxygen) and crash cart and place close at hand in case crisis occurs.
5. Check that identified client has established venous access. ▸ ***Rationale:*** IV access is necessary for infusion of fluids and administration of emergency medications.
6. Recognize deteriorating trends or patterns of signs and symptoms that require resources to stabilize the client (physician and other specialized personnel on Rapid Response Team).
7. Request a more experienced colleague to assist in validation of concerns, if indicated. ▸ ***Rationale:*** Novice nurses may be uncertain of findings and inexperienced in recognizing a "pattern" of change in clients.
8. Act upon findings and intuition by calling RRT for early intervention to stabilize the client if indicated.

Pre-Arrest Indicators

According to Ehlenbach et al. (2009), survival to discharge rates for in-hospital cardiopulmonary resuscitation averages 18.3%. Nurses must anticipate and recognize pre-arrest indicators of a serious complication and intervene before an arrest occurs. Criteria for calling the Rapid Response Team (RRT) are as follows:

Any acute change in:

- Heart rate 130 beats/min
- Systolic blood pressure, 90 mmHg
- Respiratory rate, 28
- Oxygenation saturation <90% despite O_2 supplementation
- LOC
- Urinary output <50 mL in 4 hours

Source: Ehlenbach, W. J., Barnato, A. E., Curtis, J. R., Kreuter, W., Koepsell, T. D., Deyo, R. A., Stapleton, R. D. (2009). Epidemiologic study of in-hospital cardiopulmonary resuscitation in the elderly. *New England Journal of Medicine, 361*(1), 22–31.Institute for Healthcare Improvement. Establish a rapid response team. Retrieved July 15, 2009, from http:ihi.org/IHI/Topics/CriticalCare/IntensiveCare/Changes/EstablishaRapidResponseTeam.htm

EVIDENCE-BASED PRACTICE

Benefits of Using Rapid Response Team

Statistics show the benefits of using a Rapid Response Team to intervene before a code is called or serious medical problems occur:

1. 4–month period in Australia: Cardiac arrest deaths dropped from 37 to 16, ICU days after cardiac arrest dropped from 163 to 33, and inpatient deaths dropped from 302 to 222.
2. Memphis, TN: A 28% drop in codes since implementing Rapid Response Team.

Source: Healthcare Management Council. (2006, May). http://wiki.hmcentral.com/index.php/Rapid_Response_Teams.

9. Obtain AED if client is nonresponsive.
10. Call for emergency equipment and assistance of two professional nurses, provide privacy, and remain with the client.
11. Set up O_2 and suction if not already at bedside.
12. Position client on back board.
13. *If CPR is not indicated:*
    a. Continue to assess client.
    b. Response team brings emergency supplies, establishes cardiac monitoring/AED, obtains IV access if not present.
    c. Check client's blood glucose.
14. *If CPR is indicated:*
    a. Begin CPR.
    b. Use bag–valve–mask for ventilation, establish cardiac monitoring/AED. Obtain IV access if not present.
    c. Another professional colleague retrieves supplies, supports family, accesses client's chart, and shares information with response team when they arrive.
15. Rapid Response Team takes action: orders blood tests, x-ray, medications, transfers client to intensive care setting or calls a code if indicated.

NOTE: In some hospitals, a modified RRT program is implemented, called a RAT (Rapid Assessment Team). This modified approach is directed by RNs functioning under protocols for patient management. If the team leader believes the client's condition is deteriorating, then a code is called.

Recognizing Client Changes that may Trigger Calling an RRT

- Complaints of chest pain unrelieved by nitroglycerine
- Subjective feeling that client is in danger—wary/anxious
- Sudden loss of movement or weakness in face, legs, arm
- Change in color of central or peripheral skin

Rapid Response Team Functions

Role of Rapid Response Team members:

- Airway management—MD/CRND
    - Ventilates client
    - Intubates if needed
- Airway assistant—RN/RT
    - Assists with ventilation
    - Manages oxygen and suction
- Bedside assessment—ICU RN/bedside RN
    - Assesses IV site and access
    - Administers medications
    - Applies defibrillator pads
- Crash Cart manager—ICU RN
    - Prepares medications
    - Records Code events
- Treatment leader—MD
    - Directs medical treatment
    - Determines client triage decisions
- Circulation manager—RN/MD/RT
    - Checks pulse
    - Performs chest compressions
- Procedure clinician—MD/NP/PA
    - Performs medical procedures, i.e., chest tube
    - IV central line insertion
- Data manager—RN
    - Records interventions
    - Reviews test results

Source: Scholle, C., & Mininni, N. (2006). How a Rapid Response Team saves lives. *Nursing* 2006, 36(1), 36–40.

Calling a Code

NOTE: See Procedure in Chapter 33: Advanced Skills, p. 1342.

Maintaining the Emergency "Crash" Cart

NOTE: See Procedure in Chapter 33: Advanced Skills, p. 1342.

Performing Defibrillation

NOTE: See Procedure in Chapter 33: Advanced Skills, p. 1342.

DOCUMENTATION for Emergency Life Support

- Time victim found in pre-arrest or unresponsive state
- Description of victim when found
- Time emergency measures were initiated
- Nature/description of emergency life support measures provided (CPR, use of AED, Heimlich, RRT actions, medications administered, including name, dosage, route)
- Names and titles of rescue participants (e.g., RRT)
- Duration of emergency measures provided
- Outcome of pre-arrest interventions or resuscitation efforts (client outcome)
- Recorded data from AED, monitors used, and place strips on chart per hospital policy.

CRITICAL THINKING Application

Expected Outcomes

- Basic life-support measures established within 3 minutes after arrest.
- Emergency measures performed according to established protocol.
- Client is stabilized/resuscitated with basic life support measures.
- No permanent neurologic damage is sustained.
- Obstructed airway is reestablished.
- Unresponsive client is rescued by timely intervention (calling EMS, retrieving the AED, and initiating CPR).
- Choking victim expels foreign body in response to Heimlich maneuver.
- Client has a positive outcome after emergency life support.

Unexpected Outcomes	Alternative Actions
Choking client is found on floor, Heimlich maneuver cannot be performed in usual manner.	• Initiate CPR (100 chest compressions/min), perform procedure for administering the Heimlich maneuver for unconscious client.
Client is revived but maintained on life support system.	• Assist in transferring client to ICU. Provide support for family and explain where ICU is and visitation policy.
Attempts at ventilation for rescue breathing are ineffective, chest does not rise, no air is felt.	• Reposition head. • Perform CPR, look in mouth each time rescuer opens airway. Remove object if seen.
Rescuer cannot continue efforts at what appears to be unsuccessful CPR.	• Stop CPR if exhaustion or endangerment to rescuer.
AED fails to analyze rhythm after 15 seconds.	• Resume CPR at 100 chest compressions/minute and attempt to analyze rhythm after five cycles or about 2 minutes.
Pulse does not return after AED shock.	• Resume CPR at 100 chest compressions/minute for five cycles or 2 minutes, reanalyze rhythm, check for pulse, and deliver shock if ventricular fibrillation continues.
There is no response to your EMS call for help (e.g., 911).	• Suspect that your location is not programmed into EMS system. Try local area dial for highway patrol (e.g., *55). • Be familiar with your local emergency response system's summoning directives.
Chest does not rise with delivered breaths.	• Reposition head to establish airway and try again.
AED prompt says "no shock indicated."	• Immediately resume CPR, starting at 100 chest compressions/minute; if CPR trained can start with ventilations, continue for five cycles (2 minutes) before reanalyzing heart rhythm per AED.

	• Suspect client has nonshockable rhythm such as pulseless electrical activity; hypovolemia is most common cause. • Rule out possible causes: hypovolemia, hypoxia, hypothermia, hypoglycemia.
Choking client becomes unresponsive after several attempts at Heimlich maneuver.	• Initiate CPR (30 compressions to 2 ventilations). • Look in victim's mouth each time airway is opened, but do not perform blind finger sweep to check for object. • Attempt to remove foreign body, only if seen.
Client is obese or pregnant, making abdominal thrust impossible or inappropriate to perform.	• Perform chest thrusts rather than abdominal thrusts.
Client develops complications (signs of stroke, heart attack, hypotension, altered mental status, dyspnea, tachycardia).	• Monitor client intensely, using flow chart to trend changes in status (tachypnea, decreased urinary output). • Note client's condition and document findings. • Determine and locate equipment or anticipate procedures client might require if deterioration continues. • Initiate RRT for decision making and early intervention before crisis occurs. • Be cognizant of client's advance directives regarding resuscitation measures.

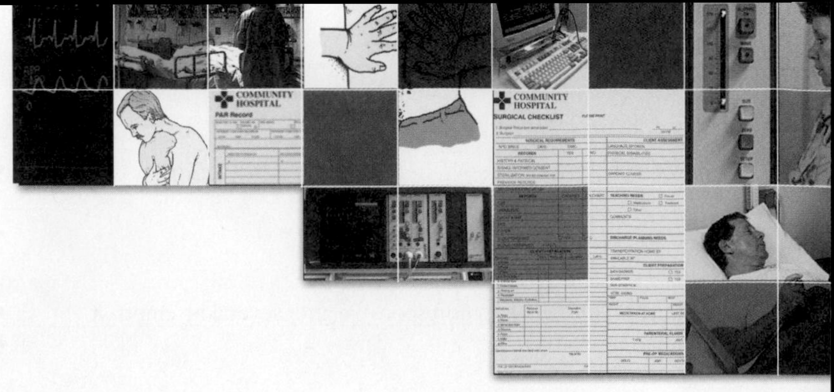

Chapter 31

UNIT 5

Pacemaker Management

Nursing Process Data

ASSESSMENT Data Base

- Assess preexisting cardiovascular status.
- Assess cardiac monitor rhythm and rate.
- Assess heart sounds.
- Observe client's general appearance for pallor, dyspnea, or edema.
- Assess for hemodynamic abnormalities related to low cardiac output, including dizziness, weakness, altered level of consciousness, low blood pressure, and decreased urinary output.
- Ensure intravenous access for administration of fluids and medications.
- Identify client's or family's knowledge of procedure.

PLANNING Objectives

- To provide temporary cardiac electrical stimulation for conditions resulting in alterations of heart rate
- To prevent bradycardia
- To overdrive fast heart rates
- To improve cardiac output

IMPLEMENTATION Procedures

EVALUATION Expected Outcomes

- Client's cardiac rate is maintained through use of a pacemaker.
- Client is prepared psychologically and physically for insertion of the pacemaker.
- Pacemaker is inserted without complications.
- Heart rate and cardiac output improve.

Pearson Nursing Student Resources

Find additional review materials at
nursing.pearsonhighered.com

Prepare for success with NCLEX®-style practice questions and Skill Checklists

Monitoring Temporary Cardiac Pacing (Transcutaneous, Transvenous, Epicardial)

Equipment

Cardiac monitor
Transcutaneous: pacing generator, pacing electrodes
Appropriate temporary pulse generator (select for single- or dual-chamber pacing)
9-volt battery for pulse generator (single- or dual-chamber)
Bridging cable for epicardial wires
Clean gloves
Established continuous cardiac monitoring—see Telemetry Monitoring skill

Preparation

1. Validate that informed consent has been obtained for temporary pacing.
2. Identify client by checking two forms of client ID.
3. Explain rationale for temporary pacing and necessary restrictions/precautions, and provide reassurance of close continuous monitoring.
4. Perform a baseline assessment: vital signs, urinary output, LOC, heart rate, rhythm, and skin color. If life-threatening dysrhythmia is assessed, prepare for pacemaker insertion. ▸ ***Rationale:*** Transcutaneous pacemakers are used for symptomatic bradycardia unresponsive to atropine or high-degree atrioventricular block causing hemodynamic compromise. If transcutaneous pacing is ineffective, then prepare for transvenous pacemaker insertion.
5. Assess IV site for patency; if no IV, establish line. ▸ ***Rationale:*** IV access is needed for drug administration.
6. Document client's cardiac rhythm according to hospital policy.
7. Perform hand hygiene.

Procedure

For Transcutaneous Pacing (TCP)

1. Sedate client. ▸ ***Rationale:*** TCP causes discomfort.
2. Clip hair, if necessary. Do not shave under electrode placement. Do not use alcohol or tincture of benzoin because they can cause burns to occur. ▸ ***Rationale:*** Improve conduction between electrode and skin. Shaving may cause nicks in skin, which may increase discomfort with pacing.
3. Ensure client is on cardiac monitoring with either lead I, II, or III. Lead II is customary as it assesses atrial activity.
4. Connect ECG cable to input connection on pacing generator.
5. Turn switch selector to "Monitor On." ECG waveform will appear.
6. Set alarm, press "Alarm On." Ensure alarm parameters are set 20 beats higher and lower than client's desired rate.
7. Record waveform by pressing "Start/Stop" button.
8. Apply pacing pads as marked, first removing posterior pad covering, then placing posterior (back) pad left of spine between the scapulas. Place anterior "front" pad to left side of lower sternum.
9. Press firmly on and around pacing electrodes. ▸ ***Rationale:*** This ensures good skin contact.
10. Attach pacing cable to pace connector on defibrillator/monitor.
11. Select "Pacer" button and green light will appear.
12. Set pacing rate to 60–80 beats/min.
13. Assess cardiac rhythm on oscilloscope and observe the QRS for sensing marker.
14. Set milliamperes (mA) threshold initially at 0. ▸ ***Rationale:*** This prevents pacemaker discharge while setting adjustment.
15. Activate pacing by depressing "Start/Stop" button.
16. Increase mA slowly, increasing it until capture appears.
17. Assess pulse and blood pressure ▸ ***Rationale:*** These parameters assess for perfusion.
18. Record ECG strip and document pacing parameters.
19. Continually assess client's need for sedation. ▸ ***Rationale:*** Pacing causes discomfort.

Clinical Alert

Transcutaneous pacing is not beneficial in asystole or pulseless electrical activity (PEA). If transcutaneous pacing fails to capture and/or increase the pulse, then transvenous pacing is required. If defibrillation is required because of ventricular defibrillation, immediately select "charge" button, as pacing will cease and defibrillation will occur.

For Epicardial Pacing

1. Don clean gloves. ▸ ***Rationale:*** Gloves are worn to prevent microshock to client.
2. Locate epicardial pacing wires on client's chest wall.
3. Securely connect pacing wires to external generator. ▸ ***Rationale:*** This promotes pacemaker impulse reception from and transmission to the myocardium.
4. Connect cable to pulse generator (positive to positive, negative to negative). ▸ ***Rationale:*** Pacing stimulus goes from pulse generator to the negative terminal and back to pulse generator by the positive terminal.
5. Remove protective cover to dial settings.

Clinical Alert

Transvenous single-chamber (ventricular) pacing is most commonly used as an emergency measure to support ventricular contraction and cardiac output. Epicardial pacing occurs when pacing electrodes are inserted into the epicardium of the right ventricle during cardiac surgery. If the physician wants to initiate atrioventricular sequential pacing, then the surgeon places an additional electrode in the right atrium. The pacing wires are then pierced through the chest wall and may be attached to the external pulse generator, which is placed on standby mode should pacing become necessary. If no pacing is indicated at this time, insert the pacing wires in either a sterile rubber glove or finger cot. Place sterile gauze and occlusive dressing over pacing wires and insertion site to prevent microshock and/or infection. Epicardial pacing electrodes provide either single-chamber atrial pacing, single-chamber ventricular pacing, or dual-chamber pacing, known as A-V sequential pacing, which is used to simulate normal pump function (atrial followed by ventricular stimulation/contraction).

6. Select pacing mode (e.g., atrial, ventricular, AV synchronous, or demand).

For Transvenous or Epicardial Pacing

1. Set dial at prescribed pacing rate (atrial and/or ventricular).
2. Set energy *output* (milliamperes or mA) on pulse generator to prescribed level (set for both atrial and ventricular pacing). ▸ ***Rationale:*** Energy output setting ensures that pacemaker stimulates the client's myocardium.
3. Return plastic cover to protect generator dial settings and hang generator from pole at client's bedside.
4. Monitor pacemaker function for *sensing* (light indicates client's QRS complexes), *capture* (pacemaker spike is followed by QRS complex), and pacemaker *rate*.
5. Monitor client's heart rhythm, vital signs, and other responses to pacing, including femoral pulsation palpable with captured beats. ▸ ***Rationale:*** These demonstrate effectiveness of pacemaker support.
6. Remove gloves and perform hand hygiene.
7. Evaluate electrode insertion/exit sites and dress according to agency protocol.

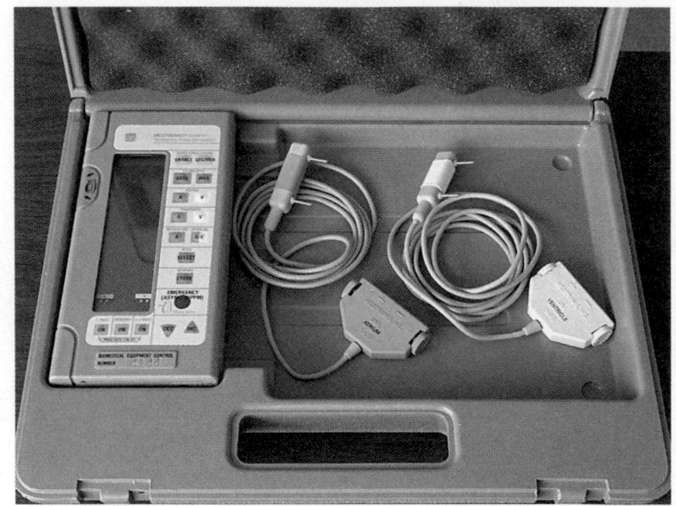

▲ Type of external pacemaker.

Assisting With Pacemaker Insertion

Equipment

Emergency cart with defibrillator
External pacemaker pulse generator
Pacing catheter electrodes
ECG monitor
Client cable
Rubber glove
Sterile antiseptic solution
Sterile gloves, gown, and mask
Sterile towels
Lidocaine, 1%–2%
Alcohol wipes
Syringe
Needles
Suture with attached needle
Sterile 4 × 4 gauze pads
Tape
Cutdown tray
Gloves

Preparation

1. Complete hand hygiene.
2. Provide sedation as necessary. Diazepam (Valium) or Versed is frequently used. Conscious sedation may be used.
3. Connect client to a continuous ECG monitor.
4. Place the client in a supine position with head flat or slightly lower than body.
5. If either the subclavian or external jugular vein is to be used, place a towel roll under the client's shoulders to provide better exposure of the insertion site.

Procedure

1. Assist physician as needed.
   a. Physician dons mask, sterile gown, and gloves.

b. Insertion site is cleansed with sterile antiseptic solution.
c. Drape area with sterile towels.
d. Break single-dose vial of lidocaine and hold at angle for physician withdrawal.
e. Physician withdraws lidocaine, using filtered needle, then changes to 25-gauge needle and injects skin.
f. Insertion is accomplished (transvenous method via cutdown or percutaneously). Catheter electrode wires are positioned, and skin sutures are applied.

2. Continuously monitor the ECG and client status during the insertion.
3. Don gloves to prevent microshock to client.
4. Connect the pacing electrode to the appropriate outlet terminal (unipolar to negative and bipolar to both the positive and negative terminals).
5. Turn on power switch on external pacemaker.
6. Set rate according to physician's orders.
7. Set milliamperes (mA) by determining threshold. To do this, observe the ECG while slowly increasing the number of milliamperes from its lowest setting to a point where each QRS complex is captured and preceded with a pacing spike.
8. Multiply the threshold level according to hospital policy (usually two to four times) to adjust the milliampere setting.
9. Set sensitivity mode according to physician's order (usually 1.5 mV).
10. Secure all connections. Put plastic cover back over pacemaker controls if required.
11. Place external pacemaker and exposed wires in a rubber glove to ensure insulation against electric shock to client.
12. Apply sterile dressings to insertion site, and tape securely.
13. Obtain chest x-ray after insertion to validate lead placement if pacemaker not inserted using fluoroscopy.
14. Obtain 12-lead ECG.

Safety Alert: Electrical

- Use only grounded equipment; use common ground.
- Remove and tag any defective equipment.
- Maintain environmental humidity at 50%–60%.
- Do not roll equipment over electrical cords.
- Avoid placing wet articles on electrical equipment.
- Insulate exposed pacing electrodes at all times.
- Wear rubber gloves when handling pacing electrodes or terminals.
- Do not touch any electric equipment while handling wire or terminals.
- Discharge static electricity by touching faucets or other metal that communicates with ground.

Safety Alert

When temporary transvenous pacemakers are used, the balloon air port is *not* to be used for IV access.

Revised NASPE/BPEG Generic Code for Antibradycardia Pacing*

I	II	III	IV	V
Chamber(s) Paced	**Chamber(s) Sensed**	**Response to Sensing**	**Rate Modulation**	**Multisite Pacing**
0 = None	O = None	O = None	O = None	O = None
A = Atrium	A = Atrium	T = Triggered	R = Rate modulation	A = Atrium
V = Ventricle	V = Ventricle	I = Inhibited		V = Ventricle
D = Dual (A+V)	D = Dual (A+V)	D = Dual (T+I)		D = Dual (A+V)
S = Single (A or V)†	S = Single (A or V)†			

NASPE policy statement: The NASPE/BPEG defibrillator code. *Pacing and Clinical Electrophysiology, 16*, 1776–1780.
Hayes, D. L. (2009). Modes of cardiac pacing: Nomenclature and selection. Retrieved July 19, 2009 from http://www.uptodate.com/online/content/topic.do?topicKey=carrhyth/26065&view=print.htm
From Bernstein, A. D., Daubert, J. C., Fletcher, R. D., Hayes, D. L., Lüderitz, B., Reynolds, D. W.,... Sutton R. (2002). The revised NASPE/BPEG generic code for antibradycardia. Adaptive-rate, and multisite pacing. *Pacing and Clinical Electrophysiology, 25*(2), 260–264.

Maintaining Temporary Pacemaker Function

Equipment

Battery
Oscilloscope

Procedure

1. Observe for failure to sense.
   a. Observe the oscilloscope for presence of pacemaker artifact (spikes): artifact before QRS complex in ventricular paced or preceding the P waves and QRS waves in AV sequential pacing.
   b. Check connections for secure, tight fit.
   c. Observe that pace–sense needle deflects to right, indicating pacing is occurring.
   d. Check sensitivity dial to determine whether sensitivity threshold is set correctly.
2. Observe for failure to pace.
   a. Check that external generator is ON.
   b. Check battery to ensure it is functioning.
   c. Check lead connector sites.
   d. Check pace–sense indicator. (Absence of or slight deflection of the pace–sense indicator reveals battery failure.)
3. Observe for failure to capture.
   a. Observe for pacing artifact not followed by QRS complex. ▸ ***Rationale:*** This indicates a failure of the stimulus to trigger a ventricular response.
   b. Check the setting of the mA, or output dial, to determine whether setting should be increased. ▸ ***Rationale:*** The myocardial threshold may be altered as a result of disease or drugs.
   c. Check all connector sites for secure, tight fit.
4. Observe that sutures are intact.
5. Assess insertion site for bleeding, hematoma formation, or infection.
6. Obtain chest x-ray post insertion.
7. Monitor client's response to therapy.
   a. Assess urine output. ▸ ***Rationale:*** Decreased urine output indicates poor cardiac output.

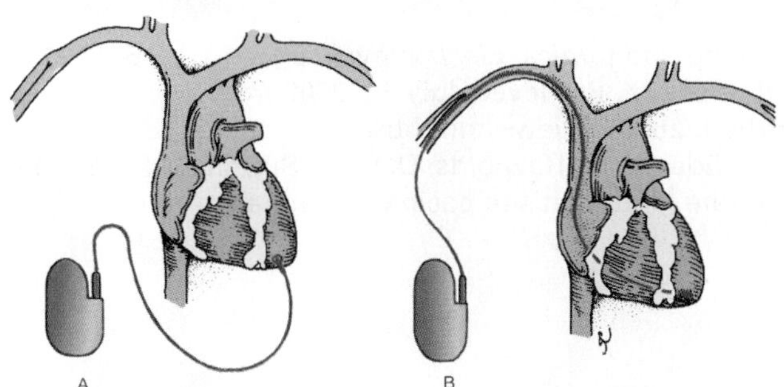

▲ Temporary pacemakers have two parts, the pulse generator and the electrode. The pulse generator is external to the body. (A) Epicardial ventricular pacemaker. (B) Transvenous ventricular pacemaker.

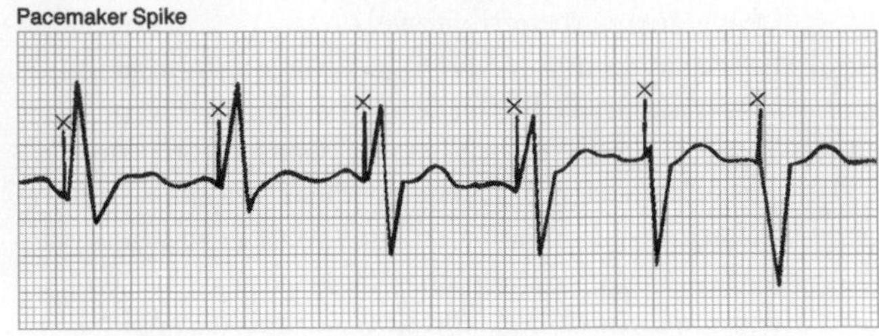

▲ ECG tracing showing pacemaker spike triggering ventricular depolarization (QRS).

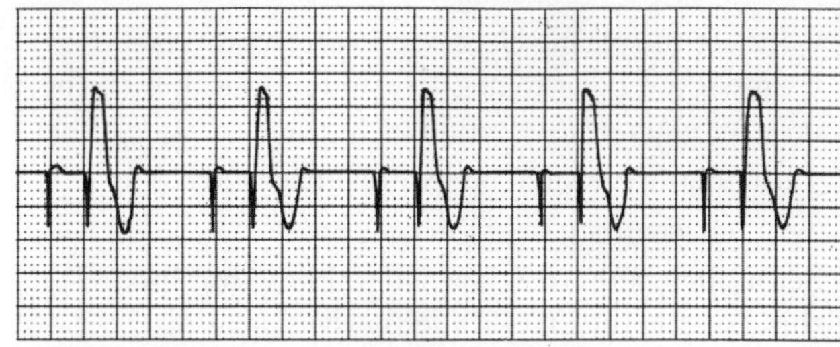

▲ ECG showing examples of pacemaker spikes.

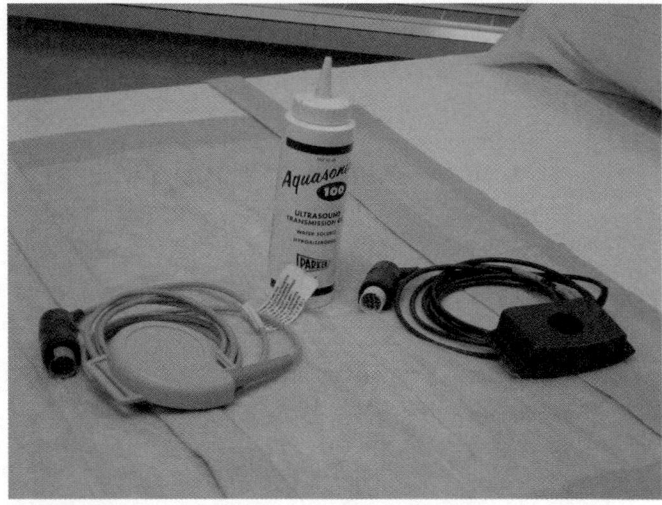

▲ Equipment for external monitoring including belts, gel, and transducers.

   b. Observe for dyspnea, crackles, heart rate, decreased blood pressure.
   c. Monitor temperature.
   d. Observe client for signs of anxiety. Complete pacemaker teaching as necessary.

Clinical Alert

Observe for pacemaker failure:

Decreased urine output
ECG pattern change
Decreased blood pressure
Bradycardia
Shortness of breath

8. Obtain and analyze a strip for functioning of pacemaker.
9. Observe for battery failure.
10. Observe for electrical interference and development of microshocks.
    a. Ground all electrical equipment in close proximity to client.
    b. Cover exposed wires with nonconductive material.
    c. Wear gloves when handling generator/lead wires.
11. Complete pacemaker teaching as necessary.

Providing Permanent Pacemaker Client Teaching

Equipment

Audiovisual aids
Written material

Procedure

1. Ascertain what client already knows and understands.
2. Determine client's ability and level of interest in learning about pacemaker.
3. Recognize client's fears, and provide opportunity to talk about them.
4. Review facts: heart anatomy and physiology and pacemaker information. Use illustrations and audiovisual aids.
5. Clarify misconceptions and allay fears.
6. Provide rationale for any mobility restrictions.
7. Answer questions and provide additional opportunities to discuss procedure.
8. Check pacemaker function regularly per instructions. With new pacemakers, physicians check them on routine visits.
9. Instruct client in clinical manifestations related to pacemaker failure and when to contact physician or pacemaker clinic.
10. Provide client with pacemaker information ID card (provided by manufacturer) and instruct to carry in wallet.
11. Suggest a Medical Alert band be worn at all times.

NOTE: Inform client of electromagnetic interference restrictions:

a. No MRI; do not place cell phone or cardiovert over generator.
b. Avoid airport hand wand, high-voltage areas, and diathermy.
c. If dizziness experienced, move away from area.

> **Pacemaker Clinics**
>
> Some clients use telephone transmission of the generator's pulse rate to determine status of pacemaker function. Special equipment is used to transmit information concerning function of the pacemaker over the telephone to a receiving system in a pacemaker clinic. The equipment converts information to electronic signals that are permanently recorded on ECG strip. Physicians monitor client's records and can intervene quickly when abnormalities appear on ECG strip. This type of clinic is very common in outlying areas where clients are unable to go to a clinic easily.

DOCUMENTATION for Pacemaker Management

- Date and time of temporary pacing
- Pacemaker settings (rate, outputs, sensitivity, AV interval)
- Client's response to treatment
- Vital signs, heart rhythm
- Rhythm strips of pacing obtained during insertion

CRITICAL THINKING Application

Expected Outcomes

- Client's cardiac rate is maintained through use of a pacemaker.
- Client is prepared psychologically and physically for insertion of the pacemaker.
- Pacemaker is inserted without complications.
- Heart rate and cardiac output improve.

Unexpected Outcomes	Alternative Actions
Temporary pacing is ineffective.	• Check for battery depletion and change if necessary (9-V batteries). • Record rhythm strip and correlate to client's signs and symptoms. • Monitor vital signs, mental status. • Check sensitivity setting. (If too high, P or T wave may be sensed; if too low, fixed-rate pacing occurs.) • Check mA setting (may be too high). • Check pace indicator for movement. • Check rate setting. • Check all connections. • Check catheter insertion site for swelling, hematoma.
Client does not understand function of pacemaker.	• If client is frightened, reassure him or her that a pacemaker is not dangerous. • If client does not understand pacemaker or procedure, use illustrated learning aids. • Allow time for questions and further explanations. • Orient your teaching to the client's intellectual and interest level.
Electromagnetic interference occurs.	• Check all electric equipment for proper grounding. Use common ground. • Remove unnecessary electric equipment from vicinity of client. • Insulate generator terminals and exposed electrodes in a rubber glove.
Inflammation occurs at insertion site.	• Provide daily site care using strict aseptic technique. • Keep dressings dry at all times. • Monitor vital signs. • Instruct client to limit extremity movement.
Diaphragmatic pacing occurs.	• Observe for hiccoughs or muscle twitching. • Change client's position. • Decrease the amperage (mA). • Notify physician that endocardial perforation may have occurred.
Failure to capture is suspected.	• Check client's heart rate. If heart rate less than the rate set on generator, and if pace indicator shows firing, suspect failure to capture. • Check all connections. • Anticipate that pacer wires are dislodged. • Check battery. • Change position of extremity. • Turn client on left side; catheter may float back to epicardial wall. • Increase amperage (mA) after checking threshold. • Obtain chest x-ray and 12-lead ECG. • Anticipate change of batteries, electrode terminals, or generator.
Battery depletion occurs.	• Have atropine and isoproterenol available. • Anticipate possible CPR. • Turn on power switch, and observe pace indicator. If there is little or no movement, replace battery immediately. • Record clock hours of battery usage. (Record should be taped to back of generator.) • Determine rate fluctuations. • Label each pacemaker with the date battery is inserted. • Store extra batteries in refrigerator and put new battery in pacemaker before use. • Disconnect catheter from pacemaker before replacing battery. Contact with battery terminal may be dangerous to the client.

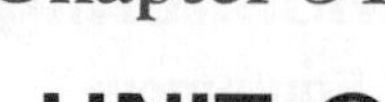

UNIT 6

Adaptations for Home Care

Nursing Process Data

ASSESSMENT Data Base

- Assess client's ability to monitor pulse accurately.
- Identify client's and/or family's knowledge of pacemaker function and safety measures.
- Assess pacemaker site for signs and symptoms of infection.
- Assess for signs and symptoms related to pacemaker dysfunction, including dizziness, weakness, altered level of consciousness, irregular pulse, low blood pressure, decreased urine output, and fatigue.
- Assess client's ability and knowledge related to contacting the pacemaker clinic.

PLANNING Objectives

- To provide client teaching related to monitoring pulse and use of magnet
- To evaluate client's knowledge base about pacemaker clinic
- To increase client's knowledge base about pacemaker function

IMPLEMENTATION Procedures

EVALUATION Expected Outcomes

- Client is able to accurately monitor pulse.
- Client's cardiac rate and rhythm are maintained through use of a pacemaker.
- Battery failure is identified early and major complications prevented.
- Client is knowledgeable about pacemaker function.
- Client is able to contact pacemaker clinic easily and comply with directions for pacemaker check.

Monitoring Pacemaker at Home

Equipment

Clock or watch with second hand

Daily record

Pacemaker magnet

Procedure

1. Instruct client in care immediately after pacemaker insertion.
   a. Keep site clean and dry for at least 2–4 days.
   b. Demonstrate daily dressing change using sterile gauze and paper tape.
   c. Do not use any ointments on incision site unless physician has instructed to do so.
   d. Assess site daily for signs of erythema, edema, or drainage. Call physician if any of these symptoms occur.
   e. Leave Steri-strips in place until they fall off.
   f. Take a bath, but keep dressing dry. Place "baggie" over dressing.
   g. Limit activity for 1 week. ▶ ***Rationale:*** To avoid damaging the pacemaker.
   h. Do not lift arm above shoulder level on side of pacemaker for 1–2 weeks.
   i. Do not hit or rub insertion site or manipulate pacemaker under skin.
   j. Avoid lifting (objects weighing more than 5 lb), running, or contact sports for at least 2 weeks.
2. Establish a daily routine check. ▶ ***Rationale:*** Battery failure can be identified in early stages by routine monitoring of pulse.
   a. Sit on side of bed.
   b. Check pulse for 1 full minute before arising.
   c. Record on daily record.
3. Contact physician if any of these symptoms occur:
   a. Sudden slowing or increasing in pulse rate.
   b. Irregular pulse.
   c. Pain or erythema over incision site.
4. Check with pacemaker magnet if ordered by physician.
   a. Sit on side of bed.
   b. Place magnet over pacemaker generator.
   c. Take pulse for 1 full minute.
   d. Record.
5. Teach safety factors to client and family.
   a. Wear Medic-Alert identification band and carry pacemaker identification card at all times. ▶ ***Rationale:*** This alerts healthcare providers to the fact that pacemaker is in place and identifies manufacturer's name.
   b. Avoid sources of electromagnetic interference (i.e., large engines, strong magnets, airport screening devices, alarm systems, radio transmitting towers, ham radios, and MRI diagnostic testing). ▶ ***Rationale:*** These devices emit intense magnetic fields that cause temporary pacemaker dysfunction.
   c. Avoid leaning over open hood of running automobile because its electrical field can interfere with pacemaker.
   d. Use microwave ovens in good working order.
   e. Use cellular phones on a different side from pacemaker or place in a shirt pocket.
   f. If dizziness occurs, check pulse. Pulse should return to normal within 5 minutes; otherwise, seek medical attention.

Clinical Alert

Instruct client to notify physician if incision site becomes painful or looks infected, or if he or she has a fever of 100.4°F or higher.

Clinical Alert

Pacemaker check with magnet should be done only if someone else is present, never if client is alone, because of possible magnet-induced ventricular arrhythmias. Newer temporary pacemakers are continuously monitored in the pacemaker clinic. They do not connect to a telephone for monitoring in physician's office.

Wireless Pacemaker

This is a pacemaker with a built-in small radio transmitter. It communicates to a base station attached to a phone line and is similar to a cordless phone. With this device physicians can monitor the client at home through the Internet.

Source: Dr. Wes (2009). Wireless home monitoring of pacemakers is here. Retrieved from http://www.medpagetoday.com/Blogs/15548

Checking With Pacemaker Clinic via Telephone

Equipment

Electrodes (e.g., finger, wrist, underarm)

Telephone

Transtelephonic transmitter

Magnet

NOTE: This is not used as often with newer devices now available.

Procedure

1. Arrange schedule of calls with nurse at pacemaker clinic.
2. Follow directions of monitoring service.
3. Place electrodes on the skin.
4. Turn on ECG transmitter.

5. Transmitter connects pulse and pacemaker data into a signal. This transmits a single-lead ECG pattern to a monitor in the clinic.
6. Instruct client to contact physician if:
   a. Pulse is five beats or more per minute less than before magnet use.
   b. ECG pattern is altered from baseline ECG on file in clinic.

NOTE: Many clinics require that you have a touch-tone phone to use services.

Instructing in Use of Holter Monitor

Equipment

Adhesive electrodes and lead wires
Magnetic recorder with cassette tape
Shoulder strap or belt clip
Paper and pencil or diary

Procedure

1. Explain that heart rate and rhythm are monitored during entire time monitor is in place. The Holter monitor is used to obtain a continuous graphic tracing of a client's pulse while ADLs are performed.
2. Explain that Holter monitor will be in place 24–48 hr; depending on symptoms, it may be in place up to seven days.
3. Place electrodes at both negative and positive poles, as directed by laboratory staff. There are either five or seven leads.
4. Assist client in strapping monitor in place. Monitor is placed in a pouch and worn on belt device or over the shoulder.
5. Connect electrodes to recorder.
6. Instruct client to record any unusual pain, abnormal signs, symptoms, activity, or stressful situations, stating the exact time. ▶ ***Rationale:*** Unusual pain, signs, symptoms, and activity are evaluated with findings from ECG tape to assist in diagnosing cardiac problems.
7. Write down the time medications are taken, when driving to work, taking a nap, or change in activity level.
8. Explain that while wearing a Holter monitor the following directions must be followed:
   a. Sleep on back, not abdomen.
   b. Take sponge bath only, avoid shower. ▶ ***Rationale:*** If pads become wet they will fall off and heart monitoring will not occur.
   c. Call for instructions if an electrode falls off.
   d. Maintain normal activity level.
   e. Instruct client to stay away from magnets, metal detectors, high-voltage areas, and electric blankets.
9. Explain to client that he or she can call the laboratory or clinic any time during the period the Holter monitor is in place if they have questions. Call if monitor lead falls off or quits working, skin erythema occurs, or client exhibits symptoms mentioned above. Provide client with phone number of appropriate facility.
10. Instruct client to take recorder, strap, and paper documentation to laboratory as directed.

NOTE: Diary should include:

a. Exact time unusual symptoms, such as pounding in chest, irregular heartbeats (fluttering in chest), shortness of breath, or trouble breathing, vertigo, or fainting occurs.
b. Time medications taken.
c. Driving to run errands or to work.
d. Stressful events or activities.
e. Exact time monitor was activated.

Clinical Alert

Two new cardiac monitors are currently in use, the Marquette and the King of Hearts recorder. These are smaller monitors, lighter in weight, and have only two leads, which provide fewer restrictions for clients.

Newer Monitoring Devices

Event Monitoring: monitors infrequent symptoms by instructing client to push a button on the device. The device records and stores electrical activity for 2 minutes of pre-activity and 2 minutes of post-event ECG tracings. The small card style unit is worn around the client's neck on a lanyard. These devices are used for weeks to months. The information is transmitted to the physician.

Signal-Averaged ECG: a painless test used to assess the client's risk of developing fatal heart arrhythmias. Test is similar to ECG, but uses sophisticated technology to test for arrhythmias.

Teaching Care of Implantable Cardioverter–Defibrillator

Procedure

1. Instruct client in the following:
   a. Call physician immediately if three shocks in a row are felt, dyspnea develops, or feet or ankle edema occurs.
   b. Take a bath whenever, but don't take a shower until incision is dry and completely healed.
   c. Do not change any medications for treating the arrhythmia unless specifically instructed by the physician.
   d. Take all medications prescribed by the physician. Carry information about medications at all times, including name and dose.
   e. Refrain from wearing tight clothing over defibrillator or lead wires if ICD is in abdomen. (Most ICDs are now implanted in the chest, so clothing restriction is not as much of an issue.) Women can wear bras.
   f. Do not participate in contact sports or activities that could damage the defibrillator.
   g. Drink caffeinated beverages in moderation. ▸ ***Rationale:*** Caffeine increases heart rate and could disturb heart rhythm.
   h. Carry medical alert band and ICD number at all times. Know settings on ICD (cutoff points in heart rate that triggers pacing and defibrillation).
2. Explain the symptoms associated with infection and instruct client to phone physician if they occur.
   a. Erythema, edema, or tenderness surrounding incision
   b. Fluid accumulation around surgical site
   c. Fever of 100°F or higher
3. Instruct client to not lift anything over 5 lb the first month after surgery. Do not excessively push, pull, or twist during this time.
4. Instruct client to not exercise arms or overuse them for at least 3 months after surgery.
5. Instruct client not to resume the following activities until approved by physician:
   a. Returning to work.
   b. Doing household chores.
   c. Traveling.
   d. Resuming sexual activity.
   e. Walking, swimming, sports.
   f. Using large electrical appliances or electrical motors in the workplace until they have been tested to determine whether there is any effect on defibrillator.
6. Remind client that he or she should not undergo an MRI test. ▸ ***Rationale:*** The equipment has a strong magnetic field and is unsafe for the defibrillator.
7. Remind client that wand metal detectors can affect the ICD, and walking through security checkpoint will set off alarms; therefore, they need to be searched by hand and allowed to enter the search area without going through scanner.
8. Explain that the following devices will not interfere with the defibrillator:
   a. Electric razor.
   b. Small kitchen appliances, including microwave ovens and small power tools.
   c. Analog cellular phones are OK but digital phones may be sensed as abnormal and affect ICD.

Clinical Alert

For an interaction between a small electromagnetic device and the defibrillator to occur, they must be within 10 cm of each other. The greater the output power of the device, the greater the possibility of an interaction with the defibrillator.

AED at Home

- FDA-approved AED (automatic external defibrillator) for home use.
- Used for adults and children 8 years and older and weighing at least 55 lb.
- Used for person believed to be in sudden cardiac arrest, does not respond when tapped, is not breathing normally, and absence of circulation.
- When activated, machine guides user through procedure.
- Defibrillator analyzes heart rate when pads attached. Low-energy biphasic therapy initiated if needed.
- Specific directions provided for CPR and calling 911.
- AED performs daily self-tests to ensure it works properly.

DOCUMENTATION for Home Care

- Complete appropriate health assessment forms, care plans, teaching forms
- Include outcomes from printouts from Holter monitor, pacemaker, or defibrillator—include number of times and type of incidents
- Symptoms that elicited graph tracings or transmission to physician's office
- Areas of erythema surrounding implanted defibrillator or pacemaker
- Document report sent to physician via phone or other means of communication
- Use of AED; necessity for use and client outcome

CRITICAL THINKING Application

Expected Outcomes

- Physician's office will keep appraised of client's condition through use of monitoring systems.
- Client is knowledgeable with use of Holter monitor and method of transmitting information to physician's office using cardiac devices.

Unexpected Outcomes	Alternative Actions
Pacemaker malfunction with magnet.	• Check pacemaker function. • Contact physician. • Check that client is not near older microwaves, large magnets, or uses excessive minutes on the cell phone. • Instruct client to use cell phone on opposite side of body from pacemaker.
Holter monitor pads come off.	• Clean and dry area for new pad application. • Instruct client to not get pads wet. • Ensure client documents in diary that pads were changed.

GERONTOLOGIC Considerations

Stressful Physical and Emotional Conditions May Have an Especially Adverse Effect on the Elderly Client.

- The heart may be unable to respond to these changes with an adequate increase in rate, which could precipitate heart failure.
- Changes in the heart lead to decreased myocardial contractility, increased left ventricular ejection time, and delayed conduction, which plays a role in this phenomenon.

Cardiac Output Is Decreased as a Result of Tachycardia or Atrial Fibrillation, Which Is Evidenced on the ECG.

- Tachycardia causes a shortened ventricular filling time.
- Atrial fibrillation causes the loss of the atrial kick (blood volume delivered to the ventricle as a result of a coordinated atrial contraction).

ECG May be Abnormal Due to a Chronic Disease Such as Heart Failure.

- Assess client for behavioral changes, changes in level of consciousness, palpitations, dyspnea, fatigue, and falls. These are indicators of a dysrhythmic heart.
- Dysrhythmias, such as PVCs and premature atrial contractions (PACs), may be very common and not cause for alarm unless they change in number or configuration.
- Pacemaker spikes are evident on ECGs for clients with pacemakers.

Geriatric Changes in Cardio Vascular System

- Exercise—↓ cardiac response.
- Cardiac valves—thicker and stiffer.
- Sino-atrial node—↓ of pacemaker cells;
- Sympathetic nervous system:
  ↓ response to physical stress
  ↓ response to emotional stress
  Less sensitive to β-adrenergic agonist drugs
- Arterial blood vessels—thicker, ↓ elasticity = ↑ BP.
- Hypertension should NOT be considered a normal consequence of aging.

Client Requiring CPR Has Dentures in Place.

- Keep dentures in place to provide for good seal around mouth.
- Bag-value breathing is more effective when tight seal around mouth is maintained.

Peripheral Vascular Assessment Is Essential When an Elderly Client Is Using Elastic Hosiery or Sequential Stockings.

- Elderly clients may very well have altered peripheral circulation before this treatment is started.
- Stockings that are too tight can interfere with the already compromised vascular blood flow, leading to ulceration of the lower extremity.
- Check color, warmth, capillary refill, and presence of pedal pulses every 4 hr when client is using these devices.

MANAGEMENT Guidelines

Each state legislates a Nurse Practice Act for RNs and LVN/LPNs. Healthcare facilities are responsible for establishing and implementing policies and procedures that conform to their state's regulations. Verify the regulations and role parameters for each healthcare worker in your facility.

Delegation

- All healthcare workers are trained in basic cardiac life support or CPR and Heimlich maneuver; therefore, anyone can initiate CPR or perform the Heimlich maneuver.
- CPR training renewal is provided frequently in the healthcare facility to ensure all employees stay current in the skill.
- RN staff assigned to the critical care units, emergency department, and operating room must also be certified in advanced cardiac life support (ACLS). These staff members can be delegated as members of the Code Team in the facility. The operating room staff does not respond to codes outside the operating room.
- RN staff may be assigned to a rapid response team for the hospital.
- It is not the usual protocol that LVN/LPNs are assigned to the critical care unit. If they do have responsibility for client care in these settings, additional education regarding ECG monitoring must be provided.
- All healthcare workers assigned to the team can measure and apply elastic hosiery.
- Ancillary staff members may have additional training in monitoring ECGs (monitoring technicians) and in taking a 12-lead ECG (ECG technician). These individuals can be delegated to perform these tasks.

Communication Matrix

- If the RN is not directly involved in monitoring the ECG, it is imperative that the technician have specific parameters for reporting the findings. These parameters must be defined during the staff report at the beginning of each shift.

- For clients on telemetry, it is critical that the staff nurse assigned to care for the client on the nursing unit be apprised of any unusual ECG findings. The telemetry nurse must place an ECG tracing on the client's chart according to hospital policy.
- During a code, the nurse caring for the client should be relieved from performing CPR duties to answer questions, obtain information, and assist others in the code team to perform the necessary skills to promote a positive outcome of the event.
- During shift report, ensure that the on-coming shift is apprised of any client who is at risk for developing cardiac complications or is considered a potential "code."
- Orders for a code or no-code status should be addressed so that all staff are aware of the client's status. The code cart should be placed near the client's room if the code is imminent.
- Call the rapid response team if client is decompensating.
- Copy of advance directives should be placed in client chart.

CRITICAL THINKING Strategies

Scenario 1

You work day shift in the transitional care unit (TCU) and have been assigned two clients who require total care. Each client is on a cardiac monitor.

Client 1: A 65-year-old male in heart failure, responding well to drug therapy of Lasix and digoxin. His lungs are clear, and he has lost 5 lb since yesterday.

Client 2: A 70-year-old female with a myocardial infarction 2 days ago. She is considered unstable and is receiving close monitoring.

1. What is your first nursing action of the morning?
2. What alterations will you expect in the assessment of Client 2? Provide rationale for your answer.
3. Which client will you attend to first? Provide rationale.
4. Complete the interpretation of the ECG for Client 1.
5. Determine the following:
   a. Heart rate
   b. Regularity of rhythm
   c. PR interval
   d. QRS duration
6. Identify the rhythm based on the information in question 5.
7. Is this a life-threatening arrhythmia?
8. What is your priority intervention?
9. Identify the rhythm strip for Client 2.
10. What are implications for the condition of this client?
11. Identify why this client may have this type of ECG reading.
12. Identify the most effective drug treatment for this arrhythmia and provide the pharmacologic action to support your answer.
13. Identify the possible side effects of the drug and the clinical manifestations you will be monitoring in your assessment.
14. As you are preparing to provide hygienic care to Client 2, you look at the monitor and see the following ECG findings.
    a. What rhythm is depicted on the above strip?
    b. Describe what is happening to the client in this rhythm.
    c. What priority intervention should be done?
    d. What is the second intervention if the priority intervention is not effective?

Scenario 2

During nursing report the nurse indicates she is very concerned about a client who has been unstable all night. You decide to check that client first on your rounds.

1. What is the initial client assessment you will make when you enter the room?
2. Is this a client who might be a candidate for the Rapid Response Team? Provide rationale for your answer.
3. Describe the function of the RRT.
4. What role does the RN taking care of the client assume on the RRT?

NCLEX® Review Questions

Unless otherwise specified, choose only one (1) answer.

1. The client you are caring for is placed on telemetry. As you assess the ECG findings, you remember the QRS complex represents
   1. Atrial depolarization.
   2. The time it takes for atrial depolarization.
   3. Depolarization of the ventricles.
   4. The time required for ventricular depolarization and repolarization.
2. An atrial dysrhythmia results from a disturbance
   1. With an SA node.
   2. In the AV node.
   3. In the Purkinje fibers.
   4. In the bundle of His.

3. A demand pacemaker is used for which one of the following cardiac needs? It
   1. Alters the rate of discharge according to changes in activity and rest.
   2. Discharges a steady electrical impulse at a certain rate regardless of the underlying heart rate.
   3. Discharges an electrical impulse only when the heart rate falls below a programmable heart rate.
   4. Discharges an electrical impulse only when a ventricular dysrhythmia occurs.
4. The morning report indicated the client you are assigned to care for is at risk for hemorrhage. When assessing the client, which one of the following symptoms would *not* lead you to suspect a hemorrhage is occurring?
   1. Urine output of 30–40 mL/hour for the last 4 hr.
   2. Diastolic pressure of 90 mmHg the last 2 hr.
   3. Respirations of 18–20 and shallow.
   4. Clammy skin and central cyanosis.
5. As you go by a client's room, the son comes running out and says, "My dad isn't breathing!" You go quickly to the bedside and determine he needs CPR. You initiate it by first
   1. Compressing the chest five times and then completing two deep breaths.
   2. Administering 30 chest compressions and two breaths.
   3. Defibrillating the client with the AED.
   4. Check for breathing by opening mouth and listening for breaths.
6. The preoperative client has an order for thigh-high graduated compression stockings before surgery. Your first action is to measure the client for the correct hosiery size. You will measure by
   1. First checking the circumference of the largest area of the calf.
   2. Measuring from the Achilles tendon to the popliteal fold.
   3. Measuring from the gluteal fold to bottom of the heel.
   4. Checking the distance between one handbreadth above the knee to the ankle.
7. The contraindications to use of sequential compression devices include which of the following conditions? ***Select all that apply.***
   1. Heart failure.
   2. Dermatitis, gangrene.
   3. Conditions that increase venous return to the heart.
   4. Pulmonary embolism.
8. While making a home visit, you find a client who seems to be choking on food. Your initial response in this emergency is to
   1. Perform an abdominal thrust.
   2. Begin CPR at the rate of 30 compressions and two breaths.
   3. Ask the client if he can speak.
   4. Strike the client on the back.
9. Which statement is incorrect?
   1. Rescue breathing is more effective when a tight seal around the mouth is maintained.
   2. Children have the same physiological reserve as adults, thus require infrequent assessment.
   3. Transcutaneous external pacemakers are used to treat symptomatic bradycardia.
   4. Pulmonary veins carry oxygenated blood.
10. A Rapid Response Team is called when
    1. A client is in imminent need of CPR.
    2. An avoidable death can be prevented.
    3. The use of AED is required during the CODE.
    4. The client needs to be transferred to the ICU.

32

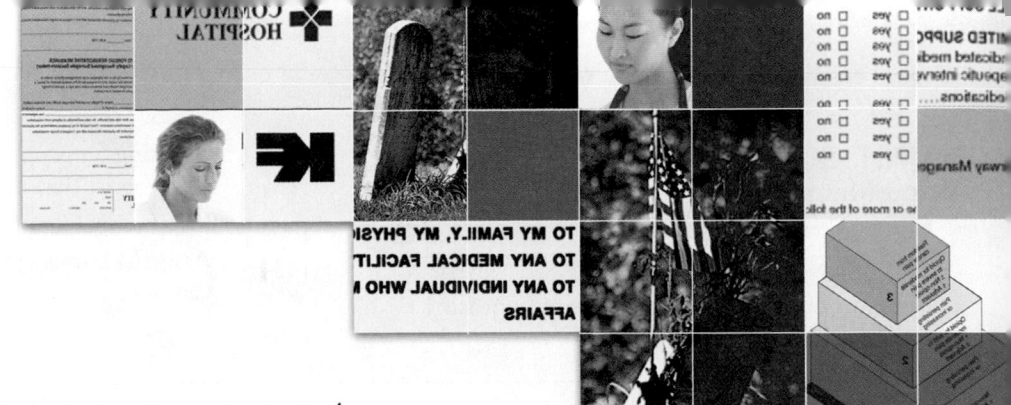

Neurologic Management

LEARNING OBJECTIVES

1. Review the structure and function of the cerebrum, cerebellum, and brainstem.
2. Describe the unique metabolic demands of the central nervous system.
3. Outline the role of structures that protect the brain.
4. Discuss the brain's ability to autoregulate cerebral blood flow.
5. Identify the three components that dictate intracranial pressure.
6. Calculate cerebral perfusion pressure (CPP) based on available data: mean arterial pressure (MAP) and intracranial pressure (ICP).
7. Discuss physiologic compensatory mechanisms that occur with an increased intracranial pressure.
8. Describe the process of assessing the neurologic client experiencing increasing intracranial pressure.
9. Discuss limitations and alternatives to the use of the Glasgow Coma Scale in comatose clients.
10. Identify various assessment tools used to evaluate pain and sedation level in the nonverbal client.
11. State criteria used to determine brain death.
12. Explain the rationale for monitoring intracranial pressure (ICP).
13. Identify components of a normal intracranial pressure (ICP) wave-form.
14. List physical and environmental/contextual factors that increase intracranial pressure.
15. Explain rationale for therapies used to treat intracranial hypertension.
16. Outline nursing responsibilities in the care of a client with an ICP monitoring system and/or ventriculostomy for cerebrospinal fluid drainage.

CHAPTER OUTLINE

TERMINOLOGY

Anisocoria pupils of unequal size.

Autoregulation ability of the brain to maintain, *within limits*, a constant blood flow despite significant changes in systemic blood pressure.

Brain Death medical–clinical diagnosis based on cessation of all brain function (unresponsiveness, absence of brainstem reflexes, apnea) when the cause is known and irreversible.

Cerebral Perfusion Pressure a calculated value derived from intracranial pressure (ICP) and mean arterial pressure (MAP) (MAP − ICP = CPP); an indirect method of evaluating adequacy of cerebral blood flow; normal CPP ranges from 60–160 mmHg.

Cognition skill for thinking and remembering, including paying attention, being aware of surroundings, reasoning, judgment, and problem solving.

Coma clinical state of altered consciousness in which a client is nonresponsive to environmental stimuli (cannot be aroused) due to diffuse bilateral cerebral hemispheric dysfunction, involvement of the brainstem, or both; coma level based on motor response to noxious stimulus.

Concussion complex pathophysiological process affecting the brain, induced by traumatic biomechanical forces (e.g., blow to the head or elsewhere with impulsive force transmitted to the head); may or may not result in loss of consciousness. Cumulative (repeated) events affect white matter (axons).

Consciousness a state of wakefulness (arousal) *and* general awareness (cognition) of self and environment, including orientation to time, place, and person. (Terminology used to describe various levels of consciousness include full consciousness, confusion, lethargy, obtundation, stupor, and coma.)

Confusion disoriented in time, place, or person; short attention span; inability to think with normal speed and clarity; impaired judgment and decision making; difficulty following commands; may have hallucinations, be agitated, restless, irritable, increasingly confused at night.

Contralateral on the opposite side.

Contusion neurologic dysfunction caused by acceleration/deceleration injury (e.g., blow to the head) often associated with coup (injury at site of impact) and contrecoup (injury at side opposite the impact) due to movement of the brain within the skull.

Craniectomy removal of a bone flap to allow decompression (expansion of edematous brain tissue) and reduce intracranial pressure.

Cushing's Triad systolic hypertension, widening pulse pressure, and bradycardia indicative of medullary ischemia.

Decerebration abnormal posturing associated with midbrain (upper brainstem) dysfunction.

Decortication abnormal posturing associated with a direct lesion of the thalamus or mass that compresses the thalamus (above the brainstem).

Diplopia seeing two separate images of the same object in visual space due to images falling on each retina at different points rather than on the same points.

Disorientation beginning loss of consciousness; impaired awareness of time, then place and memory, then recognition of self.

FOUR-Score Coma Scale "Full Outline of Un-Responsiveness" grading system (0 to 4) used to assess eye response, motor response, brainstem reflexes, and respiration.

Glasgow Coma Scale assessment tool designed to standardize observations of a patient's level of consciousness (comatose states).

Hydrocephalus progressive dilation of the ventricles due to overproduction of CSF or abnormalities of CSF circulation or reabsorption.

Intracranial Pressure (ICP) the sum of pressures exerted by intracranial contents (cerebrospinal fluid, blood, and brain tissue); normal range is 5–15 mmHg.

Ipsilateral on the same side.

Lethargy limited spontaneous movement or speech but easily aroused by speech or tactile stimulation; sluggish thought, but oriented to time, place, and person.

Level of Consciousness a continuum of responsiveness ranging from arousal/wakefulness, orientation, comprehension, and expression to nonresponsiveness to bodily or environmental stimuli.

Locked-In Syndrome state of normal level of consciousness but complete body paralysis except for vertical eye movements and ability to blink on command (paralysis below CN III).

MAP (Mean Arterial Pressure) average cardiac cycle arterial pressure:

$$MAP = \frac{(SBP) + (DBP \times 2)}{3}$$

Medial Longitudinal Fasciculus (MLF) pathway that interconnects the vestibular nuclei (CN VIII) with motor nuclei that innervate the extraocular eye muscles (CN III, IV, VI).

Microsensor fiberoptic "transducer tipped" intraventricular or intraparenchymal bolt catheter used to monitor intracranial pressure.

Neuromuscular Blockade chemical paralysis used as restraint to control increased blood pressure and ICP due to restlessness, agitation, posturing, ventilator dyssynchrony.

Nystagmus involuntary drift of the eye with rapid correction in the opposite direction; the direction of fast correction describes the nystagmus.

Obtundation state of reduced awakeness/alertness and limited response to the environment; rousable but falls asleep unless stimulated orally or by touch; responds minimally to questions.

Reticular Activating System center located in the brainstem that interacts with the cerebral hemispheres to maintain normal consciousness.

Rostrocaudal descending the long axis of the body (top downward).

Secondary Injury cascade of events including brain tissue ischemia and cerebral edema that occurs, causing damage to surrounding tissue after primary traumatic brain injury.

Stupor having minimal spontaneous movement; unresponsive except to vigorous repeated stimuli; may have unintelligible sounds or eye opening; responds appropriately to painful stimulus; may withdraw from or grab at the stimulus.

Tragus cartilaginous projection in front of the external auditory canal.

Vegetative State state in which client with bilateral hemispheric disease (metabolic encephalopathy), initially comatose, may show improvement so that the client is awake, but unaware.

Ventriculostomy a hollow ventricular catheter placed through a burr hole in the skull and advanced into the lateral ventricle of the nondominant hemisphere; used to monitor ICP, provide therapeutic CSF drainage to relieve pressure, and allow specimen sampling.

INTRODUCTION

This chapter presents a nursing process approach to care, focusing on techniques of assessing the neurologic client with altered levels of consciousness and the management of intracranial hypertension. (See chapter 11 for basic information and neurologic assessment.)

THE CONSCIOUS STATE

The nervous system includes two interdependent subsystems: the central nervous system (CNS) composed of the brain and spinal cord and the peripheral nervous system (PNS) composed of nerve fibers (cranial, spinal, and autonomic) that relay information between the CNS and other parts of the body. This complex system involves automatic feedback mechanisms that allow us to respond to stimuli from the internal and external environments through cognitive, behavioral, autonomic, and motor responses in a way that enables us to maintain a steady state, or *homeostasis*.

The brain is composed of left and right cerebral hemispheres (each divided into four functional lobes), the cerebellar lobes, and brainstem (midbrain, pons, and medulla). The conscious state includes both *wakefulness* and *awareness* of one's self and the environment (*orientation* to time, place, and person) and depends on an intact interaction between the reticular activating system (RAS) located in the brainstem and thalamus, which controls wakefulness, and the higher cerebral cortical centers, which are responsible for orientation. Altered levels of consciousness (coma) can occur with intracranial (structural) or extracranial (metabolic) disorders. The vast majority (85%) of coma cases are due to metabolic disorders, such as hypoxia, respiratory failure, hypo/hyperglycemia, uremia, or drug overdose, which cause diffuse dysfunction of both cerebral hemispheres and/or involvement of the ascending RAS. Intracranial disorders such as infection (meningitis, encephalitis) or concussion (brain trauma) can also cause coma with diffuse dysfunction.

In contrast to diffuse dysfunction, unilateral cerebral hemispheric lesions such as infarction ("brain attack"), hematoma, hemorrhage, or tumor cause *focal* neurologic signs of dysfunction related to the particular area or functional lobe involved. Focal lesions expand and, along with edema formation, increase intracranial pressure, may decrease cerebral blood flow, displace contralateral structures, and exert rostrocaudal (downward) compression on the brainstem (RAS) such that deteriorating levels of consciousness follow.

Normal function of the cerebral lobes, diencephalon (located above the brainstem), cerebellum, and brainstem and findings associated with dysfunction of these areas are reviewed in Table 32-1.

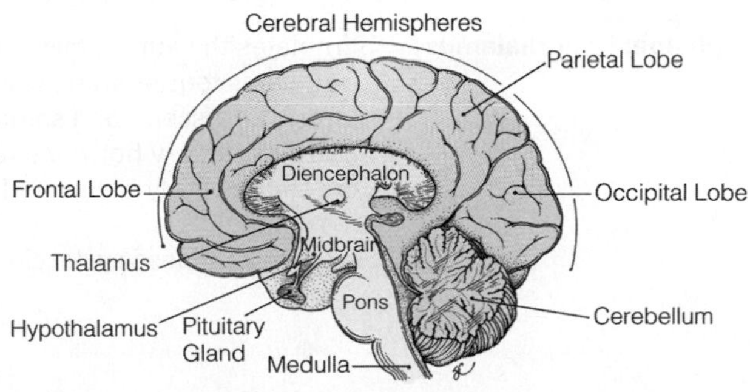

▲ Lobes of the brain.

TABLE 32-1 Functions of the Cerebral Cortex, Cerebellum, and Brainstem

Structure	Function	Dysfunctional Behaviors
Frontal Lobe Cortex	Memory, judgment, problem solving, concentration, personality, mood Initiation of motor activity and voluntary movement Expressive (motor) speech (left hemisphere)	Difficulty with attention and problem solving; inflexible thinking; personality change; behavioral changes (emotional, social, sexual) Left CVA results in contralateral hemiparesis or hemiplegia and hemisensory loss in the same distribution; expressive aphasia; contralateral homonymous hemianopsa; limited right conjugate gaze; shortened attention span; hesitancy Right CVA results in contralateral hemiparesis or hemiplegia and hemisensory loss in the same distribution; contralateral homonymous hemianopia; left visual and sensory neglect; poor left conjugate gaze; impulsive behavior; unaware of deficits.
Temporal Lobe Cortex	Memory, hearing, understanding (receptive) language Emotional affect	Short-term memory loss; may verbalize, but is unable to understand what is said by others; aggressive behavior; difficulty identifying objects; difficulty recognizing faces; disturbed selective attention; change in sexuality Auditory, visual, and sensory hallucinations
Parietal Lobe Cortex	Sense of touch, pain, position, pressure, vibration Recognition of object size, shape, texture. Spatial perceptual orientation Awareness of one's body parts Visual perception Receptive speech (written, oral) function	Difficulty naming objects; problems of reading and writing; right/left confusion; math difficulties Inability to focus visual attention; problems with eye-hand coordination; lack of awareness/inattention to body parts Receptive language dysfunction; expressive "word salad"
Occipital Lobe Cortex	Interpretation of visual stimuli (impulses from cranial nerve [CN] II)	Visual field defects; difficulty identifying colors; hallucinations/visual distortions; word blindness; difficulty reading and writing
Diencephalon: Thalamus	Relay center for all sensory and motor pathways All sensory pathways (except olfactory, CN I) gong to the brain are processed here before being sent to the cerebral cortex Awareness of pain, temperature, and light touch; reticular activating system focuses attention, stimulates cortex and ANS	Impaired consciousness Sensory and motor dysfunction Decorticate (abnormal flexor) posturing associated with a direct lesion or compression from hemispheres
Diencephalon: Hypothalamus	Stimulates the autonomic nervous system: regulates temperature, water balance, thirst, appetite, visceral and somatic activities Controls pituitary hormone release Coordinates body behavioral responses to emotion Sleep-wakefulness cycle, circadian rhythm	Impaired consciousness Alterations of body temperature Diabetes insipidus (polyuria) Syndrome of inappropriate antidiuretic hormone (water retention with hyponatremia) Cheyne-Stokes respiration (rhythmic rise and fall in rate and depth of breathing with long periods of apnea)

TABLE 32-1 Functions of the Cerebral Cortex, Cerebellum, and Brainstem (*Continued*)

Structure	Function	Dysfunctional Behaviors
Cerebellum	Maintains posture, balance Coordination of voluntary muscle activity and muscle tone Controls fine movement/skilled motor activity	Problems with fine movement/coordination; inability to make rapid movements Lack of coordination Inability to grasp objects; tremors/dizziness; slurred speech; inability to walk
Brainstem: Midbrain	Contains nuclei for CN III and IV Center for auditory and visual reflexes Lies directly beneath the diencephalon (thalamus and hypothalamus) Contains aqueduct of Sylvius Pathway between cerebral hemispheres and lower brain	Ipsilateral pupil dilation with head injury/uncal herniation Both eyes deviate medially or laterally Neurogenic hyperventilation (sustained deep breathing with no apneic periods) Decerebrate (abnormal extensor) posturing
Brainstem: Pons	Contains nuclei for CN V through VIII Medial longitudinal fasciculus tract connects CN III, IV, and VI with vestibular portion of acoustic nerve (CN VIII), allowing coordinated eye movement in response to noise, motion, position, and arousal Relays information to and from the brain Contains fourth ventricle Contains vital centers for breathing (length of inspiration/expiration, rate)	Alterations of extraocular movements *See Oculocephalic and Oculovestibular Testing* Apneustic breathing (has prolonged inspiratory or expiratory pauses)
Brainstem: Medulla	Contains nuclei for CN IX through XII Controls vital functions: swallowing, vomiting, hiccoughing, coughing, heart rate, arterial constriction, respiratory rhythm Motor tracts cross to opposite side, descend the spinal cord for contralateral voluntary movement	Cluster breathing (irregular gasping respirations with long periods of apnea) Ataxic respiration (irregular deep and shallow breathing with periods of apnea) "Cushing's Triad": bradycardia, systolic hypertension, widened pulse pressure Arrhythmias, atrioventricular block

STRUCTURES AND FUNCTIONS THAT PROTECT THE BRAIN

Skull, Meninges, and Spinal Fluid

The brain is protected by an unyielding skull, the meninges that cover the brain (dura, arachnoid, and pia mater), and cerebrospinal fluid (CSF), which circulates within the subarachnoid space to provide protective shock absorption. The ventricles produce 120 mL of CSF each day, while an equal amount is reabsorbed through arachnoid projections (villi) and returned to the venous circulation such that CSF pressure remains constant. If the villi become obstructed, the ventricles may dilate, causing a "normal pressure hydrocephalus" with a classic triad of gait instability, urinary incontinence, and altered mental status. This problem, occurring mostly in older clients, can be relieved by placement of a VP shunt that diverts CSF from the ventricles to the peritoneal cavity.

The dura mater lies close to the skull and creates a vertical fold (falx) that separates the right and left frontal lobes and a horizontal fold (tentorium) that separates the occipital and cerebellar lobes. With increasing intracranial pressure, brain tissue may herniate around these dural folds.

Fractures of the temporal and parietal bones may be associated with epidural (between the skull and dura) meningeal artery bleed that spreads freely and causes a rapid change in level of consciousness. An epidural hematoma is a surgical emergency. In contrast, a subdural bleed is venous in nature, slower, and may be associated with delayed signs of altered consciousness. This type of injury is more commonly seen in elderly clients with head injury associated with a fall that may or may not have been documented or remembered.

Fractures of the basal skull bones may be missed because they are not visible on skull or sinus x-rays but are often associated with tearing of the dura, causing CSF leakage from the ear (otorrhea) or nose (rhinorrhea) or altered CN VII function. These findings may be delayed, but should be reported immediately as they increase risk for infection. Leakage is usually self-limiting, but if it persists for 4–5 days, lumbar CSF drainage may be necessary to allow the dural tear to heal.

Autoregulation

The brain requires a continuous supply of oxygen and glucose to maintain its energy requirements. While it makes up only 2% of body weight, it receives 15% of the cardiac output and uses 20% of blood oxygen. Despite fluctuations in blood pressure, the brain is able to regulate its own blood flow by arteriolar dilation when blood pressure falls or constriction when blood pressure rises. This protective function requires a mean arterial pressure (MAP) of 50–150 mmHg and is disrupted with any increase in intracranial pressure or decrease in cerebral perfusion pressure. Then, if blood pressure rises, cerebral blood volume increases, causing an increased intracranial pressure. While hypertension must be controlled, a MAP sufficient to provide adequate cerebral perfusion must be maintained if intracranial hypertension exists. Target cerebral perfusion pressure (CPP) is 70–80 mmHg and is calculated by subtracting the intracranial pressure (ICP) from the MAP (MAP − ICP = CPP).

INTRACRANIAL HYPERTENSION

Intracranial pressure, normally 3–15 mmHg, is dictated by three components: 80% brain tissue, 10% cerebral blood volume (with 80% being venous blood), and 10% CSF. Volumes of these constituents are kept relatively constant, but pathologic conditions can cause an increase of one of these components that must be compensated for by a decrease in one or both of the other components in order to maintain a normal ICP (Monro-Kellie hypothesis).

An increase in brain tissue occurs with edema that accompanies any type of injury (trauma, CVA) or a mass such as a tumor. An increase in cerebral blood flow occurs with an intracranial bleed or subarachnoid hemorrhage, or even cerebral vasodilation due to hypoxemia, hypocarbia, or certain medications. An increase in CSF occurs with blockage of its outflow paths or obstructed reabsorption by subarachnoid villi.

The brain has limited ability to control increased ICP by: (1) shunting CSF from the intracranial to the lumbar space, where CSF reabsorption is increased; (2) by compression of the cerebral venous system to reduce cerebral blood volume; and (3) by displacement of brain tissue, but this is adaptive only with a slowly expanding mass or hematoma condition. When these compensatory mechanisms are exhausted, ICP rises exponentially, cerebral perfusion is impaired, and brain tissue displaces or herniates through available openings. (See page 1305, herniation progression.)

When ICP increases to a level that compresses arterial flow (ICP = MAP), the Cushing reflex (bradycardia, increased SBP with widened pulse pressure, erratic breathing pattern) is activated to protect the brain from inadequate blood flow. Unfortunately, these changes in vital signs are late indicators of rostrocaudal deterioration.

Intracranial pressure monitoring systems may be used to measure the mean pressure exerted in the skull and alert the nurse to increases in ICP before external signs such as altered level of consciousness or pupillary changes occur. Monitoring also guides early intervention before damage occurs, assists the nurse in determining effects that care measures have on the client's ICP responses, and serves as a basis for ongoing evaluation of goal achievement and maintenance of desired outcomes: e.g., target ICP $\leq$20 mmHg and CPP $\geq$70–80 mmHg.

A number of medical and nursing measures help to control ICP by selectively manipulating the three components that dictate intracranial pressure. Brain volume can be reduced by decreasing cerebral edema with osmotic diuretics (mannitol) and hypertonic saline, which also improve cerebral blood flow by decreasing blood viscosity and reducing serum hematocrit. During the acute phase, cerebral metabolic needs, refractory elevations of ICP, and effects of secondary brain injury can be modulated by induced hypothermia. CSF volume is reduced by continuous or intermittent external drainage of cerebrospinal fluid (ventriculostomy). Cerebral blood volume can be reduced with hyperventilation (PCO_2 25–30 mmHg), which can cause vasoconstriction with global or localized cerebral ischemia but may be used briefly as a bridge to more appropriate therapy. Blood volume can also be reduced by supporting jugular venous return with neutral head alignment, 30° bed elevation, and by preventing surges in central venous pressure associated with maneuvers that increase intra-abdominal and intrathoracic pressure. Cautious use of analgesics and sedatives is an integral component of managing ICP as these modalities blunt the ANS response to noxious stimuli, decrease O_2 consumption, and enhance psychological well-being. These agents have adverse side effects that may increase ICP and necessitate continuous assessment of the client's response to their use and impact on ventilation and oxygenation.

NURSING CARE OF THE NEUROLOGIC CLIENT

The Glasgow Coma Scale (GCS; see Glasgow Coma Scale, Chapter 11) has been used for several decades to evaluate level of consciousness (LOC) by requiring the client to hear the examiner and respond with (1) eye opening, (2) oral, and (3) motor responses. If the client is unresponsive to these, abnormal posturing response (decortication, decerebration) to shaking or noxious stimuli is assessed. Clients with a score of 8 or less are considered to be comatose and are typically intubated to protect the airway and facilitate mechanical ventilation if required. A "T" is added to their GCS score to indicate this functional limitation. Using this scale, a client with spinal cord injury who is paralyzed may receive a coma score of 8, be intubated, but not be comatose. It follows that the GCS cannot be used to assess neurologic signs in clients who are unable to respond orally (e.g., clients who are intubated, sedated, aphasic, have impaired hearing or altered level of consciousness).

The Full Outline of Un-Responsiveness ("FOUR score") coma scale is an alternative tool for assessing the comatose client, especially one with an acute metabolic or other nonstructural brain injury/disorder because it detects early changes in consciousness such as inability to follow the examiner's commands, altered brainstem reflexes, and Cheyne-Stokes breathing. It is also used to differentiate vegetative from minimally conscious states, locked-in syndrome, uncal herniation, and brain death.

Pain, general discomfort, fatigue, anxiety, restlessness, and agitation increase cerebral metabolism, heart rate, blood pressure, and intracranial pressure, but the neurologic client's inability to communicate confines the nurse to observing the behavioral and physiologic indicators of distress without the ability to identify or validate a potential cause. Since nonverbal responses have many possible stimuli that require different treatment, they may be misinterpreted and inadequately managed. For instance, failure to recognize that pain often leads to agitation may lead to excessive administration of sedatives, leaving pain untreated. It is essential to use reliable assessment tools to differentiate among distressful stimuli so that appropriate therapies can be provided. The Critical Care Pain Observation Tool and a number of sedation/agitation assessment scales have been determined to be valid and reliable to use with neurologic clients who are unable to communicate verbally.

Caring for neurologic clients challenges the nurse's insight and ability to appreciate the client's unique experience, to assess patiently, to identify distressful stimuli, and to respond empathically with informed actions. Comprehensive care also includes ongoing support of all body systems and prevention of a wide range of complications that can occur. Emotional support is provided by communicating with the client, whether or not he or she is responsive. This has been shown to help relieve anxiety and fear and serves as a means of preventing acute surges in ICP. Concerned others are also supported by answering questions and explaining how technical aspects of care contribute to the client's progress as they inform and help direct decision making. Once the client is stable, family members can be encouraged to participate in simple comforting care measures and engage in providing gentle sensory stimuli, which may enhance arousal and awareness as the client regains the conscious state.

CULTURAL AWARENESS

African Americans

May be wary of discussions of advanced directives and organ donation, especially if the client is seriously ill.

May view client's condition as God's punishment for improper behavior or as the work of the devil or that a spell has been cast. May have a fatalistic attitude about illness.

View organ donation as desecration of the body and consent may hasten one's death.

Generally do not consider organ transplantation except for immediate family members.

Believe life support should not be withdrawn, considering it a gift of God.

American Indians

Open expression is usually reserved for close of kin and friends.

May be wary of signing consents (based on historical abuse of signed documents).

Organ donation is usually not practiced.

If family members are unavailable to sign consent, procedures should be minimally invasive.

If cutting hair is necessary, ask client or family whom they prefer to do this.

May be reluctant to give up body parts. Ask client or family how hair should be disposed of; some tribes require hair to be stored by the family or to be disposed of ceremoniously.

A designated person may need to wash and style hair of seriously ill clients.

A child or family friend may be family spokesperson. Ask who should receive information.

Family should be informed if death is imminent so that arrangements can be made and loved ones can gather.

With death family may request that the body be cleansed by a special person before it is moved.

Mexican Americans

Many have special amulets (crucifix, religious medal) that should be kept near the client. Such items or special clothing should be handled carefully and given to a family member for safe-keeping if indicated.

May use a variety of home/folk remedies (teas, etc.) for symptom management.

Prefers words rather than numbers to describe intensity of symptoms.

Family unit may make decisions regarding treatment. Ask client how decisions are made.

Limited visiting policy may be viewed as attempt to hide something from the family.

May fear that speaking about death will hasten or cause it.

May be wary of nurse practitioners, thinking care is substandard, but many experience midwives as the only healthcare providers available.

May request priest or hospital chaplain to administer sacrament of the sick and may be indicated after death, before the body is removed.

Family members may be emotionally distraught and need extra time to remain with the deceased. Feelings about death and its sequel are greatly influenced by religious beliefs.

May believe the body must be buried intact and have a negative attitude about organ donation.

NURSING DIAGNOSES

The following nursing diagnoses are appropriate to use on client care plans when the components are related to clients who require focused neurologic assessment and management of increased intracranial pressure.

NURSING DIAGNOSIS	RELATED FACTORS
Aspiration, Risk for	Altered level of consciousness Airway intubation
Imbalanced Body Temperature, Risk for	Traumatic brain (hypothalamic) injury
Acute Confusion	Brain injury
Decreased Intracranial Adaptive Capacity	Increased intracranial contents (blood, tissue, spinal fluid)
Imbalanced Fluid Volume, Risk for	Traumatic brain (hypothalamic) injury
Impaired Verbal Communication	Altered level of consciousness, neuromuscular blockade, airway intubation
Ineffective Thermoregulation	Brain injury
Impaired Bed Mobility	Neuromuscular blockade; invasive monitoring
Ineffective Cerebral Tissue Perfusion, Risk for	Increased intracranial pressure
Infection, Risk for	Invasive monitoring catheters; pathologic (rhinorrhea, otorrhea) and therapeutic cerebral spinal fluid drainage
Impaired Skin Integrity, Risk for	Sedation, neuromuscular blockade (paralysis) Restricted positioning due to monitoring devices

CLEANSE HANDS The single most important nursing action to decrease the incidence of hospital-based infections is hand hygiene. *Remember to wash your hands or use antibacterial gel before and after each and every client contact.*

IDENTIFY CLIENT Before every procedure, introduce yourself and check two forms of client identification, not including room number. These actions prevent errors and conform to The Joint Commission standards.

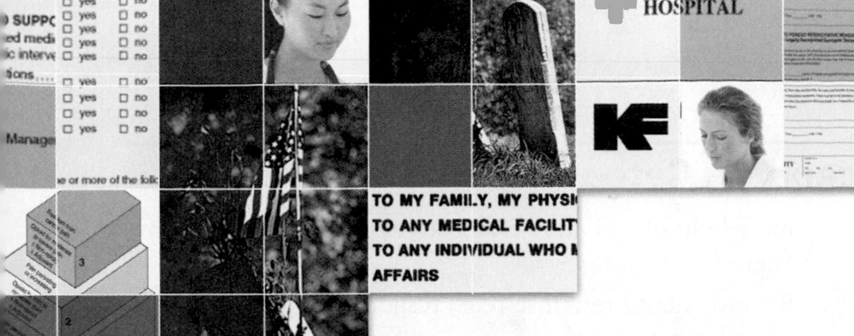

Chapter 32

UNIT 1

Assessment of the Neurologic Client

Nursing Process Data

ASSESSMENT Data Base

- Determine a neurologic client's level of consciousness
- Determine deviations and implications for care for the client with altered brainstem reflexes
- Identify signs of basilar skull fracture
- Recognize changes in vital signs that occur with altered level of consciousness
- Utilize the FOUR-Score Coma Scale for nonverbal clients
- List criteria used to determine brain death in adults

PLANNING Objectives

- To determine a neurologic client's level of consciousness
- To assess brainstem reflexes in the neurologic client
- To employ protective measures for the client with altered brainstem reflexes
- To recognize signs of basilar skull fracture and implications for care
- To identify changes in brainstem reflexes and vital signs associated with herniation syndromes
- To compare features of the Glasgow Coma Scale with those of the FOUR-Score coma scale
- To assist the physician with determination of brain death
- To support a family/caregiver of a deceased organ donor

IMPLEMENTATION Procedures

EVALUATION Expected Outcomes

- Appropriate tools are used to evaluate a neurologic client's level of consciousness.
- Ongoing assessment of brainstem reflexes and vital signs are used to identify increasing intracranial pressure in the neurologic client.
- Signs of possible basilar skull fracture are identified.
- Established criteria are used to determine brain death.
- Supportive communication is provided for family or caregiver of a deceased organ donor.

Pearson Nursing Student Resources

Find additional review materials at **nursing.pearsonhighered.com**

Prepare for success with NCLEX®-style practice questions and Skill Checklists

Assessing Levels of Consciousness (Descending Categories)

NOTE: There is no internationally accepted taxonomy of definition of LOC, no precise terminology, and no agreement on behaviors of various stages.

Procedure

1. Describe client behaviors assessed rather than using labels such as the following. ▶ ***Rationale:*** Behaviors are more helpful and allow others to easily note changes in client functioning.
2. Record client's response (e.g., responds appropriately to oral questioning).
3. See Table 32-2 below.

TABLE 32-2 Assessing Levels of Consciousness

Category	Findings and Implications for Care
Conscious	Responds immediately to minimal external stimuli. Is alert, fully awake and oriented to time, place, purpose, and person. Understands spoken and written word and expresses ideas orally or in writing. Alterations in LOC reflect cerebral and metabolic disorders very quickly.
Confused	Disoriented to time, and place, but usually oriented to person. Has short attention span, impaired memory. Has difficulty following instruction; may have hallucinations, be agitated, restless, irritable, and more confused at night. *Frequent observation/supervision is indicated.*
Lethargic	Drowsy, sluggish in speech and mental and motor responses. Requires increased stimulus to awaken. Oriented to time, place, and person. *Frequent observation/supervision is indicated.*
Obtunded	Drowsy, arouses to stimulus but with minimal response. Responds appropriately to painful stimulus. *Needs complete care.*
Stuporous	Arouses only by vigorous and continuous stimulus. Has little spontaneous movement. May appropriately localize or withdraw from stimulus. May open eyes, make incomprehensible sounds. *Needs complete care.*
Comatose	Cannot be aroused. Has no voluntary response to stimuli, including pain. Coma level is based on motor response to painful stimulus. May or may not have protective brainstem reflexes (e.g., gag). *Needs total dependent care, with airway a priority.*

Assessing Cranial Nerves (Brainstem Reflexes)

NOTE: In most clients with increasing intracranial pressure, level of consciousness deteriorates before changes in cranial nerve reflexes, motor response, and vital signs occur. See Chapter 11, Physical Assessment, for basic assessment.

Procedure

1. Record the stimulus applied and the client's response (e.g., responds appropriately to oral questioning).
2. See Table 32-3 below.

Clinical Alert

Change in pupil size, shape, or reactivity should be reported immediately. This may be an early sign of transtentorial herniation requiring immediate intervention.

- Flexor (decorticate) posturing indicates loss of all function *above* the brainstem.
- Extensor (decerebrate) posturing indicates brainstem dysfunction.
- Loss of cough, gag, or corneal (blink) reflex indicates loss of brainstem integrity.

TABLE 32-3 Assessing Cranial Nerves (Brainstem Reflexes)

Cranial Nerve	Significance of Alteration
CN II (sensory) and CN III (motor) **Pupil size, shape, and reactivity**	Normal pupils are round, usually 3–5 mm diameter, equal in size, and react (constrict) consensually (both pupils respond) and briskly to light. *Alternately, have client look at an object 4 in. from the eyes and then at something on the wall behind the observer. The pupils should constrict (accommodate) when focusing on the near object.* Anisocoria (unequal pupil size) may be found in up to 20% of healthy clients. Smaller than average pupils may occur with metabolic coma. Pinpoint pupils may indicate pontine ischemia or opiate overdose. Oval pupils are early indication of CN III compression or increased ICP (18–35 mmHg), but pupils may be round in presence of increased ICP. Ipsilateral pupil dilation with head injury indicates uncal herniation with compression of CN III. *Bilateral* dilated (small ring of iris) and fixed pupils indicate extremely increased ICP causing pontine compression with complete CN III palsy. Absence of pupillary light reflex is consistent with comatose state. Hypothermia, barbiturate coma, and opiate overdose may mimic comatose states with unreactive pupils.
CN III, IV, and VI (all motor) **Assess extraocular movements in the conscious client**	*Note: See below for assessment of the conscious client (six fields of gaze).* Inability to move the eye inward or downward may be seen with head trauma (midbrain compression of CN IV). Inability to move the eye outward (pontine compression of CN VI) may be due to intracranial hypertension. The client has diplopia (double vision) when turning the right eye, if affected, to the right and same for the left turning leftward. Consciousness with complete body paralysis except for vertical eye movements occurs with a lesion in the ventral pons as seen in locked-in syndrome.
CN III, IV, and VI (all motor) **Oculocephalic (Doll's eyes) reflex in unconscious client**	"Doll's eye reflex" is used to test extraocular movements—integrity of the pontine-midbrain level (CN III, IV, and VI) in the *unconscious* client. Damage to the reticular activating system may damage these nerves, which pass through the midbrain to innervate extraocular movements. Reflex may be absent in severe metabolic encephalopathy. *See skill that follows.*
CN V (sensory) and VII (motor) **Corneal blink reflex**	Reflex is frequently absent in the comatose client. Periorbital swelling may prevent eyelid closure. Loss of ability to blink indicates need for corneal protection (instillation of eye lubricant) to prevent corneal drying and scarring. Polyethylene film may be taped over the eyes, extending beyond the eyebrows.
CN VIII (sensory) and III, IV, VI (all motor) **Oculovestibular (Cold caloric) reflex in unconscious client** *(test performed by physician)*	Used for final assessment of brainstem function in the unconscious client and can be used when cervical spine precautions must be maintained. Test may elicit abnormal posturing in comatose client. Reflex may be temporarily absent in client with metabolic encephalopathy. *See skill that follows.*
CN IX (sensory) and X (motor) **Cough and gag reflex**	Normally this medullary reflex protects the airway; its absence places the client at high risk for aspiration. Loss of this reflex is a poor prognostic sign.

The Six Cardinal Directions of Gaze

This test assesses CNs III, IV, and VI which innervate the six extraocular muscles that move the eyes as a pair in the same direction. These eye movements interact with the internuclear pathway of the medial longitudinal fasciculus (MLF) and cerebral cortex, to coordinate focus in a given direction.

Test the six extraocular muscles (conjugate eye) movement in the conscious client:

Procedure

1. Ask the client to follow your finger through an "H" sequence: client looks rightward, leftward, left

upward, left downward, then right upward and right downward.

2. Assess that both eyes move simultaneously, symmetrically, in the same direction, and in alignment.
3. Dysconjugate movement (one eye deviating from mid position at rest), *diplopia* (double vision), impaired movement (gaze paresis or paralysis) or *nystagmus* (eye drift with rapid correction in the opposite direction) indicates cranial nerve injury.

Coordinated eye and *head movement* incorporates complex reflexes of the eyes plus *vestibular* systems (CN VIII) and the *cerebral cortex.* The **oculocephalic** reflex (doll's eyes response) and the **oculovestibular** reflex (caloric stimulation) are used to assess brainstem reflexes in the unconscious client.

Assessing the Oculocephalic (Doll's eyes) Reflex

Preparation

1. The purpose of this test is to assess extraocular movements in the unconscious client by determining presence and extent of structural damage.
   a. Cranial nerves III, IV, and VI pass through the midbrain to innervate the extraocular muscles.
   b. The medial longitudinal fasciculus (MLF) also passes through the midbrain and coordinates eye movements with head and body position changes.
   c. *If the eyes are able to cross the midline, the medial longitudinal fasciculus and midbrain through which it passes are considered to be intact.*
2. Determine that neck injury has been ruled out before this test is performed.

Procedure

1. Hold client's eyes open.
2. Briskly turn client's head to one side, then briskly turn head to the other side, noting client's eye movement. ▸ ***Rationale:*** The intact brainstem will attempt to keep the eyes looking forward even as the head is rotated laterally.
3. Assess for an intact oculocephalic reflex, when the eyes briefly remain in the direction opposite that of the head turn (positive doll's eye reflex).
4. Assess if eyes remain midline and move with the head, or if the eyes rove or move in opposite direction; this *abnormal* oculocephalic reflex indicates a lesion at the pontine-midbrain level of the brainstem.
5. *For an alternative method:* Flex the neck and note that the eyes look upward, then extend the neck and note that the eyes look downward, indicating a normal or positive "doll's eye" reflex.

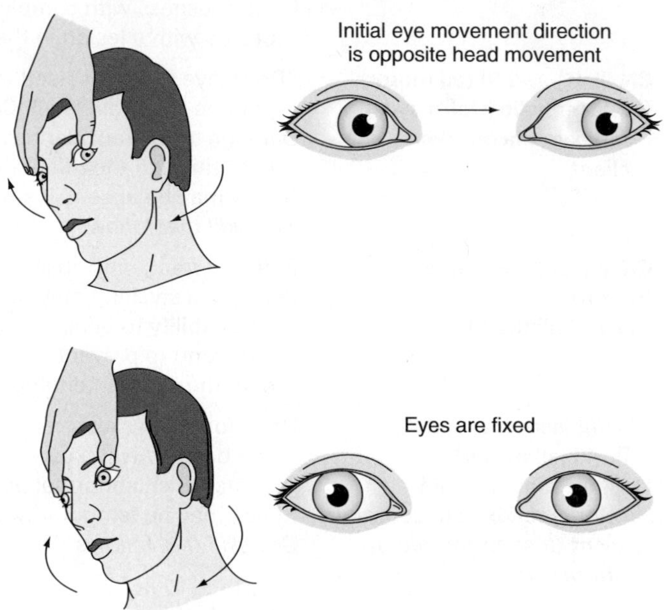

▲ Oculocephalic reflex: eyes briefly remain in the direction opposite that of the head turn (positive doll's eye reflex).

Assessing the Oculovestibular Reflex: "Cold Caloric Test"

NOTE: This test is performed by a physician. This noxious stimulation may elicit abnormal posturing in the comatose client.

Equipment

Otoscope
Catheter tip syringe
50 mL ice water

Preparation

1. Purpose of test is to assess brainstem integrity in the unconscious client.
2. Inspect to validate that client's tympanic membrane is intact.
3. Raise client's head to a 30° angle.

Procedure

1. Physician injects 20–50 mL of ice water into the external auditory canal. ▸ ***Rationale:*** This cools the mastoid bone and disturbs the endolymph flow in the inner ear. A signal passes from the medulla to the midbrain, triggering compensatory eye movements.
2. Check both eyes that tonically move toward the side of the cold water infusion, then rapidly correct back toward midline with bursts of nystagmus, indicating an intact brainstem; cortical function is overriding the tonic deviation of the eyes caused by the cold stimulation.
   a. Ipsilateral absence of eye movements despite eye deviation on the side with the intact MLF indicates unilateral dysfunction.
   b. No eye movement indicates little or no brainstem function.
3. Physician test may repeat in the other ear to test integrity of the *contralateral* side of the brainstem.

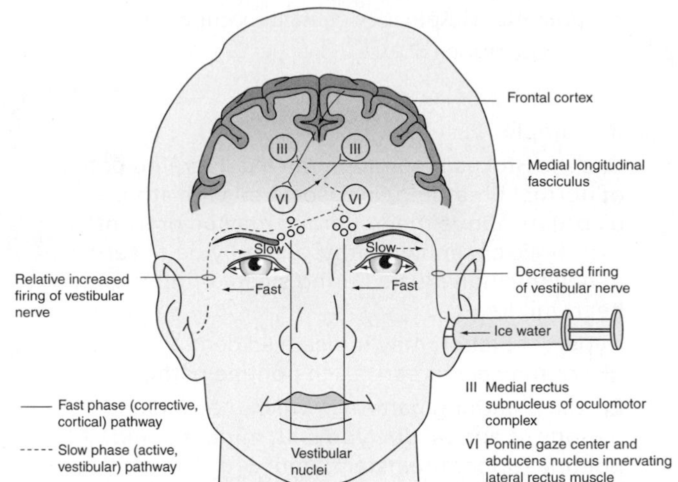

▲ Oculovestibular reflex: both eyes tonically move toward the side of cold water infusion, then rapidly back toward midline, with bursts of nystagmus (cold caloric test).

Assessing Signs of Basilar Skull Fracture

NOTE: Fractures of basal skull bones usually are not visible on skull or sinus x-rays but are often associated with tearing of the dura. A possible basilar skull fracture is suspected if the client develops leakage of CSF from the nose (rhinorrhea) or ears (otorrhea) or altered facial nerve (CN VII) function. These findings should be reported immediately as they are associated with increased risk for infection.

Procedure

1. Assess for *rhinorrhea* (leakage of blood or CSF from client's nose): Look for yellow CSF ring around bloody drainage on drip pad ("Halo sign"). ▸ ***Rationale:*** Drainage may indicate a basilar skull fracture with dural tear and risk for infection (meningitis). Drainage should not be obstructed but allowed to drip freely from the nose onto a sterile "mustache" dressing. Nasal suctioning and nose blowing must be avoided.
2. Assess auditory canal for *otorrhea* (leakage of blood or CSF from the client's ear). Look for yellow CSF ring around bloody drainage on drip pad ("Halo sign"). ▸ ***Rationale:*** Drainage may indicate a basilar skull fracture with dural tear, ruptured tympanic membrane, and risk for infection (meningitis). Drainage should not be obstructed.
3. Place client on side of drainage and allow fluid to drain freely from the ear onto a sterile towel (drip pad).
4. Assess for *Battle's sign*. Look for ecchymosis or bruising behind the ear. ▸ ***Rationale:*** May indicate a basilar skull fracture and associated with CN VII defect. Finding may be delayed and should be reported.
5. Assess for *raccoon eyes*. Look for ecchymosis or bruising around the eyes, which may be accompanied with *rhinorrhea*. ▸ ***Rationale:*** May indicate a basilar skull fracture. Finding may be delayed and should be reported.

Clinical Alert

Otorrhea and rhinorrhea are suggestive of CSF leakage, but drainage is often combined with blood, so glucose determination is unreliable to detect presence of CSF. Laboratory analysis of chloride content of drainage is more reliable because CSF chloride concentration is greater than that of serum.

If basilar skull fracture is suspected, do not insert a nasogastric tube. Orogastric placement is indicated and should be performed before orotracheal intubation in order to prevent aspiration.

Assessing Vital Signs

NOTE: Changes in vital signs are late indicators of decompensation.

Procedure

1. Measure temperature. ▸ ***Rationale:*** Hyperthermia or hypothermia may indicate hypothalamic injury, infection, or noninfectious fever.
2. Assess heart rate/rhythm. ▸ ***Rationale:*** Various arrhythmias occur with abrupt changes in ICP. Bradycardia develops in high spinal cord injury and with medullary ischemia.
3. Assess respiratory rate, and pattern.

NOTE: See Chapter 10, Vital Signs, for patterns.

▸ *Rationale:* Respiratory changes occur early, even before alterations of LOC.

For example:

- Cheyne Stokes respiration (an exaggerated pattern of normal breathing) is associated with structural disorders above the midbrain, may be present in metabolic encephalopathy, and may be observed in healthy individuals during sleep or those with heart failure.
- Hyperventilation may indicate acidemia (low blood pH) or may occur early with pontine pathology.
- Erratic breathing patterns, which may include periods of apnea, develop with midbrain and pontine (upper brainstem) injury.

NOTE: It is best to describe the breathing pattern as it is seen rather than to use names of breathing patterns. Description of the pattern clarifies the assessment finding and helps others to recognize changes.

Clinical Alert

Cushing's triad (bradycardia, systolic hypertension, and widening pulse pressure) may indicate intracranial hypertension or herniation syndrome. The presence of any component calls for further assessment and intervention.

4. Measure blood pressure. ▸ *Rationale:* Hypotension (SBP ≤90 mmHg) directly relates to cerebral ischemia and secondary brain injury.

Systolic hypertension and widening pulse pressure are responses to maintain cerebral blood flow in the presence of pressure on the brainstem (medullary ischemia).

NOTE: Loss of autoregulation occurs with any type of brain injury. If blood pressure increases, cerebral blood flow, blood volume, and ICP also increase. Systemic hypertension must be controlled, but the MAP must be maintained to support adequate cerebral blood flow (CPP near 80 mmHg) when ICP is increased.

EVIDENCE-BASED PRACTICE

Febrile patients with no evidence of infection are considered to have noninfectious fever.

Documented infections tend to be more common among febrile patients with traumatic brain injury, while noninfectious fever is more frequent among patients with subarachnoid hemorrhage associated with vasospasm.

Source: Rabinstein, A. A., & Sandhu, K. (2007). Non-infectious fever in the neurological intensive care unit: Incidence, causes and predictors. *Journal of Neurology, Neurosurgery, and Psychiatry, 78*(11), 1278–1280.

Assessing Coma in the Neurologic Client Using the Full Outline of Un-Responsiveness (FOUR) Score Coma Scale

This tool scores four components of impaired consciousness: eye response, motor response, brainstem reflexes, and respiration. It differs from the Glasgow coma scale by not requiring a verbal response. It is useful for assessing agitated and confused clients without impaired consciousness and those who are alert but unable to respond verbally, including clients who are intubated, stuporous, or comatose. It is also useful for sedated clients (since sedation affects eye opening and motor response, but not brainstem reflexes and respiration) and for clients developing early changes in consciousness who are unable to follow commands, to track examiner's finger movements, and have Cheyne-Stokes respirations.

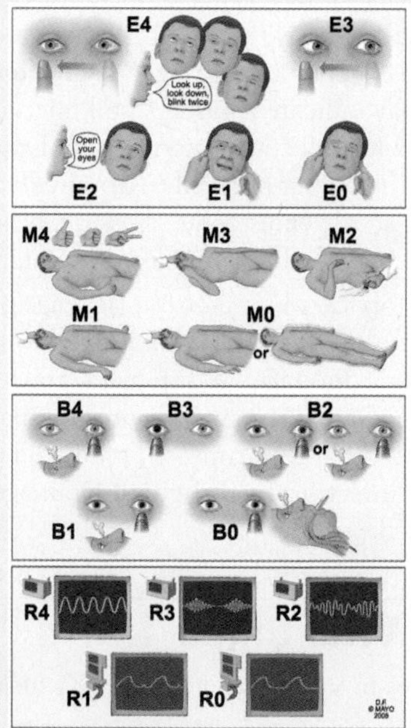

▲ FOUR (Full Outline of Un-Responsiveness) score coma scale is used to assess coma in the neurologic client.
Courtesy of and by permission of Mayo Foundation for Medical Education and Research.

Assessing Coma in the Neurologic Client (FOUR-Score Coma Scale)

Procedure

1. Determine score for each of the four components: 0 is worst response and 4 is best response. Scores are not totaled.
   a. **Assess eye response:** E4 = eyelids open or opened, tracking, or blinking to command; E3 = eyelids open but not tracking; E2 = eyelids closed but open to loud voice; E1 = eyelids closed but open to pain; E0 = eyelids remain closed with pain.
   b. **Assess motor response**: M4 = thumbs-up, fist, or peace sign; M3 = localizing to pain; M2 = flexion response to pain; M1 = extension response to pain; M0 = no response to pain or generalized myoclonus status.
   c. **Assess brainstem reflexes**: B4 = pupil and corneal reflexes present; B3 = one pupil wide and fixed; B2 = pupil or corneal reflexes absent; B1 = pupil and corneal reflexes absent; B0 = absent pupil, corneal, and cough reflex.
   d. **Assess respiratory pattern:** R4 = not intubated, regular breathing pattern; R3 = not intubated, Cheyne-Stokes breathing pattern; R2 = not intubated, irregular breathing; R1 = breathes above ventilatory rate; R0 = breathes at ventilator rate or apnea.

Determining Brain Death

The diagnosis of brain death is a medical–clinical diagnosis based on "irreversible cessation of all functions of the entire brain, including the brainstem: coma (unresponsiveness) with a known cause, absence of brainstem reflexes, and apnea."

- Recovery of neurologic function has not been reported after the clinical diagnosis of brain death has been established using these criteria.
- Minimally acceptable observation period has not been determined.
- Non–brainmediated spontaneous movements (e.g., spinal and deep tendon reflexes) can falsely suggest retained brain function.
- Ventilator triggering may falsely suggest patient-initiated breathing.

Source: Wijdicks, E. F., Varelas, P. N., Gronseth, G. S., Greer, D. M., & American Academy of Neurology. (2010). Evidence-based guideline update: Determining brain death in adults: Report of the Quality Standards Subcommittee of the American Academy of Neurology. *Neurology, 74*(23), 1911–1918.

Determining Brain Death—Assessing for Apnea (CO_2 Challenge)

NOTE: Institutional protocol may vary slightly.

Preparation

1. Determine that client lacks all evidence of responsiveness. ▸ ***Rationale:*** This confirms coma.
2. Determine that cause of coma has been established and is irreversible.
3. Before diagnosis of brain death is attempted, clinical conditions such as acid–base or electrolyte or endocrine disturbance, hypothermia, presence of CNS depressant drugs or alcohol, and recent administration of neuromuscular blockade should be normalized, if possible, since these conditions can confound making diagnosis of brain death.
4. Adjust therapies so that client is normotensive (SBP ≥100 mmHg), normothermic, euvolemic, eucapnic (PCO_2 35–45 mmHg), without history of COPD or severe obesity and has normal PO_2. ▸ ***Rationale:*** The objective of the test is to determine apnea.
5. Determine that client has absence of brainstem reflexes:
   a. Pupil, oculocephalic, oculovestibular, and corneal reflexes
   b. Pharyngeal (gag) and tracheal (cough) reflexes.
   c. Facial muscle movement to noxious stimulus.
   d. Absence of motor response to noxious stimuli in all four limbs.

Procedure

1. Preoxygenate client with 100% oxygen for 10 minutes. ▸ ***Rationale:*** To achieve a $PO_2 \geq 200$ mmHg.
2. Reduce ventilation rate to 10 breaths per minute. ▸ ***Rationale:*** To achieve eucapnia.
3. Reduce ventilator PEEP mode to 5 cm H_2O. (See Chapter 33, Advanced Nursing Skills.)
4. Obtain baseline ABGs if SPO_2 is 95%.
5. Disconnect client from ventilator. ▸ ***Rationale:*** This is the only way to determine apnea.
6. Immediately change to T-Tube with 100% FiO_2 or place small catheter through endotracheal tube to level of carina and deliver 100% O_2 at 6 L/min. ▸ ***Rationale:*** To maintain oxygenation.
7. Physician continuously observes for respiratory effort (chest, abdominal excursion) for 8–10 minutes. ▸ ***Rationale:*** If client shows *any* effort to breathe, respiratory support is reestablished according to agency protocol or consistent with measures predecided by client's family and agency's client advocate.

8. Abort test if SBP decreases to $<$90 mmHg or if SpO_2 is $<$85% for $>$30 seconds and retry procedure with T-piece, CPAP 10 cm H_2O, and 100% O_2 at 12 L/min. ▸ ***Rationale:*** Deterioration of vitals signs and oxygenation should not precede proof of apnea.
9. Repeat ABGs after 8 minutes if no respiratory drive is observed.
10. If no respiratory drive is observed and PCO_2 is 60 mmHg or 20 mmHg over baseline, apnea test result is positive. ▸ ***Rationale:*** These findings support a clinical diagnosis of brain death.
11. Brain death reexamination is not required, but may need to be repeated depending on etiology of coma. Recommended minimal time intervals between first and second clinical examinations:
    a. 6 hr after trauma or hemorrhage.
    b. 24 hr after an anoxic injury.
    c. Time interval may decrease to 12 hr if ancillary test is utilized.
    d. If there is obvious evidence of bilateral brain injury, potentially only one exam is needed to declare brain death.
12. An ancillary test may be performed to confirm brain death. ▸ ***Rationale:*** These may be indicated if uncertainty exists or apnea test cannot be fully performed, but these tests cannot replace a neurologic examination.
    a. Cerebral angiography: positive if there is no intracerebral filling at carotid bifurcation or circle of Willis.
    b. Electroencephalography (EEG): positive if there is no electrical activity throughout 30 minutes of recording.
    c. Transcranial doppler ultrasonography.
    d. Cerebral radionuclide perfusion scan: positive if there is no isotope uptake in brain tissue.
    e. CT angiogram.
    f. MRI/MRA.

Supporting the Family or Caregiver

Procedure

1. Respectfully reinforce that brain death is determined according to established and specific medical–legal criteria. ▸ ***Rationale:*** Some believe that brain death is recoverable or comparable to a coma.
2. Discontinue all medical interventions after brain death is declared. ▸ ***Rationale:*** This is ethically and legally justified.
3. Refer to the remains as a "body" rather than a "patient."
4. Avoid the words "patient," "care," and "treatment" while talking to family members. ▸ ***Rationale:*** It should not be implied that treatment or care is being provided or continued after a person has died.
5. Discontinue conversation with the "body." ▸ ***Rationale:*** Directing thoughts away from the body and toward family needs helps the family understand and accept the reality of death.
6. Encourage the family to talk, touch, and hold if they choose; allow private time.
7. Contact grief counselor or clergy as indicated.
8. Clarify concerns about the deceased donor receiving artificial support:
    a. Use the term "artificial support" in place of "life support."
    b. Clarify that the only justification for continuing artificial support is to maintain organs for transplant.
    c. Reinforce that even though artificial support continues, the equipment is not supporting life, but maintaining body organs.
    d. Reinforce that the time of death is when the client was declared dead, not when donated organs are removed.

NOTE: As many as 60% of deaths from stroke, heart disease, and traumatic brain injury may involve some kind of treatment withdrawal, making it one of the most common pathways to death in the United States.

DOCUMENTATION for Assessment of the Neurologic Client

- Level of consciousness:
  Description of stimulus applied and client's response
  Physician notification of significant changes
  Care measures provided if indicated
- Brainstem reflexes:
  Physician notification of significant changes
  Protective care measures provided if indicated
- Signs of basilar skull fracture:
  Presence of otorrhea, rhinorrhea, Battle's sign, or raccoon eyes
  Altered function of CN VII
  Physician notification
  Protective care measures implemented

- Vital signs:
  Frequency according to agency protocol
  Physician notification of significant changes
- FOUR-Score Coma Scale:
  Record score for each individual component: eye response, motor response, brainstem reflexes, and respiration.
  Scores are not totaled.
- Brain death determination: Physician completes an extensive checklist for determination of brain death, including:
  Prerequisites for brain death determination testing
  Neurologic examination
  Apnea testing
  Ancillary testing
  Time of brain death (time PCO_2 reached target value or time ancillary test is officially interpreted)

Legal Alert

- Brain death is a medical diagnosis made by a physician. State laws and hospital policy may vary on criteria for this diagnosis.
- According to the Uniform Anatomical Gift Act (revised in 2006 in many states), a donor's declared intent to be an organ donor (documented on driver's license) is sufficient evidence of consent for organs removal. Consent of spouse or family, regardless of their objections, is not necessary. This act also requires that hospital personnel ask patients on admission if they would consider being organ donors. If a person dies and didn't declare to be a donor, hospital or medical personnel must ask the person's relatives or surrogates whether they would be interested in donating the person's organs.
- The act allows medical personnel to remove organs without receiving explicit consent from a potential donor or donor's relative as long as medical personnel have made a reasonable effort to discover any objection by the donor or donor's family.

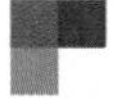

CRITICAL THINKING Application

Expected Outcomes

- Appropriate tools are used to evaluate a neurologic client's level of consciousness.
- Ongoing assessment of a client's brainstem reflexes and vital signs are used to determine compensated versus decompensating neurologic status.
- Signs of possible basilar skull fracture are identified.
- Established criteria are used to determine brain death.
- Supportive communication is provided for family or caregiver of a deceased organ donor.

Unexpected Outcomes	Alternative Actions
Neurologic client's comatose state cannot be determined using Glasgow Coma Scale due to inability to respond verbally.	• Recognize that a nonverbal client cannot respond to parameters assessed using the Glasgow Coma Scale. • Utilize the FOUR-Score Coma Scale to assess separate components of eye response, motor response, brainstem reflexes, and respiration for the nonverbal client.
Client shows signs of decreasing level of consciousness.	• Reassess to validate findings. • Notify physician of findings immediately.
Head injury client with NG tube is having watery drainage from the nose.	• Report finding of rhinorrhea as it may indicate spinal fluid leakage and unrecognized basilar skull fracture. • Change to orogastric tube placement to allow fluid drainage and prevent infection. • Request drainage fluid analysis for chloride level to determine presence of CSF. • Allow fluid to drain freely onto a drip "mustache" dressing.
Family of brain-dead organ donor has difficulty understanding why cardiac monitoring and mechanical ventilation are continued.	• Reinforce that the deceased client has been declared to be brain dead but donated organs are being maintained by supportive measures until time of removal.

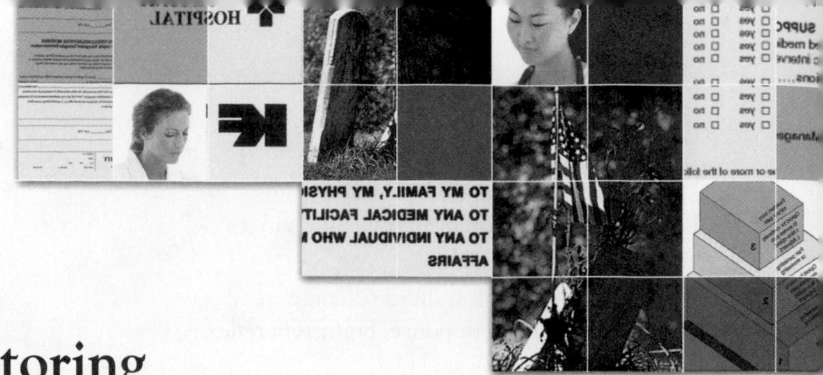

Chapter 32

UNIT ❷

Intracranial Pressure Monitoring and Management

Nursing Process Data

ASSESSMENT Data Base

- Identify signs and symptoms of increasing intracranial pressure.
- Relate signs of intracranial hypertension to rostrocaudal changes in levels of consciousness.
- Identify factors that increase/prevent/manage intracranial hypertension.
- Recognize a normal intracranial pressure waveform.
- Assess indicators of pain in the nonverbal client.
- Utilize a variety of scales to assess a client's level of sedation.
- Monitor functioning and client response to ventricular CSF drainage.

PLANNING Objectives

- To identify early signs of increasing intracranial pressure in the neurologic client
- To differentiate a normal ICP waveform from one indicating decreased cranial compliance
- To provide care that prevents/manages increased ICP.
- To respond to indicators of pain in the nonverbal client
- To provide adequate but minimal depth of sedation in the client with intracranial hypertension

IMPLEMENTATION Procedures

EVALUATION Expected Outcomes

- Signs and symptoms of increasing intracranial pressure are recognized.
- Factors that increase intracranial hypertension are identified.
- Client responds favorably to measures provided to prevent/manage intracranial hypertension.
- Microsensor displays client's intracranial pressure waveform.
- Client responses to pain management and sedation are evaluated.
- Ventriculostomy drains CSF appropriately to manage client's ICP.

Pearson Nursing Student Resources

Find additional review materials at **nursing.pearsonhighered.com**

Prepare for success with NCLEX®-style practice questions and Skill Checklists

Recognizing Signs and Symptoms of Increasing Intracranial Pressure

NOTE: Some of these changes are subtle and may be confused with contextual factors (e.g., interpreting that client is drowsy from fatigue rather than an increasing intracranial pressure).

Procedure

1. Assess change in level of consciousness (LOC). ▸ ***Rationale:*** Change in LOC is the most sensitive indicator of increasing ICP. Change may be sudden, dramatic, or very subtle.
2. Assess for headache. ▸ ***Rationale:*** Headache can be due to pressure on surrounding tissues, including the cerebral arteries, veins, and cranial nerves. Headache due to increased ICP worsens with activities that increase intrathoracic/intracranial pressure: coughing, straining, bearing down, etc.
3. Assess for vomiting. ▸ ***Rationale:*** Vomiting that is due to increased ICP typically occurs *without nausea*, is unexpected, is projectile, and is due to direct pressure on vagal motor centers located in the fourth ventricle in the medulla.
4. Assess for change in visual responses. ▸ ***Rationale:*** Altered responses of cranial nerves (II, III, IV, and VI) that are under pressure from brain swelling cause loss of visual acuity or eye movement. Altered pupillary (CN III) response, ipsilateral (same side) pupil dilation due to head injury, early sign of uncal herniation on side of injury, and altered level of consciousness may accompany or soon follow.
5. Assess for decrease in motor function. ▸ ***Rationale:*** Contralateral (opposite side) hemiparesis (weakness) and hemiplegia (paralysis) due to pressure increases in right and left hemispheres.
6. Assess for abnormal posturing that occurs due to noxious stimuli or spontaneously. ▸ ***Rationale:*** Decorticate (abnormal flexion) response indicates lesion above the brainstem (see Chapter 11, Physical Assessment, for description). Decerebrate (abnormal extension) response indicates brainstem lesion.

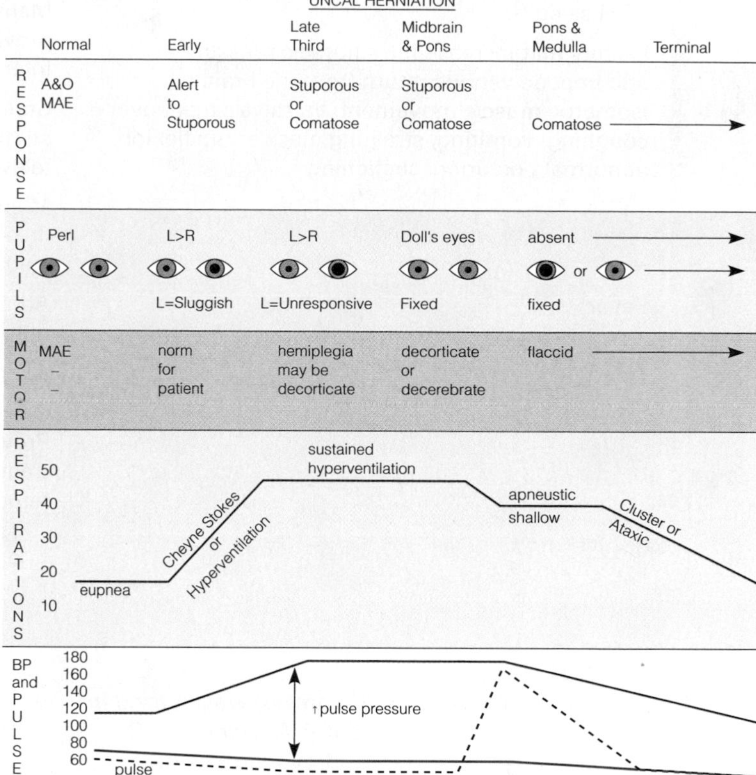

▲ Central herniation differs: deterioration of LOC precedes contralateral hemiparesis.

7. Assess for change in vital signs. ▸ ***Rationale:*** Change in vital signs can be due to increased pressure on thalamus, hypothalamus, pons, and medulla. Changes in respiratory pattern occur early. Cushing's triad: Increasing systolic blood pressure, widened pulse pressure, and slow heart rate, indicating medullary ischemia are late signs of decompensation.

Clinical Alert

It is always best to rule on the side of caution and notify the attending physician of changes so that appropriate care decisions can be made.

Factors That Affect Intracranial Pressure

Factors That Increase ICP (Goal is < 20 mmHg)	Measures to Prevent/Manage Increased ICP
Clustered nursing care activities	Note client's ICP response to various activities and space activities/procedures to allow ICP to return to baseline.
Hypotension SBP $\leq$ 90 to 120 mmHg (*goal is 140–160 mmHg*) CPP $<$ 60 mmHg (*goal is $>$ 60–70 mmHg*)	Administer IV fluids, pressor agents (norepinephrine), osmotic diuretic, hypertonic saline, CFS drainage if ICP is $>$ 20 mmHg Surgical decompressive craniectomy for ICP persistently $>$35 mmHg.
Hypoxemia (*goal is $SpO_2 > 90$ mmHg*) Increased/decreased PCO_2 (*goal is 35 mmHg*) Acidemia (low arterial blood pH) MAP $<$ 85 mmHg (*goal is to support CPP $>$60–70 mmHg*) Ventilator dyssynchrony	Promote oxygenation: Monitor and maintain $SpO_2 > 90\%$ with supplemental oxygen; determine whether desaturation occurs with a particular client position; maintain patent airway; suction PRN using prophylactic lidocaine and pre- and post-hyperoxygenation. Monitor breath sounds for atelectasis/infiltration. Provide chest percussion therapy; obtain chest x-ray; consult respiratory care practitioner regarding client/ventilator harmony.

Noxious stimuli, emotional upset	
REM sleep	Manage pain: assess for signs of pain in nonverbal client; provide analgesia; provide sedation at lowest doses with daily interruption.
Factors that increase intrathoracic pressure and impede venous return from the brain: isometric muscle movement, Valsalva's maneuver coughing, vomiting, straining, neck or hip flexion, abnormal posturing, suctioning	Control environment: maintain calm, quiet room; minimize stimulation; limit visitation; avoid prolonged hand-holding; no television Maintain positioning: head in neutral alignment without flexion or rotation. HOB elevation ≥30° if hemodynamically stable and CPP maintained; avoid hip flexion.
Fever	Administer antiemetics, antipyretics; initiate early enteral nutrition. Promote elimination: administer stool softeners; initiate a bowel program. Provide prophylactic induced hypothermia for 48+ hr for traumatic brain injury; cooling blanket for increased temperature (avoid shivering).

Clinical Alert

Hyperventilation ($PaCO_2 < 25$ mmHg) was utilized in the past to manage increased ICP. A lowered $PaCO_2$ constricts cerebral arteries, and by the rules of the Monro-Kelly Doctrine, the ICP is lowered. This is used only briefly as a bridge to move appropriate therapy because constricting the cerebral arteries leads to ischemia, further damage, and edema.

NOTE: Sensitivity to and ongoing communication with the neurologic client and family are important aspects of care. Help the family understand that a healing brain needs little stimulation (avoid constant hand-holding and stimuli such as television, limit visitation, etc.). Family members may experience an extreme feeling of powerlessness; the client's injury may result in disabilities that have far-reaching implications on family dynamics.

EVIDENCE-BASED PRACTICE

The high-tech world of the ICU has historically introduced technology before its effects on outcome could be studied. Intracranial pressure (ICP) monitoring has not been proven to clearly improve outcomes in all patient populations in which it is utilized. Further testing of ICP versus CPP as treatment goals is another area for future research.

Source: Littlejohns, L. R., & Bader, M. K. (2009). *AACN/AANN protocols for practice: "Monitoring technologies in critically ill neuroscience patients."* Sudbury, MA: Jones and Bartlett.

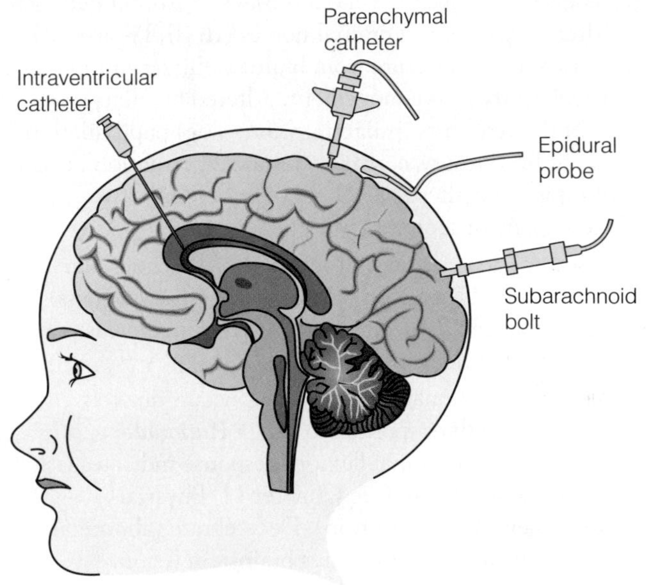

▲ Sites for ICP monitoring.

Assisting Surgeon to Insert ICP Microsensor (Fiberoptic Transducer-Tipped Catheter)

Equipment

- PPE: Sterile surgical gown, mask with face shield or eye protection, cap
- Sterile gloves for surgeon and nurse
- Sterile tray
- Prepared medication for sedation, if ordered
- Hair clippers
- Cranial access kit with hand drill
- 1% or 2% lidocaine without epinephrine
- 3-mL syringe with 18-gauge needle for withdrawal

25-gauge needle for topical anesthetic injection
Chlorhexidine-based antimicrobial scrub/wipes
Scalpel with #11 blade
Sterile drape/towels
Clean gloves
Microsensor (fiberoptic transducer-tipped bolt catheter)
External ICP microsensor monitor and monitoring cable to connect microprocessor to primary bedside monitor system
Needle drivers
2.0 silk suture
Sterile 2 × 2 gauze
Sterile clear occlusive dressing
Permanent marker

Preparation

1. Validate that client's informed consent has been obtained.
2. Perform hand hygiene.
3. Check client's identification band and have client state name and birth date, if possible.
4. Explain rationale for procedure to client.
5. Validate that client has an established peripheral IV site. ▶ ***Rationale:*** For administration of emergency fluids or medication if needed.
6. Validate that client has established arterial blood pressure monitoring. ▶ ***Rationale:*** To determine the MAP, which is used along with the ICP to calculate cerebral perfusion pressure (CPP).
7. Prepare and assemble external monitoring system following manufacturer's instructions.
8. Raise the bed height to comfortable working position.
9. Don clean gloves.
10. Clip and save client's hair and scrub selected site with antimicrobial solution. ***Rationale***: Client's hair should not be discarded, but should be returned to client or family.
11. Administer additional medication for sedation if ordered.

Procedure

1. Open sterile gloves and gown for surgeon.
2. Open sterile drape for surgeon.
3. Place cranial access kit, microsensor, and suturing materials on sterile tray within surgeon's reach.
4. Assist the surgeon to numb client's scalp.
5. Maintain cervical alignment while surgeon dissects the skin, drills the skull, and places microsensor.
   a. Before the microsensor is placed in the parenchyma, it must be zeroed. This can only be done once before the microsensor is placed and secured. ▶ ***Rationale:*** After insertion, there is no need for zero-referencing while the catheter is in use.
   b. Surgeon submerges the end of the sensor in an aqueous solution that is inside the sterile field.
   c. Zero the sensor by surgeon's request. The microsensor will give a reference number.

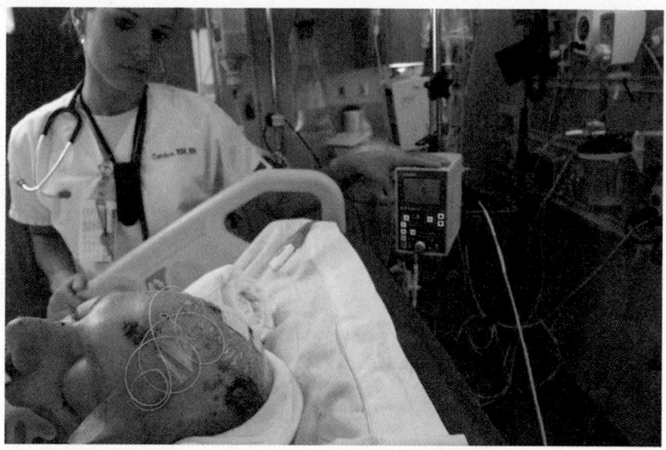

▲ ICP microsensor (fiberoptic catheter) senses changes in ICP. This system may be used to measure intraventricular parenchymal, subdural, or epidural pressure.

   d. Document reference number on the transducer using a permanent marker. ▶ ***Rationale:*** Used as reference if cables are disconnected for transport.
6. Don sterile gloves to assist surgeon as necessary.
7. After insertion, surgeon sutures microsensor in place. (Microsensor can be inserted into the lateral ventricle, subarachnoid space, subdural space, brain parenchyma, or under a bone flap.)
8. Site is covered with clear occlusive dressing (2 × 2 gauze optional).
9. Hand external monitor cable to surgeon.
10. Connect the external monitor to a central monitoring system to verify that a waveform is present.
11. Record ICP and calculated CPP (MAP − ICP = CPP).
12. Discard disposable equipment.
13. Dispose of gloves and perform hand hygiene.

Clinical Alert

Increased intracranial pressure can decrease blood flow to the brain. Pressures within various locations in the cranium vary. The closer the ventricular catheter to the pathology, the higher the ICP and more accurate and reliable the reading.

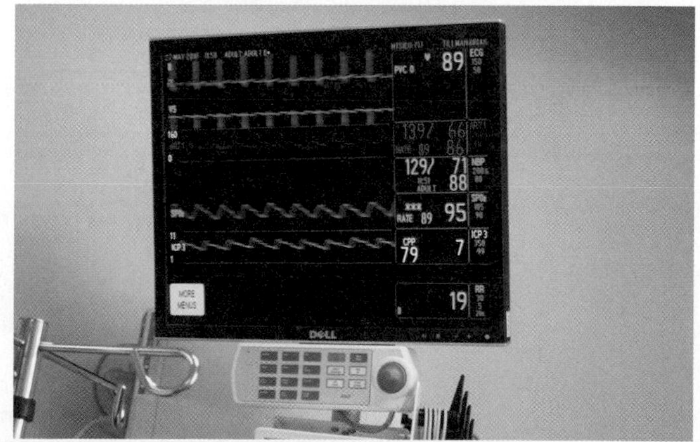

▲ Monitor displays digital readouts and pressure waveforms of the ECG, arterial BP, SPO_2 and calculated CPP (MAP–ICP = CCP).

Intracranial pressure waveforms reflect transmission of arterial and venous pressure through cerebrospinal fluid and brain tissue. A normal ICP waveform has three pressure peaks:

P1 reflects myocardial systole (arterial blood flow)

P2 reflects myocardial diastole (drop in systolic blood flow) and coincides with the arterial dicrotic notch.

P3 follows the dicrotic notch (closure of the aortic valve) and correlates with venous pressure.

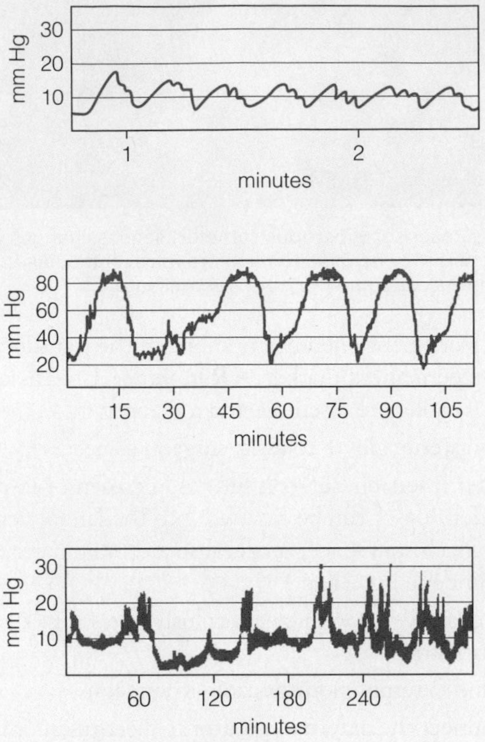

▲ Intracranial pressure waveforms.

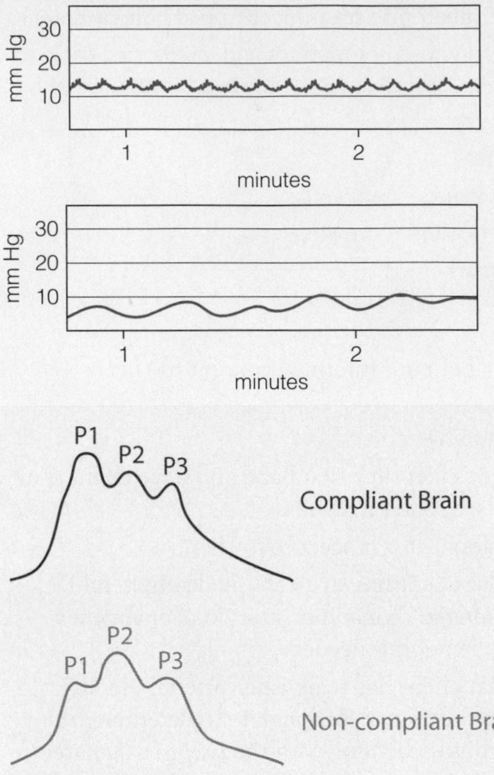

▲ Increased P2 wave.

NOTE: P2 elevation greater than P1 (P2:P1 >0.8) demonstrates an increase in intracranial pressure and loss of intracerebral compliance, especially when ICP is >10 mmHg. Frequent neurologic assessments are indicated. Changes in client status should be reported to the physician immediately.

EVIDENCE-BASED PRACTICE

This study (sample of 28 patients undergoing ICP monitoring) demonstrated that mechanical chest percussion used to treat and prevent pneumonia does not increase intracranial pressure and can be performed safely on neurologically injured patients at risk for intracranial hypertension.

Olson, D. M., Thoyre, S.M., Bennett, S. N., Stoner, J. B., & Graffagnino, C. (2009). Effect of mechanical chest percussion on intracranial pressure: A pilot study. *American Journal of Critical Care*, *18*(4), 330–335.

Monitoring Client Response to Pain

Medscape	www.medscape.com		
Indicator	**Description**	**Score**	
Facial expression	No muscular tension observed	Relaxed neutral	0
	Presence of frowning, brow lowering orbit tightening, and elevator contraction	Tense	1
	All of the above facial movements plus eyelid tightly closed	Grimacing	2
Body movements	Does not move at all (does not necessarily mean absence of pain)	Absence of movements	0
	Slow, cautious movements, touching or rubbing the pain site, seeking attention through movements	Protection	1
	Pulling tube, attempting to sit up, moving limbs thrashing, not following commands, striking at staff, trying to climb out of bed	Restlessness	2

Medscape	www.medscape.com		
Indicator	**Description**	**Score**	
Muscle tension Evaluation by passive flexion and extension of upper extremities	No resistance to passive movements	Relaxed	0
	Resistance to passive movements	Tense, rigid	1
	Strong resistance to passive movements, inability to complete them	Very tense or rigid	2
Compliance with ventilator (intubated patients)	Alarms not activated, easy ventilation	Tolerating ventilator or movement	0
	Alarms stop spontanesously	Coughing but tolerating	1
OR	Asynchrony: blocking ventilation, alarms frequently activated	Fighting ventilator	2
Vocalization (extubated patients)	Taking in normal tone or no sound	Taking in normal tone or no sound	0
	Sighing, moaning	Sighing, moaning	1
	Crying out, sobbing	Crying out, sobbing	2
Total range			0–8

NOTE: *The Critical Care Pain Observation Tool* has demonstrated acceptable validity and reliability for use with both verbal and nonverbal clients.

Source: American Association of Critical-Care Nurses. (2008). *American Journal of Critical Care.*

Monitoring Client Response to Sedation

Equipment

Sedation scales

Procedure

1. Consider nonpharmacologic interventions: (gentle touch, reassuring voice; frequent repositioning; use of distraction, music therapy, environmental control; use of complementary therapies such as massage) before sedation is initiated. ▸ ***Rationale:*** This may reduce or eliminate the need for sedation and muscle relaxation.
2. Select sedation scale to use for ongoing assessment and documentation of client response to pharmacologic intervention. ▸ ***Rationale:*** The selected scale should be used consistently and routinely by all caregivers.
   a. *Ramsay Sedation Scale* (goal 2–3) assesses rousability and is useful whenever sedative drugs or narcotics are administered, but cannot be used for the client receiving neuromuscular blocking drugs.
   b. *Riker Sedation-Agitation Scale* (goal 3–4) differs from the Ramsay Sedation Scale by defining degrees of agitation.
   c. *Richmond Agitation Sedation Scale* (goal –2 to –3) distinguishes between responses to verbal and physical stimuli. This 10-level scale has confirmed validity and reliability for use in sedated and nonsedated clients.
   d. *AACN Sedation Assessment Scale* is most comprehensive, evaluating five domains: consciousness, agitation, anxiety, sleep, and client-ventilator synchrony.
3. The Institute for Healthcare Improvement recommends "the use of dosing protocols and automatic dose reductions for benzodiazepines and other sedatives and hypnotics in target (e.g., ICU) populations." Daily sedation interruption is conducted to allow assessment of neurologic status.

Clinical Alert

Most neurologic clients have normal lungs, but may require mechanical ventilation due to lack of airway protection (swallow, cough) secondary to neuronal injury, the secondary effects of increased ICP due to the primary injury/pathology, neurogenic pulmonary edema, a concomitant pulmonary process, or management with sedative medication. ICP and CPP can be adversely affected by positive pressure ventilation and must be monitored closely. Extubation should not be delayed solely on the basis of depressed neurologic function.

EVIDENCE-BASED PRACTICE

Intermittent lightening of sedation and daily interruption of sedation (withholding all sedative and analgesic medications until patients are awake) limits excessive sedation, reduces duration of mechanical ventilation and length of ICU stay, reduces the number of neuro-diagnostic tests, and reduces frequency of complications associated with critical illness. This practice has benefits, but is underutilized due to a number of barriers that prevent its incorporation into clinical practice.

Dotson, B. (2010). Daily interruption of sedation in patients treated with mechanical ventilation. *American Journal of Health-System Pharmacy*. 67 (12). 102–1006.

Assisting Surgeon to Insert a Ventriculostomy Catheter

NOTE: ICP-lowering therapy is initiated with pressures above 20 mmHg.

Equipment

PPE: Sterile surgical gown, mask with face shield or eye protection, cap
Sterile gloves for surgeon and nurse
Clean gloves
Sterile tray
Hair clippers
Cranial access kit with hand drill
2% lidocaine with epinephrine (local anesthetic)
3-mL syringe with 18-gauge needle for withdrawal
25-gauge needle for topical anesthetic injection
Sedative to be administered if indicated
Chlorhexidine-based antimicrobial scrub/wipes
Sterile drape or towels
Twist drill and bits
Scalpel with #11 blade
Needle drivers
2.0 silk suture
Intraventricular catheter
Sterile 2 × 2 gauze (optional)
Sterile clear occlusive dressing
20-mL syringe filled with preservative-free sterile saline for flushing system
IV pole
CFS drainage system (collection tubing, chamber, and bag)
Transducer (see Chapter 33, Advanced Nursing Skills)

Preparation

1. Validate that client's informed consent has been obtained.
2. Perform hand hygiene.
3. Check client's identification band and have client state name and birth date, if possible.
4. Explain rationale for procedure to client.
5. Validate that client has an established peripheral IV site. ▸ ***Rationale:*** For administration of emergency fluids or medication if needed.
6. Prepare and assemble monitoring system (transducer and stopcocks) following manufacturer's instructions.
7. Level and zero monitoring system with air-fluid interface of zeroing stopcock level with client's foramen of Monro (level of client's tragus) or higher as determined by surgeon. ▸ ***Rationale:*** For accuracy, the same point should be used consistently for all ICP readings.

NOTE: The transducer must be releveled with any change in client's head position if continuous drainage is performed.

8. Remove tubing attached to an IV bag that establishes a pressurized flush system and discard.
9. Replace flush system with a 20-mL syringe filled with preservative-free sterile saline. ▸ ***Rationale:*** Preservatives added to medication vials are neurotoxic.
10. Flush all lumens and transducer with flush solution and leave syringe attached.
11. Raise bed to a comfortable working position.
12. Don clean gloves
13. Clip and save client's hair. ▸ ***Rationale:*** Client's hair should be returned to client or family.
14. Scrub selected site with antimicrobial solution.
15. If applicable, administer additional medications for sedation.

Procedure

1. Open sterile gloves and gown for surgeon.
2. Open sterile drape for surgeon.
3. Place cranial access kit, ventriculostomy, and suturing materials on sterile tray within surgeon's reach.
4. Don sterile gloves to assist surgeon as necessary.
5. Assist surgeon to numb client's scalp.
6. Maintain cervical alignment while surgeon dissects the skin, drills the skull, and places ventriculostomy drain.
7. Surgeon caps the drain once it is in place.
8. Surgeon sutures drain in place and applies clear occlusive dressing (2 × 2 gauze optional).
9. Hand surgeon the primed line to the drainage system to attach it to the client.
10. Position drain as directed by the surgeon.

Ventriculostomy Drainage System

This external drainage system is used to intermittently or continuously drain CSF from the ventricles of the brain or the lumbar subarachnoid space to a drainage bag. System components facilitate CSF drainage, CSF sampling, and ICP monitoring.

Components of the system include:

- Closed sterile fluid path.
- Height-adjustable, calibrated burette with stopcock which provides view of flow and clarity of the CSF, and allows reading volume of CSF before fluid enters the drainage bag.
- Drainage bag with needleless sampling site.
- Fluid-filled ICP monitoring transducer can be attached to the *red* capped port of the patient stopcock at the zero reference position to show drainage pressure.

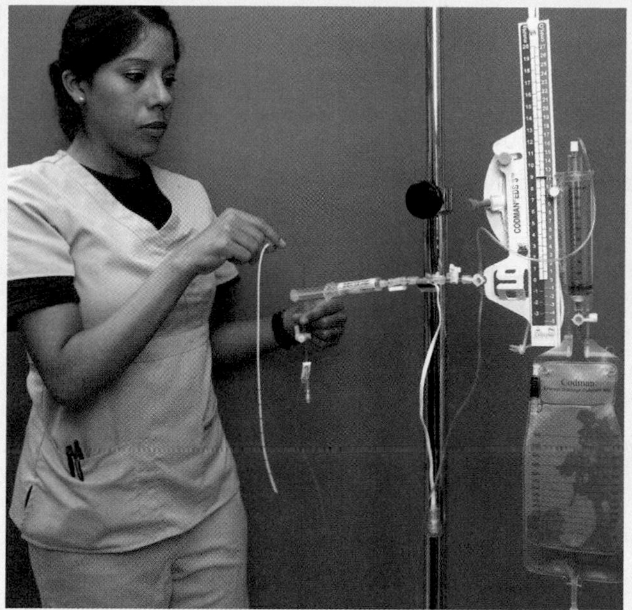

▲ Ventriculostomy catheter: nurse with drainage system.

Lumbar Subarachnoid CSF Drainage

Based on the same principles and setup as ventriculostomy drainage, lumbar puncture placement (L4–L5) of a catheter into the subarachnoid space may be performed to lower CSF pressure to allow a dural tear to heal (e.g., basilar fracture with otorrhea that persists 4–5 days).

1. The catheter is connected to a closed system to allow intermittent or continuous CSF drainage to divert CSF away from the site of the leak, lower CSF pressure, and allow the site to heal.
2. The zero reference point is the insertion site with the bed flat and client supine.
3. Drainage bag height is manipulated to drain the prescribed volume each hour (e.g., 10–20 mL/hr) based on CSF production of 20–30 mL/hr.
4. If the drainage bag is lowered, more CSF is drained.
5. The drain must be clamped if the client sits up.

11. Calculate and record ICP/CPP readings hourly. ▸***Rationale:*** To determine adequate cerebral blood flow.
12. Return drain to open position for continuous drainage of excess CSF or open closed system intermittently to drain CSF when ICP exceeds set limits. ▸***Rationale:*** Reducing CSF volume improves cerebral perfusion.
13. Discard disposable equipment.
14. Dispose of gloves and perform hand hygiene.

NOTE: If leakage persists for 4–5 days, lumbar CSF drainage may be necessary to allow resolution of dural tear. (See Lumbar Subarachnoid CSF Drainage.)

Clinical Alert

Never flush a ventriculostomy or lumbar drain toward the client. This would increase risk for infection. Additionally, instilling medications (including saline) is not within the scope of nursing practice.

EVIDENCE-BASED PRACTICE

Parenteral Nutrition in the Critically Ill Client

Bedrest and neuromuscular blockade during mechanical ventilation result in skeletal muscle wasting and inhibit protein anabolic processes. Drugs such as corticosteroids increase skeletal muscle breakdown, vasopressors decrease splanchnic blood flow, and diuretics increase excretion of electrolytes, minerals, and water-soluble vitamins. Multiple stressors increase energy expenditure and need for protein and micronutrients. Early initiation of appropriate nutrition is important for brain repair; malnutrition can contribute to cerebral edema. Most critically ill clients who require specialized nutrition (85%–90%) can be fed enterally via gastric/intestinal tube. If enteral nutrition is contraindicated (10%–15%), complete parenteral nutrition may be provided to support vital cellular and organ function, immunity, tissue repair, protein synthesis, and capacity of skeletal, cardiac, and respiratory muscles.

Source: Ziegler, T. (2009). Parenteral nutrition in the critically ill patient. *New England Journal of Medicine*, *361*, 11.

Ventilator-Associated Pneumonia

Mechanically ventilated neurologic clients are especially susceptible to ventilator-associated pneumonia (VAP) due to decreased level of consciousness, an unprotected airway, and inability to swallow properly. Monitoring devices, ventriculostomy, disease processes, and inability to temporarily stop sedation for clients with increased ICP preclude some VAP prevention strategies.

Source: Fields, L. B. (2008). Oral care intervention to reduce incidence of ventilator-associated pneumonia in the neurologic intensive care unit. *Journal of Neuroscience Nursing*, 40(5), 291–298.

Oral Care for Ventilator Clients

Oral health deteriorates significantly during intubation and improves to near baseline levels 48 hr after extubation. Intubation is associated with an increase in oral gram-negative bacteria and yeast and risk of ventilator-associated pneumonia. This study demonstrated that providing oral care does not seem to affect intracranial pressure adversely.

Prendergast, V., Hallberg, I., Jahnke, H., Kleiman, C., & Hagell, P. (2009). Oral health, ventilator-associated pneumonia, and intracranial pressure in intubated patients in a neuroscience intensive care unit. *American Journal of Critical Care*, 18(4), 368–376.

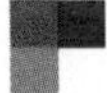

DOCUMENTATION for Intracranial Pressure Monitoring and Management

- Surgeon placing the microsensor or CSF drain (ventriculostomy)
- Location of microsensor or CSF drain placement
- Medications administered
- Client's tolerance of procedure
- Appearance of insertion site
- Dressing applied
- Client position during obtained measurements
- Obtained measurements: ICP and calculated CPP
- Amount and color of CSF drainage from ventriculostomy
- Appearance of the site, dressing, and length of monitoring/drainage catheter insertion site
- Interventions used to manipulate ICP/CPP if indicated

CRITICAL THINKING Application

Expected Outcomes

- Signs and symptoms of increased intracranial pressure are recognized.
- Factors that increase intracranial hypertension are identified.
- Measures to prevent/manage intracranial hypertension are initiated.
- Microsensor displays intracranial pressure waveform.
- Client responses to pain management and sedation are evaluated.
- Ventriculostomy drains appropriately to manage client's ICP.

Unexpected Outcomes	Alternative Actions
Client is very agitated with frequent nonpurposeful movements, despite increased frequency of sedative administration.	• Try to find a cause for the client's change in behavior. • Attempt an analgesic trial to determine whether the client's pain is managed. This trial may be therapeutic as well as diagnostic.
Microsensor fails to display a waveform.	• Verify that cable to the monitor and monitor cable are functioning appropriately and all connections are secure. • Reassess length of microsensor exiting insertion site. If microsensor has migrated from the parenchyma, it will no longer give an appropriate waveform.
Ventriculostomy drain shows a waveform but does not drain.	• Client may not have excess CSF that needs to be drained. Lower drain below the tragus until two to three drops of CSF are drained to ensure patency still remains. If patent, return drain to the ordered position. If no drops of CSF are released, notify the physician. • Do not strip tubing even if clots are visible. Stripping causes increased negative pressure and microbleeds and tears can occur.

The ventriculostomy drain fails to display a waveform.	• The drain might be clotted; lower drain as directed above to verify patency. • Verify all clamps and stopcocks are positioned in an open to the monitor position. • Verify that the cable to the monitor and monitor cable are functioning appropriately and all connections are secure. • Reassess length of drain exiting the insertion site. If the drain has become dislodged from the ventricle, it will no longer give an appropriate waveform. In this instance, it is rare that there will still be drainage of excess CSF.
Ventriculostomy drain insertion site dressing is damp.	• Inspect system for leaks. • Suspect CSF leak (test for glucose in fluid or chloride concentration if draining includes blood). • Apply new sterile occlusive dressing over insertion site. • Notify physician.
Ventriculostomy drainage bag has sudden increase in CSF.	• Immediately check for inadvertent placement of bag below prescribed level; rapid drainage can cause ventricular collapse and intracerebral hemorrhage. • Immediately reposition drainage bag to appropriate level. • Discuss benefits of intermittent rather than continuous drainage.

GERONTOLOGIC Considerations

Neurologic Disorders Are the Most Common Cause of Disability in Older Adults.

- While age-related changes do not follow a predictable course, normal neurologic system changes due to aging include:

  Decreased brain size but no decline of intelligence with age

  Alterations of thermoregulation (reduced heat production, increased heat loss)

  Slower fine-motor movement

  Diminished deep tendon and gag reflexes and vibratory sense

  Reduced ability to respond to multiple stimuli

  Slowed righting reflexes

  Smaller pupil size

  Reduced stage 3 and 4 sleep

  Modest reduction in ability to learn new things

- The brain atrophies with age, leading to an increase in space between the skull and the brain and an increase in size of ventricles. This increased space can result in greater risk for cerebral contusions and cerebral vessel damage with acceleration/deceleration injuries. Damage can also be compounded if the patient is taking an anticoagulant.
- Older clients are less likely to experience common symptoms of increased intracranial pressure (e.g., headache) and more likely to demonstrate mental status changes.
- Pathology of any organ system can precipitate neurologic dysfunction in an older client.
- As many as 60% of older hospitalized clients may experience delirium.
- Lethargy and confusion may be indications of infection among the elderly.

MANAGEMENT Guidelines

Each state legislates a Nurse Practice Act for RNs and LVN/LPNs. Healthcare facilities are responsible for establishing and implementing policies and procedures that conform to their state's regulations. Verify the regulations and role parameters for each healthcare worker in your facility.

Delegation

All personnel in the critical care setting must know how to quickly summon assistance and locate and use emergency/resuscitation equipment.

In advanced care settings, the RN simultaneously assesses, analyzes, makes decisions, intervenes, and evaluates clients on a continual basis. Complexities of care and unpredictability of outcomes necessitate *intense* ongoing client monitoring and evaluation and personal continuing education. Detection and interpretation of subtle areas of change in the client's status require the knowledge and skill of the professional nurse.

- Collaboration with the physician and respiratory care practitioner helps to support client's weaning from mechanical ventilation.
- The nurse should not assume care for any client who requires care beyond the caregiver's expertise.
- Many agencies provide emergency care protocols or standing orders of action responses to specified changes in client status. The professional nurse must be familiar with conditions for which the nurse is delegated medical care decisions guided by such protocols.
    - It is the responsibility of nursing faculty to ensure that students participating in client care (in any setting) are prepared to do so. Likewise, it is the duty of the student to refuse to perform a function he or she is not qualified or competent to perform.
    - The UAP providing personal care for the neurologic client must space activities and maintain a controlled environment to prevent overstimulation and fatigue.
    - The UAP must understand that continuous HOB elevation with the neck in neutral position is to be maintained for the neurologic client with external ventricular drainage, while the client with a lumbar drain remains supine with the bed flat.
    - The UAP must know to leave an arterial catheter site uncovered for easy observation.
- The UAP must not move tubing drainage receptacles (e.g., ventriculostomy drip chamber).
- The UAP must understand that IVs, drainage systems, and ventilator circuits and systems are closed and must be able to give care without disrupting system integrity or disconnecting components for the convenience of care (e.g., as in changing the client's gown or position).
- The UAP has a limited role in the care of clients who require invasive monitoring. The UAP can offer valued assistance in moving/positioning clients and providing personal hygiene and comfort measures under the direction of the professional nurse.
- The UAP assists the client, preserving an interface between technology and reality, by providing a human dimension of tactile presence while providing basic physical care for clients requiring sophisticated technological monitoring. This link assists all caregivers in their attempts to minimize client's feelings of alienation.

Communication Matrix

Although certain tasks may be delegated, the UAP also can provide vital data to the professional nurse by immediately *reporting*:

- Disconnected systems, loose electrodes, tubing leaks, wet/soiled dressings
- Subjective or objective change in the client's status (e.g., pain, restlessness, respiratory distress, acute change in cognition)
- Equipment alarms (e.g., ventilator alarms)
- Near-empty infusion bags
- Near-full collection devices

CRITICAL THINKING Strategies

Scenario 1

A 27-year-old male has been admitted to the neuro trauma ICU after surgical evacuation of a right parietal epidural hematoma that occurred secondary to a linear skull fracture sustained in a motorcycle accident.

1. Where does an epidural bleed occur and what is the typical source of bleeding?
2. How does an epidural hematoma differ from a subdural hematoma?
3. What behaviors/deficits might occur with injury to the right parietal lobe?
4. What signs would indicate uncal herniation due to increasing intracranial pressure?
5. List five nursing interventions that can help prevent increased intracranial pressure.

Scenario 2

A young man has been admitted to the trauma unit after evaluation in the ED and repair of a scalp laceration sustained when he was struck in the back of the head with a baseball. No cervical spine injury, internal injury, or skull fracture was identified. He had no motor or sensory deficits. Ongoing observation and neurologic assessments were indicated since the client had experienced a brief loss of consciousness and continued to have vertigo, irritability, and nausea. His Glasgow Coma Score was 13.

At 0400 the nurse awakened him for vital signs and neuro assessment and noticed a bloody stain circled by yellow discoloration on his pillowcase. It had apparently come from his ear. Drainage from the ear (otorrhea) typically results from head injury involving basal skull fracture.

1. Why was the diagnosis of basilar skull fracture missed on initial evaluation in the ED?
2. How can it be determined that the drainage includes CSF?
3. What is the major potential complication of CSF leakage?
4. How should the client be positioned?

5. How should the drainage be managed?
6. What is the typical medical management if CSF leakage persists?
7. Compare the principles of lumbar drainage and external ventricular drainage.
8. Contrast the care of a client with a lumbar drain versus one with a ventriculostomy.

NCLEX® Review Questions

Unless otherwise specified, choose only one (1) answer.

1. A client with a blood pressure of 130/80 and an intracranial pressure of 12mm Hg would have a cerebral perfusion pressure of
   1. 65.
   2. 80.
   3. 85.
   4. 97.
2. The nurse caring for a neurologic client obtains an ICP reading of 12mmHg. The nurse understands this reading reflects
   1. A severe decrease in cerebral perfusion pressure.
   2. A marked decrease in the CSF production.
   3. Normal balance of brain, blood, and CSF.
   4. A malfunction of autoregulation.
3. A client has been admitted to the hospital with a suspected brain tumor. The family report him being hateful, having outbursts of cursing, and right sided hemiparesis. These behaviors indicate that the tumor is affecting the
   1. Frontal lobe.
   2. Parietal lobe.
   3. Occipital lobe.
   4. Temporal lobe.
4. Metabolic causes of coma can be differentiated from structural causes. Metabolic causes are characterized by having
   1. Rostrocaudal deterioration.
   2. Asymmetric motor deficits.
   3. Motor deficits preceding coma.
   4. Preserved pupil reflexes.
5. Factors that lead to cerebral vasodilation and increased intracranial pressure include
   1. Hypocapnea (low PCO2).
   2. Alkalemia (low blood pH).
   3. Hypoxemia (low blood O2).
   4. Hypothermia.
6. Pressure on the midbrain would be expected to be accompanied by
   1. Loss of gag reflex.
   2. Loss of pupil response.
   3. Widening pulse pressure.
   4. Loss of blink reflex.
7. The most sensitive indicator of increasing intracranial pressure is
   1. Altered level of consciousness.
   2. Change in respiratory pattern.
   3. Lack of pupil response to light stimulus.
   4. Increase in blood pressure with slowed heart rat
8. A ventriculostomy is the most reliable system used to monitor intracranial pressure. This method includes:
   1. A subarachnoid bolt or screw.
   2. An intraventricular catheter with external drainage system and transducer.
   3. An intraparenchymal fiberoptic transducer-tipped catheter
   4. A subdural or epidural catheter.
9. ICP monitoring provides guidance in managing ICP elevations and hemodynamic status. Normal intracranial pulse waveforms are characterized by:
   1. P-2 waveform greater than P-1 and P-3.
   2. All waveforms of equal elevation.
   3. P-3 waveform greater than P-1 and P-2.
   4. P-1 waveform greater than P-2 and P-3.
10. Which of the following ancillary tests are used to confirm brain death?
    1. Spinal fluid analysis and cold calorics test.
    2. EEG and Cerebral angiography.
    3. MRI and brainstem reflexes.
    4. Deep tendon reflexes and blood pressure.

33

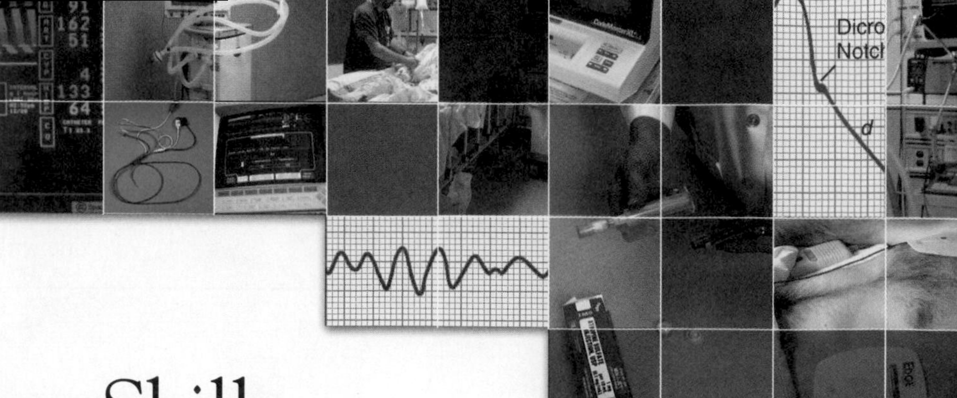

Advanced Nursing Skills

LEARNING OBJECTIVES

1. List hemodynamic information obtained by means of a pulmonary artery (balloon-tipped flow-directed) catheter.
2. Discuss the purpose and method for leveling and zeroing the monitor.
3. Differentiate waveforms for pulmonary artery and pulmonary capillary wedge pressures.
4. State three ways to troubleshoot pulmonary artery catheter problems.
5. Describe the rationale for arterial blood pressure monitoring.
6. Outline the steps in performing the Modified Allen's test.
7. Identify a normal arterial blood pressure waveform.
8. Explain the procedure for obtaining a blood sample from an arterial line.
9. Outline safety precautions for the client with an arterial line.
10. Explain how the intraaortic balloon pump assists cardiac function.
11. Describe nursing responsibilities in anticipating and responding to cardiac emergencies.
12. Ensure client and staff safety during electrical countershock procedures.
13. Differentiate various ventilator support "modes."
14. Discuss nursing care needs of the mechanically ventilated client.
15. Describe the process of weaning a client from mechanical ventilation to independent breathing.

CHAPTER OUTLINE

TERMINOLOGY

Adjunctive accessory to or assisting with.

Afterload resistance against which the heart must pump to eject blood during systole. Pulmonary vascular resistance (PVR) presents afterload to the right heart; systemic vascular resistance (SVR) presents afterload to the left heart.

Barotrauma alveolar injury and air leak due to positive pressure mechanical ventilation.

Blood conservatory process blood sampling process that requires no blood wasting.

Bolus rapid administration of a volume of fluid or a drug intravenously.

Calibrate to check or adjust a transducer to a standard measurement.

Cannulation insertion of a tube into a blood vessel for purposes of invasive pressure monitoring. The cannula is attached to a transducer which in turn converts the pressure to a monitored waveform display.

Cardiac index (CI) the cardiac output in relation to a client's body surface area.

Cardiac output (CO) amount of blood ejected by the heart per minute. Determined by multiplying heart rate by stroke volume ($HR \times SV = CO$).

Central venous pressure (CVP) reflects filling pressure of the right heart. Measures central preload.

Diastole period when ventricles are relaxed; a period of ventricular filling and coronary artery perfusion.

Dicrotic notch component of the arterial waveform that represents closure of aortic valve at the end of ventricular contraction (systole).

Diffusion movement of a gas from an area of high pressure to an area of lower pressure.

Distal area farthest away from point of reference (fingers are most distal part of upper extremity; cannulated cetheter tip is most distal).

Dysrhythmia abnormality of heart rate or rhythm.

ECC emergency cardiovascular care.

Electrical potential charges on cell membrane are separated into negative and positive charged particles.

Electrocardiogram (ECG) graphic representation of the variations in electrical potential caused by depolarization of the heart muscles.

Electrode an adhesive patch applied to the skin to transmit cardiac electrical activity to a machine for display.

Hemodynamic movement of blood.

Hypercarbia increased PCO_2 on ABGs.

Invasive involves puncturing or incising the skin for insertion of a tube or instrument into the body.

Left ventricular end-diastolic pressure (LVEDP) pressure of blood in the left ventricle at the end of diastole; a measure of left ventricular preload.

Lumen the inside, channel, or opening of a blood vessel or tube.

Mean arterial (blood) pressure (MAP) average pressure within the cardiovascular system throughout one cardiac cycle. Determined by adding systolic pressure to two times the diastolic pressure and dividing the sum by three.

Mixed venous oxygen saturation (SvO_2) hemoglobin saturation of RBCs measured in the pulmonary artery.

Modified Allen's test manual test to determine patency of the ulnar or radial artery. Digital pressure is applied directly over the radial and ulnar arteries. When pressure on one vessel is released, blood flow to palm and fingers indicates obstruction is not present in that vessel.

Oscilloscope instrument that displays a visual representation of electrical activity on a monitor screen.

Perfusion blood flow to tissues.

Phlebostatic axis the crossing of two reference lines to determine the point at which the zero mark on manometer is level with this axis.

Preload a measure of venous return; end diastolic filling pressure (stretch) in the ventricles.

Proximal refers to an area closest to the point of reference; humerus of upper extremity is more *proximal* to the body than the fingers.

Pulmonary artery pressure (PAP) waveform representing systolic and diastolic pressures in the pulmonary artery, usually displayed by hemodynamic monitoring. Pulmonary artery diastolic pressure is often used as equivalent to pulmonary artery wedge pressure.

Pulmonary artery wedge pressure (PAWP) also referred to as pulmonary artery occlusive pressure, or PAOP, an indirect indicator of left ventricular pressure—normal PAWP is 8 to 13 mmHg. Elevations are seen in left ventricular failure.

Refractory period period during which cardiac cells are not responsive to electrical stimulation (QRS and ST segment of the ECG is the absolute refractory period for the ventricles).

Repolarization period during which ionic changes restore the heart cells to resting potential.

Surfactant a phospholipid synthesized by the lungs; acts to lower alveolar tension and increase lung compliance.

Thermodilution method of calculating cardiac output by injection of solution into the proximal lumen of a pulmonary artery catheter and determining the solution's temperature change at the thermistor (distal) lumen of the catheter.

Transducer device that converts one form of energy into another (e.g., biophysical event is converted into electrical waveform, which is displayed on the oscilloscope).

Vasculature vascular system of the body.

Vasodilator causes dilation of the blood vessels. A venodilator reduces preload; an arterial vasodilator reduces afterload.

Vasopressor an agent used to increase blood pressure by constricting blood vessels.

Vasospasm intermittent constriction of a vessel due to spasm.

Ventricular systole contraction phase of the cardiac cycle during which the ventricles eject blood into receiving arteries.

Voltage electromagnetic force measured in volts.

Volutrauma iatrogenic alveolar injury due to large tidal volumes delivered by mechanical ventilation.

Waveform pictorial representation of a pressure or electrical activity of the heart, depicted on an oscilloscope.

Weaning gradual withdrawal of mechanical ventilation and the reestablishment of spontaneous breathing.

ADVANCED SKILLS IN NURSING PRACTICE

This chapter presents a nursing process framework for nursing actions used in the maintenance of homeostasis during life-threatening conditions. Provision of competent care during critical periods requires a knowledge of physiologic monitoring techniques, skill in the analysis of data, diagnostic reasoning, and decision-making. Working with monitors and providing client care at the same time can be a challenging experience for the nurse.

Monitoring techniques are useful adjunctive tools that provide the practitioner with critical information for management of select clients in intensive care settings. Interpretation and integration of this information assists in the assessment of major body systems and recognition of altered hemodynamic states (e.g., fluid deficit or fluid overload). Continuous surveillance of cardiovascular pressure readings and other dynamic measures serves as a guide for identifying appropriate nursing diagnoses, developing a plan of care, and evaluating the client's response to therapy.

In the clinical setting, nurses are constantly faced with new equipment, new techniques, and better and more sophisticated evaluative methods. To keep pace in the area of technologic advancement can be a monumental task, one that challenges the nurse's energy, patience, and abilities. The nurse's role in assessment, planning, intervention, and evaluation is based in part on the nurse's familiarity with monitoring data.

Hemodynamic monitoring has evolved over the years from continuous ECG monitoring, to measuring CVP (right heart pressure), to direct determination of cardiac output, and indirect measurements of left heart filling pressures. Hemodynamic monitoring techniques require that equipment be properly positioned and function correctly and that the monitor waveforms be representative of the client's physiologic variables and be interpreted correctly.

A multi-lumen, balloon-tipped, flow-directed catheter (e.g., Swan-Ganz VIP) is used to measure intracardiac pressures. Individual lumens reflect measures of right atrial pressure (RAP or CVP), pulmonary artery pressure (PAP), and, when advanced briefly to an occlusive position, pulmonary artery wedge pressure (PAWP or PAOP). Cardiac output (CO), systemic and pulmonary vascular resistance (SVR, PVR), and mixed venous oxygen saturation (SvO_2) are other valuable measures obtained with this catheter. It is simultaneously used for the infusion of fluids and medications. Placement of the catheter is verified by chest x-ray.

Waveforms (pressure signals) are transmitted from the catheter to a transducer by means of fluid-filled tubing. The signal is then amplified and displayed on an oscilloscope both as a visual (analog) waveform and a digital display. The client's physiologic pressure signals provide continuous data to help

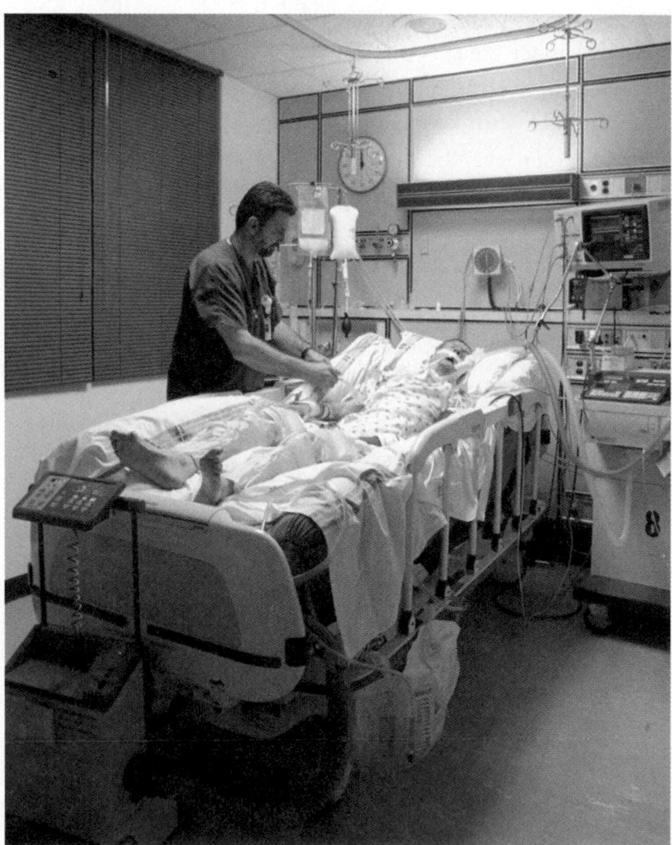

▲ Sophisticated technology facilitates the intensive care of clients.

specialized nurses make critical assessments necessary for safe and effective care decisions, such as the titration of drugs and IV fluids.

Similarly, a catheter can be placed in a peripheral artery and direct blood pressure can be monitored continuously using these same principles. Therapeutically, arterial blood pressure signals can be used to trigger timing of counterpulsation circulatory assistance (intraaortic balloon pump) in clients with compromised cardiac output, while the client's pulmonary artery catheter hemodynamic information is used to evaluate the effectiveness of intraaortic balloon pump (IABP) therapy. This is an example of the complementary power of technology and its value as an integrated aspect of care for clients receiving intensive care.

Ability to integrate all available data is essential to providing excellent nursing care. While advanced technology provides essential measures that augment more overt client data, it is important that this technology not become more important than the client. The first goal is to care for the client, not to tend the equipment. One way to achieve a balance of mastery over complex skills and the attainment of high-quality client care is to become familiar with technical equipment so that it no longer causes anxiety and uncertainty. Once this level of confidence is realized, the focus is on the client, rather than the monitoring equipment.

CULTURAL AWARENESS

Some cultures view critical illness as a curse, an imbalance of heat and cold, or disharmony with the universe rather than pathology or injury to an organ system. Western medicine's healthcare system utilizes much technology and sophisticated equipment. This approach may clash with another culture's beliefs in folk medicine, rituals, and religious healing.

Individuals of the same culture will vary in response to critical illness; therefore, the nurse must explore the meaning of the experience with each individual client in order to provide sensitive care.

NURSING DIAGNOSES

The following nursing diagnoses may be appropriate to include in a client care plan when the components are related to advanced nursing skills.

NURSING DIAGNOSIS	RELATED FACTORS
Aspiration, Risk for	Presence of tracheostomy or endotracheal tube Incompetent lower esophageal sphincter Gastrointestinal tube Tube feedings Increased gastric residual
Ineffective Breathing Pattern	Decreased minute volume Decreased vital capacity Bradypnea (respiratory rate <11) Tachypnea (respiratory rate >24)
Decreased Cardiac Output	Altered heart rate or rhythm Altered preload (increased or decreased intracardiac pressures) Altered afterload (increased or decreased systemic or pulmonary vascular resistance) Altered contractility (low stroke volume cardiac output/cardiac index)
Impaired Verbal Communication	Physical barrier (tracheostomy, intubation) Medications Lack of information
Impaired Gas Exchange	Alveolar-capillary membrane changes (barotrauma, volutrauma) Ventilation-perfusion mismatch
Infection, Risk for	Inadequate primary defenses (broken skin, decreased ciliary action, altered pH secretions, altered peristalsis) Invasive procedures Pharmaceutical agents Trauma
Imbalanced Nutrition: Less Than Body Requirements	Inability to ingest food (e.g., presence of endotracheal tube, NPO status) Difficulty chewing or swallowing Hypermetabolic state
Powerlessness	Healthcare environment Illness-related regimen Chronic or terminal illness Impaired ability to communicate

Impaired Spontaneous Ventilation	Metabolic factors Respiratory muscle fatigue
Ineffective Tissue Perfusion	Hypovolemia Shock (hypovolemic, cardiogenic, distributive) Decreased cardiac output Peripheral vascular disease
Dysfunctional Ventilatory Weaning Response	Inadequate nutrition Sleep pattern disturbance Ventilatory muscle atrophy/neuromuscular decline Inadequate pain management Oversedation without periodic interruption Anxiety or fear Inadequate preparation for weaning process Powerlessness

CLEANSE HANDS The single most important nursing action to decrease the incidence of hospital-based infections is hand hygiene. *Remember to wash your hands or use antibacterial gel before and after each and every client contact.*

IDENTIFY CLIENT Before every procedure, introduce yourself and check two forms of client identification, not including room number. These actions prevent errors and conform to The Joint Commission standards.

Chapter 33

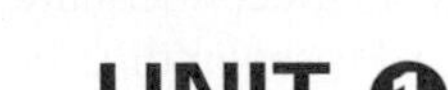

UNIT 1

Pulmonary Artery Pressure (Hemodynamic) Monitoring

Nursing Process Data

ASSESSMENT Data Base

- Determine purpose of hemodynamic monitoring and significance of data obtained.
- Evaluate client's understanding of the procedure.
- Assess for preexisting cardiovascular disease.
- Obtain baseline pulmonary, cardiovascular, hemodynamic, peripheral vascular, neurologic findings.
- Assess insertion site for inflammation or infection.
- Assess patency of all lines.
- Determine pressure on saline flush bag.
- Level and zero the monitoring system.
- Monitor PA systolic, PA diastolic, PA mean, PAWP.
- Note any laboratory data abnormalities.
- Assess cardiac output using thermodilution technique.

PLANNING Objectives

- To maintain a patent pulmonary artery monitoring system
- To administer intravenous solutions and determine response to fluid therapy
- To obtain specific hemodynamic measurements for decision making
- To measure cardiac output

IMPLEMENTATION Procedures

EVALUATION Expected Outcomes

- Pulmonary artery catheter remains patent.
- Pulmonary artery, systolic, diastolic, and pulmonary artery wedge pressure measurements are measured accurately.
- Cardiac output measurements are obtained.

Tissue oxygen consumption depends on cardiac pump performance, adequate blood volume, arterial oxygen content, and vascular distribution (perfusion). Hypovolemia, heart failure, or other conditions (e.g., sepsis) alter intracardiac pressures, tissue perfusion, and tissue oxygen consumption. Since direct measurement of left heart chamber pressures is not possible in the clinical setting, an indication of these measures is obtained by *indirect* means via the right side of the heart.

A balloon-tipped, flow-directed catheter is inserted into a central vein percutaneously or through a cut-down and advanced *transvenously* to the right atrium. Partial inflation of the balloon at the tip of the catheter allows the catheter to float through the tricuspid valve, the right ventricle, and the pulmonary valve into the pulmonary artery. Here the balloon is *deflated* and pulmonary artery pressure is monitored, permitting continuous *indirect* measurement of left ventricular function for monitoring and assisting care of hemodynamically unstable clients. Abnormal pressures can indicate changes in a client's fluid balance, heart pumping action, or vascular tone.

The pulmonary artery catheter typically has four or five lumens. Two lumens are used for pressure measurements. The proximal lumen is used to measure central venous pressure (right atrial pressure), assist in measuring cardiac output, and to inject selected solutions. The distal lumen is used to measure pulmonary artery pressure (PAP) and pulmonary artery wedge pressure (PAWP/PAOP). The third lumen is used for balloon inflation. The fourth lumen is attached to a thermistor tip that assists in the measurement of cardiac output and blood (core) temperature.

At the end of diastole (ventricular filling), the mitral valve is open, and the left ventricle, left atrium, and pulmonary vasculature momentarily act as a single chamber in which the pressure is equal throughout. Since the normal pressures of these chambers and vessels are known, pressure changes in the pulmonary artery can be used to reflect changes in left ventricular end-diastolic pressure (LVEDP). Reduced cardiac function is manifested primarily by two hemodynamic abnormalities: decreased cardiac output (or cardiac index) and increased LVEDP. The pulmonary artery catheter indirectly measures the LVEDP by directly measuring pulmonary artery and pulmonary artery wedge pressures.

If pulmonary artery wedge pressure measurement is required, the balloon is *briefly* inflated and the catheter is carried by blood flow through the pulmonary circulation until it "wedges." During this brief occlusion (wedge) time, pressure reflected back on the tip of the catheter allows indirect measurement of LVEDP. The balloon is then deflated passively and floats back to the pulmonary artery.

To calculate cardiac output, a bolus of cold or room temperature fluid is injected into the right atrial lumen. The fluid's temperature change is then detected in the pulmonary artery by the catheter-tip thermistor. The temperature change over time is computed and represents the cardiac output. Finally, mixed venous blood oxygen saturation monitoring using a fiber optic pulmonary artery catheter provides information about the balance between tissue oxygen delivery and tissue oxygen consumption (SvO_2), which is particularly valuable for monitoring clients with sepsis.

Data derived from physiologic monitoring have diagnostic and therapeutic value in the care of select critically ill (hemodynamically unstable) clients.

TABLE 33-1 Normal Pressures

Right atrial (RAP): 2–8 mmHg
Right ventricle (RV): $\frac{25}{5}$ mmHg
Pulmonary artery pressure (PAP): $\frac{25}{5}$ mmHg
PA mean $(\overline{PA}) : < 15$ mmHg
PAWP/PAOP: 10
Left atrial (LA): 5–10 mmHg
Left ventricle (LV): $\frac{130}{5-10}$ mmHg
Aorta: $\frac{130}{80}$
Mean arterial pressure (MAP):
77–90 (Diastolic × 2) + (Systolic × 1) ÷ 3
or $\frac{(SBP) + 2(DBP)}{3}$

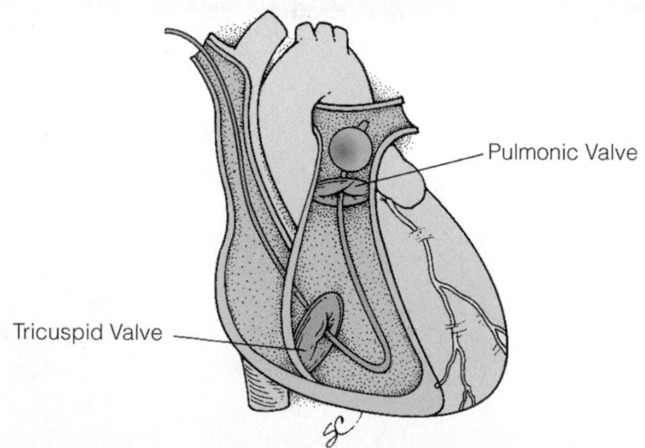

▲ Balloon-tipped, flow-directed catheter with balloon inflated briefly for pulmonary artery wedge (occlusion) pressure determination.

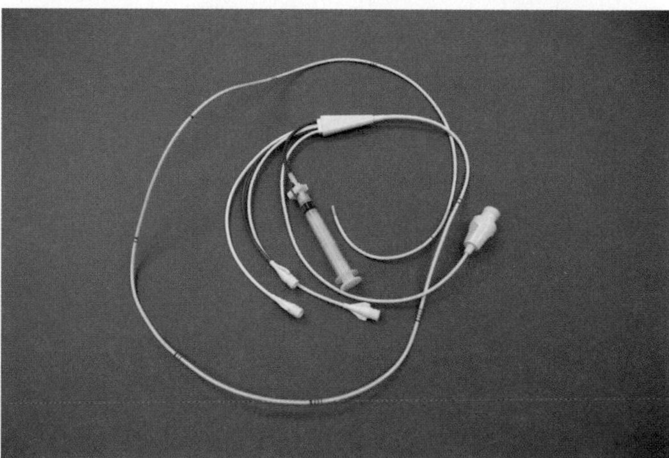

▲ Balloon-tipped catheter has multiple lumens (internal tubes) with openings used to measure intracardiac pressures and other dynamic measures.

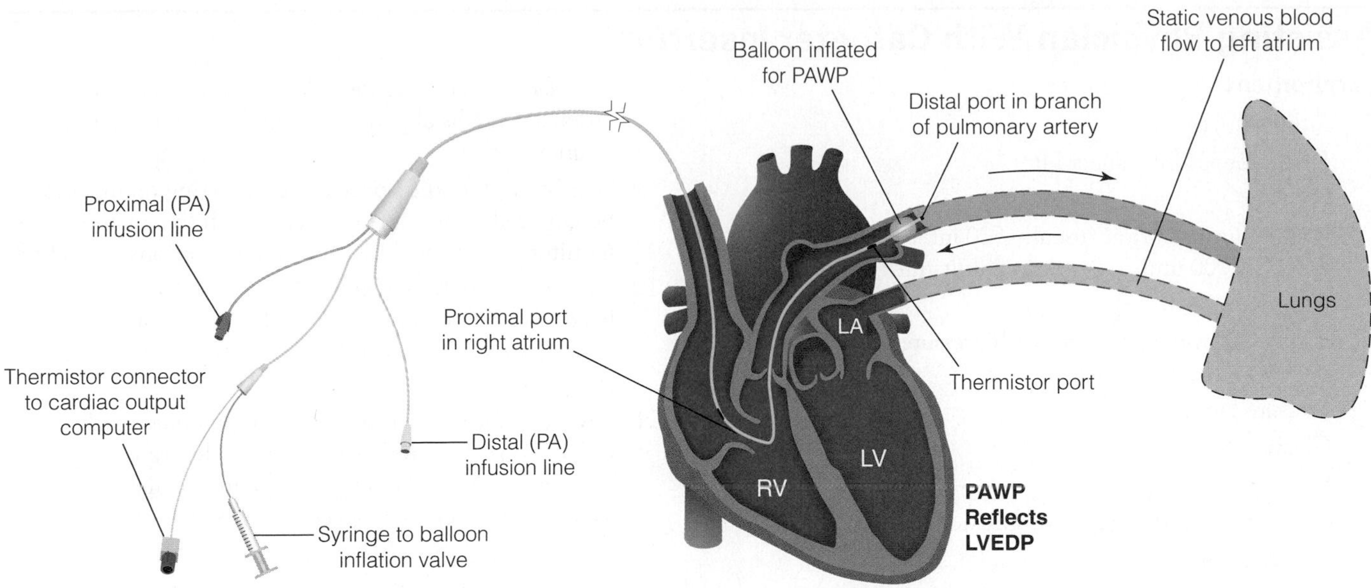

▲ Pulmonary artery catheter provides intracardiac pressure measurements—used to derive multiple cardiac function indices.

Leveling and Zeroing the Monitor System

Procedure

1. Perform hand hygiene.
2. Reassure client and explain what you are doing.
3. Calibrate system.
   a. Using carpenter's level, adjust height of transducer to level of client's atrium or phlebostatic axis. ▸ ***Rationale:*** Transducer must remain level with client's right atrium for accurate monitoring. Higher transducer position yields low readings and vice versa.
   b. To zero monitor, remove port cap (maintain sterility), open stopcock above transducer to air, closing it to the client and the flush system. ▸ ***Rationale:*** This action opens transducer to atmospheric pressure.
   c. Push the "zero" monitor button, and check if monitor reading is zero. ▸ ***Rationale:*** When reading is zero, transducer is balanced to atmospheric pressure (actually 760 mmHg).
4. Check that oscilloscope shows a flat wave at zero line. ▸ ***Rationale:*** This ensures accurate reading as it changes from zero point.
5. Recap port and close stopcock to reestablish flush system.

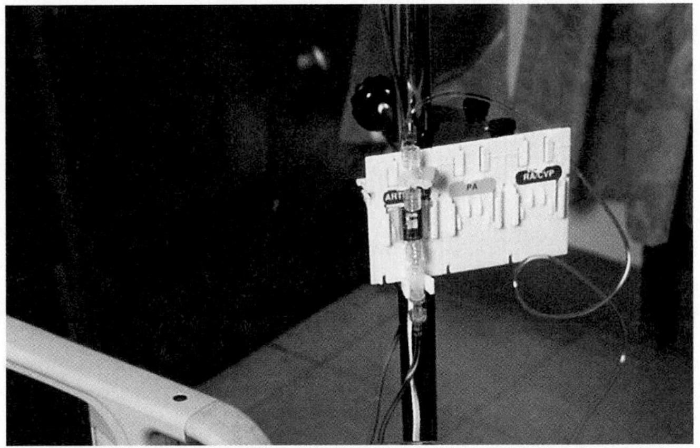

▲ Adjust height of transducer to level of client's phlebostatic axis.

Clinical Alert

Level the air/fluid interface stopcock (on top of the transducer) to client's phlebostatic axis (intersection of lines at mid anterior–posterior chest and fourth ICS) every 8 hr and any time the bed or client's position is changed.

EVIDENCE-BASED PRACTICE

Determining the Phlebostatic Axis

Since all clients' chests are not equal, the midaxillary line is not an accurate external reference point for the phlebostatic axis. Reference the intersection of two lines on the right side of the chest: one drawn vertically at the fourth intercostal space and one drawn horizontally at the midpoint between the anterior and posterior chest.

Source: McGhee, B., & Bridges, E. (2002). Monitoring arterial blood pressure: What you may not know. *Critical Care Nurse, 22*(2), 60–79.

Assisting Physician With Catheter Insertion

Equipment

- Sterile gloves
- Percutaneous introducer kit
- IV pole
- Premix flush solution (usually 500 mL of normal saline with 1,000 units of heparin 2 units/mL)
- IV tubing
- Pressure transducer system with pressure bag, tubing, flush device, and transducer
- Pressure monitor
- Clean gloves
- Sterile towels
- Antiseptic solution (2% chlorhexidine)
- Sterile 4 × 4 sponges
- Stethoscope
- Lidocaine 1%–2%
- 3-mL syringe with 18- and 25-gauge needle for topical anesthetic
- Antimicrobial wipes
- Occlusive dressing or tape
- Suture with attached needle
- Sterile needle holder or clamp
- Cutdown tray, sterile gown, mask, and cap
- Emergency cart
- Sterile syringes filled with 5 mL or 10 mL of normal saline (cardiac output)

Preparation

1. Validate that client's informed consent has been obtained.
2. Identify client's room and client's Ident-A-Band and have client state name and birth date.
3. Explain rationale for procedure to client.
4. Validate that client has an established peripheral IV site. ▸ ***Rationale:*** For administration of emergency fluids or medication if needed.
5. Perform hand hygiene.
6. Connect IV tubing to flush fluid bag.
7. Place prepared flush solution bag in pressure bag and inflate to 300 mmHg pressure. ▸ ***Rationale:*** This maintains a rate of flow through the flush device (3 mL/hr).
8. Prepare and assemble pressurized monitoring system (transducer, system flush device, and stopcocks) following manufacturer's instructions. Attach stopcocks to proximal and distal ports. Flush all lumens with flush solution.
9. Attach distal port stopcock to connecting tubing and heparinized flush solution, then attach to pressure monitoring unit, making sure all connections are tight.
10. Place client in Trendelenburg's position and turn client's head to opposite side. ▸ ***Rationale:*** This position distends central veins and prevents air embolism during the procedure.
11. Level and zero system according to manufacturer's instructions. The stopcock on top of the transducer must be at the level of client's atrium or phlebostatic axis (fourth intercostal space at the midchest line).
12. Scrub selected site with antiseptic solution.
13. Open sterile gloves for physician.
14. Open drape for physician.
15. Cleanse lidocaine vial with antimicrobial wipe.
16. Continuously monitor client's ECG throughout insertion of catheter. ▸ ***Rationale:*** Rhythm changes may occur.

Clinical Alert

By zeroing to atmospheric pressure, the system negates the effect of atmospheric pressure on the pressure being measured.

Procedure

1. Don sterile gloves to assist physician as necessary.
   a. Physician dons sterile mask, cap, gown, and gloves. Catheter is tested for leaks by inflating balloon with 0.5–1.5 mL (amount determined by catheter size) of *air* while balloon is submerged in sterile basin filled with sterile irrigating solution.
   b. Physician aspirates lidocaine with 18-gauge needle, changes to 25-gauge needle, and injects lidocaine under skin.
   c. Physician performs cutdown or percutaneous insertion. Subclavian vein usually used; however, the jugular or a peripheral vein may be selected.
   d. Physician aspirates and flushes sheath with sterile normal saline before inserting catheter. ▸ ***Rationale:*** This clears air and prevents air embolism. The use of D_5W rather than normal saline reduces risk of microshock to the client.
   e. While client performs Valsalva's maneuver or hums, catheter is attached to fluid-filled transducer system. ▸ ***Rationale:*** This prevents inhalation and possible air embolism. Continuous pressure monitoring is observed during advancement of catheter.
   f. Catheter is advanced with a balloon partially inflated until correct right atrial waveform appears on monitor (strip A).
   g. Physician inflates balloon (1–1.5 mL air) to assist in catheter's flow through tricuspid valve into right ventricle.
2. Observe for higher and more pronounced pressure waveform, indicating catheter's presence in right ventricle (strip B).

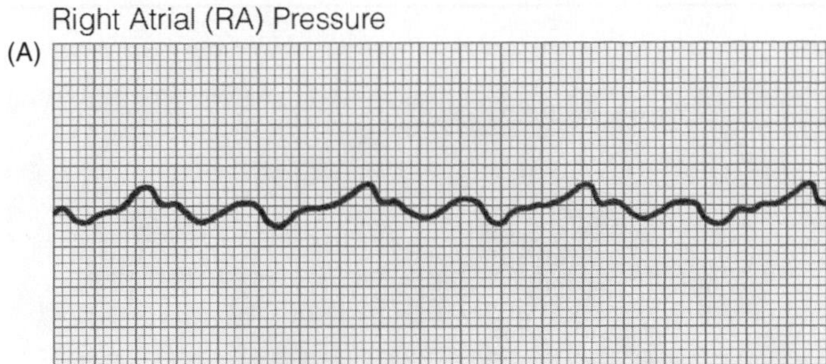

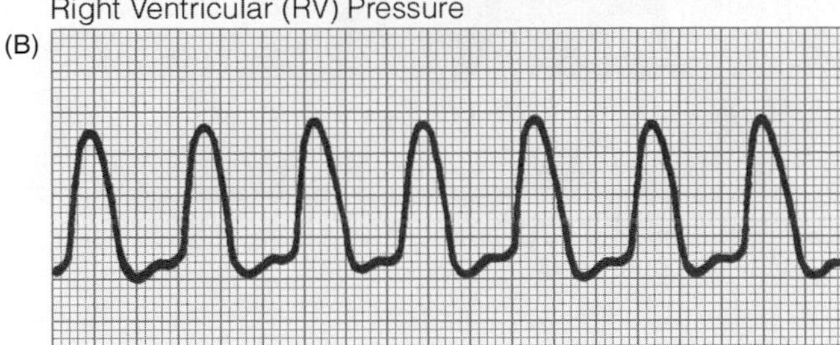

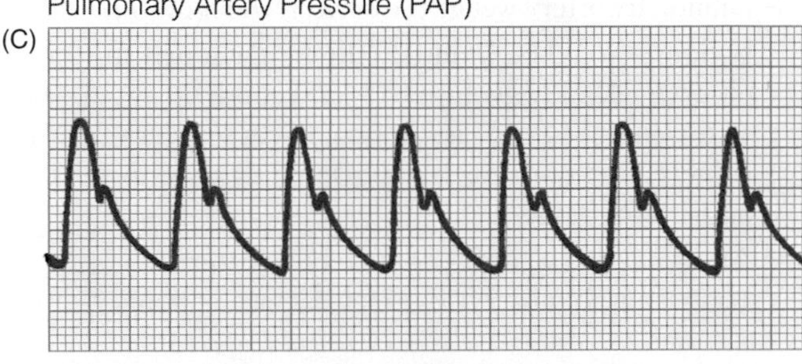

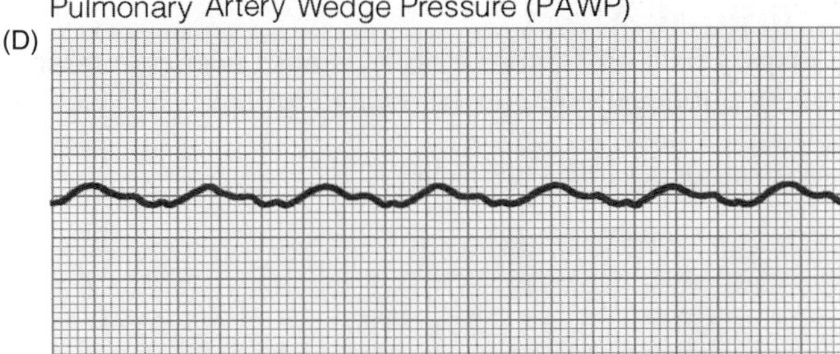

▲ Waveforms depicted on monitor correspond with right heart chambers and pulmonary artery pressures.

3. Record right ventricular pressure (systolic and diastoles reading) and observe for dysrhythmias: premature ventricular contractions (PVCs) or ventricular tachycardia.
4. Observe monitor for *higher* diastolic pressure and appearance of dicrotic notch on pulmonary arterial waveform (strip C). ▸ ***Rationale:*** Right ventricular systolic and pulmonary artery systolic pressures are similar, but pulmonary artery *diastolic* measure "steps up."
5. Remove syringe to allow balloon to deflate passively. (A special syringe is used that prevents overinflation of the balloon.)
6. Record pulmonary artery systolic (PAS), diastolic (PAD), and mean pressures.

NOTE: Measure all pulmonary artery pressures at end of expiration.

7. Inflate balloon fully (1.5 mL maximum) or until a change is seen in waveform (pulmonary artery to artery wedge pressure) (strip D). ▸ ***Rationale:*** Inflated balloon assists passage of catheter into distal pulmonary artery.
8. Record PAWP (pulmonary artery wedge pressure).
9. Deflate balloon by releasing pressure on syringe plunger or remove syringe to allow passive deflation. ▸ ***Rationale:*** Active aspiration of air from balloon with a syringe plunger can cause balloon damage.
10. Determine balloon deflation by observing return of pulmonary artery waveform. ▸ ***Rationale:*** This ensures balloon deflation. Continued occlusion of vessel can cause pulmonary infarction.
11. Repeat steps and measurements to verify function.
12. Leave balloon lumen port open at all times except during advancement for wedge pressure (PAWP) measurement.
13. Clear catheter using fast flush device.
14. Apply occlusive dressing to site after physician secures catheter with sutures.
15. Reposition client for comfort.
16. Auscultate chest for presence of breath sounds.
17. Validate catheter placement by chest x-ray. ▸ ***Rationale:*** Pneumothorax can occur with jugular or subclavian vein cannulation.
18. Dispose of equipment, remove gloves, and perform hand hygiene.

EVIDENCE-BASED PRACTICE

Confirming Digital Measurements

This study showed lack of agreement between digital and graphic measurements of CVP and PAD, which ranged from as small as 1 mmHg to as great as 40 mmHg, especially in patients with respiratory rate >20. Digital measurements should be confirmed by waveform analysis of a graphic measurement before assuming that the value is accurate.

Source: Ahrens, T., & Schallom, L. (2001). Comparison of pulmonary artery and central venous pressure waveform measurements via digital and graphic measurement methods. *Heart & Lung, 30*(1), 26–38.

Clinical Alert

For PAWP (pulmonary artery wedge pressure), inflate balloon *briefly* (8 to 15 seconds), just until PAP changes to PAWP waveform, then allow balloon to deflate by releasing pressure on syringe plunger or removing syringe.

Obtaining Pressure Readings

Preparation

1. Level transducer, and zero (calibrate) monitor at the beginning of every shift. ▸ ***Rationale:*** This ensures accurate and consistent readings.
2. Check catheter, tubing, and connection points to ensure patency and security.
3. Mark client's midchest level at fourth ICS for consistent readings.
4. Place client flat supine or up to 20° elevation.

NOTE: Consistent position is preferred for all readings.

5. Perform hand hygiene.

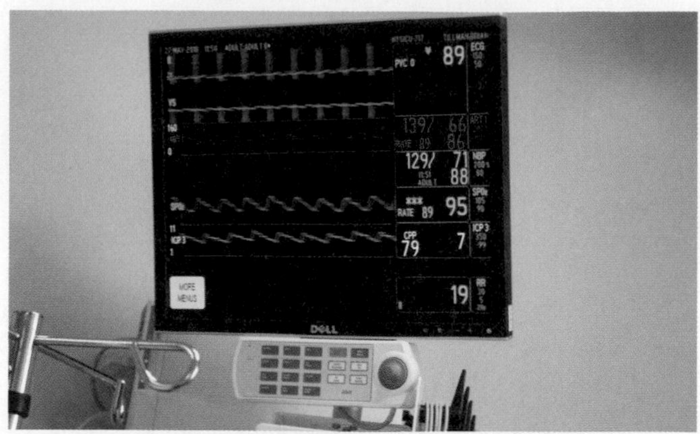

▲ Monitor display of ECG, pressure waveforms, and digital readouts for continuous client assessment.

Clinical Alert

Do not use the PA catheter for infusion of blood or other viscous fluids as they may occlude the catheter or alter pressure measurements.

Procedure

1. Check that air reference port (stopcock) of pressure transducer is at level of client's atrium (phlebostatic axis). ▸ ***Rationale:*** This ensures accurate pressure reading. Level must be adjusted if client's position is changed.
2. Expose distal port to the transducer. ▸ ***Rationale:*** All pulmonary artery pressure readings are taken from distal lumen of catheter, and right atrial pressures are taken from RA or proximal lumen.
3. Open balloon inflation port-locking device.

Clinical Alert

Pulmonary artery diastolic pressure is an acceptable equivalent of PAWP (if correlation determined) and eliminates need for occlusion (wedge) readings.

4. Attach syringe filled with proper amount of air and align stopcock to open position.
5. Slowly inject 0.8 or 1.5 mL of air into balloon. Inflate sufficient volume only to support float and change in waveform.
6. Observe waveform change from pulmonary artery to pulmonary artery wedge pressure on the monitor.
7. Balloon should be inflated only long enough to observe PAWP waveform (8–15 seconds). ▸ ***Rationale:*** Longer inflation can cause overwedging (falsely high pressure readings) and damage to pulmonary tissue.
8. Allow balloon to deflate passively. ▸ ***Rationale:*** Aspirating air with syringe may damage balloon.

Clinical Alert

Suspect balloon rupture if no resistance is encountered on inflation, syringe plunger fails to retract spontaneously, or if blood returns from balloon lumen. Mark stopcock: "DO NOT INFLATE."

9. Ensure readings are always taken at end of expiration whether or not client is on ventilator (document if client is on ventilator). ▸ ***Rationale:*** Slightly higher readings are obtained if client is on a ventilator.
10. Use analog strip chart recording to obtain the most valid pressure measurements.
11. Maintain empty syringe on balloon port.
12. Flush line with fast flush device system.
13. Record readings; verify and report unusual findings to physician if they persist.

EVIDENCE-BASED PRACTICE

Measuring Hemodynamic Pressures

Analog data (printed strip) rather than digital data or "stop-cursor" freezing the monitor screen remains the recommended method for measuring hemodynamic pressures. Mean pressures are determined by bisecting the waveform (areas above and below bisecting line are equal).

Source: Bridges, E. (2000). Monitoring pulmonary artery pressures: Just the facts. *Critical Care Nurse, 20*(6), 59–75.

Mixed Central Venous Oxygen Saturation (SvO_2) Monitoring

The SvO2 reflects a dynamic relationship between tissue oxygen delivery and tissue oxygen consumption, providing an indication of overall oxygen balance. This value has diagnostic, prognostic, and therapeutic value in the care of critically ill clients, particularly those with acute MI, heart failure, and cardiogenic, hypovolemic, or septic shock.

A fiberoptic pulmonary artery catheter analyzes light absorption reflecting RBC hemoglobin saturation (similar to a pulse oximeter). An oximeter computer with microprocessor converts this information into an electrical display (graphic trend, numeric display, or both) for continuous monitoring. Since analysis occurs in the pulmonary artery, the value reflects a measurement of overall venous oxygen saturation, reflecting oxygen consumption at the tissue level. Whereas arterial oxygen content (SaO_2) is 100%, a normal SvO_2 value is 70%–80%. Clinically significant changes in SvO_2 (±5%–10%) can be an early indicator of physiologic instability.

Low SvO_2 may be due to inadequate oxygen delivery caused by decreased cardiac output (increased heart rate or decreased stroke volume), reduced hemoglobin, low oxygen saturation, or excess tissue extraction of oxygen (e.g., due to pain or nursing procedures). Management will focus on optimizing preload, afterload, cardiac contractility, oxygen delivery, and increasing blood hemoglobin with transfusion. Adaptations in nursing care can reduce the client's oxygen requirement and utilization.

High SvO_2 occurs with low tissue extraction of oxygen, as seen in patients who are sedated, or may indicate hyperdynamic blood flow or tissue inability to utilize oxygen delivered, as occurs in sepsis.

Clinical Alert

Changes in intracardiac pressures and volumes may be altered by changes in myocardial compliance. Any pressure should be interpreted in relation to the client's clinical assessment.

14. Place client in comfortable position.
15. Change dressings per agency policy, and observe for complications at site of catheter insertion.

Measuring Cardiac Output

Equipment

Established pressure monitoring system
Closed system cardiac output set (COSET)
Includes: 500-mL bag of NS (injectate), tubing with 3-way stopcock, syringe
Cardiac output cable

Preparation

1. Check physician's orders.
2. Identify client's room, check Ident-A-Band, and ask client to state name and birth date.
3. Perform hand hygiene.
4. Spike injectate solution bag with tubing/stopcock.
5. Unclamp injectate tubing, prime tubing and stopcock, and then reclamp tubing.
6. Connect primed system to client's PA catheter proximal port.
7. Stop any medication being infused through proximal port. ▸ ***Rationale:*** To prevent medication bolus during cardiac output measurement.
8. Note pulmonary artery waveform on monitor. ▸ ***Rationale:*** To verify catheter position.
9. Connect computer cable to thermistor port of pulmonary artery catheter (according to manufacturer's instructions). ▸ ***Rationale:*** Change in injectate temperature from proximal injectate port to thermistor port at distal lumen is computer calculated and displayed as the cardiac output in L/min.
10. Obtain client's height and weight measures.

Procedure

1. Place client in position used with previous hemodynamic readings; client should be supine, but may be elevated up to 20°. ▸ ***Rationale:*** Consistency of position decreases measurement variability.
2. Slowly flush proximal injectate lumen if any medications were being infused. ▸ ***Rationale:*** To prevent bolus medication delivery during cardiac output measurement.

Clinical Alert

Vasoactive medications should not be infused through the proximal port; the Swan Ganz VIP catheter provides a separate proximal port for infusion.

3. Select *cardiac output* on bedside monitor menu.
4. Check and set computation constant to reflect size of catheter, volume (5 or 10 mL) of injectate, cold versus room temperature injectate, and injectate volume (see PA catheter manufacturer's instructions). ► ***Rationale:*** These are factored into computer-derived hemodynamic measures. A 5-mL bolus may be indicated for a fluid-restricted client.
5. Unclamp injectate solution tubing.
6. Attach syringe to stopcock and open stopcock to withdraw 10 mL of injectate into syringe.
7. Ensure that client is quiet. ► ***Rationale:*** Movement may cause inaccurate readings.
8. Open stopcock to client and inject rapidly (2–4 seconds). ► ***Rationale:*** Slower injectate results in inaccurate readings.
9. Note and record monitor display of client's cardiac output measure.
10. Repeat procedure two more times for cold injectate; repeat four more times for room temperature injectate, waiting 1–2 minutes between injections.
11. Obtain curves and discard abnormal curves or those with wandering baselines.
12. Record the average of remaining cardiac output measures.
13. Clamp injectate tubing.
14. Open stopcock to continue previous infusion to client.
15. Preserve closed cardiac output system by leaving tubing, stopcock, and syringe connections intact. ► ***Rationale:*** This eliminates need to open system each time measurements are made.
16. Determine derived values using client's cardiac output measure: stroke volume, systemic vascular resistance, pulmonary vascular resistance, cardiac index (client's height and weight factored into the cardiac output).

The value of routine use of the pulmonary artery catheter for broad groups of clients has not been substantiated. Lack of benefit may be due to ineffective or improper changes in management based on PAC data rather than to lack of potential benefit of the PAC data.

DOCUMENTATION for Pulmonary Artery Pressure Monitoring

- Physician who placed catheter
- Size of pulmonary artery catheter inserted
- Vessel placement and technique used to insert catheter (cutdown or percutaneous)
- Site care and dressing applied
- Client position during measurements
- Pressure readings obtained (specify digital or analog measures)
- Strip recordings attached
- Client's response to procedure
- Cardiac output results
- Problems arising and interventions performed

Legal Alert

A nurse caring for a client after gastric bypass surgery suspected that the client was experiencing cardiac tamponade due to displacement of the pulmonary artery catheter. In spite of the nurse's requests, the nurse manager refused to examine the client, stating that the client was agitated, restless. As the client deteriorated, the nurse attempted to contact the physician, but this was "cut off" by the manager. The client was eventually taken to emergency surgery but suffered severe brain damage and died a week later. The jury found that, with prompt reporting and medical attention, the client's condition could have been easily treated with pericardiocentesis. The jury decided against the hospital and awarded $7.3 million for the negligence of its nursing staff.

Source: Wilkinson, A. (1998). Nursing malpractice. *Nursing* 98, *28*(6), 34.

CRITICAL THINKING Application

Expected Outcomes

- Pulmonary artery catheter remains patent.
- Pulmonary artery systolic, diastolic, and pulmonary artery wedge pressure are measured accurately.
- Cardiac output measurements are obtained.

Unexpected Outcomes	Alternative Actions
Pulmonary artery catheter is not patent.	• Check that tubing is not kinked. • Ensure continuous heparinized flush or normal saline infusion. (Check hospital policy.) Check stopcock connections. (Do not use dextrose solution.) • Attempt to aspirate clotted blood through line by pulling back on plunger of a small syringe placed at proximal port. Remove clot, then flush line. • Notify physician if unable to clear line. • Fast flush system and flick tubing to eliminate tiny bubbles.
Pressure waveforms are significantly abnormal.	• Check that tubing is not kinked. • Check stopcock level. • Correlate with client for possible change in clinical condition. • Tighten all connections. • Look for air in any system port. • Eliminate added stopcocks and tubing extensions. • Ask client to cough or change position to help free catheter. • If condition persists, notify physician to reposition line, and assess client.
Analog waveform is inconsistent with digital display.	• Validate leveling at client's phlebostatic axis. • Validate zeroing of system to atmospheric pressure ("0" baseline). • Record analog strips and median measured values on chart—do not rely on digital measures.
No pressure tracing.	• Determine that power is ON. • Check for loose connections. • Check for clotted blood in line (damping is an early sign). Try to aspirate; never flush. • Check stopcocks to make sure they are turned appropriately.
No pulmonary wedge pressure tracing.	• Check and deflate balloon. • Suspect that catheter is not adequately advanced. Chest x-ray may be ordered to check placement of pulmonary artery catheter. • Reposition client. • Suspect possible balloon rupture if no resistance is felt on inflation.
Cardiac output measurements vary significantly.	• Determine whether measurements have been performed with consistent client positioning (supine or elevation degree). • Compare measurements when client is in supine and elevated position as client's hemodynamic status may account for positional differences. • Establish and document consistency in client positioning for cardiac output measurements.

Chapter 33

UNIT 2

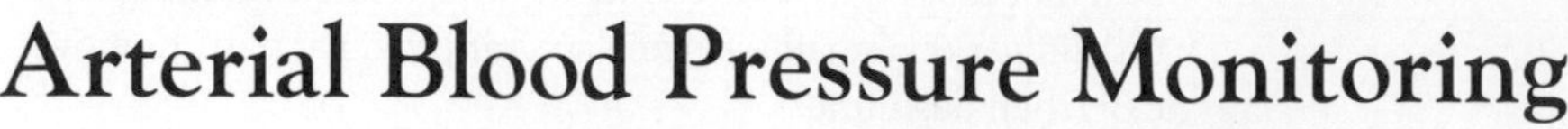

Arterial Blood Pressure Monitoring

Nursing Process Data

ASSESSMENT Data Base

- Determine need for direct arterial blood pressure monitoring.
- Assess collateral perfusion of the hand using the Modified Allen's Test.
- Measure arterial (direct) systolic and diastolic blood pressure readings.
- Observe the mean arterial pressure on the monitor and validate using analog strip measurement.
- Observe for trends in arterial pressure readings.
- Validate 300 mmHG pressure on infusion system.
- Assess catheter insertion site for signs of infection or bleeding.
- Assess circulation, temperature, motion, and sensation of extremity distal to catheter insertion site.
- Monitor systemic response to circulatory assistance (IABP)

PLANNING Objectives

- To maintain a patent arterial catheter
- To directly measure systolic, diastolic, and mean arterial blood pressures
- To provide essential information regarding fluid volume, cardiac function, and perfusion to vital organs
- To provide immediate access for arterial blood gas samples
- To provide circulatory assistance (IABP) for selected clients

IMPLEMENTATION Procedures

EVALUATION Expected Outcomes

- Blood supply to hand is adequate before and after arterial catheter placement.
- Arterial cannulation is accomplished without complication.
- Arterial blood pressure monitoring system functions reliably and accurately.
- Intraaortic balloon pump circulatory assist improves cardiac output: afterload and preload are reduced.
- Arterial blood samples are obtained.

Direct blood pressure monitoring allows continuous measurement of the client's systolic, diastolic, and mean arterial pressures (MAP) to facilitate evaluation of perfusion to vital organs. A short single-lumen catheter is placed in the client's radial artery (brachial artery may be used), then attached to a pressure transducer and high-pressure infusion system and a display monitor. Direct pressure readings are typically 10–20 mmHg higher than simultaneously measured indirect (cuff) readings.

To maintain patency of the intraarterial catheter, a continuous flush of 1–3 mL/hr of heparinized normal saline solution is administered under 300 mmHg pressure.

NOTE: The use of dextrose supports bacterial growth. Heparinized solution may be contraindicated for clients at risk for heparin-induced thrombocytopenia.

Invasive monitoring is appropriate for surgical clients, clients on mechanical ventilators, or those requiring vasodilator or vasopressor drugs or frequent arterial blood gas studies.

Continuous arterial waveforms are observed on the oscilloscope, and numerical pressures are displayed. Blood pressure deviations can immediately be detected and appropriate therapy instituted without delay. The arterial line also provides easy access to blood sampling for ABGs and other lab values. Arterial blood gas values assist in determining respiratory and metabolic acid–base status (Tables 33-2 and 33-3) as well as lung capacity to provide oxygen. The measurements serve as a guide for implementing and evaluating treatment.

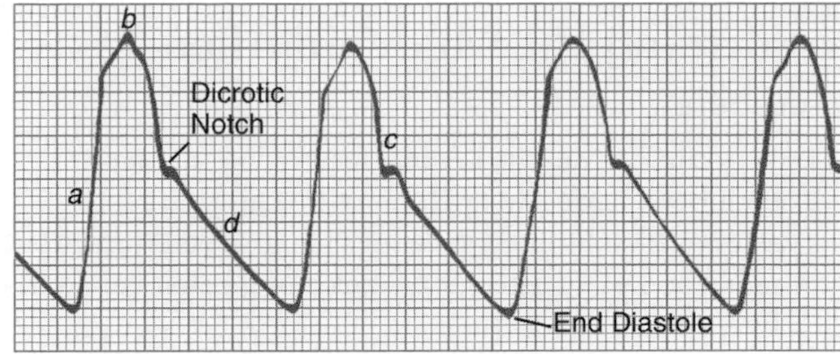

▲ Arterial pressure waveform. The dicrotic notch indicates aortic valve closure (and end of systole).

Hemodynamic Monitoring System Components

- Invasive **catheter** with high-pressure tubing connected to transducer
- **Flush/infusion system** with pressure bag at 300 mmHg maintains patency of system
- **Transducer**—converts physiologic wave to electrical energy
- **Monitor**—converts electrical energy, displays pressure waveform and digital reading in mmHg

Direct blood pressure waveform correlation to the cardiac cycle is represented by the symbols shown in the figure.

- *a* represents a sharp upstroke, correlating with ventricular systole and the QRS complex of the electrocardiogram.
- *b* represents peak systole; its numerical value is the systolic pressure recorded.
- *c* represents the notch on the downstroke of the waveform. This notch is called the *dicrotic notch* and represents closure of the aortic valve.
- *d* represents diastole and is represented by a continuous decline in pressure. The numerical value at the lowest point is the diastolic pressure.

Intraaortic Balloon Pump (IABP) Circulatory Assist Device

An example of integrative technology is the intraaortic ballon pump (IABP) which incorporates both hemodynamic and arterial blood pressure monitoring information. The IABP provides indirect short-term circulatory assistance for clients with compromised cardiac function due to myocardial infarction with complications, temporary left ventricular failure, cardiac injury, septic shock, or those awaiting cardiac transplantation. The goals are to decrease heart work, reduce afterload, improve cardiac output, enhance coronary and peripheral perfusion, and ultimately reduce preload.

The balloon catheter is inserted percutaneously into the descending aorta via the femoral artery and advanced proximally so that the balloon is positioned just below the left subclavian artery, yet above the renal artery.

The vacuum pump cyclically drives helium to inflate and deflate the balloon. Performing on the principle of counter-pulsation, the catheter balloon inflates at the onset of diastole enhancing perfusion and oxygen delivery to tissues antegrade and to the coronary arteries retrograde. The balloon deflates just before systole, creating a relatively negative suction effect, thereby reducing afterload and supporting ventricular ejection and antegrade blood flow.

Performing the Modified Allen Test

Procedure

1. Perform the Modified Allen Test to determine distal peripheral perfusion. ▸ ***Rationale:*** This procedure assesses blood supply to client's hand to determine that radial and ulnar artery are functioning before an arterial line is inserted.
2. Compress both arteries at client's wrist for about 1 minute.
3. Instruct client to clench and unclench fist several times. ▸ ***Rationale:*** This causes blanching in the hand and palm.
4. With client's hand in open, relaxed position, release pressure on ulnar artery.
5. Observe how quickly (≤7 seconds) the palm color flushes. ▸ ***Rationale:*** If color returns quickly, good collateral blood supply to the hand exists. If normal color does not return, there is insufficient collateral circulation to the hand should radial artery occlusion occur.
6. Repeat procedure with release of the radial artery.
7. Report to physician if collateral blood flow is insufficient. ▸ ***Rationale:*** A Doppler flow study may be used to help determine collateral blood flow.

Assisting With Arterial Line Insertion

Equipment

20-gauge Teflon catheter with introducer and flexible guidewire
500 mL of normal saline for flush
Heparin 1,000 units/mL
One-mL unit dose syringe
Pressure bag for flush infusion
IV tubing
Short wide-bore, high-pressure tubing
Three-way stopcocks with nonvented caps
Established pressure monitor system
Clean gloves, sterile gloves
Personal protective equipment (PPE)
Sterile towels and drape
Skin prep solution (2% chlorhexidine)
Sterile 4 × 4 gauze sponges
Lidocaine 1% (without epinephrine)
3-mL syringe with 18- and 25-gauge needles for *topical* anesthetic
Alcohol wipes
000 silk suture (if used)
Sterile transparent dressing
Atropine for reversal of bradycardia

Preparation

1. Validate that informed consent has been obtained.
2. Determine whether client has received anticoagulant therapy. ▸ ***Rationale:*** Coagulation studies may be indicated.
3. Identify client, check Ident-A-Band, and ask client to state name and birth date.
4. Explain rationale for procedure.
5. Gather equipment.
6. Perform hand hygiene.
7. Add heparin to normal saline solution and label bag with additive and date (commonly 2 units of heparin/mL fluid). Follow hospital protocols.
8. Connect IV tubing to solution bag.
9. Remove *all air* from flush solution bag.
10. Insert flush infusion bag into pressure bag and hang bag on IV pole.

> **Clinical Alert**
> **Arterial catheter alarms should always be enabled to detect disconnection, alterations in blood pressure, or pulseless electrical activity.**

11. Prepare and assemble pressurized monitoring system (transducer, continuous flush device, and stopcocks) following manufacturer's instructions.
12. Level stopcock above transducer to client's phlebostatic axis (see previous skill).
13. Inflate pressure bag to 300 mmHg using hand pump on bag.

Procedure

1. Don gloves and PPE and prepare to assist the physician as needed.
   a. Skin is prepped briskly with 2% chlorhexidine for 3 seconds.
   b. Lidocaine vial is cleansed with alcohol wipe.
   c. Physician dons sterile gloves.
   d. Sterile drape is placed over arterial insertion site.
   e. Physician aspirates lidocaine with 18-gauge needle, changes needle, and injects client's skin with 25-gauge needle. ▸ ***Rationale:*** For local anesthesia.
   f. Percutaneous insertion is made at arterial insertion site, and arterial catheter is inserted.
   g. Physician advances catheter in artery.

h. Arterial catheter is sutured in place with 000 silk suture secured with transparent dressing.

2. Observe for pulsating bright-red blood spurting retrograde into catheter. ▸ ***Rationale:*** This evidence ensures arterial catheter position.
3. Attach catheter to primed pressure-monitoring system tubing—make certain all connections are secure.
4. Press fast flush valve to clear system.
5. Observe oscilloscope for arterial waveform.
6. Apply sterile transparent dressing (with date and initials) to site after catheter is sutured into place.
7. Remove gloves and perform hand hygiene.
8. Set monitor alarms for both HIGH and LOW parameters.

Monitoring Arterial Blood Pressure

Equipment

Disposable pressure transducer, dome, and amplifier
Flush valve with flush system
Display monitor (oscilloscope)
Sterile stopcock cap
Sterile transparent dressing
Gloves
Carpenter's level
Marker

Procedure

1. Leveling and zeroing (calibrating) the system.
   a. Calibrate system at beginning of each shift. ▸ ***Rationale:*** Monitor readings are altered by changes in atmospheric pressure.
   b. Position client with HOB flat or up to 45° elevation.
   c. Using carpenter's level, align stopcock above transducer level with client's left atrium (phlebostatic axis) and mark client's chest for future readings. ▸ ***Rationale:*** Readings will be inaccurately high or low if stopcock above transducer is not level with client's phlebostatic axis.
   d. To zero ("calibrate") the system, turn stopcock near transducer off to client. Remove cap from stopcock, opening it to air.
   e. Depress "zero" button on monitor, release button, and note monitor reading is zero. ▸ ***Rationale:*** Zero reading indicates monitor is calibrated to atmospheric pressure.
   f. Replace cap or place new sterile cap on stopcock.
   g. Turn stopcock so transducer is open to client.
2. Observe waveform at eye level for the sharp systolic upstroke, peak, dicrotic notch, and end diastole.
3. Fast flush the continuous flush system and quickly release. A sharp upstroke followed by a horizontal line, then a brisk downstroke descending below, then returning to baseline indicates that the system requires no adjustment.
4. Ensure pressure bag is maintained at 300 mmHg.
5. Leave cannulated extremity uncovered for easy observation. Assess site for signs of infection every shift.

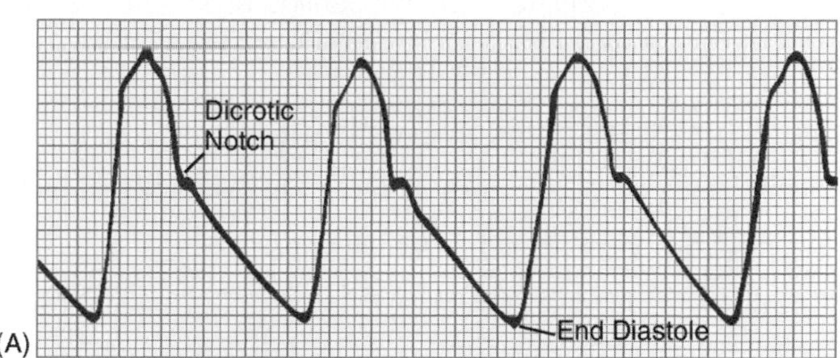

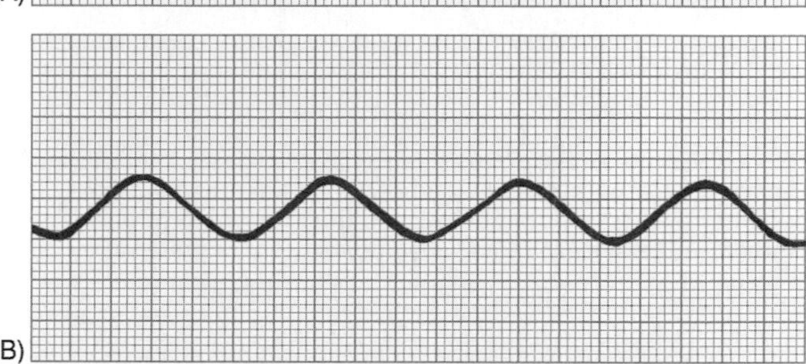

▲ (A) Arterial line—normal waveform. (B) Arterial line—flattened waveform. Flattened arterial waveform indicates damping. Damping results from obstruction in arterial line or imbalance of transducer.

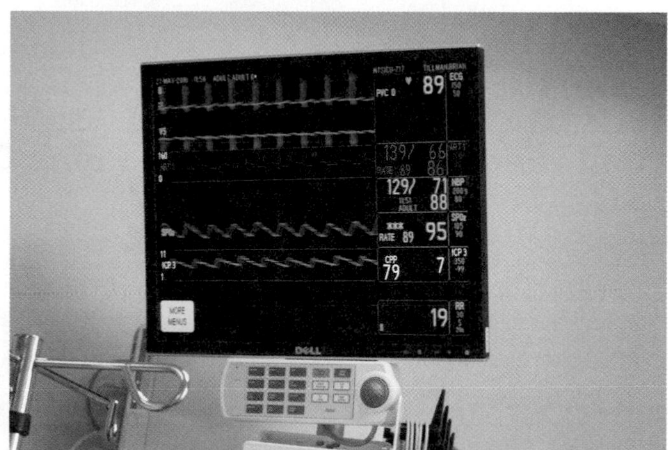

▲ Arterial line allows direct measurement of blood pressure—monitor displays digital and wave form.

6. Assess circulation, motion, and sensation of extremity distal to cannulation site every 2 hr initially, then every 8 hr.
7. Immobilize extremity if necessary.

EVIDENCE-BASED PRACTICE

Monitoring Arterial Blood Pressure

The use of an indirect brachial blood pressure measurement to determine whether an arterial pressure monitoring system is accurate is not evidence-based. It is more important to determine that technical aspects of the method are optimized and the blood pressure is adequate. In addition to obtaining an absolute measure, monitoring for trends or changes in blood pressure over time is equally important for guiding clinical decisions.

Source: Rauen, C. A, Chulay, M., Bridges, E., Vollman, K. M., & Arbour, R. (2008). Seven evidence-based practice habits: Putting some sacred cows out to pasture. *Critical Care Nurse, 28*(2), 98–123.

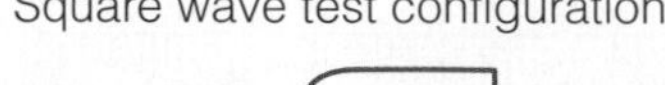

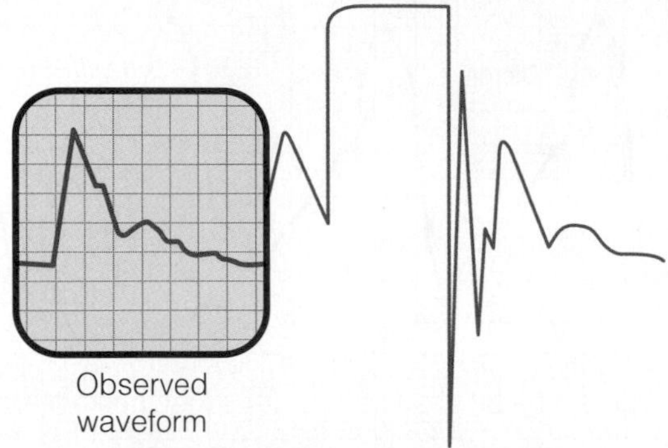

▲ Fast flush the continuous flush system and quickly release. A sharp upstroke, followed by a horizontal line, then a brisk downstroke descending below and then returning to baseline indicates the system requires no adjustment (square wave test).

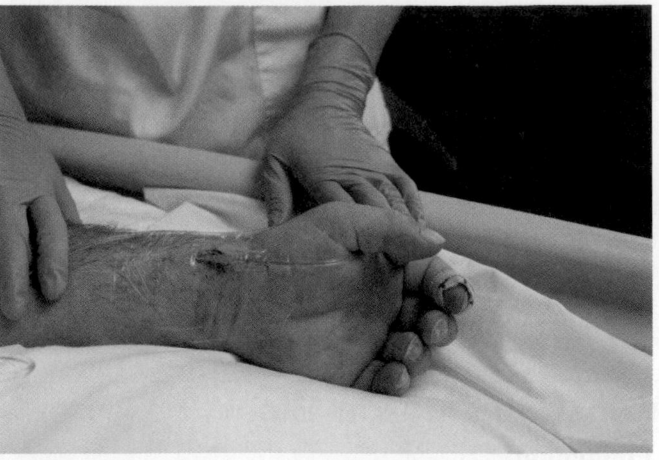

▲ Radial artery catheter provides continuous blood pressure monitoring and easy access for blood sampling.

TABLE 33-2 Causes of Acid–Base Imbalance

Acidemia	Alkalemia
Hypovolemia	
Hypoventilation	Hyperventilation
COPD	Hypokalemia
Cardiac arrest	Pulmonary embolus
Diabetic ketoacidosis	Diuretics/steroids
Severe diarrhea	Prolonged vomiting
Renal failure	NG suction

8. Change flush solution and tubing every 96 hr (according to agency policy).
9. Change dressing weekly or if it becomes loose or soiled. ▸ ***Rationale:*** Loose or soiled dressings increase risk of infection at site.
   a. Put on gloves.
   b. Remove dressing and discard in biohazard container.
   c. Apply transparent dressing, date, and initials.
10. Remove gloves and PPE and perform hand hygiene.
11. Monitor site to ensure hemostasis occurs.
12. Monitor extremity distally for adequacy of perfusion.

Monitoring Intraaortic Balloon Pump Circulatory Assistance

Procedure

For Monitoring Balloon Pump Function

1. Validate that balloon catheter tip is at second to third ICS per daily chest x-ray.
2. Assess that balloon is precisely synchronized with the client's EKG cardiac cycle or arterial wave form:
   a. Inflation starts at the dicrotic notch of the arterial wave form (closure of the aortic valve).
   b. Deflation occurs before the QRS complex (systole).
3. Maintain frequency of assist at 1:1 or other ratio as ordered.
4. Assess IABP device timing and document by recording strip of arterial pressure in 1:2 assist. ▸ ***Rationale:*** Cardiac output may decrease if timing is not precise.

For Monitoring Client Response

1. Check balloon insertion site hourly for bleeding/hematoma and signs of infection.
2. Assess circulation hourly: color, temperature, capillary refill; bilateral radial and pedal pulses. ▸ ***Rationale:*** To validate balloon position does not occlude major run-off from aorta.
3. Monitor urine output hourly; report drop in UO or <30 mL/hr $\times$ 2 hr. ▸ ***Rationale:*** To validate adequate renal perfusion.
4. Assess neurologic status every shift. ▸ ***Rationale:*** To assess effect on cerebral perfusion.
5. Note CO, CI and record every 2 hr. ▸ ***Rationale:*** To determine improved cardiac function.

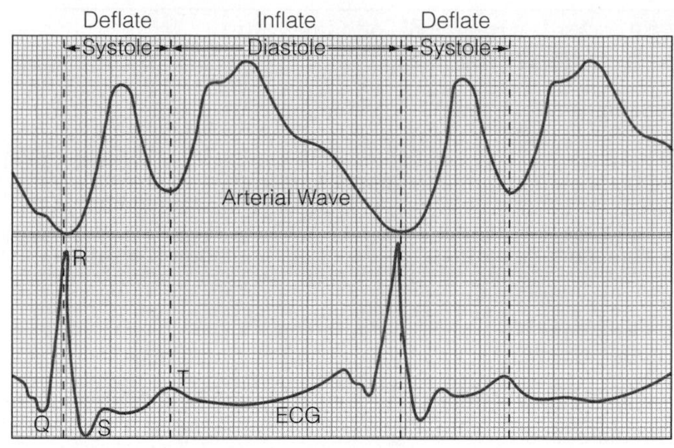

▲ Assess IABP device timing by recording strip of arterial pressure in 1:2 assist. Timing must be precise.

6. Monitor bowel sounds and assess abdomen for pain. ▸ ***Rationale:*** Abnormal findings may indicate inappropriate balloon placement and should be reported.
7. Report client experience of chest discomfort or any pain, numbness, or tingling in arms or legs.
8. Report decrease in platelet count per daily CBC. ▸ ***Rationale:*** Catheter function damages platelets.
9. Monitor coagulation profile results. ▸ ***Rationale:*** Neither clot formation nor bleeding should occur.

Withdrawing Arterial Blood Samples

Equipment

One 6-mL sterile syringe

ABG kit with one 3-mL syringe with dry lithium heparin; air filter device

Or: Vacutainer with Luer-Lok adapter cannula; blood specimen tubes

Gloves

Face shield

Container with ice (paper cup, emesis basin)

Two specimen labels

Bubble packaging

Biohazard specimen bag

Gauze sponges/pads

Preparation

1. Identify client, check Ident-A-Band, and ask client to state name and birth date.
2. Gather equipment and explain procedure to client.
3. Attach label to specimen syringe with client's name, hospital number, room number, time, and date. Also add client's current temperature and FIO_2.
4. For blood gas (ABG) specimen, maintain client's current oxygen delivery setting for 20 minutes before obtaining specimen.

EVIDENCE-BASED PRACTICE

Mean Arterial Blood Pressure

In general, the MAP (mean arterial pressure) provides a more accurate interpretation of a patient's hemodynamic status. It provides the best estimate of central aortic pressure and is less sensitive to over- and under-damping distortions.

Source: McGhee, B., & Bridges, E. (2002). Monitoring arterial blood pressure: What you may not know. *Critical Care Nurse, 22*(2), 60–79.

Clinical Alert

"In-line" blood sampling systems eliminate the need for discarding blood, thus reducing blood loss and associated risks.

5. Fill paper cup or emesis basin with ice.
6. Perform hand hygiene and don gloves.

Procedure

1. Momentarily disengage arterial alarms.
2. Turn stopcock off to client.
3. Remove protective cap from open blood sampling port on three-way stopcock closest to arterial line insertion site.
4. Attach syringe or Vacutainer with Luer-Lok adapter cannula to open port of three-way stopcock.
5. Turn stopcock off to flush solution.

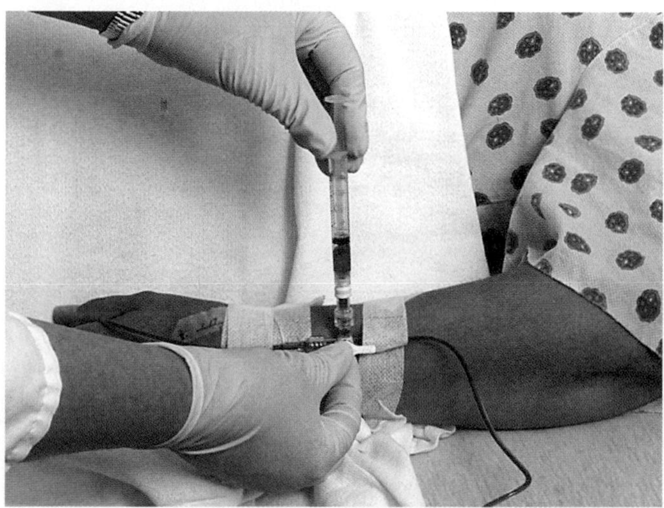

▲ Engage syringe or Vacutainer to sample port to obtain arterial blood.

6. Attach syringe or blood specimen tube into Vacutainer to establish blood draw.
7. Discard obtained sample. ▸ ***Rationale:*** This discard ensures a specimen that is free of heparin or flush solution.

NOTE: For an ABG blood sample, discard volume should be twice the dead space volume of the catheter and tubing up to the sampling site. For coagulation studies, discard volume should be six times the dead space volume.

8. Engage ABG specimen tube into Vacutainer.
9. Obtain arterial blood gas specimen.
10. Turn stopcock off to open port. ▸ ***Rationale:*** This reestablishes flow between flush solution and client.
11. Remove Vacutainers for Blood Conservatory Process.

For Blood Conservatory Process

a. Don clean gloves.
b. Aspirate blood into reservoir tubing.
c. Close stopcock to reservoir tubing.
d. Access sampling port (closest to client) using blunt cannula with tube holder (Vacutainer).
e. Engage blood collection tubes into tube holder and allow to fill. ▸ ***Rationale:*** Obtaining specimens using a blood conservatory system helps to prevent nosocomial anemia.
f. When sampling is complete, remove blunt cannula and tube holder.
g. Open stopcock to reservoir tubing and return contents to client.

12. Place arterial blood gas specimen tubes in container filled with ice.
13. Fast flush remaining blood onto gauze pad.
14. Reattach protective cap on open port.
15. Validate good arterial waveform on monitor.
16. Reactivate monitor alarms.
17. Wrap syringe/specimen in bubble packaging and place in biohazard bag with ice.
18. Remove gloves and perform hand hygiene.
19. Send specimens to laboratory immediately and notify lab that tubes are being sent.

TABLE 33-3 Arterial Blood Gas Values in Acid–Base Imbalances

Normal ABG Values		
pH	7.35–7.45	
PCO_2	35–45 mmHg	
HCO_3	22–26 mEq	
Respiratory Acidosis		**Compensation**
pH: decreased	<7.35	7.35
PCO_2: increased	>45 mmHg	
HCO_3–: normal	24	>26 mEq
Respiratory Alkalosis		**Compensation**
pH: increased	>7.45	7.45
PCO_2: decreased	<35 mmHg	
HCO_3–: normal	24	<22 mEq
Metabolic Acidosis		**Compensation**
pH: decreased	<7.35	7.35
HCO_3–: decreased	<22 mEq	
PCO_2: normal	40	<35 mmHg
Metabolic Alkalosis		**Compensation**
pH: increased	>7.45	7.45
HCO_3–: increased	>26 mEq	
PCO_2: normal	40	>45 mmHg

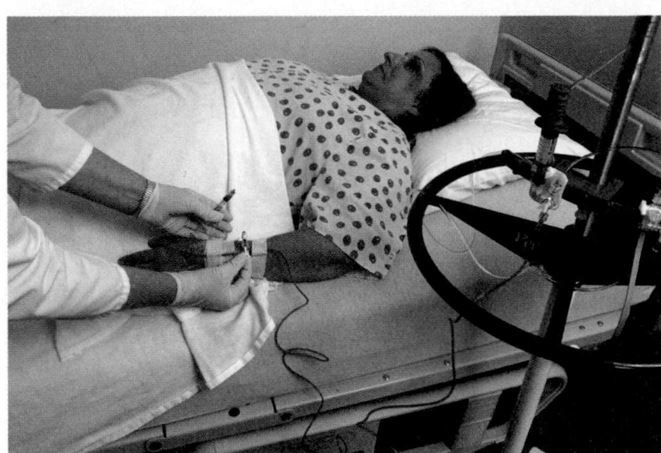

▲ When sampling is complete, open stopcock to reservoir tubing and return contents of blood conservatory system to client.

Removing Arterial Catheter

Equipment

Gloves
Personal protective equipment
Two 4 × 4 gauze pads
Suture removal set
Tape

Preparation

1. Check physician's orders.
2. Check client's coagulation lab results (values).
3. Gather equipment.
4. Perform hand hygiene.

5. Identify client; check Ident-A-Band, have client state name and birth date, and explain procedure to client.
6. Disarm monitor alarms.

Procedure

1. Don gloves and PPE.
2. Remove dressing, and discard in appropriate container.
3. Clip retaining sutures if present.
4. Apply finger pressure approximately 2 cm *above* skin puncture site. ▸ ***Rationale:*** The artery puncture site is proximal to the skin puncture site.

Clinical Alert

Apply pressure to puncture site for at least 10 minutes if client is on anticoagulation or antithrombotic therapy.

5. Place folded 4 × 4 gauze pad over cannula site with nondominant hand, and apply gentle pressure.
6. Pull arterial cannula straight out of artery with quick, even pressure.
7. Apply firm pressure over and just above cannula site for at least 5–10 minutes. ▸ ***Rationale:*** This action achieves hemostasis and prevents formation of a hematoma.
8. Place folded 4 × 4 gauze pad over puncture site, and tape tightly. ▸ ***Rationale:*** This provides additional pressure to site to prevent bleeding.
9. Discard supplies, remove gloves, PPE, and perform hand hygiene.
10. Check cannulation site frequently. ▸ ***Rationale:*** To observe for bleeding or thrombosis.
11. Check distal extremity for temperature, circulation, motion, and sensation intermittently for several hours, then routinely after catheter removal. ▸ ***Rationale:*** Delayed complications (thrombosis) may occur.

DOCUMENTATION for Arterial Blood Pressure Monitoring

- Size of arterial catheter inserted
- Name of physician inserting catheter
- Pressure readings (systolic, diastolic, and MAP)
- Direct and indirect pressure measurements
- Distal neurovascular status of cannulated extremity (temperature, color, motion, sensation)
- Position of client during readings
- Unexpected outcomes and appropriate interventions
- Client response and tolerance of procedure
- Appearance of catheter insertion site
- Monitor strip recordings

Arterial Blood Sampling

- Time specimen obtained
- Client's temperature and FIO_2 at the time blood was drawn

Arterial Site Dressing Change

- Condition of insertion site
- Type of dressing applied

IABP Circulatory Assist

- IABP assist timing ratio (e.g., 1:1)
- Femoral artery insertion site status every hour
- Peripheral circulation status every hour (pulses, color, temperature, capillary refill)
- Urine output every hour
- Abdominal and neurologic assessment every 8 hr
- Hemodynamic parameters every 2 hr (CO, CI, SVR)
- Client reports of chest or abdominal discomfort, any pain, numbness in extremities, including problem-solving interventions

Removing Arterial Catheter

- Time of removal
- Manual pressure and dressing applied
- Condition of insertion site
- Presence and quality of distal pulses
- Motion and sensation of involved extremity

CRITICAL THINKING Application

Expected Outcomes

- Blood supply to hand is adequate before and after arterial catheter placement.
- Arterial cannulation is accomplished without complication.
- Arterial blood pressure monitoring system functions reliably and accurately.
- Intraaortic balloon pump circulatory assist improves cardiac output: Afterload and preload are reduced.
- Arterial blood samples are obtained.

Unexpected Outcomes	Alternative Actions
Absence of collateral circulation noted when performing the Modified Allen Test (negative Modified Allen Test).	• Assess contralateral extremity. • Avoid radial artery. • Notify physician. (An alternate artery may be selected—femoral.)
Cannulated extremity develops diminished distal perfusion.	• Check periphery for changes in color, temperature, motion, and sensation resulting from possible thrombus occlusion or circulatory "steal." • Notify physician immediately. • Prepare for catheter removal.
Hypotension and bradycardia occur during arterial puncture or catheter removal.	• Reverse response with atropine administration.
Hematoma or bleeding occurs at arterial insertion site.	• Apply direct pressure over artery while you check for leaks in the system. • Check all stopcocks: check if catheter is inserted in artery as it should be. • Keep cannulated extremity exposed for observation. • Remove catheter if oozing continues.
Signs of infection or inflammation appear at insertion site.	• Use sterile transparent dressings exclusively. • Always use aseptic technique with dressing changes; change dressing weekly. • Cap open port on stopcock to maintain asepsis. • Do not apply ointment to insertion site. • Change tubing, flush solution and transducer every 96 hr or with catheter change using sterile technique. • Flush open port after obtaining blood specimens. • Prepare for catheter removal if infection suspected.
Arterial waveform loses definition and digital pressures drop.	• Reverse response with atropine administration. • Use low compliance (rigid) short (<3–4 ft) monitor tubing. • Check for thrombus formation by aspirating blood through stopcock and then flushing system. • Be sure to fast-flush arterial line thoroughly after arterial blood samples are obtained or system is zeroed. • Make sure all stopcocks are closed to air. • Maintain 300-mmHg pressure in pressure bag. • Ensure secure fit of all stopcocks and connections. Avoid adding stopcocks and line extensions. • Change position of extremity in which catheter is placed.
Direct blood pressure readings vary significantly.	• Flick tubing system to remove tiny air bubbles escaping the flush solution. • Recheck transducer and client position to ensure accurate data. • Recalibrate transducer. • Flush system after sampling and zeroing. • Keep flush bag adequately filled and cleared of air. • Maintain bag external pressure at 300 mmHg. • Check that connections are tightly secured.
Arterial blood sample is unobtainable.	• Suspect arterial spasm; allow spasm of artery to stop, then attempt to aspirate blood with gentle pressure using a 6-mL syringe rather than Vacutainer. • Reposition client's arm, making sure there is no pressure at catheter insertion site. • Check that catheter is in artery (note waveform on oscilloscope), flush catheter, then attempt to obtain sample.

Intra-aortic balloon ruptures.	• Turn console off and notify physician. Balloon must be removed within 30 minutes.
Console fails.	• If problem not resolved in 30 minutes, use syringe filled with 40 mL of room air to manually inflate and deflate balloon to move balloon folds in order to prevent clot formation.
Client has decreased urinary output or develops signs of radial artery occlusion.	• Suspect balloon migration. • Maintain HOB elevation at less than 45° to prevent kinking and migration of catheter. • Immobilize cannulated extremity to prevent catheter migration.

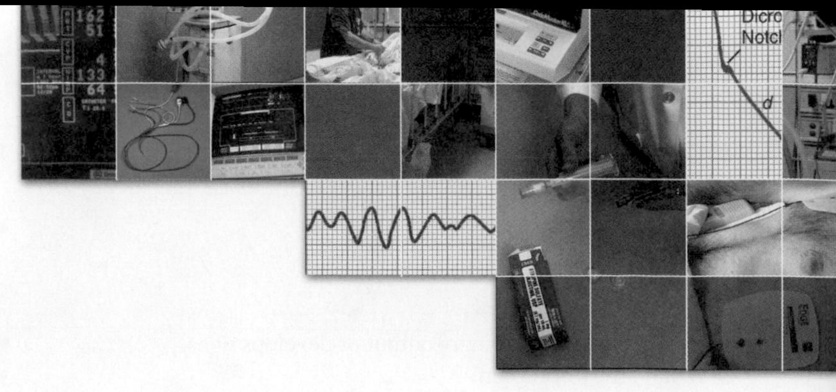

Chapter 33

UNIT 3

Cardiac Emergencies

Nursing Process Data

ASSESSMENT Data Base

- Assess client's responsiveness, breathing, and circulation.
- Identify lethal heart rhythms on the ECG recording.
- Assess availability of emergency support response and emergency supplies.
- Identify appropriate drugs needed for an emergency situation.

PLANNING Objectives

- To be prepared to respond to the needs of unstable clients
- To locate necessary supplies and appropriate medications used in emergency situations
- To provide emergency defibrillation to convert lethal arrhythmias (dysrhythmias) to normal sinus rhythm
- To assist with cardioversion to convert rapid supraventricular rhythms or unstable ventricular tachycardia to normal sinus rhythm

IMPLEMENTATION Procedures

EVALUATION Expected Outcomes

- Supplies and medications are readily available in an emergency situation.
- Client's heart rhythm is restored to normal after defibrillation or synchronized cardioversion.

Early recognition is essential for prompt and effective treatment of cardiac emergencies. Interventions for treating emergencies such as hemodynamic instability and flash pulmonary edema include measures to decrease heart work, correct lethal dysrhythmias, and remove excess body fluid.

If left untreated, symptomatic bradycardias and supraventricular or ventricular tachyarrhythmias can cause reduced cardiac output and inadequate tissue perfusion. Life-threatening tachyarrhythmias are terminated by delivering an externally applied electrical countershock to the heart. This countershock depolarizes the myocardium, interrupts the dysrhythmia, and allows the normal pacemaker (sinoatrial node) of the heart to resume control of the heart rhythm. Two types of electrical countershock applications are used: cardioversion and defibrillation.

Defibrillation is an emergency procedure in which fairly large amounts of electric current are delivered without concern for synchronization with ventricular depolarization (QRS wave) on the ECG. Defibrillation is used to terminate ventricular fibrillation or *pulseless* ventricular tachycardia.

Cardioversion is a procedure used to convert supraventricular tachyarrhythmias and ventricular tachycardia in unstable clients. The electrical countershock is synchronized with ventricular depolarization (QRS wave on ECG) to avoid discharge during the T wave (vulnerable period). This procedure may be elective (planned) or emergent.

The "crash cart" contains essential life support medications and supplies used in emergency situations in the hospital setting. Familiarity with its location and contents, including typical emergency drugs, will assist hospital staff to provide quick, competent care to clients during cardiac emergencies. The crash cart should be kept fully stocked and located in an area that is accessible and obvious to all. Nurses must have a working knowledge of the contents of each drawer of the cart to quickly find necessary supplies.

Maintaining the Emergency Cart

Equipment

- Emergency cart with locking drawers
- Emergency cart checklist
- Airway equipment
- Oxygen equipment
- Suction equipment
- Monitor leads and electrodes
- Defibrillator
- Oscilloscope
- IV equipment
- Emergency drugs

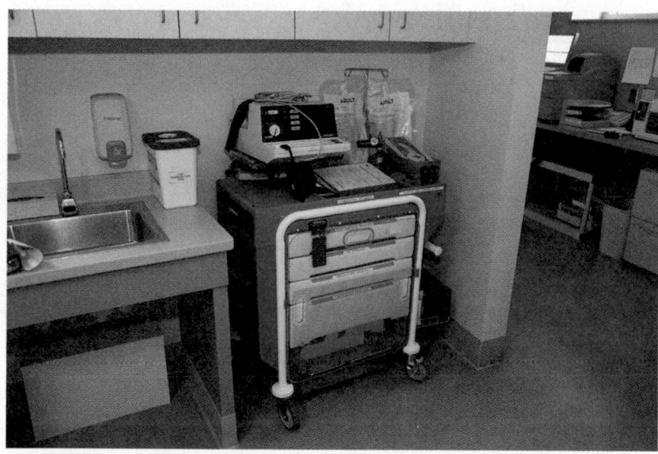

▲ Fully equipped emergency cart is placed in a readily accessible area, visible to staff. Defibrillation and respiratory supplies are kept on the top of the cart.

Procedure

1. Identify supplies and medications commonly used in emergency situations.
2. Gather equipment.
3. Maintain supplies in drawers according to priority use in the most commonly occurring emergency situations. Leave defibrillator plugged into electrical outlet at all times or check batteries every shift.
4. Lock drawers when cart is not in use. ▶ ***Rationale:*** This prevents personnel from using supplies for situations other than emergencies and not replacing it.
5. Place emergency cart checklist on outside of cart in visible area. ▶ ***Rationale:*** Cart contents are checked on a daily basis (and every 8–12 hr in critical care units) to ensure medications are not outdated, equipment is in working condition, and cart is locked.
6. Place cart in designated, easily accessible, and visible area of the nursing unit. ▶ ***Rationale:*** Provides for less confusion if the cart is needed.
7. Familiarize all personnel with location and contents of cart, function of equipment, and emergency procedures.
8. Practice retrieving and setting up equipment through mock situations. ▶ ***Rationale:*** This ensures that all personnel are able to use cart during an emergency situation.
9. Check cart daily and document; restock immediately after use. ▶ ***Rationale:*** If cart is not restocked, delays can occur during an emergency situation, jeopardizing client care.

Checking Contents of the Emergency Cart

Equipment

NOTE: Emergency cart contents vary among agencies.

Top of Cart

Defibrillator/monitor and related supplies
Respiratory supplies
Gloves, face shield

Front of Cart

Cardiac arrest board

First Drawer

Emergency medications

Second Drawer

IV access supplies
IV solutions and tubing
Syringes, special needles

Third Drawer

NG tubes
Blood pressure cuff, stethoscope
Flashlight
Suction catheter kit and supplies
Central line catheter and supplies

Side of Cart

Emergency cart checklist
Cardiac resuscitation recording sheet and clipboard
Suction unit

Calling a Code

NOTE: See procedure in Chapter 27, Circulatory Maintenance, for CPR/AED skill.

For any client who becomes unresponsive, is not breathing, and has no pulse, call a "code" and get the AED.

Clinical Alert

Summon the Rapid Response Team if noting certain "triggers": tachypnea, hypotension, signs of shock, active bleeding, chest pain, and altered level of consciousness.

NOTE: Tachypnea and hypotension frequently precede cardiac arrest.

Clinical Alert

Clinically "dead" clients may be able to hear and remember events occurring throughout resuscitation procedures.

Clinical Alert

Sudden cardiac death is the most common cause of death, outnumbering the total number of deaths from AIDS, lung cancer, breast cancer, and stroke each year.

Clinical Alert

The Joint Commission requires hospitals to track and evaluate resuscitation attempts in order to improve process and client outcomes. Development of rapid response teams and in-hospital use of AEDs as well as changes in CPR/ECC guidelines are recommendations based on this tracking data.

EVIDENCE-BASED PRACTICE

This 20-month study (including more than 24,000 patients hospitalized before and 25,000 patients hospitalized after initiation of a Rapid Response Team) showed that the RRT failed to achieve its goal of reducing hospital-wide code rates or mortality outside the ICU and raises questions about whether hospitals should devote resources to Rapid Response Teams.

Source: Chan, P. S., Khalid, A., Longmore, L. S., Berg, R. A., Kosiborod, M., & Spertus, J. A. (2008). Hospital-wide code rates and mortality before and after implementation of a rapid response team. *The Journal of the American Medical Association*, *300*(21), 2506–2513.

Performing Defibrillation*

Equipment

Defibrillator with ECG recorder
Defibrillator pads or conduction gel for paddles (do not use ultrasound gel)
(*or*)
"Hands-free" defibrillation electrodes (refer to package for product-specific instructions)
Emergency cart with:
Airway
Cardiac board
Resuscitator bag

*Skill only performed by ACLS-trained staff.

Preparation

1. Validate that client is unresponsive.
   a. Not breathing, or not breathing normally (e.g., only gasping), and
   b. No pulse is palpable within 10 seconds (no longer).

2. Call a code and get the AED and crash cart.
3. Place back board under client, deflate air-filled mattress if present, avoiding delay to initiating CPR with chest compressions within 10 seconds.
4. Immediately perform CPR (chest compressions) providing 30 compressions in 18 seconds with a depth of at least 2 inches until AED or cart and response team arrive.

Procedure

1. Plug defibrillator into electric outlet.
2. Turn defibrillator power ON and allow to warm up.
3. Attach monitor/defibrillator.
4. Dry client's chest if necessary (do not use alcohol). ▶ ***Rationale:*** To prevent skin burns.

Clinical Alert

Early defibrillation (within 3 minutes) is the key to successful resuscitation.

5. Place conducting pads on client's chest, pressing firmly for adhesion, or spread thin coat of defibrillation electrode gel evenly over surface of paddles. One pad is placed below right clavicle near sternum and second pad is placed to left of cardiac apex (below and to the left of left nipple or at the fifth to sixth intercostal space at midaxillary line). Do not place over broken skin. ▶ ***Rationale:*** Conductive medium decreases skin resistance and reduces degree of burns.

Clinical Alert

Before beginning defibrillation or cardioversion procedure, remove any transdermal medication patch on chest. Avoid placing paddles over electrodes/leads; avoid pacemaker or ICD generator by at least 8 cm.

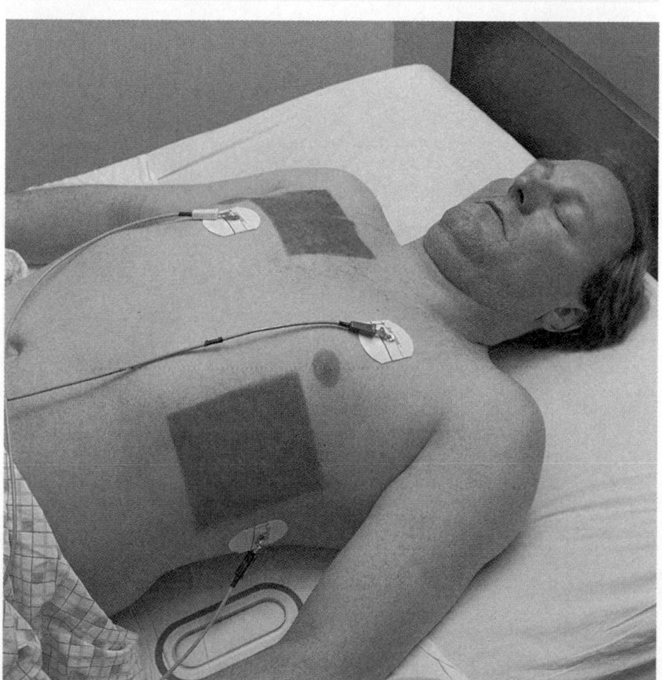

▲ Gel pads are placed below right clavicle and left of cardiac apex.

6. Alternatively, apply "hands-free" defibrillation pads.
7. Insert electrodes connector into cable. Push firmly for proper connection.
8. Turn on ECG recorder.
9. Validate that client has shockable rhythm (pulseless VT or VF is present).
10. If **nonshockable** rhythm is present (PEA, asystole), continue CPR for five cycles and administer fluids/medications before attempting defibrillation.
11. Be certain defibrillator is NOT in synchronized mode. ▶ ***Rationale:*** The machine will not respond to ventricular fibrillation if set to synchronized mode.
12. Set standard monophasic defibrillator to charge at 360 watt seconds; set biphasic device at 200 watt seconds.

Clinical Alert

During defibrillation attempts, ensure the room ventilation is adequate. An oxygen enriched atmosphere (e.g., high-flow oxygen directed across the chest) may support fire caused by spark.

13. Command all persons to move away from bed area and any equipment connected to client.
14. Stand away from bed area yourself.
15. Apply paddles with firm pressure (25 lb). ▶ ***Rationale:*** Firm pressure decreases transthoracic resistance; this is not necessary with hands-free pads.
16. Depress discharge buttons on paddles simultaneously to ensure appropriate discharge or push "shock" button on defibrillator for hands-free pads—delivering ONE shock.
17. Immediately resume chest compressions. Do not delay for rhythm reanalysis or pulse check.
18. Immediately resume CPR for five cycles.

NOTE: After advanced airway placed, breaths (8–10 per minute) are given along with *uninterrupted* chest compressions (100/min).

Clinical Alert

Gel pads may need to be replaced after three shock deliveries because of drying out.

19. Analyze ECG. If sinus rhythm is established, check for pulse, vital signs, LOC.

Defibrillation

Defibrillation is used for these lethal arrhythmias: pulseless ventricular tachycardia, ventricular fibrillation.

Synchronized Cardioversion

Synchronized cardioversion is used to convert supraventricular tachyarrhythmias and ventricular tachycardia (with pulses) if the client shows serious signs of hemodynamic instability (e.g., ventricular rate $\geq$ 150, SBP <90 mmHg).

DEFIBRILLATION ARRHYTHMIA

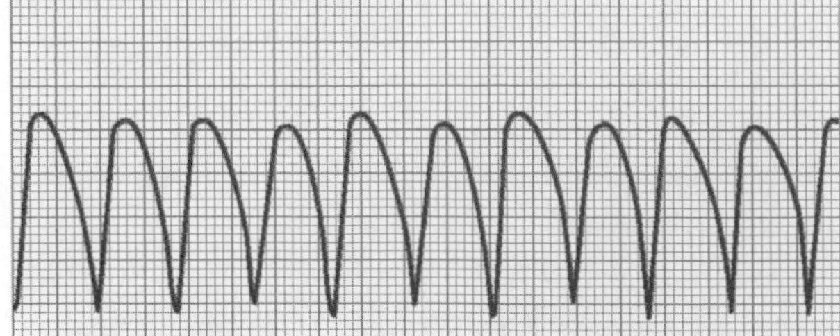

▲ Pulseless ventricular tachycardia.

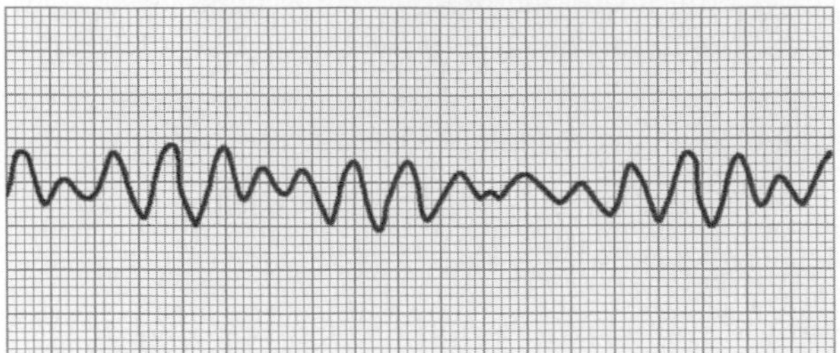

▲ Ventricular fibrillation.

20. Recharge defibrillator for second attempt at 360 watt seconds (monophasic) or 200 watt seconds (biphasic) if shockable rhythm continues.
21. Deliver ONE shock, then resume CPR immediately for five cycles.

Clinical Alert

Monophasic versus Biphasic Defibrillators

Traditional monophasic defibrillators use a single pulse of energy that travels from one electrode to the other in one direction. Biphasic defibrillators send the current from one electrode to the other, then back to the first electrode with equal success of defibrillation at lower levels of energy (120 joules for the first shock, 200 joules being the maximum). Biphasic defibrillators also adapt to the transthoracic impedance of the particular client and adjust the appropriate current accordingly (e.g., AEDs).

Advantages of the biphasic model include lower risk of skin burns, less myocardial injury, and more rapid return of heart function and MAP. Models are also smaller, weigh less, are easier to maintain, and can be used as well for synchronized cardioversion at 30 joules.

Source: Tuite, P., & George, E. (2005). Biphasic defibrillation: Know your equipment. *Nursing 2005, 35*(3), 32ccl.

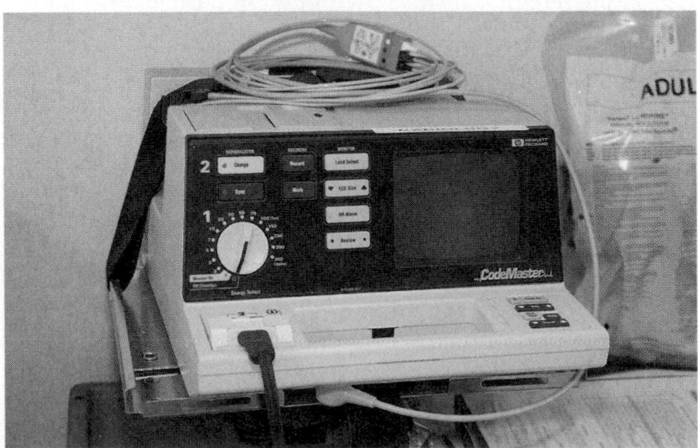

▲ CODEMASTER.

CARDIOVERSION ARRHYTHMIAS

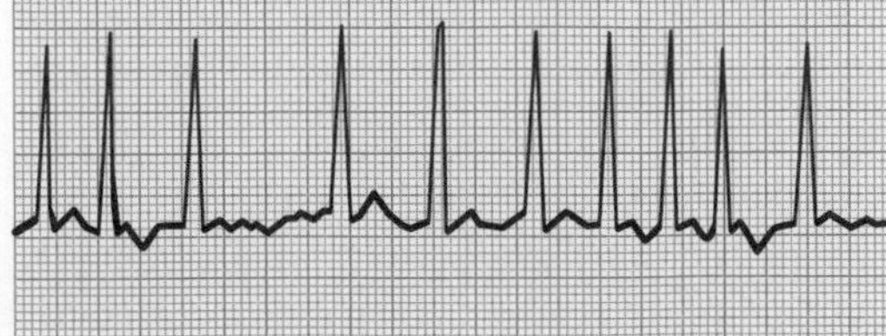

▲ Atrial fibrillation with rapid ventricular response.

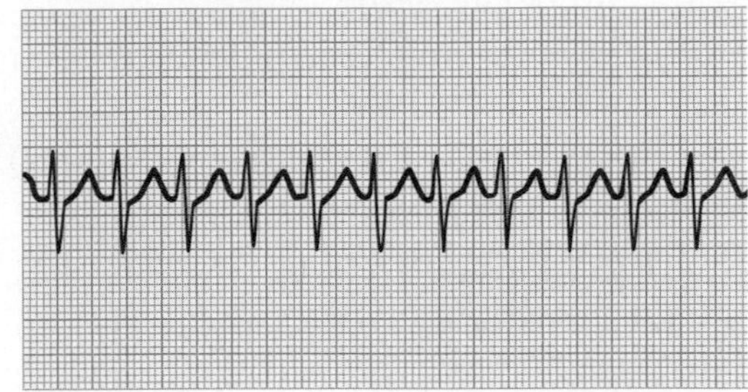

▲ Supraventricular tachycardia.

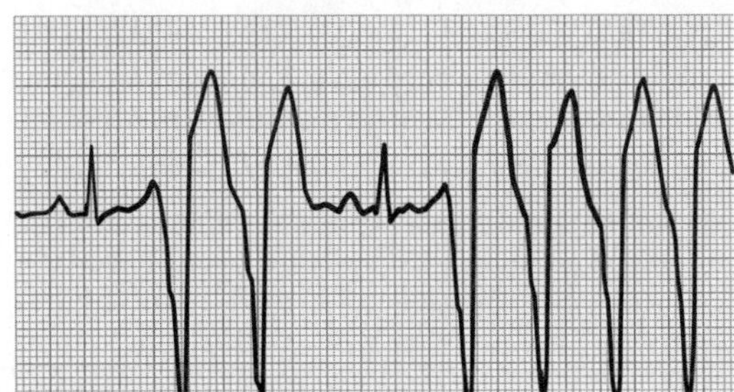

▲ Ventricular tachycardia with pulses.

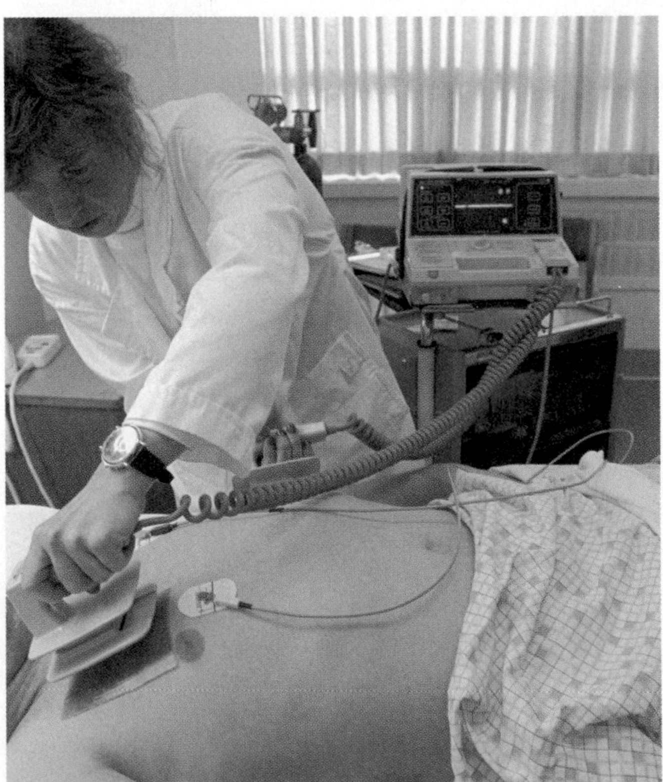

▲ Apply paddles with firm pressure over conducting pads.

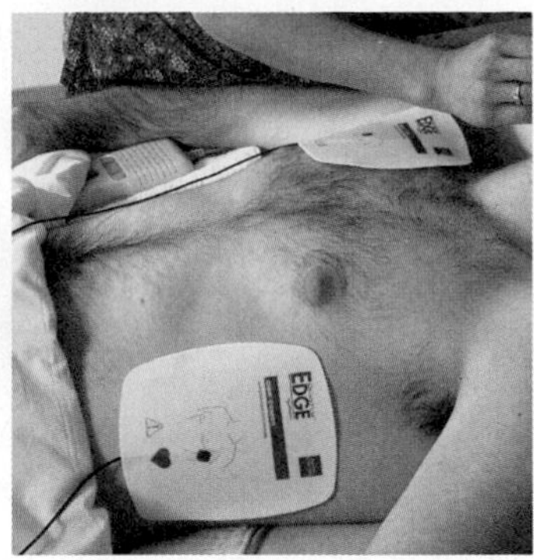

▲ Hands-free pads provide defibrillation and protect provider.

22. Give epinephrine 1 mg IV/IO during CPR; repeat every 3–5 minutes or give Vasopressin 40 units IV/IO in place of first or second dose of epinephrine.
23. Repeat steps 19, 20, and 21.
24. May administer amiodarone (300 mg IV/IO) once, or lidocaine (1–1.5 mg/kg) once, then 0.5–0.75 mg/kg IV/IO, maximum three doses, *or* magnesium (1–2 g IV/IO) for polymorphic VT (torsade de pointes).
25. Repeat steps 19–22.
26. For asystole or pulseless electrical activity (PEA), continue CPR for five cycles, administer vasopressors (see step 22). Consider treatable factors and correct (see Clinical Alert p 86).
27. Check the ECG for *shockable* rhythm, and repeat process starting with step 11 if present.
28. Continue CPR throughout entire resuscitation process.
29. Clean reusable equipment, discard used supplies, perform hand hygiene.

EVIDENCE-BASED PRACTICE

Family Support During CPR

Family members should be offered the opportunity to be present during resuscitation efforts. Ideally a staff member should be assigned to support the family and answer questions.

Source: American Heart Association Guidelines CPR/ECC 2005: *Handbook of Emergency Cardiovascular Care.*

Clinical Alert

The most common cause of PEA (pulseless electrical activity) is hypovolemia. Other contributing factors include: hypoxia, hydrogen ion imbalance (acidemia), hypo or hyperkalemia, hypoglycemia, hypothermia, toxins, tamponade (cardiac), tension pneumothorax, thrombosis (MI, PE), and trauma.

Three Phases of Cardiac Arrest

Electrical phase lasts about 5 minutes; early defibrillation is the priority intervention.

Hemodynamic phase lasts from 4 to 10 minutes; use of uninterrupted chest compressions is the priority intervention to maintain coronary perfusion (since the left heart is empty and the client is essentially in pulseless electrical activity [PEA]); use of AED can be harmful.

Metabolic phase uninterrupted chest compressions are vital to maintain coronary perfusion; medications and hypothermia may be used.

Source: Futterman, L., & Lemberg, L. (2005). Cardiopulmonary resuscitation review: Critical role of chest compressions. *American Journal of Critical Care, 14*(1), 81.

Administering Advanced Cardiac Life-Support Medications

Equipment

Client's medical record (note client's weight for drug dosage determination)

Emergency "crash" cart with medications (may be supplied in ampules, multiple dose vials, or "unit-of-use" containers [cartridge/needle units or cartridge/syringe units])

Preparation

1. Familiarize self with most commonly used medications, their action, usual dose, route and rate of administration, and side effects.

EVIDENCE-BASED PRACTICE

Induced hypothermia (32 to 34°C for 12 to 24 hours) might benefit comatose adult patients with ROSC after out of hospital arrest from a nonshockable rhythm, or cardiac arrest in hospital.

Source: 2010 AHA Guidelines for CPR and ECC. *Circulation* 2010; 122: S640-S656. part 8, p 15.

EVIDENCE-BASED PRACTICE

Vasopressors (epinephrine or vasopressin) may improve return of spontaneous circulation (ROSC), but there is insufficient evidence to suggest they improve survival to discharge.

Source: 2010 American Heart Association Guidelines for Cardiopulmonary Resuscitation and Emergency Cardiovascular Care Science. *Circulation* 2010, 122: S640–S656.

2. Review skill for Administration of Intravenous Medications (Chapter 28).
3. Client should be intubated and airway placement confirmed (see Respiratory Care, Chapter 26).
4. Establish IV access if not already present (intraosseous [IO] or bone access may be necessary in emergency situations).
5. Continue client cardiac monitoring.

Procedure

1. Prepare cartridge/syringe unit by removing caps from cartridge vial and injector.

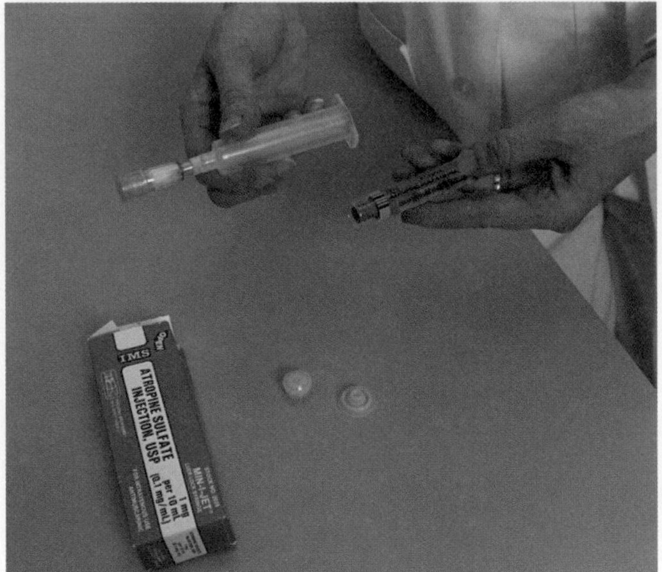

▲ Remove caps from cartridge and injector.

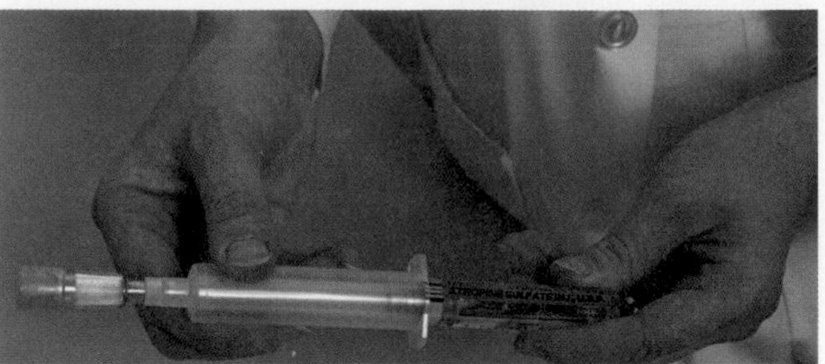

▲ Insert cartridge/vial into injector and rotate clockwise until medication enters needle.

2. Insert vial into injector, rotating clockwise until medication enters injector needle.
3. Remove protected needle or male Luer-Lok cover and gently press vial to initiate medication flow.
4. Swab IV port with antimicrobial swab and insert system for medication injection.
5. Administer emergency medications as ordered.

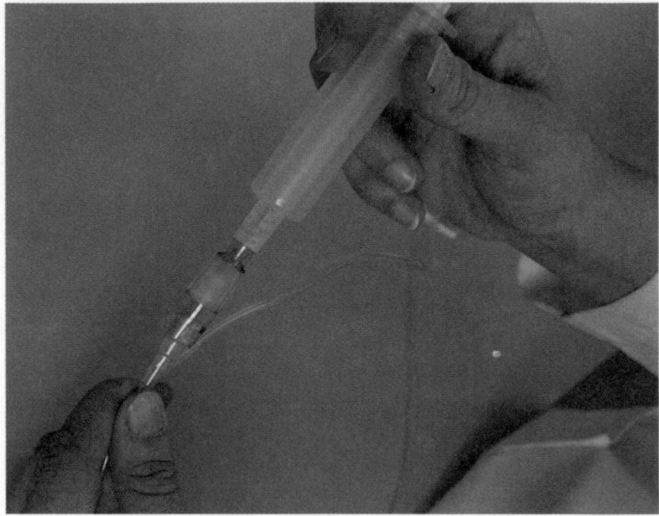

▲ Protected needle or Luer-Lok system may be used for drug administration per IV tubing port.

TABLE 33-4 Advanced Cardiac Life Support Medications May Be Given IV or IO

Medication[a]	Dose	Indication
Vasopressin	40 U IV/IO one time only in place of 1st or 2nd dose of epinephrine	For VF/pulseless VT, asystole, pulseless electrical activity
Epinephrine	1 mg IV/IO/ET; repeat every 3–5 minutes during resuscitation	Same as above, symptomatic bradycardia not responsive to atropine
Amiodarone	300 mg IV/IO, then 150 mg, only once (dilute in 20–30 mL D_5W)	Recurrent VF/VT
Lidocaine	1–1.5 mg/kg IV/IO, then 0.5–0.75mg/kg IV in 5–10 min	ET dose is 2–4/mg/kg/F for V7 pulseless VT, stable VT
Procainamide	20 mg/min to 17 mg/kg max	Stable VT, PSVT
Magnesium sulfate	1–2 g diluted in 10 mL D_5W over 5–20 minutes IV/IO	Suspected hypomagnesemia or torsade de pointes (polymorphic VT)
Atropine	0.5 mg IV/IO or ET*; repeat every 3–5 min up to 3 mg	Symptomatic bradycardia
Adenosine	6 mg *rapid* push, then in 1 to 2 minutes give 12 mg; may repeat 12 mg after 1 to 2 minutes	Terminate narrow complex AV nodal reentrant supraventricular tachycardia AVNRT in stable client
Atenolol	5 mg slow IV (over 5 minutes); may repeat after 10 minutes	Control ventricular rate in supraventricular tachyarrhythmias (atrial fibrillation, atrial flutter, PSVT)
Diltiazem	15–20 mg (0.25 mg/kg) IV over 2 minutes; after 15 minutes may give 20–25 mg over 2 minutes	Same as above

1. Follow each drug administered IV with 20-mL normal saline bolus flush, then elevate the extremity 10–20 seconds.
2. CPR and shocks are continued when drugs are administered.

Assisting With Synchronized Cardioversion

Equipment

Defibrillator monitor with ECG recorder set to SYNCHRONIZATION mode

Paddles—anteroposterior or anterolateral or hands-free pads

Conductive gel or conductive pads

Emergency cart with medications and supplies

Preparation for Elective Cardioversion

1. Review cardioversion orders and make sure consent form is signed. Check that equipment is functioning properly.
2. Review precardioversion laboratory values (electrolytes, digoxin level, ABGs). ▶ ***Rationale:*** Electrolyte imbalance, particularly hypokalemia, or digitalis toxicity may increase risk of dysrhythmias after cardioversion.
3. Check that client has been receiving anticoagulation therapy (Coumadin) for chronic atrial fibrillation.
4. Withhold food, medications, and fluids for 6–12 hr before elective cardioversion.
5. Obtain baseline 12-lead ECG, and label it "precardioversion."

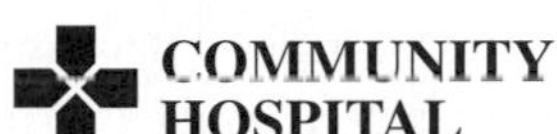

Legend:
Roc - Return of Circulation
PTA - Prior to Arrival
BVM - Bag Valve Mask

Name: ______________
Dept: ______________
Date: ______________

CODE BLUE RECORD

TIME EVENT					
DATE	RECOG TIME	LOCATION	AGE	WEIGHT	PEDS LENGTH

WAS A HOSPITAL-WIDE RESUSCITATION RESPONSE ACTIVATED? ☐Yes ☐No	CONDITION WHEN NEED FOR CHEST COMPRESSION/DEFIBRILLATION WAS IDENTIFIED ☐Pulse (poor perfusion) ☐Pulseless
WITNESSED ☐Yes ☐No	INDICATE ALL MONITORS THAT WERE PRESENT AT ONSET ☐ECG ☐Pulse Ox. ☐Apnea
PATIENT CONSCIOUS AT ONSET ☐Yes ☐No	DID THE PATIENT WITH A PULSE BECOME PULSELESS ☐Yes ☐No

AIRWAY/VENTILATION	CIRCULATION
AT ONSET ☐Spontaneous ☐Apnea ☐Assisted	FIRST DOCUMENTED RHYTHM
TYPES OF VENTILATION ☐Mouth/Mouth ☐Mouth/Mask ☐BVM ☐ETT ☐Tracheotomy ☐Other______	TIME CHEST COMPRESSIONS WERE STARTED FIRST DOCUMENTED PULSELESS RHYTHM
TIME OF FIRST ASSISTED VENTILATION	AED APPLIED ☐Yes ☐No / IF YES, TIME AED APPLIED
ETT INTUBATION TIME / SIZE	DEFIBRILLATOR TYPE(S) ☐Pads ☐Paddles ☐External Paddles
BY WHOM	
CONFIRMATION METHOD ☐Auscultation ☐Ex. CO2 ☐Other______	PACEMAKER ON ☐Yes ☐No

INTUBATED (PTA) ☐Yes ☐No; Total Amount mg.; THUMPER (PTA) ☐Yes ☐No; ATROPINE GIVEN (PTA) ☐Yes ☐No; PULSELESS (PTA) ☐Yes ☐No; DEFIBRILLATED (PTA) ☐Yes ☐No; LAST VASOPRESSIN (PTA); LAST EPI DOSE (PTA)

	CIRCULATION		O2	ELECTRICITY	IVP MEDICATIONS						DRIPS						COMMENTS
TIME	HEART RHYTHM and RATE	C = CARDIAC COMPRESSIONS SP = SPONTANEOUS	VENTILATION IA = INTUBATED AMBU AM = AMBU MASK SP = SPONTANEOUS	CARDIOVERSION/ DEFIBRILLATION (VOLTAGE/INITIALS)	EPINEPHRINE	ATROPINE	AMIODARONE	LIDOCAINE	VASOPRESIN	SODIUM BICARBONATE	IV FLUIDS/BLOOD	AMIODARONE	DOPAMINE	DOBUTAMINE	LIDOCAINE		BLOOD PRESSURE, PULSES, PROCEDURES (i.e. Periph./Central Line, Response to interventions)
					DOSAGE/INITIALS						DOSAGE/INITIALS						

OUTCOME	
RESUSCITATION EVENT ENDED	STATUS ☐Alive ☐Expired
REASON RESUSCITATION ENDED ☐Return of Circulation (> 20 min.) ☐Efforts Terminated (No sustained ROC) ☐Medical Futility ☐Advance Directive ☐Restrictions by Family	
RECORDER'S SIGNATURE	PHYSICIAN'S PRINTED NAME
ICU CODE TEAM NURSE'S SIGNATURE	PHYSICIAN'S SIGNATURE

CONFIDENTIAL INFORMATION

Provided by American Heart Association National Registry for Cardiopulmonary Resuscitation

▲ Code Blue Record.

Synchronized Cardioversion

Synchronized cardioversion is used for elective conversion of hemodynamically stable atrial fibrillation or atrial flutter.

It is also used as emergency management for hemodynamically unstable tachyarrhythmias (narrow and wide QRS complex tachycardias with pulses).

Rhythms which may require emergency synchronized cardioversion are:

- Atrial fibrillation with rapid ventricular response
- Atrial flutter 2:1
- Paroxysmal supraventricular tachycardia with signs of instability (HR > 150, SBP ≤ 90 mmHg)
- Ventricular tachycardia with pulses

6. Obtain baseline vital signs and ECG rhythms.
7. Assess peripheral pulses and neurologic status.
8. Notify anesthesiologist and physician of readiness.
9. Place emergency cart in room.
10. Perform hand hygiene.

Procedure

1. Validate client's identity: Check Ident-A-Band and have client state name and birth date.
2. Remove any jewelry. ▸ ***Rationale:*** metal conducts electricity, burns could occur.
3. Remove transdermal medication patches.
4. Establish IV line, and administer fluids at "keep open" rate.
5. Administer oxygen if ordered.
6. Plug in defibrillator and turn power switch ON.
7. Turn **synchronizer** switch ON. ▸ ***Rationale:*** Shock delivery synchronized with QRS of ECG reduces possibility of inducing ventricular arrhythmias by the electrical shock being delivered on the T wave.
8. Test synchronization by pushing manual synchronization button.
9. Disconnect all electric equipment from client except ECG monitor and cardioverter.
10. Administer sedative as ordered by physician (anesthetist/anesthesiologist may do this).
11. Charge defibrillator to level specified by physician. Note that designated charge is reached.
12. Place client in supine position.
13. Make sure client's chest is dry.
14. Apply conductive gel to surface of paddles, or use "hands-free" defibrillator pads and place on client's chest.
    a. Anterio-lateral handheld paddles are placed as in defibrillation, one below the right clavicle and the other placed to the left of the cardiac apex (below and to the left of the nipple or at the *5th* or *6th* intercostal space at the midaxillary line).
    b. Apex-posterior self-adhesive defibrillation pads are placed over the left precordium and posteriorly below the right or left scapula.

TABLE 33-5 Stepwise Energy Levels for Cardioversion

Cardioversion	Energy Level (J)*
Paroxysmal supraventricular tachycardia	50–100–200–300, then 360/J.
Atrial flutter	50–100–200–300 then 360/J.
Atrial fibrillation	200–300, then 360/J.
Unstable ventricular tachycardia (VT with pulses)	100 to 200 to 300 to 360/J.

*1 joule = 1 watt second

15. Observe ECG rhythm on monitor and start recording continuous printout using lead II to display a large R wave.
16. Discontinue oxygen. ▸ ***Rationale:*** To prevent combustion.
17. Ensure that synchronization indicator is superimposed on R wave of ECG.
18. Give command to "stand clear," and stand clear yourself.
19. The physician depresses discharge buttons on paddles and keeps them depressed until cardioversion countershock is delivered. The shock may not occur instantly, since machine waits until the next R wave in the ECG to discharge.
20. Observe postcardioversion rhythm.
21. Provide postcardioversion care.
    a. Support airway and ventilation, and oxygenate as needed.
    b. Obtain 12-lead ECG, and label it "postcardioversion."
    c. Monitor heart rhythm continuously.
    d. Evaluate vital signs, ECG, level of consciousness, peripheral pulses, and neurologic status, until stable, then routinely. ▸ ***Rationale:*** Thromboemboli to the brain, lungs, or systemic circulation may occur after cardioversion for atrial fibrillation; Coumadin therapy is continued indefinitely postcardioversion.
    e. Keep client under observation for 12 to 24 hr. ▸ ***Rationale:*** Transient hypotension and minor dysrhythmias may occur.
22. Clean reusable equipment and discard used supplies.
23. Perform hand hygiene.

Clinical Alert

If repeat cardioversion is necessary, reset defibrillator to *synchronize* mode. Most defibrillators default back to unsynchronized mode (immediate shock).

Elective cardioversion is usually not done in an acute care setting because of staff time constraints. Client is sent to cardiovascular lab where personnel use "moderate sedation" for the procedure.

DOCUMENTATION for Cardiac Emergencies

Defibrillation

- Time of event and call for code
- Time chest compressions were started
- Client assessment before and after defibrillation
- Pre- and post-defibrillation ECG rhythm printout
- Number of defibrillation attempts and watt seconds (Joules) used
- Other resuscitative measures
- Time resuscitation discontinued
- Outcome of resuscitation
- Medications administered
- Record of responses and interventions (time and personnel) on Code Record
- Family support provided

Cardioversion

- Elective cardioversion client preparation completed
- Precardioversion rhythm and vital signs
- Name of anesthetist/anesthesiologist and physician performing elective cardioversion
- Number of cardioversion attempts
- Watt seconds for each attempt
- Postcardioversion rhythm with each attempt
- Postcardioversion problems, if any
- Medications administered
- Postcardioversion monitoring

Legal Alert

In *Odem v. State ex rel Dept of Health and Hospitals* (1999), evidence supported holding nurses negligent for improperly inactivating the client's cardiac and apnea monitors. Doctors issued orders to leave monitor alarms on at all times; no nurse heard a monitor alarm, and post-death investigation indicated that the monitor alarm was not engaged. The electronic engineer from the monitor's manufacturer testified that the monitor was functional when he tested it after the incident. Had the monitor alarm sounded, the client might have lived.

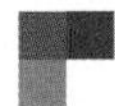

CRITICAL THINKING Application

Expected Outcomes

Supplies and medications are readily available in an emergency situation.

Client's heart rhythm is restored to normal after defibrillation or synchronized cardioversion.

Unexpected Outcomes	Alternative Actions
For Emergency Cart Equipment cannot be located promptly on cart.	• After resuscitation, suggest more logical placement of item (e.g., alphabetize or place with similar equipment). • After resuscitation, practice mock codes to retrieve items and become more familiar with cart.
Equipment malfunctions.	• Replace malfunctioning equipment immediately. • Obtain cart from the nearest unit.
For Defibrillation Electric arc crosses client's chest upon shock discharge.	• Avoid excessive gel on paddles. • Wipe off any conductive gel or perspiration between the paddle sites, and defibrillate again. • Remove transdermal medication patches.
After defibrillation, rhythm changes to asystole or rhythm shows on monitor, but carotid pulse is absent (pulseless electrical activity).	• Call a code and start CPR. • Administer IV fluids and oxygen. • Assess for treatable contributing factors. • Administer emergency medications as ordered.

For Cardioversion	
Precardioversion laboratory findings reveal electrolyte imbalance, drug toxicity, or abnormal ABGs.	• Notify physician of findings. • Reassure client that there is not a life-threatening problem. Procedure may be delayed or postponed.
Monitor shows asystole.	• Assess client for breathing and pulse. • View a different ECG lead; increase amplitude of lead. • Immediately institute CPR if indicated. • Assist physician in advanced cardiac life-support measures.
Ventricular fibrillation develops after cardioversion.	• Call a code and proceed with defibrillation CPR process.

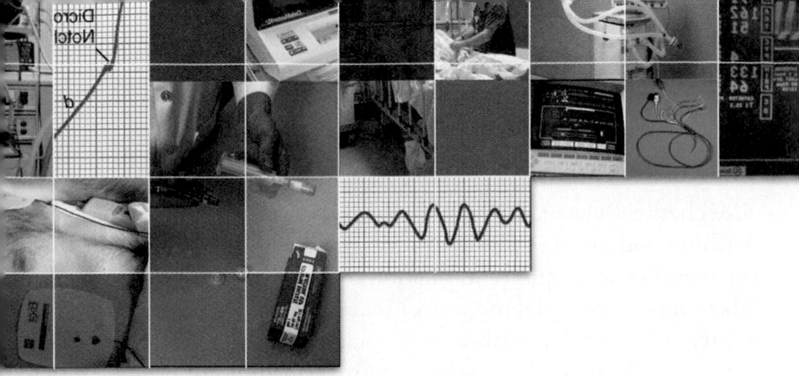

Chapter 33

UNIT 4

Mechanical Ventilation

Nursing Process Data

ASSESSMENT Data Base

- Assess client for presence of risk factors for acute respiratory distress syndrome: sepsis, massive trauma, massive fat embolism, aspiration pneumonia, and other disorders characterized by abnormal ventilation and interstitial pulmonary edema.
- Auscultate heart and lung sounds for baseline data.
- Assess vital signs and measure arterial blood gases and hemodynamic pressures if Swan–Ganz catheter is in place.
- Identify whether need for mechanical ventilation is present. Criteria for non-COPD clients:
    - Vital capacity is less than 15 mL/kg of body weight.
    - Negative inspiratory pressure is less than –25 cm H_2O.
    - PCO_2 is below 30 mmHg or above 50 mmHg.
    - Alveolar–arterial oxygen difference (A–a Δ PO_2) is greater than 350 mmHg on 100% oxygen.
    - Pulmonary shunt is greater than 30%.
    - Dead space-tidal volume (V_D–V_T) ratio is greater than 60%.
    - PO_2 is less than 60 mmHg on an FIO_2 of 1.0 (100%).
- Observe for trend of respiratory values (trend is more important than isolated measurements).
- Assess client for indications for PEEP:
    - Inability to maintain arterial PO_2 of at least 70 mmHg on 50% oxygen during continuous mechanical ventilation.
    - Failure of other methods to reduce pulmonary shunt (e.g., treatment of cardiac failure or pneumonia).
    - Normovolemia (normal blood volume).
- Check physician's orders for ventilator mode and other specified settings.
- Assess client's readiness for ventilator weaning.
- Assess client's response to ventilator weaning.

PLANNING Objectives

- To provide or augment pulmonary function
- To promote gas exchange and maintain acid/base balance
- To prevent ventilator-associated pneumonia
- To wean the client from mechanical support to independent breathing as safely and quickly as possible

IMPLEMENTATION Procedures

EVALUATION Expected Outcomes

- Mechanical ventilation maintains client's respiratory function.
- ABGs remain within an acceptable range during mechanical ventilation.
- Client does not develop ventilator associated pneumonia (VAP).
- Weaning to independent breathing is accomplished safely and as quickly as possible.

Alterations of Ventilation and Gas Exchange

Adequate gas exchange in the lungs depends on the effective ventilation of air matched with the perfusion of blood to ventilated alveoli. The thickness and permeability of the alveolar membrane, the amount of surface area available for diffusion, and the pressure gradients are also factors that affect gas exchange. The pressure gradient is the difference between the partial pressures of PO_2 and PCO_2 in the alveolar air and the pulmonary capillary blood. The pressure gradients drive the inward diffusion of oxygen from alveolar air to the blood and the outward diffusion of carbon dioxide from the blood to the alveolar air for exhalation. These pressures are obtained by arterial blood gas testing.

Ventilation replenishes the supply of oxygen in the alveoli and removes the carbon dioxide released by the capillaries. If ventilation and perfusion are not matched, blood oxygenation is reduced, resulting in a right (heart) to left (heart) "shunt." Right to left shunting is characterized by a low PO_2 (hypoxemia).

Ventilation–perfusion mismatch problems are usually the result of chronic conditions such as chronic obstructive pulmonary disease (COPD). They may also occur acutely due to perfusion failure (e.g., pulmonary embolism), ventilatory failure (e.g., drug overdose, pulmonary disease, sepsis), or pulmonary edema affecting diffusion.

Mechanical ventilation provides support for the work of breathing and ensures alveolar ventilation. This intervention, however, may require intubation of the client, interferes with normal airway defenses, and increases the risk of pulmonary injury and health-care associated infection. It is desirable to decrease the level of controlled ventilatory support as soon as possible to assist the client to extubation and the return to independent breathing. Newer techniques of ventilation allow weaning by titrating from high support to minimal support modes to facilitate the transition.

Clients (especially those with underlying disease) who require mechanical ventilation for even a day may develop "ventilator dependence." All efforts focus on identifying and addressing the physiologic and psychological factors that delay successful weaning. This complex process requires the collaborative efforts of a skilled multidisciplinary team including physician, nurse, respiratory care practitioner, dietitian, and speech pathologist. Final clinical outcomes range from successful weaning to incomplete weaning (client remains on ventilatory support at home or in a subacute setting) or terminal weaning at the client's or family's request. Terminal weaning may be facilitated with a continuous infusion of morphine or a sedative to ease the client's death.

Caring for the Mechanically Ventilated Client

Equipment

- Specific ventilator ordered (i.e., Puritan-Bennett 840, Servo 900C, Servo 300/300A, Siemens I, Dräger Evita)
- Handheld resuscitator bag connected to oxygen flowmeter
- Airway connector
- Sterile suction supplies
- Ventilator flow sheet
- Means for client communication

Preparation

1. Double-check the ventilator settings against those ordered by the physician.
2. Plug the machine in and turn it ON.
3. Familiarize yourself with location of alarm systems on the ventilator and turn on all alarm systems.
4. Validate that tube cuff inflation is appropriate with minimal occlusive volume or minimal leak (squeak heard at end inspiration) while auscultating over suprasternal notch.
5. Connect the ventilator tubing to client's endotracheal tube or tracheostomy tube.

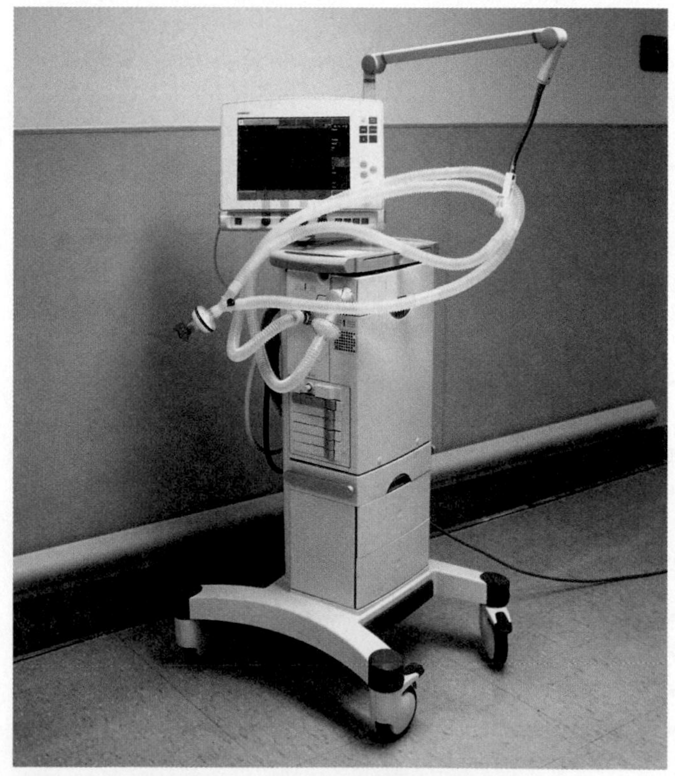

▲ Siemens 300I computerized mechanical ventilator.

EVIDENCE-BASED PRACTICE

Kinetic Rotation for Ventilatory Clients

This study examined the effect of kinetic systematic mechanical rotation of clients with 40° turns for 18 hr per day on pulmonary function and prevention of ventilator-associated pneumonia. Of the 255 client enrollees (137 in the control group who were manually turned side to supine to side every 2 hr and 118 in the kinetic therapy group), 21% of the kinetic therapy group could not tolerate bed rotation.

The study outcome supported benefits of kinetic therapy on pulmonary function and reduction of VAP, but no shorter duration of mechanical ventilation or hospitalization or improvement in survival.

The authors recommend kinetic therapy be used judiciously in clients who can tolerate it, especially neurologically depressed or sedated clients.

Source: Ahrens, T., Kollef, M., Stewart, J., & Shannon, W. (2004). Effect of kinetic therapy on pulmonary complications. *American Journal of Critical Care, 13*(5), 376–383.

Clinical Alert

Many client/ventilator systems include heat moisture filters that replace the need for external humidification of inspired gases. The use of these filters is only safe if pressure monitors are set properly so the machine can warn of impending heat moisture exchange filter occlusion.

EVIDENCE-BASED PRACTICE

Enteral Nutrition for Critically Ill Clients

While enteral nutrition is usually preferred over parenteral nutrition in critically ill clients, this study found that repeated interruptions of enteral tube feedings based on GI intolerance and elective withholding of feedings for procedures results in significant underfeeding in 68% of these mechanically ventilated clients. Thirty-eight percent of clients received less than half of their calculated daily energy requirements, 30% received adequate nutritional intake, and 1.7% were overfed due to additional kilocalories received from concomitant administration of propofol.

Source: O'Leary-Kelley, C. (2005). Nutritional adequacy in patients receiving mechanical ventilation who are fed enterally. *American Journal of Critical Care, 14*(3), 222.

Initial Ventilator Settings

- Tidal volume of 8–12 mL/kg (based on ideal body weight)

Note: Reduced volume (6 mL/kg) is indicated for clients with reduced lung compliance (e.g., ARDS) to prevent volutrauma.

- Respiratory rate of 10–15 per minute
- Inspiratory–expiratory (I:E) ratio 1:2. (I:E ratio should be less than 1:1 to prevent air trapping in the lungs.)
- Pressure limit 20% above peak airway pressures delivered.
- FiO_2 of 40%–100%.

Airway Pressure Modes

IPPB—Intermittent positive pressure breathing—inspiration by positive airway pressure; expiration is passive.

CVM/ACV—Invasive or noninvasive continuous mandatory ventilation—total support ventilation with set ventilation rate (e.g., 12) and set tidal volume (e.g., 750 mL). Client-initiated breaths receive set volume and if client does not initiate breath, set rate and volume are guaranteed (sometimes referred to as ACV, assist control ventilation).

SIMV—Synchronous intermittent mandatory ventilation—spontaneous ventilation intermittently augmented by positive pressure ventilation.

PEEP—Positive end-expiratory pressure—an expiratory airway pressure modality in which the airway pressure is maintained above atmospheric at the end of expiration. Some machines may have capability to vary the PEEP level according to a preset pattern. Stimulates surfactant production, increases FRC (functional residual capacity).

CPAP—Invasive or noninvasive continuous positive airway pressure—spontaneous ventilation with maintenance of airway pressures above atmospheric throughout the respiratory cycle.

BIPAP—Spontaneous breathing with maintenance of a bi-positive airway pressure: one set for positive inspiratory pressure and a lesser one set for positive expiratory pressure.

APRV (airway pressure release ventilation)—The ventilator maintains an inspiratory pressure throughout the inspiration time. A short pressure release at the end of the respiratory cycle allows airway pressure to return to zero for a short time.

PSV—Pressure support ventilation—in addition to other ventilator settings, 6–10 cm H_2O pressure support is provided to compensate for the added resistance imposed by artificial airways, making breathing easier; it also supports a larger tidal volume with less work of breathing. This is used as a major mode with pressure support level set to achieve optimal minute ventilation.

PCV (pressure control ventilation)—The ventilator minimizes the pressure used to deliver an acceptable tidal volume. Some machines measure the compliance of the client/ventilator interface and calculate the ideal acceptable minimum tidal volume using the least pressure necessary. The pressure control level is adjusted to some maximum number, then the machine electronically selects the appropriate tidal volume based on PCV value set and previously calculated compliance. This is also used as a major mode.

Procedure

1. Monitor client's heart rate and blood pressure until stable.
2. Obtain arterial blood gases 15 minutes after ventilation is established.

3. Monitor ventilator settings and delivered values: tidal volume, inspiratory pressure, peak pressure, rate, FIO_2, inspiratory–expiratory (I:E) ratio, ventilatory modes. Modern ventilators monitor these parameters continuously.
4. Ensure adequate heat and humidification of inspired gases.
5. Check humidifier fluid level every 8 hr and refill as necessary, if applicable.
6. Record intake, output, and daily weights.
7. Suspend ventilator tubing from an IV hook or support it on a pillow. ▸ ***Rationale:*** This reduces traction on the endotracheal or tracheostomy tube.
8. Change ventilator tubing if necessary, minimizing frequency of circuit opening. ▸ ***Rationale:*** Epidemiologic studies indicate that maintenance of a closed ventilatory/client interface is desirable.
9. Check vital signs every hour and auscultate lungs. ▸ ***Rationale:*** Positive pressure ventilation may decrease venous return and cardiac output.

NOTE: Continuous pulse oximetry facilitates constant assessment of clients receiving ventilatory assistance.

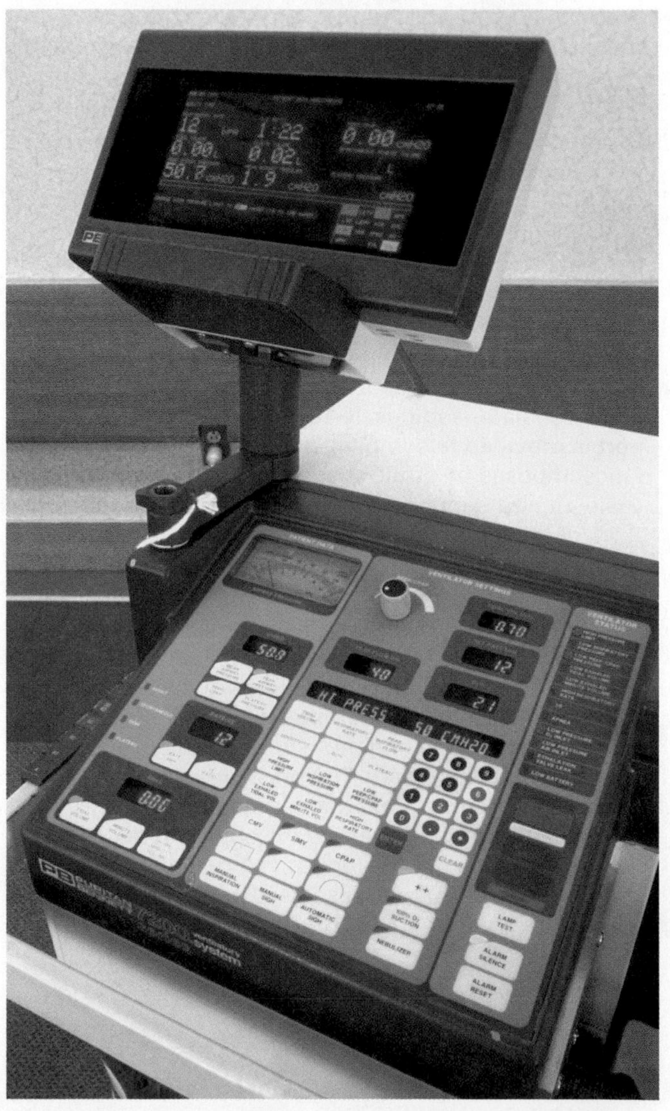

▲ Double-check all ventilator settings with physician's orders.

10. Observe and listen for possible cuff leaks around tracheostomy or endotracheal tubes.
11. If necessary, discard accumulated water in the ventilator tubing via inline closed circuit drain. ▸ ***Rationale:*** Opening circuit exposes client to environmental pathogens. Frequency of circuit opening should be minimized.
12. Provide client with call bell and method of communication, such as a "magic slate."
13. If ordered, test the gastric fluid pH, and administer medication (H_2 antagonists) as ordered. ▸ ***Rationale:*** Upper GI bleed is frequently associated with mechanical ventilation, so gastric pH should be maintained above 5.

Clinical Alert

In clients with reduced lung compliance (e.g., ARDS), tidal volume may be reduced to 6 mL/kg to prevent volutrauma. This will result in hypercarbia (increased PCO_2) and reduced blood pH (7.2 lowest acceptable). Sedation and paralytic agents may be necessary to control ventilation in these clients.

14. Test the nasogastric fluid and stool for occult blood if ordered.
15. Assess lung compliance frequently. ▸ ***Rationale:*** Lung compliance falls before changes are evident in blood gas analysis or clinical manifestations. Compliance is determined by

$$\frac{Vt}{PIP - PEEP}$$

where Vt = tidal volume; PIP = peek inspiratory pressure; and PEEP = positive end-expiratory pressure.

16. Implement methods for stress reduction, such as careful explanation of procedures, pain management, administration of sedatives, or neuromuscular blocking agents, as indicated.

Clinical Alert

Paralytic agents have no effect on wakefulness or sensory perception, including perception of pain. With complete paralysis, pain might be manifested as increased heart rate, increased blood pressure, or sweating. Never assume that a client receiving a paralytic agent is asleep. Continually inform client about care, offer reassurance, and provide pain relief while the paralyzing effect of the drug persists.

Clinical Alert

The use of sedatives in mechanically ventilated clients prolongs its duration as well as length of hospitalization and ICU stay.

Clinical Alert

Some "smart care" machines allow CPAP and PS plus an individualized weaning process based on preset client parameters, including disease process. The machine gradually decreases the degree of support as long as the client remains in a breathing comfort zone. The machine then displays a message indicating it is appropriate to extubate the client.

Cultural Awareness

Touch button voice systems are available that allow ventilated English or non–English-speaking clients to tap a touch screen that delivers preprogrammed audible words, phrases, or symbols to hold two-way communication with staff.

17. Check that ventilator alarm parameters are set.
18. Maintain appropriate "sigh" delivery. ▸ ***Rationale:*** This extra volume breath assists in preventing atelectasis and stimulates surfactant production.

NOTE: Some newer ventilators do not have "sighs"—they periodically deliver a low-level "PEEP" period to achieve the same result.

19. Monitor client frequently to detect changes in status.

Oral/Dental Care Strategies to Reduce Risk of VAP

Assess client's teeth, lips, tongue, and check oral mucosa for ulcerations; look for signs of gingival disease daily (red, spongy smooth, and shiny gingiva may be diseased).

To remove dental plaque, use a soft bristle toothbrush with antibacterial toothpaste to brush all surfaces of the teeth, gums and tongue twice daily. Rinse with alcohol-free mouth rinse.

Note: Sponge toothettes do not remove plaque, a mass that grows by layering of bacteria on the surface of teeth and surrounding soft tissues and increases over time in the ICU setting. There is a link between increases in dental plaque and the development of VAP.

Use an oral swab with 1.5% hydrogen peroxide to cleanse the oral cavity and surrounding tissues and gums every 4 hr.

Provide suctioning of subglottic secretions continuously, or intermittently every 2 hr.

Apply moisturizer to oral mucosa and lips every 2–4 hr.

Source: Garcia, R., Jendresky, L., Colbert, L., Bailey, A., Zaman, M., & Majumder, M. (2009). Reducing ventilator-associated pneumonia through advanced oral-dental care: A 48-month study. *American Journal of Critical Care, 18*(6), 523–532.

EVIDENCE-BASED NURSING PRACTICE

Delirium in Mechanically Ventilated Patients

This study validated sensitivity, specificity, and interrater reliability of an instrument (CAM-ICU) for detection of delirium in mechanically ventilated patients. Delirium occurred in 83.3% of mechanically ventilated patients, 40% of whom were in a neutral level of sedation (neither agitated nor overly sedated), while they were in the ICU.

Source: Ely, E. W., Inouye, S. K., Bernard, G. R., Gordon, S., Francis, J., May, L., ... Dittus, R. (2001, December). Delirium in mechanically ventilated patients. *Journal of the American Medical Association, 286*(21), 2703–2709.

Weaning the Mechanically Ventilated Client

Equipment

Oxygen source
T-piece adaptor or tracheostomy mask if ordered
Suctioning equipment
Arterial blood gas-sampling supplies
Continuous pulse oximetry unit
Stethoscope

Preparation

1. Validate order for weaning trial and assess client's readiness.

   Spontaneous tidal volume ≥ 7 mL/kg/ideal body weight (IBW)

   Respiratory rate between 12 and 20 breaths/min

   Minute ventilation (respiratory rate × TV) ≥ 10 L/min

   Vital signs stable (SBP ≥ 90) normal heart rate and rhythm

   Vital capacity ≥ 10 mL/kg IBW

   Negative inspiratory force is –20 cm H_2O or higher

   ABGs: pH 7.35–7.5, PO_2 ≥ 60 mmHg on FIO_2 ≤ 40% or SpO_2 90%

   Able to protect airway and responsive on minimal sedation
2. Note client's work of breathing and use of accessory muscles.
3. Note current ECG pattern for baseline.
4. Explain weaning process to client. Reassure client that transition will be based on client's responses. ▸ ***Rationale:*** When client is included in weaning process and rationale for change, anxiety is lessened.

Reducing Risk of Ventilator Associated Pneumonia (VAP)

NOTE: *Half of critically ill clients require mechanical ventilation. VAP occurs in 25% of clients who receive mechanical ventilation and is the leading cause of death from health-care associated infections.*

Perform orotracheal rather than nasotracheal intubation.

Use dual lumen ET tubes (with dorsal lumen above the cuff) to allow continuous or intermittent suctioning of subglottic secretions. This decreases VAP by as much as 20%–40%.

(See Respiratory Care, chapter 26, CASSETT tube.)

Ensure secretions are cleared from above the tube cuff before deflating the cuff.

Use only sterile fluid to flush the reusable suction catheter of secretions.

Prevent gastric reflux and oropharyngeal secretions aspiration by keeping the head of bed elevated 30–45 degrees.

Routinely verify placement of feeding tubes.

Change ventilator circuit only when visibly soiled or malfunctioning.

Drain tubing condensation away from the client.

Prevent or modulate oropharyngeal colonization with implementation of a comprehensive oral/dental hygiene program (see Box: Oral/Dental Care Strategies).

Don gloves upon entering the client's room.

Perform hand hygiene before and after putting on gloves, before and after contact with mucous membranes, respiratory secretions, or before and after contact with any respiratory device.

Use personal protective equipment as indicated.

Optimize sedation, interrupt it daily, and promote early mobilization (e.g., sitting on side of bed).

Source: Adapted from CDC Guidelines for preventing health-care associated pneumonia, 2004.

Source: Grap, M. (2009). Not-so-trivial pursuit: Mechanical ventilation risk reduction. *American Journal of Critical Care, 18*(4), 299–309.

5. Suction client. Hyperoxygenate client's lungs with 100% oxygen before and after suctioning.
6. Maintain endotracheal or tracheostomy cuff at minimal occlusive pressure (minimal leak) while mechanically ventilated.
7. Establish continuous oximetry. ▸ ***Rationale:*** Client's oxygen status should be continually assessed.

Procedure

1. Elevate head of the bed to facilitate client's diaphragmatic excursion.
2. If physician orders endotracheal tube cuff deflated during weaning, suction secretions that have accumulated above the cuff as follows:
   a. Provide positive pressure to end of tube with a handheld-resuscitation bag and 100% oxygen.
   b. Place tip of suction catheter in the posterior pharynx.
   c. Deflate cuff and apply suction to catheter. ▸ ***Rationale:*** Positive pressure blows the secretions into the pharynx, where they can be suctioned out.

NOTE: Steps a–c are not necessary if a CASSETT is in place.

   d. Hyperoxygenate lungs with 100% oxygen for three to five breaths.
3. If ordered, connect T-piece to wide-bore oxygen tubing leading to the gas source.
4. Set oxygen concentration as ordered by physician, usually 10% *higher* than the ventilator FIO_2 the client has been receiving.
5. If appropriate remove ventilator tubing from airway and connect T-piece to client's airway.
6. Cover end of ventilator tubing with sterile gauze.
7. Observe for vital sign changes, apprehension, diaphoresis, and dysrhythmias. ▸ ***Rationale:*** A mild increase in blood pressure, pulse, and respiratory rate is normal. Mild-to-moderate anxiety is also normal.

Clinical Alert

Clustering nighttime care activities to allow clients undisrupted sleep periods may facilitate the weaning process.

8. Measure arterial blood gases 1 hr after initiating weaning if client tolerates.
9. Proceed with weaning procedure as ordered. ▸ ***Rationale:*** Gradual weaning may be necessary.
10. If client tolerates no ventilator support (other than PSV), extubate client. (See Chapter 26.)
11. After weaning, continue to monitor vital signs, vital capacity, SpO_2, inspiratory pressure, blood gases, and subjective response.

DOCUMENTATION for Mechanical Ventilation

- Type of ventilator or other device used
- Ventilator or device settings; modes used in weaning process
- Time initiated
- Any problems and actions taken
- Suctioning (i.e., frequency, amount, and character of secretions)
- Indication that client is making spontaneous breathing efforts or is not triggering the machine
- Endotracheal tube location and minimal leak established
- Arterial blood gas and other lab values
- Vital signs and hemodynamic values
- Findings on pulmonary and cardiac assessment

- Ventilator modes utilized in weaning transition process
- Dental/oral care (type, frequency)
- HOB degree elevation
- Medications administered

CRITICAL THINKING Application

Expected Outcomes

- Mechanical ventilation maintains client's respiratory function.
- ABGs remain within an acceptable range during mechanical ventilation.
- Client does not develop ventilator-associated pneumonia.
- Weaning to independent breathing is accomplished safely and as quickly as possible.

Unexpected Outcomes	Alternative Actions
Client develops signs of decreased pulmonary compliance (e.g., ARDS).	• Check for signs of fluid in lungs (x-ray, increase in PAWP, crackles on auscultation, hypoxemia). • Decrease the tidal volume being delivered. • Suction client to maintain a patent airway. • Increase the level of PEEP to prevent alveolar closure. • Consider prone positioning.
Client needs to be transported for diagnostic testing.	• Start oxygen flow through handheld ventilating device. • Attach expiratory resistance, for example PEEP. • Disconnect ventilator tubing from airway at end of inspiration. • Attach handheld ventilator to airway during expiration. • Watch chest, and provide breaths with client's inspirations or at rate of 10–12/min. • Turn and deep breathe or sigh client several times an hour to reopen atelectatic alveoli.
High pressure alarm is activated.	• Check for obstructions in tubing and take corrective measures. • Suction client for possible mucous obstruction of airway.
Low pressure alarm is activated.	• Check for disconnected tubing or loose connections, and tighten them if present. • Check client for artificial airway displacement and provide emergency measures if indicated. • Deflate and reinflate the airway cuff to minimal occlusive pressure to adjust a possible cuff leak. • If unable to identify and relieve cause immediately, disconnect ventilator tubing, hand ventilate client, and summon help.
Arterial blood gases (ABGs) are not maintained within normal range.	• Notify physician of grossly abnormal ABGs, and obtain order for alteration in ventilator settings (i.e., increased percentage of oxygen, decreased tidal volume, addition of "dead space"). • Maintain mechanical ventilation. Do not attempt to wean or extubate client. • Suction client as needed to maintain airway patency.
Po_2 is not maintained at 80–100 mmHg.	• Continue delivery of PEEP as ordered. If not effective, notify MD. • Do not attempt to wean client off PEEP until desired parameters are obtained.
Cardiac output decreases significantly.	• Anticipate that client may have difficulty adjusting to increased intrathoracic pressure during weaning process. • Decrease PEEP and notify physician for weaning adjustment.

Weaning attempt is unsuccessful.	• Continue use of ventilator. • Cluster nighttime care activities to allow undisrupted sleep. • If client is extubated, consider noninvasive ventilation (CPAP). • Recruit skilled multidisciplinary team to identify and address physiologic and psychological factors that interfere with weaning success.
Decreased level of consciousness, dyspnea, severe anxiety, or fatigue occurs during weaning process.	• Note client's SpO_2 (anxiety may be due to hypoxemia). • Place client on supportive ventilation. • Provide thorough explanation, and increase reassurance. • Evaluate present use of sedatives or narcotic agents administered.
Client develops unstable vital signs.	• Place client back on more supportive ventilator mode. • Monitor vital signs more frequently, and obtain blood gases to determine oxygen concentration. • Increase FIO_2.
Client develops ventilator-associated pneumonia.	• Use a continuous aspiration subglottic secretion ET tube. • Use closed in-line system for suctioning. • Maintain HOB elevation 30–45° to prevent gastric reflux aspiration. • Discontinue mechanical ventilation as soon as possible. • Change the ventilator circuit only if soiled or malfunctioning. • Perform hand hygiene before and after contact with mucous membranes, secretions, contaminated objects. • Drain circuitry condensate away from the client. • Implement meticulous oral and oropharyngeal hygiene strategies.

GERONTOLOGIC Considerations

Elderly Clients in the Critical Care Unit Require More Intensive Observation and Consideration

- Aging is normally accompanied by a silent physiologic decline and diminished reserve in all body systems. These changes are not pathologic, but do make the elderly less adaptable to stress and illness. The elderly have a greater prevalence of chronic conditions that make them vulnerable to acute exacerbations. Over half of critical care clients are over age 65. Hospitalization is almost twice as long as that for clients under age 65 and survival is 81% compared with 98% in younger clients. However, quality of life after discharge from a critical care unit is not age-related.
- Refer to previous chapters for organ-system changes and other functional alterations as well as socioeconomic and lifestyle changes that affect care of the elderly client.

MANAGEMENT Guidelines

Each state legislates a Nurse Practice Act for RNs and LVN/LPNs. Healthcare facilities are responsible for establishing and implementing policies and procedures that conform to their state's regulations. Verify the regulations and role parameters for each healthcare worker in your facility.

Delegation

- All personnel in the critical care setting must know how to quickly summon assistance and locate and use emergency/resuscitation equipment.
- In advanced care settings, the RN simultaneously assesses, analyzes, makes decisions, intervenes, and evaluates clients on a continual basis. Complexities of care and unpredictability of outcomes necessitate *intense* ongoing client monitoring and evaluation and personal continuing education. Detection and interpretation of subtle areas of change in the client's status require the knowledge and skill of the professional nurse.
- The RN collaborates with the physician and respiratory care practitioner for ventilator settings.
- It is the responsibility of nursing faculty to ensure that students participating in client care (in any setting) are prepared to do so. Likewise, it is the duty of the student to refuse to perform a function he or she is not qualified or competent to perform.

- The nurse should not assume care for any client who requires care beyond the caregiver's expertise.
- Many agencies provide emergency care protocols or standing orders of action responses to specified changes in client status. The professional nurse must be familiar with conditions for which the nurse is delegated medical care decisions guided by such protocols.
- The CNA/UAP must know to leave arterial catheter site uncovered for easy observation.
- The CNA/UAP must not move tubing drainage receptacles (e.g., Pleur-evac) without supervision.
- The CNA/UAP must understand that IVs, drainage systems, and ventilator circuits and systems are closed and must be able to give care without disrupting system integrity or disconnecting components for the convenience of care (e.g., as in changing the client's gown or position).
- The UAP has a limited role in the care of clients who require invasive monitoring. They can offer valued assistance in moving/positioning clients and providing personal hygiene and comfort measures under the direction of the professional nurse.
- The UAP assists the client, preserving an interface between technology and reality, by providing a human dimension of tactile presence while providing basic physical care for clients requiring sophisticated technological monitoring. UAP links to the client assist all caregivers in their attempts to minimize client's feelings of alienation.

Communication Matrix

Although certain tasks may be delegated, the CNA/UAP also can provide vital data to the professional nurse by immediately *reporting*:

- Disconnected systems, loose electrodes, tubing leaks, wet/soiled dressings.
- Subjective or objective change in the client's status (e.g., pain, respiratory distress, acute change in cognition).
- Equipment alarms (e.g., ventilator alarms).
- Near-empty infusion bags.
- Near-full collection devices.
- Collaboration with an interdisciplinary team helps to support client's weaning from mechanical ventilation.

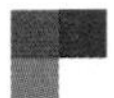

CRITICAL THINKING Strategies

Scenario 1

Mr. Jones has a history of COPD and heart failure and has been admitted to your unit with a diagnosis of acute respiratory failure. He has the following arterial blood gas values: pH 7.2, Pco_2 66 mmHg, HCO_3 25 mEq, and Po_2 49 mmHg. He is intubated and receiving mechanical ventilation to support his breathing and improve gas exchange and is being sedated with Versed.

On the third day of hospitalization, he is being weaned from mechanical ventilation, but attempts are unsuccessful due to difficulty breathing and development of pulmonary edema.

1. How does mechanical ventilation differ from the normal physiologic process of breathing?
2. How will resultant changes in intrathoracic pressure affect venous return and cardiac work?
3. What measures should be employed to help achieve successful weaning and extubation in this client?

Scenario 2

Mr. Hooper has been admitted to the coronary care unit with the diagnosis of anterior septal myocardial infarction with lateral ischemia and potential for infarct extension. He is being monitored by a balloon-tipped, flow-directed catheter for hemodynamic response to therapy. Myocardial infarction (tissue necrosis) results from an imbalance between heart work (demand for oxygen) and coronary supply of oxygen.

Mr. Hooper's hemodynamic measures include: cardiac index 1.8 (low), blood pressure 94/74, mean arterial pressure (MAP) 80 (normal), stroke volume 21 mL (low), pulmonary artery wedge pressure (PAWP) 24 (elevated), heart rate 110, systemic vascular resistance increased.

1. Explain the relationship between "heart work" and need for oxygen.
2. Discuss the parameters that can be monitored with the balloon-tipped catheter.
3. Identify two drugs that could be used to decrease "heart work" and nursing measures that would enhance their effectiveness.

NCLEX® Review Questions

Unless otherwise specified, choose only one (1) answer.

1. In the multilumen balloon-tipped flow-directed catheter, the distal lumen is used to
   1. Measure cardiac output.
   2. Measure pulmonary artery pressure.
   3. Inject solutions.
   4. Measure central venous pressure.
2. The clients' phlebostatic axis is used for the transducer level in order to obtain accurate monitoring. The phlebostatic axis is determined by joining lines at the ___________.

   Select all that apply.
   1. Midaxilla horizontally.
   2. Fourth intercostal space horizontally.
   3. Mid-anterior/posterior chest horizontally.
   4. Manubrium horizontally.
   5. Anterior axillary fold vertically.
   6. Mid-anterior/posterior chest vertically.
   7. Fourth intercostal space vertically.
3. Which of the following statements is true regarding arterial blood pressure monitoring?
   1. Measures are less accurate, but continuous, therefore more convenient.
   2. It allows intermittent sampling of venous blood.
   3. It may interfere with distal perfusion of the extremity.
   4. It can be used for calculating the heart rate.
4. Rationale for use of the blood conservatory system for arterial blood sampling is that it
   1. Eliminates the need for blood wasting.
   2. Eliminates the need to open the tubing system.
   3. Eliminates the need to disengage alarms.
   4. Is less time-consuming than standard sampling.
5. After successful cardioversion for atrial fibrillation, the client must continue
   1. Antiarrhythmic therapy.
   2. Anticoagulant therapy.
   3. Pacemaker interrogation (monitoring).
   4. Monthly cardioversion.
6. Lethal cardiac rhythms requiring defibrillation include ___________.

   Select all that apply.
   1. Pulseless ventricular tachycardia.
   2. Unstable ventricular tachycardia.
   3. Ventricular fibrillation.
   4. Atrial fibrillation with ventricular response (rate>150).
   5. Asystole.
   6. Pulseless electrical activity.
7. The most common cause of pulseless electrical activity is
   1. Peripheral vascular disease.
   2. Hyperkalemia.
   3. Hypovolemia.
   4. Heart failure.
8. Which of the following is the most supportive of all the airway pressure modes used in mechanical ventilation?
   1. PEEP (positive end expiratory pressure).
   2. SIMV (synchronous intermittent mandatory ventilation).
   3. PS (pressure support).
   4. CMV (continuous mandatory ventilation).
9. Of the following statements, the best rationale for the use of paralytic agents in the mechanically ventilated client is that they
   1. Allow the client to sleep.
   2. Eliminate the need for restraints.
   3. Allow ventilator-patient synchrony.
   4. Reduce pain perception.
10. The biggest cause of ventilator associated pneumonia is
    1. Aspiration of subglottic secretions.
    2. Accumulation of condensation in the tubing circuit.
    3. Saline injection into the airway before suctioning.
    4. Immobilization and inability to turn the client.

34

End-of-Life Care

LEARNING OBJECTIVES

1. Discuss the stages of the grief process.
2. State the main characteristics observed in a person experiencing grief.
3. Identify the factors that influence the outcome of the grieving process.
4. Explain three assessment parameters for observing psychologic and somatic symptoms that accompany the grief process.
5. Describe the stages of dying outlined by Elisabeth Kübler-Ross.
6. Discuss at least two nursing interventions for each stage of grief.
7. Explain what is meant by providing emotional care for the dying client.
8. Discuss at least four nursing interventions that assist the client during the end-of-life process.
9. Describe the three-step Analgesic Ladder for Pain Control for the Dying Client.
10. Describe the steps in providing post-mortem care.

CHAPTER OUTLINE

TERMINOLOGY

Adjuvant analgesic drugs enhance the analgesic efficacy of opioids; treat recurrent symptoms that exacerbate pain and provide independent analgesic effects.

Agitation excessive restlessness; increased mental and physical activity.

Anger a feeling of extreme displeasure, hostility, indignation, or exasperation toward someone or something.

Anorexia loss of appetite occurring from a variety of possible reasons.

Anxiety a troubled or apprehensive feeling; experiencing a sense of dread or fear.

Cope to contend with, strive, or handle.

Corneal reflex closure of eyelids resulting from direct corneal irritation or touch.

Counseling giving assistance to or guidance.

Crisis a crucial point or situation in the course of life; turning point.

Denial refusal to grant the truth of a statement or allegation.

Depression being dispirited, saddened; low in mood.

Empathy objective awareness of an insight into the feelings, emotions, and behavior of another person.

Esteem regard, respect.

Fear feeling of fright or dread related to a specific source (e.g., fear of pain or dying).

Grief intense mental anguish, deep remorse, sorrow.

Homeostasis an internal state of equilibrium or balance.

Hospice a multidisciplinary approach that focuses on client care during the last phase of life.

Idealization to regard as ideal; to make or regard someone or something as perfect.

Insomnia inability to sleep; difficulty with sleeping.

Loss the state of being deprived of or being without something that one has had, for example, the loss of a spouse or friend.

Opioids drugs such as morphine, methadone, and Numorphan, used to treat severe pain.

Pain an unpleasant sensory and emotional experience arising from actual or potential tissue damage or described in terms of such damage; whatever the experiencing person says it is, existing whenever he or she says it does.

Palliative Care client and family-centered care that optimizes quality of life by anticipating, preventing, and treating suffering throughout the continuum of illness, involving physical, intellectual, emotional, social, and spiritual needs and facilitating patient autonomy, access to information, and choice.

Psychosomatic pertaining to phenomena that are both physiologic and psychologic in origin.

Quality of Life (QOL) in the context of advanced, progressive, incurable illness, the subjective experience of an individual living with the interpersonal psychologic and existential or spiritual challenges that accompany the process of physical and functional decline and the knowledge of impending demise. A person's QOL can range from suffering associated with physical distress and/or a sense of impending disintegration to the completion of developmental work and the mastery of developmental landmarks.

Resolution the state of having made a firm determination; a course decided on.

Restitution a return to a former status.

Somatic referring to the body.

Stress a physically or emotionally disruptive or disquieting influence.

Suffering to feel pain or distress; includes fear of or actual physical distress, fear of dying, changing self-perceptions, relationship concerns, the need to find meaning in any given life experience, and past experiences of witnessing another person's distress.

Therapeutic having medicinal or healing properties.

Withdrawal to pull back or away.

LOSS AND GRIEVING

Loss is part of the experience of dying, both for the individual as well as for family members and significant others. Within the dying experience, several losses can occur including loss of health, possible loss of body parts through surgery or an accident, loss of cognitive functioning. The individual may be unable to participate in religious activities or rituals that give meaning to life and contribute to the individual's spiritual well-being. The ability to work and provide financially for self and others may lead to impoverishment and financial difficulties. In addition, the person may experience a loss of control in decision-making.

Grief is an emotion experienced in relation to loss; it can also be viewed as a behavioral response to death and dying. Human beings experience loss as the emotion of grief and must withdraw from the painful stimulus to recuperate. Emotions allow us to experience our environment—they are the means of cognition. When we are grieving, we experience the emotion of grief; this experience is accompanied by a definite syndrome with somatic and psychologic symptoms.

Stages of Grief

George Engle, in a classic article in the *American Journal of Nursing*, 1964, describes progression of the grief process in stages. These stages may occur in order, or an individual may skip a stage, become locked in a particular stage, or even return to an earlier stage already worked through.

The first stage is *shock and disbelief*, denial and numbness. The first response on learning of a death is shock and a refusal to accept or comprehend the fact. This reaction is followed by a stunned, numb feeling and does not allow the person to acknowledge the reality of death. This initial phase is characterized by attempts to protect oneself against severe stress/distress by blocking recognition of the death.

Developing awareness is the second stage. Within minutes or hours the individual becomes acutely and increasingly aware of the anguish of loss. Anger may be present during this time and may be directed toward persons or circumstances held to be responsible for the death. Behavior that frequently accompanies this stage is crying and a regression to a more helpless and childlike state. The crying and regression appear to acknowledge the loss, indicating that conscious awareness is now present.

The third stage is *restitution*, in which the various rituals of the culture, such as the funeral, attire, wake, particular folkways, and mores, help to initiate the recovery process. These rituals serve the function of emphasizing the reality of death, and the very act of experiencing them assists the mourner to face the loss.

As the reality of death becomes accepted, the *resolution* of the loss begins. This stage involves a number of steps. First, the mourner attempts to deal with the painful void created by the loss of a loved one. At this time the thoughts of the mourner are occupied almost exclusively with the deceased. Then the mourner becomes more aware of his or her own body and bodily sensations. Finally, the mourner begins to talk about the dead person, recalling the dead person's attributes and personality and reminiscing about the memories they shared. Resolving the loss is a long and painful phase that continues until the mourner remembers the positive aspects of the dead person.

The next stage that is frequently experienced is that of *idealization*. All hostile and negative feelings toward the deceased are repressed. As the process proceeds, two important changes are taking place: The recurring thoughts about the dead person bring a distinct image of the loss to mind and these memories serve to bring out the more positive aspects of the lost relationship. At the same time the grieving individual begins to assume certain admired qualities of the dead person through the mechanisms of identification or incorporation. The mourner may begin to dress, speak, or develop mannerisms or beliefs similar to the person who was lost. Often, many months are required for this process to be experienced, and as it dissipates, the mourner's preoccupation with the dead person lessens. It may be at this point that the person begins to reinvest intimate feelings toward other relationships.

The mourning process usually takes a year or more. The clearest evidence of healing is the ability to remember the deceased comfortably and realistically, with both the pleasures and disappointments of the relationship. At this stage the obsession with the loss is ended and the person accepts the responsibility of living his or her own life.

Each individual who experiences loss moves through at least some of these stages as he or she attempts to cope with loss. The stages of grief are the means human beings have of moving through the loss to resolution.

Elisabeth Kübler-Ross first introduced the five stages of dying in her 1969 book, *On Death and Dying*. It described in five discrete stages a process by which people deal with grief and loss, especially when diagnosed with a terminal illness or catastrophic event. Kübler-Ross originally applied these stages to people suffering from terminal illness and later to other forms of emotional trauma or significant life events, such as the death of a loved one, divorce, injury, infertility, or change in financial status. The stages do not necessarily come in the same order, nor are all steps experienced by all individuals. Often, people will experience several stages, going between two or more stages, returning to one or more several times before working through the stages.

The first stage, as Kübler-Ross views this process, is that of denial. The denial may be partial or complete and may occur not only during the first stages of illness or confrontation, but also later on from time to time. This initial denial is usually a temporary defense and is used as a buffer until such time as the person is able to collect himself or herself, mobilize defenses, and face the inevitability of loss or death.

The second stage is often anger. The person feels anger and questions why this is happening to them. This emotion may be directed toward persons in the environment or even projected into the environment at random. Kübler-Ross discusses this reaction and the difficulty in handling it for those close to the person by explaining that we should put ourselves in the client's position and consider how we might feel intense anger at having our life interrupted abruptly, or at experiencing this loss.

The third stage is *bargaining*. The person attempts to strike a bargain for more time to live or more time to be without pain in return for doing something for God. Often during this stage the person turns or returns to religion.

Depression is the fourth stage. Usually, when people have completed the stages of denial, anger, and bargaining, they move into depression. Kübler-Ross writes about two kinds of depression. One is preparatory depression: this is a tool for dealing with the impending loss. The second type is reactive depression. In this form of depression, the person is reacting against the impending loss of life and grieves for himself or herself.

The final stage of grieving is that of *acceptance*. This occurs when the person has worked through the previous stages and accepts his or her own inevitable death or loss. With full acceptance of impending death comes the preparation for it; however, even with acceptance, hope is still present and needs to be supported realistically.

Stages of Grief

• Shock and disbelief	• Denial
• Developing awareness	• Anger
• Restitution	• Bargaining
• Resolution	• Depression
• Idealization	• Acceptance
According to George Engle	*According to Elisabeth Kübler-Ross*

Many factors influence how individuals, at the end of life, accept death. Personal values and beliefs about life; views of personal successes, both financial and emotional; the way they look physically during the dying process; their family and friends and their families' attitudes and reactions; their past experiences in coping with difficult or traumatic situations; and, finally, the healthcare staff who are caring for them during this process—all affect an individual's attitude toward dying.

HOSPICE AND PALLIATIVE CARE

The philosophy of hospice and palliative care is based on the belief that every person has the right to die pain-free and with dignity, and that the families will receive the necessary support to ensure this happens. The word *hospice* comes from the Latin word *hospitium*, which was originally used to describe a place of shelter for weary and sick travelers. The modern hospice movements began in the 1960s by Dr. Cicely Saunders, a British physician. The first hospice in the United States was established in New Haven, Connecticut, in 1974. The National Hospice & Palliative Care Organization (NHPCO) was founded in 1978 as the National Hospice Organization and added palliative care in February 2000. Today there are more than 4,700 hospice programs with nearly 1.4 million Medicare-enrolled people cared for in 2007 alone. Eighty percent of hospice care is provided in the client's or family member's home and in nursing homes.

Hospice focuses on caring, nor curing. Hospice is not a place, but a concept of care. Hospice care addresses the needs and opportunities during the last phase of life utilizing a multidisciplinary approach that focuses on the individual's physical symptoms and the emotional and spiritual concerns of the client and his or her family. Hospice care involves a multidisciplinary team collaboration among nurses, doctors, social workers, pastoral care, family, and others. The team works together to develop a plan of care and to provide services that will enhance the quality of life and provide support for the individual and family during the terminal phases of the illness and the bereavement period.

Hospice supports the philosophy that death is an integral part of the life cycle and that intensive palliative care focuses on pain relief comfort and enhanced quality of life as appropriate goals for those at the end of life. Hospice care clients include those with AIDS and amyotrophic lateral sclerosis (ALS) or children with cardiac anomalies or other congenital conditions who have a life expectancy of 6 months. Hospice can offer any treatment necessary to

Patient-Centered Focus of Hospice Care

"As sickness progresses toward death, measures to minimize suffering should be intensified. Dying patients require palliative care of an intensity that rivals even that of curative efforts even though aggressive curative techniques are no longer indicated. Professionals and families are still called upon to use intensive measures, take extreme responsibility, and provide extraordinary sensitivity and heroic compassion."

Source: Cassel, E. (1989). The nature of suffering: Pain and Suffering (1989, March) *New England Journal of Medicine*.

Hospice and Palliative Care Information

The National Hospice and Palliative Care Organization
1731 King St.
Suite 100
Alexandria, VA 22314
(703) 837-5000
www.nhpco.org
Nonprofit membership organization representing hospice and palliative care programs and professionals in the United States.

Hospice Foundation of America
1710 Rhode Island Ave. NW
Suite 400
Washington, D.C. 20036
www.hospicefoundation.org
Provides programs for healthcare professionals and the public who cope either personally or professionally with terminal illness, death, and the process of grief.

Hospice Net
401 Bowling Ave.
Suite 51
Nashville, TN 37305-5124
www.hospicenet.org
Provides information and support to patients and families facing life-threatening illness.

National Palliative Care Research Center
Brookdale Department of Geriatrics & Adult Development
Box 1070 Mount Sinai School of Medicine
1 Gustave L. Levy Place
New York, NY 10029
www.npcrc.org
(212) 241-7447
NPCRC is a national initiative committed to stimulating, developing, and funding palliative care research directed at improving care for patients with serious illness and their families.

Children's Hospice International
1101 King St.
Suite 360
Alexandria, VA 22314
(800)-2-4-CHILD
www.chionline.org
Nonprofit organization to provide a network of support and care for children with life-threatening conditions and their families.

relieve suffering and allow a client to die peacefully and comfortably. Hospice neither speeds up nor slows down the dying process. Hospice believes that death is an integral part of the life cycle and that intensive palliative care focuses on pain relief comfort and enhanced quality of life as appropriate goals for those at the end of life.

Palliative care is central to the comprehensive treatment of serious or life-threatening illnesses. Palliative care differs from hospice care in that it is appropriate at any point on the illness continuum. The client may receive palliative care at the same time they receive treatments that are meant to improve their health. It does not depend on whether the condition can be cured or not. The purpose of palliative care is to provide relief from distressing symptoms such as pain, shortness of breath, fatigue, constipation, loss of appetite, nausea, and many others. The expected outcome of palliative care is the prevention of suffering and improved quality of life.

Clients in hospice always receive palliative care, but hospice focuses on the final months of life. To qualify for hospice programs, clients must no longer be receiving treatments to cure their illness. Most hospice care is provided in the home; however, there are hospice units in hospitals and clinic sites. The care does not vary from site to site.

CORE PRINCIPLES FOR END-OF-LIFE CARE

The Joint Commission and a significant number of specialty medical societies have endorsed, modified, or adopted a consistent set of Core Principles for End-of-Life Care. The overall philosophy was accepted by most societies, but each one amended or expanded certain issues that directly affect their practice.

The Core Principles for End-of-Life-Care, clinical policies and professional practice guidelines for end-of-life care, should:

1. Respect the dignity of both patient and caregivers.
2. Be sensitive to and respectful of the patient's and family's wishes.
3. Use the most appropriate measures that are consistent with patient choices.
4. Encompass alleviation of pain and other physical symptoms.
5. Assess and manage psychological, social, and spiritual/religious problems.
6. Offer continuity; the patient should be cared for, if so desired, by his/her primary care and specialist providers.
7. Provide access to any therapy that may realistically be expected to improve the patient's quality of life, including alternative or nontraditional treatments.
8. Provide access to palliative care and hospice care.
9. Respect the right to refuse treatment.
10. Respect the physician's professional responsibility to discontinue some treatments when appropriate, with consideration for both patient and family preferences.
11. Promote clinical and evidence-based research on providing care at the end of life.

Source: Principles for Care of Patients at the End of Life: An Emerging Consensus among the Specialties of Medicine, Castle and Foley, December 1999. Milbank Memorial Fund.

SYMPTOM MANAGEMENT

Management of debilitating symptoms has improved in recent years as a result of clinical research and new pharmacologic and behavioral therapies. Individuals who are dying experience a wide variety of symptoms, including pain, nausea, fatigue, constipation, or diarrhea. Pain and pain control has been identified as the primary concern of clients as they approach the end of life. Inadequate assessment of pain and poor pain control continue to be issues, even though much research on these topics has been done.

Assessment of pain in the dying client relies on the evaluation of level of consciousness and awareness, breathing pattern, and hemodynamics. A method to determine the amount of pain a client has is electroencephalographic signals that assess level of consciousness. This procedure has been used as an adjunctive monitor even though it is not considered an end-of-life technique. Intrusive technology and monitoring are usually discontinued during this stage.

Through routine assessments, planning of care, and administering the appropriate pharmacologic interventions, the nurse plays a critical role in the management of symptoms for clients receiving hospice and palliative care.

The World Health Organization (WHO) developed a three-step "ladder" that outlines principles of analgesic selection and titration as well as adjuvant drugs that support the effect of the analgesics or counteract adverse side effects. Each step in the ladder defines the type of pain and analgesic most effective for that level of pain. (See Chapter 16, Pain Management.)

In some clients, the pain becomes so severe that even aggressive titration of standard drugs is not sufficient to control the pain. In these cases, sedation should be considered. Sedation for end-of-life clients is considered a comfort measure when there is intractable pain and other symptoms indicate death is near. When sedation is used in this manner, the client usually loses consciousness. Family members, as well as the client, must be informed of this change in client status before sedation is started.

CULTURAL AWARENESS

Cross-Cultural Issues at the End of Life

Kagawa-Singer and Blackhall, in the article "Negotiating Cross-Cultural Issues at the End of Life," state that culture is an important part of how everyone understands their world and how this impacts their decisions, especially on healthcare issues. This includes healthcare professionals as well. Culture influences the way people make meaning out of illness and dying; therefore, it also influences how they utilize the medical community at the end of life. Each individual has a perspective that is also influenced by factors such as personal psychology, gender, and life experiences. There is a wide variation of beliefs and behaviors within any ethnic population. This leads us to realize that each client needs to be treated individually. Healthcare professionals must not influence clients with their own beliefs or cultures. Failure to take the client's cultural background seriously means we fail to understand the values held by the client.

Lack of cultural sensitivity and skills can lead to inappropriate clinical outcomes and poor interaction with clients and families at a very crucial point in their end-of-life process. Addressing and respecting cultural differences will increase trust, leading to a more satisfactory end-of-life process for both the client and the family.

Source: Kagawa-Singer, M., & Blackhall, L. J. (2001, December 19). Negotiating cross-cultural issues at the end of life. *Journal of the American Medical Association, 286*(23), 2993–3001.

Cultural Diversity at the End of Life

The 2000 census revealed that whites make up about 65% of the U.S. population; 13% are black; 13% are Hispanic; 4.5% are Asian-Pacific Islander; and 1.5% are American-Indian/Alaskan native. The remaining 2.5% list themselves as bi-ethnic. With the makeup of the United States changing, healthcare workers must become more aware of how cultural factors influence clients' reactions to serious illness and how they make decisions and cope with end-of-life issues. There are three basic dimensions in end-of-life treatment that vary culturally: communication of "bad news"; locus of decision making; and attitudes toward advance directives and end-of-life care. Many ethnic healthcare workers conceal adverse diagnoses from clients, believing that it is disrespectful, impolite, or even harmful to the client. Decisions on end-of-life care are most often made by the family or the family in consultation with the physician, not the client. Advance Directives are usually not completed by specific ethnic minority clients because they have a distrust of the U.S. healthcare system.

Source: Searight, H. R., & Gafford, J. (2005, February 1). Cultural diversity at the end of life: Issues and guidelines for family physicians. *American Family Physician, 71*(3), 515–522.

Death Rituals Vary From One Culture to Another

Death rituals occur in every culture and are practiced in a variety of ways. These rituals may be culturally related or part of a religious practice. A person affilitated with a particular cultural group may or may not practice rituals from that culture. In providing care to any individivual who is dying it is essential to learn what is important and meaningful to that person and family as well as how this need can be met. A few general examples related to culture are presented for clarification.

Arab-Americans, many of whom are Muslims, do not openly anticipate death or grieve for a dying person. Most of the Arab-American clients prefer to die in the hospital. There are special rituals after the death, such as washing the body and all orifices. The designated head of the family determines how family members will be notified of the death. Organ donation is usually not allowed out of respect for burying the body whole. They will probably not choose a DNR order; in fact, the family may lose trust in the healthcare system if this option is offered them.

Black Americans vary with respect to dying at home or in the hospital. Many families care for the clients at home until death is imminent, then bring them to the hospital. Some believe it is bad luck to die at home. There are no rituals associated with care of the body. Cremation is usually not done. Organ donation is usually not done except in cases of immediate family need.

Chinese-Americans may be fatalistic when faced with a terminal illness and death. They usually do not talk about it. Chinese believe that dying at home brings bad luck, but others believe the spirit will get lost if death occurs in the hospital. Each client and family should be supported in their belief. Organ donation and autopsy are generally not accepted, as they believe the body should be kept intact.

Native Americans embrace the present. Some tribes avoid contact with the dying, while others will want to be present 24 hours a day. Eating, playing games, and making jokes in the hospital are seen as appropriate for some tribes. Many of the tribes will bring healers to attend to the spiritual health of the dying client. Some family members will wrap the body for burial and not allow a mortuary to prepare the body, while others may avoid all contact with the body. Organ donation is generally not accepted.

Within the Mexican-American (Hispanic) culture, death is considered a family affair. Family members feel obligated to visit frequently. In the traditional Mexican family, a family member must always be with the dying client. The family members will gather in the home or hospital; therefore, it is necessary to find a place for them to congregate.

NURSING DIAGNOSES

The following nursing diagnoses are appropriate to include in a client care plan when a client is in the process of grieving or dying.

NURSING DIAGNOSIS	RELATED FACTORS
Death Anxiety	Worry about death's impact on significant others, feeling powerless over issues related to dying, anticipating pain related to death
Compromised Family Coping	Little support by family, alteration in family role
Verbal Communication, Impaired	Family has unresolved questions
Disabled Family Coping	Surgery, diagnostic tests, treatments, perceived threat to value system, lack of experience in making critical decisions
Fear	Unknown experience related to death; unfamiliarity with environment
Grieving	Loss of significant other, chronic illness, threat of death, perceived loss of biologic integrity
Ineffective Health Maintenance	Lack of motivation, lack of education, religious and cultural beliefs, cognitive impairment
Chronic Pain	Tissue, organ, or skeletal muscle damage as a result of cancer, severe pain at end of life
Spiritual Distress, Risk for	Hospital barriers to practicing spiritual rituals, loss of body part or function, terminal illness, debilitating disease, death or illness of significant other, challenge to belief or value systems

CLEANSE HANDS The single most important nursing action to decrease the incidence of hospital-based infections is hand hygiene. *Remember to wash your hands or use antibacterial gel before and after each and every client contact.*

IDENTIFY CLIENT Before every procedure, check two forms of client identification, not including room number. These actions prevent errors and conform to The Joint Commission standards.

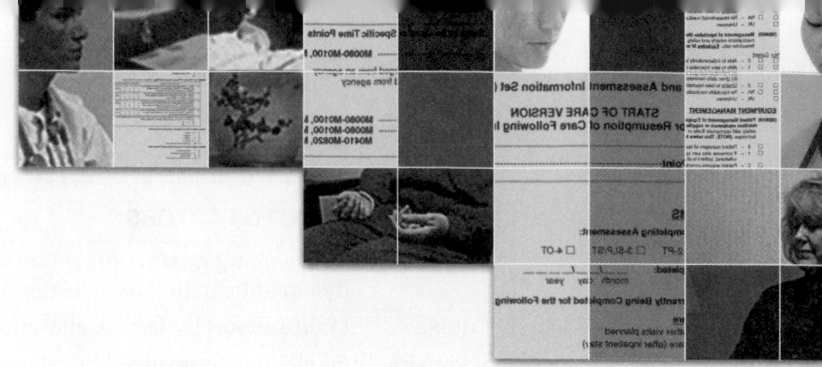

Chapter 34

UNIT 1

The Grief Process

Nursing Process Data

ASSESSMENT Data Base

- Observe for presence of psychologic symptoms:
  - Weeping
  - Guilt
  - Anger and irritability toward others and the deceased
  - Depression
  - Inability to initiate meaningful activity
- Observe for somatic symptoms:
  - Physical exhaustion
  - Insomnia
  - Restlessness and agitation
  - Digestive disturbance
  - Anorexia or overeating
- Determine client's complaints:
  - Sense of unreality
  - Sense of detachment
  - Lack of strength
- Identify stage of grief client is experiencing:
  - Denial
  - Anger
  - Bargaining
  - Depression
  - Acceptance
  - Outcome of grieving process—positive or negative
- Observe for morbid reaction to grief:
  - Delay of reaction
  - Distorted reaction—acquisition of symptoms of the deceased (e.g., psychosomatic illness or disease)
  - Atypical grief syndrome manifested by distorted pictures of grief

PLANNING Objectives

- To assist the client who is experiencing the grief process
- To intervene therapeutically and provide support
- To allow the client to express feelings of loss openly
- To understand and tolerate client's behavior that is related to loss
- To assist the client to move successfully through stages of the grief process

IMPLEMENTATION Procedures

EVALUATION Expected Outcomes

- Client is able to progress through stages of grief with support of family and nursing staff.
- Client is accepting of loss and eventual outcome of grief process.
- Cultural sensitivity is maintained throughout grief process.

Pearson Nursing Student Resources

Find additional review materials at
nursing.pearsonhighered.com

Prepare for success with NCLEX®-style practice questions and Skill Checklists

Identifying Grief

Procedure

1. Understand the importance of the deceased person as a source of support.
2. Observe the degree of dependency of the relationship between deceased and others. ▸ ***Rationale:*** The more dependent, the more difficult is the task of resolution.
3. Identify the degree of ambivalence felt toward the deceased. ▸ ***Rationale:*** When there are persistent hostile feelings, guilt may interfere with the work of mourning.
4. Identify the support system and other relationships the grieving individual has to depend on. ▸ ***Rationale:*** A client with few other meaningful relationships has a more difficult time and is less willing to give up the attachment to the deceased.
5. Identify client's cultural influence on grieving process.
6. Identify the number and nature of previous grief experiences. ▸ ***Rationale:*** Losses tend to be cumulative in their effects, and unsuccessfully resolved previous losses only aggravate the current loss.
7. Determine the degree of preparation for the loss. ▸ ***Rationale:*** In terminal illness, grief work may have begun long before the actual death of the person.
8. Determine the capacity to cope with loss. The more inner resources the client has available, the better his or her coping ability. ▸ ***Rationale:*** The physical and psychologic health of the mourner at the time of the loss determines capacity.

Assisting With Grief

Procedure

1. Become familiar with the grief process, stages of grief, and natural responses to grief.
2. Denial stage.
   a. Allow client denial of grief to give him or her time to move through shock and to mobilize defenses.
   b. Encourage client to talk when he or she is ready to do so.
   c. Understand that shock and disbelief may be first response, and anticipate that behavior may be inappropriate or disturbed.
   d. Accept client's inability to face reality, and allow mood swings and expressions of happier times (which may seem inappropriate at this time).
3. Anger stage.
   a. Allow "acting-out" of feelings and verbalization of anger.
   b. Anticipate expression of anger toward others, loved ones, and the environment.
   c. Understand that unreasonable, insatiable demands are an expression of this stage of grief, and attempt to meet the demands. Anticipate client's needs before demanded.
   d. Encourage client to take as much control as possible over care and environment, allowing the client to make as many decisions as possible. Avoid criticism and negative feedback at this time.
   e. Avoid false reassurance and false cheerfulness, which lead to distrust. Also, avoid diversion by introducing cheerful activities or stories. These actions lead client to believe you do not care about his or her feelings.
   f. Explain and clarify all procedures and treatments to decrease misinterpretation and expansion of fears.
4. Bargaining stage.
   a. Allow client to move through bargaining stage; listen to verbal expressions without judgment or pointing out reality.
   b. Encourage client to talk about bargaining with God. This may assist client to cope with guilt and not lose faith.
   c. Assist with contacting spiritual counselor or hospital chaplain.
5. Depression stage.
   a. Encourage verbalizations about loss, its meaning in client's life, and feelings about the loss.
   b. Support client's self-esteem and understand that it is affected by awareness of the loss.
   c. Encourage and reassure as appropriate; do not give false reassurance at this stage but assist client to be realistic.
   d. Be aware of your own feelings of sadness and loss so that they do not interfere with therapy.
   e. Remain with client and share on a nonverbal level.
   f. Verbalize feelings to client when they are appropriate; do not deny yourself of sadness or empathy (crying) when appropriate.
   g. Limit association with cheerful, insincere staff, friends, or family.
6. Acceptance stage.
   a. Allow client to express whatever feelings are present, knowing that he or she has moved through the above stages and may now be feeling totally empty of emotion.
   b. Spend quiet time with client, interacting on a nonverbal, nondemanding level.
   c. Encourage client to make preparations for impending death by supporting requests to finish tasks,

discussing options for plans to complete areas in his/her life.

d. Encourage client to say the things he or she wants to say to those close to him or her.

e. Honor client's requests to be alone and do not overload client with external information. Client may need a lot of quiet contemplation to prepare for death.

7. Show respect for cultural, religious, and social customs throughout stages of mourning and incorporate client's cultural, religious, and social customs when providing care during the grief process.

8. Offer support and reassurance to family.

DOCUMENTATION for the Grief Process

- Characteristics of the stage of grief client is experiencing and client's ability to cope
- Behavioral manifestations of grief
- Support systems available to client
- Measures nurse has taken to assist client to cope with grief
- Client's response to psychosocial interventions

CRITICAL THINKING Application

Expected Outcomes

- Client is able to progress through stages of grief with support of family and nursing staff.
- Client is accepting of loss and eventual outcome of grief process.
- Cultural sensitivity is maintained throughout grief process.
- Client is able to identify support system.

Unexpected Outcomes	Alternative Actions
Client experiences a morbid reaction to grief.	• Recognize distorted symptoms and be accepting but firm with client. • Request further assistance from the staff.
Family cannot support grief of client or handle their own grief.	• Know the general response to death by recognizing the stages of the grief process. • Understand that the behavior of the mourner may be unstable and disturbed. • Request assistance from nursing staff or appropriate community agencies to cope with the family.

Chapter 34

UNIT ❷

The Dying Client

Nursing Process Data

ASSESSMENT Data Base

- Assess current stage of dying.
- Observe the physical symptoms:
  - Evidence of circulatory collapse
  - Variations in blood pressure and pulse
  - Disequilibrium of body mechanisms
  - Deterioration of physical and mental capabilities
  - Absence of corneal reflex
- Observe the client's ability to fulfill basic needs without complete assistance.
- Assess the nature and degree of pain the client is experiencing.
- Observe for impending crisis or emergency situation.
- Observe for psychosocial condition:
  - Need to establish a relationship for support
  - Availability of support systems
  - Grief pattern and stage of grief the client is experiencing
  - Need to express feelings and verbalize fears and concerns
  - Determine client's awareness of terminal nature of disease
- Determine anxiety level, which may be expressed in physical or emotional behavior.
  - Sleep disturbance
  - Palpitations
  - Digestive complaints
  - Anger or hostility
  - Withdrawal
- Determine depression level that client may be experiencing:
  - High fatigue level or lethargy
  - Poor appetite, nausea, or vomiting
  - Inability to concentrate
  - Perception of unfinished business to be completed
  - Expressions of sadness, hopelessness, or uselessness
  - Assess family members' needs during the loss

PLANNING Objectives

- To assist client near the end of life to maintain comfort, if possible
- To assist the dying client to cope with end-of-life experiences
- To handle own feelings of loss and sadness that arise when caring for a client at the end of life
- To provide support for the client and the client's family during the end-of-life process
- To complete the actions necessary to care for the client who has died

IMPLEMENTATION Procedures

EVALUATION Expected Outcomes

- Client is able to progress through stages of grief with support of family and nursing staff.
- Client is accepting of loss and eventual outcome of grief process.
- Client is as pain-free as possible.
- Client's cultural beliefs are considered throughout the dying process.
- Client found internal sources to support acceptance of death.
- Family members are supported throughout the dying process.

Supporting the Client Near the End of Life

Preparation

1. Determine whether client has a Do Not Resuscitate (DNR) signed form in chart or as part of informed consent.
2. Ensure client has current Advance Directive on file in both the healthcare facility and physician's office. ▸ ***Rationale:*** Even though the Patient Self-Determination Act of 1991 requires healthcare facilities to inform clients of their right to accept or refuse health care and complete an Advance Directive, this is not always done.

NOTE: Asian-Americans, Hispanic Americans, and African Americans are less inclined to write Advance Directives, whereas 40% of whites have them. See Advance Directives, Chapter 1.

3. If client is unable to sign form, ensure that legally recognized surrogate healthcare decision maker has signed the request. ▸ ***Rationale:*** Without signed DNR orders, staff must perform CPR and begin all lifesaving measures.
4. Determine whether hospice care is appropriate for client.
5. Review agency policies and procedures related to organ procurement. Be prepared to notify the appropriate individual or organization of status of client as death is near. ▸ ***Rationale:*** Procurement team can be ready to harvest organs and tissues upon client's death.

Procedure

For Care of Client

1. Introduce yourself to client and family members.
2. Determine whether client has specific needs for comfort. ▸ ***Rationale:*** Comfort is the primary goal of therapy for dying clients. Provide daily grooming, skin and mouth care, and exercise as client can tolerate.
3. Encourage client to maintain independence by providing remote controls for TV, radio, lights, and fans. Keep ice and water at the bedside within easy reach by client.
4. Provide touch like Reiki or other therapeutic touch techniques if culturally appropriate, especially over the area of pain. ▸ ***Rationale:*** This is soothing and relaxing for client.
5. Incorporate the use of relaxation techniques in your daily nursing care of the client.
6. Serve only small portions of food that client requests. ▸ ***Rationale:*** Serving large portions only overwhelms client and he or she will not want to attempt to eat. Encourage clients to take in as much fluid as they are able.
7. Keep lemon drops or mint fresheners at bedside and within easy reach for client. ▸ ***Rationale:*** Breath fresheners make the client feel better especially if they are not eating.

For Interaction With Client and Family Members

1. Determine if and how family members may assist client during this stage and assist family members to provide care as requested. Discuss hospice care with client and family, if appropriate.
2. Provide opportunities for client and family to engage in cultural or religious practices.
3. Visiting hours for family or significant others should be unlimited. Assess if client needs rest by observing for signs of anxiety, restlessness, and voice trembling. When this occurs, ask the visitors to please leave.

TABLE 34-1 Changes During the Dying Process

Change	Signs and Symptoms
Weakness and fatigue	Inability to move self in bed, unable to perform personal hygiene
Skin breakdown	Erythema surrounding bony prominences, wounds
Decreasing appetite	Poor intake, weight loss, loss of muscle and fat, anorexia
Cardiac and renal dysfunction	Oliguria leading to anuria, tachycardia and peripheral cooling, cyanosis, in extremities, hypertension leading to hypotension.
Alterations in level of consciousness	Increasing drowsiness leading to unresponsiveness to verbal or tactile stimuli
Delirium	Agitation, moaning, groaning, nonpurposeful movements of limbs
Respiratory dysfunction	Change in respiratory rate, decreasing tidal volume with increased PCO_2 level, abnormal breathing patterns from apnea, Cheyne-Stokes, agonal breaths.
Inability to swallow	Coughing, choking, gurgling, loss of gag reflex, dysphagia
Loss of sphincter control	Incontinence of urine or bowel
Pain	Facial grimacing, moaning, agitation, tension in forehead and between eyebrows.
Inability to close eyes	Eyelids remain open with only whites of eyes showing.

Source: Emanuel, L., Ferris, F. D., von Gunten, C. F., & Von Roenn, J. H. (2010). The last hours of living: Practical advice for clinicians. Medscape Nurses. http://cme.medscape.com/viewprogram/5808.

CARDIOPULMONARY RESUSCITATION

☐ **"FULL SUPPORT"**

☐ **"LIMITED SUPPORT"**

All indicated medical care is provided except that in the event of a cardiac or pulmonary arrest, limitations of therapeutic interventions are indicated:

1. Medications	Routine	☐ yes	☐ no
	Vasopressors	☐ yes	☐ no
	Antiarrhythmics	☐ yes	☐ no
	ACLS drugs	☐ yes	☐ no
2. Airway Management	Intubation	☐ yes	☐ no
	Extubation if patient on ventilator	☐ yes	☐ no
	Reintubate after patient is weaned off ventilator or self extubation	☐ yes	☐ no
3. Chest Compressions		☐ yes	☐ no
4. Defibrillation		☐ yes	☐ no
5. Other		☐ yes	☐ no

☐ **"COMFORT SUPPORT" ***

1. New therapeutic measures contraindicated. Possible reasons may include one or more of the following:
   - 1.1 Irreversible terminal disease/coma; death is imminent.
   - 1.2 Brain death (defined by statute).
   - 1.3 Competent patient or incompetent patient with family or surrogate decision-maker expresses desire that no CPR procedures be instituted.
   - 1.4 Proposed treatment is disproportionate in terms of benefits to be gained versus burdens caused.
   - 1.5 Congenital anomalies incompatible with life.
   - 1.6 Care which is necessary to alleviate pain and suffering shall be provided.

***NOTE:** PHYSICIAN MUST ENTER INTO THE PROGRESS NOTES FOR "LIMITED SUPPORT" AND "COMFORT SUPPORT" ORDERS:

1. Diagnosis / prognosis / code status.
2. Mandatory neurological consultation for diagnosis of brain death.
3. Patient / family / surrogate decision-maker involvement in the decision.
4. Clear documentation of patient or family or surrogate decision-maker approval or support of decision to withhold future CPR procedures.

REASSESSMENT OF CPR STATUS WILL BE DONE WHEN A PATIENT'S CONDITION OR WISHES CHANGE AND/OR A REQUEST IS MADE TO RESCIND THE ORDERS.

PHYSICIAN'S SIGNATURE: ____________ DATE: ________ TIME: ________

NOTED BY: ____________ DATE: ________ TIME: ________

COMMUNITY HOSPITAL

PATIENT I.D. #
NAME
SEX AGE SS#
BIRTH DATE MED REC. #

▲ CPR form.

REQUEST TO FOREGO RESUSCITATIVE MEASURES
(Request Made by Patient)

I, ____________ (name of patient) hereby request to forego resuscitative measures. My physician, ____________, has explained to me the nature of resuscitative measures, their risks and benefits, the risks and benefits of refusing such resuscitative measures, and the alternatives to such resuscitative measures. I have had all of my questions answered by my physician.
After carefully considering all of the information my physician discussed with me, I request to forego resuscitative measures.

Signature: ____________

Date: ____________ Time: ________ A.M. / P.M.

Witness: ____________

REQUEST TO FOREGO RESUSCITATIVE MEASURES
(Request Made by Legally Recognized Surrogate Decision-maker)

NOTE: *If the patient is determined by his or her physician to be incompetent (that is, unable to understand or appreciate the nature and consequences of the medical decision at issue), a legally recognized surrogate health care decision-maker may sign a request to forego resuscitative measures on behalf of the patient.*

I, ____________ (name of legally recognized surrogate health care decision-maker) hereby request to forego resuscitative measures on behalf of ____________ (name of patient). The patient's physician, ____________, has explained to me the nature of resuscitative measures, their risks and benefits, the risks and benefits of refusing such resuscitative measures, and the alternatives to such resuscitative measures. I have had all of my questions answered by the physician.
After carefully considering all of the information the physician discussed with me, I request to forego resuscitative measures on behalf of the patient named above.

Signature: ____________

Relationship to Patient: ____________

Date: ____________ Time: ________ A.M. / P.M.

Witness: ____________

COMMUNITY HOSPITAL

PATIENT I.D. #
NAME
SEX AGE SS#
BIRTH DATE MED REC. # FIN. CLASS

▲ DNR form.

4. Assist with open communication with clients, family, and health care providers, regarding any cultural, spiritual, or religious issues they wish to discuss relative to end of life. ▸ ***Rationale:*** Understanding the client's religious or spiritual concerns will help support client and family during these times.
5. Encourage family members to communicate with clients even if unresponsive. ▸ ***Rationale:*** Clients reportedly do hear what it said even though unresponsive.

For Management of the Environment

1. Move client's bed near window so he or she can see outside vegetation, flowers, sky, etc.
2. Reduce extraneous noise. Client's room may need to be moved to accomplish this. Do not place bed near nurses' station. ▸ ***Rationale:*** Even a client who is not responding can still hear voices and noises.
3. Display cards, photos, "art work" from children, favorite objects that have special meaning for client in an area where client can see them.
4. Provide room lighting that is muted and soft, not overhead lighting.
5. Eliminate odors: perfume, cigarette smoke.
   a. Open windows when possible.
   b. Turn on fans.
   c. Use air fresheners.
   d. Use aromatherapy (oils or lotion) for massage. Provide massage with aromatherapy products if client agrees. ▸ ***Rationale:*** Massage reduces stress, decreases pain and discomfort, and stimulates blood circulation.
6. Provide soft music according to client's preference for music.
7. Use visualization and guided imagery through audiotapes if client desires.

The goal of care for the dying client changes from curative to palliative care. Helping the client achieve a measure of comfort and knowing that family members and significant others are being supported during this process is a comfort for the client.

Providing Pain Management at the End of Life*

Procedure

1. Assess client for factors that influence management of pain.
   a. Complete detailed history of the client's condition.
   b. Determine effects of pain relief measures and medications client is currently taking.
   c. Have client explain characteristics of pain and have him or her use pain scale to determine severity of pain.
   d. Ask client if there are any cultural issues related to pain that should be known by healthcare providers.
   e. Assess client's psychosocial needs.
2. Complete physical assessment of client.
3. Assess client for nonverbal clues indicating pain: restlessness, grimacing, moaning, irritability, furrowed brow, or crying, particularly if the client is sedated.
4. Assess client for physiologic signs of pain: elevated blood pressure and pulse.
5. After determining appropriate drug, dose, and route, administer drug and observe for effects of medication on pain relief and for potential side effects.

Clinical Alert

Most medications for pain are administered via oral or parenteral routes. The use of continuous subcutaneous opioid infusions in clients with chronic cancer pain is becoming more popular. High-concentration opioid medications are used with this method because the amount of drug administered must be limited to prevent tissue trauma.

Medications for persistent cancer-related pain are administered around the clock for best efficacy, not on a PRN basis. Additional PRN medications may be administered as needed.

Seventy percent to 90% of clients with advanced cancer experience pain, especially those in long-term care facilities. When properly medicated, more than 95% of the clients gain relief from the pain.

The client's verbal account of his or her pain is accepted for pain measurement. Therefore, it is important to explain the use of the pain scale so the client accurately describes his or her pain because drug therapy is based on the measurement.

WHO Three-Step Analgesic Ladder for Pain Control

Step 1: Nonopioid with or without adjuvant drugs.
Acetaminophen, aspirin, or another NSAID for mild to moderate pain.
Adjuvant drugs to enhance analgesic efficacy, treat concurrent symptoms that exacerbate pain, and provide independent analgesic activity for specific types of pain that may be used in this step as well as in the other steps.

Step 2: Opioid for mild-to-moderate pain and nonopioid drugs; may or may not use adjuvant drugs.
Add codeine or hydrocodone to the NSAID (do not substitute drugs).
Drugs are administered in fixed-dose combinations with acetaminophen or aspirin. This provides additive analgesia.
Dose-related toxicity might occur with the use of acetaminophen or NSAID.
This may limit the drug combination's efficacy.

Step 3: Opioid for moderate-to-severe pain with or without nonopioid or adjuvant drugs.
This step is used when higher doses of opioids are necessary.
Separate dosage forms of the opioid and nonopioid analgesic are used to avoid exceeding the maximum recommended doses of acetaminophen or NSAID.

Refer to Chapter 16, Pain Management, for additional information on managing pain.

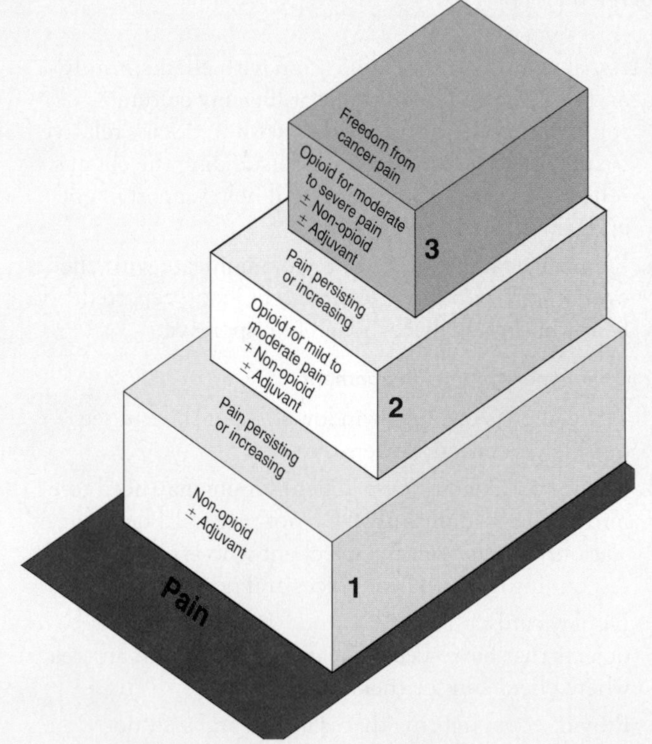

▲ WHO three-step analgesic ladder.

NOTE: The World Health Organization states that when pain is persistent or moderate to severe at the outset, it should be treated by increasing the opioid dosage or using a higher potency. Morphine, hydromorphone, methadone, fentanyl, or levorphanol can replace the codeine or hydrocodone when severe pain exists.

6. Assess client frequently for effects of pain management.
7. Maintain around-the-clock sustained-release medications for continuous pain.
8. Treat breakthrough pain with immediate-release medications.
9. Discuss a combination of medications and alternative therapies such as massage for the management of pain.

Symptom Management at the End of Life

Procedure

1. Minimize the client's discomfort as much as possible.
   a. Provide warmth.
   b. Provide assistance in moving and position client frequently.
   c. Provide assistance in bathing and personal hygiene.
   d. Administer the appropriate medications before pain becomes severe.
2. Recognize the symptoms of urgency or emergency conditions and seek immediate assistance.
3. Notify the charge nurse or team leader if there is an impending crisis and perform emergency actions until help arrives.
4. Encourage dying clients to do as much as they can for themselves so that they do not just give up—a state that only reinforces low self-esteem.
5. Provide emotional nursing care for the client.
   a. Form a relationship with the dying client. Be willing to be involved, to care, and to be committed to caring for a dying client.
   b. Allocate time to spend with the client so that not only physical care is administered.
   c. Recognize the grief pattern and support the client as he or she moves through it.
   d. Recognize that your physical presence is comforting by staying physically close to the client if he or she is frightened. Use touch if appropriate and nonverbal communication.
   e. Respect the client's need for privacy, and withdraw if the client has a need to be alone or to disengage from personal relationships.
   f. Be tuned in to client's cues that he or she wants to talk and express feelings, cry, or even intellectually discuss the dying process.
   g. Accept the client at the level on which he or she is functioning without making judgments.
6. Be aware of your own personal orientation toward the dying process.
   a. Explore your own feelings about death and dying with the understanding that until you have faced the subject of death, you will be inadequate to support the client or the family as they experience the dying process.
   b. Share your feelings about dying with the staff and others; actively work through them so that negativity does not get transferred to the client.

Supporting the Family or Caregiver

Procedure

1. Introduce yourself to the family or caregiver and explain your role in caring for the client.
2. Support the family of the dying client.
   a. Understand that the family may be going through anticipatory grief before the actual event of dying.
   b. Understand that different family members react differently to the impending death and support the different reactions.
   c. Be aware that demonstrating your concern and caring assists the family to cope with the grief process.
3. Provide honest answers to questions.
4. Reinforce client's wishes for end-of-life care related to DNR orders, living wills, and advance directive.
5. Explain each procedure/intervention you are providing for client.
6. Ask family members or caregiver how they want to participate in client care.
7. Encourage family or caregiver to take time alone to regroup.
8. Provide or obtain psychosocial support and bereavement counseling for family. ▸ ***Rationale:*** Family members may exhaust much of their energy, develop sleep deprivation, and exhibit signs of depression, anxiety, and even chronic health problems during this stressful time.
9. Encourage family members to build a support group of friends or other family members. ▸ ***Rationale:*** No one should be alone during this time.
10. Remind family or caregiver to eat properly and maintain an exercise schedule.
11. Refer family members to support groups as needed.
12. Refer family members to social services for help with issues such as insurance, living wills, funeral arrangement, and other financial constraints.
13. Prepare family for client's death.

EVIDENCE-BASED PRACTICE

Critical Care Family Needs Inventory

A meta-analysis of several studies using the Critical Care Family Needs Inventory led to a summary of the 10 most important needs of families of critically ill dying clients:

1. To be with the person.
2. To be helpful to the dying person.
3. To be informed of the dying person's changing condition.
4. To understand what is being done to the client and why.
5. To be assured of the client's comfort.
6. To be comforted.
7. To ventilate emotions.
8. To be assured that their decisions were right.
9. To find meaning in the dying of their loved one.
10. To be fed, hydrated, and rested.

Aspects of major recommendations based on the review include preparation of the client, family, and clinical team; ensuring the comfort of the client; withdrawal of life-sustaining treatments; terminal extubation versus terminal wean; special issues in communicating with families near the time of death; and special ethical issues.

Source: Truog, R. D., Cist, A. F., Brackett, S. E., Burns, J. P., Curley, M. A., Danis, M., ... Hurford, W. D. (2001). Recommendations for end-of-life care in the intensive care unit: The Ethics Committee of the Society of Critical Care Medicine. *Critical Care Medical, 29*(12), 2332–2348.

DOCUMENTATION for the Dying Client

- Client's physical symptoms
- Characteristics of the stage of dying and acceptance by client
- Support systems available to client
- Nursing care measures that make the client comfortable
- Family acceptance and interaction with client
- Comfort or limited support measure provided
- DNR orders in place
- Rituals that are being carried out during care

CRITICAL THINKING Application

Expected Outcomes

- Client is able to progress through stages of grief with support of family and nursing staff.
- Client is accepting of loss and eventual outcome of grief process.
- Client is as pain-free as possible.
- Client's cultural beliefs are considered throughout the dying process.
- Client found internal sources to support acceptance of death.
- Family members are supported throughout the dying process.

Unexpected Outcomes	Alternative Actions
Nurse is unable to care for the dying client due to her or his own emotional reaction.	• Request that other staff members take over, as the objective is to be able to give good nursing care. • Request assistance from skilled professional so you can work through your own feelings about death in order to be able to cope with the next death experience.
Client loses confidence in the healthcare team.	• Attempt to ascertain exactly what occurred to cause client to lose confidence in the team. • Report to charge nurse so that staff caring for client may be changed. Be sure to choose experienced personnel who are equipped to cope with a dying client.
Client lingers on and does not fulfill expectation that death would occur in the near future.	• Report status to staff so arrangements may be made for respite-supportive care for family who is having a difficult time coping. • Discuss hospice care with the client's family.
Pain cannot be controlled adequately with ordered medication.	• Report to physician so alternative pain relief methods may be used. • Ensure that WHO three-step analysis ladder protocols are being followed. • Ensure that around-the-clock medication administration is occurring. • Assist the client to cope by spending additional time and meeting physical needs.

Chapter 34

UNIT 3

Postmortem Care

Nursing Process Data

ASSESSMENT Data Base

- Verify that appropriate documentation is completed by the physician or other healthcare provider as required by state regulations.
- Identify cultural and/or family needs and desires.
- Identify client by name and client's belongings for labeling.
- Determine organ and tissue donation status.

PLANNING Objectives

- To prepare body for removal from clinical unit
- To acknowledge cultural and/or family rituals applicable to body preparation
- To protect the condition of the body for the purpose of respect for the deceased and his or her family during final viewing
- To document facts and time relating to death
- To identify and label client and client's belongings

IMPLEMENTATION Procedures

EVALUATION Expected Outcomes

- Postmortem care is completed, maintaining client's dignity.
- Client's family members are supported by staff during grief process.
- Appropriate procedures are carried out for organ and tissue procurement

Providing Postmortem Care

Equipment

Bathing supplies
Shroud or morgue bag
Identification tags
Protective pads, if necessary
Rolls of gauze and abdominal pads, if necessary
Paper bags or plastic bags for personal belongings
Gurney or specialized morgue cart
Clean gloves

Procedure

1. If previously determined or requested by client or family, notify appropriate clergy or support person.
2. Determine that client's death has been pronounced per agency policy and determine whether there is going to be an autopsy or a coroner involved.
3. If there are other clients or visitors in the room, carefully explain the situation and ask them to temporarily leave the room if possible. Provide privacy.
4. Collect necessary equipment. Incorporate family requests or cultural preferences when possible.
5. Follow hospital procedure regarding notification of various departments and personnel.
   a. Determine whether client has signed a donor card and/or has made a decision to donate any organs.
   b. Follow client's advance directive on file at the hospital for donor instructions.
   c. Notify appropriate hospital personnel or local procurement organization (OPO) for assistance with organ donation.
   d. Follow specific procedures for organ transplant according to hospital policy.

Signed by the donor and the following two witnesses in the presence of each other:

Signature of Donor ________ Date of Birth of Donor ________

Date Signed ________ City & State ________

Witness ________ Witness ________

This is a legal document under the Uniform Anatomical Gift Act or similar laws.

For further information consult your physician or

National Kidney Foundation
116 East 27th Street, New York, N.Y. 10016

▲ To ensure that organs are donated appropriately, instruct client to fill out and keep donor card available at all times.

6. Maintain proper alignment of the body. Raise the head of the bed 30°. Maintain head elevation throughout care and to morgue. ▶ ***Rationale:*** To prevent pooling of fluids in the head or face.
7. Don gloves.
8. Close the eyes. If necessary, use paper tape or gauze pads. You may do this after the family has visited the deceased.
9. Replace dentures and close mouth. ▶ ***Rationale:*** It is easier to insert dentures before rigor mortis begins, and this maintains the client's natural appearance.
10. Remove any external objects causing pressure or injury to the skin (e.g., oxygen mask).
11. Remove IV lines, catheters, or tubes per agency policy, unless an autopsy is to be done.

NOTE: Removing catheters and IV lines causes fluid to leak into tissues, resulting in edema and discoloration. Hospital policy may, therefore, direct that all IV lines be converted to hep locks or intermittent infusion devices to prevent fluid leaks. Follow hospital policy.

12. Cleanse the body as needed. A partial bath may be required to remove secretions, wound drainage, or stains.
13. Place protective incontinent pad under buttocks and between legs in diaper fashion.
14. If family is to visit the deceased, provide clean linen and gown for client.
15. Remove equipment used for cleansing the client.
16. Allow the family private time to view the body. Allow as much time as they desire.

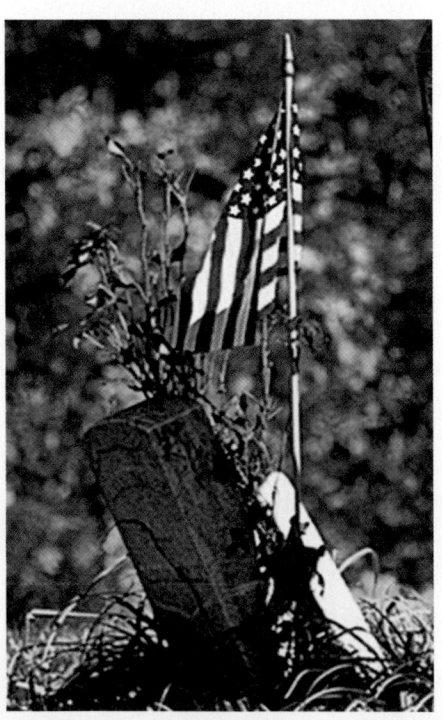

17. After family and clergy have visited, label the body, attaching ID tags to the big toe, wrist, and morgue bag or as determined by agency policy.
18. Place arms and hands loosely at side or on abdomen. ▸ ***Rationale:*** This prevents discoloration of hands.
19. Place the body in the shroud or in morgue bag.
20. Label all personal belongings and place them in a bag.
21. Remove gloves and perform hand hygiene.
22. Close doors to client's room and clear hallways in preparation to transfer the body to the morgue.
23. Transfer the body to the morgue on a gurney or a special morgue cart. Keep client's head elevated.
24. Place client's personal belongings in the appropriate place determined by hospital policy.
25. Support family members as needed. Provide for emotional and physical comfort.

NOTE: Rigor mortis begins about 4 hr after death and reaches its peak about 10 hr later. It passes from the body after 36 hr. It is best to wait until the body passes through this process before embalming. Therefore, it is not a problem to wait for relatives to view the body within a specified time frame.

Clinical Alert

Inform the funeral home if the client has tuberculosis or any other infectious disease so appropriate care can be taken to prevent contamination of the environment.

Preparing for Organ and Tissue Procurement

Procedure

1. Determine whether organs or tissues are to be "harvested" in a dying client. Check for driver's license information on transplant donor and/or check for Advance Directives or Living Will.
2. Determine appropriate procedure for securing organs and tissues. Check hospital policy and procedure.
   a. Determine time frame for collecting organs and tissues. ▸ ***Rationale:*** Organs, bones, eyes, skin, and tissues have different time frames for removal in order to preserve them appropriately. If time frame has elapsed, the organs or tissues cannot be used for transplant.
   b. If death is imminent, contact the local organ-procurement organization (OPO) according to hospital policy. Members of the organization or the coordinator will be present during the organ procurement procedures.
   c. If client is not identified as an organ donor, notify physician to determine whether client is a candidate for donation. Contact OPO to alert them about a possibility of organ donation.
   d. After evaluating client's condition, physician should contact family members to determine if they would like to donate organs or tissues. Some organs many not be appropriate for donation, but many times eyes, skin, and tissues are appropriate.
   e. Client is kept hemodynamically stable while decisions about transplantation are made by family members.
   f. When the client has been declared brain dead, the local OPO coordinator, who is a nurse or physician's assistant, will assume responsibility for the donor's management. This does include directing clinical nursing care.

DOCUMENTATION for Postmortem Care

- The exact time the physician or healthcare professional was informed and death was pronounced
- When family members or significant others were notified
- Time organ procurement team informed, if appropriate
- Consent forms signed
- Condition of the body and postmortem care delivered
- Time the body was sent to the morgue
- Mortuary contacted, if appropriate
- Disposition of client's belongings
- Disposition of organs and tissues

CRITICAL THINKING Application

Expected Outcomes

- Postmortem care is completed, maintaining client's dignity.
- Client's relatives are supported by staff during grief process.
- Appropriate procedures are carried out for organ donations.
- Appropriate disposition of patient belongings.

Unexpected Outcomes	Alternative Actions
Client is not identified properly when sent to the morgue.	• Check Ident-A-Band and shroud label before releasing client to mortician. Request another nurse to check labels.
Donated organs are needed.	• Provide support to family and give an opportunity for questions. • Obtain signatures for consent form. (Kidneys should be removed within 1 hr after death. Eyes should be removed within 6–24 hr after death.) • Examine reverse side of driver's license, or remind the charge nurse to call mortician if burial plans have been made previously, to check on permission for organ donation through a living will.

GERONTOLOGIC Considerations

Three Out of Four Elderly People Die of Heart Disease, Cancer, or Stroke

- Heart disease is leading cause of death, although it has declined since 1968.
- Death rates from cancer have decreased, but lung cancer has increased in women.
- Death statistics for people in the 65–74 age group: heart disease accounted for 38%; cancer, 30% of deaths.
- Two-thirds of hospice clients are over 65 years of age.

Death in the Life Cycle

- In American culture, the obsession with youth often results in denial of death as a natural phase of the life cycle, and death is not considered a positive process.
- Elderly may see death as an end to suffering and loneliness.
- Death is usually not feared if the person has lived a long and fulfilled life, having completed all developmental tasks.
- Spiritual beliefs or philosophy of life are important.

MANAGEMENT Guidelines

Each state legislates a Nurse Practice Act for RNs and LVN/LPNs. Healthcare facilities are responsible for establishing and implementing policies and procedures that conform to their state's regulations. Verify the regulations and role parameters for each healthcare worker in your facility.

Delegation

- Assisting the client to deal with grief may be delegated to another healthcare professional who is trained and experienced in working with grief, such as a social worker or hospice nurse. Assigning staff to work with a dying client will involve similar parameters, with the additional criteria that the nurse has worked through his or her own feelings about dying and can deal directly with the subject of death. If a client wishes to discuss dying or fears related to dying, the nurse must be able to listen and appropriately interact with the client. The nurse assigned to care for the dying client should be aware of the importance of the family in terms of support and communication.
- The nurse is responsible for reviewing the Advance Directives in the client's chart for organ donation or the living will to determine the appropriate members of the team to care for the client.
- Postmortem care may be provided by the staff. However, if there are organs to be donated, the professional nurse is responsible for carrying out the hospital policies and/or orders necessary to preserve the organs for organ transplant.

Communication Matrix

- Because nonprofessional staff are often assigned to care for the basic needs of a dying client, the RN/LVN/LPN must set up a channel of communication (both written and verbal) so the nurse is constantly aware of the status of the client and the family is informed of the client's status. The professional nurse should also provide the family with opportunities to discuss the condition of the client and plans for the future care of the client (including organ donation and hospice care). It would be inappropriate for nonprofessional staff to be assigned these activities.

CRITICAL THINKING Strategies

Scenario 1

You are assigned to care for Mrs. Garcia, an 85-year-old Hispanic client who speaks limited English. Her caregiver at home has been her daughter, who speaks somewhat more English than her mother. A son and grandson visit her often and both of them speak fluent English. Mrs. Garcia has been brought to the hospital in end-stage renal failure. Her BUN and creatinine are both very high. Her blood pressure is 210/110, pulse 110, and respirations 30 and labored. Her skin has a jaundiced appearance and she has many ecchymotic areas throughout her body. She states she "doesn't want to live like this." She is debating asking to be taken off dialysis, but that decision has not yet been made.

1. Considering her condition, what priority interventions should you consider? What is the rationale for your answer?
2. Considering her limited English skills, how will you carry out your priority interventions?
3. Her daughter asks you how long she will live without dialysis. What is your best response? Provide rationale for your response.
4. In the evening after the son has been to visit his mother in the hospital, the family discussed her wishes. It was decided that they would stop dialysis. What steps will you take to provide end-of-life care to Mrs. Garcia?
5. Identify at least four interventions you will use to assist the family in coping with the impending death of their mother and grandmother.
6. During the last day, Mrs. Garcia is complaining about mild to moderate pain. What interventions will you use to make her comfortable?

Scenario 2

You are working with a terminally ill client who is in severe pain. The client's family is considering moving the client to a hospice center.

1. What are some of the advantages for the client if this move is accomplished?
2. What are some of the barriers to hospice care that you would anticipate when discussing this decision with the family?

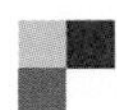

NCLEX® Review Questions

Unless otherwise specified, choose only one (1) answer.

1. Place the stages of grief, according to Elizabeth Kübler-Ross, in the order in which they progress.
    1. Anger.
    2. Depression.
    3. Acceptance.
    4. Denial.
    5. Bargaining.
2. The response in Engle's third stage of grief, restitution, is described as
    1. A time when all feelings of hostility and negative feelings toward the deceased are repressed.
    2. The beginning of the recovery process, with the onset of cultural and religious rituals that assist the mourner to face the loss.
    3. The stage in which there is a refusal to accept or comprehend the death.
    4. The mourner's attempt to deal with the painful void created by the loss of a loved one.
3. The Clinical Policies and Performance Practice Guidelines for end-of-life care include
    Select all that apply.
    1. Discontinuing alternative and nontraditional care to allow the client to rest.
    2. Allowing the client to refuse treatments.
    3. Managing spiritual/religious problems.
    4. Encouraging family members to minimize time at the bedside to prevent client and family fatigue.
4. Hospice care is recommended for which of the following clients? Those who
    1. Live alone and require rehabilitation services.
    2. Have a life expectancy of less than 6 months.
    3. Are elderly and have a short life expectancy.
    4. Require comfort care but not treatments.
5. Family members need instructions in what behaviors and/or responses they can expect by the client when he/she is in the anger stage of the grief process. The most appropriate response is
    1. "Inappropriate or disturbed behavior occurs during the stage of denial, so this would not be observed during the anger stage."
    2. "You should not expect acting out of feelings and verbalization of anger at this stage."
    3. "Clients usually yell out at God and blame him for their problems."
    4. "During this time it is helpful if you make as many decisions as possible for the client."
6. Nursing interventions carried out when the client is near death include
    1. Placing the client in a room near the nurses' station.

2. Displaying a favorite object or children's photos within easy sight.
3. Pulling the curtains around the client so he/she does not need to look at the activity outside the door.
4. Ensuring that room is well-lit to provide continuous assessment of the client's condition.

7. Which cultural group is most likely to have completed advance directives?
   1. Caucasians.
   2. Asian-Americans.
   3. African Americans.
   4. Hispanic Americans.

8. Using the WHO Three-Step Analgesic Ladder for pain control, which description best illustrates Step 2 of the ladder?
   1. Opioid drugs such as codeine are added to NSAIDs to treat mild-to-moderate pain.
   2. Nonopioid drugs, such as aspirin, are used for pain without adjuvant drugs.
   3. Opioid drugs such as morphine sulfate are used for moderate pain without adjuvant drugs.
   4. Nonopioid drugs and methadone are used for pain control only in stage II.

9. As the client is dying, the nurse needs to provide emotional nursing care for the client. This includes: ***Select all that apply.***
   1. Demonstrating caring and a willingness to be involved in his/her care.
   2. Utilizing nonverbal communications and touch, if appropriate, based on cultural and religious beliefs.
   3. Coordinating nursing care so it can be completed in a block of time to allow adequate time for communication.
   4. Recognizing that your physical presence is comforting, even if you do not talk with the client.

10. There are three basic dimensions in end-of-life treatment that vary among different cultures. Which one of the four distracters is not included in these basic dimensions?
    1. Communication between client and physician regarding treatment.
    2. Locus of decision making.
    3. Attitudes toward advance directives.
    4. Communication of "bad news."

NCLEX-RN® Answers with Rationale

Chapter 1—Professional Nursing

1. **(2)** Even though nurses do care for clients in all types of settings and they do perform ADLs and prepare the clients for home care, these statements do not define nursing (1) and (4). Not all client care is ordered by the physician; nurses have many independent actions (3).
2. **(1)** In both clinical and academic environments, ethical principles are a necessary guide to professional development. This is the rationale for adhering to the code. Answers (2) and (3) are included, but not the most important. Administering medications is not included in the code (4).
3. **(4)** Maintaining the dress code is usually part of the student nurse's responsibility for clinical practice (1). There is no relationship between what staff RNs wear and students' dress code. A professional relationship must be maintained during client care (2). It is unprofessional to call a client by his/her first name (3).
4. **(3 4 5 6)** RN responsibilities cannot be delegated to the LVN/LPN regardless of length of experience (1). (2) CNAs cannot be assigned to a newly admitted client. They cannot complete a health history.
5. **(3)** Nurses in all clinical settings function under the standards, including Advanced Practice Nurses. Each specialty group of nurses develops their specific standards, according to the same protocols.
6. **(1 2 5)** Imprisonment or compensation to cover costs to a facility is not usually associated with professional misconduct cases.
7. **(3)** Examples of malpractice are (1) and (2). (4) is not connected with a legal issue. If the nurse refuses a client assignment after the shift starts, it is considered abandonment of the client and can result in terminating the nurse's employment.
8. **(1)** The first step in providing client care is gathering the appropriate equipment. (4) is an incorrect statement. The client must be identified using two forms of identifiers, such as ID band, asking for date of birth, or asking the client to state his/her name. (2) and (3) are not appropriate actions to determine priority nursing care for a client. It is based on the assessment and by discussing the client's needs.
9. **(3)** An assessment is carried out as one of the priority interventions at the beginning of the shift. This provides the data that is used to prioritize client care throughout the shift (1)(4). A focused assessment includes a basic assessment of all systems, but more in-depth assessment of the system most affected by the diagnosis (2).
10. **(4)** Soiled linen is never placed on the linen cart. It will contaminate the entire linen cart (1). Alcohol will not decontaminate equipment. Equipment needs to be sterilized in central supply (2). Sharing client equipment is never an accepted practice. Cross contamination between clients can occur (3).

Chapter 2—Nursing Process and Critical Thinking

1. **(4 5 2 3 1)** When planning care, the steps in the nursing process are completed in this order.
2. **(1) and (2)** Nursing care is provided to clients based on their individual care needs. Critical thinking is implemented after collecting data and then determining the needs of the client by priority. In addition to the identified attributes, critical thinkers are realistic, good team players, empathetic, and open-minded. Care is not delivered in the same way for all clients.
3. **(3)** If you missed the question, it is suggested that you review nursing diagnosis statements. (4) is a medical diagnosis and (1) and (2) are written incorrectly.
4. **(1 4 6)** These choices represent nursing diagnoses, whereas the other diagnoses are medical. Nursing diagnoses can be treated by a nurse. Medical diagnoses are treated by a physician, or the nurse can collaborate on the treatment. Medical diagnoses require a physician's order before the nurse can provide specific care to the client.
5. **(1)** Nurses should make clinical decisions using the best available research and other evidence that is consistent with policies, procedures, and clinical guidelines. (2) Best practices usually are indicative of the most often used methods of providing client care. They are not necessarily based on research findings. (3) and (4) do not describe, nor are they involved in, Evidence Based Nursing. New techniques may come from EBN but would be an off-shoot of the research, rather than the goal.
6. **(2)** After a complete assessment of the client, a data base of information is then utilized to develop a nursing diagnosis, short- and long-term goals, and appropriate interventions. (1), (3), and (4) actions will take place after the assessment is completed.
7. **(3)** Compliance to client care goals is effectively carried out when the client, family, and other individuals who will be participating in the care take an active role. (4) Teaching plans are best developed using the same group of individuals. (2) The care plan is developed as soon as possible after admission; follow hospital policy and procedure on time frame for completion.
8. **(3)** The nurse would collect additional data if needed, then make the intervention. Gathering data and prioritizing clients' needs (1) are part of the assessment phase of the nursing process. (2) is an action associated with nursing diagnosis phase, and (4) is the last step of the nursing process.
9. **(4)** The major advantage of using the NIC system is that it can be electronically sent to data bases. With the implementation of the electronic health record, standardized nursing languages such as NANDA can be used to provide a broad base of nursing knowledge at the point of care. (3) NIC information can also be used as a paper-based document.
10. **(3)** LVN/LPNs can assist the RN in revising client care plans. These health care workers (1) and (2) cannot complete the tasks identified in the question. UAPs cannot develop a care plan, and CNAs are not allowed to complete tasks prior to discharge, unless it is in their scope of providing hygienic care, moving and positioning, etc. (4) Only RNs can develop the plan of care at admission.

Chapter 3—Managing Client Care: Documentation and Delegation

1. **(1 2 4 5 6)** The only function that is not a purpose of charting is (3), to remind the nurse of the care and treatments given to the client.
2. **(2)** Nurses tend to rely on data in the computer and do not question it when it may be wrong (perhaps because of wrong input of the data), so this is a major disadvantage. All other answers are positive.
3. **(3)** The correct method is to draw a single line through the entry and write "mistaken entry" above it and initial. It should remain visible.
4. **(3)** Because there may be future legal implications, it is necessary to be very specific and record all of the details, not just those considered major (1) or general (4) details.
5. **(2)** A major advantage is that this form is standardized (not individualized) and multidisciplinary. It is a tool developed to encompass all health team members, so it does not allow for complex clients to receive individual goals.
6. **(2)** The important principle here is to recognize that this is a cultural issue and that the Islamic religion requires ritual bathing after prayers

every day. Telling him to wait or that you are too busy is not acknowledging his cultural/spiritual needs.

7. (1) When making an assignment, the leader should attempt to keep the same nurse with the same client. This allows for better continuity of care. The other choices would help provide continuity of care and stability.
8. (3) Proper delegation requires that the nurse delegating tasks must make sure the person is trained to perform the task, oversees the activity, and evaluates the results. Close supervision will discourage employees and isn't necessary unless a particular problem exists (1). Delegating a task allows the employee to utilize his/her own knowledge (2).
9. (1) By witnessing the signing of a surgical consent form, the nurse is merely attesting that the client has signed the form. Answer (2) describes informed consent. Witnessing the form doesn't mean the nurse believes the client is competent (3). The nurse is not in the position to determine likelihood of success of a procedure (4).
10. (3) Some tasks may not ever be delegated, and each state sets its own requirements; for example, total assessment and evaluation may not be delegated. All other statements are correct.

Chapter 4—Communication and Nurse–Client Relationship

1. (4) Aphasia leads to feelings of frustration and discouragement. Clients require frequent praise for their efforts and encouragement to continue to try to communicate. Aphasic clients can best provide information by responding to yes or no questions.
2. (3) Termination is an ongoing process, so encouraging the client to follow through with what was learned is a good response. The nurse would *not* encourage the client to stop by, because the relationship was terminated. The last response is *not* encouraging and nontherapeutic.
3. (4) A professional relationship must remain on the professional level even though the nurse sets goals with the client, sets limits, and sets boundaries. Hospital policies are not relevent. The nurse will not necessarily maintain a distance, because a degree of emotional involvement is positive. Client needs are important but are not the focus of the relationship.
4. (3) This is a reflective response, and it opens up communication and allows the client to express whatever concerns or feelings he has without confining the discussion to dying. The other two responses cut the client off and are nontherapeutic.
5. (3) This open-ended question allows the client to further comment and expand on the subject. Answers (1) and (2) are closed ended and can be answered by a yes or no. Also, the last response is more focused, so an open-ended question is best.
6. (2) This response keeps lines of communication open so that the nurse can hear his fears and clarify any medical lack of knowledge. As he verbalizes, he can begin to more realistically cope with his condition. The remaining responses all close off communication and are nontherapeutic.
7. (4) The first intervention is to calmly set limits on the verbally abusive behavior to defuse the situation. Summoning help or sending the client away may escalate the situation, Restraints would only be a last resort.
8. (1 2 3 6 7) The age of the client and whether or not he believes in God are not components of a cultural assessment.
9. (1) The most effective mode of communication if the client is hearing impaired is to use a writing pad and gestures. Speaking, even slowly or loudly, will probably be frustrating and difficult for the client. Nonverbal communication is not as effective as writing.
10. (4) The priority is client safety, so whenever caring for a depressed client who is potentially suicidal, the intervention is to assess frequently and place the client on suicide precautions. Encouraging the client to talk about his feelings will only deepen the depression. Activity is always useful because mobilizing the client is a goal, but it is not the priority here.

Chapter 5—Admission, Transfer, and Discharge

1. (3) Only the client has the right to make decisions about resuscitation efforts. This is in compliance with the Client Self-Determination Act.
2. (2) Admitting personnel inquire about Advance Directives so that documents can be added to the client's record, updated, or executed on admission.
3. (1) The individual receives an ID bracelet during the admission process, at which time he/she becomes a client.
4. (2 4) These correlate with the client's medical record. Birth date is not an identifier, and room number may change during hospitalization.
5. (2) A strange environment causes anxiety. Familiarity with the room and equipment promotes independence and control.
6. (1 4) This information is useful and predictable. The client would not use the emergency call system, physician visits are unpredictable, and HIPAA protects against revealing client identity.
7. (1) Smoking is the most preventable cause of morbidity. Hospitalization offers an opportunity to identify clients at risk for smoking-related diseases and to offer smoking cessation counseling.
8. (3) These are the two factors used for calculating BMI.
9. (1) Mistakes in client identification are a major cause of client injury due to errors in administration of medications or procedures to the wrong client, as well as the omission of care intended for another client.
10. (2) The nurse should advocate by determining why the client wishes to leave AMA, since the client's concerns may be alleviated once identified (e.g., further explanation, social service consult, individualized accommodations).

Chapter 6—Client Education and Discharge Planning

1. (4) Nurses are the principal providers of care; therefore, they usually take the leadership role in directing the educational plan. One of the other health team members may play a major role in the teaching; however, the nurse usually directs and guides the process. (1) Physicians usually do not play a major role in education while the client is hospitalized. (3) Discharge planners are pivotal in determining placement of clients on discharge and in obtaining equipment for the home.
2. (2) Clients with multisystem issues usually require education regarding diagnosis, multiple treatments, and medications. (1) Living alone does not necessarily place a client at high risk for discharge. If the client is young, self-sufficient, and has a good support system, the client is not at high risk. Answers (3) and (4), in and of themselves do not place clients in a high-risk category.
3. (4) The first three distractors are essential to determine an appropriate educational plan. (1) The educational level determines the level and scope of information that can be presented. (2) Family members should be included in the educational plan. (3) Ethnic and cultural issues need to be taken into account, especially when discussing items such as dietary alterations. The actual employment or occupation in most cases is not necessary in developing the teaching plan.
4. (2) The amount of time the family spends at the client's beside may be dependent on their work schedule, family responsibilities at home, etc. Once the teaching needs are determined, then it is important to evaluate their active participation.
5. (4) Knowing the lifestyle and usual daily activity can assist with determining the impact of changes on this activity and the emphasis on the teaching plan. (1) This procedure is not considered a major surgical intervention. Most of the listed procedures are done on an outpatient basis; therefore, the home environment would not be evaluated. There is no need for specialized equipment. (2) All clients having outpatient or short-stay surgery must have someone take them home because of the anesthesia. It isn't important to determine who will be staying at home with the client or when they return to work. The physician will give the client directions on the return-to-work date.
6. (4) The initial teaching plan will support the client in respect to the diagnosis, treatment, medications, and expected outcomes. Teaching is a major part of this initial plan. Of course, determining the support system at home will become more essential as the teaching continues and discharge planning is discussed. (1), (2), and (3) are essential components for the teaching plan and will be integrated within the plan.
7. (1 2 3) Summarizing the teaching content or clarifying misinformation does not evaluate the effectiveness of the teaching strategies. It does provide information on retention of information, which can play a role in how effective the strategies have been. However, you do want to

evaluate the type of strategy utilized in teaching. Basically, what they are doing in (4) and (5) is reiterating information. You cannot evaluate whether they are able to utilize the information that was covered in the teaching.

8. **(1)** The client will become more agitated with you if you attempt to continue with the teaching. The other responses are all appropriate for this situation. It is best to come back at a different time (3). At that time you may be able to determine why the client is agitated and hostile. (4) Frequently, another nurse is able to establish rapport with a client, and it would be best to ask that nurse for assistance with the client.
9. **(1 2 3)** This data is important information for other health care workers to have in order to develop an appropriate plan of care for the client. Nursing interventions and I&O records are not necessary unless there is a specific issue with them. For example, if the client's urine output has been low and he/she isn't taking in fluids, that should be included in the discharge summary.
10. **(3)** Older clients frequently have hearing deficits and extraneous noise impairs their hearing. This can lead to perceiving incorrect information and directions. (2) Older clients remember about 5% of what they read. (1) They remember 50–70% of what they hear and verbalize. (4) Usually, older clients do not learn best in groups, because it can be noisy and disruptive.

Chapter 7—Safe Client Environment and Restraints

1. **(1)** Characteristics influencing adaptation to the environment are provided in (2), (3) and (4). They must be assessed to determine the client's needs and abilities to safely adjust to their immediate surroundings.
2. **(4)** A large percentage of errors occur as a result of either no communication or incomplete communication regarding client care. (2) and (3) can also lead to sentinel events, but not to the extent of a failure in communication.
3. **(2)** The order can be renewed every 4 hours for a total of 24 hours. Children between 9 and 17 must have orders renewed every 2 hours, and every 1 hour for children under 9 years.
4. **(3)** The slip knot allows for a quick release in case of a client requiring release from the restraint. (4) The least restrictive method to prevent the client from falling would be the use of sitters.
5. **(1)** Keeping the contaminated equipment in the room prevents contamination to other clients. Clients with implants do not usually receive bed baths (2). This protects health care workers from unnecessary exposure to radiation. Client care is provided by standing away from the radiation area, but the time for client care is still limited to 15 minutes/shift by one health care worker (3) and (4).
6. **(4)** Staying with the client is critical to prevent a complication related to the seizure activity. (1) The client is turned to the side to protect the airway from tongue occlusion. (2) Once a seizure has begun, tongue blades are not inserted in the mouth. (3) Clients are not restrained to prevent injury during the seizure activity.
7. **(3)** The priority is to remove the clients, if at all possible. The usual priority for fire safety can be remembered by using the mnemonic RACE. R is remove client, A is activate the fire alarm, C is confine the fire, and E is extinguish the fire if possible.
8. **(1)** Promoting ADLs and exercise will increase the clients' strength and mobility. They should be encouraged to get out of bed. (2), (3), and (4) are all safety precautions that should be practiced for elderly clients to prevent injury.
9. **(1)** Wedge-roll cushions, use of low-level beds, placing a mat on the floor by the bed can all be used to prevent injury if a client falls. (3) Environmental alterations do not include using a geri-chair; (2) placing a client near the nurses' desk does not prevent the client from falling. (4) Side rails are considered restraints, although if the client is alert and asks that they be raised to assist the client in moving, they can be left in the "up" position.
10. **(2 3 4)** The vest is placed on the client with the zipper to the back. (3) After vest tails are crossed in back of the chair, the tails are wrapped around the immovable kickspur. The tails are then tied to the kickspur using a half-bow knot.

Chapter 8—Bathing, Bed Making, and Maintaining Skin Integrity

1. **(2)** Tucking the sheet under the bed at the top of the bed and going down to the foot of the bed, would take two staff to change the bed. (1). (3) Changing only the drawsheet is not considered a complete linen change. (4) Linen changes are not made just when the bed is soiled.
2. **(5 2 3 1 4)** A bed bath is completed using the noted sequence. The nurse completes the bath using a head-to-toe approach, working from the front side to the client's back.
3. **(3)** Because the skin of the elderly client is very thin and fragile, it is imperative that it be kept moist. (2) and (4) are not correct. The bath can be a tub bath or bed bath in addition to a shower. Minimal amounts of mild soap can be used for bathing. (1) Fragrant soaps are not recommended as they can cause drying of the skin.
4. **(3)** This is considered a medication and therefore requires a physician's order. (1), (2) giving a bath in tepid water does not require an order, nor does using a hydraulic bathtub chair. (4) This type of bath is not ordered by the physician. It is the nurse's discretion based on the client's ability to assist with the bath or to ambulate to the tub or shower.
5. **(4)** The client can assist with washing his/her hands and face if the exertion is not too much. (1), (2) and (3) would not be appropriate for the client who is short of breath. It would take too much energy to perform any of these tasks.
6. **(1 2)** These activities are considered part of morning care. (3) and (4) are considered part of providing evening care. These activities are also completed when the bath is provided.
7. **(3)** Maintaining the pH of the skin prevents drying of the skin. (1) The cost is less using regular linen in most facilities, but convenience is taken into account when facilities do use disposable systems. (2) A wash cloth is also warmed, therefore this is not an advantage of the system. It is not easier or quicker to use.
8. **(3)** Cleansing the eyes first prevents water and particles from entering the lacrimal duct. (1) The head and scalp are washed last, after taking the infant out of the bath tub. (4) would be completed after the infant's ears and neck are washed.
9. **(2)** Picking up the skin is a good indicator of hydration of the client. If the skin stays tented, the client is dehydrated. (1) Checking the temperature of the skin is accomplished by placing the back of your fingers or hand on the client's skin. (3) Checking for edema is completed by firmly pressing the finger against the client's skin for several seconds and observing the indentation depth of the skin. (4) Checking the color of the skin of the hands might be done to check for peripheral circulation, not hydration.
10. **(2)** Using an adherent dressing will assist the wound to heal. (1) The skin is irrigated with normal saline solution, if needed. (3) A dry dressing will adhere to the tear and can cause the tear to open up when the dressing is removed. (4) It is not necessary to immobilize the arm.

Chapter 9—Personal Hygiene

1. **(1)** Turning the head to the side allows fluids to drain out, facilitates suctioning, and prevents aspiration. (2) is important also, but it is not the major safety action. (3) Padded tongue blades or a bite lock can be used to separate upper and lower sets of teeth to promote cleaning of inner teeth surface. Gloves are used to prevent spread of infection (4); although important, number 1 is the major safety action.
2. **(4)** Combing starts at the end of the hair shaft and works toward the scalp. (1) It is used to provide routine hair care. (2) Oil is used for coarse or curly hair that has dry or flaky areas on the scalp. (3) Hair picks are used for hair care when the client has coarse or curly hair.
3. **(2)** Nits within 6 mm of the scalp are usually viable, white in color, and indicate an active infestation. (1) Lice are light to dark brown in color, crawl, and feed on blood 3–4 times/day. (3) Lice eggs hatch in 7–10 days, not 17 days. (4) Lice have six clawed legs and crawl, but do not jump. A fine toothed comb is necessary to extract the nits from the hair.
4. **(3)** Nits witihin 6 mm of the scalp are usually viable and indicate an active infestation. (1) and (2) are incorrect. (4) Nits are not easily seen on the hair shaft.

5. **(4)** Clothing can be washed in hot water when nits or lice are found (1). Rid Home Lice Control Spray is used on furniture and mattresses, or any item that cannot be laundered. Family members are treated once lice or nits are found (2). They are usually not treated prophylactically. Launder bedding when nits or lice are found (3).
6. **(2)** Most institutions do not allow nurses to cut the nails of clients with peripheral vascular disease or diabetes (3). Skin lesions can occur with cutting nails and this can lead to infection and poor healing. Physicians, or in some instances nurses, should notify the podiatrist to see the client (4). Documentation is important, but the nurse needs to complete the assessment (1).
7. **(3)** This position prevents the client's knees from buckling. (1) can cause back injury to the nurse if the client loses balance and begins to fall, thus pulling on the nurse. (2) and (4) can lead to the nurse's injury, as it places pressure on back muscles.
8. **(3)** For uncircumcised clients, the foreskin is retracted to expose the glans penis for cleaning (1). Washing begins at the tip of the penis and proceeds to the base (2). The scrotum is washed after the penis, using a clean washcloth (4).
9. **(4)** Only rinsing or saline solution can be used to cleanse contact lenses (2). Daily wear lenses cannot be worn overnight (2).
10. **(1 2 3)** All of these responses are important when teaching care of hearing aids. Batteries should be replaced when necessary.

Chapter 10—Vital Signs

1. **(2)** Loss of peripheral pulses may indicate circulatory collapse, so a further assessment should be made. When peripheral pulses cannot be palpated, a Doppler is used. Thus, the nurse should use a Doppler ultrasound to find the pulse, then report to the physician.
2. **(1)** A pulse deficit (when apical is greater than radial rate) occurs when rhythm is irregular and atrial dysrhythmia or premature ventricular beats occur. If a significant pulse deficit is found, assess for other abnormal signs.
3. **(2)** The first intervention is to expand the assessment of vital signs so that you have more data to make a nursing diagnosis. At that point you may request orders for a cooling blanket because it is more efficient than a cool bath. After you report to the physician, there may be an order for a blood culture.
4. **(2)** If an unexpected low blood pressure is recorded, the nurse needs to first examine her technique. If the cuff is too wide, the blood pressure will be low. The client's arm should be supported horizontally at heart level.
5. **(1)** The first intervention is to use different equipment because it may be faulty. Then, if it is functioning, validate with another nurse. Finally, check his circulatory status and other vital signs, and notify the physician.
6. **(1 3 4 5)** These are the breathing patterns considered to be abnormal. Answer (2), respiratory rate 12–20, is normal for an adult.
7. **(1)** A rise in the pulse rate is one of the earliest signs of shock. A blood pressure of 110/70 and a respiratory rate of 24 are normal and do not reflect shock (2), (3). The temperature of 101 degrees F is not associated directly with a sign of shock, but may indicate other problems (4).
8. **(1)** Consistency of approach is the best, as changing position of the arm that is used may result in a different reading. The best graph is obtained by using the same approach over time.
9. **(2)** Pressure close to the tympanic membrane seals the ear canal and allows for an accurate reading. Answer (3) is not wrong, but it is not as complete an answer. Answers (1) and (4) are incorrect.
10. **(3)** Because vital signs can be assigned to any health care worker as long as their competency has been assessed, it is more man-power effective to have the nursing assistants start the shift assessment with reporting vital signs, then have the day's work assigned based on the clients' conditions. The RN and LVN would then begin caring for the most critically ill clients.

Chapter 11—Physical Assessment

1. **(4)** The basic principle to remember when auscultating lungs is to do a comparison between left and right lungs beginning at the top and alternating side-to-side.
2. **(3)** Rebound tenderness is a symptom of peritoneal irritation such as seen with appendicitis. Hold fingers at 90° angle, push fingers deeply in region away from reported tenderness, then rapidly remove fingers. Rebound of structures indented by this maneuver causes a sharp pain on the side of the inflammation. Painful areas should be examined last (1). The client should breathe normally (2). Client should have knees bent to help relax the stomach muscles (4).
3. **(1)** Macules are flat, circumscribed, and show a change in color like first-degree burns, petechiae, and purpura. Wheals are elevated, irregular shaped, and solid (2). Vesicles are elevated and fluid-filled (3). Papules are elevated, firm, and circumscribed such as a wart or mole.
4. **(3)** +2 is a normal response for deep tendon reflexes. +1 is a diminished, low normal response (1). 0 is no response (2) and +4 is brisk and hyperactive (4).
5. **(3)** IX, glossopharyngeal, is the cranial nerve assessed when testing for the gag reflex. XI, accessory, is the motor nerve that causes contractions of sternocleidomastoid and trapezius muscles (1). VII is the facial, sensory, and motor nerve (2). XII, hypoglossal, is the motor nerve that controls muscles that move the tongue (4).
6. **(4)** The S_1 heart sound can best be heard at the apex of the heart, over the mitral and tricuspid areas. The pulmonic valve is at the left second intercostal space and the aortic valve is at the right second intercostal space (1). The diaphragm is used to listen to high-pitched sounds like S_1 (2). S_1 is not loudest in the aortic area (3).
7. **(4)** Flexing the neck slightly reduces muscle tension and enhances palpation. Raising the chin tenses the neck muscles, making it more difficult to palpate nodes (1). Lying in a supine position makes it difficult to assess because access is limited (2). Swallowing water is used to assess the thyroid gland and movement of the cartilages (3).
8. **(2)** Examining the adjacent area is the next intervention because pulse locations can differ with clients. The follow-up intervention would be to use a Doppler ultrasound stethoscope to locate the pulse (3). Finally, if no pulse is found, you would notify the physician (1).
9. The normal range of specific gravity is 1.003–1.030. Abnormal specific gravity could indicate dehydration or renal failure.
10. **(3)** You are assessing the client's fund of information, so asking who is the president will reveal deteriorated or impaired cognitive processes. Asking about feelings will not reveal this information (1). With dementia, the client may remember what he did years ago, but cannot remember yesterday (2). Answer (4) is a higher level question that the client may not be able to answer, but it is not as revealing as answer (3).

Chapter 12—Body Mechanics and Positioning

1. **(4)** The newest method of preventing caregiver injuries is concentrating on handling equipment and devices. (1), (2), and (3) are older common approaches for moving and turning clients that are no longer accepted practice.
2. **(1)** 51 pounds is the standard for lifting clients, and this should be done under controlled and limited circumstances. (4) indicates the average weight of clients in the hospital. (2) and (3) are not correct responses.
3. **(3 4)** Appropriate body mechanics used when moving clients are included in correct answers. (1) is incorrect as the feet are placed flat on the floor to form a strong base of support, with one foot ahead of the other. (2) The abdomen is held firm but the buttocks is tucked in so the spine is in alignment.
4. **(1)** The most comfortable height for working is between the waist and lower level of the hip joint.
5. **(3)** It is imperative that you report any injury to your immediate supervisor so he/she can investigate the situation and provide appropriate support for you. (1) You will need to complete an unusual occurrence form; however, this is done after notifying the immediate supervisor. (4) As with any injury, the nurse is usually taken off any client care assignment and sent to the ER for an evaluation.

6. **(4)** In low-Fowler's position, the client is placed in a 15 degree position. (1) is high-Fowler's position. (2) is Fowler's position, and (3) is semi-Fowler's position.
7. **(3)** The friction-reducing sheet not only assists in turning the client but prevents skin tears. (1) A second nurse is frequently used to assist in turning, but it is not the best method to be used. (2) The lift team is used only when other methods of turning are not safe or the client is too difficult to move. (4) The client is not asked to move up in bed before the turn. This can be accomplished during the lateral turn.
8. **(4)** The client turns onto his/her back directly onto the transfer board. (1) The board is placed on the opposite side of the bed before turning the client. (2) The client is placed on his/her back, not in a side-lying position. (3) The client does not roll over the edge of the board to the gurney maintaining a side-lying position. The client remains on his/her back when using the transfer board.
9. **(3)** Clients with some arm strength and weight-bearing ability can pull themselves up by holding onto the bars. (1) is used for clients who are unable to bear any weight. (2) is used for clients who can bear weight at least on one leg. Client places foot on footrest while a sling is placed under the arms and around the back. (4) assists clients from bed to gurney.
10. **(1 2 3 4)** All responses are correct.

Chapter 13—Exercise and Ambulation

1. **(4)** Flexion is a movement that decreases the angle between two bones (1). (2) means turning outward. (3) Adduction is a movement of a bone toward the midline of the body.
2. **(1 2 4)** A client on strict bedrest with passive range-of-motion exercises ordered will not be completing the exercises independently.
3. **(3)** Raising the head of the bed slowly several times will stimulate baroreceptors and thus prevent orthostatic hypotension. (1) Client doesn't necessarily need to use a walker. (2) Vital signs are taken, but usually after the client sits up and before standing. (4) Additional assistance may be necessary to help, but this is not directly related to preventing orthostatic hypotension.
4. **(3)** The weaker side of the body is moved first by supporting body weight using the handles and then advancing the weaker leg. In (1), the client does push off the bed, but is instructed to grasp the hand grips of the walker before doing so.
5. **(4)** Cane is placed on the unaffected side of the body (1). This promotes stability. (2) Cane is placed about 12 inches in front of the foot and slightly to the outside for greater stability. (3) Cane is moved first and then the affected leg.
6. **(4)** When going upstairs, the cane and unaffected leg are placed on the step first (1). (2) The affected leg is moved to the step after the cane and unaffected leg. (3) Cane and affected leg are moved to the step after the unaffected leg is placed on the step.
7. **(2)** Client wears shoes that will be used for walking when measuring for crutches to ensure proper height of the crutches. If height is incorrect, the axilla could rest on the bar of the crutches, causing skin breakdown or nerve involvement. (1) Crutches are measured with client shoes on in bed. (3) Axilla should not rest on crutch arms. This can lead to nerve injury and skin breakdown of the axilla. (4) Client is measured while in bed, at a point 6–8 inches lateral from the heel.
8. **(3)** Three-point gait is a more rigid version of the four-point gait; therefore, the client can move and bear weight on each leg (1). (2) Client can bear little or no weight on one leg or when the client only has one leg. (4) Usually used when client's lower extremities are paralyzed.
9. **(2)** Instructions for clients going upstairs with crutches include: First place the uninjured leg and crutches on the same level. Then place crutches on first step. Next move unaffected leg to step where crutches are placed.
10. **(3 4)** Applies to a client who suffers axillary nerve pressure resulting in numbness and tingling of the fingers (1). (2) Proficiency is not what is needed to prevent slipping; it is having the tips of the crutches covered with rubber to prevent slipping on floors.

Chapter 14—Infection Control

1. **(4)** Goggles should be worn when there is a risk of contact with body fluids through spattering or splashing. The remaining three interventions would not present this risk.
2. **(2)** Standard precaution guidelines dictate that spills be cleaned immediately with 1:10 bleach or according to hospital policy. All of the other answers are incorrect because they do not meet EPA specifications.
3. **(2)** Isolation protects the immunocompromised child from the environment. The other conditions do not necessarily require isolation.
4. **(4)** Hand hygiene before giving care and after all diaper changes is an important measure in controlling and preventing the spread of infection. Using sterile technique or antibiotics are incorrect answers, and ill people should not be allowed near infants in the hospital.
5. **(2)** Placing a container in the home provides the safest means of disposing of contaminated needles. This container needs to be discarded and treated as biohazardous waste when it becomes full or is no longer needed. The needles should not be recapped, disposed of in the trash, or broken.
6. **(4)** An antiseptic solution is an effective cleansing agent for blood or body fluid contamination. This should be readily available to everyone who is at risk for exposure. Recapping the needle will risk repeated injury and exposure and should never be done (1). Breaking the needle will risk repeated injury and exposure (2). The client will not require gamma globulin, because the needle was contaminated after the injection (3).
7. **(2)** Standard precautions employ using gloves when touching body fluids containing blood. Gloves are not necessary in this instance. The nurse should continue teaching the nursing assistant by explaining the principles of infection control related to AIDS.
8. **(2)** There are three primary routes of transmission—contact, droplet, and airborne HAI (nosocomial) infections such as VRE and MRSA are usually caused by poor handwashing or hand hygiene technique by health care workers who move from client to client.
9. **(4 3 2 1)** The surface below the waist level is considered contaminated; therefore, you would untie the strings before removing gloves, which is the next step. The third step is to take off your mask; then you would perform hand hygiene.
10. **(3)** Take only needed supplies from bag and place on clean surface.

Chapter 15—Disaster Preparedness—Bioterrorism

1. **(2)** Research has shown that the triangle of safe space is beside a car or large piece of furniture. If it collapses, you will not be under it, but it will still provide you with some protection.
2. **(2)** The correct answer is an event of great magnitude that overwhelms current resources. The other answers are all characteristics.
3. **(4)** Biological agents (bacteria, viruses, or toxins) are the most difficult to identify because they have an insidious onset and symptoms may take days to develop. A nuclear attack and sarin gas would be more readily discovered, and smallpox, after an incubation period, would be easily identified by the skin eruptions.
4. **(3)** A person can absorb anything under 0.75 Gy and not experience radiation poisoning. If a victim absorbs between 0.75 and 8 Gy, he or she may develop acute radiation syndrome (ARS). A person who absorbs over 8 Gy will probably die.
5. **(1 2 4 5)** These are all agents that fall into the category of bacteria, viruses, or toxins that can cause a disease which develops into a mass casualty incident. Radiation poisoning is caused by a nuclear weapon. Sarin gas is a chemical weapon.
6. **(1)** The 5-level system of triage decreases ambiguity of the middle level of emergency care where the majority of casualties fall; thus, it is much more effective in handling large numbers of victims. The other answers are inaccurate.
7. **(2 1 4 3)** When setting up a decontamination site, first be sure it is upwind from the contamination. The next step is to find a downhill slope so that runoff can be captured. Finally, find a source of water before

supplying personnel with protection equipment and beginning to decontaminate victims.

8. (4) There are some complications such as eczema vaccinatum that can be helped by VIG. Pregnant women should not be vaccinated. Answers 1 and 2 are complications of smallpox, not helped by VIG.
9. (2) Cyanide is a chemical agent, as is chlorine (a pulmonary agent), mustard and nerve agents (sarin, VX). The other agents are biological.
10. (3) A trace of blood indicates that the needle strokes were vigorous enough to transmit the vaccine into the client. The other answers are incorrect.

Chapter 16—Pain Management

1. (3) The endorphin theory is the most accepted because it explains how the brain produces natural opiates which fit into special cells called receptors. Specificity theory suggests that sensory stimuli send pain impulses to the brain, but this theory only deals with the physiologic, not the psychologic, basis for pain. The pattern theory includes factors not explained by the specificity theory, but is not complete. The gate control theory states that there is transmission of neurologic impulses and gate mechanisms along the nervous system that control the transmission of pain. If the gate is open, pain is experienced. None of these theories, however, adequately explains pain.
2. (1 2 3 5) These are the four main factors to measure pain. Pain pathway cannot be measured, and the amount of medication needed is an indication, but not a specific measure, of the degree of pain.
3. (2) The rationale for including pain as a vital sign is that it will be assessed and documented at the same time vital signs are taken. This is important, for if the level of pain is neglected, the client's condition/safety is in jeopardy. (1) and (3) may be correct but do not adequately explain the rationale. (4) is incorrect.
4. (1) Most of the nonpharmacological methods are totally noninvasive, and thus are safer and have fewer complications than pharmacological methods. The other statements are incorrect.
5. (4) The priority safety issue is to be sure that the epidural catheter is not mistaken for an IV line. A sign must be posted over the client's bed and the catheter must be labeled clearly as an epidural catheter. All of the other issues are a concern, but they would not result in fatality.
6. (2) In order to use this method of pain control, the client must be mentally alert and able to follow the procedure instructions, because the client is in control of the narcotic administration. (1) and (3) will be part of the total assessment criteria, but not the priority assessment. (4) is incorrect because this method is commonly used for chronic pain.
7. (3) The correct intervention is to determine that the client is sedated and, because the goal of PCA is to control pain without sedation, notify the physician for new dose parameters. The other answers are incorrect.
8. (1 2 4 5) All of these answers are common dangers and should be avoided. Poor pain relief results are not a common occurrence because drugs and dosage parameters are designed for individual client pain control with the client administering the narcotic.
9. (4) Administration of an epidural must only be done by an RN and may not be delegated to a nonprofessional staff member. In many hospitals, the RN must have special certification because of the safety issues involved with this procedure.
10. (3) The preventive approach to pain control includes administration of the medication before or soon after pain begins. Smaller, more frequent doses of medication will control pain better than larger doses taken less often.

Chapter 17—Alternative Therapies and Stress Management

1. (1 2 3 4 5) All of the above are signals of stress. Fatigue and eating disorders fall into physiologic signals; anxiety and anger are psychologic signals, and restlessness is a behavioral indicator.
2. (4) The most complete definition is to consider all aspects of a person relating as an open system. (1) and (2) are accurate, but not complete. (3) is inaccurate.
3. (1) Herbal medicines are one of the most frequently used alternative treatment modes. They are much more frequently used in other parts of the world than in the United States. The other alternative practices are used, but not as frequently as herbs.
4. (1 2 3 5 6) The only adaptation factor that does not influence how the individual adapts to stress is religion. The other factors all influence these patterns.
5. (2) This is a positive suggestion for coping with stress. All of the remaining answers are exactly the opposite of a therapeutic suggestion.
6. (1) More and more research is showing that diet/nutrition is a major contributor to health and the prevention of disease. Although nutrition may influence how long we live, there is no research proving this (2). (3) and (4) may also be true, but again there is no research proving it.
7. (3) This is the most open-ended response and does not place the nurse in legal jeopardy. (1) and (2) close off communication. (4) may result in legal problems, as it may be viewed as practicing medicine.
8. (3) Stress can be controlled and coped with by a variety of methods, including physical activity and relaxation methods such as deep breathing and meditation, not just one, changing thought patterns. All of the other answers are correct and fit Selye's definition of stress.
9. (4) Although there are many signals of stress, including physical, psychologic, and behavioral, often they are difficult to identify in the client because many of them are subtle (for example, lack of interest in life, lack of concentration, irregular heartbeats). All of the other statements about stress are correct.
10. (2) Sitting quietly, clearing the mind, and deep breathing or meditation are the best methods for destressing. The other methods listed may work for certain individuals, but they have not proven to be as effective.

Chapter 18—Medication Administration

1. (3) Surveys have found that administering the wrong dose is the most common cause of injury. Route is seldom erroneous, the medication usually validated, and the client identified correctly.
2. (2) The physician would be the authority to clarify rationale for the particular medication's use based on the individual client's need/condition.
3. (4) Systolic pressures less than 90 mm Hg may be associated with decreased cardiac output or orthostatic hypotension.
4. (3 4) Alterations for oral medication administration that are acceptable include mixing liquid from capsules with food and administering sublingual tablets to a client who is NPO.
5. (1) Rapid absorption of drops such as beta blocking agents used for glaucoma can cause serious bradycardia. Pressing the inner canthus helps prevent this adverse effect.
6. (1) For adults, upward and backward pull straightens the ear canal.
7. (2 4) The anterior superior spine of iliac crest and greater trochanter are identified by using the nurse's right hand for client's left hip, or left hand for client's right hip. The acromion process is a landmark for deltoid injection and the posterior superior spine of iliac crest is used for dorsogluteal injection. The gluteal fold is not a bony landmark and is not used to identify any injection site. The upper outer quadrant of the buttocks relates to soft tissue rather than bony landmarks, is highly variable among clients, and is totally unreliable for predicting location of underlying nerves and blood vessels.
8. (3) It is not uncommon for active ingredients to be depleted while propellant remains in the canister.
9. (2 1 4 3) The cloudy insulin should never contact the clear insulin, as it would cause the clear insulin remaining in the vial to lose its intended short action.
10. (4) Pump, tubing, or needle malfunction results in failure to deliver insulin and causes risk of diabetic ketoacidosis due to elevated blood sugar.

Chapter 19—Nutritional Management and Enteral Intubation

1. (1) Transfats are polyunsaturated and monounsaturated fats that have an additional hydrogen molecule added to make the fat more saturated.

2. (2) The kidneys are the major organs for potassium excretion, so potassium intake is restricted in clients with renal failure. The other clients listed would all require an increased ingestion of potassium-rich foods or a KCl supplement because their health conditions are associated with potassium loss.
3. (3 4) Swallowing liquids, ingesting liquids and food together, or use of a straw or syringe all increase the dysphagic client's risk of aspiration.
4. (4) The blue "pigtail" allows atmospheric pressure to enter the stomach to counteract the negative pressure suction at the NG tube tip. It thus prevents the decompression tube from adhering to the gastric mucosa, which would interfere with gastric content suctioning.
5. (2) Postoperative intestinal motility is regained first by the small intestine. Bowel sounds may be present, but gastric and large bowel motility may be absent. Presence of appetite, no abdominal distention, having flatus, and bowel movement are reliable indicators of the return of bowel function.
6. (3) Since the pH of aspirate is altered because of formula presence, the best way to verify placement is to note the character of the formula aspirated; it should be curdled or bile tinged.
7. (4) Tube feeding may be continued cautiously with close client monitoring if the residual volume is ≥ 200 mL. Further client assessment is indicated if the residual volume is ≤ 200 mL. The stomach may hold from 10 to 200 mL of gastric fluid normally.
8. (3) The tube should be flushed with warm water every 4–6 hours and before and following medication administration using a gentle push/pull technique. The tube should not require replacement for 4 weeks. Acidic juices or cola curdle feeding formula will increase the incidence of clogging.
9. (3) Positioning has no beneficial effect on feeding tube advancement. The guide wire should never be replaced once removed. Administration of a prokinetic agent *before* tube insertion is the most effective intervention to promote tube advancement.
10. (3) Feeding through a surgically created tube enterostomy reduces risk of aspiration, eliminates nasal irritation, is low profile, and facilitates independent feeding.

Chapter 20—Specimen Collection

1. (1) The critical factor is to rinse the mouth before obtaining the sample. The best sputum sample is obtained before eating or drinking (2). Several deep breaths may trigger the cough reflex and raise sputum from the lungs (3). An expectorant could contaminate the sample. Chest physiotherapy is most helpful in mobilizing secretions prior to collection (4).
2. (3) Standard precautions dictate that you should wear gloves during collection of a blood specimen. IV fluid may alter the specimen (1). The skin should be cleansed with an antimicrobial wipe followed by povidone-iodine swab or use hospital policy (2). Contamination of the sample may occur if the needle is used (4).
3. (4) Ova or cysts may not be revealed in the presence of heavy metals. Barium, oil, or laxatives containing heavy metals should not be given for 7 days prior to the stool examination. The time of day to collect specimen does not matter (1). Clean catch is used to collect urine samples (2). Sample should be examined within 30 minutes and kept at body temperature to find organisms in their active state (3).
4. (3) Guaiac is used to test for occult blood in the stool that could be a sign of upper GI bleeding or cancer. A stool culture is used to detect bacteria (1). This test does not test for fat in the stool (2). A paddle test is used to determine presence of pinworms (4).
5. (3) Check with the laboratory because, based on the amount lost, time of loss, and the test to be performed, the collection may be able to be completed as scheduled. You would not stop or extend the collection. Reinforcing to the client to save urine would be done if the test is to be repeated (4).
6. (2) Urine is normally clear, not cloudy—this could be indicative of an infection. Light yellow is the normal color (1). You require at least 30 mL for an adequate sample (3). Urine is normally odorless (4).
7. (4) Cleanse the site with an antimicrobial wipe and allow to dry is the correct technique, because bacteria on the skin surface are reduced if the skin is allowed to dry. The tourniquet should be 1–2 inches above the client's elbow (1). The client should relax the fist and the tourniquet should be released before the needle is removed (2). Bending the elbow could cause a hematoma, so this is incorrect (3).
8. (4) Allen's test should precede arterial puncture to determine the adequacy of collateral perfusion. Hyperextension of the wrist will stabilize the radial artery (1). Drawing back on a syringe can cause air bubbles to fill the syringe, and inaccurate ABG results will occur (2). Pressure should be maintained for 5 to 10 minutes to prevent bleeding.
9. (3) Adding blood to the strip can cause an erroneous reading. If the meter does not show enough blood, remove the strip and begin again. This is correct—the lancet should be on the lateral side of the finger because it is less painful and prevents bruising (1). Soap and water is best for repeated sticks—alcohol can toughen the skin (2). Stroking gently increases blood flow—squeezing or applying pressure can interfere with blood flow (4).
10. (1) True because recent antibiotic or antifungal therapy may lead to false negative results. Large wounds should have separate cultures taken from different areas with a new swab (2). Specimens should be sealed in a biohazard bag (3). Specimens should not be refrigerated—they should be transported to the laboratory within 30 minutes (4).

Chapter 21—Diagnostic Procedures

1. (2) Nursing actions listed in (1), (3), and (4) are important nursing interventions, but they do not necessarily have to be completed by the nursing staff assisting the physician with interventional radiology.
2. (1) Answer (2) is related to ultrasound procedures. (3) refers to endoscopic procedures, and (4) represents the results from an MRI.
3. (3) Each x-ray has specific restrictions to food or fluids. The other interventions would be completed during preparation for x-ray studies.
4. (2 3 4) All are appropriate instructions to provide for a client having an IVP performed. (1) is incorrect. Fluids are withheld up to 12 hours. No fluids are to be taken the morning of the study.
5. (3) It is important to have a baseline value to determine potential bleeding tendencies and kidney function.
6. (1) Barium falsely increases density of the lumbar spine, therefore an inaccurate reading will be given. The client may feel embarrassed to ask a question because he did have the test before. (3) The client is not placed in a scanning machine for the test; therefore, being claustrophobic is not relevant. (4) There are no complications from the test; therefore the client will not need assistance in getting home.
7. (2) There is no need to fast or be NPO for the mammogram (1). (3) Jewelry needs to be removed from around the neck only. (4) Only the upper clothing, including the bra, needs to be removed.
8. (1) It is imperative to stop the bleeding with a pressure dressing. Then (3) elevate the extremity. (2) It is not a priority to call the lab at this time. Monitoring peripheral pulses is included in postprocedure care.
9. (2) PET scans are very useful to study seizure activity and determine spread of cancer cells because metabolic changes occur before structural changes. 60% of invasive tests or surgeries can be eliminated using the PET scan. Radioactive chemicals are administered to clients (1). PET scans can take up to 75 minutes (3). Foods and fluids are restricted for 4–6 hours (4).
10. (4) Most clients require only a local anesthetic for the procedure (1). (2) The procedure takes less than 2 hours to complete. (3) Only small incisions, large enough to accommodate the scope, are made around the knee.

Chapter 22—Urinary Elimination

1. (1) Urine production is directly related to the amount of blood pumped by the heart (cardiac output). A decreased cardiac output decreases renal perfusion and urine production and causes fluid retention and weight gain.
2. (2 4) Pregnancy and the presence of a catheter deflect ultrasound signals, thus interfering with urine volume determination by scanner.

3. **(4)** The male urethra is long. As the catheter is inserted, some nurses can feel a change as it passes through the prostatic urethra and enters the bladder.
4. **(2)** The female urethra is quite short. This renders females more susceptible to urinary tract infection.
5. **(3)** Bladder spasm and UTI may cause leakage around the retention catheter. Use of a larger catheter only increases bladder spasms and discomfort.
6. **(1 3 5)** Physicians may need to be reminded that the client has a retention catheter and long-term use is associated with increased risk for UTI. Stagnant urine in dependent draining tubing loops promotes bacterial growth and UTI, as does to/fro movement of a catheter that is not properly secured.
7. **(1)** Continuous bladder irrigation dilutes postoperative bleed and thus prevents clots from forming, as they could occlude the catheter drainage system.
8. **(1)** Protective barriers contain alcohol, may interfere with pouch sealing, and must be removed with a solvent that increases risk of skin irritation.
9. **(2)** The term end stage renal disease (ESRD) only indicates that the client is receiving renal replacement therapy (dialysis or transplant).
10. **(1)** Continuous vascular access is critical for the hemodialysis client. Clotting is the biggest cause of access failure. Stasis of blood flow due to vascular occlusion or constriction in any manner must be avoided.

Chapter 23—Bowel Elimination

1. **(1 2 4)** The MRI is usually not ordered to rule out issues with fecal incontinence (3).
2. **(2)** If you were present when the physician discussed the procedure with the client, you can reiterate the information (1). Giving this answer can upset the client as they think something is wrong, (3) and (4) are incorrect information.
3. **(1)** There is greater fluid loss with an ileostomy as a result of a more liquid stool. The fluid is not reabsorbed into the body as the ileum is resected. Clients with an ileostomy will also need to wear an appliance (2). Many clients with a colostomy do not need an appliance. (3) An ileostomy is usually performed as a result of Crohn's disease or ulcerative colitis, and the ileostomy for these conditions is not reversed. (4) There are fluid and food restrictions.
4. **(3)** Vagal stimulation as a result of fecal removal can lead to decreased pulse rate resulting from decreasing conductivity at the sino atrial node. (1), (2), and (4) are not completed before the removal occurs. Laxatives can be ordered after the removal to prevent another impaction. Fluids are infused into the lower colon prior to removal. An enema usually precedes the fecal removal, but it is not done just prior to the removal.
5. **(4)** is correct. Placing the pointed end of the suppository 3–4 inches beyond the internal sphincter will prevent expulsion of the suppository. The client is placed in a Sims position and the suppository is inserted beyond the internal sphincter (1). The client is not asked to bear down when inserting the suppository. (2) The pointed end of the suppository is generously lubricated and then the pointed side is inserted first for ease in passage through the external and internal sphincters. (3) If the suppository is inserted into fecal material, it will not dissolve.
6. **(1 2 3)** All are contraindications for the use of the BMS system. (4) A history of severe diarrhea is the condition for which the system is utilized.
7. **(2 3 1 4)** The correct sequence for inserting a BMS system.
8. **(2)** The client is placed on the left side in a Sims position (1). (3) The height is 18 inches above the rectal area. (4) Solution is instilled slowly to prevent cramps.
9. **(2)** is correct. The skin and stoma are cleansed with water. Oily substances and soap can prevent good adhesion of the pouch to the skin. The other three distractors are correct steps in applying a fecal ostomy pouch.
10. **(3)** is correct. Only an RN or an LVN/LPN can administer an enema with medications. Nursing assistants cannot perform a fecal impaction removal (1). The client can have cardiac complications that need to be assessed by an RN or LVN/LPN. (2) Many health care facilities allow UAPs to perform enema administration. (4) An LVN/LPN cannot develop a teaching plan, but he/she can implement a plan.

Chapter 24—Heat and Cold Therapies

1. **(1)** Internal stimuli (pyrogens, cytokines) cause the hypothalamus to alter the body temperature set point; therefore, a *regulated* rise in temperature occurs.
2. **(3)** Fever is caused by pyrogens.
3. **(3)** Shivering muscle activity increases heat production, thereby counteracting the goal of treatment to reduce body temperature.
4. **(3)** This water temperature is regulated as a safety measure.
5. **(1)** The surgical client would lose body heat to the environment by radiation because the surgical suite environment is cooler.
6. **(1)** Sugar-free and caffeine-free beverages are most appropriate for rehydration due to heat-induced dehydration.
7. **(2 4 6 7)** Flushing, anesthesia, burning, and numbness are expected effects of cryotherapy applications. Therapy should be discontinued on numbness. Pallor and blister formation are adverse effects.
8. **(1)** The sitz bath causes pelvic vasodilation with diversion of blood flow that could potentially result in orthostatic hypotension on standing.
9. **(4)** Nerves are sensitive to cold application and are most superficial around joints.
10. **(1)** Tissue metabolic demand increases as it is heated. If circulation is compromised, the tissue's need for oxygen will exceed what the circulation can provide.

Chapter 25—Wound Care and Dressings

1. **(3)** During the regeneration phase of wound healing, there is rapid growth of epithelial cells to produce a protective covering for a wound. The third phase, maturation (1), is the period when wound contraction takes place. The first phase, inflammatory (2), occurs immediately after an injury. Wound remodeling (4) is another term for maturation.
2. **(4)** Wounds heal by being left open, such as an infected wound or one that has dehisced. (1) refers to secondary intention. (2) is primary healing. (3) refers to a primary incision.
3. **(2)** 30–35 Cal/kg/day is required for adequate wound healing.
4. **(1)** This method is used to decontaminate hands using an alcohol rub. (2) The rub is completed until the alcohol dries, usually 15–25 seconds (2). (3) Longer times for hand scrubs are associated with the first OR scrub of the day. (4) Alcohol rubs do not require drying hands with a towel.
5. **(3)** The last flap of the wrapper is placed directly in front of the table nearest the nurse to prevent crossing over the sterile field. The first flap of the wrapper is placed away from the sterile field.
6. **(2)** Clean gloves are used (1). It is not necessary to use sterile gloves. (3) Curved tip of scissors are used and the cut is next to the knot. (4) Sutures are removed starting at the top or bottom of the incision.
7. **(1 2 3)** An advantage for the use of hydrogel dressings is (4).
8. **(3)** is correct. Wounds are not cleansed with hydrogen peroxide (1). (2) and (4) are not correct methods for obtaining a wound culture.
9. **(2)** After fluffing dressings, a moist dressing is placed over the wound.
10. **(1 2 3)** These three conditions must be present, as well as sufficient circulation to assist in healing.

Chapter 26—Perioperative Nursing

1. **(3)** A moderate sedation would not be provided in the preoperative stage. This drug is usually administered during the intraoperative stage. The other three distractors are all activities that will be performed during the preoperative stage.
2. **(4)** The physician and the entire operative team identify the correct side and site. The anesthesiologist inserts the IV if it is not already in place (2). The scrub nurse assists the physician throughout the surgical procedure (3).

3. **(1)** Nurses, both scrub and circulating, monitor sponge and instrument counts before, during and after the procedure. The entire OR staff participate in checking the side and site of the procedure, not just the nurses (2). (3) and (4) are not common malpractice actions taken against nurses.
4. **(1 2 3 4)** All distractors are correct. All of these interventions can and should be used to reduce anxiety in a preoperative client.
5. **(1)** Sharp pain under the scapula post-operatively is indicative of carbon dioxide irritation of the phrenic nerve in the diaphragm, causing the referred pain. Very infrequently is a client with a laparoscopy hospitalized to monitor pain, unless there is some extenuating circumstance (2). (3) Usually a stronger acting pain medication is administered for pain following any surgical procedure. (4) Most clients do not return to work the next day; the recovery time for anesthesia is longer than 24 hours.
6. **(4)** Check for allergies to latex, food, and medications. All latex articles must be removed from the OR, and this client should be scheduled as the first OR case for the day. (2) and (3): The surgical consent form must be signed before the preoperative medication is given. The medication is usually given at least 45 minutes before the OR transporter arrives to take the client to the OR.
7. **(3 4)** The surgical site is marked by the person performing the procedure (1). All members of the surgical team verify the site (2).
8. **(3)** A score of ≤ 9 or ± 1 point of the pre-procedural score on the Aldrete Scale must be obtained before the discharge is completed. (1) and (2) are scales used for sedation assessment parameters during the use of moderate sedation. (4) is used for assessing clients who have head injuries or who are not alert.
9. **(4)** The initial assessment/intervention is to assess for patent airway. If the client is experiencing difficulty breathing, color is pale, skin is cool, oxygen must be administered and the head of the bed slightly elevated. The other interventions should immediately follow this initial assessment and intervention.
10. **(2)** is correct. Pulmonary complications are usually evident 24–36 hours after surgery. Signs and symptoms of an ileus occur between 24–36 hours postoperatively. Urinary tract infections occur from the third to the fifth post-operative day. Wound infections can occur from 24 hours to 5 days post operatively.

Chapter 27—Orthopedic Interventions

1. **(1)** Positioning the hand higher than the elbow prevents dependent edema in the hand.
2. **(4)** Natural evaporation allows the cast to dry from inside out. External heat application may cause the cast to dry on the outside but not the inside, causing the cast to weaken.
3. **(1 2 6)** The selected items are features of synthetic casts. Additionally, they are lighter in weight, but provide less stability and can cause skin burns when drying is activated.
4. **(2 4 6)** These are early indicators of ischemia. Elevating the extremity worsens ischemia and pain. Pain is out of proportion to the injury and unrelieved by pain medication.
5. **(3)** Peroneal nerve motor function provides dorsiflexion of the foot. Peroneal nerve injury can result in permanent foot drop.
6. **(2)** Adduction or leg crossing may cause implant dislocation.
7. **(1)** Adaptive aids help prevent extremes of flexion that could result in implant dislocation.
8. **(5)** Studies show that all of the above are increased with CPM.
9. **(4)** Phantom pain is thought to be a central nervous system response to stored pain sensations from the previously intact limb.
10. **(3)** Clients have the tendency to abduct and flex the stump postoperatively. Adduction and hip extension exercises help prevent flexion contracture of the stump and help prepare the stump for walking with a prosthesis.

Chapter 28—Intravenous Therapy

1. **(1)** Ringer's lactate solution does not require an in-line filter. The other three distractors require the filters in order to filter out microorganisms and guard against inadvertent infusions of particulate matter, and endotoxins.
2. **(4)** Using the distal end of the vein reserves the more proximal areas for future IV sites. Superficial veins are palpated and used for peripheral IVs (1). The antecubital vein is not a primary site for IV placement (2). It is used as a last resort. The catheter can become kinked when placed in this area. (3) IV fluid flow will be affected if the IV is inserted in a site below the same vein that is infiltrated or where phlebitis is present.
3. **(1 2)** A warm cloth is applied to produce vasodilation that assists with insertion of the IV catheter or needle (3). The arm is placed in a dependent position to prevent venous dilation (4).
4. **(4)** Chlorhexidine swabs are recommended by the Intravenous Nurses Society to prepare the IV insertion site. The other three products have been used in the past; however, evidence-based nursing practice has identified they are not as effective as chlorhexidine.
5. **(4)** Primary and secondary tubing is changed every 72 hours (1). Primary intermittent tubing is changed every 24 hours (2). TPN and lipids are changed every 24 hours (3).
6. **(2)** The bevel of the needle is in the up position in order to check the integrity of the end of the catheter (1). (3) The needle is inserted along the side of the needle or about 1/2 inch distal to selected puncture site. (4) After hearing the "pop" sound, check for backflow of blood in the plastic hub.
7. **(2)** The answer is 15 mL. To review regulating flow rate and determine the IV drops/min. See p. 1090.
8. **(3)** The pump needs to be reprogrammed with the scanning device. The medication, client's ID, and nurse's ID badge are all rechecked. The pump cannot just be restarted when a "hard" alarm sounds, as this indicates that an error in the drug, dose, or equipment has occurred.
9. **(4)** Hypotonic solutions are (1) and (2). They hydrate cells and are used to correct dehydration. Hypertonic solutions such as dextrose 10% can be used as a nutrient source (3).
10. **(3)** One fourth of the medication is injected over a 20-second time period; therefore it takes a minimum of 80 seconds to administer the drug (1). Always check the package insert for the time frame. (2) Flushing of the IV tubing is done when an incompatible drug is being administered. (4) Check the drug compatibility chart to determine the appropriate IV solution that is acceptable for infusing the drug.

Chapter 29—Central Vascular Access

1. **(1)** PICC lines and subcutaneous ports and central catheters are termed central vascular access devices. They can be left in place for longer periods of time and with fewer complications.
2. **(1 4)** Both are correct statements related to preventing catheter-related bloodstream infections. (2) is incorrect. (3) is incorrect, 2% chlorhexidine with 70% alcohol solution is used as the antibacterial scrub.
3. **(1)** is the time used when the swab contains chlorhexidine and alcohol. (3) is the time necessary for drying povidone-iodine, and chlorhexidine alone. (4) is the time a 70% isopropyl alcohol solution is used.
4. **(3)** This is the change time for IVs for infusing parenteral nutrition and for primary and secondary IV tubing changes. The time for changing tubing when lipids are infusing is (1).
5. **(4)** A plugged filter is the most common problem that occurs when the solution is not infusing at the prescribed rate. If the hyperalimentation flow rate is not infusing at the prescribed time, you do not "catch up" by increasing the flow rate (1). This can lead to hyerglycemia as a result of increasing the amount of glucose from the IV solution. (2) Before notifying the physician, a complete assessment of the situation must occur in order to make an informed decision. (3) It is rare that the dressing is too tight to cause an occlusion of the IV flow.
6. **(1 3 2 4)** These are the steps in obtaining a central venous pressure reading. Refer to the skill if you missed this question (p. 1144).
7. **(3)** The port is inserted for long-term care, usually for clients receiving chemotherapy intermittently. The port is irrigated monthly and after each use. Normal saline is used in flushing and followed by heparin infusion.

8. (2) After stopping the IV infusion, the next step is swabbing the hub and cap with an antimicrobial swab. Then the cap is removed (3) and the syringe is flushed with normal saline (4).
9. (3) The port is swabbed with chlorhexidine. After anchoring the port site, the Huber needle is inserted at a 90-degree angle. Check for blood return, and if it is present, the drug can be infused, followed by first infusing normal saline followed by a heparin solution.
10. (4) This creates a positive pressure within the central venous access device, preventing blood from being drawn back into the catheter when the syringe is removed.

CHAPTER 30—RESPIRATORY CARE

1. (4) Slow inhalation maximizes volume; holding allows alveoli to open; and exhalation through pursed lips prevents early airway closure.
2. (2) Only those with serious retention of secretions have been found to benefit from CPT.
3. (2) The sedated client may not be able to remove the mask in the event of nausea and vomiting; there is dangerous risk of aspiration of emesis.
4. (4) The nonrebreathing mask with reservoir bag provides the greatest FiO_2 because the client inhales enriched air from the mask as well as the bag and does not rebreathe exhaled air.
5. (1 3 5) Pulse oximetry measures are not reliable in anemic clients because the decreased number of RBCs may be fully oxygenated; hypovolemic clients may be vasoconstricted; and circulating contrast can also confuse readings.
6. (2) Intubation provides a patent airway whether or not mechanical ventilation is necessary. It does not prevent aspiration and is not essential for providing oxygenation unless mechanical ventilation is used.
7. (4) A tube cuff does not prevent aspiration of secretions or food, but its inflation is necessary for ventilated air to enter the lower airways and lungs.
8. (3) This tracheostomy tube inflates passively (automatically) but must be deflated actively using a special syringe with stopcock to extract air from the cuff.
9. (2) If the tube cuff remains inflated and the tube is capped with a speaking valve, the client is unable to inhale air because both the artificial airway and the trachea are occluded.
10. (5 3 1 6 4 8 7 2) This sequence reflects necessary preparation before sterile steps are taken. Hyperoxygenation is performed before sterile equipment is handled; the catheter is advanced before suction is applied. Finally, the oropharynx is suctioned using the same catheter.

CHAPTER 31—CIRCULATORY MAINTENANCE

1. (3) The QRS complex represents the depolarization of the ventricles. Atrial depolarization is represented by the P wave. The PR interval represents the conduction time in the atria. The T wave represents ventricular repolarization.
2. (1) The SA node sends an abnormal rate of impulse generation. A normal cardiac impulse begins in the sinoatrial node. It is transmitted over myocardium; Bachman's bundle, and internodal pathways to the AV node. If there is a disturbance in this transmission, it results in an atrial dysrhythmia.
3. (3) Demand pacemakers are the most frequently used pacemakers. The electrode is triggered to stimulate the heart only when the heart's intrinsic or natural atrial or ventricular pacemaker stimulation fails.
4. (1) The urine output of 30–40 mL/hour is a normal value. When hemorrhaging occurs, the urine output will decrease because of decreased cardiac output as a result of the hemorrhage. The other distractors would be observed when hemorrhage occurs.
5. (1) After moving the client to a flat, firm surface, the next step is to begin compressions at 100/minute. The AED is used only if the client does not have a pulse.
6. (3) The appropriate thigh-hi measurement is from the bottom of the heel to the fold of the buttocks. The circumference is measured at the mid-thigh area, not the largest area of the calf (1).
7. (2 4) The use of compression devices would be contraindicated in diabetic neuropathy ulcers and arterial ischemia ulcers as well as dermatitis, gangrene, and preexisting pulmonary embolism.
8. (3) If the client can speak, you continue to allow them to cough as they should be able to expel the foreign body. The abdominal thrust is completed if the client cannot talk or coughing becomes ineffective (1).
9. (2) Frequency of the contractions are every 40–90 seconds. The contractions are mild in intensity and last 30–50 seconds. (4) is indicative of variable decelerations, (1) is indicative of early decelerations.
10. (2) The Rapid Response Team is utilized when a client is in danger and an avoidable death can be prevented by appropriate interventions. The client may be transferred to the ICU, but this is not the primary purpose of the team (4). CPR is performed by the team, but again, this is not the purpose of the team, as the nursing staff can initiate CPR as well (1).

CHAPTER 32—NEUROLOGICAL MANAGEMENT

1. (C) To determine the cerebral perfusion pressure, the ICP is subtracted from the MAP. The MAP is calculated by adding the SBP plus 2 times the DBP, divided by 3 (130 + 160 = 290, divided by 3 = 97). The ICP is 12, so 97 minus 12 = 85. This is an adequate cerebral perfusion pressure.
2. (3) An intracranial pressure of 12 is normal. Therefore, there is no increase in any one of the three intracranial components, or normal pressure has been activated by manipulation of one of the components to compensate for an increase in one of the other components.
3. (1) Frontal lobe dysfunction affects contralateral voluntary motion, and causes changes in personality and behavior.
4. (4) Signs of metabolic coma are usually diffuse, rather than unilateral, with coma preceding motor deficits and without orderly rostrocaudal deterioration, as seen with structural causes. Pupil reflexes are preserved bilaterally, while structural causes of coma are usually associated with a unilateral nonreactive pupil.
5. (3) Of the listed options, only hypoxemia (low blood O2) causes cerebral vessels to dilate and increase intracranial pressure, making ventilation a priority. Hypocapnea (hyperventilation) constricts cerebral vessels, and may be used briefly to reduce intracranial pressure. Acidemia (rather than alkalemia) causes cerebral vessels to constrict. Hypothermia does not affect cerebral vessels, but is used therapeutically to reduce cerebral metabolic demand.
6. (2) Pupil response (constriction to light) is controlled by CN III (oculomotor nerve) whose nuclei are attached to the midbrain. The nerve's location at the top of the brainstem is the first to be compressed, as intracranial pressure increases, resulting in sluggish or absent pupil response to light.
7. (1) While changes in respiratory pattern accompany neurologic deterioration, they are not specific to neurologic dysfunction. For instance, Cheyne-Stokes respirations occur in clients with heart failure and other systemic disorders. As ICP increases, neurologic deterioration progresses rostrocaudally, the diencephalon (above the brainstem) is compressed, causing impaired consciousness. This occurs before changes due to compression on the midbrain (pupil response) or alterations of blood pressure and heart rate occur. Additionally, changes in vital signs accompany many pathologic conditions.
8. (2) The ventriclostomy is the most cost-effective, accurate and reliable method of monitoring ICP. It is the only method that includes an external drainage system and transducer calibrated or zeroed against a known pressure to ensure consistent and accurate pressure measurements. The indwelling ventricular catheter allows CSF drainage to decrease ICP, is used for medication instillation, and provides access to CSF for laboratory testing.
9. (4) The P-1 waveform reflects systolic BP pulsations transmitted through the choroid plexus and is normally the highest of the 3 waveform components, while the P-3 is the lowest. The P-2 waveform reflects relative brain volume, and is often elevated in response to compromised intracranial compliance.
10. (2) The electroencephalogram is the most commonly used confirmatory test, assessing only cerebral, not brain stem function. The client must have at least 30 minutes without brainstem electrical activity. With brain death, there is absence of intracerebral blood flow from the carotid arteries and circle of Willis.

Chapter 33—Advanced Nursing Skills

1. **(2)** The distal lumen (placed in the pulmonary artery) measures pulmonary artery systolic and diastolic pressures and, when "wedged," indirectly measures the left ventricular end diastolic pressure.
2. **(6 7)** Because not all chests are equal, this is the most accurate way to determine the level of the right atrium in the supine position.
3. **(3)** Cannulation of the radial artery can result in inadequate blood flow distally. The Allen test is used to assess adequacy of distal perfusion through the ulnar artery before radial artery cannulation.
4. **(1)** Obtaining arterial blood samples using the conservatory system eliminates the need to waste blood that contains the continuous flush solution, therefore helping to prevent nosocomial anemia.
5. **(2)** Because atrial fibrillation is frequently recurrent (chronic), the client continues anticoagulation therapy (Coumadin) to prevent cardioembolic stroke.
6. **(1 3)** These lethal rhythms require immediate defibrillation to convert to sinus rhythm. The others require cardioversion or administration of fluids/medications.
7. **(3)** A functioning electrical system and a responsive pump in the presence of hypovolemia will produce an ECG without peripheral perfusion (pulseless electrical activity).
8. **(4)** This mode provides total support. It is used for the client who cannot initiate or who for a clinical situation should not initiate breathing.
9. **(3)** Asynchrony leads to wasted energy; this is especially important in infants.
10. **(1)** Accumulation of oropharyngeal secretions above the tube cuff is associated with aspiration of secretions that leads to ventilator-associated pneumonia.

Chapter 34—End-of-Life Care

1. **(4 1 5 2 3)** This is the sequencing for the stages of dying. Refer to the "Stages of Grief" in the chapter if you did not get this answer correct.
2. **(2)** The third stage of grief is the beginning of the onset of cultural and religious rituals that assist the mourner to face the loss. The stage of idealization is (1). (3) is the first stage of shock and disbelief. (4) is the stage of resolution.
3. **(3)** We continue to provide alternative and nontraditional care to improve the client's qualify of life (1). (4) Nurses should be sensitive to the need of family members and should encourage visitation as they desire.
4. **(2)** Clients requiring rehabilitative services are placed in a rehabilitation unit/facility or long-term care facility (1). (3) Unless the client is terminally ill, he/she would be cared for in a long-term care facility or at home. (4) Treatments can be provided with hospice care.
5. **(3)** Acting out and verbalizing anger is expected to occur during the anger stage of the process (2). (4) The client should be encouraged to take as much control as possible over his/her care and environment during this phase.
6. **(2)** This provides a connection with family members or memories of happy times. Clients should be placed in a calm environment, not near the busy nursing station and all the noises (1). (3) It is best to allow clients to look out windows and see activity around them, unless the client requests that curtains be drawn. (4) Lighting in the room should be muted and soft without overhead lighting being turned on.
7. **(1)** About 40% of Caucasians are more likely to have written advance directives. Other cultures have a distrust of the United States health care system and will not write advance directives.
8. **(1)** The drugs in (2) are used in Step 1 for pain control that is used for mild to moderate pain. (3) Step 3 utilizes opioid drugs at higher doses for moderate to severe pain. (4) Methadone is used in step 3 for moderate to severe pain.
9. **(1 2 4)** Nurses need to allot adequate time not only for physical care but time for just talking to the client (3).
10. **(1)** Some cultures keep adverse diagnoses regarding end-of-life care from the client. Family members discuss the treatment plan with physicians, without input from the client.

Bibliography

A.S.P.E.N. (2009). Clinical Guidelines: Clinical guidelines for the use of parenteral and enteral nutrition in adult and pediatric patients, 2009. *33*(3), 255–316.

A.S.P.E.N. (2009). Special Report: Enteral nutrition practice recommendations. *Journal of Parenteral and Enteral Nutrition*, 122–125.

AARP Bulletin (2009, March). Retrieved from www.aarpforemost.com.

Abrams, A. C. (2006). *Clinical drug therapy: Rationales for nursing practice* (7th ed.). Philadelphia: Lippincott.

Ackley, B. J., & Ladwig, G. B. (2010). *Nursing diagnosis handbook: An evidence-based guide to planning care* (8th ed.). St. Louis: Mosby.

Adams, A., & Koch, R. (2010). *Pharmacology: Connections to nursing practice*. Upper Saddle River, NJ: Pearson.

Advice PRN. (2005). Fentanyl patches. *Nursing, 35*(12), 12.

Ahmed, D. (2000). It's not my job. *American Journal of Nursing, 700*(6), 25.

Ahrens, T., et al. (2004). Effect of kinetic therapy on pulmonary complications. *American Journal of Critical Care, 13*(5), 376.

Alfaro-LeFevre, R. (2008). *Critical thinking and clinical judgment: A practical approach* (4th ed.). Philadelphia: Elsevier Health Sciences.

Alfaro-LeFevre, R. (2009). *Applying nursing process: A tool for critical thinking* (7th ed). Philadelphia: Lippincott Williams and Wilkins.

Altizer, L. (2004) Compartment syndrome. *Orthopaedic Nursing, 23*(6), 391–396.

Altizer, L. (2004). Compartment syndrome. *Orthopaedic Nursing, 23*(6), 391.

Amato-Vealey, E., & Barba, M. (2008, November). Hand-off communication: A requisite for perioperative patient safety. *AAORN Journal*, 88(5), 763–769.

Amato-Vealey, E., Barba, M., & Vealey, R. (2008). Hand-off communication: A requisite for perioperative patient safety. *AORN Journal*, 88(5)763–772.

American Diabetes Association. (2002). Clinical Practice Recommendations. *Journal of Clinical and Applied Research and Education, 25*(Suppl. 1).

American Diabetes Association. (2009). Diabetes experts issue new recommendations for inpatient glycemic control – call for systemic changes in hospitals nationwide.

American Heart Association. (2005). AHA guidelines for cardiopulmonary resuscitation and emergency cardiovascular care. *Circulation, 112* (Suppl. IV), IV1–IV203.

American Heart Association. (2005–2009). *ACLS for healthcare providers*. Chicago: AHA.

American Hospital Association. (2006–2009). *Understanding expectations: The patient care partnership*. Chicago: AHA Press.

American Hospital Association. (2009). *Patient bill of rights*. Chicago: AHA.

American Nurses' Association. (2001). *Code of ethics for nurses with interpretive statements*. Washington, DC: ANA.

American Nurses' Association. (2010). *Nursing's social policy statement: The essence of the profession*. Washington, DC: ANA.

Anderson, F., & Maloney, J. (1994, November). Taking blood pressure correctly: It's no off-the-cuff matter. *Nursing, 24*(11), 34–38.

Anderson, R. (2005, April). When to use a midline catheter. *Nursing, 35*(4), 28–30.

Andrews, M., & Boyle, S. (2008). *Transcultural concepts in nursing care* (5th ed.). Philadelphia: Lippincott.

Arbour, R. (2004). Intracranial hypertension: Monitoring and nursing assessment. *Critical Care Nurse, 24*(5), 19–32.

Armstrong, J. (2002, April). Chemical warfare. *RN Magazine*, 65(4), 32–39.

Aronoff, D., & Neilson, E. (2001). Antipyretics: Mechanisms of action and clinical use in fever suppression. *American Journal of Medicine, 111*, 304–315.

Arrich, J., (2007). Clinical application of mild therapeutic hypothermia after cardiac arrest. *Critical Care Medicine, 35*(4), 1–7.

Artz, M., Conant, R., & Lennox, C. (2006, January). The politics of caring: The Patient Safety Act of 2005 is reintroduced. *American Journal of Nursing, 106*(1), 36.

Aschenbrenner, D. (2009). Unsafe injection practices put patients at risk. *American Journal of Nursing, 109*(7), 45–47.

Aschenbrenner, D., & Venable, S. (2009). *Drug therapy in nursing* (3rd ed). Philadelphia: Wolters Kluwer/Lippincott Williams & Wilkins.

Association of Operating Room Nurses (AORN). (2008). *Perioperative standards, recommended practices, and guideline 2008*. AORN, Inc.

Astle, S., & Caulfield, E. (2003). Bedside tracheostomy: A step by step guide. *RN*, 66(10), 41.

Austin, S. (2006). Walk a fine line if your patient wants to leave AMA. *Nursing, 36*(12), 48–49.

Ayello, E., & Braden, B. (2001, November). Why is pressure ulcer risk assessment so important? *Nursing, 31*(11), 74–79.

Ayers, U. (2004). Older people and hypothermia: The role of the anaesthetic nurse. *British Journal of Nursing, 13*(7), 396.

Back, J. (1999, January). Clinical practice guidelines for chronic nonmalignant pain syndrome. *Musculoskeletal Rehabilitation, 13*, 47–58.

Baker, H. (2007). Nutrition in the elderly: An overview. *Geriatrics, 62*(7), 28–31.

Ball, J., & Bindler, R. (2006). *Child health nursing*. Upper Saddle River, NJ: Prentice Hall.

Ball, S. (2005, August). POCT (Point of care testing). *Advance for Nurses*, CA, 25–26.

Bancroft, I. (2005). Teaming up for wound care. *Nursing 2005*, 32hn1–32hn3.

Barbay, K. (2009). Research evidence for the use of preoperative exercise in patients preparing for total hip or total knee arthroplasty. *Orthopaedic Nursing, 28*(3), 127–132.

Barclay, L. (2009, January). Surgical checklist may improve outcomes for non cardiac surgery. *New England Journal of Medicine, 360*, 491–499.

Barkauskas, V. H., Baumann, L., & Darling-Fisher, C. (2002). *Health and physical assessment* (3rd ed.). St. Louis: Mosby.

Barker, E. (2008). *Neuroscience nursing: A spectrum of care* (3rd ed.). St. Louis: Mosby, Elsevier.

Barnes, P. M., et al. (2004, May). Complementary and alternative use among adults: United States, 2002. *CDC Advance Data Report*, No. 343.

Basmajian, J. V. (Ed.). (1989). *Biofeedback: Principles and practice for clinicians* (3rd ed.). Baltimore: Williams & Wilkins.

Bates, B. (2002). *Guide to physical examination and history taking* (8th ed.). Philadelphia: Lippincott Williams & Wilkins.

Beard, R., & Day, M. (2008). Fever and hyperthermia. *Nursing, 38*(6), 28–31.

Beattie, S. (2006). In from the cold. *RN*, 69(11), 22–27.

Beers, M., & Berkow, R. (2006). *The Merck manual of diagnosis and therapy* (18th ed.). Whitehouse Station, NJ: Merck Research Laboratories.

Beezhold, L., Sussman, G. L., Liss, G. M., & Chang, N. S. (1996). Latex allergy can induce clinical reaction to specific foods.*Clinical and Experimental Allergy, 26*, 416–422.

Behuniak, S. (2009, February). Semiprivate. *American Journal of Nursing, 109*(2), 11.

Berman, A., Synder, S., & Jackson, C. (2009). *Skills in Clinical Nursing* (6th ed.). Upper Saddle River, NJ: Prentice Hall.

Best Practice. (2001, February). Graduated compression stockings for the prevention of post-operative venous thromboembolism.*Evidence Based Practice Information Sheets for Health Professionals*, 5(2), 1–6.

Best Practice. (2007, April). Pre-operative hair removal to reduce surgical site infection. *Evidence Based Practice Information Sheets for Health Professionals, 11*(4), 1–4.

Best Practice. (2008, February). Pressure ulcers: prevention of pressure related damage. *Evidence Based Information Sheets for Health Professionals, 12*(2), 1–4.

Best Practice. (2008, March). Pressure ulcers: management of pressure related tissue damage. *Evidence Based Information Sheets for Health Professionals, 12*(3), 1–4.

Best practice. (2008, April). Graduated compression stockings for the prevention of post-operative venous thromboembolism. *Evidence Based Information Sheets for Health Professionals, 12*(4), 1–4.

Best, J. (2005). Revision total hip and total knee arthroplasty. *Orthopaedic Nursing, 24*(3), 174.

Billingsley. S. (2008, February). Lumbar puncture. *Advance for Nurse Practitioners, 16*(2), 36–38.

Bishop, L, Dougherty, L., Bodenham, A., Mansi, J., Crowe, P., Kibbler, C., et al. (2007, February). Guidelines on insertion and management of central venous access devices in adults. *International Journal of Laboratory Hematology, (29)*, 261–278.

Black, J., Hawkes, J., & Keene, A. (2005). *Medical–surgical nursing: Clinical management of positive outcomes* (7th ed.). Philadelphia: Saunders.

Black, L. , Persons, R., & Jamieson, B. (2009). What is the best way to manage phantom limb pain? *Journal of Family Practice*, 58(3), 155–158.

Blackwood, H. (2004, May). Obesity, a rapidly expanding challenge. *Nursing Management, 35*, 27–35.

Blaney, W. (2010, March). Taking steps to prevent pressure ulcers. *Nursing*, 40(3), 44–47.

Block, S. (2005). Otitis externa. *Journal of Family Practice, 54*(8), 669.

Blocks, M. (2005, October). *Practical solutions for safe patient handling. Nursing 2005, 35*(10), 44–45.

Board of Registered Nursing, State of California. (2003). Pain assessment: The fifth vital sign.

Boehringer, S. (2003, April). Herbal medicines. *Nurseweek California*, Sunnyvale, CA, 15–16.

Bonham, P. (2003, September). Determining the toe brachial pressure index. *Nursing, 33*(9), 54–55.

Boullata, J. (2009). Drug administration through an enteral feeding tube. *American Journal of Nursing, 109*(10), 34–41.

Bowers, S. (2000, December). All about tubes. *Nursing, 30*(12), 41–47.

Boyd, A., Benjamin, H.L., & Asplund, C. (2009). Splints and casts: Indications and methods. *American Family Physician, 80*(5), 491–499.

Boyer, M. J. (2005). *Math for nurses: A pocket guide to dosage calculations and drug preparations* (6th ed.). Philadelphia: Lippincott Williams & Wilkins.

Braden, B., & Ayello, E. (2002, March). How and why to do pressure ulcer risk assessment. *Advances in Skin and Wound Care: The Journal for Prevention and Healing, 15*(3), 125–131.

Brallier, L., (1982). *Successfully managing stress*. Los Altos, CA: National Nursing Review.

Braunwald, E., et al. (2004). *Harrison's principles of internal medicine* (16th ed.). New York: McGraw-Hill.

Brent, N. (2000). *Nurses and the law: A guide to principles and applications* (2nd ed.). Philadelphia: Saunders.

Brett, A. (2002, June). Therapeutic hypothermia for comatose survivors of cardiac arrest. *Journal Watch, 22*(6), 43.

Brettler, S. (2004). Traumatic brain injury. *RN, 67*(4), 32–37.

Bridges, E. (2001, June). Ask the experts. *Critical Care Nurse, 21*(6), 66–68.

Briggs, J. (2001, January). Graduated compression stockings for the prevention of post-operative venous thromboembolism. *Best Practice, 5*(1), 1–6.

Brooke, U. (1998, May). Legal risks of alternative therapies. *RN, 61*(5), 53–57.

Brown, I. (2002, January). When your patient wants to leave AMA. *RN*, 65(1), 71.

Brown, S. (2000, November). The legal pitfalls of home care. *RN, 63*(11), 75–80.

Bryant, G. (2001, February). Stump care. *American Journal of Nursing, 101*(2), 67–71.

Bryant, R. (2007). *Acute and chronic wounds* (3rd ed.). St. Louis: Elsevier-Mosby.

Bunce, M. (2003, December). Central lines. *RN Magazine*, 66(12), 29–32.

Burns, S. (2005). Mechanical ventilation of patients with acute respiratory distress syndrome and patients requiring weaning: The evidence guiding practice. *Critical Care Nurse, 25*(4), 14.

Bushing, J. (2006, December). Assisting with thoracentesis. *Nursing*, 36(12), 18–19.

Bushing, J. (2007, January). Assisting with lumbar puncture. *Nursing, 37*(1), 23–24.

Carpenito, I. (2009). *Nursing diagnosis: Application to clinical practice* (12th ed). Philadelphia: Lippincott Williams & Wilkins.

Carpenito-Moyet, L. (2009). *Nursing care plans and documentation: Nursing diagnosis and collaborative problems* (5th ed.). Philadelphia: Lippincott Williams & Wilkins.

Carroll, P. (2000, October). Exploring chest drain options. *RN, 63*(10), 50–54.

Carroll, P. (2005). Keeping up with mobile chest drains. *RN 2005*, 68(10).

Carroll, P. (2008, June). The transition to home care. *NurseWeek, West* 5(14), 28–31.

Carter-Templeton, J., & McCoy, T. (2008). Are we on the same page? A comparison of intramuscular injection explanations in nursing fundamental texts. *MEDSURG Nursing, 17*(4), 237–240.

Cescon, D., & Etchells, E. (2008). Barcoded medication administration. *Journal of the Aerican Medical Association, 299*(18), 2200.

Chaboyer, W., James, H., & Kendall, M. (2005). Transitional care after the intensive care unit. *Critical Care Nurse, 25*(3), 16.

Chan, P. (2009, March). Do rapid response teams save lives? *American Journal of Nursing, 109(3)*, 19.

Chan, P. S., Khalid, A., Longmore, L. S., Berg, R. A., Kosiborod, M., Spertus, J. A. (2008, December). Hospital-wide code rates and mortality before and after implementation of a rapid response team. *Journal of the American Medical Association, 300*(21), 2506–2513.

Chapman, L. (2007, May). Discharge planning: a family affair. *Nursing, 37*(5), 56hn12–56hn14.

Charlebois, D., & Wilmoth, D. (2004). Critical care of patients with obesity. *Critical Care Nurse, 24*(4), 19.

Chart Smart: Documenting a blood transfusion. (2005, January). *Nursing, 35*(1), 27.

Chart Smart: documenting peripheral I.V. therapy. (2005, July). *Nursing, 35*(7), 28.

Chenier, G. (2003). Ask the expert. *Nursing, 33*(6), 34.

Chettle, C. (2008, April). Shockingly high rates of surgical site infections remain a constant threat. *NurseWeek, CA, 4*, 24–27.

Chettle, C. (2008, August). Nurses critical as reimbursement dries up for catheter-associated UTI's. *NurseWeek*, CA, 8, 26–27.

Chulay, M. (2005). VAP prevention: The latest guidelines. *RN*, 68(3), 52.

Clemens, L. (2006, Spring). Culturally competent disaster nursing. *Minority Nurse.com, 40*, 41–43.

Clinical Rounds. (2009). Bar codes reduce errors . . . sometimes. *Nursing*, .

Clinical Rounds. (2009). Hidden hazard in transdermal patches. *Nursing*, .

Clinical Update. (2002, April). Hypothermia after brain injury. *Emergency Medicine, 34*(4), 25–27.

Clugston, D. (2007, April). Falls by older adults. *Advance for Nurse Practitioners 2007, 15*(4), 61–64.

Cohen, H., Robinson, E. S., & Mandrack, M. (2003). Getting to the root of medication errors. *Nursing, 33*(9), 36.

Cohen, M. (2001, August). Medication errors. *Nursing, 31*(8), 22.

Cohen, M. (2002, March). Double checking for errors. *Nursing, 32*(3), 18.

Cohen, M. (2004). Medication errors [column]. *Nursing, 34*(1).

Cohen, M. (2005). Medication errors. *Nursing, 35*(7), 14.

Collins, N. (2001, December). What's in that feeding formula anyway? *Nursing, 31*(12), 32hn1–32hn2.

Collins, N., & Navarre, A. (2003). Managing nutrition in an acutely ill patient. *Nursing, 33*(6), 32hn6.

Colonies, P. (2001, December). Implementing an early defibrillation program. *Nursing, 31*(12).

Colwell, J. (2005, January/February). Dealing with ostomies; good care, good devices, good quality of life. *Journal of Supportive Oncology, 3*(1), 72–74.

Complementary and Alternative Medicine. (2005, Winter). *Prayer and Spirituality in health: Ancient practices, modern science*. Washington, DC: NIH.

Consult Stat. (2005). *RN, 68*(9), 60.

Cooper, C. (2000). Reducing the use of physical restraints in nursing homes. *Postgraduate Medicine, 107*(2).

Corbett, J. (2007). *Laboratory tests and diagnostic procedures with nursing diagnoses* (7th. ed). Upper Saddle River, NJ: Pearson Prentice Hall.

Corona, G. (2004, June 21). Biphasic defibrillation. *ADVANCE for Nurses*, 33.

Cosentino, B. (2005, December). Complementary and alternative medicine in the mainstream. *Advance for Nurses*, CA, 120–122.

Craig, K., & Hopkins-Pepe, L. (2006). Understanding the new AHA guidelines, part II. *Nursing, 36*(5), 52.

D'Amico, D., & Barbarito, C. (2007). *Health & Physical Assessment Nursing* (2nd ed.). Upper Saddle River, NJ: Prentice Hall.

D'Arcy, Y. (2005). Managing phantom limb pain. *Nursing, 35*(11), 17.

D'arcy, Y. (2005). What you need to know about fentanyl patches. *Nursing, 35*(8), 73.

David, K. (2007, October). IV fluids: Do you know what's hanging and why? *RN, 70*, 35–40.

Day, M. (2006). Hypothermia: A hazard for all seasons. *Nursing, 36*(12), 45–55.

De Santis, J. (2006, March). HIV/AIDS update. *Advance for Nurses, CA*, 15–19.

DeBoer, S. (2001, April). Ipecac syrup or activated charcoal? *American Journal of Nursing, 101*(4), 75.

Deep-breathing exercises reduce atelectasis and improve pulmonary function after coronary artery bypass surgery. *Chest, 128*(5), 3482–3488.

Delaune, S., & Ladner, P. (2006). *Fundamentals of nursing: Standards and practice* (3rd ed.). Albany, NY: Delmar.

Della Rocca, J. (2007, April). Responding to atrial fibrillation. *Nursing, 37*(4), 37–41.

DelPozo, J., & Patel, R. (2009). Infection associated with prosthetic joints. *New England Journal of Medicine, 361*(8), 787–794.

Denke, M. (2002, January). Dietary retinol: A double-edged sword. *Journal of the American Medical Association, 287*(1), 102–103.

Depree, P. (2004). Six diet myths. *RN, 67*(10), 49.

Dewan, S., & Goodnough, A. (2005, September). Health challenges: Rotting food, dirty water and heat add to problems. *The New York Times*, A16.

Dietz, K, & Gares, J. (2010, February). Wound & skin care: Basic ostomy management, part 1. *Nursing, 40*(2), 61–62; part 2, May 2010, *40*(5), 62–63.

DiMaio, D., & Stevens, P. (2007). Nonvariceal upper gastrointestinal bleeding. *Gastrointestinal Endoscopy Clinics of North America, 17*(2), 253.

DiMaria-Ghalili, R., & Guenter, P. (2008). The mini nutritional assessment. *American Journal of Nursing, 108*(2), 50–59.

Dittrich, K. (2007 December) ACLS update: A new role for medications. *Nursing, 37*(12), 56cc1–56cc3.

Dochterman, J. & Jones, D. (2004, April-June). Unifying nursing languages: The harmonization of NANDA, NIC, and NOC. *International Journal of Nursing Terminologies and Classifications, 15*(2), 34.

Doenges, M., Moorhouse, M., & Geissler-Murr, A. (2006). *Nurse's pocket guide: Diagnosis, interventions, and rationales* (10th ed.). Philadelphia: Davis.

Doenges, M., Moorhouse, M., & Murr, A. (2008). *Nursing diagnosis manual: Planning, individualizing, and documenting client care* (2nd ed.). Philadelphia: Davis.

Doig, G., Simpson, F., Finfer, S., Delaney, A., Davies, A., Mitchell, I., & Dobb, G. (2008). Effect of evidence-based feeding guidelines on mortality of critically ill adults. *Journal of the American Medical Association, 300*(23), 2731–2740.

Dow, N. (2005). Intensive insulin therapy. *RN, 67*(7), 47.

Drug Watch. (2005). Warning on fentanyl patches. *AJN, 105*(11), 87.

Dubay, S. (2009, April). Insights on Infection Control, Hand Hygiene: Guideline for Hand Hygiene in Health Care Settings, CDC. Retrieved from http://community.advanceweb.com.

Duffett, K. (2005, October). Emergency care is a patient's right—insured or not. *Nurseweek California*, Sunnyvale, CA, 19–20.

Duggan, M., & Kavanagh, B. (2005). Pulmonary atelectasis: A pathogenic perioperataive entity. *Anesthesiology, 10*(4), 838–854.

Duhon, J. (2007, February). Taking the pressure out of pressure ulcer therapy. *RN, 70*(2), 25–31.

Dulak, S. (2005, December). Technology today: Smart IV pumps. *RN Magazine, 68*(12), 38–42.

Dulak, S. (2005). In-hospital CPR: Building on success. *RN, 68*(7), 53.

Dulak, S. (2005). Placing an oropharyngeal airway. *RN, 68*(2), 20ac1.

Dulak, S. (2005). Removing chest tubes. *RN, 68*(8) 28ac1.

Dulak, S. B. (2004). Hands-on help: Manual ventilation. *RN, 67*(12), 24ac1.

Dumville, K., Worthy, G., & Bland, J. (2009, June). Taking a bite out of necrotic wounds. *Nursing 2009, 39 (6), 21*.

Dunleavy, K. (2008, January). Putting a dent in pressure ulcer rates. *Nursing, 38*(1), 20–21.

Dunn, N. (2001, February). Keeping COPD patients out of the ED. *RN, 64*(2), 33–37.

Durotoye, R. (2004). How do patients determine that their metered dose inhaler is empty? *Chest, 126*, 1134–1137.

Eagan, K., & Arnold, R. (2003, September) Grief and bereavement care. *American Journal of Nursing, 103*(9), 42–52.

Eaton-Bancroft, I. (2005, April). Teaming up for wound care. *Nursing, 35*(4), 32hn1–32cc2.

Ebersole, P., Hess, P., & Luggen, A. S. (2004). *Toward healthy aging: Human needs and nursing responses* (6th ed.). St. Louis: Mosby.

Edwards, S., & Metheny N. (2000). Measurement of gastric residual volume: State of the science. *MEDSURG Nursing, 9*(3), 125.

Eliopoulos, C. (2009). *Gerontological nursing* (7th ed.). Philadelphia: Lippincott Williams & Wilkins.

Elpern, E., Borkgren Okonek, M., Bacon, M., Gerstung, C., & Skrzynski, M. (2000). Effect of the Passy-Muir tracheostomy speaking valve on pulmonary aspiration in adults. *Heart and Lung, 29*(4), 287–293.

Emanuel, L., et al. (2010, February). The last hours of living: Practical advice for clinicians. *Medscape Nurses*. Retrieved February 11, 2010, from www.mescape.com.

Engelhart, S., Glasmacher, A., Exner, M., & Kramer, M. H. (2002, May). Surveillance for nosocomial infections and fever of unknown origin among adult hematology–oncology patients.*Infection Control and Hospital Epidemiology, 23*(5), 244–248.

Environments and Health (2009). Best practices for environmental health. *American Journal of Nursing, 109*(6), 74–76.

Environments and Health. (2009). Reducing health care's ecological footprint. *American Journal of Nursing, 109*(2), 56–58.

Ericksen, A. (2010). Safety first: The Joint Commission shines the spotlight on patient safety protocols. *Healthcare Traveler*, 30–35.

Erickson, A. (2009, July). Informatics: The Future of Nursing. *RN Magazine, 7*, 34–36.

Ervin, N. (2005, November/December). Clinical coaching: A strategy for enhancing evidence-based nursing practice. *Clinical Nurse Specialist: The Journal of Advanced Nursing Practice, 19*(6), 296–301.

Evans, T., & Carroll, P. (2001, May). Rapid sequence intubation. *American Journal of Nursing, 101*(Suppl.), 16–20.

Fagan, K. (2005, September). Anticipating the big one. *San Francisco Chronicle*, Al, A15–A16.

Fain, J. (2003). Insulin pumps. *Nursing 2003, 33*(6), 51.

Fallis, W. (2005). Indwelling Foley catheters: Is the current design a source of erroneous measurement of urine output? *Critical Care Nurse, 25*(2), 44–46.

Federwisch, A. (2005, Fall). Back to basics. *Future Nurse*, 86–88.

Federwisch, A. (2005, Fall). Learning from smart pumps. *Future Nurse*, 40–41.

Feider, L., Mitchell, P., & Bridges, E. (2010). Oral care practices for orally intubated critically ill adults. *American Journal of Critical Care, 19*(2), 175–182.

Fell-Carlson, D. (2003, January). Terrorist danger. *Nurseweek California*, Sunnyvale, CA.

Fell-Carlson, D. (2003, January). The nurse's role in managing threat. *Nurseweek California*, Sunnyvale, CA.

Fellows, I., et al. (2000). Evidence-based practice for enteral feedings: Aspiration prevention strategies, bedside detection and practice change. *MEDSURG Nursing, 9*(1), 27.

Fellows, L. S, Miller, E. H., Frederickson, M., Bly, B., & Felt, P. (2000, January). Evidence-based practice for enteral feedings: Aspiration prevention strategies, bedside detection, and practice change. *MedSurg Nursing, 9*(1) 27–31.

Ferri, R., & Sofer, D. (2002, March). News. *American Journal of Nursing, 102*(3).

Fieldsmith, R., Van Sell, S., & Kindred, C. (2009, March). Home assessment. *RN, 72*(3), 26–28.

Finkelman, A. (2001). *Managed care: A nursing perspective*. Upper Saddle River, NJ: Prentice Hall.

Finkelstein, R., & Alam, H. (2010). Induced hypothermia for trauma: Current research and practice. *Journal of Intensive Care Medicine, 25*(4), 205–226.

Firth, D., & Ellerman, L. (2009, January). Legal medicine: Infection control and hand washing. Retrieved from www.legalmedicine.blogspot.com.

Fischbach, F. (2005). *Nurses' quick reference to common laboratory and diagnostic tests* (4th ed.). Philadelphia: Lippincott Williams & Wilkins.

Fitzpatrick, L. (2002, May). When to administer modified blood products. *Nursing 2002, 32*(5), 36–42.

Flasar, C. (2008 July). What is urine specific gravity? *Nursing 2008, 38*(7), 14.

Foley, A. (2005). RN + PDA IT at bedside. *2005 Future Nurse*, 34–35.

Frasco, P., Sprung, J., & Trentman, T., (2005). The impact of the Joint Commission for Accreditation of Healthcare Organizations pain initiative on perioperative opiate consumption and recovery room length of stay. *Anesthesia and Analgesia, 100*(1), 162–168.

Friedman, M. (2000, February). Improving infection control in home care: From ritual to science-based practice. *Home Healthcare Nurse, 18*(2), 99.

Friedman, M. (2000, June). The Joint Commission's "Improving Organizational Performance" Standards for Home Infusion Therapy Providers. *Journal of Intravenous Nursing, 23*(6), 352–357.

Furman, J. (2001, April). Living with dying: How to help the family caregiver. *Nursing, 31*(4), 36.

Futterman, L., & Lemberg, L. (2005). Cardiopulmonary resuscitation review: Critical role of chest compressions. *American Journal of Critical Care, 14*(1), 81.

Galvan, T. (2001). Dysphagia: Going down and staying down. *American Journal of Nursing, 101*(1), 37–43.

Garcia, R., Jendresky, L, Colbert, L., Bailey, A., Zaman, M., & Majumder, J. (2009). Reducing ventilator-associated pneumonia through advanced oral-dental care: A 48 month study. *American Journal of Critical Care, 18*(6), 523–531.

Garretson, S., & Rauzi, M. (2008, March). Implementing a rapid response team: A practical guide. *Nursing, 38*(3), 56cc1–56cc3.

Gaskill, M., (2006, September). Disaster and recovery: On their toes. *Nurseweek California*, Sunnyvale, CA, 12–14.

Gebbie, K., & Qureshi, K. (2002, January). Emergency and disaster preparedness. *American Journal of Nursing, 102*(1), 46–50.

Getting started with an insulin pump. (2009). *Consultant*, 223–224.

Gever, M. P. (1998, May). Transdermal patches. *Nursing, 28*(5), 58–59.

Gialanella, K. (2004, June). Documentation. *Advance for Nurses*, CA, 21–23.

Giuliano, KK., & Higgins, T. L. (2005). New-generation pulse oximetry in the care of critically ill patients. *American Journal of Critical Care, 14*(1), 26.

Glazer, J. (2005). Management of heatstroke and heat exhaustion. *American Family Physician, 71*(11), 2133.

Goldberg, Burton Group. (2002). *Alternative medicine: The definitive guide* (2nd ed.). Berkeley, CA: Ten Speed Press.

Goldich, G. (2006, November). Understanding 12-lead ECG part I. *Nursing, 36*(11), 36–41.

Goldsmith, C. (2005, January). Disease management empowers patients, improves lives. *Nurseweek California*, Sunnyvale, CA, 23–25.

Goldsmith, C. (2006, July). Good Things Come in Nanotech Packages. *Nurseweek, California*, Sunnyvale, CA. 19-20.

Goldsmith, C. (2009, November). Are you prepared? H1N1 Flu. *Nurseweek, California*, Sunnyvale, CA, 36–40.

Goodfellow, L., & Jones, M. (2002, January). Bronchial hygiene therapy. *American Journal of Nursing, 102*(1), 37–43.

Gorski, L. (2001, January). TPN Update: Making each visit count. *Home Healthcare Nurse, 19*(1), 15.

Gorski, L., & Czaplewski, L. (2005, June). Managing complications of midlines and PICCs. *Nursing, 35*(6), 68–69.

Gottschlich, M. (Ed.). (2001). *The science and practice of nutrition support (American Society for Parenteral and Enteral Nutrition)*. Dubuque, IA: Kendall/Hunt.

Goulette, C. (2005, June). Embracing differences: Cultural diversity enriches, strengthens nurses' role in healthcare delivery.*Advance for Nurses*, CA, 31–32.

Graf, C. (2006, January). Functional decline in hospitalized older adults. *American Journal of Nursing, 106*(1), 58–67.

Graf, C. (2008, April). The Lawton Instrumental activities of daily living scale. *American Journal of Nursing, 108*(4), 52–61.

Graf, C. (2008, August). The hospital admission risk profile. *American Journal of Nursing, 108*(8), 62–71.

Grap, M. (2009). Not-so-trivial pursuit: Mechanical ventilation risk reduction. *American Journal of Critical Care, 18*(4), 299–307.

Grap, M. J., Munro, C. L., Hummel, R. S. 3rd, Elswick, R. K. Jr., McKinney, J. L., & Sessler, C. N. (2005). Effect of backrest elevation on the development of ventilator-associated pneumonia. *American Journal of Critical Care, 14*(4), 325.

Gray, M. (2000). Urinary retention management in the acute care setting. *AJN, 100*(8), 36.

Gray-Vickrey, P. (2000, July). Combating abuse, part I: Protecting the older adult. *Nursing, 30*(7), 34.

Gray-Vickrey, P. (2010). Assessing older adults. *Nursing, 40*(3).

Greider, K. (2009, March). Battling superbugs. *AARP Bulletin*. Retrieved from http://www.aarp.org/bulletin.

Grissinger, M., & Globus, N. (2004). How technology affects your risk of medication errors. *Nursing, 34*(1), 36.

Gritter, M. (1998, September). The latex threat. *American Journal of Nursing, 98*(9), 26–32.

Gross, R. D., Mahlmann, J., & Grayhack, J. P. (2003). Physiologic effects of open and closed tracheostomy tubes on the pharyngeal swallow. *Annals of Otology, Rhinology and Laryngology, 112*(2), 143–152.

Guenter, P. , Hicks, R., & Simmons, D. (2009). Enteral feeding misconnections: an update. *Nutrition in Clinical Practice, 24*(3), 325–334.

Guido, G. (2010). *Legal and ethical issues in nursing* (5th ed.). Upper Saddle River, NJ: Prentice Hall Health.

Gusa, D., Miers, A., & Wkjdicks, E. (2007). More than meets the eye: The FOUR score is a new tool for assessing coma that won't miss licked in syndrome. *RNWEB.com*, 43–47.

Gustafson, S. (2007 November). Assess for fall risk, intervene-and bump up patient safety. *Nursing, 37*(12), 24–25.

Guterl, G. (2007, April). Cover your face. *Advance for Nurses, CA*, 22.

Guyton, A. C. & Hall, J. (2006). *Textbook of medical physiology* (11th ed.). Philadelphia: Saunders.

Haag, R., (2007, September). The basics of bioterrorism preparedness. *Advance for Nurses, CA*, 33–36.

Habel, M. (2001, October 22). Advance directives. *NurseWeek*.

Habel, M. (2005, May). The power of change: Nurses make a difference. *Nurseweek California*, Sunnyvale, CA, 36–38.

Habel, M. (2009, January). Promoting a culture of safety to prevent medical errors. *NurseWeek California*, Sunnyvale, CA, 20–21.

Hadaway, L. (2005, December). Caring for a nontunneled CVC site. *Nursing, 35*(12), 54–56.

Hadaway, L. (2006, April). Best-practice interventions: Keeping central line infection at bay. *Nursing, 36*(4), 58–63.

Hadaway, L. (2008). Targeting therapy with central venous access devices. *Nursing, 38*(5), 34–40.

Hadaway, L. (2009 March). Managing vascular access device occlusions, part 2. *Nursing, 39*(3), 13–14.

Hadaway, L., & Millam, D. (2005). On the road to successful I.V. starts. *Nursing, 35*(5), 1–14.

Hadway, L. (2009). Managing vascular access device occlusions, part 1. *Nursing, 39*(1), 10–15.

Hamage, S. (2008). Innovative bundle wipes out catheter-related bloodstream infections. *Nursing, 38*(10), 17–18.

Hamillton, S. (2001, December). Detecting dehydration and malnutrition in the elderly. *Nursing, 31*(12), 56–57.

Hark, L., & Morrison, G. (2003). *Medical nutrition and disease: A case-based approach* (3rd ed.). Malden, MA: Blackwell Science.

Harnage, S. (2008, October). Doing it better: innovative bundle wipes and catheter-related bloodstream infections. *Nursing, 38*(10), 17–18.

Harrison, B., & Roberts, J. (2005, October). Evaluating and managing pneumothorax. *Emergency Medicine*, 18.

Haydon, K., & Matthews, J. (2007, April). Safer handling saves nurses' backs. *NurseWeek, 8*(9), 16–18.

Haynes, A. B., Weiser, T. G., Berry, W. R., Lipsitz, S. R., Breizat, A. H., & Dellinger, E. P. (2009, January 29). A surgical safety checklist to reduce morbility and mortality in a global population. *New England Journal of Medicine, 360*(5), 491–499.

Health information technology is proving its merits. (2010). *American Journal of Nursing, 110*(8), 16.

Heery, K. (2000, November). Patient interview. *Nursing, 3*(6), 66–67.

Heineken, J. (2000). Establishing a bond with clients of different cultures. *Home Healthcare Nurse, 18*(1), 45.

Hellwig, K. (2000). Alternatives to restraints: What patients and caregivers should use. *Home Healthcare Nurse, 18*(6), 395.

Helwick, C. (2009, October). Postoperative sepsis rates are up but mortality is down. *Medsape Medical News*. www.medscape.com.

Hemmila, D. (2004, August). The wait is over: New rapid-results tests for HIV. *Nurseweek California*, Sunnyvale, CA, 26–21.

Henderson, D. (1999, February). The looming threat of bioterrorism. *American Association for Advancement of Science, 283*(5406), 1279–1282.

Hendey, G. (July, 2005). Seven myths of orthopedic emergencies. *Emergency Medicine*, 40.

Hendey, G. (2005). Seven myths of orthopedic emergencies. *Emergency Medicine*, 38–43.

Hendler, C. (2008, June). A perfect match: preventing blood incompatibility errors. *NurseWeek, CA*, 24–28.

Henneman, E., & Karras, G. (2004). Determining brain death in adults: A guideline for use in critical care. *Critical Care Nurse, 24*(5), 50–55.

Herkner, T., et al. (2001). Does bed rest after cervical or lumbar puncture prevent headache? *California Medical Association Journal, 165*, 1311–1316.

Hertz, J., Yocum, C., & Gawel, S. (2000). *1999 Practice analysis of newly licensed registered nurses in the U.S.* Chicago, IL: National Council of State Boards of Nursing.

Herzig, S., Howell, M., Ngo, L., & Marcantonio, E. (2009). Acid-suppressive medication use and the risk for hospital-acquired pneumonia. *Journal of the American Medical Association, 301*(20), 2120–2127.

Hess, C. (2004). *Clinical guide: Wound care* (5th ed.). Springhouse, PA: Springhouse Corporation.

Hess, C. (2009, August). Wound bed preparation. *Nursing, 39*(8), 57.

Hess, D., & Kacmarek, R. (2003). *Essentials of mechanical ventilation* (2nd ed.). New York: McGraw-Hill.

Hickey, J. (2009). The clinical practice of neurological and neurosurgical nursing (6th ed.).

Hignett, S. (2003, March). Systematic review of patient handling activities starting in lying, sitting and standing positions.*Journal of Advanced Nursing, 41*(6), 545–552.

Hoffman, R., & Norton, J. (2000, December). Lessons learned from a full-scale bioterrorism exercise. *Emerging Infectious Diseases*, 6(6), 652–653.

Hogan, S. (2004, August). How to help wounds heal. *RN Magazine, 67*(8), 26–31.

Hoggarth, A., Waring, M., Alexander, J., Greenwood, A., & Callaghan, T. (2005, December). A controlled, three-part trial to investigate the barrier function and skin hydration properties of six skin protectants. *Ostomy/Wound Management, 51*(12), 30–42.

Hohler, S. (2004, July). Hospital nursing: Tips for better patient teaching. *Nursing, 34*(7), 32hn7–32hn8.

Holden, K. (2007, March). Electronic Health Records: Useful Tools or High-Tech Headache? *American Journal of Nursing Reports, 107*(3), 25.

Holland, T. (2002). Utilizing the ankle–brachial index in clinical practice. *Ostomy/Wound Management, 48*(1), 38–43.

Hollinger-Smith, L. (2006, February). Training for disasters. *Advance for Nurses*, CA, 26–28.

Holmes, S., & Brown, S. (2005). Skeletal pin site care: National association of orthopaedic nurses guidelines for orthopaedic nursing. *Orthopaedic Nursing, 24*(2), 99–106.

Holmes, S., Brown S., with the Pin Site Care Expert Panel. (2005). Skeletal pin site care (National Association of Orthopaedic Nurses guidelines for orthopaedic nursing). *Orthopaedic Nursing, 24*(2), 99.

Holmes, T. H., & Rahe, R. H. (1967). Social readjustment rating scale. *Journal of Psychosomatic Research, 11*, 213.

Holzer, M. (2002). Mild therapeutic hypothermia to improve the neurologic outcome after cardiac arrest. *New England Journal of Medicine, 346*(8), 549–556.

How to Perform 3- or 5-lead. (2002). *Nursing, 32*(4), 50–51.

How to use transparent films. *Nursing, 30*(6), 84.

Hrouda, B. (2002). Warming up to IV infusion. *Nursing, 32*(3), 54–55.

Hudak, C., Gallo, B., & Morton, P. (2009). *Critical care nursing* (9th ed.). Philadelphia: Lippincott Williams & Wilkins.

Huether, S., & McCance, K. (2008). *Understanding pathophysiology* (4th ed). St. Louis: Mosby.

Hunt, C. (2008). Which site is best for an I.M. injection? *Nursing*, 62.

Hunt, L. W., Boone-Orke, J. L., & Fransway, A. F., et al. (1996, July). A medical center-wide, multidisciplinary approach to the problem of natural latex allergy. *Journal of Occupational Environmental Medicine, 38*(8), 765–770.

Huston, C. (2009, March). 10 tips for successful delegation. *Nursing, 39*(3), 54–55.

Infusion Nursing Standards of Practice. (2006). The Infusion Nursing Society (INS). Philadelphia: Lippincott Williams & Wilkins.

Injectable-drug errors and syringe labeling. *Nurse Advise-ERR*, 6(1), 1.

ISMP Medication Safety Alert. (2001, December). Handling verbal orders safely. *Nursing, 31*(12), 43.

Isola, S., et al. (2003, May–June). *Allergy & Asthma Proceedings, 24*(3), 193–197.

Jacobson, J. (Ed.). (2002, March). The World Trade Center children's mural. *American Journal of Nursing, 102*(3), 29–33.

Jagger, J., & Perry, J. (2002). Realistic expectations for safety devices. *Nursing, 32*(3), 72.

Jarvis, C. (2004). *Physical examination and health assessment* (4th ed.). Philadelphia: Saunders.

Johnson, A. (2009). Assessing gastric residual volumes. *Critical Care Nurse, 29*(5), 72–73.

Johnson, A., & Criddle, L. (2004). Pass the salt: Indications for and implications of using hypertonic saline. *Crictical Care Nurse, 24*(5), 36–46.

Johnson, C., Levey, A. S., Coresh, J., Levin, A., Lau, J., & Eknoyan, G. (2004). Clinical practice guidelines for chronic kidney disease in adults. Part I. Definition, disease stages, evaluation, treatment, and risk factors. *American Family Physician, 70*(5), 869–876.

Johnson, D., Lineweaver, L., & Maze, L. M. (2009). Patients' bath basins as potential sources of infection: A multicenter sampling study. *American Journal of Critical Care, 18*, 31–40.

Johnston, J, Davis, M. (2008, April). When sequential-compression devices cause falls. *American Journal of Nursing, 108*(4), 37–38.

Joint Commission on the Accreditation of Health Care Organizations. (2010). *Comprehensive Accreditation Manual for Critical Access Hospital (CAM-CAH): The Official Handbook. Sentinel Events*. Chicago: JCAHO.

Joint Commission Sentinel Event Alert (2006). Tubing misconnections – a persistent and potentially deadly occurrence. *Issue 36*, April 3.

Jolly, J. (2008, March). Laceration repair with tissue adhesives: a solution for simple wounds. *Advance for Nurse Practitioners, 16*(3), 63–64.

Jones, L., & Benthien. (2005). Putting down roots in earthquake country, adapted from editions of Southern California Earthquake Center with U.S. Geological Survey. CA, 1–30.

Kallus, C. (2009). Building a solid understanding of mechanical ventilation. *Nursing, 39*(6), 22–28.

Kaplow, R., & Hardin, S. (2007). *Critical care nursing: Synergy for optimal outcomes*. Boston: Jones & Bartlett.

Karch, A., & Karch, F. (2001). Take part in the solution: How to report medication errors. *American Journal of Nursing, 707*(10), 25.

Karch, A., & Karch, F. (2003, April). Not so fast: IV push drugs can be dangerous when given too rapidly. *American Journal of Nursing, 103*(8), 71.

Kee, J. (2009). *Laboratory and diagnostic tests with nursing implications* (8th ed.). Upper Saddle River, NJ: Prentice Hall Health.

Kee, J. L. (2010). *Laboratory and Diagnostic Tests* (8th ed.). Upper Saddle River, NJ: Prentice Hall.

Keefe, S. (2005, August 22). Postoperative ileus. *Advance for Nurses*, 29–30.

Keefe, S. (2005, October). Infusing spirituality into health education. *Advance for Nurses*, CA, 37–38.

Keefe, S. (2005, October). Inside infection control. *Advance for Nurses*, CA, 21–24.

Keefe, S. (2008, January). Community-acquired MRSA in children. *Advance for Nurses, Northern California*, 15–16.

Ketchum, K., Grass, C. A., & Padwojski, A. (2005). Medication reconciliation. *American Journal of Nursing, 105*(11), 78.

Kiekkas, P., Brokalaki, Hl, Theodorakopoulou, G., & Baltopoulos, G. (2008). Physical antipyresis in critically ill adults. *American Journal of Nursing, 108*(7), 40–50.

Kilpatrick, J. (2002, May). Nuclear attacks. *Nurseweek California*, Sunnyvale, CA, 47–51.

Knight, K., & Draper, D. (2008). *Therapeutic modalities: The art and science*. Baltimore, MD: Lippincott Williams & Wilkins.

Knutson, D. (2005, February). Chemical weapons antidotes. *BottomLine*, Boulder, CO.

Kohn-Keeth, C. (2000). How to keep feeding tubes flowing freely. *Nursing, 30*(3), 58–59.

Kohn-Keeth, C., & Frankel, E. (2004). Taking blue dye out of tube feedings. *Nursing, 34*(2), 14.

Koran, Z. (2008). Therapeutic hypothermia in the postresuscitation patient: The development and implementation of an evidence based protocol for the emergency department. *Advanced Emergency Nursing Journal, 30*(4), 319–330.

Koschel, M. (2001). Rewarming a hypothermic patient. *American Journal of Nursing, 707*(5), 85.

Kozier, B., Erb, G., Berman, A., & Burke, K. (2007). *Fundamentals of nursing: Concepts, process and practice* (8th ed.). Upper Saddle River, NJ: Prentice Hall Health.

Krueger, A. (2007). Need help finding a vein? *Nursing, 37*(6), 39–41.

Kübler-Ross, E. (1993). *On death and dying*. New York: Macmillan.

Kudzma, E. (1999). Culturally competent drug administration. *American Journal of Nursing, 99*(8), 46–51.

Kuehn, B. (2009). FDA Warning: Remove drug patches before MRI to prevent burns to skin. *Journal of the American Medical Association, 301*(13), 1328.

Kuehn, B. (2009). FDA warns against shared insulin pens. *Journal of the American Medical Association, 301*(15), 1527.

Kurtzman, E, Buerhaus, P. (2008, June). New medicare payment rules: Danger or opportunity for nursing. *American Journal of Nursing, 108*(5), 30–35.

Kushner, R., & Ognar, D. (2006, February). How to counsel patients about diet. *Consultant*, 171.

Ladden, M. (2009, July). How nurses are shaping, and being shaped by, health information technologies. *Charting Nurse's Future, a Publication of the Robert Woods Johnson Foundation*, www.rwjf.org, 1–8.

LaDuke, S. (2009). Playing it safe with bar code medication administration. *Nursing, 39*(5), 32–34.

Langan, J., & James, D. (2005). *Preparing nurses for disaster management*. Upper Saddle River, NJ: Prentice Hall.

Lattavo, K. (2001). Pinpointing postoperative hypoxemia. *Nursing, 37*(1), 32hn1–3.

Lawson, P. (2005). Zapping VAP with evidence-based practice. *Nursing, 35*(5), 66.

Leech, E. (2005). When your patient threatens to walk. *RN*, 68(9), 5.

Lehne, R. (2010). *Pharmacology for nursing care* (7th ed.). St. Louis: Saunders/Elsevier.

Leighty, J. (2004, May). Code zebra: On the frontlines, California EDs brace for action against infectious disease and bioterrorism.*Nurseweek California*, Sunnyvale, CA, 13–15.

Leininger, S. (1998, April). Caring for a patient with a hip replacement. *Nursing, 28*(4), 32H, 12–14.

LeMone, P., & Burke, K. (2007). *Medical–surgical nursing: Critical thinking in client care* (4th ed.). Upper Saddle River, NJ: Prentice Hall Health.

Lethaby, A., Temple, J., & Santy, J. (2009). Pin site care for preventing infections associated with external bone fixators and pins. *Cochrane Database of Systematic Reviews*, (4), CD004551.

Leung, A. K., Fong, J. H., Pinto-Rojas, A. (2005, November/December). Pediculosis capitis. *Journal of Pediatric Health Care, 19*, 369–373.

Lewis, A., (2007). Heatstroke in older adults. *American Journal of Nursing, 107*(6), 52–56.

Lewis, S. M., Heitkemper, M., & Dirksen, S. (2009). *Medical–surgical nursing: Assessment and management of clinical problems* (7th ed.). St. Louis: Mosby.

Lillus, K. (2005, July). Going paperless. *Advance for Nurses, CA*, 32–33.

Linde, E. (2009). Speaking up for organ donors. *Nursing, 39*(1), 28–31.

Lindgren, V., & Ames, N. (2005). Caring for patients on mechanical ventilation. *American Journal of Nursing, 105*(5), 50.

Linton, A. & Lach, H. (2007). *Matteson & McConnell's gerontological nursing: Concepts and practices* (3rd ed.). Philadelphia: Saunders.

Lipson, J., & Dibble, S. (Eds.). (2005). *Culture and clinical care*. San Francisco: UCSF Nursing Press.

Little, C. (2000). Manual ventilation. *Nursing, 30*(3), 50–51.

Littlejohns, L. & Bader, M. (Eds.). (2009): AACN-AANN protocols for practice: Monitoring *technologies in critically ill neuroscience patients*. Boston: Jones & Bartlett.

Littlejohns, L., & Trimble, B. (2005). Ask the experts. *Critical Care Nurse, 25*(3), 57–59.

Livingston, M., & Wolvos, T. (2009). *Scottsdale wound management guide*. HMP Communications, LLC.

Lo, B., Ruston, D., Kates, L. W., Arnold, R. M., Cohen, C. B., Faber-Langendoen, K., et al. (2002). Discussing religious and spiritual issues at the end of life. *Journal of the American Medical Association, 287*, 749–754.

Lowdermilk, D., & Perry, S. (2004). *Maternity & women's health care* (8th ed.). St. Louis: Mosby-Yearbook.

Lower, J. (2002). Facing neuro assessment fearlessly. *Nursing, 32*(2), 58–64.

Lynch, D. (2004). Cranberry for prevention of urinary tract infections. *American Family Physician, 70*(11), 2175.

Lynn, P. (2008). *Lippincott's photo atlas of medication administration* (3rd ed.). Philadelphia: Wolters Kluwer/Lippincott Williams & Wilkins.

Lynn-McHale Weigand, D., & Carlson, K. (2005). *AACN procedure manual for critical care*. Philadelphia: Saunders.

Mace, S. (2008, July). Getting the message. *Advance for Nurses, Northern California*, 20–21.

Madsen, D., Sebolt, T., Cullen, L., Folkedahl, B., Mueller, T., Richardson, C., et al. (2005). Listening to bowel sounds: An evidence-based practice project. *American Journal of Nursing, 105*(12), 40.

Maher, A., et al. (2002). *Orthopaedic nursing* (3rd ed.). Philadelphia: WB Saunders.

Maher, A., Salmond, S., & Pellino, T. (2002). *Orthopaedic nursing* (3rd ed.). Philadelphia: Saunders.

Management, *35*, 27–35.

Maniscalco, P., & Christem, H. (2002). *Understanding terrorism and managing the consequences*. Upper Saddle River, NJ: Pearson Education.

Manno, M. (2005). Managing mechanical ventilation. *Nursing, 35*(12), 36.

Manno, M., & Hayes, D. (2006). How medication reconciliation saves lives. *Nursing, 36*(3), 63.

Marders, J. (2005). Sounding the alarm for I.V. infiltration. *Nursing*, 18–20.

Martin, S., & Nichols, W. (2008). Does heat or cold work better for acute muscle strain? *The Journal of Family Practice, 57*(12), 820–821.

Mascioli, S, Laskowski-Jones, L.,Urban, S., & Moran, S. (2009). Improving handoff communication. *Nursing, 39*(2), 52–55.

Mattox, E. (2010). Identifying vulnerable patients at heightened risk for medical error. *Critical Care Nurse, 30*(2), 61–68.

Mayer, S., Kowalski, R., Presciutti, M., Ostapkovick, N., McGann, E., Fitzsimmons, B., et al (2004). Clinical trial of a novel surface cooling system for fever control in neurocritical care patients. *Critical Care Medicine, 32*(12), 2508–2514.

Mazanec, P., & Tyler, M. (2003, March). Cultural considerations in end-of-life care. *American Journal of Nursing, 103*(3), 50–57.

McCaffery, M. (2000, September). Pain control. *Nurseweek California*, Sunnyvale, CA, 18–19.

McCaffrey, J., Whiting, F., Bagshaw, S., & Delaney, A. (2009). Corticosteroids to prevent extubation failure: A systematic review and meta-analysis. *Intensive Care Medicine*, 35(6), 977–986.

McCaffrey, M. (1999, July). Assessing pain in a confused, nonverbal patient. *Nursing, 29*(7), 18.

McCance, K., & Huether, S. (2006). *Pathophysiology: The biologic basis for disease in adults and children* (5th ed.). St. Louis: Mosby-Yearbook.

McConnell, E. (1998, June). Clinical do's and don'ts: Applying cold treatment. *Nursing, 28*(6), 26.

McConnell, E. (2000, March). Administering an intradermal injection. *Nursing, 30*(3), 17.

McConnell, E. (2000, November). Applying a two-piece cervical collar. *Nursing, 37*(11), 24.

McConnell, E. (2001, December). Applying a hip abduction pillow. *Nursing, 37*(12), 14.

McConnell, E. (2002, February). Teaching your patient to use a metered dose inhaler. *Nursing, 32*(2), 73.

McConnell, E. A. (2000, January). Suctioning a tracheostomy tube. *Nursing, 30*(1), 80.

McConnell, E. A. (2002, January). Providing tracheostomy care. *Nursing, 32*(1), 17.

McCullough, L., & Arora, S. (2004). Diagnosis and treatment of hypothermia. *American Family Physician, 70*(12), 2325.

McCurdy, D. (2008, May). Ethical spiritual care at the end of life. *American Journal of Nursing, 108*(5), 11.

McDonald, D., Thomas, G. J., Livingston, K. E., & Severson, J. S. (2005, February). Assisting older adults to communicate their postoperative pain. *Clinical Nursing Research, 14*(2), 109.

McDonough, M. (2009, November). Mission control: Managing atrial fibrillation. *Nursing, 38*(11), 58–63.

McKenry, L., & Salerno, E. (2001). *Pharmacology in nursing* (21st ed.). St. Louis: Mosby.

McKenzie, L. (1999, February). In search of a standard for pin site care. *Orthopaedic Nursing, 78*(2), 73–78.

McPhee, S. J., & Papadakis, M. A. (Eds.) (2010). *Current medical diagnosis and treatment 2010* (49th ed.). New York: McGraw-Hill.

Meehan, M. (2009, October). Pressure ulcers: the stakes just got higher. *Nursing, 39*(10), 45–47.

Mendez-Eastman, S. (2005, May). Using negative-pressure wound therapy for positive results. *Nursing, 35*(5), 48–50.

Mercandetti, M., & Cohen, A. (2008, March). Wound healing, healing and repair: eMedicine Plastic Surgery. Retrieved from http://emedicine.medscape.com/article/1298129-overview.

Metheny, N. (2000). *Fluid and electrolyte balance: Nursing considerations* (4th ed.). Philadelphia: Lippincott.

Metheny, N. (2006). Preventing respiratory complications of tube feedings: Evidence–based practice. *American Journal of Critical Care, 15*, 360–369.

Metheny, N. (2008). Preventing aspiration in older adults with dysphagia. *American Journal of Nursing, 108*(2), 45–49.

Metheny, N., & Titler, M. (2001, May). Assessing placement of feeding tubes. *American Journal of Nursing, 101*(5), 36–46.

Metheny, N., Davis-Jackson, J., & Stewart, B. (2010). Effectiveness of an aspiration risk-reduction protocol. *Nursing Research, 59*(1), 18–25.

Metheny, W., Wiersema, M., & Clark, J. (1998, January). pH, color and feeding tubes. *RN, 61*(1), 25–27.

Metules, T. (2007). Hot and cold packs. *RN, 70*(1), 45–48.

Metules, T., & Bauer, J. (2007). JCAHO'S patient safety goals: Preventing med errors. *RN, 70*(1), 39–44.

Miller, D. (2009). Are you ready to care for a patient with an insulin pump? *Nursing*, 57–60.

Mimoz, O., Villeminey, S., Ragot, S., Dahyot-Fizelier, C., Laksiri, L., Petitpas, F., et al. (2007, October). Chlorhexidine-based antiseptic solution vs alcohol-based povidone-iodine for central venous catheter care. *Archives of Internal Medicine*. *167*(19), 2066–2072.

Mims, B., et al. (2004). *Critical care skills: A clinical handbook*. Philadelphia: Saunders.

MiniMed. (1998). *The MiniMed infusion family*. Sylmar, CA.

Miracle, V., Sims, J. (1999, July). Making sense of the 12-lead ECG. *Nursing, 29*(7), 34–39.

Mitchell, D. (2004). Vent injury: How to avoid it. *RN, 67*(7), 54.

Monachino, A. (2005, May/June). Pediatric code readiness. *Journal for Nurses in Staff Development, 21*(3), 126–131.

Monahan, F., Sands, J., Neigbors, M., Marcek, J., & Nigro-Green, C. (2007). *Phipp's medical-surgical nursing: Concepts and clinical practice* (8th ed.). St. Louis: Mosby.

Moon, L., & Backer, J. (2000, February). Relationships among self-efficacy, outcome expectancy and postoperative behaviors in total joint replacement patients. *Orthopaedic Nursing, 19*(2), 77–85.

Morris, M. (2002, January). Advice of counsel. *RN, 65*(1), 71.

Morrison,D, Smith, J. (2009, June). Taking a vested interest in a wearable cardioverter defibrillator. *Nursing, 39*(6), 31–32.

Morton, P., et al. (2005). *Critical care nursing, a holistic approach* (8th ed.). Philadelphia: Lippincott Williams & Wilkins.

Moshang, J. (2005). Making a point about insulin pens. *Nursing, 35*(2), 46.

Mueller, P. (2005, February). Advance directives. *Supplement to Mayo Clinic Women's Healthsource*.

Mullett, S. (Ed.). (2008, November). Johns Hopkins team issues disaster drill evaluation tool. *RN Magazine, 11*(3), 14.

Munoz, C., & Hilgenberg, C. (2005). Ethnopharmacology. *American Journal of Nursing, 105*(8), 40.

NANDA International. (2008). *Nursing Diagnosis: Definitions and Classification, 2009–2011* (2nd ed.). Wiley-Blackwell.

Nash, C. E., Mickan, S. M., Del Mar, C. B., Glasziou, P. P. (2004). Resting injured limbs delays recovery: A systematic review. *Journal of Family Practice, 53*(9), 706.

Nash, C., Mickan, M., DelMar, C., & Glasziou, P. (2004). Resting injured limbs delays recovery: A systematic review. *The Journal of Family Practice, 53*(9), 706–712.

National Student Nurses' Association. (2005). *Bill of rights and responsibilities for students of nursing*. Washington, DC: Author.

National Student Nurses' Association. (2009, October). *Code of academic and clinical conduct*. Washington, DC: Author.

Nelson, A., Owen, B., Lloyd, J. D., Fragala, G., Matz, M. W., Amato, M., et al. (2003, March). Safe patient handling movement. *American Journal of Nursing, 103*(3), 32–43.

Nettina, S. M. (2009). *Lippincott manual of nursing practice*. (9th ed.). Philadelphia: Lippincott Williams & Wilkins.

New national standards recommend IV safety device. (2006, January). Infusion Nurses Society (INS). INSI.org.

Ng, R., Li, X., Tu, T., & Semba, C. P. (2004). Alteplase for treatment of occluded peripherally inserted central catheters: safety and efficacy in 240 patients. *Journal of Vascular and Interventional Radiology, 15*, 45–49.

Nicoll, L., & Hesby, A. (2002). Intramuscular injection: Integrative research review and guideline for evidence-based practice. *Applied Nursing Research, 16*(2), 149–162.

Nicolson, G. (2001, December). Protection from biological warfare agents. *Townsend letter for doctors & patients*, Port Townsend, WA, 62–67.

Norris, E. H. (2005, September). *Range, magnitude, and duration of the effects of disasters on mental health*. RED/Research Education Disaster Mental Health, Dartmouth College. Retrieved from www.ncptsd.va.gov/facts/disasters/fs.

Nowlin, A. (2006). The dysphagia dilemma: How you can help. *RN, 69*(6), 44–48.

Nunnelee, J. (2005, November). Needlesticks: What you must know. *RN Magazine*, (Suppl.), 32–35.

Nurses rate first, surgeons last in operating room safety. (2006, June). *NEWS-Line for Nurses, 7*(6N), 8–9.

O'Leary-Kelley, C. M., Puntillo, K. A., Barr, J., Stotts, N., & Douglas, M. K. (2005). Nutritional adequacy in patients receiving mechanical ventilation who are fed enterally. *American Journal of Critical Care, 14*(3), 222–231.

Olds, S., Landon, M., & Ladewig, P. (2004). *Maternal-newborn nursing & women's health care* (7th ed.). Upper Saddle River, NJ: Prentice Hall Health.

Oncology Nursing Society. (2004). *Access device guidelines: recommendations for nursing practice and education* (2nd ed.). Pittsburgh, PA: Oncology Nursing Society.

Ott, L. (2008, January). Assessing blood flow with CT angiography. *Nursing, 38(1)*, 26.

Padula, C. A., Kenny, A., Planchon, C., & Lamoureux, C. (2006). Enteral feedings: What the evidence says. *American Journal of Nursing, 104*(7), 62–69.

Pagana, K. (2009, July). Mind your manners...multiculturally. *NurseWeek, Mountain West, 10*(7), 18–22.

Pagana, K., & Pagana, T. (2009). *Mosby's manual of diagnostic and laboratory tests* (4th ed.). St. Louis: Mosby.

Palatnik, A. (2009, September). Too fast, too slow, too ugly: Dysrhythmias that every nurse should know. *Nursing, 39*(9), 38–45.

Palmerchuk, L. (2007, January). Central command: making sense of central lines. *NurseWeek, CA*, 12.

Panke, J. (2002, July). Difficulties in managing pain at the end of life. *American Journal of Nursing, 104*(7), 26–33.

Pasero, C. (2002, August). Pain assessment in infants and your children: Neonates. *American Journal of Nursing, 102*(8), 61–64.

Pasero, C., & McCaffery, M. (2005, July). Authorized and unauthorized use of PCA pumps. *American Journal of Nursing, 105*(7), 30–32.

Pasero, C., & McCaffery. (1999, August). Providing epidural. *Nursing, 24*(8), 34–38.

Pasquina, P., Tramer, M., Granier, J., & Walder, B. (2006). Respiratory physiotherapy to prevent pulmonary complications after abdominal surgery. *Chest, 130*(6), 1887–1889.

Patel, C. T., Kinsey, G. C., Koperski-Moen, K. J., Bungum, L. D. (2000, December). Vacuum-assisted wound closure. *American Journal of Nursing, 100*(12), 45–48.

Pattillo, M. (2005, October). Bioterrorism. *Advance for Nurses*, CA, 15–19.

Peiffer, K. (2007, March). Brain death and organ procurement. *American Journal of Nursing, 107*(3), 58–67.

Pendergast, V. Hallaberg, I., Jahnke, H., Kleiman, C. and Hagell, P. (2009). Oral health, ventilator-associated pneumonia, and intracranial pressure in intubated patients in neuroscience intensive care unit. *Amerian Journal of Critical Care, 18*(4), 368–376.

Perrin, K. O. (2009). *Understanding the essentials of critical care nursing*. Upper Saddle River, NJ: Pearson/Prentice Hall.

Perry, J. (2004, November). How to avoid needlesticks. *RN Magazine* (Suppl.), 28ns2–28ns7.

Perry, J., Parker, G., & Jagger, J. (2001, June). Percutaneous injuries in home healthcare settings. *Home Healthcare Nurse, 19*(6), 342.

Philadelphia: Wolters Kluwer/Lippincott Williams & Wilkins.

Phillips, L. (2005). *Manual of I.V. therapeutics* (4th ed.). Philadelphia: F.A. Davis.

Physicians' desk reference to pharmaceutical specialties and biologicals (60th ed.). (2006). Montvale, MD: Medical Economics.

Poon, E., Keohane, C., Yoon, C., Ditmore, M., Bane, A., Levtzion-Korach, O., et al. (2010). Effect of bar-code technology on the safety of medication administration. *New England Journal of Medicine, 362*(18), 1698–1707.

Pope, B, Rodzen, L, Spross, G. (2007, March). Raising the SBAR: How better communication improves patient outcomes. *Nursing, 38*(3), 41–43.

Porth, C. (2006). *Pathophysiology concepts of altered health states* (7th ed.). Philadelphia: Lippincott.

Prentice, W. (2003). *Therapeutic modalities in sports medicine* (5th ed.) Boston: McGraw-Hill.

Pronovost, P., Weast, B., Schwarz, M., Wyskiel, R. M., Prow, D., Milanovich, S. N., et al. (2003). Medication reconciliation: A practical tool to reduce the risk of medication errors. *Journal of Critical Care, 18*(4), 201–205.

Pruitt, B. (2005). Clear the air with closed suctioning. *Nursing, 35*(7), 44.

Pruitt, B., & Jacobs, M. (2006). How can you prevent ventilator associated pneumonia? *Nursing, 36*(2), 36.

Pruitt, B., & Michael Jacobs (2005). Clearing away pulmonary secretions. *Nursing, 35*(7), 37.

Pullen, R. (2005). Checking for oculocephalic reflex. *Nursing, 35*(6), 24.

Pullin, R. (2007). Clinical do's and don'ts: Replacing a urostomy drainage pouch. *Nursing, 37*(6), 14.

Pullin, R. (2008, January). Transferring a patient from bed to stretcher. *Nursing, 38*(1), 43–45.

Pullin, R. (2008, March). Using a hydraulic lift for patient transfer. *Nursing, 38*(3), 54–56.

Pump up the volume – Tips for increasing error reporting (2009). *Nurse Advise-ERR, 7*(7), 1–3.

Pun, B., & Dunn, J. (2007). The sedation of critically ill adults: Part 1: Assessment. *American Journal of Nursing, 107*(7), 40–48.

Pun, B., & Dunn, J. (2007). The sedation of critically ill adults: Part 2: Management. *American Journal of Nursing, 107*(8), 40–49.

Pyrek, K. (2010, April). Catheter-related infection prevention: A review of the basics. *Infection Control Today, 14*(4), 30–32.

Rankin, S., Stallings, K. D., & London, F. (2005). *Patient education: Principles and practices* (5th ed.). Philadelphia: Lippincott Williams & Wilkins.

Ratliff, C. (2008, July). Wound exudate. *Advance for Nurse Practitioners, 16*(7), 32–35.

Rauen, C. A., Chulay, M., Bridges, E., Vollman, K. M., & Arbour, R. (2008, April). Seven evidence-based practice habits: putting some sacred cows out to pasture. *Critical Care Nurse, 28*(2), 98–124.

Rauen, C. Chuly, M., Bridges, E., Vollman, K., & Arbour, R. (2008). Seven evidence-based practice habits: Putting some sacred cows out to pasture. *Critical Care Nurse, 28*(2), 98–124.

Ray, L. (2009). A ticket to ride protects patients off the unit. *Nursing, 39*(5), 57–58.

Rea T. D., Fahrenbruch, C., Culley, L., Donohoe, R. T., Hambly, C., Innes, J., et al. (2010, July). CPR with chest compression alone or with rescue breathing. *The New England Journal of Medicine, 363*, 423–433.

Regan, E., & Dalachiesa, L. (2009). How to care for a patient with a tracheostomy. *Nursing*, 39(8), 34–39.

Registered Nurses' Association of Ontario. (2005, March). *Nursing best practice guideline: Shaping the future of nursing. Prevention of falls and fall injuries in the older adult*. 8–12.

Reising, D., & Neal, R. (2005). Enteral tube flushing. *American Journal of Nursing, 105*(3), 58–63.

Rice, R. (2005). *Home health nursing practice: Concepts and application* (4th ed.). St. Louis: Mosby.

Ringhofer, J. (2005). Meeting the needs of your ostomy patient. *RN*, 68(8), 37.

Risenberg, L., Leitzsch, J., & Cunningham, M. (2010, April). *American Journal of Nursing, 110*(4), 24–34.

Rivera, P., & Kreskow, J. (2000, February). A team approach to managing pain. *Nursing, 29*(2), 32–33.

Robinson, B., & Branson, R. (2009). Consequences of ventilator asynchrony. *Critical Care Medicine, 37*(10), 2848–2849.

Rolfes, S., et al. (2006). *Understanding normal and clinical nutrition* (7th ed). Thomson Learning.

Rolfes, S., Pinna, K., & Whitney, E. (2006). *Understanding normal and clinical nutrition* (7th ed). St. Paul, MN: Wadsworth-Thompson.

Roman, L., & Metales, T. (2005). What we can learn from the Schiavo case. *RN*, 68(8), 53.

Rosenthal, K. (2005, May). Tailor your IV insertion techniques for special populations. *Nursing, 35*(5), 37–41.

Rubenfeld, M. G., & Scheffer, B. K. (1999). *Critical thinking in nursing: An interactive approach* (2nd ed.). Philadelphia: Lippincott Williams & Wilkins.

Ruffolo, D. (2002, February). Hypothermia in trauma. *RN, 65*(2), 46–51.

Russell, J. (contributing Ed.). (2005, January). When is an MDI really empty? *Patient Care*.

Rutecki, G. (2008). Statins and stroke: A compelling reason for medication reconciliation. *Consultant*, 82.

Sakla, S. (2001). Malnutrition: A serious problem in elderly patients. *Family Practice Recertification, 23*(13), 29–39.

Salladay, S. (2009) Ethical problems, removing life support. *Nursing*, 18.

Salvatore, T. (2000, March). Elder suicide: A gatekeeper strategy for home care. *Home Healthcare Nurse, 18*(3), 180.

Salvucci, A. (2002, October). Bioterrorism safeguards. *Bottom Line*, Stamford, CT: Boardroom, Inc.

Sandau, K, Smith, M. (2009, August). Continuous ST-Segment monitoring: Protocol for practice. *Critical Care Nurse, 29*(4), 39–50.

Sarvis, C., (2007, December). Using antiseptics to manage infected wounds. *Nursing, 37*(12), 20–21.

Schears, G., et al. *Statlock catheter securement device significantly reduces central venous catheter complications: Patient safety initiative 2000*. Joint Commission on Accreditation of Healthcare Organizations, 28–36.

Schetter, J. (August 2009). A culture of safety: direct observation ensures compliance. *RN, 72*(8), 34–36.

Schulmeister, L. (2005). Medicine with muscle. *Nursing, 35*(1), 48.

Schwartz, A., & Powell, S. (2009, March). Brush up on oral assessment and care. *Nursing, 39*(3), 31–32.

Schwartz, A., & Powell, S. (2009). Brush up on oral assessment and care. *Nursing, 39*(3), 30–32.

Scoble, M., & Kinney, S. (2001, March). Effect of reusing suction catheters on the occurrence of pneumonia in children. *Heart & Lung, 30*(3), 225–233.

Scriven, M., & Paul, R. Definition of critical thinking. National Council for Excellence in Critical Thinking. Retrieved from www.criticalthinking.org/k12.

Seaver, M. (2005). A helping handheld computer—technology at the point of care. Pathways to success. *Nurseweek.com*, 46–49.

Seay, S. J., Gay, S. L., & Strauss, M. (2002). Tracheostomy emergencies. *American Journal of Nursing, 102*(3), 59.

Seery, D. (2004, November). Shifting gears from cure to comfort. *RN Magazine, 67*(11), 52–57.

Selye, H. (1965). *The stress of life*. New York: McGraw-Hill.

Selye, H. (1974). *Stress without distress*. New York: Signet.

Sepsis: Still tricky to treat: Researchers weigh measuring tissue oxygen, controlling blood glucose. (2010). *American Journal of Nursing, 110*(5), 16.

Serna, E., & McCarthy, M. (2006). Heads up to prevent aspiration during enteral feeding. *Nursing, 36*(1), 76.

Shaprio, S., Donaldson, N., & Scott, M. (2010). Rapid response teams: Seen through the eyes of the nurse. *American Journal of Nursing, 110*(6), 28–34.

Sheehan, J. (2001, November). Delegating to UAPs. *RN, 64*(11), 65–66.

Shelton, P., & Rosenthal, K. (2004, June). Sharps injury prevention: Select a safer needle. *Nursing Management, 35*(6), 25–31.

Sherman, F. (2002, January). Bedside test provides food for thought. *Geriatrics, 57*(1), 3–4.

Siela, D. (2010). Evaluation standards for management of artificial airways. *Critical Care Nurse, 30*(4), 76–77.

Skyler, J. S. (1995). *The insulin pump therapy book*. Sylmar, CA: MiniMed, Inc.

Smeltzer, S., & Bare, B. (2008). *Brunner & Suddarth's textbook of medical–surgical nursing* (11th ed.). Philadelphia: Lippincott Williams & Wilkins.

Smith, B. (2006). Peripheral intravenous catheter dwell times; a comparison of 3 securement methods for implementation of a 96-hour scheduled change protocol. *Journal of Infusion Nursing, 29*, 14–17.

Smith, J., Stevens, J., Taylor, M., & Tibbey J. (2002, February). A randomized, controlled trial comparing compression bandaging and cold therapy in postoperative total knee replacement surgery. *Orthopaedic Nursing, 21*(2), 61–66.

Smith, P. (2005, August). Tiny radiation detector could save millions. *NewsMax Magazine*, West Palm Beach, FL, 42.

Smith, S. (1998, July). RNs and UAPs: Not much difference? *RN, 62*(7), 37–38.

Smith, S. (2006). *Sandra Smith's review for NCLEX-RN* (11th ed.). Los Altos, CA: National Nursing Review.

Smith, S., Duell, D., & Martin, B. (2002). *Photo guide of nursing skills*. Upper Saddle River, NJ: Prentice Hall Health.

Smith, T., Temple, J., & Johnson, J. (2006). *Guide to clinical procedures* (5th ed.). Philadelphia: Lippincott Williams & Wilkins.

Snyder, L. (2008, August). Wound basics: types, treatment, and care. *RN, 71*(8), 32–36.

Snyder, L. (2008, August). Wound basics: types, treatment, and care. *RN, 71*(8), 32–36.

Snyder, M. (2005, February). Learn the chilling facts about hypothermia. *Nursing*, 32hn1.

Spader, C. (2006, March 13). *Diagnostic imaging; contrast counts*. *Nurseweek*, 18–20.

Spader, C. (2009, August). Cool tools, cutting edge gadgets sharpen nurses efficiency. *Advance for Nurses, Northern California*, 32–33.

Spector, R. (2008). *Cultural diversity in health and illness* (7th ed). Upper Saddle River, NJ: Prentice Hall Health.

St. John, R. (2000, April). Ask the experts. *Critical Care Nurse, 20*(4), 100–101.

St. John, R. (2004). Airway management. *Critical Care Nurse, 24*(2), 93.

Staff (2009, October). Bacteria-laden bath basins, source of contamination. *American Association of Critical Care Nurses*. Retrieved from www.aacn-boldvoicesonline.org.

Staff, Nursing Journal. (2008) *Perfecting clinical procedures*. Philadelphia: Lippincott Williams & Wilkins.

Staff. (2007). *Best practices evidenced-based nursing procedures*. (2nd ed.). Philadelphia: Lippincott Williams & Wilkins.

Stanhope M., & Knollmuller, R. (2000). *Handbook of community based and home health nursing* (3rd ed.). St. Louis: Mosby.

Stanly, M., & Beare, P. G. (1999). *Gerontological nursing* (2nd ed.). Philadelphia: Davis.

Starkey, C. (1993). *Therapeutic modalities* (2nd ed). Philadelphia: Davis.

Stein, P., & Henry, R. (2009). Poor oral hygiene in long term care. *American Journal of Nursing, 109*(6), 44–49.

Steinhauer, R. (2002, June). The emergency management plan. *RN, 65*(6), 40–45.

Steinhauer, R. (2002, May). Bioterrorism, *RN, 65*(3), 48–54.

Stevens, D., et al. (2000). Comparison of two warming interventions in surgical patients with mild and moderate hypothermia.*International Journal of Nursing Practice*, 6, 268–275.

Stewart, K., & Murray, H. (1997, May). How to use crutches correctly. *Nursing, 27*(5).

Stitik, R., & Nadler, S. (1999, December). Sports injuries: When and how to use cold most effectively. *Consultant, 38*(12), 2881–2890.

Stitik, R., & Nadler, S. (1999, January). Sports injuries: When and how to apply the heat. *Consultant, 39*(1), 144–157.

Stoessel, K. (2009,November). Hand hygiene: Challenges and strategies. *Infection Control Today, 13*(11), 26–28.

Strevy, S. R. (1998, February). Myths and facts about pain. *RN, 61*(2), 42–46.

Strowig, S. (2001, September). Insulin therapy. *RN, 64*(9), 38–44.

Sullivan-Tevault, M. (2005, June). Multicultural pain management. *Advance for Nurses, CA*, 33–34.

Sweetland, S., & Gerts, W. (2010, March). FDA warning about negative pressure wound therapy. *American Journal of Nursing, 110*(3),16-19.

Swhart, D. (2005, October). Are we safe yet? Identification of causal and contributory factors of medical errors. *Advance for Nurses, CA*, 15–18.

Taber's cyclopedic medical dictionary (21st ed). (2010). Philadelphia: Davis.

Tate, J., & Tasota, F. (2000, September). Using pulse oximetry. *Nursing, 30*(9), 30.

Taylor, C., Lillis, C., & LeMone, P. (2007). *Fundamentals of nursing: The art and science of nursing care* (6th ed.). Philadelphia: Lippincott Williams & Wilkins

Taylor, E. (2002). *Spiritual care*. Upper Saddle River, NJ: Prentice Hall Health.

Taylor, N. (2006, January). This just in: For new CPR guidelines, think 30. *Nursing Critical Care, 1*(1), 56–56.

Taylor, S. (2006, January). Research reveals the benefits of meditation. *Nurseweek California*, Sunnyvale, CA, 17–18.

The Health Insurance Portability and Accountability Act (HIPAA). (2003, April). *The privacy rule*. Washington, DC: United States Department of Health & Human Services.

The Joint Commission. (2008). Hand-off communications. NPSG.02 .05.01

The Joint Commission. (2009). Home Care National Patient Safety Goals. Retrieved from http:www.jointcommission.org/HomeCareNationaPatient SafetyGoals.

The Joint Commission. (2009). Improving America's Hospitals: The Joint Commission's Annual Report on Quality and Safety.

The Joint Commission. (2010). National Patient Safety Goals. Retrieved from http://jointcommission.org/PatientSafety/NationalSafetyGoals.

The Joint Commission. (2010). Provision of care, treatment, and services. Retrieved from http://www.jointcommission.org/AccreditationPrograms/ BehavioralHealthCare.

The V.A.C. Vacuum assisted closure: V.A.C. Therapy: Clinical guidelines. (2005, January). London: KCL.

Thew, J., & Class, P. (2005, September). Shelter from the storm. *Nurseweek California*, Sunnyvale, CA, 36–38.

Thomas Hess, C. (2000, November). Wound care: How to use transparent films. *Nursing, 30*(6), 84.

Thompson, J. (2000, November). A practical ostomy guide. *RN, 63*(1), 61–68.ok

Thompson, J. M., Hirsch, J. E., Tucker, S. M., & McFarland, G. K. (2002). *Mosby's manual of clinical nursing* (5th ed.). St. Louis: Mosby.

Thurlow, K. (2001, June). Latex allergies: Management and clinical responsibilities. *Home Healthcare Nurse, 24*(6), 369.

Tierney, K., Lindell, M., & Perry, R. (2001). *Facing the unexpected: Disaster preparedness and response in the United States*. Washington, DC: Joseph Henry Press.

Togger, D., & Brenner, P. (2001, October). Metered dose inhalers. *American Journal of Nursing, 101*(10), 26–32.

Torrey, T. Learn about Medicare's 2008 Never Events Policy. Retrieved from http://patients.about.com/od/patientempowermentissues/a/medicare08nrver.htm

Toth, P., Stricker, L., & Rijswijk, L. (2010, February). Wound wise: Peristomal skin complications. *American Journal of Nursing, 110*(2), 43–48.

Toughill, E. (2005). Indwelling urinary catheters. *American Journal of Nursing, 105*(5), 35.

Trimble, T. (2003, September). Peripheral starts: Securing and removing the catheter. *Nursing, 33*(9), 26.

Trossman, S. (2006). Hazardous conditions. *American Journal of Nursing, 106*(8), 75–77.

Troyer, E., & Thronton, S. (2005, October). Ginkgo biloba: Friend or foe. *Biosyntrx Friday Pearl*, Lexington, SC.

Trujillo, E. B., Robinson, M. K., & Jacobs, D. O. (2001, April). Feeding critically ill patients: Current concepts. *Critical Care Nurse, 21*(4), 60–67.

Tuite, P., & George, E. (2005). Biphasic defibrillation: Know your equipment. *Nursing, 35*(3), 32cc1.

Turkiski, B. (2009). Improving patient safety by improving medication communication. *Orthopaedic Nursing, 28*(3), 150–154.

U.S. Department of Agriculture. (2005). *Dietary guidelines for Americans*. Washington, DC: Author.

U.S. Department of Health & Human Services, Office for Civil Rights. (2003, May). Summary of the HIPAA privacy rule. Washington, DC: Author.

U.S. Food and Drug Administration. (2004, September). *FDA approves new extended release pain medication*. Retrieved from www.fda.gov./bbs/topics/2004/ANSO1315.

Update 2004. (2004). *Critical Care Nurse, 24*(2), 97.

Upfront Advice P.R.N. (2008). Medication administration: Don't forget to flush. *Nursing*, 10.

Urden, L., Stacy, K., & Lough, M. (2008). *Priorities in critical care nursing* (5th ed.). St. Louis: Mosby.

Valdez-Lowe, C., Ghareeb, S., & Artinian, N. (2009). Pulse oximetry in adults. *American Journal of Nursing. 109*(6), 52–59.

Vassal, T., Benoit-Gonin, B., Carrat, F., Guidet, B., Maury, E., & Offenstadt, G. (2001). Severe accidental hypothermia treated in an ICU. *Chest, 120*(6), 1998–2003.

Ventura, M. (2000, April). Chemical hazards: How to protect yourself. *RN, 63*(4) 77–80.

Veronesi, J. (2005). Heat emergencies. *RN, 68*(6), 46.

Virani, R., & Sofer, D. (2003, May). Improving the quality of end-of-life care. *American Journal of Nursing, 103*(5), 52–61.

Vollman, K., et al. (2005). Interventional patient hygiene: Proactive hygiene strategies to improve patients' outcomes. *AACN News, 22*(8).

Walker, C., Hogstel, M., & Curry, L. (2007). Hospital discharge of older adults. *American Journal of Nursing, 107*(6), 60–70.

Walker-Cillo, G. (2006, April). Bioterrorism: We put our plan to the test. *RN, 69*(4), 36–41.

Wallace, M, Shelkey, M. (2008, April). Monitoring functional status in hospitalized older adults. *American Journal of Nursing, 108*(4), 64–71.

Waters, T. (2007, August). When is it safe to manually lift a patient? *American Journal of Nursing, 107*(8), 53–58.

Weaver, S., & Marcus, J. (eds.). (2000). *Dietitian's patient education manual, Vol 2*. Gaithersburg, MD: Aspen Publishers.

Weigand, D., & Carlson, K. (Eds.). (2005). *AACN procedure manual for critical care* (5th ed.). Philadelphia: Elsevier/Saunders.

Weiner, W. J., & Goetz, C. (Eds.). (2004). *Neurology for the nonneurologist*. Philadelphia: Lippincott Williams & Wilkins.

Weinstein, R. A. (2001, March–April). Controlling antimicrobial resistance in hospitals: Infection control and use of antibiotics. *Emergency Infectious Diseases Journal, 7*(2), 188–192.

Westerdahl, E., Lindmark, B., Eriksson, T., Friberg, O., Hedenstierna, G., & Tenling, A. (2005).

Whitaker, J. (2009). *Target your health concerns with potent herbal remedies*. Baltimore, MD: Healthier News.

White, G., O'Rourke, F., Ong, B., Cordato, D., & Chan, D. (2008). Dysphagia: causes, assessment, treatment, and management. *Geriatrics, 63*(5), 15–20.

Whitney, E., Cataldo, C., & Rolfes, S. (2002). *Understanding normal and clinical nutrition* (6th ed.). Belmont, CA: Wadsworth Thomson Learning.

Whittington, A., Whitlow, G., Hewson, D., Thomas, C., & Brett, S. J. (2009, July). Bacterial contamination of stethoscopes on the intensive care unit. *Anesthesia, 64*(6), 620–624.

Whyte, J., & Marting, R. (2005, May). How to guide patients away from fad diets and toward healthy eating. *Patient Care*, 16.

Wilburn, S. (2000, February). Preventing needlesticks in your facility. *American Journal of Nursing, 100*(2), 96.

Wilkinson, J. (2006). *Nursing process and critical thinking approach* (4th ed.). Redwood City, CA: Addison-Wesley.

Willard, R., & Dreher, M. (2005). Sleep apnea. *Nursing, 35*(3), 46.

Williams, M. (2002). *Nutrition for health, fitness, and sport* (6th ed.). Boston, MA: McGraw-Hill.

Wilmoth, D., Walters, P. E., Tomlin, R., & McCray, S. F. (2001, March). Caring for adults with cystic fibrosis. *Critical Care Nurse, 21*(3), 34–44.

Wirth, J., Hudgins, J. C., & Paice, J. A. (2006, January). Use of herbal therapies to relieve pain: A review of efficacy and adverse effects. *Pain Management Nursing, 6*(4), 145–167.

Wiseman, R. (2007, September). Responding to disaster emergencies. *Advance for Nurses, Northern California*, 29–30.

Wong's Nursing care of infants and children (8th ed.). (2006). St. Louis: Mosby.

Wood, D. (2004, May). On the level(s): A five-tier triage scale system, which streamlines emergency care. *Nurseweek California*, Sunnyvale, CA, 17.

Wood, D. (2008, December). Southwest RNs stay safe with radiation while boosting outcomes. *NurseWeek, West, 15*(17), 14–15.

Woodruff, D. (2005). A quick guide to vent essentials. *RN, 68*(9), 32ac2.

Woods, A. (2005). Managing UTIs in older adults. *Nursing, 35*(3), 12.

Woolever, D. (2008). Achieve better glucose control for your hospitalized patients. *The Journal of Family Practice*, 57(12), 782–787.

Wooten, M. K., & Hawkins, K. (2001). WOCN position statement clean versus sterile: Management of chronic wounds. Wound, Ostomy Continence Nurses Society and the Association for Professionals in Infection Control and Epidemiology. Revised 2005.

World Health Organization. (2009). *Guidelines on Hand Hygiene in Health Care*. Geneva, Switzerland: WHO Press, World Health Organization, 1–3.

World, H. (2005, April). Off the charts: High-tech information systems. *Nurseweek California*, Sunnyvale, CA, 30–31.

Wygand, D. J. L., & Carlson, K. K. (Eds.). (2005). *AACN Procedure Manual for Critical Care*, 5th edition. Philadelphia: Elsevier/Saunders.

Wynne, R., & Botti, M. (2004). Postoperative pulmonary dysfunction in adults after cardiac surgery with cardiopulmonary bypass: Clinical significance and implications for practice. *American Journal of Critical Care, 13*(5), 384.

Yantis, M., & Nieman, W. (2000, April). Resting easy with PAP therapy. *Nursing, 30*(4), 62–64.

Yantis, M., Newson, K., & Ring, P. (2009, April). Leech therapy: Hirudo medicinalis has made a comeback. *American Journal of Nursing, 109*(4), 36–41.

Ziegler, T. (2009). Parenteral nutrition in the critically ill patient. *New England Journal of Medicine, 361*(11),1088–1097.

Zink, E., & McQuillan, K. (2005). Traumatic brain injury. *Nursing, 35*(9), 36–43.

Vendors

The Bair Paws® Patient Adjustable Warming System. Arizant Health care Inc. http://www.augustinemedical.com/arizanthealthcare/hp_pro_ comfort.shtml.

Central Venous Access Catheters (CVAC) and Gastrostomy (Feeding) Tubes.

Society of Interventional Radiology. http://www.sirweb.org/patPub/venousAccessCatheters.shtml.

OPIT Source Book. A Resource Guide for Products and Services Available for Intravenous Therapy. Abbott Laboratories. http://www.abbottIVsets.com.

CLC2000® for Central, Peripheral and Arterial Lines. ICU Medical, Inc. www.icumed.com.

Ports. Bard Access Systems. www.bardaccess.com.

Central Venous Catheters. Bard Access Systems. www.bardaccess.com.

Breast Cancer Diagnosis. Siemens Medical. www.medical.siemens.com.

Venous Access Devices. E-medicine Consumer Health. http://www.emedicinehealthcare/venous_access_devices/article.

Peripherally Inserted Central Catheters. Medscape from WEBMED. http://profreq.medscape.com.

Interventional Radiology. Radiology Info: The Radiology Information Resource for Patients. www.radiologyinfo.org/index.cfm?bhecp=1.

Positron Emission Tomography. RadiologyInfo: The Radiology Information Resource for Patients. www.radiologyinfo.org/indexcfm?bhecp.

Interventional Radiology. The University of Texas M.D. Anderson Cancer Center. www.mdanderson.org/department.

Point-of-Care, 8000 Series Manual. Alaris Medical Systems. www.alarismed.com.

Zassi Medical Evolutions. The Bowel Management System (BMS). http://www.ZassiMedical.com.

References Found on the Internet

www.acestar.uthscsa.edu. Evidence-Based Practice.

American College of Emergency Physicians. (2002). NBC Task Force; Office of Emergency Preparedness, Final Report: Resources for Dealing with Stress Brought on by Recent Terrorist Attacks. http://www.acep.org/advocacy.aspx?LinkIdentifier=ID&id=21354&fid=648&Mo=No&taxid=112475

American Heart Association. Cardiopulmonary Resuscitation (CPR). (2005, October). www.americanheart.org/presenterjhtml?identifier=4479.

American Hospital Association. (2002). Chemical & Biological Terrorism Preparedness Checklist; Policy Forum, Hospital Preparedness for Mass Causalities.www.hospitalconnect.com/ahapolicyforum/resources/disaster.

American Nurses Association Position statement on Elimination of Manual Patient Handling to Prevent Work-Related Musculoskeletal Disorders. (2003). www.nursingworld.org/search.

American Nurses Association. Handle with Care. www.NursingWorld.org/handlewithcare/.

American Sleep Apnea Association. http://www.sleepapnea.org

Army Regulation 40–13 Medical Services. (1985). Medical Support—Nuclear, Chemical Accidents & Incidents. www.cdc.gov/nuclear.

www.artificialeye.net/tears. Artificial Eye Information.

www.asahq.org/NEWSLETTERS. CDC Publishes New Guidelines for Prevention of Intravascular Device–Related Infections.

Association for Professionalism Infection Control and Epidemiology, Inc., Mass Casualty Disaster Plan Checklist: A Template for Healthcare Facilities. www.apic.org/bioterror/checklist.doc.

Bulletin of the American College of Surgeons. (2002, December). 12. Statement on Ensuring Correct Patient, Correct Site, and Correct Procedure Surgery. http://www.facs.org/fellows_info/statements/st-41.html.

www.c.nih.gov/nursing. SOP: Management of the Patient in Restraints.

Campbell, A. Improving Assessment and Decision Making in Predialysis Patients. www.multi-med.com/pdtoday/arto698-6.htm.

www.cbhd.org/resources. Advance Directives and "Do Not Resuscitate" Orders.

http://www.cdc.gov. Centers for Disease Control and Prevention.

Canadian Centre for Emergency preparedness. (2005). Personal Preparedness. www.ccep.ca/cceppers.html.

Center for Strategic and International Studies. Combating Chemical, Biological, Radiological, and Nuclear Terrorism. www.cis.org/home/and/reportscontactchembiorad.

Centers for Disease Control and Prevention. (2000). Biological & Chemical Terrorism: Strategic Plan for Preparedness and Response. www.cdc.gov/mmwr/preview/mmwrht/rr4901a1.htm.

Centers for Disease Control and Prevention. AIDS Information: Statistics—Cumulative Cases. www.cdc.gov/nchstp/hiv.cumulati.htm.

Centers for Disease Control and Prevention. Division of HIV/AIDS Prevention, Basic Statistics. www.cdc.gov/hiv/stats.htm.

Centers for Disease Control and Prevention. Emerging Infectious Diseases. (2002, September). Preparing at the Local Level for Events Involving Weapons of Mass Destruction. www.cdc.gov/nicdod/EID/vol8no9/01-0520.htm.

Centers for Disease Control and Prevention. Interim Recommendations for the Selection & Use of Protective Clothing & Respirators Against Biological Agents. cdc.gov/niosh/unp-intrecppe.html.

Centers for Disease Control and Prevention. Issues in Healthcare Settings, Part II. Recommendations for Isolation Precautions in Hospitals. cdc.gov/nicdod/hip/isolat/isopart2.htm.

Centers for Disease Control and Prevention. (2005). Strategic National Stockpile. www.bt.cdc.gov/stockpile/index.asp.

Centers for Disease Control and Prevention (2002). Hand Hygiene in Healthcare Settings. www.cdc.gov/handhygiene/firesafety/cmsRuling.htm.

Centers for Disease Control and Prevention. (2004–2005). Natural Disasters. Emergency Preparedness and Response. www.bt.cdc.gov/disasters/.

Centers for Disease Control and Prevention. (2004). Avian Influenza (Bird Flu). www.cdc.gov/flu/avian/gen-info/facts.htm.

Centers for Disease Control and Prevention. (2004). Bioterrorism and Public Health Preparedness. www.cdc.gov/programs/bt.htm.

Centers for Disease Control and Prevention. (2004). Preparation and Planning Emergency Preparedness and Response. www.bt.cdc.gov/planning/.

Centers for Disease Control and Prevention. (2005). Biological and Chemical Terrorism: Strategic Plan for Preparedness and Response. www.cdc.gov/mmwr/preview/mmwrhtml/rr4904.htm.

Centers for Disease Control and Prevention. (2005). Emerging Infectious Diseases (Hand Sanitizer Alert). http://www.cdc.gov/NCIDOD/EID/vol12no03/05-0955.htm.

Centers for Disease Control and Prevention. National Center for Infectious Diseases. www.cdc.gov/ncidod/publicat.htm.

Centers for Disease Control and Prevention. National Institute for Occupational Safety and Health. Chemical protective clothing.http://www.cdc.gov/niosh/topics/protclothing/.

Centers for Disease Control and Prevention. Office of Communication. CDC Radiation Studies, Nuclear Terrorism & Health Effects.www.cdc.gov/od/oc/media/9-11pk.html.

Centers for Disease Control and Prevention. Public Health Emergency Preparedness & Response FAQS About Anthrax. www.cdc.gov/documentsapp/faqanthrax.asp#Qr001.

Centers for Disease Control and Prevention. Strategic Planning Workgroup. (2002). Biological & Chemical Terrorism: Strategic Plan for Preparedness Response. www.cdc.gov/mmwr/preview/mmwrhtml/rr4904a1.htm.

Childers, L. (2005, May 23). Caring to the end. *NurseWeek*. www2.nurseweek.com/Articles/article.cfm?AID=14256.

Cleveland Clinic Health Information. What you need to know about venous leg ulcers. www.ccf.org/ed/pated/database/docs/0300/0314.htm.

Community Emergency Response Team (CERT). Training: Participant Handbook. www.cert-la.com/manuals/tc&intro.pwf.

Conor, S. (2005). What to do if a nuclear disaster is imminent. www.ki4u.com/guide.htm.

Consideration for Policy Guidelines for Registered Nurses Engaged in the Administration of Conscious Sedation. CRNA Practice: American Association of Nurse Anesthetists. (2003, June 13). http://www.aana.com/practice/conscious.asp.

Continuum of Depth of Sedation Definition of General Anesthesia and Levels of Sedation/Analgesia. American Society of Anesthesiologists .http://www.asahq.org/publications and serivices/standards/20pdf.

Criteria for Weaning from Mechanical Ventilation: Summary of Evidence Report. (2006). http://www.ahrq.gov.

Cultural Diversity in Decision Making About Care at the End of Life. www.nap.edu/readingroom.

DeBenedette, V. (2005, August 22). Drug topics: Smart pumps have huge potential to cut errors. http://www.drugtopics.com/drugtopics/content.

DeCastro, A. B. (2004, September). Handle with care: The American Nurses Association's campaign to address work-related musculoskeletal disorders. 2004 Journal of Issues in Nursing. www.nursingworld.org/ojin/topic25.tpc25_2.htm.

Disaster Preparedness and Response for Nurses. (2004). American Red Cross and Sigma Theta Tau International. www.nursingsociety.org/education/case_studies/cases/SP0004.html.

Documentation of Wounds. www.uca.edu/glenni/Wounds/wndoc.htm.

Duke University School of Nursing. Nursing Interventions Classification (NIC). www.duke.edu//goodw010/vocab/NIC.html.

Duke University School of Nursing. Nursing Outcomes classification (NOC). www.duke.edu/goodw010/vocab/NOC.html.

Duquesne Light. (2004). Storm Center, Power Outage Tips Before, During and After a Power Outage. www.duquesnelight.com/StormCenter/PowerOutageTips/Before/During/andAfteraPowerOutage.

Effective Patient Teaching. http://uuhsc.utah.edu/pated/authors/teaching.html.

Electronic Journal of Biotechnology. (1999). Biological Warfare, Bioterrorism, Biodefence and the Biological Antitoxin Weapons Convention. www.ejb.org/content/vol2/issue 3/full/.

Emedicine Consumer Health. Venous Access Devices. www.emedicinehealth.com.

Emergency Planning and Emergency Supply Kit. (2005). Department of Homeland Security. www.READY.gov.

Emergency Weapons of Mass Destruction Responses. (2001). Emergency Decontamination Triage and Treatment. www.2.sbccom. army.mil/hid.

European Guidelines for Prevention in Low Back Pain. (2004, November). WG3_Guidelines.pdf.

Evans, N. (2005, May). End-of-Life Care. Wild Iris Medical Education. http://therapyceu.com/courses/103/index_tceu.html.

www.fda.g.v/cdrh. A Guide to Bed Safety, October 11, 2000.

Federal Emergency Management Agency. (FEMA). 2001. Federal Response Plan-ESF#8. www.fema.gov/rrr/frpesf8.shtm.

Frantz, R. Identifying infection in chronic wounds. *Nursing, 73*. www.nursing2005.com.

Genentech. About Central Venous Access Devices. www.gene.com.

Graduated Compression Stockings for the Prevention of Post-operative Venous Thromboembolism. (2001). *Best Practice*, *5*(2). www.joannabriggs.edu.BPISStock.pdf.

Guidance for Radiation Accident Management. (2002). Managing Radiation Emergencies. www.orau.gove/reacts/dyndrome.htm.

Guidance for Radiation Accident Management. (2002). Oak Ridge Associated Universities Basics of Radiation Safety Around Radiation Sources. http://orise.orau.gov/reacts/.

Hepatitis Foundation International On-Line. Hepatitis Statistics. www.hepfi.org/stats.htm.

Hill, C. (2006, April). Joint Commission Issues Alert on Dangerous Tubing Misconnect. Joint Commission on Accreditation of Healthcare Organizations. http://www.jointcommission.org/NewsRoom/NewsReleases/jc_nr_040306.htm.

Hill, G., et al. Peritoneal Dialysis. www.Bgsm.edu/nursing/monitor/1996/SEP-OCT/sep-oct2.htm.

HIPAA Laws. (2003–2005). *HIPAA information*. www.hipaamanager.com/htm/laws.cfm.

Holter Monitor. Austin Heart. www.austinheart.com/tm_hlt.htm.

Hospital Infection Control Practices Advisory Committee, CDC Issues in Healthcare Settings. Evolution of Isolation Practices. www.cdc.gov/ncidod/hip/isolat/isopart/htm.

ICU Medical, Inc. CLC2000 for Central, Peripheral and Arterial Lines. www.icumed.com.

Implement the Central Line Bundle: Chlorhexidine Skin Antisepsis. Institute for Health Improvement. www.ihi.org/topics.

Interventional radiology (IR). RadiologyInfo: The Radiology Information Resource for Patients. www.radiologyinfo.org/index.cfm?bhcp=1

Issa, D. (2005). A better ending. *Advance for Nurses*. www.advanceweb.com.

IV Nurses' Society Standards. www.ins1.org.

JCAHO Standards: Patient Education (PF). http://www.wramc.army.mil/JCAHO/Division.cfm?.D_ID=26.

Joint Commission on Accreditation of Healthcare Organizations. 2005 Hospitals' National Patient Safety goals. http://www.jointcommission.org

Joint Commission on Accreditation of Healthcare Organizations. 2006 Critical Access Hospital and Hospital National Patient Safety Goals. http://www.jointcommission.org.

Joint Commission on Accreditation of Healthcare Organizations. Facts About Patient Safety 2005. http://www.jointcommission.org.

Joint Commission on Accreditation of Healthcare Organizations. JCAHO 2006 National Patient Safety Goals. Meditech on JCAHO. http://www.jointcommission.org.

Joint Commission on Accreditation of Healthcare Organizations. Universal Protocol For Preventing Wrong Site, Wrong Procedure, Wrong Person Surgery. http://www.jcaho.org/accredited+organizations/patient+safety/universal+protocol/faq_uphtm.

Kleinpell, Ruth. New Procedures Keep Radiology Nurses Charged. Nursing Spectrum. http:community.nursing.com

Knight, Catherine. Radiology Nurses Keep Pace with Interventional Technology. Nursing Spectrum. http://community.nursingspectrum.com/MagazineArticles/article.cfm?AID=4752.

100,000 Lives Campaign. How-to Guide: Preventing Catheter-Related Bloodstream Infections—Five Components of Care. www.aap.org/visit/HI.Centrallineshowtoguidefinal52505.pdf.

Kushner, F. G., et al. (2009, August). ACC/AHA guidelines for the management of patients with ST-elevation myocardial infarction and Guidelines on Percutaneous Coronary Interventions. A report of the American College of Cardiology/American Heart Association Task Force on Practice Guidelines. *Journal of American College of Cardiology*, http://www.acc.org/clinical/guidelines.

Online Library. Wiley.com

Lorenz, K., et al. End-of-Life Care and Outcomes Summary. Agency for Healthcare Research and Quality. www.ahrq.gov.

McMahon, S. (2006). Advance Directives. *Advance for Nurse Practitioners*. www.advanceweb.com.

M.D. Anderson Cancer Center. Interventional radiology. www.mdanderson.org/departments.

Medscape from WEBMD. Peripherally Inserted Central Catheters. http://profreg.medscape.com.

Medscape. Issues in Patient Education. http://www.medscape.com/viewarticle/478283_print.

Moralejo, D., & Jull, A. Handrubbing with an aqueous alcohol solution was as effective as handscrubbing with antiseptic soap for preventing surgical site infections. www.bmjjournals.com/cgi/reprintform.

Myrianthefs, P., et al. (2005, February). The epidemiology of peripheral vein complications; evaluation of the efficiency of differing methods for the maintenance of catheter patency and thrombophlebitis prevention. *Journal of Evaluation in Clinical Practice*, *11*(1), 85–89. http://www.ingentaconnect.com/content/bsc/jecp/2005.

National Center for HIV, STD, and TB Prevention. Division of HIV/AIDS Prevention. www.cdc.gov/hiv/stats.htm.

National Guideline Clearinghouse. http://www.guideline.gov

National Guideline Clearinghouse. (2002). Guideline for Hand Hygiene in Health-Care Settings. http://www.guideline.gov.

National Institutes of Health State-of-the-Science Conference Statement on Improving End-of-Life Care. National Institutes of Health State-of-the-Science Conference Statement. (2004, December 6–8). http://consensus.hih.gov/2004/2004ENDOfLifeCareSOS024html.htm.

National Kidney Foundation. http://www.kidney.org.

National Sleep Foundation. http://www.sleepfoundation.org

Nelson, A., & Baptiste, A. (2004, September). Evidence-based practices for safe patient handling and movement. *2004 Online Journal of Issues in Nursing*. Retrieved from www.NursingWorld.org.

NurseWeek: Chapter Three—The Process of Patient Education. http://nurse.cyberchalk.com/nurse/courses/nurseweek/nw0650/c3/p01.htm.

O'Grady, N.P., & Delinger, A. (2002, August). Guidelines for the prevention of intravascular catheter-related infections. Centers for Disease Control and Prevention. *MMWR. Recommendations and reports: Morbidity and mortality weekly report*, (51)RR-10, 1–29. Retrieved from www.cdc.gov/mmwr/PDF/rr/rr5110/pdf.

Ong, L., et al. (2004, January). Stress management. *Journal of Psychosomatic Research*, *56*(1), 133–137. Science Direct. www.sciencedirect.com/science.

OSHA Fact Sheet. Securing Medical Catheters. http://www.osha.gov/SLTC/bloodbornepathogens/factsheet_catheters.pdf.

OSHA. www.osha.gov.

Patients' Rights, Physical Restraint, Guide for Monitoring and Evaluating Patients in Restraints. http://www.cms.gov/default.asp?

Peterson, L. Arterial Closure Devices. Trends-in-medicine. www.trends-in-medicine.com.

Principles of Peritoneal Dialysis. Fresnius Medical Care. www.fmc-ag.com/daily/pdp_over.htm.

Proposed AORN Position Statement on Fire Prevention. Association of Peri-operative Registered Nurses. http://www.blueskybroadcast.com/Client/AORN/.

Proposed AORN Position statement on the Role of the Scrub Person. Association of Peri-operative Registered Nurses. http://www.blueskybroadcast.com/Client/AORN/.

Public Health Agency of Canada. Aging and Seniors. Evidence-Based Best Practices for the Prevention of Falls. www.phac-2spc.gc.ca/seniors.

Recommendations for Chemical Protective Clothing Database. www.cdc.gov/niosh/ncpc/ncpc2.html.

Reves, J. (2003). "Smart Pump" technology reduces errors. http://www.apsf.org/resources_center/newsletter/2003/smartpump.htm.

Searight, H. R., & Gafford, J. (2005, February 1). Cultural diversity at the end of life: Issues and guidelines for family physicians. *American Family Physician 71*(3). http://www.aafp.org/afp/20050201/515.html.

Smallpox and Smallpox Vaccines: Adverse Reactions—Thinktwice, Smallpox. www.thinktwice.com/smallpox.htm.

Sullivan, M. Multicultural pain management. Advance for nurse practitioners. www.advanceweb.com.

The University of Iowa college of Nursing. Nursing Interventions classification. www.nursing.uiowa.edu/centers/cncce/nic/niccoverview.htm.

The University of Iowa College of Nursing. Nursing Outcomes classification. www.nursing.uiowa.edu/centers/cncce/noc/nocquestions.htm.

Truog, R. D., et al. Recommendations for end-of-life care in the intensive care unit. The Ethics Committee of the Society of Critical Care Medicine. National Guideline Clearinghouse. www.guideline.gov.

VISN 8 Patient Safety Center. Safe patient handling and movement algorithms. American Nurses Association 2005. www.wisn8.med.va.gov/patientsafety.center.

Walden, J., & Kaplan, E. (2003). Estimating time and size of bioterror attack. www.gov/ncidod/eid/vol10no7/03_0632.htm.

Weapons of Mass Destruction. Information for EMS First Responders. www.oswegocountyems.org/WMD%20sheet%2ohtml.html.

Wigder, H. (2005, November 7). Restraints. EMedicine. http://www.emedicine.com/emerg/topic776.htm.

Wong-Baker (2000). Choosing a FACES Pain Scale, Revised. www.painsourcebook.ca/pdfs/pps92.

Wound Care Communication Network at Springhouse Co. First Annual OR–Acquired Pressure Ulcer Symposium: Highlights and Supplement.www.woundcarenet.com/ulcer_symp98/highlights.htm.

Zassi Medical Evolutions. The Bowel Management System (BMS). http://www.ZassiMedical.com.

Index

('t' indicates a table)

B

E

M

T

U

Index of Skills*

*This index represents the list of main skill titles found in this text. For additional skills and skill variations please see the Table of Contents in the front of the book or the Index at the end of the book for location.